MW00845016

GREEN'S

OPERATIVE HAND SURGERY

GREEN'S
OPERATIVE HAND SURGERY

SEVENTH EDITION

EDITOR IN CHIEF
SCOTT W. WOLFE, MD
Professor of Orthopaedic Surgery
Weill Medical College of Cornell University;
Emeritus Chief, Hand and Upper Extremity Surgery
Attending Orthopaedic Surgeon
Hospital for Special Surgery
New York, New York

EDITORS
ROBERT N. HOTCHKISS, MD
Associate Professor of Clinical Orthopaedic Surgery
Weill Medical College of Cornell University;
Associate Attending Orthopaedic Surgeon
Director of Clinical Research
Hospital for Special Surgery
New York, New York

WILLIAM C. PEDERSON, MD, FACS
Adjunct Professor of Surgery
The University of Texas Health Science Center;
Fellowship Director
The Hand Center of San Antonio
San Antonio, Texas

SCOTT H. KOZIN, MD
Professor
Department of Orthopaedic Surgery
Temple University School of Medicine;
Chief of Staff
Shriners Hospitals for Children
Philadelphia, Pennsylvania

MARK S. COHEN, MD
Professor
Director, Orthopaedic Education
Director, Hand and Elbow Section
Department of Orthopaedic Surgery
Rush University Medical Center
Chicago, Illinois

ELSEVIER

ELSEVIER

1600 John F. Kennedy Blvd.
Ste 1800
Philadelphia, PA 19103-2899

GREEN'S OPERATIVE HAND SURGERY, SEVENTH EDITION ISBN: 978-1-4557-7427-2

Copyright © 2017 by Elsevier, Inc. All rights reserved.
All contributors retain copyright to the original photographs and video.

No part of this publication may be reproduced or transmitted in any form or by any means, electronic or mechanical, including photocopying, recording, or any information storage and retrieval system, without permission in writing from the publisher. Details on how to seek permission, further information about the Publisher's permissions policies and our arrangements with organizations such as the Copyright Clearance Center and the Copyright Licensing Agency, can be found at our website: www.elsevier.com/permissions.

This book and the individual contributions contained in it are protected under copyright by the Publisher (other than as may be noted herein).

Notices

Knowledge and best practice in this field are constantly changing. As new research and experience broaden our understanding, changes in research methods, professional practices, or medical treatment may become necessary.

Practitioners and researchers must always rely on their own experience and knowledge in evaluating and using any information, methods, compounds, or experiments described herein. In using such information or methods they should be mindful of their own safety and the safety of others, including parties for whom they have a professional responsibility.

With respect to any drug or pharmaceutical products identified, readers are advised to check the most current information provided (i) on procedures featured or (ii) by the manufacturer of each product to be administered, to verify the recommended dose or formula, the method and duration of administration, and contraindications. It is the responsibility of practitioners, relying on their own experience and knowledge of their patients, to make diagnoses, to determine dosages and the best treatment for each individual patient, and to take all appropriate safety precautions.

To the fullest extent of the law, neither the Publisher nor the authors, contributors, or editors, assume any liability for any injury and/or damage to persons or property as a matter of products liability, negligence or otherwise, or from any use or operation of any methods, products, instructions, or ideas contained in the material herein.

Previous years copyrighted: 2011, 2005, 1999, 1993, 1988, 1982

Library of Congress Cataloging-in-Publication Data

Names: Wolfe, Scott W., editor. | Hotchkiss, Robert N., editor. | Pederson, William C., editor. |
Kozin, Scott H., editor. | Cohen, Mark S., 1960- , editor.
Title: Green's operative hand surgery / [edited by] Scott W. Wolfe, Robert N. Hotchkiss, William C. Pederson, Scott H. Kozin, Mark S. Cohen.
Other titles: Operative hand surgery
Description: Seventh edition. | Philadelphia, PA : Elsevier, [2017] | Includes bibliographical references and index.
Identifiers: LCCN 2015049498 | ISBN 9781455774272 (hardcover : alk. paper)
Subjects: | MESH: Hand—surgery
Classification: LCC RD559 | NLM WE 830 | DDC 617.5/75059—dc23
LC record available at http://lccn.loc.gov/2015049498

Executive Content Strategist: Dolores Meloni
Content Strategist: Maureen Iannuzzi
Publishing Services Manager: Catherine Jackson
Project Manager: Kate Mannix
Design Direction: Margaret Reid

Printed in China

Last digit is the print number: 9 8 7 6 5 4 3 2 1

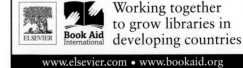

CONTRIBUTORS

Brian D. Adams, MD
Professor of Orthopedic Surgery
Baylor College of Medicine
Baylor-St. Luke's Medical Center
Houston, Texas

Julie E. Adams, MD
Associate Professor of Orthopaedic Surgery
Department of Orthopaedic Surgery
Mayo Clinic Health System
Austin, Minnesota

Nidal F. AlDeek, MD, MSc
Department of Plastic and Reconstructive
  Surgery
Chang Gung Memorial Hospital
Taipei, Taiwan

Edward A. Athanasian, MD
Clinical Professor of Orthopedic Surgery
Weill Cornell Medical College;
Chief, Hand Surgery
Hospital for Special Surgery;
Division of Orthopedics
Department of Surgery
Memorial Sloan Kettering Cancer Center
New York, New York

George S. Athwal, MD, FRCSC
Associate Professor and Consultant
HULC, St. Joseph's Health Care
University of Western Ontario
London, Ontario, Canada

Kodi Azari, MD, FACS
Professor
Orthopaedic Surgery and Plastic Surgery
David Geffen School of Medicine at UCLA
Los Angeles, California

Donald S. Bae, MD
Associate Professor of Orthopaedic Surgery
Department of Orthopaedic Surgery
Harvard Medical School;
Attending Surgeon
Department of Orthopaedic Surgery
Boston Children's Hospital
Boston, Massachusetts

Mark E. Baratz, MD
Vice Chairman
Department of Orthopaedic Surgery
Allegheny General Hospital
Pittsburgh, Pennsylvania

David P. Barei, MD, FRCSC
Professor
Department of Orthopaedic and Sports
  Medicine
University of Washington;
Director
Orthopedic Trauma Fellowship
Harborview Medical Center
Seattle, Washington

Andrea S. Bauer, MD
Pediatric Hand Surgeon
Department of Orthopaedic Surgery
Shriners Hospital for Children Northern
  California;
Assistant Clinical Professor
Department of Orthopaedic Surgery
UC Davis School of Medicine
Sacramento, California

Rolfe Birch, MChir, FRCS
Professor
Neurological Orthopaedic Surgery
University College
London, Great Britain

Allen T. Bishop, MD
Professor
Department of Orthopedic Surgery
Mayo Clinic College of Medicine;
Consultant
Division of Hand Surgery
Department of Orthopedic Surgery
Mayo Clinic
Rochester, Minnesota

Paul S. Cederna, MD
Robert O'Neal Collegiate Professor of
  Plastic Surgery
Section Head, Plastic Surgery
Professor, Department of Biomedical
  Engineering
University of Michigan School of Medicine
Ann Arbor, Michigan

Neal C. Chen, MD
The Philadelphia and South Jersey Hand
  Centers, P.C.;
Assistant Professor
Orthopaedic Surgery
Thomas Jefferson University Hospital,
Philadelphia, Pennsylvania

Mark S. Cohen, MD
Professor
Director, Orthopaedic Education
Director, Hand and Elbow Section
Department of Orthopaedic Surgery
Rush University Medical Center
Chicago, Illinois

Roger Cornwall, MD
Associate Professor of Orthopaedic Surgery
  and Developmental Biology
Clinical Director of Pediatric Orthopaedics
Cincinnati Children's Hospital Medical
  Center
Cincinnati, Ohio

**Timothy R.C. Davis, FRCS, ChM, BSc,
MB**
Honorary Professor
Nottingham University;
Hand Surgeon
Nottingham University Hospitals
Nottingham, United Kingdom

Charles S. Day, MD, MBA
Associate Professor of Orthopaedic Surgery
Director, Orthopaedic Curriculum
Harvard Medical School;
Orthopaedic Hand and Upper Extremity
  Surgery
Beth Israel Deaconess Medical Center
Boston, Massachusetts

Rafael J. Diaz-Garcia, MD
Attending Surgeon
Department of Surgery
Division of Plastic Surgery
Allegheny Health Network;
Clinical Assistant Professor
Department of Plastic Surgery
University of Pittsburgh School of Medicine
Pittsburgh, Pennsylvania

George S.M. Dyer, MD
Orthopaedic Hand Surgeon
Department of Orthopaedic Surgery
Brigham and Women's Hospital
Boston, Massachusetts

Charles Eaton, MD
Executive Director
Dupuytren Foundation
Palm Springs, Florida

Bassem T. Elhassen, MD
Assistant Professor of Orthopaedic Surgery
Department of Orthopaedics
Mayo Clinic
Rochester, Minnesota

Paul Feldon, MD
Chief, Hand Surgery Service
Newton Wellesley Hospital
Newton, Massachusetts;
Clinical Associate Professor of Orthopaedic
   Surgery
Tufts University School of Medicine
Boston, Massachusetts

Jeffrey B. Friedrich, MD, FACS
Associate Professor of Surgery and
   Orthopaedics
Department of Surgery
University of Washington
Seattle, Washington

Marc Garcia-Elias, MD, PhD
Consultant Hand Surgeon
Hand and Upper Extremity Surgery
Institut-Kaplan
Barcelona, Spain

William B. Geissler, MD
Professor and Chief, Alan E. Freeland Chair
   of Hand Surgery
Division of Hand and Upper Extremity
   Surgery
University of Mississippi Health Care
Jackson, Mississippi

Günter Germann, MD, PhD
Professor of Plastic and Hand Surgery
ETHIANUM Heidelberg Clinic for Plastic,
   Reconstructive, and Aesthetic Surgery,
   Preventative Medicine
The University of Heidelberg
Heidelberg, Germany

Vidal Haddad, Jr., MD, MSc, PhD
Associate Professor
Department of Dermatology
Botucatu Medical School
São Paulo State University
Botucatu, São Paulo, Brazil

Douglas P. Hanel, MD
Professor
Department of Orthopaedic and Sports
   Medicine
Director of Orthopaedic Education
University of Washington
Seattle, Washington

Hill Hastings, MD
Past Clinical Professor, Orthopedic Surgery
Indiana University
Telluride, Colorado

James P. Higgins, MD
Chief of Hand Surgery
The Curtis National Hand Center
MedStar Union Memorial Hospital
Baltimore, Maryland

Robert N. Hotchkiss, MD
Associate Professor of Clinical Orthopaedic
   Surgery
Weill Medical College of Cornell University;
Associate Attending Orthopaedic Surgeon
Director of Clinical Research
Hospital for Special Surgery
New York, New York

Manuel Hrabowski, MD
ETHIANUM Heidelberg Clinic for Plastic,
   Reconstructive, and Aesthetic Surgery,
   Preventative Medicine
Heidelberg, Germany

Michelle A. James, MD
Professor of Clinical Orthopaedic Surgery
Chief, Pediatric Orthopaedic Service
UC Davis School of Medicine;
Chief, Orthopaedic Surgery
Shriners Hospital for Children of Northern
   California
Sacramento, California

Neil F. Jones, MD
Chief of Hand Surgery
University of California Irvine Medical
   Center;
Professor of Orthopaedic Surgery and
   Professor of Plastic and Reconstructive
   Surgery
University of California Irvine School of
   Medicine
Orange, California;
Attending Hand Surgeon
Shriners Hospital
Los Angeles, California

Jesse B. Jupiter, MD
Hansjörg Wyss Professor of Orthopaedic
   Surgery
Harvard Medical School;
Hand and Upper Extremity Division
Massachusetts General Hospital
Boston, Massachusetts

Sanjeev Kakar, MD, MRCS
Associate Professor
Department of Orthopaedic Surgery
Mayo Clinic
Rochester, Minnesota

Morton L. Kasdan, MD
Clinical Professor of Plastic Surgery
University of Louisville
Louisville, Kentucky

**Simon P. Kay, BA, BM BCh, FRCS (Plas),
FRCSE (Hon)**
Consultant Plastic Surgeon
Department of Plastic Surgery
Leeds Teaching Hospitals NHS Trust;
Professor of Hand Surgery
University of Leeds
Leeds, Great Britain

Graham J.W. King
Director, Roth McFarlane Hand and Upper
   Limb Centre
Chief of Surgery
St. Joseph's Health Centre;
Professor of Orthopaedic Surgery and
   Biomedical Engineering
Western University
London, Ontario, Canada

L. Andrew Koman, MD
Professor and Chair
Department of Orthopaedic Surgery
Wake Forest School of Medicine
Winston-Salem, North Carolina

Scott H. Kozin, MD
Clinical Professor
Department of Orthopaedic Surgery
Temple University School of Medicine;
Chief of Staff
Shriners Hospital for Children
Philadelphia, Pennsylvania

Steve K. Lee, MD
Associate Professor of Orthopaedic Surgery
Weill Cornell Medical College;
Associate Attending Orthopaedic Surgeon
Orthopaedic Surgery
Hospital for Special Surgery
New York, New York

Fraser J. Leversedge, MD
Associate Professor and Vice-Chair
Director, Hand, Upper Extremity, and
   Microvascular Surgery Fellowship
Department of Orthopaedic Surgery
Duke University
Durham, North Carolina

Nina Lightdale-Miric, MD
Assistant Clinical Professor of Orthopaedic
   Surgery
Keck School of Medicine
University of Southern California;
Director, Hand and Upper Extremity
   Surgery
Children's Hospital Los Angeles
Los Angeles, California

Graham D. Lister, MD
Former Professor and Chief
Division of Plastic Surgery
University of Utah School of Medicine
Salt Lake City, Utah

Alberto L. Lluch, MD, PhD
Consultant Hand Surgeon
Hand and Upper Extremity Surgery
Institut-Kaplan
Barcelona, Spain

Dean S. Louis, MD
Professor of Surgery
University of Michigan
Ann Arbor, Michigan

Susan E. Mackinnon, MD, FRCSC
Schoenberg Professor and Chief
Division of Plastic and Reconstructive
  Surgery
Washington University School of Medicine
St. Louis, Missouri

David B. McCombe, MBBS, MD, FRACS
Senior Lecturer
Department of Surgery
St. Vincent's Hospital
University of Melbourne
Melbourne, Victoria, Australia

Greg Merrell, MD
Indiana Hand to Shoulder Center
Indianapolis, Indiana

Richard Meyer, MD
Associate Professor
Department of Surgery
University of Alabama
Birmingham, Alabama

Lewis H. Millender, MD[†]
Clinical Professor of Orthopaedic Surgery
Tufts University School of Medicine
Boston, Massachusetts

Peter M. Murray, MD
Professor and Chairman
Department of Orthopaedic Surgery
Consultant
Department of Orthopaedic Surgery and
  Neurosurgery
Mayo Clinic;
Staff Physician
Department of Orthopaedic Surgery
Nemours Children's Clinic
Jacksonville, Florida

Edward A. Nalebuff, MD
Emeritus Surgeon
New England Baptist Hospital;
Emeritus Professor of Orthopaedic Surgery
Tufts University School of Medicine
Boston, Massachusetts

David T. Netscher, MD
Clinical Professor of Plastic Surgery and
  Orthopedic Surgery
Baylor College of Medicine
Houston, Texas;
Adjunct Professor of Clinical Surgery
Weill Medical College;
Adjunct Professor of Clinical Surgery
Cornell University
New York, New York

Christine B. Novak, PT, PhD
Associate Professor
Division of Plastic and Reconstructive
  Surgery
University of Toronto;
Scientist and Research Associate
University Health Network
Toronto, Ontario, Canada

Mukund R. Patel, MD, FACS
Chief of Hand Surgery
Associate Clinical Professor, Orthopedic
  Surgery
New York University Medical Center;
Attending Hand Surgeon
Hospital for Joint Diseases;
Chief of Hand Surgery
Department of Orthopedics
Richmond University Medical Center
New York, New York

William C. Pederson, MD, FACS
Adjunct Professor of Surgery
The University of Texas Health Science
  Center;
Fellowship Director
The Hand Center of San Antonio
San Antonio, Texas

**Tom Quick, MB, MA(Hons)Cantab,
FRCS(Tr & Orth)**
Consultant Surgeon
Peripheral Nerve Injury Unit
Royal National Orthopaedic Hospital
Middlesex, United Kingdom;
Honorary Consultant
Defence Medical Rehabilitation Centre
Headley Court
Surrey, United Kingdom;
Honorary Consultant Surgeon
Great Ormond Street Hospital for Sick
  Children;
Honorary Senior Lecturer
Institute of Orthopaedics and
  Musculoskeletal Science
University College Hospital
London, United Kingdom

David Ring, MD, PhD
Professor of Orthopaedic Surgery
Harvard Medical School;
Chief of Hand Surgery
Massachusetts General Hospital
Boston, Massachusetts

Marco Rizzo, MD
Professor
Department of Orthopedic Surgery
Chair, Division of Hand Surgery
Mayo Clinic
Rochester, Minnesota

Trajano Sardenberg, MD, PhD
Professor of Orthopaedic, Traumatology,
  and Hand Surgery
Department of Surgery and Orthopaedics
Botucatu Medical School
São Paulo State University
Botucatu, São Paulo, Brazil

John Gray Seiler III, MD
Clinical Professor of Orthopaedic Surgery
Emory University
Georgia Hand, Shoulder, & Elbow Surgery
Atlanta, Georgia

Frances Sharpe
Assistant Clinical Professor of Orthopedics
University of Southern California, Keck
  School of Medicine;
Orthopedics and Hand Surgery
Southern California Permanente Medical
  Group
Fontana, California

[†]Deceased.

Alexander Y. Shin, MD
Professor & Consultant
Orthopedic Surgery
Mayo Clinic
Rochester, Minnesota

Beth Paterson Smith, PhD
Professor
Department of Orthopaedic Surgery
Wake Forest School of Medicine
Winston-Salem, North Carolina

Thomas L. Smith, PhD
Professor
Department of Orthopaedic Surgery
Wake Forest School of Medicine
Winston-Salem, North Carolina

Nicole Z. Sommer, MD, FACS
Associate Professor
Department of Plastic Surgery
Southern Illinois School of Medicine
Springfield, Illinois

Robert J. Spinner, MD
Chair, Department of Neurologic Surgery
Burton M. Onofrio Professor of
    Neurosurgery
Professor of Orthopedics and Anatomy
Mayo Clinic
Rochester, Minnesota

Scott P. Steinmann, MD
Professor of Orthopaedic Surgery
Department of Orthopaedic Surgery
Mayo Clinic
Rochester, Minnesota

Milan V. Stevanovic, MD
Director of the Joseph H. Boyes Hand
    Fellowship Program
Professor of Orthopedics and Surgery
Department of Orthopedics
University of Southern California Keck
    School of Medicine
Los Angeles, California

Robert J. Strauch, MD
Professor of Orthopaedic Surgery
Columbia University Medical Center
New York, New York

Andrew L. Terrono, MD
Chief, Hand Surgery Service
New England Baptist Hospital;
Clinical Professor of Orthopaedic Surgery
Tufts University School of Medicine
Boston, Massachusetts

Ann E. Van Heest, MD
Professor and Vice Chair of Education
Department of Orthopedic Surgery
University of Minnesota
Minneapolis, Minnesota

Nicholas B. Vedder, MD
Professor & Chief of Plastic Surgery
Department of Surgery
University of Washington
Seattle, Washington

Peter M. Waters, MD
John E. Hall Professor of Orthopaedic
    Surgery
Harvard Medical School;
Orthopedic Surgeon in Chief
Children's Hospital
Boston, Massachusetts

Fu-Chan Wei, MD
Department of Plastic and Reconstructive
    Surgery
Chang Gung Memorial Hospital
Taipei, Taiwan

Scott W. Wolfe, MD
Professor of Orthopaedic Surgery
Weill Medical College of Cornell University;
Emeritus Chief, Hand and Upper Extremity
    Surgery
Attending Orthopaedic Surgeon
Hospital for Special Surgery
New York, New York

Elaine Yang, MD
Clinical Instructor
Department of Anesthesiology
Weill Cornell Medical College;
Assistant Attending
Department of Anesthesiology and Critical
    Care Medicine
Hospital for Special Surgery
New York, New York

Dan A. Zlotolow, MD
Associate Professor of Orthopaedics
Temple University School of Medicine;
Attending Physician
Shriners Hospital for Children
Philadelphia, Pennsylvania

Who would have thought when the first edition of *Operative Hand Surgery* was published in 1982 that nearly three and a half decades later we would be publishing the seventh edition and the book would be sold in more than 50 countries? The success of this book has been due to three main factors: (1) Careful selection of experienced authors with recognized expertise who are willing to invest the huge time and energy commitment that it takes to write an outstanding chapter (and people who are willing to make that commitment are becoming increasingly difficult to recruit); (2) meticulous dissection and critique of each chapter by the editors, another job that requires a mammoth expenditure of hours; and (3) the worldwide explosion of interest in hand surgery and the blossoming of national hand societies throughout the world (56 at last count). In 1982, we were fortunate to be at the right place at the right time.

A huge debt of gratitude is due to the contributors of the seventh edition, who made the decision to write a chapter, which demanded that they forego more pleasurable or financially productive pursuits. I am especially grateful to Scott Wolfe, who picked up the mantle of editor-in-chief and has devoted the time and effort necessary to oversee and direct the last two editions. He has more than justified the confidence we had in choosing him for this job over many other equally qualified hand surgeons. To my good friends and former practice partners, Bob Hotchkiss and Chris Pederson, I cannot thank you enough for what you have done to stick with this book through several editions. Over many years, we have laughed, we have cried, and we have anguished together over the peaks and valleys of bringing to life this large body of work. And to the new editors, Scott Kozin and Mark Cohen, I extend my appreciation for their commitment to this demanding process. Your only reward will be knowing that someone, somewhere will benefit from your efforts.

One other person deserves credit that is long overdue. Lewis Reines was president of the American division of Churchill Livingstone in the late 1970s, and *Operative Hand Surgery* was his idea. I had wanted to do a small book on some topic in hand surgery, but Lew said, "No, do the big book." This text would never have come into being without his foresight, encouragement, and expert guidance during those early years.

David P. Green, MD
San Antonio, TX
September 2016

PREFACE

"See one, do one, teach one" was the mantra of our past generation of surgical mentors. This rubric was emblematic of a surgical apprenticeship style of learning that had been effective for centuries. But implicit in this approach is a trial and error mentality that may only have worked in a day of lower expectations and a more narrow understanding of disease. The last half century has witnessed an explosion of technological advancements, increased scientific knowledge base, and surgical complexity, coupled with parallel changes in health care financing, regulation, and work hour restrictions that challenge our ability to teach effectively.

The average adult learner requires not one, but *seven* exposures to learn a new concept, and retention becomes even more difficult if the learning occurs over a short, intense study period. Similarly, psychological theory holds that it may take as many as 10,000 repetitions to master a technique or a skill. How then can a medical student, or even an accomplished surgeon, master a surgical reconstruction of a disorder that he or she may only see twice in a career? Benjamin Franklin quipped, "Experience keeps a dear school, but fools will learn in no other." Experience alone is not a panacea, however, as one can practice and engrain incorrect techniques. Experience should be accompanied by feedback and reinforcement, such that when skill acquisition is accompanied by reading, learning, and coaching, repetition will lead to mastery.

Enter *Green's Operative Hand Surgery*, a concept that was introduced 35 years and six editions ago, and one that has remained the backbone of hand surgical learning since. David Green invited recognized masters of specific hand surgical techniques to pool their talents to create an enduring resource of expert techniques, a synthesis of current publications and novel research, and the hugely successful guide to success: the *Author's Preferred Technique*. In this book, you can immerse yourself in concise tutorials of what works and what doesn't, learn the evidence and the anecdotes that contribute to success, and enlist the surgical mentoring of nearly a hundred recognized experts in hand surgery. The electronic version of *Green's Operative Hand Surgery,* available at ExpertConsult.com, does not simply duplicate the written content but expands on it, with volumes of illustrative cases, an expert classroom of 60 video techniques, classic chapters from archived editions, and regular online updates of emerging techniques that promise to change the landscape of tomorrow's hand surgery. Through the intensely dedicated work of its five editors, *Green's* can sharpen the skills of hand surgeons worldwide and excite present and future students of hand surgery. Welcome to *Green's Operative Hand Surgery*, seventh edition.

Scott W. Wolfe, MD

ACKNOWLEDGMENTS

Publishing a multimedia reference of this magnitude requires an enormous team effort and unanimity of purpose. I'd first like to thank Dave Green for his confidence in entrusting his brainchild with me and for giving me the amazing opportunity to expand our hand educational borders across the globe. On behalf of our readership, a huge shout-out to our expert authors for their countless hours away from family and work, their exquisite attention to the details and principles of *Operative Hand Surgery*, and their dedication to education. Many of our authors wrote their chapters single-handedly, which, in the spirit of the inaugural edition of *Green's*, gives our readers firsthand exposure to their thoughts, tips, and techniques. What may be less apparent is the luster given to each chapter by our incredible editorial team, whose proficiency and dedication make *Green's* the foundational resource of hand surgery. I am indebted to my trusted colleagues Bob Hotchkiss and Chris Pederson, who have devoted their expertise in microsurgery and elbow reconstruction for more than twenty years and five editions to hone these gems to perfection. We are incredibly fortunate to have attracted Scott Kozin, a thought leader in pediatrics and congenital hand, to complete a comprehensive revision of our pediatric section in the sixth edition. With the seventh edition, I'm delighted to welcome longtime friend and colleague Mark Cohen, also a prolific writer and exemplary educator, as our newest associate editor. Special thanks as well to Jonathan Isaacs and David Dennison, whose innovative ideas and commitment will make the electronic version of *Green's Operative Hand Surgery* a true living, interactive, and fully accessible bridge between the print editions.

I'd particularly like to thank the outstanding staff of Elsevier for assuring the highest quality print and online publications. From its inception six years ago, the content strategy team of Don Scholz, Helene Caprari, and Dolores Meloni have sculpted the first fully integrated print and online edition to ensure that *Green's* is available where you are. I'm indebted to my go-to person and content strategist Maureen Iannuzzi, who choreographed the entire production from its start to its launch, gently coaxing, convincing, and cajoling our writers and editors across the finish line. Special thanks to our illustrator, Wendy Beth Jackelow, for bringing these pages to life with abundant new color drawings, and to our project manager, Kate Mannix, for transforming our concepts and documents into the published multimedia finale.

Most importantly, I want to thank my family: my incredible children, William, Elizabeth, and Christian, for giving me free passes for too many weekends holed up in the office; and most of all, my wife Missy: my best friend, historian, and trusted advisor, whose sacrifice, patience, and wisdom inspired me to complete this work.

Scott W. Wolfe, MD

CONTENTS

*Available on ExpertConsult.com

VIDEO CONTENTS

1

Anesthesia

Elaine Yang

Acknowledgments: The author wishes to recognize the work of previous authors Drs. Lauren Fisher and Michael Gordon for their contributions to Green's Operative Hand Surgery *and to this manuscript.*

There are several techniques for providing anesthesia for hand surgery. This chapter provides an overview, illustrating both the risks and benefits of each. General anesthesia will be briefly discussed and regional techniques will be addressed, as well as the unique role that regional anesthesia plays in both operative anesthesia and postoperative analgesia for hand surgery.

GENERAL ANESTHESIA

General anesthesia has long been the technique of choice for surgical procedures, using either traditional endotracheal intubation or the newer laryngeal mask airway. Considered fast and reliable, it is the standard of care at many institutions. Unfortunately, it also has its share of complications, because the systemic administration of medication can cause derangements of other organ systems, including the brain, the heart, the lungs, the airways, and the gastric, endocrine, and renal systems. General anesthesia often calls for airway manipulation, which causes additional associated complications ranging from minor sore throat and hoarseness to more feared, serious complications, including laryngospasm, aspiration, or failed airway. These serious complications are relatively rare; more prevalent are the minor complications of nausea and vomiting, grogginess, or pain requiring further treatment.[47]

REGIONAL ANESTHESIA

Regional anesthesia is the anesthetic of choice at our institution and is especially suited to upper extremity surgery, as most patients are ambulatory. For inpatients, regional anesthesia is associated with less time spent in the recovery room, improved pain control, lower opiate consumption, and less nausea and vomiting.[46] Regional blockade can be used alone as an intraoperative anesthetic or as a supplement to general anesthesia.

Contraindications
Absolute Contraindications

The two absolute contraindications to regional anesthesia are (1) patient refusal and (2) infection at the site of needle insertion. Often patients refuse regional anesthesia because they have been inadequately educated preoperatively or are misinformed about it. However, many common fears regarding regional anesthesia can be dispelled with a forthright discussion.[115] For instance, patient surveys reveal concerns regarding discomfort during needle placement or awareness of the surgical procedure.[28] These concerns are easily allayed with adequate premedication and sedation. In fact, a regional technique would be advantageous to the patient wishing to minimize sedation and remain awake.

Relative Contraindications

Need for Assessing Postoperative Nerve Status or Compartment Syndrome. Because a successful block hinders motor and sensory conduction, nerve testing in the immediate postoperative period is not possible. Therefore, if an immediate postoperative assessment of nerve function is required, a regional block should not be used.

Fear of masking postoperative compartment syndrome is another relative contraindication to regional anesthesia. Compartment syndrome is diagnosed from both the subjective history and objective findings, especially compartment pressure measurements.[49] Pain in the postoperative period is estimated to precede changes in neurovascular status by 7.3 hours but can be masked by the use of nerve blockade provided for analgesia. Even more confusing, there are also reported cases of compartment syndrome being masked by intravenous (IV) morphine administration during patient-controlled analgesia.[118] Concern for the development of compartment syndrome should be conveyed prior to the start of the case and a plan for postoperative pain control determined at that time. Appropriate vigilance is needed and measurement of compartment pressures mandatory if suspicion for increased compartment pressures exists.

Aggravating a Preexisting Nerve Injury. Another concern is the possibility that regional nerve blockade will incite further nerve injury (double-crush phenomenon) in patients with preexisting

1

nerve injury or paresthesias.[13,83] While this is an understandable concern, experience has shown that regional nerve blockade remains an appropriate option for patients undergoing uncomplicated procedures such as ulnar nerve transposition[50] and the vast majority of elective upper extremity operations.

At our institution, most surgeons and anesthesiologists, in consultation with the patient, opt for the use of regional nerve blockade, even in cases of existing nerve injury or dysfunction. The demonstrated safety of newer techniques (described in the following) and benefit of pain control outweigh the unlikely risk of nerve injury. It is important to discuss the advantages and disadvantages with the patient, allowing him or her to participate in decision making, especially when nerve dysfunction preexists. For patients who appear to fear further nerve injury, we often opt to use general anesthesia with local anesthesia at the surgical site in order to avoid adding a perceived risk and uncertainty to the fears of an already anxious patient.

Anticoagulation Therapy. A relative concern among regional anesthesiologists is performing regional blockade in patients who are taking anticoagulants. More and more patients presenting for surgery are already taking anticoagulants for treatment of underlying coronary artery disease, atrial fibrillation, or cerebrovascular disease or for prevention or treatment of deep venous thrombosis. An injury or even the stress of surgery itself, along with a prothrombotic tissue insult, places anticoagulated patients at risk for development of postoperative deep and superficial venous thrombosis and leads many practitioners to prescribe antithrombotic measures to prevent its occurrence.[90]

Regional neuraxial (spinal or epidural) anesthesia does not contribute to venous thrombosis in patients not receiving anticoagulation therapy and, in fact, has been shown to reduce the rate of blood clots following lower extremity and abdominal surgery, though this advantage has been minimized in recent years with the advent of aggressive and risk-appropriate thromboprophylaxis.[93] Postulated mechanisms include sympathetic blockade leading to improved blood flow and decreased sympathetic stimulation, as well as a direct antithrombotic effect of the local anesthetic solution. However, neuraxial regional anesthesia is contraindicated in the fully anticoagulated patient, given the risk of epidural hematoma and subsequent devastating neural injury. Performance of deep plexus blocks in this setting, though, remains practitioner-dependent. Although few case reports exist of retroperitoneal hematoma following deep lumbar plexus blockade in anticoagulated patients, the relative safety of this technique was confirmed in a large study of 670 patients who underwent continuous lumbar plexus blockade while anticoagulated with warfarin.[15]

In the anticoagulated patient, a perivascular brachial plexus nerve block has the potential to cause excessive bleeding. Yet, several case reports document the safety of peripheral nerve block in the anticoagulated patient, particularly when it is placed under ultrasound guidance.[31] Despite these reassuring findings, the most recent published regional anesthesia guidelines advocate applying the same recommendations for neuraxial anesthesia to patients undergoing deep plexus or perivascular nerve blocks.[54] Patients who have incomplete reversal of their anticoagulation or who possess mild derangements of their coagulation panel for unclear reasons must be approached on a case-by-case basis, and the risks and benefits must be discussed thoroughly with the patient.

Bilateral Procedures. Although there may be instances in which regional anesthesia could be used for bilateral procedures, there are many risks, and it should be avoided if possible. The risk of drug toxicity is higher because the dose must be nearly doubled. Using a lower amount to avoid toxicity raises the probability of block failure.[33] The type of block also influences the risk. Interscalene nerve block commonly results in phrenic nerve paralysis,[111] so bilateral interscalene nerve block is contraindicated because of the risk of respiratory failure. Even supraclavicular blockade has an estimated associated risk of diaphragmatic paralysis of around 50%[81]; this risk, compounding the associated risk of pneumothorax, makes supraclavicular blockade an unreasonable technique for bilateral regional blockade. A safer alternative may be combining techniques of proximal and distal blockade or performing the blocks using low-volume, short-acting local anesthetics in sequence (i.e., performing the block on the second limb only upon completion of the first limb).[33,53]

Relative Indications
Microvascular Surgery Patients

Regional anesthesia with the use of long-acting blocks or continuous/prolonged infusion for digital reimplantation and free flaps is discussed in a later chapter. Continuous sympathetic blockade causes vasodilation and improves blood flow to the digit at risk and reduces neurogenically mediated vasospasm.[105] Improved pain control at the graft site via an effective nerve block also reduces pain-induced sympathetic-mediated vasospasm.[120] While peripheral nerve blockade has been shown to be a safe and effective anesthetic option, it is still unclear whether continuous nerve blockade indeed results in improved graft survival.[105]

Patients with scleroderma undergoing digital sympathectomy and vascular reconstruction also benefit from prolonged anesthetic blockade.[113]

Finally, patients with complex regional pain syndrome who undergo corrective surgery are also likely to benefit from effective prolonged regional anesthesia.[25]

Pediatric Patients

Anesthesia for pediatric patients depends greatly on the age and maturity of the child and the experience of the anesthesiologist. Many techniques combine general anesthesia for the surgical procedure itself with regional anesthesia for postoperative pain control. Many practitioners are comfortable placing blocks in anesthetized children, especially under ultrasound guidance, though the dose of anesthetic agent and the anatomy must be carefully considered.[72] Regional anesthetic technique has been demonstrated to be an effective form of postoperative pain control in children with very low rates of complications[87] and it has opioid-sparing effects. A long-term study looking at the use of continuous peripheral nerve catheters in pediatric patients shows this to be a safe and effective way to provide prolonged analgesia for this population of patients.[45]

Pregnant Patients

While elective procedures are generally not performed during pregnancy, circumstances that require surgery may present.

When possible, a local or regional technique should be used to minimize the effects on maternal physiology as well as reduce the possible pharmacologic exposure of the developing fetus. Ideally, surgical procedures should be deferred to the second trimester to minimize exposure of the fetus to teratogens during the critical period of organogenesis (15 to 56 days) and also limit the risks of preterm labor more prevalent in the third trimester.[55]

An anesthetic plan must provide safe anesthesia for both the mother and the fetus. When surgery is unavoidable in a previable fetus, the American College of Obstetricians recommends monitoring the fetal heart rate by Doppler ultrasound before and after surgery. With regard to a viable fetus, fetal heart rate and contraction monitoring should occur before, during, and after the procedure. The patient should have given consent for emergency cesarean section, and obstetric staff should be on standby in the event of fetal distress.[89]

The pregnant patient has an increased cardiac output, increased minute ventilation, increased risk for gastric aspiration, and increased upper airway edema, which can increase the risk of failed intubation. Fetal safety generally relates to avoidance of teratogenicity, avoidance of fetal asphyxia, and avoidance of preterm labor. While randomized controlled trials examining teratogenicity are not ethically or clinically feasible, local anesthetics, volatile agents, induction agents, muscle relaxants, and opioids are not considered teratogenic when used in clinical concentrations when normal maternal physiology is maintained. Nitrous oxide is probably best avoided given its effects on DNA synthesis and its teratogenic effects in animals.[39]

Patients With Rheumatoid Arthritis

Patients with rheumatoid arthritis are especially suitable candidates for regional anesthesia for upper limb surgery as it decreases the need for airway manipulation and blunts the stress response to surgery. Patients with deformity associated with advanced rheumatoid arthritis require careful positioning on the operating room table to avoid injury to other areas of the body.

This patient population often carries a high potential for airway complications owing to cervical spine immobility, paradoxic atlantoaxial instability, temporomandibular joint ankylosis, and cricoarytenoid arthritis,[96] all of which make endotracheal intubation difficult. Additionally, many rheumatoid patients are maintained on antirheumatic drugs and systemic corticosteroids, which have the potential for causing immunosuppression and a decreased neuroendocrine stress response. Patients consuming at least 20 mg of prednisone a day for more than 3 weeks are considered at significant risk for hypothalamic-pituitary-adrenal suppression.[2] These patients may be considered for stress dose steroid coverage depending on the invasiveness and stress of the procedure, and steroid treatment should be provided in the event of refractory hypotension.

Advantages and Disadvantages (Box 1.1)

A common concern regarding regional anesthesia is the question of whether the block will work. Success depends on the experience and confidence of the practitioner performing the block. At our orthopedic hospital, more than 6300 upper extremity blocks are performed annually, and we are able to

---

> **BOX 1.1 Factors Limiting Use of Regional Anesthesia**
>
> In spite of the advantages of regional anesthesia, several factors may prevent its use. Each of these problems can be overcome with appropriate planning.
> - Time constraints
> - Anesthesiologist's lack of familiarity with the procedure
> - Patient's fear of anesthesia failure
> - Concern about complications
> - Patient's desire to be completely unaware during the procedure

---

achieve a surgical level of anesthesia in 94% to 98% of patients.[71,70]

While regional blockade can effectively anesthetize the upper extremity and surgical site, this does not ensure patient comfort. Patients asked to lie motionless on a hard operating room bed might be apt to move to relieve discomfort in the back or knees, therefore disturbing the operative field. We place pillows to support the head and under the knees to reduce low-back strain. Even with adequate motor and sensory blockade, some patients will experience vibration or proprioception, and even vague sensations of pressure in the operative limb. Adequate anxiolysis and sedation will minimize the sensation. Access to the airway should be maintained during surgery in case the block is inadequate or other problems ensue. If the patient's position, such as lying prone, precludes this access intraoperatively, preoperative securing of the airway may be needed.

Duration of the neural blockade is variable, anywhere from 45 minutes to 24 hours after a single injection. The duration can be extended using a peripheral nerve catheter for continuous local anesthetic administration. Catheters have been successfully inserted along various levels of the brachial plexus depending on the desired location of blockade, from above the clavicle, such as interscalene and supraclavicular locations, to below the clavicle, such as infraclavicular and axillary locations.[95] Catheters can be maintained to provide continuous-flow or patient-controlled analgesia for hospitalized patients, and many centers have started home catheter programs for their outpatient population.

Prolonged regional anesthetic blockade provides improved pain relief during immediate postoperative physical therapy, and does not necessarily preclude active participation. In a study comparing continuous patient-controlled perineural infusion with 0.2% ropivacaine with patient-controlled IV narcotic infusion following arthroscopic rotator cuff repair, regional anesthesia techniques resulted in decreased use of supplementary analgesics and had a comparable incidence of motor weakness as did IV patient-controlled analgesia.[101]

The advantages of regional nerve block have been well demonstrated in the ambulatory surgery population. These advantages include lower pain scores, decreased nausea and vomiting, and shorter stays in the postanesthesia care unit.[57,95,101] While these effects are considerable in the immediate postoperative period, studies are ongoing to demonstrate a long-term outcome difference between the different types of anesthetics.[58,103] Evidence supports the finding that in patients undergoing repair of displaced distal radius fracture, regional anesthesia offers decreased pain and improved functional outcomes at 3 and 6 months.[27]

TABLE 1.1   Characteristics of Commonly Used Drugs

Generic Name (Trade Name)	CONCENTRATION (g/dL)		Maximum Dose (mg/kg)*	Approximate Duration
	Infiltration	Nerve Block		
Procaine (Novocain)	0.75	1.5-3	10-14	45-90 min, short-acting
Chloroprocaine (Nesacaine)	0.75	1.5-3	12-15	
Lidocaine (Xylocaine)	0.5	1-2	8-11	1.5-3 hr, medium-duration
Mepivacaine (Carbocaine)	0.5	1-2	8-11	
Tetracaine (Pontocaine)	0.05	0.15-0.2	2	
Bupivacaine (Marcaine)	0.25	0.25-0.5	2.5-3.5	3-10 hr, long-acting
Ropivacaine (Naropin)	0.25	0.25-0.5	2.5-3.5	

*Higher doses with the use of 1:200,000 epinephrine.

BOX 1.2   Prevention of Systemic Toxicity

- Avoid intravascular injection.
- Use epinephrine to slow systemic absorption.
- Use benzodiazepine as a premedication.
- Use ultrasound guidance to fractionate the dose.

Equipment and Pharmacologic Requirements

Medications commonly used in regional anesthesia are listed in Table 1.1.

Regional anesthesia may be administered in a designated block room or preoperative area, in addition to in the operating room. It is crucial to have available appropriate monitoring and resuscitation equipment, including airway management supplies and resuscitative medication, should an acute complication arise. High-flow oxygen, airway management equipment, and suction capability are crucial for emergency airway management in the event of seizure or high or total spinal block. Medications including inotropes, anticholinergics, and vasopressors should be immediately available to treat symptomatic arrhythmias, bradycardias, and hypotensive episodes. Other available medications should include benzodiazepines or propofol to treat seizures and an intralipid to treat bupivacaine-induced cardiovascular collapse (Box 1.2).[4]

Local Anesthetic Additives

In recent years, the use of additives in local anesthetics to increase efficacy and onset of block, as well as overall block duration, has been readily investigated.[5] Historically, sodium bicarbonate has been used to increase onset of sensory and motor blockade in epidural anesthesia through alkalinization of the molecule, thereby facilitating its passage across lipid membranes. When used perineurally, this advantage appears to be more unpredictable for certain types of blocks and may not be clinically significant.[18] Epinephrine, on the other hand, remains one of the most popular adjuncts for prolonging the effect of short- and intermediate-acting local anesthetics by decreasing systemic uptake of the local anesthetic through vasoconstriction. It is also an excellent marker for detection of intravascular injection. The advantage of epinephrine as an adjunctive in long-acting local anesthetic peripheral nerve blocks is not as apparent, especially when juxtaposed with concerns of neurotoxicity in at-risk patients.[114]

Dexamethasone is another additive that has gained popularity in recent years because of its ability to significantly prolong peripheral nerve blockade. Through its proposed ability to inhibit nociceptive C-fibers, dexamethasone has been used with both short- and long-acting local anesthetics in upper extremity surgeries with some success, though recent randomized trials and meta-analyses suggest that this effect can be achieved just as well via IV administration, which has a well-characterized safety profile.[22,24] While investigations into concerns for neurotoxicity with dexamethasone have not yielded conclusive results, we recommend that care be taken when using this adjunct in patients with preexisting nerve injuries.

Alpha-2 selective adrenergic agonists such as clonidine and dexmedetomidine have an analgesic benefit when added to local anesthetics for peripheral blocks.[38,88] By inhibiting current channels that facilitate neurons to return to normal resting potential from a hyperpolarized state, clonidine and dexmedetomidine selectively disable C-fiber neurons from generating subsequent action potentials, resulting in analgesia. The disadvantages of using these additives include dose-dependent systemic effects of sedation, bradycardia, and hypotension.

Opioid agonists such as tramadol and buprenorphine are also used as additives to local anesthetics.[3,9] Tramadol, which acts as a weak mu-opioid agonist while stimulating serotonin release and inhibiting reuptake of norepinephrine, prolongs blockade when given perineurally but does not reliably have a clear advantage over IV or intramuscular administration.[59,61] Buprenorphine, on the other hand, has a fairly consistent record of prolonging block duration and reducing postoperative analgesia when given perineurally, an effect not related to systemic absorption of the drug. The mechanism of action of buprenorphine is an ability to inhibit voltage-gated sodium channels in a fashion similar to local anesthetics.[67] Further studies are needed to elucidate any potential neurotoxic effects of this adjunct.

Finally, additives such as ketamine, midazolam, and magnesium, while showing some promise, do not have an adequately characterized safety profile to be recommended as routine additives to local anesthetics at this time.[64-66]

Historical Techniques

Regional nerve blockade is essentially the deposition of local anesthetic near a nerve. Historically, nerve blocks were blind techniques, performed on the basis of known anatomic relationships to superficial landmarks. Practitioners noted that patients would report paresthesias as the needle advanced, leading to development of the paresthesia technique. This technique required a cooperative and conscious patient capable of providing verbal feedback, as the anesthetic practitioner would intentionally attempt to elicit a paresthesia as a means of nerve localization. Others began experimenting with the use of a nerve stimulator, applying a low-current electrical impulse through the needle near a nerve to stimulate muscle contraction.[14] Studies were unable to demonstrate outcome differences.[85] Though it was hoped that nerve localization using nerve stimulation would decrease actual needle-to-nerve contact, reducing nerve injury, a randomized prospective trial comparing the two techniques was unable to determine a difference in postoperative neurologic symptoms.[69] An advantage of the development of the nerve stimulator was decreased reliance on patient feedback and, therefore, the ability to perform the technique on sedated or even anesthetized patients.

Ultrasound was next used to improve needle placement by means of a portable device in the operating room or holding area. Ultrasound allows visualization of anatomic structures, blood vessels, and nerves, as well as of the advancement of a needle and the distribution of local anesthetic.[60] With satisfactory visualization of target structures, this technique does not require patient feedback and can be used safely after the patient has been given sedation or even general anesthesia.[78] However, when target structures are deep, needle visualization can be difficult; in such cases, it is a standard of safety to engage patient feedback whenever possible. Several studies have demonstrated improved onset and decreased dosing requirements compared with traditional techniques.[76,107] A recent metaanalysis of 16 randomized controlled trials showed that ultrasound decreased the incidence of complete hemidiaphragmatic paresis and vascular punctures and was more likely to result in a successful brachial plexus block when compared with the nerve stimulation technique.[119] Despite these benefits, ultrasound-guided blocks do not appear to decrease the incidence of neurologic injury.[71,119] Certainly, this is an area in need of further study and review as we attempt to maximize results while minimizing risks of complications for our patients.

Continuous Peripheral Nerve Catheters

The use of continuous peripheral nerve catheters has gained favor both in the inpatient setting and the outpatient setting. As mentioned before, the advantages include time-extended, opioid-sparing, and site-specific analgesia with only minimal side effects.[12] Disadvantages include increased anesthesia performance time, dislodgement or malplacement of the catheter leading to ineffective analgesia, and infection.[56] Rarely, brachial plexus peripheral nerve catheters have led to epidural and even intrathecal blockade.[40,112] The incidence of brachial plexus catheter failure on postoperative day 1 is between 19% and 26%.[1] The rate of dislodgement is low (<5%) but is directly correlated with the length of time the catheter has been in place and the extent of upper extremity movement.[74] Though there appears

to be a modest clinical benefit to the use of nerve-stimulating catheters over nonstimulating catheters to confirm tip placement, this advantage has been largely minimized by ultrasound guidance.[79] In contrast to epidural catheters, the choice of end-orifice versus multiple-orifice catheters in continuous peripheral nerve blocks does not affect analgesic quality.[35]

Once the patient is at home, peripheral nerve infusion pumps for ambulatory surgery patients are safe and effective for extending the duration of nerve blocks from hours to days. In a study of ambulatory patients comparing general anesthesia with single-shot interscalene nerve blocks with continuous interscalene blocks for 48 hours, during which time the patients went home, the catheter group had lower pain scores both at 48 hours and at 1 week.[95] Rare complications include respiratory compromise in proximal brachial plexus catheters (interscalene and supraclavicular blocks) due to ipsilateral diaphragmatic paralysis, technical problems involving the infusion pump leading to dosing inconsistency, infection due to the indwelling catheter, and catheter coiling leading to block failure or catheter retention.[56] Evidence supports the use of these catheters in children as well as adults.[45]

Minimum Effective Volume

In recent years, efforts to determine the minimum effective volume (MEV) of local anesthetic required to produce an adequate operative and postoperative anesthetic have been made in order to reduce the dose-dependent side effects and the risk of neurotoxicity and systemic absorption without sacrificing time to onset of block and overall duration of effective analgesia. These efforts have been helped enormously by the use of ultrasound. For the upper extremity, low local anesthetic volumes have been established for interscalene blocks and axillary blocks using ultrasound guidance. Although the absolute effect of type and concentration of local anesthetic on minimal volume is not yet elucidated, the MEV to elicit an interscalene blockade that is 90% to 95% successful ranges as low as less than 1 mL.[29,76] Reducing the anesthetic volume in interscalene blocks has the potential advantage of reducing the incidence of hemidiaphragmatic paresis.[92] For axillary blocks, the 90% to 95% MEV averages 1 to 2 mL per nerve.[30,42] On the contrary, the 90% to 95% MEV for supraclavicular and infraclavicular blocks averages above 30 mL.[108,109] We postulate that this discrepancy in the latter blocks may be related to increased variations in injection techniques and anatomy.

Elderly patients generally require lower local anesthetic volumes, an effect likely related to a decrease in the cross-sectional area of the brachial plexus as we age.[84] Similarly, diabetic patients are more likely to have a successful supraclavicular block than their nondiabetic counterparts for a given local anesthetic dose.[41] The authors postulate that this is due either to an increased sensitivity of diabetic nerve fibers to local anesthetic, inadvertent intraneural penetration due to decreased ability to elicit paresthesias, or a preexisting neuropathy leading to decreased sensation to surgical stimulation. Surprisingly, although associated with a higher performance difficulty, an increased body mass index does not necessitate an increased local anesthetic volume.[44,100]

In general, in the absence of additives, decreasing the dose of local anesthetic either by volume or concentration in the peripheral block results in a reduction of block duration and decreases the time until the patient first requires an analgesic.[36,99] Despite the advantage of decreasing dose-dependent complications and reducing neurotoxicity, our goal in establishing the MEV should always be juxtaposed with the surgical procedure, the patient's particular risk factors, and the expected postoperative pain. In the end, it is also important to remember that the MEV for any given block is heavily influenced by the practitioner and his or her ability to deposit local anesthetic optimally.

Specific Blocks

The goal of regional anesthesia for upper extremity surgery is to provide anesthesia in the localized area of surgery, taking into account other potential painful stimuli, including positioning and the application of a tourniquet. There are many different approaches to nerve blockade, all involving nerves encompassed in the brachial plexus and providing sensory and motor innervation to the upper extremity. The brachial plexus is formed by the ventral rami of C5-T1, occasionally with small contributions by C4 and T2 (Figure 1.1).

There are multiple approaches to blockade of the brachial plexus, beginning proximally with the interscalene approach and continuing distally with the supraclavicular, infraclavicular, axillary, and midhumeral approaches at the terminal branches. The uniting concept is the existence of a sheath encompassing the neurovascular bundle extending from the deep cervical fascia to slightly beyond the borders of the axilla.[32]

Interscalene Block

The interscalene block is the most proximal approach, performed as the brachial plexus courses in the groove between the anterior and middle scalene muscles, traditionally at the level of the cricoid cartilage (Figure 1.2).[117] This block is well suited for procedures of the shoulder, the lateral two thirds of the clavicle, and the proximal humerus. Advantages of this block include rapid and reliable blockade of the shoulder region, as well as relative ease of landmark palpation. Disadvantages of this block traditionally include incomplete coverage of the inferior trunk of the plexus; hence, insufficient anesthesia of the ulnar distribution makes it an unreliable block for forearm or hand procedures. The interscalene block commonly causes transient ipsilateral diaphragmatic paralysis and ipsilateral Horner syndrome because of the proximity of the phrenic nerve and the cervical sympathetic ganglion, respectively. Rare but serious complications include permanent phrenic nerve palsy and cervical epidural and total spinal blockade.[68]

Supraclavicular Block

A supraclavicular approach to the brachial plexus provides profound anesthesia for the entire arm, making it an appropriate block for most upper extremity procedures. Past approaches have used surface landmarks, generally lateral to the lateral border of the sternocleidomastoid muscle and superior to the clavicle, considering the first rib as the safety margin for the cupola of the lung.[63] Proximity to the brachial plexus was

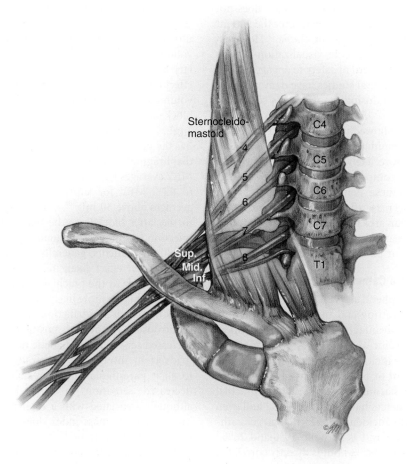

FIGURE 1.1 Brachial plexus, showing the relationship of the roots, trunks, divisions, and cords to bony landmarks. *Inf.,* Inferior; *Mid.,* middle; *Sup.,* superior. (Copyright Elizabeth Martin.)

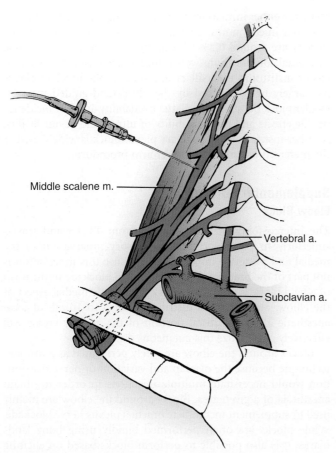

FIGURE 1.2 Interscalene technique. (From Winnie AP: Regional anesthesia. *Surg Clin North Am* 55:861–892, 1975.)

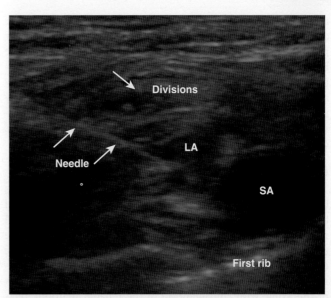

FIGURE 1.3 Ultrasound-guided supraclavicular nerve block. The brachial plexus is approached at the level of the divisions; the needle is entering the view from the lateral aspect at the top left of the screen. The pulsations of the subclavian artery (*SA*) are visualized, as is the spread of local anesthetic (*LA*).

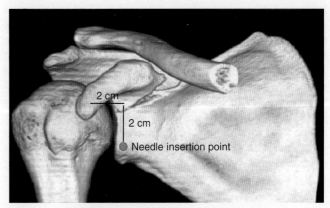

FIGURE 1.4 Landmarks for infraclavicular block.

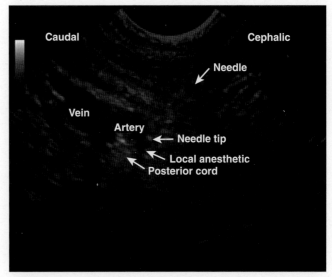

FIGURE 1.5 Ultrasound-guided infraclavicular nerve block; note the perivascular spread of local anesthetic.

determined using either paresthesia or nerve stimulator techniques.[34] Concern regarding the risk for pneumothorax with traditional techniques (estimated at 1% to 4%) led to the development of an ultrasound-guided technique for supraclavicular brachial plexus blockade (Figure 1.3).[60,116] Ultrasound guidance allows the practitioner to visualize the first rib and the border of the pleura, thereby being able to watch the approach of the needle to help ensure an appropriate distance from these vulnerable structures.[102] Advantages include a compact formation of the plexus at this level and resultant dense blockade of the entire upper extremity. Disadvantages include the remote risk of pneumothorax, suprascapular nerve palsy,[26] and potential for slower block onset.

Infraclavicular Block

The infraclavicular (or coracoid) approach is more distal still, at the level of the cords as they course circumferentially around the subclavian artery, providing dense anesthesia to the entire arm to the fingers. This block does not adequately anesthetize the shoulder but has become the block of choice at our institution for elbow, wrist, and hand surgery. Initial techniques of the infraclavicular block based needle placement on anatomic landmarks and nerve localization with a nerve stimulator,[91] but more recent approaches favor an ultrasound approach (Figures 1.4 and 1.5).[97] The consistent anatomic relationship between the cords and the vascular structures makes it a predictable and reliable block to perform under ultrasound guidance. The lower anatomic location of this block makes it unlikely to encounter phrenic blockade and therefore makes it a more appropriate block for bilateral procedures. Disadvantages include pneumothorax, a risk minimized by performing the block more laterally along the clavicle,[11] and the concern that if the subclavian artery is accidentally punctured in the infraclavicular approach, subsequent compression of the area to tamponade bleeding is difficult.

Axillary Block

The axillary block, the most distal of the brachial plexus blocks before the nerves leave the sheath and divide into their terminal branches, is perhaps one of the oldest and most traditional regional blocks for hand and wrist surgery. Various guidance techniques are described, including ultrasound, anatomic (either transarterial or paresthesia), or nerve stimulator techniques. All begin with palpation of the axillary nerve in the apex of the axilla, with consideration of the reliable anatomic relationship of the nerves to this arterial landmark (Figure 1.6). Because the musculocutaneous nerve frequently leaves the sheath proximal to the intended insertion point of this block, frequently a supplemental injection into the body of the coracobrachialis muscle is needed, especially if a forearm tourniquet is planned. This can be done easily with a blind technique as well as with ultrasound guidance, as the nerve is commonly found in the fascial plane between the coracobrachialis muscle and the biceps. A 2013 Cochrane Database Review showed that a multiple-injection technique led to more effective anesthesia than a single- or double-injection technique; however, no difference in other outcomes could be found.[16] Major risks for this block are largely related to the close proximity of the axillary artery. Risks for minor bruising and tenderness run higher with transarterial techniques, although the risk of hematoma is lower, reported from 0.2%[104] to 8%.[62] Another concern relating to the high vascularity of this area is local anesthetic toxicity

related to either intraarterial injection or rapid systemic absorption after injection near an arterial puncture. Rates of systemic toxicity are around 0.2%.[104] Although the end results of these incidental complications were minor and without lasting effect, at our institution the axillary approach to the brachial plexus has largely been replaced by the ultrasound-guided infraclavicular block because of the latter's reliability and low incidence of side effects and the availability of ultrasound at our facility. At other institutions, the axillary plexus block is widely used as the preferred technique for lower arm procedures.

Supplementary Blocks
Elbow Block

The intercostobrachial nerve arises from T1-T3 and travels superiorly to provide cutaneous sensory innervation to the medial and posterior upper arm.[82] Because this innervation is not part of the brachial plexus, additional blockade in the form of a field block is used for surgery around the medial aspect of the elbow. Subcutaneous distribution of 5 to 10 mL of local anesthetic along the distal portion of the axillary crease will effectively anesthetize this cutaneous distribution.

Blocks around the elbow are rarely performed as a primary technique because the overlap and variation of nerve distribution would necessitate multiple injections in order to obtain anesthesia of a given area. Blocks around the elbow are mainly used to supplement incomplete brachial plexus nerve blockade. While blocks are often performed blindly using bony landmarks, it is also possible to perform blocks based on eliciting paresthesias or nerve stimulation. The median, radial, and ulnar nerves are individually visualized using ultrasound as they course from the elbow to the wrist.[75]

The median nerve may be blocked as it courses posteromedial to the brachial artery superior to the antecubital crease. The nerve is typically blocked using 5 to 10 mL of local anesthetic injected slightly superior to a line connecting the epicondyles. This block can be accomplished using a blind, landmark-based technique, by eliciting paresthesias, or by using a nerve stimulator.

The radial nerve can be blocked 3 to 4 cm above the lateral epicondyle, close to the distal head of the humerus. After the lateral intramuscular septum has been pierced, paresthesias or a nerve stimulator can be used to localize the nerve. An injection of 5 to 10 mL of local anesthetic will provide an adequate nerve block in this location.

The ulnar nerve is largely missed in interscalene blocks, so supplementation is often necessary to obtain complete anesthesia of the arm. The nerve is usually blocked as it runs behind the medial epicondyle. Injection of 3 to 5 mL of local anesthetic is made between the olecranon and the medial epicondyle. Caution must be used to avoid compressing the nerve, because it runs near the bony landmarks.[94]

Wrist Block

Hand surgeons frequently use wrist blocks to produce anesthesia for surgery or supplement plexus nerve blocks. Wrist blocks are relatively simple and reliable to perform based on external landmarks. The nerve supply of the extrinsic muscles of the hand is preserved, thus allowing the patient to move the fingers of the hand, but the intrinsic muscles are paralyzed. Whereas

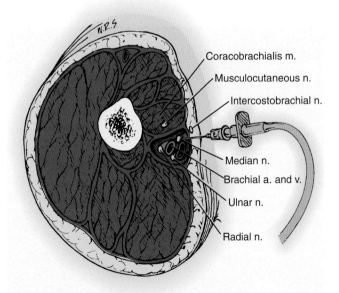

N.R.S.

Coracobrachialis m.

Musculocutaneous n.

Intercostobrachial n.

Median n.

Brachial a. and v.

Ulnar n.

Radial n.

FIGURE 1.6 Cross-sectional view of the axillary nerve block. (From Winnie AP: Regional anesthesia. *Surg Clin North Am* 55:861–892, 1975.)

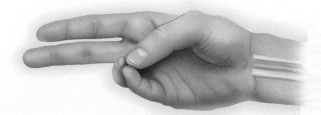

FIGURE 1.7 Surface anatomy for median nerve block at the wrist. (Reproduced with permission from Chung KC, editor: *Operative Techniques: Hand and Wrist Surgery*, Philadelphia, 2008, Saunders, p 5.)

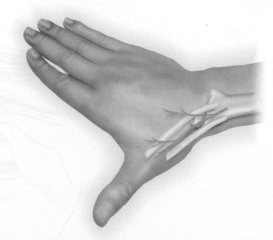

FIGURE 1.9 Surface anatomy for radial nerve block at the wrist. (Reproduced with permission from Chung KC, editor: *Operative Techniques: Hand and Wrist Surgery*, Philadelphia, 2008, Saunders, p 7).

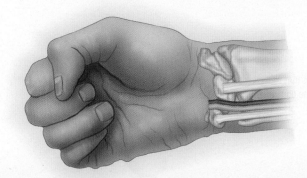

FIGURE 1.8 Surface anatomy for ulnar nerve block at the wrist. (Reproduced with permission from Chung KC, editor: *Operative Techniques: Hand and Wrist Surgery*, Philadelphia, 2008, Saunders, p 6.)

this can be an advantage in a cooperative patient, it is a potential disadvantage and distraction in an uncooperative patient. Additionally, the need for a forearm tourniquet limits the duration of surgery to 20 to 30 minutes in most instances. These blocks are especially efficacious for carpal tunnel release.[23,110]

The median nerve can be blocked as it courses between the palmaris longus and flexor carpi radialis tendons (Figure 1.7). A 1.5-cm, 25-gauge needle is inserted at the level of the ulnar styloid process or the proximal crease of the wrist. In the absence of the palmaris longus tendon, the needle is inserted on the ulnar side of the flexor carpi radialis tendon. After penetration through the flexor retinaculum at a depth of approximately 1 cm, 5 mL of local anesthetic is injected. Injecting 1 mL of local anesthetic above the retinaculum as the needle is withdrawn can block a superficial palmar branch supplying the skin over the thenar eminence.[21,94]

The ulnar nerve is blocked at the wrist at either the radial or the ulnar side of the flexor carpi ulnaris tendon (Figure 1.8). The ulnar approach is preferred so as to avoid intravascular injection, given the location of the ulnar artery on the radial side of the tendon. At the level of the distal ulna, the needle is introduced on the dorsal ulnar side of the flexor carpi ulnaris. Subsequent injection of 5 mL of local anesthetic under the flexor carpi ulnaris will result in anesthesia of this distribution. Additional subcutaneous infiltration of the dorsal ulnar area of the wrist ensures adequate blockade of the dorsal cutaneous branch of the ulnar nerve.[21]

The radial nerve is superficial and divided into branches running in the subcutaneous fat at the level of the radial styloid process (Figure 1.9). It may be blocked using 5 to 10 mL of local anesthetic injected in a subcutaneous field block at the level of the radial styloid. Initial injection is made using 2 to 3 mL of local anesthetic just lateral to the radial artery at the level of the proximal wrist crease. The needle is then redirected and advanced with subcutaneous injection of 5 to 7 mL of local anesthetic across the proximal border of the snuffbox to the midpoint of the dorsal wrist. Several injections may be necessary to follow the curvature of the wrist and block the many superficial branches.[94]

Digital Block

As the most distal innervation of the hand, four nerve branches—two dorsal and two volar—run along the sides of each digit to supply each digit (Figure 1.10). There are three main recommended approaches for performing digital nerve block—transthecal, transmetacarpal, and subcutaneous. A circumferential ring block along the base of the digit is not recommended because the subsequent pressure can result in gangrene.

Transthecal digital nerve block uses the flexor tendon sheath for anesthetic infusion. At the level of the palmar digital crease, the needle enters the flexor tendon sheath until bony contact is made (Figure 1.11). The needle is then withdrawn slowly until the local anesthetic solution is injected easily into the potential space between the periosteum and the flexor tendon. Two milliliters of local anesthetic is used for digital anesthesia. Advantages of this approach include a single injection and rapid onset[52]; however, patients often complain of prolonged discomfort in the finger after this technique.[73]

Transmetacarpal block is performed at the level of the distal palmar crease. The insertion site is approximately 1 cm proximal to the metacarpophalangeal joint, traditionally on the volar side of the hand (Figure 1.12), though some favor entering the thinner dorsal side for patient comfort. Two milliliters of local anesthetic injected on one side of the metacarpal neck effectively anesthetizes the common digital nerve supplying the finger.[98]

Subcutaneous digital nerve block is accomplished at the level of the distal palmar crease. The needle is inserted vertically into each side of the flexor tendon sheath, and 2 mL of local

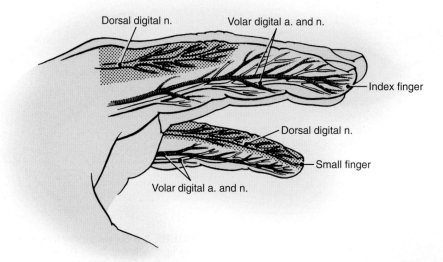

FIGURE 1.10 Relationship and distribution of the digital nerves. Note that in the small finger, the dorsal digital nerve extends to the top of the digit; in the median nerve distribution, the volar nerve supplies the dorsum of the digit distal to the proximal interphalangeal joint. (Copyright Elizabeth Martin.)

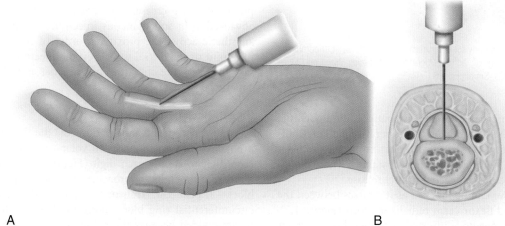

A   B

FIGURE 1.11 Transthecal digital nerve block. (Reproduced with permission from Chung KC, editor: *Operative Techniques: Hand and Wrist Surgery.* Philadelphia, 2008, Saunders, p 13.)

anesthetic is injected at each location (Figure 1.13). Alternatively, injection can be made just proximal to the web of the finger using a 1.5-cm, 25-gauge needle, creating a skin wheal superficial to the extensor hood to block the dorsal nerve. The needle is then advanced toward the palm and an additional 1-mL injection is made just under the skin on the volar side to anesthetize the volar digital nerve. The needle is then withdrawn to the skin and redirected toward the opposite side of the finger to place a superficial skin wheal, and the process is repeated on that side. Care must be taken to use small volumes of local anesthetic to avoid creating a circumferential ring. In recent years, clinicians have moved away from the traditional two injections method to a single injection method due to improved patient comfort. With this technique, 2 to 3 mL of local anesthetic are deposited into the subcutaneous space at the middle point of the palmar digital crease.

Use of Epinephrine in Digital Nerve Blockade. Long-standing debate has taken place about the use of epinephrine in digital nerve blocks because of concern regarding vasoconstriction to

the digit and subsequent ischemia and necrosis. Several studies and reviews have addressed this issue; Chowdhry and colleagues published a retrospective review in 2010 that reported no adverse events involving digital gangrene in 1111 patients.[19] The authors concluded that the use of local anesthetic with the addition of epinephrine was safe in digital nerve blockade, enabling improved hemostasis and decreasing the need for tourniquet placement.[19]

Intravenous Regional Block

Intravenous regional block, or Bier block, was one of the first techniques of regional blockade, introduced in 1908.[20] Bier block can be used for brief surgical procedures or manipulation of the distal upper extremity. Advantages of this technique include ease of use and rapid onset of anesthesia; disadvantages include the necessity of using a pneumatic tourniquet and the lack of postoperative analgesia.

This technique involves placement of an IV catheter in the dorsum of the hand, followed by exsanguination of the upper

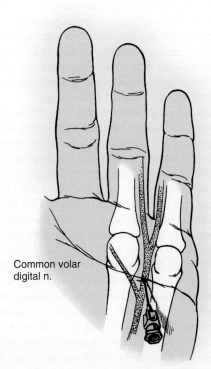

FIGURE 1.12 Transmetacarpal digital nerve block. (Copyright Elizabeth Martin.)

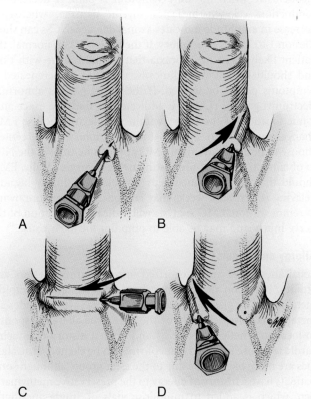

FIGURE 1.13 Subcutaneous digital nerve block. **A,** The needle is inserted along one side of the flexor tendon sheath to block the volar nerve (**B**). **C,** The dorsal digital nerve is anesthetized with a superficial skin wheal. **D,** The opposite volar nerve is blocked using the same technique. Care is taken to ensure that local anesthetic is not injected fully circumferentially around the finger. (Copyright Elizabeth Martin.)

extremity and inflation of a pneumatic tourniquet. Subsequent injection of local anesthetic into the venous system by means of the IV catheter results in rapid and profound sensory blockade. Plain lidocaine 0.5% in a dose of 3 mg/kg is the typical agent of choice, which results in a volume of 40 mL for the average adult.[20] Other agents such as prilocaine may be used instead[43]; however, bupivacaine is contraindicated in Bier block because of potential cardiac toxicity. While not well studied, additives such as acetaminophen, magnesium, narcotics, and vecuronium have been used in an effort to increase onset and efficacy of the Bier block while reducing the total local anesthetic volume needed to achieve adequate anesthesia.[77]

Contraindications include crush injuries or compound fractures in which the venous system may be interrupted or the extremity difficult to exsanguinate. Bier block is also contraindicated in patients in whom tourniquet use is contraindicated, in patients with local skin infections or cellulitis, or in those with a convincing allergy to local anesthetics. Another limitation to the use of a Bier block is duration of tourniquet application; patients tend to complain of tourniquet pain after 30 minutes. Adding a second distal tourniquet allows prolongation of the block; after tourniquet pain is experienced with the proximal tourniquet, the distal tourniquet is inflated. By using this double-tourniquet technique, the tourniquet time is prolonged up to 1 hour.[86]

Complications associated with Bier block are mainly related to drug effects of the local anesthetic, especially if there is mechanical tourniquet failure leading to early deflation of the cuff. It is recommended that the cuff stay inflated for 20 to 30 minutes after injection in order to minimize local anesthetic effects, particularly on the cardiovascular and respiratory systems.[43] Using incremental deflation, inflation, and deflation again allows for gradual release of the local anesthetic from the isolated limb. Additional complications can arise from the use of the pneumatic tourniquet, including but not limited to ischemic and mechanical crush injuries.

❖ AUTHOR'S PREFERRED METHOD OF TREATMENT: Regional Anesthesia

For surgery of the upper extremity, regional anesthesia is our standard method. Regional anesthesia is associated with decreased morbidity and shorter stays in the postanesthesia care unit.[46,57,95,101]

Our preferred blocks for regional anesthesia of the upper extremity are ultrasound-guided supraclavicular and infraclavicular blocks. They are often faster to perform in less experienced hands, have a faster onset, and allow smaller anesthetic volumes to be used.[76,106,107] Each year nearly 5000 supraclavicular and infraclavicular blocks are performed at our institution. Of these 5000, all but a few are done with ultrasound guidance. This method has proven to be very safe, rapid, and highly successful at anesthetizing the upper extremity.

The type of ultrasound-guided block chosen depends on the surgery involved. For surgery from the shoulder to the elbow and occasionally from the elbow to the hand, the block of choice at our institution is the ultrasound-guided supraclavicular block. For surgery on the more distal upper extremity, the block of choice is most frequently the ultrasound-guided infraclavicular block.

The technique for perivascular blocks involves an in-plane view of the needle at its point of entry just under the skin to its location near the plexus. The needle choice is probably less critical, although we use short-bevel, noninsulated needles, which are more echogenic. In placing the block, our goal is to keep needle movement to a minimum, thereby decreasing the chance for needle-to-nerve trauma. For the supraclavicular block, the needle is placed just inferoposterolateral to the plexus, as in "eight ball in the corner pocket" (see Figure 1.3).[102] The preferred position of the infraclavicular block is the 6 o'clock location relative to the subclavian artery (see Figure 1.4). The goal is to get close to the nerve (plexus or cord) without actually coming into contact with it. Once the fascial plane adjacent to the nerve is reached, a small amount of local anesthetic is injected. The anesthetic will hydrodissect the area and demonstrate local filling in the desired location of the nerve. Again, needle movement is kept to a minimum while injecting the full dose of local anesthetic. We find these locations to be reliable in accomplishing whole-plexus blocks while minimizing needle-to-nerve contact and trauma.

Complications
Neurapraxia (Box 1.3)

Incidence. Temporary postoperative paresthesia, or temporary sensory or motor deficit, is relatively uncommon. Injury can result from needle trauma, local anesthetic irritation, patient positioning, tourniquet compression, or surgical manipulation, to name a few of the confounding variables. Studies attempting to elucidate the relationship between neural anatomy and nerve injury, mainly correlating epineural and intraneural injections with neurologic sequelae, have been largely inconclusive.[17] The majority of these postoperative neuropathies resolve by 4 weeks, and the incidence of prolonged or permanent neurologic deficit is exceedingly rare. Certain patient risk factors have been identified that may increase the risk of neurologic injury after peripheral nerve blockade. These include old age, the use of chemotherapy, and the presence of diabetes mellitus, cervical myelopathy, multiple sclerosis, vascular disease, and any other preexisting neuropathies.[6] A review of recent literature shows the incidence of temporary neurologic complications after peripheral regional anesthesia to be 3% to 8% and of permanent nerve injury as defined by the presence of symptoms after 6 months to be between 0.04% and 0.6%.[7,37] Interestingly, the use of ultrasound guidance rather than the nerve-stimulator technique has not led to a decrease in the incidence of neurologic complications after peripheral nerve blockade.[7,37,80]

Management (Figure 1.14). It is often the surgeon who discovers the existence of residual neurapraxia postoperatively. Management of the patient's concerns and the suspected injury requires

thorough communication between the surgeon, anesthesiologist, and patient. A thorough history and physical examination are needed to determine the duration and types of symptoms and the vascular integrity, dermatomal distribution, and correlated motor or sensory deficit. It is important to investigate other confounding factors such as postoperative pain, immobility, edema, positioning, and casting or dressings.

We recommend dividing the findings into minor or major deficits. Minor deficits include positional paresthesias, defined as changes in temperature or light touch sensation without loss of motor function. Sometimes a burning sensation in a dermatomal distribution is present. For minor deficits, reassurance that the deficit will likely resolve in a few weeks will likely allay the patient's anxiety. It is important to closely follow the patient to ensure resolution of symptoms, provide reassurance, and allow early detection of a more serious problem or the need for referral to a neurologist.

Major deficits, such as complete or nearly complete palsy, should prompt early neurologic or neurosurgical consultation, which may be able to guide further diagnostic testing and treatment. If compression is suspected, ultrasound or magnetic resonance imaging should be performed to localize the lesion, followed by prompt surgical decompression.[6] Pain medication should be provided to prevent nerve sensitization and the potential for a complex regional pain syndrome. Nerve conduction studies (NCSs) can detect the presence of a lesion in myelinated nerves. However, because the nerves that transmit pain sensation are mostly unmyelinated nerves, NCSs are inconclusive when the only symptom is pain. A decrease in conduction velocity indicates myelin damage, whereas a decrease in amplitude indicates axonal damage. NCSs can show a lesion 1 to 2 days after injury. If the initial NCS is normal, the patient likely has a neurapraxia that should resolve with time and should be followed clinically, with the NCS repeated if symptoms persist or worsen. If the initial NCS is abnormal, electromyography (EMG) is indicated to find the exact anatomic location of the injury within the plexus. Because EMG changes appear 2 to 4 weeks following injury, many centers choose to perform an initial EMG at the same time as the NCS to obtain a baseline of preexisting nerve damage. Ideally, EMG should then be performed 2 to 4 weeks after injury because delaying it beyond 4 weeks may complicate the picture owing to reinnervation. EMG analysis will indicate the location of the nerve injury and may be able to pinpoint the likely cause.[48]

Allergy and Sepsis

Local anesthetics are categorized into two groups, esters and amides, based on their chemical structure. Esters are rapidly metabolized by plasma pseudocholinesterase, while amides are metabolized intracellularly by the liver. True allergic responses to local anesthetics are rare,[8,10] and often a history of a tachycardic response to added epinephrine can be elicited. True allergies are more likely to be due to the ester group, although some patients have a history of allergy to the preservative methylparaben, which is added to multidose vials of amide anesthetic. There is no evidence for cross-reactivity between the two groups, attributable to the different chemical structures.

Any injection through the skin raises concerns for infection, and regional nerve blockade is no exception. Aseptic technique is recommended, including thorough hand washing and skin

---

BOX 1.3 **Neurologic Complications**
• Neurologic complications can occur after regional or general anesthesia.
• Use of ultrasound does not appear to minimize this risk.
• The mechanisms of injury are sometimes obscure.
• With appropriate precautions the frequency of nerve injury after nerve blocks is quite low.

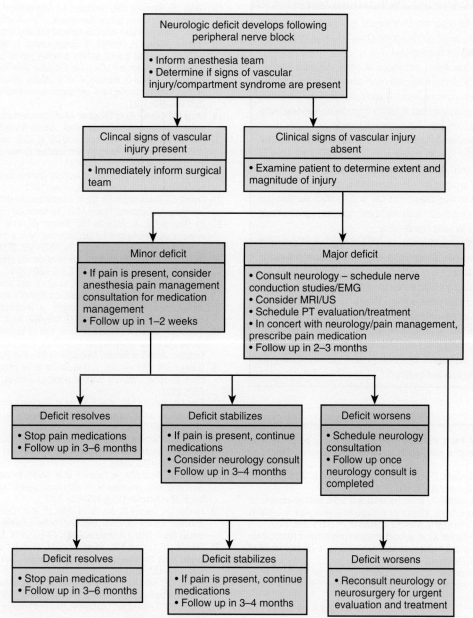

FIGURE 1.14 Management of neurologic deficit following peripheral nerve block. (Reproduced and modified with permission from Hadzic A, editor: *Textbook of Regional Anesthesia and Acute Pain Management,* New York, 2007, McGraw-Hill, p 989.)

cleansing with either povidone-iodine solution or chlorhexidine.[51] The rate of infection is exceptionally low for single-shot techniques, though sporadic case reports can be found in the literature. It is established that indwelling catheters have the potential for colonization; however, the rate of clinical infection, which positively correlates with catheter duration, is negligible.[51]

CRITICAL POINTS *Regional Anesthesia*

- Regional anesthesia for upper extremity surgery may improve the control of postoperative pain, lower opiate consumption, decrease nausea and vomiting, and decrease the hospital stay.
- Among the regional anesthesia techniques of nerve stimulator–guided, paresthesia-guided, or ultrasound-guided nerve block, there is no demonstrated improvement in outcome with any particular technique. However, ultrasound-guided blocks have been shown to improve onset and decrease dosage requirements compared with traditional techniques.
- Absolute contraindications to regional anesthesia are infection at the site of injection and patient refusal. Patient refusal often stems from fear of the unknown, which can be dispelled with a forthright discussion and promise of adequate sedation prior to administering the block.
- The use of additives to local anesthetics can prolong block duration and analgesia while reducing overall local anesthetic dose, but agents should be chosen judiciously to avoid neurotoxicity.
- Continuous peripheral nerve catheters are safe and effective for extending opioid-sparing, site-specific analgesia for adult and pediatric patients in both the inpatient and outpatient settings.
- The incidence of temporary postoperative paresthesias is between 3% and 8%; of that number, most resolve within 4 weeks.
- Prolonged neurapraxias are extremely rare, with an incidence of between 0.04% and 0.6%. In the event of a neurapraxia, a coordinated effort between the anesthesiologist and surgeon is required, as well as thorough communication with the patient. Often, early neurologic consultation will help with further diagnosis and treatment.

REFERENCES

1. Ahsan ZS, Carvalho B, Yao J: Incidence of failure of continuous peripheral nerve catheters for postoperative analgesia in upper extremity surgery. *J Hand Surg* 39(2):324–329, 2014.
2. Akkara Veetil BM, Bongartz T: Perioperative care for patients with rheumatic diseases. *Nat Rev Rheumatol* 8(1):32–41, 2012.
3. Alemanno F, Ghisi D, Fanelli A, et al: Tramadol and 0.5% levobupivacaine for single-shot interscalene block: effects on postoperative analgesia in patients undergoing shoulder arthroplasty. *Minerva Anestesiol* 78(3):291–296, 2012.
4. Aumeier C, Kasdorf B, Gruber M, et al: Lipid emulsion pretreatment has different effects on mepivacaine and bupivacaine cardiac toxicity in an isolated rat heart model. *Br J Anaes* 112(4):735–741, 2014.
5. Bailard NS, Ortiz J, Flores RA: Additives to local anesthetics for peripheral nerve blocks: Evidence, limitations, and recommendations. *Am J Health Syst Pharm* 71(5):373–385, 2014.
6. Barrington MJ, Snyder GL: Neurologic complications of regional anesthesia. *Curr Opin Anaesthesiol* 24(5):554–560, 2011.
7. Barrington MJ, Watts SA, Gledhill SR, et al: Preliminary results of the Australasian Regional Anaesthesia Collaboration: a prospective audit of more than 7000 peripheral nerve and plexus blocks for neurologic and other complications. *Reg Anesth Pain Med* 34(6):534–541, 2009.
8. Batinac T, Sotosek Tokmadzic V, Peharda V, et al: Adverse reactions and alleged allergy to local anesthetics: analysis of 331 patients. *J Dermatol* 40(7):522–527, 2013.
9. Behr A, Freo U, Ori C, et al: Buprenorphine added to levobupivacaine enhances postoperative analgesia of middle interscalene brachial plexus block. *J Anesth* 26(5):746–751, 2012.
10. Bhole MV, Manson AL, Seneviratne SL, et al: IgE-mediated allergy to local anaesthetics: separating fact from perception: a UK perspective. *Br J Anaesth* 108(6):903–911, 2012.
11. Bigeleisen P, Wilson M: A comparison of two techniques for ultrasound guided infraclavicular block. *Br J Anaesth* 96(4):502–507, 2006.
12. Bingham AE, Fu R, Horn JL, et al: Continuous peripheral nerve block compared with single-injection peripheral nerve block: a systematic review and meta-analysis of randomized controlled trials. *Reg Anesth Pain Med* 37(6):583–594, 2012.
13. Blumenthal S, Borgeat A, Maurer K, et al: Preexisting subclinical neuropathy as a risk factor for nerve injury after continuous ropivacaine administration through a femoral nerve catheter. *Anesthesiology* 105(5):1053–1056, 2006.
14. Chapman GM: Regional nerve block with the aid of a nerve stimulator. *Anaesthesia* 27(2):185–193, 1972.
15. Chelly JE, Szczodry DM, Neumann KJ: International normalized ratio and prothrombin time values before the removal of a lumbar plexus catheter in patients receiving warfarin after total hip replacement. *Br J Anaesth* 101(2):250–254, 2008.
16. Chin KJ, Alakkad H, Cubillos JE: Single, double or multiple-injection techniques for non-ultrasound guided axillary brachial plexus block in adults undergoing surgery of the lower arm. *Cochrane Database Syst Rev* (8):CD003842, 2013.
17. Choquet O, Morau D, Biboulet P, et al: Where should the tip of the needle be located in ultrasound-guided peripheral nerve blocks? *Curr Opin Anaesthesiol* 25(5):596–602, 2012.
18. Chow MY, Sia AT, Koay CK, et al: Alkalinization of lidocaine does not hasten the onset of axillary brachial plexus block. *Anesth Analg* 86(3):566–568, 1998.
19. Chowdhry S, Seidenstricker L, Cooney DS, et al: Do not use epinephrine in digital blocks: myth or truth? Part II. A retrospective review of 1111 cases. *Plast Reconstruct Surg* 126(6):2031–2034, 2010.
20. Colbern E: The Bier block for intravenous regional anesthesia: technic and literature review. *Anesth Analg* 49(6):935–940, 1970.
21. Crystal CS, Blankenship RB: Local anesthetics and peripheral nerve blocks in the emergency department. *Emerg Med Clin North Am* 23(2):477–502, 2005.
22. De Oliveira GS, Jr, Almeida MD, Benzon HT, et al: Perioperative single dose systemic dexamethasone for postoperative pain: a meta-analysis of randomized controlled trials. *Anesthesiology* 115(3):575–588, 2011.
23. Delaunay L, Chelly JE: Blocks at the wrist provide effective anesthesia for carpal tunnel release. *Can J Anaesth* 48(7):656–660, 2001.
24. Desmet M, Braems H, Reynvoet M, et al: I.V. and perineural dexamethasone are equivalent in increasing the analgesic duration of a single-shot interscalene block with ropivacaine for shoulder surgery: a prospective, randomized, placebo-controlled study. *Br J Anaesth* 111(3):445–452, 2013.
25. Detaille V, Busnel F, Ravary H, et al: Use of continuous interscalene brachial plexus block and rehabilitation to treat complex regional pain syndrome of the shoulder. *Ann Phys Rehabil Med* 53(6–7):406–416, 2010.
26. Draeger RW, Messer TM: Suprascapular nerve palsy following supraclavicular block for upper extremity surgery: report of 3 cases. *J Hand Surg* 37(12):2576–2579, 2012.
27. Egol KA, Soojian MG, Walsh M, et al: Regional anesthesia improves outcome after distal radius fracture fixation over general anesthesia. *J Orthop Trauma* 26(9):545–549, 2012.
28. Esaki RK, Mashour GA: Levels of consciousness during regional anesthesia and monitored anesthesia care: patient expectations and experiences. *Anesth Analg* 108(5):1560–1563, 2009.
29. Falcao LF, Perez MV, de Castro I, et al: Minimum effective volume of 0.5% bupivacaine with epinephrine in ultrasound-guided interscalene brachial plexus block. *Br J Anaesth* 110(3):450–455, 2013.
30. Ferraro LH, Takeda A, dos Reis Falcao LF, et al: Determination of the minimum effective volume of 0.5% bupivacaine for ultrasound-guided axillary brachial plexus block. *Braz J Anesthesiol* 64(1):49–53, 2014.
31. Ferraro LH, Tardelli MA, Yamashita AM, et al: Ultrasound-guided femoral and sciatic nerve blocks in an anticoagulated patient. Case reports. *Braz J Anesthesiol* 60(4):422–428, 2010.
32. Franco CD, Rahman A, Voronov G, et al: Gross anatomy of the brachial plexus sheath in human cadavers. *Reg Anesth Pain Med* 33(1):64–69, 2008.
33. Franco CD, Salahuddin Z, Rafizad A: Bilateral brachial plexus block. *Anesth Analg* 98(2):518–520, 2004.
34. Franco CD, Vieira ZE: 1,001 subclavian perivascular brachial plexus blocks: success with a nerve stimulator. *Reg Anesth Pain Med* 25(1):41–46, 2000.
35. Fredrickson MJ: Randomised comparison of an end-hole, triple-hole and novel six-hole catheter for continuous interscalene analgesia. *Anaesth Intensive Care* 42(1):37–42, 2014.
36. Fredrickson MJ, Abeysekera A, White R: Randomized study of the effect of local anesthetic volume and concentration on the duration of peripheral nerve blockade. *Reg Anesth Pain Med* 37(5):495–501, 2012.
37. Fredrickson MJ, Kilfoyle DH: Neurological complication analysis of 1000 ultrasound guided peripheral nerve blocks for elective orthopaedic surgery: a prospective study. *Anaesthesia* 64(8):836–844, 2009.
38. Fritsch G, Danninger T, Allerberger K, et al: Dexmedetomidine added to ropivacaine extends the duration of interscalene brachial plexus blocks for elective

shoulder surgery when compared with ropivacaine alone: a single-center, prospective, triple-blind, randomized controlled trial. *Reg Anesth Pain Med* 39(1):37–47, 2014.

39. Fujinaga M, Baden JM: Methionine prevents nitrous oxide-induced teratogenicity in rat embryos grown in culture. *Anesthesiology* 81(1):184–189, 1994.

40. Gaus P, Heb B, Tanyay Z, et al: Epidural malpositioning of an interscalene plexus catheter. *Anaesthesist* 60(9):850–853, 2011.

41. Gebhard RE, Nielsen KC, Pietrobon R, et al: Diabetes mellitus, independent of body mass index, is associated with a "higher success" rate for supraclavicular brachial plexus blocks. *Reg Anesth Pain Med* 34(5):404–407, 2009.

42. Gonzalez AP, Bernucci F, Pham K, et al: Minimum effective volume of lidocaine for double-injection ultrasound-guided axillary block. *Reg Anesth Pain Med* 38(1):16–20, 2013.

43. Guay J: Adverse events associated with intravenous regional anesthesia (Bier block): a systematic review of complications. *J Clin Anesth* 21(8):585–594, 2009.

44. Gupta PK, Pace NL, Hopkins PM: Effect of body mass index on the ED50 volume of bupivacaine 0.5% for supraclavicular brachial plexus block. *Br J Anaesth* 104(4):490–495, 2010.

45. Gurnaney H, Kraemer FW, Maxwell L, et al: Ambulatory continuous peripheral nerve blocks in children and adolescents: a longitudinal 8-year single center study. *Anesth Analg* 118(3):621–627, 2014.

46. Hadzic A, Arliss J, Kerimoglu B, et al: A comparison of infraclavicular nerve block versus general anesthesia for hand and wrist day-case surgeries. *Anesthesiology* 101(1):127–132, 2004.

47. Hadzic A, Williams BA, Karaca PE, et al: For outpatient rotator cuff surgery, nerve block anesthesia provides superior same-day recovery over general anesthesia. *Anesthesiology* 102(5):1001–1007, 2005.

48. Hadzic AE: *Textbook of regional anesthesia and acute pain management*, New York, 2007, McGraw-Hill.

49. Halpern AA, Nagel DA: Compartment syndromes of the forearm: early recognition using tissue pressure measurements. *J Hand Surg* 4(3):258–263, 1979.

50. Hebl JR, Horlocker TT, Sorenson EJ, et al: Regional anesthesia does not increase the risk of postoperative neuropathy in patients undergoing ulnar nerve transposition. *Anesth Analg* 93(6):1606–1611, 2001.

51. Hebl JR, Niesen AD: Infectious complications of regional anesthesia. *Curr Opin Anaesthesiol* 24(5):573–580, 2011.

52. Hill RG, Jr, Patterson JW, Parker JC, et al: Comparison of transthecal digital block and traditional digital block for anesthesia of the finger. *Ann Emerg Med* 25(5):604–607, 1995.

53. Holborow J, Hocking G: Regional anaesthesia for bilateral upper limb surgery: a review of challenges and solutions. *Anaesth Intensive Care* 38(2):250–258, 2010.

54. Horlocker TT, Wedel DJ, Rowlingson JC, et al: Regional anesthesia in the patient receiving antithrombotic or thrombolytic therapy: American Society of Regional Anesthesia and Pain Medicine Evidence-Based Guidelines (Third Edition). *Reg Anesth Pain Med* 35(1):64–101, 2010.

55. Humbyrd CJ, LaPorte DM: Hand surgery: considerations in pregnant patients. *J Hand Surg* 37(5):1086–1089, quiz 1089, 2012.

56. Ilfeld BM: Continuous peripheral nerve blocks in the hospital and at home. *Anesthesiol Clin* 29(2):193–211, 2011.

57. Ilfeld BM, Mariano ER, Girard PJ, et al: A multicenter, randomized, triple-masked, placebo-controlled trial of the effect of ambulatory continuous femoral nerve blocks on discharge-readiness following total knee arthroplasty in patients on general orthopaedic wards. *Pain* 150(3):477–484, 2010.

58. Ilfeld BM, Shuster JJ, Theriaque DW, et al: Long-term pain, stiffness, and functional disability after total knee arthroplasty with and without an extended ambulatory continuous femoral nerve block: a prospective, 1-year follow-up of a multicenter, randomized, triple-masked, placebo-controlled trial. *Reg Anesth Pain Med* 36(2):116–120, 2011.

59. Kaabachi O, Ouezini R, Koubaa W, et al: Tramadol as an adjuvant to lidocaine for axillary brachial plexus block. *Anesth Analg* 108(1):367–370, 2009.

60. Kapral S, Krafft P, Eibenberger K, et al: Ultrasound-guided supraclavicular approach for regional anesthesia of the brachial plexus. *Anesth Analg* 78(3):507–513, 1994.

61. Kesimci E, Izdes S, Gozdemir M, et al: Tramadol does not prolong the effect of ropivacaine 7.5 mg/ml for axillary brachial plexus block. *Acta Anaesthesiol Scand* 51(6):736–741, 2007.

62. Koscielniak-Nielsen ZJ, Hesselbjerg L, Fejlberg V: Comparison of transarterial and multiple nerve stimulation techniques for an initial axillary block by 45 mL of mepivacaine 1% with adrenaline. *Acta Anaesthesiol Scand* 42(5):570–575, 1998.

63. Kulenkampff D: Brachial plexus anaesthesia: its indications, technique, and dangers. *Ann Surg* 87(6):883–891, 1928.

64. Laiq N, Khan MN, Arif M, et al: Midazolam with bupivacaine for improving analgesia quality in brachial plexus block for upper limb surgeries. *J Coll Physicians Surg Pak* 18(11):674–678, 2008.

65. Lee AR, Yi HW, Chung IS, et al: Magnesium added to bupivacaine prolongs the duration of analgesia after interscalene nerve block. *Can J Anaesth* 59(1):21–27, 2012.

66. Lee IO, Kim WK, Kong MH, et al: No enhancement of sensory and motor blockade by ketamine added to ropivacaine interscalene brachial plexus blockade. *Acta Anaesthesiol Scand* 46(7):821–826, 2002.

67. Leffler A, Frank G, Kistner K, et al: Local anesthetic-like inhibition of voltage-gated Na(+) channels by the partial mu-opioid receptor agonist buprenorphine. *Anesthesiology* 116(6):1335–1346, 2012.

68. Lenters TR, Davies J, Matsen FA, 3rd: The types and severity of complications associated with interscalene brachial plexus block anesthesia: local and national evidence. *J Shoulder Elbow Surg* 16(4):379–387, 2007.

69. Liguori GA, Zayas VM, YaDeau JT, et al: Nerve localization techniques for interscalene brachial plexus blockade: a prospective, randomized comparison of mechanical paresthesia versus electrical stimulation. *Anesth Analg* 103(3):761–767, 2006.

70. Liu SS, Gordon MA, Shaw PM, et al: A prospective clinical registry of ultrasound-guided regional anesthesia for ambulatory shoulder surgery. *Anesth Analg* 111(3):617–623, 2010.

71. Liu SS, Zayas VM, Gordon MA, et al: A prospective, randomized, controlled trial comparing ultrasound versus nerve stimulator guidance for interscalene block for ambulatory shoulder surgery for postoperative neurological symptoms. *Anesth Analg* 109(1):265–271, 2009.

72. Lonnqvist PA: Is ultrasound guidance mandatory when performing paediatric regional anaesthesia? *Curr Opin Anaesthesiol* 23(3):337–341, 2010.

73. Low CK, Vartany A, Diao E: Comparison of transthecal and subcutaneous single-injection digital block techniques in cadaver hands. *J Hand Surg* 22(5):897–900, 1997.

74. Marhofer D, Marhofer P, Triffterer L, et al: Dislocation rates of perineural catheters: a volunteer study. *Br J Anaesth* 111(5):800–806, 2013.

75. McCartney CJ, Xu D, Constantinescu C, et al: Ultrasound examination of peripheral nerves in the forearm. *Reg Anesth Pain Med* 32(5):434–439, 2007.

76. McNaught A, Shastri U, Carmichael N, et al: Ultrasound reduces the minimum effective local anaesthetic volume compared with peripheral nerve stimulation for interscalene block. *Br J Anaesth* 106(1):124–130, 2011.

77. Mirkheshti A, Aryani MR, Shojaei P, et al: The effect of adding magnesium sulfate to lidocaine compared with paracetamol in prevention of acute pain in hand surgery patients under intravenous regional anesthesia (IVRA). *Int J Prev Med* 3(9):616–621, 2012.

78. Misamore G, Webb B, McMurray S, et al: A prospective analysis of interscalene brachial plexus blocks performed under general anesthesia. *J Shoulder Elbow Surg* 20(2):308–314, 2011.

79. Morin AM, Kranke P, Wulf H, et al: The effect of stimulating versus nonstimulating catheter techniques for continuous regional anesthesia: a semiquantitative systematic review. *Reg Anesth Pain Med* 35(2):194–199, 2010.

80. Neal JM: Ultrasound-guided regional anesthesia and patient safety: an evidence-based analysis. *Reg Anesth Pain Med* 35(2 Suppl):S59–S67, 2010.

81. Neal JM, Moore JM, Kopacz DJ, et al: Quantitative analysis of respiratory, motor, and sensory function after supraclavicular block. *Anesth Analg* 86(6):1239–1244, 1998.

82. O'Rourke MG, Tang TS, Allison SI, et al: The anatomy of the extrathoracic intercostobrachial nerve. *Aust N Z J Surg* 69(12):860–864, 1999.

83. Osterman AL: The double crush syndrome. *Orthop Clin North Am* 19(1):147–155, 1988.

84. Pavicic Saric J, Vidjak V, Tomulic K, et al: Effects of age on minimum effective volume of local anesthetic for ultrasound-guided supraclavicular brachial plexus block. *Acta Anaesthesiol Scand* 57(6):761–766, 2013.

85. Perlas A, Niazi A, McCartney C, et al: The sensitivity of motor response to nerve stimulation and paresthesia for nerve localization as evaluated by ultrasound. *Reg Anesth Pain Med* 31(5):445–450, 2006.

86. Perlas A, Peng PW, Plaza MB, et al: Forearm rescue cuff improves tourniquet tolerance during intravenous regional anesthesia. *Reg Anesth Pain Med* 28(2):98–102, 2003.

87. Polaner DM, Taenzer AH, Walker BJ, et al: Pediatric Regional Anesthesia Network (PRAN): a multi-institutional study of the use and incidence of complications of pediatric regional anesthesia. *Anesth Analg* 115(6):1353–1364, 2012.

88. Popping DM, Elia N, Marret E, et al: Clonidine as an adjuvant to local anesthetics for peripheral nerve and plexus blocks: a meta-analysis of randomized trials. *Anesthesiology* 111(2):406–415, 2009.

89. American College of Obstetricians and Gynecologists: ACOG Committee Opinion No. 474: Nonobstetric surgery during pregnancy. *Obstet Gynecol* 117(2 Pt 1):420–421, 2011.

90. Prandoni P, Temraz S, Taher A: Direct oral anticoagulants in the prevention of venous thromboembolism: evidence from major clinical trials. *Semin Hematol* 51(2):121–130, 2014.

91. Raj PP, Montgomery SJ, Nettles D, et al: Infraclavicular brachial plexus block: a new approach. *Anesth Analg* 52(6):897–904, 1973.

92. Renes SH, Rettig HC, Gielen MJ, et al: Ultrasound-guided low-dose interscalene brachial plexus block reduces the incidence of hemidiaphragmatic paresis. *Reg Anesth Pain Med* 34(5):498–502, 2009.

93. Rosencher N, Noack H, Feuring M, et al: Type of anaesthesia and the safety and efficacy of thromboprophylaxis with enoxaparin or dabigatran etexilate in major orthopaedic surgery: pooled analysis of three randomized controlled trials. *Thromb J* 10(1):9, 2012.

94. Salam GA: Regional anesthesia for office procedures: Part II. Extremity and inguinal area surgeries. *Am Fam Physician* 69(4):896–900, 2004.

95. Salviz EA, Xu D, Frulla A, et al: Continuous interscalene block in patients having outpatient rotator cuff repair surgery: a prospective randomized trial. *Anesth Analg* 117(6):1485–1492, 2013.

96. Samanta R, Shoukrey K, Griffiths R: Rheumatoid arthritis and anaesthesia. *Anaesthesia* 66(12):1146–1159, 2011.

97. Sandhu NS, Capan LM: Ultrasound-guided infraclavicular brachial plexus block. *Br J Anaesth* 89(2):254–259, 2002.

98. Scarff CE, Scarff CW: Digital nerve blocks: more gain with less pain. *Australas J Dermatol* 48(1):60–61, 2007.

99. Schoenmakers KP, Wegener JT, Stienstra R: Effect of local anesthetic volume (15 vs 40 mL) on the duration of ultrasound-guided single shot axillary brachial plexus block: a prospective randomized, observer-blinded trial. *Reg Anesth Pain Med* 37(3):242–247, 2012.

100. Schroeder K, Andrei AC, Furlong MJ, et al: The perioperative effect of increased body mass index on peripheral nerve blockade: an analysis of 528 ultrasound guided interscalene blocks. *Braz J Anesthesiol* 62(1):28–38, 2012.

101. Shin SW, Byeon GJ, Yoon JU, et al: Effective analgesia with ultrasound-guided interscalene brachial plexus block for postoperative pain control after arthroscopic rotator cuff repair. *J Anesth* 28(1):64–69, 2014.

102. Soares LG, Brull R, Lai J, et al: Eight ball, corner pocket: the optimal needle position for ultrasound-guided supraclavicular block. *Reg Anesth Pain Med* 32(1):94–95, 2007.

103. Srikumaran U, Stein BE, Tan EW, et al: Upper-extremity peripheral nerve blocks in the perioperative pain management of orthopaedic patients: AAOS exhibit selection. *J Bone Joint Surg Am* 95(24):e197, 191–113 (1–13), 2013.

104. Stan TC, Krantz MA, Solomon DL, et al: The incidence of neurovascular complications following axillary brachial plexus block using a transarterial approach. A prospective study of 1,000 consecutive patients. *Reg Anesth* 20(6):486–492, 1995.

105. Su HH, Lui PW, Yu CL, et al: The effects of continuous axillary brachial plexus block with ropivacaine infusion on skin temperature and survival of crushed fingers after microsurgical replantation. *Chang Gung Med J* 28(8):567–574, 2005.

106. Thomas LC, Graham SK, Osteen KD, et al: Comparison of ultrasound and nerve stimulation techniques for interscalene brachial plexus block for shoulder surgery in a residency training environment: a randomized, controlled, observer-blinded trial. *Ochsner J* 11(3):246–252, 2011.

107. Trabelsi W, Amor MB, Lebbi MA, et al: Ultrasound does not shorten the duration of procedure but provides a faster sensory and motor block onset in comparison to nerve stimulator in infraclavicular brachial plexus block. *Korean J Anesthesiol* 64(4):327–333, 2013.

108. Tran de QH, Dugani S, Correa JA, et al: Minimum effective volume of lidocaine for ultrasound-guided supraclavicular block. *Reg Anesth Pain Med* 36(5):466–469, 2011.

109. Tran de QH, Dugani S, Dyachenko A, et al: Minimum effective volume of lidocaine for ultrasound-guided infraclavicular block. *Reg Anesth Pain Med* 36(2):190–194, 2011.

110. Tuzuner T: Median and ulnar nerve block for endoscopic carpal tunnel release. *Adv Ther* 23(6):902–904, 2006.

111. Urmey WF, Talts KH, Sharrock NE: One hundred percent incidence of hemidiaphragmatic paresis associated with interscalene brachial plexus anesthesia as diagnosed by ultrasonography. *Anesth Analg* 72(4):498–503, 1991.

112. Walter M, Rogalla P, Spies C, et al: Intrathecal misplacement of an interscalene plexus catheter. *Anaesthesist* 54(3):215–219, 2005.

113. Ward WA, Van Moore A: Management of finger ulcers in scleroderma. *J Hand Surg* 20(5):868–872, 1995.

114. Weber A, Fournier R, Van Gessel E, et al: Epinephrine does not prolong the analgesia of 20 mL ropivacaine 0.5% or 0.2% in a femoral three-in-one block. *Anesth Analg* 93(5):1327–1331, 2001.

115. Webster F, Bremner S, McCartney CJ: Patient experiences as knowledge for the evidence base: a qualitative approach to understanding patient experiences regarding the use of regional anesthesia for hip and knee arthroplasty. *Reg Anesth Pain Med* 36(5):461–465, 2011.

116. Williams SR, Chouinard P, Arcand G, et al: Ultrasound guidance speeds execution and improves the quality of supraclavicular block. *Anesth Analg* 97(5):1518–1523, 2003.

117. Winnie AP: Interscalene brachial plexus block. *Anesth Analg* 49(3):455–466, 1970.

118. Yang J, Cooper MG: Compartment syndrome and patient-controlled analgesia in children: analgesic complication or early warning system? *Anaesth Intens Care* 38(2):359–363, 2010.

119. Yuan JM, Yang XH, Fu SK, et al: Ultrasound guidance for brachial plexus block decreases the incidence of complete hemi-diaphragmatic paresis or vascular punctures and improves success rate of brachial plexus nerve block compared with peripheral nerve stimulator in adults. *Chin Med J* 125(10):1811–1816, 2012.

120. Zor F, Ozturk S, Usyilmaz S, et al: Is stellate ganglion blockade an option to prevent early arterial vasospasm after digital microsurgical procedures? *Plast Reconstruct Surg* 117(3):1059–1060, 2006.

2

Acute Infections of the Hand

Milan V. Stevanovic and Frances Sharpe

GENERAL PRINCIPLES

Hippocrates' principles for the treatment of hand infections are fundamentally valid today. Wounds were kept clean with frequent changes of wine-soaked dressings. Dressings were kept loose "so as not to intercept the pus, but to allow it to flow away freely."[44] Coupled with these early principles is the pioneering work of Dr. Alan Kanavel, a Chicago general surgeon who treated hand infections in the preantibiotic era. Much of our current understanding of the pathogenesis and treatment of hand infections must be credited to his extensive dissections and innovative injection studies. Through these studies, he demonstrated the potential spaces of the hand and the pathogenesis of infection. From this data, he developed the surgical principles that remain the cornerstone of modern treatment of hand infections.[75]

Hand infections can result in severe disabilities, including stiffness, contracture, and amputation. These complications have been significantly reduced through the introduction of antibiotic therapy in conjunction with surgical treatment. Although antibiotics have dramatically reduced the morbidity associated with hand infections, their use does not supplant the need for expedient and proper surgical intervention. Several factors influence the outcome of hand infections. These include the location of the infection, infecting organism, timing of treatment, adequacy of surgical drainage, efficacy of antibiotics, and health status and immunocompetence of the host. In the words of one of the preeminent United States public health officials, Dr. Charles V. Chapin: "As it takes two to quarrel, so it takes two to make a disease, the microbe and the host."

Host factors play a determining role in the severity and duration of infection. Many medical conditions reduce host defenses. Malnutrition, alcoholism, autoimmune diseases, chronic corticosteroid use, hepatitis, and human immunodeficiency virus (HIV) infection are some of the comorbidities to be considered. The most prevalent disease with associated immunosuppression is diabetes mellitus, which affects up to 11% of the adult population of the United States.[140]

Early and superficial infections may respond to nonsurgical management. However, most acute infections of the hand represent surgical emergencies. Swelling and edema associated with an infection result in increased tissue pressure and can cause ischemia and tissue necrosis by a process resembling compartment syndrome.[139] Furthermore, toxins produced by the offending pathogen can cause vascular thrombosis and tissue death. Patients with necrotizing fasciitis and gas gangrene need *immediate* surgical care.

Types of Infections

Cellulitis is an infection of the subcutaneous tissue, which is often diffuse and can be associated with lymphangitis. It is caused by a single organism, usually *Staphylococcus aureus* or β-hemolytic *Streptococcus*. Lymphangitic streaking is more commonly seen with β-hemolytic streptococcal infections. It generally has a more distal nidus and spreads proximally. It is a non–pus-forming infection and as such is initially treated nonsurgically. If the cellulitis is not responding to intravenous therapy over 12 to 24 hours, this often suggests the formation of pus (*abscess*) and more serious infection. Even in the absence of abscess formation, cellulitis associated with significant swelling resolves more quickly with surgical decompression. Cellulitis often requires hospital admission and close monitoring for response to antibiotic therapy. A specific type of staphylococcal infection is the *staphylococcal scalded skin syndrome*, primarily a disease of young children that results from an exfoliative toxin-producing staphylococcal organism.[85,120] A high index of suspicion and early differentiation of this process from other skin conditions are important to treatment outcome. Although this syndrome is extremely rare in adults, it is associated with a high mortality rate, usually because of serious underlying illness, such as kidney failure or immunosuppression.[120] Detection of the exfoliative toxin is required for diagnosis. New immunologic methods allow for more rapid detection.[81] Prompt antibiotic therapy and local wound care are the mainstays of management. *Necrotizing fasciitis* is a serious life-threatening infection that may initially resemble cellulitis. Although purulence is not present, a watery discharge often described as "dishwater-like fluid" may be seen superficial to the fascia. Most other hand infections are generally pus forming and are discussed in detail throughout the chapter.

The most common infecting organisms are *Staphylococcus* and *Streptococcus* species, with staphylococcal organisms predominating. Many infections, especially those associated with bite wounds, those associated with gross contamination, or those seen in diabetics, are often caused by mixed species. *Pasteurella multocida* should be considered in most animal bites, and both streptococcal species and *Eikenella corrodens* should be considered in human bite wounds. Anaerobic infection is less common but should be considered more frequently in diabetics or intravenous drug users. Empirical antibiotic therapy should be tailored toward the most likely offending pathogen. The local prevalence of antibiotic-resistant organisms should be considered when starting empirical treatment. An infectious disease specialist is valuable in patient management because he or she is most familiar with the hospital-specific patterns of antibiotic resistance, can direct antibiotic therapy, and can follow outpatient intravenous therapy.

Methicillin-Resistant *Staphylococcus aureus* Infections

The increasing incidence of infection with methicillin-resistant *S. aureus* (MRSA) has been recognized throughout the surgical as well as infectious disease literature. A strain of *S. aureus* resistant to methicillin was mentioned in reports from the United Kingdom in 1961. This strain was soon identified worldwide and was associated with hospital-acquired infections (HA-MRSA).[113] Only a handful of successful HA-MRSA clones are responsible for the majority of infections, and different clones dominate in different geographic locations.[87] However, MRSA infections have been increasingly identified as community-acquired infections (CA-MRSA). There are unique microbiologic and genetic properties distinguishing the hospital-acquired and community-acquired strains. A community-acquired infection is defined as occurring in patients with MRSA identified by culture who have no history of a hospital or medical facility stay within the past year, who have no history of dialysis or surgery occurring within the past year, and in whom no indwelling catheters are present.

CA-MRSA is now the predominant strain in hand infections, found in up to 60% of *S. aureus* infections.[20,25,72,114] The majority of CA-MRSA infections in the United States have been caused by a single clone (USA300). One of the distinguishing features in CA-MRSA is the frequent gene sequence encoding for Panton-Valentine leukocidin (PVL), a potent toxin that leads to the characteristic tissue necrosis commonly seen in the clinical setting.

MRSA infections frequently have a characteristic appearance of a dermonecrotic skin lesion (Figure 2.1). They are often mislabeled as "spider bites" due to their dermonecrotic appearance and may not receive appropriate antibiotic therapy.[160] More recently, we have not seen the extensive tissue necrosis with MRSA infections that we have in the past. Empirical treatment of hand infections has also changed to address potential MRSA infections.[25,41,70,116] Successful treatment requires surgical débridement with excision of necrotic tissue in conjunction with appropriate antibiotic therapy.

Nosocomial Infections

The hand is a very well-vascularized region, making it less vulnerable to postoperative infection than other anatomic sites. *S. aureus* is the most common pathogen in clean surgical procedures.[21,46,141] The use of perioperative intravenous antibiotics within 1 hour preceding surgery has greatly reduced the incidence of postsurgical infections in general orthopedic practice.[27] However, the role of perioperative antibiotics in elective

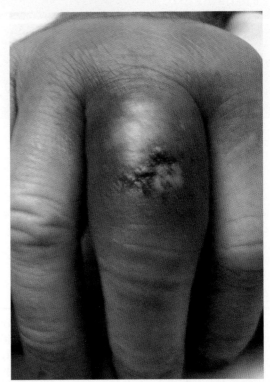

FIGURE 2.1 Characteristic appearance of MRSA infection with central skin necrosis and surrounding erythema. Purulence is not always present. Soft tissue necrosis is often more extensive than would be expected from a localized infection. (Copyright courtesy of Milan Stevanovic and Frances Sharpe.)

hand surgery is less clear. Several studies suggest that for soft tissue procedures of less than 2 hours' duration, the routine use of prophylactic antibiotics is not indicated.[19,40,64,128,154] Ultimately, the whole patient must be considered. Prophylactic antibiotics in patients with joint arthroplasties are recommended to protect the prosthesis more than to prevent surgical site infection. Patients with an altered immune response may have a potentially greater benefit from prophylactic antibiotics than an immunocompetent host. For surgical procedures that involve exposure of the bone or joint or those involving implants, we routinely give intravenous prophylaxis.*

Patient Evaluation

Clinical examination remains the hallmark of diagnosis in hand infections. Pain (dolor), and increased temperature (calor), with or without erythema (rubor), and tenderness remain the prime features of hand infection. Temperature elevation is inconsistent. Abnormalities of the white blood cell (WBC) count and C-reactive protein (CRP) level are uncommon features of a hand infection. In one study, these were normal in

---

*Editor's note (DPG): I strongly disagree with the practice of giving "prophylactic" antibiotics for all clean bone and joint cases in the wrist and hand. This is not only unnecessary but harmful in the long term, creating superresistant bacteria. In my practice, I do not administer perioperative antibiotics in clean, elective cases unless there is a specific indication to do so. Unfortunately, many orthopedic surgeons give antibiotics indiscriminately purely as a defensive measure, fearing that if the patient does get an infection and no antibiotics were given, a plaintiff's attorney will cite this as inappropriate care. In addition, many hospital policies now require the routine administration of preoperative antibiotics.

75% of patients. The erythrocyte sedimentation rate (ESR) was slightly more useful, with elevation of the ESR found in 50% of patients.[68]

The initial evaluation and management in the emergency department should include a thorough medical history, assessment of risk factors for immunocompromise, and evaluation of tetanus immunization status. Appropriate tetanus prophylaxis should be administered based on immunization history and time of the last booster shot. Tetanus immune globulin (TIG; HyperTET®) and tetanus toxoid booster are given if the patient has not had a series of tetanus immunizations. Clinical evaluation of the affected extremity should include examination for fluctuance, warmth, edema, redness, tenderness, and lymphangitis or lymphadenopathy. Areas of cellulitis should be marked on the skin so that progression or regression of the infectious process can be monitored; if an open draining wound is present, a specimen should be sent for aerobic and anaerobic culture. Blood cultures should be taken in febrile patients. Blood should be drawn for a complete blood cell count (CBC), ESR, CRP, electrolytes, and random blood glucose measurements. Hand infection may be the first presenting complaint of undiagnosed diabetes. Radiographs are obtained to evaluate for the presence of a foreign body, gas within the soft tissues, underlying fracture, septic joint, or osteomyelitis.

When a patient presents with an area of fluctuance, this should be provisionally treated with aspiration or decompression until formal surgical débridement is performed. The fluid should be sent for culture. For patients who do not clearly have an abscess, aspiration may be useful to identify a deep pyogenic infection. Swollen painful joints should be aspirated with caution. The site of aspiration should not be over an area of cellulitis, so as not to seed the joint with bacteria. The aspirated fluid should be sent for culture. Joint fluid analysis with cell count, glucose, and protein levels can be obtained if an adequate specimen is available. If the joint aspirate is not clearly pyogenic and there are not other indicators of infection, antibiotics are withheld. Nonsteroidal antiinflammatory drugs (NSAIDs) may be given to both treat the patient and help distinguish between an inflammatory process and sepsis. If the presentation is suggestive of an inflammatory process, antibiotics are withheld while the response to NSAIDs is observed. When infection is suggested, empirical antibiotic therapy should be started in the emergency department after a culture specimen has been obtained.

Differentiating between an infectious process and an inflammatory process, especially pseudogout, can be difficult. The suspicion of one process over the other depends on many factors, including the patient's history, the presence of underlying diseases, and the clinical presentation. When to withhold antibiotic therapy can be a diagnostic challenge, and the use of antibiotics in some circumstances may be done more to treat the physician's anxiety than the patient's disease. Overnight observation in the hospital while antibiotics are withheld allows the disease process to be closely monitored and allows treatment to be changed if the anticipated improvement is not evident with NSAID therapy alone. When the level of suspicion for an infectious process is low, a corticosteroid dose pack (Medrol DosePak™) may be used. The patient is reevaluated in 24 to 48 hours. The importance of seeing the patient again within 48 hours cannot be overstated. If the process is non-infectious, the symptoms will be nearly resolved. It may take years to develop the clinical experience to recognize these different processes, and even the experienced eye can mistake these two conditions.

Patients with severe infections such as necrotizing fasciitis or gas gangrene or who are immunocompromised, including diabetics, should be immediately treated with broad-spectrum antibiotic therapy and emergent surgical intervention.

Treatment Principles

Surgical drainage should be done through a large incision. The incision should be planned so that it can be extended proximally or distally. Longitudinal incisions across a flexion crease should be avoided.

Excision of all necrotic tissue is imperative for infection control. In the 1800s, Louis Pasteur noted that it is the environment and not the bacterium that allows the propagation of infection. Cultures and surgical pathologic reports should be obtained. Fungal and mycobacterial organisms are slow growing and may be more rapidly identified by staining techniques. Most wounds can be left open, with moist gauze covering the exposed surfaces. Alternatively, large wounds can be managed with a negative-pressure sponge dressing. In an acute infection, these should be changed in 48 hours. Small wounds with a tendency to heal quickly should be kept open with a gauze wick. Multiple débridements may be necessary to control infection. Amputation may be necessary to eradicate infection. Functional results may be improved by amputation of a stiff, contracted, and painful digit. In cases of severe infection such as necrotizing fasciitis or gas gangrene, amputation may be a life-saving procedure.

Postoperatively, loose soft dressings are applied. A short period of immobilization for 24 to 48 hours with a splint may afford some pain relief to the patient. Early mobilization in the first 24 hours, under the guidance of a hand therapist, reduces edema, stiffness, and contracture associated with severe hand infections.

Empirical antibiotic therapy may be started after cultures have been obtained. In the case of cellulitis, where local cultures cannot be obtained, blood cultures may identify an organism and should if possible be obtained prior to initiating antibiotic therapy. The specific empirical therapy should be based on the most commonly encountered organisms for the type of infection being treated. The patient history, such as being exposed to an aquatic or a farm environment or being bitten by an animal, may help tailor the specific treatment to the patient. The relative prevalence of MRSA is increasing in many communities, and empirical treatment for MRSA is now commonplace. An infectious disease specialist is invaluable in guiding antibiotic recommendations for both specific infections and for resistant organisms that may be relatively prevalent in one's community. Table 2.1 lists general antibiotic recommendations for common infections. Dosages should be adjusted for the patient's age, weight, renal function, and allergic status. The duration of therapy depends on the clinical response to treatment, the location and depth of the infection, and the patient's immune status. The use of peripherally inserted central venous catheters (PICC lines) can be a valuable method of providing outpatient parenteral therapy, but it comes with a risk of upper extremity venous thrombosis.

CRITICAL POINTS *Treatment Principles*

Surgical Setup and Incision
- Tourniquet control
- Elevation (not elastic) to exsanguinate the limb
- Surgical incisions long and extensile
- Planned to minimize exposure of blood vessels, nerves, or tendons
- Avoid longitudinal incisions across flexion creases

Débridement
- Excision of all necrotic tissue

Specimens
- Obtain culture specimens from the periphery of an abscess cavity
- Gram-stained smear, aerobic and anaerobic cultures
- Tissue and/or fluid to pathology department and request fungal and mycobacteria stains

Irrigation
- Copious irrigation to reduce bacterial load

Wound Management
- Wounds should be left open
- Negative-pressure dressings should be used
- Do not be overly eager for immediate wound closure
- Delayed primary wound closure or healing by secondary intention

Postoperative Care
- Frequent dressing changes for open wounds
- Dressing changes every other day for negative-pressure wound care
- Early motion to reduce the incidence of tendon adhesions and stiff joints
- Multiple débridements may be needed to control infection
- Amputation may be necessary to eradicate infection
- Empirical antibiotic therapy based on most common organisms and patient history
- Infectious disease consultation for antibiotic recommendations and management very helpful

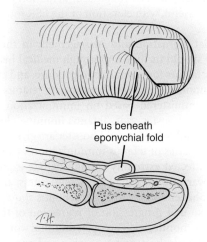

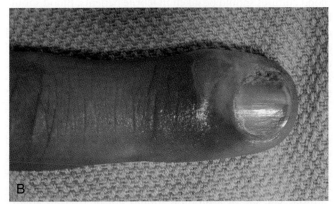

FIGURE 2.2 A, Inflamed paronychium and eponychium shown with pus extending below the eponychial fold. **B**, Clinical appearance of a purulent paronychium with partial involvement of the eponychium. (Copyright courtesy of Milan Stevanovic and Frances Sharpe.)

SPECIFIC TYPES OF COMMON HAND INFECTIONS

Acute Paronychia

Paronychia is the most common infection in the hand.[127] It is generally treated by primary care physicians, although refractory cases are often seen by the hand surgeon. Acute paronychia involves the soft tissue fold around the fingernail. It usually results from the bacterial inoculation of the paronychia tissue by a sliver of nail or hangnail, by a manicure instrument, or through nail biting. The disruption of the barrier between the nail fold and the nail plate allows the introduction of bacteria into the tissue bordering the nail (Figure 2.2). Although most paronychias are mixed infections, the most common infecting organism is *S. aureus*.

Clinical Presentation and Preoperative Evaluation

Erythema, swelling, and tenderness immediately adjacent to the nail are the hallmarks of the early clinical presentation. If left untreated, an abscess may form along the nail fold. The abscess may extend below the nail plate, either partially or completely, or it can track volarly into the pulp space. Because of the

continuity of the nail fold with the eponychial tissue overlying the base of the nail, the infection can extend into this region and may continue around to the fold on the opposite side of the fingernail. This unusual occurrence is called a "runaround infection." Infection involving the entire eponychium, as well as one lateral fold, is known as an *eponychia*. An eponychia is usually manifested as a collection of pus beneath the proximal portion of the nail in the region of the lunula. It is rare to see both lateral folds and the dorsal tissue infected in the same digit.

Radiographs and laboratory examination are not necessary in uncomplicated cases with early clinical findings. However, patients who have not responded to initial treatment or who present with significant swelling or abscess should be evaluated for underlying systemic diseases such as diabetes. The patient's history and examination will direct the need for wound cultures for atypical organisms, radiographs to evaluate for a foreign body or osteomyelitis, and laboratory evaluation. Patients who do not respond to empirical therapy with a first-generation cephalosporin may also have CA-MRSA infection and may respond to a change in antibiotic therapy.

Pertinent Anatomy

The nail complex consists of the nail bed, nail plate, and perionychium. The nail bed, which lies below the plate, consists of

TABLE 2.1 Antibiotic Recommendations for Common Infections

Infection Type	Most Common Organism	Other Considerations	Initial Antibiotic Therapy
Cellulitis	*Staphylococcus, Streptococcus*	Antibiotic synergy for streptococcal infections with clindamycin	First-generation cephalosporin or penicillin (for *Streptococcus* only)
Abscess (e.g., paronychia, felon, deep space infections)	*Staphylococcus aureus*	Methicillin-resistant *S. aureus* (MRSA) is common now in the community; start therapy for MRSA empirically and change to nafcillin or first-generation cephalosporin if infection is methicillin sensitive	**IV:** Vancomycin or clindamycin for inpatients Linezolid or tigecycline if unable to tolerate vancomycin **Oral:** Trimethoprim/sulfamethoxazole (Bactrim), clindamycin, or doxycycline
Flexor tenosynovitis	*Staphylococcus, S. aureus,* anaerobes	Polymicrobial infections have worse prognosis. Consider multimodal therapy as initial treatment until culture results are available, especially in immunocompromised patients	**IV:** Ampicillin/sulbactam (Unasyn) plus cefoxitin (second-generation cephalosporin) **Oral:** Amoxicillin/clavulanate (Augmentin) If pencillin allergic: Fluoroquinolone (ciprofloxacin or other) plus clindamycin
Pyarthrosis	*Staphylococcus*	Requires parenteral therapy MRSA is common now in the community; start therapy for MRSA empirically and change to nafcillin or first-generation cephalosporin if infection is methicillin sensitive Consider coverage for *Neisseria gonorrheae* in sexually active patients	**IV:** Vancomycin Add ceftriaxone for *N. gonorrheae* coverage Presumptive treatment for MRSA until cultures are available; then change to antibiotic appropriate to organism with the least side effect profile
Human bite	*Staphylococcus, Streptococcus, Eikenella corrodens,* anaerobes		**IV:** Ampicillin/sulbactam (Unasyn) plus cefoxitin **Oral:** Amoxicillin/clavulanate (Augmentin) If pencillin allergic: Fluoroquinolone (ciprofloxacin) plus clindamycin Alternative: Third-generation cephalosporin plus anaerobic coverage with clindamycin or metronidazole **Note:** Quinolones not indicated in children
Animal bites	*Pasteurella multocida, Staphylococcus, Streptococcus*		**IV:** Ampicillin/sulbactam (Unasyn) plus cefoxitin **Oral:** Amoxicillin/clavulanate (Augmentin) If pencillin allergic: Fluoroquinolone plus clindamycin Alternative: Third-generation cephalosporin plus anaerobic coverage with clindamycin or metronidazole **Note:** Quinolones not indicated in children
Suspected CA-MRSA (community-acquired MRSA)		Suspected based on clinical appearance and relative frequency of CA-MRSA seen in community	**IV:** Vancomycin or clindamycin **Oral:** Trimethoprim/sulfamethoxazole (Bactrim), clindamycin
Suspected HA-MRSA (hospital-acquired MRSA)			**IV:** Vancomycin, linezolid, or daptomycin
Necrotizing fasciitis	*Streptococcus* or polymicrobial infection	Treat both until organisms identified	Broad-spectrum beta-lactam (piperacillin/tazobactam; imipenem) plus vancomycin (for MRSA) plus clindamycin (for synergy for *Streptococcus pyogenes*)
Gas in soft tissues	*Clostridium. perfringens* (gas gangrene), polymicrobial infections (anaerobic and facultative anaerobes)	Intravenous drug abusers and diabetics more often have polymicrobial infections; often, gas in the soft tissues	High-dose penicillin plus clindamycin Broad-spectrum beta-lactam (piperacillin/tazobactam; imipenem) plus vancomycin (for MRSA) plus clindamycin (for synergy for *S. pyogenes*)

the germinal and sterile matrices. The germinal matrix is responsible for the majority of nail growth. The proximal portion of the nail sits below the nail fold. The border tissue surrounding the nail is the perionychium. The eponychium is the thin layer of tissue extending from the nail wall onto the nail plate. The hyponychium is the mass of keratin just distal to the sterile matrix, below the distal nail plate. This area of the nail complex is highly resistant to infection.

Treatment Options

In the very early stages, this infection can be treated by soaks in a warm solution, systemic oral antibiotics, and rest of the affected part. If there is a superficial abscess, treatment can be carried out with local anesthesia and should consist of elevation of the cuticle away from the nail plate in the area of erythema and opening the thin layer of tissue over the abscess with a sharp blade directed away from the nail bed and matrix. Drainage of

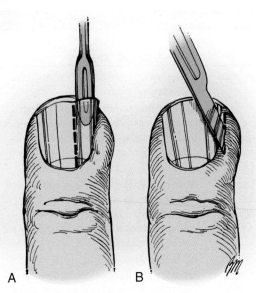

FIGURE 2.3 A, Elevation and removal of one fourth of the nail to decompress the perionychium. **B,** Incision of the perionychial fold with the blade directed away from the nail bed and matrix.

the abscess is performed where the abscess most nearly approaches the surface (Figure 2.3). The patient is counseled regarding high-risk activities, such as nail biting and manicures.

More extensive infection requires individualized treatment based on the extent of the lesion. Surgical decompression is best carried out under digital block anesthesia at the level of the metacarpal head with plain lidocaine. If the perionychial fold and the adjacent part of the eponychium are involved, the perionychium and skin adjacent to the nail fold are released. If the perionychial infection tracks volarly and involves the pulp, the incision should be deep enough to fully drain the abscess and allow evaluation of bone involvement of the distal phalanx. Infection that travels below the nail plate requires removal of a portion of the nail. If the entire nail matrix is involved, then the entire nail is removed. Purulence below the nail plate can cause pressure on the germinal matrix, resulting in ischemia of the germinal matrix and temporary or permanent arrest of nail growth.

Operative Methods. The peronychial sulcus is elevated from the nail gently by a flat, blunt instrument such as the flat portion of a malleable or metal probe or a Freer elevator. Sharp incision may be used as well. The incision is directed away from the nail bed to avoid injury to the nail bed and subsequent growth abnormality. The incision may be extended proximally along the nail fold, as far proximally as is necessary (Figure 2.4, *A* and *B*). It is generally sufficient to carry the incision only to the proximal edge of the nail, but it may extend as far proximally as the distal interphalangeal (DIP) joint.

When abscess or fluctuance is found below the eponychium and a single incision does not adequately expose or decompress the involved tissues, a parallel incision along the opposite nail fold is made, allowing the eponychium and nail fold to be elevated and reflected above the nail plate (see Figure 2.4, *C* through *E*).

When the abscess extends below the nail plate, a portion of the nail plate should be removed. The amount and location of nail removal depend on the location and extent of involvement

below the nail. If the area of fluctuance lies adjacent to the perionychium, a flat blunt probe or Freer elevator is used to separate the affected portion of the nail plate from the nail bed. The nail plate is then cut with a small scissors and removed. In the rare case where the eponychium is infected and pus is present only below the proximal portion of the nail, the eponychium and nail plate are elevated through a single or double incision. The proximal third of the nail plate is carefully removed. Only when the nail is entirely separated from the underlying matrix is it necessary to remove the entire nail plate. After decompression, the area of abscess is irrigated. The wound is left open with a small thin piece of gauze that allows the wound to stay open and drain.

❖ AUTHORS' PREFERRED METHOD OF TREATMENT

No one treatment should be used exclusively, because there are cases in which each is applicable. We prefer to treat early infections nonsurgically with oral antibiotics and soaks two to three times per day in a solution of warm water and povidone-iodine at a ratio of 10 parts water to 1 part povidone-iodine. If the patient is allergic to topical povidone-iodine, warm normal saline may be used. Antibiotic treatment should cover *S. aureus.*

CRITICAL POINTS *Acute Paronychia*

Indication
- Perionychial or eponychial infection with abscess

Preoperative Evaluation
- None required in healthy individual with acute infection
- Laboratory evaluation in diabetics or immunocompromised patients
- Radiographs if long-standing infection or no improvement with conventional therapy

Pearls
- Careful evaluation for infection residing below the nail plate or in finger pulp

Technical Point
- Incise with blade facing away from nail bed to reduce risk of injury to matrix.

Pitfalls
- Misdiagnosis as herpetic whitlow (see section on herpetic whitlow)
- Failure to recognize underlying osteomyelitis
- Underlying systemic illness or atypical organism leading to refractory infection

Postoperative Care
- Seven to ten days of oral antibiotics
- Daily soaks in dilute povidone-iodine solution
- Early finger range of motion

Surgical treatment depends on the location and extent of the perionychial infection. Generally, we release along the perionychial sulcus, extending proximally to the level of the nail base. Double incisions are reserved for more extensive eponychial involvement, or when removal of the proximal portion of the nail is planned. Removal of any portion of the nail is done only when the area of abscess extends below the nail plate. Removal of the entire nail is necessary only when the entire nail plate is separated from the nail matrix by abscess.

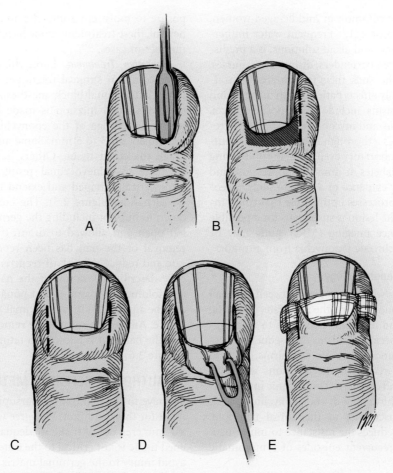

FIGURE 2.4 A, Elevation of the eponychial fold with a flat probe to expose the base of the nail. **B**, Placement of an incision to drain the paronychia and elevate the eponychial fold for excision of the proximal third of the nail. **C** to **E**, Incisions and procedure for elevating the entire eponychial fold with excision of the proximal third of the nail. A gauze pack prevents premature closure of the cavity.

Postoperative Management and Expectations

Postoperatively, the patient is given oral antibiotics for 7 to 10 days, depending on the severity of the infection. Dressings are changed two to three times per day, coinciding with soaking of the affected finger in a dilute solution of povidone-iodine for 5 to 10 minutes. We discontinue packing or wicking the wound at 3 to 4 days. Occlusive dressings can lead to skin maceration and should be avoided. Early motion is emphasized to prevent stiffness.

Improvement is noted in most acute cases of paronychia in 3 to 4 days with appropriate management; however, some tenderness and hypersensitivity around the surgical scars can be expected for several months. Nail deformity can occur either as a result of the infection or after minimal surgical injury to the nail matrix. Patients with an underlying medical illness may require a longer time for healing and recovery or require additional surgery. This population likewise has a higher risk of recurrent infection.

Complications are rare but do occur. Nail deformity can occur either from the infection itself or from inadvertent injury to the nail matrix from decompression. The risk of injury is minimized by gently separating the nail plate from the underlying matrix and by directing the scalpel blade away from the matrix when incising around the nail bed. Persistent infection despite appropriate treatment may be due to inadequate surgical decompression and drainage or inadequate antibiotic cover-

age. If the infection is not resolving at 1 week, radiographs to evaluate for osteomyelitis, cultures with antibiotic sensitivities, and repeat surgical débridement may be necessary. Robbins found that the most frequent complication of a paronychia was extension to the pulp space through a sinus at the side of the nail. This occurred in approximately 13.5% of patients treated in his series from the 1950s.[129] The occurrence of spread to the pulp space today is rare owing to improved antibiotic therapy and more aggressive surgical treatment. In children with long-standing paronychia, infection can lead to bone involvement and epiphyseal separation.

Misdiagnosis of a paronychia can occur, particularly confusion of perionychial infection with herpetic whitlow. Distinguishing herpetic whitlow from a bacterial infection is important. Incision and drainage of herpetic whitlow are contraindicated and can result in systemic viral infection and/or bacterial suprainfection.[7]

Chronic Paronychia
Clinical Presentation and Preoperative Evaluation

Chronic paronychia is characterized by chronically indurated and rounded eponychium and is a distinct clinical problem from acute paronychia. The chronic inflammation is accompanied by repeated episodes of inflammation and drainage. If left untreated, this results in thickening and grooving of the nail plate. This problem is more common in middle-aged women, with a female-to-male ratio of 4:1.[11] Frequent water immersion, particularly in detergents and alkali solutions, is a predisposing condition. Housewives, bartenders, dishwashers, nurses, swimmers, and children who suck their fingers are often affected. It also more commonly affects patients with diabetes and psoriasis.[11] Cultured organisms include gram-positive cocci, gram-negative rods, *Candida*, and mycobacterial species.[99] Preoperative evaluation includes a thorough history for contributing environmental factors, laboratory evaluation for underlying systemic diseases such as diabetes or immunosuppression, and radiographic evaluation for evidence of a foreign body, osteomyelitis, or lytic or blastic processes in the bone that could indicate a possible tumor. If the lesion is suspicious for a possible tumor, a magnetic resonance imaging (MRI) study may be helpful in distinguishing a chronic paronychia from a tumor.

Pertinent Anatomy and Pathophysiology

Chronic paronychia begins with separation between the nail plate and the dorsal soft tissue covering the nail plate, including the cuticle, eponychium, and nail fold. This leads to colonization, usually by staphylococcal organisms. Subsequent infection, by *Candida albicans* and/or colonic organisms, leads to chronic inflammation and recurrent exacerbations with episodic increased erythema and drainage. This chronic inflammation leads to fibrosis and thickening of the eponychium, with a resultant decrease in vascularity to the dorsal nail fold. The decreased vascularity reduces the resistance to minor bacterial insults, allowing for recurrent episodes of symptomatic exacerbations.[11,78]

Treatment

Conservative therapies for chronic paronychial infection have included topical corticosteroids, oral and topical antibiotics, and oral and topical antifungal agents. Although reducing exposure to moist environments and chemical irritants may be helpful, these treatments alone have been unsuccessful in a large number of cases.[11,78]

Operative Treatment. Eponychial marsupialization is the most common surgical treatment for the chronic paronychium. Under digital block anesthesia and tourniquet control, a crescent-shaped incision is made beginning 1 mm proximal to the distal edge of the eponychial nail fold and extending proximally for 3 to 5 mm. Some authors recommend removal of all thickened tissue. Others have found a 3-mm margin adequate to achieve equal results. The crescent should be symmetrically shaped and extend to the edge of the nail fold on each side (Figure 2.5). The crescent of tissue is removed down to but not including the germinal matrix. The wound is left open and allowed to drain. If nail deformity is present, removal of the nail has been reported to improve the cure rate and reduce the risk of recurrence.[11] Pabari and colleagues have described elevation of the nail fold, inverting the tissue and folding this tissue over a nonadherent gauze and anchoring the inverted skin to proximal suture with nonabsorbable suture. Anchoring sutures are removed between 2 and 7 days, and the nail fold is allowed to return to its original position[118] (Figure 2.6).

❖ AUTHORS' PREFERRED METHODS OF TREATMENT

We have found eponychial marsupialization an effective treatment for this condition. We agree with Bednar and Lane[11] that a 3-mm crescent of tissue is adequate and removal of all thickened tissue is not critical to the outcome. Special care is used to avoid injury to the germinal matrix. The removed tissue is sent for bacterial, fungal, and mycobacterial culture. The remaining tissue is sent for pathologic examination. Nail removal is performed when a nail deformity is present. Wounds are covered with Xeroform™ gauze. When the nail is removed, Xeroform gauze is placed in the nail bed and nail fold as well.

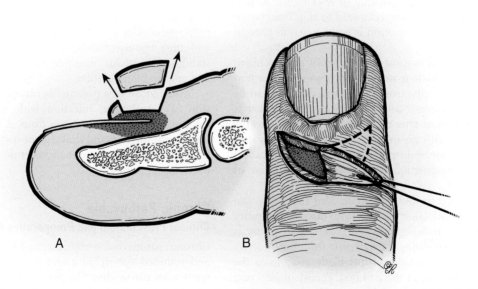

FIGURE 2.5 Eponychial marsupialization for chronic paronychia. **A**, Lateral view showing the area of wedge-shaped excision. Undisturbed matrix is stippled. **B**, Dorsal view of the crescent-shaped area of excision extending to the margins of the nail folds on each side.

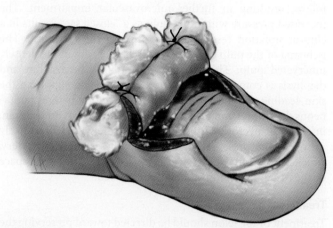

FIGURE 2.6 Alternative technique of nail marsupialization for chronic paronychia, the Swiss roll technique. (Copyright courtesy of Milan Stevanovic and Frances Sharpe.)

Patients are counseled regarding exposure to moist environments. Predisposing systemic conditions, such as diabetes and psoriasis, are medically controlled. We evaluate for activities that may lead to mycobacterial exposures, such as home aquariums or terrariums, marine work, or aviary exposure.

Postoperative Management and Expectations

The postoperative dressing is removed at 48 to 72 hours by soaking in 3% hydrogen peroxide solution. The patient is instructed to soak the area three times per day in dilute povidone-iodine solution. This continues until 2 days after all drainage has stopped. Oral antibiotics are given for 2 weeks. If cultures are negative or the organism is not sensitive, the antibiotic therapy is discontinued at 3 to 5 days.

Most chronic paronychial infections resolve with marsupialization. Systemic or topical antibiotics or antifungal agents are often not required. Wound healing by secondary intention occurs over 3 to 4 weeks. Scar sensitivity is more common than in acute paronychia and may persist for several months. Nail deformity is also more common than in treatment of acute paronychia. Six to 12 months may be required for nail growth, and residual deformity cannot be assessed until that time. Recurrence rates are higher if the patient does not correct environmental factors or if systemic diseases are not medically controlled. In the event of recurrence, re-marsupialization and nail removal should be done.

Felon

The term *felon* probably has its roots from the Latin *fel*, meaning "bile" or "venom." A felon is a subcutaneous abscess of the distal pulp of a finger or thumb (Figure 2.7). However, not all abscesses of the distal phalanx are felons. Superficial infections of the most distal part of the pulp skin are known as "apical infections." Apical infections are distinct from the felon in that the palmar pad is not involved. The term *felon* should be reserved for those infections involving multiple septal compartments and causing compartment syndrome of the distal phalangeal pulp. The most commonly cultured organism from felons is *S. aureus*. Infections from gram-negative organisms have also been reported. These are uncommon and more typically seen in immunocompromised patients or diabetics.

CRITICAL POINTS *Chronic Paronychia*

Indication
- Chronic eponychial infection

Preoperative Evaluation
- Thorough workup and social history for contributing factors
- Laboratory evaluation in diabetics or immunocompromised patients
- Radiographs

Pearls
- Nail removal in conjunction with marsupialization if nail deformity is present
- Nail removal and remarsupialization even with normal nail in setting of recurrence

Technical Point
- Protect the germinal matrix during marsupialization.

Pitfalls
- Misdiagnosis with tumor or cyst
- Unrecognized systemic illness
- Failure to correct environmental factors

Postoperative Care
- Ten to fourteen days of oral antibiotics, if cultures are positive and sensitive. Different if mycobacterial organism
- Consider oral antifungal medications
- Daily soaks in dilute povidone-iodine solution
- Early finger range of motion

Clinical Presentation and Evaluation

Felons account for 15% to 20% of all hand infections.[90] A felon is characterized by severe throbbing pain, tension, and swelling of the entire distal phalangeal pulp. The pulp space is exquisitely tender, but the associated swelling does not extend proximal to the DIP flexion crease, unless the joint or tendon sheath is involved. With the progression of swelling and tension, there is compromised venous return, leading to microvascular injury and development of necrosis and abscess formation. There is often a history of penetrating injury, such as a wood splinter, glass sliver, or minor cut, preceding a felon. "Finger-stick felons" can be seen in diabetics, who repeatedly traumatize the fingertip for blood tests. Once the felon has developed, the patient may attempt a decompression with a knife or needle. The pain and swelling usually develop rapidly. The expanding abscess breaks down the septa and can extend toward the phalanx and produce osteitis or osteomyelitis, or it can extend toward the skin and cause necrosis and a sinus somewhere on the palmar surface of the digital pulp. If such spontaneous, although inadequate, decompression does not occur, it is possible that the digital vessels will thrombose and a sloughing of the tactile pulp will result. Other complications of an untreated felon include sequestration of the diaphysis of the distal phalanx, pyogenic arthritis of the DIP joint, and flexor tenosynovitis from proximal extension, although the last is quite rare.[164]

Pertinent Anatomy

Kanavel studied the anatomy of the fingertip through multiple sagittal and coronal sections of cadaveric fingers. He described the anatomy of the distal pulp as a "closed sac connective tissue

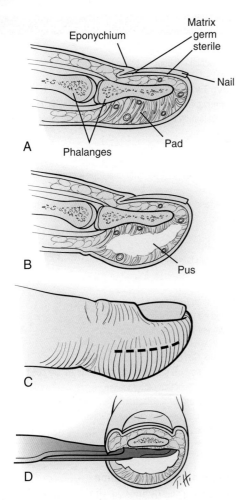

Eponychium

Matrix
germ
sterile

Nail

A

Phalanges   Pad

B   Pus

C

D

FIGURE 2.7 A, Cross section of the distal fingertip, showing the septated anatomy of the pad. **B**, Collection of pus within the finger pulp space. **C**, Incision for drainage of felon. **D**, The incision should include all of the involved septal compartments. (Copyright courtesy of Milan Stevanovic and Frances Sharpe.)

framework, isolated and different from the rest of the finger."[75] Multiple vertical trabeculations divide the pulp of the distal phalanx into a latticework of separate septal compartments. The trabeculae attach the periosteum of the distal phalanx to the epidermis, giving the fingertip structural support and stabilizing the pulp during pinch and grasp. The septal interstices are filled with fat globules and eccrine sweat glands, which open onto the epidermis and provide an access for surface bacteria to enter the pulp space. The digital arteries run parallel to the distal phalanx, giving off a nutrient branch to the epiphysis before entering the pulp space. The diaphysis is supplied principally from volar nutrient vessels from the terminal branches of the digital arteries. The terminal branches of the digital nerve are parallel and palmar to the digital arteries. They arborize extensively within the pulp of the distal phalanx, providing fine tactile discrimination. The highest concentration of sensory receptors in the hand is the volar aspect of the distal phalanx.

Felons may begin with penetrating wounds of the distal pulp or as bacterial contamination of the fat pad through the eccrine sweat glands. Inflammation and cellulitis lead to local vascular congestion, which is aggravated by the closed septal anatomy of the pulp. If left untreated, tissue necrosis and abscess formation

follow, resulting in further microvascular impairment. The increased pressure within the pulp as a "closed sac" results in a clinical situation resembling a compartment syndrome. The ischemia of the pulp causes severe ischemic pain in the densely innervated pulp. The blood supply to the periosteum and diaphysis is compromised more than the blood supply to the skin, leading to bone necrosis and sequestration before spontaneous decompression of the felon through the skin. In children, infection or necrosis of the epiphysis is rarely seen, most likely owing to the preservation of the epiphyseal nutrient artery, which arises from the digital artery proximal to the closed space of the distal pulp and is therefore preserved.

Treatment

Treatment of the felon should be directed toward preserving the function of the finger pulp. These functions include fine tactile sensibility and a stable durable pad for pinch. In the early cellulitic phase, it may be possible to treat the felon with elevation, antibiotics, and soaks. Short-term immobilization may make the patient more comfortable. Some authors recommend surgical drainage only in the presence of abscess.[152] In our hands, surgical drainage is indicated when the pulp is very tender, tense, or fluctuant. The basic tenets of all approaches are to avoid injury to the digital nerve and vessels, use an incision that will not leave a disabling scar, provide adequate drainage, and avoid inadvertent violation of the flexor tendon sheath, causing an iatrogenic tenosynovitis.

Operative Treatment. Several surgical incisions have been described (Table 2.2; Figure 2.8); some of these are of historic interest only and are no longer recommended. Surgery may be performed under digital block anesthesia or under general anesthesia. A tourniquet is helpful for visualization. Regardless of the type of incision, surgical decompression requires thorough removal of necrotic tissue, irrigation, and wound management to allow continued drainage of the abscess cavity. To keep the wound open and draining, a gauze wick is placed in the wound. The first dressing change is done at 24 to 48 hours. Authors' opinions vary as to how long the wound is kept open with a wick drainage. Two to 5 days should be adequate for most cases, depending on the severity of infection. Soaking in dilute povidone-iodine solution as described earlier is initiated after the first dressing change and continued until wound healing by secondary intention.

❖ AUTHORS' PREFERRED METHODS OF TREATMENT

Only in the very early presentation of an acute felon should nonsurgical management be considered. The felon is more typically a very rapidly developing process, and by the time of presentation, the pulp is tensely swollen and exquisitely tender. This requires surgical decompression whether fluctuance is present or not. We prefer to perform surgery under digital block anesthetic with sedation. A forearm tourniquet is used. The extremity is exsanguinated by elevation. The surgical incision is made longitudinally. When the point of maximal tenderness is located in the middle of the pulp or when a sinus is present volarly, we use the longitudinal volar incision. When the point of tenderness is on the side of the pulp, we use the unilateral longitudinal incision. Although the incision is preferably placed on the side opposite the pinching surface, the incision should always be placed on the side of maximal tenderness. When

TABLE 2.2	Surgical Incisions for the Treatment of Felon		
Incision	**Advantages**	**Disadvantages**	**Comments and Technical Points**
A: Fish-mouth incision (Figure 2.8, *A*)	None	Risks circulation leading to skin slough; unstable pulp; unsightly scar	No place in treatment
B: "J" or hockey-stick incision (Figure 2.8, *B*)	Good for extensive or severe abscess	Incision coming distally into the fingertip can cause painful scar	Adequate débridement and release of septa can be performed without crossing the fingertip (see F)
C: Through-and-through incision (Figure 2.8, *C*)	Wide access to all involved septal compartments	Additional wound; superfluous incision that can compromise circulation to the pulp	Initially described with a "J" incision on the ulnar side with a longitudinal counterincision; extension across the fingertip is *not* necessary; two dorsolateral incisions
D: Volar incision (transverse) (Figure 2.8, *D*)	Most direct access to area of abscess; easy to perform; better maintains structural integrity of palmar pad	Palmar scar; higher risk of digital nerve and vessel injury	Incision 4 to 5 mm made at site of maximal fluctuance; sharp dissection through skin and dermis only, followed by blunt dissection through the pulp; elliptical excision of sinus tract and necrotic tissue (if present)
E: Volar (longitudinal) incision (Figure 2.8, *E*)	Same as above; lower risk of digital neurovascular injury	Palmar scar	Same as above; incision should not cross DIP flexion crease
F: Unilateral longitudinal incision (Figure 2.8, *F*)			Preferred placement on the ulnar side of the index, middle, and ring fingers and on the radial side of the thumb and small fingers

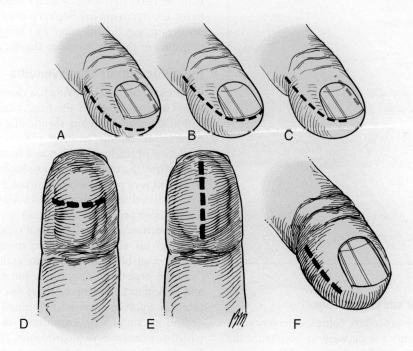

FIGURE 2.8 Incisions for drainage of felons. **A**, Fish-mouth incision. This approach is associated with significant complications and should *not* be used. **B**, Hockey-stick incision. The incision begins in the midaxial line, aims for the corner of the nail, and passes across the finger in the natural line between the skin and nail matrix (see text discussion). **C**, Abbreviated hockey-stick incision with counterincision on the opposite side. An alternative to the full hockey-stick incision is to make this incision shorter and make a second incision on the opposite side of the pulp (*faint dotted line*). **D**, Volar drainage is useful if the abscess points volarward, but this incision risks injury to the digital nerves. **E**, Alternative volar approach. There is less risk to the digital nerves, but the incision should not touch or cross the DIP joint flexion crease. **F**, Unilateral longitudinal approach. This incision is the authors' preferred method for treatment of most felons.

possible, the incision is made on the ulnar side of the second to fourth digits and on the radial side in the thumb and small finger. The incision is started dorsal to and 0.5 cm distal to the DIP joint flexion crease. It is continued distally in line with the volar margin of the distal phalanx, but it does not cross over the fingertip. The incision is deepened along a plane just volar

to the palmar cortex of the phalanx until the abscess is entered. The opening in the cavity is enlarged until adequate evacuation is achieved.

All involved septa should be opened, and a wound culture is taken. The flexor tendon sheath should not be violated, unless there are signs of tendon sheath involvement, as this can cause an iatrogenic tendon sheath infection. The distal phalanx must be examined with a probe. A rough or softened surface indicates bone involvement, which requires débridement of the softened or necrotic bone. After thorough débridement and irrigation, the wound is kept open with a thin gauze wick and a sterile dressing is applied. The first dressing change is done between 12 and 24 hours.

CRITICAL POINTS *Felon*

Indication
- Tense pulp space infection with or without fluctuance

Preoperative Evaluation
- Patient history of recent injury, medical and social history
- Laboratory evaluation in diabetics or immunocompromised patients
- Radiographs to evaluate for foreign body or osteomyelitis

Pearls
- Incision made at point of maximal tenderness

Technical Points
- Avoid incisions crossing the fingertip or DIP flexion crease.
- Protect the digital nerves and vessels.
- Do not violate the flexor tendon sheath.

Pitfalls
- Misdiagnosis as herpetic whitlow
- Unrecognized osteomyelitis
- Incomplete decompression of all involved septa
- Iatrogenic septic flexor tenosynovitis
- Creation of an unstable pulp

Postoperative Care
- Intravenous antibiotic therapy for 5 to 7 days, longer if bone is involved (in hospitalized patients)
- Patients treated in an outpatient setting usually do not require intravenous antibiotics
- Gauze wick for at least 72 hours
- Soaks three times per day in dilute povidone-iodine solution
- Early finger range of motion

Postoperative Management and Expectations

The setting of the drainage procedure (office, emergency department, or operating room) and decision to hospitalize the patient depend on the severity of the infection and the reliability of the patient. In our county hospital patients, we prefer to admit the patients and give intravenous antibiotics until a favorable response to therapy is seen. Oral antibiotics can be used when the infection is controlled. Bone involvement requires longer intravenous therapy. The choice of antibiotic depends on the cultured organism and its antibiotic sensitivity. Because most felons are caused by *S. aureus*, initial antibiotic therapy should address this organism. Factors such as underlying disease, injury mechanism, or contributing occupational or social history may influence antibiotic choice. Dressings are changed two to three times per day. At the time of dressing change, the patient soaks the affected finger in a solution of dilute povidone-iodine for 5 to 10 minutes. Packing or wicking of the wound is discontinued after 3 to 5 days. Occlusive dress-

ings are not used, because they often result in skin maceration. Early motion is emphasized to prevent stiffness.

Most felons recover in 3 to 4 weeks with appropriate management. The length of treatment and recovery depends on the severity of the infection and the presence of bone involvement. Tenderness and hypersensitivity around the surgical scars and of the entire pulp can be expected for several months after surgery. In some patients, this may be a permanent finding. Pulp deformity, most commonly pulp atrophy, occurs frequently and is permanent. Pulp instability can occur in patients where the infection has involved all of the vertical septa, regardless of the incision used. This will often resolve over time but may take 6 months to a year. In cases of osteomyelitis with large bone loss, nail deformity may occur owing to loss of underlying bone support of the nail matrix, resulting in a short finger with a short nail. Nail ablation may be necessary for painful deformities. In some cases with severe bone involvement, amputation of the distal phalanx should be considered.

Complications of treatment include recurrence of infection, usually as a result of inadequate bone débridement. In these cases, repeat surgical débridement and prolonged organism-specific antibiotic therapy will usually be sufficient. Amputation may be necessary for refractory infection. Iatrogenic septic flexor tenosynovitis has been reported. Appropriate treatment involves repeat débridement and surgical decompression and irrigation of the flexor tendon sheath, as described later.

Pyogenic Flexor Tenosynovitis

Pyogenic flexor tenosynovitis is a closed-space infection of the flexor tendon sheath of the fingers or thumb. The purulence within the flexor tendon sheath destroys the tendon gliding mechanism, rapidly creating adhesions that lead to marked limitation of tendon function and severe loss of motion. It can also destroy the blood supply, producing tendon necrosis. Early treatment is of paramount importance in limiting the morbidity associated with this diagnosis. Untreated disease and late diagnosis or presentation can lead to devastating disability in hand function. The incidence and serious sequelae of bacterial tenosynovitis are less frequent, owing to early recognition and the availability of appropriate antibiotic therapy. The most common organisms responsible for disease include *S. aureus* and β-hemolytic *Streptococcus*. *P. multocida* is frequently cultured in infections caused by animal bites. A wider host of organisms should be considered in immunocompromised patients, who have yielded positive cultures for *E. corrodens*, *Listeria monocytogenes*, and mixed gram-positive and gram-negative infections.

Clinical Presentation and Preoperative Evaluation

Most patients present with a history of penetrating trauma, typically over the volar aspect of the proximal interphalangeal (PIP) or DIP joint. A small puncture wound, often from a foreign body or animal bite, can inoculate the tendon sheath. Hematogenous septic flexor tenosynovitis is rare. When this occurs, disseminated gonococcal infections should be considered. Levy recommended that hematogenous tenosynovitis should be treated as disseminated gonorrhea until final culture results are available.[84,134]

Kanavel[74] initially described three cardinal signs of acute flexor tenosynovitis. He later added a semiflexed posture of the digit as the fourth sign.[75] All four signs need not be present, especially in the early course of the disease. Kanavel's four cardinal signs are:

1. A semiflexed position of the finger
2. Symmetric enlargement of the whole digit (fusiform swelling)
3. Excessive tenderness limited to the course of the flexor tendon sheath
4. Excruciating pain on passively extending the finger; the pain should be experienced along the flexor sheath and not localized to a particular joint or abscess.

There are different opinions as to which signs are most clinically useful. Kanavel and others believed that excessive tenderness along the tendon sheath was the most reliable and reproducible clinical sign. Neviaser believed the most reproducible clinical sign was pain with passive extension. Pang and associates noted fusiform swelling of the digit in 97% of patients. Pain on passive extension was noted in only 72% of patients.[32,75,111,119] We believe that all of these findings are useful and in combination help distinguish pyogenic flexor tenosynovitis from local abscess or pyarthrosis. Findings in the thumb and small finger may be more subtle because these fingers have a mechanism of autodecompression through the radial and ulnar bursae.

Laboratory evaluation should include a CBC. The ESR and CRP may be useful in monitoring the disease process. However, these may be elevated in noninfectious inflammatory processes, as well. Radiographs should be taken to evaluate for a retained foreign body, underlying pyarthrosis, osteomyelitis, or unrecognized trauma, such as a fracture.

There are several conditions that may mimic acute pyogenic flexor tenosynovitis. The differential diagnosis includes herpetic whitlow, felon, pyarthrosis, local abscess, and inflammatory diseases such as rheumatoid arthritis or gout or aseptic flexor tenosynovitis. Herpetic whitlow and felon, as already described, present a different clinical picture, typically with more distal findings. Herpetic whitlow is not associated with the tenseness and swelling that are found in pyogenic flexor tenosynovitis and classically presents with small skin vesicles. Pyarthrosis can more closely resemble an infection of the flexor sheath because there is commonly pain with passive joint motion and the digit is held in a flexed posture. Unlike flexor synovitis, the location of the traumatic injury is usually on the dorsal surface of the finger, the swelling is more localized around the joint, and pain with palpation is not present along the entire tendon sheath.

In cases in which the clinical presentation is not clear or there is a clinical suspicion of a nonseptic acute tenosynovitis as may be seen in gout, rheumatoid arthritis, or acute stenosing tenosynovitis, aspiration of the tendon sheath should be done. If the aspiration is negative, NSAID therapy is initiated. The patient should be closely monitored in the first 24 hours. Depending on patient reliability, this can be done on an inpatient or outpatient basis.

Pertinent Anatomy

Knowledge of the anatomy of the flexor tendon sheaths, bursae, and deep spaces of the forearm is important in understanding the presentation and possible spread of infection in the hand. The flexor tendon sheath is a double-walled structure with a visceral layer and a parietal layer. The visceral layer is closely adherent to the tendon and is essentially the epitenon. The parietal layer lies adjacent to the pulley system.[29,35] These two layers are connected proximally and distally, creating a closed system. In the fingers, the sheaths begin in the palm at the level of the metacarpal neck and end distally just proximal to the DIP joint. In the small finger, there is usually continuity between the flexor sheath and the ulnar bursa, which extends to a point just proximal to the transverse carpal ligament. In the thumb, a similar connection is seen with the radial bursa, which also extends proximal to the transverse carpal ligament.[29,35,75,136] Proximally, the radial and ulnar bursae have a potential space of communication through the Parona space, which lies between the fascia of the pronator quadratus muscle and flexor digitorum profundus (FDP) conjoined tendon sheath. This site of connection between the thumb and small fingers through the radial and ulnar bursae gives rise to the *horseshoe abscess*, in which a flexor sheath infection of the thumb or small finger tracks proximally to the wrist and then ascends along the flexor sheath on the opposite side. Although this is the most commonly described connection, many variations of flexor sheath anatomy exit. This was elegantly described by Scheldrup in 1951.[136] These potential variations and sites of interconnection should be kept in mind to direct appropriate treatment.

The flexor tendons receive their nutrient support from a direct vascular supply and diffusion from the synovial fluid. When bacteria inoculate the flexor sheath, the synovial fluid becomes the nutritional source for the bacteria. The host has limited ability to defend against the bacterial proliferation, owing to the poor vascularity within this closed system. The bacterial proliferation leads to increased volume and pressure within the tendon sheath. Schnall and colleagues demonstrated pressures exceeding 30 mm Hg in more than 50% of flexor sheath infections.[139] This high pressure likely contributes to the pathogenesis of the disease process by obstructing the arterial blood supply of the flexor tendons through the vincular system. This can quickly result in tendon necrosis and subsequent rupture. Appropriate and urgent management of flexor tendon sheath infections is imperative in preventing these unwanted complications.

Treatment

There is a narrow range of indications for nonsurgical treatment of pyogenic flexor tenosynovitis. Patients rarely present with early clinical findings, which may be managed with antibiotic therapy. Those patients who present within the first 24 hours of the onset of symptoms, have mild pain and mild swelling, and show only partial expression of one or two of Kanavel's signs may be initially treated with intravenous administration of antibiotics. A dorsal block splint is applied to place the hand at rest. The extremity is elevated. The patient is monitored with close clinical observation in an inpatient hospital setting. If the clinical symptoms are not improving in the first 12 hours, surgical treatment is indicated. Nonsurgical management should seldom be considered in the diabetic or immunocompromised patient.

Before antibiotic therapy is initiated, an aspiration of the tendon sheath is done to obtain material for culture. The aspiration is performed with a 20- to 22-gauge needle. The aspiration can be performed anywhere between the palmodigital crease and the DIP flexion crease. The aspiration should be performed away from any areas of superficial cellulitis. A small amount of saline may be necessary to lavage the sheath to obtain a specimen for culture. If frank pus is encountered on the aspiration, nonsurgical treatment should not be pursued. Patients who present with a local cellulitis along the volar surface of the finger may also have a septic flexor tendon sheath. If nonsurgical treatment is considered, aspiration should not be performed through the cellulitic subcutaneous tissue, to prevent inadvertent inoculation of the sheath.

Purulent tenosynovitis rapidly destroys the gliding mechanism within the flexor tendon sheath. Delayed or inadequate treatment increases the formation of adhesions within the sheath, permanently limiting tendon excursion and ultimately limiting the finger range of motion.

Operative Treatment. Several surgical approaches have been described for the treatment of pyogenic flexor tenosynovitis. Some of these are of historic interest only. Most describe various incisions for proximal and distal exposure of the flexor tendon sheath and various irrigation methods and solutions.

There have been two principal surgical approaches to treatment of flexor tendon sheath infections. The first is with surgical exposure of the tendon sheath through a midlateral or Brunner incision. We prefer the midlateral incision (Figure 2.9, *A*). Although this allows more direct access to the tendon sheath, it can lead to greater scarring and stiffness of the finger. In the setting of wound healing problems, this leaves the tendon or tendon sheath exposed and more typically requires return to the operating room for delayed primary wound closure.

The second approach developed because of concerns that wide exposure of the tendon sheath led to significant postoperative scarring and stiffness of the involved finger. To address this problem, a number of methods were described that were designed to limit exposure of the tendon sheath (see Figure 2.9, *B* to *D*). Variations included location of incisions, type of irrigants, and continuous methods of irrigation, but all involved limited incisions at the proximal and distal ends of the tendon sheath and proximal to distal irrigation of the sheath.

Neviaser popularized a limited midlateral incision, with opening of the tendon sheath distal to the A4 pulley. The proximal tendon sheath is exposed in the distal palm, and a catheter is placed for continuous irrigation[111] (see Figure 2.9, *D*).

In the technique of closed tendon sheath irrigation, as described by Neviaser, a zigzag incision is made in the distal area of the palm over the proximal end of the sheath. The sheath is opened at the proximal margin of the A1 pulley. A second incision is made on the ulnar midaxial side of the finger in the middle and distal segments. Access to the distal end of the sheath is obtained through a plane dorsal to the digital artery and nerve. The sheath is resected distal to the A4 pulley. A 16-gauge polyethylene catheter with a single opening at its end is inserted under the A1 pulley in the palm for a distance of 1.5 to 2 cm. The catheter is sutured to the skin, and the wound closed around it. The sheath is copiously irrigated with saline. A small drain is placed in the distal incision, making sure to be in the tendon sheath. The drain is sutured to the skin. The wound is closed around the drain. The system is flushed again to test its patency. The hand is dressed and splinted, with the catheter brought out of the dressing and connected to a 50-mL syringe. The dressing is arranged so that the drain can be seen distally. The system is tested just before the patient leaves the

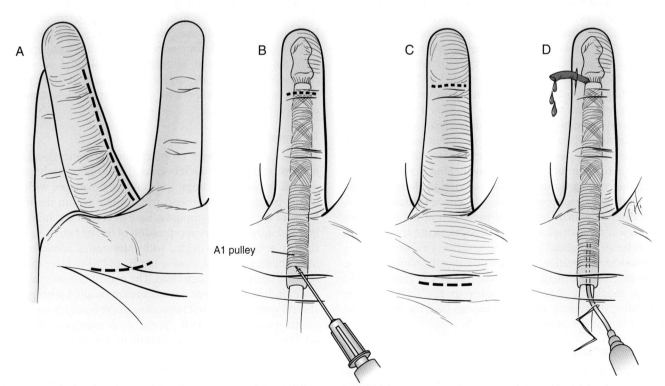

A1 pulley

FIGURE 2.9 Incisions for drainage of tendon sheath infections. **A**, Open drainage incisions through the midaxial approach. **B**, Sheath irrigation with distal opening of the sheath and proximal syringe irrigation. **C**, Incisions for intermittent through-and-through irrigation. **D**, Closed tendon sheath irrigation technique (see Neviaser R: Closed tendon sheath irrigation for pyogenic flexor tenosynovitis. *J Hand Surg* 3A(5):462–466, 1978). (Copyright courtesy of Milan Stevanovic and Frances Sharpe.)

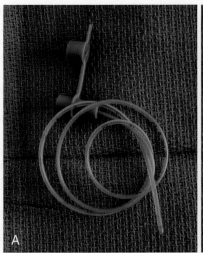
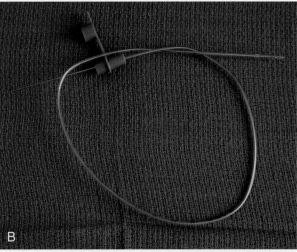

FIGURE 2.10 Cannulation of the flexor tendon sheath with a 5 Fr pediatric feeding tube can be difficult due to the flaccidity of the tube. Use of a 24-gauge wire as an obturator facilitates introduction of the feeding tube into the tendon sheath. (Technique courtesy of Dr. E. Farng.) (Copyright courtesy of Milan Stevanovic and Frances Sharpe.)

operating suite. Postoperatively, the sheath is flushed manually with 50 mL of sterile saline every 2 hours for 48 hours. At this time, the digit is inspected. If signs of infection have abated, the catheter and drain are removed. The wounds are dressed lightly to avoid impeding motion. Exercises to restore finger motion are started. If any doubt exists, the irrigation may be continued for an additional 24 hours.[111] Complete motion can be expected in a week. Several studies support the use of this technique.[32,61] Indwelling catheter placement has not been shown to be necessary and may delay active motion.[86] In our experience, we have not felt that this technique adequately decompresses the flexor tendon sheath or finger. Also, the method of continuous irrigation has often been painful to the patient, the nursing staff, and the on-call physician.

❖ AUTHORS' PREFERRED METHODS OF TREATMENT

Decompression of the septic flexor tendon sheath begins with a midlateral incision. The incisions are designed to avoid scarring on the pinching surface of the fingers. In the index, middle, and ring fingers, the incision is placed on the ulnar border, and in the thumb and small finger, it is placed on the radial side. The incision is made dorsal to Cleland's ligament (see Figure 2.9, *A*). The incision extends from the middle of the distal phalanx to just proximal to the web space. The dissection is carried out dorsal to the neurovascular bundle and down to the flexor tendon sheath. This allows decompression of the swollen finger, decreasing compartment pressure. The tendon sheath is opened distal to the A4 pulley. The sheath must be opened enough to allow the easy egress of fluid or pus, typically 4 to 6 mm. Cultures are taken from the tendon sheath effluent. A 1.5- to 2.0-cm transverse volar incision made proximal to the A1 pulley is usually sufficient to expose the proximal flexor sheath. This incision can be easily extended proximally or distally as a Brunner-type incision to allow greater exposure of the tendon sheath if it is necessary. The tendon sheath is opened proximally. If fluid for culture was not obtained distally, cultures should be taken from the proximal sheath. If hypertrophic synovitis is seen, synovial biopsy is recommended.

Pathologic examination should include fungal and mycobacterial stains.

A 14- or 16-gauge intravenous catheter or preferably a No. 5 pediatric feeding tube is introduced into the tendon sheath and advanced 1.5 to 2.0 cm into the sheath (Figure 2.10). Syringe irrigation with copious amounts of antibiotic containing normal saline is done. The fluid should be seen to egress from the distal opening in the tendon sheath. The tendon sheath should be irrigated until clear fluid is seen distally. Irrigation is discontinued if there is too much fluid extravasation into the finger.

If we encounter difficulty in irrigating, the catheter is first repositioned. Mobilizing the superficialis and profundus tendons and placing the catheter dorsal to the tendons may allow easy flow of solution. Thickened tenosynovium may impede flow, and a limited proximal synovectomy or wider exposure of the tendon sheath may be necessary.

Any wounds on the volar surface of the finger should be débrided. Even small puncture wounds, particularly those caused by cat bites, should be débrided and irrigated. In cases in which there is a large volar wound and opening in the tendon sheath at a site of abscess, the irrigant may primarily be flowing out of the abscess site. In this situation, following the débridement of the volar wound, the irrigation catheter can be placed into the tendon sheath at the site of abscess and the distal tendon sheath can be further irrigated (Case Study 2.1).

Postoperative Management and Expectations

Postoperatively, the wounds are left open. A wet gauze wick is placed into the wounds to allow continued drainage. A bulky dressing is applied. The hand is elevated, and intravenous antibiotics are continued. The first dressing change should be done at 12 to 24 hours. At this time, the patient begins soaking in a dilute solution of povidone-iodine, as described earlier. Early motion is initiated. Therapist supervision may be necessary. It is important to keep this wound open to allow drainage. If left alone, the palmar wound will close almost immediately. Therefore, moist gauze wicks are used to keep the wounds open in

CRITICAL POINTS *Pyogenic Flexor Tenosynovitis*

Indication
- Septic flexor tenosynovitis

Preoperative Evaluation
- Clinical examination is the hallmark of diagnosis.
- Laboratory evaluation may include uric acid and rheumatoid factor in addition to CBC, depending on suspicion of nonpyogenic process.
- Radiographs to evaluate for foreign body or fracture, or for joint space widening suggesting joint effusion

Pearls
- Pain with palpation along the flexor tendon sheath and pain with passive extension are most useful in diagnosing early disease.
- Urgent surgical treatment, especially in a patient with diabetes or immunocompromise, reduces the morbidity associated with this infection.

Technical Points
- Perform early decompression with complete midlateral incision of the finger.
- Incise dorsal to Cleland's ligament.
- Irrigate the sheath until the effluent is clear.
- Use wick to keep the proximal and distal incisions open.

Pitfalls
- Delayed surgical treatment
- Inadequate decompression
- Injury of the digital neurovascular structures

Postoperative Care
- Intravenous antibiotics
- Pain management to allow early range of motion
- First dressing change between 8 and 12 hours
- Soaks in dilute povidone-iodine solution three times per day with range-of-motion exercises
- Repeat débridement and irrigation in 48 hours if Kanavel's signs not resolving.

the first 48 to 72 hours. Intravenous antibiotics are continued for 7 to 10 days or until clinical improvement is seen. After this, oral antibiotics are continued to complete a 4-week course of therapy.

If the clinical signs of infection are not improving in the first 24 to 36 hours, the patient is returned to the operating room for a repeat irrigation and débridement. Repeat cultures are obtained, and organism-specific intravenous therapy is continued. A low threshold for return to the operating room should be used in diabetics and immunocompromised patients.

Most patients with pyogenic tenosynovitis, if treated promptly with adequate surgical débridement, appropriate antibiotics, and therapy, will improve rapidly. Patients usually have an almost immediate sense of relief of the severe throbbing pain that was present before treatment. Wound healing of the volar incision occurs quickly as soon as the wicking is discontinued. The midlateral incision heals by secondary intention over the course of 10 to 20 days. When the swelling subsides, Steri-Strips™ can be used to bring the wound edges together, shortening the healing time. Despite healing by secondary intention, the midlateral scar is usually painless. Over time, the scar becomes soft and essentially unnoticeable. The reported range of motion after flexor tendon sheath infection varies. Ten to 20% of patients fail to recover a full range of motion. A

more rigorous analysis of motion showed that only two thirds of normal motion was present at 6 weeks. This improved to 80% of normal motion at a 30-month follow-up.[15]

The more severe the initial presentation, the greater is the likelihood of complications and an adverse outcome. Maloon and associates identified three risk factors for a poor prognosis: 1) diabetes, 2) late presentation, and 3) association with a human bite.[94] Pang and colleagues identified five risk factors associated with a poor outcome, including 1) age over 43 years; 2) diabetes mellitus, peripheral vascular disease, or renal failure; 3) presence of subcutaneous purulence; 4) digital ischemia; and 5) polymicrobial infection. Patients with no purulence and no ischemia had no amputations and recovered 80% of the total active range of motion (TROM). Patients with subcutaneous purulence but no ischemia had an 8% risk of amputation. This group recovered 72% of the TROM. Patients with subcutaneous purulence and ischemic changes had an amputation rate of 59% and recovered only 49% of the TROM.[119] Any infection of the flexor tendon sheath may cause scarring and adhesions within the sheath, limiting flexor tendon excursion and gliding. Manipulation under local anesthesia in the first 2 to 4 weeks following treatment may have value in breaking up adhesions before dense scarring occurs. Tenolysis should not be considered until the infection has completely resolved and the patient has failed to improve with occupational therapy. Although we have not had to perform a tenolysis following pyogenic FTS, we would recommend at least 6 months of therapy following resolution of infection to allow for tendon recovery before additional procedures. Passive motion should exceed active motion for a tenolysis alone to improve function. Stiffness of the PIP or DIP joint is not uncommon, particularly if early motion is not initiated or if the patient is noncompliant with therapy. Soft tissue necrosis occurs rarely. Local débridement should be done as needed. When the infection is controlled, healing by secondary intention will occur. If the flexor tendon is exposed, local flap coverage should be considered, especially in patients who have good tendon gliding. Late treatment or severe infection may result in tendon necrosis. This requires excision of the necrotic tendons from the level of the A1 pulley to its distal insertion. In our experience, staged reconstruction of the tendon sheath and tendon grafting is difficult and often has suboptimal outcome. In the index and small finger with tendon necrosis, amputation may be considered, because this is more likely to improve functional outcome and shorten the healing time. Severe flexor tendon sheath infections with tendon necrosis in conjunction with pyarthrosis of any digit except the thumb may best be treated by amputation.

Radial and Ulnar Bursal and Parona Space Infections

Pertinent to the treatment of pyogenic flexor tenosynovitis are infections of the radial and ulnar bursae of the palm and the Perona space at the wrist. Infections in these spaces occur rarely in isolation but are more commonly associated with flexor tendon sheath infections of the small finger or thumb.

Pertinent Anatomy

Radial Bursa. The radial bursa is a continuation of the tendon sheath of the flexor pollicis longus (FPL) tendon. The sheath begins at the base of the distal phalanx of the thumb.

Technically, the sheath ends at the metacarpophalangeal (MP) joint. The radial bursa begins at this level and includes the length of the FPL tendon through the carpal canal. It ends 1 to 2 cm proximal to the proximal edge of the transverse carpal ligament. It is considered a separate bursal space from the FPL tendon sheath, even though in adults it was contiguous with the sheath in 95% of specimens.[136]

Ulnar Bursa. The ulnar bursa begins at the proximal end of the small finger flexor tendon sheath. The bursa widens more proximally, overlapping the mid fourth metacarpal and the proximal base of the third and fourth metacarpals. The bursa lies ulnar to the flexor tendons, which are invaginated into the bursa but not surrounded by it. The relationship of the small finger flexor tendon sheath with the ulnar bursa is less consistent than the relationship between the flexor tendon sheath of the thumb and the radial bursa. Early studies showed direct continuity in only 50% of specimens. Other studies have demonstrated a higher rate of communication, often with an hourglass-type narrowing between the small finger tendon sheath and the ulnar bursa. Communication between the radial and ulnar bursae occurs in 85% of specimens.[136]

Proximal to the transverse carpal ligament, the radial and ulnar bursae lie deep to the FDP tendons and above the fascia of the pronator quadratus muscle. Communication between the radial and ulnar bursae can occur across this space, known as the potential Parona space.[92]

Parona Space

The Parona space is the deep potential space in the distal volar forearm. It lies between the fascia of the pronator quadratus muscle and the sheath of the FDP tendons. It is in continuity with the midpalmar space. Although infections of the Parona space most commonly result from extension of infection from either the radial or ulnar bursa, the Parona space is not in direct continuity with these bursae. Rupture of these bursae due to infection leads to involvement of the Parona space. Also, radiocarpal joint infection may rupture through the volar capsule and spread into the Parona space. Isolated infection of the Parona space can occur after a penetrating injury or, rarely, as a spontaneous (hematogenously spread) deep space infection.

Clinical Presentation and Preoperative Evaluation

Because radial and ulnar bursal infections rarely occur in isolation, the clinical presentations of these infections are similar to those of pyogenic flexor tenosynovitis of the thumb and small finger. In addition to the cardinal signs of Kanavel, there may be swelling and tenderness along the thenar or hypothenar eminence. The adjacent fingers assume a flexed posture, as does the wrist. Although the uninvolved fingers may not be swollen, passive extension is painful. Kanavel believed that the most valuable sign of ulnar bursal infection was the presence of tenderness at the junction of the distal flexion crease of the wrist and the hypothenar eminence. In a similar manner, the most valuable sign for radial bursal infections was tenderness at the junction of the distal wrist flexion crease and the thenar eminence.[75]

Extensive swelling may not be evident, because the bursae rapidly become necrotic. Accumulation of pus does not occur, because the bursae rupture and decompress into the surrounding space. The infection can track into the adjacent bursa through intrabursal communication or across the potential space of Parona. An ascending infection along the opposite border digit can then occur, forming the so-called *horseshoe abscess*. Anatomic variations in the interconnection of the tendon sheaths occur in approximately 15% of patients.[136] Therefore, clinical examination of any flexor tendon sheath infection should include examination of the palm, wrist, and all of the adjacent fingers.

Isolated infections of the Parona space are rare but may present as swelling, tenderness, and, occasionally, fluctuance in the distal volar forearm. Digital flexion is often difficult and painful. Symptoms of numbness and tingling in the median nerve distribution may be present due to swelling or fluid present in the midpalmar space. Diagnostic ultrasound or MRI can be useful in demonstrating fluid within this space. More commonly, Parona space infections are associated with tendon sheath infections of the thumb and small finger. In a series of nine patients, the most common site of spread of infection was from the thumb flexor tendon sheath (seven of nine patients). Interestingly, in this group of patients, β-hemolytic *Streptococcus* was cultured from five of nine specimens.[142]

Treatment

Ulnar and radial bursal infections rarely occur in isolation but are a part of pyogenic flexor tenosynovitis, most commonly of the thumb and small finger. There is no role for nonsurgical treatment of this condition. These infections can cause rapid destruction of the bursal sheath, swelling within the carpal tunnel causing acute median nerve symptoms, and scarring and adhesions between the superficial and deep flexor tendons. Prompt surgical treatment is necessary. The septic flexor tenosynovitis must be treated in conjunction with the bursal infection. There is no general consensus regarding the surgical incision, use of drains, or open versus closed management with catheter irrigation. The following techniques have been described.

Open Treatment. Open treatment of ulnar bursal infections, as described by Boyes, included two separate incisions. The first incision is placed parallel to the proximal edge of the A1 pulley. It can be extended proximally along the radial margin of the hypothenar crease. The proximal end of the bursa in the forearm is exposed through a 3-inch incision, beginning just proximal to the wrist flexion crease. The incision parallels the volar edge of the distal ulna. The flexor carpi ulnaris and the dorsal sensory branch of the ulnar nerve are retracted volarward. By retracting these structures, the pronator quadratus muscle is exposed. The bulge of the ulnar bursa is easily visualized and opened. Cultures should be taken, and the wound is copiously irrigated from proximal to distal. Similarly, treatment of radial bursal infections is done through a distal incision placed at the level of the thumb MP joint. Boyes believed that the radial bursa could best be treated through the same proximal incision as the ulnar bursa, dissecting radially across the volar floor of the pronator quadratus to reach the radial bursa. He described a separate radial incision along the flexor carpi radialis; however, he believed this was superfluous when the ulnar incision was used. For advanced infections, Boyes advocated proximal extension of the palmar incision to include the decompression and drainage of the carpal tunnel. Drains are placed in the bursa and brought out through the skin; they are removed after 48 hours so that exercises can be started.[18]

For isolated Parona space infections, we prefer the incision described for the treatment of the ulnar bursa. Only the proximal incision is necessary. In cases in which there are associated carpal tunnel symptoms or an associated midpalmar infection, an extended carpal tunnel incision is necessary to drain both the midpalmar and Parona spaces.

❖ AUTHORS' PREFERRED METHOD OF TREATMENT

We treat bursal infections by first addressing the flexor tendon sheath infection when present. The exposure of the distal bursa is the same as that described by Boyes.[18] When a tendon sheath infection is present, the same incision used for exposure of the proximal tendon sheath is used for the distal exposure of the bursa. The proximal incision for ulnar bursal infections is a longitudinal incision beginning at the proximal wrist flexion crease. The incision is extended proximally for 5 cm, paralleling the radial margin of the flexor carpi ulnaris. The superficialis and profundus tendons are retracted radially. The flexor carpi ulnaris and ulnar neurovascular structures are retracted ulnarly. The bursa is exposed, opened, and drained. Cultures are taken. Proximal-to-distal irrigation with a 14- or 16-gauge angiocatheter or No. 5 pediatric feeding tube is performed using normal saline. The irrigation is continued until the distal effluent is clear. Radial bursal infections are treated in the same manner. Our incisions are the same as described under through-and-through treatment.

The incisions are left open. A ¼- to ½-inch Penrose drain is placed in the proximal incision site, at the pronator fascia. Distally, a moist gauze wick is used to keep the incision open.

For isolated Parona space infections, we prefer the incision described for the treatment of the ulnar bursa. Only the proximal incision is necessary. If carpal tunnel symptoms or a midpalmar infection are present, an extended carpal tunnel incision is necessary to drain both the midpalmar and Parona spaces.

Postoperative Management and Expectations

The postoperative management of bursal infections is the same as that described for flexor tendon sheath infections. We remove the Penrose drain at 24 to 48 hours.

Outcomes after bursal infections are generally not as favorable as for isolated flexor tenosynovitis. Tendon adhesions, flexion contracture of the fingers and wrist, and restricted motion are more likely to occur. Tenolysis for recalcitrant adhesions may be necessary if therapy does not adequately restore function.

Deep Space Infections

The hand has three anatomically defined potential spaces. These septated spaces lie between muscle fascial planes (Figure 2.11, *A*); they are the *thenar, midpalmar,* and *hypothenar spaces* in the hand. There are three more superficial spaces in the hand, the *dorsal subcutaneous space, dorsal subaponeurotic space,* and *interdigital web space.* Infections of these spaces are different from deep space abscesses in that they do not have well-defined anatomic borders; their presentations are similar to those of deep palmar space abscesses, however. Deep palmar space infections are increasingly rare, likely due to early recognition and surgical treatment of infections and improved antibiotic therapies.

Palmar Space Infections

Clinical Presentation and Preoperative Evaluation. Deep space infections are most commonly caused by penetrating trauma. In thenar and midpalmar space infections, infection can occur from spread from a septic tendon sheath (thumb, index, or long

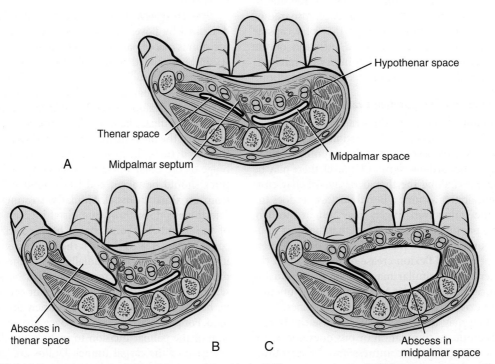

Thenar space

Midpalmar septum

A

Hypothenar space

Midpalmar space

Abscess in thenar space

B   C

Abscess in midpalmar space

FIGURE 2.11 Deep palmar spaces. **A**, Potential spaces of the midpalm. **B**, Thenar space abscess. **C**, Midpalmar space abscess. (Copyright courtesy of Milan Stevanovic and Frances Sharpe.)

TABLE 2.3	**Characteristics of Deep Palmar Space Infections**		
Space	**Thenar Space** (Figure 2.11, *A* and *B*)	**Midpalmar Space** (Figure 2.11, *A* and *C*)	**Hypothenar Space** (Figure 2.11, *A*)
Characteristics	Most common of deep space infections; can often track dorsally into space between first dorsal interosseous muscle and adductor pollicis muscle; can be confused with dorsal subcutaneous abscess if dorsal extension of abscess cavity	Rare infection	Extremely rare; distinctly separate anatomic space; is not in continuity with any of the flexor tendon sheaths
Boundaries	Dorsal: Fascia of adductor pollicis, second volar metacarpal, and first volar interosseous fascia Volar: Tendon sheath of index finger and radial palmar fascia Radial: Confluence of adductor pollicis fascia and palmar fascia at base of thumb proximal phalanx Ulnar: Midpalmar oblique septum	Dorsal: Fascia overlying second and third volar interosseous muscles and periosteum of third, fourth, and fifth metacarpals Volar: Flexor sheaths of long, ring, and small fingers and palmar aponeurosis Radial: Midpalmar oblique septum Ulnar: Hypothenar septum	Dorsal: Periosteum of fifth metacarpal and fascia of deep hypothenar muscles Volar: Palmar fascia and fascia of superficial hypothenar muscles Radial: Hypothenar septum Ulnar: Fascia of hypothenar muscles
Proximal and distal boundaries	Distal: Deep transverse fascia at level of MC head Proximal: Base of palm	Distal: Deep transverse fascia at level of MC head Proximal: Base of palm	Distal: Deep transverse fascia at level of MC head Proximal: Base of palm
Clinical findings	Swelling and exquisite tenderness of thenar eminence; thumb is abducted; pain with passive adduction	Dorsal swelling predominates; loss of palmar concavity (becomes convex); flexed posture of fingers (long and ring); pain with passive extension of fingers, but less than with septic flexor tenosynovitis	Localized tenderness and swelling of hypothenar eminence; no palmar swelling; no finger or flexor tendon sheath involvement

finger for thenar space and long, ring, or small finger for midpalmar space). Local spread from a subcutaneous abscess that tracks deep into the space can also be a route of infection.

Both thenar and midpalmar space infections often present with swelling involving the entire hand, particularly on the dorsal side. The tight fascia on the palmar surface of the hand limits the amount of volar swelling. The more loosely arranged connective tissue dorsally allows greater expansion of the soft tissue in this area. This dorsal swelling should be distinguished from local dorsal abscess and dorsal cellulitis. All of the deep palmar space infections will have areas of palmar swelling and exquisite tenderness localized over the involved palmar space. Hypothenar infections generally have less dorsal swelling.

Preoperative evaluation includes a careful history of the mechanism of injury and relevant comorbidities. Laboratory evaluation should include a CBC. Radiographs should be routinely obtained to evaluate for a retained foreign body, underlying osteomyelitis, or fracture. Aspiration, ultrasound, or MRI may be useful in identifying an abscess. If the clinical presentation strongly suggests a deep infection, a negative aspiration should not negate surgical exploration.

Pertinent Anatomy. The thenar and midpalmar spaces of the hand are located dorsal to the flexor tendons and volar to the metacarpals and interosseous muscle fasciae. They are divided by the midpalmar (oblique) septum, which extends from the palmar fascia to the volar diaphyseal ridge of the third metacarpal. The midpalmar space is separated from the hypothenar space by the hypothenar septum, which extends from the volar

ridge of the fifth metacarpal shaft to the palmar aponeurosis (Table 2.3).

Treatment. There is no role for nonsurgical management of deep space infections. These should be treated as surgical emergencies. Intravenous antibiotics are started, preferably after obtaining a culture either from the site of a draining wound or from an aspirate of the affected palmar space. If the patient cannot be taken immediately to the operating room and cultures cannot be obtained from an aspiration, then antibiotic therapy with good staphylococcal coverage should be initiated.

Thenar Space. Incisions to drain the thenar space should provide adequate exposure of the affected areas. It is also important to make incisions that will not lead to subsequent contracture. Access to the thenar space requires that an incision be placed near neurovascular structures, specifically, the recurrent motor branch of the median nerve, the digital nerves to the thumb and radial side of the index finger, the princeps pollicis artery, and the proper digital arteries. Careful dissection is necessary to avoid injury to these structures.

Drainage of the thenar space abscess has been described through dorsal, volar, or combined volar and dorsal incisions. We avoid the dorsal transverse incision owing to the risk of web space contracture. Combined approaches should not be connected through the web space, as they can also lead to contracture and/or a painful scar.

Volar Approach (Thenar Crease). An incision is made on the palmar surface of the hand just adjacent and parallel to the thenar crease (Figure 2.12, *A*). The incision begins

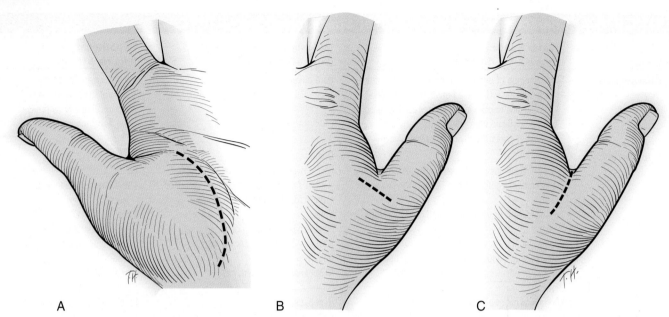

FIGURE 2.12 Incisions for drainage of the thenar space. **A**, Thenar crease approach. Motor recurrent branch of the median nerve is at risk in dissection. **B**, Dorsal transverse approach. Transverse incision is not favored as this can lead to a web space contracture. **C**, Dorsal longitudinal approach. (Copyright courtesy of Milan Stevanovic and Frances Sharpe.)

approximately 1 cm proximal to the web space and continues proximally for 3 to 4 cm. Blunt dissection through the palmar fascia is carried out toward the adductor pollicis muscle until abscess is encountered. In the proximal portion of the deep dissection, particular attention is necessary to protect the motor branch of the median nerve. After the area has been drained adequately, the dissection is extended over the distal edge of the adductor to decompress the first dorsal interosseous space.

Dorsal Longitudinal Approach. A straight or slightly curved longitudinal incision is made in the dorsum of the first web space, starting proximal to the web and extending perpendicular and proximal to the web, bisecting the interval between the first and second metacarpals (see Figure 2.12, *C*). The dissection is continued deeper into the interval between the first dorsal interosseous and the adductor pollicis, at which point pus should be encountered.

Combined Dorsal and Volar Approach. Two incisions are made: one dorsally, which is the slightly curved longitudinal approach described earlier, and one volarly, which parallels the thenar crease. Each approach is used to drain the corresponding half of the space. A separate drain is used for each incision, but through-and-through drains are not used.

Midpalmar Space. Various skin incisions have been described for decompression of the midpalmar space. These include the (1) transverse incision in the distal crease (Figure 2.13, *A*); (2) combined transverse and longitudinal approach (see Figure 2.13, *B*); and (3) curved longitudinal approach (see Figure 2.13, *C*). Whichever skin incision is used, the common digital nerves and arteries as well as superficial palmar arch are protected. The flexor tendons of the ring finger are used as a guide to the midpalmar space. The deep dissection is continued longitudinally on either side of these tendons until the abscess is opened.

Distal Palmar Approach Through the Lumbrical Canal. This approach was described by Kanavel not as a routine approach to midpalmar space infection but as treatment for a special circumstance, when a midpalmar space infection involves the lumbrical canal.[75] A longitudinal incision is made on the palmar surface of the third web space (between the middle and ring fingers). It extends from immediately proximal to the web and ends distal to the midpalmar crease. The incision should not cross the crease (see Figure 2.13, *D*). A clamp is inserted into the wound and directed proximally down the canal of the third lumbrical, dorsal to the flexor tendons, until the midpalmar space is entered and pus is encountered.

Dorsal Approach. A longitudinal incision is made between the middle and ring fingers or between the ring and small fingers. Blunt dissection is done above the periosteum on the ulnar side of the third metacarpal or along the radial or ulnar sides of the fourth metacarpal. Dissection is carried down between the metacarpal and interosseous muscles. Below the interosseous muscles lies the midpalmar space.

Hypothenar Space. The hypothenar space is decompressed through an incision in line with the ulnar border of the ring finger, starting just proximal to the midpalmar crease and continued proximally to 3 cm distal to the wrist flexion crease (Figure 2.14). The incision is deepened to the level of the hypothenar fascia. This layer is divided in the line of the incision. The abscess should be directly beneath it. After the purulence has been evacuated, a gauze dressing and/or Penrose drain is placed in the wound.

Deep Subfascial Space Infections

The deep subfascial spaces include the dorsal subcutaneous space, the dorsal subaponeurotic space, and the interdigital web space. The dorsal subcutaneous space is an extensive area of loose connective tissue without distinct boundaries, in which pus can accumulate over the entire dorsum of the hand. The dorsal subaponeurotic space lies deep to the extensor tendons, above the periosteum of the metacarpals and fascia of the dorsal interosseous muscles. The interdigital web spaces are areas of

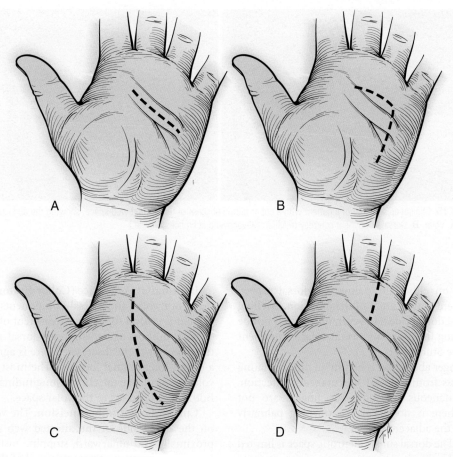

FIGURE 2.13 Incisions for drainage of the midpalmar space. **A**, Transverse incision in the distal crease. **B**, Combined transverse and longitudinal approach. **C**, Curved longitudinal approach. **D**, Distal palmar approach through the lumbrical canal. (Copyright courtesy of Milan Stevanovic and Frances Sharpe.)

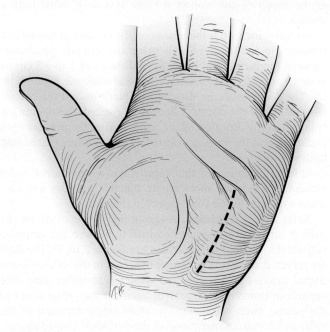

FIGURE 2.14 Approach to the hypothenar space. (Copyright courtesy of Milan Stevanovic and Frances Sharpe.)

loose connective tissue between the fingers. Infection in this area tracks both volarly and dorsally and is commonly called a *collar-button abscess*.

Clinical Presentation and Evaluation

Dorsal Subcutaneous and Dorsal Subaponeurotic Space Abscess. As with most infections of the hand, dorsal subcutaneous and dorsal subaponeurotic space infections typically result from penetrating injuries of the hand. The dorsal aspect of the hand is swollen, warm, and erythematous. The dorsal surface is tender to palpation. Fluctuance may be present. Finger extension may be difficult and is usually painful. Differentiating these infections from cellulitis or other hand infections can be difficult, because most hand infections present with dorsal swelling.

Web Space Abscess (Collar-Button Abscess). The term *collar-button abscess* refers to the hourglass shape of the abscess and the resemblance to the collar buttons used for dress shirts in the early 1900s. An infection in the web space (collar-button or collar-stud abscess) usually occurs through a fissure in the skin between the fingers, from a distal palmar callus, or from extension of an infection in the subcutaneous area of the proximal segment of a finger. The pain and swelling are localized to the web space and distal area of the palm. The adjacent fingers lie abducted from each other (Figure 2.15). The swelling may

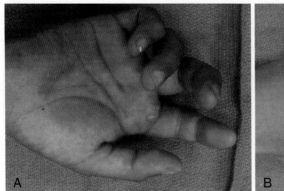
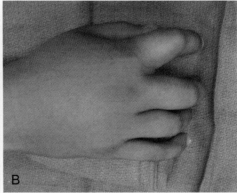

FIGURE 2.15 Clinical appearance of a patient with a collar-button abscess of the second web space, showing the abducted position of the fingers. **A**, Volar. **B**, Dorsal. (Copyright courtesy of Milan Stevanovic and Frances Sharpe.)

be more prominent on either the palmar or dorsal aspect, depending on the extent and location of the infection. Swelling is often greater on the dorsal side. However, one should not be misled into overlooking the more important volar component of this infection (Case Study 2.2).

The position of finger abduction is helpful in differentiating a collar-button abscess from a dorsal subcutaneous infection. In the dorsal subcutaneous infection, the fingers are not abducted, because there is no purulence tracking palmarly between the bases of the adjacent fingers.

Pertinent Anatomy. The dorsal subaponeurotic space is limited on its dorsal surface by the dense aponeurosis of the extensor tendons. On its volar aspect, it is limited by the periosteum of the metacarpals and the dorsal fascia of the interossei. Medially and laterally, the aponeurotic sheet merges with the deep fascia overlying the dorsal interosseous muscles, the periosteum of the first through fifth metacarpals, and the capsules of the first through fifth MP joints. Kanavel described this space as a truncated cone, with the smaller end at the wrist and the larger end toward the MP joints.

The interdigital web spaces consist of the loose areolar connective tissue between the metacarpal heads and around the deep intermetacarpal ligament. The skin of the web space is densely attached to the palmar fascia. A web space infection most commonly begins on the volar surface. The strong attachments of the palmar fascia to the skin limit the volar extension of the abscess. Therefore, the infection track is along the path of least resistance to the dorsal surface.

Treatment

Dorsal Subcutaneous and Subaponeurotic Space Abscess. Exploration of the dorsal subcutaneous and subaponeurotic spaces can be performed through one or two dorsal longitudinal incisions. The first incision is placed over the longitudinal axis of the index metacarpal. The second incision is placed between the fourth and fifth metacarpals. These incisions allow exploration of the infection to determine if this is a superficial or deep infection. The subaponeurotic space can be opened by incising along the margin of the extensor tendon. Advanced infection often involves both the dorsal subcutaneous and subaponeurotic spaces. The use of two incisions allows for good drainage of the abscess cavity, while soft tissue coverage over the extensor tendons is maintained.

Interdigital Web Space (Collar-Button Abscess). Awareness that both volar and dorsal components of infection may be present is critical for proper treatment of this abscess.

Most authors agree with both dorsal and volar incisions for treatment of these abscesses. There is agreement on the use of a dorsal longitudinal incision. The most commonly described volar incisions are the curved longitudinal and zigzag incisions. Both provide access to the volar space.

Curved Longitudinal Incision. The volar incision is begun on the radial side of the affected web space. It is continued proximally and ulnarward, stopping just distal to the midpalmar crease overlying the metacarpal of the ulnar digit involved (Figure 2.16, *A*). After the skin is divided, the subcutaneous tissue is spread with a clamp until pus is encountered. The opening in the abscess is enlarged longitudinally. Compression is applied to the dorsum of the web space by the surgeon while the volar incision is retracted. Increased drainage can be seen in the depth of the wound if there is a deep collar-button abscess.

A second incision is then made on the dorsum. It begins just proximal to the involved web space and extends proximally between the metacarpal heads for a distance of 1 to 1.5 cm or as much as is needed to decompress the abscess (see Figure 2.16, *D*). The deep tissues are divided in a plane toward the palmar abscess. When the dorsal collection is entered, the opening is enlarged in the direction of the wound. After the pus has been evacuated and the wound irrigated, gauze wicks are placed into both wounds.

One modification of this approach is a longitudinal volar incision between the metacarpals, but this provides less adequate exposure to the volar aspect of the abscess.

Volar Zigzag Approach. A zigzag incision is made on the palmar surface, starting just proximal to the web and stopping just distal to the midpalmar crease (see Figure 2.16, *B*). The flaps are reflected and the deep tissues dissected in the web while the digital arteries and nerves are retracted to either side. The superficial transverse metacarpal ligament and other fibers of the palmar fascia are divided to allow ample exposure of the volar and dorsal compartments of the dumbbell-shaped abscess. A 1.5-cm dorsal longitudinal incision is made between the bases of the proximal phalanges. Generous communication between the two incisions is established.

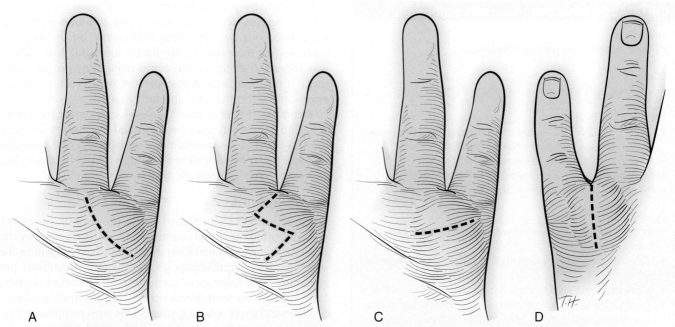

FIGURE 2.16 Incisions for web space abscesses (collar-button abscesses). **A**, Curved longitudinal incision. **B**, Volar zigzag approach. **C**, Volar transverse approach. **D**, Dorsal incision used in conjunction with any of the volar exposures. (Copyright courtesy of Milan Stevanovic and Frances Sharpe.)

Zigzag incisions provide excellent exposure for drainage of infection, but if they are left open, the flaps can retract and cause thick or tender scars. Therefore, if this incision is used, we recommend delayed primary wound closure after the infection has been controlled.

Volar Transverse Approach. Kanavel described a volar transverse incision placed parallel with the distal flexion crease of the palm over the site of maximum swelling (see Figure 2.16, *C*). He believed this was generally adequate for drainage and did not require a second incision.[75] The deep dissection is as previously described. The dorsal approach may be needed as well. One potential disadvantage of this incision is placement of the transverse limb too far distally. If this part of the incision is inadvertently carried too close to the web, a web space contracture can result.

❖ AUTHORS' PREFERRED METHOD OF TREATMENT

Thenar Space. Our preferred method of treatment for the thenar space infections is through combined dorsal and volar approaches, as described earlier. We have found that a single volar incision is not adequate to address the dorsal abscess cavity between the adductor and first dorsal interosseous muscle. Similarly, a single dorsal incision, whether it is transverse or longitudinal, can provide access to the volar abscess, but it is more difficult and we have not been satisfied with our ability to adequately decompress and irrigate the involved space. We leave the wounds open, using a moist gauze wick. We occasionally use a Penrose drain on the volar side for large areas of abscess.

Midpalmar Space. Midpalmar space infections are treated as described earlier under the curved longitudinal approach. This method provides the best exposure of the midpalmar space. It is less likely to result in a severe scar contracture, because it lies adjacent to an anatomic crease. It is an extensile incision and

can be used to simultaneously access the thenar space if necessary. We leave the incisions open, using a moist gauze wick as described earlier. Healing by secondary intention occurs rapidly provided the infection is well controlled and necrotic tissue has been removed.

Interdigital Web Space Abscess (Collar-Button Abscess). We use both a dorsal and volar approach to treat these infections. Our preferred incision is the curved longitudinal incision. We find that this incision provides excellent exposure of the abscess, reduces the risk of skin edge necrosis, and provides easier access for wound management. We try to avoid crossing the web space and do not connect the volar and dorsal skin incisions. If the web space is crossed, this should be done with a longitudinal rather than a transverse incision to avoid later web space contracture.

Postoperative Management and Expectations. The same principles of management apply for all deep space infections. Postoperatively, the wounds are left open. A wet gauze sponge is placed into the wounds to allow continued drainage. A bulky dressing is applied. The hand is elevated, and intravenous antibiotics are continued. The first dressing change should be done at 12 to 24 hours. At this time, the patient begins soaking in a dilute solution of povidone-iodine, as described earlier. Early motion is initiated. Therapist supervision may be necessary. Active finger and wrist motion is necessary to reduce problems of stiffness, contracture, and tendon adhesion. Intravenous antibiotics are continued for 14 to 21 days. After this, oral antibiotics are continued to complete a 4-week course of therapy.

If the clinical signs of infection are not improving in the first 24 to 36 hours, the patient is returned to the operating room for a repeat irrigation and débridement. An MRI may be helpful in identifying areas of abscess or joint effusion that need to be surgically assessed. Repeat cultures are obtained if the previous

CRITICAL POINTS *Deep Space Infections*

Indication
- Thenar, midpalmar, and collar-button abscesses

Etiology
- Penetrating injury is the most common source of infection.

Preoperative Evaluation
- Clinical examination features may provide a diagnosis, but diffuse dorsal swelling can cause difficulty in separating cellulitis from abscess.
- Aspiration is useful but can be misleading.
- Radiographs are necessary to evaluate for foreign body or fracture.
- MRI is very helpful in identifying localized abscess.

Pearls
- Thenar space infections present as wide abduction of the thumb and difficulty with opposition.
- Midpalmar space infections result in loss of palmar concavity; fingers are semiflexed.
- Collar-button abscesses are distinguished by abduction of adjacent fingers.
- Urgent surgical treatment, especially in a patient with diabetes or immunocompromise, reduces the morbidity associated with these infections.

Technical Points
- We prefer two incisions for thenar space infections. Use caution for the motor recurrent branch of median nerve.
- Single volar midpalmar incision. Use caution for superficial arch and digital nerves. Deep to the midpalmar space, pay attention to the deep palmar arch and motor branch of ulnar nerve.
- Two incisions are required for collar-button abscess. We prefer not to incise across the web space. If crossing the web space, keep incision longitudinal.
- Use wick to keep incisions open.

Pitfalls
- Delayed surgical treatment
- Inadequate decompression
- Injury of digital neurovascular structures

Postoperative Care
- Intravenous antibiotics
- Pain management to allow early range of motion
- First dressing change between 8 and 12 hours
- Soaks in dilute povidone-iodine solution three times per day
- Repeat débridement and irrigation in 48 hours if symptoms not improving

culture was negative, and organism-specific intravenous therapy is continued. Tissue biopsy with specific staining to diagnose fungal or atypical infections provides information more quickly than fungal and mycobacterial cultures. A low threshold for return to the operating room should be used in diabetics and immunocompromised patients.

Deep space infections are more likely to develop scarring and stiffness of the hand and fingers. With adequate treatment and rehabilitation, 70% to 80% of patients achieve full recovery. Most patients are able to return to their previous occupations.

Complications associated with deep space infections include stiffness and contracture. Extensor lag has been reported after dorsal subcutaneous and dorsal subaponeurotic space infections. Skin necrosis either dorsally or volarly can lead to exposed tendons or neurovascular structures. These problems may re-

quire secondary procedures for soft tissue coverage and contracture release. Tendon necrosis is less common with deep space infections but can occur, particularly on the extensor surface when there may be significant soft tissue loss. Painful scar formation along the incision is reduced by proper placement of the incisions and postoperative management with desensitization, scar massage, and early motion.

Nerve injury is uncommon but can occur during treatment. Infection causes soft tissue necrosis and can distort the local anatomy. This can lead to inadvertent placement of the surgical incision. It may be difficult to recognize a nerve or vessel within an ocean of pus and necrotic tissue.

Septic Arthritis

Septic arthritis is characterized by the presence of a purulent exudate within the closed confines of a joint. It is caused by the introduction and proliferation of pyogenic bacteria within the synovium in concentrations greater than 10^5 organisms per microliter, with subsequent production of a purulent exudate. Inoculation of the joint usually occurs from penetrating trauma. *S. aureus* and streptococcal species are the most common organisms. Gram-negative, anaerobic, and mixed infections also occur, especially in the immunocompromised host. A hematogenous origin of septic arthritis should raise suspicion of gonococcal infection. Expedient treatment is important to minimize articular destruction caused by infection.

Clinical Presentation and Patient Evaluation

Abscess within the joint cavity represents a cellular and immunogenic response within the synovium and reticuloendothelial system. Bacteria replicate within the joint cavity, producing toxins. This stimulates an immunogenic response. The responding leukocytes produce bactericidal enzymes that destroy the proteoglycan matrices and collagen of hyaline cartilage. Lymphocytes and related cells form immune complexes, which also can degrade articular surfaces. As the inflammatory response continues, there is increased pressure within the joint. This forces the joint into a position of maximum potential volume, producing pseudoparalysis. The increased volume within the joint further damages the articular cartilage through pressure necrosis. Untreated, pus under pressure may erode through the joint capsule and overlying skin. Alternatively, it may erode into the subchondral bone, resulting in osteomyelitis.

Patients generally present with a history of penetrating trauma, which may be caused by bites or by splinters, thorns, hooks, needles, or any of a variety of penetrating objects. The source of the injury is important in selecting empirical antibiotic therapy for the presumptive infecting organisms. Contiguous spread from an adjacent infection can occur. In the DIP joint, other common mechanisms of occurrence are from infection or direct inoculation of a mucous cyst or from contiguous spread from a felon, paronychia, or purulent flexor tenosynovitis. In the PIP joint, contiguous spread is most commonly related to a purulent flexor tenosynovitis. At the MP joint, infection from a clenched fist injury is frequently encountered. Hematogenous spread, although uncommon, has been reported and is more likely to occur in immunocompromised patients.

The clinical findings associated with septic arthritis are swelling, redness, warmth, and pain around the affected joint.

Active or passive motion produces exquisite pain. Fluctuance within the joint may be demonstrated by ballottement. Systemic signs such as fever, chills, tachycardia, malaise, sweats, and rash may be present but are not common. The presence of systemic symptoms suggesting hematogenous seeding should alert the physician to look for a primary source of infection.

Evaluation of the patient should address any history of penetrating trauma, insect bite, or animal bite or of previous therapeutic joint injection or aspiration, or the possibility of a retained foreign body. A history of immunocompromising conditions or inflammatory conditions that may mimic joint sepsis should be obtained. Many inflammatory conditions can present as an acutely swollen and painful joint of the wrist and hand. These include gout, pseudogout, rheumatoid arthritis, systemic lupus erythematosus, psoriatic arthritis, acute rheumatic fever, sarcoidosis, and Reiter syndrome. In the case of possible hematogenously spread infection, a careful review of systems may reveal the primary nidus of infection. Retained penetrating objects, in particular palm or cactus thorns or sea urchin spines, can create a chemical synovitis that resembles an infectious process. Distinction between infectious and noninfectious processes is difficult. In these circumstances, surgical treatment is necessary, with the difference that it is very important to remove the offending nidus of inflammation if still present. Identification of gout or pseudogout crystals on fluid analysis does not exclude the possibility of a commensurate infection. If the clinical picture supports infection, surgical treatment should be performed.

Laboratory evaluation should include the WBC count, ESR, and CRP. The WBC count is elevated in less than half of patients. The ESR and CRP are usually elevated in nonimmunocompromised patients. Blood cultures should be taken, particularly when systemic symptoms are present. Culture of potential distant primary sources, such as the urine or the urethra or oropharynx, should be considered in the setting of a hematogenously spread infection.

Aspiration of small joints may be difficult, especially when trying to avoid areas of cellulitis. Fluid yields may be low. If only a small volume of fluid is obtained, it is best sent for culture rather than cell count. Radiocarpal joint aspiration is more easily performed and may help differentiate acute infection from other inflammatory processes. Aspiration through cellulitic skin should be avoided. Radiocarpal aspiration is performed through the dorsal skin, just distal to the Lister tubercle. An 18-gauge needle is introduced and directed proximally to accommodate the normal palmar tilt of the distal radius. Aspiration of the midcarpal joint or distal radioulnar joint may be necessary if no fluid is obtained from the radiocarpal joint. If fluid is not easily obtained from either the radiocarpal or midcarpal joint, 1 to 2 mL of sterile saline can be injected into the joint and then aspirated for analysis. The aspirate should be sent for gram-stained smear, crystal analysis, and aerobic and anaerobic cultures. If adequate aspirate is available, cell count, fluid protein and glucose levels, and fungal and mycobacterial cultures should be obtained. The WBC count from the aspirate of more than $50,000/mm^3$ suggests joint sepsis. A lower WBC count with a high percentage of polymorphonuclear cells (>90%) can indicate an early joint infection. A high WBC count (>90,000/mm^3), regardless of the percentage of polymorphonuclear cells, should be treated as an acute infection. A synovial fluid glucose value of 40 mg/dL or less than the fasting blood glucose level also supports a septic process.

Radiographs are useful to evaluate for a retained foreign body, osteomyelitis, or gas within the joint or soft tissues indicating clostridial or other anaerobic infections. Initially, radiographs may show joint capsular distention and periarticular soft tissue swelling. Joint space narrowing on radiographs is seen as a late sequela of septic arthritis. MRI, when necessary, is a sensitive and specific technique of identifying a joint effusion.

Treatment

Septic arthritis of the hand or wrist is treated as a surgical emergency. Articular destruction from proteolytic enzymes and toxins that degrade glycosaminoglycans begins in the first 24 hours of infection. The principle of treatment for all septic joints is prompt surgical drainage. Serial aspiration has been proposed as a form of treatment for septic joint infection. In the hand and wrist, aspiration is useful diagnostically but is therapeutically unpredictable. Leslie and colleagues reported superior results with formal arthrotomy of the shoulder joint over serial aspiration. The same principle applies to the hand, where serial aspiration of small joints is more difficult and less reliable.[83] Serial aspiration should only be considered when the patient is not medically stable for formal treatment.

Infections of the Wrist Joint (Radiocarpal, Ulnocarpal, and Midcarpal Joints)

Arthrotomy of the wrist joint may include arthrotomy of the radiocarpal and ulnocarpal joints, as well as the midcarpal and distal radioulnar joints. This can be accomplished through the standard dorsal approach to the wrist joint. This is done through a longitudinal incision centered slightly ulnar to the Lister tubercle. The retinaculum between the third and fourth extensor compartments is opened. The extensor pollicis longus tendon is identified and retracted radially. The underlying joint capsule is exposed. The capsule can be opened longitudinally or with a "T" incision. A longitudinal or T-capsular incision provides adequate exposure of the joint and can easily be left open to allow continued drainage. The ligament-sparing incision is an excellent approach to the wrist joint. In the case of sepsis, the capsular flap does not have to be completed. Transverse incisions to separately open the radiocarpal and midcarpal joints can be used, and capsular windows can be created to allow ongoing drainage. Culture of the joint fluid is obtained. The joint is copiously irrigated with gravity irrigation or bulb syringe. Pulsed lavage is not used, because this can cause additional soft tissue injury. The joint is taken through flexion and extension during the irrigation to maximize removal of purulent material. Articular surfaces are inspected for discoloration, areas of thinning, or softness. Necrotic tissue and inflammatory synovium are removed as indicated. Synovial tissue should be sent for culture and histologic studies. At the completion of irrigation, the joint capsule is left open. A gauze wick is placed down into the capsule to maintain a path for continuous drainage. Alternatively, the capsule may be closed over a drain. The skin incision is left open. One or two loosely placed sutures can be used to keep the skin edges from retracting. If the skin edges are markedly retracted, Steri-Strips can be placed to gently approximate the skin edges as the swelling decreases. A transverse skin incision can also be used to approach the joint, which results in a more cosmetic scar with less skin edge retraction. However, it is not extensile and may not provide adequate exposure in all circumstances.

Arthroscopic débridement and lavage of the infected radiocarpal joint may be a useful alternative to open débridement. Viewing and working portals are established; usually the 3-4 portal is used for viewing and for fluid ingress. The working portal may be the 6R or the 4-5 portal. An 18-gauge needle attached to intravenous tubing can be placed in the 6U portal for additional fluid egress. Arthroscopic irrigation and débridement has been shown in one study to decrease the number of surgical procedures and hospital stays in those patients with a single septic joint.[133]

Metacarpophalangeal Joint

The MP joint can be opened through a dorsal longitudinal or dorsal curvilinear incision. If a wound is present, the incision is designed to incorporate the wound and excise the wound margins. The skin flaps are elevated, and the extensor mechanism is defined. The joint capsule is exposed either through longitudinal splitting of the extensor tendon hood or through an incision in the sagittal band adjacent to the tendon. The MP joint capsule is often thin and inadvertently opened through the same incision. Once the joint is open, it is copiously irrigated with saline. Longitudinal traction opens the joint space and allows better access of the irrigant to the volar recesses of the joint. The joint should be carefully inspected for any articular surface damage or a retained foreign body, especially in the scenario of MP joint infection resulting from a clenched fist injury, described later under human bite injuries. The joint capsule and wounds are left open and covered with a moist gauze dressing.

Proximal Interphalangeal Joint

Arthrotomy of the PIP joint is performed through a midaxial incision. This incision avoids exposure of an injury to the central extensor tendon slip. The midaxial incision is placed from the distal margin of the interdigital web space and continued in the midaxial line to the level of the DIP joint. In the index finger, the incision is preferentially placed on the ulnar side of the finger. In the small finger, the incision is placed on the radial side. The central two digits can be accessed through either radial or ulnar incisions. If this approach is used for the thumb MP or interphalangeal (IP) joints, a radial incision is preferred. When the incision is correctly placed, the proper digital nerves lie protected in the volar skin flap (Figure 2.17, A). However, the dorsal sensory branch of the digital nerves can be jeopardized by this approach. The transverse retinacular ligament is incised, exposing the collateral ligament complex. The PIP joint is entered by excision of the accessory collateral ligament (see Figure 2.17, B), followed by capsulectomy. Alternatively, the joint may be exposed through subperiosteal elevation of the proximal origin of the collateral ligament. The joint is thoroughly débrided and irrigated. Inspection of the articular surfaces may be difficult through this incision, but a blunt probe or Freer elevator can be used to palpate the cartilage for areas of erosion or softening. The capsule and wounds are left open and covered with a moist gauze dressing.

Wittels and associates described a combined radial and ulnar midaxial incision for drainage. In conjunction with their func-

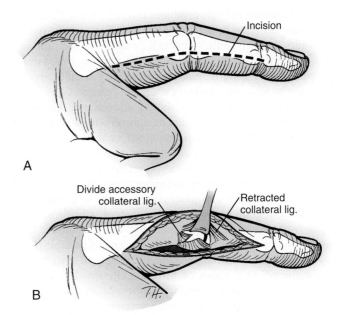

FIGURE 2.17 Lateral approach to the PIP joint. **A**, Skin incision. **B**, Arthrotomy is performed through the lateral ligamentous complex, dividing the accessory collateral ligament. (Copyright courtesy of Milan Stevanovic and Frances Sharpe.)

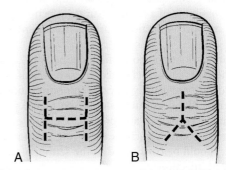

FIGURE 2.18 Dorsal approach to the DIP joint. **A**, "H" incision. **B**, Reverse "Y" or Mercedes incision. (Copyright courtesy of Milan Stevanovic and Frances Sharpe.)

tional rehabilitation, this provided very satisfactory results.[170] A dorsal arthrotomy is sometimes necessary due to the presence of a dorsal wound. In these cases, the central extensor slip and dorsal capsule are often injured or disrupted. This frequently leads to the development of a septic boutonnière deformity. When a septic PIP joint is encountered in this setting, the wound is extended proximally and distally. The arthrotomy and capsulectomy are performed adjacent to the central slip, if it is intact.

Distal Interphalangeal Joint

The DIP joint is opened through a dorsal "H" incision or through a dorsal reverse "Y" or Mercedes incision (Figure 2.18). Skin flaps are elevated over the terminal extensor tendon. The terminal tendon is retracted to the side, and the capsule is opened. It is important to protect the tendon insertion because injury can result in a mallet finger deformity. Alternatively, the midaxial incision as described for PIP joint arthrotomy can be extended distally and used to expose the DIP joint. The collateral ligament is excised to gain access to the joint. This approach may be more useful when there is an associated flexor tendon sheath infection. The joint should be adequately débrided and irrigated. The wounds are left open.

Postoperative Management and Expectations

Surgical incisions are left open, with a gauze wick to maintain patency of the capsulectomy and allow for continued wound drainage. Moist gauze dressing changes two to three times per day prevent encrustation of the wound, which results in premature wound closure. Early range of motion is critical to postoperative treatment. This provides mechanical lavage of the joint and reduces the accumulation of pus within the joint. We prefer that patients soak the affected hand in a dilute solution of povidone-iodine, as described previously. Active, active-assisted, and passive range of motion is done during the soaking period.

Empirical intravenous antibiotic therapy is started immediately after obtaining a culture from either an aspirate or surgical culture. Antibiotic selection is then tailored to treat the bacterial pathogen. There is some controversy regarding the duration of antibiotic therapy necessary for septic arthritis. Previous recommendations have included duration of intravenous therapy between 3 and 4 weeks. More recent recommendations use shorter courses of intravenous therapy, with a switch to oral antibiotics after 10 to 14 days. Oral antibiotics are continued to complete a 4- to 6-week course of therapy. We agree with others that intravenous antibiotic therapy should be continued through symptom resolution, followed by oral antibiotics for 4 to 6 weeks. The duration of antibiotic therapy should be based on surgical findings, pathogen virulence, patient compliance, and clinical response to treatment. If clinical improvement is not seen within the first 24 to 48 hours, repeat surgical irrigation and débridement should be considered, and reexamination for underlying bone involvement should be performed. Amputation may be necessary if an infection cannot be eradicated or if an affected finger has a significant negative impact on overall hand function.[18,148] Every effort should be made to preserve the thumb, even if arthrodesis, shortening, or reconstruction is required (Figure 2.19).

Symptom resolution and functional outcome after septic arthritis are correlated with the duration of symptoms before the initiation of treatment.[50,124] Some degree of joint stiffness is expected. In one study, only 13 of 33 infections of the PIP joint treated with early surgical decompression achieved full restoration of motion.[170] Early mobilization reduces the degree of postoperative stiffness but cannot reverse the changes that have occurred in the articular cartilage resulting from sepsis. Joint space narrowing is generally seen after completion of treatment. Joint arthrosis and ankylosis can occur in any setting but are more prevalent in cases in which the presentation or treatment has been delayed.

Complications associated with septic arthritis in the hand and wrist include stiffness of the affected and adjacent joints. Tendon adhesions may occur in association with the swelling and inflammation caused by the infection or as a result of the surgical incision and may require secondary surgery. Osteomyelitis of the adjacent bones may complicate or prolong the course of treatment (Case Study 2.3). Additional surgical débridement, bone resection, resection arthroplasty, or amputation may be necessary. Late complications include arthrosis and arthritis.

Pediatric patients may have associated injury to the epiphysis and growth plate. Septic arthritis of infancy may be difficult to identify and may be complicated by concurrent illnesses resulting in a delay of diagnosis. This can result in partial or complete growth arrest and stiffness.[149]

Salvage of postinfectious arthritis may include arthrodesis, resection arthroplasty, or amputation. Implant arthroplasty in previously infected joints of the hand is very controversial. At the present time, most authors do not favor this treatment.

Septic Boutonnière and Mallet Deformity

Unique complications of septic arthritis occur at the PIP and DIP joints. Septic boutonnière deformity is a complication of pyogenic arthritis of the PIP joint. It occurs in those cases in which a virulent organism has caused rapid tissue destruction or where there has been late presentation or treatment. The intraarticular collection of purulence has reached a volume that can no longer be retained within the joint. The path of least resistance for escape is dorsally. The joint is well supported palmarly by the volar plate, which blends with the accessory collateral ligaments, and by the collateral ligaments on the sides. All these structures are thick and unyielding; therefore, the pus escapes dorsally through the thin dorsal capsule. There, it can destroy the extensor mechanism over the dorsum of the joint. The central slip is attenuated or eroded, allowing the lateral bands to slip volarward. This results in a classic boutonnière deformity. Management of this problem is difficult. However, the first priority is eradication of the joint infection and preservation of full passive range of motion and active flexion. Late boutonnière reconstruction can be done when the infection is resolved and the joint is supple (see Chapter 5). Late PIP joint fusion may be appropriate in cases of severe damage to the articular cartilage or when passive range of motion cannot be recovered.

Mallet finger deformity can occur after DIP joint sepsis. The mechanism of injury is similar to that which occurs in the PIP joint. The terminal extensor tendon is attenuated or destroyed. Delayed DIP joint fusion is the most appropriate treatment after infection is eradicated.

Osteomyelitis

Osteomyelitis is an infection of the bone. Traditionally, it has been believed that once the bone has been infected, it remains infected. In the hand, it may be possible to eradicate infection, because amputation can remove the involved digit or portion of the digit. Moreover, having options for later microvascular reconstruction means that adequate bone débridement can be undertaken with less risk of permanent structural and functional loss. In the hand, osteomyelitis is rare, likely owing to the hand's abundant vascular supply. It has been reported to represent between 1% and 6% of all hand infections.[102,126] It is often related to adjacent soft tissue or joint infection. The most commonly involved bone is the distal phalanx.[8,126]

Osteomyelitis can occur after penetrating trauma, crush injuries, contiguous spread from adjacent soft tissue infections, and hematogenous seeding and in the postsurgical setting. Penetrating trauma is the most common cause of osteomyelitis.[8,90,126] Patients with immunocompromise, vascular impairment, and systemic illness are more susceptible to developing osteomyelitis.

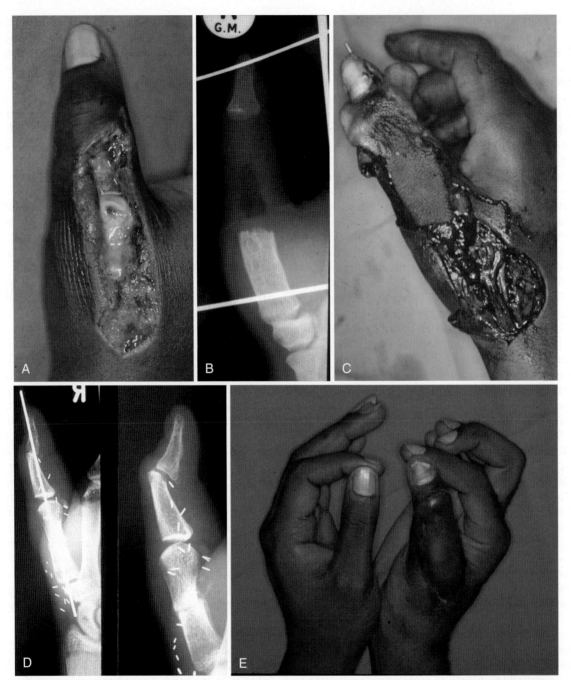

FIGURE 2.19 A 27-year-old man sustained a bite injury to his thumb during an assault. He developed a severe infection of the thumb MP joint, with subsequent spread to the metacarpal head and proximal phalanx. The volar soft tissue, flexor tendon, and neurovascular structures were intact. **A**, Open draining wound with exposed metacarpal head and necrotic proximal phalanx. **B**, Radiograph taken after resection of all necrotic bone. **C**, A free vascularized second toe transfer was used to reconstruct the bone defect, extensor pollicis longus tendon, and soft tissue defect. **D**, Radiographs immediately after surgery with Kirschner wire stabilization and at 1-year follow-up. **E**, Appearance and function of the reconstructed thumb at 1-year follow-up. There is no evidence of recurrent infection. (Copyright courtesy of Milan Stevanovic and Frances Sharpe.)

Hematogenous osteomyelitis of the hand and wrist is rare. Reilly and colleagues reported 13% of their cases were of hematogenous origin. Of those patients, half were immunocompromised.[126] Children are more susceptible to hematogenous osteomyelitis. The susceptibility to infection in the long bones in children is believed to result from the vascular arrangement around the growth plate. The long capillary loops and venous sinusoids in the metaphysis adjacent to the growth plate have a tortuous course, leading to turbulent and sluggish blood flow. These capillary loops are actually terminal branches possessing gaps that allow blood cells and bacteria to pass into the extravascular space. Once in this space, the pathogen may proliferate, causing infection. Contributing to this process is the relative acellularity of this space, decreased oxygen tension, and suboptimal phagocytic activity.[8,162] Until the age of 1 year, there is vascular continuity between the metaphysis and epiphysis via the epiphyseal plate arteries. In infants, this can lead to the spread of infection from the metaphysis into the epiphysis and subsequently into the joint space. After the age of 1 year, the epiphyseal plate capillaries disappear. This reduces the likelihood of contiguous spread of hematogenous osteomyelitis into the joint space. In immunocompetent children, these infections occur predominantly in the radial and ulnar metaphysis. In sickle cell anemia, the inciting event for hematogenous osteomyelitis is more likely bone infarction, and the location associated with hematogenous osteomyelitis favors the metacarpals and phalanges.[153]

Acute infections after closed fractures are extremely rare,[63] but open fractures of the hand can result in deep infection. McLain and colleagues reported an incidence of deep infection in 11% of patients. Factors associated with infection included grossly contaminated wounds and extensive soft tissue and skeletal injury. *S. aureus* was the dominant organism in only 30% of patients. Polymicrobial infections and enteric organisms were significant pathogens in more than 60% of cultures.[102] Fixation of open or closed fractures with Kirschner wires can lead to a local osteomyelitis along the pin track. The incidence of significant pin track infection has been reported between 0.5% and 5%.[9,16]

The most common organisms responsible for osteomyelitis are *S. aureus* and other skin organisms. Coagulase-negative *Staphylococcus* is commonly associated with infections of implants, such as hardware used for internal fixation after a fracture. Many other organisms have been isolated and reported in the literature. Often, the mechanism of injury and the environment in which the injury occurred may suggest a different infecting pathogen. For example, a penetrating injury from an animal bite would lead to empirical treatment for *Pasteurella multocida*, until definitive culture results are available. *Salmonella* remains the most common organism in hematogenous osteomyelitis in children.[153]

The classification of osteomyelitis was refined by Cierny and Mader in 1985.[26] This classification (Table 2.4) applies to long bones and describes four anatomic sites of infection and three physiologic classes of host, defining 12 clinical types of osteomyelitis (anatomic site plus physiologic class).

Clinical Presentation and Evaluation

Clinical signs of infection often include redness, swelling, warmth, and tenderness. Fluctuance and/or drainage may be present. Findings depend in part on the cause of the bone infection. When osteomyelitis has resulted from contiguous spread of infection, it is frequently difficult to differentiate bone infection from soft tissue infection, as might be seen in a felon. Systemic clinical signs such as fever, chills, and malaise are more common in hematogenous osteomyelitis. Waldvogel and colleagues reported that all patients with osteomyelitis of the hand had local signs of inflammation, but only one third of patients had fever and leukocytosis.[163] The presence of systemic symptoms should alert the examiner to the possibility of a remote source of infection. Failure of an apparent soft tissue infection to respond to appropriate treatment should suggest the diagnosis of an underlying osteomyelitis. Children can present a greater diagnostic challenge, leading to delays in diagnosis. Young children may not be able to describe their pain or its location and may present only with pseudoparalysis of a limb. Careful examination may indicate areas of increased warmth, localized bone tenderness, or joint irritability. Older children

TABLE 2.4	Classification of Osteomyelitis	
Anatomic Site		
Type 1	Medullary osteomyelitis (endosteal infection)	Associated with hematogenous osteomyelitis or intramedullary implant
Type II	Superficial osteomyelitis (periosteal and cortical involvement)	Often, overlying soft tissue is deficient
Type III	Localized infection	Both medullary and superficial bone involvement; full-thickness sequestrum
Type IV	Diffuse infection	Instability present from injury, infection, or débridement
Physiologic Class (Host Characteristics)		
A host	Normal host with good immune system	
B host	Local or systemic compromise	**Local:** Scarring, radiation, sensory compromise, lymphedema, peripheral vascular disease **Systemic:** Diabetes mellitus, liver or renal disease, malnutrition, malignancy, smoking, autoimmune disease, bariatric surgery with vitamin and mineral deficiency
C host	Markedly compromised host	Treatment of the disease is worse than the disease itself

often present with a history of trauma that may be falsely assumed to be the source of the patient's pain.

Laboratory studies are frequently normal, but evaluation should include a WBC count, ESR, CRP, and blood culture. ESR and CRP are also useful in monitoring the response to treatment. CRP normalizes more rapidly than does ESR. Both levels increase in the first 48 hours after surgery.

Radiographic findings are present in less than 5% of cases of acute osteomyelitis. Soft tissue swelling is one of the first radiographic findings. Metaphyseal rarefaction, osteopenia, osteosclerosis, and periosteal reaction are not noted until 2 to 3 weeks after the onset of infection[38,52] (Figure 2.20). Subacute or chronic osteomyelitis in the hand may be caused by a fragment of dead bone (sequestrum). Persistent drainage in the hand is uncommon and should alert the physician to the possibility of residual necrotic bone. One should always look on the radiograph for a fragment (often tiny) of bone with increased density. (See the following for information on the role of MRI in evaluating for sequestrum.)

Advanced imaging studies such as technetium-, gallium-, and indium-labeled WBC scans can be useful in identifying acute osteomyelitis. These studies are useful in the early stages of infection, when standard radiographs are normal.[52] Ultrasound can be helpful in identifying subperiosteal abscess and directing aspiration. MRI can be a very useful study in the early presentation of osteomyelitis, owing to the contrast it generally provides between the abnormal and normal bone marrow. It can also help identify areas of abscess and necrotic bone (sequestrum). MRI characteristics of osteomyelitis include high signal intensity on T_2-weighted and inversion recovery sequences, as well as regional enhancement in the bone and surrounding soft

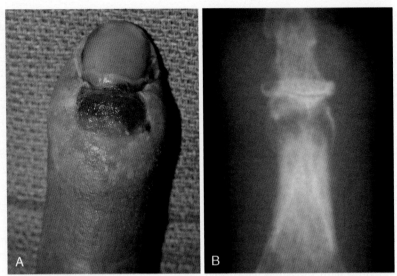

FIGURE 2.20 Osteomyelitis of the middle finger as a complication of pyarthrosis of the DIP joint. **A**, Granulation tissue overlying the DIP joint. **B**, Radiograph shows characteristic metaphyseal rarefaction and osteopenia. (Copyright courtesy of Milan Stevanovic and Frances Sharpe.)

tissues. The sensitivity of MRI in the diagnosis of osteomyelitis has been reported between 82% and 100%.[17]

Aspiration may be useful diagnostically. Subperiosteal pus may be present, typically in the pediatric patient. If pus is not obtained adjacent to bone, metaphyseal aspiration can identify the offending pathogen and direct antibiotic therapy. A negative aspirate should not stop further investigation or suspicion of bone infection.

Treatment

Early diagnosis and treatment lead to an improved functional outcome. Both surgical and medical treatments are necessary in the adult patient. Pediatric patients with osteomyelitis without subperiosteal abscess formation can be treated with antibiotic therapy alone. Adequate surgical débridement is critical to eradication of infection. Débridement of necrotic soft tissue and decompression and curettage of necrotic bone are mandatory. Repeat débridement and culture are necessary when clinical improvement is not seen in the first 72 hours. Wounds are left open and treated with frequent dressing changes or managed with negative-pressure dressings (e.g., VAC™), even though this may leave exposed bone, tendon, or implant. Repeat débridements and use of antibiotic-impregnated beads may help eradicate infection. It is better to plan bone and soft tissue reconstruction once the infection is well controlled than to inadequately débride the wound or attempt a primary closure. Treatment of osteomyelitis of the distal phalanx or of a single finger, particularly osteomyelitis associated with septic arthritis, may be best managed with amputation.[8,18,126]

Osteomyelitis can occur in the setting of an acute fracture. This may be a pin track infection or a deep infection around hardware. Pin track infections can often be managed with oral antibiotics and local wound and pin care. However, if the infection cannot be controlled, removal of the pins may be necessary. Management of deep infections around implanted hardware depends on the stage of fracture healing, host factors, and the stability of fixation. In a healthy patient with stable fixation, it is usually preferable to control the infection with débridement and intravenous or oral antibiotics until the fracture is sufficiently healed to allow hardware removal. If this cannot be achieved, hardware removal and removal of all necrotic bone and tissue are necessary. Provisional stabilization with an external fixator or with an antibiotic-impregnated methylmethacrylate spacer is used until the infection is controlled. Late reconstruction is planned based on the structural and functional deficits.

Prolonged intravenous antibiotic therapy is continued for 4 to 6 weeks and is based on the organism identified at surgical débridement and antibiotic sensitivity. Oral antibiotics that achieve therapeutic levels in bone can be used in conjunction with intravenous therapy. Resistant organisms are seen with increasing frequency. An infectious disease specialist is an invaluable resource in managing this problem.

Complications

Complications of acute osteomyelitis are common. Pain, stiffness, deformity, and loss of strength frequently persist despite successful treatment and eradication of infection. Chronic pain and cold intolerance have also been described, particularly in patients with vascular insufficiency.[8] Bone loss with shortening of the finger may occur. Fracture nonunion or malunion is not infrequent. Infection that requires amputation may result in a functional deficit. However, it is often less debilitating than preservation of a stiff and painful finger. Unresolved acute infection leads to chronic osteomyelitis and the complications associated with this process. Pediatric patients have risks of growth arrest and resultant deformity or shortening of the affected site.

SPECIFIC TYPES OF INFECTIONS AND VECTORS

Animal Bites

Domestic animal bites by dogs and cats are common. An estimated 4.5 million dog bites occur in the United States annually.

Of these, 885,000 (19%) require medical attention.[48] Dog bites represent up to 90% of all animal bites. In more than 70% of cases, the dog is known to the victim.[45,53] Children younger than age 12 years account for 50% of all dog bite injuries. Cat bites less frequently result in emergency room visits, but they are nonetheless estimated to account for 5% to 15% of emergency room animal bite injuries. The remaining 5% include various domestic and wild animal bites.[1,45,53,145]

The bacteria identified from bite wounds reflect the oral flora of the biting animal. The oral flora of the animal is also influenced by the microbiome of its ingested prey or other foods. A minority of pathogenic bacteria are from the victim's skin flora. Of the multiple organisms cultured from the dog mouth, the more common pathogens include *S. aureus, Streptococcus viridans, Bacteroides,* and *P. multocida.* Similar flora is found in the cat mouth.[1,45,48,145,151] Wound cultures often show a polymicrobial infection. Talan and associates cultured an average of five organisms per wound.[151] *P. multocida* is a frequent pathogen causing infection after dog and cat bites. It is more prevalent in cat bite infections. Cellulitis and serous or seropurulent drainage presenting in the first 12 to 24 hours after the bite injury is often caused by *P. multocida.*[1,5,48,145,167] Ulceroglandular tularemia has been reported after cat bites. The cat is thought to become a carrier of *Francisella tularensis* organisms in the mouth or claws through hunting and eating wild rodents or rabbits. The diagnosis of tularemia should be considered when patients with a history of cat bite present with pneumonia and have a soft tissue infection not responding to penicillin therapy. Cat scratch fever caused by infection with *Bartonella henselae* should also be kept in mind after feline contact. The infection typically begins with a papular skin lesion, usually 4 to 6 days after the inoculation, causing a self-limiting infection characterized by regional lymphadenopathy and fever. Symptoms usually last between 4 and 6 weeks.[1,145] *Capnocytophaga canimorsus* is a rare pathogen in dog bites. It is of particular interest because of the high fatality rate of 23% to 28% associated with this infection. A history of splenectomy, alcoholism, and chronic pulmonary disease is a significant risk factor for *C. canimorsus* infections.[1,45,107]

Although dog bites occur far more commonly than cat bites, they much less commonly become infected. In one report, cat bites were responsible for 76% of infected animal bites. Dog bites accounted for the remaining 24%.[1,45] Cat bites are produced by needle-sharp teeth, which produce a puncture wound. This allows bacteria to be injected deeply into the soft tissues. This soft tissue bed is a fertile medium for anaerobic and facultative anaerobic infections. The dog has blunt teeth and powerful masseter muscles that cause tearing of soft tissues, leaving large open wounds that are less susceptible to infection.

In general, patients present to the emergency room with a dog bite either because of a large wound or concern about the immunization status of an unknown dog. Patients presenting with cat bites are usually not there because of the wound size. They are having pain disproportionate to the wound size and should be treated as having an evolving infection. At the very least, the cat puncture wounds should be opened up and irrigated in the emergency room under local anesthesia, and oral antibiotic therapy should be initiated. Wider involvement or systemic symptoms may require formal surgical débridement and inpatient antibiotic therapy. Factors associated with hospital admissions for cat bites include location of the bite over a joint or tendon, presence of erythema or lymphangitis, wound drainage, and immunocompromised state.[6] All animal bite wounds should be thoroughly irrigated. Necrotic tissue must be débrided. All animal bite wounds should be left open. However, large gaping wounds can be loosely closed after several débridements. Primary reconstruction of soft tissue defects can be considered if the tissue bed appears healthy with no evidence of necrotic tissue or sepsis after the first 48 to 72 hours.

The initial medical treatment includes an update of tetanus immunization if necessary. The rabies immunization status of the animal should be ascertained. Prompt and thorough wound irrigation with soap or povidone-iodine solution reduces the development of rabies by up to 90%.[39,45] Infected wounds should be cultured before irrigation and débridement. Aerobic and anaerobic cultures should be sent. Failure to culture for anaerobic organisms will result in a significant number of missed pathogens and subsequent inadequate antibiotic coverage. Antibiotic treatment depends on the severity of clinical signs and symptoms. Routine prophylactic treatment for an animal bite depends on the timing of presentation and the clinical signs and symptoms.

Other domestic and wild animal bites occur much less frequently. The organisms causing infection are similar to those involved in cat and dog bites.[1,104,132] However, certain infections have been associated with particular animals, such as tularemia seen in rabbit handlers, and *Streptobacillus moniliformis* is associated with rat bites as well as contact with rat feces. *S. moniliformis* is the causative agent of rat-bite fever, which can occur through animal contact, not necessarily requiring an animal bite. Rat-bite fever presents with an eruptive fever with blisters, polyarthritis, and spectacular desquamation of the hands.[59] The increase of exotic domestic pets introduces other species-associated infections that should be considered in determining the treatment of infections.[1,104,132]

Empirical antibiotic treatment should include coverage for gram-positive, gram-negative, and anaerobic organisms. The principles of surgical treatment remain the same. The wound should be opened to expose the depth of the bite. Necrotic or crushed tissue should be sharply débrided, and the wound should be thoroughly irrigated by gravity irrigation. The wounds should be left open and managed with dressing changes. Delayed primary wound closure may be considered when swelling and erythema have subsided and healthy wound base and tissue margins are present. Wound cultures taken 12 to 24 hours after débridement may be a useful diagnostic tool in determining whether a wound should be closed.[138]

Other animal bites and stings, caused by reptiles, arthropods, and marine animals, are associated with inflammation and tissue necrosis. The soft tissue injury results from the injection of toxin-containing venom or from chemical inflammation, such as that seen with sea urchin spines. The swelling associated with these bite injuries can result in compartment syndrome. Secondary infection can occur and requires medical and surgical treatment (see Chapter 52).

Marine Organisms

Multiple pathogens have been associated with an aquatic environment. Contact may occur through occupation or hobby, including home aquariums. *Mycobacterium marinum,* although commonly associated with aquatic infections, generally presents as a chronic infection. Organisms producing acute infections include species of *Staphylococcus, Streptococcus, Pseudomonas, Aeromonas,* and *Enterobacter.* Infection often occurs through contamination of a break in the skin or through an inadvertent penetrating injury by the bones or the spines of the fish. Relatively minor wounds can be complicated by injection of venom, produced by glands on the dorsal and pectoral spines in some species, notably the catfish. When envenomation occurs, patients experience immediate severe throbbing pain, which may spread through the entire extremity. Muscle spasms and fasciculations may be noted. Over the first few hours, the site of injury may have local pallor that progresses to erythema and swelling. Occasionally, local skin necrosis and skin slough may occur. Swelling of the entire extremity may develop. Secondary infection can lead to death.[95,108]

The most serious aquatic infections associated with fresh or brackish water are the *Aeromonas* species infections. Despite aggressive surgical management, necrotizing infections associated with *Aeromonas* species have a mortality rate of up to 27%.[95,108,155] Another organism associated with brackish water is *Edwardsiella tarda.* Immunocompromised hosts, especially with underlying liver disease, are more susceptible to developing a necrotizing infection that can result in amputation or death.[31]

Serious infections associated with saltwater exposure or raw seafood ingestion are those caused by *Vibrio* species other than *Vibrio cholerae,* particularly *Vibrio vulnificus* and *Vibrio damsela.* Infections due to *Vibrio* species cause an estimated 8000 illnesses annually in the United States. The majority of these occur in the Gulf Coast states. Not all infections result in severe illness. Analysis of 4754 *Vibrio* infections identified 85% of infections with symptoms of cellulitis. Ten percent of infections resulted in amputation, and 17% resulted in death. *Vibrio* is a gram-negative, facultative anaerobic rod. *Vibrio* infections other than *V. cholerae* infections are classified into two types: primary septicemia type and localized wound type. Primary septicemia is usually acquired through the gastrointestinal tract by the ingestion of raw seafood. This typically occurs in patients with underlying liver disease or other immunocompromising disorders. The association with liver disease is thought to result from bypassing the hepatic reticuloendothelial system, as portal blood is shunted around the diseased liver. Also, high levels of serum iron associated with hepatic cirrhosis may increase the susceptibility to *V. vulnificus,* which requires iron for growth.[110] Most cases occur in males over the age of 50 years. The gender specificity has been found to be due to the protective effect of estrogen against the *V. vulnificus* endotoxin.[115] Primary septicemia can cause disseminated infection, manifesting in the extremities as a picture of necrotizing fasciitis. Patients often present with rapidly developing extremity pain, followed by skin lesions with bullae, purpura, and necrosis. The most common site of presentation is the lower extremities. It may also be seen in the upper extremities. The findings are similar to those of necrotizing fasciitis, but unlike necrotizing fasciitis, they are more commonly associated with an elevated serum creatine phosphokinase (CPK) level. In a report of eight patients with *Vibrio* septicemia, an elevated CPK level was found in seven. All patients with an elevated CPK level died. Even with aggressive medical and surgical management, these infections are associated with a very high mortality rate (67% to 88%).[110] The less common type of *Vibrio* infection, described as non-foodborne *Vibrio* infection, is increasingly recognized; it is identified in up to 25% of reported *Vibrio* infections.[33] This is typically a localized wound infection and occurs equally in immunocompetent and immunocompromised patients. The infection is a localized infection, and most are associated with a puncture wound from a fish spine or bone. *Vibrio* species as causative agents should be considered with a history of a wound infection after exposure to seawater, more specifically warm seawater. There are no distinguishing features for local infections. Diagnosis is made after culture identification of *Vibrio* species. Generally, these are self-limiting infections. Local débridement of necrotic tissue is usually adequate treatment in conjunction with antibiotic therapy. However, development of necrotizing fasciitis has been reported. Aggressive surgical débridement, including amputation, and prolonged intravenous antibiotic therapy are necessary to treat these often fatal infections.[33,115]

Leeches

Iatrogenic animal bite infections have more recently been described with the reintroduction of medicinal leeches, *Hirudo medicinalis,* which are used for salvage of tissue with venous congestion. The pseudomonad *Aeromonas hydrophila* is the organism most commonly associated with the medicinal leech and has been cultured from presumed postoperative flap infections in 18% of cases in which leeches were used.[10] It has been frequently cultured from the intestinal flora of the leech. It can result in cellulitis, myonecrosis, abscess formation, endocarditis, and sepsis. Lineaweaver and associates found that leeches that fed on antibiotic-containing blood had lower or absent intestinal cultures for *A. hydrophila.* Based on those findings, they recommended the use of broad-spectrum prophylactic antibiotics, which include coverage for *Aeromonas* species, before leech application. The increased incidence of ciprofloxacin-resistant organisms should be considered in selecting appropriate antibiotic prophylaxis.[89,91,158,168]

Human Bites

Human saliva contains nearly one billion bacteria per milliliter. It can also contain transmissible viruses, including human immunodeficiency virus (HIV) and hepatitis B and C viruses.[65] The overall incidence of human bite injuries to the hand is unknown, but such injuries are probably third in incidence below dog and cat bites. These injuries are often misdiagnosed or unreported. Frequently, it is the patient who misreports the mechanism of injury to the hand. Patzakis and colleagues reported on admissions to the orthopedic infection ward over a 5-year period: Of 2288 admissions, 10% were due to human bites, specifically clenched fist injuries.[121]

Four mechanisms of human bite injuries to the hand have been described.[36,121] The least frequent is inadvertent self-inflicted injury occurring from nail biting or secondary to sucking an open bleeding wound on the finger or thumb. The second mechanism is a traumatic amputation secondary to a bite injury. This usually occurs through the distal phalanx or the DIP joint. Full-thickness bite wounds into various parts of the hand represent the third mechanism of injury and inoculation. Although this is one of the more frequent modes of injury, it less commonly results in infection. When infection occurs, it is usually localized around the area of the penetration.[88,121] However, it has been reported to result in a rapidly spreading process continuing up to the forearm and arm, fitting a diagnosis of necrotizing fasciitis. Deaths associated with this condition were reported in the preantibiotic era.[121] The fourth mechanism of injury is a bite injury occurring when the hand strikes another person's mouth with a closed fist, more commonly known as a clenched fist injury or fight bite. The most commonly involved areas are adjacent to the third and fourth metacarpal heads of the dominant hand.[121] This type of bite injury is associated with the highest incidence of complications.

Clenched fist injuries occur as the patient strikes the mouth of another person. The area around the MP joint may be impaled by a tooth, penetrating the skin and deeper structures. At the time of contact, the skin and extensor tendons are stretched tightly over the metacarpal head and a large surface area of the metacarpal head is exposed. Deep structures, including tendons, the joint capsule, and bone, may be penetrated as well. The depth of penetration affects the location of spread of the infection. The dorsal subcutaneous space, the subtendinous space, the joint space, bone, or all of these structures may be involved. The site of the skin injury can be misleading in evaluating for injury to deeper structures. The position of the fingers at the time of impact affects the location of injury to the deeper structures. The more flexed position of the fingers at the time of penetration results in a more proximal injury to the tendon and joint capsule and a more distal injury to the metacarpal head (Figure 2.21).

Patients often present with an innocuous-appearing wound on the dorsum of the hand around the MP joint. This presentation should be considered a human bite until proven otherwise. The patient may be reluctant to provide an accurate history regarding the method of injury and often presents to the emergency department either because of a functional loss, as might be caused by fracture or extensor tendon dysfunction, or because of infection. Pain, localized swelling, and erythema may be present. Drainage from the wound is frequently seen; however, fever, lymphadenopathy, and lymphangitis are rare.

A complete blood cell count, ESR, and CRP are obtained. Often, these results are normal. Radiographs are used to evaluate for fracture, cortical violation, or the presence of a retained foreign body, such as a tooth. These radiographs also provide a baseline for comparison with subsequent films used to evaluate for osteomyelitis. In cases of late presentation, osteomyelitis may already be evident. The patient's tetanus status should be determined and updated as needed. Inquiry as to the viral status of the source should be made. Further guidance by an infectious disease specialist should be sought for those patients at risk.

The underlying injury to the hand is frequently more serious and extensive than the superficial wound and clinical presentation indicate. Patzakis and colleagues described the surgical findings in a group of 191 patients with clenched fist injuries. Seventy-five percent had injury to the deep tissue layers, including tendon, capsule, and bone. Sixty-seven percent had a violation of the joint capsule. Twenty-two percent had cartilage or bone involvement. These findings emphasize the importance of surgical exploration and débridement in the treatment of these injuries.[121] Wide exposure around the traumatic wound is

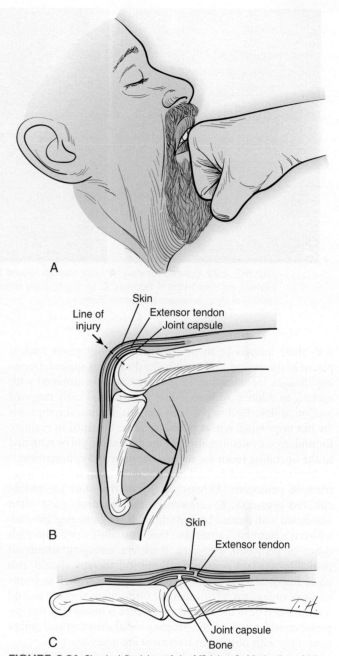

FIGURE 2.21 Clenched fist injury of the MP joint. **A,** Mechanism of injury. **B,** Linear wound track with MP joint flexed. **C,** Position of injured structures in full extension. (Copyright courtesy of Milan Stevanovic and Frances Sharpe.)

required (Figure 2.22). The tendon, joint capsule, and bone are explored with the hand in a position of flexion. Small penetrations in the joint capsule may be inconspicuous or may have become sealed off. Therefore, even when the joint capsule appears intact, we prefer to open the capsule and inspect the articular surfaces. Cultures should be taken before irrigation. Necrotic tissue must be meticulously removed. Curettage of the affected portion of bone is performed. Softened areas of bone are débrided. Loose fragments of articular cartilage are removed. The wound is left open. No attempt should be made to repair injuries to the extensor tendon or extensor mechanism. Despite the release of the sagittal band to gain access to the joint, we have not seen cases of extensor tendon subluxation associated

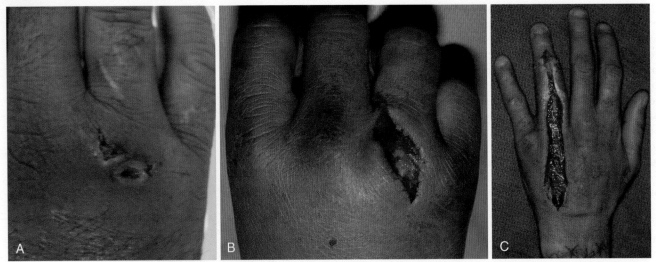

FIGURE 2.22 Clenched fist injury. **A**, Initial traumatic wound. **B**, Typical surgical extension of traumatic wound to allow adequate exposure and débridement of the injury. **C**, More extensively infected clenched fist injury requiring longer surgical exposure. (Copyright courtesy of Milan Stevanovic and Frances Sharpe.)

with these injuries or their treatment. A moist gauze wick is placed in the wound, and a soft bulky dressing is applied. Dressing changes are started at 12 to 24 hours and combined with soaking in dilute povidone-iodine solution and early range of motion as described in previous sections. If clinical symptoms are not improving, repeat radiographs are obtained to evaluate for underlying osteomyelitis, and the patient should be returned to the operating room for repeat irrigation and débridement.

Intravenous antibiotic therapy should cover a broad spectrum of pathogens. Although it is not the most commonly cultured organism, *E. corrodens* is the organism most often associated with human bite infections. It is a gram-negative rod, which is a facultative anaerobe. This is usually treated with high doses of penicillin. However, there are emerging strains of penicillin-resistant organisms. Empirical therapy should also cover *Staphylococcus* and *Streptococcus* species, as well as gram-negative organisms.[1,54,121] Inpatient intravenous therapy should be continued until the clinical appearance is improving. Appropriate consideration of the patient's social situation and ability to comply with outpatient treatment are necessary.

Complications of infected bite wounds include septic flexor tenosynovitis, septic arthritis, osteomyelitis, stiffness, and pain. Toxic shock syndrome and deaths have been reported.[36,165] Amputations or resection arthroplasty may be necessary to eradicate infection and improve function. Complications may be minimized by recognizing the human bite wound as a serious injury and treating even small seemingly innocuous wounds with early and thorough débridement and appropriate antibiotic therapy.[103,165] Educating those physicians involved in the primary care of wounds to suspect human bite infections in the appropriate clinical setting can reduce the delay to treatment and subsequent complications associated with these injuries.[96,97,165]

Prosthetic and Implant Infections

Deep infections around surgical hardware and implants are uncommon but can be difficult to treat. The eradication of infection requires removal of the implant and removal of all nonviable tissue. The presence of subclinical infection may be responsible for what has previously been labeled aseptic nonunion or aseptic loosening of the prosthesis. This presentation is due to the presence of bacterial biofilms.

Prosthetic joint replacements in the hand and wrist are more commonly performed in patients with rheumatoid arthritis. Although this patient population is generally immunocompromised, the infection rate around prosthetic implants is low, ranging from 0.5% to 4%.[37,47,73,105,112,159] When infection occurs, removal of the implant is necessary to control infection. Thorough débridement is done with removal of adjacent areas of necrotic bone. Treatment options include staged reimplantation, resection arthroplasty, or fusion, although arthrodesis after infected total elbow arthroplasty has a high failure rate.[117] In the setting of severe infection or a large dead space, temporary placement of an antibiotic-impregnated methylmethacrylate spacer can be used until the infection is controlled. The choice of intravenous antibiotic is based on the offending organism. The duration of therapy should be the same as that for treatment of osteomyelitis. Rarely is there an indication for prosthetic reimplantation. If reimplantation is considered, the patient should have a normal WBC count, ESR, and CRP. At the time of surgery, a gram-stained smear should be negative for bacteria; a frozen section with less than five polymorphonuclear cells per high-power field suggests adequate eradication of infection. Infection around Silastic® tendon rods can occur. Separate series have reported infection rates of 2% to 4%. Treatment included removal of the silicone rod, irrigation, débridement, and later reconstruction after all signs of infection were resolved and the skin and soft tissues were supple.[67,166]

Bacterial biofilms have been recognized since the 1970s. These bacterial colonies adhere to inert surfaces such as metal, plastic, nonviable bone, or living tissue. They secrete an exopolysaccharide matrix that isolates the bacterial colonies from the surrounding tissues and protects the bacteria from the host defense mechanism. Bacterial growth within the biofilm is characterized by slow growth, difficulty in culturing an organism, and triggering of an inflammatory response. They can be caused by a single or mixed species of bacteria or by fungi. The microbiologic literature refers to the sessile state of bacteria within a biofilm, which is slow growing and systemically inert. Release of bacteria from the biofilm can result in a "planktonic state," in which the bacteria can rapidly propagate and cause a systemic host response.[30] Sessile bacterial cells release antigens and stimulate the production of antibodies; however, the antibodies are not effective in killing bacteria within the biofilm. The immunologic host response contributes to the localized tissue destruction around the biofilm and can suppress the planktonic state but cannot eradicate the sessile biofilm-protected bacteria. Antibiotics are effective against the planktonic state, but bacterial or fungal cells within a biofilm are resistant to antibiotic concentrations 1000 times higher than that required to kill planktonic bacteria. Detection of bacteria within a biofilm is difficult, and bacteria are not typically identified by growth in agar media. Disturbing findings were reported in 10 cases of aseptic acetabular cup loosening. Despite negative cultures, bacteria were identified within the biofilms under electron microscopy in 8 of 10 patients.[30] This suggests that aseptic loosening may be a misnomer and should be treated as an infection, with complete removal of the implant and staged reconstruction. Newer detection methods include ELISA (enzyme-linked immunosorbent assay), PCR (polymerase chain reaction), and FISH (fluorescent in situ hybridization). More recently, diagnostic tests for biomarkers specific to infection (alpha defensin) show great promise in identifying prosthetic joint infection, with one study showing 100% specificity and sensitivity in its diagnosis.[34]

Treatment of the infection involves complete removal of the biofilm (thus, implant removal and removal of all nonviable tissue). Staged procedures with use of antibiotic-impregnated spacers in conjunction with systemic antibiotic therapy can be effective therapy against chronic infection. Newer technology with improved detection and more sophisticated antibiotic delivery systems will be part of the future treatment of these infections.[30,34]

Shooter's Abscesses: Infections Caused by Parenteral Drug Abuse

One of the most commonly encountered complications of intravenous drug abuse is infections of the skin and soft tissues. The hand and forearm provide easily accessible sites of venous access. Overall, abscesses of the upper extremity account for 40% to 80% of admissions for soft tissue infections.[57,66,137] Multiple sites of abscesses may be present. Many of these patients have underlying medical illnesses, poor medical care, and poor medical compliance. Bergstein and colleagues reported an incidence of hepatitis B seropositivity of 29%. The incidence of hepatitis C may be even higher. The incidence of HIV in patients consenting to serologic testing ranged between 9% and 50%.[13,57,109] Recent studies have correlated the incidence of abscess formation with subcutaneous or intramuscular injection rather than intravenous injection. This may occur inadvertently when the vein is missed and the injected substance extravasates into the extravascular space. It may also occur volitionally. The repeated abuse of intravenous drugs leaves hardened sclerotic veins, which are no longer accessible for injection. Subcutaneous injections (skin popping) or intramuscular injections are used when venous access is difficult. The use of cocaine or of a cocaine-heroin mixture (speedball) predisposes patients to abscess formation by inducing soft tissue ischemia.[109]

The organisms cultured from these abscesses are usually a mixed flora. Staphylococcal and streptococcal species predominate, with an increasing incidence of oxacillin-resistant S. aureus (ORSA) noted. In one study, ORSA made up 82% of S. aureus infections in 2005, compared with 5% in 1999.[3] Oral and enteric flora are also frequently present.[3,13,57,137,150] Summanen and coworkers isolated oral flora from 67% of abscesses caused by parenteral drug use. This was compared with 25% in abscesses not associated with drug use. This is likely due to the use of sputum to clean either the injection site or the needle.[150] Schnall and colleagues found that gram-negative isolates were more common in patients older than 40 years of age.[137]

The majority of these patients present to the emergency department with complaints of pain and swelling. Most patients do not have an elevated temperature and often do not have an elevated WBC count.[143] Examination may demonstrate fluctuance. Deep abscesses may be more difficult to identify. If abscess is suspected, aspiration with an 18-gauge needle in the area of suspicion may identify the presence of pus. Cultures should be sent from specimens obtained in the emergency department. Radiographs may demonstrate gas in the soft tissues or an underlying osteomyelitis.

Provisional drainage of any area of fluctuance should be performed in the emergency department. Once cultures are obtained, broad-spectrum antibiotics are given. Tetanus status is determined and updated as necessary. Hepatitis and HIV status should be investigated. The patient should be admitted to the hospital. Expedient treatment with formal irrigation and débridement in the operating room can minimize the complications associated with these infections. A longitudinal extensile surgical incision is necessary to adequately drain the abscess cavity. Removal of all necrotic tissue and copious irrigation are performed. The wounds are left open and packed with gauze soaked with dilute povidone-iodine. Wounds may heal by secondary intention. Delayed primary wound closure can also be done and has been shown to reduce the hospital stay.[138] Large wounds with associated skin loss or soft tissue fibrosis that precludes delayed primary wound closure can be skin-grafted when a healthy granulation tissue bed is present.

Large open wounds can also be managed with a vacuum-assisted wound closure (VAC) device. This technique can reduce the size of the wound, so that a smaller skin graft is required, or shorten the time needed for secondary wound healing.

Complications associated with soft tissue abscesses include spread of infection to adjacent potential spaces, such as the flexor tendon sheath or adjacent joint space. Osteomyelitis can occur with long-standing infection. Bacteria and septicemia can spread infection to distant sites. Cardiac examination for murmur suggesting endocarditis should be performed on all patients. The most serious complication of soft tissue abscess is that of necrotizing fasciitis. Although this occurs rarely, it is a life-threatening infection that requires emergent surgical and medical treatment.

Many of these patients require prolonged hospitalization, more often due to social concerns and medical compliance than because of medical necessity. Premature discharge to a situation in which the patient will not have a clean environment or be able to comply with antibiotic therapy and wound management may lead to more complications, greater morbidity, and higher social and financial costs. Releasing a patient with a history of intravenous drug abuse with an indwelling catheter for home antibiotic therapy is ill advised.

The risk of pathogen exposure to the surgeon and health care team is considerable. Although universal precautions should be exercised with every patient, greater vigilance and attention are necessary to protect the health care providers in managing this patient population.

Septic Thrombophlebitis

Suppurative septic thrombophlebitis of the upper extremity is a rare but potentially life-threatening infection of the superficial and/or deep venous system. Bacteria and purulent material are in direct communication with the vascular system, and septic emboli to distant sites (most commonly the lungs) are a common complication. Causes of peripheral septic phlebitis include venipuncture, central or peripheral venous catheters, intravenous drug abuse, and localized soft tissue lacerations or infections that are in continuity with the venous system. Treatment of these infections is typically performed by vascular surgeons. However, since the initial presentation may be similar to cellulitis or localized abscess, the hand surgeon may be the first consultant called to treat the patient. Surgical findings are characterized by purulence within the venous system. Treatment includes excision of the affected veins. Vascular surgery consultation is recommended, particularly with more proximally tracking infections. Supportive care by an intensive care team and infectious disease consultation and management help to reduce the morbidity and mortality rates of these infections.

Herpetic Whitlow (Herpes Simplex Virus Infection of the Fingers)

Herpetic viral infections of the fingers are commonly misdiagnosed as bacterial infections, such as paronychia or felon. The inappropriate treatment of these conditions as bacterial processes can result in severe complications. It is therefore important to be aware of the diagnosis and clinical presentation to avoid adverse sequelae.

The term *herpetic whitlow* is derived from the viral origin of the process and the middle English term *whitlow*. *Herpes* has a Greek origin, meaning "to creep," as this fits the general pattern of disease progression. Herpes simplex virus (HSV) types 1 and 2 are part of the alpha *Herpesviridae*. Humans are the only natural host. The term *whitlow* is believed to be a misnomer, because whitlow was generally used to describe a suppurative infection of the finger pulp, such as a felon. Other terms used to describe herpetic infection of the fingers include herpetic febrilis of the finger, herpetic paronychia, and aseptic felon. The first reported case of herpetic infection of the finger in the English literature was reported by Adamson in 1909. Since Stern's publication in 1959, this infection has been commonly named herpetic whitlow.[69]

Herpetic infections are seen in both adults and children (Figure 2.23). In a child with herpetic gingivostomatitis, the thumb or finger can become inoculated by sucking. In adults, this infection has been reported as an occupational hazard, affecting those in the medical or dental profession who come into direct contact with saliva from patients who are actively shedding HSV. This is most often infection from HSV type 1.

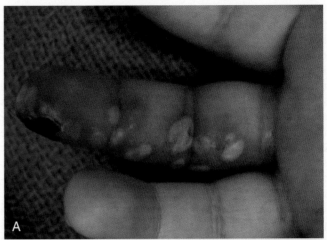

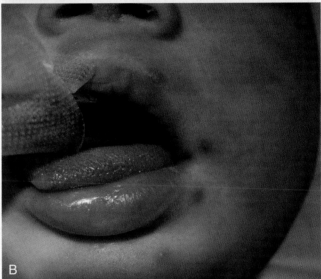

FIGURE 2.23 Herpetic whitlow in an 18-month-old child. **A,** Isolated long finger involvement. **B,** Oral lesions. (Copyright courtesy of Milan Stevanovic and Frances Sharpe.)

HSV type 1 antibodies have been detected in the saliva of up to 24% of school-aged children.[146] More recent studies emphasize the importance of autoinoculation or inoculation from a sexual partner infected with HSV type 2. HSV type 1 more commonly affects young children and the medical and dental professional in contact with saliva. HSV type 2 infections have been more common in adults.[7,49] Age and profession cannot be exclusively used to differentiate between HSV type 1 and HSV type 2 infections, and there is no difference in their clinical presentations.

Clinical Presentation and Diagnosis

The early symptoms of HSV infection of the hand mimic the presentation of herpetic lesions occurring in other locations. The incubation period of the virus ranges between 2 and 14 days, and a thorough history may provide clues to the diagnosis, possible vector, and viral type. Infection usually involves a single finger. Involvement of more than one finger may suggest another infection, such as coxsackievirus infection.

The index finger and thumb are the most frequently infected digits. However, the infection may occur on any finger or any location on the hand or integument. In the beginning of the infection, the patient has intense throbbing and pain in the affected digit. Carter reported that one of the early symptoms may be tingling in the affected digit. In the early disease process, the patient's pain is disproportionately severe to the clinical findings.[23,171] Erythema and mild swelling are present; this is followed by the development of 1- to 2-mm clear vesicles. Over several days, these vesicles creep together and coalesce. The vesicle roof usually remains intact. As the vesicles coalesce, a large confluent bulla may form. The fluid within the vesicles is initially clear. It may rapidly become turbid and appear purulent, mimicking a bacterial hand infection. Lymphangitis and adenopathy may be present but are more commonly seen with bacterial suprainfection.

Over the next 7 to 10 days, these signs and symptoms subside. Even though the symptoms are resolving, there is continued viral shedding over the next 12 to 14 days. It is during this time that the patient is most infective. The clinical course is generally self-limited and resolves over a 3-week period.

Early diagnosis depends on clinical suspicion. Distinguishing a viral infection from a bacterial infection is critical to the treatment. Suspicion of a viral infection depends on the patient history, quality and intensity of the pain, softness of the digital pulp, presence of vesicles, and a blood profile that does not fit a pattern of sepsis. Viral cultures definitively establish the diagnosis. However, the culture may take several days to become positive. The virus is sensitive to transport and cultures may be negative, even when transported in viral medium. Lesions that have crusted often do not produce positive cultures.

The Tzanck smear is performed on fresh vesicles. This microscopic examination will show multinucleated keratinocytes with steel-blue homogeneous karyoplasm. The base of the lesion is scraped vigorously with the edge of a scalpel blade. The material is touched to a glass slide and allowed to air dry. The Tzanck smear in all stages of the disease is less sensitive than viral culture. Immunofluorescent serum antibody titers, using type-specific monoclonal anti-HSV antibodies, can confirm the diagnosis and type. HSV blood testing for antibodies to the HSV type-specific G1 and G2 glycoproteins is now available and may provide a rapid diagnosis of HSV infection.[161]

Treatment of herpetic whitlow is essentially nonsurgical. The course of the disease is self-limiting. The main goal of treatment is to prevent autoinoculation or transmission of the infection. The digit should be kept covered with a dry dressing, and all contact with the lesion should be avoided. Unroofing of the vesicles may improve patient comfort. Intravenous, oral, or topical antiviral medication may be useful in shortening the natural course of the infection.[144] Partial nail excision may be indicated for a subungual herpetic lesion causing pressure below the nail plate. Surgical débridement of bacterial suprainfection must be done cautiously. Misdiagnosis of the viral infection as a paronychia or felon, which leads to surgical intervention, may result in disastrous complications. Viral encephalitis and death have been reported as a result of misdiagnosis and treatment of a herpetic infection as a felon.[7,23,77]

Once the disease resolves, the virus becomes latent in the nervous system. The responsible cell in the ganglia or the mechanism of latency is not completely understood. Twenty percent of patients will experience recurrence. The recurrent infection is usually less severe, except in immunocompromised patients, in whom the recurrence rate and infection severity are much higher.[144,146,161]

Upper Extremity Infections Associated With HIV Infection

Upper extremity infections in patients with HIV are more common in those patients with a concomitant history of intravenous drug abuse. The clinical presentation of infection is similar to patients without HIV; however, the clinical course of the infection is often more severe. Gonzalez and coworkers reported on 28 patients with HIV infection. Eight of those patients had acquired immunodeficiency syndrome (AIDS), as defined by the Centers for Disease Control and Prevention guidelines. The most common presentation was that of soft tissue abscess. Patients with AIDS were more likely to present with a spontaneous infection,[58,98] and spontaneous septic arthritis should raise suspicion of underlying immunocompromise.[51,98] The organisms most frequently isolated were streptococcal and staphylococcal species. McAuliffe and Seltzer found *S. aureus* to be the most common pathogen in 74 patients infected with HIV.[98] Pyogenic infections responded well to aggressive débridement and antibiotic therapy. Herpetic viral infections were more commonly seen than in the general population.[51,58,146] The viral infections did not run a self-limited course and often became suprainfected. Oral or intravenous antiviral therapy was necessary to resolve the infection. The incidence of necrotizing fasciitis was also disproportionately high in the patient group reported by Gonzalez and coworkers. Opportunistic infections of the hand have been reported, although less frequently than might be expected.[14]

Pyogenic infections respond well to early and aggressive surgical débridement and culture-directed antibiotic therapy. Viral infections have a prolonged course and do not resolve spontaneously. Intravenous antiviral therapy may be necessary to eradicate the infection. Amputation may be indicated for recalcitrant infection.

Diabetic Hand Infections

Approximately 7% of the adult population of the United States is diagnosed with diabetes mellitus.[22] It has been estimated that the prevalence of undiagnosed diabetes in the adult population older than the age of 50 years is 10%. Among the many complications associated with diabetes is a susceptibility to infection. Diabetics are known to have a higher rate of postsurgical infection, even after minor soft tissue procedures.[22,56] Infection may be the initial presenting complaint in patients previously undiagnosed with diabetes. Cohen and colleagues reported a 17% incidence of undiagnosed diabetes in patients treated for infections of the extremities.[28]

Several different mechanisms have been postulated for the increased susceptibility to infection in diabetics. Many studies have shown immune deficits, particularly lymphocyte dysfunction associated with elevated blood glucose levels. Deficits include decreased chemotaxis, decreased phagocytosis, decreased intracellular bactericidal activity, and decreased opsonic activity.[22,42,130] Overall, the leukocyte is less capable of performing its role of preventing infection and fighting sepsis. It has been further suggested that the local hyperglycemic environment may enhance bacterial proliferation, especially in staphylococcal infections.[42,130] Anatomic factors, notably peripheral neuropathies and diabetic angiopathy, contribute to poor wound healing and poor oxygen, leukocyte, and antibiotic delivery to the affected area. Wound healing activities, including capillary ingrowth, fibroblast proliferation, and collagen synthesis, have also been shown to be decreased in diabetics.[42]

Infections in diabetics have been separated into superficial and deep infections. The superficial infections include cellulitis and superficial localized abscess. These infections behave more like infections in nondiabetics and respond to broad-spectrum antibiotic therapy and local wound débridement.[123] Deep infections include involvement of bone, the tendon sheath, or deep palmar spaces. Francel and colleagues reported that 73% of patients in their series had deep infections.[42] Gonzalez and coworkers reported that more than 50% of patients with deep infections required more than one surgical procedure.[56] The amputation rate in diabetics with deep infection ranges from 8% to 63%.[56,79,123] Necrotizing fasciitis occurs with greater frequency in diabetics and has been associated with a higher mortality rate.[43] Diabetics with associated renal failure represent a subgroup of patients with even higher morbidity and mortality rates. Francel and colleagues reported a 100% amputation rate in this patient group with upper extremity infections.[42,146] The most common pathogen remains *S. aureus*. However, multiple organisms are present in most infections.[56,60,79,146] Gram-negative organisms were documented in up to 73% of positive cultures.[79]

Treatment includes broad-spectrum antibiotic therapy, careful monitoring and control of blood glucose levels, and aggressive surgical management. Surgical incisions should extend past the area of erythema and should include the length of the areas of indurated skin and soft tissue. Wounds should be left open to heal by secondary intention or can be treated with negative-pressure dressings. Delayed primary wound closure can be performed when the infection is controlled. Secondary procedures for repeat débridement are common. When amputation is necessary, an open amputation is performed if close to the site of infection. The bone is shortened proximal to the level of skin resection. The wound will heal readily by secondary intention as long as the infection is controlled or delayed wound closure can be performed. Primary amputation may be the most appropriate procedure to control the infection, reduce disability, and improve functional outcome.

Necrotizing Soft Tissue Infections and Gas Gangrene

Necrotizing fasciitis is a rapidly advancing necrotizing infection affecting the skin, subcutaneous tissue, and fascia. It characteristically spares the underlying muscle. It is associated with high morbidity and mortality rates and severe systemic sepsis. Whereas necrotizing soft tissue infections (NSTIs) were recognized in earlier literature, Meleney is credited with the first detailed description of the disease process and first recognized the importance of early and extensive surgical débridement. Wilson first applied the term *necrotizing fasciitis*, recognizing that the constant feature of the infection was fascial necrosis.[169]

Two types of necrotizing infections have been described based on the bacteriology of the infection. Type 1 infections are mixed aerobic and anaerobic infections. Facultative anaerobic bacteria and non–group A streptococci are present. This is the most common type and is found in approximately 80% of cases. Type 2 infections are caused by group A *Streptococcus* species alone or in combination with staphylococcal species.[55] Fungal infections are uncommon causes of necrotizing fasciitis. However, the incidence is increasing, principally in immunocompromised patients but also in previously healthy individuals.

The inciting event for the onset of infection may not be known. There may be a history of minor trauma or puncture wound. When seen in intravenous drug abusers, it is postulated that the contamination occurs through use of an unclean needle, use of saliva to clean the needle or injection site, or contamination of the street drug being injected. In the initial presentation, necrotizing fasciitis may resemble cellulitis. There is a swollen erythematous area of exquisite tenderness with an area of extensive cellulitis. Nonpitting edema is present and extends beyond the margins of the erythema, distinguishing this from cellulitis. Beyond the area of cellulitis, the skin may have an orange-peel appearance (peau d'orange skin). As the infection progresses, the skin changes from red and purple to a dusky blue-gray. The skin may become hypoesthetic or anesthetic. Later, patchy areas of frank necrosis of the skin develop. The skin may slough, owing to thrombosis of the nutrient vessels that traverse the fascial layer and supply the overlying skin and subcutaneous tissue. Bullae form and are either clear or hemorrhagic (Figure 2.24). Soft tissue crepitance may be present but is not common. Radiographs frequently demonstrate the presence of gas in the tissues.

Diagnosis begins with maintaining a high clinical suspicion in all patients, particularly patients with risk factors, including diabetes, immunocompromise, and intravenous drug abuse. (See also the previous discussion regarding *Vibrio* infections and underlying liver disease.) In the early stages, the infection appears more like cellulitis. Marking the area of both cellulitis and edema followed by reexamination within an hour for signs of progression helps distinguish a necrotizing infection from cellulitis. Tenderness beyond the area of erythema is highly suggestive of necrotizing fasciitis. If an open wound is present, the wound can be explored. A probe or finger that dissects easily along the fascia below intact skin is a hallmark finding distinguishing this process from cellulitis. When still in doubt regarding the diagnosis, an incisional biopsy can be performed at bedside. This is done proximal to the area of erythema and over the area of edema. The incision is carried down to the fascia. At least a 1-cm–square section of fascia is obtained for frozen section. Thrombosis obliterans of the perforating vessels and

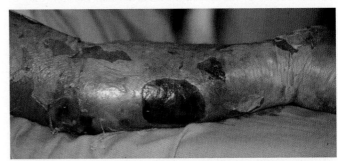

FIGURE 2.24 Characteristic appearance of necrotizing fasciitis. (Copyright courtesy of Milan Stevanovic and Frances Sharpe.)

massive infiltration of polymorphonuclear cells confirm the diagnosis. This step may delay appropriate surgical treatment. Similarly, MRI has been shown to have distinct characteristics in necrotizing fasciitis, but obtaining this study can result in further delays to treatment.[93]

Patients with necrotizing fasciitis often feel much worse than what would be expected from the initial presentation. They may experience a sense of impending doom. Fever and elevated WBC counts are not universally present. As the infection progresses, systemic signs of sepsis develop. Dehydration, electrolyte disturbance, and hypotension occur owing to the fluid shifts caused by the edema. Disseminated intravascular coagulopathy with rapidly progressing septic shock has been associated with necrotizing fasciitis.

The infection can spread rapidly over hours, involving the entire upper extremity and continuing onto the chest wall. Surgical treatment and broad-spectrum intravenous antibiotic therapy covering gram-positive and gram-negative organisms as well as anaerobic organisms are mandatory. Careful monitoring and correction of fluid and electrolyte status should be done in the intensive care setting. Intubation may be necessary as systemic signs of sepsis progress. Although the patient's medical condition should be optimized, surgical débridement should not be delayed, because this is the most important means of controlling the infection.

The surgical débridement should be extensive. Pus is not usually a component of these infections. A thin, watery exudate may be encountered, sometimes described as "dirty dishwater." The infection dissects along the fascial planes, making easy finger dissection in this plane. The fascia appears gray or grayish green and may be liquefied. Areas of normal-appearing fascia may be seen. However, under microscopic examination, these areas may be involved. Intraoperative frozen sections of the fascia can help guide the extent of débridement. Myonecrosis may be observed in cases of longer duration. In the hand, secondary thrombosis of the digital vessels results in necrotic fingers. Wide débridement of skin, subcutaneous tissue, fascia, and necrotic muscle, if present, is required. Amputation may be necessary, especially if muscle is involved or if the patient's condition is not improving despite aggressive débridement. The wounds should be left open and covered with moist gauze. Burn dressings should be used, and the patient is returned to the intensive care unit. Patient resuscitation should be the same as that used to resuscitate patients with extensive third-degree burns. These patients often require repeat débridement. However, it is the initial débridement that will most influence the treatment outcome. It is mandatory to remove all necrotic tissue at the first surgery. The wound should be reexamined no more than 24 hours after the first surgery. If the patient's clinical course is deteriorating, an earlier reexamination and repeat débridement versus amputation is indicated. The use of hyperbaric oxygen as adjunctive treatment has been reported. In centers where this facility is readily available, there may be some benefit (Case Study 2.4).

When the infection is controlled and the patient is clinically stable, wound coverage with a split-thickness skin graft is necessary. Prolonged occupational therapy is often required for functional recovery. Despite aggressive management, these infections are associated with a high morbidity and mortality rate. Mortality rates range from 9% up to 75% when chest wall involvement

is present. Factors associated with an increased mortality rate include age older than 50 years; the presence of diabetes mellitus, truncal involvement, or bacteremia on presentation; and delay to diagnosis and treatment.[43,55,76,100,101,135] Early deaths, defined as those within the first 10 days after initial débridement, were found consequent to sepsis syndrome. Late deaths were attributable to multiple organ system failure.[101]

Fungal necrotizing fasciitis is a rare cause of necrotizing infections but appears to be more common than previously recognized. Zygomycotic (mucormycotic) infections can be seen alone or in conjunction with bacterial species.[62,71] Diagnosis of mucormycosis is most rapidly made by histopathologic diagnosis, showing the characteristic abundance of broad, nonseptated hyphae invading tissue and, particularly, showing vascular invasion.[71] This highlights the importance of routinely taking tissue biopsies of necrotizing infections, as well as including cultures for fungal organisms. In our experience, we have seen three cases of fungal necrotizing fasciitis. These have all been in transplant patients who were receiving high-dose immunosuppressive therapy. Clinically, there is less erythema and swelling, but the tissue is firm and indurated with spotty areas of black necrotic lesions (Figure 2.25).

Gas gangrene is an uncommon infection of the upper extremity. These infections are rare but can be rapidly fatal. There are more than 60 species of *Clostridium*, but six types are known to cause gas gangrene. *Clostridium perfringens* is the most common, particularly in traumatic causes of infection. *Clostridium septicum* infection has been associated with spontaneous gas gangrene. The infection may "metastasize" to a site remote from the suspected portal of infection, such as the upper

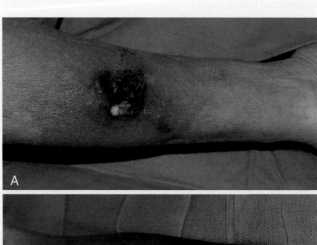
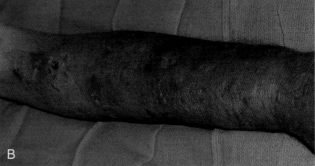

FIGURE 2.25 Fungal necrotizing fasciitis. Clinically, there is less swelling and erythema, but the tissue feels woody and indurated. There are superficial areas of black necrotic tissue. **A,** Black necrotic eschar. **B,** Indurated forearm without significant erythema or swelling. (Copyright courtesy of Milan Stevanovic and Frances Sharpe.)

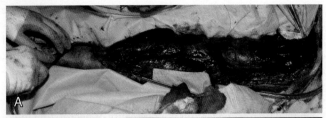
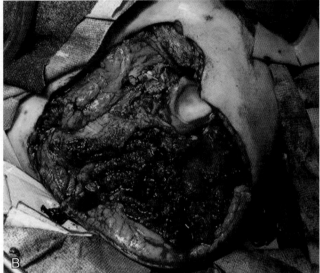

FIGURE 2.26 Spontaneous clostridial myonecrosis in a 54-year-old diagnosed with colorectal cancer 6 months prior to presentation with systemic sepsis. Despite aggressive surgical management, including left hip disarticulation and left arm disarticulation, patient survived only 12 hours after radical débridement. **A**, Myonecrosis of the arm and forearm. **B**, Following disarticulation, the resected muscles of the shoulder girdle have a healthy appearance. (Copyright courtesy of Milan Stevanovic and Frances Sharpe.)

or lower extremity.[80] Nontraumatic gangrene has an 80% association with underlying malignancy, most commonly colorectal cancers and leukemia[157] (Figure 2.26). More than 60% of gas gangrene infections also involve nonclostridial species. Clostridial organisms are obligate anaerobic gram-positive rods. They are spore forming, and the spores are highly resistant to environmental stresses. They survive for long periods and are ubiquitous in the soil. They are also found in the human gastrointestinal tract and in the female genital tract. It may be difficult to isolate *Clostridium* from a wound culture. It must be grown in an anaerobic environment in a medium with a reducing agent such as sodium thioglycolate. Clostridia produce a number of toxins. Among these, alpha toxin is responsible for the myonecrosis, hemolysis, and myocardial depression through the inhibition of the calcium pump. Theta toxin is a hemolysin and is cardiotoxic. Kappa toxin destroys blood vessels through collagenase activity.[55]

Devitalized tissue provides an excellent environment for clostridial growth. Clinical signs occur within hours of inoculation. Endotoxin production quickly produces necrosis of muscles, subcutaneous tissues, and fat. Thrombosis of local vessels further reduces the oxygen tension at the site of infection, continuing to promote a suitable environment for bacterial replication. Hydrogen sulfide and carbon dioxide gas are produced and dissect along the soft tissue planes, causing further tissue destruction. Local and systemic effects of the toxins are present as the infection continues, leading to severe hemolysis, hemoglobinuria, and, ultimately, renal failure. Death has been reported in as short a period as 12 hours after onset of infection.

The clinical findings generally include a history of trauma, often with a crush component. Infections have also occurred in postsurgical wounds and as spontaneous infections. The principal signs of clostridial infection are pain, a closed wound, tachycardia out of proportion to fever or hydration status, and subcutaneous crepitance.

Treatment requires rapid recognition of the infection and emergent surgical débridement, removing all necrotic tissue. It is imperative to leave wounds widely open. This infection is a contraindication for a negative-pressure dressing. Frequent dressing changes are initiated within 6 hours of the initial débridement. Intravenous antibiotic therapy, including high-dose penicillin therapy, is started immediately. Patient resuscitation in the intensive care unit must carefully manage fluid and electrolyte status. Hyperbaric oxygen is a valuable adjunct in the management of this devastating infection.

The principal differential diagnosis of clostridial myonecrosis includes necrotizing fasciitis and streptococcal gangrene, which also represent surgical emergencies. Gas gangrene progresses even more rapidly than necrotizing fasciitis, making early recognition imperative to patient survival. The mortality rate, despite aggressive management, remains high, approximating 25%.[131]

Cutaneous Anthrax Infections

Anthrax infection is caused by the gram-positive aerobic or facultative anaerobic bacterium *Bacillus anthracis*. The black eschar produced by the cutaneous disease gave rise to the name "anthrax," derived from the Greek word *anthrakos*, meaning "coal." The bacillus exists in a vegetative or growing state and in a spore form. In the vegetative state, it is very sensitive to environmental stress. Under these conditions, the cells undergo sporulation. The spore form is very resistant to environmental extremes, including temperature, pH, irradiation, disinfectants, sporicides, and many other stresses. The spore may remain viable in nature for up to 60 years (up to 200 years in one report).[82] Spores are present in the top 6 cm of soil and in animal products. Animals that die of anthrax release massive quantities of spores into the soil that may remain for decades before being ingested again. Burying animal carcasses is probably of little use in disrupting transmission because Pasteur showed that earthworms will carry spores back to the surface. Animal carcasses should be burned, not buried, to prevent long-term environmental contamination.

Anthrax infections have traditionally been transmitted through contaminated soil, animals, or animal products. Cases of cutaneous anthrax still occur in rural environments and in countries with a poorly developed agricultural infrastructure. Anthrax has also been used as a biologic weapon. With the potential threat of bioterrorism, it is important for clinicians to recognize the clinical manifestations of this disease. There are three main manifestations of anthrax. These are cutaneous, gastrointestinal, and inhalational. At present, the cutaneous form remains the most commonly seen, representing 95% of all reported cases worldwide. This form is also the most likely to be encountered by the hand surgeon.[156]

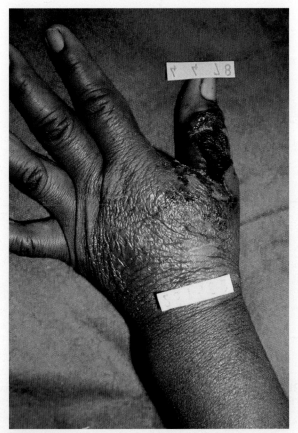

FIGURE 2.27 Cutaneous anthrax. (Courtesy of Dr. Eduardo Gotuzzo, Tropical Medicine Institute, Unversidad Peruana Cayetano Heredia, Lima, Peru.)

Clinical lesions of cutaneous anthrax usually appear within 2 to 7 days of handling sick animals or eating their meat; however, incubation periods of over 8 weeks have been reported. Cutaneous disease begins as a small, painless, red macule that progresses to a papule over 48 to 72 hours. The papule becomes vesicular and ruptures, ulcerates, and forms a brown or black eschar of 1 to 5 cm in diameter (Figure 2.27). Even when the vesicle ruptures and ulcerates, the lesion remains painless. Weeping vesicles and open ulcers should be cultured. If the patient has not received antibiotic treatment, anthrax bacilli may be cultured from the fluid. A gram-stained smear may reveal gram-positive rods. PCR and immunohistochemical staining may help confirm the diagnosis. Lesions are not purulent or painful in the absence of suprainfection. Satellite lesions and significant edema may surround the initial eschar. Depending on the location and severity of disease, edema may be extensive and life threatening, especially if the lesions are close to the chest or neck. Tender regional lymphadenopathy, fever, malaise, and chills may accompany the skin lesion.

Even with prompt antibiotic therapy, cutaneous lesions progress through the eschar phase. Progression of the cutaneous lesion occurs despite antibiotic treatment, because the tissue necrosis and ulceration occur due to the toxin, which is not neutralized by antibiotic therapy. Although antibiotics have no effect on the progression of the skin lesion, they do sterilize the ulcer. Several different antibiotics may be used, including penicillin, quinolones, or doxycycline. Intravenous therapy is used initially. Oral antibiotics are started as the patient shows clinical improvement. The duration of therapy is 60 days. *Débridement of skin lesions is contraindicated because of the risk of spreading infection.* Although 80% to 90% of lesions heal spontaneously, 10% to 20% of untreated cases may progress to malignant edema, septicemia, shock, renal failure, and death. Fatalities are uncommon with therapy.[82,156]

High-Pressure Injection Injuries

High-pressure injection injuries can result in extensive soft tissue damage, despite the often benign appearance of the entry wound. Material is injected through the skin at pressures of up to 7000 psi. The nondominant index finger is the most frequently involved digit. The extent of injury is related to the force of the injection and the type and amount of material injected. Mechanical and chemical injury results in local tissue necrosis and vascular occlusion. Oil-based paints and industrial solvents produce a greater degree of tissue necrosis than water-based paints and grease. Mirzayan and colleagues reported an amputation rate of 50% with oil-based paints. No amputations were required in water-based paint injections.[12,106] Emergent surgical decompression and débridement are necessary. Despite wide and aggressive surgical management, it is usually impossible to remove all of the foreign material. Surgical delay of more than 10 hours was found to result in higher rates of amputation.[147] Repeat surgical débridement at 48 to 72 hours may be necessary for wounds with wide contamination for removal of additional necrotic tissue and foreign material. Primary wound closure is often possible. Soft tissue reconstruction may be necessary for critical areas of soft tissue loss.[24]

Infection is not frequently a component of these injuries unless treatment is delayed. These wounds are commonly contaminated with both gram-positive and gram-negative organisms.[12,106,122] The necrotic tissue resulting from the injury provides a good culture medium for the injected bacteria. Broad-spectrum antibiotic coverage is important in the treatment of these injuries.

Mimickers of Infection

A wide range of clinical conditions may mimic an infection of the hand. It is important to recognize these conditions to provide appropriate treatment and prevent unnecessary surgery. The following conditions do not represent an exhaustive list but include those that are more commonly encountered. *Gout* and *pseudogout* represent the crystal arthropathies that may present as a pyarthrosis. Gouty tophi that erupt through the skin may have the appearance of infection with erythema of the skin and drainage. These lesions may also become secondarily infected and require surgical intervention (Figure 2.28). *Acute calcific tendinitis* presents as severe, well-localized pain overlying tendons or ligaments. Erythema and edema are often present. Other signs of infection, such as fever, lymphadenopathy, or abnormal laboratory values, are absent. Radiographs demonstrate characteristic calcific density in the area of tenderness (Figure 2.29). *Pyogenic granuloma* presents as a raised red, friable lesion (Figure 2.30). The friable tissue is sensitive to minor trauma and bleeds easily. In the hand, it is usually on the volar surface of the palm or fingers. The cause remains unclear, possibly related to repetitive irritation or minor trauma. *Pyoderma gangrenosum* is a very rare cutaneous lesion, seen principally in patients with a coexisting systemic disease, especially

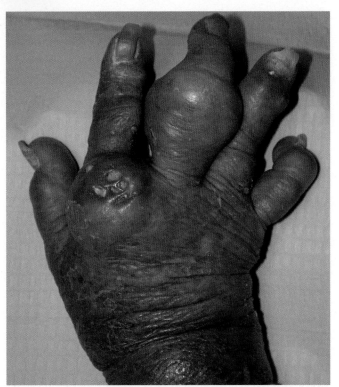

FIGURE 2.28 Tophaceous gout. (Copyright courtesy of Milan Stevanovic and Frances Sharpe.)

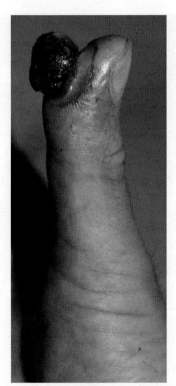

FIGURE 2.30 Pyogenic granuloma of the thumb. (Copyright Milan Stevanovic and Frances Sharpe.)

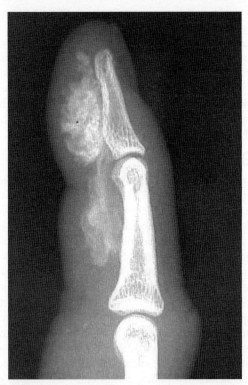

FIGURE 2.29 Calcinosis clinically presents with acute onset of severe pain, associated with swelling and, often, redness around the site of calcium deposition. (Copyright courtesy of Milan Stevanovic and Frances Sharpe.)

in patients with ulcerative colitis. The disease process begins with small papules that rapidly develop pustules. Central necrosis follows quickly, leaving a central ulcer. The border is raised and violaceous, and it advances from the center at a rate of 1 to 2 cm/day. Treatment includes local wound care. Surgical exci-

sion is contraindicated and may exacerbate the disease, resulting in a larger area of necrosis. *Retained foreign bodies* may result in an inflammatory response that mimics an infection. Woody materials can be a significant irritant. Palm thorns are known to cause a chemical irritation of the soft tissues. Intraarticular thorns or thorns that pierce the tendon sheath can result in a chemical synovitis. Removal of the offending irritant is necessary for definitive treatment. *Metastatic* or *primary tumors* on the hand are rare. However, awareness of this possibility is important to prevent a misdiagnosis and emphasizes the importance of tissue biopsy as well as tissue culture.[125] Primary lesions include squamous cell carcinoma, basal cell carcinoma, melanoma, and keratoacanthoma (see Chapter 58) (Case Study 2.5). A metastatic primary tumor is more likel to appear as a chronic infection. Metastatic lesions to the hand and wrist have been reported in all bones of the hand but are usually acral lesions, with more than 50% involving the distal phalanx. Radiographs may help distinguish between tumor and infection. Primary lung tumors are the most common metastatic lesion to the hand. Other sites of primary tumor include the breast, kidney, colon, thyroid, and prostate.[2,4,24]

For Case Studies, Videos, and more, please visit ExpertConsult.com.

REFERENCES

1. Abrahamian FM, Goldstein EJ: Microbiology of animal bite wound infections. *Clin Microbiol Rev* 24(2):231–246, 2011.
2. Afshar A, Farhadnia P, Khalkhali H: Metastases to the hand and wrist: an analysis of 221 cases. *J Hand Surg [Am]* 39(5):923–932, 2014.
3. Allison DC, Miller T, Holtom P, et al: Microbiology of upper extremity soft tissue abscesses in injecting drug abusers. *Clin Orthop Relat Res* 461:9–13, 2007.

4. Amadio P, Lombardi R: Metastatic tumors of the hand. *J Hand Surg* 12A(2):311–316, 1987.
5. Arons M, Fernando L, Polayes I: *Pasturella multocida:* the major cause of hand infections following domestic animal bites. *J Hand Surg* 7(1):47–52, 1982.
6. Babovic N, Cayci C, Carlsen BT: Cat bite infections of the hand: assessment of morbidity and predictors of severe infection. *J Hand Surg [Am]* 39(2):286–290, 2014.
7. Baran R, Haneke E: Infection of the nail apparatus: viral infection. In Krull E, Zook EG, Baran R, et al, editors: *Nail surgery: a text and atlas*, Philadelphia, 2001, Lippincott Williams & Wilkins, pp 201–205.
8. Barbieri R, Freeland A: Osteomyelitis of the hand. *Hand Clin* 14(4):589–603, 1998.
9. Battle J, Carmichael K: Incidence of pin track infections in children's fractures treated with Kirschner wire fixation. *J Pediatr Orthop* 27(2):154–157, 2007.
10. Bauters T, Buyle F, Verschraegen G, et al: Infection risk related to the use of medicinal leeches. *Pharm World Sci* 29(3):122–125, 2007.
11. Bednar M, Lane L: Eponychial marsupialization and nail removal for surgical treatment of chronic paronychia. *J Hand Surg* 16A:314–317, 1991.
12. Bekler H, Gokce A, Beyzadeoglu T, et al: The surgical treatment and outcomes of high-pressure injection injuries of the hand. *J Hand Surg Eur* 32(4):394–399, 2007.
13. Bergstein J, Baker EI, Aprahamian C, et al: Soft tissue abscesses associated with parenteral drug abuse: Presentation, microbiology, and treatment. *Am Surg* 61(12):1105–1108, 1995.
14. Biviji A, Paiement G, Steinbach L: Musculoskeletal manifestations of human immunodeficiency virus infection. *J Am Acad Orthop Surg* 10(5):312–320, 2002.
15. Boles D, Schmidt C: Pyogenic flexor tenosynovitis. *Hand Clin* 14(4):567–578, 1998.
16. Botte M, Davis J, Rose B, et al: Complications of smooth pin fixation of fractures and dislocations in the hand and wrist. *Clin Orthop* 276:194–201, 1992.
17. Boutin R, Brossmann J, Sartoris D, et al: Update on imaging of orthopedic infections. *Orthop Clin North Am* 29(1):41–66, 1998.
18. Boyes JH: Infections. In Boyes JH, editor: *Bunnell's surgery of the hand*, Philadelphia, 1970, JB Lippincott Company, pp 613–642.
19. Bratzler DW, Dellinger EP, Olsen KM, et al: Clinical practice guidelines for antimicrobial prophylaxis in surgery. *Surg Infect* 14(1):73–156, 2013.
20. Buchanan D, Heiss-Dunlop W, Mathy JA: Community acquired methicillin resistant *Staphylococcus aureus* hand infections: a South Pacific perspective: characteristics and implications for antibiotic coverage. *Hand Surg* 17(3):317–324, 2012.
21. Calkins E: Nosocomial infections in hand surgery. *Hand Clin* 14(4):531–545, 1998.
22. Calvet H, Yoshikawa T: Infections in diabetes. *Infect Dis Clin North Am* 15(2):407–421, 2001.
23. Carter S: Herpetic whitlow: Herpetic infections of the digits. Invited comments. *J Hand Surg* 4(1):93–94, 1979.
24. Chaput B, Nouaille de Gorce H, Courtade-Saidi M, et al: The role of a systematic second look at 48-72 hours in high-pressure injection injuries to the hand: a retrospective study. *Chir Main* 31(5):250–255, 2012.
25. Chung MT, Wilson P, Rinker B: Community-acquired methicillin-resistant *Staphylococcus aureus* hand infections in the pediatric population. *J Hand Surg [Am]* 37(2):326–331, 2012.
26. Cierny G, III, Mader J, Penninck J: A clinical staging system for adult osteomyelitis. *Contemp Orthop* 10(5):17–37, 1985.
27. Classen D, Evans R, Pestotnik S, et al: The timing of prophylactic administration of antibiotics and the risk of surgical wound infection. *N Engl J Med* 326(5):281–286, 1992.
28. Cohen G, Schnall S, Holtom P: New-onset diabetes mellitus in patients presenting with extremity infections. *Clin Orthop Relat Res* 403:45–48, 2002.
29. Cohen M, Kaplan L: Histology and ultrastructure of the human flexor tendon sheath. *J Hand Surg* 12A(1):25–29, 1987.
30. Costerton J: Biofilm theory can guide the treatment of device-related orthopedic infections. *Clin Orthop Relat Res* 437:7–11, 2005.
31. Crosby SN, Snoddy MC, Atkinson CT, et al: Upper extremity myonecrosis caused by *Edwardsiella tarda* resulting in transhumeral amputation: case report. *J Hand Surg* 38A(1):129–132, 2013.
32. Dailiana ZH, Rigopoulos N, Varitimidis S, et al: Purulent flexor tenosynovitis: factors influencing the functional outcome. *J Hand Surg Eur* 33(3):280–285, 2008.
33. Dechet A, Yu P, Koram N, et al: Non-foodborne *Vibrio* infections: an important cause of morbidity and mortality in the United States, 1997-2006. *Clin Infect Dis* 46(7):970–976, 2008.
34. Deirmengian C, Kardos K, Kilmartin P, et al: Diagnosing periprosthetic joint infection: has the era of the biomarker arrived? *Clin Orthop Relat Res* 4:4, 2014.
35. Doyle J: Anatomy of the flexor tendon sheath and pulley system. *J Hand Surg* 13A(4):473–484, 1988.
36. Faciszewski T, Coleman D: Human bite infections of the hand. *Hand Clin* 14(4):683–690, 1998.
37. Ferlic D, Clayton M, Holloway M: Complications of silicone implant surgery in the metacarpophalangeal joint. *J Bone Joint Surg* 57A(7):991–994, 1975.
38. Fitoussi F, Litzelmann E, Ilharreborde B, et al: Hematogenous osteomyelitis of the wrist in children. *J Pediatr Orthop* 27(7):810–813, 2007.
39. Fleisher G: The management of bite wounds. *N Engl J Med* 340(2):138–140, 1999.
40. Formaini N, Jacob P, Willis L, et al: Evaluating the use of preoperative antibiotics in pediatric orthopaedic surgery. *J Pediatr Orthop* 32(7):737–740, 2012.
41. Fowler JR, Ilyas AM: Epidemiology of adult acute hand infections at an urban medical center. *J Hand Surg* 38A(6):1189–1193, 2013.
42. Francel T, Marshall K, Savage R: Hand infections in the diabetic renal transplant patient. *Ann Plast Surg* 24(4):304–309, 1990.
43. Francis K, Lamaute H, Davis J, et al: Implications of risk factors in necrotizing fasciitis. *Am Surg* 59(5):304–308, 1993.
44. Gahhos F, Ariyan S: Hippocrates, the true father of hand surgery. *Surg Gynecol Obstet* 160:178–184, 1985.
45. Garcia V: Animal bites and *Pasteurella* infections. *Pediatr Rev* 18(4):127–130, 1997.
46. Gaston RG, Kuremsky MA: Postoperative infections: prevention and management. *Hand Clin* 26(2):265–280, 2010.
47. Gellman H, Stetson W, Brumfield R, Jr, et al: Silastic metacarpophalangeal joint arthroplasty in patients with rheumatoid arthritis. *Clin Orthop* 342:16–21, 1997.
48. Gilchrist J, Sacks JJ, White D, et al: Dog bites: still a problem? *Inj Prev* 14(5):296–301, 2008.
49. Gill M, Arlette J, Buchan K: Herpes simplex virus infection of the hand. A profile of 79 cases. *Am J Med* 84:89–93, 1988.
50. Glass K: Factors related to the resolution of treated hand infections. *J Hand Surg* 7(4):388–394, 1982.
51. Glickel S: Hand infections in patients with acquired immunodeficiency syndrome. *J Hand Surg* 13A(5):770–775, 1988.
52. Gold R, Hawkins R, Katz R: Bacterial osteomyelitis: Findings on plain radiography, CT, MR, and scintigraphy. *Am J Roentgenol* 157:365–370, 1991.
53. Goldstein E: Current concepts on animal bites. *Curr Clin Top Infect Dis* 19:99–111, 1999.
54. Goldstein E, Barones M, Miller T: *Eikenella corrodens* in hand infections. *J Hand Surg* 8(5):563–567, 1983.
55. Gonzalez M: Necrotizing fasciitis and gangrene of the upper extremity. *Hand Clin* 14(4):635–645, 1998.
56. Gonzalez M, Bochar S, Novotny J, et al: Upper extremity infections in patients with diabetes mellitus. *J Hand Surg* 24A(4):682–686, 1995.
57. Gonzalez M, Garst J, Nourbash P, et al: Abscesses of the upper extremity from drug abuse by injection. *J Hand Surg* 18A(5):868–870, 1993.
58. Gonzalez M, Nikoleit J, Weinzweig N, et al: Upper extremity infections in patients with the human immunodeficiency virus. *J Hand Surg* 23A(2):348–352, 1998.
59. Graves M, Janda J: Rat-bite fever (*Streptobacillus moniliformis*): a potential emerging disease. *Int J Infect Dis* 5(3):151–155, 2001.
60. Gunther S, Gunther S: Diabetic hand infections. *Hand Clin* 14(4):647–656, 1998.
61. Gutowski KA, Ochoa O, Adams WP, Jr: Closed-catheter irrigation is as effective as open drainage for treatment of pyogenic flexor tenosynovitis. *Ann Plast Surg* 49(4):350–354, 2002.
62. Harada A, Lau W: Successful treatment and limb salvage of mucor necrotizing fasciitis after kidney transplantation with posaconazole. *Hawaii Med J* 66(3):68–71, 2007.
63. Hardy A, Nicol R: Closed fractures complicated by acute hematogenous osteomyelitis. *Clin Orthop* 201:190–195, 1985.
64. Harness NG, Inacio MC, Pfeil FF, et al: Rate of infection after carpal tunnel release surgery and effect of antibiotic prophylaxis. *J Hand Surg* 35A(2):189–196, 2010.
65. Harrison M: A 4-year review of human bite injuries presenting to emergency medicine and proposed evidence-based guidelines. *Injury* 40(8):826–830, 2009.
66. Henriksen B, Albrektsen S, Simper L, et al: Soft tissue infections from drug abuse. A clinical and microbiological review. *Acta Orthop Scand* 65(6):625–628, 1994.
67. Honner R, Meares A: A review of 100 flexor tendon reconstructions with prosthesis. *Hand* 9(3):226–231, 1977.
68. Houshian S, Seyedipour S, Wedderkopp N: Epidemiology of bacterial hand infections. *Int J Infect Dis* 10(4):315–319, 2006.
69. Hurst L, Gluck R, Sampson S, et al: Herpetic whitlow with bacterial abcess. *J Hand Surg* 16A(2):311–313, 1991.
70. Imahara SD, Friedrich JB: Community-acquired methicillin-resistant *Staphylococcus aureus* in surgically treated hand infections. *J Hand Surg* 35A(1):97–103, 2010.
71. Jain D, Kumar Y, Vasishta R, et al: Zygomycotic necrotizing fasciitis in immunocompetent patients: a series of 18 cases. *Mod Pathol* 19:1221–1226, 2006.
72. Janis JE, Hatef DA, Reece EM, et al: Does empiric antibiotic therapy change hand infection outcomes? Cost analysis of a randomized prospective trial in a county hospital. *Plast Reconstr Surg* 133(4):511e–518e, 2014.
73. Jeon IH, Morrey BF, Anakwenze OA, et al: Incidence and implications of early postoperative wound complications after total elbow arthroplasty. *J Shoulder Elbow Surg* 20(6):857–865, 2011.
74. Kanavel A: *Infections of the hand*, ed 4, Phildelphia, 1921, Lea & Febiger.
75. Kanavel A: *Infections of the hand*, ed 7, Philadelphia, 1939, Lea & Febiger, p 503.
76. Kao LS, Lew DF, Arab SN, et al: Local variations in the epidemiology, microbiology, and outcome of necrotizing soft-tissue infections: a multicenter study. *Am J Surg* 202(2):139–145, 2011.

77. Karpathios T, Moustaki M, Yiallouros P, et al: HSV-2 meningitis disseminated from a herpetic whitlow. *Paediatr Int Child Health* 32(2):121–122, 2012.

78. Keyser J, Eaton R: Surgical cure of chronic paronychia by eponychial marsupialization. *Plast Reconst Surg* 58(1):66–70, 1976.

79. Kour A, Looi K, Phone M, et al: Hand infections in patients with diabetes. *Clin Orthop Relat Res* 331:238–244, 1996.

80. Kudsk K: Occult gastrointestinal malignancies producing metastatic *Clostridium septicum* infections in diabetic patients. *Surgery* 112:765–772, 1992.

81. Ladhani S, Cameron J, Chapple D, et al: A novel method for rapid production and purification of exfoliative toxin A of *Staphylococcus aureus*. *FEMS Microbiol Lett* 212(1):35–39, 2002.

82. LaForce F: Anthrax. *Clin Infect Dis* 19:1009–1014, 1994.

83. Leslie B, Harris J, III, Driscoll D: Septic arthritis of the shoulder in adults. *J Bone Joint Surg* 71A(10):1516–1522, 1989.

84. Levy C: Treating infections of the hand: identifying the organism and choosing the antibiotic. *Instr Course Lect* 39:533–537, 1990.

85. Li MY, Hua Y, Wei GH, et al: Staphylococcal scalded skin syndrome in neonates: an 8-year retrospective study in a single institution. *Pediatr Dermatol* 31(1):43–47, 2014.

86. Lille S, Hayakawa T, Neumeister MW, et al: Continuous postoperative catheter irrigation is not necessary for the treatment of suppurative flexor tenosynovitis. *J Hand Surg* 25B(3):304–307, 2000.

87. Lindsay JA: Hospital-associated MRSA and antibiotic resistance: what have we learned from genomics? *Int J Med Microbiol* 303(6–7):318–323, 2013.

88. Lindsey D, Christopher M, Hollenbach J, et al: Natural course of the human bite wound: incidence of infection and complications in 434 bites and 803 lacerations in the same group of patients. *J Trauma* 27(1):45–48, 1987.

89. Lineaweaver W, Furnas H, Follansbee S, et al: Postprandial *Aeromonas hydrophila* cultures and antibiotic levels of the enteric aspirates from medicinal leeches applied to patients receiving antibiotics. *Ann Plast Surg* 29(3):245–249, 1992.

90. Linscheid R, Dobyns J: Common and uncommon infections of the hand. *Orthop Clin North Am* 6(4):1063–1104, 1975.

91. Mackay D, Manders E, Saggers G, et al: *Aeromonas* species isolated from medicinal leeches. *Ann Plast Surg* 42(3):275–279, 1999.

92. Malenfant J, Walters A, Kralovic S, et al: Francesco Parona (1842-1908) and his contributions to our understanding of surgery through anatomy. *Clin Anat* 26(5):547–550, 2013.

93. Malghem J, Lecouvet FE, Omoumi P, et al: Necrotizing fasciitis: contribution and limitations of diagnostic imaging. *Joint Bone Spine* 80(2):146–154, 2013.

94. Maloon S, de V de Beer J, Opitz M, et al: Acute Flexor Tendon Sheath Infections. *J Hand Surg* 15A(3):474–477, 1990.

95. Mann J, III, Werntz J: Catfish stings to the hand. *J Hand Surg* 16A(2):318–321, 1991.

96. Mann R: *Infections of the hand*, Philadelphia, 1988, Lea & Febiger, p 190.

97. Mann R, Hoffeld T, Farmer C: Human bites of the hand: twenty years of experience. *J Hand Surg* 2(2):97–104, 1977.

98. McAuliffe J, Seltzer D, Hornicek F: Upper-extremity infections in patients seropositive for human immunodefieciency virus. *J Hand Surg* 22A(6):1084–1090, 1997.

99. McGinley K, Larson E, Leyden J: Composition and density of microflora in the subungual space of the hand. *J Clin Microbiol* 26(5):950–953, 1988.

100. McHenry C, Brandt C, Piotrowski J, et al: Idiopathic necrotizing fasciitis: recognition, incidence, and outcome of therapy. *Am Surg* 60(7):490–494, 1994.

101. McHenry C, Piotrowski J, Petrinic D, et al: Determinants of mortality for necrotizing soft-tissue infections. *Ann Surg* 221(5):563–565, 1995.

102. McLain R, Steyers C, Stoddard M: Infections in open fractures of the hand. *J Hand Surg* 16A(1):108–112, 1991.

103. Mennen U, Howells C: Human fight-bite injuries of the hand. A study of 100 cases within 18 months. *J Bone Joint Surg* 16B(3):431–435, 1991.

104. Meyer CL, Abzug JM: Domestic bird bites. *J Hand Surg* 37A(9):1925–1927, 2012.

105. Millender L, Nalebuff E, Hawkins R, et al: Infection after silicone prosthetic arthroplasty in the hand. *J Bone Joint Surg* 57A(6):825–829, 1975.

106. Mirzayan R, Schnall S, Chon J, et al: Culture results and amputation rates in high-pressure paint gun injuries of the hand. *Orthopedics* 24(6):587–589, 2001.

107. Morgan M: Prophylaxis should be considered even for trivial animal bites. *BMJ* 314:1413, 1997.

108. Murphey DK, Septimus EJ, Waagner DC: Catfish-related injury and infection: Report of two cases and review of the literature. *Clin Infect Dis* 14(3):689–693, 1992.

109. Murphy E, DeVita D, Liu H, et al: Risk factors for skin and soft-tissue abscesses among injection drug users: a case controlled study. *Clin Infect Dis* 33(July):35–40, 2001.

110. Nakafusa J, Misago N, Miura M, et al: The importance of serum creatine phosphokinase level in the early diagnosis, and as a prognostic factor, of *Vibrio vulnificus* infection. *Br J Dermatol* 145(2):280–284, 2001.

111. Neviaser R: Closed tendon sheath irrigation for pyogenic flexor tenosynovitis. *J Hand Surg* 3A(5):462–466, 1978.

112. Nydick JA, Greenberg SM, Stone JD, et al: Clinical outcomes of total wrist arthroplasty. *J Hand Surg* 37A(8):1580–1584, 2012.

113. O'Hara F, Geux N, Word JM, et al: A geographic carian of the *Staphylococcus aureus* Panton-Valentine leukocidin toxin and the origin of community-associated methicillin-resistant *S. aureus* USA300. *J Infect Dis* 197(2):187–194, 2008.

114. O'Malley M, Fowler J, Ilyas AM: Community-acquired methicillin-resistant *Staphylococcus aureus* infections of the hand: prevalence and timeliness of treatment. *J Hand Surg* 34A(3):504–508, 2009.

115. Oliver J: Wound infections caused by *Vibrio vulnificus* and other marine bacteria. *Epidemiol Infect* 133(3):383–391, 2005.

116. Otto M: Community-associated MRSA: what makes them special? *Int J Med Microbiol* 303(6–7):324–330, 2013.

117. Otto RJ, Mulieri PJ, Cottrell BJ, et al: Arthrodesis for failed total elbow arthroplasty with deep infection. *J Shoulder Elbow Surg* 23(3):302–307, 2014.

118. Pabari A, Iyer S, Khoo CT: Swiss roll technique for treatment of paronychia. *Tech Hand Up Extrem Surg* 15(2):75–77, 2011.

119. Pang H-N, Teoh L, Yam A, et al: Factors affecting the prognosis of pyogenic flexor tenosynovitis. *J Bone Joint Surg* 89A(8):1742–1748, 2007.

120. Patel GK, Finlay AY: Staphylococcal scalded skin syndrome: diagnosis and management. *Am J Clin Dermatol* 4(3):165–175, 2003.

121. Patzakis M, Wilkins J, Bassett R: Surgical findings in clenched-fist injuries. *Clin Orthop Relat Res* 220:237–240, 1987.

122. Pinto M, Turkula-Pinto L, Cooney W, et al: High-pressure injection injuries of the hand: review of 25 patients managed by open wound technique. *J Hand Surg* 18A(1):125–130, 1993.

123. Pinzur M, Bednar M, Weaver F, et al: Hand infections in the diabetic patient. *J Bone Joint Surg* 22B(1):133–134, 1997.

124. Rashkoff E, Burkhalter W, Mann R: Septic arthritis of the wrist. *J Bone Joint Surg* 65A(8):824–828, 1983.

125. Rauh MA, Duquin TR, McGrath BE, et al: Spread of squamous cell carcinoma from the thumb to the small finger via the flexor tendon sheaths. *J Hand Surg* 34A(9):1709–1713, 2009.

126. Reilly K, Linz J, Stern P, et al: Osteomyelitis of the tubular bones of the hand. *J Hand Surg* 22A(4):644–649, 1997.

127. Ritting AW, O'Malley MP, Rodner CM: Acute paronychia. *J Hand Surg* 37A(5):1068–1070, 2012.

128. Rizvi M, Bille B, Holtom P, et al: The role of prophylactic antibiotics in elective hand surgery. *J Hand Surg* 33A(3):413–420, 2008.

129. Robbins R: Infections of the hand. *J Bone Joint Surg* 34B(4):567–587, 1952.

130. Robertson H, Polk H: The mechanism of infection in patients with diabetes mellitus: a review of leukocyte malfunction. *Surgery* 75(1):123–128, 1974.

131. Roding B, Groeneveld P, Boerema I: Ten years of experience in the treatment of gas gangrene with hyperbaric oxygen. *Surg Gynecol Obstet* 134(4):579–585, 1972.

132. Rosen T, Jablon J: Infection threats from exotic pets: dermatological implications. *Dermatol Clin* 21(2):229–236, 2003.

133. Sammer DM, Shin AY: Comparison of arthroscopic and open treatment of septic arthritis of the wrist. *J Bone Joint Surg* 91A(6):1387–1393, 2009.

134. Schaefer R, Enzenauer R, Pruitt A, et al: Acute gonococcal flexor tenosynovitis in the adolescent male with pharyngitis. A case report and review of the literature. *Clin Orthop Relat Res* 281:212–215, 1992.

135. Schecter W, Meyer A, Schecter G, et al: Necrotizing fasciitis of the upper extremity. *J Hand Surg* 7A(1):15–20, 1982.

136. Scheldrup E: Tendon sheath patterns in the hand. An anatomical study based on 367 hand dissections. *Surg Gynecol Obstet* 93(1):16–22, 1951.

137. Schnall S, Holtom P, Lilley J: Abscesses secondary to parenteral abuse of drugs. *J Bone Joint Surg* 76A(10):1526–1530, 1994.

138. Schnall S, Thommen V, Allari T, et al: Delayed primary wound closure in upper extremity soft-tissue infections. *Clin Orthop Relat Res* 335:286–291, 1997.

139. Schnall S, Vu-Rose T, Holtom P, et al: Tissue pressures in pyogenic flexor tenosynovitis of the finger. Compartment syndrome and its management. *J Bone Joint Surg* 78B(5):793–795, 1996.

140. Selvin E, Parrinello CM, Sacks DB, et al: Trends in prevalence and control of diabetes in the United States, 1988-1994 and 1999-2010. *Ann Intern Med* 160(8):517–525, 2014.

141. Shapiro D: Postoperative infection in hand surgery. *Hand Clin* 14(4):669–681, 1998.

142. Sharma KS, Rao K, Hobson MI: Space of Parona infections: experience in management and outcomes in a regional hand centre. *J Plast Reconstr Aesthet Surg* 66(7):968–972, 2013.

143. Simmen H, Giovanoli P, Battaglia H, et al: Soft tissue infections of the upper extremities with special consideration of abscesses in parenteral drug abusers. *J Hand Surg* 20B(6):797–800, 1995.

144. Simmons A: Clinical manifestations and treatment considerations of herpes simplex virus infections. *J Infect Dis* 186(Suppl):S71–S77, 2002.

145. Smith P, Meadowcroft A, May D: Treating mammalian bite wounds. *J Clin Pharm Ther* 25(2):85–89, 2000.

146. Spicher VM, Bouvier P, Schlegel-Haueter SE, et al: Epidemiology of herpes simplex virus in children by detection of specific antibodies in saliva. *Pediatr Infect Dis J* 20(3):265–272, 2001.

147. Stark H, Ashworth C, Boyes J: Paint-gun injuries of the hand. *J Bone Joint Surg* 49A(4):637–647, 1967.

148. Stern P, Staneck J, McDonough J, et al: Established hand infections: a controlled prospective study. *J Hand Surg* 8A(5):553–559, 1983.

149. Strong M, Lejman T, Michno P: Septic arthritis of the wrist in infancy. *J Pediatr Orthop* 15(2):152–156, 1995.

150. Summanen P, Talan D, Strong C, et al: Bacteriology of skin and soft-tissue infections: Comparison of infections in intravenous drug users and individuals with no history of drug use. *Clin Infect Dis* 20(Suppl 2):S279–S282, 1995.

151. Talan D, Citron D, Abrahamian F, et al: Bacteriologic analysis of infected dog and cat bites. *N Engl J Med* 340(2):85–92, 1999.

152. Tannan SC, Deal DN: Diagnosis and management of the acute felon: evidence-based review. *J Hand Surg* 37A(12):2603–2604, 2012.

153. Tordjman D, Holvoet L, Benkerrou M, et al: Hematogenous osteoarticular infections of the hand and the wrist in children with sickle cell anemia: preliminary report. *J Pediatr Orthop* 34(1):123–128, 2014.

154. Tosti R, Fowler J, Dwyer J, et al: Is antibiotic prophylaxis necessary in elective soft tissue hand surgery? *Orthopedics* 35(6):e829–e833, 2012.

155. Tsai Y, Hus R, Huang T, et al: Necrotizing soft-tissue infections and sepsis caused by *Vibrio vulnificus* compared with those caused by *Aeromonas* species. *J Bone Joint Surg* 89A(3):631–636, 2007.

156. Tutrone W, Scheinfeld N, Weinberg J: Cutaneous anthrax: a concise review. *Cutis* 69(1):27–33, 2002.

157. Valentine E: Nontraumatic gas gangrene. *Ann Emerg Med* 30(1):109–111, 1997.

158. van Alphen NA, Gonzalez A, McKenna MC, et al: Ciprofloxacin-resistant *Aeromonas* infection following leech therapy for digit replantation: report of 2 cases. *J Hand Surg* 39A(3):499–502, 2014.

159. van der Lugt JC, Geskus RB, Rozing PM: Primary Souter-Strathclyde total elbow prosthesis in rheumatoid arthritis. Surgical technique. *J Bone Joint Surg* 1A(Pt 1):67–77, 2005.

160. Vetter R, Agac B, Reiland R, et al: Skin lesion in barracks: Consider community-acquired methicillin-resistant *Staphylococcus aureus* instead of spider bites. *Military Med* 171(9):830–832, 2006.

161. Wald A, Ashley-Morrow R: Serological testing for herpes simplex virus (HSV)-1 and (HSV)-2 infection. *Clin Infect Dis* 35(Suppl 2):S173–S182, 2002.

162. Waldvogel F, Medoff G, Swartz M: Osteomyelitis: a review of clinical features, therapeutic considerations and unusual aspects (first of three parts). *N Engl J Med* 282(4):198–206, 1970.

163. Waldvogel F, Medoff G, Swartz M: Osteomyelitis: a review of clinical features, therapeutic considerations and unusual aspects (second of three parts). *N Engl J Med* 282(5):260–266, 1970.

164. Watson PA, Jebson PJ: The natural history of the neglected felon. *Iowa Orthop J* 16:164–166, 1994.

165. Weber B, Rabenau H, Berger A, et al: Seroprevalence of HCV, HAV, HBV, HDV, HCMV, and HIV in high risk groups. *Zentrabl Bakteriol* 282(1):102–112, 1995.

166. Wehbe M, Mawr B, Hunter J, et al: Two-stage flexor tendon reconstruction. Ten-year experience. *J Bone Joint Surg* 68A(5):752–763, 1986.

167. Westling K, Bygdeman S, Engkvist O, et al: *Pasteurella multocida* infection following cat bites in humans. *J Infect* 40(1):97–98, 2000.

168. Whitaker IS, Kamya C, Azzopardi EA, et al: Preventing infective complications following leech therapy: is practice keeping pace with current research? *Microsurgery* 29(8):619–625, 2009.

169. Wilson B: Necrotizing fasciitis. *Am J Surg* 18(4):416–431, 1952.

170. Wittels N, Donley J, Burkhalter W: A functional treatment method for interphalangeal pyogenic arthritis. *J Hand Surg* 9A(6):894–898, 1984.

171. Zuretti A, Schwartz I: Gangrenous herpetic whitlow in a human immunodeficiency virus–positive patient. *Am J Clin Pathol* 93:828–830, 1990.

3

Chronic Infections

Mukund R. Patel

Acknowledgment: Govind Narain Malaviya was the main contributor to the section on leprosy. He was a leader in surgery for Hansen disease in the world and has now retired. I am thankful to Dr. Malaviya for his great contribution to this chapter and dedicate the leprosy section to his legacy.

GENERAL PRINCIPLES

Chronic infections of the hand and upper extremity can be caused by a variety of agents: viruses, bacteria, mycobacteria, fungi, *Prototheca*, protozoa, parasites, and insects (Table 3.1). An infection may be superficial and affect the skin or nails, or it may affect subcutaneous tissue, or it may be deep and affect the nerves, tenosynovium, joints, and bone. Chronic lesions of the hand, both superficial and deep, have a nonspecific presentation and early biopsy and cultures facilitate diagnosis. Early suspicion and diagnosis of a chronic infection is the mainstay of all ensuing treatment principles and is the primary message of this chapter.

Chronic infections of the hand and upper extremity are rare indeed and are primarily a problem of diagnosis. They often are not considered in the differential diagnosis of hand lesions. Many surgeons encounter their first case by surprise unless an unusual diagnosis is considered in the presence of unusual symptoms and signs. One must consider infection in any chronic lesion of the hand. In an immunocompromised patient, infection must always be included in the differential diagnosis. Biopsy and cultures should be considered as a part of a diagnostic workup for atypical lesions.

An infection that does not respond to antibiotics, incision, drainage, or debridement, is suspect. Because infections are rare, diagnosis is often delayed unless a high level of suspicion is maintained. "Culture a tumor and biopsy an infection," is an adage to apply when an unusual lesion is encountered[53,62,88]; otherwise, chronic and emerging infections will continue to elude physicians. With increasing numbers of international travelers, immigrants, and vacationers to endemic areas, we encounter old (i.e., tuberculosis,[46] yaws,[37] leprosy[65]) and exotic (i.e., protozoal,[18] protothecal, and parasitic gnathostomiasis[96]) infections of the hand. With more organ transplants and malignant lesions treated with chemotherapy, new and emerging infections are encountered. Recognition of all of them saves unnecessary surgery for infections that are medically treatable.

This chapter is a reservoir of rare encounters with chronic infections during hand surgery. It may serve as a reference when an unexpected or unfamiliar infection appears on a pathology or microbiology report. Moreso, I hope that it will highlight the need for early biopsy and cultures when a chronic lesion (e.g., tenosynovium, joint, bone, skin or subcutaneous tissue) of the hand and/or upper extremity eludes diagnosis.

The most common chronic hand infection traditionally has been tuberculosis (Hansen disease). Nontuberculous mycobacterial (NTM) infections—initially recognized in the 1950s as atypical or mycobacteria other than tuberculosis (MOTT)—of the hand are now more common[5,15,25,34,52,61,63,64,72,92,112,122] than mycobacterium tuberculosis infections. Tenosynovial infections of both types are far more common than joint and bone infections. In North America, the most common chronic bacterial infection is nocardiosis and the most common fungal infection is sporotrichosis. Hansen disease is the most common chronic infection affecting the hand in developing countries. It infects peripheral nerves, and the level of suspicion should be high when peripheral neuropathy of the ulnar nerve, with or without nerve enlargement, is seen in an immigrant.

Chronic hand infections caused by protozoa, *Prototheca*, and parasites are sporadically encountered in Africa, Asia, and South America but are rare in North America. Since 1981, chronic hand infections due to human immunodeficiency virus (HIV) have become increasingly common in emergency departments and consultation rooms. HIV blood testing and counseling should be considered in acute, recurrent, and chronic infections of the hand. Once a diagnosis is made, it is wise to arrange for consultation with an infectious disease specialist. Pharmacologic treatment of a chronic hand infection requires close monitoring for serious side effects and drug resistance. Recurrence of the infection due to drug resistance may occur because of poor patient compliance or prescription practices. Consultation with an infectious disease specialist, microbiology personnel, and a pathologist improves the accuracy of a diagnosis.

Diagnosis

A presumptive diagnosis of a chronic hand infection is made when one considers it as a possibility in the face of any chronic cutaneous, subcutaneous, tenosynovial, nerve, joint, or bone lesion (i.e., nodule, abscess, ulcer, sinus, fistula, or a nondescript mass) of the hand or upper extremity. Obtaining a careful history is essential and must include details about underlying diseases (e.g., leukemia, aspergillosis, diabetes, and mucormycosis), medications (e.g., corticosteroids with immigrants and reactivation of tuberculosis), occupation (e.g., barbers and interdigital sinuses[89]), immigrant status,[19] and recent travel.[37]

A history of contact with pigeons may suggest a diagnosis of cryptococcosis. A Thai immigrant's ingestion of contaminated pork may suggest a helminth infection. The initial appearance

TABLE 3.1   Etiology, Diagnosis, and Treatment of Chronic Infections of the Hand and Upper Extremity

	Organism	Predilection	Diagnosis	Chemotherapy
Bacteria	*Actinobacillus actinomycetemcomitans*	TS	Actinobacillosis	Ampicillin
	Actinomyces israelii	S, SC, J, B	Actinomycosis	Penicillin
	Bartonella henselae and *Bartonella quintana*	S	Bacillary angiomatosis/CSD	ERY
	Francisella tularensis	S	Tularemia	Streptomycin
	Nocardia species	S, SC, B	Mycetoma (actinomycetoma)	As per C&S
	Treponema pallidum	S, SC	Syphilis	Penicillin
	Treponema pertenue	S	Yaws	Penicillin
	Bacillus anthracis	S	Anthrax	Doxycycline
	Brucella	B, J	Brucellosis	RFM, TC
Fungi	*Aspergillus*	S, SC	Aspergillosis	AB, fluconazole
	Blastomyces dermatitidis	TS, B	Blastomycosis	AB, KTC
	Candida albicans	S, TS	Candidiasis	AB
	Coccidioides immitis	TS, J	Coccidioidomycosis	AB, miconazole
	Cryptococcus neoformans	TS	Cryptococcosis	AB
	Exophiala jeanselmei	Deep abscess	Chromohyphomycosis	None
	Histoplasma capsulatum	TS, J	Histoplasmosis	AB, KTC
	Madurella mycetomatis	S, SC	Mycetoma (eumycetoma)	As per C&S
	Rhizopus arrhizus	SC	Mucormycosis	AB
	Sporothrix schenckii	S, SC	Sporotrichosis	KTC, SSKI, AB
Mycobacterium leprae	*M. leprae*	N	Hansen disease	D, RFM, CFZ, ETH
Tuberculous mycobacteria	*M. tuberculosis*	S, TS, J, B	Typical tuberculosis	INH, RFM, ETH, PZA
	M. bovis	TS	Typical tuberculosis	INH, RFM, ETH, PZA
Nontuberculous mycobacteria	*M. asiaticum*	TS	Atypical tuberculosis	TC, CLAR
	M. avium (MAC or MAI)	SC, TS, J, B	Atypical tuberculosis	AZI, CLAR, ETH, RFB
	M. chelonae	TS	Atypical tuberculosis	AMK, ERY
	M. fortuitum	Deep abscess	Atypical tuberculosis	INH, RFM, MIN
	M. haemophilum	J	Atypical tuberculosis	
	M. kansasii	S, TS, J, B	Atypical tuberculosis	INH, RFM
	M. marinum	S, TS, J, B	Atypical tuberculosis	RFM, TC, MIN, AMK
	M. malmoense	TS, J	Atypical tuberculosis	INH, RFM, ETH, PZA
	M. szulgai	TS, BU	Atypical tuberculosis	INH, RFM, ETH, PZA
	M. terrae	S, SC, T, J	Atypical tuberculosis	ETH, CYCLO
Parasites (worms)	*Gnathostoma spinigerum*	SC	Gnathostomiasis	None
	Onchocerca volvulus	TS	Onchocerciasis	None
Prototheca	*Prototheca wickerhamii*	S, TS	Protothecosis	AB, TC
Protozoa	*Leishmania*	S	Leishmaniasis	Antimony, AB
Mites	*Sarcoptes scabiei*	S	Scabies	Permethrin cream
Viruses	HIV	CD4 lymphocyte	AIDS	NRTI/PI
	HPV	S (epidermis)	Warts (verruca vulgaris)	Topical salicylic acid
	Herpes simplex virus	S	Herpetic whitlow	Acyclovir
	Orf (paravaccinia) virus	S	Orf/milker's nodule	Cidofovir, imiquimod, idoxuridine cream

B, Bone; *BU*, bursa; *C&S*, culture and sensitivity; *CSD*, cat-scratch disease; *J*, joint; *MAC*, *Mycobacterium avium* complex; *MAI*, *Mycobacterium avium-intracellulare*; *N*, nerve; *S*, skin; *SC*, subcutaneous; *TS*, tenosynovium.
Chemotherapeutic drugs are abbreviated as follows: *AB*, amphotericin B; *AMK*, amikacin; *AZI*, azithromycin; *CFZ*, clofazimine; *CHL*, chloromycetin; *CLAR*, clarithromycin; *CYCLO*, cycloserine; *D*, dapsone; *ERY*, erythromycin; *ETH*, ethambutol; *GNT*, gentamicin; *INH*, isoniazid; *KTC*, ketoconazole; *MIN*, minocycline; *NRTI*, nucleoside reverse transcriptase inhibitor; *PI*, protease inhibitor; *PZA*, pyrazinamide; *RFB*, rifabutin (Mycobutin); *RFM*, rifampin (Rifadin); *SSKI*, supersaturated solution of potassium iodide; *Sulfa*, sulfonamides; *TC*, tetracycline.

of the lesion is nonspecific, and a lesion suspected to be an unusual tumor may be just a chronic infection.[54,58,88] Immunocompromised states that predispose patients to chronic hand infections include congenital hypogammaglobulinemia, HIV infection, organ transplantation, hematologic malignancies, pancytopenic anemia, systemic lupus erythematosus, and diabetes. Vascular compromise—that is, arterial injury, venous stasis, lymphangitis, severe scarring, radiation fibrosis—always increases the risk for infection.

The opposite is also true: one must suspect immunodeficiency when a certain fungus, for example, *Aspergillus*, *Cryptococcus*, *Pseudallescheria boydii*, or a Mucorales (formerly called Zygomycete), is encountered in a culture from an infected wound. An infective agent often lives in balance with an immunocompromised host. Reactivation of a latent organism in the hand can occur when malnutrition is present, cytotoxic chemotherapy is administered to treat a malignancy, and/or treatment with immunosuppressive agents (most commonly, corticosteroids) is initiated. Diagnosis is delayed until tissue (e.g., drainage, aspirate, punch biopsy, needle biopsy, open biopsy) is sent for a smear and cultured for bacteria (aerobic and anaerobic), mycobacteria (typical and atypical), and fungus.

Anaerobic organisms, such as *Actinomyces israelii* and *Nocardia* spp., do not grow well unless the specimen is properly transported to the laboratory in anaerobic medium. Organisms in chronic infections are often sparse, and they grow slowly (*M. tuberculosis* divides approximately every 24 h). Some organisms require a specific temperature for growth (e.g., *Sporotrichum schenckii*, *M. marinum*, *M. haemophilum*, *M. chelonae*, and *M. ulcerans* grow at 30°C; *M. xenopi* grows at 42°C). Some organisms do not grow at all unless ideal growth medium is provided (i.e., *M. haemophilum* requires hemoglobin). Improper collection, and/or delay in transportation of specimens, may impair growth of organisms and result in delayed treatment. There is no other area of clinical medicine where specimen selection, collection, and transportation are so important and in which close communication with the pathologist, microbiologist, and infectious disease specialist is imperative.

Laboratory Techniques

Five basic laboratory techniques can be used for the diagnosis of infectious diseases: (1) direct visualization of the organism under a microscope, (2) growth and isolation of the organism in culture, (3) serological testing by detection of microbial antigen and antimicrobial antibody, (4) detection of a specific microbial nucleotide sequence, and (5) gross and microscopic pathology. All require proper collection of the specimen and transportation to a laboratory as the following subsections detail.

Guidelines for Specimen Collection and Handling

The successful identification of a specific pathogen often depends on collection methods, transportation process, and laboratory algorithms suitable for various organisms and samples. The specimen must be kept moist and transported rapidly. In general, the more quickly a specimen is planted onto an appropriate medium, the better the chances for isolating bacterial pathogens. For ideal fungal cultures, specimens should be transported to the microbiology laboratory within 1 h of collection. If a delay is anticipated, the specimen

should be refrigerated until prompt next day delivery can be ensured. A sterile container, securely covered, is adequate; bacteriostatic saline or formalin should not be used for microbiology specimens. Biopsied tissue or pus is better as a specimen than swabs for routine anaerobic, mycobacterial, and fungal cultures.

The suspected pathogen must always be communicated to the microbiologist personally and in writing if other than routine bacteria are suspected (e.g., *Nocardia*, *Actinomyces*, *M. marinum*, *M. ulcerans*, *Sporothrix*, *Bartonella*). This facilitates the microbiologist's choice of the best incubation medium, temperature, and period. Because there are many pathogen-specific paradigms for collection–transportation procedures, it is recommended that the surgeon seek advice from the laboratory microbiologist when in doubt about a particular situation. It is absolutely essential that the microbiology laboratory be informed of the site of origin of the sample to be cultured, chronicity of the infection, and possible infectious agents suspected. This information determines the selection of culture medium, temperature of incubation, and the length of time to culture.

Swabs of superficial ulcers from the skin surface of a sinus tract or from open abscesses commonly yield a host of mixed bacterial flora and often do not reflect the organism's true infectious significance. For such infections, every effort should be made to biopsy tissue from the deeper aspects of the lesion or from the margins where the organisms are actively spreading. An adequate quantity of material should be obtained. At least 1 mL of fluid or a 1-g piece of tissue should be obtained for bacterial identification.

For mycobacterial identification, 10 mL of fluid or a tissue as large as possible should be obtained to compensate for the "paucibacillary" nature of the hand infection.[3] For example, swabs are not adequate to detect the sparse organisms of tuberculous infections. Characteristically, chronic lesions contain few organisms, so the swab is likely to obtain much serum and few organisms. To recover the most bacteria, mycobacteria, and fungi, a swab should never be submitted in lieu of curetting, biopsy material, or synovial fluid.

Tissue biopsy is more likely to show the infecting organisms than pus or necrotic detritus. If a swab is used, the patient's interests are best served by vigorous rather than gentle application of the swab to the target tissue. Biopsy from the undermined edge of an ulcer is far superior to a swab culture from the surface. Open biopsy is better than needle aspiration, punch biopsy, or superficial curettage of infected tissue. For meaningful culture results, laboratories prefer surgically obtained tissue samples, aspirates of closed abscesses, or a small amount of pus. Organism concentrations in synovial fluids and pus may be low, so as much fluid as possible should be obtained whenever mycetoma, mycobacterial, or fungal infection is a serious consideration. Specimens for smear and culture should be collected and transported in closed, leakproof, sterile containers.

Organisms are not uniformly distributed in infected tissue; thus, several parts of the lesion should be sampled for smears and cultures to find the infecting organism. Impression smears made by gently pressing a freshly cut surface of the tissue onto a slide increases the chance of organism identification and should be requested from the microbiology laboratory in addition to routine ground tissue smears. This is because tissue impression smears are easier to read and interpret than those made from material that has been ground or macerated. Gram stains, calcofluor-white, or potassium hydroxide (KOH) stains for fungi, and acid-fast stains for mycobacteria, can also be done on slide impression smears.

If results prove negative but signs and symptoms indicate otherwise, repetition of biopsy, smears, and cultures may be necessary. If antibiotic therapy has been initiated, a direct smear may be the only available guide to the etiology because growth may be inhibited. After biopsy, the tissue specimen is immediately bisected: half of it is sent to the pathologist in formalin, and the other half is sent promptly to the microbiologist for smears and cultures in a sterile container without formalin because it kills organisms.

An "eight-pack" tissue culture is sent to the microbiology laboratory for diagnosis (Table 3.2). The first three packs are sent immediately for staining: gram stain for bacteria, acid-fast stain for mycobacteria, and KOH or stains for fungi (Table 3.2). The next five packs are for cultures: two for aerobic and anaerobic bacteria, two for typical and atypical mycobacteria, and one for fungus. *M. marinum*, *M. haemophilum*, *M. ulcerans*, and *Sporothrix schenckii* grow best at 30°C. The rest of the mycobacteria grow best at 37°C; only one, *M. xenopi*, grows best at 42°C.

The microbiologist needs to know that the specimen is from a chronic lesion so that it can be incubated at an appropriate temperature. The microbiologist also should get the tissue fluid (i.e., pus, synovial fluid, serosanguineous exudate), whenever available, for eight-pack smears and cultures. The laboratory must know which antimicrobial agents, if any, the patient is taking. Whenever possible, the specimen is obtained before intraoperative antimicrobial agents are administered. A sterile

tube with a tight-fitting cap is adequate for transporting bodily fluids. A sterile bottle or a jar should be used to transport tissue specimens.

Tissue should be promptly forwarded to the laboratory. For chronic and unusual lesions, more often than not, I deliver the specimen to the microbiologist. This gives me an opportunity to communicate clinical history about the patient and tell the pathologist or microbiologist which organisms I am looking for. Fastidious organisms may not survive prolonged storage. Pus, fluid, and tissue should be placed into a transport vial in which anaerobes can survive for several hours in case the specimen is not delivered to the laboratory promptly. A simple way to collect and transport a fluid specimen, especially for anaerobes, is to aspirate at least 1 mL of it (pus, synovium) with a needle into a syringe, discharge any residual air at the top of the fluid, and seal off the syringe. It is important not to leave any air in the needle before sealing it.

Histoplasma capsulatum, *Cryptococcus neoformans*, *M. bovis*, *M. avium*, *Nocardia*, and *Bartonella* may take more than 6 weeks to grow, and it is imperative to request that the microbiology laboratory not discard the cultures for at least 4 weeks. *M. ulcerans* and *M. malmoense* may take 12 weeks to grow; so to cover all the organisms, I request that the microbiologist not discard the cultures for 12 weeks and to notify me as soon as growth is positive. It is a good idea to seek help from an infectious disease specialist who can closely follow the growth plates in the laboratory. In the care of immunocompromised patients or difficult diagnostic problems, numerous cultures or tests are often requested on the same specimen, for which there may be an inadequate quantity. The clinician should prioritize the test requests for the laboratory based on the highest clinical suspicions.

Four laboratory tests are used for identification of bacteria and mycobacteria: (1) direct visualization of the organism by staining, (2) detection of pathogenic-specific antigens and antibodies, (3) cultures in growth media, and (4) nucleic acid (DNA and RNA) amplification techniques. The fourth test is new and not widely available but is very useful for diagnosing stains, cultures, and serology tests and is very rapid.

Direct Visualization of the Organism by Staining

Gram staining is often the first step used by the hospital microbiology laboratory to identify an unknown bacterium from a clinical specimen. Gram stain differentiates between organisms with thick peptidoglycan cell walls (gram positive) and those with thin peptidoglycan cell walls that can be dissolved with acetone (gram negative). The sensitivity is such that >10^4 bacteria per mL are necessary for detection.

An acid-fast stain identifies organisms that retain red carbol fuchsin dye after washing with an acid-alcohol (i.e., "acid fast"). Ziehl-Neelsen and Kinyoun stains are carbol fuchsin-based and stain mycobacteria red. However, fluorescent stains are more sensitive for detection of mycobacteria in direct specimens. The organisms stain brightly and can be clearly distinguished from background material. Slides stained with a fluorescent dye can be examined reliably with an objective lens of lower magnification (×25′) than the oil immersion lens (×100′) required for carbol fuchsin-stained smears; in addition, reading slides is faster and more reliable. This stain is preferred by the Centers for Disease Control and Prevention (CDC). Modification of an

---

TABLE 3.2 The Eight-Pack Tissue Culture for Microbiology Covers Bacteria, Mycobacteria, and Fungi

Biopsy tissue is divided into two parts.
  I. Histopathology: 50% of tissue in formalin
  II. Microbiology: 50% of tissue *without* formalin is divided into 8 parts
Smear and stain
  1. Gram stain
  2. Acid-fast bacillus stain (Ziehl-Neelsen or Kinyoun)
  3. Fungus stains (potassium hydroxide or calcofluor-white stain)
Culture and sensitivity
  1. Aerobic (use transport medium, e.g., "Port-A-Cul™")
  2. Anaerobic (use transport medium, e.g., "Port-A-Cul")
  3. Tuberculous mycobacteria at 37°C
  4. Nontuberculous mycobacteria at 30°C (*M. marinum*) and 42°C (*M. xenopi*)
  5. Mycotic culture media (Sabouraud dextrose agar or brain–heart infusion agar)

This smear and culture protocol is useful for bacteria, mycobacteria, and fungi from the biopsy specimen. The circulating nurse sends half the biopsy specimen to the pathologist in formalin and the other half as an "eight pack" to the microbiologist in a sterile cup without formalin or saline. The specimen is delivered to the microbiologist immediately at the conclusion of surgery.

acid-fast stain also allows detection of *Actinomyces, Nocardia,* and other weakly acid-fast organisms.

Detection of Pathogenic-Specific Antigens and Antibodies (Serology)

Biochemical methods are used to detect the antigens of newer mycobacterial species from cultures. Diagnosis of cryptococcosis is confirmed by a high cryptococcal antigen titer in the purulent discharge from a cryptococcal skin ulcer. Measurement of serum antibody (i.e., IgG or IgM) provides an indirect marker for past or current infection with a specific pathogen. Testing for the presence of antibody has been successfully used for diagnosis of coccidioidomycosis and histoplasmosis in infections of the hand and elsewhere.

Detection of Specific Microbial Nucleotide Sequences

Nucleic acid amplification technology (i.e., detection and quantitation of specific DNA and RNA base sequences in clinical specimens) has gained widespread use and has become a rapid and powerful tool for diagnosis of viral, bacterial, mycobacterial, fungal, and parasitic infections. The use of nucleic acid tests generally involves lysis of intact cells and denaturation of DNA or RNA to render it single-stranded. Probes, that is, primer sequences complementary to pathogen specific base sequences, then detect the pathogen-specific sequences. Use of nucleic acid polymerase chain reaction (PCR) analysis allows very rapid DNA sequence analysis and direct identification of *M. tuberculosis* in clinical specimens. PCR can detect <10 organisms/mL in a clinical specimen, compared with 100 for cultures and the 10,000 necessary for a positive smear.

PCR analysis provides a useful method when a smear and culture are negative in the presence of a clinical presentation of tuberculosis (TB). The test is generally accessible but is skill-intense and expensive. The potential for nucleic acid amplification testing (i.e., PCR) to enhance patient care is greatest when suspicion of TB is moderate to high and specimens are acid-fast bacillus (AFB) smear negative. At least 2 g of tissue are necessary to do this test. The tissue should be set aside and preserved in 70% alcohol for later processing in case conventional smear and culture tests prove negative.

Two commercial DNA probes approved by the Food and Drug Administration (FDA) are available for the detection of organisms in the *M. tuberculosis* complex. They are used with organisms grown in culture as well as directly on patient specimens. The procedure can be performed and the organism identified within a matter of hours from the time an infection is suspected. Conventional cultures for TB generally take many weeks.

Organism Isolation in Culture and Drug-Susceptibility Testing

Several quantitative studies have shown that a minimum of 10,000 bacilli/mL of specimen is necessary to detect bacteria in stained smears. When host immunity is high and bacterial virulence is low, infected tissue may have far less organisms per mL. In such cases, acid-fast staining may be negative. In contrast, <100 organisms are necessary to grow in culture. Green and Adams suggested that when investigating chronic infections, tissue samples be cultured on blood agar, a Lowenstein-Jensen medium, and a Sabouraud glucose agar.

These three media should allow growth of most bacteria, mycobacteria, and fungi.[44] It is important that the clinician notify the laboratory if a pathogen with specific growth requirements is suspected so that special culturing media can be used. *M. haemophilum* grows best in a selective agar medium enriched with hemoglobin. A major improvement in mycobacteriology has been the development of commercial broth systems that allow for rapid growth and detection of mycobacteria within 1 to 3 weeks, compared to solid media in which growth takes 3 to 8 weeks.

Drug-Susceptibility Tests

Drug-susceptibility tests are performed on initial isolates from all patients with suspected TB to identify what should be an effective drug regimen. To generate rapid testing and faster turnaround time for better patient management, the radiometric BACTEC™ system is used to test the sensitivity of all primary antituberculous drugs (i.e., isoniazid, rifampin, pyrazinamide, and ethambutol).

Additional Evaluation

Isolation of *Aspergillus* or *Nocardia* from a patient without a known immunodeficiency should trigger a workup for an underlying host immune defect. Such a workup should include, at a minimum, evaluation of B cell-mediated humoral immunity (serum immunoglobulins and isohemagglutinins) and T cell–mediated cellular immunity (CBC count and differential, absolute lymphocyte count, peripheral smear, platelet count, and erythrocyte sedimentation rate). The most common cause of immunodeficiency currently is acquired immunodeficiency syndrome (AIDS). AIDS and iatrogenic deficiencies that result from therapies that modulate the immune system (e.g., corticosteroids, posttransplant immunosuppression, and cytotoxic chemotherapy for malignancies) are leading causes of chronic infections. Primary (congenital) immunodeficiency syndrome associated with a hand infection is rare but has been reported.[114]

An algorithm for requesting stains and cultures of biopsy material is useful in the operating room. When tenosynovitis, synovitis, or osteomyelitis is encountered during biopsy, the responsible organism is generally not discernible because the infected tissue does not have pathognomonic characteristics. Rice bodies may be found in rheumatoid arthritis, TB, and fungal infections (e.g., coccidioidomycosis, histoplasmosis, and sporotrichosis). Certain types of tenosynovitis have a high tendency of recurrence unless radical surgical excision is combined with appropriate antibiotics such as in the following infections: actinomycosis, sporotrichosis, coccidioidomycosis, *M. terrae,* and *M. avium.* Thus, complete synovectomy is reasonable at the time of biopsy or surgery because this will reduce the microbial burden for subsequent antibiotic treatment.

An exception to this approach is when the diagnosis of tuberculosis is endemic in a country (e.g., India, Hong Kong) or is known, such as in a patient with positive stains from pus, exudate, synovial fluid, sputum, or gastric washings for mycobacteria. The excised synovium should be sent for special stains (i.e., methenamine silver stains are common to many fungi) and cultures at three temperatures: *M. marinum, M. chelonae, M. hemophilum,* and *Sporothrix schenckii* grow best at 30°C;

M. xenopi at 42°C; and the rest at 37°C. *M. avium, M. fortuitum, M. terrae,* and *M. chelonae* require prolonged incubation, and some require special media—*M. hemophilum* grows only in a hemoglobin-reinforced medium, *M. malmoense* requires a pyruvate-containing medium, and *A. actinomycetemcomitans* grows in the presence of CO_2 and an aerobic as well as anaerobic environment. *Actinomyces* spp. and *Nocardia* spp. grow only in anaerobic media.

Treatment

In the war between humans and microbes, the outcome depends on the dose and virulence of the microbe and the immunity of the host. Antibiotics reduce the quantity of the invading organisms, but final elimination of them is determined by innate immunity—that is, phagocytes (neutrophils and macrophages), natural killer lymphocytes, proteins and enzymes of a complement system, and cytokines—and two arms of acquired immunity: humoral and cell mediated. Humoral immunity is conferred by B lymphocytes, which mature to plasma cells and produce immunoglobulin antibodies (i.e., IgG, IgA, IgM, IgE, IgD) that eliminate extracellular organisms. Cell-mediated immunity is mediated by T lymphocyte helper cells (CD4$^+$ T lymphocytes). The helper cells facilitate activation of phagocytes and destroy ingested microbes, and T lymphocyte cytotoxic cells (CTLs = CD^{8+} T lymphocytes) eliminate intracellular organisms by killing the cells that harbor them. Eosinophils produce antibodies against multicellular parasites, and eosinophilia is pathognomonic of a parasitic infection.

When humoral and cellular immunity is depressed, it is critical that three important components of treatment be implemented: antibiotics, surgical debridement of the infected tissue, and improved nutrition. Poor nutrition, whether from alcoholism, cancer, major trauma, or inadequate diet, predisposes the patient to infections that would otherwise be easily combated by healthy individuals. When a patient is therapeutically immunosuppressed and does not respond to adequate antibiotic therapy and surgical debridement, a reduction in immunosuppressive therapy and an improvement in nutrition may upgrade the host immunity to successfully combat the invading organisms (Table 3.3).

CHRONIC BACTERIAL INFECTIONS

Actinomycosis, botryomycosis, brucellosis, mycetoma (actinomycetoma, eumycetoma), syphilis, and yaws are rare chronic bacterial infections that have been reported to sporadically affect the hand and upper extremity. A newly emerging septic tenosynovitis of the hand is recognized to be caused by actinobacillosis. Pyoderma gangrenosum and neutrophilic dermatoses, although not infectious, are included in this section because (1) they mimic a fulminating infection that will become chronic if incorrectly diagnosed; (2) if mistakenly treated by surgery, the condition gets worse; and (3) oral prednisone remarkably and rapidly cures the conditions. With surgery, pyoderma gangrenosum spreads furiously and centrifugally (so-called pathergic reaction) and has even led to unnecessary amputations. It is important to recognize cutaneous anthrax because it has become a bioterrorism method since the 9/11 attack.

TABLE 3.3   **Ten Factors That Improve the Outcome of Chronic Infection Treatment**
1. The initial appearance of the lesion is nonspecific. Early diagnosis is made if early biopsy is done.
2. Beware of immunocompromised states, which predispose patients to chronic hand infections and may require higher doses of medication. Management of immunosuppressed patients may require upscaling antibiotic therapy and nutrition and downscaling immunosuppressive therapy to control infection.
3. Biopsy specimen should be sent to the microbiology laboratory in a sterile container.
4. Pathology specimen only should be sent in formalin.
5. Alert microbiology staff of the possibility of a chronic infection; they will require special media and may hold cultures for 12 weeks or more, especially in suspected cases of mycobacteria, fungus, or mycetoma.
6. Early consultation with an infectious disease specialist will optimize proper management of specimens and follow-up.
7. Eight-pack tissue for histopathology and cultures improves diagnostic probability (gram stain, acid-fast, KOH, aerobic, anaerobic, mycobacteria, atypical mycobacteria, fungus).
8. Request the laboratory to do cultures at 30°C (*M. marinum, M. chelonae, M. hemophilum, M. ulcerans,* and sporotrichosis), at 37°C (*M. tuberculosis*), and at 42°C (*M. xenopi*).
9. Request special media for cultures as necessary (*M. hemophilum* grows only in a hemoglobin-reinforced medium; *M. malmoense* requires a pyruvate-containing medium, actinomycetemcomitans grows in the presence of CO_2) and anaerobic environment. Actinomyces and *Nocardia* spp. grow only in anaerobic media.
10. Chemotherapy management is best done in conjunction with an infectious disease specialist because of varied and serious drug toxicity and emerging resistance to multiple drugs.

Actinobacillosis

Actinobacillosis is caused by *Actinobacillus actinomycetemcomitans,* a gram-negative bacillus that is part of the endogenous flora of the mouth and can be obtained from about 20% of teenagers and adults. It occurs in association with *A. israelii,* and it behooves physicians to look for the latter when found in infected tissue. *Actinobacillus* infections have emerged only recently.

Clinical Findings

A. actinomycetemcomitans may cause chronic tenosynovitis of dorsal wrist tendons or finger flexor tendons. After an assault, a deep hand laceration from a tooth may cause recurrent abscesses and a draining sinus at the site of original trauma in an adult patient. X-rays may show chronic osteitis of the injured metacarpal.

Diagnosis

Pus from a draining sinus may yield profuse growth of *A. actinomycetemcomitans* if grown in the presence of CO_2. Otherwise, it is difficult to grow and identify the organism.

Treatment

Incision, drainage, and ampicillin may completely eliminate the infection. Tenosynovectomy and intravenous gentamicin or oral tetracycline may also resolve the infection without further recurrence.

Actinomycosis

Etiology and Epidemiology

Actinomycosis is most commonly caused by *Actinomyces israelii*, a normal inhabitant of the oral cavity. Actinomycosis, by definition, is caused by endogenous human flora while actinomycetoma, described later, is caused by exogenous pathogenic bacteria in soil. Two percent of actinomycosis cases occur in the upper extremity. Most cases of hand actinomycosis have been noted sporadically in case reports.

Clinical Findings

In the hand, a closed-fist injury or a bite is the most common cause of actinomycosis. Oral flora may be implanted over the metacarpophalangeal joint or the metacarpal head on impact. This type of injury is designated as "punch actinomycosis." A dentist can contact it during examination of the mouth without gloves.

Clinical presentations are varied. In the early stages it may appear as nonspecific, painful induration, or as a nontender, mobile nodule. The nodule may later form a draining sinus. Any suppurative inflammatory reaction that stubbornly resists treatment and tends to discharge continuously should lead one to suspect the possibility of actinomycosis, especially if it is at the site of a human bite wound. It may start as an acute abscess, or there may be a painless and persistent swelling of the hand after the acute inflammation from the initial trauma subsides. Subcutaneous tissue may become indurated and adherent to subjacent bone. It may present as a recurrent swelling with sinuses that intermittently discharge purulent fluid.[100] When tendon sheaths are involved, purulent material may contain melon seeds, as in tuberculosis and fungus infections. A recurrent fluctuating palmar abscess may occur.

Once actinomycosis is established locally, it spreads contiguously in a slow but progressive manner, ignoring tissue planes. In the forearm, it may arise as a mass from hematogenous spread and can masquerade as a soft tissue neoplasm. Finally, contiguous invasion of subjacent bones occurs. The bones of the hand and wrist may have cystic and sclerotic or lytic changes. Isolated actinomycosis osteomyelitis is rare and may occur in the proximal phalanx or metacarpal. Infectious destruction may even cross from the dorsal-to-palmar or palmar-to-dorsal side of the hand. Infection of the upper arm can occur but is rare. Axillary nodes may become enlarged.

Diagnosis

The identification of "yellow sulfur granules" of actinomycosis organisms from a draining sinus or pus from an abscess is diagnostic. Sulfur granules are a yellow conglomeration of microorganisms that form only in vivo and characteristically are identified in bandages that cover a draining sinus. Biopsy is necessary to obtain clinical material for diagnosis if a draining sinus is not present. A specimen must be sent and cultured in anaerobic media. Cultures are positive in only 25% of the cases, perhaps because the specimen was not sent to the laboratory in anaerobic media. Histopathology of infected tissue shows the characteristic organisms and diagnosis can be firmly made in the absence of positive cultures.[80]

Treatment

Penicillin is the treatment of choice. Intravenous penicillin must be employed in high doses for several weeks followed by oral penicillin or amoxicillin for 6 to 12 months. Short-term treatment with antibiotics may result in temporary cessation of drainage. When the therapy is discontinued, however, drainage may recur. Without definitive treatment, the infection can persist for several decades and cause extensive deformities. For penicillin-allergic patients, tetracycline, erythromycin, minocycline, and clindamycin are alternatives. If infection recurs, surgical debridement is an essential component of further antibiotic treatment.

Anthrax

Etiology and Epidemiology

In the United States, the annual incidence of anthrax exposure declined from 130 cases in the early to mid 1900s to a single case reported in 1992. It reappeared in the United States as a bioterrorism method in 2001. Ten cases of cutaneous anthrax and 10 cases of pulmonary anthrax (four fatal) were reported within a month after September 11. Of the numerous biologic agents that may be used as weapons, anthrax is one of the most devastating.

Anthrax infection is caused by *Bacillus anthracis*, a grampositive, encapsulated, spore-forming bacillus. The name *anthrax* (Gk. *anthracis*, "coal") refers to the typical black eschar that is seen on affected areas. Ninety-five percent of patients with cutaneous anthrax are diagnosed when they have a relatively painless necrotic black ulcer. Humans can acquire the disease directly from contact with infected herbivores (i.e., agricultural anthrax); indirectly from contaminated meat, wool, hides, or leather from infected animals (i.e., industrial anthrax), through accidental inoculation in the laboratory (i.e., laboratory-acquired anthrax); or unexpectedly from exposure to "weaponized" spores of bioterrorism (i.e., biocriminal anthrax). The clinical forms include (1) cutaneous anthrax, which accounts for more than 95% of cases; (2) intestinal anthrax, from eating infected meat; and (3) pulmonary anthrax, from inhaling spore-laden dust. Cutaneous anthrax of the hand and upper extremity occurs in approximately one-third of all cases in an epidemic and may be presented to a hand surgeon primarily.

Clinical Findings

Cutaneous anthrax occurs after the deposition of the organism into the skin at the site of a previous cut or abrasion. The lesion may occur on a finger or hand. After an incubation period of 3 days (range, 1-12 days), the skin infection begins as an area of local edema that becomes a pruritic macule or papule. The papule progresses to a vesicle or vesicles, surrounded by erythema, in 1 to 2 days. The vesicle contains clear or bluish fluid (Figure 3.1). Patients may have a fever and regional lymphadenopathy. The vesicles rupture in 2 to 14 days and leave behind a painless black skin ulcer that becomes a black eschar (Figure 3.2). The eschar contracts into an ulcer, usually 1 to 3 cm in diameter, with small, 1- to 3-mm vesicles surrounding the ulcer. A characteristic black necrotic center develops by 4 weeks, often associated with extensive local edema. Unless the disease becomes systemic, the eschar dries, loosens, and falls off in the next 1 to 2 weeks. A lesion on the finger may heal with full mobility. The common clinical description "malignant

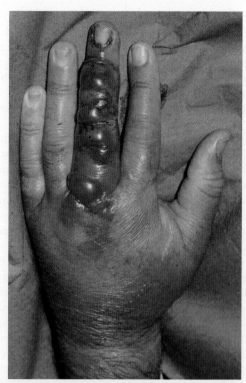

FIGURE 3.1 The initial lesion of cutaneous anthrax is a vesicle or vesicles surrounded by erythema. The vesicle contains clear or bluish fluid.

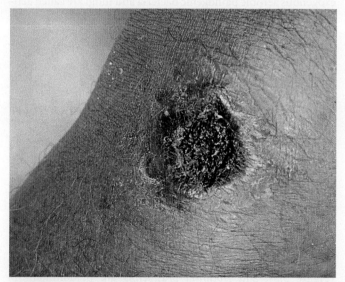

FIGURE 3.2 An anthrax skin ulcer has a black central necrosis. The local lesion is painless but the regional lymph nodes may be enlarged and tender. (From Habif TP: *Clinical dermatology: a color guide to diagnosis and therapy*, ed 5. Philadelphia, 2010, Elsevier; Figure A-3, with permission.)

pustule" is actually a misnomer because the cutaneous lesion is not purulent.

Diagnosis

Anthrax exposure is diagnosed by isolating *B. anthracis* from the vesicular fluid of skin lesions. Gram-staining reveals bacilli in the subcutaneous tissue.

Treatment

About 20% of untreated cases of cutaneous anthrax become systemic and result in death. Antibiotic therapy does not appear to change the course of eschar formation and healing; however, it does decrease the likelihood of systemic disease and death. When treated with appropriate antibiotics, the death rate is <1% and lesions resolve without complications or scarring in 80 to 90% of cases. It is rare for the black eschar on the hand to extend deeper than the dermis and over the whole of the hand's dorsum and distal forearm; if it does, soft tissue coverage may be required.[23] The eschar may extend down to the muscle fascia. In these cases, the eschar is excised, and the defect is grafted using split-thickness skin grafts. Deep eschars in the forearm have been identified to cause severe compression neuropathy of superficial nerves.

Duration of antibiotic treatment for animal-acquired and bioterrorism-acquired anthrax differs. Animal-acquired anthrax is treated with doxycycline (100 mg PO bid), ciprofloxacin (750 mg bid), or amoxicillin (500 mg tid) orally for 7 to 10 days. Lesions become sterile within 24 h and resolve within weeks. Direct person-to-person spread of anthrax is extremely unlikely. There is no need therefore to treat contacts of infected individuals unless they were also exposed to the same primary source of infection. Bioterrorism-acquired anthrax is classified either as anthrax exposure or anthrax infection. Both exposure and infection are treated for 60 days because aerosol inhalation of anthrax is presumed in instances of bioterrorism.

The case fatality rate of 11 treated cases of an inhalational bioterrorism event in 2001 was 45%.[57] A bioterrorist event should be reported to www.bt.cdc.gov, a website that also provides information about clinical diagnosis and management of anthrax and all agents of bioterrorism. In the United States, anthrax vaccine is recommended only for high-risk populations, including military combat personnel, persons who work directly with the organism in a laboratory, those who work with imported animal hides or furs, or those who handle potentially infected animal products in high-incidence areas.

Botryomycosis

Etiology and Epidemiology

Botryomycosis is a rare, chronic, granulomatous, suppurative, bacterial skin and subjacent soft tissue infection that produces loose clumps of bacteria that resemble grains. Among more than 100 cases of botryomycosis reported in the literature, three cases affecting the hand have been identified. The characteristic histologic finding of "granules" in clusters is the origin for the term *botryomycosis* (Gk. *botrys*, "bunch of grapes" in histology; mycosis for its clinical and histologic resemblance to fungal infection). The condition is in fact produced by bacteria and is truly a "granular bacteriosis." *Staphylococcus aureus*, *Pseudomonas vesicularis*, *Moraxella nonliquefasciens*, and tuberculosis have been reported to cause botryomycosis of the hand. The first case of tuberculous botryomycosis was reported in 2014 and was cured by antituberculous chemotherapy.[109]

Diagnosis

Clinically, histologically, and therapeutically this bacterial infection resembles a fungal one.

Treatment

The condition may respond rapidly to oral antibiotics, or it may be resistant to antibiotic therapy and need complete excision and skin grafting to eradicate the infection.

Brucellosis

Etiology and Epidemiology

Brucellosis is named after Sir David Bruce (1855-1931), the Scottish physician who identified the bacterium. Brucellae are gram-negative coccobacilli that chronically infect animals. Virtually all human infections derive from direct or indirect contact with cattle (*B. abortus*) or goats and sheep (*B. melitensis*). Routes of transmission to humans include cuts in the skin, inhalation of infected aerosols, and ingestion of unpasteurized milk. Brucellosis is endemic in the Middle East, South America, and the Mediterranean area. In Texas and California, the epidemiology of brucellosis has changed from a disease associated with exposure to cattle to one linked to ingestion of unpasteurized goat's milk products imported from Mexico.

Clinical Findings

The musculoskeletal system was affected in approximately one-third of 169 cases.[84] Osteomyelitis and septic arthritis involved the upper extremity. Septic arthritis occurred in the sternoclavicular joint in three cases (1.8%), shoulders in eight (5%), elbows in nine (5.3%), and wrists in six (3.5%). Osteomyelitis occurred in four (2.4%) and tendinitis was noted in one (1.2%). Dactylitis may occur with or without osteoarticular brucellosis.

Diagnosis

Diagnosis is made when blood culture or bone needle aspiration culture grow *B. melitensis*. Chronic brucellar olecranon bursitis may occur when synovial fluid and serum are positive for serologic tests and *B. melitensis* grows on chocolate agar.

Treatment

Repeated 4- to 6-week courses of rifampin and tetracycline may cure the patient without a relapse.

Mycetoma (Actinomycetoma and Eumycetoma)

Etiology and Epidemiology

Mycetoma is a twofold disease complex, caused either by large filamentous bacteria (actinomycetoma) or by fungi (eumycetoma) (synonyms: maduromycosis, Madura foot). Eumycetoma is so named because it is caused by the eumycetes group of fungi. Predictably, fungal eumycetoma is more invasive and more difficult to treat than bacterial actinomycetoma. Mycetoma is characterized by a slowly evolving, often painless, cutaneous and subcutaneous destructive inflammatory granuloma, riddled with abscesses; sinuses with interconnecting channels; and fistulas that drain characteristic colonies of the infecting organisms in the form of grains and granules.

The grains are dense clusters of organisms and are the defining characteristic of this infection. The granules, colonies of the organisms, occur in a triad of chronic infections: mycetoma (eumycetoma and actinomycetoma), actinomycosis, and botryomycosis. Only 2 to 12% of all mycetomas involve the hands, whereas the majority (70%) occur in the feet. Twenty-one cases

of the hand and arm were reviewed by Moore in 1954,[82] and since then several more hand cases have been reported. In only three recent cases was the disease diagnosed early at a nodular or abscess stage. In all other cases, diagnosis was delayed until it was in the sinusoidal or musculoskeletal stage; therefore, treatment was difficult.

A mycetoma caused by aerobic bacteria, *Actinomyces* spp., is referred to as actinomycetoma. *Actinomyces* spp. are "higher" bacteria with morphologic characteristics between bacteria and fungi. The majority of actinomycetomas in North America are caused by *Pseudallescheria boydii* (its asexual anamorph is *Scedosporium apiospermum*; previous names, *Allescheria* and *Monosporium*). *Nocardia* is another cause of mycetoma in the hand. It is important not to misdiagnose it as actinomycosis on gross and microscopic examination because of the presence of granules in both.[9]

A mycetoma caused by true fungi is referred to as eumycetoma, true mycetoma, maduromycosis, or Madura foot—named after Madura from South India where the first cases were described. More than 30 fungi are known to cause eumycetoma. Distinguishing mycetomas caused by the *Actinomyces* spp. bacteria (actinomycetoma) and fungi (eumycetoma) is extremely important. Actinomycetoma and eumycetoma both clinically look the same but the treatment and prognosis for the two are distinctly different. In contemporary medical mycology, actinomycosis is not classified as an actinomycetoma because the etiologic agents of actinomycosis are anaerobic and endogenous in the oral flora. Conventionally, only infections caused by exogenous aerobic pathogenic bacteria and fungi are called actinomycetoma and eumycetoma. This clearly differentiates actinomycosis from actinomycetoma.

Microbiology

Mycetoma of the hand has been reported to occur from a wide variety of organisms; many of them are being reported for the first time. Major mycetoma bacteria and fungi are found all over the world and are associated with woody plants and soil. The largest number of infected patients live in the tropics. In the United States, several cases of hand mycetoma have been reported, and they are equally divided between actinomycetoma and eumycetoma. Agents of mycetoma differ in various parts of the world. The most common cause of eumycetoma in the United States is *Pseudallescheria boydii* (asexual anamorph, *Scedosporium apiospermum*; previous names *Allescheria*, *Monosporium*, *Petriellidium*) and of actinomycetoma is *Nocardia*. *Madurella mycetomatis*, *Actinomadura madurae* (Figure 3.3), and *Nocardia brasiliensis* are predominant in India. *N. brasiliensis* and *A. madurae* are the most common causes of mycetoma in Mexico and Central and South America. Actinomycetomas represent 97% of mycetomas in Mexico, and 87% of them are caused by *Nocardia brasiliensis*. *Streptomyces somaliensis* and *Actinomadura pelletieri* are seen in Africa. *N. asteroides* and *Scedosporium apiospermum* are reported to predominate in Japan.

A case of hand eumycetoma caused by *Arthrographis kalrae* was reported in Japan and was successfully treated with itraconazole. A case of *S. somaliensis* hand actinomycetoma was reported in the United Kingdom and was sensitive to and treated with co-trimoxazole (trimethoprim/sulfamethoxazole,

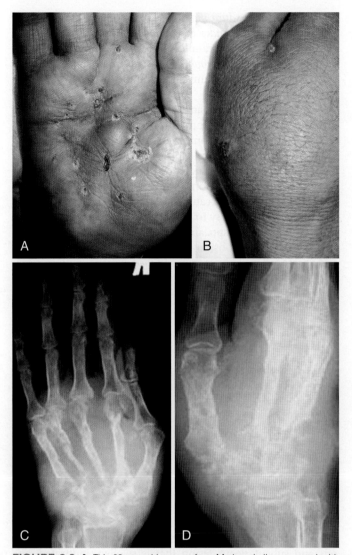

FIGURE 3.3 A, This 62-year-old woman from Madura, India, presented with a 7-year history of draining sinuses of the right hand several weeks after a scorpion bite. Multiple courses of antibiotics and other treatments helped transiently. Multiple healed sinuses in various stages can be seen on the indurated palm. **B,** Infection crosses over to the dorsum of the hand. A culture grew *Actinomadura madurae*. **C, D,** As the infection crosses from palmar side to dorsal side of the hand, osteomyelitis of the carpals and metacarpals is evident, characterized by sclerosis and lysis of bone.

Bactrim) and streptomycin. A case of actinomycetoma of the hand caused by *Gordona terrae* was reported in the Netherlands and was cured in two weeks by only doxycycline. *Phialophora jeanselmei* (*Torula jeanselmei*) hand eumycetoma was reported in Thailand. *Aspergillus nidulans* rarely causes eumycetoma of the upper extremity. *Leptosphaeria tompkinsii* is a dematiaceous fungus that is rarely reported as an agent of black-grain mycetoma. The first case of mycetoma caused by *Nocardia caviae* was reported in Brazil. At times, granules are identified in the lesion but fail to grow organisms and identification by a polymerase chain reaction is needed. In rare instances, the bacteriological origin of mycetoma cannot be ascertained.

Clinical Findings

A mycetoma is a characteristic clinical triad of tumification, draining sinuses, and granules in the discharging pus in the distal aspect of a limb. Swelling is woody and indurated (tumification), and multiple sinus tracts drain grain-filled pus; the grains are the infecting organisms. Old sinuses heal and new may grow. Characteristic grains in draining sinuses are 0.2 to 5.0 mm in diameter and may be black, white, yellow, pink, or red, depending on the causal organism. Grains may be difficult to locate in histopathologic sections and require multiple cuts through the paraffin-embedded tissue.

Mycetoma, regardless of fungal or bacterial origin, has a similar clinical presentation. The majority of the patients are males between 30 and 60 years old. The male-to-female ratio is 5 : 1. It is rare in children, and most that occur in children (80%) are eumycetoma. The disease begins following the traumatic implantation of the etiologic agent from the soil, thorn, or wood splinter into a bare hand of a healthy person. The lesions may be restricted to a finger, palm, dorsum of the hand, dorsum of the wrist, forearm, or upper arm. The lesion may be on both sides of the hand when the infection crosses the metacarpals from the dorsal-to-volar or from the volar-to-dorsal side of the hand.

Mycetomal infection begins in the skin and subcutaneous tissues as a nodule or nodules. Mycetoma tends to follow fascial planes as it spreads proximally and laterally, and with increasing depth, it progressively infects and destroys all connective tissues and eventually bone (see Figure 3.3). In the end, the untreated hand is deformed and functionless.

The annual incidence of nocardiosis in the United States has been estimated to be between 500 and 1000 cases, with 36% being cutaneous nocardiosis. The genus *Nocardia* comprises gram-positive, aerobic, acid-fast, and filamentous bacteria of which *N. brasiliensis* is usually associated with cutaneous and subcutaneous infection. The spectrum of nocardiosis of the hand manifests clinically as one of three types: (1) an acute infection consisting of cellulitis or abscesses; (2) lymphocutaneous infection with marching lymphangitis (sporotrichoid infection); (3) typical actinomycetoma stage I with nodules, stage II with purulent A0 or nonpurulent sinuses, stage III with spread to subjacent, and stage IV with metastasis proximal to the limb.

Staging

Mycetoma of the hand has been graded into five stages. Initially, the lesion is a small, firm, painless subcutaneous nodule or nodules under the skin (duration 2-3 months), which may grow to a large size (nodular, stage I). Nodules become abscesses and drain granules through sinuses to the surface of the skin or to the surface of an ulcerated nodule (duration 4-12 months) (sinusoidal, stage II). Sinuses may close after pus and granules have been discharged. Old sinuses heal and new ones crop up. If left untreated, the infection progresses to osteomyelitis (see Figures 3.3, C,D; skeletal, stage III).

Finally, limb deformity occurs over the course of a year or more (skeletal, stage IV). Lesions of the hand may metastasize to the axilla and the chest wall (metastatic, stage V). Radiographic signs include thinning of the metacarpals, bone erosions, sclerosis, and periostitis (see Figures 3.3. A,D). A network of connected sinuses is present in the soft tissues from the bone to the skin. Hand mycetoma has been reported to extend through the lymphatics to the chest wall and to the lung after many years (metastatic stage). Constitutional symptoms are absent unless there is superimposed bacterial infection. Pain is not a predominant symptom.

The patient, usually an immigrant, a rural farmer, or a laborer of lower socioeconomic status, postpones seeking medical care until the second or third stage is reached. Granules, which are aggregates of the organism, are discharged through the sinuses. Eventually, the hand and forearm become grossly enlarged, nodular, discolored, indurated, and deformed, although the patient may experience little pain or tenderness. The progression of the disease is marked by remissions and exacerbations. The period necessary for the development of the deformity varies from several months to several years. The extent of soft tissue invasion (staging) may be best evaluated with magnetic resonance imaging (MRI).

Diagnosis

Hematoxylin and eosin stain is adequate to detect the grains. Tissue-gram staining detects fine, branching hyphae within the bacteria of actinomycetoma grain, and Gomori methenamine silver, or periodic acid–Schiff stain detects the larger hyphae of fungus of eumycetoma. Species of the agent can often be recognized by the color, size, compaction, and hematoxylin-staining character of the grains when organisms fail to grow. *Actinomyces* spp. are recognized as 0.5 to 1 μm filaments and fungi by 2 to 5 μm wide hyphae. Culture should be held for at least 4 weeks.

A more exact species diagnosis is made by microscopic observation and culture of a grain, which must be as free as possible from bacterial and fungal contamination. A deep-tissue, wedge-shaped biopsy provides a good specimen for both histological and microbiologic diagnosis and avoids the bacterial contamination of surface cultures. A better strategy is the aspiration of grains directly from an unopened sinus tract because evaluation of spontaneously extruded grains may be composed of dead organisms and contaminated bacteria. Fungi that cause eumycotic mycetoma can be difficult to grow; optimizing growth is an important step. Before being inoculated onto a culture medium, the grains should be rinsed quickly in 70% alcohol and washed several times in sterile saline to eliminate contaminating bacteria.

Biopsy specimens are preferred over discharged grains because such grains may be contaminated with surface organisms or the infecting organism may already be dead. For primary isolation, actinomycetoma grains are grown on a Lowenstein-Jensen medium and fungal grains on blood agar. Sabouraud agar without antibacterial antibiotics is satisfactory for subcultures.

Two sets of cultures are prepared: one is inoculated at 37°C and the other at 26°C. Characteristic colonies are expected to develop within 10 days. Apart from *M. mycetomatis*, which secretes a brown pigment in the medium, all other organisms, both bacteria and fungi, tend to maintain the color of the original grain. Bacterial colonies are usually granular or cribriform, whereas fungal colonies are either velvety or fluffy. Further identification is made by microscopic examination of fungi in a lacto phenol blue preparation and of bacteria in gram and modified Ziehl-Neelsen stains. Actinomycotic granules may

be white (*Actinomadura madurae*), pink, or red (*A. pelletieri*); yellow (*Nocardia asteroides*, *Streptomyces somaliensis*); or orange (*N. asteroides*). Black granules are always eumycotic (*Leptosphaeria senegalensis*, *Exophilia jeanselmei*, *Madurella grisea*, *M. mycetomatis*), but eumycotic granules may also be pale (*Pseudallescheria boydii*).

In histologic sections stained with hematoxylin and eosin, involved tissue reveals a suppurative granuloma. Grains are seen embedded in an abscess composed of neutrophils accompanied by an outer epithelioid cell, plasma cell, and multinucleated giant cell reaction intermingled with areas of fibrosis. The size of various grains in sections is so characteristic that it allows specific diagnosis of the causative organism. Eumycetic hyphae within the grain are easy to see at 400× magnification, whereas those of *Actinomyces* spp. are difficult to visualize even at ×800. In electron micrographs, concentric rings of cell wall thickening and coarse cell wall fibrils around cells are seen within eumycetic grains. When stains, cultures, and histology do not help and clinical suspicion is significant, diagnosis is achieved using a panfungal polymerase chain reaction and sequencing technology.

CRITICAL POINTS *For Diagnosis of Mycetoma*

- Obvious grains should be collected and washed in alcohol to eliminate bacterial contamination.
- Deep wedge biopsy is better than collecting superficial exudate and grains.
- Request hematoxylin-eosin stain for *Actinomyces* spp.
- Request acid–Schiff stain for fungi.

Differential Diagnosis

Tentative diagnosis is made in the presence of a chronic cutaneous and subcutaneous lesion that is swollen, indurated, and riddled with nodules, abscesses, sinuses, and fistulas that discharge granules. Grains are seen in actinomycosis, botryomycosis, actinomycetoma, and eumycetoma. The linear, marching lymphangitis typical of *Nocardia* infection can also be seen with infections caused by *Sporothrix*, *M. marinum*, *M. kansasii*, *Leishmania*, *Coccidioides*, *Cryptococcus*, lupus vulgaris, and tularemia.

Treatment

The success of treatment depends not only on the differentiation between actinomycetoma and eumycetoma but also on definitive identification, culture, and sensitivity of the causal organism. Initial treatment of actinomycetoma is medical. Initial treatment of eumycetoma is a wide surgical debridement of acute and chronic necrotic tissues, followed by chemotherapy.

Actinomycetoma. In all cases of actinomycetoma, a combination of two drugs is used to prevent resistance. Streptomycin sulfate (14 mg/kg daily) may be used for the first month and on alternate days thereafter. For patients with *A. madurae* mycetoma (see Figure 3.3), dapsone is given orally (1.5 mg/kg in the morning and evening). Similarly, *S. somaliensis* mycetoma is treated by dapsone first, but if no response appears after 1 month, treatment is changed to trimethoprim-sulfamethoxazole tablets (23 mg/kg per day of sulfamethoxazole and 4.6 mg/kg per day of trimethoprim in two divided doses). *A. pelletieri* and *N. brasiliensis* mycetoma responds better to streptomycin and trimethoprim-sulfamethoxazole.

Mycetomas caused by *Nocardia* in the Americas may respond well to trimethoprim-sulfamethoxazole alone or in combination with dapsone or amikacin. Because amikacin could have deleterious side effects in patients with renal disease (and because of its high cost in developing countries), it is kept as a second-line treatment when first-line treatment with dapsone fails. Rarely has a case been cured by only doxycycline. Wide excision with skin grafting may be necessary for large lesions. The rate of cure for actinomycetoma is 63 to 95% of the cases.

Eumycetoma. Combined surgical and medical management is the currently recommended approach. Early resection with a wide margin of uninfected tissue results in the most successful outcomes. Surgery is used as a means to remove the lesion's bulk, and treatment is then supplemented with antifungal drugs. Surgical management should include excision to uninfected margins; otherwise, the recurrence rate is as high as 50%. Ketoconazole, itraconazole, and fluconazole are drugs of choice for fungi that cause eumycetoma. Eumycetoma caused by *M. mycetomatis* often responds to ketoconazole (200 mg twice daily) after debulking of the lesion. Miconazole is an option to manage mycetoma caused by *P. boydii*. Rare cases of mycetoma caused by *Acremonium falciforme*, *Aspergillus flavus*, or *Fusarium solani* have responded well to itraconazole in a dose of 200 mg twice daily.

Ketoconazole has revolutionized the treatment of fungal varieties by allowing partial resections compatible with preservation of hand function. Altman and associates successfully used oral fluconazole for 6 months to treat a eumycotic hand infection.[6] In all cases, the treatment is given for at least 6 to 12 months and has been required for up to 3 years in some cases. The cure rate is approximately 50%. Although side effects are few, patients are regularly monitored to assess hematologic, kidney, and liver function.

Syphilis

Etiology
Syphilis has vast and varied clinical presentations and Osler's adage remains relevant: "He who knows syphilis, knows medicine." It has often been called "the great imitator" because so many of the signs and symptoms are indistinguishable from those of other diseases. The illness is caused by slender, motile, spiral bacteria—*Treponema pallidum*. Syphilitic lesions of the hand may be congenital, primary, secondary, or tertiary, and all affect the hand as the following subsections describe.

Clinical Findings
Congenital syphilis may present as bilateral dactylitis and metacarpitis in a newborn. Syphilitic dactylitis is characterized by edema of the hands and fusiform swelling of digits. Metacarpals and phalanges show new bone formation (i.e., reactive sclerosis), bone destruction (i.e., patchy rarefaction), and periosteal new bone formation. Syphilitic dactylitis in the infant may resemble tuberculous *spina ventosa*. Pathologic fractures of the metaphysis can masquerade as pseudoparalysis. Syphilis should be considered in the differential diagnosis of infantile osteomyelitis.

Primary syphilis of fingers is seldom seen now and usually occurs in men who have had contact with genital or anal lesions during sexual encounters. It may be contracted by physicians when examining an infected lesion on a patient. Examination of patients, deliveries, pelvic examinations, needle punctures, and tonsillectomies are the most common procedures performed by physicians who subsequently became infected. Extragenital syphilitic ulcers in adults occur in at least 5% of primary syphilis patients and mostly affect fingers, lips, and nipples. The hand constitutes 14% of extra genital chancres during syphilitic epidemics.

Syphilis may present as syphilitic dactylitis with generalized swelling, induration, and erythema of a finger, or as a painless ulcer within 2 to 3 weeks after exposure. The lesion begins as a rapidly growing solitary nodule on the nail or nail bed, pulp, paronychium, finger, hand, or arm that soon ulcerates and appears as nodular-ulcerative chancre. Early on, the ulcer (chancre) is red and oozing (Figure 3.4, *A*). The base of the ulcer has a firm or "cartilaginous" consistency and is surrounded by erythema and scaling (Figure 3.4, *B*). Edges of the ulcer may be rounded. Paronychia may present as a "discharging horseshoe ulcer" around the nail fold or as inflammatory periungual and

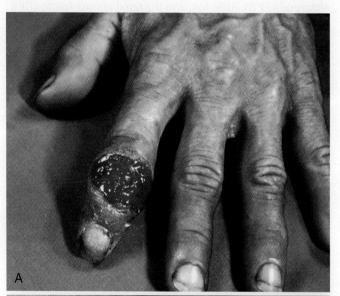

A

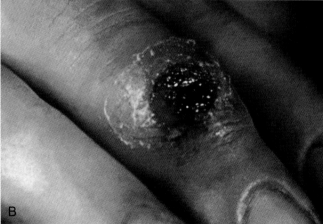

B

FIGURE 3.4 A, Acute syphilitic chancre is red and oozes infected serous fluid. **B,** As the chancre heals spontaneously or with treatment, peripheral skin peels and the chancre shrinks.

subungual papules. Lesions on multiple fingers can occur. A concurrent lesion on the hand and genitalia (i.e., bipolar syphilis) may or may not be present. Enlarged, painless, and nontender epitrochlear and axillary nodes are almost always palpable but rarely unpalpable. There is generally no fever or constitutional symptoms.

Differential Diagnosis of a Hand Ulcer

Differential diagnosis of an ulcer on the hand, in addition to syphilis (Figure 3.4, *A,B*), includes (A-Z) anthrax (see Figure 3.2), aspergillosis, buruli ulcer, *Candida albicans*, cryptococcosis, leishmaniasis (see Figure 3.34), mucormycosis, neutrophilic dermatoses (e.g., classical pyoderma gangrenosum) (see Figures 3.6-3.9), protothecosis, sporotrichosis (see Figures 3.12 and 3.15), tularemia, tuberculosis, and yaws. Interdigital ulcers are typical of a *C. albicans* infection. (Figures 3.6-3.9, 3.12, 3.15, and 3.34 are shown later in this chapter.)

Diagnosis

Diagnosis is confirmed by dark-field microscopic examination of ulcer exudate which almost always shows spirochetes. Diagnosis of syphilis made by using a Venereal Disease Research Laboratory (VDRL) test, a fluorescent treponemal antibody absorption (FTA-ABS) test, and the rapid plasma reagin (RPR) test are presumptive because the tests may be false positive in nonvenereal treponemal infections such as yaws. The nucleic acid amplification test for *T. pallidum* is positive and useful when microscopic examination is negative.

Secondary syphilis may develop 6 to 8 weeks later if a primary syphilitic lesion is not treated. Paronychia or panaritium of the finger may present during secondary syphilis. Secondary syphilitic lesions in the hand may consist of exuberant ulcerated lesions on the palms or hand and wrist. Tertiary syphilis, now relatively rare in the United States, develops after 10 years in about 10% of untreated patients. Tertiary lesions of syphilis in the hand present as gummas—nonspecific, chronic granulomatous lesions that may involve tissues from skin to bone. The skin gumma is a superficial nodule or deep granulomatous lesion that appears as a punched out ulcer. Diagnosis is facilitated by concurrent cardiovascular or neurological syphilis that may be present in 10% of untreated patients after 10 years of onset.

Treatment

Pathologic fractures and dactylitis in congenital syphilis are treated with protective splints in addition to an appropriate dose of penicillin. In primary syphilis, a single dose of 2.4 million units of intramuscular benzathine penicillin G resolves the lesion in 2 weeks without residual scarring. This long-acting antibiotic can be detected in blood up to 4 weeks after injection. The regimen for penicillin-allergic patients is doxycycline (100 mg), administered orally two times daily for 2 weeks. Secondary and tertiary syphilis are treated with benzathine penicillin G, 2.4 million units intramuscularly, given 1 week apart for 3 consecutive weeks. As the lesion heals, it shrinks, skin around it peels away, and the ulcer is covered by crust.

Tularemia

Etiology and Epidemiology

Tularemia, a bacterial zoonosis, is caused by *Francisella tularensis*, one of the most infectious pathogenic bacteria known. It requires inoculation or inhalation of as few as 10 organisms to cause disease. *F. tularensis* is a small, nonmotile, aerobic, gram-negative coccobacillus.

Rabbits, hares, and rodents are especially susceptible. Humans can become infected through several routes, including tick and deer fly (i.e., yellow fly) bites, skin contact with infected animals, ingestion of contaminated water, laboratory exposure, and inhalation of contaminated dusts or aerosols. In addition, humans can be exposed as a result of bioterrorism. In the United States, naturally occurring infections have been reported in all states except Hawaii.

Clinical Presentation

The main form of this disease is ulceroglandular (70%), usually occurring following a tick or deer fly bite or after handling of an infected animal. A skin ulcer appears at the site where the organism entered the body. The ulcer is accompanied by swelling of regional lymph glands, usually in the armpit or groin. Untreated, the disease may progress to include a moderate to high fever, inflammation of the face and eyes, ulcerating lymph nodes, extreme fatigue, loss of appetite, and sepsis; in approximately 1% of cases the disease is fatal.

Diagnostic Testing

Growth of *F. tularensis* in culture is the definitive means of confirming the diagnosis of tularemia. Appropriate specimens include swabs or scrapping of skin lesions, lymph node aspirates or biopsies, pharyngeal washings, sputum specimens, or gastric aspirates, depending on the form of the illness. Paradoxically, blood cultures are often negative.

Physicians who suspect tularemia should promptly alert the laboratory about the need for special diagnostic and safety procedures. Rapid diagnostic testing for tularemia is not widely available and help from the CDC should be sought; check its website for current contact information.

A presumptive diagnosis of tularemia may be made through testing of specimens using direct fluorescent antibody, immunohistochemical staining, or PCR. The diagnosis of tularemia can also be established serologically by demonstrating a fourfold change in specific antibody titers between acute and convalescent sera. Convalescent sera are best drawn at least 4 weeks after illness onset; thus, this method is not useful for clinical management.

Treatment

Streptomycin is the drug of choice. Tetracyclines may be a suitable alternative for patients who are less severely ill. Tetracyclines are static agents and should be given for at least 14 days to avoid relapse.

Yaws

Etiology and Epidemiology

Yaws is an infectious, chronic, relapsing, nonvenereal, treponemal disease caused by *Treponema pallidum* ssp. *pertenue* (*T. p. pertenue*). It is transmitted by direct skin contact with the contagious exudate of an exposed and infected skin lesion. About 75% of those affected are children under 15 years of age, and the peak incidence occurs in children 5 to 10 years old. It is endemic in tropical regions of the world. Humidity and constant warm temperatures are necessary for the treponema to flourish. It occurs "where the highways end," and there is poverty, overcrowding, low levels of collective hygiene, poor sanitation, scanty clothing, and minimal health care; all of which facilitate the spread of yaws. Many areas of Africa, Southeast Asia, South America, and Oceania are included, and any area of exposed skin is at risk. Yaws is categorized into early and late stages of infection; early yaws consists of the primary and secondary stages and late yaws consists of the tertiary stage.

Clinical Findings

The primary yaws lesion arises in the skin at the site of inoculation. It usually appears 9 to 90 days (average, 21 days) after inoculation and begins as an erythematous papule that turns into a nodules or papillomas. Nodules and papillomas subsequently enlarge into highly infectious, raspberry colored, friable ulcers containing numerous *Treponema*. The lesions may be multiple and bilateral. At initial presentation, papilloma is more common (80%) than the ulcerative lesion (20%). This ulcerative lesion, also called mother yaws, usually heals spontaneously after several weeks to months, leaving an atrophic scar.

The secondary stage of infection typically occurs weeks to months after the appearance of mother yaws. Secondary lesions (called daughter yaws) are smaller than mother yaws but are more widespread. They exude highly infectious serum. The soft tissue skin and subcutaneous lesion eventually invades bone and cartilage. The striking feature of secondary yaws is osteoperiostitis, involving the phalanges, metacarpals,[36] and forearm bones. Periostitis occurs with increased bone density, sclerosis, thickening, and enlargement of the cortex and an increase in the width of the entire shaft (Figure 3.5).[36] Proximal, middle, and distal phalanges are involved in yaws dactylitis in that order of frequency. Tender and fusiform or spindle-shaped soft tissue and bone swelling of fingers and metacarpals is a characteristic clinical presentation in secondary yaws.[36] It may be bilateral and symmetric[36] with considerable finger, hand, and forearm pain. Yaws osteoperiostitis is similar clinically to osteoperiostitis in tuberculous, syphilitic, blastomycotic, and brucellosis dactylitis.

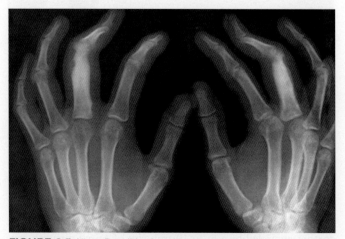

FIGURE 3.5 Yaws. Dactylitis of proximal phalanges of both middle fingers is characterized by osteoperiostitis. There is periosteal reaction, cortical thickening, sclerosis, and scalloping of proximal phalanges of both middle fingers.

Tertiary lesions appear after a latency period of 5 to 10 years in 10% of the cases. Gummas may involve skin and subcutaneous tissues over areas of underlying osteitis. Nodules may develop in the vicinity of joints. The disease is rarely fatal; however, without treatment, it can lead to chronic disfigurement and disability.

Diagnosis

The diagnosis of yaws is primarily based on clinical findings in an epidemiological context.[37] A painless ulcer, in a child below 15 years who lives in an endemic area or who has immigrated from an endemic area, may be diagnosed as yaws.[37] Morphological and serological tests are identical to those for syphilis and are used to diagnose yaws as well. The clinical diagnosis can be confirmed by examining a sample of serum from an ulcerative skin lesion under a microscope with dark field examination. A VDRL test, rapid plasma reagin (RPR) test, a fluorescent treponemal antibody absorption test (FTA-Abs), an agglutination assay for antibodies to *T. pallidum* (TPHA), and a microhemagglutination assay for *T. pallidum* (MHA-TP) can be done and are positive for yaws the same as for syphilis.

Treatment

Penicillin remains the drug of choice. Yaws can be treated with a single dose of benzathine penicillin injection, which cures both the early and late versions. Relapse is very rare. The dose for adults is 1.2 million units and for children <10 years old is 600,000 units. Resistance to penicillin has emerged in rare cases. For those who are allergic or resistant to penicillin, tetracycline, erythromycin, and doxycycline can be used. Spirochetes are usually not detectable by dark-field microscopy within 8 to 10 h of treatment and the lesions resolve in 90% of cases within a month. However, 25% of children show clinical and/or serological evidence of either relapse or reinfection within 2 years.

Neutrophilic Dermatoses and Pyoderma Gangrenosum

Etiology and Epidemiology

Neutrophilic dermatoses are ulcerative dermal diseases in which the ulcer edges are full of neutrophils. Su et al[113] classified ulcers of neutrophilic dermatoses into four types: (1) pyoderma gangrenosum (PG), the classic ulcerative PG[55]; (2) bullous or atypical PG[12]; (3) pustular PG; and (4) vegetative PG.[68] The ulcerative classic form is the most common and the pathognomonic lesion is an ulcer with purplish overhanging border. PG is a progressive, necrotizing, noninfectious, autoimmune, and ulcerative dermatosis that commonly mimics an acute or chronic infection. It is an indicator of an underlying immunological or inflammatory bowel disease (ulcerative colitis, Crohn syndrome) in more than 50% of cases.[55]

Pyoderma gangrenosum was first described as a fulminant streptococcal infection, but it has subsequently been proved to be a noninfectious ulcer. However, the name "pyogenic granuloma" persisted because of the original assumed etiology. It is most common in the lower limbs (70-80%) and rare in the hands and upper extremity (16%).[55] Only 20 cases in the hand and upper extremity were reported in the English literature between 1983 and 2001; all were misdiagnosed initially as

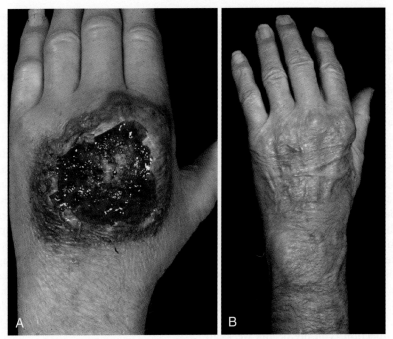

FIGURE 3.6 Pyoderma gangrenosum. **A,** The ulcer is a centrifugally creeping one surrounded by a rough, serpentine, undermining black-blue rim, which is further encircled by a 5- to 10-mm rim of raised purplish erythema and covered by a thin, translucent, graying epidermis. The central portion undergoes wet gangrenous necrosis, oozes, and impersonates infection. **B,** With oral cortisone, skin returns to normal because the deep layers of dermis are still intact.

infections.[55] Since then the condition has been classified under ulcerative neutrophilic dermatoses.[113] The prevalence of PG in ulcerative colitis is about 5%, and in Crohn syndrome it is about 2%.

Bullous or atypical PG is associated with hematological neoplasms (i.e., myeloproliferative diseases[55] such as acute myeloid leukemia, hairy cell leukemia, myelodysplastic syndrome) in 70% of cases.[81] Miyata reviewed 17 cases of bullous PG that have been reported over 20 years, from 1991 to 2011.[81] Unlike the reddish or violaceous halo of classic PG, bullous PG has bulla and bluish-gray halo surrounding the ulcer.[113] Pustular PG is associated with arthralgia, inflammatory bowel disease, and monoclonal gammopathy in 70% of cases.[81] It is considered a *forme fruste* of ulcerative PG in which pustules do not evolve into frank ulcers. Histologically, it shows pustular vasculitis. When bullous PG, pustular PG, and bullous sweet syndrome occurred on the dorsum of both hands, Galaria called it "neutrophilic dermatosis of the dorsal hands"[39] in 2000, and reports of more than 100 cases since then have validated this condition.

Vegetative PG is the most benign, localized, and nonaggressive form of PG and is not associated with systemic diseases, has superficial verrucous and ulcerative lesions, a granulomatous histologic appearance, and responds to minor treatment measures that do not require corticosteroids in most cases. Mixed types of PG also occur,[81] showing that different forms are part of a single clinical spectrum from the nonaggressive vegetative PG to the rapidly destructive classical PG. In all cases, the margin of the ulcer is packed with "noninfectious" neutrophils. In 25% of patients with a generalized category of neutrophilic dermatoses, no known underlying medical condition was found.

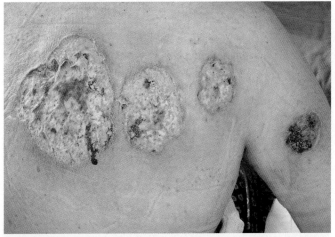

FIGURE 3.7 Pyoderma gangrenosum can occur in the upper arm and posterior chest wall. (From en.wikipedia.org/wiki/Pyoderma_gangrenosum #mediaviewer/ File:Pyoderma_gangrenosum_01.jpg.)

Clinical Findings

Neutrophilic dermatoses characteristically affect the dorsal surface of a single finger,[55] rarely multiple fingers, hand[55] (Figure 3.6, *A*), wrist, forearm, elbow, or upper arm[55,81] (Figure 3.7). Patients are most often between their third and fourth decades and 4% are children. A centrifugally creeping and weeping ulcer is surrounded with a rough, serpentine, undermining, burrowing, black-blue, violaceous, or gunmetal gray border, which is further encircled by a 5- to 10-mm rim of raised purplish erythema and covered by a thin, translucent graying epidermis (see Figure 3.6, *A*). It spreads 1 to 2 cm/day in a centrifugal pattern.

Pain is a significant symptom in 75% of cases. The central portion undergoes wet gangrenous necrosis, oozes, and impersonates infection. PG does not respond to traditional antibiotics or surgical intervention.

Diagnosis

Neutrophilic dermatosis (mostly characterized by PG) is a clinical diagnosis, and a high clinical suspicion prompts correct diagnosis and treatment. If it is on the dorsum of both hands, the condition is designated as neutrophilic dermatosis of dorsal hands (Figures 3.8 and 3.9) If after debridement of a supposedly infected wound (with pustules, bullae, or ulcerations) there is no improvement, but there is centrifugal extension of the lesions with a "sepsis-like" syndrome and persistent negative cultures, PG is highly probable; in that case, corticosteroids (not antibiotics) are the definitive treatment. Rarely, PG may masquerade as necrotizing fasciitis. PG ulcers appear similar to other cutaneous ulcers, such as aspergillosis, and may lead to misdiagnosis.

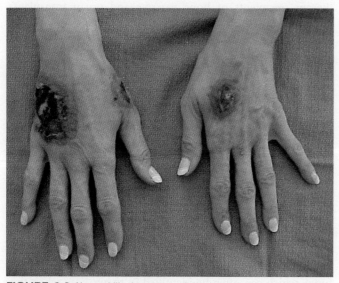

FIGURE 3.8 Neutrophilic dermatoses of the dorsal is characterized by pyogenic granuloma-like lesions on the dorsal side of both hands.

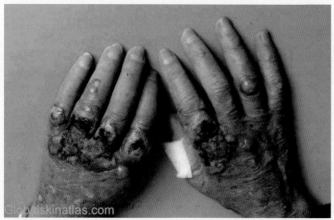

FIGURE 3.9 Neutrophilic dermatoses of dorsal hands may extend into the fingers.

Biopsy is of limited diagnostic value as it accelerates the ulcerative process; however, in cases where biopsy is done, "a sea of neutrophils" are characteristic in the marching edge of the ulcer. No laboratory test is confirmatory. In a clinical setting, when an ulcer does not yield infectious organisms and biopsy aggravates the ulceration, a diagnosis of PG is paramount. Dermal neutrophilia in the advancing border of the ulcer confirms that diagnosis.

In a review of 13 cases in the literature and 7 cases added by Huish and colleagues, every patient initially had a misdiagnosis of infection.[55] In a later review of 35 cases of the hand by Wong, 29 were initially treated for infection and 13 were debrided with further deterioration of ulceration. Thirteen misdiagnoses in Huish's series resulted in 16 unnecessary surgeries, including 2 failed skin grafts and 4 amputations. No surgical procedure resulted in clinical improvement, and all were followed by unrelenting extension of the ulcer. Five physicians on an average examined each patient before the final diagnosis of PG was made by a dermatologist. Clinical improvement after correct medical treatment with oral prednisone, azathioprine, or dapsone was dramatic and occurred within a week.[55]

Treatment

Biopsy or wound debridement consistently leads to deterioration of the condition; this so-called idiopathic pathergic response is a hallmark of this disease.[55] Pathergy, first described by Blobner, is a violent inflammatory response of the skin after any intradermal trauma. It is seen in both PG and neutrophilic dermatoses. Pathergic response also explains the occurrence of PG in patients who sustain occupationally induced trauma or develop PG following a hand injury or surgery.

Management includes (1) immunosuppressive therapy with oral administration of corticosteroids (i.e., prednisone, 100 mg/day); (2) treatment of associated medical conditions (i.e., ulcerative colitis, Crohn syndrome, myeloproliferative conditions, or myelodysplastic syndrome); (3) local wound care; and (4) the most important, avoidance of surgical intervention. The administration of corticosteroids is tapered when the ulcers show signs of healing. There is dramatic improvement within 24 h, and within 6 weeks the lesion is completely epithelialized because the deeper layers of the dermis, sweat glands, and hair follicles remain intact (see Figure 3.6, B).

PG responds to oral dapsone, azathioprine, topical glucocorticoid ointment, or intralesional steroid injections when oral corticosteroids are contraindicated. Corticosteroid-resistant PG associated with Crohn syndrome rapidly responds to cyclosporine or infliximab. Before the advent of these drugs, the skin lesions healed with an atrophic scar when the underlying disease, such as ulcerative colitis, was controlled.

FUNGAL INFECTIONS

Etiology, Epidemiology, and Classification

Given the increasing number of immunocompromised individuals throughout the world, the incidence of infection caused by fungal and unusual organisms has increased. Fungal (*L. fungosus*, "mushroom") infections are classified into categories based on anatomic location of infection and epidemiology. Anatomic categories that affect the hand are: cutaneous, subcutaneous, and deep. Cutaneous and subcutaneous infections can cause serious morbidity but are rarely fatal. Deep infections are often fatal without treatment. The epidemiologic categories are endemic and opportunistic.

The endemic mycoses are exogenous infections (e.g., coccidioidomycosis) and are caused by fungal organisms that are not part of the normal human microbial flora and are acquired from the external environment. Endemic mycoses cause severe illness in immunocompetent individuals and more serious infections in immunocompromised patients. Patients acquire infection with endemic fungi almost exclusively by inhalation. The soil is the natural reservoir for the vast majority of endemic mycosis. In contrast, the opportunistic mycoses (e.g., *Candida*, *Aspergillus*) are endogenous and are caused by organisms that are components of normal human flora. Opportunistic fungi cause serious infections when immunity of the host is depressed, allowing the organisms to transition from harmless commensals to invasive pathogens.

The incidence of fungal infections has risen as a consequence of intentional immunosuppression (e.g., organ and stem cell transplantation), administration of cytotoxic chemotherapy for cancers, corticosteroid therapy, and liberal use of antibacterial agents. *Any yeast or mold recovered from an immunocompromised patient should not be dismissed as a "contaminant" or colonizer without first ruling out its role in the patient's disease.* Fungi commonly associated with immunodeficiencies are shown in Table 3.4.

Diagnosis

Three terms used to describe fungi are yeast, mold, and dimorphic varieties. Yeasts (e.g., *Candida* and *Cryptococcus*) are typically round and reproduce by budding. Molds (e.g., *Aspergillus*, Mucorales) are filamentous and grow by branching both at room and body temperature. Dimorphic fungi (e.g., blastomycosis, coccidioidomycosis, histoplasmosis, sporotrichosis) are fungi that grow as yeasts in human tissue but as filamentous forms in the environment at room temperature.

There are two fungal infections, aspergillosis and mucormycosis, that need special cautionary mention because they infect the blood vessels and cause avascular necrosis of dermis and deep tissues. They cause rapid necrosis of the dermis, resulting in a black eschar that may progress to gangrene. Rapid and progressive black eschar formation in an immunocompromised patient should arouse suspicion of angioinvasive fungus and warrant prompt biopsy rather than a culture because the host tissue grows the fungus faster than the petri dish. The definitive diagnosis of these fungal infections requires histopathologic identification of them in the infected tissue, and early diagnosis can prevent unnecessary amputation or mortality. Evidence of inflammatory response in the biopsy tissue is critical for diagnosis of infection by *Aspergillus*, as these species are ubiquitous in air and can contaminate biopsy material, causing false-positive microscopic identification. A high level of suspicion is necessary to make diagnosis of a fungal infection, especially in immunocompromised patients.

Any unusual swelling of the upper extremity should raise suspicion of the more common chronic infections, such as fungus infection, tuberculosis, and actinomycetoma, in addition to aerobic infections (e.g., actinomycosis) and anaerobic infections (e.g., botryomycosis). Fungal hand infections have been reported in patients with AIDS, hematologic malignancies, cancer patients on chemotherapy, those on corticosteroid therapy, recipients of bone marrow and organ transplants, patients with prosthetic finger joint implants, patients with prosthetic arteriovenous shunts and distal steal phenomena, patients with chronic renal failure, diabetics, rheumatoid patients on disease-modifying drugs, alcoholics, and those with severe burns.

Identification of *Aspergillus*, *Nocardia*, *Cryptococcus*, or Mucorales from a patient without a known immunodeficiency is sufficient grounds for pursuing the probability of an underlying immune defect. A biopsy to identify the infecting organism and an appropriate workup to identify the immunodeficiency are then warranted. When a soft tissue, joint, or bone infection presents as a chronic draining sinus that has not responded to usual antibiotics, deep fungal infection should be considered. Surgical wound cultures from chronic lesions that are repeatedly negative for the usual bacteria also raise the possibility of a fungal infection. The main role of the surgeon is to perform an adequate biopsy and request smears and cultures that include fungi, which can often be identified in tissue, even when they do not grow in culture.

The stains most commonly used to identify fungi are periodic acid–Schiff and Gomori silver. India ink preparation is diagnostic for cryptococcosis. Most laboratories now use calcofluor-white staining coupled with fluorescent microscopy to identify fungi in fluid specimens. The histologic finding of a fungus in a biopsy tissue specimen can be more rapidly diagnostic than culture when the mycosis is caused by a slow-growing fungus, which can take weeks to a month or more to grow in the laboratory and may require a special growth medium. Again, a biopsy may provide proof that the fungus is invading tissue and is not just a contaminant (e.g., a saprophyte growing on a skin ulcer). It is important to rapidly transport the specimen to the microbiology laboratory to minimize overgrowth of contaminating bacteria. Most fungi grow within 4 weeks but occasionally take 8 weeks (as is the case with *Sporothrix schenckii* and some of the filamentous fungi); it is wise to request that the microbiology laboratory not discard, usually after 4 weeks, the cultures when fungi are suspected.

TABLE 3.4	Risk Factors and Commonly Associated Fungi
Predisposing Host Risk Factors	**Fungi/Infection**
Neutropenia (hematogenous malignancies)	*Aspergillus*, mucormycosis
Cell-mediated immune defects, including AIDS	*Cryptococcus*
Malnutrition	*Aspergillus*, mucormycosis
Diabetes	Mucormycosis
Corticosteroids	*Cryptococcus*, *Pseudallescheria boydii* (*Allescheria boydii*, *Petriellidium boydii*), mucormycosis
Cytotoxic chemotherapy	*Aspergillus*
Exposure to pigeons	*Cryptococcus*

The only mycosis for which serodiagnosis (i.e., testing for the presence of antibody) has established a role is coccidioidomycosis. This test is the most frequent means for diagnosis and is highly specific for active coccidioidomycosis. Detection of cryptococcal polysaccharide antigen in serum is the most reliable for diagnosis of cryptococcosis. Correlation of clinical and microbiologic results is always necessary. Some fungi (e.g., *Blastomyces dermatitidis, Coccidioides immitis, Histoplasma capsulatum*) usually infect immunocompetent hosts while other fungi (e.g., *Aspergillus, Rhizopus, Cryptococcus, Pseudallescheria*) infect immunocompromised hosts. However, the endemic fungi are important causes of infection in seriously immunocompromised hosts such as those with AIDS or heart transplant recipients. Recovery of *Aspergillus* or *Candida* from an otherwise immunocompetent host may not be indicative of invasive disease, but the burden is to consider these seriously before ruling out infection. Many risk factors are specific to certain fungal infections. The differential diagnosis can often be narrowed on the basis of the specific immune defect present (see Table 3.4).

The diagnostic laboratory should be alerted when specimens from patients suspected of having coccidioidomycosis or histoplasmosis are sent for culture. Once these cultures grow in mold form, they can be easily aerosolized if the cultures are not maintained in a biohazard hood. Infection of the laboratory with *H. capsulatum* or *C. immitis* is a well-documented occurrence and can lead to considerable morbidity and even mortality of the infected laboratory worker. With a rare exception (e.g., ringworm), mycoses are not transmissible from patient to patient.

Treatment

Prompt surgical debridement of infected tissue is the keystone of treatment in aspergillosis and mucormycosis, irrespective of the host's immunocompetence. Due to their angioinvasive predilection, these two fungi cause severe and often progressive tissue infarction, necrosis, and gangrene.[93] Removal of nonviable tissue is critical to prevent further invasion and infection of neighboring viable tissue and to increase the success of treatment. If possible, reversal of the underlying immunocompromising predisposition should be vigorously attempted by reducing immunosuppressive therapy.

Amphotericin B (AmB, Fungizone) has been the treatment of choice for patients with fungal diseases from the time of its introduction in 1958 and by default became the gold standard for antifungal therapy of invasive mycoses. It is given intravenously and has serious toxic effects on kidney, liver, and blood. The availability of lipid formulations of AmB, such as Abelcet and AmBisome, has resulted in the ability to administer higher doses of it with significantly fewer side effects.

Currently, there is some controversy concerning whether the lipid formulations should replace Fungizone for most indications. Because these lipid formulations of AmB are rather expensive, many physicians are hesitant to prescribe them, especially when the much less expensive conventional amphotericin B can be used. Consultation with experts in the treatment of invasive fungal diseases is encouraged so that the most effective and least toxic regimen can be recommended. Echinocandins (micafungin, caspofungin) now offer broad spectrum activity against all *Candida* species and has relatively low toxicity. Turbinafine has been as effective as itraconazole in the treatment of onychomycosis and more effective than griseofulvin in the treatment of ringworm infections.

Use of effective oral antifungal therapy with little or no nephrotoxicity for the treatment of invasive mycoses is a relatively recent development. Since the FDA approval of ketoconazole (Nizoral in 1983), fluconazole (Diflucan in 1990), itraconazole (Sporanox in 1994), voriconazole in 2002, and posaconazole in 2006, these synthetic oral antifungal azoles have been increasingly and effectively used as therapy for various systemic mycoses. Unlike AmB, these drugs are fungistatic, not fungicidal. In certain circumstances, they have equivalent efficacy, improved safety, and ease of administration when compared with AmB. Itraconazole has emerged as a possible alternative to amphotericin B in treating several fungal infections, including blastomycosis, coccidioidomycosis, histoplasmosis, pseudallescheriasis, and sporotrichosis. Voriconazole has now superseded AmB as a drug of choice for treatment for aspergillosis.

Posaconazole is uniquely effective against Mucorales and is the only antifungal agent with clinically relevant activity against this group of pathogens. Antifungal agents in current use are shown in Table 3.5. Because of the infrequency of these

TABLE 3.5 Spectrum of Antifungal Agent Activity and Preferred Agent(s) for Most Clinical Infections

	Amphotericin B	Flucytosine	Ketoconazole	Fluconazole	Itraconazole
Aspergillus	+	+	−	−	+
Blastomyces	+	+	+	+	
Candida albicans	+	+	+	+	+
Chromomycosis		+	+	−	+
Cryptococcus	+	+	+	+	+
Coccidioides	+	−	+	+	+
Histoplasma	+	−	+	+	+
Mucormycosis	+	−	−	−	−
Pseudallescheria			+		+
Sporothrix	+	−	+	+	+

In general, acutely ill patients with life-threatening mycosis should be treated with AmB. Azole therapy can follow once the patient's condition is stabilized.

infections, potential hepatotoxicity and the emergence of resistant strains, an infectious disease consultation is advisable. Some drugs (e.g., itraconazole capsules) are erratically absorbed and can have multiple drug interactions. When antifungal agents are used for chronic therapy, serum blood concentration monitoring is necessary and doses adjusted as necessary. The use of flucytosine has diminished in recent years as newer antifungal drugs have been developed.

Cutaneous Fungal Infections

Etiology and Epidemiology

The most common fungal infections of the hand are cutaneous (skin and nail) infections and are commonly treated by dermatologists and primary care physicians. Nail infections (onychomycosis) can be diagnosed by direct smear in 75% and by histology in 80% of the cases.

Cutaneous (superficial) infections are caused by fungi that infect and metabolize keratin (e.g., skin, hair, and nails). Because these organisms depend on keratin for nutrition, they do not invade beneath the skin. Most of the clinical manifestations of skin infections are a consequence of host reaction to fungal metabolic products. Patients with skin and nail infections usually seek medical care from dermatologists. *Candida albicans* and dermatophytes (*Trichophyton*, *Microsporum*, and *Epidermophyton*) are the cause of the majority of chronic cutaneous and nail infections.

Chronic cutaneous *C. albicans* infection occurs in the moist palms and webs of a "clenched fist" in patients with spasticity. Trichophytosis ("ringworm") is the most common cutaneous (and nail) infection. It is more often treated by a family physician or dermatologist, although hand surgeons are now consulted by patients directly and often. The skin diseases associated with *Trichophyton* ringworms in interdigital spaces are also commonly referred to as "tinea." It may occur on the dorsum of the hand (Figures 3.10 and 3.11) and may have typical rings within the lesion (Figure 3.11). Other fungi that infect the skin are *Epidermophyton* and *Microsporum*. "Wristwatch ringworm" occurs in moist skin under a watch or its strap. Tinea nigra palmaris has been reported to be misdiagnosed as malignant melanoma.

Diagnosis

Most of cutaneous fungi are easily identified on wet KOH preparations. They grow hyphae (Greek *hyphos*, "a web") readily on a Sabouraud medium. Skin or nail scrapings from the suspected area are placed in 10% KOH on a glass slide, which can be heated over an alcohol lamp until bubbles are seen. Spores or branching mycelia under the microscope confirm the presence of fungus. Definitive diagnosis requires fungal cultures because the infections caused by *Trichophyton* and *C. albicans* may not be clinically distinguishable and respond to various antifungal agents.

Treatment

Uncomplicated cases of tinea are easily treated with cream or lotion of tolnaftate (Tinactin), miconazole (Monistat), or ciclopirox (Loprox). Widespread lesions require treatment with oral griseofulvin, ketoconazole, fluconazole, or itraconazole. It is probably not necessary to use the newer broad-spectrum triazole derivatives, such as voriconazole, for the treatment of

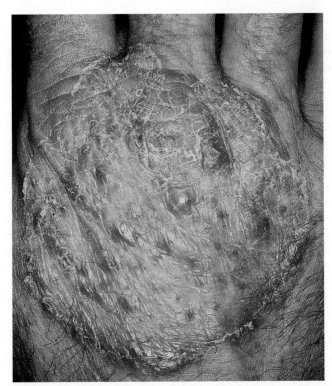

FIGURE 3.10 Ringworm infection on the dorsum of the hand. (From Habif TP: *Clinical dermatology: a color guide to diagnosis and therapy*, Philadelphia, 2010, Elsevier; Figure 13.29, with permission.)

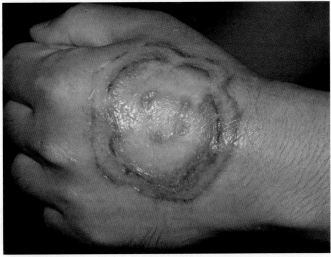

FIGURE 3.11 Concentric rings can be seen in some lesions of ring worm.

these infections. For the cerebral palsy patient with a clenched fist, tendon or fascial lengthening may be necessary to prevent recurrent infections if routine hand hygiene fails to keep the skin dry.

Subcutaneous Fungal Infections

Classification

There are three major subcutaneous fungal infections of the hand: chronic paronychia, sporotrichosis, and phaeomycotic cysts. Chronic paronychia is usually initially misdiagnosed as a bacterial infection. Lack of response to repeated courses of the usual antibiotics is an important clue to the fungal etiology of this infection. Drainage and debridement may be needed if medical management fails. Sporotrichosis is rare but responds readily to medical treatment. A phaeomycotic cyst is a deep dermal or subcutaneous infection that results from the traumatic implantation of a dematiaceous (pigmented) fungus such as *Exophiala* or *Phialophora*. A subcutaneous soft tissue abscess of the forearm can occur in a patient with refractory acute myeloid leukemia caused by *Scedosporium apiospermum*.

Chronic Paronychia

Etiology and Epidemiology. Chronic paronychia is characterized by a relatively well-localized area of skin inflammation proximal to the cuticle. The skin becomes pink, warm, indurated, glistening, and tense and extends to the cuticle. The cuticle is chronically retracted, rounded, and detached from the nail plate, allowing free passage of moisture and water under the eponychium. It usually affects a female patient who frequently soaks her hands in water, as required either by her job or her domestic duties. Mechanical trauma that damages the cuticle at modern nail salons is responsible for bacterial and fungal invasion of the nail fold. Patients with chronic paronychia have a higher incidence of *Candida* colonization of the mouth, bowel, and vagina than controls. Patients do not routinely have a history of acute paronychia, and surgical exploration does not identify pus deep to the nail plate. Unless the disease process is stopped, secondary thickening, ridging, and discoloration of the nail can occur, eventually resulting in nail loss. Specific diagnosis can be made by gram stain, KOH preparation, and culture.

C. albicans is responsible for the majority (70-97%) of cases of chronic paronychia. Stone and Mullins first reproduced this entity in 1964 by soaking fingers in water until the skin macerated and inoculated either viable or nonviable *Candida* into the cul-de-sac between the base of the nail and eponychium. Inflammatory reaction in the presence of dead *C. albicans* indicated that the exogenous byproducts of fungal organisms caused local chronic inflammation. Chronic maceration of the fingers is accompanied by separation of the cuticle from the nail so that a pocket of water is entrapped under the proximal nail fold. Once this pocket is formed, capillary action retains water in it and transient flora (e.g., *C. albicans* and gram-negative rods) thrive in it. As Stone refers to it, the process forms a "dermatologic cesspool" and cultures yield *C. albicans* and mixed bacterial flora, including *Proteus*, *Streptococcus*, and gram-negative rods (usually *Escherichia coli* and *Pseudomonas*). The condition has been reported in up to 9% of diabetic and in 3% of nondiabetic women older than 20 years. Thumb sucking can be the etiology of chronic paronychia in children. In men, the condition may be occupational. For barbers, chronic paronychia can occur when hair is embedded in the paronychium.

Clinical Findings. The lateral nail fold may show the first signs of chronic swelling, with a separation of this fold from the nail's lateral margin. After weeks or months, the process may progress to the posterior nail fold, the eponychium. The cuticle separates from the nail plate and allows moisture and *C. albicans* to reside in the subeponychial cul-de-sac. Germinal matrix in the eponychial area is eventually invaded and causes irregularities of the dorsum of the nail plate, usually grooving. In 30% of cases, the nail plate becomes greenish owing to secondary colonization by *Pseudomonas aeruginosa*, which are normal

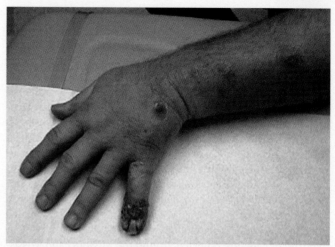

FIGURE 3.12 Sporotrichosis of fifth finger in a gardener simulates a paronychial lesion. Note marching lesions in hand and forearm.

colonizers of the hyponychial space between the skin and free edge of the nail. Subacute intermittent flare-ups by secondary bacterial infection may require treatment with oral antibiotics but do not cure the underlying chronic hyponychial candidiasis.

Differential Diagnosis. Other causes of paronychia include syphilis (see Figure 3.4), sporotrichosis (Figure 3.12), blastomycosis, tuberculosis, and herpetic paronychia. Squamous cell carcinoma, subungual keratoacanthoma, leukemia cutis, amyloidosis, and pilonidal sinus around the nail have been reported to mimic chronic paronychia.

Diagnosis. Chronic paronychia is entirely a clinical diagnosis; the visual picture presented is so characteristic as to present no diagnostic difficulties. Ninety-two percent of patients are women; of affected men, 25% are chefs, bartenders, or fishmongers. A chronically indurated, retracted, and rounded eponychium is the hallmark of diagnosis of chronic paronychia. Recurrent episodes cause inflammation, followed by thickening, transverse grooving, and nail deformity. Patients with chronic paronychia complain of a long history of annoying and disfigured thickening of the eponychial skin. If smears of skin and nail scrapings are negative for *C. albicans*, the diagnosis can be established with a culture.

Treatment. Keeping the area as dry as possible and prolonged application of a topical azole antifungal agent, such as clotrimazole (Lotrimin, Mycelex) or econazole, may adequately treat a *C. albicans* infection. Oral therapy with fluconazole, 200 to 400 mg/day, is a more effective alternative, but long-term prognosis of either topical or oral therapy remains unsatisfactory. Approximately 40% of patients remain free of paronychia, 40% heal periodically, and 20% have continuous disease after a year. When medical management does not succeed, eponychial marsupialization should be considered. In this operation, the fibrotic cutaneous and subcutaneous tissue of the eponychium is excised to permit unrestricted drainage of the fungi and their exogenous byproducts so that the infectious and inflammatory processes are reversed.

For additional information on marsupialization, see eFigure 3.1 and the online version of this chapter at www.Expert Consult.com.

Sporotrichosis (Rose Thorn Disease)

Etiology and Epidemiology. Sporotrichosis is the most common cutaneous and lymphatic (lymphocutaneous) fungal infection in North America. If sporotrichosis is promptly diagnosed, it can usually be cured with medical treatment. If unrecognized, the disease can result in progressive disability. Sporotrichosis was first diagnosed by Schenck in 1898 at Johns Hopkins Hospital in a patient with a primary lesion in his finger and secondary lymphatic lesions in the forearm. The infecting organism was a dimorphic fungus and was termed *Sporothrix* (or *Sporotrichum*) *schenckii*. In the United States, the infection in humans is an occupational hazard of rose growers, gardeners, and florists, as well as farmers, horticulturists, and nursery workers. The organism is ubiquitous in soil and frequently inoculated into the skin and subcutaneous tissues by a rose thorn. The majority of cases are reported around the Missouri and Mississippi rivers, but the disease occurs worldwide. The fungus has been recovered from nails of cats, so sporotrichosis should be considered following cat scratches. It is common in Brazil but rare in the United States; only 36 cases were treated at the Mayo Clinic in the 29 years between 1957 and 1986.

Clinical Findings. The infection may be solitary or multiple with marching lymphocutaneous lesions. Solitary cutaneous lesion, so-called a fixed lesion, remains localized to the site of infection, perhaps due to a higher degree of immunity. Lymphocutaneous marching infection accounts for 50 to 80% of cases of sporotrichosis (Figures 3.12 and 3.13), and 80% of infections occur in the upper extremity (see Figures 3.12 through 3.15). It should be suspected in any patient with painless, ulcerative lesions of the skin that are unresponsive to antibacterial treatment. Infection can start at the tip of a finger as paronychia (see Figure 3.12) or as nonhealing ulcer of the pulp, finger, or the hand (see Figures 3.14 and 3.15). The lesion is usually unilateral; however, Haruna et al reviewed 15 cases of bilateral upper extremity sporotrichosis in Japan (see Figure 3.14).[48]

Bilateral cases may be due to autoinoculation or multiple inoculations. The infection is usually nonopportunistic and affects healthy subjects and is rare during childhood. Infection begins when the fungus is inoculated into a site of skin injury on the exposed part of hand or forearm. It produces an erythematous or verrucous nodule that gradually ulcerates. The ulcers develop raised borders. The ulcer closely resembles a syphilitic chancre.

The infection is characterized by linear marching nodules on the forearm and arm, which represent spread through local lymphatic channels (see Figure 3.13). Regional lymph nodes become enlarged, and seropurulent drainage may occur from both the primary lesion and the involved nodes. The lymphocutaneous lesions are typically painless, and a chronic cyclical process of spontaneous healing, nodule formation, ulceration, and drainage may continue for years if untreated. Infection can result in exposure of the tendons and require skin grafting (see Figure 3.15).

Diagnosis. Diagnosis of sporotrichosis is often missed owing to the relative rarity of the disease. The average delay in diagnosis is 4 months.[33] The standard histologic stains may not show the organism. Periodic acid–Schiff or silver staining will highlight the fungus as red or black, respectively. Examination of biopsy specimens reveals a pyogranulomatous response and

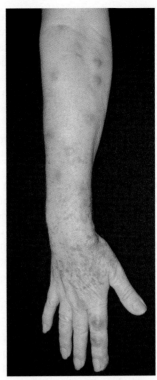

FIGURE 3.13 Lymphocutaneous sporotrichosis. A 68-year-old Brazilian housewife presented with a 2-week history of a small ulcer on her right forefinger and palpable erythematous nodules on her right forearm of 4 weeks duration; this occurred after a bite from a domestic cat that had a lesion on its hind foot. The patient had taken an antibiotic (cephalexin) without improvement. An ulcer measured 1 cm in diameter with erythematous borders on her right forefinger. Subcutaneous erythematous nodules extended in a linear and ascending distribution on her right hand and forearm. The fungal culture, performed at 25°C using Sabouraud dextrose agar for 5 days, showed a creamy white-colored colony. Microscopy demonstrated *Sporothrix schenckii*. (From *Dermatology Online Journal* 14(7), 2008.)

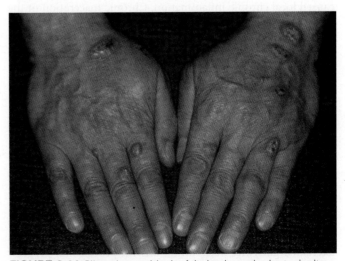

FIGURE 3.14 Bilateral sporotrichosis of the hands may be due to simultaneous infection or contralateral inoculation. (From Haruna K, Shiraki Y, Hiruma M, et al: A case of lymphangitic sporotrichosis occurring on both forearms with a published work review of cases of bilateral sporotrichosis in Japan. *J Dermatol* 33:364–367, 2006, with permission.)

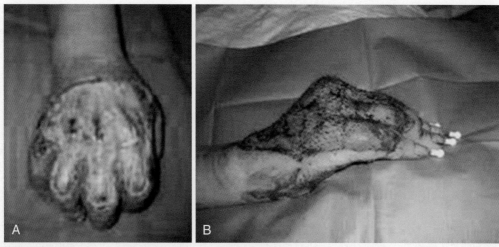

FIGURE 3.15 Sporotrichosis. **A,** Skin loss due to cutaneous sporotrichosis can be devastating when it is not diagnosed and treated early. **B,** Skin loss was treated by skin grafting.

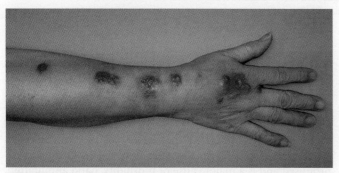

FIGURE 3.16 Sporotrichoid erythematous nodular and pustular marching lymphangitis in a Chinese woman during a 2014 *M. marinum* outbreak in New York City. The women cleaned fish without gloves.

is diagnostic if characteristic cigar-shaped yeast forms are seen. Unfortunately, the yeast can be difficult to detect unless multiple sections are examined because characteristically there are very few organisms in infected tissue. A diagnosis is best made by culture of the infected site, although repeated attempts at culture may have to be made. Aspirates or deep cultures are preferable to swabbed specimens because the organisms are sparse. Cultures become positive in a few days to a month and must be incubated at 30°C or room temperature in a modified Sabouraud agar fungal medium. False-negative cultures may result if the specimens are cultured at 37°C. Sporotrichosis should be included in the differential diagnosis of a chronic ulcerated skin lesion (see Figures 3.12 and 3.15).

Among the differential diagnoses of the nodular marching lymphangitis pattern of lymphocutaneous sporotrichosis are nocardiosis, leishmaniasis, and atypical mycobacterial infections, especially *M. marinum* (Figure 3.16 and Table 3.6). The ulceroglandular form of tularemia is usually accompanied by systemic symptoms. Much less often, botryomycosis, *Blastomyces dermatitidis*, *Coccidioides immitis*, *Cryptococcus neoformans*, *Histoplasma capsulatum*, *Mycobacterium kansasii*, *Staphylococcus aureus*, *Streptococcus pyogenes*, *Burkholderia pseudomallei*, *Bacillus anthracis*, and *Vaccinia virus* may also be characterized by nodular lymphangitis.

Treatment. Itraconazole is the drug of choice for lymphocutaneous sporotrichosis. Treatment with 200 mg/day for 3 to 6 months results in complete resolution for most patients. The drug should be administered with a fatty meal or carbonated beverage to enhance absorption. Heat (warm soaks) is considered a useful adjunct to medicinal therapy because the organism grows at temperatures below 37°C. Cutaneous sporotrichosis was treated in the past with a saturated solution of potassium iodide (SSKI, 1 g/mL) and this may still be considered if itraconazole causes hepatotoxic side effects. SSKI may not be convenient because it causes a bitter taste and gastrointestinal upset. It is still the mainstay of treatment in developing countries because SSKI is effective and inexpensive.

Oral terbinafine (125 mg/day) has been shown to be effective against sporotrichosis in Japan. Fluconazole, 400 to 800 mg/day, can also be used. Isolated cutaneous sporotrichosis responds well to medication and has an excellent prognosis. Rarely, sporotrichosis can present as a deep fungal infection in immunocompromised hosts; it is described later. da Rosa et al reviewed 304 cases of sporotrichosis in Brazil over a period of 35 years between 1967 and 2002.[27] Duran et al reviewed 23 cases of sporotrichosis in the United States.[33]

CRITICAL POINTS *Sporotrichosis*

- Sporotrichosis is a cutaneous mycotic infection caused by the dimorphic organism *Sporothrix schenckii*.
- Clinically, sporotrichosis classically presents as subcutaneous nodules at the primary inoculation site and spreads linearly along the lymphatic channels on the hand and forearm.
- Biopsy rarely reveals fungal organisms, but when present, rounded or budding spores, cigar-shaped fungal elements, and asteroid bodies are characteristic.
- Histology alone cannot identify the causative organism, but fungal culture or PCR analysis can confirm a diagnosis of sporotrichosis.
- Itraconazole is used as a first-line treatment for lymphocutaneous or fixed-cutaneous sporotrichosis.
  - Alternative treatment options include other antifungal agents, SSKI, and hyperthermia.

TABLE 3.6 **Differential Diagnosis and Treatment for Major Causes of Multiple, Marching, Linear Nodular Lymphangitis**

Organism	Exposure History	Diagnosis	Preferred Therapy	Alternative Therapy	Duration of Treatment
Sporothrix schenckii	Gardening, soil contamination, splinters, animal scratches or bites	Biopsy and culture	Itraconazole (Sporanox), 200 mg daily	SSKI, 5 drops in water three times daily, slowly increased to 40-50 drops three times daily as tolerated Terbinafine (Lamisil), 250 mg twice daily	Two months after resolution of lesions
Nocardia brasiliensis	Gardening, soil contamination, splinters	Biopsy and culture	TMP-SMX (Bactrim, Septra), 2 double-strength tablets three times daily	Minocycline (Minocin), 200 mg twice daily See text for additional alternatives	Three months
Mycobacterium marinum	Aquariums; fish handling; swimming in oceans, lakes, or pools	Biopsy and culture	Minocycline, doxycycline	TMP-SMX Rifampin, 10-15 mg/kg daily, with clarithromycin (Biaxin), 30 mg/kg daily	Two to three months after resolution of symptoms
Leishmania brasiliensis	Residence in or travel to endemic areas	Biopsy and culture	Stibogluconate sodium, 20 mg/kg daily, or meglumine antimonate, 20 mg/kg daily	AmB (Fungizone IV), 0.25-1.00 mg/kg daily See text for additional alternatives	20 days

SSKI, Supersaturated potassium iodide; *TMP-SMX*, trimethoprim-sulfamethoxazole.

Phaeomycotic Cysts

A phaeomycotic cyst is a rare deep dermal and subcutaneous cystic infection due to a darkly pigmented fungus such as *Exophiala*, *Phialophora*, or *Bantalis*. It most commonly results from the traumatic implantation of a wood splinter, but it may be nosocomially acquired at the site of an intravenous catheter in an immunocompromised patient. In a review of phaeomycotic cysts from the Armed Forces Institute of Pathology, 25 cases were seen over 19 years.[121] Eleven were on the upper extremity, 12 on the lower extremity, and 2 on the face. The standard of care for this infection is surgical removal. It is not clear whether antifungal therapy alone could be successful.

Deep Fungal Infections

Deep fungal infections are serious clinical problems that often result in significant morbidity and even mortality. Several of the organisms described in the following subsections can also present as cutaneous or superficial infections; both superficial and deep infections are presented together under each fungal infection. Fortunately, deep infections are rare in the hand and upper extremity but may affect the tenosynovium, joints, or bone. The only way to make a diagnosis of hand or upper extremity fungal infection is to include fungal stains and cultures in the biopsy for every presentation of chronic tenosynovitis, arthritis, or osteomyelitis. Infectious disease consultation is recommended for diagnosis and treatment of deep fungal infections. They are difficult to treat because drug therapy is prolonged, drug toxicity is often severe, and recurrences are common in both immunocompetent and immunocompromised patients. The infections are presented in alphabetic order next.

Aspergillosis

Etiology. Aspergillosis of the upper extremity, like cryptococcosis and mucormycosis in an immunocompromised patient, is a devastating disease. Prompt and timely biopsy and treatment prevents serious morbidity. *A. fumigatus* is the most common species recovered from patients with aspergillosis. *A. ustus* was found in a case of forearm abscess in a cardiac transplant patient.

Clinical Findings. *Aspergillus* infections of the hand are rarely encountered in a healthy person and are reported and occur as localized dermal nodules. It may be seen as a necrotic ulcer in a finger, hand, or forearm. As a rule, it infects the immunocompromised and is a major cause of morbidity, hand amputation, and mortality in immunosuppressed patients because it infects blood vessels and causes devastating tissue necrosis as in mucormycosis. Hand infection has been reported in immunocompromised adults with diabetes, in immunocompromised children with acute leukemia,[45] and in cardiac and/or liver transplant patients.

In the upper extremity, primary cutaneous aspergillosis is often associated with burns,[101] sites of IV or catheter insertion in leukemic children, and surgical wounds. It typically presents as minor erythema and induration that rapidly progresses to devastating skin and deep necrosis. Granulocytopenia (<500 polymorphonuclear leukocytes per mL) that results from cytotoxic chemotherapy predisposes children to invasion by *Aspergillus*. A hemorrhagic vesicle, bleb, or necrotic ulcer on the finger, hand, forearm, or arm of a child who is undergoing chemotherapy for acute leukemia should alert the hand surgeon to aspergillosis. Puncture wounds after intravenous infusion are common sites of infection. Infection in an organ transplant patient should arouse a strong suspicion.

Diagnosis. Biopsy is essential to establish a diagnosis; blood cultures fail to reveal the diagnosis. *Aspergillus* species are common contaminants in the bacteriology laboratory but should not be dismissed when the culture is obtained from an immunosuppressed patient. Biopsy of the necrotic lesions shows numerous fungal hyphae on a wet KOH preparation. Definitive diagnosis of *Aspergillus* infection depends on identification of the organism in cultures of the infected biopsy tissue.

Treatment. Rapid radical surgical debridement, intravenous or oral voriconazole, and reversal of underlying host immune defect with reduction of high doses of immunosuppressive therapy are the mainstays of treatment. Repeated debridement may be necessary due to its invasiveness and tissue necrosis caused by vascular infection. This may be followed by skin grafting. Itraconazole was successful in the treatment of a localized cutaneous *Aspergillus* infection of the hand; however, voriconazole is now considered the drug of choice against aspergillosis. It has replaced AmB because it is more potent and has fewer side effects. Transient and reversible visual disturbance occurs in 30% of patients receiving voriconazole. Without treatment, aspergillosis metastasis to different sites occurs rapidly and generally proves fatal. When necrosis of tendons, joints, and neurovascular bundles occurs, ray amputation may be necessary. In an immunocompetent subject, excision of the lesion is curative.

Blastomycosis

Etiology and Epidemiology. Blastomycosis is caused by *Blastomyces dermatitidis*. It is reported mostly in North America's Ohio and Mississippi River valleys and has a similar distribution as histoplasmosis. It is a disease of immunocompetent hosts who work in contact with soil. The fungus is inhaled and causes a clinical or subclinical lung infection. Primary cutaneous blastomycosis can be caused by direct implantation into the skin or secondarily by dissemination of the fungus from the lungs. Hand infections are rare and only sporadically reported. Traumatic implantation of *B. dermatitidis* may occur in the hand of a veterinarian who handled an infected necropsy specimen. Blastomycosis can occur as a primary infection of the upper extremity[47] or secondarily as part of a systemic infection.[47] Primary inoculation blastomycosis in a finger can occur when there is an accidental inoculation of *Blastomyces dermatitidis*. It can occur in AIDS patients.

Clinical Findings. Clinical findings are nonspecific and multifarious. It may appear as a plaque, ulcer, or nodules on a finger, hand, or forearm.[43] Skin lesions can be in the form of subcutaneous nodules and can be solitary[43] or multiple; they may appear concurrently in the hand or wrist[43] or on separate regions of the same upper extremity, or another extremity, or elsewhere on the body. Blastomycosis may appear as paronychia, nodules on a finger, dorsum of the hand, or forearm. It may appear as a painless soft tissue mass on the forearm. Subcutaneous nodules can develop into abscesses with draining fistulas and finally into ulcers. Lesions may be exudative, suppurative, or granulomatous. Contiguous spread to bone, joint, or flexor tendon of a finger can occur. It may present as a blastomycotic phalangeal osteomyelitis (dactylitis). A localized osteomyelitis of the distal radius that simulates a sarcoma may occur in an otherwise asymptomatic patient. Osteoarticular lesions occur in 60% of patients who have systemic blastomycosis and may include septic arthritis and osteomyelitis in the hand and elbow. Lymphangitis and lymphadenitis may occur.

Diagnosis. Histopathologic diagnosis of biopsy tissue may require special stains, including periodic acid–Schiff or silver stain. The fungus has a characteristic histologic appearance with a double refractile cell wall and broad-based buds between the mother/daughter cells.

Treatment. Ketoconazole and itraconazole are highly effective against *B. dermatitidis*. Surgery is necessary only for diagnostic biopsy. The value of surgical debulking is questionable.

Candidiasis

Etiology and Epidemiology. The increasing incidence of HIV infection and the implantation of prosthetic devices are important in the increasing incidence of local and systemic candidiasis. The most common species recovered from clinical specimens include *C. albicans*, *C. tropicalis*, *C. glabrata*, and *C. parapsilosis*. Many other less common species have also been described. *C. albicans* can cause an interdigital web ulcer.

Clinical Findings. Flexor and extensor tenosynovitis of the hand has been reported in newborns and in AIDS patients. Osteomyelitis and septic arthritis of the wrist with *C. parapsilosis* has been reported. Silicone arthroplasty of the metacarpophalangeal joint may become infected with *C. albicans*.

Diagnosis. Infected prosthetic joints may be aspirated or opened, and staining and culture for the fungus should be included in microbiologic studies.

Treatment. Fluconazole and AmB are the drugs of choice for use in patients with deep candidiasis. For periprosthetic infection, radical synovectomy, tenosynovectomy, and removal of the implant are recommended in addition to chemotherapy combined with amphotericin B and 5-fluorouracil.

Coccidioidomycosis

Etiology and Epidemiology. Coccidioidomycosis is caused by *Coccidioides immitis*. It is a highly infectious fungus that is found only in hot and arid regions of the San Joaquin Valley in California and the US deserts of the southwest, where the infection is endemic.

Clinical Findings. This fungus has a predilection for synovium, and 10% of coccidioidal infections occur in the wrist and hand. Coccidioidal tenosynovitis,[29] joint infection, and osteomyelitis[53] of the hand have been reported. All four cases of coccidioidal osteomyelitis were in children. Coccidioidal osteomyelitis of a metacarpal has been reported to mimic an enchondroma.[53] Patients with tenosynovitis present with chronic diffuse swelling over the dorsal or volar side of the wrist or palm. If untreated, tenosynovitis can lead to extensor tendon rupture and mimic rheumatoid arthritis. Rarely has concurrent pulmonary coccidioidomycosis been diagnosed. Coccidioidomycosis of the hand may occur as a part of disseminated coccidioidomycosis or after traumatic implantation of the fungus.

Diagnosis. Clinical, gross histopathologic (rice bodies and melon seed bodies), and microhistopathologic similarities (noncaseating granulomas) between coccidioidal and other fungal and tuberculous infections are well recognized. Diagnosis is made from positive complement fixation titer, presence of chronic granuloma, microabscesses in the synovial biopsy, and identification of *C. immitis* in synovial stains and cultures. The organism has a characteristic appearance in tissue and can be identified in many cases under a microscope. Histopathology of excised synovium shows the characteristic *C. immitis* spherules in synovium, and the dimorphic fungus grows in synovium culture. The fungus in its hyphal form is highly infectious. The laboratory should be alerted to the presumed diagnosis so that it can handle the specimens and cultures in an appropriate biohazard hood to prevent airborne dissemination.

Treatment. Coccidioidomycosis is one of the most difficult to treat among invasive mycoses because the nonpulmonary infection often requires years to cure, and lifelong antifungal suppressive therapy may be needed. The infection resists aggressive treatment with synovectomy, tenosynovectomy, and high doses of AmB. Patients may have multiple recurrences of tenosynovitis, even when they are treated with adequate tenosynovectomy and intravenous amphotericin B. The infection flares up during periods of immunosuppression or lowered host resistance. Preexisting and dormant tenosynovitis may suffer flare-up of infection during chemotherapy for leukemia. Complement fixation titers correlate closely with clinical response to therapy and are useful in detecting subclinical recurrences.

Therapy with fluconazole, itraconazole, or AmB may be indicated depending on the patient's condition. The azoles are particularly useful for long-term therapy and have provided many patients with chronic suppression of otherwise relapsing manifestations of the disease. Consultation with a knowledgeable infectious disease consultant is highly recommended because a long-term commitment to therapy and attention to drug side effects, drug interactions, and possibly disease flareups is frequently necessary.

Cryptococcosis

Etiology and Epidemiology. Cryptococcosis of the upper extremity, like aspergillosis and mucormycosis, in an immunocompromised patient is a devastating disease and prompt and timely biopsy and treatment will prevent serious morbidity. In immunocompetent patients, primary infection in the lung is rare and is typically asymptomatic and self-limited. In immunocompromised patients, *Cryptococcus* from the lung may be disseminated to many sites, commonly to the skin, brain, and meninges. Cryptococcosis (European blastomycosis, torulosis) is an infection caused by the opportunistic fungus *Cryptococcus neoformans*. It is usually associated with avian habitats and, in particular, with pigeons and pigeon's droppings. There are two varieties of neoformans: *C. neoformans* and *C. gattii*.

Clinical Findings. The skin is the third most common organ affected in *C. neoformans* infections, after the lung and central nervous system. Cutaneous cryptococcosis can present in a variety of ways, including papules, pustules, plaques, cellulitis, abscesses, nodules, sinuses, and ulcers—all of which may present diagnostic problems for the hand surgeon. Opportunistic cryptococcal infections of the hand are reported in patients who are immunodeficient because of renal failure or end-stage renal disease, in renal allograft recipients, in diabetics, in patients with malignancy, and in patients receiving long-term corticosteroids. With HIV, cryptococcosis is listed as an AIDS-defining disease. The hand and entire forearm may be bullous in an immunocompromised patient.

Cryptococcal tenosynovitis may present as a sausage finger and was reported in a rheumatoid patient treated with the disease-modifying drug adalimumab. *Cryptococcus* species very rarely cause disease of the upper extremity in an immunocompetent patient, and having it is an exception to the rule. Primary cutaneous cryptococcosis presenting as a hemorrhagic pustular lesion and an abscess and osteomyelitis of the proximal phalanx are reported in immunocompetent patients.[4] A patient may develop a finger infection after accidental inoculation with an cryptococcal-contaminated needle. The most common radiological presentation of cryptococcal osteomyelitis is a lytic lesion with or without a periosteal reaction. Thick and tenacious pus in the wound should arouse suspicion of cryptococcal infection, especially when thorough surgical debridement fails to clear the infection.

Diagnosis. The simple procedure of mixing together India ink and biologic fluids from sinus, ulcer, or abscess identifies capsulated yeast and remains a rapid and effective method for identifying *Cryptococcus* infection. Diagnosis is confirmed by a high cryptococcal antigen titer and growth of the fungus from biopsy specimens within 48 h on most routine agar media. Histology is an effective way to establish diagnosis of cryptococcosis as the organism is easily and readily identified in the biopsy specimen. Draining material, deep skin biopsy, or curettage from the bone show granulomatous inflammation and encapsulated yeasts.

Treatment. Fluconazole, itraconazole, and flucytosine are all effective in eradicating the infection. Treatment of hand infections with a minimum of 12 weeks of therapy with fluconazole (400 mg/day or more) should control most of these infections. Alternatives include flucytosine, itraconazole, or the newer azoles (e.g., voriconazole). If the patient is immunosuppressed, long-term antifungal therapy is recommended. Patients with diabetes, end-stage renal failure, and uremia who develop infection of the hand with ipsilateral synthetic arteriovenous fistula do not resolve with AmB, 5-flucytosine, and repeated surgical drainages until the graft is removed. Early therapy with fluconazole prevents infection in injuries incidentally caused by needles contaminated with viable *C. neoformans*.

Histoplasmosis

Etiology and Epidemiology. Histoplasmosis is caused by *Histoplasma capsulatum*. It is a highly infectious fungus endemic in the Mississippi and Ohio River valleys.

Clinical Findings. Histoplasmosis may present as cutaneous infection, tenosynovitis, tendon ruptures, carpal tunnel syndrome, arthritis, and in severe burns of the upper extremity with fatal necrotizing myofasciitis. A case of recurrent osteomyelitis of capitate bone with 10-year latency between initial inadequate curettage and clinical recurrence has been reported. African histoplasmosis may cause fungating shoulder and elbow swellings with lytic destruction of lateral clavicle and distal humerus, respectively. Infected synovial tissue is red-brown, contains many rice bodies, and undergoes active caseous granulomatous inflammation.

Diagnosis. The diagnosis of histoplasmosis is difficult because the clinical syndrome is nonspecific, and it may be difficult to isolate *H. capsulatum* from clinical specimens. It is revealed in the biopsy tissue if Grocott silver stain is specified. *H. capsulatum* is difficult to grow; it can take several weeks. Close collaboration between surgeon, rheumatologist, infectious disease specialist, pathologist, and microbiologist is paramount in the diagnosis and treatment of these cases. Since the late 1940s, serology has been important in the diagnosis of infection with *H. capsulatum*. Complement fixation test is reliably and commonly used in the clinical laboratory. For complement fixation of antibodies, a titer of 1:8 is considered presumptive and a titer of more than 1:32 is significantly suggestive of active infection. Sensitivity of antibody tests may be lower in immunocompromised hosts. An antigen test can help in diagnosis of histoplasmosis and gauge the efficacy of antifungal therapy.

Treatment. Combined medical and surgical treatment is critical to prevent recurrence. A combination of complete tenosynovectomy, bone debridement, and prolonged systemic antifungal therapy (e.g., oral ketoconazole or itraconazole or intravenous AmB) is used. The drug of choice for long-term therapy is 200 mg of itraconazole twice daily. Fluconazole, 400 to 800 mg/day, can serve as an alternative. The histoplasmosis reference laboratory in Indianapolis, Indiana (histodgn @indyunix.lupui.edu), provides services in histoplasmosis antigen testing and itraconazole serum levels.

Mucormycosis

Etiology and Epidemiology. Mucormycosis of the upper extremity in an immunocompetent (in context of trauma) as well as immunocompromised patient (especially diabetes) is a devastating disease, and prompt biopsy and earliest possible treatment prevent serious morbidity (amputation) and mortality. Mucormycosis is an acute and chronic fungal infection characterized by vascular infection, arterial and venous thrombosis, and gangrenous tissue infarction and necrosis. These infections are highly invasive and relentlessly progressive and among the most aggressive, destructive, and necrotizing of all fungal infections. It has a higher rate of morbidity and mortality (>40%) than many other infections. In mucormycosis, necrotizing fasciitis carries a mortality rate approaching 80%. It rapidly infects the blood vessels at the site of infection and quickly spreads to adjacent and subjacent soft tissues all the way to the bone. There is rapid onset of local and widespread tissue necrosis and gangrene, all while the physician struggles to make a diagnosis because of its rarity.

Recent reclassification has abolished the class Zygomycetes. Although called phycomycosis and zygomycosis in the past, the infection is caused by fungi of the class Mucoromycotina and order Mucorales and is now called mucormycosis. *Rhizopus* species are the most commonly isolated agents of mucormycosis, followed by *Rhizomucor*. *Mucor* species, despite its name, is a rare cause of mucormycosis. *Mucor hiemalis*, a common soil inhabitant, was recovered from a diabetic gardener with a localized subcutaneous infection of a finger.

Mucorales are opportunistic fungi that are angioinvasive like *Aspergillus*. Cutaneous mucormycosis can result from external implantation of the fungus or conversely from hematogenous dissemination. External implantation–related infection has been described in the setting of heavy soil contamination of open wounds (e.g., in high-energy severe motor vehicle accidents), penetrating injury from plant material (e.g., a thorn), injections of medications (e.g., insulin or corticosteroids), catheter insertion, contaminated surgical dressings, and use of tape to secure endotracheal tubes or oxygen-monitoring devices. Cutaneous mucormycosis is a common infection in immunocompromised patients and remains rare in the immunocompetent patient outside the setting of major trauma.[83] Cutaneous infections represent <10% of all *Mucor* cases. Cutaneous mucormycosis predominantly involves the epidermis and dermis (eschar), and tissue necrosis and gangrene develop secondary to vascular invasion of subcutaneous tissues and major arteries, respectively.

Clinical Findings. *Rhizopus* and *Mucor* infection of the hand is usually cutaneous and subcutaneous. The upper extremity is involved in 24% of all cutaneous and subcutaneous cases. As an isolated lesion it can occur in the hand,[111] forearm, upper arm,[111] or shoulder.

Fifty percent of cases of primary cutaneous mucormycosis occur in immunocompetent patients with severe trauma where a large and open extensive soft tissue wound is heavily contaminated by soil. Moran et al. have wisely warned that hand surgeons should have a high level of suspicion of *Mucor* infections in high-energy automobile and agricultural injuries with open, contaminated, extensive soft tissue wounds involving the upper extremity in immunocompetent patients.[83] All seven of their patients had an average of 10 surgical debridements (range, 4-20) and four resulted in amputations: one partial hand amputation, one below the elbow, one above the elbow, and one at the glenohumeral joint. Cutaneous mucormycosis of the wrist can occur after an arterial puncture in an immunocompetent host. Infection may start as a blister at the puncture site and progress to a large eschar that needs a large skin graft. If the diagnosis is not made with biopsy, waiting for cultures may result in an amputation and/or loss of life.

The other 50% of the *Mucor* infections occur in immunodeficient patients. Of the 50%, most patients have diabetes (20%), leukemia or aplastic anemia (9%), chronic kidney failure (5%), organ transplants (4%), and rarely alcoholic encephalopathy.[93] An infection of the forearm may occur at an intravenous infusion site, at the arterial line,[93] or follow an intramuscular corticosteroid injection in immunocompromised patients. Persistent and progressive thrombophlebitis at the site of an intravenous line in an immunocompromised diabetic should arouse suspicion of mucormycosis.

The disease occurs as a devastating and often fatal infection in severe burns of the upper extremity. Whereas some mild and localized cases have been described in the hand, the disease more often results in devastating tissue necrosis. Al-Qattan rightly recognized cutaneous and subcutaneous infections of the upper extremity in three stages: dermal plexus (black eschar), subcutaneous vessels (bleeding ulcer), and deep extension to major subjacent arteries (digital and hand gangrene).[2] It is critical to recognize the infection when it is limited to the dermal plexus as a black eschar with progressive necrosis of the wound margin.

Diagnosis. The most important criteria to remember that may point to diagnosis of mucormycosis is a triad of rapid cutaneous and subcutaneous gangrenous destruction, diabetes, and blood vessel thrombosis (i.e., arterial or venous). Enlarging black skin eschars and gangrene should lead one to consideration of advanced mucormycosis, both in immunocompetent and immunocompromised hosts. The diagnosis may be difficult to make because the infectious lesions can be confused with ischemic pathology in patients with multiorgan failure.[93] It may behave like necrotizing fasciitis with rapid necrosis of subcutaneous tissue. Progressive gangrene has prompted finger, hand, below-elbow, above-elbow, and shoulder amputation.

Mucormycosis is notorious for its tendency to invade deep tissues, although mucormycosis osteomyelitis in the hand is rare. Extension of pathology across tissue planes, dermis-to-subcutaneous tissue to vascular invasion of a major artery strongly suggests a mucoral etiology and urgent need for a biopsy. Biopsy and histopathologic examination remain the most sensitive and specific modality for definitive diagnosis. Cultures are positive in less than half of the cases of mucormycosis.

Biopsy specimens taken from the center of the lesion down to the subcutaneous fat are most likely to reveal presence of fungus. The organisms are scattered within a large area of necrosis. Biopsy and smears often reveal the organisms when cultures are negative. Cultures from an excised ulcer may grow *Rhizopus*, *Mucor*, or *Absidia*, as well as other Mucorales (e.g., *Cunninghamella* and *Apophysomyces*). They grow abundantly in 1 to 7 days on routine fungal media when the biopsy material is sampled from deep tissue.

Histopathology for diagnosis of fungus in the infected tissue is immediate and reliable and waiting for cultures may be too late to prevent extremity amputation or death. For histopathologic examination, the laboratory must be alerted as to the nature of the lesion because certain fungal media contain cycloheximide, which suppresses growth of Mucorales species. Yield on superficial swab cultures is low and not recommended.

Treatment. Rapid diagnosis and radical debridement of all necrotic tissues are essential to preserve tissues and prevent limb amputation and loss of life, both in immunocompetent and immunocompromised patients. Successful treatment of mucormycosis requires four steps:

1. Early biopsy
2. Prompt and aggressive surgical debridement of necrotic tissue
3. Rapid initiation of effective, high-dose systemic lipid formulation of amphotericin B
4. Reversal of any underlying predisposing systemic factors; that is, rapid restoration of euglycemia in diabetes, and reducing the dose of immunosuppressive medications if possible helps eliminate the infection

With older patients, tissue necrosis may be so extensive that major debridement and multiple skin grafts are necessary. Intravenous lipid formulations of AmB remain the drugs of choice for the treatment of mucormycosis and should be given in full dose without the delay of increasing dose titration. High doses of these agents are necessary for patients who are at risk of dying of this infection, despite their known nephrotoxicity.

Cutaneous and subcutaneous mucormycosis that is more localized has a much better prognosis (mortality, 15%) than deep-seated infections (mortality, 40%). Mortality of cutaneous mucormycosis is higher in immunocompromised patients than immunocompetent patients, especially when early and aggressive surgery is undertaken.[83] For patients receiving immunosuppressive therapy, secondary antifungal prophylaxis is continued for as long as the immunosuppressive regimen is administered. *Mucor* and *Aspergillus* infection of burns and bones is devastating and is considered separately in the following. Al-Qattan,[1] Prabhu et al,[90] Moran et al,[83] and Spellberg et al[108] recently reviewed mucormycosis comprehensively.

Deep (Extracutaneous) Sporotrichosis

Etiology and Epidemiology. Extracutaneous sporotrichosis is rare and usually occurs within the musculoskeletal system of an immunocompromised host. The organism frequently enters the body through the lungs, and a concomitant pneumonia is often present. Deep sporotrichosis infection may localize to the bones, joints, or tenosynovium in the hand. Sporotrichal osteomyelitis may present as multifocal subchondral and periarticular erosions of the hand's bones. Among articular lesions, wrist joint and hand joints are the most commonly involved.

Diagnosis. A joint infection with a sinus should arouse suspicion. Tenosynovial lesions can occur on the dorsal wrist tendons. Extensor tenosynovitis may cause rupture of an extensor tendon. Sporotrichal flexor tenosynovitis can result in carpal tunnel syndrome or ulnar nerve entrapment. Bursal sporotrichosis can occur in the olecranon bursa. Sporotrichal myositis of the biceps muscle can occur without skin or lymphatic involvement.

A high level of suspicion is needed to make the diagnosis of sporotrichal arthritis, osteomyelitis, and tenosynovitis. The diagnosis of sporotrichal arthritis is often delayed for two reasons: (1) *Sporothrix schenckii* is an uncommon cause of arthritis and (2) sporotrichal arthritis often occurs in the absence of the clinically familiar cutaneous lesions. Eighty-four percent of sporotrichal joint infections presented as monoarthritis. Sporotrichosis should be considered in the differential diagnosis when granulomatous synovitis is recognized by histologic examination.

Sporotrichal osteomyelitis is equally rare. Infected patients have localized swelling, local sinus tract formation, and concomitant arthritis. Roentgenographic findings in osseous sporotrichosis are nonspecific and include destruction of bone without reactive sclerosis or periosteal reaction. Tenosynovial swelling of sporotrichosis is clinically similar to rheumatoid tenosynovitis and on gross examination proliferative tenosynovium is similar to rheumatoid tenosynovium. Rice bodies may be found in the inflamed tenosynovium, as is common in tenosynovitis due to rheumatoid arthritis, tuberculosis, and many other causes.

Olecranon bursal sporotrichosis has been reported.*** Even when biopsy is done expeditiously, diagnosis can be missed on histopathologic examination unless multiple sections are diligently examined. *S. schenckii* may grow from aspirated pus or from tenosynovium, or not grow on repeated cultures. Delay in diagnosis can range from 2 to 12 months. Repeated synovial fluid cultures and synovium biopsies may be necessary before a diagnosis is made. Cultures usually grow in 4 weeks, but growth may be delayed up to 8 weeks.[30] Histologic examination typically reveals a nonspecific pyogranulomatous response or a noncaseating granuloma. It is diagnostic only when characteristic cigar-shaped yeasts are seen and *Sporothrix schenckii* grow on culture.

Treatment. Aggressive chemotherapy in combination with surgical debridement is necessary to cure deep sporotrichosis. For bone, joint, and tenosynovial sporotrichosis, SSKI is not adequate because it is for the treatment of cutaneous and lymphocutaneous sporotrichosis. Amphotericin B is the drug of choice, and 2-hydroxystilbamidine, ketoconazole, itraconazole, and fluconazole have all been used successfully. If surgical debridement in conjunction with chemotherapy does not eradicate the infection, arthrodesis or amputation may be necessary. Appropriate use of antifungal agents, however, should make such radical surgery less likely. Osteoarticular sporotrichosis may require prolonged therapy but is not life threatening.

Fungal infections of burns and fungal osteomyelitis are described separately in the following subsection because they are exceedingly devastating, resulting in morbidity and mortality.

CRITICAL POINTS *Diagnosis and Treatment of Mucormycosis*

- Beware of an eschar (mucormycosis, aspergillosis).
- Fungus grows faster in host than in petri dish.
- Biopsy gives faster diagnosis than cultures.
- Waiting for culture result can cost limb or life.
- Excise infected tissues to healthy margins.

Fungal Infections Following Large Upper Extremity Burns

Fungal infections following large upper extremity burns are rare but devastating. They are best reviewed by Salisbury et al.[101] Seven out of 16 patients died in spite of correct diagnosis and treatment with AmB and radical surgery including amputations in four. The extent of the burns in the patients averaged 50%. The presence of invasive fungal infection was diagnosed from 3 to 27 days from the occurrence of the burns. There were only two invading organisms: mucormycosis (Phycomycetes) in 13 and *Aspergillus* species in 3. Suspicious signs included: (1) inflammation, (2) a rapidly progressive change in color of the wound to violaceous or black, and (3) earlier separation of eschar.

There was rapid progression of clinical disease, compared to slow and inconsistent growth of fungi on cultures. Thus, histological examination of a burn wound suspected of fungal invasion should be carried out promptly because the fungus is easily visible in biopsy tissue. The fungus may be on the surface of the wound (contamination), may colonize on the wound surface, may colonize partial eschar, may colonize entire eschar, may infect subeschar, and finally may invade the muscle locally or extensively. Prompt and radical excision of infected tissue including muscle combined with AmB is the treatment of choice. Three levels of invasion necessitated amputation: (1) widespread muscle invasion, (2) bone involvement, and (3) vascular invasion.

Fungal Osteomyelitis

Clinical aspects of mycotic infections of bone are well reviewed by Rhangos and Chick.[97] The three major causes of fungal osteomyelitis are blastomycosis, coccidioidomycosis, and histoplasmosis. Coccidioidomycosis and histoplasmosis are asymptomatic or moderate in 75% of the infections. Bone lesions due to *C. immitis* may be expected in 10% of severe infections caused by it.

The most important factor in diagnosis of a mycotic infection is a high level of suspicion. Without this, the proper diagnostic steps may never be taken. The skin tests done with fungal antigens of *H. capsulatum* and *C. immitis* are simple diagnostic tools and are performed in the same way as the Mantoux PPD test for tuberculosis. Five millimeters or more of induration after 48 h indicates present or past infection. A negative test rules out infection by either of these two organisms. Serologic tests provide useful information in that the presence of a positive titer indicates active infection.

Serial determinations are a precise method of following the extent of the infection. The complement fixation test is most widely applied with *Histoplasma*, *Coccidioides*, and *Blastomyces*. Skin and serologic tests provide a presumptive diagnosis. Diag-nosis is verified by demonstration of fungus in a culture, but that takes up to 4 or more weeks. A more rapid diagnosis of *B. dermatitidis*, *C. immitis*, and *C. neoformans* is provided by biopsy material in which the fungus is identified. The best all-purpose stain is methenamine silver, which will demonstrate all of the preceding fungi that involve bone.

In blastomycosis, about half the cases infect bone, and carpal bone infection has been reported. Radiologically, there is sharp, well-defined bone destruction. In *Coccidioides*, about 20% of the cases involve bones and joints. Infection of the wrist and elbow are favorite sites in the upper extremity. Radiologic examination shows sharply demarcated cystic lesions. In cryptococcosis, 20% of 200 cases had bone involvement. Radiologically, lesions resemble osteomyelitis with eventual breakdown of soft tissues and formation of a draining sinus. The radiographic appearance is again that of a discrete osteolytic lesion surrounded by a zone of dense bone.

Mucormycosis osteomyelitis in the hand is a rare occurrence, but occurs commonly in diabetics. Inoculation happens from trauma with soil contamination, burns, and intramuscular injection. Zygomycotic *Apophysomyces elegans* fungus was the infecting organism in 3 of Stevanovic's 9 cases. They are angio-invasive and lead to tissue necrosis by vascular thrombosis and amputation was necessary in 4 of 9 cases reviewed by Stevanovic et al.[111]

Newly Emerging Hand Fungal Infections
Etiology and Epidemiology

In recent years, a number of emerging fungal infections have become apparent. This category includes resurgent organisms that had previously declined in prevalence, as well as newly identified organisms. Such fungal infections are generally rare and often of low grade, causing encapsulated cysts localized to subcutaneous tissue.

Hand infections with several new fungi have been reported. Pheohyphomycosis (i.e., chromomycosis, chromohyphomycosis, chromoblastomycosis) is the general term for infections caused by dematiaceous (e.g., pigmented, yellow-brown, light brown, black) fungi, commonly seen in tropical and subtropical climates. These infections should be suspected in a visitor from or traveler to such regions. Such infections are being reported at an increasing rate. Pheomycotic cyst or subcutaneous pheohyphomycosis is the most common type of pheohyphomycosis.

Among the pheohyphomycosis cases reported in the hand, many rare fungi have been reported, including *Phaeoacremonium aleophilum*, *Curvularia*, *Pyrenochaeta romeroi*, *Exophilia dermatitidis*, *Exophiala jeanselmei*, *Geotrichum candidum*, *Phialophora richardsiae*, *Cladophialophora carrionii*, *Alternaria alternata*, *C. bantiana*, *Fonsecaea pedrosoi*, *Rhinocladiella aquaspersa*, *Cladosporium*, *Actinomucor elegans*, *Microsporum persicolor*, *Scedosporium apiospermum*, *Fusarium oxysporum*, *Moraxella lacunata*, and *Paecilomyces lilacinus*. *Pseudallescheria boydii* is known to cause mycetoma in immunocompetent subjects. Rare *Leptosphaeria tompkinsii* was reported to cause mycetoma of the hand. *P. richardsiae* is a rare fungus found in wood pulp and has been known to cause two infections in the upper extremity, one in the hand, and one in the olecranon bursa. Splinters may cause pheomycotic cysts of the finger.

Treatment

These fungi are relatively less virulent and invoke minimal inflammation and result in formation of a thick capsule that allows easy excision, which is generally curative. No antibiotics are necessary if the entire encapsulated mass of fungus is excised. The cysts should not be opened while dissecting them because the fungus from within them will spill into virgin tissue and cause recurrence. If a cyst filled with fungus is opened, it is essential to irrigate the wound before the tourniquet is released to prevent hematogenous dissemination of live fungi.

One case recurred when surgical excision was not complete. *Pseudallescheria boydii* is known to cause infection of hand, wrist joint, tendons, and soft tissues of the forearm in immunocompromised patients. The infections respond to itraconazole, although surgical excision is an important adjunct for treatment of this infection. These fungi are inherently resistant to AmB and may be less sensitive to azoles as well. Treatment with voriconazole, high-dose fluconazole, or itraconazole is the preferred strategy. Long-term therapy (>3 months) is likely to be necessary.

Consultation with the CDC's mycotic disease branch in Atlanta (www.cdc.gov) or fungus testing laboratory at the University of Texas, Health Sciences Center, San Antonio (rinaldi@uthscsa.edu), may help with choosing the latest diagnostic and therapeutic laboratory tests and treatment.

MYCOBACTERIAL INFECTIONS (TUBERCULOUS AND NONTUBERCULOUS)

Tubercle bacillus was identified, isolated, and grown in 1872 by Robert Koch, for which he received a Nobel Prize in 1905. Almost 150 years after Koch, *M. tuberculosis* continues to affect an estimated 2 billion people (i.e., one-third of the world's population). Worldwide, it is second only to AIDS as a cause of death resulting from a single infectious agent. Globally, in 2012, approximately 8.6 million became ill with TB, and 1.3 million died from the disease.

In the United States, after the resurgence of it during 1985 to 1992 as a result of the AIDS epidemic, the annual TB rate decreased steadily. In 2011, a total of 10,528 new US cases (3.4/100,000) were reported. This represents a decline of 60.5% from 1992 due to retroviral treatment of AIDS. Unfortunately, multidrug-resistant TB (MDR TB) has become a threat, and extensively drug-resistant TB (XDR TB) is an emerging threat. Racial and ethnic minorities and foreign-born individuals continue to account for the largest number of TB cases in the United States. In 2011, 84% of all reported cases occurred in racial and ethnic minorities: 30% in Asians, 29% in Hispanics, 23% in African Americans, whereas 16% of cases occurred in non-Hispanic whites.

The percentage of recorded TB cases for foreign-born people increased from 28% in 1990 to 62% in 2011. Among the foreign-born, 46% were Asian, 34% were Hispanic or Latino, 13% were non-Hispanic black or African American, and 5% were non-Hispanic white. In 2011, the seven top countries reported 61% of the total cases, with Mexico having 22%, the Philippines 11.6%, Vietnam 8.4%, India 7.7%, China 5.8%, Haiti 2.9%, and Guatemala 2.5%. People from more than 135 other countries accounted for the rest (39%) of US foreign-born individuals with TB. Approximately 65% of the immigrants affected developed tuberculosis in the United States within 5 years of their arrival. Five states (i.e., California, Florida, Illinois, New York, and Texas) recorded for more than half of all TB cases. Understandably, the most common chronic infection of the hand is tuberculosis.

The number of MDR TB cases (i.e., resistant to >1 agent and at least isoniazid or rifampin) worldwide was about a half million in 45 countries. In the United States, primary drug resistance was first reported in 1993. Resistance to at least isoniazid in 2011 was 9.2%. Multidrug-resistant TB in 2011 was 1.3%. Drug resistance is also higher in foreign-born individuals; the percentage of isoniazid resistance was approximately two times higher among the foreign-born than among US-born individuals in 2010. Cases of XDR TB (i.e., resistant to isoniazid and rifampin, plus resistant to any fluoroquinolone and at least 1 of 3 injectable second-line anti-TB drugs) have been reported in 17 countries almost every year, including the United States and all G8 countries. Six cases of XDR TB were reported in the United States in 2011. (For further information about the preceding discussion, see www.cdc.gov/tb/statistics/surv/surv2011/slides/surv21.htm.)

Tuberculous tenosynovitis, arthritis, and bursitis simulate rheumatoid synovitis but are localized to a few tendons, a joint, or a bursa. Absence of generalized findings of rheumatoid arthritis or proliferative tenosynovitis of unknown origin should alert the clinician to the possibility of tuberculosis. Biopsy for histopathology and microbiology is always necessary for definitive diagnosis. The sine qua nonhistologic hallmark of a tuberculous infection is the granuloma (tubercle). A granuloma is a minute aggregation of cell-mediated T lymphocytes, macrophages, epithelioid cells, and Langhans giant cells that limit the multiplication and spread of the tubercle bacillus. The tuberculosis granuloma can be distinguished from those of NTM by its characteristic central necrosis or caseating granuloma.[24]

NTM, however, in rare cases can cause a caseating granuloma, and organism identification is necessary for definitive diagnosis.[24,122] Caseated material represents host cells composed of tubercle bacilli that are killed by cytotoxic lymphocytes (CTLs) and a chronic delayed type hypersensitivity immune reaction (type 2 hypersensitivity reaction) to the residual and persisting dead tubercle bacillus wall antigens. If an initial biopsy does not yield a positive culture, a repeat biopsy may help to establish a diagnosis because the organisms are often sparse and grow with difficulty. Ultrasonography can detect soft tissue extension of the bony lesions and can guide drainage or biopsy procedures.

All mycobacterial hand infections reported before 1960 were attributed to *M. tuberculosis*. Since 1960, reported cases of *M. tuberculosis* of the hand are few and reported hand infections caused by NTM[5,15,34,52,64,72,92] are more frequent. Nontuberculous mycobacteria may be either slow growing (>7 days to grow) or fast growing (<7 days to grow) (Table 3.7). Currently there are more than 120 species of NTM, of which approximately 60 are human pathogens. Of the 60 known human NTM, only 19 have been reported to cause hand infections. *M. marinum* is the most widespread cutaneous tuberculosis and *M. avium*, *M. chelonae*, and *M. haemophilum* are the most common AIDS-related mycobacterial infections in the United States.

The clinical presentation of tuberculous and NTM infections is indistinguishable. Mycobacterial identification is paramount

TABLE 3.7	**Growth Rates of Mycobacteria**	
Slowly Growing	**Intermediately Growing**	**Rapidly Growing (<7 days)**
M. avium complex (M. avium and M. intracellulare)	M. marinum	M. fortuitum
M. kansasii	M. gordonae	M. chelonae
M. xenopi		M. smegmatis
M. szulgai		M. abscessus
M. scrofulaceum		
M. malmoense		
M. terrae		
M. haemophilum		
M. asiaticum		

Growth rates have become a practical means of grouping the species within laboratories.

because the virulence, growth requirements, drug sensitivity, and treatment of the various species differ greatly. The constitutional symptoms present in pulmonary tuberculosis are notoriously lacking in extrapulmonary tuberculosis. The erythrocyte sedimentation rate (ESR) may be normal or only slightly elevated in infection with *M. tuberculosis* but is almost invariably normal in immunocompetent patients with NTM infections.

A higher ESR occurs in patients with lower immunity with more inflammatory disease and indicates a more severe infection. It may necessitate diagnostic workup for an active primary focus and multicentric tuberculosis. Regional lymphadenopathy is usually absent. A positive tuberculin skin test is not indicative of a currently active infection, is positive in people who had BCG vaccination or subclinical infection, is negative in debilitated and anergic patients, and is not useful for diagnosis. Pulmonary disease does not generally accompany mycobacterial infection of the hand[11] unless immunity is low in an inadequately nourished patient.

Surgical findings of TB and NTM infection are indistinguishable. Acid-fast bacillus (AFB) smears of sampled granuloma may not show any organisms or reveal only sparse bacilli after painstaking scrutiny. The purulent aspirate from an infected joint often shows the organisms on a smear. Cultures most often grow the organism in 1 to 12 weeks on a Lowenstein-Jensen medium. *M. marinum, M. haemophilum, M. chelonae,* and *M. ulcerans* grow at 30°C (room temperature), whereas *M. tuberculosis* and other NTM grow at 37°C (body temperature). *M. xenopi* grows best at 42°C. It is wise and critical to request incubation at three temperatures in a suspected chronic hand infection because many laboratories do not routinely incubate mycobacterial cultures at 30°C and 42°C.

The TB and NTM infections differ in their prognosis, and their sensitivity to antimicrobial drugs varies widely. The clinical course of NTM infections varies from self-healing cutaneous lesions to highly resistant deep lesions, resistant both to surgical debridement and chemotherapy. *M. avium, M. chelonae,* and *M. malmoense* infections are tenacious, resistant, and recurrent, often requiring amputation. Some grow readily on cultures and others (e.g., *M. avium, M. chelonae,* and *M. malmoense*) do not. Some grow quickly in 7 to 10 days (fast-growing mycobacteria) and others take 7 to 12 weeks (*M. avium, M. malmoense*).

Sites of tuberculous and NTM infections in the upper extremity are the skin, subcutaneous tissues, tenosynovium, bursa, joints, and bone. A combination of the preceding may be seen in immunocompromised patients. The three most common *M. tuberculosis* infections of the hand are flexor tenosynovitis, wrist joint infection, and phalangeal osteomyelitis (dactylitis). Of 32 cases of the tuberculosis of the hand seen over a 4-year period by Kotwal et al,[66] 12 had bony infection and 20 had soft tissue infection. Out of the 20 soft tissue infections, 14 had flexor or extensor tenosynovitis. Out of the 12 bony infections, about half had dactylitis (i.e., phalangeal or metacarpal infections). Of the 6 joint infections, all involved the wrist.[66]

Rarely, mycobacterial infections can cause a midpalmar space abscess, a large soft tissue forearm abscess, fasciitis, compartment syndrome in the forearm due to expanding purulent caseation, or a cold abscess in a muscle. Cold abscess of muscle may occur in deltoid, brachialis, or biceps brachii muscles. Corticosteroids can cause reactivation of a latent focus of extrapulmonary tuberculosis in an immigrant from an endemic country or after organ transplantation.

Cutaneous Tuberculosis
Clinical Findings
The most common TB infection of the hand involves the skin; 80% of cutaneous tuberculosis affects the hand and the upper extremity. It is rare in childhood even in countries with a high burden of tuberculosis. It may be acquired in the skin in one of the following ways: by inoculation from an exogenous source through a breach in the skin, inoculation by tattoo needles, by acupuncture needles, by BCG vaccination, by contiguous spread from bone to skin (scrofuloderma), or by hematogenous spread to skin from a pulmonary or extrapulmonary focus (lupus vulgaris). *M. marinum* (*M. balnei*) is the most commonly reported NTM skin infection of the hand in Western countries and *M. tuberculosis* in Eastern countries. An underlying disease that compromises host immunity may be found in up to 30% of cases. Cutaneous tuberculosis of the hand in AIDS patients occurs in rare cases.

Skin infections can be caused in medical personnel by accidental primary inoculation with a cannulated needle withdrawn from an infected patient, primary inoculation of a surgeon from a blade that operated on tuberculous tissue, accidental injection of infected fluid in the laboratory, or mycobacterial infection from autopsy material (i.e., prosector's paronychia). Tuberculous paronychia has been reported in a nurse caring for a patient with active pulmonary tuberculosis. The disease is usually self-limited if host immunity is high, but chemotherapy expedites cure and reduces morbidity. Surgical excision of the lesion is clearly indicated for one caused by accidental inoculation by a known drug-resistant organism.

The most common nontuberculous mycobacterial skin infection is caused by *M. marinum* (see Figure 3.16). Fish tank exposure is the most frequent source of cutaneous *M. marinum* infections and can be prevented by use of waterproof gloves by anyone with an open skin lesion. The cutaneous infections by *M. kansasii* may heal spontaneously over a period of time, but chemotherapy may be given to expedite healing and prevent scarring. A TB skin gumma can occur on the hand after a contaminated skin venipuncture. *M. bovis* skin infection can occur occupationally in butchers (butcher's wart).

Diagnosis

The most common presentation is a node, abscess, ulcer, or a plaque lesion on the finger, hand, or forearm. A nontender nodule gradually progresses to single or multiple abscesses that drain clear liquid. Nodules do not heal with antibiotics and soaks. Less common presentations include erythema, swelling, cellulitis, crusting, verrucous plaque, verrucous nodule, sporo-trichoid lesion, and ulceration. Cortisone exacerbates the disease. Signs of lymphatic spread are evident in 70% of cases. Multiple, marching, linear lesions may be seen along the lymphatics on the hand, wrist, and forearm (i.e., sporotrichoid type) (see Figure 3.17).

Most patients have lesions for 2 months or more before they seek care, and there is usually a substantial delay between initial consultation and correct diagnosis because of the rarity of the condition. Patients infected with *M. marinum* give a history of a puncture wound involved with a fish, fish tank, or swimming pool in more than half the cases. Such a lesion is aptly known as "fish tank granuloma," "fish tank finger," "fish fancier's finger," "swimming pool granuloma," and "fish breeder's granuloma." To this list we can add "fish cleaner's finger."

An outbreak of *M. marinum* occurred in 2014 in New York among Chinese housewives who cleaned fish without gloves (see Figure 3.16). A pustular or nodular phase may subsequently ulcerate to form a "tuberculous chancre"; rarely it may present as marching plaques. Regional lymphadenopathy develops in 3 to 4 weeks after the primary skin lesion is noted. The tubercu-lous chancre and affected regional lymph nodes constitute the "tuberculous primary complex" of the skin, akin to the classic Ghon lesion in the lung. Organisms may not be seen on AFB staining, and cultures may not grow mycobacteria. Under these circumstances, the detection of mycobacteria by PCR to analyze nucleic acid sequences is recommended, useful, and diagnostic.

Differential Diagnosis

The linear, marching lymphangitis typical of *Sporothrix* infec-tion can also be seen with infections caused by *M. marinum*, *M. kansasii*, *Leishmania*, *Coccidioides*, *Cryptococcus*, *Nocardia*, and tularemia. Tuberculous cutaneous infection of the hand can also be confused with infection by blastomycosis, histoplasmo-sis, syphilis, and yaws. Final diagnosis of TB infection requires skin biopsy with mycobacterial culture.

Treatment

The US researcher Selman Waksman was awarded a Nobel Prize in 1952 for his discovery of streptomycin—the first antibiotic demonstrated to be effective against tuberculosis. To avoid resistance, *M. tuberculosis* infection is treated with a combina-tion of bactericidal drugs, including isoniazid and rifampin taken daily for at least 6 months, as well as ethambutol and pyrazinamide for the first 2 months. Prompt chemotherapy is curative.

Treatment of NTM infection differs from treatment of tuberculosis. Optimal treatment of cutaneous *M. marinum* infection is not well established. Mild infection resolves spon-taneously but complete resolution may take up to 2 years. A two drug combination is recommended to prevent resistance. *M. marinum* is sensitive to clarithromycin, rifampicin, etham-butol, minocycline, and levofloxacin. Resistance to tetracy-cline, minocycline, doxycycline, and rifampin is emerging. Thus, results of antimicrobial sensitivity tests are essential in guiding chemotherapy. Treatment of *M. kansasii* cutaneous infection is usually effective with the standard antituberculous drugs, erythromycin and cotrimoxazole. Drug sensitivity test-ing against *M. kansasii* is recommended because resistance to rifampin is known.

Current concepts of cutaneous *M. tuberculosis* treatment have been reviewed by Sehgal.[103] Large series of *M. marinum* and *M. kansasii* skin infections of the hand have been reviewed by Breathnach et al.[15] When the infection is caused inadver-tently by inoculation of drug-resistant *M. tuberculosis*, surgical excision of the lesion is important.

Subcutaneous Tuberculosis

Mycobacterium Ulcerans (Buruli Ulcer)

Etiology and Epidemiology. By far the most common cause of subcutaneous infection is *M. ulcerans* (buruli ulcer). After *M. tuberculosis* and *M. leprae* infections, *M. ulcerans* infection is the third most common TB disease in the world. It has been diag-nosed in US immigrants from endemic countries. Buruli ulcer was first described in 1948 in six Australian patients, who each had a single ulcerative lesion on an arm or leg. In the 1960s, many patients in the Buruli district of Uganda, near the Nile River, had ulcers that were caused by *M. ulcerans*.

The disease has since become known as buruli ulcer (BU) and is prevalent in West and Central Africa; however, it has been reported to occur in 32 other countries. In Japan, about half of the 19 cases appeared in the upper extremity. The first case in the United States was reported in 1974 in an immigrant physician from Nigeria who developed a chronic ulcer around the elbow. Necrosis of subcutaneous fat is the pathologic hall-mark of BU. Inoculation into subcutaneous tissue usually occurs through penetrating skin trauma. Secretions of toxins by the organisms (e.g., mycolactone, phospholipase C) cause extensive subcutaneous fatty tissue necrosis resulting in exten-sive fibrosis.

Clinical Findings. A lesion usually starts as a painless subcu-taneous edema and progresses to a subcutaneous nodule that secondarily ulcerates with a characteristic undermined edge. The ulcers may vary from few centimeters to a large part of the arm. The ulcers may be very large because the entire ulcerative phase is painless and available medical facilities are limited. The disease progresses in four stages: edema, subcutaneous nodule, ulceration, and end-stage scar formation with deformity. A painless ulcer that has undermined edges and a necrotic center with hyperpigmented and shiny surrounding skin is pathognomonic of a buruli ulcer. If untreated, the infection can invade all subjacent tissues including the bones. Infections invading phalanges, metacarpals, and ulna have been reported (Figure 3.17).

Diagnosis. There are five laboratory methods to confirm the disease.

- *Direct smear examination*—An examination done on swabs from ulcers or smears from tissue biopsies that can be promptly conducted at local health facilities where TB microscopy is also done. The exam is conducted using the acid-fast (Ziehl-Neelsen) stain procedure. Nevertheless, the sensitivity of this method is low (~40%) because *M. ulcerans* numbers tend to decrease over time. It is important to

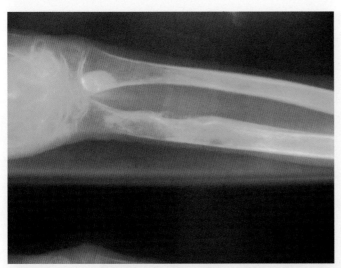

FIGURE 3.17 Buruli osteomyelitis of radius and ulna. The patient's absence of pain and inadequate health care access led in this case to advanced lesions. Note osteolysis, osteosclerosis, scalloping, and periosteal reaction.

emphasize that the positivity of the test varies with the clinical form of the disease. It is more useful in the ulcerative stage, but if the lesion is not ulcerated, a skin biopsy of the nodule is sufficient for the examination. In the nodular form, positivity can reach 60% and in the edematous form, it can reach up to 80%, both in the direct examination and culture. It is considered by many the easiest and most accessible method to arrive at a diagnosis.

- *Culture of* M. ulcerans—A procedure done on swabs from ulcers or tissue biopsies through the Lowenstein-Jensen medium that takes 6-8 weeks or more; sensitivity is approximately 20 to 60%. It is especially difficult to culture *M. ulcerans* when the sample is taken from bone tissue. *M. ulcerans* grows at 30°C. It is difficult to grow and up to 3 months of incubation are required, and the laboratory should be alerted not to discard the medium prematurely.
- *Polymerase chain reaction (PCR)*—This is a test from which results can be obtained within two days on swabs of ulcers or tissue biopsies; sensitivity is around 98%.[2,7] The positivity of PCR and histopathological tests does not vary with the clinical form of the disease.
- *Histopathology*—Tissue biopsies are sensitive in about 90% of cases and are useful for differential diagnoses when the results of other methods are negative. It should be done with a scalpel, thus avoiding the use of punches. The incision should cover the border of the lesion and extend into the subcutaneous tissue.
- *Fine-needle aspiration*—This technique is used in cases of nodular lesions and allows the collection of material for direct examination and culture.

Treatment. Current WHO recommendations for treatment are as follows. A combination of rifampicin and streptomycin/amikacin for eight weeks as a first-line treatment for all forms of the active disease. Clarithromycin and rifampin were successfully used in 19 cases in Japan. Nodules or uncomplicated cases can be treated without surgery. Surgery is done mainly to remove necrotic tissue, cover skin defects, and correct deformi-

ties. A necrotic ulcer should be excised to normal healthy tissue to prevent recurrence from residual bacilli and the defect can be skin grafted.

Deep Infections

Deep infections most commonly involve tenosynovium, less commonly joints, and least commonly bone.

Mycobacterial Tenosynovitis

Etiology and Epidemiology. Mycobacterial tenosynovitis is rare. However, it is the most common form of tuberculosis of the hand. Mycobacteria have more predilection for tenosynovium than joints, bone, subcutaneous tissue, or nerve. Flexor tendons of the fingers (Figure 3.18, *A,B*), palm, wrist, and forearm are affected more often than extensor tendons (Figure 3.19, *A-C*). Tuberculous tenosynovitis of flexor carpi ulnaris, abductor pollicis longus, and biceps tendon are rare. Nontuberculous mycobacterial tenosynovitis is more common than TB mycobacterial tenosynovitis.[122] More than half of the reported hand NTM tenosynovial infections are due to *M. marinum* (see Figure 3.18).

The second most common infecting organism is *M. kansasii*, and the ratio of *M. kansasii* and *M. marinum* is 1:5. The third most frequent infecting organism is *M. avium-intracellulare* complex. The less common tenosynovial infections caused by NTM are *M. scrofulaceum* (Figure 3.20), *M. szulgai*,[112] *M. terrae*,[71] *M. fortuitum*,[95] *M. chelonae*,[67] *M. abscessus, M. malmoense*,[38] and *M. xenopi*.[26] Reports of *M. tuberculosis* tenosynovitis since 1960 have been sporadic compared with a larger series in prior years. Infection may follow cortisone injection due to reactivation of dormant infection or proliferation of an active infection.

Clinical Findings. Nontuberculous mycobacterial tenosynovitis is more common than tuberculous tenosynovitis and appears to occur more frequently during the fourth to seventh decades of life. Tenosynovitis caused by tuberculous mycobacteria and nontuberculous mycobacteria is clinically similar. The most common presentation of all mycobacterial tenosynovitis is digital flexor tenosynovitis. The physician may feel rice bodies, millet seeds, or melon seeds glide beneath the examining fingers. Flexor tenosynovitis produces three classic presentations: a sausage finger (see Figures 3.18, *A,B*), compound palmar ganglion, and rice body-laden carpal tunnel syndrome (see Figure 3.20). Of the TB tenosynovitis in the carpal tunnel, 90% show thick synovium laden with large rice bodies. The patient is generally healthy and constitutional symptoms are lacking. Inflammatory signs (e.g., erythema, warmth, tenderness) are absent (cold abscess).

Coexistent pulmonary or extrapulmonary tuberculosis is rare. Wrist and hand radiographs are almost always normal. Late in the disease, tendons may rupture and the infection can spread to adjacent joints or bone. The ESR may be elevated in multifocal *M. tuberculosis* infection and is almost always normal in NTM infections but rarely may be elevated. The delay between the onset of symptoms and diagnosis is lengthy—one year in a survey of 32 cases by Kozin et al.[67] Early diagnosis is important because tendon rupture, wrist infection, or secondary osteomyelitis can be prevented. When treatment with steroid injection aggravates the condition, it should raise suspicion of tuberculosis or fungal infection.

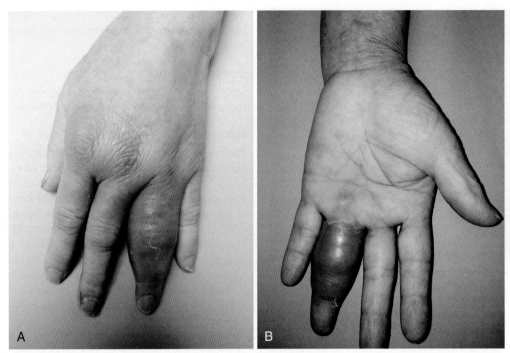

FIGURE 3.18 *Mycobacterium marinum* flexor tenosynovitis caused a sausage finger in a Chinese housewife during an outbreak in New York City. This finger was completely stiff in extension. **A,** Dorsal view. **B,** Volar view.

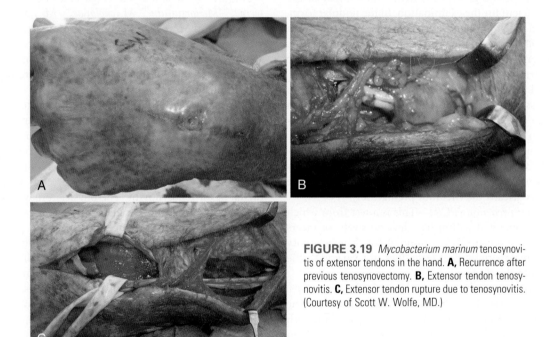

FIGURE 3.19 *Mycobacterium marinum* tenosynovitis of extensor tendons in the hand. **A,** Recurrence after previous tenosynovectomy. **B,** Extensor tendon tenosynovitis. **C,** Extensor tendon rupture due to tenosynovitis. (Courtesy of Scott W. Wolfe, MD.)

Diagnosis. The old dictum that tuberculosis (and syphilis) can mimic almost any other disease entity remains true today. Hand surgeons who are aware of this and perform an early biopsy are more likely to make a correct diagnosis, treat early on, and prevent a bad outcome.

Delay in diagnosis and misdiagnosis can cost the patient an amputation. Lau described two patients with *M. chelonae* infection that required amputation owing to the delay in diagnosis and treatment.[69] Three patients underwent finger amputations

for a missed diagnosis of *M. marinum* infection. Delay in diagnosis occurs for several reasons. Clinically, the disease pattern is nonspecific. Pain is conspicuously absent until late in the disease. It starts insidiously and becomes indolent. Other than the hand lesion, the patient is healthy. The diagnosis is not suspected because the tenosynovitis resembles nonspecific or rheumatoid tenosynovitis. Carpal tunnel syndrome can be an initial manifestation of tuberculosis and when proliferative tenosynovitis with or without rice bodies or melon and millet

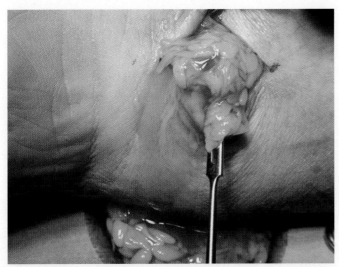

FIGURE 3.20 *Mycobacterium scrofulaceum* tenosynovitis and rice bodies in flexor tendons of the palm. (Courtesy of Scott W. Wolfe, MD.)

seeds is encountered, biopsy and cultures most likely will reveal the correct diagnosis. Smears of fluid aspirated from the lesion may provide the first clue to diagnosis, but this is often not done. Tenosynovial biopsy is often not done at the time of carpal tunnel release. When biopsy is done, tissue is often sent for histopathology but not for microbiology.

Histopathology shows poorly or noncaseating granuloma and may be misinterpreted as sarcoidosis. When biopsy tissue is sent for culture, it can be mistakenly sent in formalin. Even when properly done, histopathology studies reveal only scanty bacilli after painstaking scrutiny. Hand tuberculosis is a paucibacillary lesion and smears and cultures are frequently negative. When tenosynovitis is not clinically visible or palpable, MRI of fingers, hand, and wrist show inflammation around the flexor and extensor tendons. Inflammatory changes are demonstrated and margins of the extensor tendons lose clear delineation compared to those of adjacent fingers. Cultures may not be requested for or not done at 30°C for *M. marinum* at some hospitals. Polymerase chain reaction to confirm tuberculosis is essential to make a diagnosis when stains and cultures are negative. The disease may present in one of four stages depending on the duration of the infection and host immunity.

1. A thin synovitis with free synovial fluid may be seen.
2. For up to 2 years, granulation tissue, thick tenosynovial proliferation, and rice bodies appear.
3. Infection invades the tendon; they may be frayed, infiltrated, ruptured, or caseated into a fungoid mass. Fraying of tendons occurs at an average of 3 years and rupture of tendons occurs at an average of 4 years from the onset of tenosynovitis.
4. Only very late, the infection spreads to the adjacent joints or bone and a sinus may be present with or without superimposed pyogenic infection.

Histologic sections are first examined with the hematoxylin and eosin stain. This is best done as a rapid intraoperative biopsy (frozen section). If granulomas are observed, even if poorly formed, additional stained specimens with Ziehl-Neelsen stain (for AFB) and Gomori methenamine silver stain (for fungi) are examined. *M. tuberculosis* forms caseated granulomas but nontuberculous mycobacteria form mostly noncaseated granulomas.

Failure to demonstrate AFB by staining the synovium does not rule out tuberculosis because cultures may be positive when smears are negative. Only 30% of patients with NTM infection have positive acid-fast stains. Definitive diagnosis can be made by culturing infected synovium or rice bodies. Rice bodies are tubercles in the synovial tissue that become detached and contain live mycobacteria that grow on culture, but only 40% of 166 patients with *M. marinum* yielded positive cultures. Rice bodies are a feature of both *M. tuberculosis* and NTM. A bacteriologic diagnosis can often be made by smearing and culturing drainage from a sinus.

Treatment. The treatment algorithm suggested by Zenone et al is useful.[122] The first step in it is to treat chronic tenosynovitis with thorough tenosynovectomy because tenosynovitis due to pernicious mycobacteria (i.e., *M. avium*, *M. chelonae*, *M. malmoense*, and *M. terrae*) is indistinguishable from other mycobacterial infections. If the patient is immunocompromised, "aggressive synovectomy" becomes essential and helps to reduce the mycobacterial load. Tenosynovectomy should be done from musculotendinous junction to the tendon insertion into the bone.

Chow and colleagues recommend that the role of synovectomy in an immunocompetent patient, in areas where *M. tuberculosis* is endemic, is a "minimal" biopsy to make a diagnosis with removal of enough synovium for histopathology, smears, and cultures.[22] If the diagnosis is established through a "minimal" biopsy or through culture of drainage material, treatment may be successful with chemotherapy without synovectomy. When the patient is on immunosuppressive therapy, in addition to chemotherapy and thorough synovectomy, the physician may be forced to decrease the dose of immunosuppressive drugs to control the infection.

It is reasonable to start chemotherapy based on positive smear staining or histopathology and revise chemotherapy if necessary when results of culture and sensitivity become available. Multidrug therapy with four antituberculous antibiotics remains the cornerstone of treatment for *M. tuberculosis*. Before the development of effective antituberculous therapy, fewer than one half of patients with tuberculous tenosynovitis were cured by complete surgical extirpation of all infected synovium if immunity was adequate.

The most effective empirical combination of chemotherapy for NTM infections is rifampin, isoniazid, and ethambutol. Because of extensive resistance of many nontuberculous mycobacteria, the empirical addition of clarithromycin in a multidrug regimen would probably be appropriate for most nontuberculous mycobacteria causing tenosynovitis[122] (see Figure 3.18, *A,B*). A variety of antibiotic regimens have been used successfully in the treatment of *M. marinum* in two of the largest series. A rifampicin and ethambutol combination was successfully used by Cheung and colleagues in 70 of 75 patients.[20]

Clarithromycin in combination with doxycycline or minocycline or rifampin or ofloxacin or ethambutol is the drug of choice for treatment of *M. marinum* infections. It is important to remember that *M. marinum* is resistant to isoniazid and can be discontinued once culture results or identification by PCR are available. The optimum duration of treatment is unknown and controversial. Average duration of therapy was 7.2 months according to Cheung[20] and 10 months in a survey from the Mayo Clinic.[67] The worst outcome was in patients who were misdiagnosed for more than 2 months and were mistakenly treated with cortisone injections preoperatively.

Untreated, tuberculous tenosynovitis in the finger and wrist eventually leads to painless tendon attrition and rupture. Flexor tendon grafting restores finger flexion, if the infection is contained within the flexor tendon sheath and the sheath and underlying joints are spared. When a tendon ruptures in the palm or carpal tunnel or distal forearm, the ruptured tendon's distal end can be "piggybacked" to an adjacent functional tendon. When infection spreads from a tendon sheath in a finger to adjacent joint and bone, chemotherapy controls the infection but mobility is lost. Reactivation of a dormant tuberculous infection of the hand may recur many years after it is successfully treated with tenosynovectomy and multidrug therapy (MDT) if the patient's immunity is decreased for any reason, such as immunosuppressive therapy or cytotoxic therapy.

Tuberculous Bursitis

Tuberculous bursitis is uncommon. Most frequent bursa infected by tuberculosis in the upper extremity is subdeltoid bursa followed by olecranon bursa and bicipitoradial bursa. Calcification of the bursal sac is seen in approximately one third of the cases. If the diagnosis is delayed, an adjacent joint may become infected. Early incision and drainage facilitates diagnosis and chemotherapy is curative.

Tuberculous Arthritis

Osteoarticular tuberculosis of the extremities is rare and occurs in only 1% of patients with extrapulmonary tuberculosis. The wrist is the most commonly infected joint by *M. tuberculosis* in the upper extremity. Tuberculous infection of the wrist can be seeded by a blood-borne infection or may spread from untreated flexor tenosynovitis. The infection has been demonstrated to spread from flexor tendons across the wrist joint to the dorsal tenosynovium and result in a swelling on both sides of the wrist. The elbow and interphalangeal joint infections are less common. Wilson[118] published results of 31 cases of elbow tuberculosis in adults. Dix-Peek et al[31] published facts from 10 cases of tuberculosis of the elbow in children between the ages of 1 and 11 and concluded that elbow infections generally start from the olecranon, the lower end of the humerus, or the olecranon bursa.

Clinical Findings. The earliest manifestation of tuberculous arthritis is pain, swelling, and limitation of joint motion. The joint may be held in flexion. Tuberculous arthritis may be suspected when drainage persists from an infected elbow, wrist, or finger joint despite multiple courses of antibiotics and multiple drainage procedures. Most joint infections are monoarticular and may strongly resemble a case of monoarticular rheumatoid arthritis. Concurrent pulmonary or extrapulmonary tuberculosis is uncommon. Skoll and Hudson have classified and graded the radiological findings in osteoarticular tuberculosis.[107]

Roentgenographic hallmarks of early joint infection are soft tissue swelling and periarticular osteoporosis (Figure 3.21, *A*). In the second phase, the hyaline cartilage is invaded, and joint space is reduced or lost (Figure 3.21, *B*) and pannus causes subchondral cysts on both sides of the joint. Finally, in the third stage, there is gross destruction, deformity, dislocation, or ankylosis of the joint (Figure 3.21, *C,D*). The Phemister triad of radiographic findings—juxtaarticular osteoporosis, subchondral cysts, and gradual narrowing of the cartilage space—are part of this classification.

NTM also causes joint infection. The clinical difference between joint infections with *M. tuberculosis* and *M. marinum* is that *M. marinum* infections are positively associated with traumatic exposure to a fish bone, saltwater, a fish tank, or a swimming pool in 80% of the cases. Of the 166 patients treated by Cheung, 50% were fishermen or fishmongers and 15% were seafood handlers at work or home.[20] Diagnosis is made with biopsy and culture. Cultures are positive between 2 and 6 weeks of incubation at 30°C on a Lowenstein-Jensen medium. In *M. marinum* infections, a finger joint is infected in three-fourths of the cases and the wrist is infected in the rest. Infections are typically monoarticular. Symptoms usually begin within 1 to 2 weeks after the initial trauma.

The mean time from onset of symptoms to bacteriologic diagnosis is 8 months (range, 3 months to 3 years). The pain is mild, but swelling of the involved joint is marked and boggy. Organisms may be stained from draining joint fluid, aspirated joint fluid, or synovial biopsy in 75% of cases. Mycobacterial cultures are positive in almost all (95%) of synovial fluid and synovial biopsy specimens. A severely immunocompromised patient (e.g., from chemotherapy, corticosteroids, systemic lupus) may develop a multicentric *M. marinum* mycobacteriosis that may include bones, joints, tendons, and skin.

Diagnosis. In the absence of coexistent extraarticular tuberculosis, diagnosis of *M. tuberculosis* joint infection almost always requires arthrocentesis or biopsy. Synovial fluid aspirate may show AFB on smear, and cultures are generally positive. Granulomas with caseation are present in three-fourths of the biopsy specimens. Clinical confusion may occur when *M. tuberculosis* infects joints previously involved with rheumatoid arthritis or gouty arthritis.

Treatment. Treatment of *M. tuberculosis* septic arthritis consists of chemotherapy and prevention of deformity by splinting during the first and second stages. Intermittent active exercises for the elbow, forearm, wrist, and finger joints should be encouraged as pain permits. Although total or partial synovectomy has been performed at the time of biopsy, the value of it is controversial. Some favor chemotherapy after debridement once diagnosis is confirmed. Benkeddache and Gettesman[11] recommend biopsy only for diagnosis and chemotherapy for treatment. In its earliest stage almost all infected joints recover fully with chemotherapy and without surgical debridement. In the second stage, painful joints are fused.

If the source of pain can be localized to the distal radioulnar joint, resection of the distal end of the ulna, synovectomy of distal radioulnar joint, and chemotherapy may be required. In patients with an unfavorable response within 3 months, or with recurrence of infection, Tuli recommends surgical debridement.[116] Unfavorable therapeutic response can occur if the organism is marginally sensitive to drugs or if host resistance is low due to malnutrition, drug immunosuppression, or an underlying immune deficiency disease. In the third stage, a painful, dislocated, unstable, ankylosed, or deformed joint requires fusion, excisional arthroplasty, or corrective osteotomy. Fusion is delayed until progressive bone destruction is halted and bone is sufficiently vascularized after chemotherapy. Chemotherapy is given for 9 months.

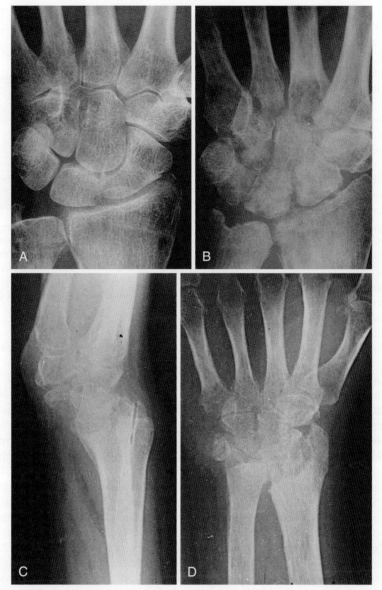

FIGURE 3.21 A, Tuberculosis of the wrist joint can start in the synovium and cause subchondral erosions in the carpal bones. **B,** Gradually the hyline cartilage is destroyed, the joint space is reduced, and the bones become osteopenic. **C, D,** Finally, there is destruction of supporting ligaments and volar subluxation of the radiocarpal joint. (Courtesy of S. M. Tuli, New Delhi, India.)

Successful outcome with this method (i.e., biopsy for diagnosis and chemotherapy for treatment) has been confirmed in the treatment of tuberculosis of the elbow and the wrist.[116] *M. marinum* arthritis does not have as favorable a therapeutic response to chemotherapy as *M. marinum* tenosynovitis. A combination of chemotherapy and synovectomy is preferred in the treatment of *M. marinum* arthritis. Patients with involvement for more than 6 months had worse results. *M. marinum* strains are uniformly resistant to isoniazid but are sensitive to rifampin, ethambutol, and ciprofloxacin. Monotherapy with minocycline and trimethoprim-sulfamethoxazole has been effective for superficial infections, but combination chemotherapy is recommended for *M. marinum* arthritis to prevent resistance. Rifampin–ethambutol combination is the most successful in past reports. Chemotherapy for a minimum of 6 months, or for at least 2 months after complete resolution of joint infection, is recommended for all NTM joint infections.

Brashear et al[14] and Tsai et al[115] reviewed *M. tuberculosis* infections of the wrist joint. Wilson and Dix-Peek et al[31] reviewed the largest number of elbow tuberculosis. The largest numbers of deep NTM infections of the hand are reported and reviewed by Hurst,[56] Chow,[22] Kozin,[67] Hellinger,[52] and Zenone.[122] The largest number of cases of *M. marinum* joint infections of the hand have been reviewed by Alloway and colleagues.[5]

Tuberculous Osteomyelitis

Etiology and Epidemiology. Extrapulmonary tuberculosis accounts for almost 20% of all cases of tuberculosis in the general population and 72% of all cases in US AIDS patients. In the United States, skeletal tuberculosis is 1% of all tuberculosis and 10% of all extrapulmonary tuberculosis. Of skeletal tuberculosis, approximately 50% occurs in the spine, 33% in the lower extremity (12% in pelvis, 10% in hip and femur, 10% in knee and tibia, 1% in ankle and foot), 7% in the ribs, and 10% in the upper extremity; that is, 1% in shoulder and humerus, 2% in elbow, forearm, and wrist, 4% in hand and fingers, and an additional 3% in the hand accompanied by multifocal sites elsewhere.[11] Tuberculosis of the bones of the hand is less common than tuberculosis of the tenosynovium and joints of the hand. It typically occurs in the phalanges (i.e., tuberculous dactylitis) and metacarpals.

Diagnosis. Clinical presentation of skeletal tuberculosis of the hand in children and adults is different and has changed in character over the years based on health and immunity of the affected group.

Tuberculous Osteomyelitis of Children's Hands. The highest incidence of skeletal tuberculosis of the hand before the era of antituberculous therapy was in infants and children. In children, two-thirds of the patients were age 2 or younger. It was uncommon after age 5 and scarce after 10 years. The natural course of the disease was often self-limiting but was accompanied by residual deformity. *M. bovis* was then the main infecting organism, and with pasteurization of milk it is rarely reported in children today. Adult cases currently are reported more often and are caused by *M. tuberculosis* or NTM.[116] Concurrent pulmonary infection and multifocal skeletal tuberculosis was common in the past but is rare today both in children and adults.[116]

Of 37 cases of tuberculous dactylitis reviewed by Ritz et al, only 20% had concurrent pulmonary tuberculosis.[98] It also may follow previously treated pulmonary tuberculosis. Tuberculosis of phalanges (tubercular dactylitis) and metacarpals is the most common form of skeletal tuberculosis in infants and children. The proximal phalanx, middle phalanx, distal phalanx, and metacarpals are involved in that order. The second, third, and fourth fingers are involved most frequently. From a clinical viewpoint, there are three types of dactylitis.

- One group consists of those individuals who have generalized tuberculous infection and tuberculous dactylitis is a manifestation of the whole.
- The second group consists of patients whose dactylitis is the presenting symptom and who have no evidence of generalized tuberculous infection.
- The third group consists of multifocal tuberculous dactylitis with coexistent musculoskeletal tuberculosis in additional fingers of the same hand (Figure 3.22) and/or opposite hand, or in other parts of the same extremity or in another extremity.[46]

Thirty percent of children who have tuberculous dactylitis have multifocal tuberculosis. In all cases, symptoms begin with a painless, nonsuppurative, and insidious swelling on the fingers (phalangeal infection) or the hand (metacarpal infection). On examination, there is a typical fusiform swelling of a finger or a diffuse swelling on the dorsum of the hand. There is practically no tenderness or local heat, but the part may appear taut and shiny. It is not easily diagnosed at this early stage because the presentation is nonspecific and may simulate a tumor.[49,58]

The swelling often reaches considerable size, doubling the digital girth. In late cases, an abscess may form with skin discoloration and fluctuation. The abscess may burst and leave a sinus that drains a cheesy, yellowish exudate. Multiple discharging sinuses occur with disseminated dactylitis. Where secondary infection of a sinus occurs, the condition closely resembles a subacute osteomyelitis of pyogenic origin. Radiographs are

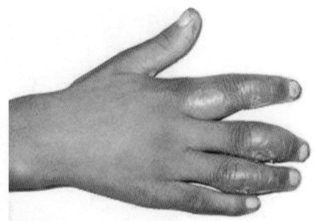

FIGURE 3.22 Tuberculous dactylitis can be single-digital or multidigital in the same hand, bilateral, or associated with tuberculosis of other joints in the same or other extremities. This child has tubercular dactylitis of the proximal phalanx of index finger and middle phalanges of index, middle, and ring fingers. (From Kumar V, Kumar M: Multiple discharging sinuses with disseminated dactylitis. *Indian Pediatr,* 48:583–584, 2011, with permission.)

characterized by endosteal resorption of bone and progressive subperiosteal hyperplasia.

During infancy and childhood, the short tubular bones have a lavish blood supply through a large nutrient artery entering in the middle of the bone. The agent lodges in the center of the marrow cavity, and the interior of the short tubular bone is converted into a virtual granuloma. This leads to a spindle-shaped expansion and inflated shape of the bone. Endosteal resorption of bone is followed by progressive subperiosteal hyperplasia and has been termed as *spina ventosa* by Dupuytren (Latin *spina,* "spine"; *ventosa,* "distended with air").[32]

Metaphyseal tuberculous osteomyelitis may be the initial pathology and then the infection crosses the epiphyseal plate into the joint and there may be telltale enlargement of epiphysis. Transphyseal spread of infection is more commonly seen in tuberculous than in nontuberculous osteomyelitis. Syphilitic dactylitis has a similar radiographic appearance, but serology distinguishes the two clinically. Early in the course of a TB infection, the epiphysis is spared because of its rich blood supply, but in late cases it is invaded and causes shortening or deformity of the digit. Radiographic findings of tuberculosis in children include joint effusion, periarticular osteopenia, joint space narrowing, endosteal thinning with cortical irregularity, lytic lesions, periosteal new bone formation, and advanced epiphyseal maturity.

Diagnosis cannot be made without a biopsy. Singh et al showed that fine-needle aspiration cytology reveals granulomas with or without necrosis in a third of cases and staining showed AFB in all their eight cases of tuberculous dactylitis.[105] If the biopsy shows granulomatous inflammation on frozen section, AFB staining of the tissue should be requested because it may show tubercle bacilli. A high level of suspicion for tuberculosis in a chronic bone lesion and an eight-pack culture at the time of biopsy expedite the diagnosis.

Tuberculous Osteomyelitis of Adult Hands. Tuberculosis osteomyelitis in the adult occurs more commonly in fingers than metacarpals; more in middle and ring fingers than index and small fingers; and more in the proximal, middle, and distal

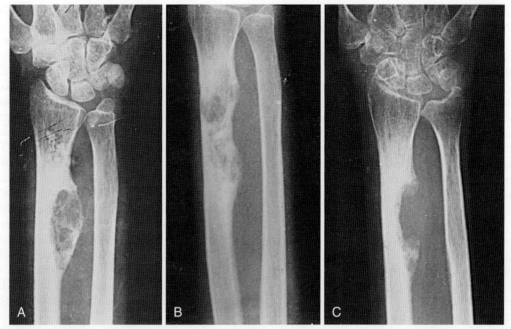

FIGURE 3.23 Tuberculous osteomyelitis of the radial shaft. **A,** This resembles a tumorous lesion of the bone; there is bone destruction and cultures grew *Mycobacterium tuberculosis*. **B,** Mixed cystic-sclerotic pattern. **C,** The lesion heals with reossification in response to oral antituberculous chemotherapy. (Courtesy of S. M. Tuli, New Delhi, India.)

phalanges in that order. Tuberculosis osteomyelitis of carpal bones is rare. A single bone lesion that appears to be a bone tumor (e.g., a GCT of distal radius[88]) may be tuberculosis. In patients with skeletal tuberculosis, only 20% have a pulmonary lesion and 10% have abdominal disease. In 70% of the patients with skeletal tuberculosis, no primary focus can be demonstrated. Therefore, the presence of osteoarticular lesions without pulmonary or abdominal lesions does not exclude diagnosis of tuberculosis.

Multifocal tuberculosis involving the hand may include multiple digits or it may be part of generalized multifocal and systemic tuberculosis. Failure to consider tuberculosis in the differential diagnosis of multifocal skeletal lesions can substantially delay diagnosis. It may be suspected in a patient coming from a region endemic for tuberculosis. Constitutional symptoms, rare in solitary skeletal tuberculosis, may be present in multifocal tuberculosis with fever, chills, anorexia, and loss of weight. Discharging lesions are more common in multiple lesions than in solitary lesions. Multifocal lesions are more common in immunosuppressed patients, including those with AIDS. Elevated ESR and positive PPD, rare in solitary lesions, may also be present. Technetium-99m helps to detect multifocal tuberculosis when radiographs have not yet become positive. ESR is elevated in multifocal cases more than solitary ones, presumably because multifocal disease occurs with reduced immunity. In multifocal tuberculosis, pulmonary and abdominal lesions are more common than in solitary skeletal tuberculosis. Multicentric tuberculosis can be mistaken for a malignant metastatic disease. Tuberculous dactylitis may coexist with another extrapulmonary nonskeletal focus of tuberculosis such as tuberculosis of the cervix.

Local discomfort and swelling are the usual presenting findings. A pathologic fracture of a metacarpal or a phalanx may

occur. A draining sinus or fistula forms in untreated cases. Al-Qattan et al,[3] who reviewed the literature on radiological patterns of tuberculous osteomyelitis in the hand and wrist, found six patterns:

1. In early cases, there is soft tissue swelling followed by periosteal reaction and metaphyseal osteoporosis. This is followed by a well-defined cystic lesion that simulates a bone cyst.
2. Bone destruction with honeycombing, shown in Figure 3.23, A. It may resemble a GCT when it is near the metaphysis.[88]
3. A mixed cystic-sclerotic pattern with a lytic lesion that is surrounded by a sclerotic rim (Figure 3.23, B).
4. A diaphyseal lytic lesion that crosses the epiphyseal plate; this pattern is classic of pediatric tuberculous osteomyelitis.
5. Spina ventosa, as described earlier.
6. Bony lytic lesion with bone destruction that resembles bacterial osteomyelitis.[3]

Increased bone density and sequestra may be seen if staphylococcal osteomyelitis is superimposed. MRI of the digit can show that the draining sinus is continuous with the bone marrow through a cortical defect. Radiographically, the cystic lesion is replaced by bone with antibiotics (Figure 3.23, C). Osteomyelitis as a result of *M. marinum*, *M. kansasii*, and *M. scrofulaceum* is clinically and radiologically similar but treatment should be different.

Diagnosis is made by biopsy, which should be taken from the granulomatous area where a cyst is apparent on the radiograph or the histological results may be equivocal.

Differential diagnosis of tuberculous dactylitis should include other causes of dactylitis; it can occur in infections that include yaws,[35,36] syphilis, leishmaniasis, brucellosis, blastomycosis,[40] leprosy, and blistering distal dactylitis. Noninfectious causes of dactylitis are sarcoidosis, sickle cell anemia, and celiac disease. Spondyloarthritis causes dactylitis that looks like a sausage digit.[85] Osteomyelitis may be caused by nontuberculous mycobacteria in AIDS and has been reported to be caused by *M. szulgai*.[72]

Treatment. Tuli's approach of "do not operate when antibiotics can do the job and operate when you must" is based on experience with thousands of cases of musculoskeletal tuberculosis treated over three decades. MDT is the keystone of treatment of tuberculosis.[116] Curettage is chosen by the treating surgeon at the time of biopsy because it is easy and removes pathologic tissue. It does reduce the bacterial dose when chemotherapy begins. Because of the efficacy of available chemotherapy today, curettage is not essential if a diagnosis is established with biopsy or staining and culture of draining material. On the other hand, if the organism is resistant, or if the host is immunosuppressed or there is evidence of bone sequestrum, surgical debridement of infected bone is essential. Histological findings compatible with tuberculosis (i.e., chronic granuloma, with or without caseation) in the presence of negative fungal cultures warrant MDT.

Before the advent of chemotherapy, many infants and children with localized TB dactylitis without generalized active tuberculosis recovered without surgical debridement in 1 to 3 years. When tuberculous dactylitis occurs in an infant or a child as a part of severe generalized tuberculosis, it does not resolve spontaneously. When it occurs in an adult patient and remains untreated, it progresses slowly and may necessitate amputation. Benkeddache and Gettesman treated all their skeletal cases with surgical biopsy for diagnosis and antimycobacterial drugs for treatment without further surgical debridement.[11] Kotwal et al had success with biopsy and conservative treatment in 75% of their 32 tuberculous hand infections.[66] In early stages, treatment with chemotherapy results in complete resolution. The immune status of the host is an overwhelming predictor of eventual outcome. In the immunocompromised patient population, less than half of the patients have resolution of a deep infection with surgery as well as chemotherapy.[67]

Antituberculous Drugs and Multidrug Therapy Regimens

The modern era of tuberculosis began in 1944 with the demonstration of the efficacy of streptomycin in humans by Waksman in New Jersey. In 1952, the more effective bactericidal drug isoniazid (INH) became available at Seaview Hospital on Staten Island in New York, making tuberculosis curable in the great majority of patients. In 1970, the bactericidal drug rifampin (RMP) attained equal status to INH. In 1993, rifabutin (RFB) became available for *M. tuberculosis* associated with HIV infection.[51] Rifapentine is the latest (1999) rifamycin that is not only long-acting but also more potent, allowing less frequent dosage and a shorter duration of therapy for *M. tuberculosis*. The duration of chemotherapy progressively decreased from approximately 2 years with streptomycin and INH, to 9 months with INH and RMP given together, to 6 months using MDT that includes INH, RMP, pyrazinamide (PZA), and ethambutol (EMB).

INH is bactericidal and is the cornerstone of therapy. It is included in all regimens until resistance is established on cultures. It can cause hepatitis and peripheral neuropathy. Pyridoxine (50 mg PO daily) is given conjointly with INH to minimize

peripheral neuropathy. RMP is also bactericidal and is the second major antituberculous agent. The most important complication of RMP is hepatitis. Rifabutin is a semisynthetic derivative of rifamycin that shows good activity against *M. intercellulare* and about one-third of rifampin-resistant strains of *M. tuberculosis*. PZA is an essential component of all MDT regimens. It is bacteriostatic, and its beneficial effect is mostly limited to the first 2 to 3 months of treatment. It can cause hepatitis and hyperuricemia. EMB is also bacteriostatic and is an initial component of most regimens. The most important complication of EMB is optic neuritis, which may require its removal from the regimen. Blurring and acuity of vision are determined at baseline and reviewed monthly.

Because of side effects and emerging resistance to the first line of antituberculous drugs, tuberculosis should be treated in collaboration with an infectious disease specialist. Second-line agents (e.g., fluoroquinolones, three injectable drugs [amikacin, kanamycin, capreomycin], ethionamide, and cycloserine) are less efficacious and more toxic than the first-line drugs. Drug resistance to one or more antituberculous drugs has developed and remains a challenge. Multiple drug-resistant strains of tuberculosis both to RMP and INH have been seen. Directly observed therapy (DOT) is the five-component treatment strategy developed by the World Health Organization to prevent emergence of drug-resistant strains and is now the US standard of care. In 2009, 60% of all the patients received their therapy entirely as DOT and 90% received at least some portion of their treatment as DOT in the United States.

Indications for Treatment

Histologic findings compatible with tuberculosis (i.e., granulomatous synovitis, with or without caseation) warrant chemotherapy, although other chronic infections can cause an identical clinical and histologic picture. This is best to establish it on a frozen section of biopsy material. The differential diagnosis of granulomatous synovitis includes TB and NTM infections, fungus, foreign bodies, brucellosis, sarcoidosis, and Crohn syndrome, among others. In the presence of negative fungal smears and cultures, a diagnosis of tuberculosis is presumed when caseating granuloma is histologically confirmed with an intraoperative frozen section. Once sensitivity results are reported by the laboratory, chemotherapy is revised to use appropriate drugs. In early stages, treatment with chemotherapy results in complete resolution.

Regimens

Modern tuberculosis therapy guidelines by the CDC and the American Thoracic Society are summarized in Table 3.8. The basic principles that underlie treatment of pulmonary tuberculosis apply to extrapulmonary forms of the disease. Although relatively few studies have examined treatment of extrapulmonary tuberculosis, increasing evidence suggests that 4 months of INH and RMP or 6 months of INH and ethambutol are effective for soft tissue infections. In bone and joint disease, 9 to 12 months of cumulative chemotherapy is advised. The first 2 months include a four-drug regimen of INH, RMP, PZA, and EMB. After the initial regimen, a two-drug regimen (i.e., INH and RMP or INH and ethambutol) may be resumed if the bacillus is sensitive to both RMP and ethambutol. Patients with initial resistance to RMP or INH (XDR TB) are treated with at

TABLE 3.8   Antituberculous Drugs Used in the United States

Drug	Adult Daily Dosage	Pediatric Daily Dosage	Main Drug Toxicity
First-Line Drugs			
Isoniazid[a,d]	300 mg PO, IM	10-20 mg/kg (max, 300 mg)	Hepatic toxicity, peripheral neuropathy
Rifampin[a,b,c] (rifadin, rifocin, rimactane) or rifapentine	600 mg PO, IV	10-20 mg/kg (max, 600 mg)	Hepatic toxicity, flu-like syndrome
Pyrazinamide[e]	1.5-2.5 g PO	15-30 mg/kg (max, 2 g)	Arthralgia, hepatic toxicity, hyperuricemia
Ethambutol (Myambutol)	15-25 mg/kg PO	15-25 μγ per κγ ΠΟ	Optic neuritis
Second-Line Drugs (in Alphabetical Order)			
Capreomycin (Capastat)	15 mg/kg IM	15-30/μγ per κγ	Auditory, vestibular, and renal toxicity
Cycloserine[g] (Seromycin)	250-500 mg bid PO or 1 g in a single dose	10-20 mg/kg	Psychiatric symptoms, seizures
Ethionamide/prothionamide (Trecator-SC)	250-500 mg bid PO or 1-g single dose	15-20 mg/kg	Gastrointestinal and hepatic toxicity
Gatifloxacin			
Kanamycin (Kantrex)	15 mg/kg IM, IV (max, 1 g/day)	15-30/μγ per κγ	Auditory and renal toxicity
Levofloxacin			
Moxifloxacin			
Para-aminosalicylic acid	4-6 g bid PO or 12-g single dose	75 mg/kg bid	Gastrointestinal disturbance
Streptomycin	15 mg/kg IM	20-30 mg/kg	Vestibular toxicity, renal toxicity

[a]Intravenous preparations of isoniazid and rifampin are available.
[b]Pyridoxine, 10-25 mg, should be given to prevent neuropathy in malnourished or pregnant patients and in those with HIV infection, alcoholism, or diabetes. For intermittent use after initial daily therapy for a few months, the dosage is 15 mg/kg (max, 900 mg) twice a week for adults.
[c]For intermittent use after a few months of daily therapy, the dosage is 600 mg twice a week.
[d]Rifabutin is effective against 30% of rifampin-resistant *M. tuberculosis*. It is the drug of choice against *M. avium* infections.
[e]For intermittent use after the first 8 weeks of daily therapy, the dosage is 2.5-3.5 g twice a week.
[g]May recommend pyridoxine, 50 mg for every 250 mg of cycloserine, to decrease the incidence of adverse neurologic effects.

least four drugs that are shown by culture to be effective and should be continued for at least 18 months. All patients with organisms resistant to either INH or RMP should receive DOT.

The four-drug regimen can be administered three times a week for 6 months if the therapy is directly observed. Only ~30% of XDR cases can be cured using combinations of the previously described medications for 24 months. Concurrent pulmonary tuberculosis with chronic tuberculous hand infection is rare but infrequent concurrent pulmonary tuberculosis must be ruled out in every case because cases with positive sputum smears or positive sputum cultures are highly infectious. Every patient who has hand tuberculosis must have chest radiography. Patients receiving chemotherapy become noninfectious within 2 weeks. If the chest radiograph and sputum are positive, isolation for the first 2 weeks of treatment is recommended to control the spread of tuberculosis. No isolation is necessary for extrapulmonary tuberculosis without active pulmonary tuberculosis.

Special Features and Treatment of Nontuberculous Mycobacteria

Of the more than 100 species of NTM mycobacteria that are currently considered to be potential sources of disease, only 18 have been reported to cause infection of the hand and upper extremity (Table 3.9). NTM infection occurs in both immunocompetent and immunodeficient patients. When NTM infec-

tion is encountered, a cause for underlying immunodeficiency should be sought. *M. marinum* is an increasingly common opportunistic infection in patients treated by anti-TNF-α biologic therapy. Postmarketing FDA surveillance through January of 2007 noted 239 atypical mycobacterial infections in patients on anti-TNF-α therapy, and 12 different species of mycobacterium were implicated. There is a wide range of clinical presentation, virulence, and drug sensitivity among NTM species, which makes chemotherapy and treatment of NTM different from that of *M. tuberculosis*. Atypical mycobacterial infections in immunosuppressed patients may show delayed response to antibiotics and surgery and portend serious morbidity.

❖ AUTHOR'S PREFERRED METHOD OF TREATMENT

The most common manifestation of tuberculosis and mycosis in the hand is chronic tenosynovitis. Arthritis and osteomyelitis come next in that order of frequency.

If chronic tenosynovitis is nonspecific (i.e., no indication of rheumatoid arthritis), is made worse by cortisone injection, reoccurs after tenosynovectomy, or is accompanied by sinus formation, tuberculosis or fungal infection may be ruled out with biopsy. At the time of biopsy, the specific diagnosis may not be discernible because the tissues do not have pathognomonic characteristics. Rice bodies may be found in rheumatoid arthritis, tuberculosis, and fungal infections such as coccidioidomycosis, sporotrichosis, and histoplasmosis.

TABLE 3.9   Diagnosis and Treatment of Nontuberculous Mycobacterial Hand Infections

NTM	Year Identified	Tissue Affected	Growth	Effective Chemotherapy
M. abscessus		T	Takes 6 weeks to grow	Clarithromycin, ciprofloxacin
M. asiaticum	1965	T	Radical tenosynovectomy	Minocycline, clarithromycin
M. avium-intracellulare complex[89]	1943	T	Most resistant, tenacious, and troublesome May take 8 weeks to grow Radical tenosynovectomy necessary	Clarithromycin, rifabutin, and ethambutol
M. chelonae		T, SQ	Difficult growth delays diagnosis Multiple biopsies may be necessary for diagnosis	Clarithromycin, erythromycin, doxycycline, kanamycin
M. fortuitum	1972	T		
M. gordonae		T		
M. haemophilum	1978	S	Grows at 30°C with hemoglobin media Fastidious, slow growing Occurs in AIDS	Difficult to treat because of underlying immune deficiency
M. kansasii	1953	T, S	Generally low-grade infections	Erythromycin, ethambutol, rifampin, isoniazid
M. malmoense	1977	T, SQ	Diagnosis delayed because organism takes 12 weeks to grow	Isoniazid, rifampin, ethambutol, pyrazinamide
M. marinum	1926	C, T, S	Grows at 30°C. Easily treated with antibiotics alone[81]	Clarithromycin, minocycline, trimethoprim-sulfamethoxazole, ethambutol, rifampin
M. monacense	2008	SQ		Clarithromycin, levofloxacin
M. scrofulaceum	1956	T, B		
M. simiae		C		
M. smegmatis (M. goodii)	2001	OB		
M. terrae complex (M. terrae, M. nonchromogenicum, M. triviale, radish bacillus)	1950	SQ, T, S, B		
M. ulcerans (buruli ulcer)	1930	SQ	Grows at 30°C. Difficult to grow, failure in more than half of all cases Up to 3 months of incubation required	None
M. xenopi	1957	T	Grows at 42°C	
M. szulgai	1972	T, OB		Isoniazid, rifampin, ethambutol, pyrazinamide

B, Bone; C, cutaneous; OB, olecranon bursitis; S, synovium; SQ, subcutaneous; T, tenosynovium.

Certain chronic infections have a high tendency of recurrence unless radical surgical excision is combined with appropriate antibiotics, as with M. avium, M. chelonae, M. malmoense and M. terrae, Sporothrix, Actinomyces, and Coccidioides. Thus, complete synovectomy is reasonable at the time of biopsy or surgery because this will reduce the microbial burden for subsequent antibiotic treatment. An exception to this approach is when the diagnosis is known, as in a patient with positive stains from pus, exudate, synovial fluid, sputum, or gastric washings for mycobacteria.

At surgery, I divide the excised tissue and save half the specimen without formalin for the microbiology laboratory; the other half is sent to the histopathology laboratory in formalin. The pathologist is asked to look for granuloma in the frozen section and permanent sections. If a granuloma is reported on frozen section, the need for multiple smears and cultures is reinforced. In addition to biopsy, I send the fluids (e.g., pus, synovial fluid, exudates) for smears and cultures and request three smears (gram, AFB, and KOH fungus) on the biopsy tissue as well as the fluid. I request six cultures (i.e., aerobic and anaerobic bacteria [Actinomyces spp. and Nocardia spp. are anaerobic], tuberculous and NTM, and fungi and mycetoma) on the tissue specimen as well as fluids. The cultures need to be done at three temperatures, held for more than three months, and inoculated on special media for M. haemophilum.

I request the mycobacterial cultures at 30°C for M. marinum, M. haemophilum, M. ulcerans, and Sporothrix, at 37°C for the rest of the mycobacteria, and at 42°C for M. xenopi. More often than not, I personally take the specimen to the microbiology laboratory and urge the microbiologist not to discard the cultures for 4 to 6 months because that covers the slowest-growing M. ulcerans species. I alert the microbiologist and the pathologist of possible chronic infections in the hand and request the infectious disease specialist to participate in the identification and treatment of the infectious agent. This partnership improves the chances of laboratory diagnosis of these rare, unexpected, and newly emerging infections.

Treatment. If there is histopathologic evidence of granuloma, caseating, or noncaseating, I start treatment for tuberculosis with four drugs (i.e., isoniazid, rifampin, pyrazinamide, ethambutol) until the cultures and sensitivities become available. Pyridoxine is added to combat INH neurotoxicity. Histologic findings compatible with tuberculosis warrant MDT, although other chronic infections (e.g., mycetoma, fungi, and NTM) can cause identical clinical and histologic pictures. It may be difficult to distinguish between granuloma of various mycobacteria and fungi, and it is reasonable to start treatment for nontuberculous mycobacterial infection because this is the most common granulomatous hand infection.

Cultures may take 1 to 12 weeks depending on the organism (e.g., *T. ulcerans*). Once the sensitivity of the organism is determined, I revise the chemotherapy. Wounds generally heal without complications while mycobacteria are being cultured. It is important to seek the help of an infectious disease specialist because the drugs are toxic to liver and kidneys among other tissues, and drug resistance may develop at any time owing to inadequate drug compliance. I monitor therapy with monthly examinations. Bone and joint lesions on chemotherapy are monitored with radiographs every 3 months for improvement or deterioration. If improvement is not seen, surgical debridement is considered again, especially in immunocompromised patients. I consider surgical treatment of a tuberculous mass for certain cases of XDR TB when chemotherapy is not an option.

Additional Information on *M. Tuberculosis*. Recent recommendations on treatment of tuberculosis are available from the CDC, Division of Tuberculosis Elimination at www.cdc.gov. For management of drug-resistant tuberculosis, the website lists current contact information.

HANSEN DISEASE (LEPROSY)

Hansen disease (HD) is a chronic neurologic and dermatologic disease with immunological overtones. The ulnar, median, and radial nerves, usually in that order, are affected in the upper extremity in 70% of active and relapsing cases of leprosy. The nerves suffer a triple blow from *M. leprae*: infective neuropathy, immunologic neuropathy, and compressive neuropathy (intraneural and extraneural compression). The bacteria preferentially infect nerves in the cooler parts of the body: the fine terminal dermal nerves, small subcutaneous nerves, and the superficially located large nerve trunks. Sensory loss almost always precedes motor loss because superficial dermal nerve damage precedes deeper nerve trunk damage. Nonmyelinated and thinly myelinated fibers are affected before myelinated fibers. Untreated peripheral neuropathy leads to the characteristic deformities of Hansen disease. Sensory damage and sensory loss lead to gradual and progressive absorption and autoamputation of fingers from recurrent injury and infection; autonomic damage causes loss of protective sudomotor and vasomotor functions, and, finally, motor damage causes

muscle imbalance, leading to flexible and subsequently fixed deformities.

Etiology

Gerhard Armauer Hansen from Norway identified the acid-fast bacillus *M. leprae* in 1873, 10 years before Robert Koch, his contemporary, described *M. tuberculosis*. *M. leprae* was the first bacterium to be implicated as a cause of a human infection. Leprosy is now officially called Hansen disease to remove the stigma of the words "leper" and "leprosy." HD is curable with outpatient oral chemotherapy. Fear of the disease is no longer justified by the lay public or the medical profession. Dapsone renders the patient noncontagious in less than 6 weeks and rifampin in 2 days. Treated early, it is cured; treated late, infection is cured but the nerve damage lingers. The care of HD patients is now firmly integrated into general outpatient health care services.

Epidemiology

Leprosy, one of the most ancient, feared, and disabling diseases of humankind, is almost on the verge of elimination (<1 new case/10,000 population), if not eradication. Since 1985, the prevalence rate of the disease has dropped by 90%—from 21.1/10,000 inhabitants to <1/10,000 inhabitants in 2000. This is because treatment with MDT has been successful without discernible resistance and is provided by WHO free to all. There has been a dramatic decrease in the global disease burden from 5 million cases in 1985 to 180,000 at the end of 2011. Leprosy has been eliminated from 119 countries out of 122 where the disease was considered as a public health problem in 1985. India (134,000), Brazil (38,000), and Indonesia (17,000) had the highest number of cases in the world in 2010.

In the United States, there are approximately 6500 cases of leprosy, 90% of which are in immigrants from countries where leprosy is endemic. Asians and Latinos comprise the majority of the cases. The number of cases with active disease that require drug treatment is approximately 600. There are 200 to 250 new leprosy cases reported each year, with about 175 of these being first-time occurrences; 80% of US cases were reported in Hawaii, Puerto Rico, California, Texas, Louisiana, Florida, and New York. The island populations in Hawaii and Puerto Rico have the highest incidence and prevalence of HD in the United States. The National Hansen's Disease Program in Baton Rouge, Louisiana, is exclusively devoted to the disease. Most patients in the United States are treated under US Public Health Service grants at clinics in major cities.

In terms of reservoirs, most consider that HD is largely a human disease. In Texas and Louisiana, 15% of wild armadillos are infected with *M. leprae*. One-quarter of 175 new cases of Hansen disease in the United States occur in US-born people who have never traveled to endemic countries; the cases are thought to be a result of contact with infected armadillos because the genomes of *M. leprae* in them and the native whites match in 80% of the cases. The most commonly held view of transmission of HD is that it spreads from human to human, primarily as a nasal droplet infection. Skin-to-skin contact is unproven. Incidence rates rise to a peak between 10 and 20 years of age and then decline. About 20% of HD patients are children who develop the disease below the age of 10 and 50% as young adults.

Clinical Pathology

HD is essentially an infection of the peripheral nerves—the only bacillary infection of the nerves. Only a few cases of tuberculoma (i.e., tubercular infection of ulnar nerve) have recently been described.[94] Schwann cells are where *M. leprae* preferentially proliferate in the peripheral nerve. Some patients develop peripheral neuropathy before the appearance of skin lesions (pure or primary neuritic leprosy), some develop it after starting therapy (infectious and immunologic neuritis), and others continue to develop neuropathies well after therapy is stopped (immunologic neuritis or relapse). HD causes mononeuritis or mononeuritis multiplex. There is always nerve damage with HD because there is no such thing as nonneural leprosy.

From onset, the cutaneous nerves and fine intradermal nerve fibers are involved in all forms of HD, and sensory loss is the first and most devastating manifestation of it. Skin lesions and sensory loss develop more or less simultaneously; when skin lesions are present, the underlying dermal nerves are always infected. Although it is the skin lesions that bring one to the doctor, it is the nerve lesions that cripple the patient. About 30% of sensory fibers must be destroyed before evidence of sensory impairment can be detected. Thus, by the time an anesthetic skin patch is detected, the nerve infection is well advanced. According to Ridley and Jopling, if a skin lesion is found to be insensitive, and/or an adjacent subcutaneous nerve is visible or palpable, HD can confidently be suspected.[59]

The bacillary load in the nerves is always higher than that observed in the skin in all stages and all types of HD. The first and the earliest change observed in lepromatous (LL) HD is the presence of *M. leprae* inside the Schwann cells. In tuberculoid HD, the bacilli are found in 70% of the nerves but are almost never found in the skin. At the time of diagnosis of HD, 50% of patients have nerve impairment or disability, both motor and/or sensory. An additional 10 to 20% develop nerve impairment during and after completion of treatment. Of new patients who have no nerve disability at diagnosis, 10% develop it within 2 years of treatment.

Nerve lesions are the result of infection of the nerves and are compounded by the immune reactions that continue in them long after the patient is rendered free of living bacteria. Dead bacterial remnants persist in the nerves after a full course of antibiotic treatment. The presence of these antigens causes intraneural inflammation and fibrosis indefinitely.

The maximum concentrations of bacilli, and thus the greatest damage, are found in the fine dermal nerves, subcutaneous nerves, and the superficially located nerve trunks. In all types of HD, the infected nerve is ultimately replaced by hyalinized fibrous tissue. *M. leprae* conveniently hide in the fibrous tissue and are not reached by drugs. There is the possibility of relapse of the disease from persistent *M. leprae* in the fibrosed nerves. Profound loss of sensation allows uncontrolled and progressive tissue damage from unrecognized injury and infection. With repeated tissue necrosis and self-debridement, the fingers and toes may shorten to form mitten hands and feet. Antia has described three patterns of sensory loss in HD[7]: (1) anesthetic patch from infection of a dermal or subcutaneous nerve, (2) regional loss from infection of a nerve trunk in tuberculoid disease, and (3) a glove-and-stocking pattern due to confluent involvement of sensory nerves in lepromatous disease.

The incubation period of HD is not accurately known; 2 to 7 days is considered usual. Ninety percent of the people who are exposed to *M. leprae* infection have a natural immunity to it. Most who are infected with *M. leprae* develop a subclinical infection and recover naturally without having symptoms or signs of disease. In the remainder, HD progresses slowly over months and years.

Most of the serious sequelae are the result of infection of the peripheral nerves. Bacterial multiplication occurs within Schwann cells, and they spread intraneurally to adjacent Schwann cells. A stage is reached when intraneural infection is "recognized" by the host immune system and the nerve is invaded by lymphocytes and macrophages to combat *M. leprae*. A granuloma forms and fibrosis occurs within the epineurium, perineurium, and endoneurium. Enlargement of peripheral nerves results not from initial infection but instead from subsequent immunologic reaction and caseation. Enlarged nerves are pathognomonic of HD. They are present in 25% of newly diagnosed cases, and neurologic deficit is present with 95% of patients with enlarged nerves. Outside the peripheral nerves, the pathology of HD is largely confined to the skin, eyes, upper respiratory tract, and testes.

Classification

The clinical manifestations of HD vary, depending on the host's resistance or immunity. At one end of the spectrum, a patient may have high cell-mediated immunity and ability to resist, fight, and contain bacteria. Of infected patients, 95% do not develop a clinically diagnosable disease. At the other end of the spectrum, a patient may have complete tolerance to *M. leprae* due to lack of any detectable cell-mediated immunity against the microbe. These patients are actually teeming with bacteria, so the host becomes a perfect culture medium for *M. leprae*. Between these two ends of the spectrum, the borderline group encompasses most patients.

The three main clinical types of HD are tuberculoid (TT, high immunity), lepromatous (LL, low immunity), and borderline (BB, intermediate immunity); BB can fluctuate in either direction. In tuberculoid HD, a cell-mediated immune response to *M. leprae* rapidly destroys both the bacillus and the host Schwann cell in which it resides and leads to early caseous necrosis with total destruction of the nerve. In lepromatous HD, because there is very little immune response to the bacillus, *M. leprae* multiply freely in the Schwann cells, producing a slow fibrosis over many years. Histoid leprosy and Lucio leprosy are variants of lepromatous leprosy. For research purposes, in 1966 Ridley and Jopling divided the borderline cases into three immunologic subsets: BL, BB, and BT (Table 3.10).[59]

Ridley further divided TT and LL into polar (LLp, TTp) and subpolar (LLs, TTs) groups. In 1982, the World Health Organization recommended a simplified, clinical, and operational classification of HD into paucibacillary (PB) and multibacillary (MB) for treatment purposes based on the result of slit-skin smears. When a skin smear is positive, the disease is classified as MB. Under this classification, most of indeterminate (I), TT, and BT cases are PB, but any of them showing smear positivity are classified as MB for purposes of drug therapy. The smears are positive in LL, BL, and usually in BB cases and are classified as multibacillary. The number of drugs and length of therapy are more for multibacillary than for paucibacillary disease.

TABLE 3.10 Clinical, Bacteriologic, Histologic, and Immunologic Features of HD

Lesions and Tests	TYPE OF HANSEN DISEASE				
	TT	BT	BB	BL	LL
Number of skin lesions	Usually single	Single or few, may be distant	Several	Many	Very many
Size of skin lesions	Variable	Variable	Variable, mixed large and small lesions	Variable	Small
Surface of skin lesions	Very dry, sometimes scaly	Dry	Slightly shiny	Shiny	Shiny
Sensation in skin lesions	Absent	Moderately to markedly diminished	Slightly to moderately diminished in large lesions	Slightly diminished in large lesions	Not affected
Loss of hair and sweating in skin lesions	Absent	Markedly diminished	Moderately diminished	Slightly diminished	Not affected
AFB in skin lesions	Nil	Nil or scanty	Moderate numbers	Many	Very many (plus globi)
AFB in nasal scrapings or nose blows	Nil	Nil	Nil	Usually nil	Very many (plus globi)
Nerve lesions	Nerve may be thickened (one or two nerves only)	Thickening of several nerves	Thickening of several nerves	Thickening of several nerves, bilateral	Nerve thickening mild; may not be obvious until late stages
Histology	Dermal nerves are destroyed and cannot be recognized AFB not seen Foci of lymphocytes, epithelioid cells, and giant cells invading the skin indicative of host cell-mediated immunity Cutaneous nerves are greatly swollen because of epithelioid cell granuloma; they may caseate or are destroyed Nerve abscess more common	In BT there is a tuberculoid reaction more diffuse than in TT AFB may or may not be seen	In BB there is a diffuse epithelioid cell granuloma with occasional foam cells AFB in small numbers	In BL there is a granuloma composed of macrophages with lymphocytes in clumps or sheets AFB present	Diffuse leproma of foamy macrophages with few lymphocytes and plasma cells indicative of poor cell-mediated immunity Cutaneous nerves may show slight cellular infiltrate with foam cells AFB seen in clumps Nerve abscess less common
Lepromin test	Strongly positive (+++)	Moderately or weakly positive (++ or +)	Negative	Negative	Negative

AFB, Acid-fast bacillus; *BB*, borderline; *BL*, borderline lepromatous; *BT*, borderline tuberculoid; *LL*, lepromatous; *TT*, tuberculoid.

When a slit smear is not possible, a patient can be classified clinically by the number of skin lesions, but this is not ideal. A patient with >6 lesions is classified as MB, and one with less than six lesions as PB, with a reasonable balance between sensitivity and specificity. PB patients are further classified into those with a single lesion and those with 2 to 6 lesions because the treatment of the two differs in drugs used. The limitation of using a purely clinical classification is that a single-lesion, or paucilesional smear-positive, case may be falsely classified as PB and will receive inadequate chemotherapy, with the risk of relapse and resistance, because approximately 3% of single-lesion patients and 1% of paucilesional smear-positive cases are multibacillary.

Clinical characteristics, skin and nerve lesions, bacteriology, histology, and immunology of HD in its spectrum are summarized earlier in Table 3.10. It remains unknown why certain individuals develop HD and others do not.

Early Diagnosis

Early diagnosis of HD can usually be made by clinical examination supported by slit-skin smear and is conducive to cure and normal life.

Cardinal Signs

WHO has emphasized three cardinal signs for clinical diagnosis of HD: an anesthetic skin patch, nerve thickening, and a hypopigmented skin lesion. The diagnosis must be confirmed by bacteriologic examination. A skin smear positive for HD bacilli confirms the diagnosis. At least two of the first three cardinal signs, or the fourth (positive bacteriological examination), should be present for the diagnosis of HD to be made. Sensory loss in hands and feet should be accompanied with nerve trunk thickening for diagnosis of leprosy. In the absence of nerve thickening one has to be cautious to label a patient suffering from leprosy because of the emotional trauma associated with it. Such cases are kept under observation and periodically examined for the confirmation of disease.

Anesthetic Skin Patch. There are numerous diseases that produce patches on the skin, and there are varied neurologic conditions that cause sensory loss. Demonstrable loss of sensation restricted to a skin patch is unique and pathognomonic of HD. The tests (slit-skin smears) help further treatment classification of the disease.[7] Patients seldom complain of numbness because they adapt to gradual loss of sensation. Anesthesia may be patchy in the distribution of the dermal and cutaneous nerves, regional in the distribution of the peripheral nerve trunks, or in a diffuse glove-and-stocking pattern when damage has occurred to the dermal, subcutaneous, and the main nerve trunk, as seen in lepromatous HD.

The first tests to show and quantitate sensory nerve function impairment are moving two-point discrimination and Semmes-Weinstein monofilament testing. A painless burn may be the presenting symptom or sign of HD. In lepromatous HD a period of pruritus (formication) may precede all other symptoms very early in the course of the disease.

Thickened Nerves. Thickened nerves at the site of predilection are pathognomonic of HD (Figure 3.24). The ulnar nerve is always the first nerve trunk to be involved in the upper extremity and is the most commonly affected with or without skin lesions. In an immigrant from an endemic region of the world who presents with an ulnar nerve enlargement or carpal tunnel syndrome,[65] one must consider HD as a possible diagnosis.[86]

There are four clinical stages of nerve infection in HD:

I. *Parasitization*—Bacteria invade the Schwann cells; clinically the nerve is normal but 50% of the patients have neurologic deficit.
II. *Inflammation*—Adhesion of the nerve to the perineurium is noted with inability to roll the nerve during palpation.[8]
III. *Enlargement*—The nerve is palpably enlarged (nerve caseation without or with an abscess). Ninety-five percent of these patients have a neurologic deficit.
IV. *Destruction*—The nerve is irreversibly damaged and converted to a cord of scar tissue.

Of the newly identified cases, 25% have one or more enlarged nerves. The enlarged nerves may be palpable but not visible, palpable and visible, or palpable and fluctuant. The nerve may be soft (parasitization), not rollable (inflammation), firm (caseation), or hard (fibrosed).

Thickening of nerve trunks occurs most often in the borderline, lepromatous, and pure neuritic types of HD. Pain in one or several nerves may be the presenting symptom even before skin lesions appear. In the beginning, the nerve may be normal in size but may be tender. As granuloma, edema, and fibrosis occur in the nerves, they become enlarged and firm. Enlarged nerves may or may not be tender. Caseation may follow and progress to a solitary tuberculoid nerve lesion or a cold nerve abscess with or without sinus formation. Finally, the nerve is calcified.[75]

If the body's cellular immunity anchors the infection within one or more nerves, the patient may present initially with clinical nerve deficit but no skin lesions and negative slit-skin smears. This is called "pure neuritic" or "primary neuritic" HD.[59,117] Mean prevalence rate of pure neuritic HD varies from 0.8 to 18%. In pure neuritic HD, commonly one nerve is involved, typically the ulnar nerve at the elbow, or the patient may have polyneuropathy. The most common clinical presentation is with numbness or weakness; wasting, deformity, and pain/tingling can also be presenting symptoms in a small minority of cases. The nerve is palpable or visible in 80% of patients with pure neuritic HD.

An early and accurate diagnosis of pure neuritic HD is essential to avoid mismanagement and should be suspected in an immigrant with an enlarged nerve from an endemic region. In absence of anesthetic skin patches or AFB in slit-skin smears, fine-needle nerve aspiration or an open nerve biopsy can establish a diagnosis. Histopathology of pure neuritic lesions reveals a spectrum from paucibacillary (tuberculoid) to multibacillary (lepromatous) type. When it is not possible to biopsy a nerve in pure neuritic HD, three factors help to decide the classification and choice of treatment regimen. First, a pure mononeuritic case generally responds well to a PB regimen. However, it is reasonable to consider HD involving multiple nerves on both sides of the body (i.e., mononeuritis multiplex) as multibacillary. Second, a clinically mononeuritic case may show multiple nerve involvement on electrophysiologic studies, indicating a more widespread involvement and need for a MB regimen. Third, the lepromin reaction is helpful in both mononeuritis and mononeuritis multiplex in determining the patient's position on the immunologic spectrum.

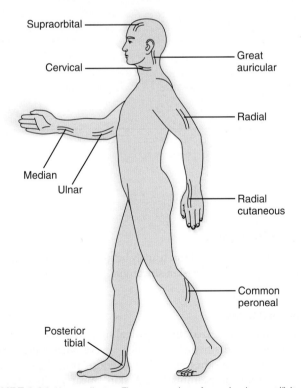

FIGURE 3.24 Hansen disease. The common sites of nerve involvement ("sites of predilection") in the upper extremity are the ulnar nerve at the elbow, the median nerve just proximal to the carpal tunnel, and the sensory branch of the radial nerve. These nerves are closer to the skin and thus reside in colder temperatures. *M. leprae* preferentially infect nerves in the cooler parts of the body. (From Hastings RC: *Leprosy,* ed 2, New York, 1994, Churchill Livingstone, with permission.)

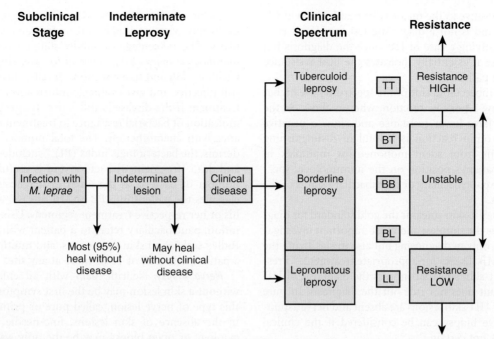

FIGURE 3.25 The course of leprosy after infection with *Mycobacterium leprae*. Clinical disease manifests in <5% of the infected individuals. Clinical spectrum of the disease depends on the immunity of the patient.

Skin Lesions. Skin lesions may become visible at any time during the course of primary neuritic HD. The patient's body should be examined for pigmented or hypopigmented patches and nodules in light that should preferentially fall on the patient from behind the shoulders of the examiner. Classically, the first lesion is a symptomless, ill-defined, slightly hypopigmented macule that is commonly seen on the face, trunk, or limbs. Sensation is only slightly impaired or normal. Bacilli are difficult to find, and diagnosis depends on careful, continuing observation. This lesion is called "indeterminate"; it may heal or progress to one of the three determinate types: tuberculoid, borderline, or lepromatous HD. An I lesion most often heals spontaneously. Only about 30% of indeterminate lesions progress to a determinate type (Figure 3.25).[59] Only 5% of all infected people ever develop clinical symptoms.

The most common and earliest clinical manifestation in HD is a hypopigmented, numb patch of the skin. Discolored skin lesions occur in numerous diseases and numbness of skin occurs in many nerve disorders, but a discolored skin lesion that is anesthetic occurs only in HD. When such a lesion is encountered, diagnosis of HD is clinically confirmed. Increasing anesthesia and elevation of the margins of the skin lesion indicate movement toward the tuberculoid pole. An increase in the number of the lesions and central elevation of the skin lesion indicate movement toward the lepromatous pole. On light skin, the lesions are copper colored; on dark skin, they are hypopigmented. In MB disease the skin lesions are multiple and symmetrical whereas in PB disease the lesions are fewer and asymmetrical (Figure 3.26). A hyperpigmented palmar lesion is a rare presentation of HD.

The diagnosis of HD occasionally can be difficult, as in the following three situations: (1) there is a skin lesion without sensory loss, (2) there is a sensory loss without a skin lesion, and (3) there is an enlarged nerve without motor or sensory loss and a skin lesion is absent (i.e., primary neuritic HD).

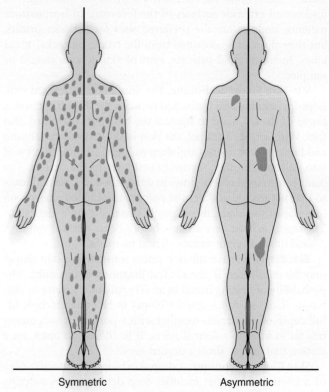

Symmetric   Asymmetric

FIGURE 3.26 The lesions of MB Hansen disease are multiple and symmetrical and those of PB disease are few and asymmetric. (From Hastings RC: *Leprosy*, ed 2, New York, 1994, Churchill Livingstone, with permission.)

Diagnostic Tests

Lepromin Skin Test. A majority of individuals exposed to *M. leprae* get infected but only a small percentage of these go on to develop the disease. The lepromin test is positive in people who develop subclinical infection because their inherent resistance is high. It is thus positive in the majority of healthy individuals in endemic areas and is not a diagnostic test for HD. It is of great value in classifying a case of HD once the diagnosis has been made because it essentially indicates the host resistance (immunity) of the patient.

Patients on the tuberculoid side of the spectrum have higher resistance and show a positive reaction, whereas those on the lepromatous side have lower resistance and show a negative reaction. The lepromin reaction is helpful in distinguishing silent mononeuritis from silent mononeuritis multiplex in determining the patient's position on the immunologic spectrum to determine paucibacillary or multibacillary status of the HD and treatment.[8]

Slit-Skin Smears. Slit-skin smear is the gold standard for diagnosis of HD. This is the simplest and most important investigation that helps not only in diagnosing but also in classifying the HD into PB and MB disease for appropriate treatment.[59] Presence of AFB in slit-skin smears confirms the diagnosis of HD but a negative result does not rule out the diagnosis. In pure (primary) neuritic HD, skin lesions are absent and nerve aspiration or open nerve biopsy can be considered if the clinical diagnosis of HD is not certain.[117]

Slit-skin smears are made from a suspect lesion, as well as from sites commonly affected in lepromatous HD, which include skin from the dorsum of proximal phalanges of fingers and extensor surfaces of the forearms. In lepromatous patients, nodules are the preferred sites for slit-skin smears, but they also can be obtained from the trunk, buttocks, or ear lobes. In tuberculoid patients, rims of skin lesions should be sampled.

Slit-Skin Smear Technique. The skin lesion is cleansed with isopropyl alcohol and is pinched between the thumb and index finger of the left hand to squeeze the blood off the raised skin fold. With a No. 15 scalpel, the skin is slit between the thumb and finger (~5 mm long) and deep enough (~3 mm) to get well into, but not through, the infiltrated layer of the dermis. The blade is then used several times to scrape the cut edges of dermis so that tissue fluid and dermal pulp, but not blood, collects on one side of the blade; this is gently smeared onto a glass slide. The smear is fixed over a flame before being sent for staining. A total of six or eight smears should be made.

Skin Biopsy. When a slit-skin smear is negative, a skin biopsy may be considered if the clinical diagnosis is in doubt. The probability of finding bacilli in an HD patient is greater in skin biopsy than slit-skin smears. A biopsy in HD must include the full depth of the dermis together with a portion of subcutaneous fat to include a dermal nerve. It is difficult to opine on a section that fails to show a dermal nerve.

Skin Biopsy Technique. A deep skin biopsy at the active edge of a lesion is done that includes deep dermal nerves entering the deep surface of the dermis and/or a nerve in the subcutaneous tissue. The biopsy can be preserved in a suitable preservative (e.g., 10% formaldehyde) for further processing. A portion of the skin can be saved in 70% ethyl alcohol so that PCR can be done if bacilli are not found in the skin. PCR can detect as few as 10 to 100 bacilli in a skin sample of an early or TT lesion. When a biopsy is being sent for a mouse footpad test, it should be placed in a small sterile bottle without any additive and kept at 4°C in a flask containing ice.

Viable *M. leprae* are solid, are nonfragmented, and stain uniformly, whereas dead bacilli are fragmented and stain irregularly. The percentage of solidly staining bacilli, termed the *morphologic index* (MI), is useful for assessing viability of the bacilli in skin and tissue sections. It tells whether the patient is still infective and gives valuable information as to response to treatment if the disease is still active. It also provides an early indication of bacterial resistance to treatment or of noncompliance with chemotherapy. The total number of bacilli in the dermis, the bacteriologic index (BI),[59] includes both live (solid) and dead (fragmented) bacteria and is useful in assessing the number of bacteria at the onset of diagnosis (Table 3.11); it classifies the patient into PB or MB disease, which determines his or her respective treatment regimens. Using the WHO definition, paucibacillary refers to a patient with a BI of 0 on the Ridley scale at all skin smear sites, and multibacillary refers to a patient with a BI of 1+ or more at any site.

Nerve Biopsy. Neuritic pain with an enlarged nerve and without a skin lesion may be the first symptom/sign of HD. In this type of nerve lesion, called pure or primary neuritic HD, in the absence of skin lesions, fine-needle nerve aspiration cytology or open biopsy may be the only way to confirm the diagnosis of HD. Nerve aspiration cytology is simple and rapid; material obtained is abundant, absence of trauma and scarring are appreciated by the patient, and an operating room visit for nerve biopsy is avoided. A thickened pure sensory nerve with minimal functional deficit (e.g., sural, radial sensory, supraclavicular) is suitable. When *M. leprae* is not visible on microscopy in the nerve, as in pure neuritic HD or TT disease, PCR, which is positive in 80% of cases, is the last resort to find *M. leprae* in the nerve or the skin.

Fine-Needle Nerve Aspiration Technique. The nerve is palpated and the most obvious site is noted. Skin is anesthetized 1 cm proximal to the site of aspiration. A 22-gauge, 4-cm needle fixed to a 10-mL disposable syringe is used, and aspiration is

TABLE 3.11 Method of Grading the Bacteriologic Index in a Slit-Skin Smear or in a Skin or Nerve Biopsy Specimen

Bacterial Index	Average Number of Bacilli per (100>) Field	WHO Classification
0	0 in 100 fields	Paucibacillary
1	1-10 in 100 fields	Multibacillary
2	1-10 in 10 fields	Multibacillary
3	1-10 per field	Multibacillary
4	10-100 per field	Multibacillary
5	100-1000 per field	Multibacillary
6	>1000 per field	Multibacillary

Classification of patients into paucibacillary (BI = 0) and multibacillary (BI > 0) for treatment purposes makes detailed computing unimportant in diagnosis. The index is nevertheless useful in monitoring improvement or deterioration of the disease (drug compliance and drug resistance). The morphologic index calls for consistently high standards of staining, fixation, and microscopy, which are rarely available outside research and scientific units.

performed using a single puncture. The direction of the needle is always kept parallel to the length of the nerve. The material aspirated is smeared on glass slides. Hematoxylin and eosin and AFS are done. Of the aspirated nerves, 65% showed inflammatory cells, 25% showed granulomas consistent with the diagnosis of HD, and 24% showed AFB. No neurologic deficit was identified at 1-year follow-up.

Open Nerve Biopsy Technique. Biopsy of one or two fascicles of a palpable, thickened, and superficially placed sensory nerve is recommended, preferably under magnification so as to select the most likely affected fascicles. If the nerve is severely damaged and fascicles are obliterated, a small longitudinal wedge of nerve can be removed. A 2-cm-long nerve biopsy provides enough length for histology and electron microscopy.[8] It is important to identify proximal and distal ends of the nerve for the pathologist. The excised portion is immediately immersed in a fixative (10% buffered formalin or 70% alcohol).

Electrophysiological Studies. Nerve conduction studies and electromyography are not specific in the diagnosis of HD but are useful in confirming the site of compression neuropathy before surgery and in assessing the extent of nerve damage in early stages of leprosy.

Imaging Studies. Magnetic resonance imaging can localize a mass, fluctuating or not, in a nerve and facilitate early diagnosis of a nerve abscess or calcification.

Treatment

The patient is classified based on the lepromin test, skin smears, skin biopsy, or nerve biopsy. Based on this, chemotherapeutic agents and duration of treatment are decided. The primary aim in managing patients with HD is to prevent deformities in those who do not have them and to reduce disabilities or arrest their progression in those with them. If treated early, the disease leaves no residual marks. The diagnosis should not be made by exclusion or by therapeutic trial. No one should be treated for HD unless a diagnosis is established. A mistaken diagnosis may cause severe social complications. The objectives of treatment of HD include:

- Elimination of infecting bacteria (multidrug therapy)
- Relief of pain (antiinflammatory medications and nerve decompression)
- Preservation of sensation (corticosteroids, thalidomide, and nerve decompression)
- Restoration of sensation (innervated skin flaps, nerve transfer, nerve decompression, sensory reeducation)
- Treatment of deformities: flexible and fixed (hand therapy and reconstructive surgery)
- Rehabilitation (psychological, social, vocational, and avocational)

Elimination of Infecting Bacteria With MDT

In the 1940s, dapsone was shown to cure patients with HD and was the first landmark in its treatment. Monotherapy with dapsone led to drug resistance. In 1982, WHO recommended multidrug therapy to combat resistance to drugs. Dapsone, which is bacteriostatic, makes the patient noninfective in 6 weeks, and rifampin, which is bactericidal for *M. leprae*, makes the patient noninfective in 2 days. MDT is very effective in the prevention of drug resistance in leprosy, but it has not been possible to reduce the length of treatment substantially and resistance of *M. leprae* to rifampin is emerging.

Since the mid-1980s, bactericidal activities of ofloxacin, minocycline, and clarithromycin have provided treatment for rifampin-resistant *M. leprae*. Mouse footpad antibiotic sensitivity testing should be done on all MB patients whenever possible. In vitro techniques are being developed to identify resistant strains of *M. leprae* in suspected cases. Lately, mouse footpad and genomic studies on *M. leprae* obtained from leprosy patients have begun to show occurrence of *M. leprae* resistance to more than one drug. Isolation of *M. leprae* resistant to a combination of dapsone, rifampicin, ofloxacin and sparfloxacin has been reported.

Paucibacillary Hansen Disease. Paucibacillary HD is treated with two drugs: dapsone, 100 mg once daily, orally, unsupervised; and rifampin, 600 mg once a month, orally, supervised. The drugs are given orally on an ambulatory basis, and WHO recommends treatment for 6 months. In developing countries, rifampin is given once a month because it is very expensive. US recommendations include rifampin in a "full" dosage of 600 mg daily.

A single dose of a three-drug bactericidal combination of rifampin, 600 mg, plus ofloxacin, 400 mg, plus minocycline, 100 mg (i.e., the ROM regimen) is shown to kill 99% of viable *M. leprae*. In 1997, WHO endorsed the use of single-dose ROM for the treatment of patients with single-lesion paucibacillary HD but some reports are now challenging the efficacy of this drug schedule.

Multibacillary Hansen Disease. Multibacillary HD is treated with three drugs: dapsone, 100 mg daily, orally, unsupervised; rifampin, 600 mg once monthly, orally, supervised; and clofazimine, 300 mg once a month, orally, supervised and 50 mg daily, orally, unsupervised. WHO recommends treatment for 12 months. If the skin smears remain positive, the treatment is continued until the smears become negative. Patients in the urban United States often refuse to take clofazimine because it discolors the skin. Rifampin is hepatotoxic, and its use must be monitored with periodic liver function tests. An elevation of serum bilirubin and serum aspartate transaminase (AST or SGOT) is an indication to stop rifampin. It should not be prescribed during the first 3 months of pregnancy.[16]

Drug resistance, persistence of viable *M. leprae* in the tissues for many years after effective therapy (persisters), and resulting relapses after release from treatment (RFT) make eradication of HD difficult. Persisters relapse when their immunity falls for any reason. Relapse rate after MDT is about 0.6% 5 years after RFT. Relapses are more often in MB than PB patients after both monodrug therapy and MDT. Relapses in multibacillary patients occur more often in patients who have a higher bacillary load (BI >4 before MDT).

Relief of Pain

Neuritic pain in HD occurs secondary to nerve infection, nerve reactions due to immunologic defense mechanisms,[16] nerve compression in fibroosseous tunnels, and nerve abscess. Nonneuritic pain in HD may arise from dermatitis, tenosynovitis (Figure 3.27, *A,B*), arthritis, dactylitis (Figure 3.27, *C*), and myositis. Chronic regional pain syndrome has been described as a cause of pain in leprosy that responds effectively to

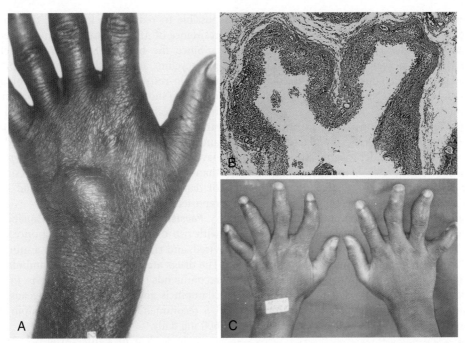

FIGURE 3.27 Rare initial presentations of Hansen disease. **A,** Tenosynovitis is manifested as a moderately painful swelling on the dorsum of one or both wrists, hands, or fingers. By comparison, idiopathic and rheumatoid extensor tenosynovitis is often painless. **B,** Histology shows proliferative tenosynovial tissue. **C,** Arthritis and joint deformities in type 2 reaction in fingers. (Courtesy of G. N. Malaviya, India.)

sympathetic blocks and drugs traditionally used for complex regional pain syndrome (CRPS).

Reactions. The term *reaction* is used to describe the sudden exacerbations in the manifestations of HD that may occur before, during, or after a course of MDT. Reactional episodes are said to be brought about by alterations in immunologic balance. They are antigen-antibody reactions to *M. leprae* polysaccharides and proteins. In the upper extremity, they manifest with acute inflammation in the skin, nerves, tenosynovium, and joint. The patient suffers pain from tender nerves, skin, joints, and tenosynovitis. Swelling of the joints is symmetric and occurs mainly in the wrist, metacarpophalangeal joints, and proximal interphalangeal joints and resembles rheumatoid arthritis. All are precursors to edema and stiffness. The shoulder–hand–finger syndrome can develop in the reactive phases of HD as an edematous, painful, stiff upper extremity and has been called the "stasis hand" of leprosy.

Much of the nerve damage in HD takes place during the reactive phase, which produces intraneural caseous necrosis in tuberculoid disease and microabscesses in lepromatous disease. Reaction neuritis is a medical emergency. Unless it is treated immediately, sensory loss can become devastating and irreversible. A reaction may be the initial manifestation of HD. Reactions plague the patient before treatment, during treatment, and long after MDT has practically eliminated all viable organisms from the body. New deformity or disability occurs in 5% of MB patients during therapy and 2.5% after RFT during the surveillance period as a result of leprae reactions. They continue to disable and deform the patient for life. HD is thus truly an immunologic peripheral nerve disease. Three types of reactions occur in HD: reversal reaction (type 1), erythema nodosum leprosum (type 2), and the Lucio reaction (Table 3.12).

Reversal Reaction (Leprae Type 1). Sometimes there is a rapid increase in cell-mediated immunity when a patient is under adequate and regular treatment, which increases the immunologic resistance, and is associated with a reaction characterized as an "upgrading reaction" or "reversal reaction" (RR). These type 1 reactions are most common in borderline and tuberculoid patients. Clinically, reaction is manifested in the skin, nerves, and tendons. It may be mild and manifested by dull pain or with severe neuritic pain, skin lesions, and tenosynovitis.

ENL Reaction (Leprae Type 2). Leprae type 2 reactions affect mainly lepromatous (LL > BL) patients. In contrast to a reversal reaction, erythema nodosum leprosum is a generalized process involving several organ systems, concurrently or sequentially. The patient is often ill with fever and granulocytosis. The process takes its name from crops of painful, red, cutaneous, and subcutaneous nodules that develop all over the face, limbs, and trunk. Joints may become swollen and tender. Neuritis occurs in 20% of cases owing to formation of microabscesses. Periostitis, tendinitis, and myositis are sometimes observed. It has been hypothesized that a high bacterial antigen load leads to an immune reaction in which immune complexes cause vasculitis—the histologic hallmark of ENL (see Table 3.12).

Lucio Reaction. The Lucio reaction is a necrotizing skin reaction associated with nonnodular diffuse lepromatous HD. The Lucio reaction is common in Mexico and Central America. Large recurrent, sloughing cutaneous ulcerations occur that heal inadequately. It may present as intense hand and foot edema. Necrosis, ulceration, and purulent exudate are superimposed on purpuric cutaneous plaques on hands and feet. There may be rapid and profound deterioration of health, and delay in diagnosis causes high morbidity and mortality. This is

TABLE 3.12 Classification of Lepra Reaction in Leprosy

Type	Type of Leprosy Involved	Main Clinical Features	Main Histologic Features	Main Hematologic Findings
Type 1	1. Borderline (BT < BB < BL)	Erythema and swelling of some or all leprosy skin lesions	With an upgrading reaction there is edema, reduced bacilli, and increased defensive cells (e.g., lymphocytes, epithelioid, and giant) With a downgrading reaction there is an increase in bacilli and defensive cells are replaced by macrophages	Nil
Reversal (RR)		New lesions may appear		
Increased hypersensitivity to *M. leprae*		Edema of extremities Neuritis		
Type 2 (ENL reaction) Immune complex formation	1. LL 2. BL	Fever, skin eruptions, ENL with any of the following, singly or in various combinations: *Hand*—neuritis, bone pain, joint pain, dactylitis, tenosynovitis, lymphadenitis *Systemic*—fever, malaise, rhinitis, epistaxis, iritis, epididymo-orchitis, proteinuria	In ENL lesions there is edema, neutrophil infiltration, and vasculitis (veins and arterioles)	Polymorphonuclear leukocytosis Raised ESR Thrombocytosis Raised IgG, IgM, complement 2, and complement 3 Normocytic normochromic anemia
		In severe cases (e.g., erythema necroticans), skin lesions may become vesicular or bullous and break down	In erythema necroticans there is obliterative angiitis and endarteritis Bacilli are fragmented and granular	
Lucio	Lucio leprosy (in Mexico and South America)	Small pink lesions on the skin become large; bullae develop, become necrotic, and cause large painful ulcers	Necrosis of superficial blood vessels Deposits of immunoglobulin and complement in vessel walls Abundant AFBs	High titers of circulating immune complexes and cryoglobulins

AFB, Acid-fast bacillus; *BL*, borderline lepromatous; *ENL*, erythema nodosum leprosum; *ESR*, erythrocyte sedimentation rate; *LL*, lepromatous.

TABLE 3.13 Treatment of Lepra Reaction

Type	Corticosteroids	Clofazimine	Thalidomide
1	At least 60-80 mg prednisone daily Initially attempt to taper over a 2-3-month period For chronic reactions, try to taper to every other day	300 mg daily until controlled without corticosteroids; then taper to 100 mg daily Increase as needed if reaction recurs	Ineffective
2	Usually 60 mg of prednisone daily Initially attempt to taper over a 2-3-month period For chronic reactions, try to taper to every other day	300 mg daily until controlled without corticosteroids; then taper to 100 mg daily Increase as needed if reaction recurs	100 mg four times daily tapered after reaction controlled For chronic reaction, maintenance level of 100 mg every other day to 100 mg twice daily Try to discontinue after 6 months
Lucio	At least 60 mg of prednisone daily Initially attempt to taper over a period of several weeks For chronic reactions, try to taper to every other day	Value questionable except as antileprosy therapy	Ineffective

considered to be a type of HD reaction associated with necrosis of arterioles, the endothelium of which is massively invaded by *M. leprae* (see Table 3.12).

Treatment of Reactions. Leprosy is cured but nerves die, unless reactions are prevented or treated early (Table 3.13).

Mild reactions are accompanied by nagging pain without neurologic deficit. Aspirin is adequate for this type of mild to moderate pain and is the drug of choice. More severe reactions are best managed by resting the nerve (i.e., splinting the affected joint) and oral corticosteroid therapy. Prednisone reduces edema virtually overnight and decreases postinflammatory scarring.

In reversal reactions, corticosteroids may be needed for 6 months or longer to prevent relapses, and use for up to 5 years has shown very beneficial results. In ENL, clofazimine and thalidomide help to reduce the corticosteroid dose once acute pain subsides. Acute tenosynovitis is treated with oral cortisone, hand elevation, and a balanced combination of splinting and mobilization of the joints.

In the Lucio reaction, debridement of sloughing skin and skin grafting are indicated early, particularly when joints are exposed. It is also necessary to provide immunosuppressive drug therapy and MDT. Hands affected by reactive phases of HD do well if occupational and physical hand therapists prevent "frozen hands" and "frozen shoulders."

Compression Neuropathy. There may be internal compression of the nerves where the nerve fibers are strangulated by the thickened epineurium because of intraneural edema ("acute nerve compartment syndrome") or intraneural granuloma formation and caseation ("chronic nerve compartment syndrome") or external compression from the fibroosseous tunnel that contains it. Surgical decompression is complementary to, and not a substitute for, treatment of acute neuritis. Nerve compression is surgically decompressed (1) when nerve pain is severe even after function may have been lost for months or years and (2) when there is recent and/or progressive loss of nerve function (motor or sensory) after adequate cortisone treatment from 3 days to 3 weeks.

Those with extensive surgical experience in HD, including Brand,[13] Antia,[8] and Srinivasan,[110] found that when unrelenting pain was the main problem, ulnar nerve decompression was a satisfying operation for the patient and the surgeon. Both extraneural pressure release (fibroosseous tunnel) (Figure 3.28, *A*)

and intraneural pressure release (epineurotomy) (Figure 3.28, *B*) are essential parts of the surgery. Varying grades of motor and sensory recovery were additional benefits in 50% of the patients when surgery was done early.

Results of carpal tunnel release are mixed. The decompression of the median nerve is beneficial. Pain relief is dramatic, sensory recovery is seen in 90% of cases, and muscle strength improves in 45% of cases. Srinivasan and Palande observed motor recovery in 75% of patients with median nerve palsy if operated on within 2 months of paralysis.[110] Results of radial nerve release in the nerve groove of humerus are equivocal. The number of cases requiring any nerve decompression have been significantly reduced after using cortisone, clofazimine, and thalidomide to control acute leprous reactions.

Nerve Abscess. Nerve abscess may be (1) the initial presenting problem in HD, (2) seen during therapy, or (3) appear during post-MDT surveillance after RFT. A nerve abscess may appear as a single swelling (Figure 3.29), multiple swellings on a single nerve (Figure 3.30), or multiple swellings on multiple nerves. Children and teenagers accounted for 47% of 145 nerve abscesses and occur across the entire spectrum of HD. The abscess may be fluctuant, nonfluctuant, subcutaneous, deep, painless, painful, collar-stud, moderate in size, giant in size, without a sinus, with an impending sinus (see Figure 3.30), with a draining sinus, with a dried sinus, without calcification, or with calcification (Figure 3.31, *A,B*).[75] It is most frequently seen in the ulnar nerve (58%) and rarely in the median (7%) or the radial nerves and can be unilateral or bilateral. Abscesses may occur along one or more cutaneous nerves of the arm and forearm (Figure 3.32). Medial cutaneous nerves of arm and forearm account for 35% of abscesses.

Treatment of a Nerve Abscess. A painless abscess may subside with oral corticosteroid therapy. If a painful and

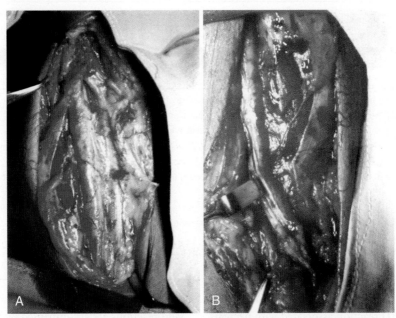

FIGURE 3.28 Surgical exposure of the ulnar nerve at the elbow in a case of Hansen disease. **A,** The incision is made in the upper arm over the palpable nerve at least 10 cm proximal and distal to the medial epicondyle. Extraperineurial pressure over the fibroosseous tunnel containing the enlarged nerve is decompressed. **B,** More importantly, intraepineurial pressure in the ulnar nerve due to infection is released by longitudinal epineurotomy along the entire enlarged nerve. Epineurotomy is limited to the exposed side of the nerve and the nerve is left intact in the bed to preserve compromised circulation to the nerve due to perineurial fibrosis. (Courtesy of G. N. Malaviya, India.)

fluctuating abscess does not respond to oral corticosteroid therapy, it is drained to debulk the caseous granulation tissue and to decompress the surviving nerve fascicles. This relieves pain and may prevent further deterioration of nerve function.[76]

Nerve Abscess Drainage Technique. A painless and fluctuating abscess without progressive nerve deficit can simply be aspirated under sonography. An abscess with progressive neurologic deficit is drained with a single longitudinal epineurotomy. Caseous material is drained and nerve fascicles are not disturbed, and the epineurium is not closed. The skin can be primarily closed over a drain that is removed 24 to 48 h after surgery. A chronic sinus secondary to a discharged nerve abscess can be treated by excision of the sinus tract along with necrotic nerve tissue. In cases of complete nerve trunk palsy, a course of rifampin and isoniazid may heal the sinus in about 6 months.

Preservation of Sensation

Infection of the peripheral nerve in HD impairs pain perception. Loss of pain allows the patient to injure himself or herself. Fingertips undergo "terminal absorption" due to recurrent trauma and infection. Shortening of the fingers results in "mitten" hands.

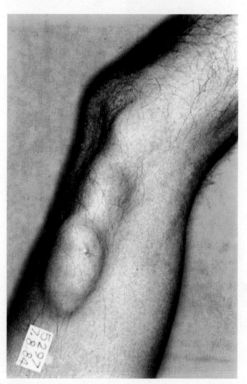

FIGURE 3.30 There are two abscesses on one nerve shown here. A nerve abscess with an impending sinus may need early incision and drainage to prevent formation of a chronic sinus and more perineurial fibrosis. (Courtesy of G. N. Malaviya, India.)

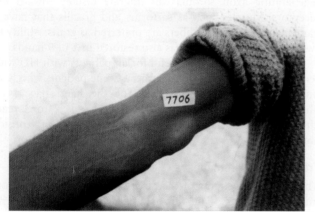

FIGURE 3.29 Clinical features of a nerve abscess caused by Hansen disease are highly variable. A single swelling is the most common finding. Ultrasound is helpful for making a diagnosis of nerve abscess. Of abscesses, 58% are seen in the ulnar nerve. (Courtesy of G. N. Malaviya, India.)

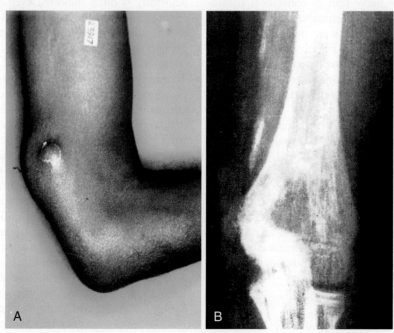

FIGURE 3.31 A, A nerve abscess can become calcified. **B,** Calcified nerve can be seen on a radiograph as a longitudinal opacity corresponding to the location of the nerve. (Courtesy of G. N. Malaviya, India.)

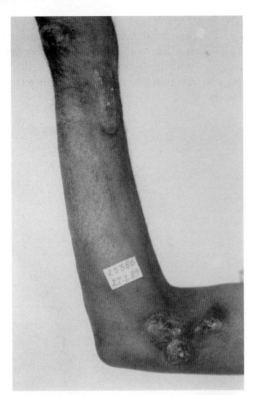

FIGURE 3.32 Cutaneous nerve abscesses can be seen along one or more cutaneous nerves in the upper arm and forearm. The medial cutaneous nerve of the upper arm and of the forearm account for 35% of nerve abscesses. (Courtesy of G. N. Malaviya, India.)

Sensory loss occurs in HD from several causes, but the basic pathology is a varying mixture of segmental demyelination and axonal degeneration. There is swelling of vascular endothelium in leprous vasculitis and this causes narrowing of lumina and nerve ischemia. Progressive nerve fibrosis converts it into a fibrous cord. Complete and early elimination of bacteria by MDT may cure the patient. Reactions are treated by prompt administration of corticosteroids. For patients with recent loss of sensation who do not respond to corticosteroids, surgical decompression of the involved nerve is indicated.[8] Surgery done no later than 3 months after the onset of nerve damage has been shown to be beneficial.

Silent Neuritis. Silent neuritis occurs with neurologic loss (sensory and motor) but without neuropathic pain or tenderness and in absence of a leprae reaction (i.e., types 1, 2, or Lucio) in a large HD population. In 67 to 75% of those who developed deformities, patients gave no history of reactions; 95% of those with pure neuritic HD did not give a history of neuritic pain. The nerves are silently damaged by Schwann cell destruction and segmental demyelination during continuous or recurrent subclinical types 1 and 2 reactions. In silent neuritis, corticosteroids are beneficial in reversing motor weakness, but their benefit in impaired sensibility is not known.

Restoration of Sensibility

Antia reported that 20 to 30% of patients develop irreversible nerve damage in HD.[8] Restoring sensibility in anesthetic extremities of HD patients is the next surgical frontier. The minimum desirable level of sensibility in Hansen disease is protective sensibility. This prevents self-mutilation of the hand. Surgery is successful if the patient can resume "injury-free" hand activities. The recovery of sensory abilities therefore will help in "normalization" of the activities of the patients.[73,74] Procedures to restore sensibility should be delayed until all indicated tendon transfers have been done and the patient has supple tissues with an established range of motion. The following possibilities have currently been used in HD with varying success.

Ozkan and associates have described restoration of sensibility in leprosy-affected hands by transferring a sensory branch of the radial nerve to appropriate median or ulnar nerve branches.[87] Frozen skeletal muscle bridge grafts have been used to replace damaged nerve segments. After freezing, muscle fibers degenerate and leave their sarcolemmal tubes intact. These tubes act as a framework, along and through which the regenerating axon sprouts can migrate distally toward the receptors. Muscles such as sartorius and gracilis that have a parallel arrangement of fibers are preferred as grafts. Ability to sweat in the affected area was also restored in 1 of 9 hands.

Sensory reeducation is useful for all patients with HD with sensory loss, with or without surgery. Some patients who have undergone reconstructive surgery of the hand have been observed to get some "feeling" in their hands 2 to 3 years after surgery, especially when the hand has been put to considerable use.

Treatment of Deformities

The horror and stigma of the disease are rooted in the deformity it can cause. The normal-appearing but infected HD patient moves about freely in society. The deformed but noncontagious patient is an outcast. To the deformed patient, appearance means the difference between being an outcast and having a normal work and social life. With HD, the appearance of the hand is as important as its function. The correction of deformity is often indicated even if it does not substantially restore hand function because it restores a patient's dignity.

The ulnar nerve damage is responsible for 50% of the primary hand deformities. The ulnar claw hand is the most common paralytic deformity in HD. The second most common deformity is because of a combined ulnar and median nerve paralysis, the complete claw hand, with simian deformity. Deformities that are a result of radial nerve paralysis are rare, occurring only in 1 to 2% of the deformed cases. Radial nerve palsy is usually a part of a "triple nerve paralysis." Pure median and radial nerve involvement is rarely encountered in HD. Surgical treatment of hand deformities from muscle imbalance due to nerve palsy is reviewed extensively in Chapter 31.

In cases of ulnar palsy, the atrophy of first dorsal interosseous muscle results in a deep gutter in the first web space. Although it does not lead to any functional deficit, patients at times request that this gap be filled for cosmetic reasons. This problem has not been given much attention by hand surgeons. Several attempts have been made in the past to fill it with silicone gel, dermal grafts, dermofat grafts, and structured autologous fat grafts with varying success. An adipofascial flap raised from the forearm, based on cephalic vein and distal perforators of the radial artery, has been satisfactory for correcting this deformity because it is a vascularized substitute.[91]

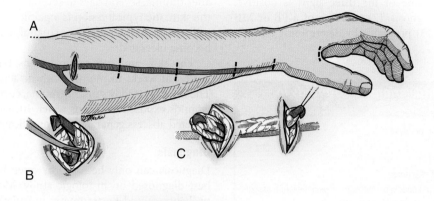

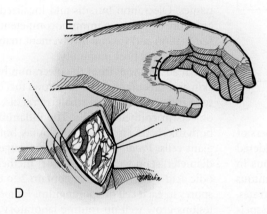

FIGURE 3.33 Reconstruction of first dorsal interosseous gutter. **A,** Dorsal first web space gutter as a result of atrophy of the first dorsal interosseous muscle. **B,** Incisions used to design an adipofascial flap. **C,** Dissection of the adipofascial flap. **D,** Dissected flap. **E,** Thumb web space after in-setting of the flap. (Copyright © Elizabeth Martin.)

Overcorrection is required because 50% of the bulk may be lost in about 6 months to a year, as reported by the authors (Figure 3.33, *A-E*).

Rehabilitation

Psychiatric morbidity is common in HD patients. One must therefore evaluate the deformity a patient has as well as the person who has it. For them to make a decision about treatment, it is essential that patients know what kind of surgery is available and what is expected during the postoperative period. Patients with HD have to face three different sets of problems: overuse, misuse, and protected use. The entire rehabilitation process depends on patients' understanding of those problems, acceptance of residual disability, and desire to adapt to the new situation. Among these, acceptance of disability is the most important and the most difficult. It is patients who need rehabilitation, not the hand alone.

It is important that the surgeon assemble a multidisciplinary team to follow the patient, including an infectious disease specialist, a physical and occupational therapist, and a social worker. Rehabilitation of the patient's psychological, social, vocational, and avocational life restores his or her self-esteem. These are the final and most important milestones in restoring social acceptability and dignity to the dejected and stigmatized HD patient. In his enthusiasm for surgery and research, Brand never forgot the person behind the disease.[13]

Resource Materials

For the latest guidelines on diagnosis and treatment of HD, National Hansen's Disease Program (Baton Rouge, LA) maintains a referral service to several federally funded ambulatory HD centers; they are located in Boston; Chicago; Los Angeles, Martinez, and San Diego, California; Miami; New York; Phoenix; Puerto Rico; Seattle; and Dallas, Harlington, Houston, and San Antonio, Texas.

Several texts on medical and surgical treatment have been published by physicians[16,50,59] and surgeons[7,8,110] experienced in HD. Two journals (*Indian J. Lepr.* and *Lepr. Rev.*) are dedicated to basic and clinical HD research in English. The publication of the *International Journal of Leprosy* and *Acta leprologica* has been discontinued. The International Congress of Leprosy first met in 1897 and convenes every fifth year under the auspices of the International Leprosy Association to update research and clinical information; it last met in 2012 in New York.

CRITICAL POINTS *For Diagnosis of Hansen Disease*

Two of the following three clinical signs are needed for clinical diagnosis:
- A hypopigmented skin patch
- An anesthetic skin patch
- An enlarged nerve (ulnar nerve at elbow, median nerve at wrist, sensory branch of radial nerve)

A smear positive for *M. leprae* from the skin or nerve biopsy is diagnostic when only one of the three signs is positive. Smear is done for (1) diagnosis, (2) selection of a PB or MB treatment regimen, and (3) prognosis by determining bacteriological level.

CRITICAL POINTS *Indications for Steroids in Leprosy Reactions*

- Impending or recent muscle paralysis
- Recent loss of sensation
- Painful neuritis
- Moderate to severe type 1 reactions
- Moderate to severe erythema nodosum leprosum, especially when associated with neuritis, arthritis, and orchitis or uveitis

---

PROTOTHECAL, PROTOZOAL, AND PARASITIC INFECTIONS

Protothecosis (Algae Infections)

Etiology and Epidemiology

Human protothecosis is a rare infection caused by members of the genus *Prototheca*. *Prototheca* species are generally considered to be achlorophyllous (colorless) algae and are ubiquitous in nature. *Prototheca* spp. exist in the environment as ubiquitous detritus inhabitants and contaminants of various substrates. *Prototheca wickerhamii* and *Prototheca zopfii* have been associated with human disease. It is often classified as a fungus because the organisms are frequently preliminarily identified in tissue biopsy as yeast. It was first identified in 1894, but the first case of human protothecosis was not described until 1964. Since then, 50 cases have been reported and reviewed up to 1992 and 80 cases up to 2006.[120] Of the first 50 cases, 28 were in the upper extremity (i.e., 3 in fingers, 1 in palm, 1 on dorsum of hand, 2 in wrist, 2 in forearm, 16 in olecranon bursa, and 4 in upper arm).

About half the cases were cutaneous/subcutaneous and the other half were bursitis, tenosynovitis, and fasciitis. The cutaneous/subcutaneous cases occurred in immunocompromised patients, mainly due to systemic corticosteroid administration, diabetes, renal failure, and topical application of corticosteroids at the site of infection.

Clinical Findings

The most common form of protothecosis in the upper extremity is olecranon bursitis. *P. wickerhamii* is the most frequent alga infection in the upper extremity. The occurrence of protothecosis can be local or disseminated and acute or chronic, with the latter being more common. Diseases have been classified as (1) cutaneous lesions, (2) olecranon bursitis, and (3) disseminated-systemic manifestations. Infections can occur in both immunocompetent and immunosuppressed patients. More severe and disseminated infections tend to occur in immunocompromised individuals.

The most common presentations of protothecosis in the upper extremity are olecranon bursitis and tenosynovitis. Protothecosis deserves to be included in the differential diagnosis of recurrent olecranon bursitis. Most olecranon bursitis occurs after trauma, several days to several weeks prior to infection. In the skin, the typical lesion is a painless, slowly progressive, and well-circumscribed plaque or papulonodular lesion that may become ulcerated.

The skin and soft tissue lesions typically enlarge over a period of weeks to months with no tendency for self-healing. The infection follows minor trauma, corticosteroid injection, or wounds exposed to soil or water. Incision and drainage of an infected abscess generally are complicated by recurrence.

Diagnosis

Diagnosis can only be made by open biopsy. Protothecosis is best diagnosed on histologic study. Most such infections are probably caused by traumatic inoculation into subcutaneous tissues. Olecranon bursitis and localized cutaneous infections are more common in immunocompetent patients, whereas dissemination and visceral involvement mainly affect patients with compromised host immunity.

An abscess wall from the olecranon bursa, tenosynovitis, or skin and subcutaneous tissue shows foci of chronic granulomatous inflammation and small, refractile, and morula-like oval objects in epithelioid cells. The inflammatory response shows both microabscesses and granulomas, both with multinucleated giant cells. *Prototheca* cells usually range from 8 to 20 mm in diameter, stain well with Gomori methenamine silver or periodic acid–Schiff, and often contain 2 to 8 tightly packed endospores in each cell or sporangium. *Prototheca* species from skin lesions grow well on routine laboratory media such as a Sabouraud dextrose agar; however, only half of the synovial protothecosis can be isolated by culture.[78,106] When the organisms grow, white opaque colonies appear in a few days on a Sabouraud agar. Recognition of *Prototheca* cells in host's living tissue is essential to making the diagnosis of protothecosis. When histopathologic material is not available, repeated isolation from clinical material may be necessary to confirm protothecal etiology.

Treatment

Usually, treatment involves combined medical and surgical approaches; treatment failure is not uncommon. Protothecosis has little, if any, tendency toward self-healing. Surgical excision of lesions is successful when it is meticulous and complete. Prolonged therapy with ketoconazole, itraconazole, or fluconazole should be added in immunosuppressed patients. A case of cutaneous protothecosis of the hand in an immunocompromised patient that did not respond to high doses of itraconazole treatment showed complete resolution in 2 months after thermal adjuvant therapy with a disposable body warmer; it provided 55°C average heat over clothes used every day without recurrence at 2 years.

Protozoal Infections

Leishmaniasis Infection

Etiology and Epidemiology. Leishmaniasis is transmitted by the bite of small insects called sand flies. Exposed hands, feet, and face are thus sites of infection. Leishmaniasis threatens 350 million people in 88 countries where the disease is endemic. The estimated yearly incidence is 1 to 1.5 million cases of the cutaneous variety and 500,000 cases of visceral leishmaniasis (kala azar). Of these cases, 90% occur in Saudi Arabia, Afghanistan, Peru, Brazil, and Iran. From 2002 to 2004, 522 new cases of cutaneous leishmaniasis were reported among troops stationed in Afghanistan, Iraq, and Kuwait, mostly due to *L. major*. More than 80% of a total of 12 million infected patients live in Brazil (New World leishmaniasis) and 20% live in Tunisia, Syria, Iran, and Afghanistan (Old World leishmaniasis).

Kabul is considered to be the largest center of cutaneous leishmaniasis in the world, with approximately 67,500 cases in 2004. The disease is endemic in southern Texas because of its proximity to Mexico. Travelers to Costa Rica and Central America are the most common importers of leishmanial ulcers to the United States. It should be included in the differential diagnosis of skin lesions on exposed upper extremity in personnel returning from the military in endemic areas. Leishmaniasis is an intracellular infection caused by the protozoa *Leishmania*. Rodents and canines are the normal reservoirs, humans are the hosts, and the vector is the sandfly. Humans can also act as reservoirs when they are actively infected. The parasite multiplies in the macrophages, which then rupture and release the *Leishmania* organisms into the bloodstream.

Clinical Findings. There are three anatomic sites affected by leishmaniasis: cutaneous, mucocutaneous, and visceral. Cutaneous leishmaniasis (e.g., Baghdad boil, Delhi boil, tropical sore, oriental sore, Balkan sore, chiclero ulcer, Saldana) is the most common form and of interest to upper extremity surgeons because 80% of the lesions are located on exposed body sites of the upper extremity and the lower extremity and face.

In the finger, it may present as a node, whitlow,[4] chronic paronychia, or an ulcer that has not responded to a variety of treatments. It may occur on the finger, hand, wrist, forearm, elbow, or upper arm. In an AIDS patient, uncontrolled infection of a fingertip can cause necrosis of the distal phalanx. The initial lesion is a red-brown papule or a nodule at the bite site. It gradually enlarges to a 2- to 4-cm painless, chronic ulcer within 6 months. The ulcer has a necrotic base and indurated margin and is covered by a firmly adherent crust. It has a "pizza-like" appearance with a raised outer margin.

A solitary lesion occurs in 76% of cases, two lesions in 15%, three lesions in 6%, and four lesions in 1%. Multiple ulcers occur in immunocompromised patients. Without treatment, the ulcer begins to heal over the course of a year, eventually leaving a characteristic cribriform scar. Lymphadenopathy is absent. The lesion may present as a marching lymphocutaneous sporotrichoid abscesses. Basal cell carcinoma or squamous cell carcinoma may develop in an untreated, neglected, chronic leishmaniasis ulcer.

Diagnosis. A chronic nonhealing ulcer in the exposed part of the upper extremity of a traveler, immigrant, or military personnel from an endemic country (e.g., Brazil, Middle East) should arouse suspicion of a leishmanial ulcer. A nonhealing nodular ulcer is an indication to carry out a smear, culture, or biopsy. Final diagnosis is usually delayed unless the level of suspicion is high. In a series of 28 patients, the diagnosis of leishmaniasis was delayed an average of 125 days despite an average of three physicians' examinations.

Diagnosis is made by identification of the parasite from smear, fine-needle aspiration cytology, or biopsy specimen. The first smear may be positive in 80% of cases, and a second smear may be positive in an additional 10% of cases. Smears taken from the center of the ulcer have a greater sensitivity than those from its edge. Before a biopsy sample is immersed in formaldehyde, an impression smear of tissue should be made and a prolonged Giemsa stain (45 min) should be performed on the smear. PCR is the most accurate test for identification of the *Leishmania* species but is limited to specialized laboratories. The microorganism has to be cultivated from biopsy material on a special medium (i.e., Novy-MacNeal-Nicolle) and a positive culture can take a month to grow.

Treatment. Treatment minimizes scar formation and may ultimately avert formation of carcinoma. Topical therapy with paromomycin and methylbenzethonium chloride has been used successfully for the treatment of Old World leishmaniasis in a randomized, controlled, double-blind study. Intralesional injection of antimony compounds is successful in 76% of cases. Therapy was carried out using intralesional injection of 1 mL/cm^2 of meglumine antimoniate or sodium stibogluconate once a week. The average number of injections was 11.

As a preventive measure for travelers to endemic countries, the CDC recommends (1) avoidance of outdoor activities from dawn to dusk when sand flies are most active, (2) wearing long sleeve shirts and pants when out between dawn and dusk, and (3) application of repellent with diethyltoluamide (DEET) to exposed skin and edges of clothing to prevent sand flies from biting.

Parasitic Worm (Nematode) Infection

Parasitic worm (nematode) infections of the upper extremity have been reported due to three worms: two roundworms, *Gnathostoma spinigerum* and *Onchocerca volvulus*, and a tapeworm, *Taenia solium*. The T_H^2 subsets of helper T lymphocytes recognize helminthic antigens and stimulate IgE antibodies. Eosinophils adhere to and attain defenses against helminths, and Eosinophilia is pathognomonic of helminthic infections.

Gnathostomiasis (Round Worm) Infection

Gnathostomiasis is a subcutaneous infection caused by a roundworm (nematode), Gnathostoma spinigerum. It is a chronic, cutaneous "migrating" larval infection. It is common in Thailand, Southeast Asia, and Japan, where people eat uncooked fish or raw pork. Daengsvang et al alluded to five cases of gnathostomiasis occurring in the fingers.[28] In the United States, a patient is likely to be an immigrant. Multiple migrating episodes of swelling and pain can occur in the hand, foot, shoulder, and face over several years as larva migrate subcutaneously. Eosinophilic count is typically high because eosinophils are specifically effective against helminthic parasites. A skin test and a serum precipitin test are useful in confirming the clinical diagnosis. Exploration, recognition, and removal of the larva that are 1 cm × 1 mm from the infected part of the hand is curative. Drug therapy is not necessary once the larvae are removed.

Onchocerciasis (Onchocercosis, Filarial, Round Worm) Infection

Onchocerciasis is a rare parasitic infection of the soft tissues caused by a roundworm (nematode), *Onchocerca volvulus*.

Onchocerciasis of the flexor tendons of finger, wrist, carpal tunnel, and forearm have been reported in North America. Eosinophilia is pathognomonic of parasitic infestations. Synovectomy is curative. Drug therapy is not necessary if all the parasites are removed with the infected tissue.

Tapeworm (Cysticercosis, *Taenia Solium*) Infection

The tapeworm (*Taenia solium*) can infect a muscle and present as a mass that can be mistaken clinically for malignant sarcoma. Tapeworm infections of the upper extremity have been reported in the triceps muscle and flexor digitorum profundus muscle. Tapeworm infection is acquired by ingestion of inadequately cooked and infected pork. The differential diagnosis of a muscle mass should include cysticercosis. The diagnosis is made by fine-needle aspiration of the cyst. Simple surgical excision cures the condition.

OCCUPATIONAL INFECTIONS

Barber's interdigital pilonidal sinus, shearer's disease, milker's interdigital granuloma, and slaughterer's interdigital granuloma are foreign-body occupational hand infections caused by penetration of human or animal hair into skin. Anthrax, *M. marinum*, tuberculous paronychia, herpetic paronychia, prosector's wart, milker's nodule, human orf, and viral warts are also infectious occupational diseases of the hand and are described in detail in the bacterial, tuberculous, and viral infection sections.

Barber's Interdigital Pilonidal Sinus

Etiology and Epidemiology
Barber's interdigital pilonidal sinus of the hand is a foreign-body hair granuloma.[89] The term *pilonidal* is derived from the Latin terms *pilos*, which means "hair," and *nidus*, which means "nest." Interdigital pilonidal sinus in barbers was first described in 1942 as a foreign-body reaction or a granuloma of the customer's hair implanted in the barber's interdigital skin. Since then, cases have been described as hair-bearing sinus, barber's interdigital pilonidal sinus, barber's disease, and interdigital sinus. Interdigital pilonidal sinus is a disease of male barbers and hairdressers only. It has never been reported in female hairdressers. It rarely affects the pulp of a finger. The condition is not a congenital cyst because hair roots are not seen in the sinus or the cyst, and the hairs are not immature, curly, or fine like those found in a congenital pilonidal cyst.

Clinical Findings and Diagnosis
Clinically, a pit or sinus develops in the interdigital web space dorsally. The sharp snipped hair ends enter the soft skin of the digital webs when barbers or hairdressers use their fingers to comb the customer's hair. Constant rubbing of the fingers against each other exacerbates the problem. Once inside the web space the hairs cause a foreign-body reaction and sinus formation. As more hairs enter the web space through the sinus, a cyst can form. In time, the sinus or the cyst becomes infected and an abscess forms that intermittently discharges purulent fluid with pieces of hair. Histologically, the lesion reproduces the features of a nonspecific inflammatory granuloma.[89]

Several loose and easily removable hairs, of different lengths, color, and texture, generally protrude from the sinus. They have sharp, pointed ends and are consistently thick, stiff, and straight, essentially the male type. This may explain why the condition occurs in men's hairdressers. Women's hair is generally soft and thin, and the ends are more likely to bend rather than penetrate. Rarely is more than one interdigital web space affected. The order of predilection is the third web space followed by the second and fourth. The first web space has been reported to be involved only once.

Treatment
Excision of the lesion and primary wound closure results in a less obvious scar than incision and drainage.

Shearer's Disease
A similar and related condition to barber's interdigital sinus occurs in the interdigital spaces of sheep shearers and is caused by wool. Small tufts of wool may protrude from the sinus. Symptoms are made worse after shearing lambs because newer, finer wool tufts enter the open sinus with ease. It can result in a recurrent subungual pilonidal sinus and can cause chronic osteomyelitis of the subjacent phalanx. The foreign-body hair granuloma is a well-recognized occupational hazard in dog groomers in the United Kingdom as well.

Milker's Interdigital Granuloma
The hairs of cattle, barbed at an angle, can penetrate skin of milker's hands and migrate slowly and deeply under the skin and cause a foreign-body reaction. Milker's interdigital granuloma is a painful, red, granulating, discharging, vegetating lesion found in the hands of milkers. It can vary from pea size to nut size, and the surface may be irregular and riddled with sinuses. The second and third interdigital spaces of the dominant hand are the usual location. Treatment is removal of all hair and control of the inflammatory process. A persistent granuloma should be excised.

Slaughterman's Interdigital Granuloma
Slaughterhouse employees can develop a pilonidal sinus in the interdigital space from hair of the animals they slaughter. The lesion persists with conservative treatment until it is completely excised.

SCABIES

The discovery of the itch mite in 1687 marked scabies as the first disease of humans with a known cause.

Etiology and Epidemiology
Scabies is not an infection but an infestation of the epidermis and dermis by a microscopic eight-legged mite, the *Sarcoptes scabiei*. Each mite is less than half a millimeter long, and under a magnifying glass mites can be seen on skin as black dots. Typically, an affected host is infested by only about 10 to 12 adult mites. After mating, the male dies. The female mite burrows into the epidermis and dermis of the skin where she lives, lays up to 3 eggs each day for her 1- to 2-month lifetime, and dies.

Development from egg to adult scabies mite takes 10 to 21 days. They are highly contagious and can be spread by close, skin-to-skin contact. Institutions (e.g., nursing homes, extended-care facilities, and prisons) are often sites of scabies outbreaks. People who have a decreased immune system sometimes develop a more severe form of scabies known as Norwegian scabies, which refers to a particularly severe form of scabies that is also known as crusted scabies. Crusted scabies is called Norwegian scabies because the condition was first described in Norway in the mid-19th century.

Clinical Findings

Any area of the body can be affected, but the interdigital regions of hands and feet, the groin, and popliteal fossa are the more common sites. Infected individuals usually develop a pimple-like rash and intense itching. If it is the first time a person has had scabies, he or she may not develop symptoms for up to 6 weeks. During this period, those infected are contagious despite not having symptoms. Scabies can spread easily among people who have close physical contact with an infected person; the longer the skin-to-skin contact, the more likely the spread. Crusted (Norwegian) scabies is a more severe, more contagious form of infestation that occurs in people who are debilitated or have a weak immune system.

Diagnosis

Each mite is less than half a millimeter long and this makes them very difficult to spot. To the naked eye, they may look like tiny black dots on the skin. A microscope can identify mites, eggs, or fecal matter from a skin scraping.

Treatment

Treatment is needed to get rid of scabies and prevent it from spreading to others. It will not go away on its own. Treatment consists of killing the mites, symptom control, and decontamination. In the United States, permethrin cream, 5% (Elimite), is used to treat scabies by killing the mites. Treatment should be considered for all those who have had skin-to-skin contact with an infected individual. Vigorous scratching can lead to a bacterial infection requiring treatment with an antibiotic. Although the rash may not be present all over the body, patients are usually instructed to apply the cream to all areas of the body except the face. If infants are being treated, directions may include application of the cream to the scalp and head. A second application of medication may also be needed in some cases. Attention to the area under the fingernails is necessary. If the scabicide medication is used correctly, it usually kills the mites relatively quickly.

A particular danger of scabies is that these lesions often predispose to the development of secondary infections, as with *Staphylococcus* bacteria. Like typical scabies, Norwegian scabies is treated with topical permethrin cream and the oral medication ivermectin (Stromectol). Treatment of crusted scabies can require oral medications along with multiple applications of scabicide cream. After effective treatment, no new rashes will develop. Although the mites are killed, itching can still persist for a few weeks.

Prevention

Home care involves cleaning and removing the mites from areas of the home that the infected person may have come into contact with. This helps prevent reinfection and spreading of the infection to others. Clothes, bedding, and towels need to be washed in hot water to kill mites. The infected person should avoid skin-to-skin contact with others until after treatment. With the correct use of medication and proper home care, scabies can be effectively treated and spread of the condition prevented.

VIRAL INFECTIONS

Chronic viral infections of the hand include AIDS, human orf, milker's nodules, and warts. AIDS is associated with infections and tumors of the hand secondary to suppressed immunity. Orf is self-limiting in immunocompetent subjects but in an immunodeficient patient attains "giant" size and can be misdiagnosed and mistreated as a malignancy. Warts are often seen by hand surgeons and most are managed conservatively. Larger warts, those that do not respond to conservative treatment, and pariungual and subungual warts may need surgical excision. I consider surgery on patients who wish immediate eradication of warts and do not want prolonged conservative treatment.

Acquired Immunodeficiency Syndrome

Etiology and Epidemiology

Although two serotypes of human immunodeficiency virus (HIV) are currently recognized, namely HIV-1 and HIV-2, the term *HIV* is generally used to designate HIV-1, which is the major virus. Less than 100 cases of HIV-2 infections are reported in the United States. AIDS syndrome is defined by the development of serious opportunistic infections, neoplasms, or other life-threatening manifestations that result from progressive HIV-induced immunosuppression. AIDS has affected approximately 60 million people globally. In 2010, approximately 1.1 million over the age of 13 were living with AIDS in the United States alone. To learn more about the etiology and epidemiology and classification and clinical diagnosis, please visit Expert-Consult.com.

Clinical Manifestations of AIDS Infection in the Hands

Ching and coworkers,[21] Gonzalez and coworkers,[42] McAuliffe et al,[79] and Seltzer and associates[104] described hand infections in patients with HIV disease in the late 1990s. Approximately 10% of the patients who presented with hand infections in metropolitan hospital emergency departments had HIV infection. Of the intravenous drug users who presented with hand and upper extremity infections, 80% had HIV infection. Glickel suggests that diagnosis of AIDS should be considered when there is an unusual hand infection.[41] It should be taken into consideration for any patient who needs a repeat drainage or debridement procedure. Fingers of those with AIDS may be red with painless erythema and periungual telangiectasia. Nails may be blue or show clubbing. Ching and colleagues noted that among 14 AIDS patients with hand infections, almost one-third needed multiple debridements and resulted in amputation of a finger or hand.[21]

McAuliffe et al,[79] in a review of 74 HIV-seropositive patients who were treated for upper extremity infections, found that intravenous drug use was the most common risk factor for HIV infection as well as the most common cause of the infection necessitating admission. These 74 patients were admitted a total of 97 times for treatment of 89 different infections and underwent 120 surgical procedures. Twenty-six (29%) infections required more than 1 operation, and 11 (12%) resulted in amputation. Patients with AIDS were significantly more likely to present with spontaneous infection than were those who were HIV seropositive. The infections may be seen early in the course of the disease, and in one-half of the patients, they preceded the diagnosis of AIDS. Gonzalez et al, in a study of 28 patients, found 5 who had necrotizing fasciitis; all needed more than one debridement, and one required forequarter amputation.[42]

Herpes Simplex Virus. Herpes simplex virus type 2 (HSV-2) infection of the hand is clinically diagnosed when characteristic multiple vesicular lesions on an erythematous base are present. It generally resolves within 3 weeks in non-HIV infected patients. Although HSV-2 can recur in nonimmunosuppressed hosts, it recurs more frequently and for prolonged periods in patients with HIV infection. When it lasts longer than 3 weeks, a level of suspicion for immunosuppression or AIDS should be raised. In an occult or overt HIV infection, herpes simplex may present as a chronic granulating hand infection that does not respond to routine antibiotics and may progress to finger necrosis or gangrene. Staining of scrapings from the base of the lesions with Wright, Giemsa (Tzanck preparation), or Papanicolaou stain demonstrates characteristic giant cells or intranuclear inclusions of HSV infection. These cytological techniques are often useful as quick procedures to confirm the diagnosis.

Direct immunofluorescent antibody and indirect immunoperoxidase staining are equally sensitive and specific for the detection of HSV antigen. In the eyes of most virologists, viral cultures remain the gold standard by which other methods of diagnosis of HSV are judged. For treatment of cutaneous HSV infections, acyclovir and its related compounds, famciclovir and valacyclovir, have been the mainstay of therapy. Treatment with intravenous acyclovir is followed by oral acyclovir (200 mg q 4-5 h) to prevent recurrences. Famciclovir and valacyclovir have more convenient dosing schedules (three times daily) compared with acyclovir (five times daily). Necrotic and gangrenous parts of the hand are excised. Acyclovir-resistant strains of HSV are being identified with increasing frequency in HIV-infected individuals.

Isolation of HSV from persisting lesions despite adequate dosages of acyclovir should raise the suspicion of acyclovir resistance. Therapy with the intravenous foscarnet (Foscavir) and topical cidofovir gel (Forvade), trifluorothymidine ointment, and vidarabine speeds healing of acyclovir-resistant herpes. Herpetic infections of the pulp in AIDS patients should not be mistaken for felons or paronychia and should not be violated with incision and drainage. If inappropriately treated with surgery, local secondary bacterial bone lysis or metastatic viral encephalitis can occur.

Bacillary Angiomatosis. Bacillary angiomatosis was first described in 1983 in AIDS patients and is an infectious, cutaneous, vascular, tumor-like disorder found almost exclusively in HIV-positive individuals. The lesion may be a pea-sized nodule with or without plaques when first noticed (Figure 3.34). It may be nonpedunculated or pedunculated, and the lesions can occur anywhere on the body and have solitary (Figure 3.34) or multiple nodules. When punctured by a needle or scalpel, the lesion may bleed profusely. It may resemble a benign pyogenic granuloma or present as an ulcer (Figure 3.35).

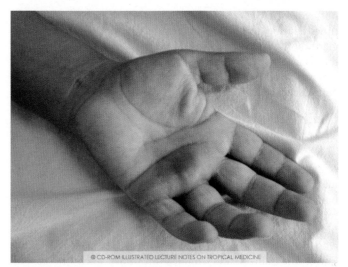

FIGURE 3.34 Early lesions of bacillary angiomatosis in an AIDS patient may be nodular.

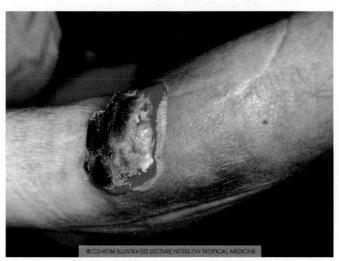

FIGURE 3.35 Bacillary angiomatosis can present as a large ulcer with necrotic areas in an AIDS patient.

Histologically, it is characterized by vascular perforation, hemorrhage, and necrosis of skin. The disease is caused by the bacteria species *Bartonella henselae* and *Bartonella quintana* and is transmitted by cats, ticks, fleas, and lice. The diagnosis of bacillary angiomatosis is best made by fine-needle aspiration biopsy. Warthin-Starry stains show perivascular accumulations of bacilli; these findings may be confirmed by electron microscopy, although this is not usually necessary. The diagnosis can also be established by culture of the organism in several special media or by detection of *Bartonella* DNA by polymerase chain reaction. Serologic assays for anti-*Bartonella* antibodies are available through the special pathogens branch of the CDC.

If left untreated, bacillary angiomatosis follows a progressive and potentially fatal course. Once it is properly identified, treatment consists of prolonged therapy with erythromycin or doxycycline, which prevents recurrence of bacillary angiomatosis. Fluoroquinolones, other macrolides, and trimethoprim-sulfamethoxazole also have activity against *Bartonella*.

Kaposi Sarcoma. Kaposi sarcoma (KS) is a vascular disorder that in the United States is seen predominantly in HIV-infected men. Human herpes virus type 8 is transmitted sexually. It may present as a solitary nodule or multiple nodules or as plaques. Lesions of KS are often difficult to distinguish from those of bacillary angiomatosis; biopsy is required for diagnosis.

KS may occur in the hand[60] and may need punch or open biopsy or excision for histologic confirmation. The skin is the most common first site of presentation. The lesions are generally painless and nonpruritic and appear as firm, slightly raised nodular tumors. In light-skinned individuals, the lesions are typically violaceous in color. In dark-skinned individuals, the lesions appear more brownish or black. More information about Kaposi sarcoma can be found online at ExpertConsult .com.

Treatment. The natural history of AIDS-related KS is variable and difficult to predict. Kaposi sarcoma does not commonly cause death of patients with HIV infection. Despite the relative lack of mortality associated with KS, morbidity associated with a more advanced disease is considerable. KS is staged as (1) cutaneous, locally indolent; (2) cutaneous, locally aggressive with or without regional lymph node enlargement; (3) generalized mucocutaneous with or without regional lymph node enlargement; and (4) visceral. The patient with limited disease and controlled HIV infection does reasonably well. In the setting of uncontrolled HIV viral replication, KS progresses rapidly. It is a systemic disease and mandates a systemic approach with MDT (highly active antiretroviral therapy).

Vascular lesions other than KS occur as serious complications of the hand in HIV infection. Symptoms of Raynaud phenomenon develop in HIV-infected patients when treated with bleomycin and vincristine. Digital gangrene can occur from vasculitis, obliteration of digital arteries, and vascular injury resulting from chemotherapy. HIV-induced thrombocytopenia may cause compartment syndrome of the forearm.

Treatment of AIDS

Currently most patients on their initial antiretroviral regimen take a combination of two nucleoside reverse transcriptase inhibitors with either a protease inhibitor or a nonnucleoside reverse transcriptase inhibitor. Before the availability of these drugs, the median survival after the diagnosis of AIDS was 12 to 18 months. Now antiretroviral treatment leads to a near-normal life expectancy.

Warts

A wart is a cauliflower-like, raised, demarcated, grayish mass with an irregular surface traversed by many projections. It was a century ago that warts were first provoked in the skin of volunteers by injection of appropriately filtered wart tissue, suggesting that it is a viral infection. Half a century ago the causal virus was demonstrated under an electron microscope and was subsequently included under the group of human papillomaviruses (HPVs).

Classification

Two types of cutaneous warts are widespread in hands. Common verrucated warts, *Verruca vulgaris* (*L. verruca*, "a little hill"), represent 95% of cutaneous hand warts. The second most common warts are flat or plane (verruca plana) (5%). Both types are seen predominantly in children but also affect adolescents and young adults. Adults at high risk for the development of warts are veterinary surgeons, butchers, meat packers, fowl handlers, poultry processors, and fish handlers—all occupations in which hands are frequently exposed to moisture.

Pathogenesis of Human Papillomavirus

The incubation period of HPV disease is 1 to 3 months. The virus infects only the epidermis. Warts have a characteristic histologic appearance, showing acanthosis, papillomatosis, hyperkeratosis, and parakeratosis.

Diagnosis

Common Verrucated Wart. The clinical appearance of a common verrucated wart is quite characteristic and usually consists of a single lesion on the hand, fingers, or around the nail. It is a cauliflower-like, raised, demarcated, and grayish mass, with an irregular surface traversed by many projections (Figure 3.36, *A*). It is often painless, and the adjacent skin is healthy. Warts in the palm may be painful because of pressure during grip. If untreated, the common wart can multiply and infect the surrounding skin or the opposite hand. When multiple, there may be several dozen "seed lesions" surrounding a larger and older "mother wart." A cluster of closely spaced papules can coalesce into a large "mosaic wart." "Kissing warts" are seen in areas of skin contact (web spaces) and may represent direct inoculation. Filiform warts are slender, finger-like papules. Periungual warts can extend into the nail bed under the nail plate (subungual warts) and can persist for many years in spite of conservative treatment.

Flat (Plane) Warts. Flat (plane) warts are minimally elevated papules that are 2 to 5 mm in diameter. They appear as multiple lesions with a smooth surface. They have an enhanced likelihood of spontaneous involution. Flat warts in adults are more common in women.

Multiple Warts. Common warts rarely if ever transform into squamous cell carcinoma. Immunosuppressed patients with an inherited defect, such as epidermodysplasia verruciformis, acquired defects in immunity (renal transplant recipients), lymphoproliferative disorders, or those on chemotherapeutic drugs may develop multiple warts. These warts can transform into squamous cell carcinoma. Biopsy is indicated when the diagnosis is doubtful.

Treatment

No antiviral chemotherapy is available for HPV warts. They are a cosmetic nuisance in most cases and often disappear spontaneously; this seems to occur in 50% of children within a year and 90% within 5 years. Fluctuations in immunity to human papillomavirus may be responsible for spontaneous regression or resurgence of preexisting warts. If left untreated, however, some may persist for many years and become larger. A periungual wart can lead to bone destruction of distal phalanx. Rarely does a wart transform into a carcinoma.

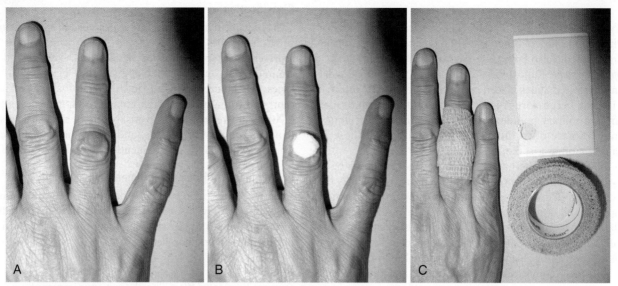

FIGURE 3.36 A, Typical wart in the hand of a woman who frequently immerses her hands in water. **B,** A piece of medicated adhesive tape (Mediplast) slightly larger than the diameter of the wart is applied over the lesion. **C,** The tape is secured in place with waterproof tape (Coban).

Conservative treatment remains the hallmark for management of common warts. When they do not respond to conservative treatment or are too large and cosmetically unacceptable, surgical excision is a good option that cures the problem. Multiplicity of treatments for warts attests to the lack of any single satisfactory therapy method. Cooperation and preference of the patient or parent and experience of the physician determine the appropriate treatment modality.

Most therapeutic modalities consist of chemical or physical destruction of warts. Surgical excision of large isolated lesions can be successful. In contrast, warts in immunosuppressed adults are likely to be progressive, recalcitrant, recurrent, and unresponsive to all but the most aggressive therapy and are more likely to become malignant. Infectious disease and dermatology specialists should be consulted for treatment recommendations. Patients with verrucated warts usually seek treatment for cosmetic reasons. Patients with flat warts usually do not seek treatment.

Keratolytic Therapy. Keratolytic therapy is simple, inexpensive, painless, and preferred because it is as effective as cryotherapy, with a success rate of approximately 70% and a minimal recurrence rate of 4%. Treatment is just as successful as more invasive methods. Less aggressive therapy for common warts in childhood is preferred because of the increased likelihood of spontaneous resolution[77] and lack of tolerance to painful ablative treatments. Salicylic acid is the most commonly used ingredient in the chemical destruction of the lesion and the virus it harbors. Local applications of keratolytic agents result in chemical debridement of the infected epidermal cells. The most used method is a self-applied paint of salicylic acid with lactic acid in collodion (1:1:4). A drop of the solution (e.g., Duofilm, Occlusal, Paplex) is placed over the wart and left in place for a few minutes. The area is then soaked in warm water, and white sloughing keratin is mechanically debrided gently with a cloth. This is repeated daily; it takes a few days to a few weeks to "melt" a wart.

A cure rate of 70% within 12 weeks was reported in a randomized trial by Bunney,[17] and the treatment was as effective as cryotherapy. Compliance is a major limitation. A high-potency 26% salicylic acid can reduce the treatment period to 2 weeks. Forty percent salicylic acid is available as a thin layer applied on a tape (Mediplast) and is an excellent alternative in my experience. A small piece of the tape, which is a little larger than the wart, is cut, then the protective plastic that covers the salicylic acid on the tape is peeled off. The tape firmly adheres to the wart (Figure 3.36, *B*) and is left in place for a day or two. On a finger, it may be reinforced with waterproof 3M tape (Figure 3.36, *C*). When taking a shower, it is removed, sloughed epidermis is scrubbed off, and a new tape is applied over dry skin. Slow tissue necrosis removes the infected epidermis over a few days to few weeks. Irritation of normal skin surrounding the wart rarely occurs. This treatment is painless, convenient, and safe. Patient compliance is good, and self-treatment is inexpensive.

Periungual warts are difficult to treat when they extend under the nail plate and are inaccessible to salicylic acid treatment. Application of plain adhesive tape to the entire finger distal to the proximal interphalangeal joint is another option. The patient is instructed to remove the tape in 6.5 days, scrub off the necrotic skin, and reapply the tape after 12 h. The process is repeated for 6 to 9 weeks. Additional fingers with warts can be taped similarly.

Cryotherapy. Liquid nitrogen or carbon dioxide without local anesthesia has been used for the management of warts. Burning pain associated with cryotherapy is well tolerated by adults but not children. Children's adverse reactions have included premature closure of the distal phalangeal physis, angular deviation of the distal interphalangeal joint, and destruction of the proximal interphalangeal joint.

Intralesional Injection of Bleomycin. Intralesional injection of bleomycin (0.1-0.2 mL of 1 unit/mL) has been used in the treatment of recalcitrant warts and found to be successful in 88% of patients.[3] The Raynaud phenomenon is reported in digits injected with bleomycin.

Electrosurgery. Electrosurgery includes electrocautery, electrocoagulation, electrodesiccation, and laser ablation. Ablation of the wart can be done with a diathermy knife under local anesthesia or under general anesthesia for multiple lesions. There is risk of recurrence of warts in and around the site of treatment. Concerns about laser therapy include risk to the operator and paramedics from the dispersion of virus in the plume of vapor generated by the laser.

Surgical Excision. A wart can be curetted out with a small curette. No controlled studies have been published, but gratifying results have been reported. To prevent recurrence, it is safe to apply a tape with a keratolytic agent (e.g., Mediplast) to debride the curetted margins of the wart. Simple surgical excision has not been prospectively studied. I have had success with it and have not encountered recurrences after removal of more than 30 warts in 5 years. It is important to excise the wart through a wide margin, generally at least 1 mm, to prevent recurrence. If the excision is incomplete, recurrence in the suture tracts can occur. Periungual warts creeping under the nail plate infect the nail bed (subungual warts); they respond poorly to keratolytic therapy, cryotherapy, and electrosurgery due to inaccessibility and often require removal of nail plate and surgical excision.

Prognosis. Prognosis in general depends in part on the age and immunity of the patient, as well as on the type, location, number, and chronicity of warts. Warts in children respond to treatment more readily than in adults. Immunodeficiency inhibits the response to treatment. Mosaic and plane warts are more resistant to treatment. Single warts disappear more rapidly than multiple warts, and chronic warts tend to be more recalcitrant to treatment. Warts should not be considered cured until at least a 6-month period has elapsed.

❖ AUTHOR'S PREFERRED METHOD OF TREATMENT

I use 40% acetylsalicylic acid keratolytic therapy with Mediplast as my first choice of treatment. It is acceptable to patients, is simple to execute, and is effective for a large percentage of patients. When a patient does not want to undertake prolonged treatment and the wart is large, I surgically excise it with a 1- to 2-mm margin. In cases of periungual and subungual warts, I remove the nail plate and excise the superficial surface of the infected nail bed.

Human Orf (Farm Yard Pox, Milker's Nodule, Ecthyma Contagiosum, Contagious Pustular Dermatitis)

Human orf infection is important to a hand surgeon because it causes a large tumor-like lesion in immunodeficient hosts that resolves with simple topical cidofovir application. Misdiagnosis has led to unnecessary excisions, multiple excisions, and even amputation.[102] Four cases of human orf were reported in the United States between 2009 and 2011 from household exposure to lamb and goat slaughter.

The word "orf" is an old Anglo-Saxon name for cattle, and the disease is endemic in sheep and goats. Orf is caused by a large paravaccinia DNA virus that belongs in the subgroup of pox viruses. It is common in humans who have direct contact with infected sheep and goats or with products or objects that come in contact with sheep and goats. The virus can persist for long periods on such objects as fences, barn doors, and feeding troughs from which the disease is indirectly transmitted to a susceptible host. In one year, 1.4% of 16,484 sheep and goat handlers in New Zealand were infected.[99] The risk was highest (4%) with mutton slaughterers. It occurs on the exposed parts of the body, especially the hands. Human orf is an occupational disease in "risk populations" such as shepherds, sheep shearers, butchers, and veterinary surgeons.

There is a yearly outbreak of orf infection of the hand in Saudi Arabia. Two million people visit there for "Hajj" every year, and hundreds of thousands of sheep are slaughtered by nongloved hands at the end of the ceremony. Inoculation occurs in preexisting or incidental new injuries of the hand from the infected animals. Outbreaks in Turkey and Belgium occur 2 to 3 weeks after the Islamic "Feast of Sacrifice" (Aid el-Kebir or Eid el-Adha) in men who bleed the sheep and in women who handle their skin and meat. The epidemic is predictable 9 weeks after the end of Ramadan every year and 75% of patients are Islamic.

Clinical Findings

Ninety-five percent of the lesions are on the finger (Figure 3.37, A,B), hand, wrist, or forearm—the area of contact with infected animals. The lesion is usually unilateral, rarely bilateral. The lesions may be single (Figure 3.37, A) or multiple (Figure 3.37, B). It may occur as paronychia and is distinguished from bacterial paronychia by the presence of a nodule with central red discoloration, a middle bluish-white ring, and peripheral erythematous or violaceous halo (Figure 3.37, A). There is a history of exposure to sheep or goats, a goat/sheep bite, or handling of goat/sheep for "sacrifice." After an incubation period of 3 to 7 days, the infected skin lesion erupts clinically. In humans, orf is commonly known as ecthyma contagiosum or contagious purulent dermatitis (CPD), but this is in part a misnomer because pustules are not purulent (ecthyma = purulent pustules) in human orf.

Leavell described the lesion in six clinical stages in a study of 19 cases of human orf.[70] Each stage lasts approximately a week, and the disease resolves without treatment in approximately 6 weeks (range, 14-72 days). The first stage is characterized by an erythematous macule or papule. In the second (target stage) the lesion turns into a nodule. The lesion may be bullous at this stage (Figure 3.37, B). The third, or the weeping, stage is characterized by a weeping surface on a nodule. The fourth stage consists of a thin yellow crust with underlying black dots over the nodule. The fifth (papillomatous stage) consists of small surface papillomas and finger-like projections of the epidermis. The sixth and final stage is characterized by reduction in the size of the lesion and formation of a thick crust that looks like an ulcer before final healing. Lesions do not always correspond to these stages and may present as an erythematous nodule, a tense bullous lesion, a giant lesion, or a felon. In a felon there is an absence of local pain and drops of clear fluid may exude from the lesion.

Diagnosis

The diagnosis is based on clinical features and contact with goats or sheep. Orf may be confirmed by electron microscopy

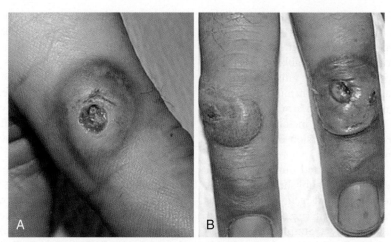

FIGURE 3.37 Orf can infect one or two fingers simultaneously. **A,** The lesion has an umbilicated red center, a white middle, and a peripheral violaceous halo. **B,** The lesion may be bulbous and affect multiple fingers. (**A,** From Karabay O, Goksugur N: Red-blue, umbilicated nodules on the fingers. *Am Fam Physician* 76:119–120, 2007, with permission. **B,** From http://quizlet.com/8107530/viruses-flash-cards/.)

of negatively stained suspensions from lesions, which is the most rapid laboratory method available. Provisional diagnosis can be made in an hour compared with several weeks when tissue culture techniques are used. The virus survives without preservatives in crusts, vesicular fluid, or biopsy of suspected lesions for as long as 30 days and can be safely saved and mailed to a distant electron microscopic facility for identification. A scab from the surface of the lesion is usually sufficient to establish the diagnosis because these contain large amounts of orf virus and characteristic large multiple oval viral particles can be seen within the keratinocytes under an electron microscope. In most cases, however, the clinical appearance of the lesion on a finger, hand, wrist, or forearm and a history of contact with sheep or goats are sufficient to make a diagnosis of human orf.

In an immunocompromised patient, the lesion may attain a large size. Immunosuppressed patients with chronic lymphatic leukemia, patients on immunosuppressive medication for a lymphoma, and renal and heart-lung transplant patients have been reported with "giant" orf lesions on their fingers or palms. The lesion may recur several times after thorough excision, and skin grafting may be necessary. It may assume giant proportions in atopic dermatitis. Giant orf in a normal individual is rare, and immunologic workup is in order when one is encountered. A giant orf on dorsum of proximal interphalangeal can weaken the extensor mechanism and cause swan neck deformity. It has been erroneously stated that infection with the orf virus confers lifelong immunity. Many cases of reinfection in immunocompetent patients have been reported. Person-to-person transmission is rare.

Differential Diagnosis

Orf and milker's nodule are essentially identical on clinical, histologic, and virologic examination. Orf is diagnosed if the patient has been in contact with sheep or goats, whereas milker's nodule is suspected if the patient has been manually milking cows or buffaloes. Frequently the patient can remember seeing

a scabby mouth lesion on a sheep or a crusting pseudocowpox lesion on an udder. In the absence of such history, diagnosis of "farmyard pox" or "parapox infection" affords the clinician a diagnosis based on common clinical and electron microscopic findings. Arnaud et al have wisely warned that orf infection of pulp that is superinfected must be differentiated from a felon. Presence of drops of clear liquid from the lesion and absence of local pain contribute to a correct diagnosis of orf.

Treatment

An orf lesion is self-limiting in 6 weeks and does not require antiviral treatment in immunocompetent patients. If an orf nodule does not undergo spontaneous healing in 6 weeks, the nodule continues to rapidly evolve into an ulcer or a pyogenic granuloma-like lesion, assumes tumoral proportion, or recurs after multiple and radical excisions and skin grafts, immunocompromise should be suspected and investigated. If the patient is immunosuppressed due to organ transplantation (kidney or heart–lung) or has hematogenous malignancy (e.g., lymphoma, lymphocytic leukemia), treatment should include local antiviral therapy (e.g., cidofovir cream, imiquimod cream, idoxuridine 40% cream) and a reduction in immunosuppression or cytotoxic chemotherapy to control the infection.[119] Otherwise, the lesion may grow and become more resistant to treatment.

Multiple surgical excisions and even an amputation[102] have been described when (1) correct diagnosis is not made, (2) correct antiviral treatment is not initiated, and/or (3) immunosuppression has not been reduced in an immunocompromised patient. With correct diagnosis and treatment, the nodular lesion in an immunocompetent patient or even the giant lesion in an immunodeficient patient resolves in 6 weeks without further recurrence.

Milker's Nodule (Paravaccinia Virus, Pseudocowpox)

Paravaccinia virus that infects sheep and goats also infects cows. In humans, nodules on the hand caused by this virus are called milker's nodules because milkers acquire hand infections from the cow's infected udder through direct contact or indirectly through contaminated objects. Milker's nodule is usually regarded as an occupational disease of dairy farm workers.

The initial lesion is on the exposed part of the hand and upper extremity in more than 50% of cases. The incidence of milker's nodule has fallen since the majority of cows are now milked by machine. It has been reported in a healthy young cattle veterinarian. The bovine virus is morphologically indistinguishable from the ovine orf virus. When the animal source is unknown, it is not possible to clinically differentiate between ovine (sheep and goat) and bovine (cow) nodular lesions on the exposed hand and upper extremity and under the electron microscope. Diagnosis of the disease is based for the most part on knowledge of the animal source. Rarely, the lesion of pseudocowpox presents as a black necrotic ulcer clinically indistinguishable from anthrax. Large eosinophilic intracytoplasmic inclusions within epidermal cells and DNA sequencing to match paravaccinia can quickly distinguish the two when anthrax has to be ruled out promptly.

Treatment

Milker's nodule is easily recognized by those working with cows. The understanding that the disease spontaneously resolves in 6 weeks inclines many workers not to seek medical attention. When a physician who is unaware of such a lesion encounters one, misdiagnosis and unnecessary treatment may occur.

CONCLUSION

In the coming years, physicians will continue to see four types of chronic infections of the hand.

- There will be infections of known organisms that have not yet caused chronic infections of the hand. As an example, atypical mycobacterial hand infections were not recognized until the 1960s. These are, however, easy to diagnose as long as biopsy, staining, serology, cultures, and sequencing methods are routinely used for diagnosis.
- More elusive infections may be those that arise from organisms that have not been previously suspected. Herpes virus was not recognized as a cause of Kaposi sarcoma until 1986 because detection and quantitation of specific DNA and RNA base sequences in clinical specimens had not yet became available.
- Physicians will see chronic infections that are caused by newly recognized organisms. Fungal infections are on the rise and recently identified fungal infections are reported more frequently. Many of these fungal infections respond inadequately to currently available antifungal antibiotics.
- Finally, chronic infections will continue to increase as worldwide travel and immigration brings older and exotic organisms into the United States.[37] Cases of leishmaniasis trickle into Texas from Mexico and into all parts of the United States from those who vacation in Costa Rica.

Awareness of the characteristics of chronic hand infections, and vigilant use of biopsy and culture techniques, should be able to reveal and control such infections in the upper extremity.

For Case Studies, Videos, and more, please visit ExpertConsult.com.

REFERENCES

1. Al-Qattan MM: Opportunistic mycotic infections of the upper limb. A review. *J Hand Surg* 21B:148, 1996.
2. Al-Qattan MM, al Mazrou AM: Mucormycosis of the upper limb. *J Hand Surg [Br]* 21:261, 1996.
3. Al-Qattan MM, Bowen V, Manktelow RT: Tuberculosis of the hand. *J Hand Surg [Br]* 19:234, 1994.
4. Allegue F, de Lis MP, Perez-Alvarez R: Primary cutaneous cryptococcosis presenting as a whitlow. *Acta Derm Venereol* 87:443, 2007.
5. Alloway JA, Evangelisti SM, Sartin JS: *Mycobacterium marinum* arthritis. *Semin Arthritis Rheum* 24:382, 1995.
6. Altman DT, Lubahn JD, Kuhn PJ: A case report and review of mycetoma of the hand: a diagnostic and therapeutic challenge. *J Hand Surg* 19A:998, 1994.
7. Antia NH, Enna CD, Daver BM: *The surgical management of deformities in leprosy*, Bombay, 1992, Oxford University Press.
8. Antia NH, Shetty VP: *The peripheral nerve in leprosy and other neuropathies*, New Delhi, 1997, Oxford University Press.
9. Becton J, Neibauer J: Nocardia infection of the hand. *J Bone Joint Surg* 52A:1443, 1970.
10. Bednar MS, Lane LB: Eponychial marsupialization and nail removal for surgical treatment of chronic paronychia. *J Hand Surg* 16A:314, 1991.
11. Benkeddache Y, Gettesman H: Skeletal tuberculosis of the wrist and hand: a study of 27 cases. *J Hand Surg* 7:593, 1982.
12. Bennett ML, Jackson JM, Jorizzo JL, et al: Pyoderma gangrenosum. A comparison of typical and atypical forms with an emphasis on time to remission. Case review of 86 patients from 2 institutions. *Medicine (Baltimore)* 79:37, 2000.
13. Brand PW, Fritschi E: Rehabilitation in leprosy. In Hastings R, editor: *Leprosy*, New York, 1985, Churchill Livingstone.
14. Brashear HR, Winfield HG: Tuberculosis of the wrist: a report of ten cases. *South Med J* 68:1345, 1975.
15. Breathnach A, Levell N, Munro C, et al: Cutaneous *Mycobacterium kansasii* infection: case report and review. *Clin Infect Dis* 20:812, 1995.
16. Bryceson A, Pfaltzgraff RE: *Leprosy*, New York, 1990, Churchill Livingstone.
17. Bunney MH, Benton C, Cubie HA: *Viral warts. Biology and treatment*, Oxford, 1992, Oxford University Press.
18. Charters AD, Staer PA: Cutaneous leishmaniasis of long incubation period in an Italian immigrant in Western Australia. *Med J Aust* 2:278, 1970.
19. Charters AD, Staer PA: Cutaenous leishmaniasis of long incubation period in an Italian immigrant in Western Australia. *Med J Aust* 2:278, 1970.
20. Cheung JP, Fung B, Ip WY, et al: *Mycobacterium marinum* infection of the hand and wrist. *J Orthop Surg (Hong Kong)* 20:214, 2012.
21. Ching V, Ritz M, Song C, et al: Human immunodeficiency virus infection in an emergency hand service. *J Hand Surg* 21A:696, 1996.
22. Chow SP, Ip FK, Lau JH, et al: *Mycobacterium marinum* infection of the hand and wrist. Results of conservative treatment in twenty-four cases. *J Bone Joint Surg* 69:1161, 1987.
23. Coban YK, Balik O, Boran C: Cutaneous anthrax of the hand and its reconstruction with a reverse-flow radial forearm flap. *Ann Plast Surg* 49:109, 2002.
24. Collins RJ, Chow SP, Ip FK, et al: Synovial involvement by *Mycobacterium marinum*. A histopathological study of 25 culture-proven cases. *Pathology* 20:340, 1988.
25. Colville A, Ispahani P: Non-tuberculous mycobacterial tenosynovitis. *Lancet* 2:1161, 1989.
26. Coombes GM, Teh LS, Denton J, et al: *Mycobacterium xenopi*—an unusual presentation as tenosynovitis of the wrist in an immunocompetent patient. *Br J Rheumatol* 35:1008, 1996.
27. da Rosa AC, Scroferneker ML, Vettorato R, et al: Epidemiology of sporotrichosis: a study of 304 cases in Brazil. *J Am Acad Dermatol* 52:451, 2005.
28. Daengsvang S, Sangsingkeo P, Ayudhya BSN: A case of gnathostomiasis of a finger. *Southeast Asian J Trop Med Pub Health* 4:260, 1973.
29. Danzig LA, Fierer J: Coccidioidomycosis of the extensor tenosynovium of the wrist. *Clin Orthop* 129:245, 1977.
30. Dehaven KE, Wilde AH, O'Duffy JD: Sporotrichosis arthritis and tenosynovitis: report of a case cured by synovectomy and amphotericin B. *J Bone Joint Surg* 54-A:874, 1972.
31. Dix-Peek SI, Vrettos BC, Hoffman EB: Tuberculosis of the elbow in children. *J Shoulder Elbow Surg* 12:282, 2003.
32. Dupuytren G: The Classic: On osteo-sarcoma, spina-ventosa, and tubercles in bone. Injuries and Diseases of Bones; 1847: 416-433. *Clin Orthop Relat Res* 450:17, 2006.

33. Duran RJ, Coventry MB, Weed LA: Sporotrichosis: a report of 23 cases in the upper extremity. *J Bone Joint Surg* 39A:1330, 1957.
34. Edwards MS, Huber TW, Baker CJ: Mycobacterium terrae synovitis and osteomyelitis. *Am Rev Respir Dis* 117:161, 1978.
35. Engelkens HJ, Ginai AZ, Jadanarso J, et al: Case report 274. *Skeletal Radiol* 21:194, 1992.
36. Engelkens HJ, Ginai AZ, Judanarso J, et al: Radiological and dermatological findings in two patients suffering from early yaws in Indonesia. *Genitourin Med* 66:259, 1990.
37. Engelkens HJ, Orange AP, Stolz E: Early yaws imported in the Netherlands. *Genitourin Med* 65:316, 1989.
38. Gabl M, Pechlaner S, Hausdorfer H: Tenosynovitis in the hand caused by *Mycobacterium malmoense*: a case report. *J Hand Surg* 22:338, 1997.
39. Galaria NA, Jenkins-Hopkins JM, Kligman D, et al: Neutrophilic dermatosis of the dorsal hands: pustular vasculitis revisited. *J Am Acad Dermatol* 43:870, 2000.
40. Gelman MI: Blastomycotic dactylitis. *Radiology* 107:331, 1973.
41. Glickel SZ: Hand infections in patients with acquired immunodeficiency syndrome. *J Hand Surg* 13:770, 1988.
42. Gonzalez MH, Nikoleit J, Weinzweig N, et al: Upper extremity infections in patients with the human immunodeficiency virus. *J Hand Surg [Am]* 23:348, 1998.
43. Graham WR, Callaway JL: Primary inoculation blastomycosis in a veterinarian. *Am Acad Dermatol* 7:785, 1982.
44. Green WO, Adams TE: Mycetoma in the United States. *Am J Clin Pathol* 42:75, 1964.
45. Grossman ME, Fithian EC, Behrens C, et al: Primary cutaneous aspergillosis in in six leukemic children. *J Am Acad Dermatol* 12:313, 1985.
46. Haider N, Khan AQ, Zulfiqur M: Tubercular dactylitis and multifocal osteoarticular tuberculosis—two rare cases of extrapulmonary tuberculosis. *BMJ Case Reports* 10:1, 2011.
47. Hankins CL: Blastomycotic hand infections. *Scand J Plast Reconstr Surg Hand Surg* 43:166, 2009.
48. Haruna K, Shiraki Y, Hiruma M, et al: A case of lymphangitic sporotrichosis occurring on both forearms with a published work review of cases of bilateral sporotrichosis in Japan. *J Dermatol* 33:364, 2006.
49. Hassan FO: Tuberculous dactylitis pseudotumor of an adult thumb: a case report. *Strategies Trauma Limb Reconstr* 5:53, 2010.
50. Hastings RC: *Leprosy*, New York, 1994, Churchill Livingstone.
51. Hauser AR: Antibiotic basics for clinicians. Philadelphia, Wolters Kluwer, 2013.
52. Hellinger WC, Smilack JD, Greider JL, Jr, et al: Localized soft-tissue infections with *Mycobacterium avium / Mycobacterium intracellulare* complex in immunocompetent patients: granulomatous tenosynovitis of the hand or wrist. *Clin Infect Dis* 21:65, 1995.
53. Huang JI, Seeger LL, Jones NF: Coccidioidomycosis fungal infection in the hand mimicking a metacarpal enchondroma. *J Hand Surg* 25B:475, 2000.
54. Huang JI, Seeger LL, Jones NF: Coccidioidomycosis fungal infection in the hand mimicking a metacarpal enchondroma. *J Hand Surg [Br]* 25:475, 2000.
55. Huish SB, de la Paz EM, Ellis PR, III, et al: Pyoderma gangrenosum of the hand: a case series and review of the literature. *J Hand Surg* 26A:679, 2001.
56. Hurst LC, Amadio PC, Badalamente MA, et al: *Mycobacterium marinum* infections of the hand. *J Hand Surg* 12:428, 1987.
57. *Iowa State University, The Center for Food Security and Public Health*. <www.cfsph.iastate.edu/Factsheets/pdfs/anthrax.pdf>, March 2007.
58. Jensen CM, Jensen CH, Paerregaard A: A diagnostic problem in tuberculosis dactylitis. *J Hand Surg* 16B(2):202, 1991.
59. Jopling WH, McDougall AC: *Handbook of leprosy*, New Delhi, 1996, CBS Publishers.
60. Keith JE, Jr, Wilgis EF: Kaposi's sarcoma in the hand of an AIDS patient. *J Hand Surg* 11A:410, 1986.
61. Kelly PJ, Weed LA, Lipscomb PR: Infection of tendon sheaths, bursae, joints and soft tissues by acid-fast bacilli other than tubercle bacilli. *J Bone Joint Surg* 45A:327, 1963.
62. Khan K, Bandyopadhyay A: A rare case of chondromyxoid fibroma mimicking spina ventosa. *J Surg Tech Case Rep* 4:43, 2012.
63. Kiely JL, O'Riordan DM, Sheehan S, et al: Tenosynovitis due to mycobacteria other than tuberculosis: a hazard of water sports and hobbies. *Respir Med* 89:69, 1995.
64. Kim JE, Sung H, Kim MN, et al: Synchronous infection with *Mycobacterium chelonae* and Paecilomyces in a heart transplant patient. *Transpl Infect Dis* 13:80, 2011.
65. Koss SD, Reardon TF, Groves RJ: Recurrent carpal tunnel syndrome due to tuberculoid leprosy in an Asian immigrant. *J Hand Surg* 18:740, 1993.
66. Kotwal PP, Khan SA: Tuberculosis of the hand: clinical presentation and functional outcome in 32 patients. *J Bone Joint Surg Br* 91:1054, 2009.
67. Kozin S, Bishop A: Atypical Mycobacterium infections of the upper extremity. *J Hand Surg* 19A:480, 1994.
68. Langan SM, Powell FC: Vegetative pyoderma gangrenosum: a report of two new cases and a review of the literature. *Int J Dermatol* 44:623, 2005.
69. Lau JHK: Hand infection with *Mycobacterium chelonei*. *Br Med J* 292:444, 1986.
70. Leavell UW, McNamara MJ, Muelling R: Orf. Report of 19 human cases with clinical and pathological observations. *JAMA* 203:657, 1968.
71. Love GL, Melchior E: *Mycobacterium terrae* tenosynovitis. *J Hand Surg* 10:730, 1985.
72. Luque AE, Kaminski D, Reichman R, et al: *Mycobacterium szulgai* osteomyelitis in an AIDS patient. *Scand J Infect Dis* 30:88, 1998.
73. Malaviya GN: Towards restoring sensibility in anesthetic extremities of leprosy patients. *Acta Leprol* 9:111, 1995.
74. Malaviya GN: Rehabilitation of insensitive hands. *Indian J Lepr* 74:151, 2002.
75. Malaviya GN, Mishra B, Girdhar BK, et al: Calcification of nerves in leprosy—report of three cases. *Indian J Lepr* 57:651, 1985.
76. Malaviya GN, Mukherjee A, Ramu G: Nerve abscess in lepromatous leprosy. *Lepr India* 54:123, 1982.
77. Massing AM, Epstein WL: Natural history of warts. A two year study. *Arch Dermatol* 87:306, 1963.
78. Matsuda T, Matsumoto T: Protothecosis: a report of two cases in Japan and a review of the literature. *Eur J Epidemiol* 8:397, 1992.
79. McAuliffe JA, Seltzer DG, Hornicek FJ: Upper-extremity infections in patients seropositive for human immunodeficiency virus. *J Hand Surg [Am]* 22:1084, 1997.
80. Mert A, Bilir M, Bahar H, et al: Primary actinomycosis of the hand: a case report and literature review. *Int J Infect Dis* 5:112, 2001.
81. Miyata T, Yashiro M, Hayashi M, et al: Bullous pyoderma gangrenosum of the bilateral dorsal hands. *J Dermatol* 39:1006, 2012.
82. Moore M: Mycetoma of hand and arm caused by *Madurella*; report of a case with a review of the literature. *Am J Trop Med* 3:303, 1954.
83. Moran SL, Strickland J, Shin AY: Upper-extremity mucormycosis infections in immunocompetent patients. *J Hand Surg [Am]* 31:1201, 2006.
84. Mousa AR, Muhtaseb SA, Almudallal DS, et al: Osteoarticular complications of brucellosis: a study of 169 cases. *Review Infect Dis* 9:531, 1987.
85. Olivieri I, Scarano E, Padula A, et al: *Dactylitis*, a term for different digit diseases. *Scand J Rheumatol* 35:333, 2006.
86. Ooi WW, Moschella SL: Update on leprosy in immigrants in the United States: status in the year 2000. *Clin Infect Dis* 32:930, 2001.
87. Ozkan T, Ozer K, Gulgonen A: Restoration of sensibility in irreparable ulnar and median nerve lesions with use of sensory nerve transfer: long-term follow-up of 20 cases. *J Hand Surg [Am]* 26:44, 2001.
88. Pan KL, Ibrahim S: Tuberculosis of the distal end of the radius mimiking a giant-cell tumor. *Med J Malaysia* 55:105, 2000.
89. Patel MR, Bassini L, Nashad R, et al: Barber's interdigital pilonidal sinus of the hand: a foreign body hair granuloma. *J Hand Surg* 15A:652, 1990.
90. Prabhu RM, Patel R: Mucormycosis and entomophthoramycosis: a review of clinical manifestations, diagnosis and treatment. *Clin Microbiol Infect* 10:31, 2004.
91. Prakash V, Husain S, Malaviya GN: Adiposubcutaneous flap for reconstruction of first web space depression in ulnar paralysis in leprosy patients. *Plast Reconstr Surg* 102:2519, 1998.
92. Raffi F, Moinard D, Drugeon HB: Non-tuberculous mycobacterial tenosynovitis. *Lancet* 335:613, 1990.
93. Raizman NM, Parisien M, Grafe MW, et al: Mucormycosis of the upper extremity in a patient with alcoholic encephalopathy. *J Hand Surg [Am]* 32:384, 2007.
94. Ramesh Chandra VV, Prasad BC, Varaprasad G: Ulnar nerve tuberculoma. *J Neurosurg Pediatrics* 11:751, 2013.
95. Randall G, Smith PW, Korbitz B: Carpal tunnel syndrome caused Mycobacterium fortuitum and Histoplasma capulatum. *J Neurosurg* 56:299, 1982.
96. Raturi U, Burkhalter W: Gnathostomiasis externa: a case report. *J Hand Surg* 11A:751, 1986.
97. Rhangos WC, Chick EW: Mycotic infections of bone. *South Med J* 57:664, 1964.
98. Ritz N, Connell TG, Tebruegge M, et al: Tuberculous dactylitis—an easily missed diagnosis. *Eur J Clin Microbiol Infect Dis* 30:1303, 2011.
99. Robinson AJ, Peterson GV: Orf virus infection of workers in the meat industry. *N Z Med J* 96:81, 1983.
100. Rushforth GF, Susannah JE: Actinomycosis of the hand. *Hand* 14:194, 1982.
101. Salisbury RE, Silverstein P, Goodwin MN, Jr: Upper extremity fungal invasions secondary to large burns. *Plast Reconstr Surg* 54:654, 1974.
102. Savage J, Black MM: "Giant" orf of finger in a patient with a lymphoma. *Proc R Soc Med* 65:766, 1972.
103. Sehgal VN: Cutaneous tuberculosis. Current concepts. *Int J Dermatol* 29:237, 1990.
104. Seltzer DG, McAuliffe J, Campbell DR: AIDS in the hand patient: the team approach. *Hand Clin* 7:433, 1991.
105. Singh S, Gupta R, Jain S, et al: Tubercular dactylitis: Fine needle aspiration cytology as a diagnostic modality. *Acta Cytol* 50:669, 2006.
106. Sirikulchayanonta V, Visuthikosol V, Tanphaichitra D, et al: Protothecosis following hand injury. *J Hand Surg* 14B:88, 1989.

107. Skoll PJ, Hudson DA: Tuberculosis of the upper extremity. *Ann Plast Surg* 43:374, 1999.

108. Spellberg B, Ibrahim A: Mucormycosis. In Kasper DL, Fauci AS, editors: *Harrison's infectious diseases*, New York, 2013, McGraw-Hill Education.

109. Sreekanth R, Pallapati SCR, Thomas BP: Tuberculous *Botryomycosis* of the hand: case report. *J Hand Surgery* 39(9):1810–1812, 2014.

110. Srinivasan H, Palande DD: *Essential surgery in leprosy. Techniques for district hospitals*, Geneva, 1997, World Health Organization.

111. Stevanovic MV, Mirzayan R, Holtom PD, et al: Mucormycosis osteomyelitis in the hand. *Orthopedics* 22:449, 1999.

112. Stratton CW, Phelps DB, Reller LB: Tuberculoid tenosynovitis and carpal tunnel syndrome caused by *Mycobacterium szulgai*. *Am J Med* 65:349, 1978.

113. Su WP, Davis MD, Weening RH: Pyoderma gangrenosum: clinicopathologic correlation and proposed diagnostic criteria. *Int J Dermatol* 43:790, 2004.

114. Tan ST, Blake GB, Chambers S: Recurrent orf in an immunocompromised host. *Br J Plast Surg* 44:465, 1991.

115. Tsai MS, Liu JW, Chen WS, et al: Tuberculous wrist in the era of effective chemotherapy: an eleven-year experience. *Int J Tuberc Lung Dis* 7:690, 2003.

116. Tuli SM: *Tuberculosis of the skeletal system*, New Delhi, 1991, Jaypee Brothers Medical Publishers (P) Ltd.

117. Uplekar MW, Antia NH: Clinical and histopathological observations on pure neuritic leprosy. *Indian J Lepr* 58:513, 1986.

118. Wilson JN: Tuberculosis of the elbow; a study of thirty-one cases. *J Bone Joint Surg Br* 35-B:551, 1953.

119. Zaharia D, Kanitakis J, Pouteil-Noble C, et al: Rapidly growing orf in a renal transplant recipient: favourable outcome with reduction of immunosuppression and imiquimod. *Transpl Int* 23:e62, 2010.

120. Zaitz C, Godoy AM, Colucci FM, et al: Cutaneous protothecosis: report of a third Brazilian case. *Int J Dermatol* 45:124, 2006.

121. Zeifer A, Connor DH: Pheomycotic cyst: a clinicopathologic study of twenty-five patients. *Am J Trop Med Hyg* 29:901, 1980.

122. Zenone T, Boibieux A, Tigaud S, et al: Non-tuberculous mycobacterial tenosynovitis: a review. *Scand J Infect Dis* 31:221, 1999.

Dupuytren Disease

Charles Eaton

> These videos may be found at
> *ExpertConsult.com:*
> 4.1 Collagenase injection for Dupuytren contracture

Dupuytren disease (DD) is the most common heritable disorder affecting connective tissues. It is an inherited, benign, chronic progressive condition that results in fibrotic changes of the palmar and digital fascia and adjacent soft tissues. DD causes tissues to shorten along lines of mechanical tension, limiting digit extension. *Dupuytren contracture* (DC) is the end result of DD. There is not yet an effective treatment for DD. Primary treatment options for DC range from soft tissue release (i.e., collagenase injection, open or percutaneous needle fasciotomy) to excision (i.e., fasciectomy, dermofasciectomy). Because current treatments address only the contracture not its cause, both *recurrence* (reappearance of clinical disease in a treated area) and *extension* (posttreatment appearance of disease in untreated areas) are common.

Treatment of both primary and recurrent disease should be individualized, based on a person's risk factors and disease history. Treatment is empiric, and many aspects of DD lack clarity: enigmatic biology; unpredictable natural history; lack of standard terminology either for severity, outcome, recurrence, or patient satisfaction; lack of an animal model; lack of a unique biomarker; variation in biologic aggressiveness; or slow progression, often over the course of years. Proper management can be very rewarding, and treatment options have grown in the last decade, yet "… two issues remain unsolved relevant to Dupuytren's disease: its cause and its cure."[87]

DEMOGRAPHICS

DD has the highest prevalence in senior Caucasian men with blue or green eyes[13] who have a family history of the condition. DD is uncommon in those under the age of 40, but prevalence increases with age, as shown in Figure 4.1. Mean prevalence in Western countries is 12% at age 55, 21% at age 65, and 29% at age 75.[63] Pediatric DD has been reported sporadically,[56] but the diagnosis cannot be confirmed with certainty because of a lack of a unique biomarker. The most common age range at diagnosis is early fifties to early sixties. Incidence in women parallels that of men, but lags by an average of 10 to 15 years,[65] resulting in a male:female prevalence ratio that decreases with age.

Some studies have reported that prevalence in men decreases after the age of 70 and in women after the age of 80, thought to reflect attrition from increased mortality rates of patients with DD compared to the general population,[39] as well as higher mortality rates of men compared to women in the general population. The average patient has two or three affected rays; the ring or little finger are most commonly involved.[26] Overall, half of patients have bilateral disease,[64] but this varies with age; DD presents bilaterally in only 20% of patients, but over time increases to at least 70%.[48] The overall prevalence of Dupuytren *contracture* accounts for less than one-fifth of all patients with Dupuytren disease.[64]

Clinical behavior stratifies patients into four biologic groups. In order of increasing risk of needing future treatment for DC, these groups are those *without* clinical DD, those *with* DD but no contracture, those with *untreated* DC, and those with *treated* DC. Unfortunately, because diagnostic codes prior to the 10th revision of the International Statistical Classification of Diseases and Related Health Problems (ICD-10) did not differentiate Dupuytren *disease* from *contracture*, data for these groups have often been mingled.

Heritability

Inheritance patterns of DD appear to follow an autosomal dominant pattern with variable penetrance.[52,65] Despite reports of a northern European concentration, recent studies suggest that it is common in Caucasians in general, common throughout Europe and less common in Asia, as shown in Figure 4.2. Definitive prevalence data are lacking from Africa, Russia, India, and China. African Americans have just less than one-fifth the prevalence of Caucasian Americans,[92] similar to the average percent Caucasian heritage of African Americans.[83] Hispanic Americans have one-third and Asian Americans one-tenth the prevalence of Caucasian Americans.[92] Prevalence reported in family history studies is often underestimated because of the combination of late onset and lack of awareness of mild involvement in senior relatives.[65] Nearly half of patients with DD have a relative who is known to have the disease.[65,48]

Positive family history is the single strongest predictor of the disease and is associated with both earlier age of onset and earlier age of first treatment.[7,48] A family history involving both parents is associated with younger age of onset than a history of only one affected parent.[7] An affected sibling triples one's risk of developing DD.[48] Although these findings strongly suggest a genetic basis, a specific locus has yet to be identified. It is not clear whether DD is one condition or, like diabetes, the common destination of several different starting points.

Associated Conditions

DD has been associated with comorbidities including hypercholesterolemia, diabetes,[37] smoking tobacco,[14] excessive alcohol use, epilepsy, antiepileptic medication, regional trauma,[33]

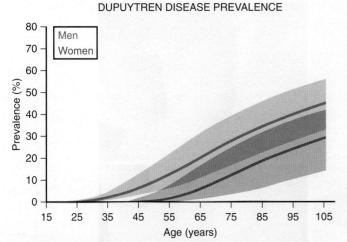

FIGURE 4.1 Summary of Dupuytren disease prevalence data in 11 high-quality studies selected from 199 reviewed publications.[63] Lines represent mean values; shaded areas are 95% confidence intervals. Prevalence in women parallels that of men, but lags by about 15 years.

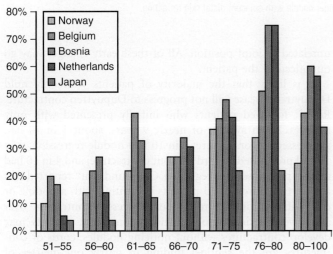

FIGURE 4.2 Prevalence of Dupuytren disease in men reported in studies from five different countries.[23,32,64,73,118] In these, prevalence in northern and southern Europe is similar; both are greater than the incidence in Japan.

chronic heavy manual labor,[25] and a lower-than-average body mass index.[41] The literature is far from clear on this topic and lack of association has also been reported for each of these factors. False association bias with other medical disorders may exist in that DD is more likely to be diagnosed in patients who have more medical office visits for other conditions.[37] The volume of evidence suggests that these conditions are probably *associated but not causative* of DD.

GENETIC BIOMARKERS

Efforts to characterize gene expression associated with disease activity have identified cellular regulatory abnormalities associated with DD. Dupuytren tissue is *not* a monoclonal neoplastic process.[16] The largest genome-wide association study to date identified nine genetic loci associated with genetic susceptibility

to DD.[30] Genetic markers specific to DD have been identified in profibrotic pathways involving regulation of transforming growth factor beta one (TGFβ1); cell differentiation; proliferation and apoptosis[85]; metalloproteinase activity[115]; fibroblast growth factor[3]; vascular endothelial growth factor[50]; hypoxia inducible factor alpha[50]; and, in particular, proteins in the Wnt-signaling pathway.[30] HLA studies have identified an increased incidence of HLA-DRB1*01 genotype[58] in Caucasians with DD, and HLA-B7 haplotype in both Peyronie disease and DD.[80]

DD gene expression studies face many challenges. The *physical setup* of cell culture affects gene expression and cytokine response[94] and may not replicate the mechanical environment that influences gene expression in vivo.[111] The *site of tissue origin* affects mechanoregulation of gene expression in otherwise similar tissues.[51] Finally, the *genetic relationship of DD and gender* is complex: palmar fascia has overexpression of androgen receptors[82]; *TIMP-1*, the gene that expresses tissue inhibitor of metalloproteinase 1 (a collagenase implicated in DD), is located on the X-chromosome[82]; estrogen suppresses both collagen synthesis[43] and matrix metalloproteinase gene expression in response to acute mechanical stress.[101] Compared to men, incidence in women is delayed until after the average age of menopause.

PREOPERATIVE EVALUATION

Physical Examination

Early Dupuytren disease is commonly overlooked and underreported.[28] The earliest signs of Dupuytren *disease* takes the form of skin tightness (i.e., exaggerated blanching with finger extension), contour changes (i.e., skin crease deformation, dimples), nodules, cords without contractures, or prominence of the palmar monticuli, as shown in Figure 4.3. Nodules are the first change noticed by about 6 out of 10 patients.[28] Nodules are flattened round or ovoid areas of subdermal firmness, fixed to the dermis, typically 0.5 to 1.5 cm in diameter with indistinct peripheral margins. The dermal papillae overlying nodules may be prominent or may be longitudinally compressed, different from the type of papillary ridge stretching and flattening seen with other slowly growing tumors (Figure 4.4). Uncommonly, nodules are initially erythematous, tender, or itchy. Skin crease deformation or dimples are the first change noticed in about 1 out of 10 patients.[28]

Dorsal Dupuytren nodules (DDN), also called *Garrod pads* or *knuckle pads*, are firm masses on the extensor aspect of the digital joints, and histologically resemble palmar nodules (Figure 4.5). DDN most commonly affect the proximal interphalangeal (PIP) joints, but occasionally the distal interphalangeal (DIP), metacarpophalangeal (MCP), or interphalangeal (IP) joint of the thumb, or rarely the extensor mechanism.[53] DDN are fixed to the superficial paratenon of the extensor mechanism and involve overlying subcutaneous tissue and retinacular fibers to a variable degree. Secondary skin involvement may occur. DDN can be confused with *dorsal cutaneous pads*: local dorsal joint skin thickening and hyperkeratosis that only involves the skin. DDN are found in one in five DD patients, often precede palmar DD, and are associated with more aggressive biology.[54]

In contrast, dorsal cutaneous pads are *not* associated with Dupuytren disease and are equally common with and without

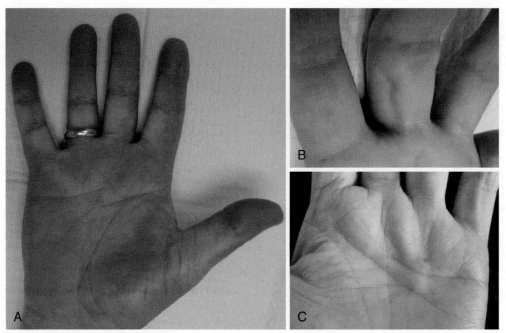

FIGURE 4.3 Earliest signs of Dupuytren disease in patients with Dupuytren contracture on the opposite hand. **A,** Palmar skin tightness, blanching in the digits with neutral extension; **B,** dimpling of the lateral digit; **C,** prominence of the interdigital palmar monticuli in the distal palm from central band tightness. This hand also demonstrates a ring finger nodule with adjacent distal skin retraction.

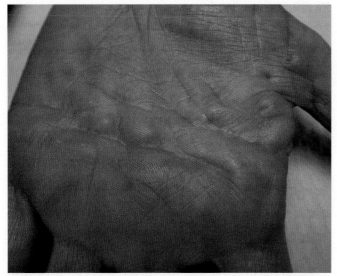

FIGURE 4.4 This patient has diffuse nodular skin involvement of Dupuytren disease, but no contractures. The dermal papillae are abnormally prominent over the nodules of the middle and ring rays, almost resembling fingerprints. Dimples and nodules are also visible at the base of the index finger and thumb as well as the first-web space.

DD.[86] Occasionally, the earliest sign of a DDN is a tethered depression of the extensor skin creases[54] (see Figure 4.5). Palpated *cords* feel like strings beneath the skin, and vary from a few millimeters to greater than a centimeter in width. Although they may be found independent of each other, nodules and cords are usually arranged as beads on a string. Nonnodular cords, unlike nodules, feel firm only when placed under tension, have well-defined margins, and are not fixed to the dermis. There is often overlap of nodules and cords[112]; that is, nodular cords share nodular aspects of dermal adherence and firmness

unrelated to joint position. All of these early changes may go unnoticed by the patient.

It is likely that the majority of patients with only mild Dupuytren disease will not progress to Dupuytren contracture. Reilly[89] followed patients who initially presented with only nodules. At an average of nearly 9 years, about 1 in 10 had progressed to contracture; 1 in 10 had nodule regression; 4 in 10 had progressed to cord without contracture; and 4 in 10 had neither progressed nor regressed. Gudmundsson[40] reported that almost two-thirds of 75 patients presenting with a nodule or cord without contracture did not progress to contracture over an 18-year period of observation. Conversely, patients may develop contractures without noticing nodules: cords or contractures are the sentinel finding in nearly one-quarter of patients.[28]

Because the diagnosis is made by clinical examination, the differential diagnosis of palmar nodules also includes fibrosarcoma, fibrous histiocytoma, giant cell tumor, synovial sarcoma, calcifying aponeurotic fibroma, epithelioid sarcoma, and other less common tumors. For this reason, the patient presenting with an isolated palmar mass diagnosed as DD should be seen for scheduled follow-up to confirm that the mass does not undergo unexpected changes.

The earliest appearance of Dupuytren *contracture* is passive extension deficit due to a contracted cord, most often affecting the MCP and PIP joints of the fingers. Almost all cords can be palpated with fingertip pressure. Because nonnodular cords feel firm only when under tension, the key to cord palpation is to feel for a change from soft to firm as the finger is passively ranged from flexion to extension. Most cords develop along recognizable lines of mechanical tension produced by passive extension or abduction. Patients with aggressive Dupuytren biology or who have had prior treatment are more likely to vary from these common patterns.

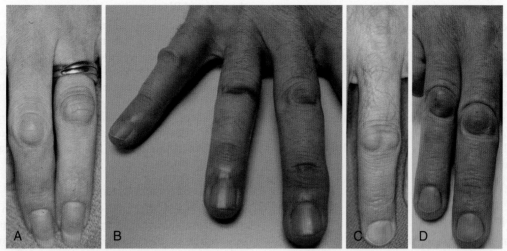

FIGURE 4.5 Variations of dorsal Dupuytren nodules. **A,** No skin involvement; **B,** dimpling with or without nodule; **C,** prominence over the condyles; **D,** inflammatory with diffuse skin tethering.

Cords may result in isolated flexion contractures of the MCP, PIP, or DIP joints or combinations of these. Thumb involvement may result in carpometacarpal (CMC) MCP or IP flexion contractures and/or radial or palmar adduction contractures. Natatory ligament contractures that adduct the fingers may be masked by the adducting effect of MCP joint contractures. Contractures on the ulnar border of the palm may produce little finger MCP flexion/abduction contractures.

Staging

There is no universally accepted system for either describing the quality or quantifying the severity of DC. Objective multifactorial tests, such as the Sollerman test and Rosenbloom joint mobility assessment, and other measures have been used for evaluation of DD but are not disease-specific. Because DC is usually painless, the inclusion of pain questions dilutes the value of subjective tests such as the Disabilities of the Arm, Shoulder, and Hand (DASH) and Michigan Hand Outcomes (MHQ); neither correlate well with range-of-motion measurements.[120] Range-of-motion measurements are the most common assessment, but often cannot be compared because of incompatible formats such as individual versus multiple joints, active versus passive measurements, and other author-defined measures. Range-of-motion measurements alone do not correlate well with hand function.[31,57]

Other systems exist, incorporating grip strength, flexion deficit, sensibility, scarring, improvement, satisfaction, and other measures specific to postoperative evaluation. The Unité Rhumatologique des Affections de la Main scale (URAM) questionnaire[6] and Southampton Dupuytren's Scoring System (SDSS)[77] have been developed as disease-specific staging systems, but neither has yet gained wide adoption. Each of the following subsections focuses on common classification schemes for a specific portion of the overall picture.

Luck Classification and Related Histology

Luck[67] described a progression of three histologic stages: *proliferative, involutional,* and *residual,* roughly corresponding to nodules, nodular cords, and nonnodular cords, respectively.

The *key cell* is the *myofibroblast*, which under light microscopy resembles a fibroblast but has ultrastructural differences: stress fibers, cell membrane adhesion complexes, fibronectin fibers, smooth muscle α-actin, and other unique characteristics. The *proliferative* cellular stage is characterized by highly cellular, mitotic histology with randomly oriented myofibroblasts and sparse, randomly oriented collagen fibrils. Specimens of the *involutional* fibrocellular stage are less cellular with no mitoses, and show some parallel orientation of myofibroblasts and collagen fibrils. *Residual* fibrotic stage histology is characterized by relatively acellular collagen with flattened cells within areas of uniformly oriented densely packed collagen bundles. Occluded microvessels and basal lamina thickening are also present in cords, nodules, and perinodular areas.

Luck staging correlates with collagen type. Normal palmar fascia has little or no type III collagen. Abnormally high levels of type III collagen exist in the palmar fascia of DD patients even in the absence of contracture.[11] The ratio of type III to type I collagen is highest in the proliferative stage (>35%).[62] This ratio decreases to the range of 20 to 35% in involutional specimens, and to less than 20% in residual specimens.[62] Type III collagen persists in affected tissues: the involutional stage is static, but not normal.

Luck staging correlates with recurrence rate after fasciectomy. Balaguer et al[4] analyzed outcomes at 8 to 9 years after fasciectomy and reported that proliferative histology more than doubled recurrence compared to involutional histology and more than tripled recurrence compared to residual histology. This Luck stage parallels clinical assessment of nodularity and may prove applicable for preoperative recurrence prediction or for procedures performed without tissue sampling.

Tubiana Staging

The Tubiana stage is an index of composite flexion contracture. The composite MCP + PIP joint flexion contracture of each ray is placed in a group of 45-degree increments:
- Stage 0: no contracture
- Stage 1: 0 to 45 degrees
- Stage 2: 45 to 90 degrees

- Stage 3: 90 to 135 degrees
- Stage 4: greater than 135 degrees

DIP joint angles are not included.

This classification has been modified to include notations for the presence of nodules or distal IP hyperextension for each ray, and a summary number for the entire hand as well as other notations[46]; however, the most common use is as a quick descriptor—the stage number of the affected finger. This classification has the unique advantage of summarizing contractures from cords that span both MCP and PIP joints and complements individual joint measurements. A variation of the Tubiana stage is the total contracture index (TCI), which is the composite MCP + PIP flexion contracture in degrees.

Individual Joint Measurements

Range-of-motion measurement of individual joints using a goniometer might seem to be the most objective documentation. However, two DD-specific issues can result in a pattern of bias affecting individual joint measurements. First, limited joint motion from Dupuytren cords may produce static or dynamic contractures. Cords spanning sequential joints produce *dynamic contractures* via fasciodesis: measurements at one joint are linked to the position of the adjacent spanned joint. Grotesman[38] found dynamic contractures in more than one-third of rays having combined MCP + PIP contractures, primarily affecting a PIP joint.

This is consistent with the report of correction of untreated PIP contractures in more than one-third of combined MCP + PIP contractures in which only the MCP joint was treated with collagenase clostridium histolyticum (CCH) injection.[44] Cords extending to the proximal palm are affected by CMC joint position, which cannot easily be measured and can affect both MCP and PIP joint measurements in a zigzag fashion (Figure 4.6). Second, although cords themselves are inelastic, they arise from soft tissues that have elastic attachments: passive range-of-motion measurements are subject to examiner bias from the force applied to the finger.

Location of Disease

Although much has been written regarding the anatomical basis of cords, not all cord areas have been named, and published reports lack a precise, standard system to tag cord and nodule locations in the palm based on physical examination. A diagram developed for this purpose based on skin landmarks and common patterns of DD is shown in Figure 4.7. Forms based on this are available at http://dupuytrens.org/research-publications/forms-for-documentation, and these allow documentation of initial evaluation disease location, joint measurements, and treatment details.

Diathesis Score and Severity

Biologic severity affects the clinical course both before and after treatment. Biologic severity is reflected both in the rate of progression from diagnosis to the need for treatment and the risk of recurrence, extension, stiffness, and inflammatory reaction after treatment. Biologic severity varies greatly between individuals and is *not* simply contracture severity. One index of biologic severity is association with specific fibrotic conditions: that is, DDN, Peyronie, Ledderhose, frozen shoulder. Despite conflicting reports, each of these is probably associated with increased risk of DD and vice versa. Why is this?

Each of these conditions occurs where *inelastic fascial structures* are subjected to *high peak shearing* or *traction forces*. The author's opinion is that there is an underlying connective tissue disorder triggered by the mechanics at each of these sites, which would explain the observed overlap of risk factors; *family history* of DD increases the risk both of Ledderhose and of DDN.[42] In contrast, other fibrotic conditions, such as keloid or scleroderma, are *not* associated with increased DD risk and appear to have different molecular pathways.[9,55]

Diathesis factors predict biologic severity. Diathesis factors include bilateral palmar disease, DDN, Ledderhose disease, positive family history, age of onset younger than 50, male gender,[47] first ray disease,[1] and involvement of more than two digits.[22] There has not been full agreement on the relative

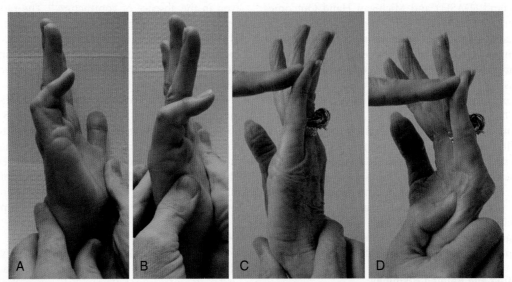

FIGURE 4.6 Demonstration of dynamic contractures with carpometacarpal (CMC) fasciodesis. **A,** Patients use a trick motion to compensate for tight fascia, flexing their ring and small CMC joints to allow metacarpophalangeal (MCP) extension. **B,** CMC flexion allows 10 degrees of active MCP hyperextension. **C,** When CMC flexion is blocked, active MCP extension is limited to 20 degrees, which in turn improves active proximal interphalangeal extension by 10 degrees. **D,** blocking CMC flexion changes passive MCP extension from 0 to 65 degrees.

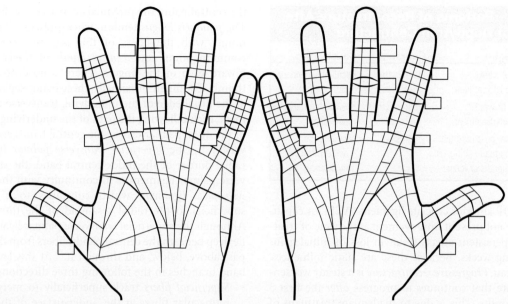

FIGURE 4.7 This diagram is based on common zones of involvement and allows standard documentation of the location of physical findings, procedures, and joint measurements. PDF versions of this as evaluation and procedure forms are available at http://dupuytrens.org/research-publications/forms-for-documentation.

importance of each, but in general, the greater the number of diathesis factors, the higher the recurrence rate after surgery. The strongest predictor of greater biologic severity is younger age of onset.[7,29]

Similarly, rate of recurrence drops with greater age at the time of first treatment.[109] Some factors, such as frozen shoulder[99] and Peyronie disease,[79] increase the incidence risk of DD but not the rate of recurrence after surgery.[22,47] This paradox might be explained by the effect of index event bias on interpretation of recurrence data,[100] and more clarification is needed. Diathesis factors share genetic markers. Patients with early age of onset, DDNs, and a positive family history were found to have a greater likelihood of having a high genetic risk score based on a profile of single nucleotide polymorphisms associated with DD.[29]

Documentation of DD biologic severity should include diathesis factors: family history of DD in siblings or parents; gender; age of onset of DD; current age; age of first treatment; bilaterality of DD; number of digits involved; thumb involvement; presence of nodules; presence of DDNs; presence of Ledderhose disease; presence of Peyronie disease; and history of frozen shoulder. A high diathesis score implies three or more of these factors: age of onset younger than 50, positive family history, DDN, bilateral disease, Ledderhose.

Treatment Outcome Score

Outcome assessment is most meaningful in the context of the initial contracture. Two useful objective comparative outcome measures are the *Thomine coefficient* ([degrees of improvement]/[degrees of initial contracture]) and *CCH success* ([number of joints corrected to 5 degrees or less]/[number of treated joints]). The fact that neither adequately reflects functional change in all patients reflects the difficulty of this issue. Consider, for example, a patient with a 40-degree contracture

and a patient with a 140-degree contracture. For these patients, complete correction would give the same outcome score by either measure, despite very different changes in function. A 30-degree improvement would not be considered a CCH success for either, but the first patient would likely be happier than the second. Patient satisfaction correlates poorly with range-of-motion measurements regardless. Roush and Stern[90] reported results of surgery for recurrence in which 95% of patients were "unconditionally satisfied and stated that they would have the procedure again" despite lack of improvement in average total active motion.

Recurrence Assessment

Because recurrence is a lifetime issue, recurrence percentages are meaningless unless duration is also specified. Recurrence is most accurately described as a *percent per year rate*, not simply a percent, and also not an average of a broad range of follow-up intervals. Many definitions of recurrence exist. Quantitative definitions include need for repeat treatment, loss of a defined percent of initial correction, or loss of a defined number of degrees of correction. Different metrics cannot be easily compared. For example, recurrence as defined in CCH studies excludes the subset of treated patients not corrected to within 5 degrees of complete extension, a group known to have a higher recurrence rate[84]; this skews recurrence results favorably compared to other recurrence definitions. In addition, many published studies define recurrence qualitatively or not at all.

Not all contracture recurrence is Dupuytren recurrence. Contracture recurrence falls into three categories: early, progressive, and late (Table 4.1). *Early recontracture* develops during the first 3 postoperative months, followed by a plateau.[27] This pattern is not recurrent Dupuytren contracture. It is due to incomplete correction of secondary pathology at the time of treatment. Central slip laxity, oblique retinacular ligament

TABLE 4.1   Patterns of Recontracture After Treatment of Dupuytren Contracture

Type	Begins	Course	Cause
Early	1–2 weeks posttreatment	Plateau after 6–12 weeks	Residual secondary pathology
Progressive	6–12 weeks posttreatment	Progressive	Residual primary pathology
Late	After posttreatment plateau lasting 12 months or longer	Progressive	New disease activity (true recurrence)

tightness, mild PIP anterior cruciate ligament (ACL), or capsular tightness may not prevent improvement at the time of treatment, but their persistent effects result in loss of initial gains over the following weeks. Because these are static influences, their effects plateau. *Progressive recontracture* is a steady worsening of contracture that continues to progress *after* the first 3 postoperative months. This is due to inadequate treatment of primary pathology: inadequate fasciotomy/ectomy of all mechanically important cord(s).

Both severe contractures and diffuse disease are more likely to have multiple cords affecting the same joint,[105] some of which may escape treatment. Residual cords with soft tissue attachments may stretch without becoming discontinuous and remain biologically active and contractile during the early postoperative period. *Late recontracture* develops after an initial period of stability lasting a year or more after treatment.

Similar to extension of disease after treatment, late recontracture is due to progression of new Dupuytren activity and represents *true recurrence*. Failure to clearly separate these groups has led to confusion regarding outcomes. The author recommends the definition of recurrence published by the international Dupuytren Delphi group: "an increase in joint contracture in any treated joint of at least 20 degrees at 1 year posttreatment compared to 6 weeks posttreatment."[59]

Diagnostic Imaging

Diagnosis is made by physical examination. Although there are objective findings *consistent* with Dupuytren disease, there is neither laboratory result, imaging finding, nor a biomarker *unique* to DD. Plain x-rays may be helpful in determining presence and extent of degenerative joint changes or heterotopic ossification of cords.[93] Ultrasound imaging[106] or Doppler ultrasound examination may help identify neurovascular displacement from a spiral cord.[35] MRI can be used to evaluate the cellularity of disease[117] and, in theory, the Luck stage—however, it has not yet been widely adopted for this use.

◼ PERTINENT ANATOMY

Normal Anatomy

DD produces progressive changes in the palmar fascia, its attachments, adjacent subcutaneous tissues, and dermis. Normal anatomy is diagrammed in Figure 4.8.

Palm

The *superficial palmar fascia* lies in a coronal plane deep beneath the palmar subcutaneous tissue and covers a triangular area of

the central palm, the proximal corner facing directly proximal. The *palmaris longus* tendon, when present, terminates in continuity with the fibers of this proximal corner. From this common point, four *central bands* of fascia extend distally toward each of the fingers. There is no central band for the thumb. Confluent proximally, these bands separate and diverge at the distal edge of the underlying transverse retinacular ligament, each following the path of the underlying ray. At the level of the distal palmar crease, the central bands are bridged transversely by the *superficial transverse palmar ligament*. At the radial border of the index central band, the superficial transverse palmar ligament is in continuity with the *proximal first-web-space ligament*, which continues to a point roughly superficial to the radial sesamoid of the thumb MCP joint. Although the superficial transverse palmar ligament appears to lie deep beneath the central bands, fibers from the central bands pass above, below, and through it.[49] At this level, each central band branches in the following three directions.

- *Superficial fibers* track superficially to merge with vertical retinacular fibers at the undersurface of the dermis in the distal palm in areas between skin flexion creases, where nodules commonly arise.
- *Intermediate fibers* split transversely into two sections, which extend toward the lateral border of the base of the digit. This track of fibers is called the *spiral band* because fibers track *around* the neurovascular bundle: proximally, they are central and superficial to the bundle; distally, lateral and deep beneath it. Neurovascular spiral bundles result from involvement of these fibers.
- *Deep fibers* continue dorsally to merge with the sagittally oriented interosseous fascia and pierce the transverse MP ligament to merge with fibers of the sagittal bands of the extensor mechanism. These fibers are rarely involved in contractures.

Web Spaces

A subdermal fascial layer borders the periphery of the web spaces from thumb to little finger. Fascial fibers follow the direction of this layer. The section of this structure spanning the fingers is referred to as the *natatory ligament*; its continuation across the first-web space is referred to as the *distal first-web-space ligament*. It crosses the thumb to join fibers of the proximal first-web-space ligament over the radial sesamoid area. Fibers from the natatory ligament extend distally at the lateral base of each finger in continuity with the Grayson ligament and the lateral digit dermis.

Digits

Contradictory descriptions exist of the digital fascia anatomy because of difficulties inherent in dissecting fascial structures in the digits[119]: fibrous strands less than 1-mm thick follow oblique curved paths; distortion from release of skin attachments are needed for exposure; distortion when fingers preserved in flexion are later straightened for dissection. Zwanenburg et al.[119] recently reported a clarification of anatomy, as shown earlier in Figure 4.8. The digital neurovascular structures are circumferentially enveloped within thin layers of fascia.

The traditional name for components of this envelope *dorsal* to the neurovascular bundle is *Cleland ligament*, and the traditional name for components *palmar* to the neurovascular

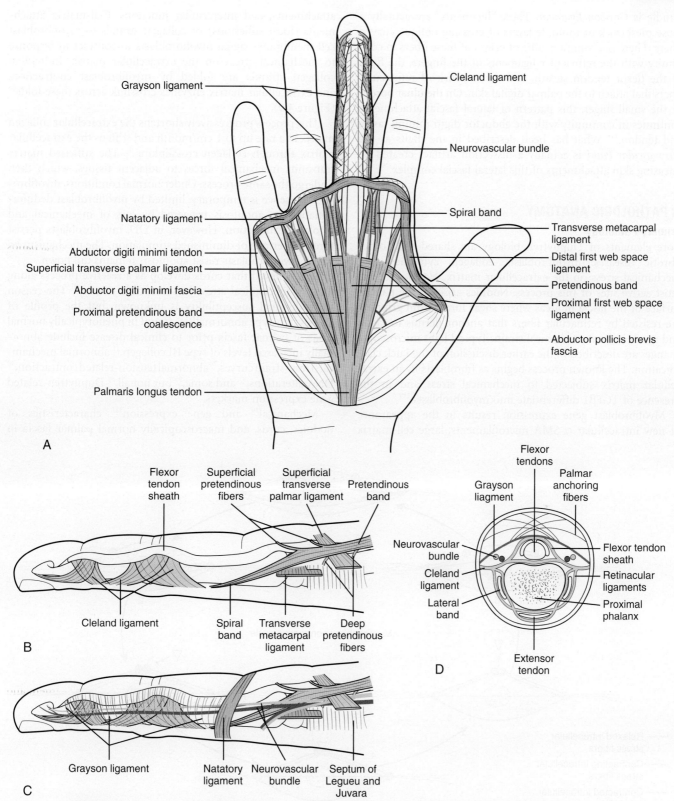

FIGURE 4.8 Normal fascial anatomy. **A,** Palmar view of structures beneath skin and subcutaneous tissues of the palm and finger. **B,** Lateral view of the deeper structures of the distal palm and finger. **C,** Lateral view of the more superficial structures of the distal palm and finger. **D,** Axial cross sectional view of finger proximal to the proximal interphalangeal joint.

bundle is *Grayson ligament*. These "ligaments" are actually a loose meshwork of multiple layers of crossing oblique curved fibers. There is a common zone of origin of these fibers in continuity with the retinacular ligaments of the fingers, the floor of the flexor tendon sheath, and the network of retinacular fibers that attach to the palmar digital skin. On the ulnar border of the small finger, this pattern of lateral fascial attachments continues in continuity with the abductor digiti minimi fascia and tendon.[114] What has been described in the digits as the *retrovascular band* is actually a dissection artifact created by releasing skin attachments of this lateral fascial complex.

◣ PATHOLOGIC ANATOMY

Primary Pathology

Core elements of Dupuytren biology are shared with other fibrotic diseases: myofibroblasts, collagen, cytokines, and mechanical stress on the extracellular matrix. *Nodules* are the most active sites of this process. Nodules arise on the palmar surface of the fascia in areas where shear forces from gripping are resisted by retinacular fibers that anchor dermis to fascia and result in local mechanical strain. Typical light microscopic changes are described in the earlier discussion of the Luck classification. The known process begins as fibroblasts in an extracellular matrix subjected to mechanical stress and in the presence of TGFβ1 differentiate into myofibroblasts.[110]

Myofibroblast gene expression results in the appearance of new intracellular α-SMA microfilaments, large cell-matrix

attachments, and intercellular junctions. Cell-matrix attachments (focal adhesions) of collagen strands to myofibroblast cell membranes signal myofibroblasts to contract in response to mechanical stress on the extracellular matrix. Individual collagen strands are folded by myofibroblast contraction, and extracellular matrix enzymes crosslink across these folds[15] (Figure 4.9).

This process progressively shortens the extracellular collagen matrix at a rate up to 1 cm/month and stiffens the extracellular matrix through collagen crosslinking.[15] The stiffened matrix transmits mechanical forces to adjacent tissues, which then undergo the same process. Under normal conditions, myofibroblast presence is temporary, limited by myofibroblast dedifferentiation or apoptosis triggered by loss of mechanical and cytokine stimulation. However, in DD, myofibroblasts persist through periods of diminished stimulation. The mechanism by which myofibroblasts resist apoptosis remains unknown.

It is believed that cords develop as a reactive process along lines of mechanical stress in susceptible tissues.[60] The reason for individual susceptibility is unknown, but the profile of Dupuytren-type abnormalities found in phenotypically normal areas of palmar fascia prior to clinical disease include abnormally increased levels of type III collagen,[11] abnormal mechanical stress–strain curves,[74] abnormal tension-related contraction,[10] DNA alterations,[97] and some,[95] but not all,[88] Dupuytren-related gene expression markers.

Mechanical[10] and gene expression[111] characteristics of nodules, cords, and macroscopically normal palmar fascia in

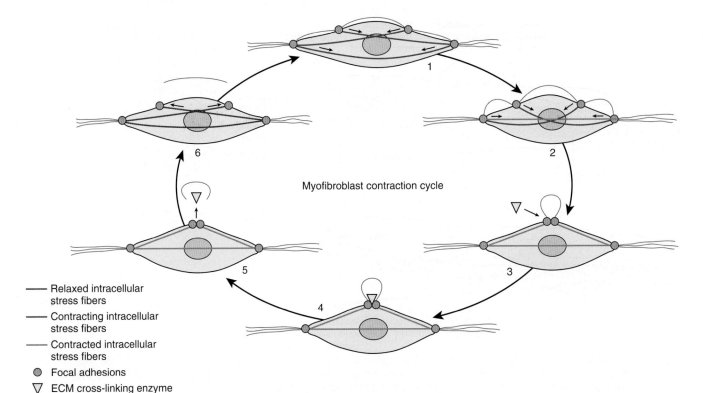

Myofibroblast contraction cycle

—— Relaxed intracellular
    stress fibers
—— Contracting intracellular
    stress fibers
—— Contracted intracellular
    stress fibers
● Focal adhesions
▽ ECM cross-linking enzyme

FIGURE 4.9 Myofibroblast cycle of extracellular matrix (ECM) remodeling.[15] Relaxed (*green lines*) and contracting (*red lines*) intracellular stress fibers are joined to extracellular collagen strands via focal adhesions (*green circles*) in the cell membrane. *1:* Mechanical stress on the ECM triggers global contraction of all stress fibers. *2:* This generates slack in individual collagen strands along lines of mechanical tension. *3:* The slack collagen strands are repositioned by individual stress fibers, creating a loop. *4:* ECM crosslinking enzymes (yellow triangle) join the base of the loop and trim the redundant strand. *5:* The strand is released into the ECM. *6:* The shortened strand then stress shields the stress fibers, allowing the cell to return to its prior state and repeat the cycle.

Dupuytren patients are all abnormal, but to different degrees. There is growing understanding of the biomechanics of fascial response to strain,[96] age,[61] and the cause-and-effect relationships of type III collagen to DD. The starting point could be the abnormal presence of type III collagen, mechanically different than type I, triggering abnormal mechanoregulatory stimulation of gene expression. Alternatively, the priming event might be abnormal mechanoregulation of gene activation resulting in overexpression of type III collagen.[51]

Patterns of contracture may have more to do with collagen crosslinking than myofibroblast contraction. Some locations (i.e., distal palm, palmar digit) produce clinical contractures, but other common locations (i.e., DDN, Ledderhose) do not, despite the fact that biopsy tissue from each contracts similarly in vitro. A possible explanation is that Dupuytren biology fixes tissues in their resting position.[72] The biology of collagen deposition and remodeling is activated by mechanical stress, but then continues during periods of rest. At rest, activated myofibroblasts and collagen crosslinking enzymes in the extracellular matrix shorten redundant collagen fibrils. At rest, this process remodels collagen length to match the resting dimension—similar to contracture of the PIP volar plate, which occurs after injury and prolonged flexion.

Such a process would be expected to produce contractures resembling the resting posture of the hand—flexion and adduction—which is what is seen in the vast majority of cases.

It would also explain why knuckle pads and Ledderhose rarely develop contractures, because the IP joints rest in flexion and the metatarsophalangeal joints of the toes rest in extension.

Most patterns of DC can be explained as transformation of existing fascial structures through Luck's stages into fibrous cords, guided by stress and stress shielding. In the process of cord formation, there is a reorientation of collagen fibers parallel to lines of mechanical stress. Any palmar fascial structure subjected to mechanical stress may contribute to Dupuytren cords. Stress shielding reduces the risk of contracture of certain locations, some of which have only minimal case reports of involvement. Structures rarely involved because of stress shielding include the Cleland ligament (shielded by adjacent phalanx); longitudinal fibers deep beneath the transverse superficial palmar ligament (shielded by the central band); transverse superficial palmar ligament (shielded by the transverse metacarpal ligament); and the septa of Legueu and Juvara (shielded by adjacent metacarpal). Stress shielding also provides the endpoint for disease progression.

As contractures progress, stress shielding from lack of use or from secondary capsuloligamentous joint contractures permanently removes mechanical stress from the cord; in the end, this allows myofibroblast apoptosis and progression to the final, involutional, static stage of disease.[112]

Common cord patterns are shown in Figure 4.10. Cords may be confined to the palm, the digit, or span both. Unlike cords

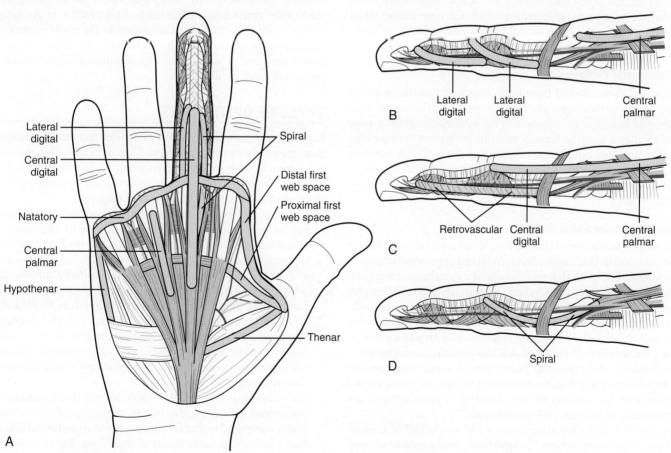

FIGURE 4.10 Common cord patterns. **A,** Central digital, central palmar, distal first-web space, hypothenar, **(B)** lateral digital, **(C)** retrovascular, **(D)** spiral.

that arise in the palm, cords isolated to a digit may have both proximal and distal bony attachments, making them more difficult to palpate.

Common *central palm cords* are *central palmar*, *spiral*, and *proximal first web*. Common *border palm cords* are *natatory*, *distal first web*, *hypothenar*, and *thenar*. Thenar and hypothenar cords are uncommon and are usually associated with diffuse disease or aggressive biology. The majority of MCP joint contractures are a result of the effect of an isolated central cord. In contrast, the majority of PIP contractures are due to multiple *digital cords*, which, in order of frequency, are *central digital*, *retrovascular*, and *spiral* or *lateral*.[105] Multiple cords can exist at the same longitudinal level in either palm or digit.

Secondary Pathology

Over time, flexed posture results in anatomic changes of joints and tendons independent of the causative cord. These issues are more likely to develop with more severe primary contractures. The PIP joint is particularly vulnerable to such changes. Contractures of the accessory collateral ligament are more common in PIP joint contractures greater than 45 degrees.[105] Central slip attenuation contributes to extension deficit for PIP contractures greater than 60 degrees,[98] which are less likely to achieve full correction than those with less severe contractures.[75] Boutonnière, sagittal band rupture, or mallet deformity may develop secondary to chronic contractures. Sagittal band rupture can be difficult to diagnose in the context of a fixed MCP flexion contracture, but a key clue is MCP abduction–supination in the absence of a responsible palmar cord. Chronic rotational or lateral deformities from digital cords often persist after treatment of the primary disease.

Synergistic Pathology

Postural abnormalities from prior injury, chronic flexor tendinitis, osteoarthritis, peripheral neuropathy, intrinsic weakness, or mild spasticity are common in the senior demographic population and must be kept in mind in evaluation because they affect outcome expectations. Dupuytren disease is less common in rheumatoid patients,[2] but it can coexist. This author has seen all of these conditions concurrent with DC, often not previously diagnosed.

Neurovascular Spiral Bundle

A neurovascular spiral bundle (i.e., spiral cord, or spiral nerve) is common in DC. Tissues that form a cord may initially describe a longitudinal path that spirals around a straight neurovascular bundle (see Figure 4.10). When this path tightens and straightens, the neurovascular bundle is displaced into a spiral path, raising a section of the bundle into a subcutaneous position that is superficial to the cord. If the neurovascular fat pad surrounding the bundle is displaced as well, this presents as an area where a palpable subdermal cord passes beneath a soft subcutaneous mass beneath soft skin. Such a finding is associated with a spiral bundle in the majority of cases, but lack of this finding is not predictive of absence of a spiral bundle.[108]

Spiral bundles have been reported in nearly half of Dupuytren finger contractures.[108] Superficial displacement is most common between the distal palmar crease and the flexion crease of the PIP joint. Variations occur, including cords that pass

between the digital nerve and a dorsal branch, double spirals,[45] and spirals at the level of the middle phalanx. Spiral bundles are at risk for inadvertent injury during open or percutaneous procedures.

Little Finger PIP Joint

Little finger PIP joint contractures have a worse prognosis and higher recurrence rate than other PIP joints, independent of surgical technique. Abductor digiti minimi (ADM) tendon involvement, common in little finger contractures, is *not* an independent risk factor for either inferior outcome or higher recurrence,[113] and similar intrinsic tendon involvement can occur in any digit. ADM fascia involvement may explain loss of little finger supination frequently seen by this author with mild contractures.

HISTORICAL REVIEW

Percutaneous fasciotomy and open fasciotomy were the most common procedures performed for DC in the early 1800s. Fasciectomy became the dominant procedure in the late 1800s, facilitated by the introduction of general anesthesia and then sterile technique. Radical fasciectomy, developed in the early 1900s, became the recommended procedure until the mid-1900s, when it became clear that it led to more morbidity but was not more effective. A trend to conservative treatment followed, paralleling development of minimally invasive techniques in all surgical specialties. Percutaneous needle fasciotomy and enzymatic fasciotomy, both pioneered in France during the mid-1900s, entered the mainstream of US practice in the early 2000s. As of this writing, fasciectomy is the most common procedure performed in the United States for DC, and by extension is the current standard of care. Additional historical data points are listed in Table 4.2.

TYPES OF OPERATIONS

Current treatments fall into four categories: minimally invasive, fasciectomy, dermofasciectomy, and salvage. Choice is based on the desires of both patient and surgeon. All existing DC procedures are palliative and prone to recurrence. The following are three unsolved issues with Dupuytren surgery:

1. The core *biology* resembles that of wound contracture and can be provoked by the wounding process of fasciectomy. One consequence of this is the postfasciectomy *flare reaction*: disproportionate and prolonged swelling, stiffness and pain, and worsening several weeks after an initially uneventful postop course and continuing for months thereafter. Postfasciectomy flare reaction occurs in about 1 in 10 patients and leads to permanent stiffness in about 1 in 20.[24] Average postfasciectomy edema and stiffness are greater both after more extensive dissection and in overweight patients.[5] Minimally invasive procedures are not commonly associated with flare reaction.

2. The *anatomy* is distorted and some normal tissue planes are obliterated, increasing the risk of iatrogenic neurovascular injury compared to that for other elective procedures. Digital nerve injury has been reported in at least 3% of primary fasciectomy procedures; the risk is more than five times greater in fasciectomy for recurrence.[24]

TABLE 4.2 Historical Points in the Treatment of Dupuytren Contracture

Year	Author	Significance
1614	Plater	Clinical description
1777	Cline	Suggested fasciotomy
1822	Cooper	Percutaneous fasciotomy
1831	Dupuytren	Open fasciotomy
1834	Goyrand	Fasciectomy
1875	Busch	Open fasciotomy and skin graft
1906	Keen	Radical fasciectomy
1908	Ombrédanne	PIP arthrectomy for PIP contracture
1919	Griffith	Fasciectomy and transposition flaps
1919	Davis	Fasciectomy and full-thickness skin graft
1922	Eckstein	Proximal phalanx-shortening osteotomy for PIP contracture
1931	Lexer	Radical dermofasciectomy and full-thickness skin graft
1932	Palmén	Fasciectomy and Y–V-plasty
1948	McIndoe	Fasciectomy and Z-plasty
1957	De Seze and Debeyre	Steroid injection and needle fasciotomy
1959	Luck	Histologic staging
1963	Hueston	Diathesis concept
1964	McCash	Open palm technique
1965	Bassot	Enzymatic fasciotomy with trypsin and other enzymes
1972	Gabbiani	Myofibroblast identified in DC
1996	Moermans	Segmental fasciectomy
2002	Agee	Skeletal extension torque for PIP contractures
2009	Degreef	Tamoxifen reduces recurrence after fasciectomy in high-risk patients
2010	Hurst and Badalamente	CCH approved by FDA as contracture treatment

CCH, Collagenase clostridium histolyticum; *DC,* Dupuytren contracture; *PIP,* proximal interphalangeal.

3. Optimum *timing* of surgery for best outcome is unknown.
   a. Operations should be performed before the severity of contracture compromises the chance of an excellent result, which is about 40 degrees at the PIP joint.[105]
   b. For lesser contractures, defer procedures until the patient has functional problems to minimize the number of lifetime procedures. A commonly recommended window of opportunity is between the tabletop test (cannot place the palm flat on a table) and the pocket test (difficulty slipping a hand into one's pants pocket).
   c. Ideally, avoid treatment during the proliferative phase to reduce postoperative recurrence rate.[4] This parallels historical advice to postpone surgery until disease is no longer "active" (nodular). Unfortunately, activity may persist until contractures are past the point of expectation of a satisfactory surgical result, which explains why there is also traditional advice that contradicts this—that is, to operate if the contracture is rapidly getting worse.

The three procedures for primary disease have similar outcomes in terms of initial correction of deformity[78,81,104] but differ in terms of cost effectiveness, length of recovery, morbidity, and recurrence (Table 4.3). Relative indications for different procedures are listed in Table 4.4.

Patient choice of DC treatment is influenced by social networking. Individuals may seek treatment for early DD because they fear progression or have heard that someone was told by their surgeon that they had "waited too long" for treatment. Conversely, patients may avoid treatment for advanced DC because of fear or have heard of a long, difficult ordeal after fasciectomy. Patients are deterred by the memory of fasciectomy: patients with recurrence after fasciectomy are less likely to opt for repeat treatment than those with recurrence after minimally invasive treatment.[109] Patients who seek treatment but are put off by the prospect of fasciectomy will choose minimally invasive treatment with full knowledge that recurrence rates are higher.

Minimally Invasive Procedures

The most commonly performed minimally invasive procedures are enzymatic fasciotomy and percutaneous needle fasciotomy. These are indicated when the benefit of shorter recovery

TABLE 4.3 Comparison of Various Procedures

Procedure	Cost Effectiveness	Length of Recovery	Most Common Treatment-Specific Complications	Recurrence (%/year)
Needle fasciotomy	Best	Week–weeks	>1%: skin tears <1%: nerve, tendon injury	10–20
Enzymatic fasciotomy	Next best	Week–weeks	>1%: extensive bruising, skin tears <1%: tendon rupture, pulley rupture	10–20
Local fasciectomy, ± skin graft	Worse	Month–months	>1%: prolonged inflammation, delayed healing, nerve injury, loss of flexion <1%: amputation for ischemia	5–10
Dermofasciectomy	Worse	Months	>1%: prolonged inflammation, delayed healing, nerve injury, loss of flexion <1%: amputation for ischemia	2

TABLE 4.4 **Indications and Options for Various Clinical Scenarios**

Indication	Best Options
Nodule only	Observe *or* steroid injection
Primary presentation + low diathesis score	Minimally invasive procedure
Recurrence + low diathesis score	Repeat initial procedure *or* fasciectomy
Multiple recurrence/severe recurrence	Dermofasciectomy
High diathesis score	Dermofasciectomy
Insufficient longitudinal skin or diffuse skin involvement	Fasciectomy + skin flap/graft *or* dermofasciectomy
Isolated MCP *or* MCP + PIP contracture	Any procedure
Primary isolated PIP contracture	Any procedure
Recurrent isolated PIP contracture	Stronger consideration of skeletal extension torque ± fasciectomy/ dermofasciectomy *or* skeletal shortening
Composite contracture < 90 (Tubiana I or II)	Any procedure
Composite contracture > 90 (Tubiana III or IV)	Consider staged procedures: staged releases *or* preliminary skeletal extension torque followed by definitive procedure

MCP, Metacarpophalangeal; *PIP,* proximal interphalangeal.

outweighs the disadvantage of higher recurrence rate. These two approaches have similar outcomes[81] and compared to fasciectomy are similar in terms of length of recovery (shorter), morbidity, complication rate (less), and recurrence rate (greater). (See Video 4.1 for a review of collagenase injection.)

Percutaneous Needle Fasciotomy

Indications. The minimum requirement for percutaneous needle fasciotomy (PNF) is a cooperative patient with joint contracture(s) due to a palpable, tensionable cord with adequate skin reserve.

Contraindications. PNF is contraindicated for patients who cannot tolerate an awake procedure or who have tight skin or scars preventing extension, diffuse skin involvement, lack of a palpable cord, rapid recurrence in a young patient, or healing wounds or infection in the area of the procedure.

Preoperative Planning. PNF can be performed as a single visit office procedure under local anesthesia. Cords are identified by inspection and palpation.

Technique. Local prep and field sterility (as for IV cannula insertion) are used. Needle entry sites ("portals") are injected with *intradermal anesthetic.* A small gauge hypodermic needle is inserted through a portal and, with the cord maintained under tension, the needle tip is used to progressively sever cord fibers until the cord "gives" at that level. The procedure is then repeated for all areas of palpable cords, ideally in a distal to proximal sequence. Nerve status and tendon status are checked repeatedly throughout the procedure.

After all palpable cords have been released, final passive extension is performed and light bandages are applied. The patient may discontinue bandage use when wounds are dry, usually the same day. The other hand can be treated the following day. Neither therapy nor splinting is routinely used. Strenuous gripping and forceful use of the hand are to be avoided for 1 week.

Enzymatic Fasciotomy With Collagenase Clostridium Histolyticum

Indications. Indications are the same as for PNF.

Contraindications. Collagenase clostridium histolyticum (CCH) is contraindicated for patients with a history of severe allergic reaction to CCH or to collagenase used in any other therapeutic application or application method. The safety of CCH is unknown in patients who are pregnant, plan to become pregnant, are breastfeeding, plan to begin breastfeeding, have a bleeding problem, have other medical conditions, are on any anticoagulant medications, or are less than 18 years old.[116] Otherwise, contraindications are the same as for PNF.

Preoperative Planning. CCH injection is performed over the course of two closely spaced office visits, typically 2 consecutive days per hand, with additional injections spaced a minimum of 30 days apart. An area of clearly palpable cord responsible for a specific joint contracture is chosen for injection. For the little finger, the manufacturer recommends limiting needle penetration to a maximum depth of 3 mm and avoiding injection more than 4 mm distal to the palmar flexion crease at the base of the finger. The drug must be maintained under constant refrigeration until use.

Technique. Of all procedures, CCH is the easiest and least time-consuming option for the surgeon. CCH is reconstituted with the accompanying diluent solution immediately before use according to package directions. Using a sterile technique, the central substance of the chosen cord segment is injected at three closely spaced points with the recommended dose of the reconstituted drug. After injection, the hand is wrapped in a soft immobilizing bandage. The patient is instructed to keep the hand elevated and avoid moving the fingers until the next office visit. Manipulation is performed by the physician on postinjection days 1 through 4, optionally using local anesthetic. The patient is then fitted with a static extension splint to wear for 1 month while sleeping, given a set of active range-of-motion exercises to perform during the day, and instructed to avoid strenuous activities with the treated hand until instructed otherwise, usually after several weeks.

Open Surgical Procedures

Fasciectomy

There are two current approaches to fasciectomy. *Segmental fasciectomy* involves minimal dissection to remove short segments of cords. *Regional fasciectomy* (also called local fasciectomy) is removal of all diseased fascia. Currently, segmental fasciectomy is more popular in Europe than in the United States. These two procedures have similar outcomes.[76] *Radical fasciectomy* is removal of *all* palmar fascia, including paratendinous septa, subcutaneous and subfascial fatty tissue, and fat pads of the palmar monticuli. Radical fasciectomy is no longer recommended because of greater morbidity and lack of any

TABLE 4.5 Comparison of Fasciectomy Technical Options

Technique		Pros	Cons
Incision	Longitudinal zigzag (either primary zigzag or straight incision converted to zigzag with Z-plasties at closure)	Most extensile exposure for a single ray	Greater risk of marginal wound ischemia; challenging for multiple adjacent rays in palm
	Transverse	Wide exposure for adjacent rays in the palm; closure optional; can be converted to zigzag	Visibility more challenging; not extensile
	Combined: finger zigzag + transverse palm	Most extensile for multiple rays	No advantage for single ray
Adding skin	Local flap (Z-plasty, Y–V-plasty)	Lowers recurrence vs. longitudinal closure[19]	Risk of flap loss
	Regional flap (homodigital lateral digit, cross finger)	More durable than skin graft	Limited donor sites
	Skin graft addition for closure	Allows closure	Doesn't change recurrence rate, requires immobilization
	Dermofasciectomy: skin excision and replacement with skin graft	Lowest recurrence rate[12,103]	Longest recovery
Ligament or pulley release	Flexor tendon sheath	May avoid need for joint release	May require coverage: FTSG if <1 cm^2, flap, or dermal substitute followed by skin graft
	Accessory collateral	Does not destabilize joint	Does not correct the dorsal joint changes that result in early recontracture
	Checkrein/volar plate	Often allows full intraoperative correction	Same as ACL and destabilizes joint, risks postop snapping swan neck
Immobilization	Delayed until a few days postop	More comfortable	Not applicable for skin graft
	Intraoperative splint	Stabilize skin graft	May increase risk of flap or wound-margin ischemia
	PIP transarticular pin	Stabilize skin graft spanning PIP joint	Does not improve outcome of joint release[8]
Closure	Open	Less pain	Appearance stressful for some patients
	Closed	Shorter bandage duration	Suture removal; increased risk of marginal necrosis

ACL, Anterior cruciate ligament; *FTSG,* full-thickness skin graft; *PIP,* proximal interphalangeal.

additional benefit. Relative indications for different technical choices in fasciectomy are listed earlier in Table 4.5.

Indications. Fasciectomy is indicated for failed minimally invasive treatment, for diffuse disease, for concurrent treatment of secondary pathology, or surgeon/patient preference.

Contraindications. Fasciectomy is contraindicated for patients for whom a long operation, a long recovery, or proper postoperative therapy is not possible. Segmental fasciectomy is contraindicated for cases in which skin shortage itself is severe enough to limit extension or if treatment of secondary pathology requires wide exposure. Regional fasciectomy is contraindicated for hands that have diffuse skin tightness or skin shortage greater than what local flaps could be expected to correct. Dermofasciectomy and skin grafting should be considered for such cases and for patients with a high diathesis score.

Preoperative Planning. Fasciectomy is performed as an outpatient procedure in a surgical setting. The procedure is performed either under general or regional anesthesia with tourniquet control or use of the wide awake local anesthetic no tourniquet (WALANT) technique. Provisional incisions should be considered for skin graft, lateral digital, or cross finger flap coverage of exposed flexor tendons in the event that a flexor tendon sheath breach results in a large area of exposed flexors that cannot be covered by primary wound closure. An alternative is to have available acellular dermal matrix to cover exposed tendons, followed by skin grafting as a secondary procedure.[34] Splinting is scheduled for fabrication during the first postoperative week.

Technique

Segmental Fasciectomy. This is performed using multiple short transverse or longitudinal "C"-shaped incisions (Figure 4.11). If nodules exist in continuity with cords, incisions are planned directly over the nodules. Otherwise, incisions are centered over points of maximum cord bowstringing. Nodules and cord segments are excised through these incisions to restore extension. No attempt is made to remove all cord pathology. The skin is closed, and a soft bandage is applied.

Regional Fasciectomy. This is performed through either longitudinal, longitudinal zigzag, or transverse incisions. Combinations of incisions are used for exposure of multiple fingers that converge in the palm (see Figure 4.11). Local flaps (Z- or Y–V-plasty) can be incorporated into the primary skin incisions (Figure 4.11). Incisions can be either contiguous or separate, but deep dissection is contiguous across the entire length of each excised cord and all visibly diseased tissue is removed. Helpful tips to minimize neurovascular injury consequences include the following:

- Search for spiral cords preoperatively.
- Transect cord(s) proximally to allow extension and improve early exposure.
- Follow neurovascular structures from uninvolved areas—proximal, distal, or retrovascular[66]—toward the diseased areas ("known to unknown").
- Use sharp rather than spreading (tearing) dissection: neurovascular structures will tear before cords.

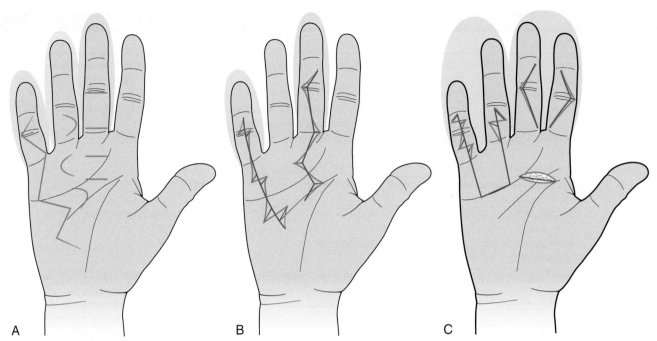

FIGURE 4.11 Common fasciectomy incisions. For flaps, initial incisions are red; blue lines are final closure. **A,** Incisions without skin rearrangement: zigzag (*little finger*), C (*ring finger*), transverse (*middle finger*); the C and transverse incisions are typical for segmental fasciectomy. **B,** Z-plasty (*little finger*), Y–V-plasty (*middle finger*). **C,** Combined incisions for multiple fingers: in continuity, with closure (*ring and little fingers*), discontinuous, with open palm technique (*index and middle fingers*).

- Don't skeletonize or strip the fat from the neurovascular bundles.
- Have microvascular equipment and microscope available.

Longitudinal incisions should always be converted to zigzag ones using Z-plasties at the time of closure. Zigzag incisions and flap insets are sutured. The *open palm* method is regional fasciectomy through transverse incisions, which are not closed, healing by wound contracture over the next 3 to 4 weeks.

Following this principle, transverse incisions or transverse limbs of zigzags may be closed or left open. Flaps or grafts may be used to achieve full closure, but the addition of small gap-filling skin grafts do not improve early outcome or later recurrence rates.[107] Splints are incorporated into the operative dressing to protect skin grafts; transarticular PIP joint pins may be placed to immobilize grafted joints. Otherwise, only a soft bandage is applied and splinting is initiated during the first postoperative week.

Dermofasciectomy

Dermofasciectomy is not simply fasciectomy augmented with skin graft, but rather functional unit replacement of skin and regional nonessential palmar soft tissues with full thickness skin graft. Recurrence rates are lower for dermofasciectomy than fasciectomy.[12] Replacement of skin with full thickness skin graft both changes soft tissue mechanics and inhibits myofibroblast activity.[91] Duration of recovery after dermofasciectomy averages 50% longer than fasciectomy.[103]

Indications. Dermofasciectomy is indicated for:
- Longitudinal skin shortage beyond the capacity of local flaps to correct
- Recurrent contracture with diffuse skin involvement or extensive scarring

- Skin irretrievably devascularized during surgery
- First procedure in selected young patients with strong diathesis profile

Contraindications. Dermofasciectomy is contraindicated in patients for whom a long operation, a long recovery, or proper postoperative therapy is not possible and in patients for whom skin grafting is not advisable.

Preoperative Planning. Setting and anesthesia are the same as for fasciectomy. In primary dermofasciectomy, skin excision in the palm is planned as a truncated ellipse centered over the distal palmar crease, and in the fingers as a rectangular palmar hemicircumference of the pulp space (Figure 4.12). Incisions can be left separate or connected with access incisions planned in tension-free lines for wide extensile exposure. Plans are modified as needed to incorporate scarred or shortened skin. If possible, skin graft is avoided over the palmar prominences of the metacarpal heads to avoid durability and sensitivity issues.

Incisions are planned such that the healed junctions of graft and normal skin will follow tension-free lines. *Full thickness* skin graft donor sites are planned in hairless areas, if available (e.g., the proximal medial ipsilateral forearm or the groin crease lateral to the femoral triangle). Full thickness skin grafts may be used to cover up to 1 cm² of exposed flexor tendon if the periphery of the graft lies on a well-vascularized bed. Larger areas of flexor tendon exposure should be covered with a local flap or acellular dermal matrix, as described for fasciectomy.

Technique. Dermofasciectomy as a primary procedure is styled after regional fasciectomy with wide extensile exposure. Dermofasciectomy for recurrence after fasciectomy can be performed similar to segmental fasciectomy, limiting exposure to the areas planned for excision, avoiding dissection through scarred tissues other than as needed for exposure for skin

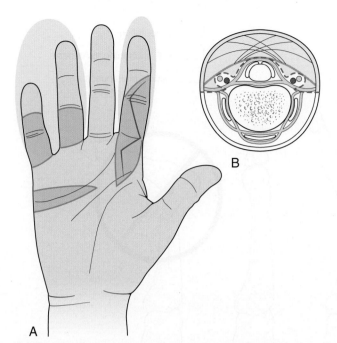

FIGURE 4.12 Dermofasciectomy variations. **A,** Segmental replacement (*ring and little fingers*), extensile, excising prior scarred skin (*index finger*). **B,** Block of tissue excision including Cleland ligaments for digital dermofasciectomy.

excision. In the digit, all lateral digital fascia including Cleland ligament tissues are excised (see Figure 4.11). For little finger involvement, the abductor digiti minimi fascia is also excised.

After all zones of skin replacement are excised, the tourniquet is released, hemostasis is achieved, vascularity is confirmed, and access incisions are closed. Transarticular PIP joint pins can be placed to immobilize grafted joints. Skin graft templates of the defects are then created and used to plan and harvest full thickness skin grafts. After donor site closure, skin grafts are inset, and the hand is bandaged, incorporating a resting splint.

Special Cases

Dorsal Dupuytren Nodules. Most DDN do not require treatment, but occasionally are tender, painful, or a cosmetic concern. They may tether the extensor mechanism, limiting flexion, or they may spontaneously regress. Steroid injections are particularly helpful for relieving symptoms of pain, tenderness, and extensor tightness, for example, 5 mg triamcinolone or equivalent using a lateral approach, angling the needle tangential to the skin, aiming for the center of the nodule. Steroid injections have a high response rate, but also at least 50% recurrence and a common finding of temporary poststeroid pink shiny skin at the injection site. Because there is no plane between the extensor mechanism and the similar appearing nodule tissue, attempts at excision risk extensor tendon injury with secondary boutonnière. Most patients do well after excision, but recurrence or persistent tenderness is common. DDN excision is indicated only in selected cases.

Severe PIP Contracture. Fixed PIP contractures greater than 60 degrees are often associated with secondary extensor mechanism laxity, capsuloligamentous tightness, and flexor tendon sheath tightness. Surgery often results in palmar skin tightness even if scars are well planned. Treatment of severe PIP contrac-

tures with inadequate palmar skin reserve requires either *soft tissue lengthening* or *skeletal shortening*.

A staged approach with preliminary *skeletal extension torque* followed by fasciectomy or dermofasciectomy has been shown to have better outcomes than single-stage release and fasciectomy.[20] Boutonnière associated with severe recurrent PIP contractures is most predictably managed with DIP arthrodesis in addition to treatment of the PIP contracture. Skeletal shortening (i.e., PIP arthrodesis, middle phalangectomy, amputation) (Figure 4.13) is an option when soft tissue lengthening is not possible. PIP arthrodesis is predictable, but results in a flexion arc mismatched with the rest of the fingers. *Middle phalangectomy* constructs an IP joint between proximal and distal phalanges, which maintains a normal flexion arc at the PIP level.[102]

Amputation is an option for patients who have failed results with other options. DC is the most common indication for elective finger amputation, and has high patient satisfaction for those who request, rather than simply consent to the procedure. If amputation is selected, *ray amputation* is indicated for combined PIP + MCP contractures, and *PIP disarticulation* is appropriate for isolated PIP contractures with full MCP extension. *PIP implant arthroplasty* and fasciectomy has been reported as a salvage procedure, but has not achieved popularity. Middle phalanx extension osteotomy is not recommended; the author's experience is that gains made by osteotomy are negated by additional joint flexion, which simply reduces the flexion arc without improving extension.

Severe Composite Contracture. Composite MCP + PIP contractures greater than 135 degrees (Tubiana stage IV) present unique problems beyond secondary joint and tendon changes.

Skin maceration is common and may not be obvious without thorough examination. If present, the affected areas should be treated to reduce risk of postoperative infection. An effective routine is cleansing with rubbing alcohol, using cotton-tipped applicators for inaccessible areas, and drying with a thin towel and a hair dryer set on cool, four times a day for several days preoperatively.

Limited access to the digits may be addressed in stages, first to open the palm and MCP joints and second to treat the digits 3 months later. This approach is appropriate for both open and minimally invasive procedures and may be necessary for intractable skin maceration. Alternatively, PNF may be used as a first step to improve exposure for fasciectomy at the same setting.[36]

Cortical reorganization may occur with chronic severe contractures. In such cases, when the patient attempts to straighten his or her fingers, the "reorganized" digits actively flex as the others actively extend. Functionally, this mimics amputation—an improvement for fingers that otherwise only extend enough to be a nuisance. This is a contraindication to treatment aimed at restoring function of the affected digit(s).

❖ AUTHOR'S PREFERRED METHOD OF TREATMENT

PNF is the least expensive and least complicated treatment option, and has high patient satisfaction. PNF should be considered as the first intervention for Dupuytren disease in patients with a low diathesis score for whom a shorter recovery is more important than early recurrence. PNF can be performed as an office procedure and does not require changes in medication or diet. With proper planning, it may be performed at the

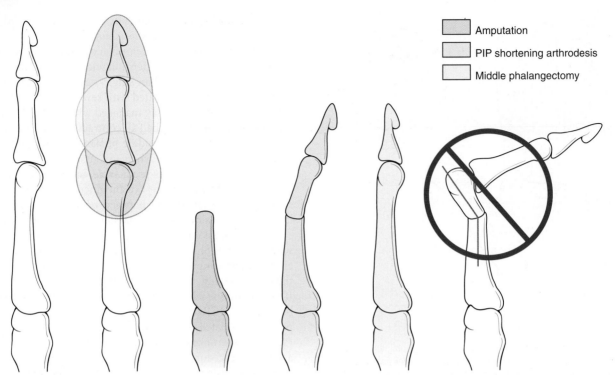

Amputation

PIP shortening arthrodesis

Middle phalangectomy

FIGURE 4.13 Skeletal-shortening procedures for severe recurrent proximal interphalangeal (PIP) contractures includes amputation (*red*), PIP-shortening arthrodesis (*blue*), and middle phalangectomy (*green*). Extension osteotomy (*far right*) results in increased PIP joint flexion, which limits its usefulness.

time of the patient's first office visit and does not require scheduled follow-up.

Patient Instructions

Before the Procedure

If PNF is planned for the first office visit, patients should have a previsit screening to confirm suitability for PNF. For patients traveling to have PNF on their first office visit, the diagnosis of Dupuytren contracture and suitability for PNF should be assessed by having them send or email images of their hands for review prior to booking a date. When setting a procedure date, patients should be instructed that on arrival, the hand to be treated must be free of recent or healing injuries; they should plan to avoid strenuous gripping for 1 week postprocedure. Prior to the office visit, rings should be removed from affected fingers. Patients who normally take an anxiolytic medication for routine dental work should plan to do the same for this procedure.

During the Procedure

Best results require the patient to follow these guidelines as an active participant during the procedure.

1. Patients should be instructed to consciously relax their fingers while you are working. This aids your ability to palpate tethering cords and avoids bowstringing the flexor tendons in the areas where the work is being done.
2. Patients should be instructed to report any uncomfortable sensations and to describe both their location (whether it's where the needle is or out at the fingertip) and quality (sharp vs. electrical). This will help you assess whether or not the sensation represents digital nerve stimulation from needle proximity.

3. Patients should be instructed and asked to demonstrate "scratching" movement (short arc active finger flexion and extension), as you may ask them to do this again during the procedure to check proximity of the needle to flexor tendons. This also serves as a preoperative check for active finger flexion, which might otherwise be missed in the evaluation of a severe contracture or boutonnière deformity.
4. Patients should be asked to alert you if at any point they feel any numbness or tingling during the procedure.

After the Procedure

Expectations discussed with the patient prior to the procedure should include the following. The patient should remove bandages the same day to prevent maceration. Skin tears occur in a minority of patients, but on occasion can be dramatic. Skin tears are managed with bandages changed frequently enough to avoid maceration and can be expected to heal within a week or two. Patients are encouraged to chill and elevate the operated hand for the first 36 hours after the procedure. Strenuous or sports-related gripping should be avoided for 1 week, including golf, tennis, biking, rowing, gripping during weight training, push-ups, pull-ups, shoveling, and so on. It's important to be very specific about this because there is often little or no pain with these activities, but they may provoke a delayed inflammatory reaction that can mimic infection and may last for days.

Typical immediate outcome is up to 90 degrees improvement of composite (MCP + PIP) extension and an average of 50% improvement of PIP extension. It is common for partial corrections to improve for several months after release, with or without splinting. Recurrence significant enough to require a repeat procedure occurs at a rate of 8% per year.[68] Repeat procedures are usually possible and reasonable if the initial release worked well, the release lasted at least one year, the recontracture is due to a palpable cord, or adequate skin reserve remains. Repeat release can be expected to result in similar improvement as the prior release, with some diminishing returns and less predictability. There are no clear data to either support or discourage splinting after PNF. Soft indications for splinting include preoperative isolated PIP with MCP hyperextension, preoperative composite contracture of 90 degrees or greater, postoperative extensor lag, and patient request.

Planning

Planning Portals

Ideal needle entry areas are over tensionable cords palpable beneath mobile skin. Portals may be marked preoperatively or intraoperatively. Single portals are best planned directly over the most prominent area of the cord. Dual portals on each side of the cord are used for broad cords in the palm and for bowstringing lateral digital cords to improve safe access, and in areas where skin tethering is thought to pose an increased risk for skin tear. Avoid planning portals in areas of poor skin reserve, including areas in which the skin blanches on stretch. Avoid portals in areas of skin tethering from skin creases, scars, dimples, or nodules.

Some nodules resemble cords, but can be distinguished by lack of softening when the finger is flexed. Cords may have nodular involvement, and it may not be possible to avoid nodules altogether. Portals proximal to Kaplan's line should also be avoided if possible because this area may remain sensitive for weeks, similar to "pillar pain" after open carpal tunnel release. Proximal or distal interphalangeal portals are planned a few millimeters offset from the flexion creases, and oblique needle paths may be used to detach the crease dermis from the underlying cord, which improves release gains and reduces the chance of a crease tear.

Dimples

Skin dimples are due to traction from retinacular fibers attached to contracted cords. The depth of dimples should be confirmed by direct inspection or with the use of a probe. A disposable dental floss passer works well as a probe and can be used as a dipstick: povidone iodine is placed into the dimple, and the level of iodine remaining on the withdrawn probe indicates depth. Dimples may be associated with deep needle sensitivity, as discussed in the following. Dimple sinuses may extend deep and follow a path tangential to the skin, posing a risk for transection by needle release adjacent to the visible dimple.

Digital Cords

The biggest concern in treating digital cords is the location of the neurovascular bundle. In most cases, the neurovascular bundle lies deep beneath cords at the PIP joint. Away from the PIP joint, the neurovascular bundle usually lies central to lateral and spiral cords and lateral to central cords[70] (Figure 4.10). Doppler ultrasound is useful in this context.

Spiral Bundles

Spiral bundles should be suspected if there are areas in which a subdermal cord is in continuity with a cord segment lying beneath bulky subcutaneous tissue. The vascular pulse of a spiral cord is occasionally palpable, and the displaced digital nerve is occasionally tender to firm, direct pressure while passively tensioning the cord. Doppler probe is a more definitive examination tool of these fleshy areas and should be pointed to areas where the neurovascular bundle should not normally lie. For example, the Doppler tip may be angled tangential to the skin to listen to areas more superficial than the normal course of the neurovascular bundle. Portals should not be used at the direct level of an identified spiral cord, but taking advantage of the spiral anatomy, may be planned 8 to 10 millimeters proximal or distal to the area in which the bundle has been identified as most superficial. Ultrasound imaging may also be useful in this context.

Procedure

Positioning

During the procedure, the patient may rest in a supine or semi-recumbent position. If the patient is seated, there should be a simple mechanism to either have the chair recline or transfer the patient to a supine position in the event of a vasovagal reaction.

Assistance

Because sterile gloves are not required, this is not mandatory, but an assistant is helpful.

Antisepsis

Immediately prior to the procedure, the patient should wash his or her hands to clean and degrease the skin. The procedure may be performed using *field sterility*, similar to starting an intravenous line. The area of interest is prepped with a povidone iodine solution or other topical antiseptic solutions. Sterile drapes and sterile gloves are not needed. Needles are handled in a manner to preserve sterility of the metal portion of the needle. A mask and eye cover are recommended to protect the surgeon in the event of backspray during anesthetic injection or joint manipulation.

Anesthetic

The goal is *superficial intradermal anesthetic injection*, avoiding subcutaneous spread and potential digital nerve conduction block. Plain lidocaine buffered 1:10 with sodium bicarbonate given via a 30-gauge needle on a 3-cc syringe reduces injection pain. To confine anesthetic to the dermis, the needle tip is placed about 1 mm into the dermis and injection is given as the needle is withdrawn. Pinpoint local anesthesia develops immediately with this technique and lasts 15 to 30 minutes. Lidocaine with epinephrine or bupivacaine may be used, but their prolonged effect is a disadvantage if a conduction block develops. If a block develops that precludes desired work, plain lidocaine effect usually wears off rapidly enough to resume during the same setting; long-lasting anesthetics may require deferring completion to the following day.

Bleeding during the procedure is minimal and does not justify the need for epinephrine. Ideally, digital nerve block is avoided and the fingertip remains sensate throughout the procedure. Tip sensitivity is checked prior to each anesthetic injection, prior to beginning each new portal, and at regular intervals between injections. Anesthetic joint injections and management of finger numbness are discussed in later sections.

Needle Size

The tip of a hypodermic needle has two short scalpel-sharp cutting edges. Needle-tip proportions are such that the length of each cutting edge measures slightly less than twice the diameter of the needle. Any needle gauge can be used; the author recommends a short 25-gauge needle. An 18-gauge needle has a terminal blade length of 2.6 mm; a 25-gauge needle has a diameter of 0.5 mm and a terminal blade length of 0.8 mm.

Smaller-gauge needles require more passes to divide cords but have the advantage of greater control and less likelihood of inadvertently severing a digital nerve with a single pass. Smaller needles are more flexible, and using the shortest possible needle gives the best control of the tip. Some surgeons hold a hypodermic needle directly with their fingertips, but mounting the needle on a 3-cc Luer-lock syringe is recommended for control and sterility.

Portal Sequence

An important safety factor of needle aponeurotomy is the ability to monitor digital nerve function through the procedure. For this reason, the safest approach is to begin distally and work proximally. That way, if a digital nerve block develops, the procedure may be continued at the more proximal portal level, where the nerve is still sensitive to local irritation. By the same logic, if several fingers are being treated at the same sitting, completing all work on the digits before moving into the palm prevents an unexpected common digital nerve block from affecting an adjacent digit before its release.

Needle Maneuvers

Needle bevel alignment should be maintained perpendicular to the cord; otherwise the needle may not cut the fibers. It's helpful to note the bevel orientation in relation to the syringe markings to reference while the tip is inserted and out of view. The three basic needle maneuvers are (1) clear, (2) perforate, and (3) sweep (Figure 4.14). After initial needle insertion through the dermis, a local exploration is performed to define the surface of the cord by feel. The needle is used to divide vertical retinacular fibers and clear a path superficial to the cord the width of the cord. The needle is then used to perforate into the cord a millimeter or two in depth at multiple points across this transverse line. This divides fibers and also reveals unexpectedly displaced nerves. If no unexpected tenderness is encountered with perforation, the needle is then used to graze or sweep the surface of the cord transversely to the previously perforated depth.

It is possible to divide cords entirely by continuing to perforate through the depth of the cord, but sweeping is more efficient, requires fewer needle passes, and leaves the smallest internal wound. The process of perforating and then sweeping is then repeated to divide the cord progressively from superficial to deep. While sweeping, needle depth insertion is critical (Figure 4.15). If the needle tip is inserted to a depth beyond the terminal cutting edge, the blunt needle shaft proximal to the tip will engage the cord, preventing the needle edge from cutting until enough force is exerted that the needle tip suddenly pops out of the area of cord entry, cutting as it exits. This type of uncontrolled motion can be avoided by estimating the depth of insertion by feel and using a light touch. The syringe should be

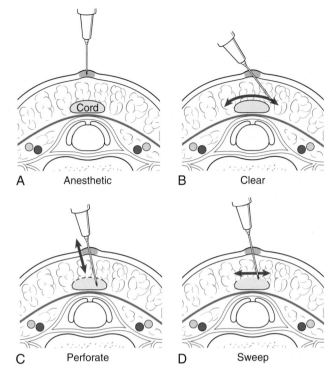

FIGURE 4.14 Maneuvers for percutaneous fasciotomy. **A,** Anesthetic is limited to the dermis to reduce the chance of a conduction block. **B,** The needle tip is used to clear a working area superficial to the cord. **C,** The needle perforates a line of points across the cord using a reciprocating motion. **D,** The bevel of the needle scores the surface of the cord to progressively divide fibers from superficial to deep.

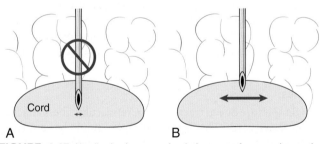

FIGURE 4.15 Needle depth penetration is important for sweeping motion. **A,** Cord penetration beyond the bevel prevents lateral motion. **B,** Optimum placement for scoring the surface of the cord is with only the distal needle bevel engaged.

held with a light grip to avoid an unexpected shish-kabab event if the patient makes a sudden move.

Cord Traction

Cord fibers are cut most efficiently while under constant tension, which also provides constant feedback regarding the status of cord division. Cords may be tensioned by pulling the finger into extension, but this also tensions the flexor tendons, potentially pulling them into harm's way. There are two alternatives to passive composite pull. The first is to passively extend the most affected joint, but flex the adjacent joint (or, at least, not pull on it). For example, while working on a cord contracting the MCP joint, flex the PIP joint and extend the MCP joint; for cords affecting the PIP joint, flex the DIP joint while extending the PIP joint.

The second option is to take advantage of the anatomic fact that cords are tethered to the dermis: using your fingertip to create traction on the skin proximal or distal to the portal in a direction away from the portal will also tension the cord from its attachment to the skin. This is also a helpful alternative if joints are painful to passive extension. Finally, it's worth checking that the patient isn't unconsciously flexing his or her fingers against your pull, which both bowstrings flexors and prevents assessment of cord release.

Needle Problems

If the needle bends, you are using too much force, most likely because the needle tip is inserted too deeply, as previously described. An advantage of using a 25-gauge needle is that it is the most sensitive indicator of this. Replace the needle. Needle edges dull quickly and can burr easily; expect to replace the needle for every portal or two. Signs of a dull needle edge include slow progress dividing the cord, drag, catching, and unexpected tenderness. When in doubt, replace the needle. A 25-gauge needle costs 11 cents.

Flexor Tendon Issues

Flexor tendons are at risk for injury. The patient should be reminded to relax his or her fingers ("just let them go limp") to avoid tensioning the flexors. Bowstring the cord, not the flexors. In addition, active posturing by the patient—either flexion or extension—makes it more difficult to palpate cords and contractures. If there is any question regarding flexor proximity, check by having the patient gently perform short arc "scratching motion" finger flexion and extension with the needle in place, cautioning the patient to not make a fist.

Needle contact with a moving tendon will either produce a gritty feel of the needle or will visibly move the needle, depending on whether the needle tip is on or in the tendon. If there is a confirmed breach of the flexor tendon sheath, use of that portal should be discontinued, and the tendon should be checked for continuity, triggering, and pain with flexion against resistance. If there is evidence or strong suspicion of a mechanically significant tendon injury, that issue assumes management priority. If not, the procedure may be continued at a different level and the patient should be cautioned to avoid strenuous gripping for 1 month to reduce the chance of provoking tendinitis.

Nerve Issues

Distal to proximal portal sequence should be followed, including finishing the fingers before starting in the palm, as described previously. Fingertip sensitivity should be checked: prior to each anesthetic injection, prior to starting each new portal, and at regular intervals in between. Even with careful technique, digital nerve block may develop from anesthetic diffusion or digital nerve contusion and may appear without any precedent event or patient awareness of it developing. If the patient develops a digital nerve block, the safest step is to continue only *proximal* to the last anesthetized portal.

Pain or Paresthesia With Needle Movement

Patients may experience pain with needle maneuvers, and this should always be evaluated. Cords are insensate and do not require anesthetic. The capsuloligamentous structures and associated cruciate pulleys of the proximal[18] and distal[17] interphalangeal joints have at least proprioceptive sensory innervation, which may confer sensitivity to needle contact. It is not known if there is sensory innervation of the other zones of the flexor tendon sheath or of the annular pulleys.

Following intradermal injection, needle maneuvering is usually painless. Pain during the procedure may be due to contact of the needle tip with unanesthetized adjacent deep dermis; joint capsule or cruciate pulley areas, neurovascular bundle or adjacent Pacinian corpuscles; or pressure on any of these structures from the needle shaft with lateral motion. If the patient has unexpected pain with needle maneuvering, follow the evaluation protocol shown in Figure 4.16. Traction on deep dermis from retinacular fiber involvement may result in subdermal tenderness deep beneath or adjacent to skin creases or dimples. If so, anesthetic injection into the dermis at the level of the crease or dimple usually relieves this needle tenderness (Figure 4.17).

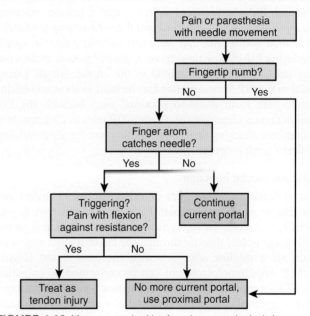

FIGURE 4.16 Management algorithm for pain or paresthesia during percutaneous fasciotomy.

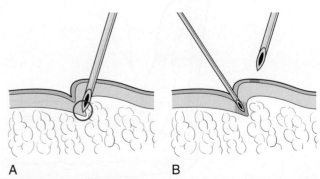

A   B

FIGURE 4.17 A, Deep tenderness adjacent to a dimple may be due to innervated deep dermis of a dimple pulled into the path of the needle. **B,** After checking the depth of the dimple to confirm that there is not a dimple sinus in harm's way, the dermis at the depth of the dimple may be anesthetized and the procedure continued without pain.

Uncommonly, a cord may remain tender to needle penetration despite these steps. If there is no possibility of dimple-related tenderness, this may represent nerve end organ or digital nerve tethering from the cord. An option in this situation is to inject the cord itself with 0.1 to 0.2 cc local anesthetic directly in the area of sensitivity. Following this, check the fingertip for sensibility, and if the fingertip is not numb, return to cord division at the current portal. If a conduction block develops, discontinue work at this level and proceed to the next most proximal level (Figure 4.16).

Portal-Level Goal

Release at a given portal level is continued until the cord releases or the cord is no longer tensionable or palpable. Progress is often incremental, a few degrees at a time: a definitive "pop" or "snap" may or may not occur.

Needling the PIP

PIP contractures have concurrent involvement of multiple structures more often than MCP contractures.[105] It's helpful to approach PIP release in a stepwise sequential fashion, releasing the most obvious palpable cord and then reassessing to identify additional constraints that were not initially palpable. Cords producing PIP contractures traverse the PIP flexion creases but may only be palpable proximal to the crease. Portals placed distal to the PIP flexion creases may be used to allow an oblique needle path from distal to proximal deep beneath the PIP flexion creases (Figure 4.18). During PIP release, it's important to continue checking fingertip sensibility and for the possibility of flexor tendon contact.

Joint Anesthetic Injection

Intraarticular anesthetic joint injection improves comfort and the effectiveness of interphalangeal joint manipulation. A predictable technique for interphalangeal joint injection is to use a 30-gauge needle directly through the flexor tendon and volar plate via a midline approach with the joint flexed (Figure 4.18).[69] Anesthetic placement can be confirmed by palpating dorsal joint capsule distention during injection. The advantages of this approach are greater predictability of achieving intraarticular infiltration and less likelihood of inadvertent digital nerve or sheath block. Joint anesthesia usually develops within 2 minutes of injection.

Manipulation

Final manipulations are performed after all releases are complete and interphalangeal anesthetic joint injections are performed. Because multiple cord locations are common at the PIP joint, a series of stretching maneuvers are performed in sequence. Because cords are midpalmar and palmar-lateral, the joint is stretched in the opposite directions of each: straight dorsal, dorsal–ulnar, and dorsal–radial. These maneuvers are first performed individually on each joint, leaving the adjacent joints slack, and then performed as composite stretches of all joints.

Postprocedure

Postprocedure care was described earlier, in the "Patient Instructions After the Procedure" section.

> **CRITICAL POINTS**
>
> - The ideal patient has well-defined cords, supple skin, and is able to tolerate an awake procedure.
> - Preoperative discussion should include the patient's role in relaxing, reporting pain or numbness, and moving his or her fingers when asked.
> - Portals are planned at cord levels where the skin is soft and the cord is subdermal.
> - Use intradermal anesthetic, avoiding subcutaneous injection.
> - Release through distal-to-proximal portals, and avoid working in an area with a nerve block.
> - Check nerve and tendon status before each portal and regularly in between.
> - Caution patient to avoid strenuous gripping for 1 week postprocedure, even if the patient has no pain (which is usually the case).

THE FUTURE

Dupuytren disease has parallels with rheumatoid arthritis. Both are systemic conditions that commonly lead patients to hand surgeons. Both have inspired a diverse array of innovative procedures with impressive early outcomes but high long-term

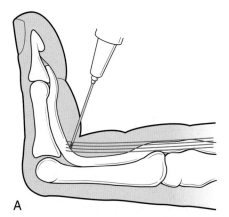
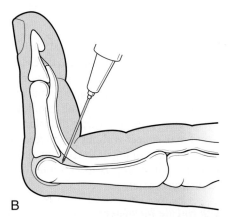

FIGURE 4.18 Palmar approaches to the proximal interphalangeal (PIP) joint. **A,** Cords producing PIP contractures often cross beneath the PIP skin flexion crease and may be approached distal to this crease. **B,** Intraarticular anesthetic may be given with a small gauge needle through the flexor tendon and volar plate to anesthetize the joint, but not the rest of the finger, helpful to reduce pain during manipulation.

failure rates. Senior hand surgeons will recall when this resemblance abruptly changed: anti-TNF drugs suddenly reduced the need for rheumatoid hand surgery, proof that they modified the disease biology—a first. A parallel change is needed for Dupuytren disease, which is a medical, not a surgical, condition.

Minimally invasive treatments have recently gained popularity despite higher recurrence rates, largely because the morbidity of fasciectomy makes it an unpopular choice with patients, a scenario that also occurred in the late 1800s and again in the mid-1900s. This is change without progress, a persistent theme in the history of this disease. Collagen is not the culprit; it is simply the footprint left by the primary biology.

A 1990 treatment review included diagrams of 67 different incisions recommended for fasciectomy,[71] and many more have been described since. This alone is testimony that local treatment is the wrong focus of effort. Because hand surgeons are the primary caregivers for this disease, the responsibility to our patients is to change this focus to the development of disease-modifying interventions by engaging colleagues in the fields of molecular biology, genomics, and fibrosis research. Tamoxifen has been shown to reduce recurrence rates[21] after fasciectomy in high-risk patients, proof that it is possible to modify DD biology—a first.

Treatment with microRNA or SiRNA to downregulate the production of TGFβ1 or its receptors, identification of molecules that inhibit or bind to TGFβ1 or other implicated cytokines (the strategy used to develop anti-TNF drugs), and molecular stenting to prevent excessive collagen crosslinking are the types of approaches that must be explored to change the landscape of Dupuytren disease. Absent this, the cycle will continue to repeat.

For Case Studies, Videos, and more, please visit ExpertConsult.com.

REFERENCES

1. Abe Y, Rokkaku T, Ofuchi S, et al: An objective method to evaluate the risk of recurrence and extension of Dupuytren's disease. *J Hand Surg [Br]* 29:427–430, 2004.
2. Arafa M, Steingold RF, Noble J: The incidence of Dupuytren's disease in patients with rheumatoid arthritis. *J Hand Surg [Br]* 9:165–166, 1984.
3. Baird KS, Crossan JF, Ralston SH: Abnormal growth factor and cytokine expression in Dupuytren's contracture. *J Clin Pathol* 46(5):425–428, 1993.
4. Balaguer T, David S, Ihrai T, et al: Histological staging and Dupuytren's disease recurrence or extension after surgical treatment: a retrospective study of 124 patients. *J Hand Surg Eur* 34:493–496, 2009.
5. Barclay TL: Edema following operation for Dupuytren's contracture. *Plast Reconstr Surg Transpl Bull* 23(4):348–360, 1959.
6. Beaudreuil J, Allard A, Zerkak D, et al: Unité rhumatologique des affections de la main (URAM) scale: development and validation of a tool to assess Dupuytren's disease-specific disability. *Arthritis Care Res (Hoboken)* 63:1448–1455, 2011.
7. Becker K, Tinschert S, Lienert A, et al: The importance of genetic susceptibility in Dupuytren's disease. *Clin Gen* 87:483–487, 2015.
8. Belusa L, Buck-Gramcko D, Partecke BD: Results of interphalangeal joint arthrolysis in patients with Dupuytren disease. *Handchir Mikrochir Plast Chir* 29(3):158–163, 1997.
9. Bhavsar S, Nimigan A, Hackam DG, et al: Keloid scarring, but not Dupuytren's contracture, is associated with unexplained carotid atherosclerosis. *Clin Invest Med* 32:E95–E102, 2009.
10. Bisson MA, Mudera V, McGrouther DA, et al: The contractile properties and responses to tensional loading of Dupuytren's disease-derived fibroblasts are altered: a cause of the contracture? *Plast Reconstr Surg* 113:64–611, 2004.
11. Brickley-Parsons D, Glimcher MJ, Smith RJ, et al: Biochemical changes in the collagen of the palmar fascia in patients with Dupuytren's disease. *J Bone Jt Surg Am* 63:787–797, 1981.
12. Brotherston TM, Balakrishnan C, Milner RH, et al: Long-term follow-up of dermo-fasciectomy for Dupuytren's contracture. *Br J Plast Surg* 47(6):440–443, 1994.
13. Brouet JP: Etude de 1000 dossiers de maladie de Dupuytren. In Tubiana R, Hueston JT, editors: *La maladie Dupuytren*, ed 3, Paris, 1986, Expansion Scientifique, pp 98–105.
14. Burge P, Hoy G, Regan P, et al: Smoking, alcohol and the risk of Dupuytren's contracture. *J Bone Joint Surg Br* 79(2):206–210, 1997.
15. Castella LF, Buscemi L, Godbout C, et al: A new lock-step mechanism of matrix remodelling based on subcellular contractile events. *J Cell Sci* 123:1751–1760, 2010.
16. Chansky HA, Trumble TE, Conrad EU, et al: Evidence for a polyclonal etiology of palmar fibromatosis. *J Hand Surg [Am]* 24(2):339–344, 1999.
17. Chikenji T, Berger RA, Fujimiya M, et al: Distribution of nerve endings in human distal interphalangeal joint and surrounding structures. *J Hand Surg [Am]* 36(3):406–412, 2011.
18. Chikenji T, Suzuki D, Fujimiya M, et al: Distribution of nerve endings in the human proximal interphalangeal joint and surrounding structures. *J Hand Surg [Am]* 35(8):1286–1293, 2010.
19. Citron N, Hearnden A: Skin tension in the aetiology of Dupuytren's disease: a prospective trial. *J Hand Surg [Br]* 28(6):528–530, 2003.
20. Craft RO, Smith AA, Coakley BB, et al: Preliminary soft-tissue distraction versus checkrein ligament release after fasciectomy in the treatment of Dupuytren proximal interphalangeal joint contractures. *Plast Reconstr Surg* 128:113–1107, 2011.
21. Degreef I, De Smet L: Dupuytren disease: on our way to a cure? *Acta Orthop Belg* 79:243–249, 2013.
22. Degreef I, De Smet L: Risk factors in Dupuytren's diathesis: is recurrence after surgery predictable? *Acta Orthop Belg* 77:27–32, 2011.
23. Degreef I, De Smet LA: High prevalence of Dupuytren's disease in Flanders. *Acta Orthop Belg* 76(3):316–320, 2010.
24. Denkler K: Surgical complications associated with fasciectomy for Dupuytren's disease: a 20-year review of the English literature. *Eplasty* 10:e15, 2010.
25. Descatha A, Jauffret P, Chastang JF, et al: Should we consider Dupuytren's contracture as work-related? A review and meta-analysis of an old debate. *BMC Musculoskelet Disord* 12:96, 2011.
26. Dias JJ, Braybrooke J: Dupuytren's contracture: an audit of the outcomes of surgery. *J Hand Surg [Br]* 31(5):514–521, 2006.
27. Dias JJ, Singh HP, Ullah A, et al: Patterns of recontracture after surgical correction of Dupuytren disease. *J Hand Surg [Am]* 38:1987–1993, 2013.
28. Dibenedetti DD, Nguyen D, Zografos L, et al: Prevalence, incidence, and treatments of Dupuytren's disease in the United States: results from a population-based study. *Hand* 6(2):149–158, 2011.
29. Dolmans GH, de Bock GH, Werker PM: Dupuytren diathesis and genetic risk. *J Hand Surg [Am]* 37:2106–2111, 2012.
30. Dolmans GH, Werker PM, Hennies HC, et al: Wnt signaling and Dupuytren's disease. *N Engl J Med* 365(4):307–317, 2011.
31. Draviaraj KP, Chakrabarti I: Functional outcome after surgery for Dupuytren's contracture: a prospective study. *J Hand Surg [Am]* 29:88–804, 2004.
32. Egawa T, Senrui H, Horiki A: Epidemiology of the oriental patient. In *Dupuytren's dis. biol. treat*, New York, 1990, Churchill Livingstone, pp 239–245.
33. Elliot D, Ragoowansi R: Dupuytren's disease secondary to acute injury, infection or operation distal to the elbow in the ipsilateral upper limb—a historical review. *J Hand Surg [Br]* 30(2):148–156, 2005.
34. Ellis CV, Kulber DA: A cellular dermal matrices in hand reconstruction. *Plast Reconstr Surg* 130(5 Suppl 2):256S–69S, 2012.
35. Elsahy NI: Doppler ultrasound detection of displaced neurovascular bundles in Dupuytren's contracture. *Plast Reconstr Surg* 57:104–105, 1976.
36. Erne HC: Downgrading severe stages of Dupuytren's contracture to simplify partial aponeurectomy using percutaneous needle fasciotomy. *Plast Reconstr Surg* 133:79e–80e, 2014.
37. Geoghegan JM, Forbes J, Clark DI, et al: Dupuytren's disease risk factors. *J Hand Surg [Br]* 29(5):423–426, 2004.
38. Grotesman A: *Clinical assessment in Dupuytren's disease. Presentation at Dupuytren's Disease Symposium*, New York, Stony Brook University Medical Center, Stony Brook. 4/17/2010.
39. Gudmundsson KG, Arngrímsson R, Sigfússon N, et al: Increased total mortality and cancer mortality in men with Dupuytren's disease: a 15-year follow-up study. *J Clin Epidemiol* 55(1):5–10, 2002.
40. Gudmundsson KG, Arngrimsson R, Jónsson T: Eighteen years follow-up study of the clinical manifestations and progression of Dupuytren's disease. *Scandinavian J Rheumatol* 30(1):31–34, 2001.
41. Gudmundsson KG, Arngrimsson R, Sigfusson N, et al: Epidemiology of Dupuytren's disease: clinical, serological, and social assessment. The Reykjavik Study. *J Clin Epidemiol* 53(3):291–296, 2000.
42. Gudmundsson KG, Jónsson T, Arngrimsson R, et al: Association of Morbus Ledderhose with Dupuytren's contracture. *Foot Ankle Int* 34(6):841–845, 2013.

43. Hansen M, Koskinen SO, Petersen SG, et al: Ethinyl oestradiol administration in women suppresses synthesis of collagen in tendon in response to exercise. *J Physiol* 586:316–3005, 2008.

44. Hayton MJ, Bayat A, Chapman DS, et al: Isolated and spontaneous correction of proximal interphalangeal joint contractures in Dupuytren's disease: An exploratory analysis of the efficacy and safety of collagenase clostridium histolyticum. *Clin Drug Investig* 33(12):905–912, 2013.

45. Hettiaratchy S, Tonkin MA, Edmunds IA: Spiralling of the neurovascular bundle in Dupuytren's disease. *J Hand Surg Eur Vol* 35:103–108, 2010.

46. Hindocha S, Stanley JK, Watson JS, et al: Revised Tubiana's staging system for assessment of disease severity in Dupuytren's disease-preliminary clinical findings. *Hand (NY)* 3:6–80, 2008.

47. Hindocha S, Stanley JK, Watson S, et al: Dupuytren's diathesis revisited: Evaluation of prognostic indicators for risk of disease recurrence. *J Hand Surg [Am]* 31:1626–1634, 2006.

48. Hindocha S, John S, Stanley JK, et al: The heritability of Dupuytren's disease: familial aggregation and its clinical significance. *J Hand Surg [Am]* 31(2):204–210, 2006.

49. Holland AJ, McGrouther DA: Dupuytren's disease and the relationship between the transverse and longitudinal fibers of the palmar fascia: a dissection study. *Clin Anat* 10:97–103, 1997.

50. Holzer LA, Cor A, Pfandlsteiner G, et al: Expression of VEGF, its receptors, and HIF-1α in Dupuytren's disease. *Acta Orthop* 84(4):420–425, 2013.

51. Hsieh AH, Tsai CM, Ma QJ, et al: Time-dependent increases in type-III collagen gene expression in medical collateral ligament fibroblasts under cyclic strains. *J Orthop Res* 18:220–227, 2000.

52. Hu FZ, Nystrom A, Ahmed A, et al: Mapping of an autosomal dominant gene for Dupuytren's contracture to chromosome 16q in a Swedish family. *Clin Genet* 68(5):49–424, 2005.

53. Hueston JT: Dorsal Dupuytren's disease. *J Hand Surg [Am]* 7:384–387, 1982.

54. Hueston JT: Some observations on knuckle pads. *J Hand Surg [Br]* 9(1):75–78, 1984.

55. Igarashi A, Nashiro K, Kikuchi K, et al: Connective tissue growth factor gene expression in tissue sections from localized scleroderma, keloid, and other fibrotic skin disorders. *J Invest Dermatol* 106:729–733, 1996.

56. Izadpanah A, Viezel-Mathieu A, Izadpanah A, et al: Dupuytren contracture in the pediatric population: A systematic review. *Eur J Pediatr Surg* 25:151–154, 2015.

57. Jerosch-Herold C, Shepstone L, Chojnowski A, et al: Severity of contracture and self-reported disability in patients with Dupuytren's contracture referred for surgery. *J Hand Ther* 24:6–10, 2011.

58. Jónsson T, Gudmundsson KG, Bjarnadóttir K, et al: Association of HLA-DRB1*01 with Dupuytren's disease. *Scandinavian J Rheumatol* 42(1):45–47, 2013.

59. Kan HJ, Verrijp FW, Hovius SER—the Dupuytren Delphi Group: *An international multidisciplinary Delphi-based consensus definition of recurrence after Dupuytren treatment*. Presentation A-0655 at XIXth FESSH Congress Paris, France 18th-21st June 2014.

60. Kim A, Lakshman N, Petroll WM: Quantitative assessment of local collagen matrix remodeling in 3-D culture: the role of Rho kinase. *Exp Cell Res* 312(18):3683–3692, 2006.

61. LaCroix AS, Duenwald-Kuehl SE, Brickson S, et al: Effect of age and exercise on the viscoelastic properties of rat tail tendon. *Ann Biomed Eng* 41:1120–1128, 2013.

62. Lam WL, Rawlins JM, Karoo ROS, et al: Re-visiting Luck's classification: a histological analysis of Dupuytren's disease. *J Hand Surg Eur Vol* 35:37–312, 2010.

63. Lanting R, Broekstra DC, Werker PMN, et al: A systematic review and meta-analysis on the prevalence of Dupuytren disease in the general population of Western countries. *Plast Reconstr Surg* 133:593–603, 2014.

64. Lanting RR, van den Heuvel ER, Westerink BB, et al: Prevalence of Dupuytren disease in the Netherlands. *Plast Reconstr Surg* 132:394–403, 2013.

65. Ling RS: The genetic factor in Dupuytren's disease. *J Bone Joint Surg Br* 45(4):709–718, 1963.

66. Lo S, Pickford M: Retrovascular fasciectomy: an approach that facilitates dissection of the neurovascular bundles in Dupuytren's fasciectomy. *J Hand Surg Eur Vol* 36:705–707, 2011.

67. Luck JV: Dupuytren's contracture: a new concept of the pathogenesis correlated with surgical management. *J Bone Joint Surg Am* 41A:635–664, 1959.

68. Matton A: *Long-term retreatment rate of Dupuytren's disease after percutaneous needle fasciotomy*, Thesis, 2012, University of Groningen.

69. McClelland WB, Jr, McClinton MA: Proximal interphalangeal joint injection through a volar approach: anatomic feasibility and cadaveric assessment of success. *J Hand Surg [Am]* 38(4):733–739, 2013.

70. McFarlane RM: Patterns of the diseased fascia in the fingers in Dupuytren's contracture. Displacement of the neurovascular bundle. *Plast Reconstr Surg* 54(1):31–44, 1974.

71. McGrouther DA: An overview of operative treatment. In McFarlane RM, McGrouther DA, Flint MH, editors: *Dupuytren's disease biology and treatment*, Edinburgh, 1990, Churchill Livingstone, pp 295–310.

72. Meinel AG: Dupuytren contracture—how fibromatosis remodels the palmar subcutaneous tissue and its fibrous environment. *Adv Surg Sci* 1:11–16, 2013.

73. Mikkelsen OA: The prevalence of Dupuytren's disease in Norway. A study in a representative population sample of the municipality of Haugesund. *Acta Chir Scand* 138(7):695–700, 1972.

74. Millesi H: Basic thoughts on Dupuytren's contracture. In Eaton C, et al, editors: *Dupuytren's disease and related hyperproliferative disorders*, Berlin, 2012, Springer-Verlag, pp 21–26.

75. Misra A, Jain A, Ghazanfar R, et al: Predicting the outcome of surgery for the proximal interphalangeal joint in Dupuytren's disease. *J Hand Surg [Am]* 32:240–245, 2007.

76. Moermans JP: Long-term results after segmental aponeurectomy for Dupuytren's disease. *J Hand Surg [Br]* 21:797–800, 1996.

77. Mohan A, Vadher J, Ismail H, et al: The Southampton Dupuytren's Scoring Scheme. *J Plast Surg Hand Surg* 48:28–33, 2014.

78. Naam NH: Functional outcome of collagenase injections compared with fasciectomy in treatment of Dupuytren's contracture. *Hand* 8(4):410–416, 2013.

79. Nugteren HM, Nijman JM, de Jong IJ, et al: The association between Peyronie's and Dupuytren's disease. *Int J Impot Res* 23:15–142, 2011.

80. Nyberg LM, Bias WB, Hochberg MC, et al: Identification of an inherited form of Peyronie's disease with autosomal dominant inheritance and association with Dupuytren's contracture and histocompatibility B7 cross-reacting antigens. *J Urol* 128(1):48–51, 1982.

81. Nydick JA, Olliff BW, Garcia MJ, et al: A comparison of percutaneous needle fasciotomy and collagenase injection for Dupuytren disease. *J Hand Surg [Am]* 38(12):2377–2380, 2013.

82. Pagnotta A, Specchia N, Greco F: Androgen receptors in Dupuytren's contracture. *J Orthop Res* 20:163–168, 2002.

83. Parra EJ, Marcini A, Akey J, et al: Estimating African American admixture proportions by use of population-specific alleles. *Am J Hum Genet* 63(6):1839–1851, 1998.

84. Peimer CA, Blazar P, Coleman S, et al: Dupuytren contracture recurrence following treatment with collagenase clostridium histolyticum (CORDLESS study): 3-year data. *J Hand Surg [Am]* 38:12–22, 2013.

85. Ratkaj I, Bujak M, Jurišic D, et al: Microarray analysis of Dupuytren's disease cells: the profibrogenic role of the TGF-β inducible p38 MAPK pathway. *Cell Physiol Biochem* 30(4):927–942, 2012.

86. Rayan GM, Ali M, Orozco J: Dorsal pads versus nodules in normal population and Dupuytren's disease patients. *J Hand Surg [Am]* 35:1559–1571, 2010.

87. Rayan G: Dupuytren's disease. *Hand Clin* 15(1):xiii, 1999.

88. Raykha C, Crawford J, Gan BS, et al: IGF-II and IGFBP-6 regulate cellular contractility and proliferation in Dupuytren's disease. *Biochim Biophys Acta* 1832:1511–1519, 2013.

89. Reilly RM, Stern PJ, Goldfarb CA: A retrospective review of the management of Dupuytren's nodules. *J Hand Surg [Am]* 30:1014–1018, 2005.

90. Roush TF, Stern PJ: Results following surgery for recurrent Dupuytren's disease. *J Hand Surg [Am]* 25:291–296, 2000.

91. Rudolph R: Inhibition of myofibroblasts by skin grafts. *Plast Reconstr Surg* 63:473–480, 1979.

92. Saboeiro AP, Porkorny JJ, Shehadi SI, et al: Racial distribution of Dupuytren's disease in Department of Veterans Affairs patients. *Plast Reconstr Surg* 106(1):71–75, 2000.

93. Sadideen H, Athanasou N, Ashmore A, et al: Heterotopic ossification in Dupuytren's disease: clinical and histological significance. *J Bone Joint Surg Br* 93:1676–1678, 2011.

94. Satish L, LaFramboise WA, Johnson S, et al: Fibroblasts from phenotypically normal palmar fascia exhibit molecular profiles highly similar to fibroblasts from active disease in Dupuytren's contracture. *BMC Med Genomics* 5:15, 2012.

95. Satish L, O'Gorman DB, Johnson S, et al: Increased CCT-eta expression is a marker of latent and active disease and a modulator of fibroblast contractility in Dupuytren's contracture. *Cell Stress Chaperones* 18:397–404, 2013.

96. Schleip R, Duerselen L, Vleeming A, et al: Strain hardening of fascia: static stretching of dense fibrous connective tissues can induce a temporary stiffness increase accompanied by enhanced matrix hydration. *J Bodyw Mov Ther* 16:94–100, 2012.

97. Shih BB, Tassabehji M, Watson JS, et al: Genome-wide high-resolution screening in Dupuytren's disease reveals common regions of DNA copy number alterations. *J Hand Surg [Am]* 35:1172–1183, 2010.

98. Smith P, Breed C: Central slip attenuation in Dupuytren's contracture: a cause of persistent flexion of the proximal interphalangeal joint. *J Hand Surg [Am]* 19:840–843, 1994.

99. Smith SP, Devaraj VS, Bunker TD: The association between frozen shoulder and Dupuytren's disease. *J Shoulder Elbow Surg* 10:149–151, 2001.

100. Smits LJM, van Kuijk SMJ, Leffers P, et al: Index event bias—a numerical example. *J Clin Epidemiol* 66:192–196, 2013.

101. Sullivan BE, Carroll CC, Jemiolo BB, et al: Effect of acute resistance exercise and sex on human patellar tendon structural and regulatory mRNA expression. *J Appl Physiol* 106:75–468, 2009.
102. Teboul F, Sabri E, Goubier J-N: Case report: middle phalanx resection as an alternative treatment to amputation of recurrent Dupuytren's contracture of the fifth digit. *Eur J Plast Surg* 35:901–903, 2012.
103. Tonkin MA, Burke FD, Varian JP: Dupuytren's contracture: a comparative study of fasciectomy and dermofasciectomy in one hundred patients. *J Hand Surg [Br]* 9:156–162, 1984.
104. Toppi JT, Trompf L, Smoll NR, et al: Dupuytren's contracture: an analysis of outcomes of percutaneous needle fasciotomy versus open fasciectomy. *ANZ J Surg* 1–5, 2014.
105. Trickett RW, Savage R, Logan AJ: Angular correction related to excision of specific cords in fasciectomy for Dupuytren's disease. *J Hand Surg Eur* 39:472–476, 2014.
106. Uehara K, Miura T, Morizaki Y, et al: Ultrasonographic evaluation of displaced neurovascular bundle in Dupuytren disease. *J Hand Surg [Am]* 38:23–28, 2013.
107. Ullaha S, Dias JJ, Bhowal B: Does a "firebreak" full-thickness skin graft prevent recurrence after surgery for Dupuytren's contracture? a prospective, randomised trial. *J Bone Jt Surg Br* 91:374–378, 2009.
108. Umlas ME, Bischoff RJ, Gelberman RH: Predictors of neurovascular displacement in hands with Dupuytren's contracture. *J Hand Surg [Br]* 19:664–666, 1994.
109. van Rijssen AL, ter Linden H, Werker PMN: Five-year results of a randomized clinical trial on treatment in Dupuytren's disease: percutaneous needle fasciotomy versus limited fasciectomy. *Plast Reconstr Surg* 129:469–477, 2012.
110. Vaughan MB, Howard EW, Tomasek JJ: Transforming growth factor-beta1 promotes the morphological and functional differentiation of the myofibroblast. *Exp Cell Res* 257:180–189, 2000.
111. Verhoekx JS, Beckett KS, Bisson MA, et al: The mechanical environment in Dupuytren's contracture determines cell contractility and associated MMP-mediated matrix remodeling. *J Orthop Res* 31(2):34–328, 2013.
112. Verjee LS, Midwood K, Davidson D, et al: Myofibroblast distribution in Dupuytren's cords: correlation with digital contracture. *J Hand Surg [Am]* 34:194–1785, 2009.
113. Walton MJ, Pearson D, Clark DA, et al: The prognosis of fasciectomy for abductor digiti minimi and pretendinous cords in Dupuytren's disease of the little finger. *Hand Surg* 14(2–3):89–92, 2009.
114. White S: Anatomy of the palmar fascia on the ulnar border of the hand. *J Hand Surg [Br]* 9:50–56, 1984.
115. Wilkinson JM, Davidson RK, Swingler TE, et al: MMP-14 and MMP-2 are key metalloproteases in Dupuytren's disease fibroblast-mediated contraction. *Biochim Biophys Acta* 1822(6):897–905, 2012.
116. Xiaflex.com: *Xiaflex Prescribing Information.* <www.xiaflex.com/_assets/pdf/XIAFLEX-PI-and-MedGuide-Combined-20131206-ver-e.pdf>.
117. Yacoe ME, Bergman AG, Ladd AL, et al: Dupuytren's contracture: MR imaging findings and correlation between MR signal intensity and cellularity of lesions. *Am J Roentgenol* 160:813–817, 1993.
118. Zerajic D, Finsen V: Dupuytren's disease in Bosnia and Herzegovina. An epidemiological study. *BMC Musculoskelet Disord* 5:10, 2004.
119. Zwanenburg RL, Werker PMN, McGrouther DA: The anatomy and function of Cleland's ligaments. *J Hand Surg Eur* 39:482–490, 2014.
120. Zyluk A, Jagielski W: The effect of the severity of the Dupuytren's contracture on the function of the hand before and after surgery. *J Hand Surg Eur* 32:326–329, 2007.

5

Extensor Tendon Injury

Robert J. Strauch

Acknowledgments: The author gratefully acknowledges the outstanding previous chapters on these topics in prior editions of Green's Operative Hand Surgery, written by James R. Doyle, Richard I. Burton, Julie A. Melchior, Mark E. Baratz, Christopher C. Schmidt, and Thomas B. Hughes.

▶ These videos may be found at
ExpertConsult.com:
5.1 Subluxation of extensor carpi ulnaris

In contrast to zone 2 flexor tendon injuries, most extensor tendon repairs are liberated from the confines of a fibroosseous tunnel. Conversely, standard core flexor tendon sutures become technically impossible when dealing with the thin, flat extensor mechanism over the phalanges. These are just some of the differences between injuries of the flexor and extensor tendons. This chapter reviews issues concerning the evaluation and treatment of acute and chronic extensor tendon injuries.

⬚ ANATOMY

As in most areas of the hand, an understanding of extensor tendon anatomy is crucial to analyzing and treating injuries to this system.

Muscles

The extensor tendons originate from the finger extensor muscle bellies of the extensor digitorum communis (EDC), extensor indicis proprius (EIP), extensor pollicis longus (EPL), extensor digiti minimi (EDM), abductor pollicis longus (APL), and extensor pollicis brevis (EPB); the radial wrist extensor muscle bellies of the extensor carpi radialis longus and brevis (ECRL and ECRB); and the extensor carpi ulnaris (ECU). All of these muscles are innervated by branches from either the radial nerve or the posterior interosseous nerve.

Anatomic Variations of Extensor Muscles

Wrist Extensors. The most common anatomic variations are accessory muscles and tendons associated with the wrist extensors. The extensor carpi radialis intermedius, reported to be found in 12% of limbs, may arise superficial and radial to or between the ECRL and ECRB.[122] The significance of this accessory muscle is that it may be harvested for use as a tendon transfer in paralytic disorders when donor muscles are lacking. Anomalous tendons originating from the radial wrist extensors have been described inserting on the index or middle metacar-

pal base. These accessory tendons and interconnections may need to be released during tendon transfer procedures to achieve full excursion.

Finger Extensors. The extensor medii proprius can be considered to be an EIP of the middle finger, found in 10% of hands, and has recently been used in reconstruction of chronic sagittal band injuries.[6] The insertion is typically ulnar to the EDC insertion on the middle finger, as is the usual arrangement of the EIP with respect to the EDC index tendon and the EDM with respect to the small finger EDC tendon. The extensor indicis et medii communis is a variation of the EIP that inserts into the middle and index fingers.[113]

The extensor digitorum brevis manus muscle (EDBM) is an anomalous muscle on the dorsum of the hand, found in 3% of hands, usually arising between the index and middle finger metacarpals and inserting on the extensor hood of the index or middle fingers with or without anomalies of the EIP. Ogura and associates[73] described five types of EDBMs, depending on the insertion and relationship to the EIP. The clinical significance of the EDBM is that it can be mistaken for a dorsal wrist ganglion cyst; it becomes firm when the wrist is slightly flexed and the fingers are extended. It may also be a source of dorsal wrist pain and can be completely excised if needed (Figure 5.1).

Tendons at the Wrist Level

The musculotendinous junction is usually approximately 4 cm proximal to the wrist joint, although muscle fibers of the EIP often continue to the wrist joint level. At the level of the wrist, the tendons course through six individual, synovial-lined, fibroosseous sheaths, known as the six extensor tendon compartments (Figure 5.2, *A*). The fifth extensor compartment is technically a fibrous tunnel only because it does not insert on bone. The sixth extensor tendon compartment, containing the ECU tendon, has a subsheath that maintains the relationship of the tendon to the underlying ulna, and rupture or injury of this subsheath may result in symptomatic ECU tendon subluxation (Figure 5.3 and Video 5.1).[100] (Case Study 5.1; also see Chapter 13.)

Juncturae Tendinum

Proximal to the metacarpophalangeal (MP) joint level, stout interconnecting bands exist between the ring EDC and the small and middle fingers, and there is a less substantial band from the middle to the index finger. The importance of these juncturae tendinum is that finger extension can be preserved if the EDC is lacerated proximal to a junctura tendinum that connects that finger to an intact extensor tendon.[117] The juncturae tendinum also restrict independent extension of the ring and

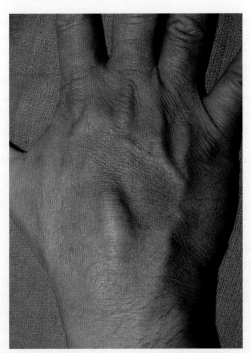

FIGURE 5.1 Extensor digitorum brevis manus (EDBM) muscle. Extension of the fingers increases the prominence of this anomalous muscle.

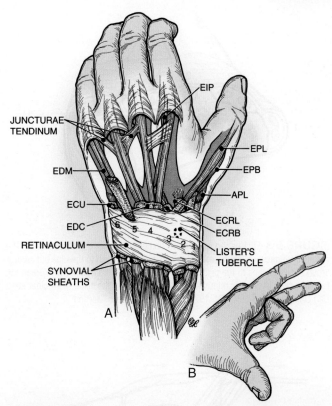

FIGURE 5.2 A, Extensor tendons gain entrance into the hand from the forearm through a series of six canals, five fibroosseous canals and one fibrous canal (the fifth dorsal compartment, which contains the EDM). The first compartment contains the APL and EPB; the second, radial wrist extensors; the third, the EPL, which angles around the Lister tubercle; the fourth, the EDC to the fingers and EIP; the fifth, the EDM; and the sixth, the ECU. The communis tendons are joined distally near the MP joints by fibrous interconnections called juncturae tendinum. These juncturae are found only between the communis tendons and may aid in surgical recognition of the proprius tendon of the index finger. The proprius tendons are usually positioned to the ulnar side of the adjacent communis tendons, but variations may be present that alter this arrangement (see text discussion). Beneath the retinaculum, the extensor tendons are covered with a synovial sheath. **B,** Proprius tendons to the index and little fingers are capable of independent extension, and their function may be evaluated as depicted. With the middle and ring fingers flexed into the palm, the proprius tendons can extend the ring and little fingers. Independent extension of the index finger is not always lost after transfer of the indicis proprius, however, and is less likely to be lost if the extensor hood is not injured; and is probably never lost if the hood is preserved and the junctura tendinum between the index and middle fingers is excised. This figure represents the usual anatomic arrangement found over the wrist and hand, but variations are common, and the reader is referred to the section on anatomic variations. (Copyright Elizabeth Martin.)

middle fingers when the other digits are flexed at the MP joints. Varying morphologic views of juncturae tendinum have been described by Hirai and colleagues[36] (see Figure 5.2).

Independent Extension of the Index and Small Fingers

The EIP and EDM allow independent extension of the index and small fingers, although loss of the EIP because of tendon transfer or injury does not eliminate the ability to extend the index finger independently at the MP joint. This is true as long as the extensor hood at the index MP joint level is not injured. Isolated loss of the EDM can lead to loss of independent extension of the small finger, however, because the anatomic structure of the EDC to the small finger is highly variable, and it may be replaced exclusively by a junctura tendinum from the ring finger (see Figure 5.2).

Variations of Extensor Tendons of the Fingers

The typical arrangement of finger extensor tendons is as follows: (1) single EIP inserting ulnar to the EDC tendon of the index finger; (2) single tendon from the EDC to the index and middle fingers; (3) double tendon from the EDC to the ring finger; (4) absent EDC to the small finger but usually a substantial junctura tendinum from the ring EDC to the EDM; and (5) double EDM tendon to the little finger with a double insertion into the MP joint hood (see Figure 5.2).[113] Variations of extensor tendons have been noted, including a double slip of the EIP; an EIP inserting volar or radial to the EDC; and, rarely, absence of the EDC and junctura tendinum to the small finger, in which case harvesting the EDM would lead to small finger MP joint extensor lag.

Sagittal Bands

The extensor tendon at the MP joint level is maintained in a central position by the sagittal bands, which arise from the volar plate of the MP joint and the intermetacarpal ligaments, to insert on the extensor hood. Injury to the sagittal bands may result in subluxation of the EDC.

Extensor Digitorum Communis Insertion

The mechanism by which extension of the MP joint is achieved by the pull of EDC tendons is not related to a direct insertion of the tendon on the base of the proximal phalanx. Van Sint Jan and colleagues[112] showed that although there is a "central slip" on the base of the middle phalanx, there is no such structure on the base of the proximal phalanx. Instead, there is loose connective tissue between the EDC and the base of the proximal

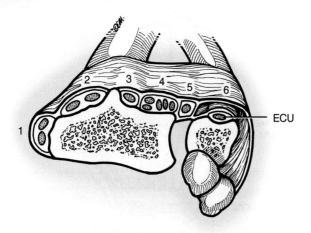

FIGURE 5.3 ECU lies in a separate fibroosseous tunnel, or subsheath. The extensor retinaculum lies superficial to and does not attach to the ulna but swings around and attaches to the pisiform and triquetrum. (From Spinner M, Kaplan EB: Extensor carpi ulnaris: its relationship to the stability of the distal radio-ulnar joint, *Clin Orthop Relat Res* 68:124, 1970. Copyright Elizabeth Martin.)

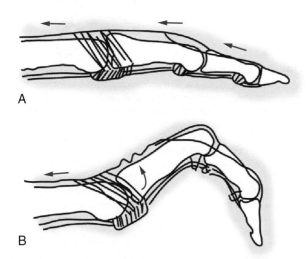

FIGURE 5.4 **A**, EDC allows extension of MP joint via insertion onto the sagittal bands, which "lasso" around the base of the proximal phalanx. There is usually no tendinous insertion of EDC to the dorsal base of the proximal phalanx. When MP joint hyperextension is prevented, EDC is capable of extending MP, PIP, and DIP joints even in the absence of intrinsic muscle function. **B**, When MP joint hyperextension is allowed, as with intrinsic paralysis, "slack" develops in EDC system distal to the sagittal bands, in addition to increased tone in the flexor system, all producing a flexion posture at the PIP and DIP joints, or claw finger.

phalanx. Extension of the MP joint is transmitted by the pull of the EDC tendon through the sagittal bands (Figure 5.4). When the sagittal band system is damaged, and the EDC tendon subluxates or dislocates off the central axis of the finger, MP joint extension is compromised.

Anatomy of the Extensor Mechanism Over the Proximal Phalanx

The anatomy of the extensor mechanism is an intricate and layered system that changes geometry as the finger flexes and extends, allowing the lateral bands to displace volarly in flexion

and return to the dorsum of the finger in extension. The intrinsic tendons from the lumbricals and interossei form the lateral bands, which join the extensor mechanism at the proximal third of the proximal phalanx. The lumbrical muscle functions both to flex the MP joint and to extend the IP joints owing to its insertion on the lateral band. The lumbrical also contracts during IP and MP extension in order to "relax" the profundus tendon by pulling it distally through its proximal origin from the FDP.[120] The EDC trifurcates proximal to the proximal interphalangeal (PIP) joint, with the central component becoming the central slip and the lateral components joining up with the lateral bands.[88] These conjoined lateral bands coalesce over the middle phalanx and continue distally to become the terminal tendon (Figure 5.5).

Anatomy of the Extensor Mechanism Over the Middle Phalanx

The lateral bands are maintained in position by the triangular ligament, which unites them dorsal and distal to the PIP joint, and the transverse retinacular ligaments, which stabilize them to the flexor tendon sheath. The primary function of the triangular ligament is to prevent palmar subluxation of the lateral bands during PIP joint flexion, which can occur in the boutonnière deformity as a result of triangular ligament incompetence. The primary function of the transverse retinacular ligament is to prevent dorsal subluxation of the lateral bands during extension, as can occur in a swan neck deformity. There is a normal dorsal-palmar translation of the lateral bands with respect to the PIP joint axis of rotation during flexion and extension, which must be preserved to retain normal extensor function. The central slip insertion on the base of the middle phalanx helps to initiate extension of the PIP joint; however, PIP joint extension is possible even in the absence of the central slip, provided that the triangular ligament, lateral bands, and transverse retinacular ligaments are functioning normally (Figures 5.6 and 5.7). Distal to the triangular ligament, the lateral bands converge to form the terminal tendon, which inserts onto the base of the distal phalanx. The germinal nail matrix, which creates the nail plate, arises approximately 1.2 mm distal to the terminal tendon insertion.[94]

Extension of the Fingers

Extension of the fingers at the MP joint is exclusively a function of the extrinsic extensor tendons. Extension of the PIP joints, although primarily a function of the intrinsic interossei and lumbrical muscles, can also occur through the extrinsic tendon extensor system, provided that MP joint hyperextension is blocked. When intrinsic palsy allows the MP joint to hyperextend, the extrinsic extensor system becomes insufficient to extend the interphalangeal (IP) joints, and a "claw finger" results. This deformity occurs because of "slack" in the extensor mechanism distal to the sagittal bands and the increased flexor tone in this position (see Figure 5.4).

Extension at the MP joint is possible regardless of the position of flexion of the PIP and distal interphalangeal (DIP) joints, so the "intrinsic plus" and "hook grip" are both tenable positions. It is physically impossible, under normal circumstances, to extend or flex the PIP and DIP joints independent of one another (i.e., to extend the PIP joint without simultaneously extending the DIP joint). Only in individuals who can

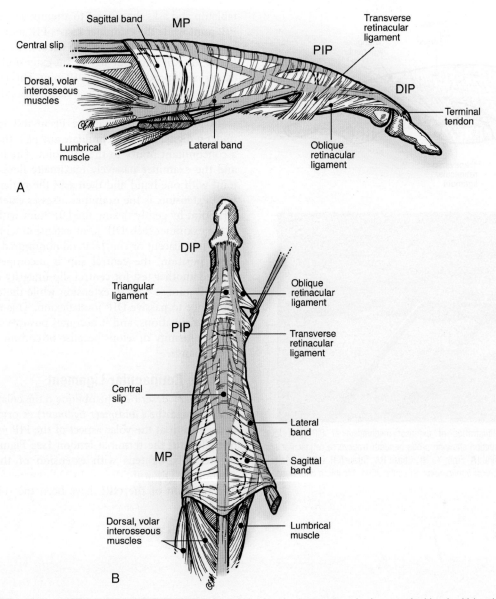

FIGURE 5.5 A and **B**, Extensor tendon at MP joint level is held in place by the transverse lamina or sagittal band, which tethers and centers the extensor tendons over the joint. This sagittal band arises from the volar plate and the intermetacarpal ligaments at the neck of the metacarpals. Any injury to this extensor hood or expansion may result in subluxation or dislocation of the extensor tendon. Intrinsic tendons from lumbrical and interosseous muscles join the extensor mechanism at about the level of the proximal portion and midportion of the proximal phalanx and continue distally to the DIP joint of the finger. Extensor mechanism at PIP joint is best described as a trifurcation of the extensor tendon into the central slip, which attaches to the dorsal base of the middle phalanx, and the two lateral bands. These lateral bands continue distally to insert at the dorsal base of the distal phalanx. Extensor mechanism is maintained in place over PIP joint by transverse retinacular ligaments. (Copyright Elizabeth Martin.)

voluntarily or involuntarily lock their PIP joints in hyperextension or when the PIP joint is passively held in full extension, can DIP joint flexion be accomplished independently using the flexor digitorum profundus tendon.

Testing the Anatomic Integrity of the Central Slip: Elson Test

When the PIP joint is passively flexed completely, the central slip insertion is pulled distally along with its proximal attachments, and "slack" is created between the lateral band insertions on the terminal tendon and the lateral connections of the central slip to the lateral band. This slack can be easily appreci-

ated by manually assessing the resistance to passive flexion of the DIP joint with the PIP joint fully extended versus fully flexed. This elegant mechanism permits full flexion of the DIP joint when the PIP joint is maximally flexed (Figure 5.8, *A* and *B*). A corollary is that active extension of the DIP joint becomes impossible when the PIP joint is fully flexed because of the slack in the lateral bands (see Figure 5.8, *C* and *D*).

When the central slip is injured or incompetent, it is possible to generate extensor force at the DIP joint with maximal passive PIP joint flexion, which is the basis of the Elson test for detecting acute central slip rupture.[23] As described by Elson,[23] the examiner passively flexes the PIP joint to 90 degrees over a

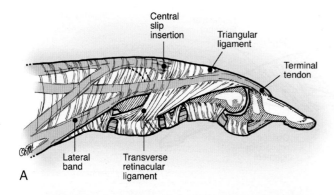

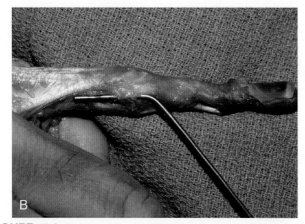

FIGURE 5.6 A, Illustration of extensor mechanism at PIP joint level. **B**, Cadaver finger dissection showing probe beneath transverse retinacular ligament at level of PIP joint. (**A**, From Yu HL, Chase RA, Strauch B, editors: *Atlas of Hand Anatomy and Clinical Implications,* St Louis, 2004, Mosby, p 343. Redrawn by Elizabeth Martin.)

tabletop and asks the patient to attempt active extension of the PIP joint while the examiner resists PIP joint extension. When acute rupture of the central slip occurs, no extension power is felt at the PIP joint but significant extension power, or hyperextension, is produced at the DIP joint. This test has been found to be the most sensitive physical examination test to detect acute central slip rupture.[87]

In practice, I find that the Elson test is best performed under a digital block to eliminate any pain that may arise from a concomitant injury to the PIP joint. The hand is supinated, and the examiner passively maximally flexes the injured PIP joint with one hand and then asks the patient to attempt PIP joint extension as the examiner assesses extension force at the DIP joint by gently flexing the DIP joint with the other hand. If the examiner feels DIP joint extension with force compared with the adjacent or contralateral noninjured digits held in the same position, the central slip is incompetent. Boyes[11] described another test for central slip integrity in 1970, in which the PIP joint is held in extension while the examiner assesses resistance to passive DIP joint flexion. This test is not helpful in acute situations, and it becomes positive only as a boutonnière deformity develops because of chronic retraction of the lateral bands.

Oblique Retinacular Ligament

Landsmeer[55] described the oblique retinacular ligament (ORL) (also termed the *Landsmeer ligament*) as originating from the flexor sheath at the volar aspect of the PIP joint and inserting dorsally into the terminal tendon (see Figure 5.5). The ORL theoretically tightens with extension of the PIP joint and extends the DIP joint during PIP joint extension. The existence and function of the ORL have been the subject of debate.[89]

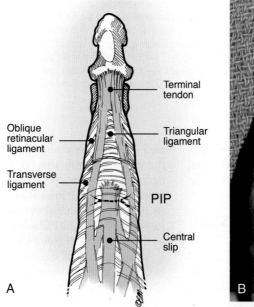

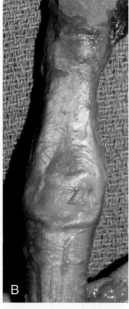

FIGURE 5.7 A, Triangular ligament. **B**, Cadaver triangular ligament. (**A**, Copyright Elizabeth Martin.)

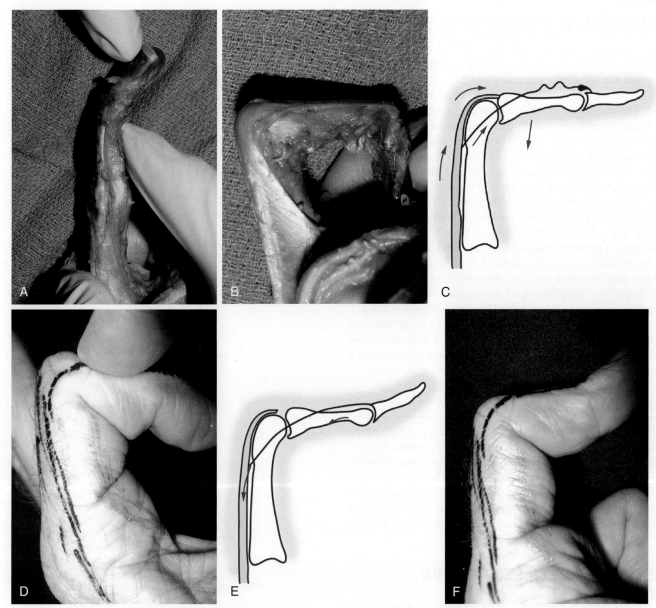

FIGURE 5.8 A, Maximal passive PIP joint extension prohibits full DIP joint flexion by normal tension in lateral bands. **B**, Full PIP joint flexion allows slack in the lateral bands, permitting full DIP joint flexion. **C**, Maximal passive flexion of PIP joint induces slack in the lateral bands via proximal interconnections, resulting in loss of power of active DIP joint extension and increased DIP joint flexion. **D**, Finger maximally flexed prohibits any ability to extend DIP joint actively. **E**, Injury to central slip eliminates the slack in the lateral bands produced by passive PIP joint flexion and allows extensor tension to be generated at DIP joint. This is the basis for the Elson test. **F**, With central slip injury, DIP joint can be actively extended with maximum PIP joint flexion.

Shrewsbury and Johnson[92] showed that it is present less than 50% of the time except on the ulnar side of the ring finger, where it is found more than 90% of the time. Excision of the ORL has not been shown to cause an extensor deficit at the DIP joint.

An alternative explanation to Landsmeer's theory is that the collateral ligaments of the DIP joint alone can account for the "spring back" tendency of the DIP joint in the absence of an ORL. Shrewsbury and Johnson[93] noted that a complete extensor lag does not occur when the terminal tendon is intentionally sectioned, as in the treatment of the DIP joint hyperextension posture of a boutonnière deformity. In practice, identification

and preservation of the ORL, if present, would be prudent. Shrewsbury and Johnson[93] believed the presence of a functioning terminal tendon alone is sufficient to account for full extension of the DIP joint, and that the ORL was of no practical functional importance. Ueba and colleagues[110] found the ORL present in 38 of 40 cadaver fingers in an anatomic and biomechanical study; the ORL contributed up to 30% of passive resistance to DIP joint flexion, with a maximum at 30 degrees of PIP joint flexion. Regardless of its presence or absence, the *concept* of the ORL is useful in surgically creating a passive tendon "checkrein" to enable simultaneous DIP and PIP joint extension in the setting of a chronic mallet finger.

BIOMECHANICS OF FINGER EXTENSION

Boyes[11] suggested that the amplitude of tendon excursion for the wrist extensors is 3.3 cm and the amplitude of tendon excursion for the finger extensors and EPL is 5 cm; however, most of this excursion occurs over the forearm, wrist, and dorsal hand. The amplitude of tendon excursion over the dorsum of the finger is extremely small; this explains why small tendon gaps, overtightening of tendon repairs, or small amounts of bony shortening or angulation can lead to dramatic extensor lags or restriction of flexion at the PIP and DIP joints. Vahey and associates[111] found that an experimental 12-degree PIP joint extensor lag was produced with every 1 mm of tendon lengthening over the proximal phalanx. Schweitzer and Rayan[90] showed that 1 mm of terminal tendon lengthening resulted in a 25-degree DIP joint extensor lag and that 1 mm of terminal tendon shortening severely restricted DIP joint flexion.

Over the dorsum of the hand, it has been shown experimentally that relative lengthening of the extensor tendon by 2 mm produces an extensor lag of approximately 7 degrees at the MP joint. Because most MP joints had a "reserve" of hyperextension ability of about 35 degrees, however, 5 to 6 mm of relative extensor tendon lengthening in this zone may not produce a clinically relevant lack of extension.[102]

ZONES OF INJURY

The classification of extensor tendon injuries proposed by Kleinert and Verdan[51] ended at zone 8 (the forearm). Doyle[21] added a ninth zone for the muscular area of the extensor mechanism at the middle and proximal forearm. The classification is easy to recall if one remembers that the joints are odd numbered; from distal to proximal, the DIP joint is zone 1, PIP joint is zone 3, and so forth. The thumb IP joint is zone 1, and the MP joint is zone 3 (Figure 5.9).

TREATMENT OF EXTENSOR TENDON LACERATIONS

Suture Repair Techniques

There are few published studies on the strength of various suture techniques for extensor tendon injuries compared with the plethora of studies concerning flexor tendon repair techniques. One problem concerns the variability in the thickness of the extensor tendon as it changes from proximal to distal. Proximally, at the forearm and wrist level, the tendons are thicker and more capable of holding core sutures, and at the finger level, the tendons become broader but quite thin, and are incapable of holding standard core sutures. Doyle[21] measured the thickness of the extensor mechanism in the fingers to be within a range of 1.75 mm in zone 6 (dorsal hand) to 0.65 mm at zone 1. A similar range was found at the thumb level.

In 1992, Newport and Williams[72] found the Kleinert modification of the Bunnell repair to be the strongest technique in a cadaver study of zone 6 extensor tendon repairs performed with 4-0 polypropylene (Prolene) suture material. In 1995, Newport and coworkers[71] reported that the Kleinert-modified Bunnell technique and the modified Kessler techniques were the stron-

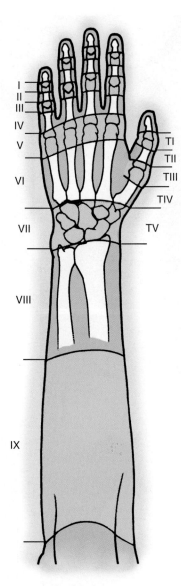

FIGURE 5.9 Zones of extensor tendon injury.

gest techniques for zone 4 injuries, and were suitable for dynamic or active range of motion under controlled conditions and in short arcs.

In 1997, Howard and colleagues[38] compared the MGH, modified Bunnell, and modified Krackow-Thomas repairs in cadaveric zone 6 extensor tendon lacerations and found the MGH technique to be superior. In a 2005 study of zone 4 extensor tendon repairs with 4-0 nonabsorbable, braided polyester (Ticron) suture, Woo and coworkers[121] found the modified Becker technique to be the strongest repair, with a significantly greater resistance to a 1- and 2-mm gap and the greatest ultimate strength. Lee and colleagues[56] compared the augmented Becker technique, the modified Bunnell technique, and a new, running interlocking horizontal mattress technique and found the newer technique to be stiffer, to produce less shortening, and to be faster to accomplish than the other techniques, without a significant difference in the ultimate load to failure. This newer technique, termed the *corset suture,* does not require the placement of core sutures and was found to have good to

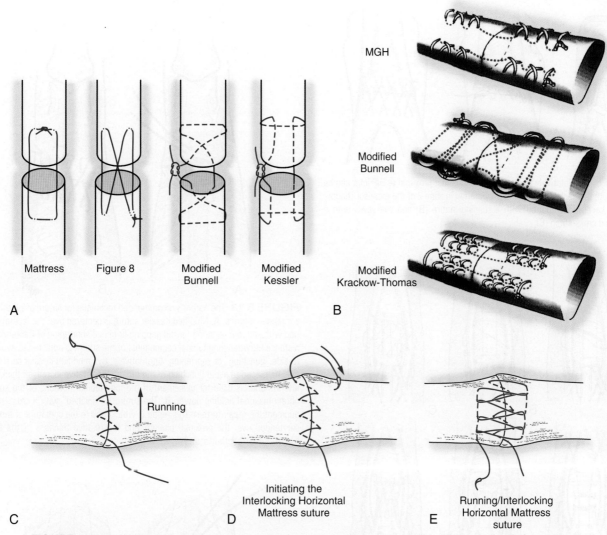

FIGURE 5.10 A, Modified Bunnell suture was the strongest suture with the least loss of MP or PIP joint motion. **B,** Schematic representation of four-strand MGH, modified Bunnell, and modified Krackow-Thomas repairs. **C,** Starting running suture of corset suture. This suture configuration was evaluated in zone 6 but may be used in any zone. It does not employ any core sutures. **D,** Initiating the interlocking horizontal mattress suture. **E,** Completed running interlocking horizontal mattress suture. (**A,** From Newport ML, Williams CD: Biomechanical characteristics of extensor tendon suture techniques. *J Hand Surg Am* 17:111–119, 1992, with permission from The American Society for Surgery of the Hand; **B,** From Howard RF, Ondrovic L, Greenwald DP: Biomechanical analysis of four-strand extensor tendon repair techniques. *J Hand Surg Am* 22:838–842, 1997, with permission from The American Society for Surgery of the Hand; **C** to **E,** From Lee SK, Dubey A, Kim BH, et al: A biomechanical study of extensor tendon repair methods: introduction to the running-interlocking horizontal mattress extensor tendon repair. *J Hand Surg Am* 35:19–23, 2010, with permission from The American Society for Surgery of the Hand.)

excellent clinical results in a study of zones 4 and 5 extensor tendon lacerations[3] (Figure 5.10).

Doyle[21] proposed the following techniques for extensor tendon repair:

Zone 1 (DIP joint): Running suture incorporating skin and tendon.

Zone 2 (middle phalanx): Running 5-0 stitch near cut edge of tendon, completed with a "basket-weave" or "Chinese finger trap" type of cross-stitch on the dorsal surface of the tendon (Figure 5.11).

Zones 3 through 5 in fingers, and zones 2 and 3 in thumb: Modified Kessler suture of 4-0 synthetic material in the thickest portion of the tendon. A 5-0 cross-stitch tied to itself at the beginning and end is run on the dorsal surface of the tendon (Figures 5.12, 5.13, and 5.14).

Zones 6 and 7: Same as for zones 3 through 5, except the cross-stitch is run around the entire circumference of the tendon, if feasible.

❖ AUTHOR'S PREFERRED TREATMENT

I agree with Doyle's recommendations except that I usually use two modified Kessler core suture repairs for zones 3 through 5 complete tendon lacerations, on either side of the tendon, to avoid "bunching up" of the tendon. For zone 1 injuries, I do a running suture of 5-0 polypropylene supplemented by a transarticular Kirschner wire in full extension for 6 weeks, instead of a "roll" suture incorporating skin and tendon; sometimes I will use several interrupted and buried figure-of-eight 5-0 polypropylene sutures to anatomically reapproximate the tendon in zones 1 to 4, if the tendon laceration is jagged.

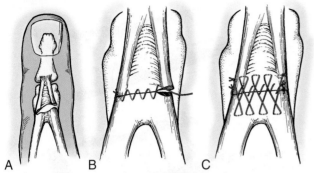

FIGURE 5.11 Relatively thin extensor tendon just proximal to DIP joint can be repaired with this technique. **A**, Sharp laceration in zone 2 of the extensor tendon. **B** and **C**, Laceration repaired with a running suture (**B**) and oversewn with a Silfverskiöld cross-stitch (**C**).

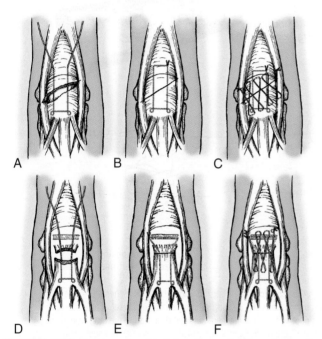

FIGURE 5.12 Doyle's preferred technique for repair of zone 3 lacerations. **A** to **C**, Central slip laceration with sufficient tendon to repair with core suture and oversew with Silfverskiöld epitendinous stitch. **D** to **F**, Core stitch can be passed through trough in the base of the middle phalanx when the tendon laceration is distal, leaving a small stump of central slip.

Postoperative Management

The traditional postoperative program for extensor tendon repairs in zones 1 and 2 is 6 weeks of immobilization with either splint or Kirschner wire fixation of the DIP joint, and this generally remains the preferred regimen. Zones 3 through 5 repairs have historically been protected with the wrist in 40 degrees of extension, slight flexion at the MP joint, and extension at the PIP joints for 4 weeks. Zones 6 and 7 repairs have usually been managed with similar wrist and MP joint extension, allowing full active motion at the IP joints for 4 weeks.[21] As in the rehabilitation of flexor tendon injuries, the main concern after repair is to maintain the integrity of the repair while limiting adhesion formation. The concept of early protected range of motion has been investigated for extensor tendon injuries, as it has been for flexor tendon injuries.

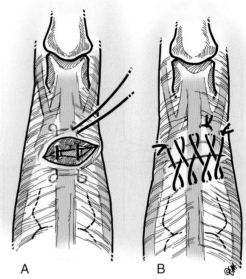

FIGURE 5.13 The author's recommended technique for suture of zone 4 extensor tendon injuries. **A**, Modified Kessler suture is centered over the laceration and tied with suitable tension to avoid gapping or undue shortening of the tendon. The distance between longitudinal components of the suture is adjusted to avoid side-to-side "bunching" or shortening. Alternatively, two modified Kessler core sutures may be placed to avoid bunching of the repair. The relative increased thickness of lateral bands is used for placement of the longitudinal portions of the suture to obtain maximal holding power. **B**, The suture is "finished" with a cross-stitch to augment the repair further. This repair is well suited to the curvature of the extensor tendon over the proximal phalanx and the relative thinness of the tendon. (Copyright Elizabeth Martin.)

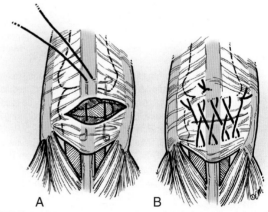

FIGURE 5.14 Lacerations over MP joint (zone 5) are in a region of increased thickness and substance compared with the extensor tendon mechanism distally. **A** and **B**, The author's preferred technique for repair of lacerations in this zone includes the modified Kessler (**A**), followed by the cross-stitch (**B**). (Copyright Elizabeth Martin.)

The ideal candidate for early range of motion (dynamic splinting) is a motivated patient with a complex injury involving more than one structure (e.g., tendon, bone, nerve). The concept of early passive motion for extensor tendon rehabilitation is that by moving joints through a controlled arc of motion, extensor tendon gliding of 3 to 5 mm may limit adhesion formation. Evans and Burkhalter[24] found that 30 degrees of MP joint flexion created 5 mm of EDC glide in zones 5 through 7. The EPL glides approximately 5 mm at the Lister tubercle with 60 degrees of thumb IP joint flexion. The Evans and Burkhalter

TABLE 5.1		Studies of Postoperative Dynamic, Static, or Active Splinting		
Study	**Year**	**Zones of Injury**	**Comparison**	**Results**
Browne and Ribik[11a]	1989	Zones 4-7	Dynamic splinting only	Full flexion in all. No tendon ruptures
Hung et al[39]	1990	Zones 2-5; prospective study	Dynamic splinting only	Poor results distal to MP joint
Saldana et al[87b]	1991	Zone 3 only	Dynamic splinting only	Most good or excellent. One mild boutonnière deformity
Evans[23a]	1994	Zone 3	Static extension splinting versus early active short arc motion	Short arc motion is better
Sylaidis et al[103a]	1997	Zones 4-7	CAM; not dynamic splinting	Excellent results in 22 of 24 cases
Purcell et al[80a]	2000	All zones	Static splinting only	76% excellent, 24% good results
Khandwala et al[48a]	2000	Zones 5-6	Dynamic splinting versus CAM	No difference between groups. Prefer CAM as simpler and less expensive
Chester et al[16a]	2002	Zones 4-8; prospective randomized study	Dynamic splinting versus CAM	Dynamic splinting better
Russell et al[87a]	2003	Zones 5-8	Dynamic splinting versus static splinting	Prefer static splinting because results similar
Mowlavi et al[57]	2005	Zones 5-6; prospective randomized study	Dynamic versus static splinting	Dynamic better at 4, 6, and 8 weeks but not at 6 months
Bulstrode et al[12]	2005	Zones 5-6; prospective comparative trial	Static splinting of MP and IP joints versus static splinting allowing IP motion only versus Norwich regimen	Motion in static group worse at 4 weeks but equal at 12 weeks
Kitis et al[50]	2012	Zones 5-7; prospective randomized trial	Dynamic versus static splinting	Dynamic better at 12 weeks and 6 months
Patil and Koul[78]	2012	Zone 5-8; prospective randomized trial	Static versus early active motion	Active better at 12 weeks but equal at 6 months

CAM, Controlled active mobilization.

method of postoperative rehabilitation for extensor tendon repair in zones 5 through 7 starts with dynamic splinting 3 days postoperatively to allow MP joint flexion to about 30 degrees, keeping the wrist in 45 degrees of extension. Dynamic splinting involves passive joint extension with a dynamic outrigger device, with flexion limited by the confines of the palmar splint (see Figure 5.27). Controlled active mobilization involves active joint extension, limiting joint flexion with a palmar splint. Short arc motion protocol involves passive extension splinting with intermittent, splint-assisted passive flexion and active extension. Table 5.1 summarizes studies done on various postoperative splinting protocols.

Outcomes

In 1942, Miller[67] suggested criteria for assessing extensor tendon repair outcomes, which were later endorsed by Newport and associates[70] (Table 5.2). This rating system takes into account extension lag and loss of flexion secondary to extensor adhesions and stiffness in terms of total active motion. In 1990, Newport and colleagues[70] reported on the long-term results of extensor tendon repair treated with static splinting. Of patients without associated injury, 64% achieved good or excellent results, whereas only 45% of patients with associated injuries achieved good or excellent results. More fingers lost the ability to flex fully than lost the ability to extend. Injuries in zones 1 through 4 had a worse outcome than injuries in the more proximal zones. Fair or poor results were found in 7 of 12 zone 1 injuries, 6 of 6 zone 2 injuries, 10 of 14 zone 3 injuries, and 4 of 7 zone 4 injuries. These injury zones were associated with total extensor lags of the PIP and DIP joints of 11 to 45 degrees or more, and loss of flexion of 21 to 45 degrees or more. Zones 5 through 7 usually regained approximately 80% or more of normal motion.[58] In a prospective randomized trial of dynamic

TABLE 5.2	Miller Criteria for Assessing Extensor Tendon Function	
Result	**Total Extension Lag (degrees)**	**Total Flexion Loss (degrees)**
Excellent	0	0
Good	≤10	≤20
Fair	11-45	21-45
Poor	≥45	≥45

From Miller H: Repair of severed tendons of the hand and wrist. *Surg Gynecol Obstet* 75:693–698, 1942.

versus static splinting for uncomplicated zones 5 and 6 lacerations, Mowlavi and coworkers[68] found total active motion of 250 degrees for both groups at 6-month follow-up, with grip strength of 80% of normal in the dynamic group and 73% of normal in the static group. A systematic review of the literature in 2012 noted that both static and early motion protocols resulted in favorable results, but neither technique could be shown to be superior owing to variability in outcome measure reporting.[33]

I employ dynamic splinting and controlled active motion for extensor tendon injuries in zones 4 through 7 in compliant patients, or when multiple structures are involved in certain patients with injuries in zones 2 and 3. There is no level I evidence that accelerated rehabilitation confers any long-term advantage in outcome over static splinting.

Complications After Extensor Tendon Repair

Adhesions are the most frequent complication of extensor tendon repair and can cause an extension lag and loss of flexion. An extensor tenolysis may be considered if, after 6 months, progress is considered to be unsatisfactory by the patient. Tenolysis of the extensor mechanism over the hand and finger may require concomitant joint releases and flexor tenolysis, either simultaneously or in a staged fashion. In the ideal situation, full passive motion should be present before tenolysis because this implies that there are no secondary capsular or ligamentous contractures. Lack of full passive motion after an appropriate course of therapy is not a contraindication to surgery, but the patient should be aware of the diminished expectations when joint release and mobilization are necessary. Creighton and Steichen[18] reported the results of tenolysis after fracture and found only a 31% improvement in total active motion overall, 50% improvement in extensor lag if only a tenolysis was required, and 21% improvement in total active motion if a dorsal capsulotomy was required with no improvement of the active extensor lag.

CRITICAL POINTS *Extensor Tendon Repair*

- "Bunching up" the flat extensor tendon over the phalanges with one large core suture should be avoided.
- Repairs in zones 1 through 3 are not usually amenable to early motion protocols.
- Dynamic splinting may be used for injuries proximal to the PIP joints, but may not produce better outcomes than static or early active motion rehabilitation.

Expected Outcomes

- Loss of digital flexion may be greater than residual loss of extension.
- Repairs in zones 1 through 4 typically have worse motion than more proximal injuries.

SPECIFIC EXTENSOR TENDON INJURIES

Acute Mallet Finger Injury (Zone 1: Distal Interphalangeal Joint Level) (Case Study 5.2)

Mallet finger injury is characterized by discontinuity of the terminal extensor tendon resulting in an extensor lag at the DIP joint with or without compensatory hyperextension at the PIP joint (*swan neck deformity*). The injury has also been termed *drop finger* or *baseball finger*. Mallet fingers are classically described as "soft tissue" (tendon rupture) or "bony" (avulsed fragment of bone). For a seemingly simple injury, a lengthy, tedious treatment course is often required to obtain a satisfactory result. Poor outcomes are not unusual and can be a considerable source of frustration for the patient and the surgeon.

Mechanism of Injury

Mallet finger may be caused by open injuries or more commonly by closed rupture of the terminal tendon with or without associated fracture of the distal phalanx. Closed injuries are more common and are typically unnoticed at the moment of injury. Snagging the extending finger on a pants cuff, a bedsheet, or other object that suddenly flexes the extending DIP joint is a frequent cause. Less commonly, a forceful hyperextension injury of the DIP joint may result in a large fracture of the base of the distal phalanx involving one third or more of the articular surface. Elderly patients with osteoarthritis of the DIP joint may have "mallet" deformities that are not related to trauma, and individuals with hyperlax joints may have multiple pseudomallet swan neck postures that are unrelated to trauma.

Incidence

The most frequently involved digits are the small, ring, and middle fingers of the dominant hand, with a male predominance.[32] Tendinous mallet fingers have been reported to occur from age 11 onward. In skeletally immature individuals, a transepiphyseal plate fracture may be seen. According to Jones and Peterson,[44] who noted 20 mallet fingers in 7 family members, there may be a familial predisposition to mallet fingers.

◆ ANATOMY

The radial and ulnar lateral bands merge to form the terminal tendon distal to the triangular ligament over the dorsum of the middle phalanx. Warren and associates[115] suggested that an area of avascularity in the area of the terminal tendon may predispose it to rupture. The extensor mechanism over the dorsum of the middle phalanx is proximally tethered by its anatomic connections. Katzman and colleagues[47] showed that PIP joint motion and intrinsic tendon tension did not cause a tendon gap in a transected terminal tendon. If the DIP joint is fully extended, the gap closes; if the DIP joint is flexed, the gap opens. The position of the DIP joint alone dictates the gap at the site of healing of a torn terminal tendon, regardless of the position of the PIP joint. Theoretically, PIP joint flexion should advance the extensor mechanism distally through interconnections between the central slip and lateral bands, and some historical treatments did immobilize the PIP joint in flexion along with DIP joint extension. PIP joint flexion is not currently recommended in the treatment of mallet fingers.

The posture of the DIP joint is exquisitely sensitive to changes in the length of the terminal tendon. Lengthening of the extensor mechanism over the middle phalanx or DIP joint by 1 mm may result in a DIP joint extensor lag of 25 degrees, and lengthening of 0.5 mm results in a lag of 10 degrees.[90] This finding helps to explain why mallet finger injuries frequently result in residual extensor DIP joint lags and why such prolonged immobilization is required. Twenty percent of patients may have a residual extensor DIP joint lag of 10 degrees or more.[17]

Individuals with the ability to hyperextend the PIP joint because of volar plate laxity (either traumatic or congenital) may develop a secondary swan neck deformity after a mallet injury, as the central slip overcompensates at the PIP joint. The small finger is especially prone to this deformity.

Mallet fingers associated with large fragments of bone from the dorsal base of the distal phalanx may result in volar subluxation of the distal phalanx because the collateral ligaments remain attached to the fracture fragment and are incapable of resisting the volar translation moment of the flexor profundus. Fracture fragments that are less than 43% of the distal phalanx articular surface usually do not allow volar subluxation, whereas fragments involving more than 52% of the joint surface consistently allow subluxation.[40]

Classification

Doyle[21] has classified mallet finger deformities as four types (Table 5.3). The most common injury is type I. Patients presenting within 4 weeks of injury are considered to have acute injuries; patients presenting later than 4 weeks are considered to have chronic injuries. X-rays are always recommended for mallet injuries to assess for fractures.

TABLE 5.3 Classification of Mallet Fingers

Type I	Closed injury, with or without small dorsal avulsion fracture
Type II	Open injury, laceration of tendon
Type III	Open injury with loss of skin, subcutaneous cover, and tendon substance
Type IV	Mallet fracture
A	Transepiphyseal plate fracture in children
B	Hyperflexion injury with fracture of articular surface of 20% to 50%
C	Hyperextension injury with fracture of the articular surface >50% and with early or late volar subluxation of distal phalanx

From Doyle JR: Extensor tendons: acute injuries. In Green D, editor: *Green's operative hand surgery.* ed 4, New York, 1999, Churchill Livingstone, pp 195–198.
Doyle, JR: Extensor tendons: acute injuries. In Green DP, Hotchkiss RN, Pederson WC, et al, editors: *Green's operative hand surgery.* ed 5, New York, 1999, Churchill Livingstone, pp 195–197.

Management of Type I Acute Mallet Injuries

The DIP joint is splinted in full extension for 6 to 8 weeks, followed by progressive weaning of the splint. Mallet fingers manifesting several months after injury have been found to be amenable to successful splint treatment.

Nonoperative Treatment. Methods of immobilizing the DIP joint in extension include aluminum foam splints applied palmarly or dorsally, premade plastic splints, or custom-molded thermoplastic splints. Using a premade plastic splint, Okafor and colleagues[75] noted an average DIP joint extensor lag of 8.3 degrees at 5-year follow up in 31 patients. Using a dorsal DIP joint thermoplastic splint, Foucher and colleagues[26] noted an extensor lag of 5 degrees at 5 years after the injury. Using a premade plastic splint for 8 weeks, Crawford[17] noted that 20% of patients had an extensor lag of more than 10 degrees, and these tended to be patients who were noncompliant with proper splinting. Pike and colleagues[79] found no difference in clinical outcomes in a blinded, prospective randomized trial comparing volar or dorsal aluminum foam splints and custom splints; increased extensor lags were seen after discontinuation of splinting.

Historical methods of treatment involved plaster casting the finger with the PIP joint in flexion and DIP joint in extension, although now it is appreciated that the PIP joint need not be immobilized to obtain tendon coaptation. Plaster casting has been reported to be helpful with children or noncompliant patients, but this technique has largely fallen out of favor.

Operative Treatment

Tendon Suture. In 1930, Mason[63a] recommended immediate operative repair of closed mallet finger injuries; however, treatment has evolved such that immediate repair is neither necessary nor desirable for type I mallet injuries. This change in thinking is due to the difficulty of obtaining adequate tendon repair at the level of the paper-thin terminal tendon and the relative success of nonoperative treatment. Even with operative repair, prolonged immobilization of the DIP joint in extension is still required to allow tendon healing without gapping.

Kirschner Wire Fixation. Kirschner wire fixation has historically been recommended for patients who are unable to work wearing a splint, such as surgeons. Axial or oblique Kirschner wire fixation of the DIP joint, without directly repairing the

tendon, has been advocated in these cases for 6 to 8 weeks, followed by 2 to 4 weeks of part-time splinting. Typically, 0.045- or 0.035-inch Kirschner wires are used depending on the size of the joint. The advantage of oblique Kirschner wires is that if they are passed through the opposite cortex of the middle phalanx, they may be extracted in the event of breakage, as opposed to a broken centrally placed Kirschner wire in the DIP joint, which is quite difficult to extricate. Instead of Kirschner wire fixation, surgeons with acute mallet fingers may use the aluminum foam splint without the foam portion (moleskin applied to the aluminum), creating a thin splint that can be protected with a sterile wrap and easily fits into a sterile glove.

Management of Types II and III Open Mallet Finger Injuries

Open lacerations of the terminal tendon are typically managed by débridement and tendon suture. Type III injuries involving loss of skin and tendon substance may require skin coverage procedures, with or without tendon grafts. Theoretically, there is no reason why closed treatment for type II injuries should not be successful (suture skin only and splint the DIP joint), and in late presentations of open injuries this may be preferable. So long as the tendon ends are approximated, an equally successful result with closed treatment should be expected. The open nature of the acute injury necessitates surgical cleansing of the contaminated joint and lends itself well to immediate tendon repair.

Management of Type IV Mallet Finger Injuries

Mallet fractures in children differ from their adult counterparts because the fractures are transepiphyseal rather than articular (Seymour fracture).[91] The extensor tendon inserts on the epiphysis and the flexor tendon inserts on the metaphysis and spans the fracture. Al Qattan[2] noted, as did Seymour, that most of these injuries were located 1 to 2 mm distal to the growth plate, and he recommended fixing the fracture with a longitudinal Kirschner wire spanning the DIP joint. I concur with axial Kirschner wire fixation of this injury. The physician should be vigilant for the frequent open nature of this injury; the nail plate can be avulsed proximally from beneath the eponychial fold. Failure to recognize this injury and treat with appropriate irrigation and antibiotic coverage can result in osteomyelitis of the terminal tuft.

The treatment of large fracture fragments in adults with or without volar subluxation of the DIP joint is controversial.[7,21,118] Intuitively, operative anatomic restoration of a large articular fragment at the DIP joint would seem preferable to nonoperative treatment and acceptance of a gap of several millimeters in the joint surface. Experience has shown that successful results are obtainable with splint treatment of these injuries.

Nonoperative Treatment. Wehbe and Schneider[118] recommended nonoperative treatment for all mallet fractures, including injuries with volar subluxation of the distal phalanx, citing the complications of operative treatment and the satisfactory results obtained with closed treatment. They found that remodeling of the articular surface occurred even with volar subluxation, leading to a near-normal painless joint despite persistent joint subluxation and a dorsal prominence. King, Shin, and Kang[49] noted a 41% incidence of complications following operative treatment of mallet fractures, the most common of which was skin necrosis.

Crawford[17] found that splint treatment of mallet fractures was usually successful, but that in some cases with large fracture fragments, the DIP joint should not be immobilized in hyperextension because this might encourage volar subluxation of the distal phalanx. Operative treatment was recommended by Crawford only for cases involving volar subluxation of the distal phalanx.[17] Kalainov and associates[45] reviewed 22 mallet fractures involving more than one third of the articular surface treated with 5.5 weeks of splinting; 13 were associated with volar DIP joint subluxation. An average DIP joint extensor lag of 9 degrees and flexion of 59 degrees resulted, and most had degenerative joint changes. All patients expressed some dissatisfaction with the final appearance of the digit because of residual dorsal joint prominence, swan neck deformity, or extensor lag. Pain was negligible, but there was overall high satisfaction with finger function and minimal difficulties with work and activities of daily living. A delay in treatment of 1 month after initial injury did not adversely affect outcome.[45] A Cochrane analysis of four randomized clinical trials found insufficient evidence to support operative over nonoperative treatment of mallet fractures.[34]

Operative Treatment. Open and closed methods of reduction of large articular fragments have been described. Open operative reduction is technically difficult and frequently results in comminution of the small piece of bone. Closed reduction and Kirschner wire pinning or "extension block pinning" has been described by several authors with different techniques.[65,105] The DIP joint is maximally flexed, and a 0.045- or 0.035-inch Kirschner wire is introduced into the head of the middle phalanx at a 45-degree angle to create an extension block for the bony fragment. Alternatively, the Kirschner wire may be inserted using a Kapandji-like technique, to lever the fragment down into flexion. A second Kirschner wire is placed axially from distal to proximal across the DIP joint to maintain extension and reduction. The pins are removed at 4 to 6 weeks postoperatively. Tetik and Gudemez[105] reported all fractures healed with this technique, and a congruent joint was obtained in 17 of 18 patients (Figure 5.15).

Complications. Stern and Kastrup[101] reported a 45% complication rate in digits treated with extension splinting and a 53% complication rate in digits treated surgically. Splinting complications were minor and included skin-related problems, whereas most of the surgical complications were major, including four DIP joint fusions and one amputation.

❖ AUTHOR'S PREFERRED METHOD OF TREATMENT OF ACUTE MALLET INJURIES

Type I Injuries. I prefer aluminum foam splints with or without the foam, applied dorsally for 8 weeks of full-time splinting, followed by 4 weeks of night-time splinting; during this time, for the first 2 weeks the splint is worn half-time during the day. If the foam portion of the splint is completely removed, moleskin may be applied to the aluminum for skin comfort; alternatively, the foam portion can be thinned with a scissors. Slight hyperextension is built into the splint to improve tendon coaptation. I have not seen skin problems with slight hyperextension of the DIP joint, although some authors have reported vascular compromise of the skin as a complication.[82] The splint is changed every 3 days or so to check the skin, with care taken to ensure the DIP joint remains extended. Active flexion is allowed

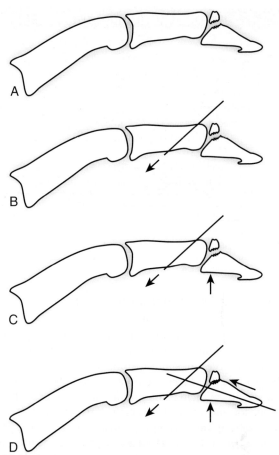

FIGURE 5.15 Extension block pinning of mallet fractures. **A,** Large mallet fracture in preparation for extension block pinning. **B,** A 0.045- or 0.035-inch Kirschner wire introduced at 45-degree angle to "block" the fragment and enable the volar piece to be reduced to it, after "levering" it down in a Kapandji-like technique, or after maximally flexing DIP joint. **C,** Volar fracture piece is reduced to dorsal fragment. **D,** Axial or oblique Kirschner wire is introduced from the distal to the middle phalanx to maintain the reduction.

after splint removal, and passive manipulation of the DIP joint into flexion is avoided to prevent elongation of the healed tendon. Full DIP joint flexion may require 4 additional months. The skin over the DIP joint and the distal middle phalanx may remain swollen and slightly red for several months after splint cessation, which may be a reaction to the prolonged splinting and underlying tendon thickening (Figure 5.16). Patients are counseled that a 5- to 10-degree extension lag is common, and that unsatisfactory results may occur in 10% of patients despite optimal splint treatment.

Types II and III Injuries. Open repair of the extensor tendon with a running 5-0 polypropylene suture, or placement of multiple interrupted and buried figure-of-eight 5-0 polypropylene sutures, is performed; an oblique or axial 0.045-inch Kirschner wire is placed across the DIP joint in full extension to protect the repair and removed 1 month later, followed by full-time splinting for 2 weeks and night-time splinting for 1 month.

Type IV Injuries (Mallet Fractures). Unless volar subluxation is present, extension splinting for 5 to 6 weeks is my treatment of choice. I currently recommend treating large fragments associated with volar subluxation with extension block pinning as described previously, although I have had success with

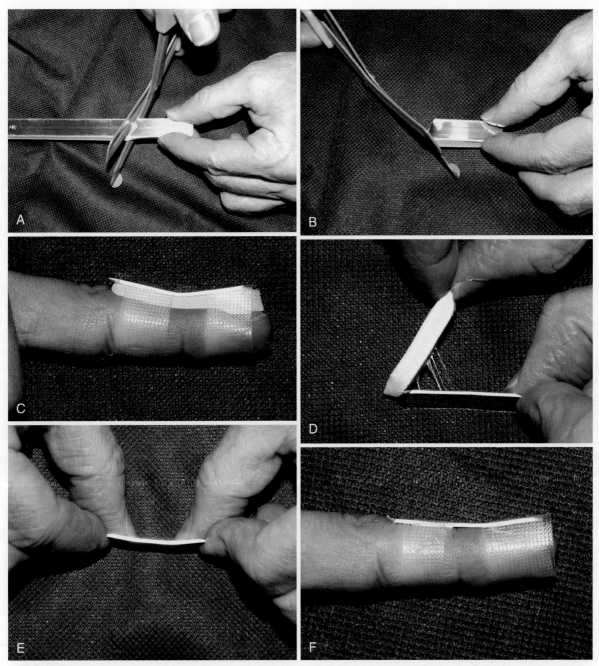

FIGURE 5.16 Author's preferred splinting regimen for mallet fingers. **A**, Cutting aluminum foam finger splint. **B**, It is important to ensure that sharp edges on the splint edge are trimmed off. **C**, Slight hyperextension is applied to splint to encourage tendon approximation. **D**, For compliant patients desiring a thinner splint, the foam can be removed. The "shiny," nonsticky side faces the skin. **E**, Slight bending of the splint into extension is performed. **F**, The "thin" splint easily fits into gloves. Care must be taken to ensure that the skin tolerates the splint in all cases using padded or nonpadded splints.

operative and nonoperative treatment of these injuries. Either splint treatment or extension block splinting is acceptable based on the current literature for mallet fractures, including fractures with volar subluxation. Patients are always advised that they may have a permanent dorsal bump with either surgical or nonsurgical treatment.

Chronic Mallet Injuries

Mallet deformities manifesting several months after the injury have been successfully treated with an extension splinting pro-

tocol.[28] Surgical options involve direct tendon repair or skin imbrications (or both),[42] tendon rebalancing with a central slip tenotomy (Fowler tenotomy),[10,31] or creating an ORL using a lateral band or tendon graft.[52,106] Arthrodesis is a salvage procedure for patients with resistant fixed or painful mallet deformities associated with arthritic changes. Tendon grafting has also been recently reported with a tendon-bone construct harvested from the ECRB–third metacarpal junction with a mean residual extensor lag of 4 degrees in 28 fingers.[114] Suh and Wolfe[103] reviewed the outcomes of various treatment options for chronic

CRITICAL POINTS *Acute Mallet Finger Splinting*

- A splint is worn full-time for 8 weeks, with weaning off of the splint over 1 month.
- Night-time splinting is implemented for 4 weeks after full-time splint wear.
- Full PIP joint flexion exercises are encouraged to prevent stiffness and to slacken lateral band tension.
- Mallet fractures may be treated nonoperatively with 5 to 6 weeks of splinting. Acute mallet fractures associated with volar subluxation of the DIP joint are treated with extension block pinning, although excellent functional results can also result from splint treatment.

Expected Outcomes
- A 10-degree residual extensor lag is common.
- The dorsal skin may remain pink and tender for 1 to 2 months after splint cessation.

mallet finger and noted generally less than 10 degrees of residual extensor lag in small studies involving splinting, tenodermodesis, palmaris longus grafting, central slip tenotomy, and ORL reconstruction.

Technique of Skin Imbrication

Tenodermodesis involves an elliptical wedge resection of skin and scarred tendon with suturing of the skin and tendon as a single unit.[42] A Kirschner wire is used to maintain the DIP joint in full extension for 4 to 6 weeks.

Technique of Fowler Tenotomy

The Fowler central slip tenotomy relies on a mature terminal tendon that has healed with slight elongation resulting in a persistent extensor lag. Typically, at least 6 to 12 months have passed since injury to allow full tendon maturation. The passage of time also allows most patients to realize that they no longer desire surgical correction because finger function is adequate. The procedure allows the extensor mechanism to slide proximally at the PIP joint by removing the tethering effect of the central slip insertion; this effectively takes up the "slack" induced by elongation at the terminal tendon. A boutonnière deformity is not created, because the triangular ligament is not injured, so long as the central slip is released from *underneath* the extensor mechanism, as described subsequently.

The finger is exposed via a midlateral incision centered over the PIP joint, performed under a local digital block with sedation. The transverse retinacular ligament is incised, and a Freer elevator is inserted under the extensor mechanism proximal to the central slip and underneath the lateral bands distal to the central slip. A tenolysis may need to be performed over the middle phalanx to break up any adhesions of the tendon to bone. The triangular ligament is left intact. The insertion of the central slip is visualized deep to the extensor mechanism. The insertion is divided by sliding a scalpel from proximal to distal underneath the extensor mechanism, and active extension of the DIP joint is attempted. A dorsal view of the extensor mechanism would not reveal any discontinuity in the tendon anatomy. Usually a near-full correction is obtained with preoperative extensor lags of up to 35 degrees.[16] The ability to extend the DIP joint actively is now better with the PIP joint held passively in flexion as opposed to extension (the reverse of normal, where

DIP joint extension is limited by PIP joint flexion—the basis of the Elson test) owing to increased tension in the extensor mechanism.

The skin is closed, and a dorsal splint is applied over a thin dressing to hold the PIP joint in about 20 degrees of flexion and the DIP joint fully extended, the idea being to maximize tension on the extensor mechanism at the DIP joint. Two separate dorsal aluminum splints are applied 2 to 3 days postoperatively, one to keep the DIP joint in full extension and the second as an extension block splint for the PIP joint of about 20 degrees. The dorsal blocking splint over the PIP is discarded 2 weeks postoperatively (although PIP joint hyperextension should not be allowed), and the DIP joint extension splint is removed several times daily to allow active flexion exercises, although it is worn full-time otherwise. At 4 weeks postoperatively, the DIP joint extension splint is removed all day, although it is still worn at night for another month (Figure 5.17).

Results of Fowler Tenotomy. In a series of 20 patients, Grundberg and Reagan[31] noted an average preoperative DIP joint extensor lag of 37 degrees corrected to an average of 9 degrees at most recent follow-up using an immediate motion postoperative protocol. Houpt and colleagues[37] noted that 26 of 35 patients regained full extension, 8 patients had a residual 10- to 20-degree lag, and 1 patient had a residual 30-degree lag using an immediate motion postoperative protocol. Lucas[61] reported 11 cases of which 8 had an extensor lag of 10 degrees or less; one patient who had a mallet deformity for only a few weeks had a poor result with a 30-degree lag. Lucas[61] used a postoperative protocol of splinting the PIP joint in flexion and the DIP joint in extension for 2 weeks, followed by a Stack splint for another 2 weeks, then full motion. Bowers and Hurst[10] reported five patients; four obtained full DIP joint extension, and one had a residual lag of 10 degrees. One patient had a PIP joint lag of 12 degrees. Preoperative DIP joint extension lags ranged from 45 to 70 degrees. The postoperative splinting protocol involved splinting the PIP joint at 45 degrees of flexion and the DIP joint in full extension for 2 weeks, followed by full motion except for PIP joint flexion, which was not allowed past 45 degrees for an additional 2 weeks. I have been more pleased with respect to maintenance of the mallet correction with a progressive postoperative splinting regimen (as described previously) than by allowing full active immediate motion without any splinting, which was my previous postoperative protocol.

Treatment of Swan Neck Deformity Associated With Chronic Mallet Injury

Swan neck deformity may result from chronic mallet injury provided that the PIP joint is capable of hyperextension. PIP hyperextension results from innate or acquired laxity of the volar plate combined with increased tension in the central slip and lateral bands owing to elongation of the terminal tendon. The swan neck deformity may also arise (not due to terminal tendon injury) from overactivity of the extrinsic or intrinsic extensor mechanism due to spasticity or intrinsic contracture, and can result from insufficiency of the volar stabilizers of the PIP joint, such as volar plate incompetence or flexor digitorum superficialis injury.[108] Swan neck deformity may become symptomatic due to locking of the PIP joint in hyperextension (pseudotriggering) upon initiating PIP flexion from the hyperextended position, as well as the cosmetic deformity of the

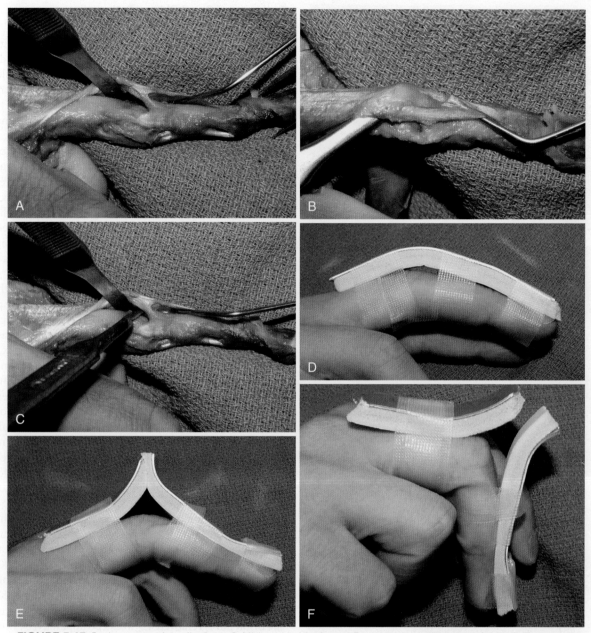

FIGURE 5.17 Fowler tenotomy for mallet finger. **A**, Midlateral incision is used. Transverse retinacular ligament is incised. The extensor mechanism over the proximal and middle phalanges is freed from any adhesions, and the central slip is identified. **B**, Dorsal view showing that the triangular ligament and dorsal extensor mechanism are not violated when the central slip insertion is transected. **C**, Central slip is transected with scalpel at its insertion into the middle phalanx base, allowing the extensor mechanism to slide proximally, reliably correcting up to a 35-degree extensor lag. **D**, Postoperatively, the finger is immobilized in PIP joint flexion and DIP joint extension for approximately 3 days. **E**, At 3 days postoperatively, a dorsal PIP joint extension block splint is applied until 2 weeks postoperatively. During this time, the DIP joint is kept in full extension. **F**, PIP joint flexion is allowed in the splint. At 2 weeks postoperatively, the proximal splint is removed, and full PIP joint motion is allowed, restricting hyperextension at PIP joint, if it was present preoperatively. The DIP joint extension splint is removed three to four times daily to allow motion; otherwise, it is kept on all the time. At 4 weeks postoperatively, the DIP joint splint is left off all day but used at night for another month.

finger. Some individuals are able to voluntarily put the finger in the swan neck position and this is physiologic in the absence of symptoms.

If PIP laxity is the primary cause, preventing PIP hyperextension will correct the DIP extensor lag associated with the swan neck deformity. A physical examination maneuver that will distinguish between swan neck deformity caused primarily by PIP laxity or mallet finger is to manually block PIP hyperextension; if full DIP extension is possible, blocking PIP hyper-

extension will suffice to correct the swan neck deformity (Figure 5.18). This may be considered a "distal Bouvier-type maneuver." If this maneuver corrects the mallet deformity, restricting PIP hyperextension may be accomplished through figure-of-eight splinting or surgical means, such as volar plate imbrication, flexor digitorum superficialis (FDS) tenodesis, or lateral band translocation.[108] Should this maneuver not result in correction of the DIP extensor lag, surgically increasing the extensor force at the DIP joint is required in addition to restricting PIP

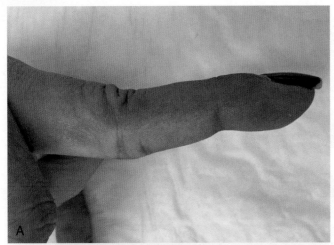

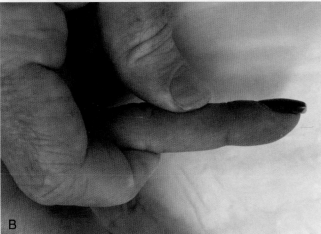

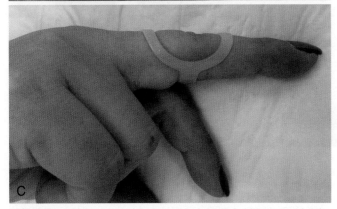

FIGURE 5.18 Physical examination maneuver to distinguish swan neck deformity due to mallet finger from other causes. **A**, Swan neck deformity due to congenital PIP joint laxity. Note the PIP hyperextension with DIP extensor lag. **B**, Manual blocking of PIP hyperextension by the examiner eliminates the DIP extensor lag, indicating that the primary problem is at the PIP joint. **C**, Figure-of-eight splint that blocks PIP hyperextension eliminates the swan neck deformity while allowing full finger flexion. This was sufficient for this patient; after wearing the splint for a few months, her symptomatic locking in hyperextension was no longer bothersome.

hyperextension. Both of these goals can be achieved by surgical reconstruction of an ORL, either by using one of the existing lateral bands[58,108] or by tendon graft procedures.[52,106] Correction of the swan neck deformity can also be accomplished via the Fowler tenotomy, which reduces central slip tone while increasing extensor force at the DIP joint.[10]

Technique of Spiral Oblique Retinacular Ligament Reconstruction

The concept of the ORL as a dynamic tenodesis linking the volar flexor sheath to the lateral aspect of the terminal tendon provides a mechanism for automatic DIP joint extension with active PIP joint extension. An ORL can be surgically created in several ways. Littler[58] described a technique to correct the swan neck deformity that divided the lateral band proximally and rerouted it palmar to the axis of PIP joint rotation, securing it to the flexor tendon sheath. Theoretically, if bridging scar tissue is stable enough to support the Fowler tenotomy concept for mallet fingers, it should work for the Littler procedure as well, although in this situation a much thinner piece of scar tissue is being relied on to extend the DIP joint. Oh and colleagues[74] found no clinical differences with the use of one lateral band (Littler's original procedure[58]) or a tendon graft (spiral ORL reconstruction) in the treatment of mallet finger in a series of 27 patients.

In 1978, Thompson and colleagues[106] described the spiral ORL, which is a procedure creating an ORL with a free palmaris or plantaris tendon graft (Figure 5.19). The tendon graft was placed through gouge holes in the distal phalanx and then directed in a spiral fashion around the middle phalanx, deep to the neurovascular bundles, over the flexor sheath, and transversely through the base of the proximal phalanx. Graft tension was adjusted with the PIP and DIP joints in neutral extension by securing the proximal end with a button or hemoclips, or both. Care is taken to avoid overtightening, which could create a boutonnière deformity. Kirschner wire fixation was not used, and active motion was begun 3 weeks postoperatively. Most patients fully corrected their preoperative mallet deformities, and one patient required slight graft lengthening for 20 degrees of DIP joint hyperextension.

In 1984, Kleinman and Petersen[52] modified the Thompson procedure, terming it the *ORL reconstruction*, and demonstrated its efficacy in 12 patients, 8 of whom had a concomitant swan neck deformity. The modifications involved axial Kirschner wire pinning of the DIP joint in neutral and pinning of the PIP joint in 10 to 15 degrees of flexion with an oblique Kirschner wire. The proximal pin is removed 3 weeks postoperatively, and the distal pin is removed 4.5 weeks postoperatively, with splinting of the DIP joint in extension for another 1.5 weeks. Additionally, Kleinman and Petersen[52] secured the graft to the dorsal distal phalanx with a 4-0 Bunnell steel pull-out wire, and the proximal juncture was attached to the palmar flexor tendon sheath with nonabsorbable sutures. This technique resulted in normal DIP joint extension in 9 of 12 cases, and slight active hyperextension of 10 to 25 degrees was seen in 3 of 12 patients. One patient required flexor tenolysis for adhesions, and one patient developed a 35-degree PIP joint flexion contracture that responded to step-cut lengthening of the graft (see Figure 5.18).

❖ AUTHOR'S PREFERRED TREATMENT OF CHRONIC MALLET INJURY

Because there is little downside to a trial of splinting, I attempt an 8-week trial of full-time extension splint treatment for neglected mallet deformities of up to 6 months' duration. For patients with an extensor lag of less than 35 to 40 degrees, more than 6 months after the injury, I find Fowler's central slip tenotomy effective; greater degrees of extensor lag may not correct

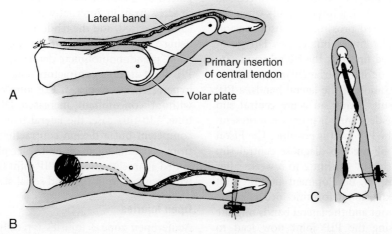

FIGURE 5.19 Spiral oblique retinacular ligament reconstruction. **A,** Schematic representation of the mallet deformity with compensatory swan neck deformity. **B** and **C,** The tendon graft is fixed to the distal phalanx, in this case using a pull-out suture. The graft is passed between the flexor sheath and the neurovascular bundles palmar to the PIP joint. The graft is tensioned and anchored into the shaft of the proximal phalanx.

as well, and alternative procedures should be considered.[16] Fowler's tenotomy also reduces PIP joint extension moment by disinserting the central slip and usually improves a swan neck deformity. For mallet fingers with extensor lags greater than 45 degrees, when there is an associated swan neck deformity, or where there is no tendon continuity at all between the retracted terminal tendon and the distal phalanx, I recommend the ORL reconstruction procedure, with or without a tendon graft.

Mallet Thumb Injury

Excellent results have been reported with nonoperative (splint) and operative treatment of closed mallet thumb injuries.[1,77] Generally, I treat closed mallet thumbs with the same splinting protocol used for type I mallet fingers and repair open tendon injuries. I have successfully treated several cases with late presentation of open mallet thumb injuries (1 to 2 weeks following the injury) with a splinting protocol in patients who have refused surgical repair.

Zone 2 Extensor Tendon Injuries

Lacerations over the dorsal aspect of the middle phalanx involve injury to one or both lateral bands or the triangular ligament that unites them (or both). One functioning lateral band is sufficient to achieve full extension of the DIP joint, and lacerations involving 50% of the extensor mechanism may be treated without tendon repair.[21] Local wound care for 1 to 2 weeks followed by active motion is sufficient. Lacerations involving more than 50% of the extensor mechanism may be repaired using a running suture of 5-0 polypropylene followed by a cross-stitch of 5-0 polypropylene, as described by Doyle[21] (see Figure 5.12). Core sutures are not technically feasible in this zone, because the tendon is too thin. Postoperatively, static splinting or pinning of the DIP joint in extension for 6 weeks is recommended, allowing PIP joint motion. Thumb zone 2 lacerations are treated in a similar manner. Chronic zone 2 injuries may be treated with a tendon graft as described previously, using the spiral ORL reconstruction.[52]

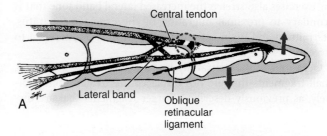

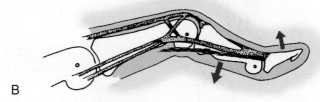

FIGURE 5.20 Pathomechanics of the boutonnière deformity. **A,** Attenuation of the central slip results in unopposed flexion at the PIP joint. **B,** With PIP joint flexion, the lateral bands drift palmar to the axis of rotation at the PIP joint. The lateral bands stay in the palmar position owing to loss of dorsal support from the attenuated triangular ligament and contracture of the transverse retinacular ligament.

Zone 3 (Proximal Interphalangeal Joint) Injuries (Case Study 5.3)

Closed or open injury to the extensor mechanism over the PIP joint may injure the central slip or the lateral bands (or both) and result in a PIP joint extensor lag and DIP joint hyperextension, termed a *boutonnière deformity* (Figure 5.20). Causes of a closed boutonnière deformity include blunt trauma to the dorsum of the PIP joint and volar dislocation of the PIP joint that results in an avulsion of the central slip, with or without a piece of bone.[99]

As noted earlier in the section on the Fowler tenotomy, an isolated, surgically created, central slip injury would not cause a PIP joint extensor lag, although it would allow increased proximal extensor tension at the DIP joint, especially when the PIP joint is flexed. This increased proximal extensor tension permits correction of a mallet finger but causes DIP joint hyperextension in an uninjured finger. If the lateral bands are also cut over the PIP joint, or if the triangular ligament is injured, allowing volar subluxation of the lateral bands, a PIP joint extensor lag would result.[10] After an acute central slip injury, the classic boutonnière deformity is usually not present, and full range of motion of the PIP joint is possible. The Elson test (see Figure 5.8) should be used to diagnose central slip disruption in suspected injuries.[23,87] Within 2 to 3 weeks after untreated central slip disruption, development of PIP joint flexion and DIP joint hyperextension deformities occurs as the triangular ligament stretches out and the lateral bands migrate palmarly. All tendons crossing the PIP joint now lead to increased PIP joint flexion (the two flexor tendons and the two lateral bands) (see Figure 5.20).

Treatment of acute central slip injury consists of splinting or pinning the PIP joint in full extension for approximately 6 weeks to allow the central slip to heal, during which time active DIP joint flexion exercises are performed hourly to draw the lateral bands into the correct dorsal alignment (Figure 5.21). The exercises also stretch the increased lateral band tone that is secondary to proximal migration of the extensor apparatus. Intermittent and night splinting follows for an additional 4 to 6 weeks.

Occasionally, the central slip is avulsed with a piece of bone. Small fragments that are not displaced are treated nonoperatively, as previously described. Larger fragments that are dis-

placed by 2 mm or more can be repaired with Kirschner wire or screw fixation. Alternatively, small or comminuted fragments can be excised, and the tendon can be repaired directly to bone using a pull-out wire or suture anchor.[21]

A "pseudoboutonnière deformity" is one in which there is a PIP joint flexion contracture that typically follows PIP joint hyperextension injury, or PIP joint collateral ligament sprains, without concomitant increased DIP joint extensor tendon tone.[55] In this case, the lateral bands and central slip remain competent but a flexion contracture of the joint has resulted from collateral ligament and volar plate scarring. Treatment is aimed at ameliorating the PIP joint flexion contracture, usually with dynamic splinting and serial static casting techniques.

Open Injuries

Acute open zone 3 injuries typically enter the PIP joint, and appropriate wound management and irrigation should be performed. Injury to one lateral band or 50% or less of the central slip does not require operative repair and may be treated with wound care and early motion. Complete transection of the central slip warrants open repair. Surgical repair of central slip lacerations may be done with reattachment to bone using a suture anchor, to a bone tunnel, or to the insertion itself, if sufficient tendon remains distally. A cross-stitch may be used to supplement the repair (see Figure 5.12). Doyle and Atkinson[22] noted that although the average thickness of the central slip just proximal to the PIP joint is 0.5 mm, this thickness doubles as a result of the fibrocartilaginous dorsal plate at the insertion of the central slip, providing better suture purchase. If there is sufficient tendon remaining distally, one or two core sutures of 4-0 or 5-0 followed by a 5-0 cross-stitch may be performed. The PIP joint must be maintained in extension during healing, and often this is facilitated by use of a transarticular 0.045-inch Kirschner wire.

❖ AUTHOR'S PREFERRED METHOD OF TREATMENT OF ZONE 3 INJURIES

In the setting of an injured, acutely tender PIP joint, the Elson test is performed with a digital block, as previously described, to evaluate for the presence of central slip injury. If the central slip is found to be injured, splinting the PIP joint in extension using an aluminum foam splint similar to mallet treatment (except placed over the dorsal PIP joint) is employed for 6 weeks, followed by part-time and night-time wear for another 4 to 6 weeks. DIP joint active and passive flexion exercises are performed hourly with the PIP joint fully extended during the entire splinting and rehabilitation course.

When treating subacute open zone 3 injuries, if the wound was sutured in the emergency department and the extent of tendon injury is unknown at the time of presentation (a common scenario), there are several options. An obvious PIP joint extensor lag would indicate the need for open repair. If there is no PIP joint extensor lag but the history indicates that a tendon was noted to be lacerated, surgical exploration generally provides the best method to assess the extent of injury (e.g., 90% laceration of the central slip versus 5%) and guide the necessity for tendon repair. The Elson test, performed in the office (under digital block), assesses the integrity of the central slip; if disruption is evident, operative repair is recommended. Because closed central slip disruptions are treated

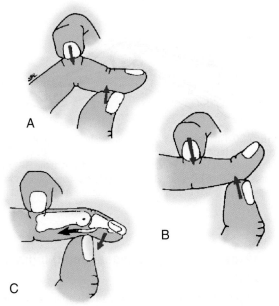

FIGURE 5.21 Exercise program for boutonnière deformity. Many patients with boutonnière deformity respond well to a carefully structured exercise and splinting program. The exercise is done in three steps. **A,** The patient is instructed to place the index finger of the opposite hand on the dorsum of PIP joint of the involved finger. The thumb of the uninvolved hand is placed on flexor aspect of DIP joint. **B,** PIP joint is passively extended by the patient as far as can be tolerated. This passively corrects the deformity at the proximal joint but increases the tone in the lateral bands and ORL, increasing hyperextension at DIP joint. **C,** The patient actively flexes DIP joint over the thumb of the opposite hand, stretching the ORLs and lateral bands (see text discussion).

nonoperatively, an argument could be made for splint treatment of open central slip injuries as well; however, I prefer open surgical repair of the lacerated tendon in this situation using a suture anchor or cross-stitch suture. If the central slip is intact based on the Elson test and the patient has full active extension against resistance (a digital block may be necessary to assess the strength of resistance free of pain), active motion is allowed, with a reexamination in 1 week to ensure that a partial tendon laceration did not propagate. If a PIP joint lag or loss of extension power develops, surgical exploration is recommended.

After operative repair, I usually place a 0.045-inch Kirschner wire obliquely across the joint in full extension to protect the repair for 5 to 6 weeks, followed by pin removal and range-of-motion exercises with interval splinting for another 2 to 4 weeks. Some authors recommend early motion or dynamic splinting. Lateral band lacerations may be repaired and rehabilitated similarly. Gentle active DIP joint motion is permitted if motion on the operating table does not stress or gap the lateral band repair. When there is loss of tendon substance, the gap in the tendon may be overcome using a graft, or the method of Snow, who used a proximally based flap of central slip tendon and rotated it distally to reconstruct the central slip (Figure 5.22).[97,96]

Open Thumb Metacarpophalangeal Joint Lacerations (Zone 3 Lacerations). Zone 3 lacerations over the MP joint of the thumb may involve the EPL or EPB, or both. In this location, a standard core type of suture may be used (I use a 4-0 or 3-0 locked Kessler suture on either side of the tendon to avoid bunching), augmented by a 5-0 cross-stitch. The underlying MP joint capsule is repaired separately. I either place a 0.045-inch Kirschner wire across the joint in full extension or splint the MP and IP joints in full extension for 4 weeks. If the EPB only is lacerated, the IP joint may be left free.

Congenital absence of the EPB occurs without thumb MP joint extensor lag, and if an isolated EPB laceration occurs in the setting of an intact EPL with full extension of MP and IP thumb joints, EPB repair may not be required. In patients presenting late to the office in this situation, the EPB laceration is likely to be overlooked; however, if a complete EPB laceration is noted acutely during the course of wound exploration, I recommend repairing the EPB to avoid potential late MP joint extensor lag.

CRITICAL POINTS *Acute Boutonnière Deformity Treatment*

- Recognize the injury by using the Elson test.
- Splint the PIP joint in full extension for 6 weeks.
- Perform active and passive DIP joint flexion exercises hourly to stretch out the lateral bands.

Expected Outcome

- Some tendency toward DIP joint hyperextension usually remains, along with a slight PIP joint extensor lag, even if splint treatment is initiated promptly.

Chronic Zone 3 Closed Injuries (Chronic Boutonnière Deformities)

Flexible boutonnière deformities can be successfully managed with splints several months after injury.[59] It is postulated that

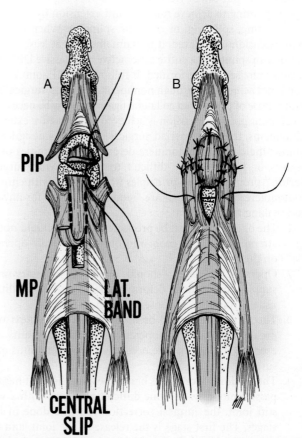

FIGURE 5.22 Acute boutonnière deformities associated with loss of substance of the extensor mechanism at PIP joint are difficult to treat. **A** and **B**, In an attempt to solve this problem, Snow took a retrograde flap from the central slip of the extensor (**A**) and applied it as a reinforcing batten over the central slip repair. The retrograde flap is carefully sutured into place over the repair site to act as a reinforcement in the area of repair. The defect in the central slip is closed with interrupted sutures (**B**). (Copyright Elizabeth Martin.)

late splint treatment allows the lateral bands to realign themselves by stretching out the tight transverse retinacular ligaments, resulting in correction of the deformity despite central slip discontinuity. Chronic boutonnière deformity is distinguished by the presence of fixed PIP joint or DIP joint contractures (or both). The central slip may have been traumatically disrupted or may have attenuated because of inflammatory synovitis, because of osteoarthritis, or through prolonged flexion contracture as is seen with Dupuytren contracture, flexor pulley disruptions, or burns.[62] In the presence of fixed contractures, treatment and successful results are far more difficult because both flexor tendons and the subluxated lateral bands are deforming forces. Despite the PIP joint contracture, however, many patients have functional complaints related to the inability to flex the DIP joint.

Burton[13] classified chronic boutonnière deformity into three stages:

Stage I: Supple, passively correctable deformity
Stage II: Fixed contracture, contracted lateral bands
Stage III: Fixed contracture, joint fibrosis, collateral ligament and palmar plate contractures
Stage IV is added to this classification, which is stage III plus PIP joint arthritis.

Stages I and II can be treated with a therapy regimen consisting of splinting to achieve full PIP joint extension by means of serial casting, splinting, or dynamic splinting. When full PIP joint extension is achieved, it is maintained for at least 6 to 12 weeks with splints. The entire time, active and passive DIP joint flexion exercises are performed. If full passive PIP joint extension is not achievable through nonoperative means, surgical PIP joint release of contracted collateral ligaments may be necessary. If PIP joint passive extension is achieved but an active extensor lag remains, there are myriad surgical procedures designed to address the chronic boutonnière deformity. Deformities of 30 degrees or less are quite difficult to improve with surgery. Burton[13] proposed seven principles when dealing with chronic boutonnière deformity that are "required reading" for anyone undertaking this problem:

1. The operations must be precisely done and should not be attempted by a surgeon who only occasionally operates on the hand.

2. Operative treatment should rarely be necessary in a supple boutonnière deformity because this condition usually responds to conservative management.

3. The procedure should be done within the context of a preoperative and postoperative exercise program. The exercises and splints are needed for several months after surgery.

4. The tendon procedure is best done after the joint has full passive mobility. In some difficult problems with a very stiff joint, the surgical correction must be done in two stages. The first stage is the release of the joint, and the second is the tendon reconstruction. In many patients, after the joint release is completed and the exercise program is resumed, the extensor mechanism rebalances with the conscientious performance of the two-stage exercise program and the splinting or cast support of the PIP joint. In these patients, the second stage is not required.

5. If radiograph shows significant arthritic changes, extensor mechanism rebalancing must be combined with implant arthroplasty or with PIP joint fusion.

6. Most patients with a boutonnière deformity retain full flexion and full grip function; even with this deformity, most patients have good function. As surgery is planned, the surgeon must be constantly aware of the need not to jeopardize flexor function in an attempt to gain extension.

7. All procedures involve a rebalancing of the extensor system, decreasing the tone at the distal joint and diverting it to the proximal joint.

Surgical Techniques to Correct Supple Boutonnière Deformity

Terminal Tendon Tenotomy (Distal Fowler or Dolphin Tenotomy). The concept of terminal tendon tenotomy is that operatively creating a "mallet finger" would decrease the extensor tone at the DIP joint, allowing DIP joint flexion and permitting the extensor mechanism to slide proximally to increase the extensor tension at the PIP joint. This procedure is designed for patients with full passive PIP joint extension and is contraindicated in patients with a fixed PIP joint flexion deformity. A dorsal incision is made over the middle phalanx, and the extensor

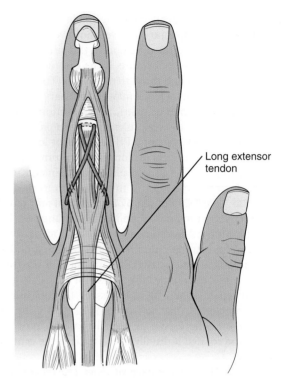

FIGURE 5.23 The Littler tendon graft technique. A thin graft is woven through the base of the middle phalanx and through the extensor tendon to restore extensor tone to the PIP joint.

mechanism is divided transversely over the junction of its middle and proximal thirds, distal to the triangular ligament. Care is taken to identify and preserve ORLs, if present (see Case Study 5.4). Why a mallet finger does not usually develop is unknown. It is possible that the DIP joint capsule and ligaments have chronically tightened so that rebound joint extension occurs after the joint is flexed. Postoperatively, a DIP joint extension splint is removed for active range-of-motion exercises several times a day for 6 to 8 weeks.[20,27,69]

Tendon Grafts. Tendon grafts have been employed, as in the figure-of-eight tendon graft through the extensor mechanism into the base of the middle phalanx described by Littler[57] (Figure 5.23). Full passive mobility of the PIP joint is required for success.

Lateral Band Mobilization and Relocation. The lateral bands normally move in a dorsal-palmar direction with PIP joint flexion and extension. Dividing them distally and suturing them to the central slip insertion has been used to restrict PIP joint flexion, with mixed results.[30,59,64,98,116]

❖ AUTHOR'S PREFERRED METHOD: The Curtis Staged Reconstruction

There are three stages of the Curtis procedure, depending on the correction obtained at each step (Figure 5.24).[19] All are done under a local anesthetic, and all rely on full passive preoperative PIP joint motion. The use of local anesthetic allows the surgeon to test active extension at each stage.

In stage I, a lazy "S" incision is made centered on the PIP joint. The transverse retinacular ligament is freed distally and proximally, and a tenolysis of the extensor tendon is performed. If full extension is present, the operation stops.

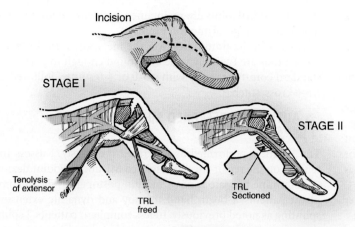

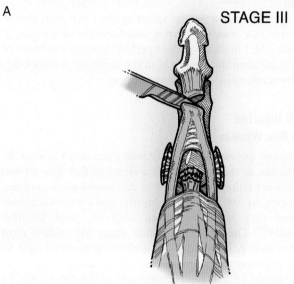

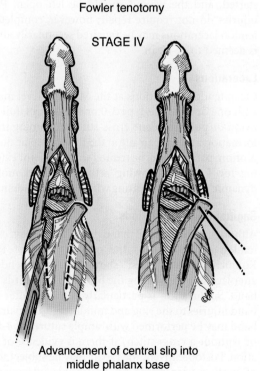

FIGURE 5.24 The Curtis staged reconstruction of boutonnière deformity. This operation relies on full preoperative passive mobility of PIP joint. **A,** Stages I and II: The transverse retinacular ligament is freed and transected if necessary, allowing the lateral bands to swing dorsally. **B,** Stage III: If full correction is not obtained after stage II but PIP joint extensor lag is less than 20 degrees, a Fowler tenotomy is performed. If PIP joint extensor lag is significant and more than 20 degrees after stage II, this step is skipped, and one proceeds directly to stage IV. **C,** Stage IV: The central slip is advanced into the middle phalanx base after removing 4 to 6 mm of intervening scar tissue between the native tendon and its insertion. (From Curtis RM, Reid RL, Provost JM: A staged technique for the repair of the traumatic boutonniere deformity, *J Hand Surg Am* 8:167–171, 1983. Copyright Elizabeth Martin.)

In stage II, if full extension is not achieved, the transverse retinacular ligament is sectioned, allowing the lateral bands to swing dorsally. If full extension is achieved (seen in 30% to 40% of cases), the MP joint is splinted at 70 degrees of flexion, the PIP and DIP joints are splinted at 0 degrees for 1 week, and then dynamic PIP joint splinting is performed.

In stage III, if there is still a 20-degree or smaller lag after stage II, a distal Fowler tenotomy is performed. Curtis recommended a "step-cut lengthening" of the lateral bands to prevent a mallet finger. I usually just obliquely transect the extensor mechanism distal to the triangular ligament. If full extension is present, the operation stops.

If an extensor lag of more than 20 degrees is still present after stage II, Curtis recommended proceeding directly to stage IV (necessary in 38% of his cases). The central tendon is dissected free and advanced about 4 to 6 mm into a drill hole in the dorsal base of the middle phalanx. The lateral bands, now slack, are loosely sutured to the central tendon.

Curtis's results at 1 year of follow-up revealed a 10-degree PIP joint lag, with an average 31-degree improvement from the preoperative status.[19] For patients requiring stage IV reconstruction with an average PIP joint preoperative lag of 55 degrees, a 17-degree lag persisted postoperatively. All but 3 of 23 patients showed improved flexion after the procedure.

CRITICAL POINTS *Treatment of Chronic Boutonnière Deformity*

- Exhaust the splinting protocol before surgical correction.
- Ensure full passive PIP joint motion before embarking on any tendon rebalancing or reconstructive procedure.
- A stepwise approach (Curtis procedure) is a rational solution to the problem.

Expected Outcomes

- A 20-degree persistent extensor lag is common, and surgery for PIP joint extensor lags of 20 to 30 degrees may not result in significant improvements. Although flexion loss is possible postoperatively, it is uncommon using the stepwise approach (Curtis procedure).

Zone 4 Injuries

Because of the convex bony contour of the proximal phalanx, dorsal lacerations are frequently associated with partial tendon injuries. Fractures of the proximal phalanx are commonly seen in association with these injuries. Similar to tendon injuries in other locations, the ideal method of evaluating the extent of injury is by surgical exploration. Partial lacerations of greater than 50% and complete tendon lacerations are repaired with one or two modified Kessler 4-0 core braided polyester sutures and a 5-0 cross-stitch on the dorsal side of the tendon.[5,21] The core suture should be placed into the relatively thicker area of the lateral bands to obtain maximal purchase (see Figure 5.13). Early motion protocols to prevent adhesions to the proximal phalanx involve the use of a dynamic extension splint to allow PIP joint flexion. The postoperative splint includes a dorsal outrigger with elastic straps to provide passive PIP joint extension (see Figure 5.29). The degree to which the PIP joint can be safely flexed is determined during surgery by observing repair site tension. Accelerated rehabilitation protocols generally begin within the first week of repair. If treated with immobilization,

the PIP and MP joints are maintained in extension for 4 weeks, followed by range-of-motion exercises.

Zone 4 in the thumb lies over the metacarpal. In this zone, the tendons are typically wide and round enough to perform a standard core-type repair with a 3-0 or 4-0 suture, followed by a 5-0 cross-stitch.

❖ AUTHOR'S PREFERRED METHOD OF ZONE 4 REPAIRS

The repair is performed as described previously. I assess the tension on the repair site with isolated MP and PIP joint flexion to determine the safe zone of motion postoperatively. In compliant patients, I begin hand therapy and dynamic extension splinting as noted previously. In less compliant patients, I splint the wrist in 20 degrees of extension, splint the MP joints in full extension, and mold a palmar splint to allow PIP joint flexion to a degree that does not permit visual tension or gapping at the repair site; I have the patient perform passive extension of the PIP joint, limiting flexion with the splint for 4 weeks, followed by active range-of-motion exercises.

Zone 5 Injuries
Human Bite Wounds

Open tendon injuries over the MP joint often result from striking someone in the mouth with a clenched fist. The tendon laceration is frequently partial, and the wound often communicates with the MP joint. These injuries initially appear innocuous and may be unrecognized until the joint becomes infected.[29,63,109] The dominant middle finger MP joint is most often involved. A high index of suspicion is required, and an x-ray is required to exclude a fracture or foreign body. The wound should be irrigated, appropriate antibiotics should be started, and the wound should be left open. Partial tendon injuries do not require repair; however, complete or complex tendon lacerations may be repaired secondarily after the wound is deemed to be clean.

Lacerations

Clean tendon lacerations at the MP joint level may be repaired with one or two core-type 3-0 or 4-0 sutures, followed by a 5-0 nylon or polypropylene cross-stitch. Assuming there is no gap formation at the repair site at the time of repair during PIP joint motion, patients may be treated with MP joint extension splinting for 4 weeks, allowing active PIP joint motion, or with dynamic extension splinting within the limits defined at surgery.

Sagittal Band Lacerations

Although rare, sagittal band lacerations may cause extensor tendon subluxation to the opposite side of the MP joint. Koniuch and associates[54] showed extensor tendon instability after laceration involving the proximal two thirds of the sagittal band. Subluxation is particularly common after radial sagittal band injuries to the ring and middle digits. Repair of the sagittal band may be performed with simple sutures of 4-0 or 5-0 (with or without a cross-stitch) if there is evidence of EDC subluxation. Postoperatively, the repair may be subject to gentle range of motion (depending on the visible intraoperative tension caused by flexion and extension) and "buddy taping" the finger to the adjacent finger.

Closed Sagittal Band Rupture

Closed sagittal band ruptures are more common than open lacerations and usually involve the radial sagittal band of the middle or ring finger following resisted extension ("flicking") of the finger, or direct trauma to the dorsum of the MP joint.[43] The condition may be mistaken for a trigger finger because of a snapping sensation that occurs when the extensor tendon shifts back and forth between the ulnar groove and its normal position over the metacarpal head. Consequently, early treatment may be delayed. Often, MP joint extension cannot be initiated from the flexed position of the joint, and the involved finger is abducted ulnarly. When passively positioned in full extension, the reduced position can be actively maintained. The middle finger may be more frequently involved because of its exposed position and the looser anchoring of the middle EDC tendon to the sagittal band. Rarely, radial extensor tendon subluxation secondary to ulnar sagittal band injury has been reported.[86] Individuals with hyperlaxity may have nonpathologic subluxation of the middle and ring finger EDC tendons at the MP joints with flexion, and this does not warrant treatment; it is important to evaluate the opposite side for comparison when dealing with this condition to ensure that an actual injury is not present (Figure 5.25).

Ishizuki[43] identified superficial and deep layers of the sagittal band and noted disruption of the superficial layer only in "spontaneous" cases caused by "flicking" of a finger or "crumpling" up of paper. The deep and superficial layers were disrupted in traumatic cases involving a direct blow or forced MP joint flexion from a contusion or fall (Figure 5.26).

Rayan and Murray[83] classified sagittal band injuries into three types. Type I is a contusion without tear of the sagittal bands and without instability. Type II involves tearing of the sagittal bands with snapping of the extensor tendon but without complete dislocation. Type III consists of tendon dislocation into the groove between the metacarpal heads.

Sagittal band injuries that do not cause EDC subluxation may be treated with buddy taping to an adjacent digit for 4 weeks, but pain in the area may persist for 1 year.[83] If pain, swelling, and loss of MP joint motion persist for 3 months after direct MP joint trauma, consideration should be given to surgical exploration. Koniuch and colleagues[54] reported nine patients undergoing exploration because of persistent MP joint pain and swelling without EDC subluxation and repaired a partial tear of the ulnar sagittal band in seven and radial sagittal band in four; 25% of the patients also had MP joint pathologic conditions, including synovitis, loose bodies, chondral injuries, and palmar plate disruption. Postoperatively, patients were begun on dynamic passive extension and active flexion splinting, with eight of nine patients returning to full activities. All patients experienced pain relief. Posner and Ambrose[80] termed this entity *boxer's knuckle* and noted that sagittal band injuries without instability could be a cause of chronic pain in the area of the involved MP joint.

Sagittal band injuries with EDC subluxation that are seen within 3 weeks of injury may be treated nonoperatively.[4,14,39,83,86] An MP joint flexion block splint, or "sagittal band" splint, may be used to limit MP joint flexion of the involved finger and allow healing of the torn tendon. The splint is applied to hold the injured MP joint in 25 to 35 degrees of hyperextension compared with the adjacent MP joints. It is recommended that the splint be worn full-time for 8 weeks.[15] Active motion of the MP and IP joints is permitted with the splint in place (Figure 5.27). Using this technique, Catalano and colleagues[15] found a full range of flexion and extension in 10 patients; 8 patients had no pain, and 3 had moderate pain. Three of the 10 patients had persistently symptomatic EDC subluxation, and one required sagittal band reconstruction. Alternatively, the involved and neighboring fingers can be casted or splinted for 4 weeks with the MP joints extended and the IP joints free.

Patients presenting later than 2 to 3 weeks after injury or patients in whom splinting has been unsuccessful are candidates for surgical repair. The ulnar sagittal band may need to be partially released to allow the tendon to be centralized. The involved (usually radial) sagittal band is examined to see whether or not it is amenable for repair. If a primary repair is impossible, there are many methods of sagittal band reconstruction (Figure 5.28).[14,48,66,119]

Atraumatic, acquired, ulnar subluxation of the EDC at the MP joints has been described predominantly in elderly women. If the subluxation is symptomatic, extensor tendon reconstruction may be required.[60]

❖ AUTHOR'S PREFERRED METHOD OF TREATMENT OF CLOSED SAGITTAL BAND DISRUPTION

Patients with EDC subluxation who present within 3 weeks of injury are treated with a sagittal band splint, as described previously. Patients presenting late or who remain symptomatic despite a trial of splinting are candidates for sagittal band reconstruction. I have no experience with late repair of the radial sagittal band for these injuries, and I prefer the reconstructive technique described by Carroll and associates,[14] wherein a distally based radial slip of tendon is harvested from the EDC, passed around the radial collateral ligament of the involved MP joint, and sutured to itself to centralize the EDC mechanism. I also use this technique for elderly women with chronically attenuated radial sagittal bands of the middle and ring fingers, resulting in symptomatic EDC subluxation (see Figure 5.28, *E*).

Thumb Zone 5 Injuries (Carpometacarpal Joint)

Lacerations in zone 5 involve the EPB, APL, and, rarely, EPL. Repair at this level is by core suture and a cross-stitch. Either static splinting or active motion may be employed postoperatively. Imai and colleagues[41] described closed ulnar subluxation of the EPB at the MP joint level (zone 3), resulting from gripping a racquet tightly. Persistent flexion at the thumb MP joint resulted and was effectively treated with EPB centralization.

Finger Zone 6 Injuries at the Metacarpal Level (Case Study 5.5)

Zone 6 injuries over the dorsal hand area usually have a favorable prognosis for several reasons, as noted by Doyle[21]:

1. They are unlikely to be associated with a joint injury.
2. There is greater tendon excursion, which means that slight limitation of motion would not lead to the significant loss of joint motion seen with injuries over the phalanges.
3. Increased subcutaneous tissue lessens the chances of adhesion formation.
4. Core sutures may be easily placed.
5. Dynamic splinting can be easily performed.

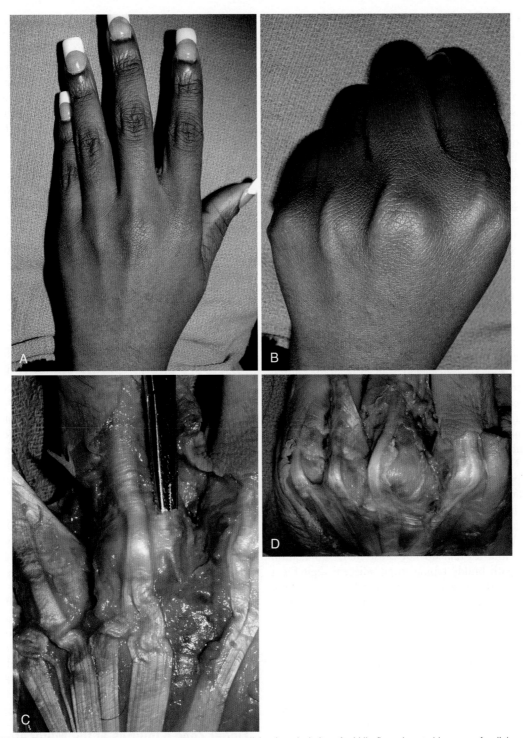

FIGURE 5.25 Closed sagittal band rupture. **A**, In extension, slight ulnar deviation of middle finger is noted because of radial sagittal band rupture of middle finger MP joint. **B**, In flexion, middle finger sagittal band subluxates into the groove between the middle and ring fingers. **C**, Cadaver dissection showing probe underneath intact radial sagittal band of middle finger. **D**, Cadaver dissection showing dislocation of extensor mechanism after sectioning of radial sagittal band.

As noted in the anatomy section, complete EDC lacerations may not result in MP joint extensor lag because of the tethering effect of the juncturae tendinum connections. As is the case for all extensor tendon lacerations, exploration is helpful to guide treatment, and a laceration of 50% or more may be repaired with core sutures of 3-0 nonabsorbable material. A 5-0 cross-stitch may be performed at the discretion of the surgeon.

Postoperatively, either static or dynamic splinting may be employed. Static splinting involves wrist extension of 30 to 45 degrees, MP joints at neutral to 15 degrees of flexion, and IP joints free for active range of motion. Dynamic splinting involves wrist extension, dynamic rubber band MP joint extension, and passive MP joint flexion to the level of repair tension determined at the time of surgery (Figure 5.29).

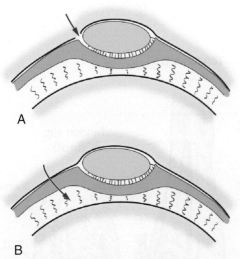

FIGURE 5.26 Anatomy of sagittal band injury. **A**, The Ishizuki interpretation of a spontaneous dislocation, in which the superficial layer of the sagittal band is disrupted. **B**, Traumatic dislocation is shown in which superficial and deep layers are torn. (From Ishizuki M: Traumatic and spontaneous dislocation of extensor tendon of the long finger. *J Hand Surg Am* 15:969, 1990, with permission from The American Society for Surgery of the Hand.)

❖ AUTHOR'S PREFERRED METHOD OF TREATMENT OF ZONE 6 INJURIES

I have employed various core sutures over the years and found equal success with a Newport modified Bunnell repair or a modified locked Kessler (Strickland) repair, as described earlier (see Figures 5.12 through 5.14). The tendons at this level are usually large enough to accommodate a core suture of 3-0 caliber. A cross-stitch may be used to supplement the repair. Dynamic splinting is employed in compliant patients.

Chronic Zone 6 Injuries

Lacerations. Lacerated extensors over the metacarpal may remain tethered in position by the juncturae tendinum, permitting delayed repair several weeks after injury. If direct repair is impossible, side-to-side transfer or intercalary tendon grafts may be performed. In severe cases of tendon loss, a two-stage reconstruction with silicone rods may be considered when the soft tissue envelope is adherent.[107] In long-standing cases of tendon loss, scar tissue may intervene, and some individuals may have adequate function even with total loss of the EDC over the dorsum of the hand, especially if the MP joints are stiff in extension.[81,107]

Chronic Blunt Trauma to the Dorsal Hand: Secretan Disorder. A factitious illness characterized by dorsal hand edema and fibrosis, *Secretan disorder* is a self-inflicted condition in which the patient is intentionally causing the signs and symptoms.[84,85,95] The cause is likely repetitive intentional blunt trauma[17] or other self-inflicted trauma to the dorsal hand area. It may sometimes mimic EDC tenosynovitis. Recognition of the disorder is paramount. After exclusion of underlying rheumatic or neoplastic conditions with magnetic resonance imaging (MRI), the condition characteristically responds temporarily to full-hand casting, but it often recurs when the behavior is repeated after cast

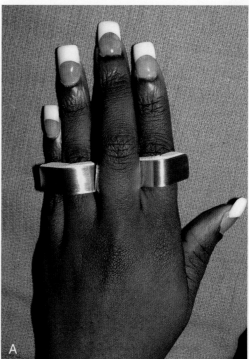

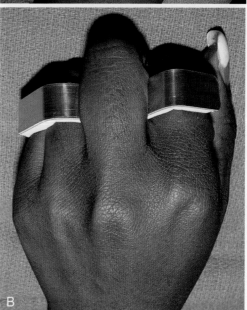

FIGURE 5.27 Sagittal band splint. **A**, Aluminum foam finger splint or splint custom made by a hand therapist is used for 8 weeks full-time to allow the injured sagittal band to heal. Splint should hold injured MP joint in about 25 degrees of extension relative to adjacent digits. **B**, Full active motion of MP and IP joints is allowed with splint in place.

removal. Confrontation is usually not helpful and may lead to violent outbursts on the part of the patient. Psychotherapy is encouraged, although this is often not accepted by the patient. Surgery must be avoided because nonhealing wounds and multiple reoperations may ensue. Factitious illnesses such as Secretan disorder are extremely frustrating and difficult conditions for the physician to treat because the patient is actively contributing to the problem.

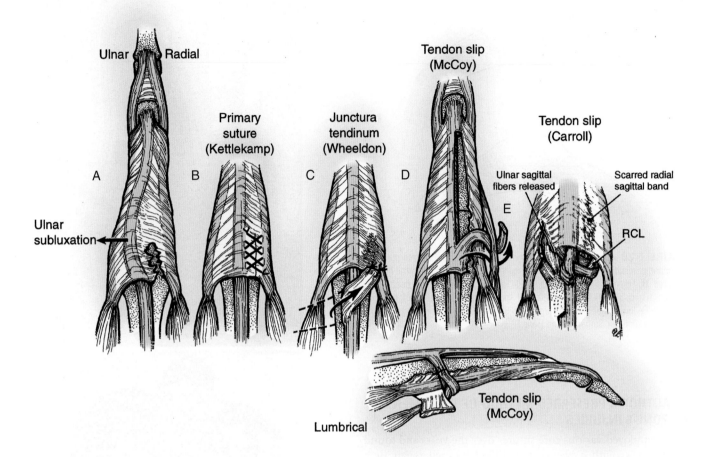

FIGURE 5.28 Methods of sagittal band reconstruction (left middle finger). **A**, Ulnar subluxation of EDC tendon caused by torn radial sagittal band. **B**, Primary suture of radial sagittal band centering EDC tendon. **C**, Ulnar junctura tendinum is released from the adjacent tendon and sutured to the palmar radial sagittal band remnant of the deep intermetacarpal ligament. **D**, Distal tendon is splinted on the radial side and wrapped around the lumbrical muscle. **E**, Ulnar, distally based slip of EDC is looped around the radial collateral ligament (RCL). (Copyright Elizabeth Martin.)

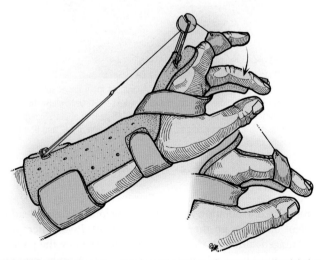

FIGURE 5.29 Dynamic splint for early motion of extensor tendon injuries. Elastic traction maintains fingers in extension. Excursion of the repaired extensor tendon is achieved by active flexion. Splinting is started 3 to 5 days after surgery and is maintained for 5 weeks. Active flexion is performed 10 times an hour. See text for details. (Copyright Elizabeth Martin.)

Zone 7 Injuries (Dorsal Wrist Injuries)

Zone 7 injuries are similar to zone 2 flexor tendon injuries in that the repaired tendon may lie in a synovial-lined tunnel beneath the extensor retinaculum. Although the extensor retinaculum prevents extensor tendon bowstringing, excision of portions of the retinaculum overlying the extensor tendon repair site do not seem to cause harm and may facilitate tendon gliding. In contrast to A2 and A4 pulleys, which are nearly impossible to repair if they are sacrificed during the course of flexor tendon repair, the extensor retinaculum may be incised to allow exposure and repaired primarily or by means of relaxing incisions. It is usually also possible to preserve sufficient retinaculum to prevent bowstringing while excising the retinacular portion over the repair site to prevent adhesions.

In contrast to lacerations over the metacarpals, tendon lacerations in this zone frequently retract into the forearm, and patients should be advised that counterincisions in the forearm or longer extensions of the original incision may be required to retrieve retracted proximal stumps. In this zone, core sutures of 3-0 or 2-0 diameter are easily placed, and a cross-stitch may be added at the surgeon's discretion.

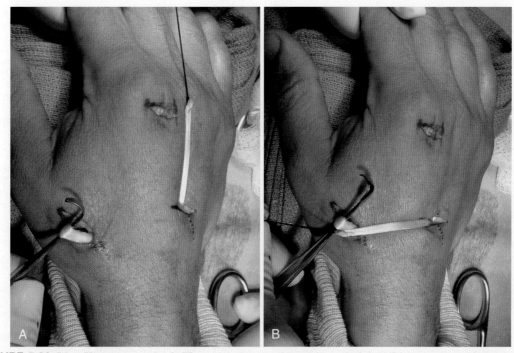

FIGURE 5.30 EIP to EPL tendon transfer. **A**, EIP, which is the most ulnar tendon at the index MP joint, is transected proximal to the sagittal bands. It is withdrawn through a transverse incision located at the distal edge of the extensor retinaculum. **B**, EIP is tunneled subcutaneously (shown here on top of the skin for demonstration) to the distal end of nonfunctioning EPL tendon. It is unnecessary to dissect out proximal EPL tendon. A Pulvertaft weave is performed with the thumb in full extension and the wrist in 20 degrees of extension. It is important to ensure that the transferred tendon does not "wrap up" EDC of the index MP joint during its passage.

Chronic Injuries and Ruptures in Zone 7

Nondisplaced distal radius fractures may be associated with late rupture of the EPL tendon. The cause for this rupture is unclear, but it has been suggested that extravasation of blood and fracture debris into a tight third dorsal compartment may constrict the EPL and lead to late attritional rupture.[35] It has been postulated that there exists a relative "watershed" zone of intrinsic vascular supply to the tendon beneath the extensor retinaculum, which may predispose the tendon further to rupture. The condition is usually treated by transfer of the EIP tendon to the EPL tendon with excellent results (Figure 5.30).

Transfer of the Extensor Indicis Proprius Tendon to the Extensor Pollicis Longus Tendon. A transverse incision is made just proximal to the index MP joint, and the EIP tendon, which is the ulnar tendon, is identified and freed up subcutaneously to the level of the wrist retinaculum. It is transected proximal to its insertion on the extensor hood. A second transverse incision is made overlying the EIP tendon just distal to the retinaculum, and the tendon is withdrawn to this location. A third incision is made longitudinally overlying the EPL tendon at the metacarpal level, close to the MP joint. The EIP tendon is passed subcutaneously to the EPL tendon, with care taken not to ensnare any EDC tendons in the passage. The EIP tendon is sutured in a Pulvertaft weave with several 3-0 nonabsorbable sutures. The repair is tensioned with the wrist in 30 degrees of extension and at the thumb in extension at the carpometacarpal and IP joints and in neutral at the MP joint. A thumb spica splint is placed full-time for 4 weeks, at which time active motion is allowed with a removable thumb spica splint for another 2 weeks.

❖ AUTHOR'S PREFERRED METHOD OF TREATMENT OF ZONE 7 INJURIES

I prefer to window the extensor retinaculum over the extensor tendon repair site to prevent adhesion formation. I prefer sutures of 2-0 caliber for the wrist extensors and of 3-0 caliber for the digital extensors. I usually employ a four-strand core suture repair using either a locked modified Kessler suture plus a horizontal mattress or a locked four-strand cruciate repair. A 5-0 circumferential cross-stitch may be added. Postoperative splinting with the wrist in extension and the MP and IP joints free is done for wrist extensor lacerations for 4 weeks, followed by active range of motion, and finger extensors are splinted with the MP joints in extension and IP joints free. I employ dynamic extension splinting in well-motivated patients.

Zone 8 Injuries (Distal Forearm Injuries) (Case Study 5.6)

Injuries in zone 8 involve the musculotendinous junction, and repairs in this zone may have tenuous holding power in the muscle tissue. Musculotendinous juncture closed ruptures are rare but have been reported as a consequence of violent resisted wrist or finger extension.[104] The EDC tendons to the middle and ring fingers are reported to be the most commonly injured. When repair to the muscle fascia is flimsy, a side-to-side tendon transfer may be the best option.[104]

Zone 9 Injuries (Proximal Forearm Injuries)

Zone 9 is the site of the muscle bellies of the extensor tendons in the proximal half of the forearm. Penetrating trauma, as with knife or glass injuries, is the most frequent cause of injury in this zone. Loss of finger or wrist extension may result from muscle transection or nerve injury, or both.[25] Surgical exploration reveals the extent of injury, and muscle belly wounds may be repaired with multiple figure-of-eight sutures. Botte and colleagues[9] noted that tendon grafting was an effective method of overcoming defects in this area and used the palmaris longus or toe extensors as graft material. Indications for this procedure were laceration of two or more muscle bellies with laceration of at least 50% of the muscle substance. Patients with less severe lacerations had epimysial repair with interrupted figure-of-eight sutures using absorbable sutures. Most patients in Botte's series had lacerations with 100% of the muscle substance disrupted, a gap of 2 cm at the laceration site, and concomitant nerve and arterial injuries.[9] Patients who present a week or two after injury and who demonstrate mild to moderate extensor lag of one or more digits may be considered for extension splinting for 3 to 4 weeks, as this may allow muscle healing and return to function.

Nerve injuries to the posterior interosseous nerve may be difficult to localize and repair in the substance of the muscle bellies. Chronic nerve injuries may be treated with tendon transfers.

For Case Studies, Videos, and more, please visit ExpertConsult.com.

REFERENCES

1. Abouna JM, Brown H: The treatment of mallet finger. The results in a series of 148 consecutive cases and a review of the literature. Br J Surg 55:653–667, 1968.
2. Al-Qattan MM: Extra-articular transverse fractures of the base of the distal phalanx (Seymour's fracture) in children and adults. J Hand Surg [Br] 26:201–206, 2001.
3. Altobelli GG, Conneely S, Haufler C, et al: Outcomes of digital zone IV and V and thumb zone TI to TIV extensor tendon repairs using a running interlocking horizontal mattress technique. J Hand Surg [Am] 38:1079–1083, 2013.
4. Araki S, Ohtani T, Tanaka T: Acute dislocation of the extensor digitorum communis tendon at the metacarpophalangeal joint. A report of five cases. J Bone Joint Surg Am 69:616–619, 1987.
5. Baratz ME, Schmidt CC, Hughes TB: Extensor tendon injuries. In Green DP, Hotchkiss RN, Pederson WC, et al, editors: Green's operative hand surgery, ed 5, New York, 2005, Churchill Livingstone.
6. Beck JD, Riehl JT, Klena JC: Anomalous tendon to the middle finger for sagittal band reconstruction: report of 2 cases. J Hand Surg [Am] 37:1646–1649, 2012.
7. Bendre AA, Hartigan BJ, Kalainov DM: Mallet finger. J Am Acad Orthop Surg 13:336–344, 2005.
8. Blue AI, Spira M, Hardy SB: Repair of extensor tendon injuries of the hand. Am J Surg 132:128–132, 1976.
9. Botte MJ, Gelberman RH, Smith DG, et al: Repair of severe muscle belly lacerations using a tendon graft. J Hand Surg [Am] 12:406–412, 1987.
10. Bowers WH, Hurst LC: Chronic mallet finger: the use of Fowler's central slip release. J Hand Surg [Am] 3:373–376, 1978.
11. Boyes JH, editor: Bunnell's surgery of the hand, ed 5, Philadelphia, 1970, Lippincott.
11a. Browne EZ, Jr, Ribik CA: Early dynamic splinting for extensor tendon injuries. J Hand Surg [Am] 14:72–76, 1989.
12. Bulstrode NW, Burr N, Pratt AL, et al: Extensor tendon rehabilitation: a prospective trial comparing three rehabilitation regimes. J Hand Surg [Br] 30:175–179, 2005.
13. Burton RI: Extensor tendons: late reconstruction. In Green DP, Hotchkiss RN, Pederson WC, et al, editors: Green's operative hand surgery, ed 5, New York, 1988, Churchill Livingstone, pp 2073–2116.
14. Carroll C, 4th, Moore JR, Weiland AJ: Posttraumatic ulnar subluxation of the extensor tendons: a reconstructive technique. J Hand Surg [Am] 12:227–231, 1987.
15. Catalano LW, 3rd, Gupta S, Ragland R, 3rd, et al: Closed treatment of nonrheumatoid extensor tendon dislocations at the metacarpophalangeal joint. J Hand Surg [Am] 31:242–245, 2006.

16. Chao JD, Sarwahi V, Da Silva YS, et al: Central slip tenotomy for the treatment of chronic mallet finger: an anatomic study. J Hand Surg [Am] 29:216–219, 2004.
16a. Chester DL, Beale S, Beveridge L, et al: A prospective, controlled, randomized trial comparing early active extension with passive extension using a dynamic splint in the rehabilitation of repaired extensor tendons. J Hand Surg [Br] 27:283–288, 1984.
17. Crawford GP: The molded polythene splint for mallet finger deformities. J Hand Surg [Am] 9:231–237, 1984.
18. Creighton JJ, Jr, Steichen JB: Complications in phalangeal and metacarpal fracture management. Results of extensor tenolysis. Hand Clin 10:111–116, 1994.
19. Curtis RM, Reid RL, Provost JM: A staged technique for the repair of the traumatic boutonniere deformity. J Hand Surg [Am] 8:167–171, 1983.
20. Dolphin JA: Extensor tenotomy for chronic boutonnière deformity of the finger: report of two cases. J Bone Joint Surg Am 47:161–164, 1965.
21. Doyle JR: Extensor tendons: acute injuries. In Green DP, Hotchkiss RN, Pederson WC, et al, editors: Green's operative hand surgery, ed 5, New York, 1999, Churchill Livingstone, pp 195–1987.
22. Doyle JR, Atkinson RE: Rupture of the radial collateral ligament of the metacarpophalangeal joint of the index finger: a report of three cases. J Hand Surg [Br] 14:248–250, 1989.
23. Elson RA: Rupture of the central slip of the extensor hood of the finger. A test for early diagnosis. J Bone Joint Surg Br 68:229–231, 1986.
23a. Evans RB: Early active short arc motion for the repaired central slip. J Hand Surg [Am] 10:991–997, 1994.
24. Evans RB, Burkhalter WE: A study of the dynamic anatomy of extensor tendons and implications for treatment. J Hand Surg [Am] 11:774–779, 1986.
25. Fischer CR, Tang P: Lacerations to zones VIII and IX: it is not just a tendon injury. Adv Orthop 2010. [Epub September 14, 2010].
26. Foucher G, Binhamer P, Cange S, et al: Long-term results of splintage for mallet finger. Int Orthop 20:129–131, 1996.
27. Fowler SB: The management of tendon injuries. J Bone Joint Surg Am 41:579–580, 1959.
28. Garberman SF, Diao E, Peimer CA: Mallet finger: results of early versus delayed closed treatment. J Hand Surg [Am] 19:850–852, 1994.
29. Gonzalez MH, Papierski P, Hall RF, Jr: Osteomyelitis of the hand after a human bite. J Hand Surg [Am] 18:520–522, 1993.
30. Grundberg AB: Anatomic repair of boutonniere deformity. Clin Orthop Relat Res 153:226–229, 1980.
31. Grundberg AB, Reagan DS: Central slip tenotomy for chronic mallet finger deformity. J Hand Surg [Am] 12:545–547, 1987.
32. Hallberg D, Lindholm A: Subcutaneous rupture of the extensor tendon of the distal phalanx of the finger: "mallet finger": brief review of the literature and report on 127 cases treated conservatively. Acta Chir Scand 119:260–267, 1960.
33. Hammond K, Starr H, Katz D, et al: Effect of aftercare regimen with extensor tendon repair: a systematic review of the literature. J Surg Orthop Adv 21:246–252, 2012.
34. Handoll HH, Vaghela MV: Interventions for treating mallet finger injuries. Cochrane Database Syst Rev (3):CD004574, 2004.
35. Helal B, Chen SC, Iwegbu G: Rupture of the extensor pollicis longus tendon in undisplaced Colles' type of fracture. Hand 14:41–47, 1982.
36. Hirai Y, Yoshida K, Yamanaka K, et al: An anatomic study of the extensor tendons of the human hand. J Hand Surg [Am] 26:1009–1015, 2001.
37. Houpt P, Dijkstra R, Storm van Leeuwen JB: Fowler's tenotomy for mallet deformity. J Hand Surg [Br] 18:499–500, 1993.
38. Howard RF, Ondrovic L, Greenwald DP: Biomechanical analysis of four-strand extensor tendon repair techniques. J Hand Surg [Am] 22:838–842, 1997.
39. Hung LK, Chan A, Chang J, et al: Early controlled active mobilization with dynamic splintage for treatment of extensor tendon injuries. J Hand Surg [Am] 15:251–257, 1990.
40. Husain SN, Dietz JF, Kalainov DM, et al: A biomechanical study of distal interphalangeal joint subluxation after mallet fracture injury. J Hand Surg [Am] 33:26–30, 2008.
41. Imai S, Kikuchi K, Matsusue Y: Posttraumatic recurrent dislocation of extensor pollicis brevis tendon over the metacarpophalangeal joint. J Hand Surg [Am] 30:147–150, 2005.
42. Iselin F, Levame J, Godoy J: A simplified technique for treating mallet fingers: tenodermodesis. J Hand Surg [Am] 2:118–121, 1977.
43. Ishizuki M: Traumatic and spontaneous dislocation of extensor tendon of the long finger. J Hand Surg [Am] 15:967–972, 1990.
44. Jones NF, Peterson J: Epidemiologic study of the mallet finger deformity. J Hand Surg [Am] 13:334–338, 1988.
45. Kalainov DM, Hoepfner PE, Hartigan BJ, et al: Nonsurgical treatment of closed mallet finger fractures. J Hand Surg [Am] 30:580–586, 2005.
46. Katzman SS, Gibeault JD, Dickson K, et al: Use of a Herbert screw for interphalangeal joint arthrodesis. Clin Orthop Relat Res 296:127–132, 1993.

47. Katzman BM, Klein DM, Mesa J, et al: Immobilization of the mallet finger. Effects on the extensor tendon. *J Hand Surg [Br]* 24:80–84, 1999.

48. Kettelkamp DB, Flatt AE, Moulds R: Traumatic dislocation of the long-finger extensor tendon. A clinical, anatomical, and biomechanical study. *J Bone Joint Surg Am* 53:229–240, 1971.

48a. Khandwala AR, Webb J, Harris SB, et al: A comparison of dynamic extension splinting and controlled active mobilization of complete divisions of extensor tendons in zones 5 and 6. *J Hand Surg [Br]* 25:140–146, 2000.

49. King HJ, Shin SJ, Kang ES: Complications of operative treatment for mallet fractures of the distal phalanx. *J Hand Surg [Br]* 26:28–31, 2001.

50. Kitis A, Ozcan RH, Bagdatli D, et al: Comparison of static and dynamic splinting regimens for extensor tendon repairs in zones V to VII. *J Plast Surg Hand Surg* 46:267–271, 2012.

51. Kleinert HE, Verdan C: Report of the Committee on Tendon Injuries (International Federation of Societies for Surgery of the Hand). *J Hand Surg [Am]* 8:794–798, 1983.

52. Kleinman WB, Petersen DP: Oblique retinacular ligament reconstruction for chronic mallet finger deformity. *J Hand Surg [Am]* 9:399–404, 1984.

53. Deleted in review.

54. Koniuch MP, Peimer CA, VanGorder T, et al: Closed crush injury of the metacarpophalangeal joint. *J Hand Surg [Am]* 12:750–757, 1987.

55. Landsmeer JM: Anatomy of the dorsal aponeurosis of the human finger and its functional signficance. *Anat Rec* 104:31–44, 1949.

56. Lee SK, Dubey A, Kim BH, et al: A biomechanical study of extensor tendon repair methods: introduction to the running-interlocking horizontal mattress extensor tendon repair technique. *J Hand Surg [Am]* 35:19–23, 2010.

57. Littler JW: The digital extensor-flexor system. In Converse J, editor: *Reconstructive plastic surgery*, Philadelphia, 1964, WB Saunders, pp 1612–1632.

58. Littler JW: Restoration of the oblique retinacular ligament for correcting hyperextension deformity of the proximal interphalangeal joint. In Tubiana R, editor: *La main rheumatoide*, Paris, 1966, Expansion Scientifique Francaise, pp 159–167.

59. Littler JW, Eaton RG: Redistribution of forces in the correction of Boutonniere deformity. *J Bone Joint Surg Am* 49:1267–1274, 1967.

60. Love GJ, MacLean JG: Ulnar subluxation of the extensor tendons in elderly osteoarthritic females: a neglected diagnosis. *J Hand Surg Eur Vol* 32:45–49, 2007.

61. Lucas GL: Fowler central slip tenotomy for old mallet deformity. *Plast Reconstr Surg* 80:92–94, 1987.

62. Maisels DO: The middle slip or boutonniere deformity in burned hands. *Br J Plast Surg* 18:117–129, 1965.

63. Mann RJ, Hoffeld TA, Farmer CB: Human bites of the hand: twenty years of experience. *J Hand Surg [Am]* 2:97–104, 1977.

63a. Mason ML: Rupture of the tendons of the hand. *Surg Gynecol Obstet* 50:611–624, 1930.

64. Matev I: Transposition of the lateral slips of the aponeurosis in treatment of longstanding "boutonnière deformity" of the fingers. *Br J Plast Surg* 17:281–286, 1964.

65. Mazurek MT, Hofmeister EP, Shin AY, et al: Extension-block pinning for treatment of displaced mallet fractures. *Am J Orthop (Belle Mead NJ)* 31:652–654, 2002.

66. McCoy FJ, Winsky AJ: Lumbrical loop operation for luxation of the extensor tendons of the hand. *Plast Reconstr Surg* 44:142–146, 1969.

67. Miller H: Repair of severed tendons of the hand and wrist. *Surg Gynecol Obstet* 75:693–698, 1942.

68. Mowlavi A, Burns M, Brown RE: Dynamic versus static splinting of simple zone V and zone VI extensor tendon repairs: a prospective, randomized, controlled study. *Plast Reconstr Surg* 115:482–487, 2005.

69. Nalebuff EA, Millender LH: Surgical treatment of the boutonniere deformity in rheumatoid arthritis. *Orthop Clin North Am* 6:753–763, 1975.

70. Newport ML, Blair WF, Steyers CM, Jr: Long-term results of extensor tendon repair. *J Hand Surg [Am]* 15:961–966, 1990.

71. Newport ML, Pollack GR, Williams CD: Biomechanical characteristics of suture techniques in extensor zone IV. *J Hand Surg [Am]* 20:650–656, 1995.

72. Newport ML, Williams CD: Biomechanical characteristics of extensor tendon suture techniques. *J Hand Surg [Am]* 17:1117–1123, 1992.

73. Ogura T, Inoue H, Tanabe G: Anatomic and clinical studies of the extensor digitorum brevis manus. *J Hand Surg [Am]* 12:100–107, 1987.

74. Oh JY, Kim JS, Lee DC, et al: Comparative study of spiral oblique retinacular ligament reconstruction techniques using either a lateral band or a tendon graft. *Arch Plast Surg* 40:773–778, 2013.

75. Okafor B, Mbubaegbu C, Munshi I, et al: Mallet deformity of the finger. Five-year follow-up of conservative treatment. *J Bone Joint Surg Br* 79:544–547, 1997.

76. Patel MR, Desai SS, Bassini-Lipson L, et al: Painful extensor digitorum brevis manus muscle. *J Hand Surg [Am]* 14:674–678, 1989.

77. Patel MR, Lipson LB, Desai SS: Conservative treatment of mallet thumb. *J Hand Surg [Am]* 11:45–47, 1986.

78. Patil RK, Koul AR: Early active mobilisation versus immobilisation after extrinsic extensor tendon repair: a prospective randomised trial. *Indian J Plast Surg* 45:29–37, 2012.

79. Pike J, Mulpuri K, Metzger M, et al: Blinded, prospective, randomized clinical trial comparing volar, dorsal, and custom thermoplastic splinting in treatment of acute mallet finger. *J Hand Surg [Am]* 35:580–588, 2010.

80. Posner MA, Ambrose L: Boxer's knuckle: dorsal capsular rupture of the metacarpophalangeal joint of a finger. *J Hand Surg [Am]* 14:229–236, 1989.

80a. Purcell T, Eadie PA, Murugan S, et al: Static splinting of extensor tendon repairs. *J Hand Surg [Br]* 25:180–182, 2000.

81. Quaba AA, Elliot D, Sommerlad BC: Long term hand function without long finger extensors: a clinical study. *J Hand Surg [Br]* 13:66–71, 1988.

82. Rayan GM, Mullins PT: Skin necrosis complicating mallet finger splinting and vascularity of the distal interphalangeal joint overlying skin. *J Hand Surg [Am]* 12:548–552, 1987.

83. Rayan GM, Murray D: Classification and treatment of closed sagittal band injuries. *J Hand Surg [Am]* 19:590–594, 1994.

84. Reading G: Secretan's syndrome: hard edema of the dorsum of the hand. *Plast Reconstr Surg* 65:182–187, 1980.

85. Redfern AB, Curtis RM, Wilgis EF: Experience with peritendinous fibrosis of the dorsum of the hand. *J Hand Surg [Am]* 7:380–383, 1982.

86. Ritts GD, Wood MB, Engber WD: Nonoperative treatment of traumatic dislocations of the extensor digitorum tendons in patients without rheumatoid disorders. *J Hand Surg [Am]* 10:714–716, 1985.

87. Rubin J, Bozentka DJ, Bora FW: Diagnosis of closed central slip injuries. A cadaveric analysis of non-invasive tests. *J Hand Surg [Br]* 21:614–616, 1996.

87a. Russel RC, Jones M, Grobbelaar A: Extensor tendon repair: moblise or splint? *Chir Main* 22:19–23, 2003.

87b. Saldana MJ, Choban S, Westerbeck P, et al: Results of acute Zone III extensor tendon injuries treated with dynamic extension splinting. *J Hand Surg [Am]* 16:1145–1150, 1991.

88. Schultz RJ, Furlong J, 2nd, Storace A: Detailed anatomy of the extensor mechanism at the proximal aspect of the finger. *J Hand Surg [Am]* 6:493–498, 1981.

89. Schweitzer TP, Rayan GM: The terminal tendon of the digital extensor mechanism: Part I, anatomic study. *J Hand Surg [Am]* 29:898–902, 2004.

90. Schweitzer TP, Rayan GM: The terminal tendon of the digital extensor mechanism: Part II, kinematic study. *J Hand Surg [Am]* 29:903–908, 2004.

91. Seymour N: Juxta-epiphysial fracture of the terminal phalanx of the finger. *J Bone Joint Surg Br* 48:347–349, 1966.

92. Shrewsbury MM, Johnson RK: A systematic study of the oblique retinacular ligament of the human finger: its structure and function. *J Hand Surg [Am]* 2:194–199, 1977.

93. Shrewsbury MM, Johnson RK: Ligaments of the distal interphalangeal joint and the mallet position. *J Hand Surg [Am]* 5:214–216, 1980.

94. Shum C, Bruno RJ, Ristic S, et al: Examination of the anatomic relationship of the proximal germinal nail matrix to the extensor tendon insertion. *J Hand Surg [Am]* 25:1114–1117, 2000.

95. Smith RJ: Factitious lymphedema of the hand. *J Bone Joint Surg Am* 57:89–94, 1975.

96. Snow JW: Use of a retrograde tendon flap in repairing a severed extensor in the PIP joint area. *Plast Reconstr Surg* 51:555–558, 1973.

97. Snow JW: A method for reconstruction of the central slip of the extensor tendon of a finger. *Plast Reconstr Surg* 57:455–459, 1976.

98. Souter WA: The problem of boutonniere deformity. *Clin Orthop Relat Res* 104:116–133, 1974.

99. Spinner M, Choi BY: Anterior dislocation of the proximal interphalangeal joint. A cause of rupture of the central slip of the extensor mechanism. *J Bone Joint Surg Am* 52:1329–1336, 1970.

100. Spinner M, Kaplan EB: Extensor carpi ulnaris. Its relationship to the stability of the distal radio-ulnar joint. *Clin Orthop Relat Res* 68:124–129, 1970.

101. Stern PJ, Kastrup JJ: Complications and prognosis of treatment of mallet finger. *J Hand Surg [Am]* 13:329–334, 1988.

102. Strauch RJ, Rosenwasser MP, Lunt JG: Metacarpal shaft fractures: the effect of shortening on the extensor tendon mechanism. *J Hand Surg [Am]* 23:519–523, 1998.

103. Suh N, Wolfe SW: Soft tissue mallet finger injuries with delayed treatment. *J Hand Surg [Am]* 38:1803–1805, 2013.

103a. Syladis P, Youatt M, Logan A: Early active mobilization for extensor tendon injuries: the Norwich regime. *J Hand Surg [Br]* 22:594–596, 1997.

104. Takami H, Takahashi S, Ando M, et al: Traumatic rupture of the extensor tendons at the musculotendinous junction. *J Hand Surg [Am]* 20:474–477, 1995.

105. Tetik C, Gudemez E: Modification of the extension block Kirschner wire technique for mallet fractures. *Clin Orthop Relat Res* 404:284–290, 2002.

106. Thompson JS, Littler JW, Upton J: The spiral oblique retinacular ligament (SORL). *J Hand Surg [Am]* 3:482–487, 1978.

107. Tomaino MM, Plakseychuk A: Two-stage extensor tendon reconstruction after composite tissue loss from the dorsum of the hand. *Am J Orthop* 29:122–124, 2000.

108. Tonkin MA, Hughes J, Smith KL: Lateral band translocation for swan-neck deformity. *J Hand Surg [Am]* 17:260–267, 1992.
109. Tonta K, Kimble FW: Human bites of the hand: the Tasmanian experience. *ANZ J Surg* 71:467–471, 2001.
110. Ueba H, Moradi N, Erne HC, et al: An anatomic and biomechanical study of the oblique retinacular ligament and its role in finger extension. *J Hand Surg [Am]* 36:1959–1964, 2011.
111. Vahey JW, Wegner DA, Hastings H, 3rd: Effect of proximal phalangeal fracture deformity on extensor tendon function. *J Hand Surg [Am]* 23:673–681, 1998.
112. Van Sint Jan S, Rooze M, Van Audekerke J, et al: The insertion of the extensor digitorum tendon on the proximal phalanx. *J Hand Surg [Am]* 21:69–76, 1996.
113. von Schroeder HP, Botte MJ: Anatomy of the extensor tendons of the fingers: variations and multiplicity. *J Hand Surg [Am]* 20:27–34, 1995.
114. Wang L, Zhang X, Liu Z, et al: Tendon-bone graft for tendinous mallet fingers following failed splinting. *J Hand Surg [Am]* 38:2353–2359, 2013.
115. Warren RA, Norris SH, Ferguson DG: Mallet finger: a trial of two splints. *J Hand Surg [Br]* 13:151–153, 1988.
116. Weeks PM: The chronic boutonniere deformity: a method of repair. *Plast Reconstr Surg* 40:248–251, 1967.
117. Wehbe MA: Junctura anatomy. *J Hand Surg [Am]* 17:1124–1129, 1992.
118. Wehbe MA, Schneider LH: Mallet fractures. *J Bone Joint Surg Am* 66:658–669, 1984.
119. Wheeldon FT: Recurrent dislocation of extensor tendons in the hand. *J Bone Joint Surg Br* 36:612–617, 1954.
120. Whillis J, Channell GD: The action of the lumbrical and interosseous muscles in some of the movements of the digits. *J Anat* 83:60, 1949.
121. Woo SH, Tsai TM, Kleinert HE, et al: A biomechanical comparison of four extensor tendon repair techniques in zone IV. *Plast Reconstr Surg* 115:1674–1681, discussion 1682–1683, 2005.
122. Wood VE: The extensor carpi radialis intermedius tendon. *J Hand Surg [Am]* 13:242–245, 1988.

6

Flexor Tendon Injury

John Gray Seiler III

Acknowledgments: The author would like to acknowledge the assistance of Dr. Mihir Desai in the preparation of these works on flexor tendon repair and flexor tendon grafting.

The author acknowledges the work of Drs. James Strickland, Lawrence Schneider, and Martin I. Boyer, whose outstanding chapters in previous editions have been modified, combined, and updated. Their contributions to our understanding of repair and reconstruction of the damaged flexor tendon system have greatly advanced our ability to care for these injuries.

The author also acknowledges the contributions of Mr. Daniel Acker, OT, CHT, to the rehabilitation portion of this chapter.

> These videos may be found at
> *ExpertConsult.com:*
> **6.1** Flexor tendon repair
> **6.2** Paneva-Holevich technique for chronic tendon laceration

REPAIR OF ACUTE FLEXOR TENDON INJURIES

In the 1960s, initial clinical reports began to emerge that suggested primary tendon repair was possible and desirable.[112-115,134,136,236] Since that time, there have been major advances in the understanding of intrasynovial flexor tendon anatomy, biology, mechanisms of response to injury, and methods of repair.[*] Pioneering work by Lundborg validated primary adhesion-free intrasynovial tendon repair in experimental and clinical studies.[†] More recent research has focused on improvements in surgical and aftercare methods that can achieve a reliable flexor tendon repair site and are associated with satisfactory digital motion.[‡] These advances coupled with improvements in suture design, optical magnification, and rehabilitation methods have made primary flexor tendon repair the preferred operative treatment for lacerated tendons in zone 2.[§] Table 6.1 summarizes research relevant to flexor tendon repair.

The goals of surgical treatment of a lacerated intrasynovial flexor tendon have remained constant: accurate coaptation of the tendon ends in such a manner as to allow application of a postoperative rehabilitation protocol that encourages tendon gliding, inhibits the formation of peritendinous adhesions, stimulates restoration of the gliding surface, allows for primary healing of the repair site, and ultimately restores normal range of motion to the finger.[214-218]

Preoperative Evaluation

A thorough patient history and physical examination of the injured hand are performed as a part of the initial evaluation and before the administration of local anesthesia or sedation so that any potential neurologic or vascular injuries can be accurately detected. Generally, a systematic method of examining each system in the hand is most effective in documenting the components of the injury. This primary evaluation is important to planning the nature and timing of future medical and surgical treatments.

Systematic Examination

Integument Examination. The integrity of the skin on the volar and dorsal aspects of the injured digit is examined to ascertain the presence or absence of additional injuries. The nature of each skin injury should be recorded.

Musculoskeletal Examination. Obvious angular or rotational deformity of the digit signifies either a fracture or a ligamentous injury that requires further assessment. Realignment of a fracture or reduction of a dislocation may be required before the evaluation of flexor tendon integrity or the presence of digital neurovascular injury. If the flexor tendons are lacerated, the digit loses its inherent flexor tone and assumes an extended posture at the proximal interphalangeal (PIP) and distal interphalangeal (DIP) joints. If the tendons are completely transected, there is no active flexion and the tenodesis effect (normal increase in flexor tone) is lost with passive wrist extension.

The tendons should be examined individually in each finger. To isolate the flexor digitorum superficialis (FDS) tendon (Figure 6.1), the adjacent digits are held in full extension or in mild hyperextension by the examiner at the metacarpophalangeal (MP), PIP, and DIP joints. Active flexion of the PIP joint is evaluated for each digit, and its presence indicates that the fibers of the FDS tendon are intact. The presence of active flexion does not rule out partial FDS tendon injury, however. Pain on active flexion may suggest a partial tendon injury. The flexor digitorum profundus (FDP) tendon examination is done by positioning the finger in full extension, stabilizing the middle phalanx against the examining surface, and asking the patient to flex the DIP joint actively.

Neurologic Examination. An assessment of light touch and static two-point discrimination is preferred; loss of sensation in

---

*References 1, 4-6, 16, 18, 32, 36, 45-49, 67-76, 78, 97, 126-131, 141, 162-166, 185, 187, 197, 225, 226, 240, 245-248, 250.

†References 11-13, 20-23, 42-44, 51, 85, 90, 92, 143-159.

‡References 73, 75, 111, 135, 137, 138, 142, 168, 174, 220.

§References 78, 80, 203-218, 223, 251, 252.

TABLE 6.1		**Contributions to Our Understanding of Flexor Tendon Repair**	
Author	**Publication Activity**	**Main Area of Contribution**	**Significance**
Bunnell	1918-1951	Surgical technique of tendon repair, grafting	Stressed importance of gentle, precise surgical technique as having a direct effect on results
Mason et al	1932-1959	Animal model study of repair site healing	Classic in vivo study of repair site healing and accrual of strength
Boyes et al	1947-1989	Surgical technique of tendon repair, grafting	Detailed techniques and results of intrasynovial flexor tendon grafts
Peacock et al	1957-1987	Tendon biology, healing	Stressed contribution of surrounding sheath to tendon repair site healing
Verdan et al	1960-1987	Primary tendon repair	First report of successful primary tendon repair within digital sheath
Potenza et al	1962-1986	Tendon biology, healing	Stressed the contribution of surrounding sheath to repair site healing
Kleinert et al	1967-present	Early motion rehabilitation	Reported technique of reliable and reproducible postoperative "rubber band" rehabilitation. Also first valid report in United States of primary zone 2 repair
Burner	1967-1975	Skin incisions	Zigzag volar approach to digital sheath
Kessler et al	1969-1987	Primary tendon repair	Core suture technique
Ketchum et al	1971-1985	Biology and biomechanics of tendon repair	Experimental study of tendon repair and healing
Lundborg et al	1975-present	Tendon healing, vascularity, nutrition	Advocated concept of "intrinsic" tendon healing, detailed vascularity of flexor tendon
Duran et al	1975-1990	Early motion rehabilitation	Passive motion rehabilitation protocol
Manske et al	1977-present	Tendon biology, biomechanics	Classic studies of tendon nutrition, repair site biology, and biomechanics
Leddy et al	1977-1993	FDP avulsion injuries	Classification of FDP avulsions
Lister et al	1977-1986	Rehabilitation, pulley reconstruction	Clinical studies of pulley reconstruction and handling of digital sheath
Gelberman et al	1980-present	Tendon biology, biomechanics, rehabilitation	Classic experimental and clinical studies of tendon repair site biology, biomechanics, vascularity, and rehabilitation
Strickland et al	1982-present	Tendon repair, rehabilitation	Classic clinical and experimental studies of flexor tendon repair and rehabilitation
Silfverskiöld et al	1983-1994	Tendon repair, rehabilitation	Clinical and experimental study of repair site gap formation and rehabilitation
Amadio et al	1984-present	Tendon and pulley biology, biomechanics, rehabilitation	Classic experimental studies of tendon repair site biology, biomechanics, and rehabilitation
Hitchcock et al	1987	Tendon biology, rehabilitation	Experimental study of biologic effect of passive motion rehabilitation
Doyle	1988	Flexor pulley system	Relative importance of each pulley
Mass et al	1989-present	Tendon biomechanics	Experimental study of in vitro repair site biomechanics
Abrahamsson et al	1989-present	Growth factors in tendon healing	In vitro studies of growth factor synthesis during repair site healing and their effects
Seiler et al		Biology of tendon repair	Identification of growth factors in repair, suture methods in tendon repair
Schuind et al	1992-present	In vivo flexor tendon forces	Classic study documenting in vivo flexor forces during digital motion
Diao et al	1996-present	Core and circumferential suture techniques	Experimental study of role of circumferential suture in time-zero repair site strength
Sandow and McMahon	1996-present	Core suture technique	Improved time-zero core suture technique
Boyer et al	1997-present	Tendon biology, biomechanics, rehabilitation	Experimental studies of tendon repair site biology, biomechanics, vascularity, and rehabilitation
Wolfe et al	1999-present	Core suture technique	Core suture technique
Taras	1999-present	Core suture technique	Core suture technique
Leversedge	2000-present	Tendon vascularity and neovascularization after repair	Experimental studies of tendon repair site and insertion site vascularity

a digital nerve dermatome after a sharp laceration represents a nerve transection until proven otherwise.

Vascular Examination. Capillary refill of the volar digital pulp and the nail bed is assessed. When necessary, a digital Allen test can be done. Delayed capillary refill or poor turgor may suggest a digital artery laceration.

After a complete evaluation of the skin, skeleton, tendons, nerves, and vascular supply, the evaluating physician can make a judgment regarding the timing and nature of the anticipated surgical repair. The surgeon must be prepared, however, to treat any findings that could be encountered during surgical exploration.

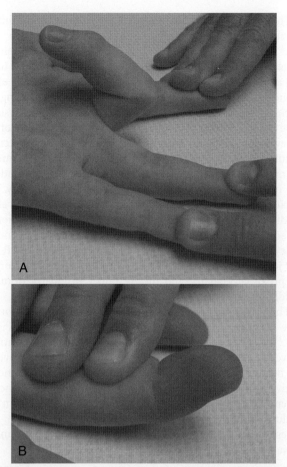

FIGURE 6.1 A, Continuity of FDS tendon is evaluated by asking the patient to flex the finger actively while holding MP joints of the uninvolved fingers in hyperextension, and PIP and DIP joints of the uninvolved fingers in full extension. This effectively eliminates the profundus and allows the superficialis action to be evaluated. **B,** Middle phalanx is held firmly, and active flexion at DIP joint is carried out. This shows continuity of FDP tendon.

Diagnostic Imaging

Plain radiographs are usually obtained at the time of initial assessment while the patient is in the emergency department. Diagnostic ultrasound may be useful when the continuity of a flexor tendon is in question, or to assess a suspected partial laceration. Intraoperative fluoroscopic images may be useful, especially if indicated by the findings of surgical exploration.

ANATOMY

The FDS muscle has two heads of origin. The ulnar head arises from the anterior aspect of the medial epicondyle, the ulnar collateral ligament of the elbow, the medial aspect of the coronoid process, and the proximal ulna. The radial head arises from the proximal radius immediately distal to the insertion of the supinator muscle and lies deep to the pronator teres. The median nerve is loosely adherent to the deep surface of the FDS muscle. At the level of the midforearm, the FDS muscle divides and sends tendons to the middle and ring fingers (superficial) and the index and small fingers (deep). The innervation of the FDS muscle is from the median nerve. The blood supply is from the radial and the ulnar arteries.

The FDP muscle belly arises from the volar and medial aspects of the proximal three fourths of the ulna and from the

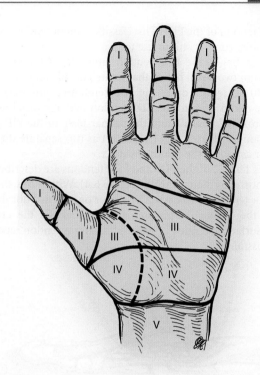

FIGURE 6.2 Flexor system has been divided into five zones or levels for the purposes of discussion and treatment. Zone 2, which lies within the fibroosseous sheath, has been called "no man's land" because it was previously believed that primary repair should not be done in this zone. (Copyright Elizabeth Martin.)

interosseous membrane. In the deepest layer of the volar forearm, the FDP muscle lies adjacent to the flexor pollicis longus muscle. The ulnar nerve innervates the muscle-tendon units of the ring and small fingers. The anterior interosseous branch of the median nerve innervates the FDP muscle-tendon units of the index and middle fingers. The blood supply to the FDP muscle is largely from the ulnar artery.

The flexor pollicis longus (FPL) tendon arises from the volar aspect of the middle third of the radial shaft and from the lateral aspect of the interosseous membrane. The anterior interosseous branch of the median nerve innervates the FPL muscle belly in the proximal forearm or midforearm. The blood supply of the FPL muscle is predominantly from the radial artery.

The tendons of the nine digital flexors enter the proximal aspect of the carpal tunnel in a fairly constant relationship. The most superficial tendons are the FDS tendons to the long and ring fingers. Immediately beneath them are the FDS tendons to the index and little fingers. In the deepest layer are four FDP tendons and the FPL.

Kleinert and colleagues[115] and Verdan[236] used their knowledge of anatomy to facilitate classification of tendon injuries into five anatomic zones (Figure 6.2). Zone 5 extends from the muscle-tendon junction to the proximal aspect of the carpal tunnel, and zone 4 describes the flexor tendons within the carpal tunnel. Distal to the transverse carpal ligament at approximately the level of the superficial palmar vascular arch, the lumbrical tendons take their origin from the FDP tendons. Zone 3 denotes the origin of the lumbricals from the FDP tendon. The proximal aspect of the A1 pulley is the entrance to zone 2, or "no man's land." Zone 1 is distal to the insertion of the FDS tendon. A laceration in zone 1, by definition, injures only the tendon of the FDP. This classification of tendon injury, by anatomic zone, is still in use today.

In each finger, the FDS tendon enters the A1 pulley and divides into two equal halves that rotate laterally and then dorsally (180 degrees) around the FDP tendon (Figure 6.3). The two slips rejoin deep to the FDP tendon over the distal aspect of the proximal phalanx and the palmar plate of the PIP joint at the Camper chiasm, and then insert as two separate slips on the volar aspect of the middle phalanx.

Zones 1 and 2 of the FDS and FDP tendons are described by the fibroosseous digital sheath (Figure 6.4). Within this sheath, the flexor tendons are covered by a layer of flattened fibroblasts termed the *epitenon*. This specialized surface is the crucial gliding surface that must be restored for flexor tendon repair to be successful.

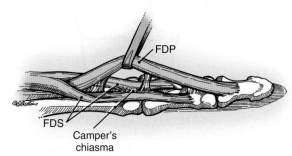

FIGURE 6.3 In the proximal part of the flexor sheath, FDS tendon divides into two slips, which encircle the FDP tendon first at the volar aspect, then at the radial and ulnar aspects, and finally at the dorsal aspect. The two portions of the FDS tendon reunite at the Camper chiasm and redivide before inserting onto the middle three fifths of the volar aspect of the middle phalanx, forming the floor of the flexor sheath in this area. (Copyright Elizabeth Martin.)

The pulley mechanism of the flexor sheath consists of thicker annular pulleys and thinner, more flexible cruciform pulleys.[39,40,45] The annular pulleys are stiffer and keep the tendon closely applied to the underlying bone.[175] Their form and function allow an economical amount of tendon excursion to effect a significant amount of joint angular rotation, improving the efficiency of the flexor apparatus.[230,231] Structural analysis of these pulleys has suggested that each of the three layers of the pulley has a strategic purpose. The innermost layer secretes hyaluronic acid and is designed to facilitate gliding. The middle layer, rich in collagen, resists palmar translation of the tendons. The outer areolar layer facilitates nutrition of the pulley. The cruciform pulleys are collapsible and can "accordion" to allow for digital flexion to occur without significant deformation of the annular pulley system (see Figure 6.4). The A1, A3, and A5 pulleys take origin from the palmar plates of the MP, PIP, and DIP joints. The A2 pulley originates from the proximal third of the proximal phalanx, and the A4 pulley originates from the middle phalanx.

The dual nutritional supply of the digital flexor tendons in zone 2 is from vascular perfusion and synovial diffusion (Figure 6.5).[140,240] The parietal paratenon[230] allows for passive nutrient delivery to, and waste removal from, the flexor tendon within the flexor sheath by means of diffusion. The flexor tendons receive a direct arterial supply from the well-developed vincular system, osseous bony insertions, reflected vessels from the tendon sheath, and longitudinal vessels from the palm. The system of blood supply allows delivery of nutrients and removal of wastes.

Surgical Treatment
Preoperative Considerations

Optimal timing of flexor tendon repair depends on the findings of a thorough history and physical examination. Emergency repair of the lacerated tendons is indicated only in the setting of altered digital perfusion that requires microvascular repair

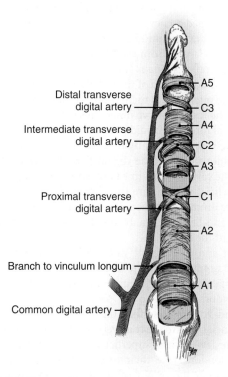

Distal transverse digital artery — C3
— A5
— A4
Intermediate transverse digital artery — C2
— A3
Proximal transverse digital artery — C1
— A2
Branch to vinculum longum
Common digital artery — A1

FIGURE 6.4 Fibrous retinacular sheath starts at the neck of the metacarpal and ends at the distal phalanx. Condensations of the sheath form the flexor pulleys, which can be identified as five heavier annular bands and three filmy cruciform ligaments (see text). (Copyright Elizabeth Martin.)

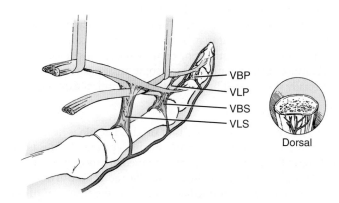

Dorsal

VBP
VLP
VBS
VLS

FIGURE 6.5 Blood supply to flexor tendons within the digital sheath. The segmental vascular supply to the flexor tendons is via long and short vincular connections. The vinculum brevis superficialis (VBS) and the vinculum brevis profundus (VBP) consist of small triangular mesenteries near the insertion of the FDS and FDP tendons. The vinculum longum to the superficialis tendon (VLS) arises from the floor of the digital sheath of the proximal phalanx. The vinculum longum to the profundus tendon (VLP) arises from the superficialis at the level of the PIP joint. *Cutaway view* depicts relative avascularity of the palmar side of the flexor tendons in zones 1 and 2 compared with the richer blood supply on the dorsal side, which connects with the vincula.

or reconstruction. If digital perfusion is compromised, or if the mechanism of injury is consistent with injury to arteries, urgent exploration and tendon repair with microvascular digital artery and nerve repair are indicated.

Primary repair done within days of the injury allows for preparation of the patient and ensures optimal conditions for the procedure. Basic science and clinical evidence suggest that it is preferable to perform tendon repair early after injury. Undue delay can be associated with changes in the tendon ends and proximal muscle that make primary tendon repair difficult. Done promptly after injury, the wound is easier to manage and the tendon ends are fresh for the repair.

In some cases of delayed presentation, or when the patient provides an unreliable history, the interval between injury and diagnosis may be unknown. In these cases, adequate preoperative consideration should be given to the possible need for tendon reconstruction and tendon repair. These more complicated cases may require the use of a primary tendon graft or placement of a tendon spacer.

In some settings, repair of both tendons is impossible. If the tendon ends are severely injured, unclean, or ragged, or if there is insufficient tendon for repair, excision of the FDS tendon and isolated repair of the FDP tendon may be the best alternative.[52,118,245] Isolated repair of the FDP tendon creates a simpler finger and is generally associated with diminished adhesion formation in a severely traumatized digit. In cases where only repair of the FDS tendon is possible, FDP tenodesis to the middle phalanx or DIP joint fusion may be necessary. Generally, repair of both tendons is preferable for optimal gliding and strength. In select cases, excision of one slip of the FDS tendon may be necessary to diminish the bulk of the repair and facilitate gliding through the tendon sheath. The need for repair of the flexor sheath is controversial.[168,223]

Repair of Zone 1 Tendon Lacerations or Avulsions

Laceration of the FDP tendon distal to the insertion of the FDS tendon or avulsion from its insertion at the base of the proximal aspect of the distal phalanx is a zone 1 injury. If the tendon is lacerated and the distal tendon stump is less than 1 cm long, FDP tendon advancement and primary repair to bone is usually indicated. If more than 1 cm of FDP stump is available for suture, primary tenorrhaphy is usually done because shortening of the FDP tendon by more than 1 cm may result in a "quadriga effect" on the intact FDP tendons. The term *quadriga* (*quadri* meaning "four" and *jungere* meaning "to yoke") refers to a Roman chariot pulled by four horses abreast. When excessive advancement of a tendon is done for the purpose of repair, it also creates tension in the other "yoked" tendons of the FDP muscle. Because of this increased tension, diminished flexion occurs in the other fingers when the injured finger is flexed.

Tendon-to-Bone Repair. The many techniques for tendon-to-bone repair can be divided into two general types: traditional pull-out suture methods and internal suture methods. Traditional methods of FDP tendon repair to bone call for the placement of a core suture in the proximal tendon and using the free ends of the suture to secure the cut end of the tendon into a small trough in the distal phalanx. The free ends of the sutures are passed through or around the distal phalanx and through the sterile matrix and nail plate, and tied over the dorsum of the fingernail (see Figure 6.11, *C*, and Figure 6.27). This

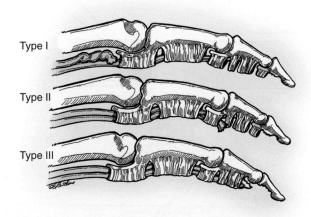

FIGURE 6.6 Leddy and Packer classification of profundus avulsions. *Type I:* The FDP tendon is avulsed from its insertion and retracts into the palm. *Type II:* The profundus tendon is avulsed from its insertion, but the stump remains within the digital sheath, implying that the vinculum longum profundus is still intact. *Type III:* A bony fragment is attached to the tendon stump, which remains within the flexor sheath. Further proximal retraction is prevented at the distal end of the A4 pulley. (Copyright Elizabeth Martin.)

"pull-out suture" usually is removed approximately 6 weeks after the procedure. All internal suture methods use suture anchors or other methods to affix the tendon directly to the bone. The development of miniature anchors, appropriate for deployment into the distal phalanx, has improved our ability to use newer core suture types, that is, four-strand tendon repairs, so as to fix the tendon to the distal phalanx in a stable manner. Whatever technique is used, it is essential that the FDP stump be secured directly to the footprint in the distal phalanx when the knot is secured.

Flexor Digitorum Profundus Avulsion. Leddy and Packer[123] classified FDP avulsions into three types (Figure 6.6). In type I avulsions, the FDP tendon retracts into the palm and the vincular blood supply of the tendon has been disrupted. These injuries are best treated by urgent surgical repair. In type II avulsions, the tendon stump retracts to the level of the PIP joint and some vincular blood supply is preserved. In some type II cases, a primary tendon repair may be done 6 weeks after injury. A large bone fragment is attached to the stump of the FDP tendon in type III injuries. This fragment usually prevents tendon retraction proximal to the distal edge of the A4 pulley. Fracture repair using Kirschner wire or miniature screw fixation is necessary for treatment of this injury. Since Leddy and Packer's description was created, a fourth type of injury has been identified.[229] A type IV injury is defined as a fracture *and* avulsion of the FDP tendon from the fracture fragment. The stump may be located either within the tendon sheath or within the palm. Suspicion of this injury can be confirmed with advanced digital imaging; either ultrasound or magnetic resonance imaging (MRI) is appropriate. Repair of the fracture is done first, after which the tendon is advanced and affixed to the distal phalanx. In some cases with a small fracture fragment, the bone may be excised, and the tendon may be advanced and sutured into the distal phalanx. Generally, this type IV injury is more severe and may be associated with a less optimal outcome. Because the initial radiographic findings may be inconsistent with the proximal location of the flexor tendon, I recommend

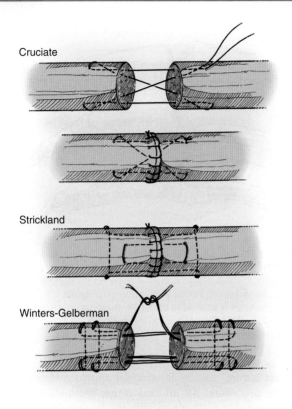

Cruciate

Strickland

Winters-Gelberman

FIGURE 6.7 Commonly used techniques for end-to-end flexor tendon repair. (Copyright Elizabeth Martin.)

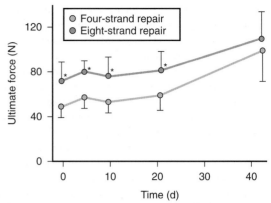

FIGURE 6.8 Comparison of ultimate force versus time between suture techniques from 0 to 21 days. The repairs with the eight-strand technique were significantly stronger than the repairs that used the four-strand technique. *Asterisks* denote a significant difference between the eight-strand and four-strand techniques at *P* < .05. (Redrawn from Boyer MI, Gelberman RH, Burns ME, et al: Intrasynovial flexor tendon repair: an experimental study comparing low and high levels of in vivo force during rehabilitation in canines, *J Bone Joint Surg [Am]* 83:891–899, 2001.)

that all flexor tendon avulsion injuries be treated by early repair when possible.

Repair of Zone 2 Tendon Lacerations

Attempts to improve the strength of flexor tendon repairs have focused on strategies to vary the material properties of the suture, the suture caliber, and the suture technique to coapt the tendon ends accurately. A smooth tendon suture is important for restoration of a low-friction gliding surface and facilitates tendon rehabilitation. Generally, surgeons need to master a method that allows for atraumatic suture placement and stable, accurate coaptation of the tendon ends. The method of tendon coaptation must be strong enough to allow early digital mobilization.

Core Sutures. Ex vivo and in vivo investigations in clinically relevant models have suggested that core suture configurations with the greatest tensile strength are those in which there are multiple sites of tendon-suture integration. Although two-strand suture methods (Kessler and modified Kessler and Tajima techniques) still enjoy widespread acceptance, newer multistrand suture methods (Strickland, cruciate, Becker, Savage, and Winters) are being used with increasing frequency because they are stronger and have increased resistance to repair site gapping (Figures 6.7 and 6.8 and Video 6.1). These more modern methods of core tendon suture placement have not only been shown to offer greater initial repair site tensile strength but also to improve strength 6 weeks postoperatively.

It is well accepted that core suture strength is related to the type of suture material, the caliber of the suture, and the number of suture strands crossing the repair site. This concept holds

true in time-zero mechanical studies and in clinical studies for the first 6 weeks after repair. The practical limitation of the more esoteric repairs is the time required and the complexity of suture placement in a small space using a minimally traumatic technique. Most surgeons choose the suture size based on the caliber of the tendon to be repaired because a 3-0 suture shows increased strength compared with a 4-0 suture. Ex vivo studies have shown that the loop of the core suture that is positioned to "lock" rather than "grasp" the tendon stumps shows greater time-zero strength. Similarly, increasing the number of locks or grasps increases the time-zero tensile strength (Figure 6.9).

The placement of the suture knot either within or away from the repair site has not been shown to have an independent effect on tensile strength. Greater quantity of suture within the repair site may increase repair site bulk, increase the work of flexion, and diminish the surface area available for repair.[167] External knot placement distant to the repair site may also adversely affect tendon gliding within the flexor tendon sheath by causing increased friction or knot trapping between tendon and sheath.[166,175]

Epitendinous Suture. Initially proposed as a method to smooth the site of tendon repair, epitendinous, or *circumferential*, suture has been shown to augment repair site strength. Diao and colleagues[43] and others have shown that by making the suture deeper or by altering the configuration, there is some improvement in repair site strength.[117,238] Although the circumferential suture can increase the initial and early postoperative strength of the repair site, it remains an adjunct to core tendon suture. In some cases, placement of the circumferential suture first (at least in the dorsalmost aspect of the tendon repair) can facilitate tendon orientation and make placement and tensioning of the core suture easier.[182]

Gap Formation. There is a negative effect of early repair site gap formation on tendon healing and accrual of repair site strength. An in vivo canine study showed that tendons healing without repair site gaps, or with gaps of less than 3 mm, acquire strength 6 weeks after repair. In this same study, if there was a

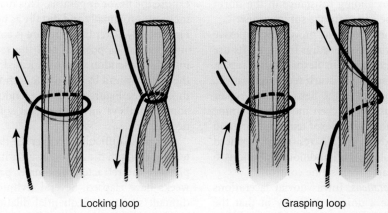

Locking loop   Grasping loop

FIGURE 6.9 Relationship between the longitudinal and transverse intratendinous components of the core suture defines whether the suture is "locking" or "grasping." When the transverse component passes within the tendon superficial to the longitudinal component, the suture "locks" a bundle of tendon fibers. When the transverse component passes deep to the longitudinal component, however, the suture does not "lock" a bundle of tendon fibers but pulls through the tendon. (Copyright Elizabeth Martin.)

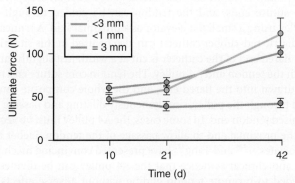

FIGURE 6.10 Ultimate tensile strength is plotted as function of time. Tendons with repair site gaps less than 3 mm accrue strength during the fourth to sixth week postoperatively, whereas tendons with repair site gaps greater than 3 mm show no significant increase in ultimate tensile strength during the early postoperative period. (Redrawn from Gelberman RH, Boyer MI, Brodt MD, et al: The effect of gap formation at the repair site on the strength and excursion of intrasynovial flexor tendons: an experimental study on the early stages of tendon-healing in dogs, *J Bone Joint Surg [Am]* 81:965–982, 1999.)

repair site gap greater than 3 mm, significant accrual of repair site strength did not occur. Repair site gaps that develop early in the postoperative period pose a greater risk of rupture as rehabilitation progresses after 3 weeks (Figure 6.10).

Biologic Considerations. Since Lundborg's important observation that intrinsic tendon healing was possible, large strides have been made in the investigation of the biologic processes occurring at the repair site during the postoperative period. The process of flexor tendon repair can be divided into three general phases: early inflammatory, intermediate active repair, and late remodeling. The area within 1 cm of the repair site is the most active and is characterized by early cellular proliferation and migration to the repair site. Although suture methods maintain the position of the tendon ends, the biology of the repair response is the ultimate arbiter of outcome. Increased synthesis of type I collagen mRNA and protein has been shown within repair site cells and cells within the adjacent epitenon early in the postoperative period. Fibronectin, an abundant extracellu-

lar matrix protein involved in cell-matrix communication, and $\alpha_5\beta_1$ and $\alpha_v\beta_3$ integrins, cell surface compounds involved in the binding of fibroblasts to extracellular matrix, are also upregulated during the early postoperative period.[21-23]

Role of Postoperative Passive Motion Rehabilitation. Despite advances in suture methods and understanding of the biology of the repair site, the formation of adhesions between the tendon and the surrounding fibroosseous sheath with resultant digital stiffness remains one of the most common complications after intrasynovial flexor tendon repair. In vivo studies have suggested that the formation of these restrictive intrasynovial adhesions at the repair site and at remote sites between tendon and sheath may be obviated if a sufficient amount of tendon excursion is achieved during passive motion rehabilitation. In vivo canine studies have shown that repaired tendons need only be moved passively 1.6 mm or more during postoperative rehabilitation to prevent clinically relevant adhesion formation.[22,23]

In an effort to improve the accrual of strength at the tendon repair site, investigators have advocated rehabilitation methods that generate increased levels of applied in vivo force across the repair. Although some level of force application is valuable, Boyer and colleagues[22,23] showed that increasing levels of applied force during postoperative rehabilitation from 5N to 17N did not accelerate the accrual of repair site strength after placement of a multistrand repair and may risk gap or rupture.

Future Concepts. Recent studies have explored the use of fibrin glue in the flexor tendon repair. Fibrin glue has been used in a variety of surgical procedures to promote hemostasis and tissue bonding and as a cell carrier for stem cells on tendons. Using a rabbit model, He and associates[87] reported improved range of motion in digits following zone 2 tendon repair augmented with fibrin glue at 3 weeks compared with controls. At 8 weeks there was no difference in the range of motion between the two groups. There was no change in the biomechanical properties of the repair in the experimental group. A recent cadaveric study examined the effect of fibrin glue augmentation following zone 2 repairs. The authors compared a standard four-strand core repair plus fibrin glue augmentation with a standard four-strand core repair with epitendinous sutures. They reported a significantly higher gliding resistance in the fibrin glue group compared with the epitendinous suture group.[256]

Vitamin C has become a hot topic in preventing reflexive sympathetic dystrophy following distal radius fractures. Its use as an antioxidant has been examined in flexor tendon repair. Tissue damage and hemorrhage can disturb redox regulation, thereby favoring fibrotic responses in the flexor tendon repair site. Hung and colleagues[96] used a chicken model to examine the effects of local vitamin C following flexor tendon injury and repair. They reported improved gliding resistance, reduced fibrotic size, and fewer histologic peritendinous adhesions 6 weeks following repair compared with saline controls.

Flexor Pollicis Longus Lacerations. Intrasynovial lacerations of the FPL tendon may pose a unique difficulty in that the proximal tendon stump frequently retracts deep to the thenar musculature, making retrieval of the proximal end more difficult.[23,79,114] If the proximal stump has retracted proximal to the distal edge of the thenar musculature, it can be localized through a separate incision in the carpal canal or distal forearm.

Repair of Tendon Lacerations in Zones 3, 4, and 5

The principles for operative exploration and repair of flexor tendon injuries proximal to the A1 pulley are similar to injuries in zone 2, though the potential for disruptive adhesion formation postoperatively is considerably reduced. Generally, repair of lacerations in these zones has an improved prognosis. The preoperative planning for these repairs should account for the possible need for microsurgical nerve and arterial repair. Techniques and considerations for the placement of the core and circumferential sutures and postoperative rehabilitation are the same as those described for zone 2 injuries.

Repair of Partial Tendon Lacerations

There has been considerable debate about the appropriate management of partial tendon lacerations. Partial flexor tendon lacerations can progress to late tendon rupture and tendon entrapment or triggering. For lacerations that are more than 50% of the tendon cross-sectional area, I usually repair the tendon using a core suture method and a circumferential suture. If the cross-sectional area lacerated is less than 50%, the tendon is either repaired or débrided to avoid entrapment and triggering of the tendon. My preference is to explore wounds where there is high probability on physical examination that a tendon injury has occurred. Advanced imaging can be useful in select cases for decision making but is unlikely to take the place of exploration in the majority of cases.

❖ AUTHOR'S PREFERRED TECHNIQUE: Zone 1 Tendon-to-Bone Repair

The patient is placed supine on the operating table, and the arm lies at a right angle to the long axis of the body. A well-padded brachial tourniquet is placed on the arm. The arm is prepared using a povidone-iodine (Betadine) scrub and paint. A surgical pause or "time out" is done. The limb is exsanguinated using an elastic bandage, and the tourniquet is inflated to a pressure that is 100 mm Hg greater than the systolic blood pressure. Prior to insufflation of the tourniquet, a first-generation cephalosporin or other appropriate antibiotic(s) is administered as determined by the nature of the injury.

When possible, an extensile midlateral incision is used to expose the flexor apparatus. This may be extended with Bruner incisions proximally and distally as needed (Figure 6.11; see also Figure 6.14). After the exposure is completed, assessment of the entire injury is possible and the sequence of repair is determined. The tendon stump is located proximally and drawn into the distal wound by any of the techniques described for zone 2 injuries (see Figure 6.11). The tendon is then transfixed to the annular pulleys and the digital soft tissues with a 25-gauge needle.

It is often difficult to deliver the flared-out stump of the FDP tendon through the A4 pulley after it has avulsed from the distal phalanx and retracted proximally, particularly if several days or weeks have elapsed. Several techniques are available for this difficult situation. Sequential dilation of the A4 pulley using pediatric cervical sounds or dilators can be effective. The edges of the stump may be trimmed so that the width of the stump does not exceed that of the pulley. After sequential dilation of the pulley, a core suture is placed in the stump, and the suture strands are delivered in a proximal-to-distal direction through the pulley. With the sutures placed, gentle traction is applied to the suture ends, and the tendon can be guided through the pulley using a small flat elevator as a proximal skid. A truncated pediatric red-rubber catheter can also be used in this situation; the flared end of the catheter is cut at a width just slightly larger than the tendon and A4 pulley. The tendon core suture end may be drawn into the flared end, and the whole composite can be slid through the pulley, simultaneously dilating and passing the avulsed tendon end. In some cases, the A4 pulley must be vented at the proximal end to allow passage of the tendon. Lieber and associates[128,129] and Tang[222] have presented convincing mechanical and clinical evidence that the A4 pulley can be divided as needed to promote tendon gliding without adverse effects on work of flexion or functional outcome.

The bone at the volar base of the distal phalanx is exposed to establish a repair footprint for the tendon reinsertion. If the distal phalanx is large enough to accept a miniature suture anchor, I place an anchor in the center of the distal phalanx.[29] Next, I place two corner sutures at the edge of the phalanx in the osteoperiosteal sleeve using 5-0 polypropylene. I use these sutures to seat the tendon into the footprint, and then secure the tendon into final position using the anchor suture ends. Using this technique, the tendon can be seated securely and then the grasping core suture can be more easily placed and appropriately tensioned. Two- or four-strand core suture methods can be used with this technique,[125] and I prefer incorporating a Becker type of suture (Figure 6.12).[174] When the distal phalanx is not large enough to accommodate an anchor, I use a traditional pull-out suture. Placement of the corner sutures is still useful, however, to guide and reinforce the repair site. The pull-out sutures (a modified Kessler type of 3-0 polypropylene suture) are passed through the distal phalanges using straight Keith needles that are drilled through the footprint at the base of the distal phalanx and are tied over a button placed on the nail plate dorsally (see Figure 6.25). It is preferable to have the needles exit the nail plate beyond the lunula (and beyond the germinal matrix) to avoid nail deformity or eponychial injury. The button and suture are left in place for 6 weeks.

The rehabilitation protocol generally follows the same progression as described for zone 2 injuries (see later).

CRITICAL POINTS *Zone 1 Repair*

Surgical Timing
- Leddy type I injuries require early (within 3 weeks) diagnosis and treatment.
- Although all flexor tendon avulsion injuries are best treated early, Leddy type II and III injuries may be amenable to later repair. Careful exploration is useful here.

Pearls
- Direct tendon repair is preferable if there is at least 1 cm of distal tendon stump.
- Tendon repair to bone is done if there is less than 1 cm of distal tendon stump. Either suture anchors or pull-out suture and button constructs may be used.
- The tendon-bone site should be observed directly before final knot-tying to ensure the tendon is well seated on the repair footprint (distal phalanx).

Pitfalls
- A tendon that is advanced too far and inserted too tightly leads to quadriga.
- Two-strand repair techniques may be insufficient for rehabilitation programs that employ early active range of motion.

Technical Points
- Identify and prepare the bony insertion site.
- Ensure the tendon is seated in the footprint when the knot is secured.
- Place additional peripheral sutures that guide and secure the tendon.

Postoperative Care
- Apply a dorsal splint with wrist and MP joints flexed and PIP and DIP joints at 0 to 10 degrees.
- Use a graded rehabilitation protocol under supervision of a qualified therapist.

Return to Activities
- The patient may return to full activity at 4 to 6 months after surgery.

❖ AUTHOR'S PREFERRED TECHNIQUE: Primary Tendon Repair in Zones 1 and 2

After the initial evaluation has been done and a decision has been made in favor of early repair, the wound is irrigated with an antibiotic solution and closed with a fine monofilament suture. For clean wounds and healthy patients, I administer a weight-based dosage (1-2 g) of a first-generation cephalosporin and a tetanus toxoid when necessary. For patients who have not been immunized and for patients whose immunization status is uncertain, passive immunization may be indicated. Passive immunization is not a substitute for wound débridement. Patients who are at risk for methicillin-resistant *Staphylococcus aureus* or have a highly contaminated injury may require a more formal irrigation and débridement and/or broader-spectrum antibiotic coverage. A dorsal splint that includes all digits is applied. For cases that do not require urgent repair, I prefer to repair the tendon within 7 days of injury.

The patient is prepped and draped as above. The initial wound is examined, and then incisions are planned that would predictably allow access to both tendon ends. A midlateral incision is preferred because it gives wide exposure and places intact skin and subcutaneous fat directly over the flexor tendon sheath. When the laceration is complex, a midlateral approach may not

be practical, and in those instances I incorporate the existing laceration into the approach to the tendon sheath (Figures 6.13 and 6.14). The goal of the exposure should be to provide maximum visualization while maintaining useful durable skin flaps over the area of the tendon repair. The skin and subcutaneous fat are raised off of the tendon sheath as a single thick layer. Separation of these tissues must be avoided because skin perfusion is by random vascular supply, and thinning of the skin flap can cause decreased perfusion at the distalmost aspect of the flap. I generally design the longitudinal limb of the incision to be associated with the nerve and artery that may require repair.

The wound is completely examined to define the nature and elements of the injury. After a thorough lavage, the sequence of repairs can be determined. The laceration of the sheath is identified, and a limited débridement of the hemorrhagic ends of the sheath is performed. Exposure of the tendons is done by reflecting a radial- or ulnar-based flap of sheath within repair "windows" between the A2 and A4 annular pulleys. Sheath venting and excision should be limited to that necessary for visualization and repair, as excessive sheath division can lead to bowstringing.

If the digit was in a position of significant flexion at the time of injury, the distal stump usually lies distal to the skin laceration and may rest beneath or distal to the A4 pulley with the finger in extension. The distal tendon stump may often be delivered by passive flexion of the DIP and PIP joints. If the tendon does not pass readily, gentle sequential dilation of the A4 pulley with pediatric cervical sounds or dilators may be beneficial. Often, I place half of the core suture in the tendon distal to the pulley, and then pass the sutures and tendon end proximally beneath the pulley to complete the repair. Partial or complete A4 pulley division, pulley venting, and pulley lengthening may occasionally be necessary. I prefer to obtain a smooth repair, with full excursion on intraoperative range-of-motion testing without additional alteration of the annular pulleys when possible. Some newer studies find that this is easily done with local anesthetic methods that may facilitate intraoperative examination of tendon excursion and digital range of motion.[89]

The proximal tendon stumps may be visible within the fibro-osseous sheath. The proximal tendon end may be retrieved using a variety of methods. If the tendon is immediately accessible, I gently grasp the endotenon of the FDP and pull the tendons distally; usually the FDS tendon comes into the wound with distally applied traction on the FDP tendon.[252] The tendon position is maintained by placement of a 25-gauge, 5/8-inch needle through the tendon and one of the proximal annular pulleys.

For tendons that are not locally accessible, I milk the tendon ends into the wound using a proximal-to-distal massage of the digit. The tendon is grasped directly on its cut end (the endotenon) with nontoothed forceps and is held in position using a 25-gauge needle. If the proximal tendon stump is not visible and cannot be delivered by milking into the wound, the wound is extended or a counterincision is made in the palm to retrieve the proximal tendon end. Repeated blind passes into the digital sheath using a hemostat or similar device in an attempt to grasp the tendon end can be associated with additional injury to the tendon sheath and should not be done. Because there is some evidence that epitendinous injury can be associated with peritendinous adhesion formation, I try to limit contact with the

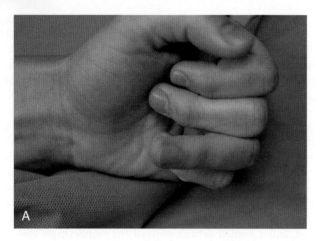

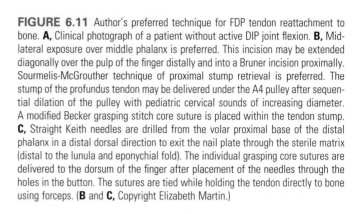

FIGURE 6.11 Author's preferred technique for FDP tendon reattachment to bone. **A,** Clinical photograph of a patient without active DIP joint flexion. **B,** Mid-lateral exposure over middle phalanx is preferred. This incision may be extended diagonally over the pulp of the finger distally and into a Bruner incision proximally. Sourmelis-McGrouther technique of proximal stump retrieval is preferred. The stump of the profundus tendon may be delivered under the A4 pulley after sequential dilation of the pulley with pediatric cervical sounds of increasing diameter. A modified Becker grasping stitch core suture is placed within the tendon stump. **C,** Straight Keith needles are drilled from the volar proximal base of the distal phalanx in a distal dorsal direction to exit the nail plate through the sterile matrix (distal to the lunula and eponychial fold). The individual grasping core sutures are delivered to the dorsum of the finger after placement of the needles through the holes in the button. The sutures are tied while holding the tendon directly to bone using forceps. (**B** and **C,** Copyright Elizabeth Martin.)

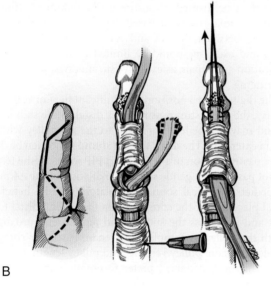

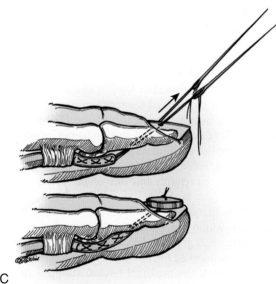

epitenon during tendon repair and grasp the tendon by the endotenon whenever possible.

Although there are several methods for acquisition of the proximal tendons, the method advocated by Sourmelis and McGrouther[209] is reliable and effective. A small pediatric feeding tube or similar device is passed in a retrograde manner through the digital sheath. The tube should enter at the site of the laceration and exit in the palm proximal to the A1 pulley. The flexor tendons are left in situ in the sheath, and, through a midpalmar incision, the catheter is sutured to both tendons several centimeters proximal to the A1 pulley. The catheter is pulled distally, delivering the tendon stumps into the distal repair site easily. A 25-gauge, 5/8-inch needle is used to secure the tendons to adjacent soft tissues at the repair site. In situations in which the tendons have retracted proximal to the A1 pulley, an incision is made just proximal to the A1 pulley and the lacerated tendons and adjacent neurovascular structures are identified. The proximal stumps are delivered distally by the catheter method when possible. A Freer elevator or one of several commercial instruments may be used to "shoehorn" the tendon atraumatically into the flexor sheath beneath the A1 pulley.

It is crucial to reestablish the proper anatomic relationship of the FDS and FDP tendons in the palm and at the site of the repair. In some complex lacerations, orientation of the tendons and repair of all injured tendons may be impractical. In those cases, I resect one slip of the FDS tendon and repair one slip. This repair strategy facilitates gliding of the repairs within the sheath and simplifies tendon orientation.

If the tendon is lacerated proximal to the FDS decussation, a core suture is often used (see Figure 6.7). I base the core suture method on the caliber of the tendon that is available for repair. The more robust, thicker FDP tendon is ideal for core suture placement within zones 1 and 2. I prefer a 3-0 braided caprolactam looped (double-strand) suture affixed to a curved, tapered needle end. A four-strand modified Kessler core suture with locked loops offers a substantial improvement in time-zero repair site tensile strength and stiffness over traditional two-strand core suture techniques.

For smaller tendons, I use a four-strand modified Kessler suture that is placed with a 4-0 braided caprolactam looped suture. The suture may be placed simply in both ends and results in a strong four-strand repair. For larger tendons or

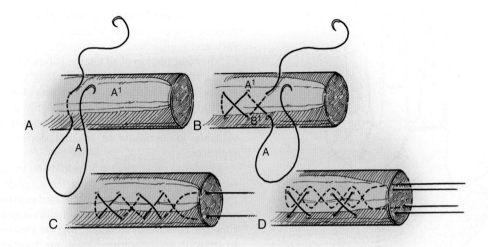

FIGURE 6.12 A to D, Four-strand modified Becker repair (see text). (Copyright Elizabeth Martin.)

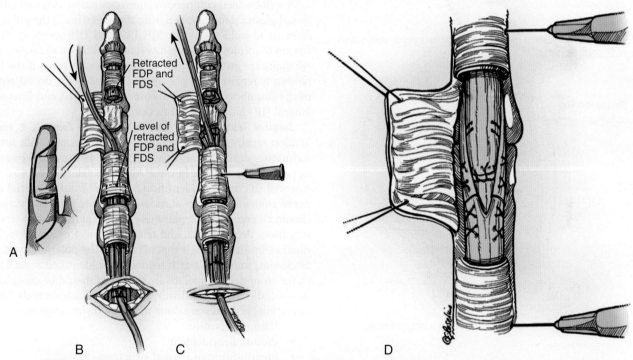

Retracted
FDP and
FDS

Level of
retracted
FDP and
FDS

A   B   C   D

FIGURE 6.13 Author's technique of flexor tendon repair in zone 2. **A,** Knife laceration through zone 2 with digit in full flexion. The distal stumps retract distal to the skin incision with digital extension. **B,** Radial and ulnar extending incisions are used to allow wide exposure of the flexor tendon system. Note appearance of the flexor tendon system of the involved fingers after the retraction of skin flaps. The laceration occurred through the C1 cruciate area. Note the proximal and distal position of the flexor tendon stumps. Retraction of small flaps (windows) in the cruciate portion of synovial sheath allows the distal flexor tendon stumps to be delivered into the wound by passive flexion of DIP joint. The profundus and superficialis stumps are retrieved proximal to the wound by passive flexion of DIP joint. The profundus and superficialis stumps are retrieved proximal to the sheath by the use of a small catheter or infant feeding gastrostomy tube. **C,** Proximal flexor tendon stumps are maintained at the repair site by means of a transversely placed small-gauge hypodermic needle, allowing repair of the FDS slips without tension. **D,** Completed repair of FDS and FDP tendons is shown with DIP joint in full flexion. Extension of DIP joint delivers the repair under the intact distal flexor tendon sheath. Wound repair is done at the conclusion of the procedure. (Copyright Elizabeth Martin.)

where a stronger repair is desirable, I use two continuous modified Kessler sutures placed with a 3-0 looped suture made of braided caprolactam (eight strands). Using this method, the sutures lie side by side within the tendon. Because of the increase in suture volume, care must be taken to prevent impaling the transverse suture limb when passing the suture out of the cut end of the tendon. Locking loops of suture are not used. When using a single suture, the core suture is tensioned to bring the stumps together before beginning the second core component. When using looped suture, care must

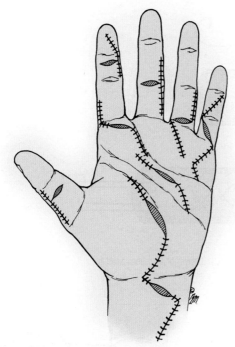

FIGURE 6.14 Incision options for wound extension during flexor tendon repair. (Copyright Elizabeth Martin.)

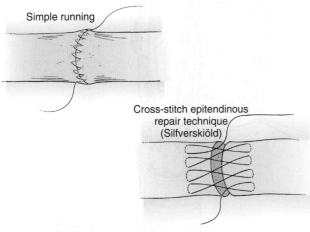

Simple running

Cross-stitch epitendinous repair technique (Silfverskiöld)

FIGURE 6.15 Circumferential epitendinous suture techniques.

be taken to maintain even tension in all limbs of the suture; this allows the setting of an evenly tensioned suture knot. To finish the repair, a 6-0 polypropylene suture is used for a deep, running circumferential suture. This suture is started on a volar corner of the repair site and is placed circumferentially around the tendon over the repair site. When the stitch is started, I invert the first pass to facilitate inversion of the suture knot into the repair site. I leave one tail long when the suture is cut so that the running suture may be tied to itself when the suture is completed (Figure 6.15).

More distally, the FDS tendon repair is made difficult by the thin, flat shape of the tendon slips as they wrap around the FDP tendon. A traditional core suture may not be possible in the flattened FDS tendon slips near the PIP joint; these tendons may best be repaired using one of the zone 2 to 4 extensor tendon techniques.[124] It is preferable to use a smaller needle along with

a smaller-caliber suture to minimize tissue trauma. A 4-0 or 5-0 braided polyester suture affixed to a small, tapered needle at each end is effective.

After completion of all tendon sutures, I evaluate the stability of the repairs throughout a full range of digital motion and ensure satisfactory gliding of the repairs through the fibroosseous tunnel. Sheath closure is done only if it does not impair tendon gliding. These intraoperative observations may be valuable to clinicians in making decisions about aftercare regimens.

I prefer to repair the tendons first and then repair the injured nerves and arteries. Often the arterial repair is done last, with the tourniquet deflated using standard microsurgical dissection and repair methods. This also provides a satisfactory length of time for hemostasis to occur. Bipolar electrocautery is critical to prevent postoperative hematoma formation, and primary wound closure is performed in clean wounds using simple 5-0 nylon sutures. I believe that meticulous hemostasis limits postoperative swelling, diminishes postoperative pain, and facilitates rehabilitation.

A well-padded compressive, nonconstrictive dressing with a dorsal plaster slab is applied from the fingertips to the proximal forearm to hold the wrist, MP, PIP, and DIP joints in slight flexion to minimize passive myostatic tension on the repair site. All digits are included in the postoperative dressing. If the FPL tendon is repaired, the plaster splint overlies the dorsal aspect of the thumb to hold the carpometacarpal, MP, and interphalangeal (IP) joints in slight flexion.

Surgical Techniques for Tendon Repairs in Zones 3, 4, and 5. Tendon repairs in zones 3, 4, and 5 are performed with suture techniques similar to those used in zone 2. Because of the nature of penetrating injuries in these zones, an extensile approach is essential to complete identification of the injury. Arterial and nerve injuries in these areas are common, and the surgeon should be prepared to repair these injuries at the time of wound irrigation, débridement, and tendon repair. I prefer a longitudinal extensile approach that allows for the potential need for fasciotomy and allows each tendon to be identified at each end of the wound. Intraoperatively, the digits should be completely flexed and extended to identify the lacerated tendon ends. These operations generally are done in the following sequence:

- Wound exposure
- Wound débridement
- Identification of injured structures
- Repair of injured structures

For the forearm, I prefer to perform the arterial repairs first, the tendon repairs second, and the nerve repairs last. The tendon repairs are started from the deepest tendon that is lacerated, and the progression of repairs is to the most superficial tendon that is lacerated. If arterial repair is necessary or if the swelling in the forearm seems significant, I will consider a forearm fasciotomy prior to skin closure. For the specific repair method, I use a 3-0 looped, braided caprolactam suture and a modified Kessler four-strand technique. In these zones, it is often useful to place a simple suture in the corners of the tendon ends to begin the approximation and then place the core suture. This simple step eliminates the need to set the tension in the suture after suture passage and limits any gap formation between the tendon ends. I do not routinely use epitendinous sutures in these areas.

CRITICAL POINTS *Zone 2 Repair*

Surgical Timing
- Emergency repair is indicated if both digital nerves and arteries are lacerated. Tendon repair is done in conjunction with digit revascularization.
- Routine tendon repairs are preferably done no later than 7 days after injury.
- After 6 weeks, primary repair is unlikely to be possible.

Pearls
- A multistrand core suture method with a running circumferential suture is preferred when the caliber of the tendon is sufficient.
- A pediatric No. 8 feeding tube should be ready if retrieval is required (Sourmelis technique).
- Knowledge of the patient's history and the nature of the injury and observation of the repair should guide the approach to rehabilitation.

Pitfalls
- The importance of patient compliance with aftercare strategies should be emphasized.

Technical Points
- Enter sheath between distal A2 pulley and proximal A4 pulley.
- Retrieve proximal stump by milking, feeding tube, or direct exposure.
- Deliver distal stump by passive DIP hyperflexion.
- Stabilize the tendon ends for repair by transfixation using a 25-gauge, 5/8-inch needle. For some cases, single inverted simple sutures can provide temporary tendon alignment while the core suture is being placed.
- The caliber of the tendon and the probable method of aftercare determine the choice of repair method.
- Use at least a four-strand core suture technique (3-0 or 4-0 suture) with a running 6-0 polypropylene circumferential suture (nonlocked, deep bites into tendon).
- Repair both the FDS and FDP tendons. Excise a single slip of the FDS tendon if it is excessively bulky or gliding is impaired.
- Examine the intraoperative range of motion to guide therapy considerations.
- Sheath repair is optional.
- Ensure adequate hemostasis before closure.

Postoperative Care
- The postoperative dressing should be applied to position the wrist in flexion (20 to 30 degrees), the MP joints in flexion (50 to 70 degrees), and the PIP and DIP joints at zero or slight flexion. Apply the dressing so that it is well padded and nonconstricting and does not have any fulcrum effect in the palm.
- Use a graded rehabilitation protocol under supervision of a qualified hand therapist.
- Use synergistic wrist motion to increase excursion.

Return to Activities
- The patient may return to unrestricted activity at 4 to 6 months after surgery.

Expected Outcomes of Flexor Tendon Repair

The outcome after flexor tendon repair is variable and depends on the nature of the injury, the patient's individual biologic response to injury, the timing of repair, the method of repair, and the ability of the patient to participate in a program of postoperative occupational therapy. If satisfactory tendon repair can be obtained and if the patient can participate in a tendon repair aftercare program, forearm tendon repair is generally associated with a good functional outcome.

The most common complication after tendon repair is digital stiffness related to peritendinous adhesion formation or digital joint contracture. Repair site rupture occurs uncommonly and can often be related to noncompliance with the suggested aftercare program. An early second attempt at repair can be performed successfully with the anticipation of good outcome, provided the patient is compliant and has access to supervised hand therapy. Pulley rupture with resultant tendon bowstringing, quadriga, digital triggering, swan neck digital deformity, and lumbrical-plus fingers can occur but are less common provided the mechanical and anatomic relationships of the tendons and the pulley system are maintained.

Postoperative Management: Rehabilitation

❖ AUTHOR'S PREFERRED TECHNIQUE: Postoperative Rehabilitation of Repairs in Zones 1 and 2

Philosophically, I believe the tendon rehabilitation program has to be constructed to try to improve the function of the entire hand and facilitate differential incorporation of the injured soft tissues (Figures 6.16 to 6.18). Generally, the method of rehabilitation is significantly influenced by the compliance of the patient, the nature of the wound, and the method and location of the repair. Although we still employ general time guidelines for implementation of various therapeutic interventions, we also accelerate and decelerate patients' regimens based on their individual response to treatment. In this environment, there is no substitute for an experienced, energetic, meticulous hand therapist.

Therapists are encouraged to choose a postoperative program that controls the amount of *force* to the repair site, while promoting *excursion* of the tendon proximally and distally. Improvements in tendon excursion are thought to be associated with improvements in range of motion and patient outcome. The rationale for applying any force to the healing tendon during a postoperative rehabilitation program is to promote a small amount of proximal excursion and not to accelerate healing.[38,253] Excessive force during rehabilitation can lead to tendon gapping or rupture. The force that is applied to the repair site is controlled during an aftercare program by exercise and the position of the wrist, MP, and IP joints.

Excursion, measured in millimeters, is best described as the total amount of glide that a point on the tendon travels during range of motion. In the original Duran and associates protocol,[51] the authors reported that 3 to 5 mm of tendon excursion was sufficient to prevent restrictive adhesions after repair. This concept has been widely accepted and incorporated into tendon rehabilitation programs over the last 30 years. More recently, authors have concluded that 6 to 9 mm of excursion was the maximal limit of therapeutic excursion during a postoperative program, and that further excursion was not beneficial.[202] Low force and moderate excursion programs have traditionally been effective and should continue to be effective in the future.

The first 4 weeks of therapy are the most important phase in the patient's rehabilitation. Although each patient's situation is generally similar, the particular therapy program must be individualized. Many factors influence decision making in the aftercare regimen, including patient compliance, edema (which increases the work of flexion), suture size and configuration,

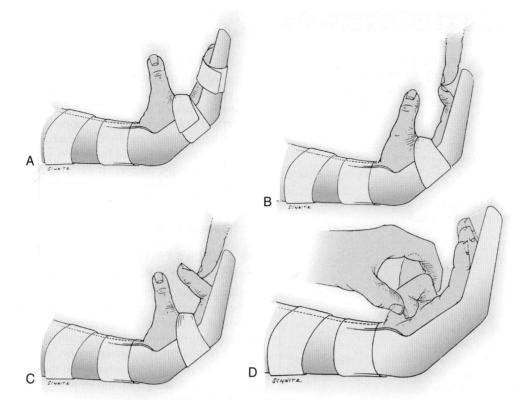

FIGURE 6.16 Controlled passive motion method. **A,** Orthoplast dorsal blocking splint is used to hold wrist in mild flexion, MP joints in about 45 degrees of flexion, and PIP and DIP joints in nearly full extension. **B,** Full isolated passive flexion of DIP joint. **C,** Full isolated passive flexion of PIP joint. **D,** Full passive flexion of MP, PIP, and DIP joints.

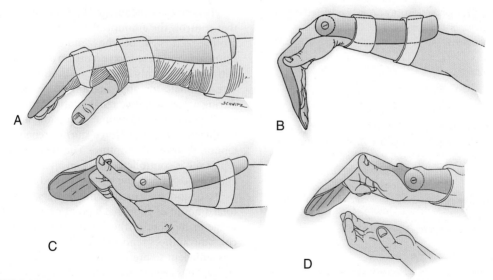

FIGURE 6.17 Controlled place-and-hold motion after flexor tendon repair protocol. **A,** After removal of the surgical bandage, a traditional dorsal blocking splint that positions the wrist in 20 degrees of palmar flexion, MP joints in 50 degrees of flexion, and IP joints in extension is applied. **B,** A tenodesis splint with a wrist hinge is fabricated to allow for full wrist flexion, wrist extension of 30 degrees, and maintenance of MP joint flexion of at least 60 degrees. **C,** After composite passive digital flexion, the wrist is extended and passive flexion is maintained. **D,** The patient actively maintains digital flexion and holds that position for about 5 seconds. Patients are instructed to use the lightest muscle power necessary to maintain digital flexion.

wound complications, tight wound dressings, systemic conditions, or concomitant injury. With these factors in mind, our center categorizes and treats postoperative patients in two general categories: patients who are appropriate for an accelerated rehabilitation program, and patients who are not. That decision is usually made with the input of the surgeon and the therapist.

Before beginning therapy, it is important for the therapist to have information from the operating surgeon about the type of repair that was done and whether other structures were injured.

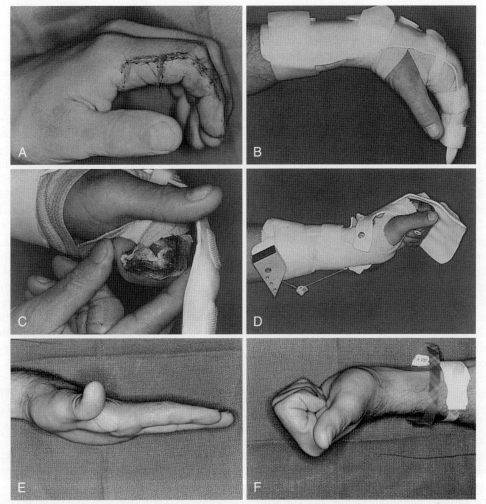

FIGURE 6.18 Clinical examples of the author's program following flexor tendon repair. **A,** Index finger after a four-strand repair of FDS and FDP tendons. **B,** Resting splint with wrist and MP joints flexed and IP joints extended. **C,** Finger is passively flexed with the wrist in flexion. **D,** Wrist is extended while maintaining passive digital flexion. The patient holds this position with light active flexion. **E,** Extension at 3 years. **F,** Flexion at 3 years. (Courtesy of James W. Strickland, MD.)

If a high-strength tendon repair technique was successfully performed in a compliant patient, the patient is placed in a more aggressive early motion program that employs individual decision making based on patient progress. Therapy typically begins 1 to 5 days after surgery. On the initial visit, a wrist-neutral dorsal blocking orthosis is applied. The MP joints are positioned at 50 degrees of flexion, a position that promotes gentle stretch on the collateral ligaments of the MP joints and prevents excessive stretch on the flexor tendons.

The patient is taught an hourly home exercise program that consists initially of passive positioning of the fingers in a fist for 3 minutes, with the splint in place. Next, within the confines of the orthosis, the patient performs the exercise of passive flexion of the affected finger to the palm, followed by actively extending the finger to the orthosis: 15 passive flexion and active extension movements to the bib of the splint are done in each hour. Finally, the patient removes the splint and performs a tenodesis program. The fingers are passively flexed into the palm using the unaffected hand, and the wrist is actively extended to a comfortable end range. The patient gently contracts the flexor muscles, removes the unaffected hand, and actively holds the fist position for 5 seconds. After 5 seconds, the patient releases

wrist extension and the wrist falls into flexion, and as it does, the fingers passively extend. The tenodesis cycle is repeated 10 times.

When not exercising, the patient straps the fingers into the bib of the splint, positioning the MP joints in flexion and the IP joints at −10 to 0 degrees of extension. Based on the patient's comfort with the program and any complicating factors, components of the program can be decelerated, accelerated, or discontinued by the therapist. The patient is counseled to stretch the PIP joint gently and passively with the MP joints held in flexion to avoid joint contracture. Wounds are dressed with loose-fitting 1/2-inch tube gauze. Edema is addressed in the first 2 weeks with elevation, the gentle pumping action of the exercises, and the gentle compression of the gauze. After 2 weeks postoperatively, compressive bandages can be applied as needed.

At 3 weeks postoperatively, the dorsal protective splint is removed for isolated and composite active joint range-of-motion exercises that are done hourly. The timing and type of active exercises prescribed at this point in the aftercare program are based on the physiologic healing response of the injured hand. Our decision to prescribe more forceful exercises has been adapted from the work of Groth,[80] who analyzed and reported the results of differing wrist and hand positions coupled with passive and active movements to create a pyramid of progressive force application to the healing tendon. Groth defined "high" or "low" physiologic tissue responses and suggested clinical approaches to each. Accelerated wound healing, edema, and dense scar resulting in the formation of peritendinous adhesions characterize a "high" physiologic response. Ultimately with a "high" physiologic response, there is significant loss of flexor tendon excursion. Patients who exhibit a "high" response are progressed through the pyramid of exercises quickly to promote force and prevent further adhesions. During this time, the clinical evaluation for the formation of peritendinous adhesions that limit tendon excursion is done. The nonresistive exercises of the pyramid are ranked in ascending order of increased force, which includes place-and-hold, composite-fist, straight-fist, and isolated joint motion with joint blocking exercises.

Conversely, a "low" physiologic response is characterized by slower wound healing, limited edema, and minimal discrepancy between the patient's active and passive finger flexion measurements. These patients generally have improved flexor tendon excursion, and less risk is required in therapy to maintain the range of motion. These patients may not have as robust a repair response, so progression to resistive exercises may be delayed, and patients are counseled not to use the hand in strength activities until cleared to do so by their surgeon.

The dorsal protective splint usually is discontinued at approximately 6 to 8 weeks postoperatively. If any flexion contractures of the IP joints are present, they are addressed with a static progressive device at that time. Isolated strength exercises are gradually introduced at 10 weeks postoperatively.

For more complicated cases, for patients with limited understanding, or for cases where compliance with the program is questionable, we use a passive mobilization program. The same dorsal protective splint is used, with the wrist in neutral and the MP joints in 50 degrees of flexion. A passive range-of-motion program (Duran type of program) of isolated IP and MP joint passive motion is taught. This program requires that the patient passively flex and extend the PIP joint of the affected finger while holding the DIP and MP joints flexed, and then passively move the DIP joint into extension and flexion with the MP and PIP joints flexed. All of the exercises are performed within the confines of the splint. The patient's wounds and edema are addressed as described previously. The progression of force application after 4 weeks of passive motion is similar to that described previously, but delayed for 2 to 3 weeks.

When children or adolescents have sustained a lacerated tendon and subsequent repair, the surgeon must make a decision with help from the parents and treating therapist as to whether or not the patient is a candidate for an early motion program. A basic tenet of any early motion flexor tendon rehabilitation program is that the patient be an active participant in aftercare. For this reason, the surgeon, parents, and child all must agree that the child is mature enough to perform the essential functions of rehabilitation safely. If the decision is not to allow an early motion program, the patient's wrist and hand are immobilized for 4 to 6 weeks in a cast positioning the wrist in neutral, the MP joints in 70 degrees of flexion, and the IP joints straight. After the initial period of immobilization, the patient is referred to therapy for careful initiation and progression of range-of-motion exercises for the next 6 weeks. Although

the advantages of increased repair site tensile strength, decreased peritendinous adhesions, and better functional outcomes associated with early motion programs are well documented, immobilizing a child's hand after flexor tendon repair has not been found to be as deleterious as it is for adults.[162]

If participants agree that the patient is a candidate for an early protected range-of-motion program, the tenodesis aftercare program discussed previously is employed. The treating therapist must frequently monitor the patient's compliance by having the patient attend therapy at least two times a week for the first 6 to 8 weeks. If more complicated forceful movements need to be eliminated from the child's aftercare program, movements such as tenodesis with place-and-hold therapy or simply place-and-hold therapy alone can be reduced to passive flexion/active extension movements within the splint. Progression through the phase of therapy is done based on both the injury and the patient's individual physiologic response to the injury.

Recent research has described the use of ibuprofen at anti-inflammatory doses (2400 mg/day) to decrease peritendinous adhesions following zone 2 flexor tendon repairs. In their study, Rouhani and colleagues[183] found that patients who received ibuprofen following tendon repair had a better range of motion compared with their control group. There were no reported complications.

Complications Following Flexor Tendon Repair

Despite continued improvement in surgical care and rehabilitation of flexor tendon injuries, complications still occur and may have devastating effects on hand function.[139,216] Infection, skin flap necrosis, tendon repair rupture, and tendon adherence all adversely affect digital function after injury. The greatest protection against repair site rupture is a well-done multistrand core suture, complemented by a running circumferential repair, and early institution of high-quality hand therapy. Should rupture occur up to 3 weeks postoperatively, repeat repair is done. At time periods longer than 3 weeks postoperatively, the chance of a successful repeat repair is less likely. If rupture occurs, it is crucial that the condition be diagnosed and treated within days of the event, before scarring and retraction prevent successful repeat repair. Patients should be counseled regarding the possibility of tendon reconstruction with a silicone rod or tendon graft.

The repaired tendons may become adherent and fail to glide sufficiently to restore unimpeded digital function. The decision to proceed with tenolysis is made after serial joint measurements fail to show improved active digital motion despite continued therapy.[251] A prerequisite for successful tenolysis is that full or nearly full passive digital flexion has been achieved. Tenolysis is a surgical strategy that should be considered 4 to 6 months after tendon repair for patients who have significant loss of tendon excursion.

Interphalangeal joint contracture can occur after flexor tendon repair, especially among patients treated with elastic traction. Early identification and treatment of the contracture usually result in satisfactory outcomes using nonsurgical strategies. Generally, these contractures can be resolved using passive stretching exercises and static progressive splints as needed. Patients with recalcitrant contractures that limit hand function at 4 to 6 months after tendon repair can be considered for small joint release.

CRITICAL POINTS *General Principles of Flexor Tendon Repair*

- Extensile exposure in a controlled setting with optical magnification allows the extent of the injury to be defined.
- Tendon retrieval is done using atraumatic techniques and windows through noncrucial areas of the flexor tendon sheath.
- Handling of the tendon should be minimal.
- The tendon must be accurately oriented.
- The core tendon sutures should be placed to allow for accurate coaptation of the tendon ends. The suture method should provide a stable, smooth repair that is freely gliding within the tendon sheath.
- Circumferential suture is used to "finish" the repair and add strength to the repair.
- Sheath closure is necessary only if it improves tendon gliding.

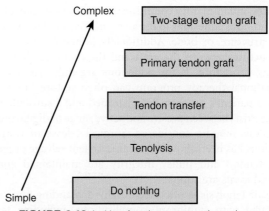

FIGURE 6.19 Ladder of tendon reconstruction options.

Acknowledgments: The authors acknowledge the work of Dr. John S. Taras and Dr. Robert A. Kaufmann, whose outstanding chapters in previous editions have been modified, combined, and updated. Their contributions to our understanding of repair and reconstruction of the damaged flexor tendon system have greatly advanced our ability to care for these injuries. The authors also acknowledge the contributions of Mr. Daniel Acker, OT, CHT, to the rehabilitation portion of this chapter.

FLEXOR TENDON RECONSTRUCTION

With improvements in flexor tendon repair methods, the need for flexor tendon reconstruction has substantially diminished. Still, flexor tendon reconstruction is a necessary and important procedure for failed and neglected tendon repairs. Prior to Lister's report detailing a successful method for zone 2 flexor tendon repair, tendon transection in the finger had been treated using tendon grafting as the preferred method for the reconstruction of finger flexion. Restoration of satisfactory digital function after an unrepaired flexor tendon laceration or a failed repair remains one of the most difficult challenges in hand surgery.[105,152-154,157,158,217]

In this section, we review the indications and methods for primary tendon grafting, staged tendon grafting, select tendon transfers, pulley reconstruction, and tenolysis. These cases remain among the most challenging in hand surgery; advances in repair methods and postoperative rehabilitation strategies have improved the results of flexor tendon reconstruction, however. Research that focuses on surface cell modulation, scaffold seeding, other tissue engineering methods, and biochemical agents that may decrease adhesion formation and facilitate graft survival will likely improve surgical strategies in the future.

Patient Selection

Proper patient selection is essential for the success of flexor tendon reconstruction. Before proceeding with surgery, the nature and number of procedures as well as the extent of postoperative therapy should be outlined for the patient. Finsen[61] reported that a significant number of patients underestimate the impact of the reconstruction process. The patient must be willing and able to adhere to the aftercare regimen to optimize outcome. A number of patient variables have been identified that affect the need for and outcome after tendon grafting:

1. *Age of the patient.* Younger patients typically do better than elderly patients; however, in very young patients, technical difficulties and difficulties with rehabilitation compliance may compromise the outcome.
2. *Mechanism and extent of trauma.* Crushing injuries, fractures, joint disruption, nerve and artery damage, skin loss, and infection contribute to a poorer prognosis after reconstructive surgery.
3. *Level of tendon laceration.* As a rule, tendons injured outside the digital flexor sheath yield better results than tendons injured within zone 2.
4. *Healing response of the patient.* The patient's innate healing response to injury is likely to influence the end result more than the actual technique of suturing, the type of suture material chosen, or the timing of the procedure.

The timing of and nature of reconstructive procedures play a role in contributing to the success of the care plan. Reconstruction of the flexor tendon system can be viewed as a management ladder, with each rung representing a need to address greater impairment (Figure 6.19). For patients with early tendon repair site disruption, we still recommend an early reattempt at repair if possible. For patients who have previously undergone repair, we recommend 4 to 6 months of occupational therapy and rehabilitation to restore normal tendon gliding and joint mobility prior to considering tenolysis and joint release. If, upon exploration, tendon grafting is necessary, primary tendon grafting can be done from palm to fingertip when the palm and fibroosseous tunnel are satisfactory. If extensive adhesions have formed in the fibroosseous tunnel, a staged tendon grafting procedure should be started using a temporary silicone spacer to recreate a gliding space and the tendon graft implanted at a second procedure.

Flexor Tenolysis
Preoperative Evaluation

Full smooth finger motion is, in part, the result of normal flexor tendon excursion within the digital sheath. Any source of significant peritendinous adhesion formation will limit tendon excursion and, consequently, active digital motion. Tendon adhesions occur whenever the surface of a tendon has been compromised either by the injury itself or by surgical manipulation.[145,146] Failed primary tendon repairs, crush injuries, fractures, inflammatory conditions, and infections can all cause peritendinous adhesions to the adjacent tendon, skin, neurovascular structure, or bone. Additionally, adhesions may form at the juncture between the graft and the native tendon after a grafting procedure. If the adhesions are mild, an organized occupational therapy program can often restore full gliding. When a patient's progress has plateaued and a substantial difference exists between passive and active range of digital motion, a tenolysis may be considered. Surgical release of restrictive adhesions has been shown to be an excellent salvage procedure when tendon and pulley integrity are maintained and the involved joints are supple.[25,58,109,190,213,217,246]

Flexor tenolysis is often technically demanding and can be associated with significant complications, including tendon repair site and graft juncture rupture. If unsuccessful, the patient's hand function may be even worse than before surgery. Tenolysis is usually considered approximately 4 to 6 months after the index procedure and when the soft tissues have recovered sufficiently to allow another attempt at restoration of motion. The best candidate for tenolysis is a patient with limited active but full passive range of motion, supple soft tissues, and a tendon repair with localized adhesions that limit tendon gliding (Figure 6.20). It is paramount that the patient can begin occupational therapy immediately. When surgical release of this region has been accomplished successfully, full or near full range of motion is usually regained. Commonly, adhesions have formed over a long segment of the involved tendon and require extensive exposure for release.

Because optimizing results after tenolysis requires immediate mobilization, any concomitant surgery that requires immobilization (i.e., repair of nonunion or skin coverage) in the postoperative period should be done in a staged manner prior to tenolysis. Joint contracture is frequently seen in patients requiring tenolysis. These patients may also require a capsulectomy, which complicates the problem further and results in diminished gains.[235] Prognostic indicators that are associated with a poorer outcome include patient age older than 40 years, nerve repair or graft, late tenolysis (>1 year postoperatively), and tenolysis requiring a prolonged operative time.[235]

Although opinions vary on the best timing of tenolysis, almost all surgeons agree that a reasonable time should be

allowed for durable tendon repair, wound softening, and spontaneous remodeling of adhesions and scar tissue. Fetrow,[60] after reviewing Pulvertaft's cases, stated that 6 months should elapse before tenolysis after a free tendon graft to lessen the risk of graft rupture and suggested that a minimum of 3 months of healing be allowed before tenolysis after primary tendon repair. Rank and Wakefield[180] originally waited 3 months, but later advocated a delay of 6 to 9 months before considering tenolysis. Weeks and Wray[242] reported that most of the active digital function obtained after a tendon graft occurred by the 22nd postoperative week. Based on these reports, we usually consider tenolysis at 4 postoperative months in motivated patients with loss of active motion, full passive motion, stable soft tissues, and healed fractures. The patients need to be both willing and able to work with an occupational therapist after the surgery to obtain the best outcome and must accept the potential risk of tendon rupture following surgery.

The effect of patient age on functional improvement after tenolysis in children was investigated in a report by Birney and Idler.[17] These authors noted that tenolysis in children younger than 11 years resulted in only minimal gains, whereas older children benefited from tenolysis even when it was done more than 1 year after the original operation.

Agents That May Limit Adhesion Formation

Several authors have investigated the use of agents to block restrictive adhesion formation after tenolysis or tendon repair.[109] Steroid preparations have been locally instilled to alter wound healing in the belief that adhesion formation would be less robust. Whitaker and colleagues,[246] James,[108] Carstam,[33,34] Rank and associates,[181] and Wrenn and coworkers[255] suggested locally administered steroids to be of some value, whereas Verdan[235] and Fetrow[60] concluded that steroids do not improve the results of tenolysis. Bora and colleagues[19] found that many of these materials promoted additional scarring. Using a rabbit model, Tan and associates[221] reported that oral ibuprofen administration limited adhesion formation after FDP repair. Other authors have reported on the potential benefits of 5-fluorouracil[2,260] and hyaluronic acid[31] surface treatments in limiting adhesion formation following tenolysis and tendon repair in animal models.

❖ AUTHORS' PREFERRED TECHNIQUE: Tenolysis

Schneider and Hunter and coworkers[101,102,193,195] advocated local anesthesia and intravenous sedation to allow the patient's active participation during tenolysis (see the section on neuroleptanalgesia in Chapter 2). In our practice we often use local blocks for tenolysis. After the procedure is completed, the patient can easily demonstrate the range of motion that can be the postoperative goal. Recently, Lalonde and colleagues[119] have advocated "wide-awake" surgery done without tourniquet (WALANT). These methods of anesthesia have improved our ability to verify that the tenolysis is complete and the extent to which the patient can activate the tendon.

We reserve regional or general anesthesia for anxious patients and patients with extensive scarring where the procedure time would be extended. When a patient is under a regional nerve block or general anesthesia, the surgeon must be certain to extend the tenolysis proximal and distal to the zone of injury to ensure that all adhesions are released. Whitaker and

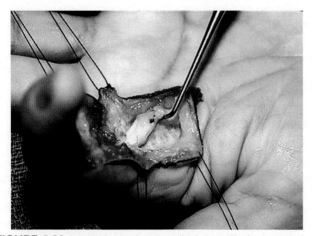

FIGURE 6.20 Localized area of tendon adhesion permits simple tenolysis to restore full tendon gliding.

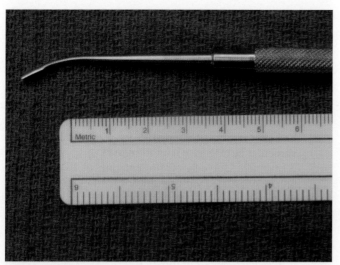

FIGURE 6.21 Specially designed tenolysis blades are invaluable in cleaving dense tendon adhesions.

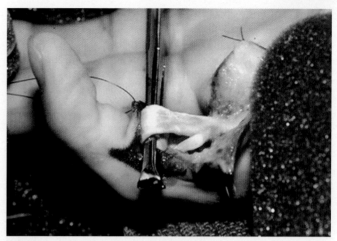

FIGURE 6.22 By gently twisting the tendons with an Allis clamp, tendon excursion can be confirmed during tenolysis.

colleagues[246] recommended a "traction flexor check" by pulling on the involved tendon through a separate incision at the wrist; this provides an estimate of the potential range of motion and has the additional benefit of breaking up any adhesions that may have been missed.

The involved flexor system is approached through an incision sufficiently long to uncover the entire length of the adhesions. Preoperative planning should ensure that the entire flexor apparatus can be exposed if necessary. Flexibility of the surgical approach may be required to use previous surgical scars. Beginning in a proximal area without adhesion formation and using careful dissection methods, all peritendinous adhesions are methodically excised. The tendon surface should be carefully identified proximally and distally to make it easier to define the areas of dense scar tissue formation. Optical magnification and specialized instrumentation may facilitate this process. Fine Beaver blades (Beaver-Visitec, Waltham, MA) (#6300, 6400, and 6900) or specialized tenolysis knives (Meals Tenolysis Knives; George Tiemann and Company, Hauppauge, NY) are particularly useful to cleave tendon adhesions (Figure 6.21). The dissection is continued along the tendon surfaces until all adhesions are removed or a need for tendon grafting is determined. Traction on the proximal end of the tendon and finger flexion and extension during the procedure will help the surgeon evaluate for additional areas of adhesion formation (Figure 6.22). It is imperative to preserve crucial elements of the pulley system, especially the A2 and A4 pulleys. If this preservation is impossible, new pulleys can be constructed at the time of tenolysis,[133] but we believe that this practice greatly reduces the probability of success.

A staged tendon implant should be considered when the tendon sheath is obliterated over a long section or an adequate pulley system cannot be preserved and must be reconstructed at the time of tenolysis. A poor-quality tendon can rupture during a tenolysis, forcing the surgeon "up the reconstructive ladder" to consider tendon grafting (see Figure 6.19).

After the tourniquet is released, intraoperative hemostasis is helpful in limiting hematoma formation, which facilitates aftercare. Wound closure is also a critical step. Using fine sutures to evert the skin edges for a nice closure is important to the success of the operation. A major benefit of using anesthesia that allows the patient to remain awake or using the WALANT method is the opportunity to allow the patient to witness the improved active digital flexion gained at surgery and establish rehabilitation goals. Final intraoperative range-of-motion measurements are useful to both the patient and occupational therapist as a method of setting the goals for rehabilitation.

Postoperative Care Following Tenolysis

After closure, a nonconstrictive dressing is placed so that immediate flexion can be performed within the bandage to maintain the gains made at surgery. Active finger motion is begun under the supervision of a hand therapist on the first postoperative day. Active range-of-motion exercises must be the primary therapeutic modality after tenolysis.[59,62] To help the patient get through the difficult and often painful first week after tenolysis, an indwelling polyethylene catheter can be left in the involved area at the time of surgery. The catheter is inserted percutaneously so that the catheter tip lies below the proximal extent of the incision. A specialized continuous inflow device (ON-Q pump, Halyard Health, Alpharetta, GA) can provide up to 5 days of local anesthesia. Alternatively the catheter can be injected or a new block administered prior to therapy on the first few visits to improve discomfort during the session.

Continuous passive motion devices can be useful when joint contracture releases are performed concomitantly after tenolysis,[149] but passive motion devices cannot substitute for immediate active pull-through exercises of the lysed tendon system. Continuous passive motion devices may impart a false impression of success if they are used without active-assisted exercises.

Expectations Following Tenolysis

Tenolysis is a tedious and complicated procedure that, if successful, has a high likelihood of improving the discrepancy between the patient's active and passive ranges of motion. The procedure has the following risks: neurovascular injury; tendon rupture; impaired healing; development of a cold, insensitive, and/or painful finger; and recurrence of adhesion. Some of these complications could provoke a need for digit amputation.

Having cautiously optimistic patients who understand the complexities and expect the unexpected is perhaps the healthiest mind-set for the treating surgeon and the patient. One series reported an increase in active PIP joint and DIP joint range of motion of 70 degrees in 80% of patients, no change in 10% of patients, and loss of motion of 25 degrees in 10% of patients.[62]

CRITICAL POINTS *Tenolysis*

Indication
- Tendon adhesions

Preoperative Evaluation
- A discrepancy exists between passive (full) and active (limited) range of motion after progress at hand therapy has plateaued.

Pearls
- Do not operate earlier than 4 months following repair or grafting.

Technical Points
- Use a block, the WALANT method, or neuroleptanesthesia, if possible. Perform a proximal "traction check" through an additional wrist incision.
- Use an extensile approach that allows for exposure of the entire flexor apparatus.
- Start in an area of normal tendon to help with identification of the tendon surface when scar tissue is thick.
- Specialized tenolysis blades may help divide adhesions without compromising pulley function.

Pitfalls
- Concurrent capsulectomy, concurrent osteotomy, age older than 40 years, and a 1-year delay contribute to a worse prognosis.

Postoperative Care
- Maintain digital anesthesia with a lidocaine pump for several days.
- Supervised occupational therapy and active range-of-motion exercises should begin immediately.

Single-Stage Flexor Tendon Grafting: Flexor Digitorum Profundus and Flexor Digitorum Superficialis Tendons Disrupted

Single-stage free tendon grafting after flexor tendon injury remains one of the most elegant and difficult procedures in the hand surgeon's armamentarium. The injured tendons are excised and replaced with a suitable tendon graft secured to the base of the distal phalanx at the FDP insertion and joined to a proximal motor in the palm or distal forearm. The palm-to-fingertip tendon graft (Figure 6.23) is usually performed in fingers that have had both flexor tendons severed in zone 2. Important surgical principles include the following:
- Reconstruct only one tendon in each finger.
- Never sacrifice an intact FDS tendon.
- Use a graft of small caliber.
- Perform the junctions outside of the tendon sheath.
- Ensure adequate graft tension.

Indications for Tendon Grafting

Flexor tendon grafting is indicated in the following clinical situations[10,81,24,83,239]:

1. Failure of flexor tendon repair.
2. Injuries resulting in segmental tendon loss.
3. Delay in repair that obviates primary repair. Late referral or a missed diagnosis may preclude primary treatment. Lacerations that have been neglected for more than 3 to 6 weeks show tendon degeneration accompanied by scarring within the tendon sheath.
4. Patients in whom the surgeon believes delayed grafting is the better treatment alternative for a zone 2 injury (e.g., segmental or extensive tendon injury).
5. Occasionally, for delayed presentation of FDP avulsion injuries associated with significant tendon retraction.

Before flexor tendon reconstruction surgery is considered, the soft tissues should be healed, mobile, and stable; the joints should be free of contracture; and the finger should, ideally, have full passive motion (Boyes' grade 1) (Table 6.2).[25] Pulvertaft[178] emphasized that "The hand [must be] in good overall condition. There is no extensive scarring. Passive movements are full or nearly full. The circulation is satisfactory. At least one digital nerve in the affected digit is intact." Prior to considering flexor tendon reconstruction, the surgeon should be prepared for and the patient advised of the need for additional reconstruction procedures after initial exploration. For example, at the time of initial exploration joint release, pulley reconstruction, tenolysis, and nerve reconstruction may be necessary, in addition to silicone rod implantation.

Initial Exploration

Initial exploration is usually done using a midlateral incision. This incision allows wide exposure of the digit and allows a nice thick flap of skin to be placed over the flexor tendon sheath. Sometimes, prior incisions dictate the operative approach. At the time of exploration it is crucial to make full assessment of the condition of the digit and reconstruct any injury that will facilitate the ultimate outcome of the reconstructive effort. For example, joint release, tenolysis, and pulley reconstruction should be done at the time of initial exploration. After exploration the surgeon can determine the best method for distal tendon juncture and the location and method for proximal tendon juncture. The length of the tendon graft can then be determined by measuring the extended finger from the distal juncture to the proximal juncture and adding 4 to 6 cm depending on the method of juncture that is anticipated.

TABLE 6.2 Boyes' Preoperative Classification

Grade	Preoperative Condition
1	Good: Minimal scarring with mobile joints and no trophic changes
2	Cicatrix: Heavy skin scarring because of injury or prior surgery; deep scarring because of failed primary repair or infection
3	Joint damage: Injury to joint with restricted range of motion
4	Nerve damage: Injury to digital nerves resulting in trophic changes in finger
5	Multiple sites of damage: Involvement of multiple fingers with combination of above problems

From Boyes JH: Flexor tendon grafts in the fingers and thumb: an evaluation of end results, *J Bone Joint Surg Am* 32:489–499, 1950.

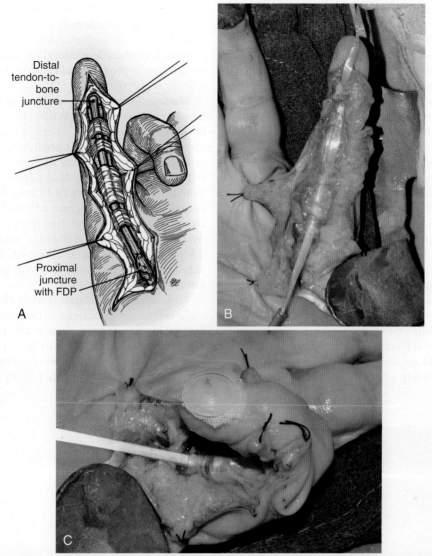

FIGURE 6.23 A, Flexor tendon graft. Tendon junctures are placed outside the confines of the flexor sheath (zone 2). **B,** In this clinical case, the graft has been passed from distal to proximal using a red-rubber catheter beneath the intact pulley system. **C,** Following distal junction repair with an "around-the-bone" pull-out suture, the graft is tensioned before the proximal juncture. (**A,** Copyright Elizabeth Martin; **B** and **C,** Copyright Scott W. Wolfe.)

In the figure labels: Distal tendon-to-bone juncture; Proximal juncture with FDP

Biology of Tendon Graft Incorporation

Using a clinically relevant canine model, basic science investigators have reported on the incorporation of free tendon grafts when placed into the specialized environment of the digital synovial sheath. They have found that intrasynovial donor tendons seem adapted to survive transplantation to the digital sheath and can incorporate without the formation of peritendinous adhesions. This adhesion-free or minimal adhesion incorporation is associated with improved functional characteristics (tendon excursion and angular joint range of motion). In contrast, extrasynovial donor tendons undergo considerable peritendinous necrosis, which is associated with the formation of dense peritendinous adhesions during tendon graft incorporation. These adhesions limit tendon graft excursion and joint range of motion.[127,199]

Obtaining Donor Tendon Grafts

The most popular tendon grafts are the palmaris longus for palm-to-fingertip reconstruction and the plantaris for forearm-to-fingertip reconstruction. Other sources of graft material include the long extensors of the three middle toes, the toe flexors, the extensor indicis proprius, and one slip of the extensor digiti minimi. The selection of a graft in any specific case is determined by the particular demands of the surgical procedure. Several authors have investigated the use of intrasynovial toe flexor grafts. These grafts healed with fewer adhesions in animal models compared with extrasynovial grafts, but their clinical superiority has not been shown to date. All tendon grafts should be harvested and handled with the utmost care. A harvested tendon should be placed in a sponge moistened with saline or lactated Ringer solution to protect it from drying. Allis-type clamps or suture on each end can be used to facilitate handling of the graft.

Palmaris Longus Tendon. Generally, we prefer the palmaris longus tendon for use in the palm-to-fingertip graft because it is in the same field of surgery and is accessible.[160] The presence of the palmaris longus tendon is easily determined during preoperative examination. The patient is asked to oppose the thumb to the little finger while flexing the wrist against resistance. The palmaris longus tendon should be readily visible, superficial, and palpable in the midline of the wrist. While there is some difference among populations, the palmaris longus tendon is present in at least 75% to 85% of the population.

Technique of Palmaris Longus Tendon Harvest. A 1- to 2-cm transverse incision is made at the wrist crease that is centered over the long axis of the long finger. The palmaris longus tendon is identified just beneath the skin. Care is taken to identify and protect the immediately subjacent median nerve and its palmar cutaneous branch during harvest of the palmaris longus tendon. Inadvertent median nerve harvest during this procedure has been reported.[241] If there is any question as to the identification of the palmaris longus versus the median nerve, a counterincision is made in the midforearm to confirm the structure prior to harvest. After its identification and distal dissection, the tendon may be harvested through several transverse forearm incisions or with the use of a tendon stripper that allows the entire tendon to be removed with only one or two small incisions. After transection at the wrist crease, the distal end of the graft is held with a 4-0 suture or Kocher clamp. The tendon is mobilized, under direct vision, for 6 to 8 cm and threaded through a circular tendon stripper (Figure 6.24). With firm, gentle tension held on the graft at its distal end with a clamp, the stripper is slowly advanced with a slight twisting

motion. As the stripper advances into the proximal region of the forearm, the muscle belly fills the circular cutting blade and is divided; this allows the tendon to be withdrawn through one incision. Occasionally, a second proximal incision is made over the stripper in the proximal forearm if undue resistance to the stripper is experienced.

Plantaris Tendon. When multiple grafts are needed, or one long distal forearm-to-fingertip graft is required, it is necessary to harvest tendons in the lower extremity. The presence of the plantaris tendon cannot be predicted clinically, but ultrasound or MRI can reliably identify its presence. Although it is said to be absent in only 7% of cadavers, Harvey and associates[84] found that the tendon was present in only 80% of limbs. It is also unusable sometimes because of variations in its girth or by virtue of attachments to the triceps surae, which make its removal in one length impossible. When robust, the plantaris tendon is an excellent graft, however, and can supply two and occasionally three palm-to-fingertip grafts or one long distal forearm-to-fingertip graft.

Technique of Plantaris Tendon Harvest. A 5-cm vertical incision is made just anterior to the medial aspect of the Achilles tendon, starting at the insertion and proceeding proximally.[27] The tendon is identified, bluntly dissected anterior to the Achilles tendon, and divided near its insertion (Figure 6.25, *D*). With a holding suture securely fixed in its cut end, the tendon is

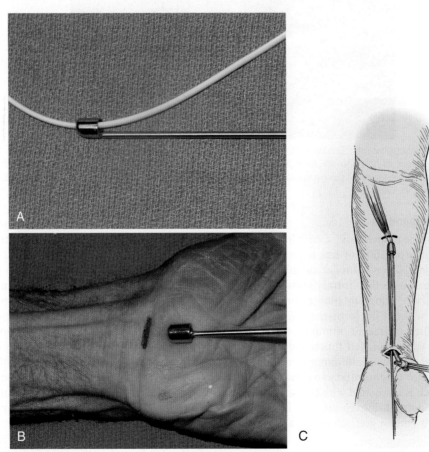

FIGURE 6.24 Palmaris longus graft. Our preferred technique for obtaining the graft uses a tendon stripper, which is a circular knife passed along the surface of the tendon. **A,** Tendon stripper. **B,** Placement of stripper. **C,** Stripper is advanced until it cuts off the graft at the muscle belly, or a second proximal incision can be used to obtain the proximal end of the tendon graft. (**A** and **B,** Copyright John Seiler; **C,** Copyright Elizabeth Martin.)

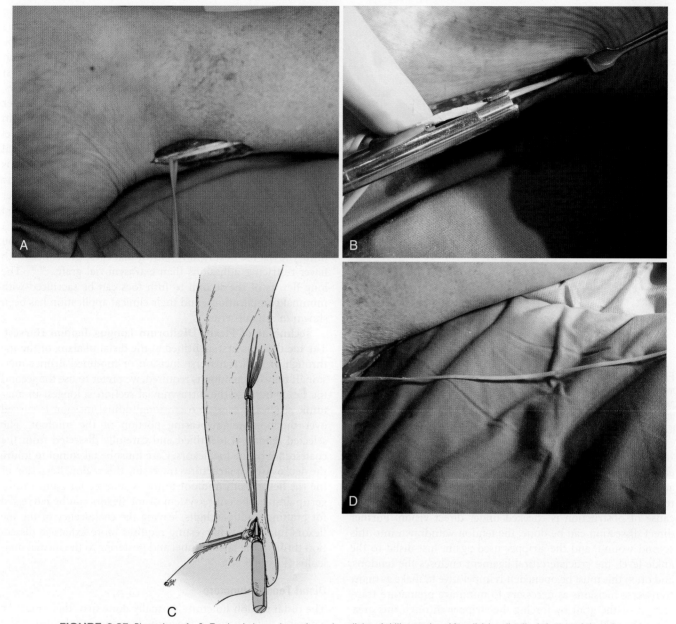

FIGURE 6.25 Plantaris graft. **A,** Tendon is located anterior and medial to Achilles tendon. After division distally, it is passed through circular stripper. **B,** Stripper is advanced up the leg. **C,** When stripper engages the muscle belly, it divides it, and the surgeon can withdraw the tendon. **D,** Plantaris graft can supply two fingertip-to-palm grafts. (**A, B,** and **D,** Copyright Scott W. Wolfe; **C,** Copyright Elizabeth Martin.)

mobilized as far as possible under direct vision; this gives the tubular stripper through which the tendon is threaded a straight course up the leg. The stripper should be held parallel to the leg and advanced with a gentle twisting motion while the tendon graft is held under tension. The knee should be extended. When the belly of the plantaris muscle fills the stripper, the muscle is divided to allow the entire plantaris tendon to be withdrawn from the wound. Alternatively, the tendon stripper can be palpated in the proximal leg and then a second incision made to allow for direct section of the proximal tendon. Care must be taken to keep the stripper parallel to the long axis of the tendon, or the tendon may be severed prematurely. Compartment syndrome after plantaris harvest has been reported; therefore, we recommend palpation of the calf at the conclusion of the procedure to assess for bleeding and excessive calf swelling.[227]

Long Toe Extensor Tendon. The long toe extensors can provide excellent grafts. Their presence is never in doubt, and their diameter is adequate for most needs. Three long tendon grafts can be acquired when the tendons to the second, third, and fourth toes are harvested. A frequent problem is that the individual tendons may fuse distal to the ankle, and three long grafts may be unobtainable. Although some authors advise their removal through a large longitudinal incision, we recommend the use of a tendon stripper and/or multiple transverse incisions to harvest these tendons.

Technique of Long Toe Extensor Tendon Harvest. A generous transverse incision is made on the dorsum of the forefoot at the level of the metatarsophalangeal joint (Figure 6.26). The long toe extensor is isolated proximal to the extensor hood and prepared for harvest by placing a holding suture in the tendon

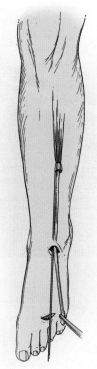

FIGURE 6.26 Long toe extensors. These tendons are best obtained through multiple transverse incisions on the foot. Graft is obtainable when the long toe extensor is used. When proximal to ankle, stripper can be advanced up the leg until the muscle is severed. More incisions than the two shown may be required. (Copyright Elizabeth Martin.)

and transecting it. After mobilization, a small stripper is advanced proximally, but stopped when resistance is encountered. A second transverse incision is made at this level, and the cause of obstruction is checked under direct vision. Further direct dissection can be done, the tendon withdrawn into this second wound, and the stripper used again. Just distal to the ankle level, the cruciate crural ligament encloses the tendons, and often this must be opened. It is imperative to make as many transverse incisions as necessary to minimize premature transection of the graft by forcing the stripper through this area. From the ankle proximally, the tendon can be stripped up into the lower leg. In some cases, all the long extensors will become confluent in the lower leg or ankle area, making it impossible to obtain a high-quality, long graft. When this problem is encountered, extensile incisions are used, and the tendons are dissected out individually. This approach creates "raw" or cut surfaces along the sides of the graft which may be associated with increased peritendinous adhesion formation after placement of the graft.

Extensor Proprius Tendons. The extensor indicis proprius and extensor digiti minimi tendons are both suitable as grafting material, and have the advantage of ease of access to the operative site. Each tendon is long enough for one palm-to-fingertip graft.

Technique of Extensor Indicis Proprius Tendon Harvest.
The tendon is exposed through a transverse incision over the MP joint of either the index or the little finger. The extensor indicis proprius tendon is ulnar to the index extensor digitorum communis tendon and is transected about 1 cm proximal to the extensor hood. The tendon is mobilized subcutaneously, and a

second incision is made over the musculotendinous junction proximal to the wrist (often the tendon can be identified as the lowest-lying muscle belly here). The tendon can usually be pulled into the second wound and transected. If the tendon does not withdraw easily, an interval incision between the first and second incisions may be necessary. Using these windows, any synovial connections or juncturae can be released under direct vision. The extensor digiti minimi tendon is harvested in a similar manner. At the metacarpophalangeal joint (MPJ) level it is the ulnar of the two tendons and is released just proximal to the extensor hood of the MPJ. The proximal dissection is similar to that for the extensor indicis proprius tendon. The extensor digiti minimi tendon is smaller in caliber and shorter in length. It is composed of two slips; Snow has recommended that only the ulnar half be used as a graft.[206]

Flexor Digitorum Longus Tendon of the Foot. Experiments on intrasynovial toe flexors have shown that these grafts heal with fewer restrictive adhesions than extrasynovial grafts.[199,201] The long flexors of the second to fifth toes can be sacrificed with minimal complications, and their clinical application has been shown in a small series.[127]

Technique of Flexor Digitorum Longus Tendon Harvest.
The toe flexor is first identified at the distal phalanx of the toe through a small transverse incision or modified Bruner incision. If only one tendon is required, we prefer to use the second toe flexor because the intrasynovial section is longest in anatomic studies.[200] Next, a 6-cm longitudinal incision is curved over the non–weight-bearing portion of the midfoot. The selected tendon is identified and carefully dissected from the coalescence of the toe flexors. Care must be taken not to injure the neurovascular structures traversing this region. Resection of the toe flexor from midfoot to toe is suitable for palm-to-fingertip grafts. The entire system of toe flexors can be harvested for grafting multiple digits, leaving the coalescence of the toe flexors intact. This harvesting requires more extensive dissection through the tarsal tunnel and posterior to the medial malleolus (Figure 6.27).

Distal Tendon Juncture

The distal tendon juncture is usually done first; there must be a durable union between the grafted tendon and the distalmost FDP stump or volar base of the distal phalanx. If the distal juncture is completed first, the graft length and graft tension may be adjusted when the proximal juncture is completed. There are several techniques for attaching the tendon graft to the distal phalanx, and these are based primarily on the length and condition of the distal FDP stump. If enough profundus stump is available, the graft can be sutured to the profundus stump or woven through the stump as in an end-weave juncture.

When there is not sufficient profundus tendon available for primary repair, the traditional method is a modification of the classic Bunnell tendon-to-bone pull-out technique (Figure 6.28). A drill hole is made in the volar cortex of the distal phalanx into which Keith needles are passed through the nail plate. Many surgeons employ a sterile button tied over a stent on top of the nail plate for securing the pull-out suture. Currently, suture anchors are commonly used in patients with good bone quality and may be combined with a pull-out suture for the increased strength of a multistrand repair.

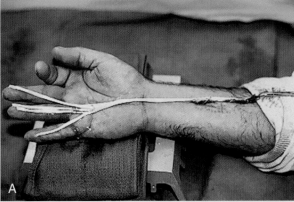

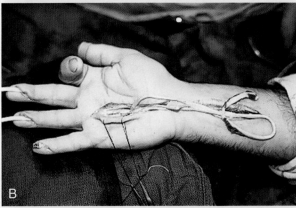

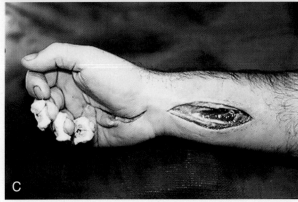

FIGURE 6.27 A to C, Toe flexor grafts. Multiple digits can be grafted using toe flexors, as illustrated by this case. The ulnar three digits were grafted using the entire long toe flexor tendons after silicone implants. (Courtesy of David Zelouf, MD.)

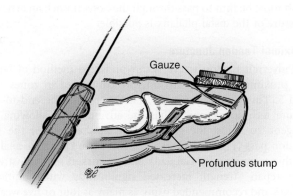

Gauze

Profundus stump

FIGURE 6.28 Modified Bunnell distal juncture technique. Pull-out sutures are passed through the distal phalanx. (Copyright Elizabeth Martin.)

CRITICAL POINTS *Obtaining Tendon Grafts*

Indications
- The need for a tendon graft is noted during flexor tendon reconstruction.
- Graft selection is determined by the donor's presence, the anticipated length of graft material necessary to secure the graft, and the demands of the procedure.

Preoperative Evaluation
- The presence of the palmaris longus tendon is easily determined through opposition of the thumb to the little finger as the wrist is flexed against resistance.
- The most common donor tendon for palm-to-fingertip reconstruction is the palmaris longus tendon, and the most common donor tendon for forearm-to-fingertip reconstruction is the plantaris tendon.
- Prior to use of the plantaris tendon, consider preoperative imaging to determine its presence.
- Other graft options are long extensors of the three middle toes, toe flexors, extensor indicis proprius tendon, and extensor digiti minimi tendon.

Pearls
- Intrasynovial grafts are associated with fewer adhesions in animal models.
- Keep harvested graft material in a moist saline sponge and handle it with the utmost care.

Technical Points
- Make a transverse incision just proximal to the wrist crease and in line with the long finger metacarpal centered over the palmaris longus tendon. The dissection is subcutaneous at this point, and the tendon is readily identifiable.
- Underneath this incision, use direct inspection to mobilize the tendon proximally 6 to 8 cm.
- Place a suture in the free distal tendon end, and thread the tendon through a circular tendon stripper.
- If a stripper is unavailable, use a multiple-incision method.

Pitfalls
- Identify and protect the median nerve at the time of palmaris longus tendon graft harvest. Careful subcutaneous dissection just proximal to the wrist flexion crease should allow identification of the tendon and, if necessary, the median nerve. The palmaris longus tendon is present in only 75% to 85% of people.
- Consider preoperative imaging for identification of the plantaris tendon. It is difficult to identify on physical examination, and imaging can confirm its presence prior to the procedure. The plantaris tendon is present in about 80% of people.

Pull-Out Sutures (Around the Bone)

Some surgeons prefer passing the pull-out suture around instead of through the distal phalanx (Figure 6.29, *A* to *D*). If the distal profundus stump has been preserved, it is reflected to its insertion on the volar lip of the distal phalanx. A 3-0 polypropylene pull-out core suture is placed in one end of the graft using a crisscrossed Bunnell technique. The sutures and graft are passed through the FDP stump and the pull-out sutures are threaded onto Keith needles. With the use of a needle holder, the Keith needles are passed around both sides of the distal phalanx and through the middle third of the nail plate (see Figure 6.29, *C*). An effort should be made to avoid the germinal nail matrix; the ideal point of exit through the nail plate should be 3 to 4 mm distal to the lunula and approximately 2 mm from the midline. The tails of the suture may be tied directly over the

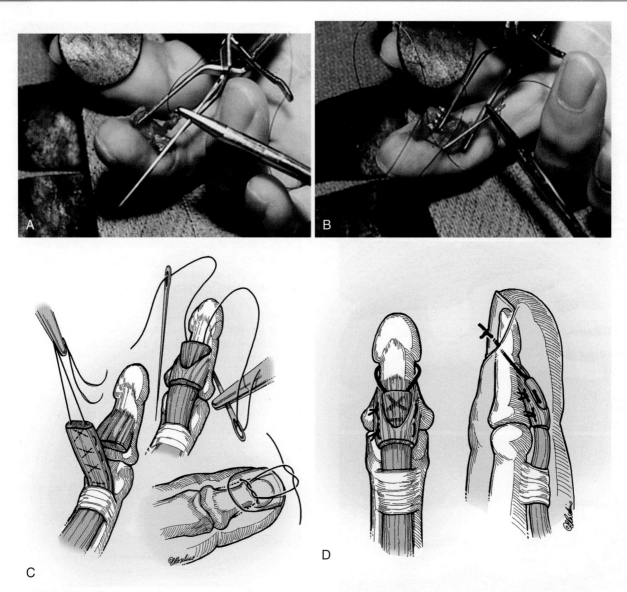

FIGURE 6.29 A and **B,** Pull-out suture for distal juncture of securing a tendon graft is passed around both sides of distal phalanx with aid of Keith needles. **C,** Diagram of technique. The sutures pass through the nail bed and are tied directly over the nail plate. **D,** Completed repair. (**C** and **D,** Copyright Elizabeth Martin.)

nail plate (see Figure 6.29, *D*) or over a button (see Figure 6.27). At least two 3-0 or 4-0 nonabsorbable mattress sutures reinforce the FDP-graft juncture.

When the distal FDP stump is insufficient to allow braiding, or in children with open physes, the distal stump may be split longitudinally and the graft laid within the split. The graft is drawn through the pulp with a large needle, and the projecting graft is temporarily clamped at the fingertip (Figure 6.30, *A*), allowing for precise tension adjustment. Nonabsorbable 3-0 or 4-0 sutures are placed between the graft and the FDP stump through which it was passed. If the surgeon is confident in the strength of the horizontal mattress sutures, the tendon may be trimmed (see Figure 6.30, *B*). For additional strength and security, the tendon may also be temporarily fixed at the fingertip with a padded button for 4 to 6 weeks (see Figure 6.30, *C*).

Another technique places a transverse drill hole across the base of the distal phalanx, with the graft threaded through and sutured to itself (Figure 6.31).[156,176] This technique allows for graft tension judgment but is technically more difficult, as the graft must be thin to pass through the bony tunnel; an articular fracture of the distal phalanx is possible.

Proximal Tendon Juncture

A Pulvertaft tendon weave is our preferred method of repair for proximal tendon graft juncture completed in zones 3, 4, and 5. This type of juncture is stronger than the end-to-end suture techniques, and it has the advantage of allowing the surgeon to adjust the graft tension at the time of the first tendon pass (Figure 6.32).[176,177,228] A human cadaveric analysis of this technique by Gabuzda and coworkers[65] demonstrated that repair strength increased significantly with additional weaves and recommended using as many as four or five weaves. We prefer to use at least two passes to create a strong juncture.

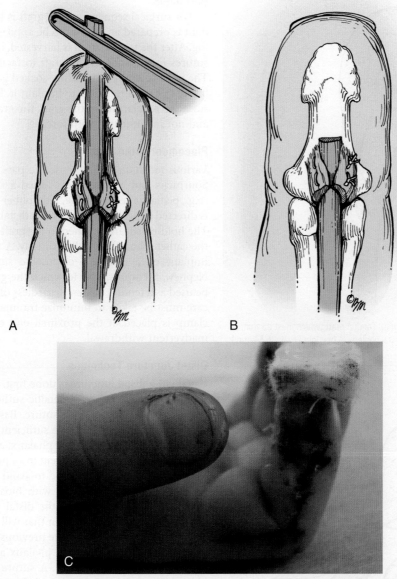

FIGURE 6.30 Distal juncture technique. **A,** Graft is drawn through the pulp, and after tension adjustments are made, is sutured to profundus stump. **B,** In this tendon-to-tendon technique, an interweave suture is used to fix graft to stump of FDP tendon. **C,** In this 6-year-old child, the graft was temporarily secured to the fingertip with a padded button. (**A** and **B,** Copyright Elizabeth Martin; **C,** Copyright Scott W. Wolfe.)

❖ AUTHORS' PREFERRED TECHNIQUE: Single-Stage Grafting Technique

All flexor tendon surgery should be done under tourniquet control. When possible, we prefer a midlateral incision for several reasons: This exposure gives wide access to the digital sheath, it places a thick flap of essentially normal skin over the tendon sheath at the time of wound closure, and it is durable during the rehabilitation process. After exposure, a thorough assessment of the injury is performed. The proximal and distal ends of the remaining tendon are identified. If the digital sheath is in good condition and a suitable proximal motor tendon can be identified, we prefer to proceed with single-stage tendon graft reconstruction. If the tendon sheath is severely damaged or contracted, making tendon graft passage impractical, staged

tendon reconstruction is indicated. At this time, a decision must also be made about the need for nerve repair or reconstruction, pulley reconstruction, joint release, and arterial repair or reconstruction. The area of tendon rupture and interval tendon is excised from the digital sheath. The margins of the resection should allow the tendon graft junctures to be done distal to the A4 pulley and proximal to the A2 pulley. Approximately 1 to 2 cm of the FDP stump is preserved distally to strengthen the distal juncture. Proximally, the FDP tendon is sectioned just distal to the lumbrical origin in the palm.

In most cases, neither of the digital flexor tendons is functioning. When this is true, the proximal stump of the FDS tendon is pulled distally and the tendon is transected, allowing the remaining stump to retract proximally. The distal FDS tendon is excised sharply, but 1 to 2 cm of its insertion is left

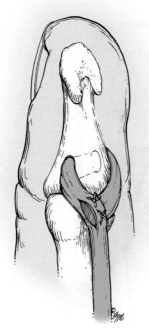

FIGURE 6.31 Distal juncture technique. Tendon graft, which must be thin, is passed through transverse drill hole in distal phalanx. (Copyright Elizabeth Martin.)

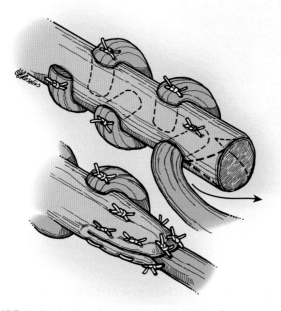

FIGURE 6.32 Modified Pulvertaft end-weave technique. The graft is secured to the proximal motor tendon via multiple weaves through the motor tendon held in place with 3-0 polyester sutures. (Copyright Elizabeth Martin.)

undisturbed because this provides a more favorable dorsal bed for the graft; also, the presence of the FDS tail provides stability at the PIP joint, helping to prevent a hyperextension (swan neck) deformity, a problem occasionally seen in fingers without an FDS tendon.[232]

The intact proximal FDP tendon is preferred as the graft "motor," unless it is of poor quality, in which case the transected FDS tendon of the injured digit may be used. Occasionally, the FDP tendon of an uninjured neighboring digit may be used as

an end-to-side proximal transfer if both proximal motors are unsuitable.

For surgical sequencing, the graft is harvested only after the digit is prepared and found to be appropriate for tendon grafting. After the tendon graft is harvested, it is prepared by placing sutures in the ends of the graft to facilitate passing the graft. The graft is wrapped in saline-soaked gauze and placed on the back table until it is time to implant it. In an effort to limit any surface irregularities in the graft, the graft is handled with care and not manipulated with forceps.

Placement of the Graft

Various techniques can be used to pass the graft. Leddy[122] and Sourmelis and McGrouther[209] used a flexible rubber catheter (e.g., pediatric feeding tube, red-rubber catheter) as a passer. It is directed beneath the pulleys in a distal-to-proximal direction. The holding suture attached to the grafted tendon is sutured to the catheter and then pulled distally. A flexible silicone tendon implant or a Swanson disposable suture passer (Smith & Nephew, Memphis, TN) to which the graft is sutured can also be used as a tendon passer. Regardless of which method is used, care must be taken to minimize trauma to the intact sheath. A clamp is placed at the proximal end of the graft to prevent inadvertent withdrawal.

Distal Juncture Technique

Usually the distal juncture is done first. For patients with good bone quality, we prefer a metallic suture anchor method and the use of a nonabsorbable suture. Basic science studies have shown metallic anchors to be sufficient to provide stable fixation of the graft to the distal phalanx, and this method avoids potential complications inherent in all pull-out suture methods. Metallic anchors are preferred to avoid the possible complication of osteolysis associated with bioabsorbable anchors. By measuring the thickness of the distal phalanx on the lateral view, an anchor can be chosen that will fit within the bone. To prepare the distal phalanx, the previous FDP stump is lifted to expose the base of the distal phalanx and the cortical surface roughened to bleeding bone. A suture anchor hole is drilled obliquely and the anchor embedded into the distal phalanx. The end of the tendon graft is passed through the previous FDP stump. The anchor sutures are passed through the tendon using one of the locking suture techniques and secured. Horizontal reinforcing sutures are passed between the FDP stump and the tendon graft. For patients with poor bone quality, a pull-out suture method is advised (see Figure 6.28).[15,66,121,144]

Proximal Juncture Technique

For proximal repairs in zones 3 and 5, we prefer to join the graft to the FDP tendon (just distal to the lumbrical origin in zone 3) using a Pulvertaft end-to-side weave method with three mattress sutures of 3-0 nonabsorbable suture material (see Figure 6.32). We perform the proximal repair after the distal repair is complete.[53] This repair sequence allows stable repair of the tendon ends and also allows the graft to be tensioned appropriately. The tension in the graft (and flexor positioning of the finger) is best set after the first pass of the graft through the proximal "motor" tendon. After the tension is established, the finishing sutures can be inserted and the Pulvertaft weave completed. General recommendations have been (and we agree)

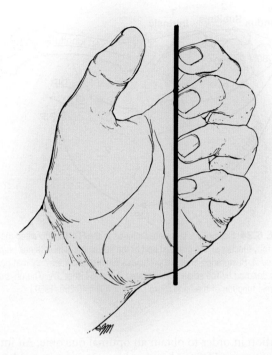

FIGURE 6.33 Determining tension in a reconstructed flexor system at the time of suturing the proximal juncture. With the wrist in neutral position, each finger falls into slightly less flexion than its ulnar neighbor. (Copyright Elizabeth Martin.)

that the tendon graft tension should be such that the digital flexor cascade is reproduced or slightly increased for the finger requiring tendon grafting (Figure 6.33).

Postoperative Care

Postoperative care of tendon grafts has undergone a transformation[10] that favors early motion protocols[212] over the more traditional cast immobilization.

Accelerated rehabilitation protocols are as valuable in the setting of tendon grafting as they are in primary flexor tendon repair because they improve tendon excursion and also joint mobility in the early postoperative period. Our early active motion protocol is used for compliant patients with secure tendon junctures and is directed by an occupational hand therapist. The protocol should be used only when the surgeon is confident that the graft junctures are strong enough to withstand the additional tensile stresses of this regimen. The postoperative splint that we prefer is a static dorsal blocking splint, with the wrist positioned in neutral, the MP joints in 45 degrees of flexion, and the IP joints in neutral. This splint is applied early in the postoperative period and worn for protection until 6 weeks after surgery.

Therapist-guided protected passive range-of-motion exercise can be instituted at the first postoperative visit 2 to 3 days after surgery. At 2 weeks after surgery, gentle place-and-hold flexion exercises and active short-arc digital flexion and extension exercises are added to the therapy program. Blocked flexion of the MP or PIP joint enables increased active flexion at the distal joints but puts additional stress on the junctures. Despite this tensile stress, the blocked flexion exercise method optimizes tendon gliding and is instituted actively at 4 weeks and with resistance at 6 weeks. Flexion contractures are treated with

protected passive stretching and specific splinting techniques. Patient education is of paramount importance, and judgment must be used in restraining more active patients and prodding reluctant patients.

Graft Incorporation

If a grafted tendon is explored after 6 or more months, it often has a normal appearance and may resemble a histologic replica of the original tendon. Whether the tendon is, in reality, the original graft or a repopulation of a tendon scaffolding is a question studied by a number of basic science research efforts. Seiler and Gelberman and colleagues have reported on the incorporation of various types of tendon grafts in a clinically relevant canine model.[199] Traditional extrasynovial grafts, such as palmaris longus or plantaris tendon grafts, undergo a significant cellular necrosis when transplanted to the digital sheath and are repopulated by fibroblasts donated through the formation of peritendinous adhesion or through the proximal tendon juncture sites. Similarly, studies of tendon graft neovascularization show new vessels growing to the tendon graft through adhesion formation and also through the tendon junctures. These newly donated fibroblasts are responsible for producing collagen that will strengthen the graft over time. Intrasynovial grafts have, in basic science study and limited clinical study, showed an improved capacity to survive transplantation to the digital sheath. They have a surface that is designed to allow for synovial fluid imbibition and that may promote nutrition and cellular survival. It may also explain the ability of these grafts to incorporate with much less cellular necrosis or adhesion formation and with maintenance of the critical gliding surface.[199]

Single-Stage Flexor Tendon Grafting: Flexor Digitorum Profundus Tendon Disrupted, Flexor Digitorum Superficialis Tendon Intact
Indications

In patients with transection of the FDP tendon but an intact FDS tendon, early direct FDP repair is the preferred treatment method. When more than 4 weeks have elapsed from the time of injury, tendon grafting may be necessary and, depending on the status of the tendon sheath, can be done as a one- or two-stage procedure. When the FDS tendon is functional, caution must be exercised in offering a free tendon graft to restore distal joint function.[192]

Useful digital motion is maintained when the FDS tendon is functional (Figure 6.34). Most patients with a severed FDP tendon but an intact FDS tendon adapt nicely and may require no treatment; this is especially true if the DIP joint is stable. An appropriate preoperative explanation of the considerable risk of worsening function after attempted reconstruction of the isolated FDP laceration is essential. Most surgeons advise nonoperative treatment, especially in older patients or heavy laborers.[91] In patients troubled by instability at the DIP joint or weakness of grip, stabilization of the DIP joint by tenodesis or arthrodesis is a good solution. Despite the difficulties and considerable risks, outstanding results with FDP grafting in carefully selected patients have been reported.[35,77,106,107,150,177,184,211] Some of the variability in patient results may be attributed to different methods of patient evaluation.[192]

CRITICAL POINTS *Single-Stage Tendon Grafting: Flexor Digitorum Profundus and Flexor Digitorum Superficialis Tendons Disrupted*

Indication
- Definitive repair has been delayed or ruptured, and direct repair is impossible or impractical.

Preoperative Evaluation
- Joint contractures need correction before grafting.

Pearls
- The Pulvertaft weave technique allows easy graft tensioning when creating the proximal juncture.
- Graft tension is correct when, with the wrist in neutral, the grafted finger shows a slight increase in flexor tone (or slightly more flexion in the flexor cascade).

Technical Points
- Use a midlateral incision.
- Preserve the crucial pulleys.
- When flexor tendon grafting is chosen, clear the flexor sheath of unnecessary tendon but preserve the FDP tendon distal to the A4 pulley for the distal juncture.
- Pass the graft using a small pediatric feeding tube or silicone rod.
- Create the distal juncture with a suture anchor or suture pull-out technique.
- Proximally, use the FDP tendon of the involved finger as the graft motor. The proximal juncture should be just distal to the lumbrical origin when possible
- Set the tension in the graft by passing the graft through the motor and creating the desired flexor cascade.
- Use two or more right angle passes of the graft by means of a Pulvertaft technique and nonabsorbable sutures to complete the proximal juncture.

Pitfalls
- A two-stage tendon graft is needed if there is extensive scarring, pulley incompetence, or joint contracture.
- Handle the graft carefully. Careless handling, pinching, or probing of the graft may increase surface irregularities and, therefore, the number and density of adhesions.

Postoperative Care
- Use an early range-of-motion protocol if graft junctures are strong.
- Apply a static dorsal blocking splint (4 to 6 weeks) with the wrist in neutral position, the MP joints at 45 degrees, and the IP joints in neutral position.
- Treat flexion contractures with passive stretching and splinting (6 to 8 weeks).

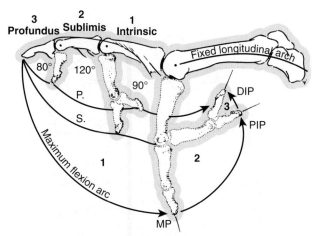

FIGURE 6.34 Flexion arc. In isolated injuries to the FDP tendon when the FDS tendon is fully functional, the greatest part of the flexion arc is maintained (*stippled areas 1 and 2*). Restoration of active profundus function provides only that portion of the arc denoted by the small *stippled area 3*. (From Littler JW: The physiology and dynamic function of the hand, *Surg Clin North Am* 40:259, 1960.)

decussation in order to obtain an optimal outcome. An intact, fully functioning FDS tendon should not be removed, although concomitant tenolysis may be useful to improve independent tendon excursion. Harrison[82] suggested removal of one tail of the FDS tendon to facilitate graft passage and gliding. The procedure occasionally has been performed in two stages,[41,77,237,249] with a tendon implant placed at the first stage, particularly if there has been some element of injury to the FDS tendon, flexor tendon bed, or pulley system. A staged tendon graft has been gratifying when appropriately used in fingers with a poor sheath.[41,219]

Postoperative Care of Tendon Grafts With an Intact Flexor Digitorum Superficialis Tendon (Zone 1 Injuries)

We favor early active range-of-motion protocols to maintain normal FDS tendon function, particularly because Schneider[192] noted that, despite careful preoperative patient selection, numerous patients required subsequent tenolysis. To help limit tendon adhesion formation, we favor exercises designed to facilitate independent tendon gliding, including short-arc active extension and finger flexion exercises. Within the first postoperative week, we begin gentle place-and-hold and straight-fist flexion exercises in compliant patients.

Expectations

We counsel patients that grafting to restore FDP tendon function when the FDS tendon is intact can be associated with significant digital stiffness and is usually best done to meet specific functional demands, such as playing a musical instrument or doing specialized work.

We restrict this procedure to young patients with supple joints and a reasonable need for active DIP joint function. The graft may have more potential benefit to patients with ring and small finger injury who require a power grip (Figure 6.35).

Single-Stage Grafting Technique With an Intact Flexor Digitorum Superficialis Tendon (Zone 1 Injuries)

The technique is similar to the technique for free tendon grafting described in the previous section. A thinner graft is easier to pass, making a palmaris longus, extensor digiti quinti, or plantaris graft an excellent choice. The graft must be passed accurately and glide easily through the intact FDS tendon

Two-Stage Flexor Tendon Reconstruction
Indications

In 1965, Hunter first published his personal experience with tendon implants; in 1971, Hunter and Salisbury[100] presented more than 10 years' experience with staged tendon reconstruction using an implant reinforced with silicone and Dacron. The

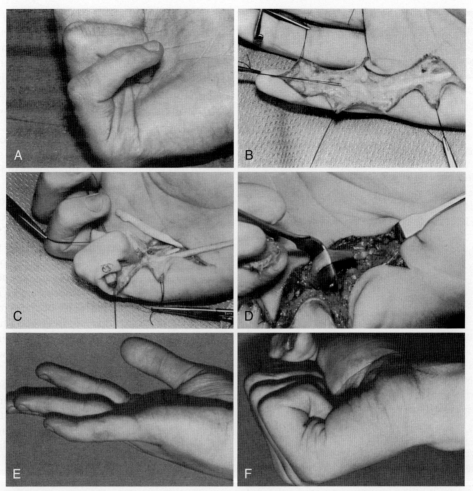

FIGURE 6.35 Tendon graft through intact FDS tendon. **A,** A 17-year-old boy had ruptured the FDP tendon and had incomplete function of the FDS tendon 3 months after injury. **B,** FDP tendon was retrieved and mobilized, but it was impossible to advance it to the insertion. A tendon graft was placed. **C,** The graft in place. The finger is to be closed before completing the proximal juncture. **D,** Interlace juncture in the palm using the FDP tendon as the motor. **E** and **F,** End result at 1 year. There is a flexion deformity at the tip, but 50 degrees of strong flexion has been gained at the DIP joint.

next four decades witnessed significant advances in the ability to restore flexor tendon function to badly scarred digits. The first procedure of a staged reconstruction employs a thorough digital exploration, reconstruction of associated injuries, and placement of a passive silicone tendon implant. This allows for correction of any joint contracture, reconstruction of critical pulleys, and formation of a pseudosheath around the silicone rod. The index procedure is followed by placement of a tendon graft at a second operation, which is usually done 6 to 12 weeks after the index operation.

Tissue Response to a Silicone Implant. The nature of the sheath formed by silicone and other materials has received significant investigation. Hunter's group,[103,104] working in the late 1960s, observed an orderly pattern of cellular organization on the surface of the implant when silicone implants were placed in the paravertebral soft tissues of dogs. A parallel study evaluated the response to an actively gliding implant in the extensor system of dogs and showed that the system could function as a physiologic sheath capable of supporting a long tendon graft initially by synovial fluid nutrition and subsequently via mobile vascular adhesions. Urbaniak and colleagues[232] performed experiments in the flexor system and confirmed revasculariza-

tion of tendon in dogs by intratendinous vessels within the sheath. Farkas and colleagues[58] reported ultrastructural evidence of a normal-appearing reconstituted tendon sheath in chickens, and also concluded that motion was important for remodeling.

The nature of the sheath created in response to a flexible silicone implant used in a passive-gliding program in humans is still debated. Some of the varying observations may be a result of different species and experimental conditions. Most commonly the silicone rod placement is associated with the formation of a soft, flexible, translucent sheath, which is suitable for supporting the purpose of tendon grafting. In a series of 109 digits, the reported complications from silicone rod implantation during stage 1 included rod buckling, rupture of the distal end of the rod, rod migration, synovitis, and infection.[208]

Alternative Techniques. Other researchers have investigated alternative techniques for reconstruction.[257] In the staged technique published by Paneva-Holevich in 1969,[169] the damaged tendons are removed from the flexor sheath and transected in the palm (Video 6.2). The cut ends of the FDS and FDP tendons are sutured in the palm to create the proximal tendon juncture. Approximately 6 weeks later at a second stage, the FDS tendon

CRITICAL POINTS *Single-Stage Tendon Grafting: Flexor Digitorum Profundus Tendon Disrupted, Flexor Digitorum Superficialis Tendon Intact (Chronic Zone 1 FDP Injury)*

Indications
- Young person with supple joints and a reasonable need for active DIP joint function.
- More useful on the ulnar side of the hand for power grip.
- DIP joint that is unstable but supple.

Preoperative Evaluation
- Document absence of FDP function.
- Evaluate the DIP joint for instability.
- If on exploration the FDP tendon position is maintained, early direct repair is indicated.
- Later repair is possible if a short vinculum to the FDP tendon maintains the tendon in a distal location.
- MRI or ultrasound may be useful to determine the location of the proximal FDP stump.

Pearls
- Never remove an intact, fully functioning FDS tendon in an effort to place a graft.
- Tenolysis of the FDS tendon may be necessary.
- The procedure may be done in one or two stages, depending on the condition of the flexor tendon sheath.
- The graft must be accurately oriented through the decussation of the FDS tendon.
- The proximal motor for the graft is usually the FDP tendon of the same finger, with the proximal juncture done just distal to the lumbrical origin.
- For some cases a more proximal tenolysis of the FDP motor must be done to improve the tendon excursion.

Technical Points
- Use a similar technique as in free tendon grafting.
- Know that a thinner graft is easier to pass (plantaris).
- Pass the graft through the FDS tendon decussation.
- One FDS tail can be removed for tendon graft passage if the graft is too bulky to pass.

Pitfalls
- Patients should be selected for the goal of restoring the specific function of grip.
- Patients with an intact FDS tendon usually adapt nicely and require no treatment.
- Digital scarring can be heavy and result in adhesions, loss of motion, and further functional impairment.

Postoperative Care
- Apply a static dorsal blocking splint (4 to 6 weeks) with the wrist in neutral position, MP joints at 45 degrees, and IP joints in neutral position.
- Use an early motion protocol if the graft juncture is strong.
- Treat flexion contractures with passive stretching and splinting (6 to 8 weeks).

is severed at the muscle-tendon junction in the forearm and passed distally through the tendon sheath to be attached to the distal phalanx or distal FDP tendon. Although this procedure results in a finger with one tendon, it has the advantage of requiring a single distal repair at the second stage and may transplant an intrasynovial tendon segment of the FDS to the digital sheath. This can be a good solution for severely injured fingers, especially in patients with limited tendon donor options. Later, this method was combined with implantation of a silicone prosthesis during the first stage to prepare a bed for the subsequent distal pedicle transfer[3,14,28,161] (Figure 6.36). The relatively larger size of the FDS tendon compared with a conventional tendon graft may require the use of a silicone rod with a larger diameter.

Composite Tissue Transfer Methods. Peacock[171] showed that a transplanted allograft of the entire flexor system, tendon, and sheath was well tolerated in three digits in four patients, but no range-of-motion details were provided. Hueston and colleagues[94] also presented a clinical series of three cases using homografts, although no clinical results were reported, and the technique was not widely adopted. In 1974, Chacha[35] used autologous composite grafts from the toe to the flexor system of the hand with only modest results. More recently, Asencio and associates[9] implanted human composite flexor tendon allografts into two fingers with irreparable injuries of the flexor tendon system. Although none of these methods has current clinical applicability, they are interesting to consider and may represent fertile ground for future tissue engineering research. Some of the biggest future improvements will likely come from tissue engineering strategies.

Permanent (active) tendon implants varying in size, shape, material, and type of end device for distal and proximal fixation have been reported in the literature. Unfortunately, biologically durable bonding between the tendon implant distal to bone and proximal to native tendon has not been reliably achieved. Basic science researchers continue to search for a permanent active tendon implant.[84]

❖ AUTHORS' PREFERRED TECHNIQUE: Staged Tendon Grafting: Stage I

The flexor system of the involved finger is exposed through a midlateral incision. The annular pulleys are dissected and preserved. An assessment is made as to the need for pulley reconstruction. The injured flexor tendons are excised. If a 2-cm FDS tail can be preserved, it is left attached to the middle phalanx for stability. A second curvilinear incision is made proximal to the wrist crease in the ulnar half of the volar forearm. The involved FDS tendon is identified, drawn into the wound, and divided near the musculotendinous junction. Excised tendon material is set aside in moist sponges for possible use in pulley reconstruction.

The proximal FDP tendon is transected at the lumbrical origin level; if the lumbrical is scarred, it is also excised. Fixed flexion deformities are corrected with capsulectomy and volar plate and accessory collateral ligament release.

A trial set of silicone tendon implants is useful to determine the appropriate size needed. Men generally can accommodate a tendon implant of up to 5 or 6 mm, but we usually use a smaller 4-mm implant. This implant is closer in size to the expected tendon graft and creates a nice fit through the tendon sheath. When threaded into the pulley system, the implant should glide freely. The integrity of the pulley system is assessed. A minimal requirement is the presence of A2 and A4 pulleys; however, when possible, a four-pulley system is preferable. The pulleys must be strong and snug but not binding, so that passive gliding of the implant is possible.

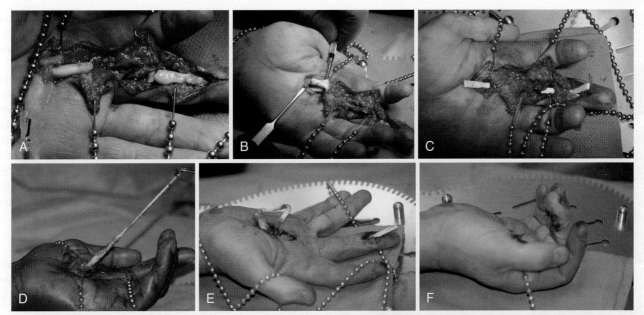

FIGURE 6.36 FDS-FDP Paneva-Holevich reconstruction. **A,** Tendon injury requiring graft reconstruction. **B,** *Stage I:* FDS and FDP loop sewn together with four-strand repair. **C,** Silastic spacer placed in finger, preserving critical pulleys. **D,** *Stage II:* FDS tendon cut at musculotendinous junction and withdrawn into site of previous FDS-FDP juncture. Tenolysis of juncture is required. **E,** FDS tendon tied to Silastic spacer and drawn into finger. **F,** FDS tendon tension set slightly greater than natural cascade of digits.

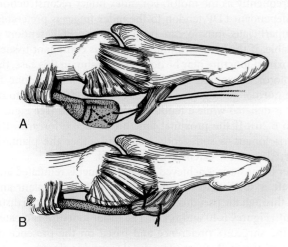

FIGURE 6.37 Stage I flexor reconstruction. **A** and **B,** In the distal juncture wire suture technique, a figure-of-eight suture of 3-0 polypropylene is placed in the implant and sutured to the profundus stump. Additional sutures are placed on each side of the implant. (Copyright Elizabeth Martin.)

The silicone implant is removed from its sterile package, and care is taken to handle the implant with smooth forceps using a "no touch" technique. Handling the rod with standard surgical gloves may lead to talc adherence to the implant and increase the likelihood of an inflammatory reaction. The silicone tendon spacer is placed in the tendon sheath and affixed distally to the distal phalanx with 3-0 polypropylene sutures or wire (Figure 6.37). Proximally, the spacer is placed adjacent to the intended motor for the tendon graft and may be trimmed to end in the palm or threaded across the carpal tunnel and into the distal forearm. At this point the pulley integrity is assessed by traction on the implant (Figure 6.38). Bowstringing of the implant indicates the need for pulley reconstruction. Pulley reconstruction is done over the silicone rod using a variety of pulley techniques

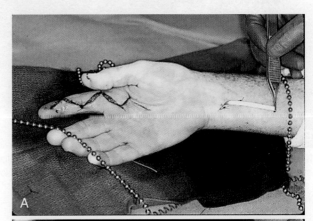

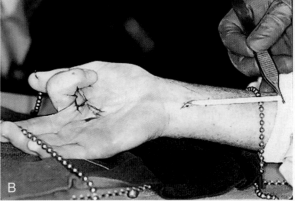

FIGURE 6.38 A and **B,** Potential of the planned graft is tested by pulling the implant proximally. A bowstring posture of the implant indicates the need for pulley reconstruction.

and using excised tendon material whenever possible (Figure 6.39, *A* and *B*). The A2 pulley is reconstructed on the proximal half of the proximal phalanx. If a tendon belt loop technique is used, the graft is passed beneath the dorsal extensor apparatus. The A4 pulley is reconstructed on the middle of the middle

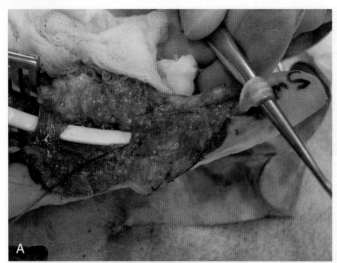

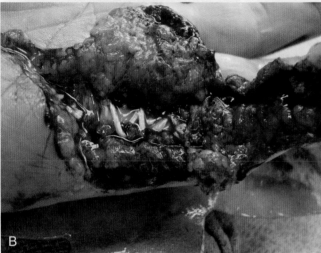

FIGURE 6.39 At the time of implant placement, deficiencies in the pulley system are addressed by pulley reconstruction. **A,** A2 to A3 pulley reconstruction in small finger. **B,** A Weilby repair of the pulley system is performed over the silicone rod. (Copyright Scott W. Wolfe.)

phalanx, and if a belt loop technique is used, it is passed dorsal to the extensor apparatus.

Postoperative Care

After wound closure, a bulky dressing is applied with a posterior plaster splint, so that the wrist is maintained in about 35 degrees of flexion. This splint ensures more proximal placement of the implant, which creates a longer proximal extension of the sheath, giving the implant more room to move without buckling during the passive range-of-motion program between stages I and II. The splint should extend past the fingertips, with the MP joints kept in 60 to 70 degrees of flexion and the IP joints relaxed in the extended position.

Passive motion is started on the first postoperative visit 2 to 3 days after surgery. Patients are taught passive range-of-motion exercises, including the use of trapping with adjacent normal fingers to regain passive range of motion of the operated finger. When there is a concomitant nerve laceration, we prefer nerve reconstruction that allows for full digital motion. Often this can be done with a conduit or allograft to avoid tension at the repair site, allowing immediate mobilization of the digit. Patients who

also require contracture release will require intensive occupational therapy. The goal is to recover full passive range of motion and to have a stable soft tissue environment prior to implantation of the tendon graft.

The appropriate interval between stages I and II is the time needed for wound healing and the development of a gliding sheath in response to the implant. We usually wait 6 weeks before considering stage II tendon graft implantation and prefer that the patient has maintained full passive range of motion. Because these cases are complex, the specific timing of the second procedure is individualized to the needs of the patient. Any inflammatory reaction to the implant should be controlled prior to stage II, and patients should have achieved full passive range of motion of the involved digit.

Stage II

Technique. After approximately 6 weeks, the second stage can be done and smaller incisions are necessary. The silicone rod is identified using a small incision at the distal phalanx, and care is taken not to disrupt the A4 pulley.

If the proximal juncture is to be done in the forearm, the proximal incision is opened and the soft, thin, translucent pseudosheath identified. The sheath is incised; the proximal implant is exposed; and the common profundus mass tendon is selected most frequently as the motor. For index finger reconstruction, the independent FDP tendon to the index finger is preferable. The superficialis muscle can be used if the FDP tendon is unsuitable. If the hand is uninjured and has compliant tissues, the proximal juncture may be done in the palm; in this case, the FDP motor is exposed in the palm and a tenolysis done to ensure normal gliding. The wounds are packed, and the tourniquet is deflated while a tendon graft is obtained (see Figures 6.24 to 6.26). If the proximal juncture is in the forearm, the palmaris longus is sufficiently long, and either the plantaris (preferred) or a toe extensor must be used.

After hemostasis is achieved, the tourniquet is reinflated and the graft is sutured to the proximal end of the implant and pulled through the pseudosheath by gentle traction on the distal implant (Figures 6.40 and 6.41). The distal juncture is created using the surgeon's preference and based on the presence or absence of the FDP stump. The distal wound is closed.

Attention is now directed to the proximal juncture. The graft is woven into the motor tendon or tendons (see Figure 6.39, *B*). When only one motor is used, an end-weave technique is advised (see Figure 6.30). In cases in which the profundus mass of the long, ring, and little fingers is chosen as a common motor, an interweave juncture (see Figure 6.39, *B*) is created to the common origin of these tendons. It is important to choose a juncture site that enables full simultaneous extension of the digits and wrist without impingement on the flexor retinaculum. Tensioning is performed following the first weave to gain an appropriate flexion cascade (eFigure 6.1).

In the less common instance in which the palm is not compromised by trauma or through prior surgery, a shorter graft can be used, motored by the FDP tendon at the lumbrical origin. A sufficiently proximal juncture is necessary to avoid impingement on the flexor tendon sheath when the finger is in full extension. The option of using an adjacent FDS tendon as a motor is also available within the palm if the FDP tendon is deemed inadequate. The wound is closed by careful eversion of

CRITICAL POINTS *Two-Stage Flexor Tendon Reconstruction: Stage I*

Indications
- Extensive peritendinous adhesion and failure of tendon repair.
- Crush injuries associated with an underlying fracture or overlying skin damage.
- Failure of previous operations.
- Damaged pulley system.
- Joint contracture.
- Nerve or artery reconstruction.
- Repair of nonunion.

Contraindications
- Recent or remote septic tenosynovitis.
- Patients with severe neurovascular impairment are poor candidates.
- Arthrodesis or amputation may be a better alternative.

Preoperative Evaluation
- The patient must understand the necessity of the prolonged postoperative therapy program.

Pearls
- A range-of-motion and scar-softening therapy program is important to attain maximal preoperative passive range of motion and to evaluate the patient's willingness to participate in postoperative therapy.

Technical Points
- Preserve potential pulley material, injured or uninjured.
- Transect the proximal FDP tendon at the level of the lumbrical origin.
- Correct joint flexion deformities.
- Make a second incision in the distal forearm.
- Identify the involved FDS tendon, draw it into the wound, and transect it near the musculotendinous junction.
- Determine the appropriate size of the silicone implant.
- Assess the integrity of the pulley system; the presence of the A2 and A4 pulleys is a minimum requirement.
- Affix the silicone implant to the distal phalanx with 3-0 polypropylene sutures.
- Exert traction on the proximal end of the implant to observe the range of motion.
- If there is significant bowstringing at A3, it must be corrected at this stage with additional pulley reconstruction.

Pitfalls
- Ensure that the tendon implant does not buckle with passive flexion.

Postoperative Care
- Apply a splint with the wrist in 35 degrees of flexion, MP joints at 60 to 70 degrees of flexion, and IP joints extended.
- Start passive motion on the first postoperative visit.
- Contracture releases may benefit from dynamic splinting (6 to 8 weeks).

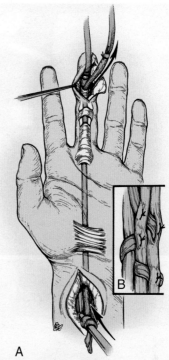

FIGURE 6.40 Stage II flexor reconstruction. **A,** Distal portion of finger wound and distal forearm wound are opened, and both ends of the implant are located. Tendon graft is now sutured to the proximal end of the implant and drawn into the newly created sheath. **B,** Proximal juncture is either an interweave of the graft into the adjacent FDP motor in the case of the long, ring, and little fingers or an interlace into the FDP tendon of the index finger. (See Figure 6.33 for the Pulvertaft end-weave technique.) (Copyright Elizabeth Martin.)

the repair and the degree of adhesion formation. Dynamic splinting may also be employed at 6 to 8 weeks to combat joint contracture. Therapy must be more aggressive, with active and resisted exercises being instituted earlier in cases where tendon adhesion is observed. Therapy should be supervised and reinforced on a regular basis.

For less compliant patients and children, the hand may be immobilized initially, followed by active and passive range-of-motion exercises at 3 weeks and blocking at 4 weeks. The program is continued as in the early mobilization program described previously.

Thumb Flexor Tendon Reconstruction

The flexor system of the thumb is less complicated than the flexor system of the fingers. The thumb contains one fewer joint than the fingers, and only one tendon (the FPL tendon) is involved. When the FPL tendon is reconstructed, a more modest recovery of 30 to 40 degrees of active IP joint flexion is associated with excellent thumb function. For these reasons, reconstruction of the FPL is often indicated after failure of repair or neglected injury.

Indication

Direct repair at all levels of injury may be possible 3 to 6 weeks after injury and even later in cases in which the tendon ends have not widely separated.[7,151,233] Reconstruction for FPL tendon injuries is indicated when satisfactory passive IP joint motion is established and primary repair is no longer possible.

the skin edges, and a short-arm dorsal blocking splint is applied, with the wrist in neutral position, the MP joints flexed 45 degrees, and the IP joints in neutral position.

Postoperative Care. Protected passive range of motion and an early controlled active motion program are begun within days of surgery. At 2 weeks after surgery, short-arc active extension and flexion and place-and-hold flexion exercises can be added to the therapy program. Resistance is added to the exercise regimen at 4 to 6 weeks after surgery based on the strength of

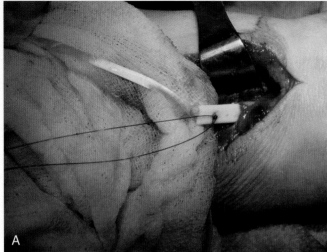

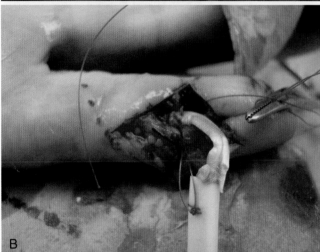

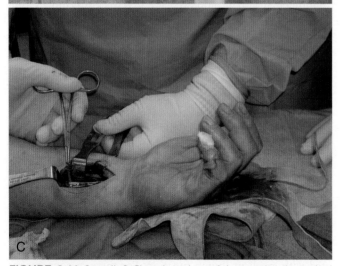

FIGURE 6.41 Stage II. **A,** Plantaris tendon graft is secured to the proximal end of the implant in the distal forearm. **B,** Implant is removed from distal incision, pulling the graft into place. The graft is sutured distally and proximally. **C,** Tension is adjusted following distal fixation with a pull-out suture and before completing the proximal Pulvertaft weave to attain an appropriate flexion cascade. (Copyright Scott W. Wolfe.)

CRITICAL POINTS *Two-Stage Flexor Tendon Reconstruction: Stage II*

Indication
- Patient who underwent stage I of flexor reconstruction process.

Preoperative Evaluation
- The interval between stages I and II is at least 6 weeks.
- The hand wounds should be soft and durable, and the joints should be fully mobile.

Pearls
- The newly formed sheath is disturbed as little as possible.
- Proximal juncture is placed in the forearm: a longer graft is needed (plantaris or toe extensor), motored by the FDP tendon.
- Proximal juncture is placed in the palm (palm not involved in trauma): a shorter graft can be used (palmaris), motored by the FDP tendon at the lumbrical origin.

Technical Points
- Open the distal portion of the finger incision to the middle of the middle phalanx.
- Locate the implant at its attachment to the distal phalanx.
- Reopen the proximal incision in the distal forearm or the midpalm.
- Excise the forearm fascia, and incise the sheath.
- Select the motor.
- Obtain the tendon graft.
- Suture the graft to the proximal end of the implant and pull it distally through the sheath. It should pass smoothly.
- Fix the distal juncture.
- Create the proximal juncture with a slight increase in the flexor cascade for the grafted finger.

Pitfalls
- Proper tension on the graft and proximal tendon excursion are essential for success.

Postoperative Care
- Apply a short-arm dorsal blocking splint (wrist in neutral position, MP joints at 45 degrees, and IP joints in neutral position).
- Begin therapy in a formal setting.
- Start protected passive range-of-motion and early controlled motion program.
- Use dynamic splinting for contractures.

Reconstruction can be done by intercalary tendon grafting (single- or two-stage grafting) or by tendon transfer.

Thumb Free Tendon Graft

Technique. The same basic technique is used as has been described for free tendon grafting in the fingers. The flexor system is approached through a volar zigzag incision from the distal phalanx to the MP joint. The essential oblique pulley is preserved with care, and the injured tendon is excised. Incompetence of the pulley system is an indication to proceed to a two-stage grafting procedure with a silicone tendon spacer. A second 6-cm incision is made in curvilinear fashion at the volar-radial aspect of the distal end of the forearm. The musculotendinous junction of the FPL tendon is identified, and the transected tendon is pulled into this incision. The palmaris longus or plantaris tendon is obtained and threaded through the pulley system with a tendon passer. The distal juncture is performed, preferably using a weave or docking repair to bone with suture anchors. A distal pull-out suture technique can also be employed when necessary. The distal wound is closed. The graft is interwoven into the proximal tendon of the FPL using a Pulvertaft weave (see Figure 6.32). The graft tension should be adjusted at the time of forming the proximal juncture such that with the wrist in neutral, the thumb IP joint is in approximately 30 degrees of flexion.

After wound closure and dressing, a dorsal splint is applied with the wrist in neutral to 5 degrees of flexion and the thumb protected in about 30 degrees of abduction at the carpometacarpal joint. The MP and IP joints are positioned in 20 to 30 degrees of flexion in the dorsal splint. We use a similar program of immediate passive mobilization and early active mobilization for the grafted tendon when the repairs are durable and the patient is compliant with the hand therapy program. At 6 weeks, more strenuous activities, including blocking techniques, are allowed.

Flexor Digitorum Superficialis Tendon Transfer

An alternative method to tendon grafting, particularly indicated when the FPL muscle is not a useful motor, is use of the ring finger FDS tendon transfer.[173,196]

This method of tendon reconstruction can be particularly useful after rupture of the FPL tendon following treatment of distal radius fractures by plate fixation.

Technique. The zigzag volar approach to the flexor system of the thumb is used, along with a second vertical incision in the distal region of the forearm (eFigure 6.1). The injured tendon is removed with preservation of as much of the pulley system as possible. A transverse incision is made at the base of the ring finger, and the FDS tendon is identified, a tagging suture is placed in one tail, and the tendon is transected about 2 cm proximal to the PIP joint. The tendon is located as the ulnarmost of the two superficial digital flexors in the forearm wound and withdrawn proximally; this may be difficult because of synovial thickenings and tendinous interconnections. A second incision in the palm is used as needed to free these connections. The proximally retracted FDS tendon is passed distally into the thumb flexor sheath, and a distal juncture is done (see earlier in this chapter). Critical tension is more difficult to establish at the distal juncture, especially if a tendon-to-bone technique is planned. For this reason, we prefer the distal juncture interweave technique, in which the graft is woven through the stump of the FDP, allowing more precise distal juncture tensioning (see Figure 6.29).

The repair is fixed with one suture, and tension is evaluated before completion of the juncture. After confirming that satisfactory tension has been established, the distal repair is completed. The rehabilitation protocol postoperatively is similar to that used in free tendon grafting. Mobilization of the transfer by combining active ring finger flexion with thumb flexion helps patients who are learning to use the transfer.

Staged Tendon Reconstruction in the Thumb

In patients in whom it is imperative to restore active thumb flexion and in whom prior surgery has failed, or in whom there is a severely scarred tendon bed, staged flexor tendon reconstruction offers an opportunity to salvage thumb function. This approach becomes even more of a necessity when the retinacular pulley system has been destroyed. Pulley reconstruction over the implant at the level of the proximal half of the proximal phalanx usually suffices if the oblique pulley has been destroyed.

Technique. Details of the technique are similar to those of the technique performed in the fingers. In the thumb, the surgeon can use either a free graft or an FDS transfer at stage II.[127,199]

Other Options After Loss of Flexor Pollicis Longus Function

In patients who have lost FPL tendon function but have a stable distal joint, no additional treatment may be necessary, especially if the carpometacarpal and MP joints are functioning normally. This approach is reasonable in less active patients. When more stable pinch is required, especially in the presence of articular damage at the IP joint or in patients with a hyperextensible IP joint, arthrodesis is a useful alternative.

Secondary Reconstruction of Tendon Injuries in Zones 3, 4, and 5
Indications

When flexor tendons are injured in the palm, wrist, carpal tunnel, or distal forearm, direct repair at an early date is desirable. When primary repair fails, secondary reconstruction carries a more favorable prognosis for these proximal levels than does reconstruction in zone 2. Before secondary tendon surgery, the wounds should be well healed and the hand should be soft and fully mobile. Generous longitudinal, curvilinear incisions are needed to identify and repair the injured structures. The operation is technically easier to do through ample exposure, and the likelihood of additional damage is lessened if all structures are first identified proximally and distally in unscarred areas of normal anatomy and then carefully dissected into the zone of injury using optical magnification. If synovial connections and adhesions have prevented proximal migration of the tendons, direct end-to-end repairs can occasionally be performed. When the tendons cannot be brought together without undue tension, three techniques have proved useful for zones 3, 4, and 5.

Interposition Graft

When trying to reunite the FDP tendon ends in the palm or wrist after delay, the surgeon often finds that a gap of 2 to 5 cm needs to be bridged to bring the tendons to normal functional length. A short tendon graft may be interposed using a segment of the injured FDS or palmaris longus tendon and a bridging suture technique (Figure 6.42).[210] In this setting there is no particular advantage to any particular donor tendon, so the

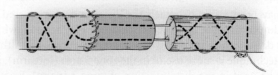

FIGURE 6.42 Interposition graft. By using short segments of available graft material, a gap can be closed in the late repair of zone 3, 4, or 5 injuries. (Copyright Elizabeth Martin.)

CRITICAL POINTS *Thumb Flexor Tendon Reconstruction*

Indications
- Repair of the FPL tendon is delayed or soft tissue trauma does not allow repair.
- Satisfactory preoperative range of passive IP joint motion.

Preoperative Evaluation
- Free tendon graft: similar indications as for fingers.
- Assess the patient for the presence of a suitable donor tendon.
- Superficialis transfer: alternative to free tendon graft.
- Two-stage tendon reconstruction: severely scarred synovial sheath or destroyed pulley system, or both.
- IP joint arthrodesis: when stable pinch is required, especially in the presence of articular damage at the IP joint or in patients with hyperextensile IP joint.

Pearls
- Recovery of 30 to 40 degrees of active IP joint flexion may provide a well-functioning thumb.
- Tension is crucial.
- Tension is estimated by placing the wrist in neutral position, the thumb in palmar abduction in front of the index metacarpal, and the IP joint in 30 degrees of flexion.
- Pulley reconstruction over the implant at the level of the proximal half of the proximal phalanx usually suffices if the oblique pulley has been destroyed. This pulley reconstruction is usually done as a belt loop method passed dorsally underneath the extensor apparatus.

Technical Points
Free Tendon Graft
- Extensile exposure of the thumb is crucial to assess the nature of the injury and the preferred reconstructive method.
- Preserve the pulleys as the damaged tendon tissue is removed.
- Preserve enough distal FPL tendon to allow for a tendon weave method for the distal juncture when possible.
- Make a second incision in the distal forearm.
- Identify the musculotendinous junction of the FPL tendon.
- Obtain the graft, and thread it through the pulley system.
- Fashion the distal juncture by means of a distal pull-out suture technique.
- Interweave the graft into the FPL tendon to create the proximal juncture.

Superficialis Tendon Transfer
- Use a zigzag volar approach to the thumb.
- Make a longitudinal incision in the distal forearm.
- Remove the injured tendon with preservation of the uninjured pulley system.
- Make a transverse incision at the base of the ring finger.
- Flex the finger and divide the FDS tendon distally to allow for sufficient tendon harvest to reach to the distal phalanx of the thumb.
- Transect the FDS tendon 2 cm proximal to the PIP joint.
- Withdraw the tendon into the proximal wound.
- Create a distal juncture as in a free tendon graft.

Pitfalls
- Proper tension is difficult to create with FDS transfer.

Postoperative Care
- Apply a dorsal splint with the wrist in neutral position, the thumb in 30 degrees of abduction at the carpometacarpal joint, and the MP and IP joints in 20 to 30 degrees of flexion.
- Limit passive flexion and active extension with a splint for the first 2 weeks.
- Begin active flexion and extension at 2 weeks.
- At 6 weeks, begin blocking techniques.

---

most expendable and available donor tendon is selected. Pulvertaft weave methods can also be used for bridging larger gaps with tendon graft and are tensioned so that the appropriate resting posture of the finger is obtained. Proper tension is crucial here, and local or WALANT anesthesia with active cooperation of the patient can facilitate determination of appropriate tension.

Flexor Digitorum Superficialis Tendon Transfer

A tendon gap at the palm or wrist level can be overcome by intercalary tendon grafting or by transfer of an adjacent intact FDS tendon passed deep to the neurovascular bundle or median nerve and sewn to the distal segment of the injured tendon (Figure 6.43 and eFigure 6.2). Any of the techniques described for end-to-end tendon repair can be used. Tension is crucial, and the use of regional or local anesthesia can be helpful for this process.

End-to-Side Flexor Digitorum Profundus Tendon Juncture

It may be possible to attach the distal end of a severed FDP tendon to the side of an intact adjacent FDP tendon, which is best done with an interweave technique (Figure 6.44). Although the technique is more useful in the zone 5 area (forearm), it can also be used in the distal portion of zone 3 (palm). Excursion must be carefully assessed in all positions because the juncture can impinge on the A1 pulley in extension. A1 pulley division should be formed as needed.

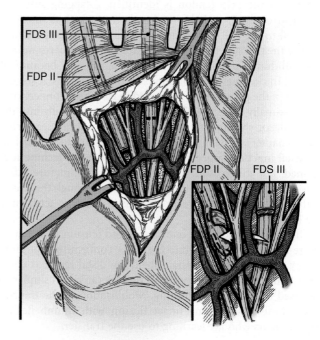

FIGURE 6.43 FDS transfer for FDP injuries in another finger. See eFigure 6.2. (**A,** Copyright Elizabeth Martin.)

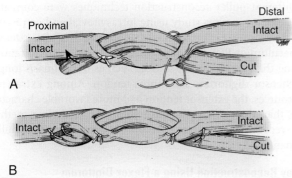

FIGURE 6.44 A and **B,** End-to-side interweave suture technique useful in zone 5 injuries. (Copyright Elizabeth Martin.)

Postoperative Care

A short-arm posterior molded plaster splint is applied from the fingertips to below the elbow. The wrist is maintained in neutral position, the MP joints in 40 to 50 degrees of flexion, and the IP joints in neutral position. A program of controlled active range of motion (passive flexion followed by active extension to the limits of the dorsal splint) and protected passive range of motion is begun at the first postoperative visit. Flexion contractures can develop rapidly if full extension at the PIP joint is not achieved early. The patient should be followed closely for development of contractures so that adjustments can be made to the splint and therapy regimen. Active range of motion is introduced early after surgery. Often these repairs are more durable and we will start active motion sooner in the rehabilitation program. Splint protection is discontinued at 4 weeks. Resisted exercise and blocking techniques at each of the IP joints are allowed 4 to 5 weeks after the repair.

Expectations

In general, the outcomes after flexor tendon grafting are inferior to the results of primary flexor tendon repair. Using intrasynovial tendon grafts and early active range-of-motion rehabilitation, Leversedge and colleagues[127] reported that the active motion recovery was 64% for single-stage reconstructions and 55% for multiple-stage reconstructions. Single-digit reconstructions had the best outcomes, with a total active motion recovery of 73% of normal. Coyle and Leddy[41] reported on a fingertip-to-palm reconstruction using a two-stage method and reported an active motion recovery that averaged 91% of the preoperative range of motion. The differences in reporting methods and in the nature of the injury likely account for the differences reported in these two series. Finsen reported on a cohort of 43 patients treated with a two-stage tendon grafting method and found the time away from work was 44 days after the first procedure and 104 days after the second procedure. Furthermore, the author reported that tertiary procedures were needed in 42% of patients and that 28% of patients would not have had the procedure done if they had had to do it again. By their estimation, 28% of patients had a poor outcome. These series highlight the difficult nature of these procedures.[24,41,61,120,127,205,243]

Reconstruction of the Pulley System

Successful reconstruction of the flexor tendon system depends not only on treatment of the tendon itself but also on the important structural aspects of the pulley system.[4,172,242] Because the flexor muscles have a maximum shortening capability, only a certain amount of tendon excursion can be created. The purpose of the annular pulleys is to maintain the tendons in proximity to the joint center of rotation such that an economical amount of tendon excursion can create the desired amount of angular joint rotation. Competent pulleys prevent palmar tendon translation (clinically referred to as "bowstringing"), which may lead to a fixed flexion contracture and limited flexion of the finger. When two or more contiguous annular pulleys are disrupted, decreased range of motion and a PIP joint flexion contracture generally results.

The relative importance of the individual pulleys has been studied by Doyle and Blythe,[45-47] Hunter and colleagues,[98,99] and others.[26,50,130,132,186,207] They confirmed the work of Barton, who stated that at least two pulleys (A2 and A4) need to be retained or reconstructed. If it is determined by direct inspection that flexor tendon bowstringing has occurred despite intact A2 and A4 pulleys, consideration should be given to pulley reconstruction to optimize the efficiency of digital flexion.[95]

Indications

Intraoperative assessment of pulley function during flexor tendon reconstruction is crucial. If a one-stage tendon graft is planned, all uninjured pulley material is retained[100] to encourage flexor tendon healing within the uninjured sheath. If pulley material is absent because of injury or prior surgery, reconstruction must be done, at which time a two-staged tendon reconstruction is recommended.[194] During a two-stage reconstruction, it may be acceptable to repair an injured pulley by suturing the ends over the implant. Damaged pulleys that are structurally intact are also useful in two-stage reconstructions because they would not adhere to the implant as they would to a tendon graft. For this reason, all pulley material is saved at the first stage of the two-stage reconstruction. If a pulley is constricted, the tissue may be dilated, often using a cylindrical probe or small uterine sound so that it can be enlarged sufficiently to accept the implant.

Pulley Reconstruction Using a Free Tendon Graft

When doing a two-stage tendon reconstruction, sufficient tendon material generally may be available after tendon graft harvest to reconstruct the annular pulleys (Figure 6.45). If additional donor material is necessary for pulley reconstruction, we usually use the palmaris longus tendon. There may be a theoretical advantage to the use of the intrasynovial section of the flexor digitorum longus tendon for tendon gliding in a heavily scarred bed.

Many pulley reconstruction techniques have been proposed and tested mechanically. Bunnell advocated encircling the phalanx with a free tendon graft.[30] In his original description, the pulley graft was placed superficial (dorsal) to the extensor apparatus in the middle phalanx and deep to the extensor mechanism in the area of the proximal phalanx. Although this type of pulley reconstruction may be bulky, it has the advantage of being easier to tension and, in our experience, does not seem to have an adverse effect on the extensor system.

Several methods can facilitate wrapping of tendon graft around the phalanx. A curved suture passer may be used to pull sutures placed into the tendon graft around the phalanx. A

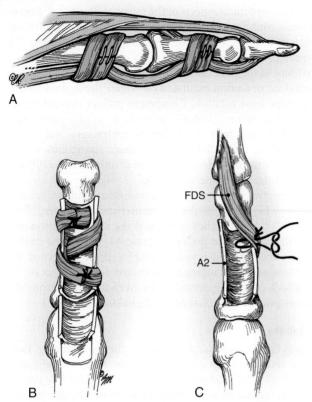

FIGURE 6.45 Methods of reconstruction of pulley system. **A,** Free tendon graft pulleys encircling the phalanx deep to the extensor mechanism at proximal and middle phalanges. **B,** Free tendon graft pulley can be constructed by suturing graft material to the rim of the destroyed pulley. This can take the form of an interweave into the rim, or if the rim is inadequate, the graft can be sutured through drill holes in the bone (not shown). **C,** Tail of FDS tendon, when left attached to its insertion, can be sutured over implant to the periosteum or to the rim of the original A2 pulley. (Copyright Elizabeth Martin.)

Penrose drain that is passed with a right-angled hemostat can also be used. We use a custom instrument designed for this purpose to facilitate both dissection and passage of the tendon graft (Seiler personal data).

Given that the double-loop method has been considered strong enough for early active protected motion,[66,254] encircling the phalanx and tendons twice is a reasonable balance between pulley strength and pulley width. In a study by Lin and coworkers,[130] it was reported that this type of reconstruction using three loops around the proximal phalanx approached the strength of a normal annulus in vitro.[66,254] After the graft is passed, an assessment of the finger is made in both flexion and extension to ensure that the pulley is both appropriately tensioned and approximates the flexor tendon to the phalanx. The reconstructed pulley should be sufficient to resist palmar translation of the flexor tendon when proximal traction is placed on the tendon.

Other methods proposed for pulley reconstruction include Kleinert and Bennett's[116] "ever-present rim" technique. This method weaves a thin graft back and forth through the remaining rim of the pulley system (see Figure 6.45, *B*). Doyle and Blythe[47] described a technique in which the graft is passed through a drill hole in the phalanx and then sutured back to itself. While durable, this technique may weaken the phalanx, creating a possibility for intraoperative or postoperative phalangeal fracture.

Different pulley reconstruction techniques were compared in an elegant in vitro study using intrasynovial and extrasynovial tissue sources. Intrasynovial grafts such as the extensor retinaculum or FDS tendon showed lower resistance to tendon gliding than extrasynovial sources such as the palmaris longus or extensor digitorum communis tendon. Among extrasynovial sources, the extensor tendon had more favorable characteristics than the palmaris longus tendon. An encircling method was recommended over tendon weaving through pulley remnants.[163]

Pulley Reconstruction Using a Flexor Digitorum Superficialis Tendon

The FDS tendon tail may be used as a pulley if it is long enough (see Figure 6.45, *C*). In this technique, the distal attachment is preserved, and the free proximal end is sutured over the implant onto the contralateral side. It may be sutured to either periosteum or the original pulley rim, or fastened via small holes drilled into bone. This makes an excellent pulley in the A3 area.

Pulley Reconstruction Using the Extensor Retinaculum

Lister[133] described good results with a technique in which a segment of the extensor retinaculum from the dorsum of the wrist is passed around the phalanx for pulley reconstruction. The advantages of this technique are that (1) the undersurface of the retinaculum is an ideal gliding surface (the broad fourth dorsal compartment segment of the retinaculum is rotated into a position overlying the flexor tendon or silicone implant), and (2) the new pulley is strong enough to allow early motion (e.g., after tenolysis). The major disadvantage is that harvesting the 6- to 8-cm length of retinaculum is technically difficult and time-consuming and requires a separate incision. Tang and associates[224] used the sheath of the first dorsal compartment to reconstruct the digital sheath with good results in delayed tendon repairs.

Pulley Reconstruction Using the Volar Plate

Karev[110] described a technique that creates slits in the volar plate for pulley reconstruction. More recent articles have suggested that this "belt-loop" technique is nearly as strong as a normal annular band but does not attain normal joint motion.[66,254] Widstrom and coworkers[247] published an excellent comparison of different pulley reconstruction techniques. They showed that among six methods studied in cadaver limbs, the technique of Karev was the most mechanically effective, but an encircling technique was the strongest and most resistant to failure.

Pulley Reconstruction Using Artificial Materials

Artificial materials have been used in the reconstruction of pulleys. These materials include knitted Dacron arterial graft,[254] silicone rubber sheeting, xenograft materials, polytetrafluoroethylene, woven nylon and fascia lata, and porcine collagen and peritoneum. The use of artificial materials is not routine at this time.

❖ AUTHORS' PREFERRED TECHNIQUE: Pulley Reconstruction

We prefer to create a circumferential pulley using the method of Bunnell. Our choice, however, is to place the graft deep to the extensor at the proximal and middle phalangeal levels (see

Figure 6.45, *A*). We prefer to use the palmaris longus tendon for our donor tendon and consider using the flexor digitorum longus tendon in complex cases.

At the proximal phalanx level, the tendon graft is placed inside the neurovascular bundles and deep to the dorsal extensor mechanism to prevent compression of the intrinsic system. To best simulate the biomechanics of the A2 and A4 pulleys, we use a minimum of two circumferential wraps for A2 and A4. Each wrap is passed around the phalanx under direct vision, and the repair is finished and tensioned using a modified Pulvertaft-type method, passing the graft through itself and tensioning it sufficiently to maintain the tendons in position. The repair is secured with a nonabsorbable mattress suture, and then the entire repair can be rotated away from the volar surface of the digit to minimize the impact of the repair on the volar tendon reconstruction. If the entirety of the A2 pulley requires reconstruction (which is normally 18 to 20 mm in length), this may require three to four tendon wraps. In the A4 region, two wraps create a pulley approximately 10 mm in length and should adequately simulate the biomechanics of the native pulley (Figure 6.46). For severely damaged tendon sheaths, a combination of strategies and donor grafts may be necessary to reconstruct the pulleys sufficiently to withstand the stresses of digital flexion. For reference, approximately 6 to 8 cm of graft is required to encircle the phalanx one time.

Postoperative Care

Postoperatively, splinting should include an external protective pulley ring, worn for 4 to 6 weeks. This ring can be rigid and fabricated from moldable plastic or flexible and formed from a simple elastic wrap. The therapist should be apprised of the pulley reconstruction so that this area can be supported manually during active and resisted exercise.

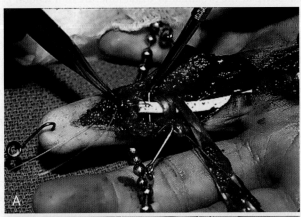
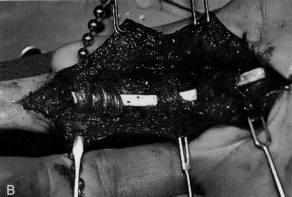

FIGURE 6.46 A and **B,** Pulley reconstruction. Resected FDS tendon is used to create a circumferential-type pulley around the silicone tendon implant by the phalanx technique.

CRITICAL POINTS *Pulley Reconstruction*

Indication
- Inadequate pulley function or bowstringing.

Preoperative Evaluation
- During a two-stage reconstruction, it may be acceptable to repair an injured pulley by suturing the ends over the implant.
- The most popular method of pulley reconstruction is the Bunnell encircling method.
- Other options include the Kleinert technique of weaving the graft into a remnant of the pulley rim, the Karev volar plate belt-loop technique, and the Lister extensor retinaculum pulley reconstruction.

Pearls
- The reconstructed pulley must be vigorously tested under direct visualization on the operating table.
- The tendon must be held as close to underlying bone as possible without restricting gliding.

Technical Points
- The encircling method requires a 16-cm graft for A2 reconstruction (phalanx encircled twice).
- Place the graft inside the neurovascular bundles and deep to the extensor mechanism at all levels.

Pitfall
- When encircling the phalanx with the graft, protect the neurovascular bundle.

Postoperative Care
- Wear a protective external ring for 4 to 6 weeks to protect the reconstruction.

Flexor Tendon Reconstruction in Children
Indications

Flexor tendon injuries in children can be particularly difficult to diagnose and treat. Careful observation and the use of various tricks geared to stimulate withdrawal of the fingers into flexion assist in the diagnosis of flexor tendon disruption. Children heal rapidly, and contractures rarely develop unless the joint has been directly injured. Generally, if wound conditions permit, direct early repair at all ages and all levels of injury is encouraged.[55,88,191] Flexor tendon grafting in young children is particularly difficult, and the appropriate timing for this procedure has been debated. Although loupe magnification helps eliminate technical difficulties, the physically small size of the tendon or silicone graft does not always hold sutures well, and repair site gapping may occur after primary repair. The inability of children to cooperate in postoperative care and rehabilitation has also been cited as a reason for poorer results.[176] Although one study concluded that age was not a contraindication to grafting,[61] and grafts have been successfully placed in young children,[8] we advocate a conservative approach and encourage waiting until the patient is age 7 years or older.

❖ AUTHORS' PREFERRED TECHNIQUE: Tendon Graft in Children

The technique for tendon graft in children is essentially the same as that in adults except that the distal juncture is not generally placed through the distal phalangeal bone. Our method in children and adults is the "around-the-bone technique," woven through the FDP stump, if available. Another technique involves placement of the graft through a split in the FDP stump that is then passed through the fingertip (see Figure 6.30, *C*). If no distal stump is present, the graft may be secured directly to bone with nonabsorbable sutures through drill holes placed *distal* to the physeal plate.

The preferred graft material is the palmaris longus or FDS tendon of the injured finger. A plantaris tendon in a child may be too thin to hold sutures adequately, so informed consent should enable use of other sources. As the child grows, a successfully placed flexor tendon graft is likely to grow with the child's hand. This clinical observation was questioned by Hage and Dupius,[81] however, who reported that, despite good function, the involved finger remained slightly smaller than the uninjured fingers.

Flexor tendon injuries are difficult problems for the child and the surgeon. The difficulties encountered with grafting make direct repair a better procedure than late reconstruction.[25,170] As with hand injuries in other children, the use of absorbable skin sutures makes aftercare more pleasant.

CRITICAL POINTS *Tendon Reconstruction in Children*

Indication
- Same as in adults.

Preoperative Evaluation
- Direct repair is preferable to late reconstruction.
- Reconstruction should be deferred until the patient is 7 years old or older.

Pearls
- Skin suture is done with absorbable material.
- Children heal rapidly, and contractures rarely develop unless the joint is directly injured.
- The plantaris tendon is too thin.

Technical Points
- Use the same technique in children as in adults except for distal juncture.
- Do not violate the distal phalanx epiphysis.
- Pass distally out of the fingertip and/or weave into the distal FDP stump.
- For graft material, the palmaris longus or FDS tendon of the injured finger is preferred.

Pitfalls
- Children present difficulties with diagnosis.
- Because of its small size, the tendon or silicone graft does not hold sutures well.
- Young children cooperate poorly in postoperative care and rehabilitation.

Postoperative Care
- The flexor tendon graft should grow with the child's hand.
- The involved finger may remain slightly smaller than uninjured fingers.

Complications Following Flexor Tendon Grafting

Adhesion Formation

The most common problem after flexor tendon grafting, as in all flexor tendon surgery, is adhesion formation. This formation may occur at any level of the graft reconstruction. To help reduce this problem, the surgeon must practice gentle handling of the tissues, use fine instruments, and adhere to proven surgical indications. Each injury to the surface of the tendon results in an adhesion at that level. The assistance of a good hand therapy program often helps mobilize adhesions and guide the patient through the critical 8-week period after surgery. Tenolysis (stage III) can improve tendon graft excursion in patients with adhesion formation, provided that the patient has reached a plateau and at least 3 to 6 months have elapsed since the grafting procedure.[60] Tenolysis can also be associated with tendon graft failure.

Mechanical Failure of the Implant

Breakdown of the distal juncture during stage I of a two-stage reconstruction is rare.[249] Dacron-reinforced silicone is recommended to prevent suture pull-out. The proximal end should not be sewn to a muscle motor in an attempt to create an "active" implant. This juncture usually disrupts and creates additional irritation and scarring in the forearm. If this unnecessary proximal juncture is stronger than the distal juncture, the distal end may rupture.

Graft Rupture

Breakdown at the proximal or distal juncture of a tendon graft has been seen in primary tendon grafting and staged tendon reconstruction. Adherence to excellent surgical technique and a closely supervised hand therapy program has made this a rare complication. When rupture at the graft juncture does occur, the patient can usually determine the location of the rupture. If recognized early, the situation can be salvaged by early reoperation. This complication occurs more frequently at the distal juncture. If the tendon cannot be advanced to the original insertion, the end of the graft can be attached to the middle phalanx, and an FDS-only finger can be created. Attenuation of the graft interweave can manifest as a proximal graft rupture. Early exploration of the distal forearm often leads to successful reattachment. Although most failures occur within the first few months after surgery, late intratendinous rupture has been reported.[57]

Pulley Disruption

Pulley failure is confirmed by a reduction of previously regained range of motion combined with bowstringing of the tendon graft. Early blocking support of the flexor tendon using the patient's contralateral hand, a wooden block, or an external ring helps maintain necessary tendon gliding while consideration for secondary pulley reconstruction is undertaken. The complication of reconstructed pulley disruption has been virtually eliminated in our practice with the use of an encircling method.

Quadriga Syndrome

Quadriga syndrome manifests as a decrease in flexion of an adjacent normal finger when an FDP tendon has been shortened or becomes adherent due to injury, repair, or reconstruction.[189] It was first described by Bunnell[30] and later by Verdan[234]; the term *quadriga* is derived from the Roman four-horse chariots driven by one charioteer who controlled all four horses with a common rein. If injury or a surgical procedure prevents normal proximal excursion of a single FDP tendon, a tethering effect is experienced by the other FDP tendons that share a common musculotendinous origin. The adjacent FDP tendons cannot fully flex their respective digits, and the injured finger develops a flexion deformity.

The quadriga syndrome may occur in numerous settings, as when one FDP tendon is advanced too far distally in a reattachment procedure in zone 1. Other causes include a tendon graft that is too short, a distal finger amputation in which the flexor is sutured over the tip to the extensor tendon, or an amputation in which the FDP tendon adheres to the proximal phalanx. Treatment is tendon lengthening, tenolysis, or severing of the offending tendon to allow the other normal adjacent fingers to flex fully.

Hyperextension of the Proximal Interphalangeal Joint

Absence of the FDS tendon in a grafted finger may result in a hyperextension deformity at the PIP joint.[170] It manifests as a swan neck deformity with difficulty initiating flexion at the PIP joint and is more apt to occur in patients with hyperextensile, loose joints. A tenodesis with one slip of the FDS tendon across the PIP joint may prevent or resolve the deformity.

Lumbrical-Plus Finger

The reverse of the quadriga effect is the lumbrical-plus finger described by Parkes,[170] seen when a graft is placed with insufficient tension.[54,56] This complication occurs because the lumbrical origin is normally pulled proximally with proximal movement of the FDP tendon. If an FDP tendon graft is too long, traction is exerted on the lumbrical muscle, which paradoxically causes extension of the IP joints. This problem can be avoided by ensuring proper length at the time of placement of the graft.

Synovitis

Synovitis after stage I is characterized by increased warmth, crepitus, and swelling secondary to fluid accumulation within the sheath. It is associated with a thickened, less pliable sheath at stage II (eFigure 6.3). Its incidence was initially believed to be 15% to 20%, but more recently synovitis was identified in 8% of patients after stage I surgery.[14] This serious complication is often, but not always, followed by a less successful end result after stage II. Cultures for bacteria in the fluid found within these sheaths have consistently shown no growth.

Although the inciting cause for this inflammatory reaction is not always apparent, certain circumstances are implicated. Breakdown of the distal juncture after stage I is often followed by a clinical picture of synovitis. Rigid fixation of the tendon implant to the distal FDP stump and use of a Dacron-reinforced implant have all but eliminated this cause of mechanical sheath irritation. Buckling or binding of the implant because of tight or inadequate pulleys is another cause for synovial irritation. Appropriate pulley reconstruction should eliminate this problem. Intraoperative finger motion at the time of stage I surgery usually shows the need for either further dilation or reconstruction of a pulley. Postoperative lateral radiographs in

flexion and extension identify the amount of implant excursion and often show buckling if present.

An effort to minimize implant handling and careful cleansing of the surgeon's gloves reduce the likelihood that foreign materials such as talc may induce synovitis. When synovitis is recognized, the patient's exercise program should be limited to short periods of passive range of motion, and resting splints should be employed. An earlier stage II procedure may be advisable if the problem is not controllable.

Infection

As in any implant procedure, postoperative infection after stage I is a disastrous complication. When confronted with infection in the sheath, antibiotic irrigation with small-bore catheters has been attempted. Established infection generally necessitates removal of the implant, with a healing period of 3 to 6 months and then, if feasible, placement of a new implant.

Late Flexion Deformity

A late flexion deformity may develop in the postoperative period and may be related to an incompetent pulley system, splinting difficulties, or wound contracture. These problems require early intervention and are rarely seen in patients with good initial motion after stage I. When noticed early, splinting the digits in extension between therapy sessions and at night can correct this problem. This program combined with gentle stretching exercises may continue for 1 year. Chronic deformities may require capsular release and flexor tenolysis. Flexion deformity may also be caused by an inadequate annular pulley system and resultant bowstringing. Joint contracture release at stage I and the construction of strong pulleys are of paramount importance.

Future Concepts

Investigators reporting on current concepts in tissue engineering have found that the flexor tendon is a tissue type amenable to various methods of tissue engineering. Allograft tendons and engineered tissue avoid any potential complications with autograft harvest and address the issue of graft availability in multiple-digit tendon reconstructions. Chong and colleagues, using a rabbit model, found that grafts can be satisfactorily acellularized and that acellularized tendon grafts provide high-strength scaffolding for tendon grafting.[37] Furthermore, it may be possible to seed these grafts with cells and to modify their surfaces, which creates a tendon graft optimized for gliding within the specialized synovial spaces of the hand.[93] Chang has worked extensively with stem cells derived from adipose tissue and with certain growth factors to delineate their use in seeding allografts for tendon grafting.[179,188] With improvements in these methods, it may be possible to engineer tissue that is optimized for the purpose of tendon grafting. Numerous investigators are examining the use of surface modifications to allograft tendons to reduce adhesions and gliding ability following tendon reconstruction. Using a canine model, Zhao, Amadio, and colleagues found that carbodiimide-derivatized hyaluronic acid and gelatin-modified intrasynovial allografts had less mean work of flexion and reduced gliding resistance compared with saline controls.[259] Follow-up in vivo canine studies have shown that resurfacing allograft tendons with carbodiimide-derivatized hyaluronic acid combined with lubricin resulted in fewer adhesions, less resistance, and less work of flexion. This surface modification resulted in inferior healing at the tendon-bone repair site as seen on histologic studies, however.[258]

With growing concerns about failure at the tendon-bone interface at the distal juncture, bone-block tendon allografts theoretically allow bone-to-bone healing versus tendon-to-bone healing. Biomechanical studies have addressed the ability to use bone-block tendon grafts for distal repair. Using a cadaveric model, Wei and colleagues compared the mechanical force of three distal juncture techniques: a suture pull-out technique, a suture anchor technique, and a suture pull-out with an FDP allograft with the distal bony attachment intact.[244] The authors found no difference in the load to failure and the stiffness in reconstructions using the suture pull-out or suture anchors. The group treated with the bony attachment had a significantly higher tensile strength compared with the group treated with tendon-to-bone attachment. Other cadaveric studies have shown no significant difference in the tensile strength of these tendon-to-bone composite allografts even after decellularization processes.[63]

Flexor Digitorum Superficialis Finger: Salvage Procedure

In flexor tendon reconstruction, an effort is usually made to restore active motion in the PIP and DIP joints. Occasionally, under specific conditions, efforts are directed at regaining motion only in the PIP joint in a more modest attempt to salvage function. This procedure has been called the FDS finger, although most of these reconstructions, in our experience, have been motored by the FDP tendon inserted into the middle phalanx. Perhaps the term *PIP joint finger* would be more appropriate.

The following three clinical scenarios involve flexor tendon disruption without reasonable likelihood of achieving acceptable DIP joint motion. Under these circumstances, restoration of motion at the PIP joint alone might be considered:

- *Type I*: Digits in which the DIP joint is inadequate because of either articular damage or extensor mechanism dysfunction (i.e., DIP arthrodesis).
- *Type II*: Digits with a poorly functioning flexor system because of tendon bowstringing secondary to pulley absence or failure despite one or more attempts at pulley reconstruction.
- *Type III*: Digits in which the distal insertion ruptured after tendon grafting.

Technique

In type I, a standard tendon graft is performed as described earlier, but the graft is inserted into the middle phalanx by the pull-out technique as used in the standard tendon graft. Particular attention is directed to padding placed between the button and the skin to distribute skin pressure over as wide an area as possible. Alternatively, the graft can be sutured by various techniques: to the middle phalanx via use of the pulley remnants; to the FDS tail, through the use of suture anchors; or to the local periosteum (Figure 6.47). With the patient anesthetized, tension must be adjusted so that with the wrist in neutral, the finger adopts a flexion posture at the PIP joint similar to that of the adjacent fingers. Whenever possible, we prefer to do this procedure with local sedative anesthesia so that the patient

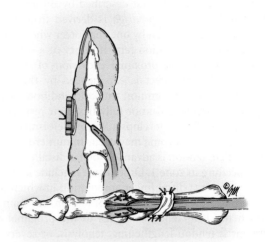

FIGURE 6.47 FDS finger. Graft is inserted into middle phalanx by one of several techniques. If the distal joint is unstable, tenodesis or arthrodesis of the DIP joint can be carried out at the same operation. (Copyright Elizabeth Martin.)

can cooperate directly in the setting of distal juncture tension at the middle phalangeal level. In situations in which the distal joint is unstable, arthrodesis or tenodesis in 20 to 30 degrees of flexion is also done.

In types II and III, the FDP tendon is identified through a volar approach to the finger and reattached, preferably to bone. The technique is the same as in type I cases except that pulley reconstruction is needed in type II cases. The use of local anesthesia to allow active participation of the patient is useful.

Postoperative Care

Tendon grafts (type I) are treated exactly as a standard graft would be treated. In types II and III, early unresisted motion is allowed in a protective dorsal splint, which may be combined with gentle rubber band traction on the fingernail, according to the surgeon's preference. The MP joints are placed in 70 degrees of flexion, with the posterior splint allowing full PIP joint extension. The wrist is flexed approximately 30 degrees. When a pulley is reconstructed, a molded plastic ring splint measuring about 2 cm in width is fabricated and worn to protect the pulley. At 3 to 4 weeks, the splint is removed, but the rubber band, attached to a wrist cuff, is continued for a total of 6 weeks. The ring is worn for at least 8 weeks postoperatively.

For Case Studies, Videos, and more, please visit ExpertConsult.com.

REFERENCES

1. Abrahamsson SO: Matrix metabolism and healing in the flexor tendon: experimental studies on rabbit tendon. *Scand J Plast Reconstr Surg Hand Surg Suppl* 23: 1–51, 1991.
2. Akali A, Khan U, Khaw PT, et al: Decrease in adhesion formation by a single application of 5-fluorouracil after flexor tendon injury. *Plast Reconstr Surg* 103: 151–158, 1999.
3. Alms A: Pedicle tendon graft for flexor tendon injuries of the fingers. *J Bone Joint Surg Br* 55:881, 1973.
4. Amadio PC, Hunter JM, Jaeger SH, et al: The effect of vincular injury on the results of flexor tendon surgery in zone 2. *J Hand Surg [Am]* 10:626–632, 1985.
5. Amiel D, Ishizue K, Billings E, Jr, et al: Hyaluronan in flexor tendon repair. *J Hand Surg [Am]* 14:837–843, 1989.

6. Aoki M, Manske PR, Pruitt DL, et al: Work of flexion after tendon repair with various suture methods: a human cadaveric study. *J Hand Surg [Br]* 20:310–313, 1995.

7. Apfelberg DB, Maser MR, Lash H, et al: "I-P flexor lag" after thumb flexor reconstruction: causes and solution. *Hand* 12:167–172, 1980.

8. Arons MS: Purposeful delay of the primary repair of cut tendons in "some man's land" in children. *Plast Reconstr Surg* 53:638–642, 1974.

9. Asencio G, Abihaidar G, Leonardi C: Human composite flexor tendon grafts. *J Hand Surg [Br]* 21:84–88, 1996.

10. Bakalim G: Primary mobilization after secondary flexor tendon surgery. *Scand J Plast Reconstr Surg* 9:240–244, 1975.

11. Barrie KA, Tomak SL, Cholewicki J, et al: The role of multiple strands and locking sutures on gap formation of flexor tendon repairs during cyclical loading. *J Hand Surg [Am]* 25:714–720, 2000.

12. Barrie KA, Wolfe SW, Shean C, et al: A biomechanical comparison of multistrand flexor tendon repairs using an in situ testing model. *J Hand Surg [Am]* 25:499–506, 2000.

13. Becker H: Primary repair of flexor tendons in the hand without immobilization: preliminary report. *Hand* 10:37–47, 1978.

14. Beris AE: Two-stage flexor tendon reconstruction in zone II using a silicone rod and a pedicled intrasynovial graft. *J Hand Surg [Am]* 28:652–660, 2003.

15. Bertelli JA, Santos MA, Kechele PR, et al: Flexor tendon grafting using a plantaris tendon with a fragment of attached bone for fixation to the distal phalanx: a preliminary cohort study. *J Hand Surg [Am]* 32:1543–1548, 2007.

16. Bidder M, Towler DA, Gelberman RH, et al: Expression of mRNA for vascular endothelial growth factor at the repair site of healing canine flexor tendon. *J Orthop Res* 18:247–252, 2000.

17. Birney HB, Idler RS: Flexor tenolysis in children. *J Hand Surg [Am]* 20:254–257, 1995.

18. Boardman ND, 3rd, Morifusa S, Saw SS, et al: Effects of tenorrhaphy on the gliding function and tensile properties of partially lacerated canine digital flexor tendons. *J Hand Surg [Am]* 24:302–309, 1999.

19. Bora FW, Lane JM, Prockop DJ: Inhibitors of collagen biosynthesis as a means of controlling scar formation in tendon injury. *J Bone Joint Surg Am* 54:1501–1508, 1972.

20. Boulas HJ, Strickland JW: Strength and functional recovery following repair of flexor digitorum superficialis in zone 2. *J Hand Surg [Br]* 18:22–25, 1993.

21. Boyer MI, Ditsios K, Gelberman RH, et al: Repair of flexor digitorum profundus tendon avulsions from bone: an ex vivo biomechanical analysis. *J Hand Surg [Am]* 27:594–598, 2002.

22. Boyer MI, Gelberman RH, Burns ME, et al: Intrasynovial flexor tendon repair: an experimental study comparing low and high levels of in vivo force during rehabilitation in canines. *J Bone Joint Surg Am* 83:891–899, 2001.

23. Boyer MI, Strickland JW, Engles D, et al: Flexor tendon repair and rehabilitation: state of the art in 2002. *Instr Course Lect* 52:137–161, 2003.

24. Boyes JH, Stark HH: Flexor tendon grafts in the fingers and thumb: a study of factors influencing results in 1000 cases. *J Bone Joint Surg Am* 53:1332–1342, 1971.

25. Boyes JH: Flexor tendon grafts in the fingers and thumb: an evaluation of end results. *J Bone Joint Surg Am* 32:489–499, 1950.

26. Brand PW, Cranor KC, Ellis JC: Tendon and pulleys at the metacarpophalangeal joint of a finger. *J Bone Joint Surg Am* 57:779–784, 1975.

27. Brand PW: Tendon grafting. *J Bone Joint Surg Br* 43:444–453, 1961.

28. Brug E, Stedtfeld HW: Experience with a two stage pedicled flexor tendon graft. *Hand* 11:198–205, 1979.

29. Buch BD, Innis P, McClinton MA, et al: The Mitek Mini G2 suture anchor: biomechanical analysis of use in the hand. *J Hand Surg [Am]* 20:877–881, 1995.

30. Bunnell S: Reconstructive surgery of the hand. *Surg Gynecol Obstet* 34:259–274, 1924.

31. Burns JW, Skinner K, Colt MJ, et al: A hyaluronate based gel for the prevention of postsurgical adhesions: evaluation in two animal species. *Fertil Steril* 66:814–821, 1996.

32. Bynum DK, Gilbert JA: Avulsion of the flexor digitorum profundus: anatomic and biomechanical considerations. *J Hand Surg [Am]* 13:222–227, 1988.

33. Carstam N: Prevention of experimental tendon adhesions by cortisone. *Acta Orthop Scand* 22:15–24, 1953.

34. Carstam N: The efforts of cortisone on the formation of tendon adhesions and on tendon healing. *Acta Chir Scand Suppl* 182:1–111, 1953.

35. Chacha P: Free autologous composite tendon grafts for division of both flexor tendons within the digital theca of the hand. *J Bone Joint Surg Am* 56:960–978, 1974.

36. Chang J, Thunder R, Most D, et al: Studies in flexor tendon wound healing: neutralizing antibody to TGF-beta1 increases postoperative range of motion. *Plast Reconstr Surg* 105:148–155, 2000.

37. Chong AK, Riboh J, Smith RL, et al: Flexor tendon tissue engineering: acellularized and reseeded tendon constructs. *Plast Reconstr Surg* 123:1759–1766, 2009.

38. Chow SP, Stephens MM, Ngai WK, et al: A splint for controlled active motion after flexor tendon repair: design, mechanical testing, and preliminary clinical results. *J Hand Surg [Am]* 15:645–651, 1990.

39. Coert JH, Uchiyama S, Amadio PC, et al: Flexor tendon-pulley interaction after tendon repair: a biomechanical study. *J Hand Surg [Br]* 20:573–577, 1995.

40. Cohen MJ, Kaplan L: Histology and ultrastructure of the human flexor tendon sheath. *J Hand Surg [Am]* 12:25–29, 1987.

41. Coyle MP, Jr, Leddy TP, Leddy JP: Staged flexor tendon reconstruction fingertip to palm. *J Hand Surg [Am]* 27:581–585, 2002.

42. Cribb AM, Scott JE: Tendon response to tensile stress: an ultrastructural investigation of collagen:proteoglycan interactions in stressed tendon. *J Anat* 187(Pt 2):423–428, 1995.

43. Diao E, Hariharan JS, Soejima O, et al: Effect of peripheral suture depth on strength of tendon repairs. *J Hand Surg [Am]* 21:234–239, 1996.

44. Dinopoulos HT, Boyer MI, Burns ME, et al: The resistance of a four- and eight-strand suture technique to gap formation during tensile testing: an experimental study of repaired canine flexor tendons after 10 days of in vivo healing. *J Hand Surg [Am]* 25:489–498, 2000.

45. Doyle JR: Anatomy of the finger flexor tendon sheath and pulley system. *J Hand Surg [Am]* 13:473–484, 1988.

46. Doyle JR, Blythe W: The finger flexor tendon sheath and pulleys: anatomy and reconstruction. In *AAOS symposium on tendon surgery in the hand*, St. Louis, 1975, Mosby, pp 81–87.

47. Doyle JR, Blythe WF: Anatomy of the flexor tendon sheath and pulleys of the tendon sheath and pulleys of the thumb. *J Hand Surg [Am]* 2:149–151, 1977.

48. Duffy FJ, Jr, Seiler JG, Gelberman RH, et al: Growth factors and canine flexor tendon healing: initial studies in uninjured and repair models. *J Hand Surg [Am]* 20:645–649, 1995.

49. Duffy FJ, Seiler JG, Hergrueter CA, et al: Intrinsic mitogenic potential of canine flexor tendons. *J Hand Surg [Br]* 17:275–277, 1992.

50. Dunlap J, McCarthy JA, Manske PR: Flexor tendon pulley reconstructions: a histological and ultrastructural study in non-human primates. *J Hand Surg [Br]* 14:273–277, 1989.

51. Duran R, Houser R, Coleman C, et al: A preliminary report in the use of controlled passive motion following flexor tendon repair in zones II and III [abstract]. *J Hand Surg [Am]* 1:79, 1976.

52. Elliot D, Khandwalla A, Ragoowansi R: The flexor digitorum profundus demitendon: a new technique for passage of the flexor profundus tendon through the A4 pulley. *J Hand Surg [Br]* 26:422–426, 2001.

53. Engles D, Diao E, Seiler, JG, III, et al: Reconstruction after flexor tendon injury: state of the art. *Instr Course Lect* 58:561–572, 2009.

54. Enna CD, Dyer RE: Tendon plasticity: a property applicable to reconstructive surgery of the hand. *Hand* 8:118–124, 1976.

55. Entin MA: Flexor tendon repair and grafting in children. *Am J Surg* 109:287–290, 1965.

56. Entin MA: Flexor tendon surgery in children. In *AAOS symposium on tendon surgery in the hand*, St. Louis, 1975, Mosby, pp 132–144.

57. Eshman SJ, Posner MA: Intratendinous rupture of a flexor tendon graft many years after staged reconstruction: a report of three cases. *J Hand Surg [Am]* 25:1135–1139, 2000.

58. Farkas LG, McCain WG, Sweeney P, et al: An experimental study of the changes following Silastic rod preparation of a new tendon sheath and subsequent tendon grafting. *J Bone Joint Surg Am* 55:1149–1158, 1973.

59. Feldscher SB, Schneider LH: Flexor tenolysis. *Hand Surg* 7:61–74, 2002.

60. Fetrow KO: Tenolysis in the hand and wrist: a clinical evaluation of two hundred and twenty flexor and extensor tenolyses. *J Bone Joint Surg Am* 49:667–685, 1967.

61. Finsen V: Two-stage grafting of digital flexor tendons: a review of 43 patients after 3 to 15 years. *Scand J Plast Reconstr Surg Hand Surg* 37:159–162, 2003.

62. Foucher G, Lenoble E, Ben Youseff K, et al: A post-operative regime after digital flexor tenolysis. *J Hand Surg [Br]* 18:35–40, 1993.

63. Fox PM, Farnebo S, Lindsey D, et al: Decellularized human tendon-bone grafts for composite flexor tendon reconstruction: a cadaveric model of initial mechanical properties. *J Hand Surg [Am]* 38:2323–2328, 2013.

64. Franko OI, Lee NM, Finneran JJ, et al: Quantification of partial or complete A4 pulley release with FDP repair in cadaveric tendons. *J Hand Surg [Am]* 36(3):439–445, 2011.

65. Gabuzda GM, Lovallo JL, Nowak MD: Tensile strength of the end-weave flexor tendon repair. *J Hand Surg [Br]* 19:397–400, 1994.

66. Galano GJ, Jiang KN, Strauch RJ, et al: Inflammatory response with osteolysis related to a bioabsorbable anchor in the finger: a case report. *Hand* 5:307–312, 2010.

67. Gelberman RH: Flexor tendon physiology: tendon nutrition and cellular activity in injury and repair. *Instr Course Lect* 34:351–360, 1985.

68. Gelberman RH, Amiel D, Harwood F: Genetic expression for type I procollagen in the early stages of flexor tendon healing. *J Hand Surg [Am]* 17:551–558, 1992.

69. Gelberman RH, Botte MJ, Spiegelman JJ, et al: The excursion and deformation of repaired flexor tendons treated with protected early motion. *J Hand Surg [Am]* 11:106–110, 1986.

70. Gelberman RH, Boyer MI, Brodt MD, et al: The effect of gap formation at the repair site on the strength and excursion of intrasynovial flexor tendons: an experimental study on the early stages of tendon-healing in dogs. *J Bone Joint Surg Am* 81:975–982, 1999.

71. Gelberman RH, Khabie V, Cahill CJ: The revascularization of healing flexor tendons in the digital sheath: a vascular injection study in dogs. *J Bone Joint Surg Am* 73:868–881, 1991.

72. Gelberman RH, Manske PR, Akeson WH, et al: Flexor tendon repair. *J Orthop Res* 4:119–128, 1986.

73. Gelberman RH, Nunley JA, 2nd, Osterman AL, et al: Influences of the protected passive mobilization interval on flexor tendon healing: a prospective randomized clinical study. *Clin Orthop* (264):189–196, 1991.

74. Gelberman RH, Siegel DB, Woo SL, et al: Healing of digital flexor tendons: importance of the interval from injury to repair: a biomechanical, biochemical, and morphological study in dogs. *J Bone Joint Surg Am* 73:66–75, 1991.

75. Gelberman RH, Vande Berg JS, Lundborg GN, et al: Flexor tendon healing and restoration of the gliding surface: an ultrastructural study in dogs. *J Bone Joint Surg Am* 65:70–80, 1983.

76. Gelberman RH, Vandeberg JS, Manske PR, et al: The early stages of flexor tendon healing: a morphologic study of the first fourteen days. *J Hand Surg [Am]* 10(6 Pt 1):776–784, 1985.

77. Goldner JL, Coonrad RW: Tendon grafting of the flexor profundus in the presence of a completely or partially intact flexor sublimis. *J Bone Joint Surg Am* 51:527–532, 1969.

78. Greenwald DP, Randolph MA, Hong HZ, et al: Augmented Becker versus modified Kessler tenorrhaphy in monkeys: dynamic mechanical analysis. *J Hand Surg [Am]* 20:267–272, 1995.

79. Grobbelaar AO, Hudson DA: Flexor pollicis longus tendon injuries in children. *Ann R Coll Surg Engl* 77:135–137, 1995.

80. Groth G: Pyramid of progressive force exercises to the injured flexor tendon. *J Hand Ther* 17:31–42, 2004.

81. Hage J, Dupius CC: The intriguing fate of tendon grafts in small children's hands and their results. *Br J Plast Surg* 18:341–349, 1965.

82. Harrison SH: Repair of digital flexor tendon injuries in the hand. *Br J Plast Surg* 14:211, 1961.

83. Harrison SH: Delayed primary flexor tendon grafts. *Hand* 1:106–107, 1969.

84. Harvey FJ, Chu G, Harvey PM: Surgical availability of the plantaris tendon. *J Hand Surg [Am]* 8:243–247, 1983.

85. Hatanaka H, Zhang J, Manske PR: An in vivo study of locking and grasping techniques using a passive mobilization protocol in experimental animals. *J Hand Surg [Am]* 25:260–269, 2000.

86. Hatano I, Suga T, Diao E, et al: Adhesions from flexor tendon surgery: an animal study comparing surgical techniques. *J Hand Surg [Am]* 25:252–259, 2000.

87. He M, Gan AWT, Lim AYT, et al: The effect of fibrin glue on tendon healing and adhesion formation in a rabbit model of flexor tendon injury and repair. *J Plast Surg Hand Surg* 47:509–512, 2013.

88. Herndon JH: Treatment of tendon injuries in children. *Orthop Clin North Am* 7:717–731, 1976.

89. Higgins A, Lalonde DH, Bell M, et al: Avoiding flexor tendon repair rupture with intraoperative total active movement examination. *Plast Reconstr Surg* 126(3):941–945, 2010.

90. Hitchcock TF, Light TR, Bunch WH, et al: The effect of immediate constrained digital motion on the strength of flexor tendon repairs in chickens. *J Hand Surg [Am]* 12:590–595, 1987.

91. Honnor R: The late management of the isolated lesion of the flexor digitorum profundus tendon. *Hand* 7:171–174, 1975.

92. Howard RF, Ondrovic L, Greenwald DP: Biomechanical analysis of four-strand extensor tendon repair techniques. *J Hand Surg [Am]* 22:838–842, 1997.

93. Huang D, Balian G, Chhabra AB: Tendon tissue engineering and gene transfer: the future of surgical treatment. *J Hand Surg [Am]* 31:693–704, 2006.

94. Hueston JJ, Hubble B, Rigg BR: Homografts of the digital flexor tendon system. *Aust N Z J Surg* 36:269–274, 1967.

95. Hume EL, Hutchinson DT, Jaeger SA, et al: Biomechanics of pulley reconstruction. *J Hand Surg [Am]* 16:722–730, 1991.

96. Hung LK, Fu SC, Lee YW, et al: Local vitamin-C injection reduced tendon adhesion in a chicken model of flexor digitorum profundus tendon injury. *J Bone Joint Surg Am* 95:e41–e47, 2013.

97. Hunter J: Anatomy of flexor tendons: pulley, vincular, synovia, and vascular structures. In Spinner M, editor: *Kaplan's functional and surgical anatomy of the hand*, Philadelphia, 1984, JB Lippincott, pp 65–92.

98. Hunter JM, Cook JF, Jr: The pulley system: rationale for reconstruction. In Strickland JW, Steinchen JB, editors: *Difficult problems in hand surgery*, St. Louis, 1982, Mosby, pp 94–102.

99. Hunter JM, Cook JF, Ochiai N, et al: The pulley system. *Orthop Trans* 4:4, 1980.

100. Hunter JM, Salisbury RE: Flexor tendon reconstruction in severely damaged hands: a two-stage procedure using a silicone Dacron reinforced gliding prosthesis prior to tendon grafting. *J Bone Joint Surg Am* 53:829–858, 1971.

101. Hunter JM, Schneider LH, Dumont J, et al: A dynamic approach to problems of hand function using local anesthesia supplemented by intravenous fentanyl-droperidol. *Clin Orthop* 104:112–115, 1974.

102. Hunter JM, Seinsheimer F, Mackin EJ: Tenolysis: pain control and rehabilitation. In Strickland JW, Steinchen JB, editors: *Difficult problems in hand surgery*, St. Louis, 1982, Mosby, pp 312–318.

103. Hunter JM, Steindel C, Salisbury R, et al: Study of early sheath development using static non-gliding implants. *J Biomed Mater Res* 5:155, 1974.

104. Hunter JM, Subin D, Minkow F, et al: Sheath formation in response to limited active gliding implants (animals). *J Biomed Mater Res* 5:155, 1974.

105. Hunter JM, Taras JS, Mackin EJ, et al: Staged flexor tendon reconstruction using passive and active tendon implants. In Hunter JM, Mackin EJ, Callahan AD, editors: *Rehabilitation of the hand: surgery and therapy*, St. Louis, 1995, Mosby, pp 477–514.

106. Ipsen T, Barfield T: Early mobilization after flexor tendon grafting for isolated profundus tendon lesions. *Scand J Plast Reconstr Surg* 22:163, 1988.

107. Jaffe S, Weckesser E: Profundus tendon grafting with the sublimis intact: the end result of thirty patients. *J Bone Joint Surg Am* 49:1298–1308, 1967.

108. James JIP: The use of cortisone in tenolysis. *J Bone Joint Surg Br* 41:209–210, 1959.

109. James JIP: The value of tenolysis. *Hand* 1:118–119, 1969.

110. Karev A: The "belt loop" technique for the reconstruction of pulleys in the first stage of flexor tendon grafting. *J Hand Surg [Am]* 9:923–924, 1984.

111. Kato H, Minami A, Suenaga N, et al: Long-term results after primary repairs of zone 2 flexor tendon lacerations in children younger than age 6 years. *J Pediatr Orthop* 22:732–735, 2002.

112. Ketchum LD, Martin NL, Kappel DA: Experimental evaluation of factors affecting the strength of tendon repairs. *Plast Reconstr Surg* 59:708–719, 1977.

113. Kleinert H, Cash S: Management of acute flexor tendon injuries in the hand. *Instr Course Lect* 34:361–372, 1985.

114. Kleinert H, Cash S: Current guidelines for flexor tendon repair within the fibroosseous tunnel: indications, timing and techniques. In Hunter J, Schneider L, Mackin E, editors: *Tendon surgery in the hand*, St. Louis, 1987, Mosby, pp 118–125.

115. Kleinert H, Kutz J, Ashbell T, et al: Primary repair of lacerated flexor tendons in "no man's land." *J Bone Joint Surg Am* 49:577, 1967.

116. Kleinert HE, Bennett JB: Digital pulley reconstruction employing the always present rim of the previous pulley. *J Hand Surg [Am]* 3:297–298, 1978.

117. Kubota H, Aoki M, Pruitt DL, et al: Mechanical properties of various circumferential tendon suture techniques. *J Hand Surg [Br]* 21:474–480, 1996.

118. Kwai Ben I, Elliot D: "Venting" or partial lateral release of the A2 and A4 pulleys after repair of zone 2 flexor tendon injuries. *J Hand Surg [Br]* 23:649–654, 1998.

119. Lalonde DH, Martin AL: Wide-awake flexor tendon repair and early tendon mobilization in zones 1 and 2. *Hand Clin* 29:207–213, 2013.

120. LaSalle WB, Strickland JW: An evaluation of the two-stage flexor tendon reconstruction technique. *J Hand Surg [Am]* 8:263–267, 1983.

121. Latendresse K, Dona E, Scougall PJ, et al: Cyclic testing of pullout sutures and micro-mitek suture anchors in flexor digitorum profundus tendon distal fixation. *J Hand Surg [Am]* 30:471–478, 2005.

122. Leddy JP: Flexor tendons: acute injuries. In Green DP, editor: *Operative hand surgery*, Edinburgh, 1982, Churchill Livingstone, pp 1347–1373.

123. Leddy JP, Packer JW: Avulsion of the profundus tendon insertion in athletes. *J Hand Surg [Am]* 2:66–69, 1977.

124. Lee SK, Dubey A, Kim BH, et al: A biomechanical study of extensor tendon repair methods: introduction to the running-interlocking horizontal mattress extensor tendon repair technique. *J Hand Surg [Am]* 35(1):19–23, 2010.

125. Lee SK, Fajardo M, Kardashian G, et al: Repair of flexor digitorum profundus to distal phalanx: a biomechanical evaluation of four techniques. *J Hand Surg [Am]* 36(10):1604–1609, 2011.

126. Leversedge FJ, Ditsios K, Goldfarb CA, et al: Vascular anatomy of the human flexor digitorum profundus tendon insertion. *J Hand Surg [Am]* 27:806–812, 2002.

127. Leversedge FJ, Zelouf D, Williams C, et al: Flexor tendon grafting to the hand: an assessment of the intrasynovial donor tendon: a preliminary single-cohort study. *J Hand Surg [Am]* 25:721–730, 2000.

128. Lieber RL, Amiel D, Kaufman KR, et al: Relationship between joint motion and flexor tendon force in the canine forelimb. *J Hand Surg [Am]* 21:957–962, 1996.

129. Lieber RL, Silva MJ, Amiel D, et al: Wrist and digital joint motion produce unique flexor tendon force and excursion in the canine forelimb. *J Biomech* 32:175–181, 1999.

130. Lin GT, Amadio PC, An KN, et al: Biomechanical analysis of finger flexor pulley reconstruction. *J Hand Surg [Br]* 14:278–282, 1989.

131. Lin GT, Amadio PC, An KN, et al: Functional anatomy of the human digital flexor pulley system. *J Hand Surg [Am]* 14:949–956, 1989.

132. Lin G-T, Cooney WP, Amadio PC, et al: Mechanical properties of human pulleys. *J Hand Surg [Br]* 15:429–434, 1990.

133. Lister GD: Reconstruction of pulleys employing extensor retinaculum. *J Hand Surg [Am]* 4:461–464, 1979.

134. Lister GD, Kleinert HE, Kutz JE, et al: Primary flexor tendon repair followed by immediate controlled mobilization. *J Hand Surg [Am]* 2:441–451, 1977.

135. Lundborg G: Experimental flexor tendon healing without adhesion formation: a new concept of tendon nutrition and intrinsic healing mechanisms: a preliminary report. *Hand* 8:235–238, 1976.

136. Lundborg G, Rank F: Experimental intrinsic healing of flexor tendons based upon synovial fluid nutrition. *J Hand Surg [Am]* 3:21–31, 1978.

137. Lundborg G, Rank F: Experimental studies on cellular mechanisms involved in healing of animal and human flexor tendon in synovial environment. *Hand* 12:3–11, 1980.

138. Lundborg G, Rank F: Tendon healing: intrinsic mechanisms. In Hunter J, Schneider L, Mackin E, editors: *Tendon surgery in the hand*, St. Louis, 1987, Mosby, pp 54–60.

139. Mackin E: Flexor tenolysis. In Hunter J, Schneider L, Mackin E, editors: *Tendon surgery in the hand*, St. Louis, 1987, Mosby.

140. Manske P, Lesker P: Diffusion as a nutrient pathway to the flexor tendon. In Hunter J, Schneider L, Mackin E, editors: *Tendon surgery in the hand*, St. Louis, 1987, Mosby, pp 86–90.

141. Manske PR, Gelberman RH, Vande Berg JS, et al: Intrinsic flexor-tendon repair: a morphological study in vitro. *J Bone Joint Surg Am* 66:385–396, 1984.

142. Manske PR, Lesker PA, Gelberman RH, et al: Intrinsic restoration of the flexor tendon surface in the nonhuman primate. *J Hand Surg [Am]* 10:632–637, 1985.

143. Mass DP, Tuel RJ: Intrinsic healing of the laceration site in human superficialis flexor tendons in vitro. *J Hand Surg [Am]* 16:24–30, 1991.

144. Matsuzaki H, Zaegel MA, Gelberman RH, et al: Effect of suture material and bone quality on the mechanical properties of zone I flexor tendon-bone reattachment with bone anchors. *J Hand Surg [Am]* 33:709–717, 2008.

145. Matthews P, Richards H: Factors in the adherence of flexor tendons after repair. *J Bone Joint Surg Br* 58:230–236, 1976.

146. May H: Tendon transplantation in the hand. *Surg Gynecol Obstet* 83:631–638, 1946.

147. May EJ, Silfverskiöld KL, Sollerman CJ: Controlled mobilization after flexor tendon repair in zone II: a prospective comparison of three methods. *J Hand Surg [Am]* 17:942–952, 1992.

148. May EJ, Silfverskiöld KL: Rate of recovery after flexor tendon repair in zone II: a prospective longitudinal study of 145 digits. *Scand J Plast Reconstr Surg Hand Surg* 27:89–94, 1993.

149. McCarthy JA, Lesker PA, Peterson WW, et al: Continuous passive motion as an adjunct therapy for tenolysis. *J Hand Surg [Br]* 11:88–90, 1986.

150. McClinton MA, Curtis RM, Wilgis EFS: 100 tendon grafts for isolated flexor digitorum profundus injuries. *J Hand Surg [Am]* 7:224–229, 1982.

151. McCollough FH: Repair of the flexor pollicis longus tendon. *U S Armed Forces Med J* 2:1579–1591, 1951.

152. McCormack RM, Demuth RJ, Kindling PH: Flexor tendon grafts in the less-than-optimal situation. *J Bone Joint Surg Am* 44:1360–1364, 1962.

153. McFarlane RM, Lamon R, Jarvis G: Flexor tendon injuries within the finger: a study of the results of tendon suture and tendon graft. *J Trauma* 8:987–1003, 1968.

154. McKenzie AR: Function after reconstruction of severed long flexor tendons of the hand: a review of 297 tendons. *J Bone Joint Surg Br* 49:424–439, 1967.

155. McLarney E, Hoffman H, Wolfe SW: Biomechanical analysis of the cruciate four-strand flexor tendon repair. *J Hand Surg [Am]* 24:295–301, 1999.

156. McNally TA, Hamman JJ, Heminger H, et al: The strength of distal fixation of flexor digitorum profundus tendon grafts in human cadavers. *J Hand Surg [Am]* 27:599–604, 2002.

157. Meals RA: Flexor tendon injuries: current concepts review. *J Bone Joint Surg Am* 67:817–821, 1985.

158. Millar R, Dickie WR, Colville J: The results of long delayed flexor tendon grafting. *Hand* 4:261–262, 1972.

159. Miller L, Mass DP: A comparison of four repair techniques for Camper's chiasma flexor digitorum superficialis lacerations: tested in an in vitro model. *J Hand Surg [Am]* 25:1122–1126, 2000.

160. Morrison WA, Schlicht SM: The plantaris tendon as a tendon osseous graft. II: Clinical studies. *J Hand Surg [Br]* 17:471–475, 1992.

161. Naam NH: Staged flexor tendon reconstruction using pedicled tendon graft from the flexor digitorum superficialis. *J Hand Surg [Am]* 22:323–327, 1997.

162. Nietosvaara Y, Lindfors N, Palmu S, et al: Flexor tendon injuries in pediatric patients. *J Hand Surg [Am]* 32:1549–1557, 2007.

163. Nishida J, Amadio PC: Flexor tendon-pulley interaction after pulley reconstruction: a biomechanical study in a human model in vivo. *J Hand Surg [Am]* 23:665–672, 1998.

164. Nishida J, Amadio PC, Bettinger PC, et al: Flexor tendon-pulley interaction after pulley reconstruction: a biomechanical study in a human model in vitro. *J Hand Surg [Am]* 23:665–672, 1998.

165. Nishida J, Seiler JG, Amadio PC, et al: Flexor tendon-pulley interaction after annular pulley reconstruction: a biomechanical study in a dog model in vivo. *J Hand Surg [Am]* 23:279–284, 1998.

166. Noguchi M, Seiler JG, 3rd, Gelberman RH, et al: In vitro biomechanical analysis of suture methods for flexor tendon repair. *J Orthop Res* 11:603–611, 1993.

167. Norris SR, Ellis FD, Chen MI, et al: Flexor tendon suture methods: a quantitative analysis of suture material within the repair site. *Orthopedics* 22:413–416, 1999.

168. O'Connell SJ, Moore MM, Strickland JW, et al: Results of zone I and zone II flexor tendon repairs in children. *J Hand Surg [Am]* 19:48–52, 1994.

169. Paneva-Holevich E: Two-stage tenoplasty in injury of the flexor tendons of the hand. *J Bone Joint Surg Am* 51:21–32, 1969.

170. Parkes A: The "lumbrical plus" finger. *J Bone Joint Surg Br* 53:236–239, 1971.

171. Peacock EE: Homologous composite tissue grafts of the digital flexor mechanism in human beings. *Plast Reconstr Surg* 25:418–421, 1960.

172. Peterson WW, Manske PR, Bollinger BA, et al: Effect of pulley excision on flexor tendon biomechanics. *J Orthop Res* 4:96–101, 1986.

173. Posner MA: Flexor superficialis tendon transfers to the thumb: an alternative to the free tendon graft for treatment of chronic injuries within the digital sheath. *J Hand Surg [Am]* 8:876–881, 1998.

174. Pribaz JJ, Morrison WA, Macleod AM: Primary repair of flexor tendons in no-man's land using the Becker repair. *J Hand Surg [Br]* 14:400–405, 1989.

175. Pruitt DL, Aoki M, Manske PR: Effect of suture knot location on tensile strength after flexor tendon repair. *J Hand Surg [Am]* 21:969–973, 1996.

176. Pulvertaft RG: Tendon grafts for flexor tendon injuries in the fingers and thumb: a study of technique and results. *J Bone Joint Surg Br* 38:175–194, 1956.

177. Pulvertaft RG: The treatment of profundus division by the free tendon graft. *J Bone Joint Surg Am* 42:1363–1371, 1960.

178. Pulvertaft RG: Indications for tendon grafting. In *AAOS symposium on tendon surgery in the hand*, St. Louis, 1975, Mosby, p 123.

179. Raghavan SS, Woon CY, Kraus A, et al: Optimization of human tendon tissue engineering: synergistic effects of growth factors for use in tendon scaffold repopulation. *Plast Reconstr Surg* 129:479–489, 2012.

180. Rank BK, Wakefield AR: *Surgery of repair as applied to hand injuries*, ed 2, Edinburgh, 1960, E & S Livingstone.

181. Rank BK, Wakefield AR, Hueston JJ: *Surgery of repair as applied to hand injuries*, ed 4, Baltimore, 1973, Williams & Wilkins.

182. Rispler D, Greenwald D, Shumway S, et al: Efficiency of the flexor tendon pulley system in human cadaver hands. *J Hand Surg [Am]* 21:444–450, 1996.

183. Rouhani AR, Barzgar H, Ghavidel E, et al: Effects of non-steroidal anti-inflammatory drugs on flexor tendon rehabilitation after laceration repair. *J Am Sci* 9:98–100, 2013.

184. Sakellarides HT, Papadopoulos G: Surgical treatment of the divided flexor digitorum profundus tendon in zone 2, delayed more than 6 weeks, by tendon grafting in 50 cases. *J Hand Surg [Br]* 21:63–66, 1966.

185. Sandow M, McMahon M: Single cross-grasp six-strand repair for acute flexor tenorrhaphy: modified Savage technique. *Atlas Hand Clin* 1:41–64, 1996.

186. Savage R: The mechanical effect of partial resection of the digital fibrous flexor sheath. *J Hand Surg [Br]* 15:435–442, 1990.

187. Schlenker JD, Lister GD, Kleinert HE: Three complications of untreated partial laceration of flexor tendon-entrapment, rupture, and triggering. *J Hand Surg [Am]* 6:392–398, 1981.

188. Schmitt T, Fox PM, Woon CY, et al: Human flexor tendon tissue engineering: in vivo effects of stem cell reseeding. *Plast Reconstr Surg* 132:567e–576e, 2013.

189. Schneider LH: *Flexor tendon injuries*, Boston, 1985, Little, Brown.

190. Schneider LH: Flexor tenolysis. In Hunter JM, Schneider LH, Mackin EJ, editors: *Flexor tendon surgery in the hand*, St. Louis, 1986, Mosby, pp 348–361.

191. Schneider LH: Injuries to tendons in children. In Bora FW, editor: *The pediatric upper extremity*, Philadelphia, 1986, WB Saunders, pp 91–119.

192. Schneider LH: Treatment of isolated flexor digitorum profundus injuries by tendon grafting. In Hunter JM, Schneider LH, Mackin EJ, editors: *Flexor tendon surgery in the hand*, St. Louis, 1986, Mosby, pp 518–525.

193. Schneider LH, Hunter JM: Tendon injuries in the hand. In Cotler J, editor: *Cyclopedia of medicine, surgery and specialities*, Philadelphia, 1975, FA Davis, p 723.

194. Schneider LH, Hunter JM: Flexor tendons: late reconstruction. In Green DP, editor: *Operative hand surgery*, New York, 1982, Churchill Livingstone, pp 1375–1440.

195. Schneider LH, Mackin EJ: Tenolysis. In Hunter JM, Schneider LH, Mackin EJ, et al, editors: *Rehabilitation of the hand*, St. Louis, 1978, Mosby, pp 229–234.

196. Schneider LH, Wiltshire D: Restoration of flexor pollicis longus function by flexor digitorum superficialis transfer. *J Hand Surg [Am]* 8:98–101, 1983.

197. Schuind F, Garcia-Elias M, Cooney WP, 3rd, et al: Flexor tendon forces: in vivo measurements. *J Hand Surg [Am]* 17:291–298, 1992.

198. Seiler JG, Chu CR, Amiel DA, et al: Autogenous flexor tendon grafts: biologic mechanisms for incorporation. *Clin Orthop Relat Res* 345:239–247, 1997.

199. Seiler JG, Gelberman RH, Williams CS, et al: Autogenous flexor-tendon grafts: a biomechanical and morphological study in dogs. *J Bone Joint Surg Am* 75:104–114, 1993.
200. Seiler JG, Reddy AS, Simpson LE, et al: The flexor digitorum longus: an anatomic and microscopic study for use as a tendon graft. *J Hand Surg [Am]* 20:492–495, 1995.
201. Seiler JG, Uchiyama S, Ellis F, et al: Reconstruction of the flexor pulley: the effect of tension and source of the graft in an in vitro dog model. *J Bone Joint Surg Am* 80:669–703, 1998.
202. Silfverskiöld KL, May EJ: Gap formation after flexor tendon repair in zone II: results with a new controlled motion programme. *Scand J Plast Reconstr Surg Hand Surg* 27:263–268, 1993.
203. Silfverskiöld KL, May EJ, Oden A: Factors affecting results after flexor tendon repair in zone II: a multivariate prospective analysis. *J Hand Surg [Am]* 18:654–662, 1993.
204. Silfverskiöld KL, May EJ, Tornvall AH: Flexor digitorum profundus tendon excursions during controlled motion after flexor tendon repair in zone II: a prospective clinical study. *J Hand Surg [Am]* 17:122–131, 1992.
205. Smith P, Jones M, Grobbelaar A: Two-stage grafting of flexor tendons: results after mobilization by controlled early active movement. *Scand J Plast Reconstr Surg Hand Surg* 38:220–227, 2004.
206. Snow JW: Ulnar half of extensor digiti-quinti proprius tendon for flexor grafts. *Plast Reconstr Surg* 42:603–604, 1968.
207. Solonen KA, Hoyer P: Positioning of the pulley mechanism when reconstructing deep flexor tendons of the fingers. *Acta Orthop Scand* 38:321–328, 1967.
208. Soucacos PN, Beris AE, Malizos KN, et al: Two-stage treatment of flexor tendon ruptures: Silicon rod complications analyzed in 109 digits. *Acta Orthop Scand Suppl* 275:48–51, 1997.
209. Sourmelis SG, McGrouther DA: Retrieval of the retracted flexor tendon. *J Hand Surg [Br]* 12:109–111, 1987.
210. Stark HH, Anderson DR, Boyes JH, et al: Bridge grafts of flexor tendons. *Orthop Trans* 7:44, 1983.
211. Stark HH, Zemel NP, Boyes JH, et al: Flexor tendon graft through intact superficialis tendon. *J Hand Surg [Am]* 2:456–461, 1977.
212. Steelman P: Treatment of flexor tendon injuries: therapist's commentary. *J Hand Ther* 12:149–151, 1991.
213. Strickland JW: Flexor tenolysis: a personal experience. In Hunter JM, Schneider LH, Mackin EJ, editors: *Tendon surgery in the hand*, St. Louis, 1987, Mosby, pp 216–233.
214. Strickland JW: Flexor tendon injuries. I: Foundations of treatment. *J Am Acad Orthop Surg* 3:44–54, 1995.
215. Strickland JW: Flexor tendon injuries. II: Operative technique. *J Am Acad Orthop Surg* 3:55–62, 1995.
216. Strickland JW: Flexor tendon repair. *Hand Clin* 1:55–68, 1985.
217. Strickland JW: Flexor tendon surgery. II: Free tendon grafts and tenolysis. *J Hand Surg [Br]* 14:368–382, 1989.
218. Strickland JW, Glogovac SV: Digital function following flexor tendon repair in zone II: a comparison of immobilization and controlled passive motion techniques. *J Hand Surg [Am]* 5:537–543, 1980.
219. Sullivan DJ: Disappointing outcomes in staged flexor tendon grafting for isolated profundus loss. *J Hand Surg [Br]* 11:231–233, 1986.
220. Szabo RM, Younger E: Effects of indomethacin on adhesion formation after repair of zone II tendon lacerations in the rabbit. *J Hand Surg [Am]* 15:480–483, 1990.
221. Tan V, Nourbakhsh A, Capo J, et al: Effects of nonsteroidal anti-inflammatory drugs on flexor tendon adhesion. *J Hand Surg [Am]* 35:941–947, 2010.
222. Tang JB: Indications, methods, postoperative motion and outcome evaluation of primary flexor tendon repairs in zone 2. *J Hand Surg Eur Vol* 32(2):118–129, 2007.
223. Tang JB, Ishii S, Usui M, et al: Flexor sheath closure during delayed primary tendon repair. *J Hand Surg [Am]* 19:636–640, 1994.
224. Tang JB, Zhang QG, Ishii S: Autogenous free sheath grafts in reconstruction of injured digital flexor tendon sheath at the delayed primary stage. *J Hand Surg [Br]* 18:31–32, 1993.
225. Taras J: Primary flexor tendon repair. *Oper Tech Orthop Surg* 3:270–277, 1993.
226. Taras J, Skahen J, James R, et al: The double-grasping and cross-stitch for acute flexor tendon repair: applications with active motion. *Atlas Hand Clin* 1:13–28, 1996.
227. Taras JS, Fitzpatrick MJ: Compartment syndrome of the leg after plantaris tendon harvest: a case report. *J Hand Surg [Am]* 26:1135–1137, 2001.
228. Taras JS, Marion M, Culp RW: Staged flexor tendon reconstruction with Hunter implants. In Osterman AL, editor: *Atlas of hand clinics: flexor tendon repair*, St. Louis, 1996, Mosby, pp 129–152.
229. Trumble TE, Vedder NE, Benirschke SK: Misleading fractures after profundus tendon avulsions: a report of 6 cases. *J Hand Surg [Am]* 17:902–906, 1992.
230. Uchiyama S, Amadio PC, Coert JH, et al: Gliding resistance of extrasynovial and intrasynovial tendons through the A2 pulley. *J Bone Joint Surg Am* 79:219–224, 1997.
231. Uchiyama S, Amadio PC, Ishikawa J, et al: Boundary lubrication between the tendon and the pulley in the finger. *J Bone Joint Surg Am* 79:213–218, 1997.
232. Urbaniak JR, Bright DS, Gill LH, et al: Vascularization and the gliding mechanism of free flexor tendon grafts inserted by the silicone rod method. *J Bone Joint Surg Am* 56:473–482, 1974.
233. Urbaniak JR, Goldner JL: Laceration of the flexor pollicis longus tendon: delayed repair by advancement, free graft or direct suture. *J Bone Joint Surg Am* 55:1123–1148, 1973.
234. Verdan C: Syndrome of the quadriga. *Surg Clin North Am* 40:425, 1960.
235. Verdan C: Tenolysis. In Verdan C, editor: *Tendon surgery of the hand*, Edinburgh, 1979, Churchill Livingstone, pp 137–142.
236. Verdan CE: Half a century of flexor-tendon surgery: current status and changing philosophies. *J Bone Joint Surg Am* 54:472–491, 1972.
237. Versaci AD: Secondary tendon grafting for isolated flexor digitorum profundus injury. *Plast Reconstr Surg* 46:57–60, 1970.
238. Wade PJ, Wetherell RG, Amis AA: Flexor tendon repair: significant gain in strength from the Halsted peripheral suture technique. *J Hand Surg [Br]* 14:232–235, 1989.
239. Wakefield AR: Late flexor tendon grafts. *Surg Clin North Am* 40:399, 1960.
240. Weber E: Nutritional pathways for flexor tendons in the digital theca. In Hunter J, Schneider L, Mackin E, editors: *Tendon surgery in the hand*, St. Louis, 1987, Mosby, pp 91–99.
241. Weber RV, Mackinnon SE: Median nerve mistaken for palmaris longus tendon: restoration of function with sensory nerve transfers. *Hand* 2:1–4, 2007.
242. Weeks PM, Wray RC: Rate and extent of functional recovery after flexor tendon grafting with and without silicone rod preparation. *J Hand Surg [Am]* 1:174–180, 1976.
243. Wehbe MA, Hunter JM, Schneider LH, et al: Two-stage flexor-tendon reconstruction: ten-year experience. *J Bone Joint Surg Am* 68:752–763, 1986.
244. Wei Z, Thoreson AR, Amadio PC, et al: Distal attachment of flexor tendon allograft: a biomechanical study of different reconstruction techniques in human cadaver hands. *J Orthop Res* 31:1720–1724, 2013.
245. Weidrich T: Acute repairs of zone II flexor digitorum profundus lacerations, with excision of the flexor digitorum superficialis. *Atlas Hand Clin* 5:131–148, 2000.
246. Whitaker JH, Strickland JW, Ellis RK: The role of flexor tenolysis in the palm and digits. *J Hand Surg [Am]* 2:462–470, 1977.
247. Widstrom CJ, Doyle JR, Johnson G, et al: A mechanical study of six digital pulley reconstruction techniques. II: Strength of individual reconstructions. *J Hand Surg [Am]* 14:826–829, 1989.
248. Widstrom CJ, Johnson G, Doyle JR, et al: A mechanical study of six digital pulley reconstruction techniques. I: Mechanical effectiveness. *J Hand Surg [Am]* 14:821–825, 1989.
249. Wilson RL, Carter MS, Holdeman VA, et al: Flexor profundus injuries treated with delayed two-staged tendon grafting. *J Hand Surg Am* 5:74–78, 1980.
250. Winters SC, Gelberman RH, Woo SL-Y, et al: The effects of multiple-strand suture methods on the strength and excursion of repaired intrasynovial flexor tendon: a biomechanical study in dogs. *J Hand Surg [Am]* 23:97–104, 1998.
251. Winters SC, Seiler JG, 3rd, Woo SL, et al: Suture methods for flexor tendon repair: a biomechanical analysis during the first six weeks following repair. *Ann Chir Main Memb Super* 16:229–234, 1997.
252. Woo SL, Gelberman RH, Cobb NG, et al: The importance of controlled passive mobilization on flexor tendon healing: a biomechanical study. *Acta Orthop Scand* 52:615–622, 1981.
253. Wray RC, Jr, Moucharafieh B, Weeks PM: Experimental study of the optimal time for tenolysis. *Plast Reconstr Surg* 61:184–189, 1978.
254. Wray RC, Weeks PM: Reconstruction of digital pulley. *Plast Reconstr Surg* 53:534–536, 1974.
255. Wrenn RN, Goldner JL, Markee JL: An experimental study of the effect of cortisone on the healing process and tensile strength of tendons. *J Bone Joint Surg Am* 36:588–601, 1954.
256. Xu NM, Brown PJ, Plate JF, et al: Fibrin glue augmentation for flexor tendon repair increases friction compared with epitendinous suture. *J Hand Surg [Am]* 38:2329–2334, 2013.
257. Yajima H, Inada Y, Shono M, et al: Radical forearm flap with vascularized tendons for hand reconstruction. *Plast Reconstr Surg* 98:328–333, 1996.
258. Zhao C, Hashimoto T, Kirk RL, et al: Resurfacing with chemically modified hyaluronic acid and lubricin for flexor tendon reconstruction. *J Orthop Res* 31:969–975, 2013.
259. Zhao C, Sun YL, Ikeda J, et al: Improvement of flexor tendon reconstruction with carbodiimide-derivatized hyaluronic acid and gelatin-modified intrasynovial allografts: study of a primary repair failure model. *J Bone Joint Surg Am* 92:2817–2828, 2010.
260. Zhao C, Zobitz ME, Sun YL, et al: Surface treatment with 5-fluorouracil after flexor tendon repair in a canine in vivo model. *J Bone Joint Surg Am* 91:2673–2682, 2009.

7

Fractures of the Metacarpals and Phalanges

Charles S. Day

Acknowledgment: I would like to acknowledge Dr. Peter Stern for all of his contributions to this chapter in this and previous editions of Green's Operative Hand Surgery.

Fractures of the metacarpals and phalanges are the most common fractures of the upper extremity, totaling approximately 600,000 in 1998.[22,69] Roughly 70% of all metacarpal and phalangeal fractures occur between the ages of 11 and 45.[112]

Until the early part of the 20th century, these fractures all were managed nonoperatively, and most continue to be managed successfully without surgery today. Most fractures are functionally stable either before or after closed reduction and fare well with protective splints and early mobilization.[99] Certain fractures require operative fixation (Box 7.1). Selection of the optimal treatment depends on many factors, including fracture location (articular versus extraarticular), fracture geometry (transverse, spiral or oblique, comminuted), deformity (angular, rotational, shortening), whether the fracture is open or closed, whether osseous and soft tissue injuries are associated, and intrinsic fracture stability. Additional considerations include the patient's age, occupation, and socioeconomic status; the presence of systemic illnesses; the surgeon's skill; and the patient's compliance. Despite the numerous treatment options, Swanson[116] aptly stated, "Hand fractures can be complicated by deformity from no treatment, stiffness from overtreatment, and both deformity and stiffness from poor treatment."

Over the past three decades, operative fixation of hand fractures has gained increasing popularity[11,114] for the following reasons:

1. Improved materials, implant designs, and instrumentation: Traditionally, implants have been made of 316L stainless steel. Although this metal is fully acceptable for fracture fixation, some surgeons prefer titanium, which has a modulus of elasticity that approximates bone. Self-tapping and miniature screws, with an outer diameter of 1 mm, are now available and in selected cases can be inserted percutaneously. Plates for the metacarpals and phalanges are low profile, easy to contour and cut, and available in various configurations.
2. Better understanding of the biomechanical principles of internal fixation
3. More demanding public expectations
4. Radiographic imaging: Cross-sectional imaging, particularly computed tomography (CT), permits multiplanar analysis of any fracture and may be useful in the assessment of articular fractures. In the operating room, portable minifluoroscopy units have been shown to reduce operating time substantially. Such units have eliminated much of the guesswork in fracture reduction, are helpful when inserting pins and screws (especially percutaneously), and allow assessment of fracture reduction and fixation in multiple planes. Radiation exposure is minimal.
5. Availability of specialists in hand surgery
6. Anesthesia: Many fractures, particularly of the phalanges, can be managed by local nerve blocks and sedation with monitored anesthesia care. In addition, a sterile forearm tourniquet with appropriate sedation can be comfortably inflated for 60 to 75 minutes.
7. Therapy: Hand therapists play an integral role in the operative and nonoperative management of hand fractures. Wound management, edema and scar control, fabrication of thermoplastic splints, supervision of therapeutic modalities, and structuring an exercise program all contribute to improved outcomes.

Prolonged immobilization should be avoided because of the risk of permanent stiffness; however, overly aggressive attempts at internal fixation may lead to soft tissue damage, tendon adhesions, infection, and the necessity for a secondary procedure for implant removal. Operative fixation must be used judiciously and with the expectation that the ultimate outcome will be as good as, and optimally better than, the outcome after nonoperative management.

METACARPAL FRACTURES (EXCLUDING THE THUMB)

Metacarpal Head Fractures

Fractures of the metacarpal head are rare and are usually articular. McElfresh and Dobyns[87] reported on 103 metacarpal head fractures. The injury involved the index metacarpal most frequently, presumably because it is a border digit, and its carpometacarpal (CMC) joint is relatively immobile. Fractures were classified into several categories (Box 7.2). Comminuted fractures occurred most commonly. Half of the comminuted fractures had loss of more than 45 degrees of flexion at the metacarpophalangeal (MP) joint. Articular defects may remodel with time; in contrast to weight-bearing joints, an incongruous MP joint may function satisfactorily with painless motion.

Articular fractures of the metacarpal head can also occur with complex dorsal MP dislocations. These fractures may need open reduction and internal fixation (ORIF) through a dorsal approach.

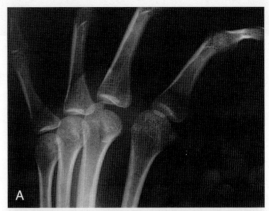

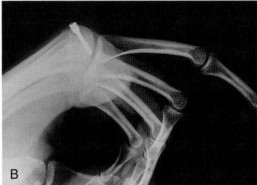

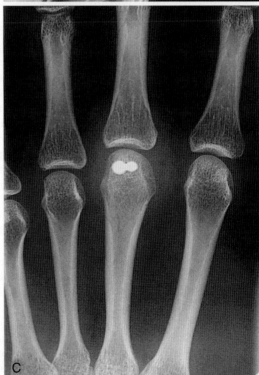

BOX 7.1 Indications for Fixation of Metacarpal and Phalangeal Fractures

Irreducible fractures
Malrotation (spiral and short oblique)
Articular fractures
Subcapital fractures (phalangeal)
Open fractures
Segmental bone loss
Polytrauma with hand fractures
Multiple hand or wrist fractures
Fractures with soft tissue injury (vessel, tendon, nerve, skin)
Reconstruction (i.e., osteotomy)

BOX 7.2 Types of Fractures of the Metacarpal Head

Epiphyseal fractures (all nondisplaced Salter-Harris type III fractures)
Ligamentous avulsions
Osteochondral shear fractures
Three-part fractures occurring in different planes (sagittal, coronal, axial)
Comminuted fractures
Boxer fractures with articular extension
Fractures with substance loss
Occult compression fractures with subsequent avascular necrosis

Radiographic evaluation requires three views: posteroanterior, lateral, and oblique. The lateral view is difficult to interpret because of the adjacent overlying metacarpal heads. The Brewerton view (MP joint flexed 65 degrees with the dorsum of the fingers lying flat on the x-ray plate and the tube angled 15 degrees in an ulnar-to-radial direction) profiles the articular contour better.

Treatment of these fractures must be individualized. Displaced ligament avulsion fractures and osteochondral fractures can be satisfactorily managed by ORIF (Figure 7.1).[85] Kumar and Satku[73] emphasized that small osteochondral fragments should not be discarded or independently fixed with hardware, but instead "trapped in place" by larger fragments. Two-part coronal, sagittal, and oblique articular fractures are best managed by ORIF with Kirschner wires or interfragmentary screws.[55,87] Shewring and Thomas[108] examined 19 patients with collateral ligament avulsion fractures from the metacarpal heads, including displaced and nondisplaced fractures, and found that the fractures are prone to symptomatic nonunion even when treated conservatively and may require subsequent surgery. Good results were seen for internal fixation of displaced fractures using a single lag screw through a dorsal approach. A 3-month delay in operative treatment of nondisplaced fractures can still lead to good radiographic and functional outcomes.

Occasionally, an injury occurs with partial loss of a metacarpal head. Boulas and colleagues[11] reported successful short-term results in five patients with osteochondral autografts taken from a similarly sized metatarsal.

A comminuted articular fracture is the most difficult fracture to treat. It is often associated with soft tissue injuries and metaphyseal impaction or bone loss. ORIF may be frustrating, if not impossible. Alternative forms of treatment include skel-

FIGURE 7.1 A, Displaced, articular sagittal slice fracture of middle finger metacarpal head. **B** and **C,** Postoperative posteroanterior (**B**) and lateral (**C**) views show anatomic reduction and fixation with headless screw. Full MP mobility was restored.

etal traction or joint arthroplasty. The most common complication of articular metacarpal head fractures is stiffness. This stiffness may result from extensor tendon adhesions, collateral ligament or dorsal capsular contracture, devascularization of small articular fragments, or articular incongruity.

❖ AUTHOR'S PREFERRED METHOD OF TREATMENT

Noncomminuted, displaced fractures that constitute more than 25% of the articular surface or exhibit more than 1 mm of articular step-off are treated operatively. We approach these fractures through a dorsal longitudinal incision that splits the extensor tendon to expose the joint. Two-part articular fractures are usually amenable to fixation with headless screws. Fixation with Kirschner wires, although easier, is less rigid and requires immobilization for 3 to 4 weeks.

Open fractures of a metacarpal head secondary to a clenched fist injury should be presumed to have oral contamination and are treated by formal irrigation and débridement. The wound is generally left open, and internal fixation, if necessary, is delayed until the wound shows no sign of infection.

Comminuted fractures are problematic. Direct fracture fixation with multiple Kirschner wires or cerclage wires can be effective in stabilizing tenuous reductions of these fractures. Unstable reductions may require immobilization for 2 to 3 weeks before range-of-motion exercises are begun. Often these joints need a delayed tenolysis and capsulotomy procedure to improve the functional outcome. If Kirschner wires or cerclage wires fail to stabilize the fracture and maintain the reduction, we prefer immobilization for 2 to 3 weeks with the MP joint flexed 70 degrees, followed by intensive range-of-motion exercises. Skeletal traction or external fixation may be needed if there are associated comminuted fractures of the adjacent base of the proximal phalanx. For open comminuted head fractures, especially fractures with bone loss, prosthetic arthroplasty is a reasonable alternative, but it should not be done under the following circumstances:

1. Fracture of the head of the index finger because shear stresses from pinch predictably result in implant failure
2. Inadequate soft tissue coverage
3. Excessive metacarpal bone loss because excessive shortening and instability occur

MP arthrodesis is a salvage procedure and should seldom be done acutely because of the risk of excessive shortening or nonunion.

Metacarpal Neck Fractures

Metacarpal neck fractures (boxer's fracture) are common and usually involve the ring and small metacarpals. "Boxer's fracture" is really a misnomer. Fractures of the fifth metacarpal neck are rarely seen in professional boxers; they are far more common in brawlers and in people who hit solid objects such as walls. The term *boxer's fracture* seems to be deeply ingrained in the orthopedic literature, however. These fractures invariably occur when a clenched MP joint strikes a solid object and angulates with its apex dorsal. Apex dorsal angulation occurs because (1) the impact occurs on the dorsum of the metacarpal head and causes comminution of the volar metacarpal neck, and (2) the intrinsic muscles that cross the MP joint lie volar to its axis of rotation and maintain a flexed metacarpal head posture.

Controversy exists regarding the optimal treatment of this fracture, which varies from nonoperative treatment to various internal fixation techniques. Nonunion is uncommon; however, malunion occasionally can be a problem. Patient complaints may include a loss of prominence of the metacarpal head,

diminished range of motion, a palpable metacarpal head in the palm, and, occasionally, rotatory malalignment.

When deciding on treatment, the following factors must be considered: (1) which metacarpal neck is fractured, (2) the degree of angulation, and (3) presence of a rotational deformity. The ring and small finger CMC joints have 20 to 30 degrees of mobility in the sagittal plane, whereas the index and middle CMC joints have less mobility. Angulation can be better compensated for in the ring and small fingers.

Although the reliability of measurement of angulation on plain films is low, it may be unimportant, because several surgeons believe that considerable angulation of a small finger metacarpal neck fracture is acceptable without compromising hand function. Hunter and Cowen[61] and Kuokkanen and colleagues[74] noted no significant disability with 70 degrees of angulation. Hunter and Cowen[61] did not attempt manipulation of fractures with less than 40 degrees of angulation and noted no increase in angulation during healing. Hansen and Hansen[53] prospectively compared casting, a functional brace, and an elastic bandage in patients with less than 60 degrees of angulation. They found no difference in patient satisfaction, but recommended a functional brace because patients became mobile faster and experienced less pain. Statius Muller and associates[113] prospectively treated 40 patients exhibiting angulation less than 70 degrees with either an ulnar gutter plaster cast for 3 weeks followed by mobilization or a pressure bandage for 1 week and immediate mobilization. They found that immediate mobilization yielded satisfied patients. There were no statistical differences with regard to range of motion, pain perception, and patients' satisfaction between these two treatments for boxer's fractures.

In a prospective series of 73 small finger metacarpal neck fractures, Lowdon[82] noted no relationship between the presence of symptoms and residual angulation. McKerrell and associates[88] studied two statistically comparable groups of patients with fifth metacarpal neck fractures treated conservatively and operatively. Failure to correct dorsal angulation was not associated with functional disability despite residual dorsal angulation in the nonoperative group. Tavassoli and coworkers[118] examined the difference between immobilizing the MP joint in extension or flexion for metacarpal neck fractures and found no significant functional and radiographic difference between the two casting groups. Because of the lack of compensatory CMC motion, there is almost universal agreement that residual angulation greater than 10 to 15 degrees in fractures of the index and middle metacarpal necks should not be accepted.[66]

Closed Reduction of Metacarpal Neck Fractures

Jahss[64] recognized that flexing the MP joint to 90 degrees relaxed the deforming intrinsic muscles and tightened the collateral ligaments, allowing the proximal phalanx to exert a dorsal force on the metacarpal head. He applied a cast in two parts: first immobilizing the proximal metacarpal fragment with the MP flexed, and subsequently pushing dorsally on the flexed proximal interphalangeal (PIP) joint while applying the second part. The Jahss maneuver (Figure 7.2) remains the best technique of closed reduction; however, fingers should never be immobilized in the "Jahss position" (MP and PIP joints flexed 90 degrees) because of the risk of skin necrosis over the dorsum of the PIP joint or permanent PIP stiffness.

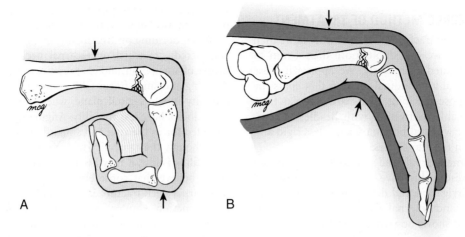

FIGURE 7.2 A, Jahss maneuver for reduction of metacarpal neck fracture. *Arrows* indicate direction of pressure application for fracture reduction. **B,** After reduction, fingers are held in intrinsic-plus (safe) position in ulnar gutter splint with molding as indicated by *arrows*.

With regard to cast immobilization, Hofmeister and colleagues[58] demonstrated that immobilization of the fifth metacarpal fracture in extension rather than flexion (as in the Jahss maneuver) did not affect fracture healing. However, the extension cast was faster to apply and showed greater improvement of angulation.

Maintenance of closed reduction by percutaneous longitudinal or crossed Kirschner pin fixation of the fractured metacarpal neck is a popular method of treatment for metacarpal neck and shaft fractures. Percutaneous transverse Kirschner wire fixation to the adjacent metacarpal has also been used for these fractures. Percutaneous fixation has the advantage of being minimally invasive, with a decreased likelihood of postoperative swelling and stiffness that may follow ORIF. The disadvantage is that it does not provide rigid fixation and requires some form of external immobilization for $2\frac{1}{2}$ to 3 weeks. Galanakis and associates[42] reported excellent functional and anatomic outcomes in treatment of closed metacarpal neck fractures by transverse percutaneous pinning, using two Kirschner wires distally and one proximally. Active flexion-extension exercises of the fingers were started at 1 week after surgery. These investigators reported no fixation failures. Transarticular Kirschner wire fixation may be also used to hold a reduction adequately.

Foucher[35] reported excellent results with the use of "bouquet" osteosynthesis in the management of displaced small finger metacarpal neck fractures (Figure 7.3). The fracture is reduced in closed fashion; a hole is made in the proximal ulnar metaphysis of the metacarpal; and three blunt prebent Kirschner wires are passed antegrade down the medullary canal, across the fracture, and into the subchondral bone of the metacarpal head. This antegrade fixation technique has the advantage of avoiding the fracture site, but it can be technically difficult, and pins can migrate either proximally or distally. Using a similar antegrade intramedullary Kirschner wire fixation technique, Kelsch and Ulrich[68] reported satisfactory 1-year radiographic and functional results in 35 patients. The fractures were immobilized for 2 to 6 weeks, depending on patient compliance.

As the antegrade intramedullary fixation technique has gained in popularity, multiple studies have compared this

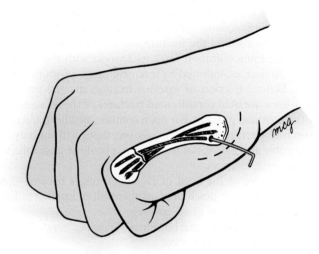

FIGURE 7.3 Technique for antegrade fixation of metacarpal neck fracture with multiple prebent Kirschner wires. Exposure of fracture site is avoided.

technique with traditional Kirschner wire fixation. In a retrospective study of 30 patients with displaced neck fractures of the fifth metacarpal that compared retrograde crossed pinning with antegrade intramedullary fixation, Schadel-Hopfner and colleagues[105] found significantly decreased motion of the MP joint in the retrograde cohort. There was decreased shortening of the metacarpal after antegrade fixation, suggesting that intramedullary fixation was preferable. When comparing antegrade intramedullary pinning with transverse Kirschner wire fixation, Wong and associates[134] found no statistical difference in the effectiveness, functional outcome, or complications, concluding that both methods are comparable in treating small finger metacarpal neck fractures.

Facca and colleagues[30] demonstrated no benefit of locked dorsal plate fixation and immediate motion when compared with intramedullary fixation. Both techniques had a high complication rate (>30%), and the authors concluded that the intramedullary pinning technique should be continued as the fixation standard for displaced fractures of the fifth metacarpal neck.

Open Reduction of Metacarpal Neck Fractures

Malunions of the fifth metacarpal neck rarely result in significant disability. Open reduction is occasionally indicated when manipulation fails to restore acceptable angulatory or rotational alignment. Following reduction, any number of techniques can stabilize the reduction adequately, including wires or tension band or miniplate fixation.

❖ AUTHOR'S PREFERRED METHOD OF TREATMENT

Most closed metacarpal neck fractures (especially of the ring and small fingers) should be treated nonoperatively. In the absence of pseudoclawing or rotational malalignment, metacarpal neck fractures produce minimal, if any, functional problems despite angulation on the lateral radiograph and shortening in the frontal projection. The term *pseudoclawing* refers to compensatory hyperextension of the MP joint and flexion of the PIP joint caused by excessive metacarpal neck flexion; the relative metacarpal shortening creates an imbalance between the longer extrinsic extensors and the short intrinsics. If pseudoclawing is not present on attempted digital extension, we prefer to use a functional brace. A forearm-based, dorsal-ulnar gutter splint using thermoplastic material is fabricated such that the wrist is extended 30 degrees, and the proximal phalanges of the ring and small fingers are splinted in approximately 70 degrees of flexion. "Buddy taping" is used to secure the digits to one another. Active range of motion is encouraged. The splint is worn for 2 weeks and is discontinued when pain has resolved.

Reduction of metacarpal neck fractures is clinically indicated when there is pseudoclawing or when there is a rotational deformity. After appropriate anesthesia, a closed manipulation of the metacarpal neck fracture is performed by the Jahss maneuver (see Figure 7.2). This maneuver is accomplished by flexing the MP and PIP joints to 90 degrees and exerting upward pressure through the flexed proximal phalanx and simultaneous downward pressure on the metacarpal shaft. Particular attention is paid to correcting any rotational deformity by using the flexed proximal phalanx as a crank. A forearm-based ulnar gutter plaster cast is applied and includes the adjacent, stable finger. The wrist is placed in 30 degrees of extension, the MP joints are maximally flexed, and the PIP joints are held extended (see Figure 7.2, *B*).

Radiographs are obtained to check the accuracy of reduction. Angulation greater than 15 degrees is unacceptable for fractures of the index and middle metacarpal necks. Angulation of 30 to 40 degrees is acceptable in the ring finger, and angulation of 50 or 60 degrees is acceptable in the small finger. Patients who use their hands extensively for gripping (e.g., professional athletes, carpenters) may generate discomfort, however, from the flexed metacarpal head of the small finger in their palm. In these patients, we would typically not accept flexion greater than 40 degrees. Immobilization usually can be discontinued after 12 to 14 days, and a program of active range of motion and intermittent splinting is initiated. The patient may return to sports and unrestricted activity at 4 to 6 weeks. Manipulation is not usually worth attempting if the fracture is older than 7 to 10 days.

In fresh metacarpal neck fractures, closed reduction is usually possible; however, reduction may be difficult to maintain because of volar comminution and intrinsic muscle pull. If an acceptable reduction cannot be maintained, we prefer percutaneously inserted crossed Kirschner wires (Figure 7.4) or antegrade intramedullary fixation under fluoroscopic guidance. After closed reduction, the pins are inserted into the nonarticular portion of the metacarpal head and drilled proximally into the metacarpal shaft. Alternatively, two pins can be percutaneously inserted in a transverse fashion from the fractured metacarpal head and fixed to the adjacent intact metacarpal (Figure 7.5). Care should be taken not to induce lateral translation of the fractured metacarpal head.

If open reduction is necessary, we prefer crossed Kirschner pins. Alternatively, a dorsal tension band wire with a supplemental Kirschner pin or a laterally applied minicondylar plate

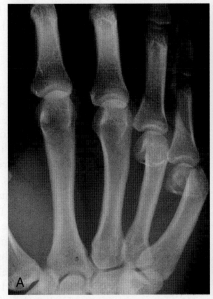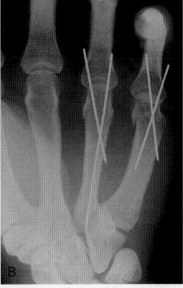

FIGURE 7.4 A, Severely displaced neck fractures of ring and small metacarpals. **B,** Closed reduction using Jahss maneuver and percutaneous crossed pins.

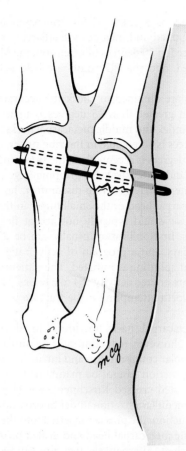

FIGURE 7.5 Percutaneous transverse pinning of displaced metacarpal neck fracture. After closed reduction, significantly angulated metacarpal neck fracture can be held with two percutaneous pins extending into adjacent intact metacarpal.

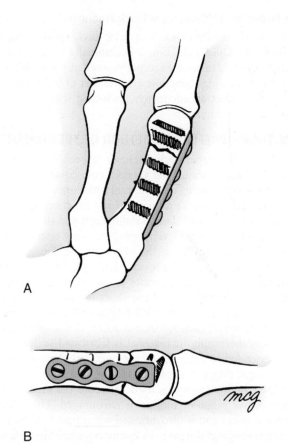

FIGURE 7.6 Laterally applied 2-mm minicondylar plate for stabilization of metacarpal neck fracture. **A,** Anteroposterior view. **B,** Lateral view.

(Figure 7.6) can be applied. Plate application requires more dissection, however, which may result in tendon adherence and MP stiffness, and should be used as a last resort. Plates require intracapsular positioning and may interfere with tendon gliding and collateral ligament function, all of which can adversely affect MP joint mobility.

Postoperatively, the operated digit is immobilized in an intrinsic-plus position for 5 to 7 days. Radiographs are taken to verify hardware position and fracture alignment, and, if satisfactory, protected active range-of-motion exercises are initiated after internal fixation. Immobilization in an ulnar gutter splint is usually maintained for 2 to 3 weeks after percutaneous pin fixation. If MP joint transarticular pins have been placed, immobilization is maintained until the pins are removed at 3 weeks postoperatively. Edema control with an elastic garment is also recommended.

Metacarpal Shaft Fractures

Metacarpal shaft fractures are broadly classified into three types: transverse, oblique/spiral, and comminuted. Each fracture type presents characteristic deformities that may lead to complications if unrecognized or improperly treated. Although most metacarpal fractures are readily diagnosed with standard biplanar views, oblique views may be helpful when there is clinical suspicion of a fracture.

Transverse fractures are usually produced by axial loading and angulate with the apex dorsal; the interosseous muscles are the deforming force. Dorsal angulation is better tolerated in the ring and small metacarpals. Dorsal angulation has several undesirable effects, however, as follows:

1. The metacarpal head becomes prominent in the palm and may cause pain on grasping.
2. There may be compensatory hyperextension at the MP joint that results in a secondary pseudoclaw deformity with digital extension.
3. Patients find the dorsal prominence aesthetically displeasing.
4. There is metacarpal shortening; if great enough, the intrinsic muscles may be unable to accommodate and are consequently weakened.

Although opinions vary, reduction generally is required for angulation greater than 30 degrees in the small finger, angulation greater than 20 degrees in the ring finger, and any angulation in the middle and index fingers. Likewise, opinions vary as to the degree of acceptable shortening. Most surgeons accept shortening of 2 to 5 mm, provided there is no pseudoclawing.

Oblique and spiral fractures are usually the result of torsional forces and can cause rotational malalignment. Malrotation is poorly tolerated and is difficult to assess on plain radiographs. It is best judged clinically by asking the patient to flex all the fingers *simultaneously*.[16] If scissoring or malrotation is present with composite digital flexion, open reduction should be considered.

CRITICAL POINTS *Operative Management of Boxer's Fractures*

Indications
- Angulation greater than 60 degrees (small finger) on lateral view
- Rotatory malalignment
- Associated fractures in fifth ray of hand
- Open fractures with associated soft tissue injury (excluding human bites)
- Presence of pseudoclawing

Preoperative Evaluation
- Inquire as to the mechanism of injury (e.g., human bite).
- Obtain anteroposterior and true lateral radiographs.
- Assess active range of motion, and check for presence of pseudoclawing (compensatory MP hyperextension and PIP flexion).

Pearls
- Less invasive techniques are preferred.
- Use closed reduction and percutaneous pinning.
- Many patients with this fracture are unreliable, and this may compromise outcome.

Technical Points
- Reduction is accomplished with the Jahss maneuver (see Figure 7.2).
- Under fluoroscopic guidance, insert two 0.9-mm retrograde crossed Kirschner wires from the lateral or dorsal (nonarticular) portion of the metacarpal head into the shaft (see Figure 7.4). The pins may cross the joint surface if necessary.
- Pins should exit through the dorsal metacarpal shaft.

Other Options
- Two transverse pins from small to intact ring metacarpal head (see Figure 7.5)
- "Bouquet" osteosynthesis: percutaneous antegrade insertion of prebent Kirschner wires from small finger metacarpal base into head (see Figure 7.3)
- ORIF with a lateral minicondylar plate (see Figure 7.6); least desirable treatment option because stiffness may occur

Postoperative Care
- Immobilize in ulnar gutter cast for 3 weeks.
- Begin protected active range-of-motion exercises stressing MP flexion. Extension of the MP joint may be impossible because of the location of the wires.
- Control edema with use of an elastic garment.

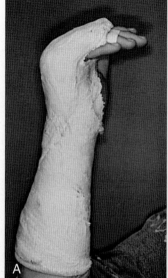 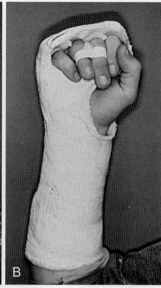

FIGURE 7.7 A and **B,** Clam-digger cast for metacarpal shaft fracture. Wrist is extended 30 degrees, MP joints are flexed 80 to 90 degrees, and IP joints are extended. Active range of motion is encouraged, and supplemental "buddy taping" can help control rotation.

Comminuted fractures are usually produced by direct impact, are often associated with soft tissue injury, and may produce shortening. There is considerable controversy regarding the amount of shortening that is acceptable. Regardless of fracture geometry, certain situations may influence the surgeon to perform operative fixation (eTable 7.1). These include the presence of multiple fractures (especially spiral and oblique); open fractures, especially with bone loss or concomitant soft tissue injury; and fractures in polytrauma victims who cannot cooperate or tolerate cast immobilization.

Closed Reduction and Plaster Immobilization
Closed reduction with plaster immobilization works well for most metacarpal shaft fractures, and overtreatment is to be avoided. Many metacarpal fractures are inherently stable and

may be treated with minimal or no immobilization. In athletes, Rettig and associates[103] reported that 82% of the fractures were minimally displaced or nondisplaced, and the average time lost from practice or competition was 13.7 days. Burkhalter[15] advocated closed treatment for fractures that showed no rotational malalignment on clinical examination. He used a short-arm cast with the wrist in 30 to 40 degrees of extension and added a dorsal extension block to hold the MP joints flexed 80 to 90 degrees and the interphalangeal (IP) joints extended. Composite active MP and IP flexion was initiated, and the cast was maintained for 4 weeks.

When the PIP joints are extended in this splint, the hand assumes the intrinsic-plus or clam-digger[132] position (Figure 7.7). This position limits joint contractures and maintains the intrinsics in a relaxed position. In a retrospective study examining 263 patients, Tavassoli and coworkers[118] compared three different casting techniques for metacarpal neck or shaft fractures and found that positioning the MP joints in flexion or extension or the IP joints free or immobilized resulted in no difference in motion, grip strength, or fracture alignment. They recommended immobilizing the MP joints in extension and allowing full motion of the IP joints. A recent study performed by Westbrook and colleagues[130] in Britain examined the functional and aesthetic outcomes of operative and nonoperative treatment of little finger metacarpal fractures in 262 patients. The authors concluded that up to 40 degrees of flexion of the metacarpal shaft can be safely managed nonoperatively, although the patient must be warned that a visible deformity is possible.

Closed Reduction and Percutaneous Pinning
Antegrade or retrograde percutaneous pinning can be successfully employed as above; if cut and bent outside the skin, short-term immobilization is necessary. Buried intramedullary Kirschner wire fixation for unstable metacarpal fractures has

been advocated and is greatly facilitated by the use of image intensification.[31,45] Using an awl, a cortical window is made at the ulnar base of the fifth metacarpal 1 cm distal to the CMC joint. Three or four prebent (≈30 degrees) 0.9-mm pins are inserted and buried within the medullary canal (Figure 7.8).

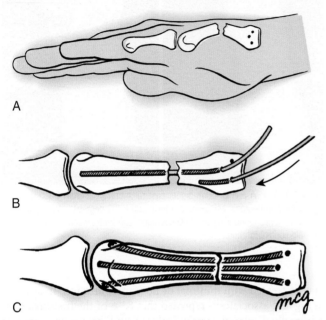

FIGURE 7.8 Intramedullary pins are inserted in antegrade fashion through multiple drill holes. Technique is facilitated by fluoroscopy. **A,** Fifth metacarpal shaft fracture. **B,** Antegrade pin insertion. **C,** Pins cut so that they are buried within medullary canal.

Open Reduction

A small percentage of metacarpal fractures were irreducible by closed manipulation or percutaneous pinning and require open reduction. Absolute indications for open reduction include the following:

1. Open fractures are associated with bone loss, contamination, or soft tissue injury.
2. Multiple fractures: In such cases, the stabilizing effect of the adjacent metacarpals is lost.
3. Unstable fractures: Fractures of the border metacarpals tend to be more unstable and more difficult to control than fractures of the central metacarpals because of the lack of support for soft tissue on both sides.
4. Malalignment: Rotational malalignment is unacceptable and is characteristically seen in spiral and oblique fractures. When correction of a rotational deformity by closed techniques or percutaneous pinning is unsatisfactory, open reduction is indicated.

Techniques of Open Reduction. See eTable 7.1.

Kirschner Wires. Kirschner wires may be used in nearly any fracture pattern (Figure 7.9). Pin fixation is technically easy, requires minimal dissection, and is universally available. Pin configurations can be either single or multiple and may be crossed,[29] transverse, longitudinal (intramedullary), or in combination. They can be used to supplement other forms of fracture fixation and can be used as a "bailout" if more complicated fixation has failed. Kirschner wires are not rigid; may loosen or even migrate; and, if improperly inserted, may distract fracture fragments. Pin track infections may develop secondary to skin irritation or loosening, and pin protrusion may make therapy and splinting awkward. Botte and associates[10] reviewed a series

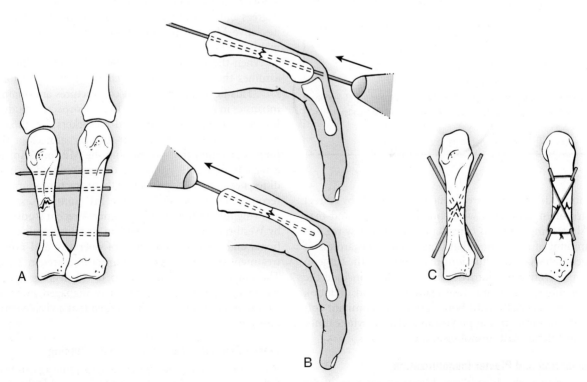

FIGURE 7.9 Techniques for Kirschner pin fixation of metacarpal shaft fractures. **A,** Transverse pins may be inserted percutaneously or open. **B,** Retrograde intramedullary fixation. Pin can be backed out so that they do not remain in MP joint. **C,** Crossed pins (*left*) and supplemental 25-gauge stainless steel wire (composite wiring) (*right*).

of 422 Kirschner wires placed in the hand and wrist and reported an 18% complication rate.

For longitudinal fixation, the pin can be drilled in antegrade fashion from the fractured end out the dorsal radial aspect of the metacarpal head. After reduction, the pin can be drilled in a retrograde fashion back down the shaft through the reduced fracture. Antegrade drilling of the proximal fragment through the fracture site is also possible with the wrist acutely flexed. Retrograde pins can also be introduced directly into the metacarpal head on either side of the extensor tendon and driven down the metacarpal shaft to engage subchondral bone at the CMC joint. Transarticular pins are generally bent outside the skin and left in place for 3 weeks. One or more supplemental transverse pins are generally recommended for unstable or transverse fractures in border digits when using this technique.

Composite (Tension Band) Wiring. Composite wiring for metacarpal fractures is a combination of Kirschner wires (0.035-inch or 0.045-inch diameter) and monofilament stainless steel wire (24-gauge or 26-gauge). The stainless steel wire is inserted as a tension band through a small transverse drill hole in the distal fragment and crossed around the Kirschner wires at the bone interface proximally (see Figure 7.9, *C*). Composite wiring provides additional stability and fracture compression and superior strength, stiffness, and approximation compared with crossed Kirschner wires alone. Little, if any, additional dissection is necessary. The technique is rigid enough to permit early motion. The technique is contraindicated when there is bone loss, comminution, or osteopenia.

Cerclage and Interosseous Wiring. Cerclage (circumferential) wiring with 24-gauge stainless steel wire can be successfully employed for oblique and spiral metacarpal shaft fractures (see Figure 7.38), but the technique is not widely popular. The technique was originally described to include scoring of the cortical bone with a side-cutting bur so that wire migration would not occur.[80] Al-Qattan and Al-Lazzam[3] showed that cerclage wire fixation can be sufficient without scoring of bone or finger immobilization for midshaft oblique or spiral fractures in 19 cases.

Gingrass and colleagues[44] achieved six excellent or good results in seven metacarpal fractures treated by double 26-gauge interosseous wires placed in a dorsal-volar direction. A single Kirschner pin was added in five of seven cases to augment stability. These authors suggest that interosseous wiring done without supplemental Kirschner pin fixation is generally unsuitable for metacarpal shaft fractures because wire loosening and subsequent loss of reduction are real possibilities. In contrast, Al-Qattan[2] reported treatment of 36 metacarpal shaft fractures with interosseous loop wire fixation alone and concluded that interosseous wiring without Kirschner wire fixation is rigid enough for immediate postoperative finger mobilization. Of 36 patients, 34 regained full range of motion. It is prudent to use supplementary Kirschner wires if the fracture is comminuted or if bone is missing.

Intramedullary Fixation. Open reduction and intramedullary fixation are applicable for transverse fractures, are easy to perform, and allow early active motion (Figure 7.10). There are no exposed pins, and secondary removal is unnecessary. In 1981, Grundberg[51] reported one nonunion in 27 metacarpals treated by open reduction and permanent intramedullary fixation with a large Steinmann pin. Potential disadvantages include rotational instability, pin migration, and occasional fracture distraction. The technique is not recommended for spiral or long oblique fractures.

The technique involves determining the diameter of the medullary canal using a smooth Steinmann pin and drilling one size larger. Next, the pin is introduced into the proximal fragment (blunt end first to avoid penetration of the subchondral

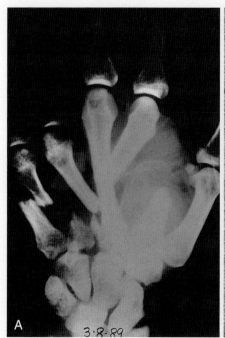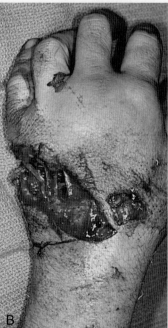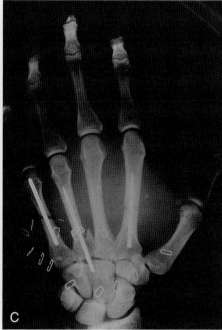

FIGURE 7.10 Intramedullary fixation. **A,** Displaced open metacarpal shaft fractures. **B,** Clinical appearance of dorsum of hand. **C,** Intramedullary Steinmann pin fixation. Pin in ring metacarpal extends into carpus for more secure fixation.

bone) and cut so that it protrudes 1.5 cm. The fracture is distracted, and the pin is introduced into the distal fragment. Finally, the fracture is impacted to achieve rotational stability.

When segmental bone loss is present and the soft tissue sleeve is largely intact, locked intramedullary fixation with rods[5,45] or plates with bone grafting is recommended.[5] In this situation, the rod or plate acts as an internal spacer while the defect is bridged with corticocancellous autogenous bone graft. One or more supplementary Kirschner wires may be necessary.

Interfragmentary Compression Screws. Interfragmentary compression screws provide stable fixation and are primarily indicated for long oblique and spiral shaft fractures (Figure 7.11). Interfragmentary screw fixation is stable enough to allow early active range of motion. To ensure success, the fracture length must be a minimum of twice the bone diameter. The fracture is reduced by manipulating it into alignment and holding the reduction with provisional Kirschner wires or a fracture reduction forceps, followed by placement of two or three interfragmentary compression screws (see Figure 7.11). A dorsal miniplate can be applied to neutralize the fracture if stability of the fracture is questionable.

To optimally resist axial and torsion loading, the screw should be placed in a plane bisecting the fracture plane and longitudinal axis. In large patients, at least two 2.7-mm screws are necessary, and in smaller individuals three 2.4-mm or 2-mm screws are necessary. To avoid fragmentation, the screw hole should be a minimum of two screw diameters from the fracture margin.[56]

Interfragmentary screw fixation (2.7-mm) of a metacarpal fracture involves six sequential steps (see Figure 7.11). There is little tolerance for technical error with this technique; if the screw is inserted through the near cortex and is misdirected such that it strikes the endosteal surface of the far cortex, the fracture is distracted, and the reduction lost. Any resistance to screw tightening should alert the surgeon to stop and redirect the screw.

Plate Fixation. Dorsal metacarpal plating with or without an interfragmentary screw provides more stable fixation than crossed Kirschner wires, an interosseous wire loop alone, or an

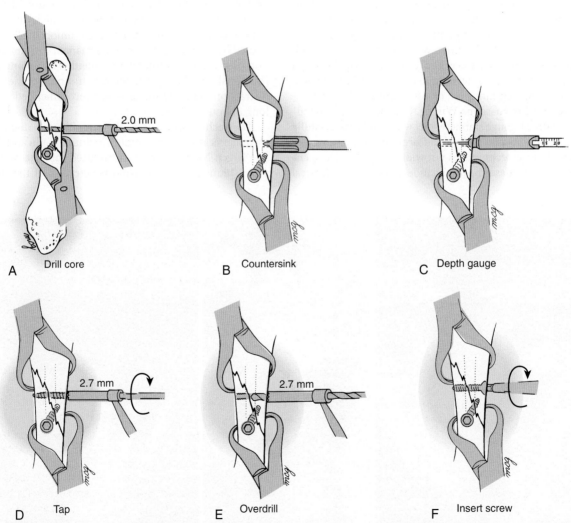

FIGURE 7.11 Fixation of spiral metacarpal fracture with 2.7-mm lag screws. **A,** A 2-mm bicortical hole is drilled. **B,** Near hole is countersunk to accept truncated screw head and distribute compression. **C,** Screw length is determined with depth gauge. **D,** Precision use of the 2.7-mm tap is critical, as failure to engage the far cortical drill hole can disrupt fracture reduction. Most modern screws are self-tapping. **E,** The near (gliding) hole is overdrilled with a 2.7-mm drill bit. **F,** Insertion of screw, engaging far hole and compressing the fracture.

interosseous wire with a Kirschner pin. The amount of strength required for stable fixation in the clinical setting has not been determined; fixation should be customized to the particular fracture.

Page and Stern[93] reported multiple complications of metacarpal fracture plating, however, including malunion, nonunion, and stiffness (articular and tendon adhesions). Complications were more frequent when there was associated bone loss, soft tissue injury, and open fractures. Fusetti and colleagues[41] assessed 81 patients treated with plate fixation and reported complications in 28 (35%). Complications included difficulty with fracture healing (15%), stiffness (10%), plate loosening or breakage (8%), complex regional pain syndrome, and infection. In another study, Fusetti and Della Santa[40] reported significant correlation between a transverse fracture pattern and nonunions when treated with plate fixation.

Most implants are made of either stainless steel or titanium. Although titanium is more expensive, some advantages of titanium include generally lower incidence of corrosion and allergic reactions, ease of contouring, and a modulus of elasticity that approaches that of bone.[83] Some studies have shown, however, that use of titanium plates may still lead to significant corrosion and release of metal debris.[70] No clinical difference in outcomes has been shown with the use of titanium implants. Great care must be taken when using titanium implants; screws may break, especially when being removed, and plates can break if excessively contoured before application.

Successful use of small titanium maxillofacial plates has been reported.[20] Screws are self-tapping, and diameters range from 0.8 to 1.7 mm. Because the plates are low profile ($\approx$1 mm), the periosteum can often be closed over the plate to reduce adhesion formation. Fracture stabilization was adequate to allow early mobilization with a low incidence (3%) of hardware failure or plate breakage in a series of 36 patients treated for metacarpal and phalangeal fractures after acute and complex hand injury.[20]

Bioabsorbable plates and screws are not widely used in the United States, and clear advantages of such plates over metal implants have not been demonstrated.

External Fixation. The advantages of external fixation were enumerated by Schuind and coworkers[107]: "There is respect of bone biology." Fracture fragments are not stripped of periosteal blood supply and further devascularized. External fixators are adjustable, and there is adequate stability to permit early mobilization. When there has been concomitant soft tissue injury, external fixation permits ready access to the wound for débridement and for reconstruction of tendons, nerves, and blood vessels.[4]

Hastings[54] identified numerous complications of external fixation, including pin track infection, osteomyelitis, fracture through pin holes after removal, neurovascular injury during insertion, overdistraction with subsequent nonunion, loss of reduction, impairment of tendon gliding and motion, and interference with adjacent digits by the fixator. In weighing the advantages and disadvantages of external fixation, the technique is primarily indicated for severe fractures when anatomic reconstitution of the skeleton is not feasible. Examples include highly comminuted open shaft fractures with or without bone loss; displaced, comminuted articular fractures; and fractures with injury or loss of soft tissue structures. In addition, external

fixation can be used to stabilize septic nonunions after débridement.[4]

❖ AUTHOR'S PREFERRED METHOD OF TREATMENT

Most metacarpal shaft fractures can be managed nonoperatively. Stable fractures that do not require reduction can be treated in a clam-digger cast or thermoplastic splint until the fracture is clinically nontender. The fractured finger is "buddy taped" to an adjacent finger, and immediate finger flexion is initiated.

Transverse shaft fractures are usually easy to reduce, but maintenance of acceptable alignment may be difficult. To achieve reduction, a palmarly directed load is applied to the dorsal apex at the fracture site with a dorsally directed force to the flexed MP joint (see Figure 7.2). A well-molded, forearm-based cast extending to the IP joints and holding the MP joints in 60 degrees of flexion is applied. Special attention must be paid to ensure satisfactory rotational alignment. The fracture is monitored with radiographic imaging at weekly intervals, and guarded active range-of-motion exercises can be initiated at 3 to 4 weeks. Marked swelling, which is often present in acute metacarpal shaft fractures, does not preclude manipulation and casting. The cast should be changed at 5 to 7 days when the swelling subsides.

Closed manipulation and percutaneous treatment are indicated when the fracture can be reduced but cannot be maintained in plaster or when concomitant soft tissue injury requires dressing changes and inspection. Fluoroscopy is invaluable to confirm fracture reduction and assist in placement of fixation devices. Reduction can sometimes be facilitated by placing a small incision over the fracture and inserting an elevator to manipulate the fragments. I pin transverse fractures of the fifth or fourth metacarpal to the neighboring intact metacarpal using two parallel transverse pins into the distal fragment and one through the proximal fragment (see Figure 7.9, A).

Open reduction is indicated for transverse shaft fractures that either are significantly displaced or have residual angulation of more than 10 degrees in the second and third metacarpals, 20 to 30 degrees in the ring metacarpal, and 30 to 40 degrees in the small finger metacarpal. ORIF using Kirschner wires or interfragmentary screws is indicated for most spiral and oblique fractures, particularly if there is evidence of a rotational deformity on physical examination, because fracture reduction is difficult to maintain by closed techniques. ORIF is nearly always indicated when there are multiple metacarpal fractures or when the fracture is open and associated with soft tissue injury or bone loss.

Fracture exposure is accomplished through a longitudinal incision just to one side of the extensor tendon overlying the involved metacarpal. If all four metacarpals require reduction, two longitudinal incisions are used: one between the fourth and fifth metacarpals and one between the second and third metacarpals. Care is taken to preserve cutaneous nerves and the paratenon surrounding the extensor tendons. Occasionally, one of the juncturae tendinum requires division for better fracture visualization; if this is necessary, the junctura should be repaired after fixation. The fracture ends are exposed, and fracture hematoma is removed. Reduction is accomplished by applying longitudinal traction and is maintained with reduction clamps.

Fixation options include Kirschner wires, composite wiring, an intramedullary rod, multiple interfragmentary screws, or a plate and screws. The choice of implant is dictated by the fracture configuration and experience of the surgeon (see eTable 7.1).

Kirschner wire fixation can be used for nearly all fracture configurations. Kirschner wire fixation alone is not rigid and may require immobilization postoperatively. If wire placement or fracture alignment is initially unacceptable, reinsertion is a simple matter. Multiple passes with the wires should be avoided, however, because this may lead to thermal necrosis of bone and increase the incidence of pin track infection. In addition, wires may loosen or distract a fracture, and pin track infection may necessitate premature removal.

I prefer K-wire fixation for isolated short oblique and transverse fractures and when possible supplement the pins with composite wiring to increase rigidity of fixation.[49] The pins, when placed percutaneously, are left in place for 3.5 to 4 weeks, and protected range of motion is initiated at the first postoperative visit (5 to 7 days after fixation). Patients should be instructed that if there is drainage, early pin removal may be necessary.

I find intramedullary fixation using precut Steinmann pins or commercially available rods particularly useful for multiple open transverse shaft fractures (see Figure 7.10). In this situation, there may be injury to the intrinsic muscles that allows the fracture to be easily distracted, facilitating pin insertion. Intramedullary fixation is easy and takes little time, but rotational stability may be a problem, particularly if the fracture ends fail to interdigitate. If the adjacent metacarpal is not fractured, a transverse wire can be added to control rotation.

Spiral and long oblique fractures are well suited for interfragmentary fixation. The fracture length should be at least twice, and preferably three times, the diameter of the bone at the level of the fracture. Reduction is achieved by anatomically interdigitating the proximal and distal apex of the fracture into its corresponding fragment under direct visualization. The reduction is held with two bone clamps, and the screws are inserted. Fixation may be achieved by using two 2.7-mm screws or three 2-mm or 2.4-mm screws. The diameter of the bone and configuration of the fracture may dictate mixing screws of different diameters in the same fracture.

I generally reserve plate and screw fixation for complex situations such as open fractures, multiple metacarpal shaft fractures, or when there is a combination of diaphyseal bony loss or comminution associated with significant soft tissue injury (Figure 7.12). Successful plate application is technically gratifying, provides stable fixation, and maintains length when there has been comminution or bone loss. Plate application is demanding, however, and there is no margin for error. Application requires considerable soft tissue mobilization, and the plates are bulky. Removal is often necessary, and a fracture can occur through a screw hole or at the "original" fracture site. I prefer a 2-mm or 2.4-mm plate that allows screw fixation of at least four cortices, proximal and distal to the fracture, to ensure

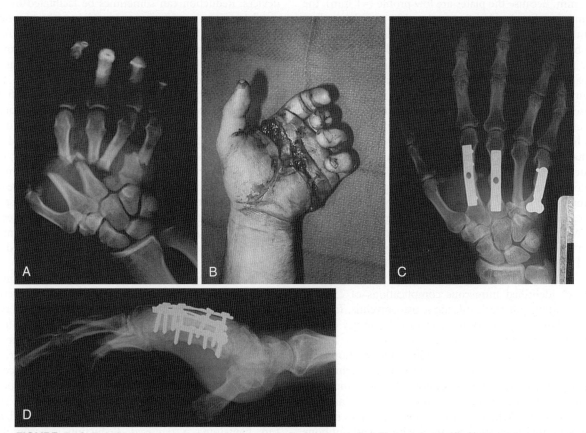

FIGURE 7.12 Plate fixation for metacarpal shaft fractures. **A,** Shaft fractures of all four metacarpals. **B,** Fractures were open, and revascularization was required. **C,** Anteroposterior radiograph showing healed fractures. Plate fixation provided stable framework for microvascular repairs. **D,** Lateral view.

stable fixation. Supplemental fixation with an interfragmentary screw (for transverse and short oblique fractures) placed either through a hole in the plate or obliquely across the fracture significantly enhances fracture stability. Larger 2.7-mm locking plates are not routinely indicated. Such plates may be indicated in osteopenic bone or for reconstruction of nonunions or malunions. Plate fixation is undesirable if the fracture cannot be covered by local soft tissue or flaps. In such situations, I prefer external fixation.

Whenever possible, after ORIF the periosteum is approximated with an absorbable suture. A forearm-based plaster splint with bulky dressing is applied for 4 to 7 days. Assuming stable reduction, active range of motion is initiated. The wrist is splinted in a slightly extended position. Restoration of full MP flexion may be difficult because of edema, intrinsic muscle injury, and subsequent MP collateral ligament contracture. To maximize MP flexion, elastic garments are worn for edema control, and the IP joints are splinted in extension during MP flexion exercises.

Hardware removal depends on the type of implant. Kirschner wires may be removed 3 to 6 weeks after fixation. The AO-ASIF group recommends screw and plate removal approximately 6 months after fixation. Despite the aforementioned admonitions, I do not routinely remove plates. If the plate is perceived as bulky or is irritating, or if there are restrictive adhesions and a tenolysis and capsulotomy procedure is indicated, I remove the plate. Patients should be informed that refracture may occur after plate removal.

Expected Outcomes: Metacarpal Shaft Fractures

Most metacarpal shaft fractures are inherently stable and can be treated conservatively with acceptable functional outcomes. In a comparison study of three casting techniques, no difference was found in motion, grip strength, or fracture alignment between the treatments.[116] Open reduction and internal fixation can be accomplished using numerous techniques, including Kirschner wire fixation, composite and cerclage wiring, intramedullary fixation, screw fixation, and plate fixation. Kirschner wire fixation has been reported to result in an 18% complication rate.[10] Outcomes of cerclage wiring (although more technically demanding) have generally been positive, with full range of motion reported in 34 of 36 patients.[2] Intramedullary fixation allows for early active motion, with only one nonunion in 27 fractures reported in a single cohort study.[51] Screw fixation also typically results in successful outcomes, especially in long oblique and spiral shaft fractures. Plate fixation shows good to excellent outcomes, but has been associated with a complication rate of 35%.[41] Cerclage wiring, screw fixation, and plate fixation are typically rigid enough to allow for early range of motion. Generally, the least invasive method that can reliably restore and maintain anatomic alignment of metacarpal shaft fractures is preferable for successful outcomes.

Segmental Metacarpal Loss

Restoration of metacarpal stability and function after segmental bone loss is a challenge. This situation occurs after an open injury and is nearly always associated with varying degrees of soft tissue injury or loss. Restoration of hand function is usually staged and begins with thorough débridement of devitalized tissue. A discussion of the timing of the soft tissue

reconstruction is beyond the scope of this chapter, but it should not begin until a stable osseous framework has been achieved.

There are two philosophies regarding the management of acute metacarpal bone loss. The traditional viewpoint advocates maintaining metacarpal length with transverse intermetacarpal Kirschner wires or external fixation devices, with soft tissue coverage performed as a primary or delayed procedure. Bone grafting is performed only after joint motion is regained and healed wounds have matured. External fixation has been used successfully, but little information has been provided to help surgeons choose the most appropriate construct for a specific injury.

Freeland and Jabaley[36,37] believed that the best time to restore osseous stability with a bone graft and internal fixation is within the first 10 days of injury ("the golden period of wound repair"). Initial wound care consists of débridement and temporary skeletal stabilization. The wound is reinspected 3 to 7 days later, and if it is judged to be ready for closure or coverage, definitive fracture stabilization, bone grafting, and skin flap coverage (if required) are performed. Calkins and colleagues[18] reported satisfactory functional results in 9 of 10 patients who had traumatic segmental bone defects of the hand. Corticocancellous grafts were inserted within 2½ weeks of injury. The soft tissue wounds were left open, there were no cases of infection, and all grafts went on to incorporate. The authors believed that stable fixation combined with bone grafting promoted optimal return of function by allowing for early mobilization to minimize chronic swelling, pain, tendon adhesions, and articular stiffness.

Along similar lines, Gonzalez and colleagues[46] reported excellent results in the treatment of 64 metacarpal fractures secondary to low-velocity gunshot wounds treated with early débridement and stabilization (1 to 7 days). Fracture fixation was performed with an intramedullary rod, and the bone void was filled with autogenous iliac graft. There were no deep infections. The average range of motion at the MP joint was 65 degrees.

Reconstitution of osseous stability involves two steps:
1. Provisional stabilization (Figures 7.13 and 7.14): Maintenance of metacarpal length can be accomplished by numerous techniques, including transfixation pins,[76] external fixation,[4,36] methyl methacrylate spacers,[79] and combinations of these techniques.
2. Bone grafting with or without internal fixation (Figure 7.15): Most defects can be bridged with autogenous iliac corticocancellous graft. If more than one metacarpal has segmental loss, a single curved iliac crest graft designed to fit the defects in all metacarpals is useful.

❖ AUTHOR'S PREFERRED METHOD OF TREATMENT: Segmental Loss

Generally, when there is metacarpal bone loss, there are associated soft tissue defects and contamination. After thorough débridement, osseous stability is achieved with an external fixator. Additional débridements are carried out over the next 2 to 5 days until the wound is surgically clean. At that time, a corticocancellous or cancellous bone graft is harvested from the iliac crest and fashioned to fit into the defect. Stabilization is accomplished with an appropriately contoured dorsal plate.

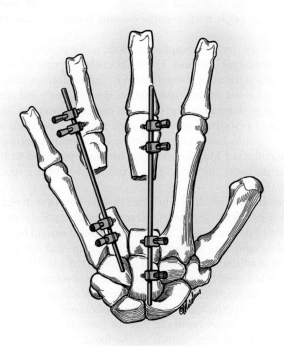

FIGURE 7.13 External fixator is ideal treatment for metacarpal bone loss. Pins may be placed in carpus or phalanges when necessary. (Copyright Elizabeth Martin.)

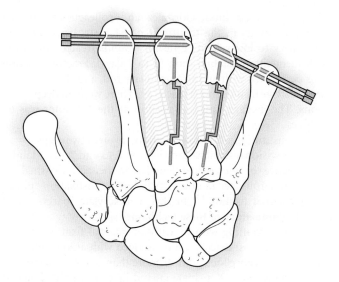

FIGURE 7.14 Transfixation pins and spacer wires are useful as temporary treatment for metacarpal bone loss.

When there is bone loss from multiple metacarpals, I prefer to use a monoblock of corticocancellous or pure cancellous graft, rather than individual metacarpal bone reconstruction. Soft tissue coverage is obtained with a regional, distant, or free flap. I prefer staged tendon reconstruction in which silicone rods are inserted at the time of flap coverage and replaced later with free tendon grafts.

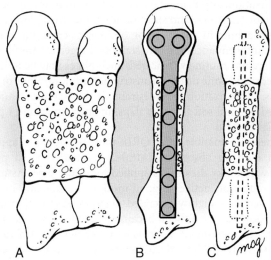

FIGURE 7.15 Techniques of corticocancellous or cancellous bone graft after metacarpal loss. **A,** A block of iliac crest graft is especially useful when there is bone loss in more than one metacarpal. **B,** Corticocancellous graft and plate fixation. **C,** Littler's technique using corticocancellous dowel and intramedullary Kirschner pin.

Metacarpal Base Fractures and Carpometacarpal Fracture-Dislocations

Avulsion Fractures of the Second and Third Metacarpal Bases

Isolated articular fractures of the base of the second and third metacarpals are rare because of the lack of motion in these joints, and there is no consensus regarding optimal treatment. These fractures are usually the result of a fall on a flexed wrist. Avulsion fractures from the dorsal base of the index or middle metacarpals have been successfully managed operatively and nonoperatively. Justification for surgical reattachment includes restoration of the integrity of the extensor carpi radialis longus or brevis, reconstitution of the articular surface of the CMC joint, and elimination of a potentially irritating fragment of dorsal bone.

Fracture-Dislocations of the Ring Finger Carpometacarpal Joint

Ring finger CMC joint dislocations are uncommon, may be associated with a metacarpal fracture, and may be missed at presentation. Isolated ring finger metacarpal fractures should raise the possibility of an associated CMC joint injury and prompt careful examination of various radiographic views. Computed tomography may be helpful to better delineate articular fragments.

Fracture-Dislocations of the Small Finger Carpometacarpal Joint

Articular fractures of the hamate–fifth metacarpal joint are common and are usually associated with proximal and dorsal subluxation of the metacarpal. The hamate articulates with the ring and small metacarpals by two concave facets separated by a ridge. The base of the fifth metacarpal consists of a concave-convex facet that articulates with the hamate and a flat radial facet that articulates with the fourth metacarpal base. Dorsal and palmar intermetacarpal ligaments and an interosseous ligament stabilize the intermetacarpal joint. The injury results from a longitudinally directed force along the fifth metacarpal resulting in proximal and dorsal subluxation of the metacarpal base. The displacement is accentuated by the pull of the extensor carpi ulnaris.

Because the extent of the injury is frequently missed on routine radiographs, Bora and Didizian[7] recommended an anteroposterior view with the forearm pronated 30 degrees from the fully supinated position. A 30-degree pronated lateral view is also helpful to profile the subluxated metacarpal. For difficult visualization or assessment of articular comminution, CT scan is occasionally warranted.

There is no consensus regarding optimal treatment of these fractures. Options run the gamut from closed reduction and cast immobilization to ORIF. Bora and Didizian[7] found that weakness of grip was the major functional disability resulting from inadequate reduction or lost reduction. These authors recommended closed reduction and percutaneous pin fixation of the fifth metacarpal to the fourth metacarpal or carpus for maintenance of reduction.

Petrie and Lamb[94a] treated 14 fracture-dislocations of the fifth metacarpal–hamate joint by immediate, unrestricted motion and reviewed them at 4.5 years. Despite persistent metacarpal shortening, incongruity in the articular surface, and widening of the joint, only one patient had enough pain to affect work. These investigators believed that the case for surgical treatment was not strong because arthrodesis of the joint could always be performed for persistent pain. Kjaer-Petersen and colleagues[71] reported that regardless of the method of treatment (closed, percutaneous, or open), 19 of 50 (38%) patients had some symptoms at a median follow-up of 4.3 years. They believed that restoration of the articular surface should be the goal of treatment. Cain and associates[17] noted that fracture-dislocations of the fourth and fifth CMC joints, in association with comminuted dorsal hamate fractures or coronal shear

fractures through the hamate, were particularly unstable, and ORIF was uniformly necessary. For single large hamate shear fractures, screw fixation to the body serves to treat the fracture and the dislocation.

Multiple Carpometacarpal Dislocations

Multiple CMC dislocations are high-energy injuries that nearly always require ORIF.[78,116] Lawlis and Gunther[78] reported on 20 patients, 14 of whom had multiple CMC dislocations. Closed reduction was uniformly unsuccessful because of redislocation or subluxation, and reduction with Kirschner pin fixation was recommended. Open reduction is necessary only if closed reduction is unsuccessful. At 6.5 years' follow-up, patients with isolated second and third CMC dislocations or concomitant ulnar nerve injury did poorly. Lawlis and Gunther[78] indicated that it was unclear why these patients did poorly compared with patients with dislocations of all four CMC joints. It is possible that these patients had fractures that were unreduced or had recurrent subluxation. Clendenin and Smith[23] reported relief of symptomatic arthritis of the hamate–fifth metacarpal joint when treated by arthrodesis using an iliac crest bone graft.

❖ AUTHOR'S PREFERRED METHOD OF TREATMENT

Fracture-dislocations of the fifth CMC joint are inherently unstable, and closed reduction and cast immobilization can be risky. Redislocation may not be appreciated because radiographic imaging is difficult as a result of bony overlap and plaster artifact. For unstable fracture-dislocations of the fifth CMC joint, we prefer closed reduction and percutaneous pinning. With appropriate anesthesia, longitudinal traction is applied, and palmar pressure is exerted on the base of the fifth metacarpal. Under image intensification, the fifth metacarpal shaft is pinned into the fourth metacarpal. A second pin can be obliquely directed across the fifth metacarpal–hamate joint (Figure 7.16). When multiple fragments or comminution exists, preoperative CT may be useful.

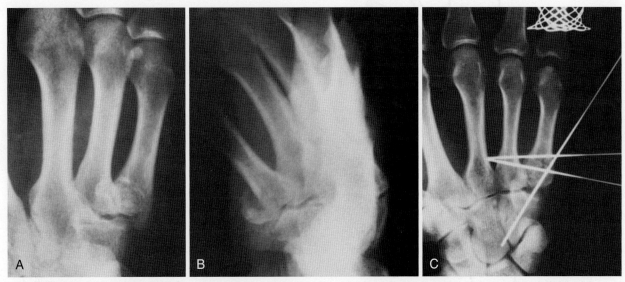

FIGURE 7.16 A, Articular fracture of base of fifth metacarpal with proximal and dorsal subluxation of carpometacarpal (CMC) joint. **B,** Oblique view taken with hand pronated 30 degrees from fully supinated position shows extent of articular injury. **C,** Reduction was obtained by longitudinal traction and lateral pressure on displaced bone. Firm fixation with transarticular pin and transfixation pins into adjacent metacarpal allowed early motion.

If ORIF is elected, a dorsal ulnar incision is used to visualize the joint. Care must be taken to protect the dorsal sensory branch of the ulnar nerve. The joint is débrided of loose fracture fragments, the articular surface is reduced, and reduction is maintained with multiple Kirschner wires or small screws. Articular comminution may be so extensive that ORIF is impossible; in such cases, percutaneous reduction of the dislocated metacarpal may be a safer option. Postoperatively, a forearm-based ulnar gutter splint is applied. Digital motion is started at 10 to 14 days, and the internal fixation pins are removed at 6 weeks.

For multiple CMC joint dislocations, closed reduction and percutaneous pinning or ORIF is nearly always indicated. The dislocated joints are well visualized through a dorsal longitudinal incision. Reduction is usually simple and can be maintained with Kirschner wires extending from the metacarpals into the carpus.

If a fracture-dislocation of the fifth CMC joint is seen more than 3 weeks after the injury, we prefer to accept the alignment. If symptomatic arthritis develops, secondary arthrodesis can be performed.

For patients with symptomatic CMC joint arthritis, the arthrodesis is accomplished by removing the articular surfaces down to subchondral cancellous bone, and fixation is accomplished with Kirschner wires extending from the hamate to the fifth metacarpal shaft. If graft is needed for the arthrodesis, we prefer using a corticocancellous slot graft from the iliac crest (Figure 7.17). Fusion of this joint does not significantly compromise hand function.

Complications of Metacarpal Fractures
Malunion

Extraarticular malunions may be angulatory, usually as a result of a malunited transverse shaft fracture; rotational, as a result

of a spiral or oblique fracture; or shortened, as a result of a crush injury with bone loss. After crush injuries or open fractures, there may be shortening and associated soft tissue problems, such as tendon adhesions, poor skin coverage, and neurologic deficit. In such cases, one may elect to perform an osteotomy and correct the soft tissue problem simultaneously.

Dorsal Angulation. Metacarpal malunion after a transverse fracture results in apex dorsal angulation in the sagittal plane. Healing of second and third metacarpals with moderate to severe angulation is particularly bothersome cosmetically (pseudoclawing) and functionally (i.e., prominent metacarpal head in the palm resulting in painful and weak grip). With the use of plates and screws, corrective osteotomies have union rates that approach 100% and result in a high degree of clinical satisfaction for isolated malunions and fractures that involve an adjacent joint or extensive soft tissue injury, or both.[122] Correction can be accomplished through either an opening or a closing wedge osteotomy. A closing wedge osteotomy (Figure 7.18) is simpler[47] than an opening wedge osteotomy, and geometrically little, if any, shortening results because length is gained by correction of the angulation. Preoperatively, the size of the wedge is calculated by using a template, and the volar periosteum is left intact to act as a hinge intraoperatively. We prefer fixation with a 2.4-mm or 2.7-mm dorsal plate and supplemental cancellous bone graft. In malunions with metacarpal osteoporosis or insufficient bone stock to achieve at least four cortices of screw fixation proximally and distally, a locking plate should be considered.

If the metacarpal is appreciably shortened because of bone loss, an opening wedge osteotomy (Figure 7.19) with a trapezoid interpositional iliac crest bone graft is preferable. Stable fixation to allow early motion is accomplished with a dorsal plate.

Malrotation. Rotational malunion of a metacarpal results in overlapping of the affected finger over an adjacent finger (scissoring). It usually results from a malunited spiral or oblique fracture. The cosmetic deformity is often marked, and grip

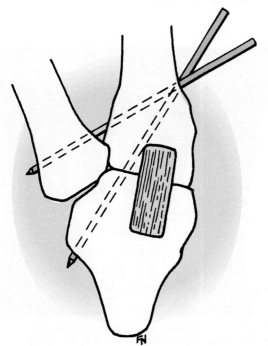

FIGURE 7.17 Method of arthrodesis of fifth carpometacarpal (CMC) joint with inlay graft and pins.

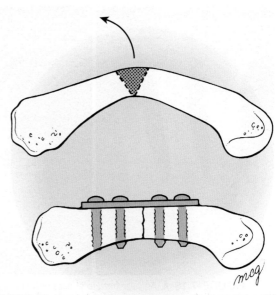

FIGURE 7.18 Metacarpal closing wedge osteotomy for malunion. Volar periosteum is left intact, a precisely calculated triangular wedge is removed, and fixation is provided with dorsal plate.

is impaired. Weckesser[128] advocated a corrective osteotomy through the base and was able to correct 25 degrees in each direction. Fixation was accomplished with Kirschner wires. Gross and Gelberman[50] noted that the maximal correction obtained in fresh cadaveric metacarpal osteotomies was 18 to 19 degrees for the index, long, and ring fingers and 20 to 30 degrees for the small finger. The transverse metacarpal ligament limited the maximal rotation obtained, but the orientation of the MP joint did not limit its motion.

We have been pleased with the results achieved when the osteotomy is performed through the metaphyseal base with the technique (Figure 7.20) described by Weckesser.[128] After rotational correction, the osteotomy is transfixed with a provisional Kirschner pin. Correction is assessed by observing the tenodesis effect of passive wrist flexion and extension, evaluating the plane of the fingernails, and checking for alignment of the fingertips to the scaphoid tuberosity. Final fixation is performed with multiple pins. This fixation technique is appealing because it is simple and forgiving, and union usually occurs rapidly. Alternatively, fixation can be secured with a T-plate, L-plate, or minicondylar plate. This procedure is technically more demanding, and care must be taken not to lose correction when the plate is being applied and to ensure that there is good contact between the bony surfaces.

Articular Malunions. Articular malunions are rarely amenable to corrective osteotomy. If the fracture line can be visualized, and bone quality is satisfactory, osteotomy with reconstitution of the articular surface is the optimal treatment.

Osteomyelitis

Osteomyelitis occurring after metacarpal fracture fixation is uncommon, and treatment must be individualized. In a review of osteomyelitis of the tubular bones of the hand, delay in treatment of more than 6 months or performance of more than three procedures was associated with a very high amputation rate.[102] For metacarpal shaft osteomyelitis, the following is recommended:

1. Obtain cultures, remove loose implants, and generously débride bone and soft tissue. Stabilize the proximal and distal segments with an external fixator. The void can be filled with a block of antibiotic-impregnated polymethyl methacrylate, which also provides a spacer for insertion of a future bone graft.
2. Appropriate systemic antibiotics are recommended for at least 4 to 6 weeks. Débride the wound repeatedly until it is surgically clean, and allow wound closure by secondary intention.
3. When sepsis has cleared, insert cancellous or corticocancellous bone graft, preferably with plate and screw fixation.

Nonunion

Nonunion after closed metacarpal fractures is uncommon. Hypertrophic nonunions are rare in the hand; most are atrophic and hypovascular. Recommended treatment in these cases

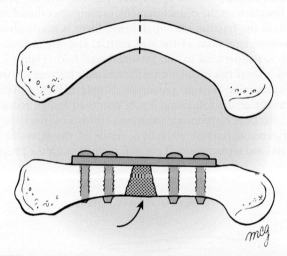

FIGURE 7.19 If there is significant metacarpal shortening, opening wedge osteotomy and plate fixation would reconstitute metacarpal length, although a bone graft would be required.

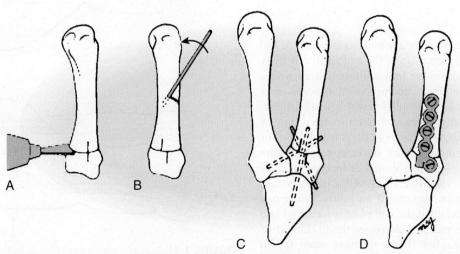

FIGURE 7.20 Metacarpal osteotomy for rotational malunion. **A,** Before osteotomy, a longitudinal mark is placed on metaphysis with osteotome. Osteotomy is made with oscillating saw perpendicular to mark. **B,** Kirschner pin in the shaft acts as joystick for correction. **C** and **D,** Fixation is accomplished with multiple Kirschner wires (**C**) or plate (**D**).

requires resection of the pseudarthrosis, bone grafting, and stable internal fixation.

Nonunions usually occur after bone loss, osteomyelitis, inadequate immobilization, or poor fixation (i.e., a metacarpal fracture pinned in distraction).[67] Jupiter and associates[67] reported 25 nonunions in 23 patients, and advised surgical intervention at 4 months. Nine nonunions occurred in metacarpals, most of which had previously been fixed with Kirschner wires. Six of nine nonunions were treated, and all healed after bone grafting. Three were fixed with a plate and screws, two were fixed by Kirschner wires, and one had no fixation. Rigid internal fixation was preferred because it enabled early active motion and permitted concomitant procedures such as capsulotomy and tenolysis.

Other Complications

Complications are the result of the fracture itself, treatment of the fracture, or a combination of both. Tendon adhesions occurring after closed metacarpal fractures are uncommon. Usually, adhesions follow tendon lacerations or crush injuries and are most frequently seen between the extensor tendons and the underlying bone. Initial treatment should consist of therapy and include dynamic MP flexion splinting. If initial treatment fails, tenolysis with or without MP capsulotomy is indicated.

Intrinsic muscle dysfunction can occur under the following circumstances: loss of innervation, loss of muscle substance, or secondary to contracture. Significant loss of intrinsic muscle substance or denervation can result in clawing, and treatment may require tendon transfers. Intrinsic contractures may also occur, especially after a closed crushing injury associated with an unrecognized hand compartment syndrome, and may require intrinsic releases to improve function (see Chapter 32).

PHALANGEAL FRACTURES

Fractures of the Distal Phalanx

Distal phalangeal fractures are the most commonly encountered fracture in the hand. Distal phalangeal fractures are classified as tuft fractures, shaft fractures, or articular injuries (eTable 7.2).

Tuft Fractures

Tuft fractures usually occur secondary to a crushing injury and are often associated with laceration of the nail matrix or pulp, or both. Closed tuft fractures are frequently associated with a painful subungual hematoma. Decompression provides dramatic pain relief and can be accomplished with a small drill bit, heated paper clip, or battery-powered electrocautery unit. A short period of immobilization (10 to 14 days) is indicated for symptomatic relief. Comminuted tuft fractures rarely require internal fixation. Instead, attention should be focused on carefully approximating associated lacerations of the pulp and nail matrix. The nail should be removed if an injury to the nail matrix is suspected, especially if the nail plate is fractured and displaced. Repair of the nail bed decreases the likelihood of subsequent nail abnormalities. These fractures often fail to unite but are invariably stabilized by a fibrous union. If the nail plate is intentionally perforated to decompress a hematoma or removed to perform a nail bed repair, a closed fracture is

theoretically converted to an open fracture, and a short course of oral antibiotic therapy can be considered.

Shaft Fractures

There are two types of shaft fractures: transverse and longitudinal. Nondisplaced transverse fractures are sufficiently stabilized by the surrounding soft tissue and do not require internal fixation. Displaced transverse fractures may be open and are often associated with a transverse laceration of the overlying nail matrix. Longitudinal Kirschner pin fixation and nail matrix repair should be considered.

Epiphyseal Fractures of the Distal Phalanx

Epiphyseal injuries of the distal phalanx result from hyperflexion. Failure to recognize and treat this injury, especially in a toddler, can result in a foreshortened digit that has decreased range of motion at the distal interphalangeal (DIP) joint.[127] The injury may be manifested as an open mallet deformity and mistaken for DIP joint dislocation. The terminal tendon is attached to the proximal epiphyseal fragment and the profundus insertion on the distal fragment, causing apex dorsal angulation at the fracture site. In children, there is nearly always a transverse laceration of the nail matrix, and the avulsed nail plate lies superficial to the proximal nail fold (Figure 7.21). There is some risk in discarding the nail plate because it is useful in maintaining fracture reduction. Simple reduction without treatment of the soft tissue injury results in loss of reduction and infection. Appropriate treatment consists of irrigation and débridement, fracture reduction, repair of the lacerated nail matrix, and replacement of the nail plate beneath the proximal

SEYMOUR FRACTURE

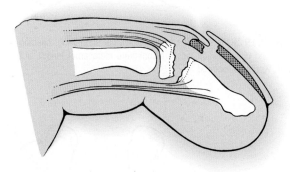

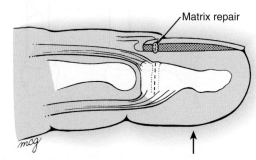

FIGURE 7.21 Open epiphyseal fracture of distal phalanx in a child. *Top,* Note matrix disruption (*stippled*); nail plate has been avulsed and is dorsal to proximal nail fold. *Bottom,* Reduction requires matrix repair and replacement of nail plate beneath proximal nail fold.

nail fold to act as a stent in maintaining the reduction. Failure to recognize the injury or inadequate primary treatment may result in acute osteomyelitis or septic arthritis, or both. Postoperatively, a splint is applied to hold the distal fragment in extension.

Complications of Distal Phalangeal Fractures

Symptomatic nonunion of distal phalangeal fractures occurs occasionally. Itoh and coworkers[63] reported six patients with nonunions of the waist of the distal phalanx successfully treated with crossed Kirschner wires and bone graft with exposure through a palmar midline approach. Late presentation of a pediatric epiphyseal fracture is characterized by a dorsal bump secondary to continued growth of the dorsally displaced epiphysis.

Fractures of the Middle and Proximal Phalanges

Phalangeal fractures that are stable and nondisplaced can be effectively managed by "buddy taping" or splint immobilization. Improper treatment of unstable fractures often leads to stiffness and deformity.

In studies by Strickland and colleagues,[115] several factors had a deleterious effect on ultimate digital mobility (eBox 7.1). These investigators pointed out that if an extraarticular fracture occurred in persons in the first 2 decades of life, 88% of the mobility was restored; however, in persons in the sixth and seventh decades, less than 60% of total active motion was restored. In addition, older patients are more likely to have chronic diseases or underlying osteoarthritis that could contribute to residual stiffness. Uncooperative and noncompliant patients must be identified. These patients require heavy-duty splints and casts that are not removable, and if surgery is performed, rigid fracture fixation is recommended.

Articular injury has a major influence on the ultimate result. Because these joints are not subjected to heavy loads, stability and alignment are likely more important than articular congruency in determining outcome. There is a low incidence of late symptomatic osteoarthritis in conservatively treated articular fractures; articular reconstitution over time is often observed in the small joints of the hand. Likewise, comminuted fractures, fractures associated with bone loss, and unstable fractures with considerable deformity are also prone to residual disability regardless of the method of treatment.

Injury to the soft tissue sleeve, usually the result of a crushing injury, may severely compromise digital mobility.[62,99] Duncan and coworkers[28] reviewed 140 open fractures at an average time past surgery of 17 months. They found that there was a direct correlation between the severity of the soft tissue injury and the final range of motion at follow-up. In addition, they found that fractures located in flexor tendon zone 2 had the worst prognosis. Huffaker and coworkers[60] concluded that flexor tendon injuries have a more serious effect on recovery of digital mobility than do extensor tendon injuries, and prolonged immobilization has a detrimental influence. Strickland and colleagues[115] pointed out that if immobilization after a phalangeal fracture was less than 4 weeks, final active motion was 80% of normal. If immobilization exceeded 4 weeks, total active motion declined to 66% of normal. A successful outcome depends on selection of the appropriate treatment and must be tailored to the individual patient and fracture.

It is convenient to divide phalangeal fractures into articular and nonarticular injuries. Articular fractures include condylar fractures; comminuted fractures; dorsal, volar, or lateral base fractures; fracture-dislocations; and shaft fractures extending into the joint. Nonarticular fractures include fractures of the neck, shaft, or base.

Articular Fractures of the Phalanges

Condylar Fractures. Condylar fractures can be classified into three categories. Type I fractures consist of stable fractures without displacement; type II fractures include unicondylar, unstable fractures; and type III fractures are bicondylar or comminuted fractures. In addition to standard anteroposterior and lateral radiographs, oblique radiographs are mandatory to visualize the fracture geometry properly and assess stability and displacement better.

Weiss and Hastings[129] developed a useful classification for unicondylar fractures of the proximal phalanx (Figure 7.22) and made two important observations. First, even initially nondisplaced fractures are inherently unstable (Figure 7.23). Nonoperative management warrants extremely close follow-up. Second, fixation with a *single* Kirschner pin is inadequate. Displaced unicondylar fractures usually require ORIF.[55,65] The two most popular techniques of fixation are (1) Kirschner wires and (2) a lag screw. Of these, multiple Kirschner wires provided the best final range of motion at the PIP joint. Postoperatively, a 20- to 30-degree PIP extensor lag was frequent. Some correction of this problem can be obtained by dynamic extension splinting.

Bicondylar fractures and comminuted articular fractures can be very difficult to fix. Buchler and Fischer used a minicondylar plate.[12] Regardless of the fixation method, PIP joint stiffness frequently occurs.

Other Fractures of the Head of the Phalanx. Displaced collateral ligament avulsion fractures of the head of the proximal phalanx may be symptomatic if nonunion or fibrous union results. Open reduction or repair of these injuries should be done if the injuries are associated with lateral instability.

Extensively comminuted phalangeal head fractures may preclude satisfactory open reduction. These fractures are frequently associated with considerable damage to the soft tissue sleeve and are best treated nonoperatively. Treatment must be individualized.

Dorsal, Volar, or Lateral Base Fractures. Avulsion fractures of the dorsal base of the middle phalanx represent detachment of the insertion of the central tendon and are usually the result of an anterior PIP joint dislocation. If the avulsed fragment is displaced more than 2 mm, accurate reduction and internal or percutaneous pin fixation are necessary to prevent extensor lag and subsequent boutonnière deformity (Figure 7.24).

Fractures of the lateral volar base of the proximal or middle phalanx usually represent collateral ligament avulsion injuries. Minimally displaced lateral corner fractures that do not compromise joint stability or result in an incongruous articular surface can be treated by splinting for comfort measures only and accompanied by early range of motion. Significantly displaced lateral corner fractures may compromise joint stability and may need ORIF. Kuhn and colleagues[72] recommended a volar approach for internal fixation of proximal phalangeal base fractures. They reported 11 avulsion fractures; at final follow-up,

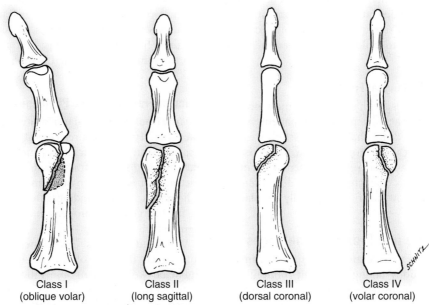

Class I	Class II	Class III	Class IV
(oblique volar)	(long sagittal)	(dorsal coronal)	(volar coronal)

FIGURE 7.22 Weiss-Hastings classification of unicondylar fractures of proximal phalanx. These fractures are nearly all unstable and nearly always require operative fixation. (From Weiss APC, Hastings HH: Distal unicondylar fractures of the proximal phalanx, *J Hand Surg [Am]* 18:594–599, 1993.)

CRITICAL POINTS *Operative Management of Unicondylar Fractures of the Proximal Phalanx*

Indication
- Any displaced condylar fracture

Preoperative Evaluation
- Evaluate for angulation or malrotation with flexion.
- Obtain an anteroposterior radiograph to assess articular step-off.
- Check a lateral radiograph to see if the fractured condyle is displaced palmarly.
- Check an oblique radiograph for orientation of the fracture line.

Pearls
- This is a highly unstable fracture; err on the side of operative intervention.
- Internal fixation *always* requires two screws or two Kirschner wires, or one of each.

Technical Points
- Closed reduction by application of longitudinal traction is worth a try.
- If reduction is achieved, provisionally hold it with one or two towel clips.
- Confirm reduction with fluoroscopy.
- Percutaneously fix the fracture with two Kirschner wires (0.7 mm or 0.9 mm).
- If closed reduction fails, proceed to open reduction.
- Make a dorsal longitudinal incision on the side of the fracture.
- Enter the PIP joint by incising between the lateral band and central tendon.

- Take care not to detach the central tendon.
- Expose the condylar fragment from its apex proximally to its articular surface distally.
- When mobilizing the condylar fragment, take care not to detach the collateral ligament.
- Reduction must be anatomic at the articular surface and proximally so that the condylar apex keys into the phalanx.
- Provisionally maintain reduction with a Kirschner pin or drill bit to be replaced later by a screw.
- Fix with two Kirschner wires (0.7 mm or 0.9 mm) or two (lag) screws (2 mm or 1.5 mm [1.3 mm]).
- Confirm reduction with radiographs (three views).

Pitfalls
- One screw or pin may result in loss of reduction from either rotation or loosening.
- Detachment of the collateral ligament may produce instability or osteonecrosis of the condylar fragment.

Postoperative Care
- At 5 to 7 days, initiate active range of motion.
- Splint the PIP joint in full extension when not exercising.
- Remove Kirschner wires at 3 to 4 weeks.

---

all digits had full range of motion and a stable MP joint. To expose the fracture, the A1 and proximal portion of the A2 pulley are completely divided, and the flexor tendons are retracted to expose the volar plate (Figure 7.25). The volar plate is longitudinally split in its midline and detached distally from the proximal phalanx on the side of the fracture. The avulsed fragment is now well visualized and reduced. Fixation is accomplished with either 1.5-mm screws or Kirschner wires. The volar plate is repaired, and the digit is splinted in partial flexion. With secure screw fixation, protected active range of motion is initiated at the first postoperative visit.

Hastings and Carroll[55] brought attention to lateral plateau fractures of the base of the middle phalanx. They postulated that these are compression injuries that result in articular depression and metaphyseal bony compaction. Open reduction with cancellous bone grafting and tension band fixation demonstrates satisfactory results.[133]

Comminuted articular fractures, particularly fractures at the base of the middle phalanx, have been termed *pilon fractures*. The fracture is the result of an axial load that causes central articular depression and variable splay of the articular margins. Stern[114] reported 20 injuries treated in three ways: splinting, time. Hamilton and coworkers[52] evaluated nine patients who were retrospectively identified as having been treated with open reduction and screw fixation for unstable dorsal fracture–dislocations to the PIP joint. Their results indicated that PIP range of motion is usually compromised, and they advised careful selection of candidates for ORIF screw fixation.

Because of the unpredictable outcome associated with treatment of this injury, various dynamic external fixation devices have been developed.[55] These devices are hinged and span the PIP joint to allow early protected range of motion, while maintaining reduction of the joint. Majumder and associates[85] reported their experience with the "pins and rubber traction system," originally introduced by Slade and colleagues,[109] for the treatment of articular base fractures in 14 patients. The traction system was left in for 4 to 7 weeks, and range-of-motion exercises began early. Majumder and associates[85] found an average of 74 degrees at the PIP joint and total active motion of 196 degrees.

As an alternative to dynamic distraction-fixation, ORIF with an autologous "hemihamate" osteoarticular graft can be performed for PIP joint fracture-dislocations in which more than 50% of the base of the middle phalanx is fractured with an intact dorsal cortex. Williams and associates[131] achieved satisfactory results after treating 13 patients with PIP joint fracture-dislocations using a hemihamate autograft and screw fixation. Motion was initiated approximately 1 week after surgery.

Shaft Fractures Involving the Joint. A long spiral fracture of the proximal (and sometimes middle) phalanx may project into the retrocondylar space of the IP joint and can be a mechanical block to flexion. ORIF is usually necessary. If the fracture is unreduced and heals with a residual spike that blocks PIP flexion, the bony projection can be removed to improve flexion.

❖ AUTHOR'S PREFERRED METHOD OF TREATMENT: Articular Fractures

Nondisplaced unicondylar fractures are potentially unstable. Immobilization in a splint is risky, and displacement should be anticipated. If nonsurgical treatment is selected, careful and frequent radiographic follow-up is mandatory to avoid a malunion with articular incongruity.

Displaced unicondylar fractures of the proximal phalanx are best managed operatively (Figure 7.27). The fracture is exposed through either a dorsal radial or dorsal ulnar longitudinal incision. The joint is entered between the central tendon and lateral band. The central tendon should not be detached from its insertion into the dorsal base of the middle phalanx. Fracture hematoma is removed, with care taken not to detach the condyle from its attachment to the collateral ligament. Under direct visualization, the fracture is anatomically reduced with a bone tenaculum, and the reduction is confirmed fluoroscopically. The condylar fragment is fixed with two parallel Kirschner wires (0.028-inch or 0.035-inch) drilled through the fragment into the intact bone. Interfragmentary screw fixation with two 1.5-mm or 1.3-mm screws can be used if the fracture fragment is two and a half to three times the external diameter of the screw. The dorsal extensor apparatus is reapproximated. Postoperatively, early active motion is initiated, and the PIP joint is splinted in extension to avoid extensor lag. Kirschner wires are removed at 3 to 4 weeks. Screws do not require removal unless they are symptomatic.

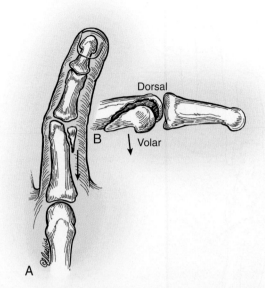

FIGURE 7.23 Inherent instability of a unicondylar fracture. **A,** Anteroposterior appearance of a condylar fracture. Note the articular step-off. **B,** Lateral view. Note volar displacement of the condylar fragment. (Copyright Elizabeth Martin.)

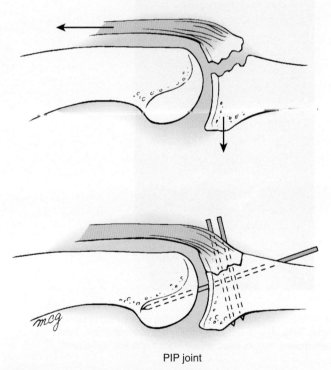

PIP joint

FIGURE 7.24 Anterior PIP fracture-dislocation. *Top,* Avulsion fracture from dorsal base of middle phalanx results in anterior displacement of middle phalanx. *Bottom,* Open reduction with Kirschner wires and transarticular pinning (for 3 weeks) is necessary for fracture and joint reduction.

traction through the middle phalanx, and open reduction. Splinting resulted in considerable stiffness. Skeletal traction through the middle phalanx (Figure 7.26) and ORIF had similar results. Anatomic articular restoration was not accomplished in any case, and no patient regained full mobility. Regardless of the treatment, there was significant articular remolding over

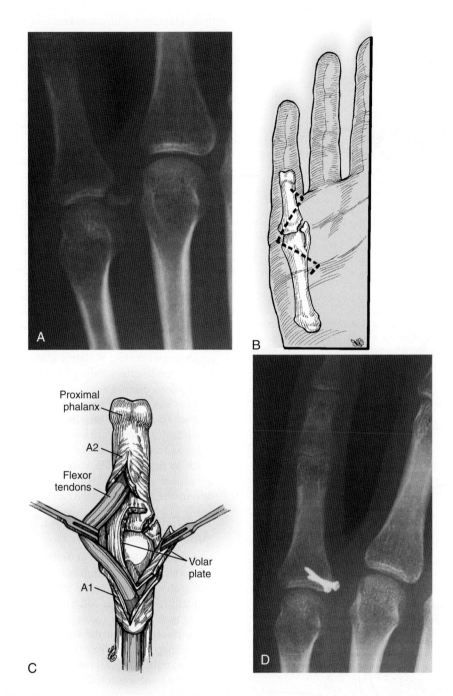

FIGURE 7.25 A, Radiograph showing displaced avulsion fracture from radial base of proximal phalanx. **B,** Zigzag incision used to expose fracture. **C,** A1 pulley (not shown) and proximal part of A2 pulley are divided. Volar plate is split longitudinally and detached distally from its insertion on base of proximal phalanx to expose fracture. **D,** Radiograph showing fracture reduction and fixation with two mini-screws. (**B** and **C,** Copyright Elizabeth Martin.)

Although ORIF is the standard of care for the management of condylar fractures, closed reduction and percutaneous pin fixation can also be considered within 5 days from the injury (Figure 7.28). Using a mini C-arm, a pin is placed into the condylar fragment and used as a joystick to manipulate the fragment into its anatomic position. Finger trap traction is sometimes helpful to assist in reduction and to free the surgeon's hands for fragment manipulation and fixation. The reduction is provisionally maintained with a bone tenaculum, and the reduction is verified radiographically. Fixation is secured with two to three appropriately sized Kirschner wires. Small cannulated screws are also available for percutaneous management of these fractures. This technique has the advantage of minimizing soft tissue damage, but can be tedious and does not allow direct visualization of the fracture to verify anatomic reduction. One must also be cautious that the joystick pin and the bone tenaculum do not inadvertently fragment the fractured condyle.

Bicondylar fractures of the proximal phalangeal head are nearly always displaced and often comminuted. Anatomic

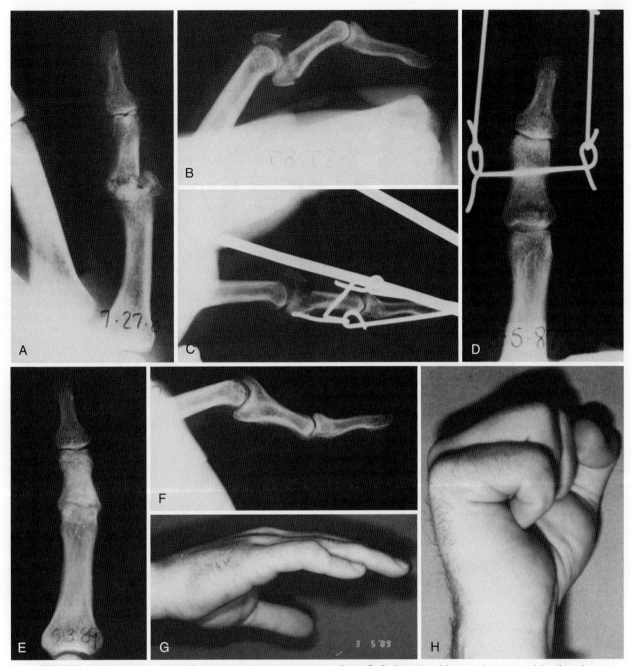

FIGURE 7.26 Pilon fracture of PIP joint treated by skeletal traction. **A** and **B,** Radiographs of fracture show severe joint disruption. **C** and **D,** Radiographs after 7 days of skeletal traction. Note correction of palmar subluxation but persistent displacement of dorsal fragment. **E** and **F,** There has been consolidation of fracture fragments and articular remodeling 21 months after injury. **G** and **H,** At 21 months' follow-up, there is excellent flexion. There is persistent PIP joint swelling and loss of extension, however. (From Stern PJ, Roman RJ, Kiefhaber TR, et al: Pilon fractures of the proximal interphalangeal joint, *J Hand Surg [Am]* 16:844–850, 1991.)

restoration of articular congruency usually cannot be accomplished by closed manipulation. Open reduction using the same approach as for unicondylar fractures is advised (Figure 7.29). First, the two condyles are reduced and fixed to each other with either a screw or Kirschner wires. Next, the head fragment is secured to the shaft in a similar fashion. Postoperatively, range of motion within 3 weeks is encouraged; however, residual stiffness or extensor lag, or both, are common. When there is significant comminution, open reduction may be frustrating, and restoration of the articular surface may be impossible. In such circumstances, skeletal traction or external fixation can be applied for 3½ to 4 weeks. Fracture consolidation can be anticipated, and some articular remodeling occurs. Restoration of full motion is unlikely. Primary arthrodesis is unpredictable and may result in excessive shortening.

Untreated displaced (>2 mm) fractures of the dorsal base of the middle phalanx can lead to a boutonnière deformity. Open reduction through a dorsal approach between the central tendon and the lateral band is recommended. Fixation can be accomplished with two small Kirschner wires or miniscrews. The fixation should be protected with a transarticular Kirschner pin for 3 weeks.

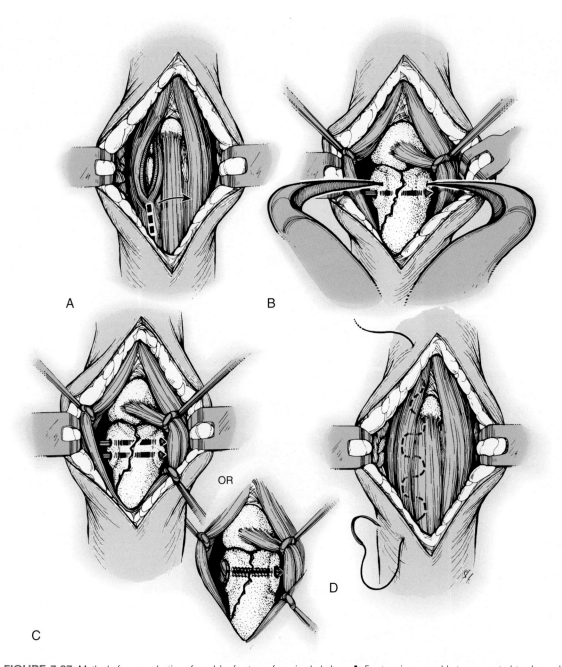

FIGURE 7.27 Method of open reduction of condylar fracture of proximal phalanx. **A,** Fracture is exposed between central tendon and lateral band. Care must be taken not to disrupt insertion of central slip from middle phalanx and origin of collateral ligament from condylar fragment. **B,** Fracture is reduced and held with towel clips (specially designed cannulated clamp may also be used). **C,** Internal fixation is accomplished with two transverse Kirschner wires or small screws. **D,** Central slip and lateral band are reapproximated with running 4-0 suture. (Copyright Elizabeth Martin.)

Displaced fractures of the base of the proximal phalanx require open reduction. I prefer a volar approach in which the A1 and proximal portion of the A2 pulley are divided followed by splitting the volar plate longitudinally. The fracture is easily visualized, and anatomic reduction can usually be achieved and preferably held with small screws. Isolated fractures of the base of the middle phalanx are unusual. There can be an impaction fracture to the articular surface, however, resulting in a depressed plateau type of fracture. These fractures typically need ORIF, with or without subchondral bone grafting.[133]

Pilon fractures of the base of the middle phalanx involve articular impaction and splay of the dorsal/palmar and radial/ulnar margins of the bone. I do not believe that ORIF is possible, and autograft replacement (hemihamate autograft) is precluded because the dorsal cortex is usually fractured. I prefer dynamic distraction fixation for these injuries combined with supervised range of motion of the IP joints. PIP joint arthritis or stiffness can be addressed surgically at a later time.

Because loss of DIP joint mobility is less disabling, bicondylar fractures of the head of the middle phalanx can sometimes

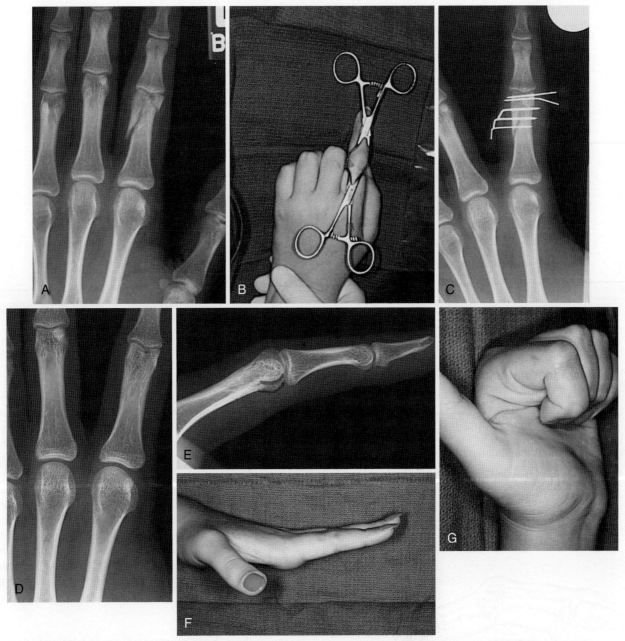

FIGURE 7.28 Percutaneous fixation of unstable bicondylar proximal phalangeal fracture. **A,** Preoperative radiograph. **B,** Fluoroscopically assisted reduction held with towel clips. **C,** Percutaneous pin fixation. **D,** Anteroposterior view of healed fracture. Note small central-radial depression. **E,** Lateral view. Volar condylar surfaces (*outlined*) should be colinear. They were not in this case. **F** and **G,** Final extension and flexion.

be treated by closed reduction, molding, and early protected motion at around 2 weeks, especially if minimally displaced. If open reduction is necessary, a dorsal lateral approach with mobilization of the conjoined lateral bands allows sufficient exposure to perform ORIF with either Kirschner wires or screws. Diminished motion of the DIP joint should be anticipated.

Nonarticular Fractures of the Phalanges

Neck Fractures. Neck fractures (subcapital or subcondylar) of the phalanges are uncommon in adults and can usually be managed in closed fashion by reduction and splinting or by percutaneous crossed Kirschner wires. Neck fractures of the

proximal or middle phalanx are common in toddlers and result when the child violently attempts to withdraw a finger trapped in a closing door (Figure 7.30). The serious nature of the neck fracture may be missed unless a true lateral radiograph is obtained. In this view, displacement of the head fragment is best visualized. With lack of tendon attachment, the head fragment displaces dorsally and rotates 90 degrees such that the fracture surface faces palmarly and the cartilaginous surface faces dorsally. These fractures are deceptive and have little capacity to remodel.

Displaced neck fractures usually require open reduction. Fractures involving the head of the middle phalanx can be approached radial or ulnar to the conjoined lateral band,

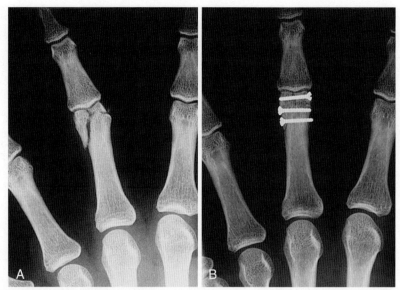

FIGURE 7.29 Open reduction of displaced bicondylar proximal phalangeal fracture. **A,** Note articular component and angular deformity. **B,** Anatomic reduction with three lag screws. (Courtesy T. R. Kiefhaber.)

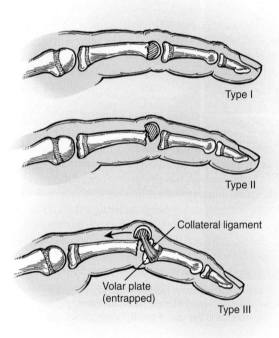

FIGURE 7.30 Classification of fractures of neck of proximal phalanx in a child. *Type I*: Nondisplaced fracture. *Type II*: Displaced with some bone-to-bone contact. *Type III*: Completely displaced, no bone-to-bone contact; may rotate 180 degrees. (Modified from Al-Qattan MM: Phalangeal neck fractures in children: classification and outcome in 66 cases, *J Hand Surg [Br]* 26:112-121, 2001. Redrawn by Elizabeth Martin.)

reduced, and pinned with a single Kirschner pin extending longitudinally from the distal phalanx, across the DIP joint and head fragment, and into the middle phalanx. Fractures of the proximal phalanx are approached between the lateral band and central tendon, reduced, and immobilized with one or two Kirschner wires, preferably avoiding the base of the middle phalanx. In either case, the pins are left in place for 4 to 5 weeks. Complications[1] include persistent angulation in either the

frontal plane or the sagittal plane, limited extension secondary to injury to the extensor tendon, limited flexion secondary to a bony block, and nonunion.

Delayed open reduction can be successfully done 4 weeks after injury; a Freer elevator is used to pry the fracture apart, followed by reduction and pin fixation. If the fracture is healed but PIP flexion is lacking, an ostectomy (Figure 7.31) of the protruding spike of the proximal fragment can be done through a lateral approach.

Shaft Fractures. Phalangeal fractures can be transverse, oblique or spiral, and comminuted. Spiral and oblique fractures are more common in the proximal phalanx, whereas transverse fractures tend to be more common in the middle phalanx. Proximal phalangeal fractures have apex volar angulation, the proximal fragment being flexed by the strong interosseous muscle insertion. Angulation of middle phalangeal fractures is variable.

Healing Time

Many authors have commented on the lack of correlation between radiographic and clinical signs of union of phalangeal fractures. Smith and Rider[110] studied phalangeal (toes and hands) fracture healing and found that the average time for complete bony healing was approximately 5 months, and that the clinical healing time when the patient could return to work was about one fourth of this.

Closed Reduction With a Cast or Splint

Traditionally, digital stiffness was an almost inevitable sequela of phalangeal fractures. James[65] realized the importance of maintaining 70 degrees of MP flexion to avoid the contracture of the collateral ligaments that occurs with MP extension. The PIP joints are held in nearly full extension to prevent collateral ligament and volar plate contracture that may otherwise occur in flexion (Figure 7.32).

Burkhalter and Reyes[16] advocated treatment of proximal phalangeal shaft fractures by closed reduction and positioning in a short-arm cast with the wrist held in 30 to 40 degrees of

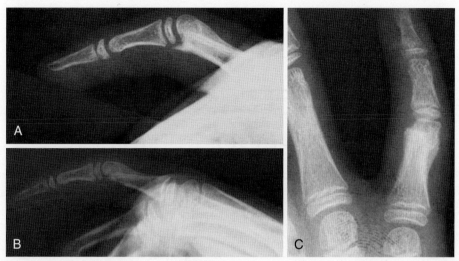

FIGURE 7.31 A and **B,** Malunion of neck fracture of proximal phalanx in an adolescent. Flexion was blocked by volar spike at 30 degrees. **C,** Ostectomy of volar spike restored 95 degrees of flexion.

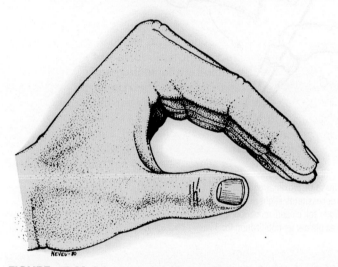

FIGURE 7.32 Safe or intrinsic-plus position of James for hand immobilization.

extension. A dorsal plaster extension block is added to hold the MP joints in maximal flexion and to allow full IP extension (intrinsic-plus position). These authors believed that the dorsal apparatus overlying the proximal phalanx acted as a tension band, and similar positioning of the adjacent digits controlled rotation and angulation. A program of immediate active flexion was then initiated. Reyes and Latta[104] reported 92% satisfactory results using this technique. Rajesh and associates[101] also implemented an MP block splint in a dynamic mobilization program and reported excellent or good results in 94% of patients. Borgeskov[8] stressed the value of early motion and recorded a good functional result in 68% of 485 metacarpal and phalangeal fractures treated without internal fixation.

Closed Reduction and Percutaneous Pinning

Percutaneous Kirschner pin fixation[6] has the advantage of stabilizing the fracture and allowing early motion while minimizing injury to the soft tissue sleeve. This technique is particularly useful in shaft fractures that are transverse, spiral, or oblique in orientation.

Various pin configurations have been described to stabilize transverse fractures (Figure 7.33). Belsky and colleagues[6] used a technique for extraarticular transverse shaft fractures at various levels of the proximal phalanx with wrist block anesthesia. The fracture is reduced by flexing the MP joint. Next, an anterograde pin is driven through the metacarpal head across the MP joint and across the fracture. The fracture is immobilized for approximately 3 weeks, at which time the pin is removed; however, PIP joint motion can be initiated within the first week. Good and excellent results were reported in 90% of fractures treated within 5 days of injury. Green and Anderson[48] achieved full range of motion in 18 of 22 patients with 26 long oblique fractures of the proximal phalanx treated by closed reduction and two or three percutaneous pins (midlateral) perpendicular to the fracture (Figure 7.34). They left the pins in for 3 weeks and protected the finger by "buddy taping" for an additional 3 weeks.

Freeland and Sennett[38] introduced the technique of percutaneous screw fixation for spiral phalangeal fractures. After closed reduction (maintained with bone tenaculum), a self-tapping screw is inserted with fluoroscopic guidance through a very small incision. The value of this technique is that it minimizes soft tissue dissection and provides more stable fixation than Kirschner wires. The technique is exacting and difficult given the small fragments; cannulated screws simplify the process by simultaneously fixing the fracture and aligning the screw for maximum purchase.

Open Reduction and Internal Fixation

If an unstable proximal and middle phalangeal fracture cannot be reduced, or if percutaneous pinning is impossible, ORIF becomes an option. Ip and colleagues[62] showed that if operative fixation is undertaken, rigid constructs have significantly better outcomes than nonrigid constructs because immediate mobilization is possible.

Surgical Approaches

Many authors[62] have stressed the desirability of exact anatomic reduction and solid internal fixation to permit early motion. Pratt[97] exposed the shaft of the proximal phalanx by splitting

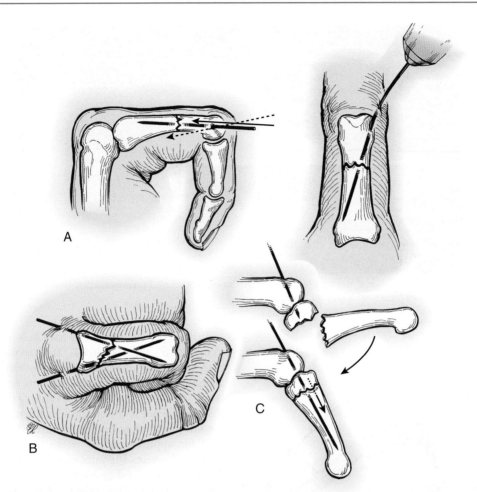

FIGURE 7.33 Three methods of closed reduction and percutaneous pinning of transverse phalangeal fracture. **A,** Fracture is reduced in 90-90 fixed position, and Kirschner wire is introduced in retrocondylar fossa of proximal phalanx. Slight reverse bowing of pin while it is being drilled is often necessary. Normal dorsal bow of proximal phalanx necessitates slight dorsal direction of pin. **B,** Alternative method of percutaneous pinning for fractures of proximal half of shaft. **C,** Technique for closed reduction and percutaneous pin fixation useful for extraarticular fractures near base of proximal phalanx. This method requires plaster immobilization for 3 weeks because Kirschner pin crosses MP joint.

the dorsal apparatus longitudinally and closing it with a running pull-out wire suture (Figure 7.35). This approach has the potential disadvantage of causing scarring of the dorsal apparatus to the skin and bone. Posner[96] used a midlateral incision and excised one of the lateral bands to expose the fracture. He opened the finger on the side to which the distal fragment had shifted (Figure 7.36). Field and associates[33] recommended a midaxial approach to the proximal phalanx. They argued that scarring of the dorsal apparatus is less likely and PIP extensor lag is minimized.

Open Reduction With Pin Fixation

Smooth Kirschner wires have been the most popular technique of maintaining fracture reduction. A pin can be inserted with minimal soft tissue stripping, preserving the blood supply to bone and enhancing the potential for healing. In addition, Kirschner wires are less bulky compared with a plate or screws, may be inserted so that the dorsal apparatus is not impaled, and allow for easy closure of soft tissue.

Pins are acceptable for nearly all fracture configurations. They have been used longitudinally or obliquely in the medullary canal for transverse or short oblique fractures.

Placement perpendicular to the fracture or bone is recommended for long oblique fractures, and crossed Kirschner wires are best for transverse fractures; however, distraction may be a problem if the bone ends are not firmly impacted during pin insertion.

Considerable disagreement exists regarding whether the ends of the pins should be allowed to protrude through the skin or should be cut off beneath the skin. In a series of 590 Kirschner pin fixations, Stahl and Schwartz[111] noted no difference in the infection rate between buried and protruding pins. The authors did not indicate the method of immobilization for these cases.

Kirschner wires are not a panacea. Pins do not provide stable fixation, and the necessary cast or splint immobilization may result in tendon adhesion and stiffness after open reduction. Pun and coworkers[99] prospectively reported on 109 unstable digital fractures treated with Kirschner pin fixation. Nearly 70% had fair or poor results. Open fractures, comminuted fractures, and associated significant soft tissue injuries were unfavorable prognostic signs. These authors did not condemn Kirschner wire fixation but emphasized that there are many determinants of outcome, including stable fracture fixation.

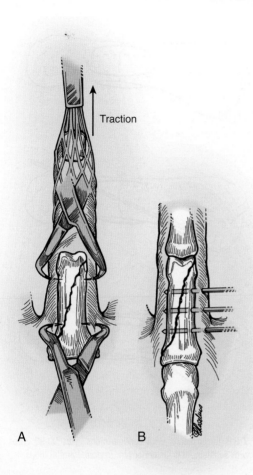

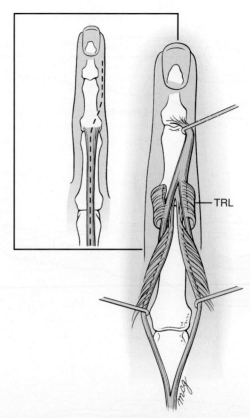

FIGURE 7.35 Author's preferred incision for exposure of proximal and middle phalangeal fractures. For proximal phalangeal exposure, central tendon is longitudinally split. Care must be taken not to detach its insertion into dorsal base of middle phalanx. For middle phalangeal exposure, transverse retinacular ligament (TRL) is divided at its insertion into dorsal apparatus, and fracture is exposed by retracting conjoined tendon radially or ulnarly.

FIGURE 7.34 A, Closed reduction and percutaneous pinning of oblique phalangeal fracture. Fracture is reduced by longitudinal traction and compressed with towel clip or reduction clamp. **B,** Next, Kirschner wires are drilled transversely across fracture. (Copyright Elizabeth Martin.)

through the base of the fractured phalanx in an antegrade direction. Phalangeal fractures were treated with either two nonlocked nails or one locked nail. They found a residual angulation of 9 degrees and shortening of 1.5 mm in the nonlocking group compared with 10 degrees and 1.6 mm in the locking group. Orbay and Touhami[91] concluded that intramedullary nailing is a minimally invasive technique that provides good functional results; they advised locked nails for unstable spiral and comminuted fractures.

Screw Fixation

Because a single, longitudinal Kirschner pin does not provide rotational stability, and crossed pins may distract the fracture, more rigid methods of fixation have been sought. Interfragmentary screw fixation enhances stability by using the lag technique to achieve compression. A minimum of two screws is necessary, and they should be inserted at least two screw diameters from the fracture edge. Generally, 2-mm and 1.5-mm screws are used in the proximal phalanx and 2-mm, 1.5-mm, and 1.3-mm screws are used in the middle phalanx. Even smaller-diameter self-tapping screws of 1 mm to 0.75 mm may be useful.

In a prospective randomized study, Horton and associates[59] compared treatments for spiral or long oblique fractures of the proximal phalanx. One group was treated by closed reduction

Greene and colleagues[49] showed that fracture stability is enhanced when Kirschner wires are supplemented with stainless steel (26-gauge) composite (or tension band) wiring (Figure 7.37). This technique is particularly useful in spiral and oblique fractures; it should be avoided in comminuted fractures. As the stainless steel wire, which is looped under the pins, is cinched down, compression at the fracture site can be achieved. The Kirschner wires are cut so that there is a 2-mm to 3-mm tail. Pehlivan and coworkers[94] used tension band wiring of unstable phalangeal shaft fractures in 20 patients, and all fractures healed. The mean range of motion for a proximal phalanx fracture was 92%, and the mean range of motion for a middle phalanx fracture was 76%.

Interosseous wiring (Figure 7.38) can be used alone or as a supplement to Kirschner pin fixation (eTable 7.3). It requires minimal exposure, is less prominent than screws and plates, and theoretically minimizes the risk of adhesions to overlying tendons. The technique is most frequently used for transverse phalangeal fractures and in digital replantation.[44,80,133]

Intramedullary Fixation

Orbay and Touhami[91] retrospectively reviewed 150 cases involving flexible intramedullary nails inserted percutaneously

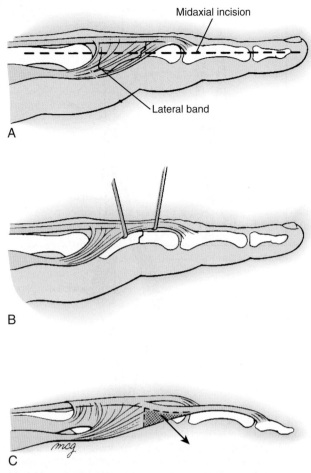

FIGURE 7.36 **A,** Midaxial incision is an approach to proximal phalanx. **B,** Lateral band is retracted dorsally to expose fracture. **C,** Alternatively, triangular portion of distal lateral band can be excised to facilitate exposure.

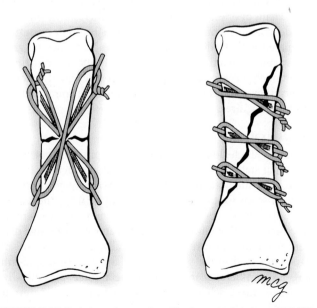

FIGURE 7.37 Technique of composite wiring in proximal phalanx with 0.035-inch Kirschner wires and 26-gauge to 28-gauge stainless steel wire. Pins are left protruding from bony cortex 2 to 3 mm. *Left,* Transverse fracture. *Right,* Spiral fracture.

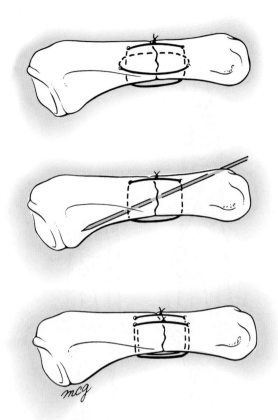

FIGURE 7.38 Intraosseous wire configurations. *Top,* 90-90 wires. *Middle,* Single loop with supplemental Kirschner pin. *Bottom,* Parallel loops.

and Kirschner pin fixation, and the other was treated by open reduction and lag screw fixation. They found no statistical difference in outcomes.

Plate Fixation

Plate and screw stabilization of phalangeal fractures has the advantage of providing stable fixation, permitting early range of motion. Page and Stern[93] reported frequent complications, however, after plate fixation with AO (Arbeitsgemeinschaft für Osteosynthesefragen) minifragment plates for phalangeal fractures. Total active digital motion was less than 180 degrees in 62% of fractures, and open fractures carried a particularly poor prognosis.

Pun and colleagues[99] prospectively analyzed 42 unstable fractures treated by AO minifragment plate fixation. Results were good in 26%, fair in 33%, and poor in 41% of the fractures. When there was considerable soft tissue injury, good results were seen in only 5% of the fractures. When the investigators compared these results with results of a similar series from their institution treated by Kirschner pin fixation,[99] there was no statistically significant difference in the outcome of these two fixation techniques. In 1987, Buchler and Fischer[12] introduced a laterally placed minicondylar plate for the stabilization of periarticular phalangeal (1.5-mm) and metacarpal (2-mm) fractures. Technical errors occurred in 18% of the cases, and secondary surgery was frequently necessary. Subsequent biomechanical studies showed that lateral application of this plate resulted in less PIP flexion loss than dorsally applied plates.[90] Ouellette and Freeland[92] used this plate for metacarpal and phalangeal fractures and noted a high complication rate secondary to technical errors and the severity of the fractures they treated.

Puckett and colleagues[98] applied thinner maxillofacial miniplates and microplates (0.8-mm screws) with excellent results. The screws are self-tapping; less periosteal stripping is required for application; and the plates are low profile, which may result in less interference with extensor tendon excursion. Supplemental Kirschner pin fixation can be used if the construct is deemed unstable.

External Fixation

External fixation is indicated for open fractures, especially fractures with concomitant soft tissue injury, such as gunshot wounds, highly comminuted diaphyseal fractures, severely comminuted articular fractures, and fractures with significant loss of bone stock.[4] Advantages include ease of insertion, minimal dissection and devascularization of soft tissue and bone, and preservation of bony length. External fixation provides access for additional soft tissue care.

Ashmead and coworkers[4] reported a 90% union rate when using external fixation for acute hand fractures. There were no cases of hardware failure and no iatrogenic tendon or neurovascular injuries; there was one pin track infection; and the device was well tolerated psychologically. Freeland[36] emphasized that external fixation is particularly useful in comminuted fractures that require concomitant management of soft tissue injury.

❖ AUTHOR'S PREFERRED METHOD OF TREATMENT: Phalangeal Shaft Fractures

I consider four factors when determining appropriate fracture management:

1. *Stability.* Phalangeal fracture stability is determined clinically and radiographically. Fractures with the potential to rotate, angulate, or shorten are unstable. Rotation is difficult to judge radiographically and is best assessed clinically by having patients actively flex their fingers simultaneously while the examiner looks for digital overlap (scissoring). Angulatory malalignment is radiographically apparent in either the coronal or the sagittal plane. Clinical angulation in the coronal plane results in digital overlap on flexion. Angulation (apex volar) in the sagittal plane of the proximal phalanx produces compensatory hyperextension at the MP joint and an extensor lag at the PIP joint (pseudoclawing). Shortening, typically seen in comminuted fractures, is assessed radiographically and clinically.

2. *Open versus closed.* Open phalangeal shaft fractures usually result from direct high-energy trauma and tend to be unstable.

3. *Associated injuries.* Fractures with injuries to adjacent structures, such as nerves, vessels, the soft tissue sleeve, or tendons, are usually open and generally require internal stabilization. Concomitant fractures either in the same ray or in the hand also necessitate operative fixation because it is difficult to maintain satisfactory alignment of multiple fractures by closed means.

4. *Fracture geometry.* Three basic fracture patterns occur: transverse, oblique and spiral, and comminuted. Transverse fractures tend to produce angulatory deformities in the lateral and frontal views. Oblique fractures produce rotational deformities, but they may also angulate or shorten. Comminuted fractures nearly always shorten and may also malrotate or angulate.

Nondisplaced and Stable Fractures of the Phalanges

Management of nondisplaced and stable fractures is nonoperative. The "safe" position of 70 degrees of MP flexion and nearly full IP extension should be used whenever possible when treating phalangeal fractures. A forearm-based splint with the wrist extended facilitates maintenance of this position. Protected range of motion should be initiated within 3 weeks. If there is minimal pain, immediate motion with "buddy splinting" can be initiated. Follow-up radiographs should be obtained at weekly intervals to ensure that alignment remains satisfactory.

Displaced Fractures: Stable After Closed Reduction

Displaced fractures that are malaligned can often be manipulated into alignment and stabilized. Transverse fractures of the proximal and middle phalanx are especially amenable to closed reduction. First, flex the MP joint maximally to stabilize the proximal fragment, and then flex the distal fragment to correct the volar angulation. Particular attention should be paid to rotation by comparing the planes of the nails. The reduction can be maintained with a clam-digger or short-arm cast (wrist in neutral or slightly extended), with a dorsal plaster extension block holding the MP joints flexed 70 to 90 degrees and the IP joints extended (see Figure 7.7). The extension block splint should include the adjacent digits with "buddy taping" to help control fracture alignment. Serial x-rays should be taken to monitor for fracture displacement. Active flexion of the digit should begin approximately 3 weeks after reduction and should include supervised hand therapy with customized splinting to optimize the final outcome. The splint is maintained for approximately 3 weeks; "buddy taping" is continued an additional 2 weeks after splint removal.

Spiral and oblique fractures often displace and shorten after reduction and casting and frequently require fixation. These fractures require careful scrutiny if treated with splinting alone. Radiographs can be especially deceptive and difficult to interpret. In addition, after the digit has been immobilized, rotational malalignment is almost impossible to assess.

The position for immobilization of spiral fractures is similar to the position for transverse fractures. Initiation of early motion often results in loss of reduction, however. For the rare stable spiral fracture, immobilization for 3 to 3½ weeks is recommended, followed by mobilization in an extension block cast or "buddy taping" for approximately 2 weeks. Repeated attempts at closed treatment are not warranted. If loss of reduction occurs or if anatomic alignment cannot be realized, we recommend operative fixation.

Displaced Fractures: Unstable After Closed Reduction

Spiral and Oblique Fractures. Closed pinning works particularly well for spiral and oblique fractures treated within 3 to 4 days of injury. We prefer wrist block anesthesia with conscious sedation so that the patient can actively flex the digits to assess rotational alignment after pinning. Provisional reduction is accomplished by applying longitudinal traction and squeezing the fracture fragments together with reduction clamps (see Figure 7.34). Fluoroscopy greatly facilitates fracture reduction and pin placement. Two or three 0.035-inch or 0.045-inch Kirschner wires are inserted at right angles to the fracture and should be placed as far apart as possible and engage both sides of the fracture. For additional stability, the pins should not be placed precisely parallel to one another.

After pin insertion, rotational alignment should be checked by asking the patient to actively flex and extend the digits. If malalignment persists (clinically or radiographically), either the pins should be removed and another effort should be made at closed reduction or open reduction should be pursued. It is unwise to make more than two or three attempts at closed pinning. In such situations, we proceed to open reduction.

A straight dorsal skin incision is our preferred method for exposure of proximal and middle phalangeal shaft fractures (see Figure 7.35). A midaxial incision may make visualization of the other side difficult and may necessitate either a second midaxial incision or more soft tissue mobilization, including a longer incision (see Figure 7.36). Generous skin flaps can be elevated, with care taken to preserve the dorsal longitudinal venous system. The extensor tendon is split longitudinally for exposure of proximal phalangeal fractures. Fractures of the middle phalanx are satisfactorily approached by dividing the transverse retinacular ligament and mobilizing the dorsal apparatus without splitting it. Next, the periosteum is longitudinally incised and elevated to expose the fracture.

To reduce spiral and oblique fractures anatomically, one must expose the sharp proximal and distal fracture spikes, key them into the corresponding fragment, and provisionally maintain the reduction with reduction clamps or towel clips. Fixation is accomplished with either interfragmentary screws or Kirschner wires. Acceptable results can be achieved with both techniques, and I have no preference as long as a stable anatomic reduction is achieved. If interfragmentary screws are used, two or three 2-mm screws are placed in proximal phalanx fractures, and two 1.5-mm or 1.3-mm screws are used for middle phalangeal fractures. Ideally, the screws should be inserted in the plane that bisects the long axis of the bone and the fracture plane and at least two screw diameters from the fracture line. The screws should be lagged for interfragmentary compression and countersunk to prevent interference with tendon gliding. After screw or pin insertion, an attempt is made to close the periosteum with absorbable sutures. If the dorsal apparatus over the proximal phalanx has been divided, it is reapproximated with either a running 4-0 nonabsorbable suture or interrupted inverted sutures.

Postoperatively, after stable fixation of the fracture, a bulky dressing is applied for 3 to 5 days and is followed by active mobilization. When not exercising, a splint maintaining the MP joint in flexion and the IP joints extended is preferred to counteract extrinsic deforming forces and minimize extensor lag at the PIP joint. Soft tissue swelling is minimized with an elastic sleeve or Coban self-adherent wrap. If pins have been inserted, the patient is immobilized in a protective gutter splint, and I begin active motion of joints proximal to the fracture within a week. Pins are removed 3 to 4 weeks after insertion, and supervised motion of joints distal to the fracture is initiated.

Transverse Fractures. Percutaneous cross-pinning of unstable transverse fractures is difficult even with an image intensifier.

The goal is to insert two pins in crossed fashion and avoid the MP and PIP joints. Closed percutaneous cross-pinning of these fractures can be frustrating. An alternative percutaneous technique is to insert the pin through the flexed MP joint into the medullary canal of the proximal phalanx (see Figure 7.33, *C*). The pin penetrates the metacarpal head to either the radial or the ulnar side of the extensor tendon and should be driven into the subchondral region of the proximal phalangeal head. Although this technique does not provide rotational stability, it is simple and effective. The hand should be splinted or casted in the intrinsic-plus position. Active range of motion of the IP joints is encouraged. At $3\frac{1}{2}$ to 4 weeks, the pin is removed, and range of motion of the MP joint is initiated.

Some unstable phalangeal shaft fractures require open reduction to facilitate management of concomitant injuries, or because closed reduction and percutaneous pinning failed. In such cases, the fracture can be fixed with two bicortical Kirschner wires inserted in the coronal plane by one of two methods: retrograde cross-pinning or cross-pinning of the reduced fracture. Regardless of the technique, image intensification greatly facilitates the procedure.

In the retrograde cross-pinning method, after the fracture surfaces are exposed, a trial reduction is accomplished (Figure 7.39). A preview pin held over the dorsal surface of the reduced fracture before pinning helps plan the entrance site of the first pin in one fragment and the exit site of the pin in the other fragment. Either the proximal or the distal fragment may be drilled first; however, the distal fragment is usually easier to pin because the adjacent digits can be flexed out of the way of the distally protruding pin. An elevator placed beneath the volar cortex is used to lift the fragment up and make the medullary canal accessible. The pin is drilled in the coronal plane through the middle of the medullary canal. Care must be taken not to angle the pin more than 30 degrees from the long axis of the phalanx because it would not engage adequate cortex of the proximal fragment. Sometimes the pin bounces off the endosteal cortex when drilling the first fragment. The pin is drilled through the cortex and out through the skin, and, ideally, the extensor mechanism is retracted dorsally so that it is not impaled. A second pin is inserted on the other side of the first fragment in a similar fashion; both pins are backed up flush to the fracture surface, and the fracture is reduced. To prevent distraction, the fracture ends are compressed firmly together while the two pins are drilled retrograde into the fragment. It helps to stabilize the proximal fragment by holding it with a towel clip while the pins are drilled.

In another method, the fracture is held reduced while two crossed Kirschner wires are drilled obliquely from the outside across the fracture (Figure 7.40). This method is more difficult because it is challenging to maintain fracture reduction and drive pins simultaneously. Regardless of the technique, pin placement and fracture reduction are confirmed with biplanar radiographs, and closure is accomplished as noted earlier.

Intraosseous wires (25-gauge or 26-gauge) work well for the fixation of unstable transverse shaft fractures (see Figure 7.38). The holes for the wire should be drilled at least 3 to 4 mm from the fracture edge so that the wire does not cut out when it is being tightened. In addition, caution should be exercised to avoid kinking because tightening becomes impossible. Intraosseous wire fixation is particularly useful in open or severely

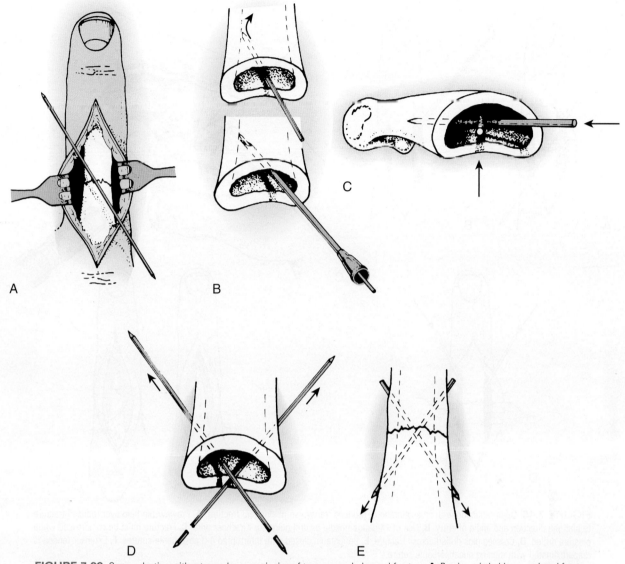

FIGURE 7.39 Open reduction with retrograde cross-pinning of transverse phalangeal fracture. **A,** Preview pin held over reduced fracture helps plan pin direction and angle of entry. **B,** Use of 14-gauge needle as drill guide to prevent pin from sliding off endosteal surface of cortex. **C,** Pins are drilled so that they are through middle of medullary canal in coronal plane. **D,** Pins are drilled through cortex and backed up flush to fracture surface. **E,** Fracture is reduced and fracture ends are compressed, while two pins are drilled retrogradely into other fragment. (From Edwards GS Jr, O'Brien ET, Heckman MM: Retrograde cross pinning of transverse metacarpal and phalangeal fractures, *Hand* 14:141-148, 1982.)

displaced fractures in which the fracture has already been circumferentially exposed (secondary to the trauma) because wire passage is facilitated. Supplemental fixation with an oblique Kirschner pin may provide additional stability, particularly in the phalangeal diaphysis, where the bending moment is greatest.

Occasionally, we employ a 1.5-mm minicondylar plate[12,92] (Figure 7.41) or a T-plate to stabilize periarticular phalangeal fractures. The technique is exacting and should not be attempted without full knowledge of the implant system.

Plate fixation of noncomminuted unstable transverse phalangeal shaft fractures is technically demanding, and there is no margin for error. Considerable exposure is necessary, there is a considerable complication profile, including tendon excursion and stiffness, and secondary removal may be necessary. Despite

the secure fixation that plates provide, Kirschner wires, intraosseous wires, and combinations of the two are my preferences for such fractures.

Displaced Fractures: Unstable and Comminuted

Unstable and comminuted fractures are usually open and often associated with soft tissue injury. Instability patterns include angulation, malrotation, and shortening. Fracture stabilization is necessary to restore length and alignment and to facilitate management of concomitant soft tissue injuries. Operative intervention is necessary in nearly all cases.

My preferred treatment is application of a mini–external fixation device. It provides stabilization, allows access to open wounds, and does not risk devitalization of small fracture fragments, which may have a tenuous blood supply. Two transverse

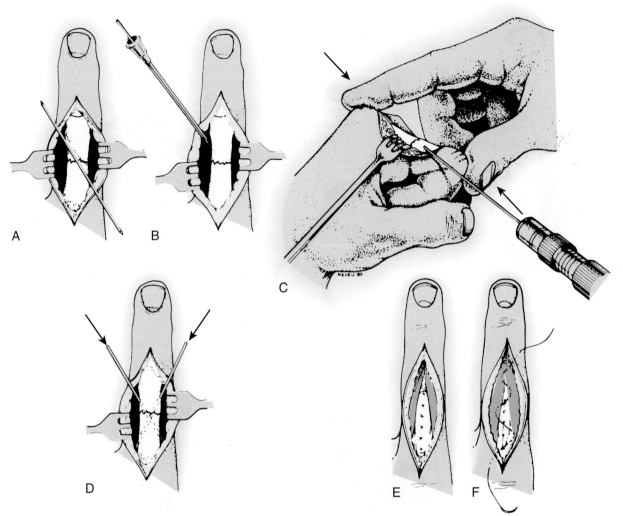

FIGURE 7.40 Open reduction with cross-pinning of reduced transverse phalangeal fracture. **A,** Preview pin held over reduced fracture to plan pin direction and angle of entry. **B,** Use of 14-gauge needle as drill guide for Kirschner wire. **C,** Fracture must be compressed while pins are drilled. **D,** Crossed pins drilled across fracture. **E,** Periosteum closed with interrupted 4-0 absorbable sutures. **F,** Extensor tendon is reapproximated with running nonabsorbable suture.

pins are placed proximal and distal to the fracture and inserted through midaxial or dorsolateral incisions. Fluoroscopy facilitates pin insertion, minimizes the risk of articular penetration, and diminishes the chance of further fracture comminution during multiple drill passes. After insertion of the transverse pins, the connecting rods and swivel clamps are applied. With the image intensifier, the fracture is reduced, and the swivel clamps are tightened to maintain reduction. Usually, stability can be maintained with a single half-frame; if necessary, a second half-frame can be applied. Supplemental Kirschner wires and intraosseous or cerclage wires may also increase stability. If there is an osseous void, bone grafting can be considered, assuming that the wound is clean and there is adequate soft tissue coverage. The fixator is left in place for 4 weeks, during which time active mobilization of uninvolved joints is encouraged. In fractures with extensive comminution or instability, the fixator may need to remain in place an additional 2 to 3 weeks. On removal, an intensive hand therapy program is initiated. Secondary surgery, including tenolysis and capsulot-

omy, is frequently necessary, but should be delayed until there is solid bony union and the soft tissue sleeve is mature and pliable.

Plates and screws are a popular alternative to external fixation. Several caveats are warranted: Additional soft tissue mobilization is usually necessary, the plate may interfere with tendon gliding, and soft tissue coverage (without a flap) may be impossible. For these reasons, plate fixation is not my first choice for stabilization of comminuted or open phalangeal shaft fractures.

Expected Outcomes: Phalangeal Shaft Fractures

The time for complete bony healing of phalangeal shaft fractures is typically 5 months, although patients can return to work in about 6 weeks.[110] A satisfactory treatment rate of 92% to 94% has been reported with closed reduction and casting or splinting of these fractures.[101,104] Most closed reduction and casting procedures provide sufficient stability to enable early mobilization. Mobilizing the finger within the first 4 weeks is critical to

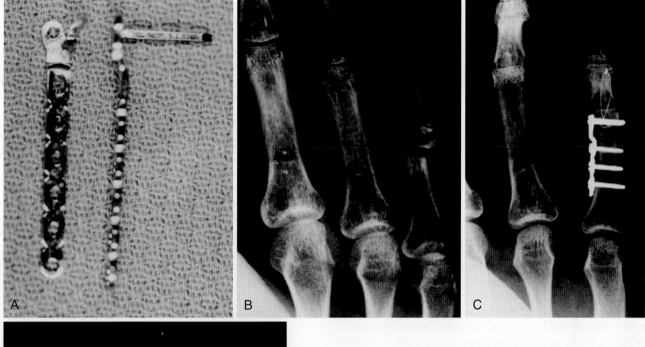

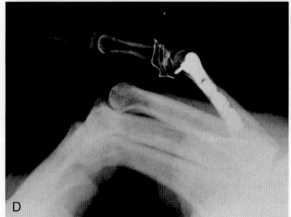

FIGURE 7.41 A, Minicondylar plate. **B,** Open transverse fracture through proximal phalangeal neck. **C** and **D,** Blade plates are low profile, provide stable fixation, and do not interfere with tendon excursion, but require exacting technique. Pull-out wire was used for concomitant volar plate avulsion. (Courtesy P. R. Fassler.)

preventing hand stiffness. Closed reduction percutaneous pinning has led to 90% good and excellent results when fracture was treated within 5 days of injury.[6] Active range of motion was fully restored in 82% of patients treated using this technique.[48] In patients treated using tension band wiring, range-of-motion recovery was 92% for the proximal phalanx and 76% for the middle phalanx.[94] Screw fixation typically enhances stability and is associated with earlier mobilization. Intramedullary fixation is a minimally invasive procedure that has been reported with 84% recovery of range of motion and 89% recovery of grip strength.[91] Finally, although plate and screw fixation provides the stability to permit early range of motion, it has also been associated with frequent complications. In a prospective study of fractures treated using miniplates, results were good in 26% and fair or poor in 74%.[100]

Base Fractures of the Proximal Phalanx

Extraarticular fractures at the base of the proximal phalanx occur at the metaphyseal-diaphyseal junction. The fracture is usually comminuted dorsally, is impacted, and has apex volar angulation. There also may be mild angulation in the frontal plane; rotational deformity is rare.

Oblique views may be deceptive and may lead the surgeon to underestimate the severity of the fracture. Coonrad and Pohlman[24] pointed out that malunion was associated with loss of reduction, secondary to immobilization of the digit in insufficient flexion at the MP joint. A malunion may produce pseudoclawing (see Author's Preferred Method of Treatment: Phalangeal Shaft Fractures). In younger children, 30 degrees of apex volar angulation is acceptable, but uncorrected angulation of 25 degrees or more in adults causes loss of motion and may necessitate corrective osteotomy. This fracture is reduced by flexing the MP joint maximally to stabilize the proximal fragment and relax the intrinsic muscles and then correcting the volar angulation by flexing the distal fragment. Immobilization with the MP joint flexed 70 degrees and the PIP joint extended for 3 to 4 weeks is recommended. Closed reduction with intermedullary pinning, as described by Belsky and colleagues,[6] is an excellent technique to maintain reduction. A Kirschner pin is drilled through the flexed MP joint into the proximal fragment to stabilize it. After the distal fragment is reduced onto the proximal fragment, the Kirschner pin is drilled across the fracture into the distal fragment. This percutaneous pinning for extraarticular base fractures can also be performed with crossed

K-wires inserted percutaneously. Faruqui and colleagues[32] retrospectively compared the outcomes of 25 patients using each technique and found no differences in range of motion between the two cohorts. Both methods were equally effective in maintaining radiographic alignment; however, both methods were also associated with a high rate of complications and an average loss of flexion arc at the PIP joint of 35 degrees.

Complications of Phalangeal Fractures
Malunion

Malunion (eBox 7.2) is a common complication of phalangeal fractures and may involve several different planes of deformity: malrotation, apex volar angulation, lateral angulation, and shortening.

Malrotation

Malrotation is usually seen after oblique or spiral fractures of the proximal and middle phalanges. It may be difficult to assess radiographically and is best assessed by having the patient make a fist and looking for digital overlap. Small amounts of malrotation may be acceptable to many patients. Greater degrees of malrotation result in functional impairment, pain from joint malalignment, and diminished grip strength.[13] Osteotomy is usually required, preferably through the phalanx. Phalangeal osteotomy offers the advantages of correcting the malunion at its site of origin, allowing for multiplanar correction and permitting concomitant soft tissue procedures such as tenolysis and capsulotomy. The risk of postoperative adhesions between the dorsal apparatus and phalanx is considerable and may result in digital stiffness. It is simplest to create a transverse osteotomy[39] with a power saw with a thin blade. Transverse osteotomies can be held with a miniplate or Kirschner wires.

Before the development of secure internal fixation, malrotation was corrected by an osteotomy through the metacarpal base. Gross and Gelberman[50] experimentally determined that correction of 18 to 19 degrees can be obtained by osteotomy of the index, long, and ring fingers and that 20 to 30 degrees of correction can be achieved in the small finger. Although this osteotomy is technically easier, the amount of rotational correction is limited, and multiplanar correction is impossible. If concomitant tenolysis and capsulotomy are planned, exposure of the malunion is necessary anyway, which may obviate the simplicity of a metacarpal correction.

I prefer phalangeal osteotomy using plate fixation. The use of a supplemental bone graft is individualized. Postoperatively, an early and intensive range-of-motion program is necessary to minimize stiffness.

Apex Volar Angulation

Malunion of adult basilar proximal phalangeal fractures of more than 25 to 30 degrees results in pseudoclawing. This deformity may compromise dexterity, is often aesthetically unacceptable, and can result in a fixed PIP flexion contracture.[47] An osteotomy may be performed with an oscillating saw by making an opening or closing wedge at the level of the malunion. If shortening is a concern, an opening osteotomy with insertion of a corticocancellous wedge-shaped graft is recommended. Otherwise, a closing wedge osteotomy (apex dorsal, base volar) is preferred because it is simpler than an opening

osteotomy and does not require an intercalated bone graft. Preoperatively, a template of the malunited phalanx is made to assess accurately the dimensions of the wedge to be removed. Fixation is accomplished with Kirschner wires, plates and screws, or intraosseous wires. We prefer to use plates and screws (Figure 7.42) for this procedure, with early range of motion initiated at 5 to 7 days postoperatively.

Lateral Angulation

Lateral angulation can be corrected by either an opening or a closing wedge osteotomy. A closing osteotomy can be done with an oscillating saw or power burs, as described by Froimson.[39] Alternatively, corrective opening wedge osteotomy can be accomplished (Figure 7.43). It is preferable to leave the opposite cortex intact, use either a pure cancellous or a corticocancellous graft, and obtain fixation with a laterally applied

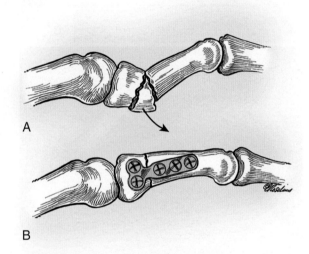

FIGURE 7.42 Closing wedge osteotomy for correction of malunion of the proximal phalanx with volar angulation. **A,** Demonstrating the osteotomy lines for correcting the volar angulation of the malunion. **B,** Plate and screw fixation once the wedge osteotomy bone is removed.

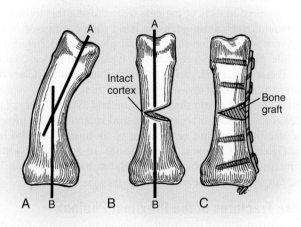

FIGURE 7.43 Technique for lateral opening phalangeal osteotomy. **A,** Angulatory deformity in frontal plane. Lines *A* and *B* show alignment of proximal and distal portions of phalanx. **B,** Corrective osteotomy leaving opposite cortex intact. **C,** Corticocancellous graft inserted with lateral plate fixation. (Copyright Elizabeth Martin.)

plate. Although closing wedge osteotomy is technically easier and does not require bone grafting, I lean toward opening wedge osteotomy if there is concern for loss of phalangeal length and extensor lag.

Shortening

Shortening may occur after a comminuted fracture that is allowed to heal in a collapsed fashion or after a long spiral fracture. Restoration of phalangeal length alone is rarely indicated because of the inherent risks of osteotomy and interposition bone grafting. When there is a concomitant rotational or angular deformity, diaphyseal osteotomy with an appropriately fashioned intercalated graft may be indicated.

Occasionally, a spiral fracture of the proximal phalanx heals in a shortened position such that the distal spike on the proximal fragment protrudes into the retrocondylar space of the PIP joint and acts as a flexion block. In such instances, digital flexion can be restored by removing the spike through a volar approach. This procedure is best performed by using local anesthesia with sedation so that the patient can actively flex the affected digit intraoperatively to ensure that full digital flexion has been restored. Care must be taken not to be overzealous in bony removal because an iatrogenic fracture can occur. Malunited subcondylar fractures through the neck of the proximal phalanx can result in a block to active and passive PIP flexion. Correction can be attained through a volar approach by removing the bony block. We recommend against osteotomy because of its difficulty and the increased risk of avascular necrosis of the head fragment.

Articular Malunion

Unreduced condylar fractures that extend into the PIP joint may produce pain, angulatory deformity, stiffness, and, ultimately, degenerative arthritis. Treatment options include corrective articular or juxtaarticular osteotomy, arthrodesis, or arthroplasty. Juxtaarticular osteotomy corrects alignment but does not address the articular step-off.

In young patients who do not have posttraumatic arthritis, I prefer an articular osteotomy for uniplanar deformities. Patients should be informed that proper alignment can be corrected but restoration of full mobility is unlikely. Degenerative arthritis can develop in the future.

Outcomes. Buchler and colleagues[13] reviewed 59 extraarticular phalangeal malunions treated by phalangeal osteotomy. Full correction was achieved in 76% of the digits, and 89% showed increased range of motion. For digits with an isolated malunion, 83% had excellent results and 13% had good results. For digits with additional soft tissue injuries, there were only 45% excellent results and 19% good results. Along similar lines, Trumble and Gilbert[120] reported excellent results in 11 patients using an in situ closing wedge osteotomy to correct either uniplanar or multiplanar deformities. They used a 1.3-mm or 1.5-mm dorsally applied plate for fixation and reported no major complications. More recently, Del Pinal and associates[26] treated 10 patients with malunited phalangeal base fractures with an opening wedge osteotomy, insertion of a distal radius bone graft, and fixation using titanium lag screws or cerclage wires, or both. All patients had good results and achieved functional range of motion in the PIP joint, although decreased DIP joint motion was common.

CRITICAL POINTS *Osteotomy for Phalangeal Malunion*

Indications
- Angulatory or rotatory deformity with or without stiffness
- Pain, weakness

Preoperative Evaluation
- Assess the plane of deformity.
- Assess the integrity of the soft tissue sleeve and flexor and extensor tendons.
- Obtain anteroposterior, lateral, and oblique radiographs.
- Assess bone loss (determine whether opening wedge and bone graft are necessary).

Pearls
- Use miniplate and screw fixation whenever possible.
- Maintain phalangeal length rather than shorten it.
- Consider other options (arthrodesis or amputation) when associated with joint stiffness, unstable soft tissue coverage, or history of osteomyelitis.

Pitfalls
- Inadequate correction
- Poor fixation precluding early range-of-motion exercises
- Shortening more than 3 mm is unacceptable.

Technical Points
- Use template to assess length, opening versus closing wedge, or rotational osteotomy.
- Make a dorsal incision; preserve veins in skin flaps.
- Place longitudinal line on phalanx to assess rotational correction or temporary Kirschner wires perpendicular to coronal and sagittal planes.
- Create an osteotomy with a thin saw blade or osteotome.
- If lateral or volar angulation is present, consider an incomplete opening wedge (leave opposite cortex intact) and bone graft.
- Adjust alignment and temporarily hold with Kirschner pin.
- Apply low-profile plate (minimum four cortices above and below osteotomy) on lateral surface if possible.
- Perform tenolysis and/or capsulotomy if necessary.

Postoperative Care
- Apply bulky dressing for 4 to 7 days.
- Begin intensive active and gentle passive range-of-motion exercises.
- Edema control is done with an elastic garment.
- Splint IP joints in extension when not exercising.

Nonunion

Nonunion of phalangeal fractures is uncommon, although delayed union is seen quite often. Jupiter and colleagues[67] advised operative intervention for fractures that had not healed within 4 months of injury. They reported eight nonunions of the proximal phalanx, four of which were treated with plate fixation. Union was achieved in all patients. The earlier motion allowed in the rigid fixation (plate) group resulted in significantly greater total range of motion than in the group fixed with Kirschner wires. Two phalangeal nonunions were treated by arthrodeses, and one required a ray deletion. These procedures were performed in patients with substantial soft tissue problems or joint contractures.

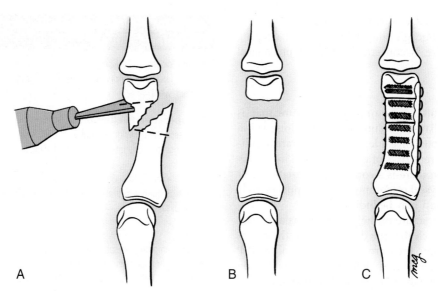

FIGURE 7.44 Technique for treatment of atrophic nonunion. **A,** Nonunion is resected with oscillating saw. **B,** Osseous gap after resection. **C,** Gap is filled with corticocancellous graft, and stabilization is accomplished with laterally applied plate.

Surgical preparation of the nonunion site is just as important as the method of fixation for phalangeal nonunions (Figure 7.44). Fibrous tissue must be removed until there are freshened fracture ends. If a resultant gap produces unacceptable shortening, intercalated corticocancellous bone grafting is indicated. Plate fixation has the advantage of being stable and affords the opportunity for concomitant tenolysis and capsulotomy when indicated (Figure 7.45). It is nevertheless a difficult procedure and requires exacting technique.

Loss of Motion

Stiffness of the PIP joint may result from intraarticular incongruity, arthrofibrosis, tendon adherence, or ligament contracture. Stiffness may be exacerbated by the choice of fixation. Kurzen and colleagues[75] retrospectively reviewed 54 patients who had plate fixation for phalangeal fractures and found that stiffness was the most frequent complication. Immobilization for longer than 4 weeks, associated joint injury, more than one fracture per finger, crush injury, and soft tissue injury all are contributing factors to decreased mobility of a fractured digit. In a prospective study of 245 open phalangeal fractures, Chow and colleagues[21] noted that the results directly correlated with the extent of injury to soft tissue, tendon, and nerve. If the fracture was associated with a laceration or isolated digital nerve injury, 40% of the results were good and 25% were poor. If there was an associated extensor tendon injury or extensive skin loss, 18% of the results were good and 50% were poor. If there was an injury to the flexor tendon or more than one component of soft tissue damage, 80% of the results were poor and good results were rare.

The treatment of stiffness should include an intensive program of hand therapy, with active and passive motion exercises and dynamic splinting. In addition, swelling should be controlled with compressive garments. When there has been a plateau in motion and soft tissue induration and edema have been minimized, surgical intervention can be considered. Extensor tendon adhesions restrict passive PIP joint flexion and limit active extension. Passive extension is not usually limited. Extensor tendon adherence is best treated by tenolysis of the dorsal apparatus.

Schneider[106] pointed out that the use of tenolysis and capsulotomy after phalangeal fractures must be individualized. He recommends using local anesthesia with sedation. Initially, extensor tenolysis over the proximal phalanx is performed; if PIP passive flexion is limited (<90 degrees), a dorsal PIP capsulotomy and collateral ligament release are usually needed. When full passive PIP flexion has been achieved, the patient is asked actively to flex and extend the digit. If there is a discrepancy between active and passive flexion (i.e., if passive flexion exceeds active flexion) flexor tenolysis is performed. Creighton and Steichen[25] found that addition of a dorsal PIP capsulotomy to an extensor tenolysis did not improve the gains in active PIP extensor function.

When there is combined joint stiffness and tendon adhesions, surgical results can be disappointing. Arthrodesis of the PIP joint in a functional position or ray deletion is an option when severe contractures or stiffness persists.

Proximal Interphalangeal Joint Extensor Lag

Extensor lag at the PIP joint is commonly encountered after proximal phalangeal fracture. Causes include adhesions of the dorsal apparatus to the proximal phalanx, shortening of the proximal phalanx, and an angulatory (apex volar) deformity of the proximal phalanx. Vahey and colleagues[121] noted in a cadaveric study that for an average apex volar angulation of 16 degrees, 37 degrees, and 46 degrees, a PIP lag resulted of 10 degrees, 24 degrees, and 66 degrees, respectively. With respect to proximal phalangeal shortening, for each 1 mm of shortening, there was a 12-degree lag. Clinically, the intrinsic and extrinsic muscles are capable, however, of compensating for some degree of bone shortening.

Ideally, prevention of extensor lag is the management of choice. Isolated fractures of the proximal phalanx treated operatively and nonoperatively should have the PIP joint statically

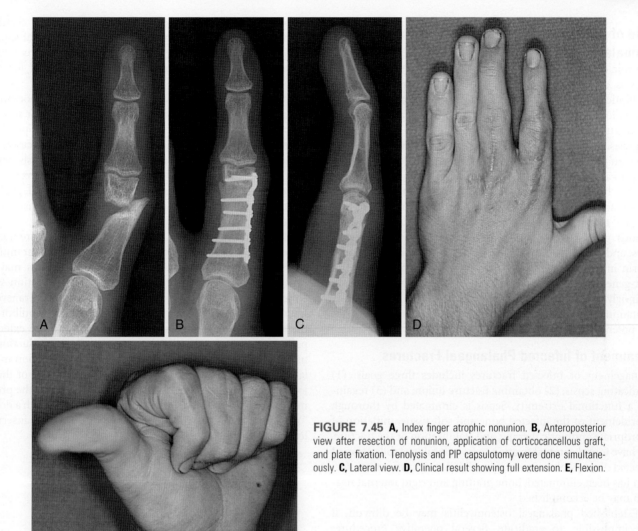

FIGURE 7.45 A, Index finger atrophic nonunion. **B,** Anteroposterior view after resection of nonunion, application of corticocancellous graft, and plate fixation. Tenolysis and PIP capsulotomy were done simultaneously. **C,** Lateral view. **D,** Clinical result showing full extension. **E,** Flexion.

splinted in extension. If an extensor lag is noted, a dynamic PIP extension splint, including a lumbrical bar to prevent metacarpophalangeal joint hyperextension, should be applied.

Late management of an extensor lag depends on the cause and the degree of the lag. Most individuals tolerate a lag of less than 15 to 20 degrees. The Elson test should be performed to rule out disruption of the central slip. A dynamic ultrasound may be helpful to identify the site and degree of tendon adherence. If the lag is symptomatic, the central slip is intact, and adhesions are suspected, extensor tenolysis should be considered.

Flexor Tendon Rupture or Entrapment

Flexor tendon rupture is uncommon and usually iatrogenic, secondary to attritional rupture from screws that penetrate the fibroosseous sheath. Entrapment of flexor tendons between fracture fragments is likewise unusual.

Infection

Infection after fracture treatment is rare. The incidence of infection in open fractures ranges from 2.04%[21] to 11%.[89] Infection usually occurs after an open injury in which there has been a delay in treatment, a comminuted fracture, immune compromise, or contamination.

Swanson and associates[117] reviewed 200 open hand fractures in 121 patients. They classified fractures into two types, as follows:

Type I
A. Clean wounds without significant contamination or delay in treatment
B. No significant systemic illness

Type II
A. Gross contamination (animal bite, grossly dirty, or barnyard injury)
B. Delay in treatment of more than 24 hours
C. Significant systemic illness

The infection rate in type I injuries was 1.4% and in type II injuries was 14%. The incidence of infection was not related to the presence of internal fixation, high-energy injury, or concomitant soft tissue injuries. Swanson and associates[117] recommended primary closure for type I injuries and delayed closure for type II injuries.

Role of Antibiotics in the Management of Phalangeal Fractures

The role of antibiotics in the management of phalangeal fractures is controversial. Hoffman and Adams[57] recommended antibiotic treatment in situations involving open wound contamination, extensive soft tissue and bony injury, and soft tissue reconstructive procedures with large flaps. For elective hand surgeries, Platt and Page[95] recommended prophylactic antibiotics when procedures are more than 2 hours long, when surgery involves implants or percutaneous Kirschner wires, or when patients have certain preexisting conditions such as diabetes. I use broad-spectrum antibiotics for open phalangeal fractures because the organisms isolated from open fractures include various gram-positive and gram-negative organisms, anaerobes, and occasional fungi. I prefer a first-generation cephalosporin in the emergency department and a combination of a first-generation or second-generation cephalosporin with an aminoglycoside for the first 24 postoperative hours. For grossly contaminated fractures (farm injuries), penicillin is added for the potential of anaerobic contamination.

Treatment of Infected Phalangeal Fractures

Management of infected fractures includes three goals: (1) eradicating sepsis, (2) obtaining fracture union, and (3) regaining a functional extremity. Sepsis is eliminated by thorough débridement of the infected bone and soft tissue, initiation of appropriate antibiotic therapy, and stabilization of the fracture. We have found external fixation to be helpful in stabilization of infected diaphyseal fractures after débridement. After the infection has been eliminated, bone grafting and rigid internal fixation may be accomplished.

Established phalangeal osteomyelitis may be difficult, if not impossible, to eradicate. Several operative procedures may be necessary, and the final result is often a painful, stiff, useless digit. In such circumstances, amputation must be considered.

FRACTURES OF THE THUMB

Because of the compensatory movement of the adjacent joints, the thumb is more forgiving of residual deformity than the fingers. Malrotation is rarely a problem. Angulatory deformities in the frontal plane of less than 15 to 20 degrees are functionally acceptable, although cosmetically they may be bothersome. Likewise, angulation of less than 20 to 30 degrees in the lateral plane usually causes no functional deficit. Articular fractures must be reduced anatomically to avoid loss of motion and post-traumatic arthritis.

Thumb Phalangeal Fractures
Extraarticular Thumb Fractures

Fractures of the proximal and distal phalanx of the thumb are often the result of direct trauma and are less common than fractures of the thumb metacarpal. These fractures can be divided into tuft, transverse shaft, and longitudinal shaft fractures.

Tuft fractures are usually comminuted and are nearly always associated with an injury to the nail matrix or pulp,

or both. The fracture rarely requires reduction or fixation. Treatment should consist of evacuation of the painful subungual hematoma and repair of dermal and nail matrix lacerations when indicated. Splint immobilization is used for 3 to 4 weeks.

Distal phalangeal transverse shaft fractures are potentially unstable. The fracture angulates with its apex anterior secondary to the pull of the flexor pollicis longus on the proximal fragment. If reduction cannot be held in a splint, it is reasonable to insert a longitudinal Kirschner wire percutaneously across the fracture and into the head of the proximal phalanx.

Longitudinal extraarticular fractures of the distal phalanx are uncommon. When displaced, the fracture can usually be reduced and percutaneously pinned.

Head and neck fractures of the proximal phalanx are treated according to the same principles used in treating similar injuries in the fingers. Displaced spiral or oblique fractures may be treated by percutaneous pinning or by open reduction with either Kirschner wires or interfragmentary screws. Transverse fractures angulate the apex volarly secondary to the pull of the thenar intrinsics on the proximal fragment and the extensor pollicis longus on the distal fragment. Closed reduction is usually stable. More than 20 to 30 degrees of angulation in the lateral plane is unacceptable because an extensor lag of the IP joint would result. If open reduction of a fracture of the proximal phalanx is required, the fracture is exposed through a dorsal "Y"-shaped incision with the extensor pollicis longus insertion left intact (Figure 7.46).

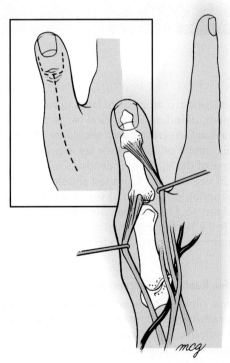

FIGURE 7.46 Exposure of thumb metacarpal and phalanges. Interval between extensor pollicis longus and extensor pollicis brevis is divided, with both tendons left intact. When exposing thumb, care must be taken not to injure terminal branches of superficial radial nerve or radial artery in anatomic snuffbox.

Articular Fractures and Avulsions of the Thumb

Articular fractures of the IP or MP joint may constitute a single fragment (a sign of a ligament or avulsion injury) or may be significantly comminuted. Comminuted fractures usually occur after blunt trauma. Ideally, articular congruity should be restored. If symptomatic arthritis ensues, IP or MP arthrodesis can be accomplished with little functional impairment.

Avulsion fractures of the dorsal base of the distal phalanx are designated a "mallet thumb." Unless there is volar subluxation of the distal phalanx, treatment should consist of continuous extension splinting of the IP joint for 6 weeks. Avulsion fractures of the volar lip of the base of the distal phalanx usually represent impaction fractures after a dorsal IP dislocation or, rarely, avulsion of the flexor pollicis longus. Avulsion fractures from the ulnar base of the proximal phalanx usually represent disruption of the ulnar collateral ligament (gamekeeper's or skier's thumb). If the fragment is displaced more than 2 mm and the MP joint is unstable to stress, stability needs to be restored surgically. If the fracture fragment is small or breaks during internal fixation, it can be removed and the ligament reinserted with a pull-out wire or suture anchor. Larger fragments can be fixed with either Kirschner wires or a small screw. The repair is protected with a transarticular smooth K-wire and thumb spica cast immobilization for 4 to 6 weeks. Avulsion fractures of the radial side represent a radial collateral ligament injury. When the fracture is displaced, open reduction is necessary to ensure joint stability.

Fractures of the Thumb Metacarpal

Metacarpal Head Fractures

Metacarpal head fractures are unusual because the longitudinally directed force that produces them is usually dissipated at the proximal metaphysis or trapeziometacarpal joint. Displaced articular fractures require anatomic reduction. Fixation can be obtained with percutaneous Kirschner wires or by open reduction. The fracture is approached by splitting the dorsal apparatus between the extensor pollicis longus and extensor pollicis brevis (see Figure 7.46) With pin fixation, the thumb is immobilized for 2 to 3 weeks before initiating motion. With screw fixation, motion is initiated at 5 to 7 days postoperatively.

Shaft Fractures of the Thumb

Fractures of the thumb metacarpal occur in three locations: shaft, base, and articular fractures. Extraarticular fractures through the base are common and are usually transverse or mildly oblique. They generally occur at the proximal metaphyseal-diaphyseal junction and are referred to as *epibasal*. The fracture is angulated with its apex dorsal such that the distal fragment is adducted and flexed (Figure 7.47). A true lateral radiograph is necessary to evaluate the degree of angulation, and radiographs must be carefully evaluated to rule out an articular component. Adequacy of the lateral radiograph should be verified by superimposition of the thumb MP joint sesamoids.

Closed reduction of epibasal thumb fractures is usually easy to accomplish by longitudinal traction, downward pressure on the apex of the fracture, mild pronation of the distal fragment, and thumb extension. The reduction is often unstable because

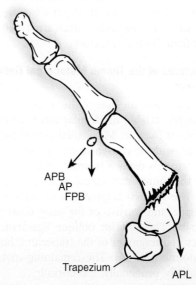

FIGURE 7.47 Deforming forces of thumb metacarpal shaft fracture. Abductor pollicis brevis (*APB*), adductor pollicis (*AP*), and flexor pollicis brevis (*FPB*) flex distal fragment, and abductor pollicis longus (*APL*) extends proximal fragment.

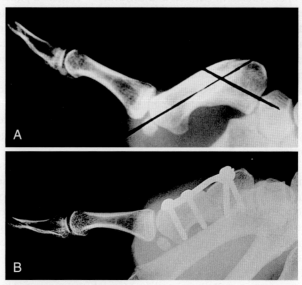

FIGURE 7.48 A, Hyperextension deformity after malunion of thumb metacarpal shaft fracture. **B,** Correction by closing wedge osteotomy and plate fixation. Note postural correction of previously hyperextended MP joint.

of the deforming force of the abductor pollicis. If cast treatment is chosen, the reduction should be closely monitored for displacement. Angulation of less than 30 degrees is usually well compensated because of the abundant motion at the trapeziometacarpal joint. Angulation of more than 30 degrees results in compensatory hyperextension of the MP joint, however, and may be unacceptable (Figure 7.48). In fractures angulated more than 30 degrees, I prefer closed reduction and percutaneous pinning. Open reduction for these epibasal fractures is rarely necessary.

Comminuted thumb metacarpal shaft fractures are usually the result of direct trauma and are often associated with soft tissue injury. Fracture stabilization must be individualized.

Open shaft fractures may require an external fixator to prevent metacarpal shortening and to allow soft tissue healing. Extension of the frame to the index metacarpal helps prevent a thumb/index finger web contracture.

Articular Fractures of the Thumb Metacarpal Base: Bennett Fracture

An articular fracture of the base of the thumb metacarpal consisting of a single, variable-sized, volar-ulnar fracture fragment is termed *Bennett fracture*. Many methods of treatment have been advocated, with no consensus on the best technique.

Bennett fracture is really a fracture subluxation. The injury occurs when the thumb metacarpal is axially loaded and partially flexed. The Bennett fragment is of variable size, is pyramidal in shape, and consists of the volar-ulnar aspect of the metacarpal base. The anterior oblique ligament, which runs from the fractured fragment to the trapezium, holds the fragment in anatomic position. The remaining metacarpal base subluxates radially, proximally, and dorsally.

Before the 1970s, nonoperative management was the rule, and controversy regarding the need for anatomic reduction persists today. Most authors recommend an attempt at improvement of the metacarpal subluxation with percutaneous or open reduction. Cannon and coworkers[19] evaluated patients nearly 10 years after nonoperative management and noted little evidence of symptomatic arthritis despite imperfect reduction. Kjaer-Petersen and colleagues[71] noted a higher incidence of symptomatic arthritis when articular incongruity persisted after reduction. Livesley[81] observed 17 patients for 26 years after closed reduction and casting. All patients had diminished mobility and strength, and most had radiographic evidence of degenerative arthritis and joint subluxation. Livesley[81] concluded that this fracture should not be managed conservatively.

Numerous techniques for closed reduction and percutaneous fixation have been recommended. Closed reduction and fluoroscopically guided percutaneous pinning from the thumb metacarpal into the trapezium without anatomic restoration of the metacarpal articular surface has become increasingly popular. Another technique is Kirschner pin fixation between the first and second metacarpals (intermetacarpal pinning) as advocated by van Niekerk and Ouwens.[123]

Timmenga and associates[119] observed patients nearly 11 years after percutaneous or open reduction of a Bennett fracture. They concluded that exact reduction should be the aim of treatment. Most of their patients had some degenerative changes radiographically, but there was no correlation with symptoms. Lutz and associates[84] assessed the long-term functional outcome of 32 patients with Bennett fractures with an articular step-off of less than 1 mm. They noted no difference in clinical outcome or incidence of osteoarthritis between percutaneous and open reduction in treatment of Bennett fractures. They recommended percutaneous reduction for fracture-dislocations with a large beak fragment and open reduction for irreducible fractures. If the Bennett fragment is of adequate size, internal fixation with a screw can be performed.

❖ AUTHOR'S PREFERRED METHOD OF TREATMENT

Although some patients with malunited Bennett fractures remain relatively asymptomatic despite radiographic incongru-

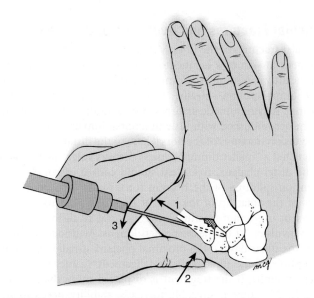

FIGURE 7.49 Percutaneous pin fixation of a Bennett fracture. Reduction is performed by longitudinal traction (*1*), pressure at thumb metacarpal base (*2*), and pronation (*3*). Pin is passed from metacarpal to trapezium. It is unnecessary to pin the Bennett fragment.

ity and degenerative changes, anatomic reduction is the most reliable method of achieving a satisfactory result. When the Bennett fragment is less than 15% to 20% of the articular surface, we prefer closed reduction and percutaneous pinning of the CMC joint. Under regional or general anesthesia, the thumb metacarpal is extended and pronated, while longitudinal traction and downward pressure are applied to the metacarpal base (Figure 7.49). While the reduction is held, a Kirschner wire is drilled obliquely across the trapeziometacarpal joint under fluoroscopic guidance. The reduction, articular congruity, and pin position are checked with the image intensifier. If the metacarpal is reduced to the Bennett fragment and there is less than 2 mm of articular step-off, we accept the reduction and immobilize the digit in a thumb spica cast.

If the Bennett fragment is irreducible, we prefer ORIF. The joint is approached through a Wagner[125] incision (Figure 7.50, *A*). The longitudinal limb of this incision is over the subcutaneous border of the thumb metacarpal (between the abductor pollicis longus and the thenar muscles) and is extended proximally and ulnarly to the radial border of the flexor carpi radialis. The thenar muscles are reflected subperiosteally, the joint capsule is incised, and the fracture is visualized. When articular congruity has been restored, the articular fragment is held reduced with either reduction forceps or a small bone hook. Fixation of large fragments is secured with either a 1.5-mm or 2-mm lag screw (Figure 7.51), as suggested by Foster and Hastings.[34] For smaller fragments, 0.035-inch Kirschner wires can be placed across the fracture (see Figure 7.50, *B*). With pin fixation, it is advisable to protect the reduction with an additional transarticular pin.

Postoperatively, if pins are used, the thumb is immobilized in a thumb spica cast for 4 weeks, and the transarticular pin is removed. The pins holding the fracture fragment are removed at 6 weeks. Screw fixation, although technically more demanding, is more secure, and active range of motion may be initiated 5 to 10 days postoperatively.

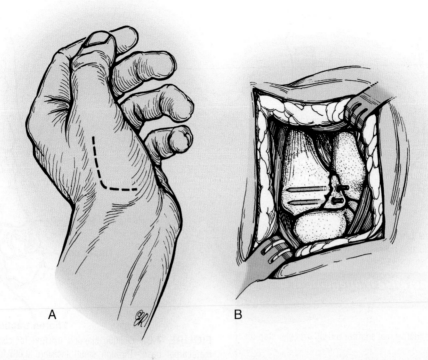

FIGURE 7.50 Incision (**A**) and technique (**B**) of open reduction and pin fixation of a Bennett fracture. (Copyright Elizabeth Martin.)

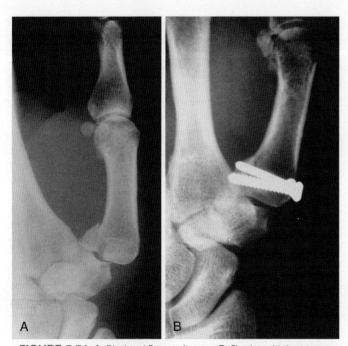

FIGURE 7.51 A, Displaced Bennett fracture. **B,** Fixation with lag screws.

Complications. Long-standing instability with painful arthritis is best treated by a trapeziometacarpal joint arthrodesis. Nonunion is practically unknown. A contracture of the first web can result if the thumb metacarpal has been immobilized in an adducted position.

Expected Outcomes for Bennett Fractures. There is some controversy over the outcomes of imperfect reduction resulting from nonmanagement of Bennett fractures. A low incidence of symptomatic arthritis has been reported in a 10-year follow-up study of conservatively treated fractures.[19] In a 26-year follow-up of patients with closed reduction and casting, the authors reported diminished mobility and strength, degenerative arthritis, and joint subluxation.[81] Surgical techniques for treatment of Bennett fractures include closed reduction and percutaneous pinning and ORIF. There is typically no significant difference in clinical outcome between the two techniques, as long as anatomic alignment can be achieved.[84] Long-term degenerative changes may become evident radiographically after closed percutaneous or open reduction of Bennett fractures.[118]

Rolando Fractures of the Thumb

The term *Rolando fracture* includes any comminuted articular fracture of the base of the thumb metacarpal. Techniques of open reduction include multiple Kirschner wires and plate fixation.[34] Successful closed reduction with percutaneous pinning is usually difficult to accomplish in this fracture because of the difficulty of reducing all the articular fragments. Articular reduction is most likely to be successful when there are two fragments with minimal comminution. The surgical exposure for plate fixation is the same as for Bennett fractures. Longitudinal traction is applied, and a provisional reduction of the two articular fragments is held with Kirschner wires or a reduction clamp, or both. Articular congruity of the metacarpal base is verified by radiographs and by direct visualization. A 2.4-mm to 2.7-mm L-plate or T-plate is applied (Figure 7.52).

For comminuted articular fractures, Gelberman and coworkers[43] recommended oblique traction (Figure 7.53) through the thumb metacarpal. This technique is appealing for its simplicity and low complication rate. A 1-cm incision is made just distal to the abductor pollicis longus insertion and radial and volar to

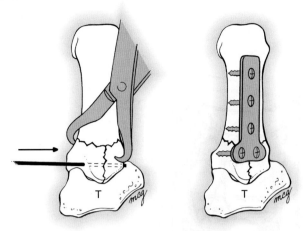

FIGURE 7.52 Rolando fracture. *Left,* Provisional reduction is held with clamp and Kirschner pin. *Right,* Final reduction maintained with T-plate.

CRITICAL POINTS *Operative Management of Bennett Fracture*

Indications
- Displacement of the Bennett metacarpal shaft or a CMC articular step-off of more than 2 mm.

Preoperative Evaluation
- Obtain *true* anteroposterior (Betts and Roberts views) and lateral radiographs.
- CT is unnecessary unless comminution is suspected.

Pearls
- Anatomic articular restoration is probably unnecessary, but reduction of dislocation is mandatory.

Technical Points
- For a reducible Bennett fracture-dislocation, use closed reduction and percutaneous pinning.
- Use general or regional anesthesia.
- Apply longitudinal traction, and with downward pressure at base of the thumb metacarpal, position the metacarpal in pronation.
- Fluoroscopy greatly facilitates accurate pin placement.
- Insert two or three 0.9-mm or 1.1-mm pins from thumb metacarpal into trapezium or index metacarpal.
- For irreducible fracture-dislocation, use ORIF.
- Use Wagner (volar) approach along subcutaneous border of metacarpal.
- Elevate thenar musculature off thumb metacarpal.
- Anatomically reduce fracture with skin hooks or dental probe.
- Provisionally pin in a reduced position with 0.7-mm pin.
- Fix the Bennett fragment to the metacarpal with two 2-mm or 1.5-mm screws using lag technique if feasible.
- Verify articular reduction with fluoroscopy.
- Ensure screws have not penetrated articular surface.

Pitfalls
- Avoid inappropriately placed pins or fracture malreduction.
- Use radiography to properly classify the fracture and extent of comminution.

Postoperative Care
- If percutaneous pin fixation is used, immobilize for 4 to 5 weeks in thumb spica cast before removing pins.
- If ORIF is used, begin range-of-motion exercises at first postoperative visit.

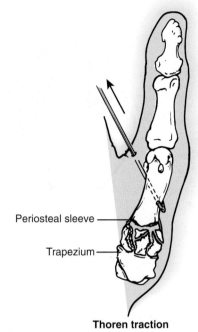

Thoren traction

FIGURE 7.53 Oblique skeletal traction for comminuted fracture of thumb metacarpal base. Through small incision, 0.062-inch Kirschner pin is drilled obliquely through proximal metacarpal shaft; it exits distally through thumb web. Pin is crimped proximally, and distal traction is applied through banjo outrigger.

the extensor pollicis brevis tendon. A 0.062-inch Kirschner pin is drilled obliquely through the thumb metacarpal in a distal and ulnar direction with a slight volar tilt so that it exits in the thumb/index finger web space. The proximal end of the pin is bent 90 degrees, and the incision is closed. A forearm cast with a banjo outrigger is applied with exclusion of the thumb web, and rubber band traction is maintained for 4 to 6 weeks. A satisfactory outcome can usually be anticipated.

For comminuted fractures, Buchler and colleagues[14] recommended the application of a quadrilateral mini–external fixation device placed between the thumb and index metacarpal, followed by limited open reduction with Kirschner wires or screws and a cancellous bone graft as needed (Figure 7.54). At nearly 3 years later, nine patients had a good result and one had a fair result. Focal articular incongruity was common.

❖ AUTHOR'S PREFERRED METHOD OF TREATMENT
The choice of treatment depends primarily on the degree of comminution. Rolando fractures can appear deceptively benign on plain radiographs. CT may be helpful in assessing the comminution and extent of articular disruption. If a classic three-part Rolando fracture exists, we prefer ORIF with either multiple Kirschner wires or a plate. One should be prepared to use bone graft if there is a metaphyseal void secondary to compaction of the cancellous subchondral bone. If there is significant comminution, open reduction may be frustrating and unproductive. Buchler's technique of using quadrilateral external fixation, articular reduction with Kirschner wires, and cancellous bone grafting is a reasonable alternative. Anatomic reduction is not usually possible, and prolonged attempts to attain perfect reduction may result in devascularization of the osteochondral fragments and further articular injury.

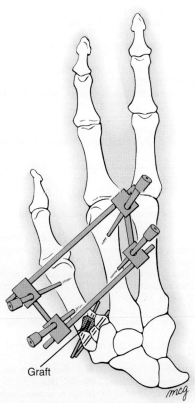

Graft

mcg

FIGURE 7.54 Quadrilateral frame for comminuted fracture of base of thumb. Two pins each are inserted into thumb and index finger metacarpals and interconnected with rods and swivel clamps. Thumb metacarpal articular surface is reduced and held with Kirschner wires, and metaphysis is grafted with cancellous bone.

After operative management, if there is persistent pain, we prefer no further intervention for a minimum of 6 months. If pain persists and there is radiographic evidence of articular incongruity, we recommend an arthrodesis of the trapeziometacarpal joint.

For Case Studies, Videos, and more, please visit ExpertConsult.com.

REFERENCES

1. Al-Qattan MM: The cartilaginous cap fracture. *Hand Clin* 16:535–539, 2000.
2. Al-Qattan MM: Metacarpal shaft fractures of the fingers: treatment with interosseous loop wire fixation and immediate postoperative finger mobilisation in a wrist splint. *J Hand Surg [Br]* 31:377–382, 2006.
3. Al-Qattan MM, Al-Lazzam A: Long oblique/spiral mid-shaft metacarpal fractures of the fingers: treatment with cerclage wire fixation and immediate post-operative finger mobilisation in a wrist splint. *J Hand Surg Eur Vol* 32:637–640, 2007.
4. Ashmead DT, Rothkopf DM, Walton RL, et al: Treatment of hand injuries by external fixation. *J Hand Surg [Am]* 17:954–964, 1992.
5. Bach HG, Gonzalez MH, Hall RF, Jr: Locked intramedullary nailing of metacarpal fractures secondary to gunshot wounds. *J Hand Surg [Am]* 31:1083–1087, 2006.
6. Belsky MR, Eaton RG, Lane LB: Closed reduction and internal fixation of proximal phalangeal fractures. *J Hand Surg [Am]* 9:725–729, 1984.
7. Bora FW, Jr, Didizian NH: The treatment of injuries to the carpometacarpal joint of the little finger. *J Bone Joint Surg Am* 56:1459–1463, 1974.
8. Borgeskov S: Conservative therapy for fractures of the phalanges and metacarpals. *Acta Chir Scand* 133:123–130, 1967.
9. Bostman OM: Absorbable implants for the fixation of fractures. *J Bone Joint Surg Am* 73:148–153, 1991.
10. Botte MJ, Davis JL, Rose BA, et al: Complications of smooth pin fixation of fractures and dislocations in the hand and wrist. *Clin Orthop Relat Res* 276:194–201, 1992.
11. Boulas HJ, Herren A, Buchler U: Osteochondral metatarsophalangeal autografts for traumatic articular metacarpophalangeal defects: a preliminary report. *J Hand Surg [Am]* 18:1086–1092, 1993.
12. Buchler U, Fischer T: Use of a minicondylar plate for metacarpal and phalangeal periarticular injuries. *Clin Orthop Relat Res* 214:53–58, 1987.
13. Buchler U, Gupta A, Ruf S: Corrective osteotomy for post-traumatic malunion of the phalanges in the hand. *J Hand Surg [Br]* 21:33–42, 1996.
14. Buchler U, McCollam SM, Oppikofer C: Comminuted fractures of the basilar joint of the thumb: combined treatment by external fixation, limited internal fixation, and bone grafting. *J Hand Surg [Am]* 16:556–560, 1991.
15. Burkhalter WE: Closed treatment of hand fractures. *J Hand Surg [Am]* 14(2 Pt 2):390–393, 1989.
16. Burkhalter WE, Reyes FA: Closed treatment of fractures of the hand. *Bull Hosp Jt Dis Orthop Inst* 44:145–162, 1984.
17. Cain JE, Jr, Shepler TR, Wilson MR: Hamatometacarpal fracture-dislocation: classification and treatment. *J Hand Surg [Am]* 12(5 Pt 1):762–767, 1987.
18. Calkins MS, Burkhalter W, Reyes F: Traumatic segmental bone defects in the upper extremity: treatment with exposed grafts of corticocancellous bone. *J Bone Joint Surg Am* 69:19–27, 1987.
19. Cannon SR, Dowd GS, Williams DH, et al: A long-term study following Bennett's fracture. *J Hand Surg [Br]* 11:426–431, 1986.
20. Chen SH, Wei FC, Chen HC, et al: Miniature plates and screws in acute complex hand injury. *J Trauma* 37:237–242, 1994.
21. Chow SP, Pun WK, So YC, et al: A prospective study of 245 open digital fractures of the hand. *J Hand Surg [Br]* 16:137–140, 1991.
22. Chung KC, Spilson SV: The frequency and epidemiology of hand and forearm fractures in the United States. *J Hand Surg [Am]* 26:908–915, 2001.
23. Clendenin MB, Smith RJ: Fifth metacarpal/hamate arthrodesis for posttraumatic osteoarthritis. *J Hand Surg [Am]* 9:374–378, 1984.
24. Coonrad RW, Pohlman MH: Impacted fractures in the proximal portion of the proximal phalanx of the finger. *J Bone Joint Surg Am* 51:1291–1296, 1969.
25. Creighton JJ, Jr, Steichen JB: Complications in phalangeal and metacarpal fracture management: results of extensor tenolysis. *Hand Clin* 10:111–116, 1994.
26. Del Pinal F, Garcia-Bernal FJ, Delgado J, et al: Results of osteotomy, open reduction, and internal fixation for late-presenting malunited articular fractures of the base of the middle phalanx. *J Hand Surg [Am]* 30:1039, 2005.
27. Dumont C, Fuchs M, Burchhardt H, et al: Clinical results of absorbable plates for displaced metacarpal fractures. *J Hand Surg [Am]* 32:491–496, 2007.
28. Duncan RW, Freeland AE, Jabaley ME, et al: Open hand fractures: an analysis of the recovery of active motion and of complications. *J Hand Surg [Am]* 18:387–394, 1993.
29. Edwards GS, Jr, O'Brien ET, Heckman MM: Retrograde cross-pinning of transverse metacarpal and phalangeal fractures. *Hand* 14:141–148, 1982.
30. Facca S, Ramdhian R, Pelissier A, et al: Fifth metacarpal neck fracture fixation: locking plate versus K-wire? *Orthop Traumatol Surg Res* 96(5):506–512, 2010.
31. Faraj AA, Davis TR: Percutaneous intramedullary fixation of metacarpal shaft fractures. *J Hand Surg [Br]* 24:76–79, 1999.
32. Faruqui S, Stern PJ, Kiefhaber TR: Percutaneous pinning of fractures in the proximal third of the proximal phalanx: complications and outcomes. *J Hand Surg [Am]* 37(7):1342–1348, 2012.
33. Field LD, Freeland AE, Jabaley ME: Midaxial approach to the proximal phalanx for fracture fixation. *Contemp Orthop* 25:133–137, 1992.
34. Foster RJ, Hastings H, 2nd: Treatment of Bennett, Rolando, and vertical intraarticular trapezial fractures. *Clin Orthop Relat Res* 214:121–129, 1987.
35. Foucher G: "Bouquet" osteosynthesis in metacarpal neck fractures: a series of 66 patients. *J Hand Surg [Am]* 20(3 Pt 2):S86–S90, 1995.
36. Freeland AE: External fixation for skeletal stabilization of severe open fractures of the hand. *Clin Orthop Relat Res* 214:93–100, 1987.
37. Freeland AE, Jabaley ME: Stabilization of fractures in the hand and wrist with traumatic soft tissue and bone loss. *Hand Clin* 4:425–436, 1988.
38. Freeland AE, Sennett BJ: Phalangeal fractures. In Peimer CA, editor: *Surgery of the hand and upper extremity*, New York, 1996, McGraw-Hill, pp 921–937.
39. Froimson AI: Osteotomy for digital deformity. *J Hand Surg [Am]* 6:585–589, 1981.
40. Fusetti C, Della Santa DR: Influence of fracture pattern on consolidation after metacarpal plate fixation. *Chir Main* 23:32–36, 2004.
41. Fusetti C, Meyer H, Borisch N, et al: Complications of plate fixation in metacarpal fractures. *J Trauma* 52:535–539, 2002.
42. Galanakis I, Aligizakis A, Katonis P, et al: Treatment of closed unstable metacarpal fractures using percutaneous transverse fixation with Kirschner wires. *J Trauma* 55:509–513, 2003.
43. Gelberman RH, Vance RM, Zakaib GS: Fractures at the base of the thumb: treatment with oblique traction. *J Bone Joint Surg Am* 61:260–262, 1979.

44. Gingrass RP, Fehring B, Matloub H: Intraosseous wiring of complex hand fractures. *Plast Reconstr Surg* 66:383–394, 1980.

45. Gonzalez MH, Hall RF, Jr: Intramedullary fixation of metacarpal and proximal phalangeal fractures of the hand. *Clin Orthop Relat Res* 327:47–54, 1996.

46. Gonzalez MH, McKay W, Hall RF, Jr: Low-velocity gunshot wounds of the metacarpal: treatment by early stable fixation and bone grafting. *J Hand Surg [Am]* 18:267–270, 1993.

47. Green DP: Complications of phalangeal and metacarpal fractures. *Hand Clin* 2:307–328, 1986.

48. Green DP, Anderson JR: Closed reduction and percutaneous pin fixation of fractured phalanges. *J Bone Joint Surg Am* 55:1651–1654, 1973.

49. Greene TL, Noellert RC, Belsole RJ, et al: Composite wiring of metacarpal and phalangeal fractures. *J Hand Surg [Am]* 14:665–669, 1989.

50. Gross MS, Gelberman RH: Metacarpal rotational osteotomy. *J Hand Surg [Am]* 10:105–108, 1985.

51. Grundberg AB: Intramedullary fixation for fractures of the hand. *J Hand Surg [Am]* 6:568–573, 1981.

52. Hamilton SC, Stern PJ, Fassler PR, et al: Mini-screw fixation for the treatment of proximal interphalangeal joint dorsal fracture-dislocations. *J Hand Surg [Am]* 31:1349–1354, 2006.

53. Hansen PB, Hansen TB: The treatment of fractures of the ring and little metacarpal necks: a prospective randomized study of three different types of treatment. *J Hand Surg [Br]* 23:245–247, 1998.

54. Hastings H, 2nd: Open fractures and those with soft tissue damage: treatment by external fixation. In Barton NJ, editor: *Fractures of the hand and wrist*, Edinburgh, 1988, Churchill Livingstone, pp 145–172.

55. Hastings H, 2nd, Carroll CT: Treatment of closed articular fractures of the metacarpophalangeal and proximal interphalangeal joints. *Hand Clin* 4:503–527, 1988.

56. Hastings H, 2nd, Cohen MS: Screw fixation of the diaphysis of the metacarpals. In Blair WF, editor: *Techniques in hand surgery*, Baltimore, 1996, Williams & Wilkins, pp 246–254.

57. Hoffman RD, Adams BD: The role of antibiotics in the management of elective and post-traumatic hand surgery. *Hand Clin* 14:657–666, 1998.

58. Hofmeister EP, Kim J, Shin AY: Comparison of 2 methods of immobilization of fifth metacarpal neck fractures: a prospective randomized study. *J Hand Surg [Am]* 33(8):1362–1368, 2008.

59. Horton TC, Hatton M, Davis TR: A prospective randomized controlled study of fixation of long oblique and spiral shaft fractures of the proximal phalanx: closed reduction and percutaneous Kirschner wiring versus open reduction and lag screw fixation. *J Hand Surg [Br]* 28:5–9, 2003.

60. Huffaker WH, Wray RC, Jr, Weeks PM: Factors influencing final range of motion in the fingers after fractures of the hand. *Plast Reconstr Surg* 63:82–87, 1979.

61. Hunter JM, Cowen NJ: Fifth metacarpal fractures in a compensation clinic population: a report on one hundred and thirty-three cases. *J Bone Joint Surg Am* 52:1159–1165, 1970.

62. Ip WY, Ng KH, Chow SP: A prospective study of 924 digital fractures of the hand. *Injury* 27:279–285, 1996.

63. Itoh Y, Uchinishi K, Oka Y: Treatment of pseudoarthrosis of the distal phalanx with the palmar midline approach. *J Hand Surg [Am]* 8:80–84, 1983.

64. Jahss SA: Fractures of the metacarpals: a new method of reduction and immobilization. *J Bone Joint Surg Am* 20:178–186, 1938.

65. James JI: Fractures of the proximal and middle phalanges of the fingers. *Acta Orthop Scand* 32:401–412, 1962.

66. Jupiter JB, Belsky MR: Fracture and dislocations of the hand. In Browner BD, Jupiter JB, Levine AM, et al, editors: *Skeletal trauma*, Philadelphia, 1992, WB Saunders, pp 925–1024.

67. Jupiter JB, Koniuch MP, Smith RJ: The management of delayed union and nonunion of the metacarpals and phalanges. *J Hand Surg [Am]* 10:457–466, 1985.

68. Kelsch G, Ulrich C: Intramedullary K-wire fixation of metacarpal fractures. *Arch Orthop Trauma Surg* 124:523–526, 2004.

69. Kelsey JL, Pastides H, Kreiger N, et al, editors: *Upper extremity disorders: a survey of their frequency and cost in the United States*, St. Louis, 1980, Mosby.

70. Kim YK, Yeo HH, Lim SC: Tissue response to titanium plates: a transmitted electron microscopic study. *J Oral Maxillofac Surg* 55:322–326, 1997.

71. Kjaer-Petersen K, Langhoff O, Andersen K: Bennett's fracture. *J Hand Surg [Br]* 15:58–61, 1990.

72. Kuhn KM, Dao KD, Shin AY: Volar A1 pulley approach for fixation of avulsion fractures of the base of the proximal phalanx. *J Hand Surg [Am]* 26:762–771, 2001.

73. Kumar VP, Satku K: Surgical management of osteochondral fractures of the phalanges and metacarpals: a surgical technique. *J Hand Surg [Am]* 20:1028–1031, 1995.

74. Kuokkanen HO, Mulari-Keranen SK, Niskanen RO, et al: Treatment of subcapital fractures of the fifth metacarpal bone: a prospective randomised comparison between functional treatment and reposition and splinting. *Scand J Plast Reconstr Surg Hand Surg* 33:315–317, 1999.

75. Kurzen P, Fusetti C, Bonaccio M, et al: Complications after plate fixation of phalangeal fractures. *J Trauma* 60:841–843, 2006.

76. Lamb DW, Abernethy PA, Raine PA: Unstable fractures of the metacarpals: a method of treatment by transverse wire fixation to intact metacarpals. *Hand* 5:43–48, 1973.

77. Lane CS: Detecting occult fractures of the metacarpal head: the Brewerton view. *J Hand Surg [Am]* 2:131–133, 1977.

78. Lawlis JF, 3rd, Gunther SF: Carpometacarpal dislocations: long-term follow-up. *J Bone Joint Surg Am* 73:52–59, 1991.

79. Levin LS, Condit DP: Combined injuries—soft tissue management. *Clin Orthop Relat Res* 327:172–181, 1996.

80. Lister G: Intraosseous wiring of the digital skeleton. *J Hand Surg [Am]* 3:427–435, 1978.

81. Livesley PJ: The conservative management of Bennett's fracture-dislocation: a 26-year follow-up. *J Hand Surg [Br]* 15:291–294, 1990.

82. Lowdon IM: Fractures of the metacarpal neck of the little finger. *Injury* 17:189–192, 1986.

83. Lowka K: Plates and screws. In Bruser P, editor: *Bone and joint injuries*, London, 1999, Martin Dunitz, pp 17–22.

84. Lutz M, Sailer R, Zimmermann R, et al: Closed reduction transarticular Kirschner wire fixation versus open reduction internal fixation in the treatment of Bennett's fracture dislocation. *J Hand Surg [Br]* 28:142–147, 2003.

85. Majumder S, Peck F, Watson JS, et al: Lessons learned from the management of complex articular fractures at the base of the middle phalanges of fingers. *J Hand Surg [Br]* 28:559–565, 2003.

86. Massengill JB, Alexander H, Langrana N, et al: A phalangeal fracture model—quantitative analysis of rigidity and failure. *J Hand Surg [Am]* 7:264–270, 1982.

87. McElfresh EC, Dobyns JH: Articular metacarpal head fractures. *J Hand Surg [Am]* 8:383–393, 1983.

88. McKerrell J, Bowen V, Johnston G, et al: Boxer's fractures—conservative or operative management? *J Trauma* 27:486–490, 1987.

89. McLain RF, Steyers C, Stoddard M: Infections in open fractures of the hand. *J Hand Surg [Am]* 16:108–112, 1991.

90. Nunley JA, Kloen P: Biomechanical and functional testing of plate fixation devices for proximal phalangeal fractures. *J Hand Surg [Am]* 16:991–998, 1991.

91. Orbay JL, Touhami A: The treatment of unstable metacarpal and phalangeal shaft fractures with flexible nonlocking and locking intramedullary nails. *Hand Clin* 22:279–286, 2006.

92. Ouellette EA, Freeland AE: Use of the minicondylar plate in metacarpal and phalangeal fractures. *Clin Orthop Relat Res* 327:38–46, 1996.

93. Page SM, Stern PJ: Complications and range of motion following plate fixation of metacarpal and phalangeal fractures. *J Hand Surg [Am]* 23:827–832, 1998.

94. Pehlivan O, Kiral A, Solakoglu C, et al: Tension band wiring of unstable transverse fractures of the proximal and middle phalanges of the hand. *J Hand Surg [Br]* 29:130–134, 2004.

94a. Petrie PW, Lamb DW: Fracture-subluxation of base of fifth metacarpal. *Hand* 6:82–86, 1974.

95. Platt AJ, Page RE: Post-operative infection following hand surgery: guidelines for antibiotic use. *J Hand Surg [Br]* 20:685–690, 1995.

96. Posner MA: Injuries to the hand and wrist in athletes. *Orthop Clin North Am* 8:593–618, 1977.

97. Pratt DR: Exposing fractures of the proximal phalanx of the finger longitudinally through the dorsal extensor apparatus. *Clin Orthop* 15:22–26, 1959.

98. Puckett CL, Welsh CF, Croll GH, et al: Application of maxillofacial miniplating and microplating systems to the hand. *Plast Reconstr Surg* 92:699–707, discussion 708–709, 1993.

99. Pun WK, Chow SP, So YC, et al: A prospective study on 284 digital fractures of the hand. *J Hand Surg [Am]* 14:474–481, 1989.

100. Pun WK, Chow SP, So YC, et al: Unstable phalangeal fractures: treatment by A.O. screw and plate fixation. *J Hand Surg [Am]* 16:113–117, 1991.

101. Rajesh G, Ip WY, Chow SP, et al: Dynamic treatment for proximal phalangeal fracture of the hand. *J Orthop Surg (Hong Kong)* 15:211–215, 2007.

102. Reilly KE, Linz JC, Stern PJ, et al: Osteomyelitis of the tubular bones of the hand. *J Hand Surg [Am]* 22:644–649, 1997.

103. Rettig AC, Ryan R, Shelbourne KD, et al: Metacarpal fractures in the athlete. *Am J Sports Med* 17:567–572, 1989.

104. Reyes FA, Latta LL: Conservative management of difficult phalangeal fractures. *Clin Orthop Relat Res* 214:23–30, 1987.

105. Schadel-Hopfner M, Wild M, Windolf J, et al: Antegrade intramedullary splinting or percutaneous retrograde crossed pinning for displaced neck fractures of the fifth metacarpal? *Arch Orthop Trauma Surg* 127:435–440, 2007.

106. Schneider LH: Tenolysis and capsulectomy after hand fractures. *Clin Orthop Relat Res* 327:72–78, 1996.

107. Schuind F, Cooney WP, 3rd, Burny F, et al: Small external fixation devices for the hand and wrist. *Clin Orthop Relat Res* 293:77–82, 1993.

108. Shewring DJ, Thomas RH: Collateral ligament avulsion fractures from the heads of the metacarpals of the fingers. *J Hand Surg [Br]* 31:537–541, 2006.

109. Slade JF, Baxamusa TH, Wolfe SW: External fixation of proximal interphalangeal joint fracture-dislocations. *Atlas Hand Clin* 5:1–29, 2000.

110. Smith FL, Rider DL: A study of the healing of one hundred consecutive phalangeal fractures. *J Bone Joint Surg Am* 17:91–109, 1935.

111. Stahl S, Schwartz O: Complications of K-wire fixation of fractures and dislocations in the hand and wrist. *Arch Orthop Trauma Surg* 121:527–530, 2001.

112. Stanton JS, Dias JJ, Burke FD: Fractures of the tubular bones of the hand. *J Hand Surg Eur Vol* 32:626–636, 2007.

113. Statius Muller MG, Poolman RW, van Hoogstraten MJ, et al: Immediate mobilization gives good results in boxer's fractures with volar angulation up to 70 degrees: a prospective randomized trial comparing immediate mobilization with cast immobilization. *Arch Orthop Trauma Surg* 123:534–537, 2003.

114. Stern PJ: Management of fractures of the hand over the last 25 years. *J Hand Surg [Am]* 25:817–823, 2000.

115. Strickland JW, Steichen JB, Kleinman WB, et al: Phalangeal fractures: factors influencing digital performance. *Orthop Rev* 11:39–50, 1982.

116. Swanson AB: Fractures involving the digits of the hand. *Orthop Clin North Am* 1:261–274, 1970.

117. Swanson TV, Szabo RM, Anderson DD: Open hand fractures: prognosis and classification. *J Hand Surg [Am]* 16:101–107, 1991.

118. Tavassoli J, Ruland RT, Hogan CJ, et al: Three cast techniques for the treatment of extra-articular metacarpal fractures: comparison of short-term outcomes and final fracture alignments. *J Bone Joint Surg Am* 87:2196–2201, 2005.

119. Timmenga EJ, Blokhuis TJ, Maas M, et al: Long-term evaluation of Bennett's fracture: a comparison between open and closed reduction. *J Hand Surg [Br]* 19:373–377, 1994.

120. Trumble T, Gilbert M: In situ osteotomy for extra-articular malunion of the proximal phalanx. *J Hand Surg [Am]* 23:821–826, 1998.

121. Vahey JW, Wegner DA, Hastings H, 3rd: Effect of proximal phalangeal fracture deformity on extensor tendon function. *J Hand Surg [Am]* 23:673–681, 1998.

122. van der Lei B, de Jonge J, Robinson PH, et al: Correction osteotomies of phalanges and metacarpals for rotational and angular malunion: a long-term follow-up and a review of the literature. *J Trauma* 35:902–908, 1993.

123. van Niekerk JL, Ouwens R: Fractures of the base of the first metacarpal bone: results of surgical treatment. *Injury* 20:359–362, 1989.

124. Viegas SF, Ferren EL, Self J, et al: Comparative mechanical properties of various Kirschner wire configurations in transverse and oblique phalangeal fractures. *J Hand Surg [Am]* 13:246–253, 1988.

125. Wagner CJ: Method of treatment of Bennett's fracture dislocation. *Am J Surg* 80:230–231, 1950.

126. Waris E, Ashammakhi N, Happonen H, et al: Bioabsorbable miniplating versus metallic fixation for metacarpal fractures. *Clin Orthop Relat Res* 410:310–319, 2003.

127. Waters PM, Benson LS: Dislocation of the distal phalanx epiphysis in toddlers. *J Hand Surg [Am]* 18:581–585, 1993.

128. Weckesser EC: Rotational osteotomy of the metacarpal for overlapping fingers. *J Bone Joint Surg Am* 47:751–756, 1965.

129. Weiss AP, Hastings H, 2nd: Distal unicondylar fractures of the proximal phalanx. *J Hand Surg [Am]* 18:594–599, 1993.

130. Westbrook AP, Davis TR, Armstrong D, et al: The clinical significance of malunion of fractures of the neck and shaft of the little finger metacarpal. *J Hand Surg Eur Vol* 33(6):732–739, 2008.

131. Williams RM, Kiefhaber TR, Sommerkamp TG, et al: Treatment of unstable dorsal proximal interphalangeal fracture/dislocations using a hemi-hamate autograft. *J Hand Surg [Am]* 28:856–865, 2003.

132. Wilson RL, Carter MS: Management of hand fractures. In Hunter JM, Schneider LH, Mackin EJ, et al, editors: *Rehabilitation of the hand*, St. Louis, 1978, Mosby, pp 180–194.

133. Wolfe SW, Katz LD: Articular impaction fractures of the phalanges. *J Hand Surg [Am]* 20:327–333, 1995.

134. Wong TC, Ip FK, Yeung SH: Comparison between percutaneous transverse fixation and intramedullary K-wires in treating closed fractures of the metacarpal neck of the little finger. *J Hand Surg [Br]* 31:61–65, 2006.

135. Zimmerman NB, Weiland AJ: Ninety-ninety intraosseous wiring for internal fixation of the digital skeleton. *Orthopedics* 12:99–103, discussion 103–104, 1989.

8

Dislocations and Ligament Injuries of the Digits

Greg Merrell and Hill Hastings

This chapter will cover the following injuries in order, divided into subsections based on the joint involved:

Proximal interphalangeal joint
- Proximal interphalangeal (PIP) joint dislocations (dorsal, lateral, and volar)
- PIP joint fracture-dislocations, acute
- Chronic PIP joint injuries
- Flexion contractures of the PIP joint

Distal interphalangeal joint
- Finger distal interphalangeal (DIP) joint injuries

Thumb interphalangeal joint
- Thumb interphalangeal (IP) joint injuries

Metacarpophalangeal joint of the fingers
- Metacarpophalangeal (MP) joint dislocations of the fingers
- MP collateral ligament injuries of the finger
- Locked MP joints

Metacarpophalangeal joint of the thumb
- Thumb ulnar collateral ligament (UCL) injury, acute
- Thumb UCL injury, chronic
- Thumb radial collateral ligament (RCL) injury
- Thumb MP joint dislocations

Carpometacarpal joint
- Carpometacarpal (CMC) joint dislocations
- Thumb CMC joint dislocation

PROXIMAL INTERPHALANGEAL JOINT

▪ PERTINENT ANATOMY

The PIP joint is a hinge joint with stability derived from the bony articular contours, collateral ligaments, and volar plate. Slight asymmetry of the condyles imparts up to 9 degrees of supination through the complete arc of PIP motion.[78]

The collateral ligaments arise from a concave fossa on the lateral aspect of each condyle and pass obliquely and volarly to their insertions. The collateral ligaments have proper and volar accessory components. They are anatomically confluent but distinguished by their points of insertion. The proper collateral ligament, which has both a dorsal and a volar component, inserts on the volar third of the base of the middle phalanx, whereas the accessory collateral inserts on the volar plate.[78] The collateral ligaments are the primary restraints to radial and ulnar joint deviation.

The volar plate forms the floor of the joint and is suspended laterally by the collateral ligaments. The thick fibrocartilaginous distal portion inserts across the volar base of the middle phalanx. This insertion is only densely attached at its lateral margins,

where it is confluent with the insertion of the collateral ligament. It is thinner centrally and blends with the volar periosteum of the middle phalanx.[12] Laterally, the proximal part of the volar plate thickens to form a pair of checkrein ligaments. The checkrein ligaments originate from the periosteum of the proximal phalanx, just inside the walls of the second annular (A2) pulley at its distal margin, and are confluent with the proximal origins of the first cruciate (C1) pulley.[12] The resulting paired, cordlike structures prevent hyperextension of the joint while permitting full flexion, thereby providing remarkable stability with minimum bulk. The volar plate is a secondary stabilizer against lateral deviation, especially with the PIP joint extended, but only when the collateral ligaments are incompetent or torn.[71]

The key to PIP joint stability is this boxlike complex, secured laterally by the collateral ligaments and volarly by the volar plate and volar base of the middle phalanx (Figure 8.1). This configuration produces a three-dimensional construct that strongly resists PIP displacement. For displacement of the middle phalanx to occur, the ligament-box complex must be disrupted in at least two planes.

Typically, collateral ligaments fail proximally while the volar plate avulses distally, although variable failure patterns have been reported.

Preoperative Evaluation of the Injured PIP Joint

PIP joint injury is the most common ligamentous injury in the hand. The spectrum of injury can vary from a simple sprain and jammed finger to very challenging fracture-dislocations. Radiographic and clinical evaluation will help differentiate the following differential diagnoses: collateral ligament sprain, volar plate avulsion, central slip disruption, dislocations (which may include disruptions of collateral ligaments or the volar plate, or both), fracture-dislocations, and impacted pilon-type injuries.

Radiographic Evaluation

Dedicated posteroanterior and true lateral radiographs of the digit or magnified views of the joint itself must be obtained to determine if recent or preexisting articular involvement is present. Radiographs of the hand alone are not adequate. A subtle fracture or subluxation may otherwise be missed. Keep in mind that the joint may have spontaneously reduced, masking the pathologic situation of a dislocation. Look for the "V" sign dorsally to identify incongruent or dorsally subluxated joints (Figure 8.2). Pronated and supinated oblique radiographs can

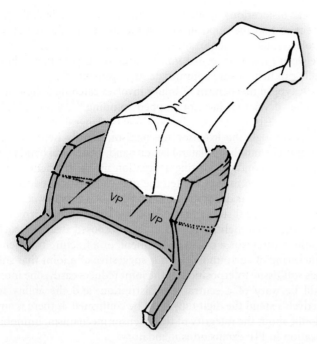

FIGURE 8.1 Three-dimensional ligament-box complex provides strength with minimal bulk. At least two sides of this box must be disrupted for displacement of the joint to occur. *VP,* Volar plate.

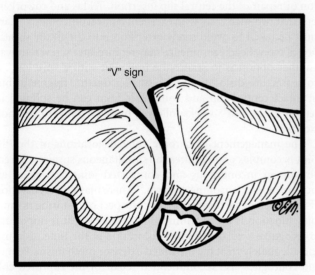

FIGURE 8.2 Subtle proximal interphalangeal joint subluxation is recognized by dorsal joint widening known as the "V" sign. (Copyright © Elizabeth Martin.)

also be helpful in evaluating fractures at the base of the middle phalanx.

Clinical Evaluation

The ultimate determinant of treatment is whether the joint remains concentrically reduced with active motion. This requires adequate pain control from a digital block. Functional stability may be determined by the following two-phase test, after a nerve block.[30]

1. *Active stability.* The patient voluntarily moves the digit through its normal range of motion. Completion of a full or nearly full range indicates that, despite ligament dis-

ruption, adequate joint stability remains. Redisplacement with motion, however, indicates significant ligament disruption (i.e., at least two sides of the "box"). The position at which displacement occurs is a clue to the specific site of ligament injury, as well as the optimum position for joint immobilization.

2. *Passive stability.* A final assessment of stability is determined by passive manipulation. Examine the uninjured side first to establish the baseline level of ligamentous laxity in the patient. Gentle lateral stress is applied to each collateral ligament in full extension and 30 degrees of flexion. The flexion examination tests primarily the collateral ligaments. The examination in extension gives an indication of the secondary stability afforded by the bony anatomy, accessory collateral ligaments, and volar plate. Dorsovolar stability is tested by shearing the joint surfaces dorsally and volarly.

Collateral ligament injury with the corresponding stability is classified into three grades:

Grade I: Pain, but no laxity
Grade II: Laxity, but a firm end point and stable arc of motion
Grade III: Gross instability, but no firm end point

Dislocations of the Proximal Interphalangeal Joint

The PIP joint may dislocate in one of three directions: dorsal, lateral, or volar. The terms refer to the position of the middle phalanx with respect to the proximal phalanx.

Acute Dorsal Proximal Interphalangeal Dislocations

The mechanism of injury in dorsal dislocations is usually PIP joint hyperextension combined with some degree of longitudinal compression, most frequently exemplified by a ball striking a fingertip. The greater the longitudinal force, the more likely it is that the volar lip of the middle phalanx will be sheared off or impacted, producing a fracture-dislocation. In a pure dislocation, the collateral ligaments are torn, but after reduction they remain functionally intact whereas the volar plate is sheared off the base of the middle phalanx. A small avulsion fracture of the base of the middle phalanx is common with dorsal dislocations (44% in one series of 57 hyperextension dislocations)[64] and does not change the diagnosis or treatment.

A simple dorsal dislocation presents in one of two ways: A type I injury is a hyperextension deformity with joint surfaces still touching, and a type II injury is in a bayonet position. Type III injuries are fracture-dislocations and are discussed later. The hyperextension deformity typically reduces very easily with a small amount of force directed volarly and in flexion after a digital block. In a bayonet dislocation, after digital block, extension stress should be applied to the middle phalanx and the examiner's thumb can be used to hook the base of the middle phalanx back over the head of the metacarpal. If pure longitudinal traction is used, it can trap the condyles by the collateral ligaments and pull the volar plate into the joint, turning a reducible dislocation into an irreducible dislocation. The stability examination, as described previously, is performed after reduction. If the joint is stable through a full range of motion, immediate motion should be encouraged with protection via buddy taping. Stiffness from prolonged immobilization is the most common complication from treating these injuries.

If the joint is unstable, it is placed in an extension block splint at 10 degrees more flexion than the point at which it begins to subluxate. Each week the splint is extended 10 degrees. The goal is to have patients out of splints by 3 weeks or sooner. A cadaveric study suggests that extension block splinting in slight flexion reliably places the avulsed volar plate in a nearly anatomic position to facilitate healing.[80] If the digit requires flexion past 30 degrees to maintain congruency and stability, operative repair should be considered. Patients should be counseled to expect occasional pain, swelling, and stiffness for at least 6 months because recovery is typically prolonged.

Open Reduction. On rare occasions, the volar plate ruptures proximally and can become interposed between the head of the proximal phalanx and the base of the middle phalanx. This can result in an irreducible dislocation requiring an open reduction.[37] Open reduction can sometimes be performed through a limited dorsal incision. A dorsal incision of 5 to 10 mm can be made between the central slip and the lateral band. The capsule can be incised with just enough space to pass a Freer elevator. The Freer elevator can be used to push the volar plate out of the joint and gently lever the joint into a reduced position. If this works, it can speed recovery and minimize the risk of flexor adhesions. If this fails, the injury is best approached through a Bruner extensile volar incision, with reflection of the A3 pulley and flexor tendons and removal of the volar plate from the joint. If possible, the volar plate is repaired to provide immediate improvement in stability and prevent reentrapment. Positioning in the immediate postoperative period is dictated by the degree of stability identified intraoperatively.

Lateral Proximal Interphalangeal Dislocations

The critical anatomic lesions in a lateral dislocation of the PIP joint are rupture of one collateral ligament and at least partial avulsion of the volar plate from the middle phalanx. More than 20 degrees of deformity on gentle static lateral testing in extension indicates complete collateral ligament disruption and injury to at least one other secondary stabilizer.[71] This is a major disruption of the four-sided ligamentous box, but with few exceptions the ligaments heal when the joint is reduced and early controlled motion begun.[111] The joint should be protected with buddy tapes to an adjacent uninjured digit. Irreducible lateral dislocations typically demonstrate interposition of the lateral band on operative exploration.

Repair of the ruptured collateral ligaments has been frequently reported after PIP dislocations in general and lateral dislocations in particular. Most of these series involve athletes, and it has been suggested that surgery will enable a faster return to sport. Kato and colleagues reported on 11 primary repairs of acute PIP joint collateral ligament tears in athletes and manual laborers.[68] Suture anchors were used in the repair, active motion was initiated at 2 to 3 weeks, and unlimited activities were allowed at 6 weeks. Nevertheless, because the usual sequela of ligament injury of the PIP joint is stiffness and not instability, the surgical trauma of ligament repair may have an adverse effect on the ultimate range of motion after lateral dislocations.

Volar Proximal Interphalangeal Dislocations

Volar dislocations of the PIP joint are rare injuries. The base of the middle phalanx may dislocate volarly without rotation (volar dislocation) or may rotate on one intact collateral ligament so that the opposite side subluxates in a volar direction (volar rotatory subluxation). Appreciating the difference between these two related injuries and identifying them clinically can help ensure appropriate management.

A typical mechanism of injury involves catching a digit in a clothes dryer that has not stopped spinning.[12] As the middle phalanx displaces volarly, the proximal phalangeal condyle ruptures through the extensor mechanism, usually between the central slip and the ipsilateral lateral band. The lateral band may entrap the condyle, creating a situation in which traction and joint extension further tighten the noose and block reduction.

When a volar dislocation occurs without a rotatory component, the central slip is ruptured. If the dislocation is irreducible, there is a high likelihood of an interposed structure such as the central slip, a collateral ligament, or a fracture fragment. Puckering of surrounding skin is suggestive of a joint that still has soft tissue interposition. If the joint reduces easily, one must still be wary of a central slip disruption, and the ability to actively extend the digit fully must be confirmed. If there is any doubt about the integrity of the extensor mechanism, immobilization in PIP extension is mandatory.

Volar fracture-dislocations are quite rare. Injuries with a large dorsal fragment should be treated with open reduction and internal fixation (ORIF) via minifragment lag screw fixation to allow early motion. Open reduction will permit inspection or repair of the central slip insertion. Tekkis and coworkers reported two such cases with excellent clinical outcomes.[116] Care must be taken to avoid screw extension into the flexor sheath. Dorsal screw head prominence may require later screw removal. Another option is to secure the fragment with a wire loop.[126] Volar fracture-dislocations with smaller fracture fragments but an intact central slip and concentric joint can be splinted in extension for 1 to 3 weeks followed by active range-of-motion exercises.

The management of chronic volar dislocations of the PIP joint is complex and requires the simultaneous surgical correction of an incongruous and contracted joint as well as an incompetent extensor mechanism.[94] There may be degeneration of the articular cartilage; if so, the prospect of restoring normal joint function is greatly diminished. Therefore, it is important to recognize a volar PIP joint dislocation at the time of injury and adequately treat the disrupted extensor mechanism. Peimer and colleagues also recommended repair of the ruptured collateral ligament.[94] In this relatively large series of 15 patients with volar PIP dislocation, inspection at the time of surgery revealed disruption of the extensor mechanism, the volar plate, and one collateral ligament in all patients. In each, the extensor mechanism and collateral ligament were repaired, the joint was pinned in extension, and motion with therapy was started at 4 weeks after removal of the Kirschner wire. Although all patients had painless, stable PIP motion, no patient achieved preinjury PIP motion.

❖ AUTHORS' PREFERRED METHOD OF TREATMENT OF VOLAR ROTATORY DISLOCATION

Technique of Closed Treatment of Volar Rotatory Proximal Interphalangeal Dislocation. The management of volar rotatory dislocations of the PIP joint is controversial. Volar rotatory dislocation has been described as irreducible or trapped by many authors and one that necessitates open reduction.[43,63,97] Open reduction is advocated not only to reduce the interposed extensor mechanism but also to repair the rent in this mechanism. Others have reported that it is necessary to repair the torn ligaments and volar plate as well.[83] However, I believe that open reduction is necessary only if closed reduction fails.

The reduction can be done with a digital anesthetic block. The majority of volar rotatory dislocations can be reduced without surgery by applying gentle traction while holding both of the MP and PIP joints flexed. This maneuver relaxes the volarly displaced lateral band so that with a gentle rotatory motion the intraarticular portion can be disengaged from behind the condyle and reduction accomplished. If necessary, relaxation of the extensor mechanism can be achieved by moderate wrist extension. Once the joint is reduced, active motion is tested. When the joint is reduced, the ligaments are usually restored to their anatomic alignment. Postreduction radiographs should confirm congruous reduction. After reduction of a volar rotatory dislocation, full active extension is usually possible because the contralateral lateral band and at least a portion of the central slip usually remain intact. If the patient cannot actively extend to neutral, the PIP joint should be immobilized in full extension for 6 weeks, just as one would treat a closed boutonnière deformity. The only indication for open reduction, therefore, would be failure to obtain a completely congruous reduction, confirmed by radiographs, and presumably due to the presence of a ligament, capsule, or extensor mechanism trapped within the joint.

In volar dislocations without a rotatory component, the reduction is easily accomplished under a digital block. Typically there is a central slip injury. If extension cannot be maintained, the patient is similarly treated in full PIP extension for 6 weeks, allowing and encouraging active DIP flexion.

Technique of Open Reduction of Volar Rotatory Proximal Interphalangeal Dislocation. Open reduction is approached through a dorsolateral incision on the side of the ligament disruption. The lateral band is atraumatically extricated from the joint and reduction is easily accomplished. With the patient under local or wrist block anesthesia, it is possible to test active extension. If the lateral band is torn but not severely traumatized, it may be carefully repaired. Should the band be ragged, it is best to excise it because the normal contralateral lateral band is sufficient to provide intrinsic extensor power. If full extension and a stable joint are demonstrable on examination, active range of motion can be initiated. Repair of the extensor mechanism would require a zone 3 tendon repair protocol (see Chapter 5). I avoid cross-pinning of the joint if the soft tissue repair/reduction provides adequate stability.

Expected Outcomes. The literature contains only a few case reports and results vary substantially, but an 80-degree arc of motion with a 10-degree extensor lag would be a reasonable expectation.[94]

Dorsal Dislocations and Fracture-Dislocations of the Proximal Interphalangeal Joint

There are two fundamental parameters that guide treatment of these injuries: stability and joint congruity. These parameters are the basis for the treatment algorithm seen in Figure 8.3.

Stable fracture-dislocations have a volar fragment that represents less than 30% of the volar articular surface and a

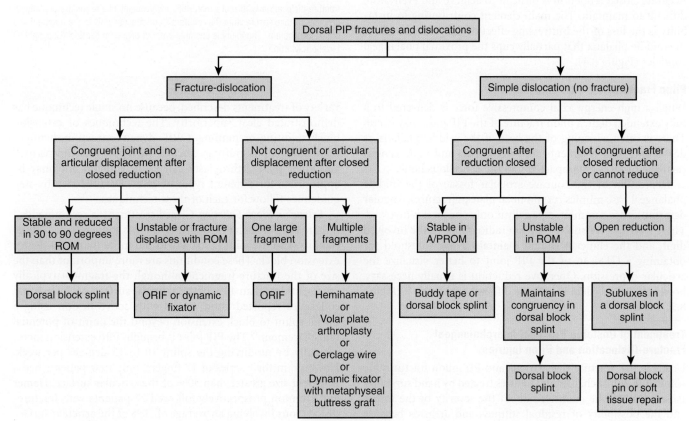

FIGURE 8.3 Treatment algorithm for proximal interphalangeal (PIP) joint fractures and dislocations. *A/PROM,* Active/passive range of motion; *ORIF,* open reduction and internal fixation; *ROM,* range of motion.

concentric joint after reduction. In this case, the disruption occurs through the base of the phalanx rather than at the insertion of the volar plate. Sufficient volar bone remains to render the joint stable. The collateral ligaments, torn or not, do not influence the stability of the reduction other than by contributing to lateral stability on stress. These usually behave like a simple dorsal dislocation. Radiographs tend to underestimate the percentage of volar fracture involvement, as frequently the fracture will involve a greater amount of one middle phalanx articular facet than the other. Stable fracture-dislocations can generally be treated conservatively with 3 weeks of dorsal block splinting, allowing range-of-motion exercises while the splint is worn. It is important to check both active and passive motion (described in the previous examination section) because the volar fracture fragment may become trapped within the flexor sheath and inhibit motion.[34] Fluoroscopy after a digital block can help determine how much extension is possible while fracture and joint reduction is maintained. Many patients will require formal hand therapy to regain full motion and function.

Tenuously stable fracture-dislocations involve 30 to 50% of the volar buttress and reduce with less than 30 degrees of flexion. In cases with less than 40% of volar articular involvement, the joint is usually stable in all positions. With 40 to 60% volar articular involvement, progressively greater flexion is required to render the joint stable.[49]

Unstable fracture-dislocations demonstrate greater than 60% involvement of the volar articular surface. Beyond 60% involvement, joints tend to be unstable in all positions or require more than 60 degrees of flexion to obtain a congruent reduction.[49] Accurate closed reduction is difficult to achieve and even more difficult to maintain. The main element contributing to instability is the loss of the buttressing effect of the volar margin of the middle phalanx that partially cups the proximal phalangeal condyles (Figure 8.4).

Pilon Fracture

When a high-energy axial compressive force is delivered to a fully extended digit, a pilon fracture of the PIP joint may occur. There is often widening of the base of the middle phalanx as dorsal and volar fragments are driven apart and more central cartilage surfaces are impacted into the cancellous bone.

Depression of the concave articular fossae of the middle phalangeal base mimics certain tibial plateau fractures. Angular deformities are common, especially if only one facet is involved. These fractures are subtle on plain radiographs of the involved digit, and the clinician should maintain a low threshold for obtaining a CT scan of the PIP joint to better visualize the articular depression. Operative reduction is usually necessary, however, and excellent results are difficult to achieve[123] (Figure 8.5, *A* and *B*).

Treatment of Unstable Proximal Interphalangeal Fracture-Dislocation and Pilon Injuries

Unstable PIP fracture-dislocations and PIP pilon fractures are some of the most challenging injuries treated by hand surgeons. Patients should be counseled about the severity of the injury and the possibility of residual stiffness and arthritis because they often consider a "broken finger" to be a relatively minor injury from which they will recover completely. There are a

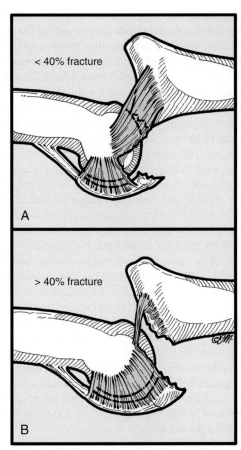

FIGURE 8.4 A, Fracture-dislocation with less than 40% of proximal articular surface allows some collateral ligament attachment to middle phalanx. **B,** A fracture-dislocation with more than 40% involvement of the middle phalangeal articular surface ensures that the collaterals are attached only to the fragment and not to the phalanx. The injury is unstable without operative fixation. (Copyright © Elizabeth Martin.)

variety of treatments described, because no single technique has demonstrated clear superiority. The techniques of extension block splinting or pinning, ORIF, dynamic traction, hemihamate autogenous grafting, cerclage wiring, hemiarthroplasty,[50] and volar plate arthroplasty can all be difficult and may be appropriate for different types of cases. Detailed step-by-step guidelines follow for each of these techniques.

Extension Block Splinting. Closed treatment is recommended if there is no articular incongruity, there is some retained lateral stability, and the joint is stable with no more than a 30-degree extension block. These conditions are more important than the size of the fracture fragment, although the fragment typically represents less than 40% of the articular surface. McElfresh and colleagues reported good results with active flexion using a dorsal splint to block extension beyond the point of potential redisplacement.[84] The PIP joint is brought into extension incrementally by modifying the splint 10 to 15 degrees per week. However, in their series of 17 fingers, only four patients had a fragment size greater than 30% of the articular surface. Hamer and Quinton prospectively followed 27 patients with fracture-dislocations involving an average of 50% of the articular surface treated by extension block splinting for less than 2 years.[44] They reported a mean of 87 degrees of active PIP motion and good

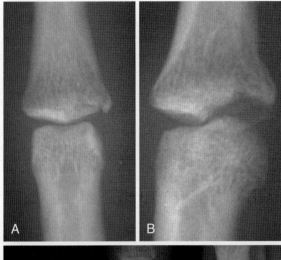
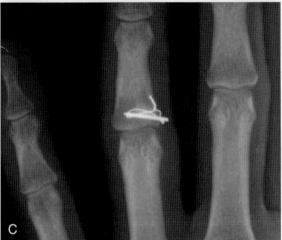
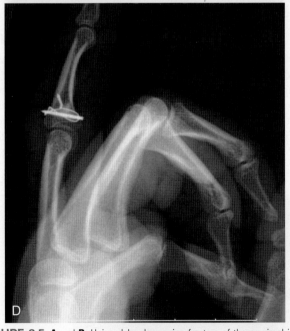

FIGURE 8.5 A and **B,** Unicondylar depression fracture of the proximal interphalangeal joint. **C** and **D,** The depressed phalangeal "plateau" was elevated with a Kleinert/Kutz elevator, supported by bone graft, and fixed with a Kirschner wire tension band construct. (Courtesy Scott W. Wolfe, MD.)

results in 70% of patients. If more than 30 degrees of flexion is required to achieve stability, the risk for late flexion contracture is dramatically increased; consequently, other treatment options should be considered. Short, small, or very swollen fingers make the fixation of the extension block splint more difficult and may increase the risk of subluxation. Serial radiographs must be obtained to document the ongoing efficacy of this technique.

Extension Block Pinning. This technique is advocated in rare cases when the injury might be amenable to closed treatment but either the digit is too short and swollen to maintain a splint or there are questions with splint compliance. The technique involves placement of a Kirschner wire into the head of the proximal phalanx at an angle that mechanically blocks extension of the PIP joint and prevents dorsal subluxation of the middle phalanx.[118] The pin must be placed obliquely between the central tendon and lateral bands to allow gentle active motion. Even with a pin in place the joint should be splinted in a single-digit or hand-based splint to decrease the risk for pin migration, loosening, or pin tract infection. Reports of this technique include only a small number of cases, and its clinical efficacy must be substantiated through further study. A modification of this technique has been reported using intramedullary fixation,[120] and the technique has been combined with percutaneous volar pin fixation of the middle phalanx.[119]

Dynamic Skeletal Traction. This technique refers to the use of ligamentotaxis to achieve joint and fracture reduction by the application of Kirschner wire external fixators or various commercial fixators. We use dynamic skeletal traction most frequently in pilon injuries and in tenuously unstable injuries with several small fragments constituting 30% to 50% of the joint surface. When ligamentotaxis is insufficient to achieve an adequate reduction (seen commonly with pilon injuries with depressed fragments), it can be combined with either an open reduction or a percutaneous reduction of the joint surface. The fixator can also be combined with volar plate arthroplasty, ORIF, or hemihamate reconstruction to allow earlier active motion with those reconstructions.[75] A fixator can help maintain joint reduction while allowing motion and can neutralize joint reaction forces to minimize the potential for settling of articular fragments that may not be amenable to fixation. A relative contraindication is serious injury to adjacent digits. The fixators can be somewhat cumbersome to wear and can interfere with the care and mobilization of adjacent swollen digits.

Open Reduction With Internal Fixation. ORIF has many advocates and is most likely to be successful in acute cases with a single, large volar fragment. Anatomic restoration of the articular surface is technically difficult, especially because the remaining articular contour may be disrupted secondary to impaction of subchondral cancellous bone. Even excellent anatomic reduction can still lead to problems of flexion contracture, decreased arc of motion, and cold intolerance.[5] The joint can be approached from either a dorsal or a volar direction. The dorsal technique is described well by Lee and colleagues.[77] The volar technique is described in detail in the following. Results vary widely in reported series. It is advisable to caution patients that there will be decreased flexion, an extensor lag, and possibilities of persistent pain, swelling, and cold intolerance.

Cerclage Wiring. For pilon or comminuted fractures with fragments too small for individual screw fixation, one may consider elevation and grafting of depressed fragments followed by cerclage wiring to prevent widening of the articular surface (Figure 8.6). This technique is most appropriate for the rare case where there is minimal joint subluxation but significant comminution of the joint surface. In a series of 12 patients, Weiss demonstrated an average range of motion of 89 degrees with an 8-degree extensor lag.[121] The technique is described in detail in the following text.

Volar Plate Arthroplasty. Multiple authors have reported on the technique and efficacy of using the distal aspect of the fibrocartilaginous volar plate to resurface the comminuted volar articular surface of the middle phalanx, especially when other techniques are not feasible.[26,81] There is little consensus on the percentage of volar articular involvement that is amenable

to volar plate arthroplasty. As a variation on the theme of volar plate arthroplasty, Wiley proposed débridement of the fragments and insertion of a slip of flexor superficialis tendon into the defect to reduce the displacement by active tendon tone.[122] The irregularity of the articular surface was not specifically corrected in his series. Volar plate arthroplasty is most likely to succeed in cases with less than 40% volar articular involvement or when there is minimal impaction of the volar rim, in which case thickness of the interposed volar plate may correct for the buttress effect that has been lost. It is not recommended when volar articular involvement exceeds 40% of the joint surface. A full description of the technique follows.

Hemihamate Autogenous Grafting. Using a novel technique introduced by Hastings in 1999,[48] Williams and associates reported on 13 consecutive patients treated with a hemihamate autograft. The autograft is harvested from the dorsal distal aspect of the hamate centered at the fourth and fifth CMC articulations, spanning approximately half of each in both the radioulnar and dorsovolar planes. The graft is rotated 180 degrees in two planes, keyed into the prepared bed at the volar base of the middle phalanx, and stabilized with two or three minifragment lag screws. The authors expressed cautious optimism as to the longevity of the procedure. Calfee and associates[15] reported 4.5-year follow-up results on 22 patients and found little functional impairment. Disabilities of the Arm, Shoulder, and Hand (DASH) scores and visual analog scale (VAS) measurements of pain and function were slightly inferior for cases reconstructed for chronic deformity compared with acute cases. The authors concluded that the hemihamate graft is a viable alternative to volar plate arthroplasty for PIP volar fracture-dislocations with extensive articular comminution, and demonstrates a decreased risk of resubluxation. The technique is described in detail in the following.

❖ AUTHORS' PREFERRED METHODS OF TREATMENT

For less severe fracture-dislocations, we have found extension block splinting to be quite effective for cases where there is a congruent joint following reduction and the articular involvement is less than 40% (Figure 8.7). Care must be taken to ensure that dorsal subluxation (loss of reduction) does not occur during the course of treatment with the splint in place. If the PIP joint injury is amenable to extension block splinting but

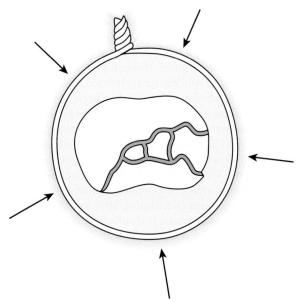

FIGURE 8.6 After shotgun exposure of joint, fragments are managed with elevation and bone graft as needed. Cerclage wire is passed around proximal end of phalanx, preventing typical dorsal/volar expansion in pilon-type injuries and holding small fragments that otherwise may not be amenable to interfragmentary fixation. (Technique courtesy of Dr. A.P.C. Weiss. From Weiss AP: Cerclage fixation for fracture dislocation of the PIP joint, _Clin Orthop Relat Res_ (327):21–28, 1996.)

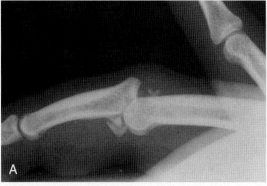
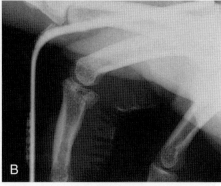

FIGURE 8.7 A, Type III fracture-dislocation of proximal interphalangeal (PIP) joint in which approximately 40% of volar articular surface is displaced with fracture fragment. **B,** Fracture-dislocations with 40% or less of articular surface involved may be successfully treated with dorsal extension block splinting. The patient is allowed to actively flex the PIP joint, which is progressively extended over approximately 4 weeks. The key to this mode of treatment is concentric reduction of the PIP joint.

the digit is too short, stocky, or swollen for such treatment, I will occasionally use an extension block pin. In general, if a fracture is unstable enough to warrant pinning over a simple splint, the fracture fragment is likely large enough to warrant operative fixation.

Several satisfactory options exist for the treatment of unstable PIP joint fracture-dislocations, but none is perfect. The authors are not wedded to a particular modality of treatment and allow the injury characteristics to guide the approach (see algorithm in Figure 8.3).

The hand surgeon will often see a PIP fracture-dislocation after it has been initially treated elsewhere, and the true nature of this complicated injury may not have been appreciated or conveyed to the patient. The patient must understand from the outset that while normal PIP joint function is possible, it is highly unlikely. Patients must also be told that the best functional result will only be possible with extensive and dedicated compliance with postoperative hand therapy. Overall results diminish as the time from injury to treatment increases, even with a delay beyond 2 weeks, but especially beyond 6 weeks.[22,42]

Dynamic Skeletal Traction. Dynamic skeletal traction is useful in select cases, especially with increased comminution and fracture lines extending dorsally (pilon) or distally through the base of the middle phalanx. The fracture is viewed under traction using fluoroscopy to get a sense of the amount of reduction possible and to consider whether the fracture may be more amenable to a different technique (Figure 8.8). Although many fixators have been described, in the authors' opinion the easiest, least expensive, and most effective is a fixator constructed in the operating room using three Kirschner wires and dental rubber bands. The fixator requires 9-inch Kirschner wires (check ahead of time because many centers stock only short Kirschner wires). The fixator is assembled by placing two Kirschner wires perpendicular to the digit along the midaxial plane through the proximal and middle phalangeal condyles (Figure 8.9). It is critical for the initial wire to be placed in the center of rotation of the proximal phalangeal condyles. The proximal phalanx wire is bent distally and fashioned into hooks. The second wire is inserted through the center of rotation of the middle phalangeal head, and this condylar wire is also bent

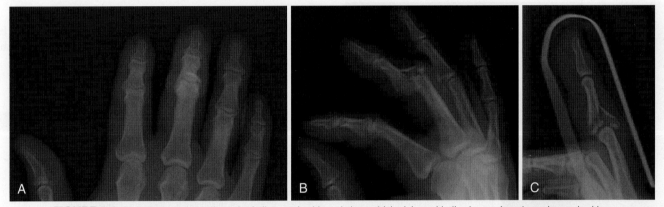

FIGURE 8.8 A, Anteroposterior radiograph of pilon proximal interphalangeal joint injury with distal extension, shortening, and subluxation. **B,** Lateral radiograph of same injury before traction. **C,** Lateral radiograph after closed reduction.

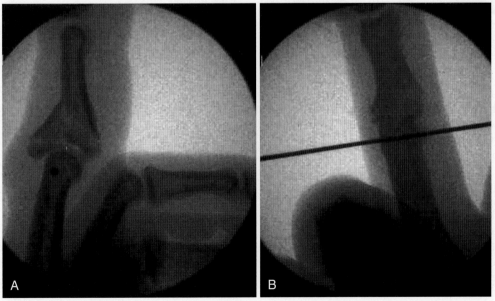

FIGURE 8.9 A, Lateral radiograph of proximal wire placement in center of rotation. **B,** Anteroposterior radiograph of proximal wire placement transverse to longitudinal axis of finger.

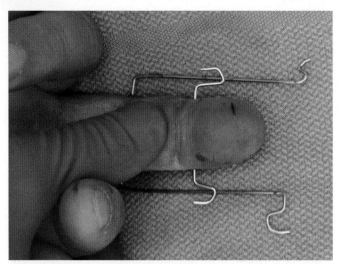

FIGURE 8.10 Demonstration of wire placement with hooks made for dental rubber bands.

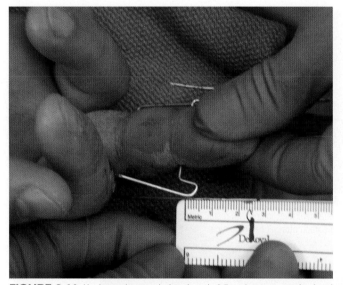

FIGURE 8.11 Hooks are bent such that there is 2.5 cm between proximal and distal hooks, a typically reliable amount of traction.

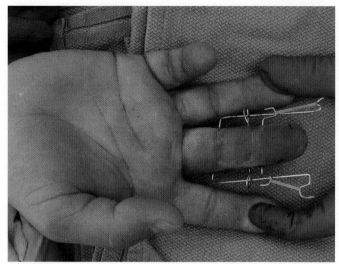

FIGURE 8.12 A third wire is added in middle axial line through middle phalanx. By placing this dorsal to the proximal phalangeal wire, a volar-directed moment is applied to the joint to prevent dorsal subluxation without excessive traction.

or alternatively, an 18-gauge needle or Kirschner wire can be directed fluoroscopically into the fracture site to tamp up the impacted fracture fragment (Figure 8.14).

CRITICAL POINTS *Dynamic Skeletal Traction*

Preoperative Planning
- The construct requires long 0.045-inch Kirschner wires; short Kirschner wires are insufficient.
- Sterilizable dental rubber bands of 3/8 inch are used.
- Less effective if neighboring digits are injured, given width of the construct
- Excellent technique for unstable injuries with comminuted fragments

Technical Points
- Careful placement of the proximal phalanx Kirschner wire in the center of rotation of the condyle is needed, as viewed on posteroanterior and lateral radiographs.
- Add a third Kirschner wire to prevent dorsal subluxation and minimize the needed distraction force.
- Measure 2.5 cm between anchor points for rubber bands on proximal and distal wires.
- Confirm motion and reduction in flexion and extension (it helps to advise the hand therapist).

Postoperative Planning
- Give the patient extra rubber bands to take home in case some break.
- Patient dedication is required in the rehabilitation process.

---

and fashioned into hooks (Figure 8.10). The distance between the proximal and distal hooks is approximately 2.5 cm (Figure 8.11), which allows for an adequate but not excessive distraction force by dental rubber bands. Give extra rubber bands to the patient to take home in case one ruptures. Prior to applying the rubber bands, a third midaxial wire is placed in the middle phalanx, which acts as fulcrum, blocking dorsal dislocation of the PIP joint (Figure 8.12). This third wire is not seen in all publications on the subject but is crucial in unstable pilon-type fractures to provide joint reduction in the sagittal plane without excessive distraction force. Typically, two rubber bands are applied to each set of hooks. Intraoperative fluoroscopy is used to confirm concentric reduction through a full arc of motion (Figure 8.13), and additional rubber bands are applied as necessary to tailor the distraction. If impacted central fragments remain, one can consider open reduction and bone grafting,

Postoperative protocol. Patients are instructed to elevate and rest the hand for 2 to 3 days to decrease swelling before beginning hand therapy. Patients are permitted both active and passive range of motion as tolerated. Postoperative motion with the fixator in place is typically less than what was demonstrated in the operating room. Pins are swabbed with half-strength

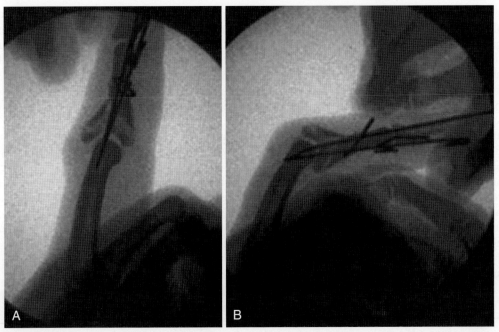

FIGURE 8.13 Full extension is typically the most unstable position. **A,** Lateral radiograph shows some overall widening or cupping at the joint, but no subluxation or secondary incongruity. **B,** Lateral view with joint flexed also shows congruity.

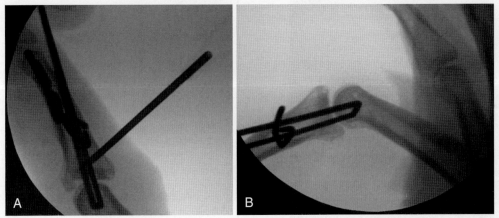

FIGURE 8.14 A, Percutaneous introduction of 18-gauge needle to elevated impacted fragments. **B,** Reduction after tension is applied to the dynamic fixator and joint is reduced percutaneously.

peroxide for the first week twice a day and thereafter only if they have drainage. Patients are permitted to get the fixator wet in the shower once wounds are sealed and benign in appearance. Pin tract redness, swelling, or drainage is treated with antibiotics and rest. Radiographs are taken at 1 week to ensure that fracture and joint reduction are maintained. Distraction can be adjusted with rubber band application or removal as indicated by radiographs; ideally, the joint should be only minimally distracted when compared with neighboring PIP joints. After 4 weeks, adequate healing is confirmed by removing the dental rubber bands and obtaining lateral radiographs of the digit in flexion and extension. Fixator removal as early as 3 weeks has been reported with successful results.[23] If there is evidence of fracture healing and the joint stays congruent, the fixator is removed; otherwise, it is rechecked in 1 to 2 weeks.

Expected outcomes. A review of several recent reports showed an average range of motion of approximately 85 degrees

at follow-up after 1 to 2 years.[23,33,61,88,100,114] Superficial pin tract infections are present in 10 to 30% of cases, but they typically resolve without incident. Patients demonstrate 92% grip strength on average. Only a few patients in these series have reported residual pain. On subset analysis, patients with significant joint comminution or a delay to surgery perform less well.

Our own results, although good for this difficult injury, have had more instances of residual pain than these case series may suggest. Perhaps the degree of joint comminution was more than the case examples shown in radiographs presented in these papers.

Open Reduction and Internal Fixation. ORIF is an excellent form of treatment when there is a single large volar fragment. The procedure is performed through a volar zigzag incision; the flap is based radially in the index and long fingers and ulnarly in the ring and small fingers to reduce the potential for contact hypersensitivity. The A3 pulley is excised or everted for later repair. The flexor tendons are retracted. A self-retaining operative tray with ball-and-chain hooks or an aluminum or lead hand may be helpful to retract the neighboring digits. The PIP joint is entered in the A2 to A4 interval between the flexor sheath, and the sheath is excised or everted for later reattachment. It is important to fully visualize the articular surface to ensure anatomic reduction, which may require a "shotgun" hyperextension approach (Fig 8.15, *A* and *B*). To do this, the neurovascular bundles are mobilized to prevent traction injury, the flexor tendons are protected and retracted with a Penrose drain, and the collateral ligaments that remain attached to the middle phalanx are excised except for the most volar remnants. These are preserved for later use in the procedure to suture each corner of the volar plate margin. The volar plate is generally left attached to the volar fracture fragment but can be detached as necessary. Although preservation of the volar plate insertion on the fragment will maintain the blood supply, fracture healing is usually not dependent upon this. Detaching the collateral ligaments allows the joint to be maximally hyperextended, as one would open a shotgun. With both articular surfaces completely exposed, the feasibility of reduction and fixation of the fragments can be determined. Impacted fragments of the dorsal articular surface may be elevated with a dental pick or Freer elevator, and the subchondral void filled with a small autologous or allograft cancellous crouton.

If the volar fragment is large, the joint is reduced and the fragment held with one or two 1-mm lag screws, the goal being an anatomic, stable reduction. In hard bone, the small screw head(s) are countersunk to minimize flexor sheath irritation, and care is taken to avoid screw tips extending beyond the dorsal cortex where they may irritate the extensor mechanism. Release of the collateral ligament attachments to the fragment greatly improves visualization and eases manipulation. When there is comminution of the volar fragment(s), a 1.3-mm volar buttress plate can be applied. The flexor digitorum superficialis inserts laterally, so a centrally placed plate is well tolerated. Protected early motion is the goal.

CRITICAL POINTS *Open Reduction and Internal Fixation*

Preoperative Considerations

- Have a backup plan (i.e., hemihamate autograft or dynamic skeletal fixation) because comminution is often worse than demonstrated on preoperative radiographs.
- The technique is best for a single, large fragment pattern, but smaller implant systems with 1-mm screws and 1.3-mm plates can render stable reduction with certain fracture types.

Technical Points

- Sharp dissection with meticulous handling of soft tissues cannot be overemphasized.
- Inspect the dorsal surface carefully to make sure it is anatomic, and elevate impacted fragments and bone graft as needed.
- After fixation, check a lateral in flexion and extension to make sure the joint maintains a congruent reduction and does not subluxate in extension.

Postoperative Planning

- Construct must be sufficiently stable to permit early motion. If unstable, consider adding an additional Kirschner wire fixator to maintain stability during early motion. Avoid overdistraction.

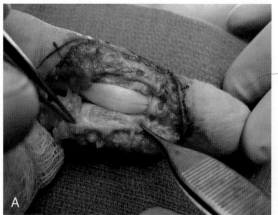
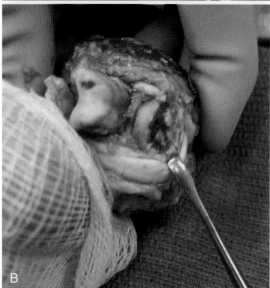

FIGURE 8.15 Shotgun approach for proximal interphalangeal joint exposure. **A,** Flexor sheath between A2 and A4 pulleys is incised along one edge and elevated. When closing, it can be passed under the tendon to prevent adhesions at repair site. **B,** After recession of collaterals, joint can be "shotgunned" open. (Courtesy Hill Hastings, MD.)

Postoperative protocol. Patients begin immediate active range-of-motion movements of the joint. Between exercises the digit is immobilized in a gutter splint with the PIP joint maintained in full extension (as long as there is no joint subluxation) to prevent flexion contracture. Passive range-of-motion movements and dynamic splints are started based on the surgeon's assessment of the integrity of the repair; we prefer to start as soon as possible.

Expected outcomes. Four recent case series of 54 patients who had undergone volar miniscrew ORIF demonstrated PIP motion of 55 to 115 degrees (average, 80 degrees) with a 10-degree flexion contracture. Strength averaged 85% of the uninjured side.[20,42,45,60]

Volar Plate Arthroplasty. The PIP joint is exposed using a radially based flap through a chevron-shaped incision with its apex at the ulnar midaxial point. The flexor sheath is excised between the A2 and A4 pulleys, and the flexor tendons are atraumatically retracted with a Penrose drain. The articular surfaces are very difficult to assess with the joint reduced. Hyperextension of the joint will usually expose the distal edge of the fracture fragment, facilitating entrance into the joint. A shotgun joint is exposed using a radially based flap through to gain access and to release any preexisting joint contracture.

Congruous reduction may not be possible if the fracture fragments are markedly comminuted or impacted. Loose bone fragments and the segment attached to the volar plate are excised and saved for potential bone graft material. The defect in the volar rim of the middle phalanx is shaped into a transverse groove perpendicular to the long axis of the phalanx. Deeply impacted fragments should be left undisturbed to serve as a buttress for the volar plate. The interval between the volar plate and both collateral ligaments is incised, and the fibrocartilaginous plate is mobilized if necessary to allow its advancement 4 to 6 mm distally into the defect in the middle phalanx. The more recent the injury, the more easily the plate will advance. In late cases, it is usually necessary to partially release (Figure 8.16) the proximal checkrein ligaments to gain sufficient length for advancement.

The volar plate is advanced into the middle phalangeal defect by means of a pull-out wire or suture, which spirals along the lateral margins of the volar plate and is passed through drill holes in the lateral margins of the middle phalangeal defect (Figure 8.17). The holes are made by drilling a Keith needle from volar to dorsal, and the needles are threaded with the suture and pulled out dorsally. These holes should be as proximal as possible (immediately deep to the remaining dorsal subchondral plate) to draw the plate against the edge of the remaining articular cartilage. They should exit the dorsum of the middle phalanx more centrally through the triangular ligament of the extensor mechanism to avoid binding down the

lateral bands. The DIP joint should be flexed 30 degrees as the suture is passed through the extensor mechanism to avoid tethering the tendon. Traction on the sutures emerging from the dorsum of the middle phalanx facilitates reduction of the joint as the plate is advanced into the defect.

Lateral radiographs are obtained before tying the sutures, to confirm that a congruous reduction throughout a full arc of motion has been achieved. Maintenance of the reduction with

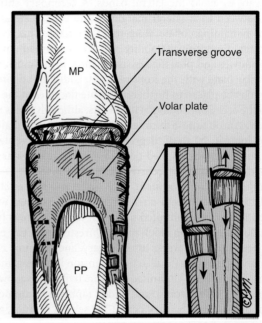

FIGURE 8.16 Step-cuts can be made along checkrein ligaments to allow distal advancement of volar plate into the defect. *MP*, Metacarpophalangeal; *PP*, proximal phalanx. (Copyright © Elizabeth Martin.)

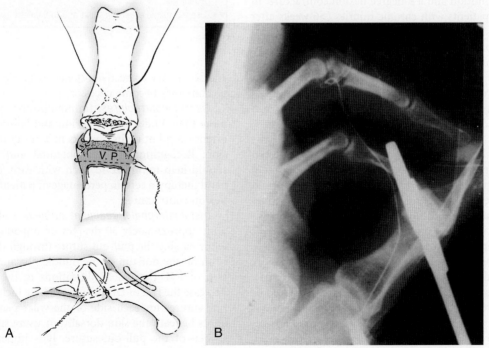

FIGURE 8.17 A, Volar plate advanced into defect of reduced joint and held with pull-out wires over a button. **B,** Radiograph showing a reduced joint with volar plate advancement.

articular gliding through the flexion arc (as opposed to hinging on the dorsal articular surface) must be documented. This is particularly true in chronic fracture-dislocations with dorsal adhesions. If hinging is present, additional release is necessary, usually of the dorsal capsule, which may have become scarred and inelastic over time. Once a congruous reduction and arc of motion are ensured, the pull-out sutures are tied over felt and a button. Alternatively, a small incision can be made dorsally and sutures tied down just distal to the central slip insertion, taking care to avoid the lateral bands. A secondary suture is placed between each lateral margin of the volar plate and its adjacent remaining collateral ligament remnant. This reestablishes three-dimensional stability and ensures broad coverage of the condyles and phalangeal base. If there is too much laxity in the volar plate with the joint reduced, additional tightening sutures may be placed to further imbricate the sides of the volar plate to the accessory collateral ligaments, although this is rarely necessary. An oblique Kirschner wire is used to maintain the reduced joint in 20 to 30 degrees of flexion. In large defects, bone graft should be applied deep to the advanced volar plate to reduce the chance for recurrent subluxation.

Postoperative management. DIP joint motion is started immediately. Three weeks after surgery, the Kirschner wire is removed and active, unlimited flexion of the PIP joint is begun using a dorsal extension block splint. Unrestricted active extension is permitted at 4 weeks after surgery, and dynamic extension splinting is begun if full active extension is not regained by 5 weeks after surgery. Unlimited sports activities are allowed at 8 weeks with buddy taping, and buddy taping is continued for 4 to 6 months. Swelling may persist for several months, and it may take up to 6 to 8 months to achieve final range of motion.

Eaton and Malerich reported on 24 patients who underwent volar plate arthroplasty for both acute and chronic PIP fracture-dislocations, with a 10-year average follow-up.[31] The seven procedures performed within 6 weeks of injury attained an average of 95 degrees of motion and a 6-degree flexion contracture. In contrast, the 17 patients with chronic injuries (>6 weeks after injury) achieved 78 degrees of motion and 12 degrees of contracture. Only 3 patients reported pain, and only with strenuous use. Other reports have also noted good results in most patients.[10,28] Our own experience has not been as optimistic. The procedure is more appropriate for patients with volar articular involvement of less than 40 to 50%, and it has failed when we have used it for joints with greater involvement.

Complications

Redisplacement. Failure to achieve a stable reduction, pull-out suture failure, or inadequate protection during mobilization may result in recurrent dorsal subluxation. One cause of pull-out suture failure is damage from the transarticular Kirschner wire fixation. This complication may be obviated by prepositioning of the wire in the middle phalanx after Keith needle passage but before the sutures are pulled through. With close clinical and radiographic follow-up, such problems can be more expeditiously addressed and their effects minimized.

Angulation. Asymmetric impaction of the base of the middle phalanx or failure to create a trough for the volar plate that is perpendicular to the long axis of the middle phalanx will occasionally result in angulation of the middle phalanx. Although postoperative angular deformity is usually mild and not functionally significant, patient satisfaction may be compromised

---

> ### CRITICAL POINTS *Volar Plate Arthroplasty for Dorsal Fracture-Dislocations of the Proximal Interphalangeal Joint*
>
> **Preoperative Evaluation**
> - Determine whether the remaining dorsal articular surface is anatomic or impacted.
> - Appropriate for unstable fracture-dislocations unsuitable for ORIF; indicated for fractures in which 40% or less of the articular surface is involved and in occasional cases with articular depression of more than 40% but less than 1.5 to 2 mm; not advised for volar fracture involvement exceeding 40% to 50%
>
> **Technical Points**
> - Use volar approach with chevron incision
> - "se volar approach with chevron incisionnatomic or impact
> - Excise comminuted fragments and elevate dorsal, impacted articular surface
> - Place holes for pull-out sutures as proximal as possible and avoid lateral bands dorsally
> - Establish ideal length of volar plate with joint reduced
> - Reduce joint, tie sutures with DIP flexed, and document congruency radiographically in flexion and extension
> - Pin in 20 to 30 degrees of flexion for 3 weeks only
>
> **Pitfalls**
> - Leaving stable but impacted dorsal articular surface unaddressed
> - Impaling lateral bands with pull-out sutures
> - Failing to spread volar plate broadly across condyles
> - Failing to identify hinged versus gliding flexion via dorsal adhesions
> - Applying technique to fracture-dislocations with more than 40% volar articular involvement (failure is likely)
>
> **Postoperative Care**
> - Immobilize joint with Kirschner wire and splint for 3 weeks.
> - Remove pin at 3 weeks and obtain radiographs after pin removal.
> - Use extension block flexion for 1 to 3 weeks and then unlimited extension.
> - Use a dynamic extension splint at 5 to 6 weeks as needed.

and secondary corrective osteotomy at the base of the middle phalanx may become necessary.

Flexion contractures. Immobilization of the PIP joint in more than 30 degrees of flexion and failure to begin dynamic extension splinting by 5 weeks may result in lack of full extension. Recognition of this potential and common problem should help minimize it. Even with early motion and formal hand therapy, a certain percentage of patients will develop a PIP flexion contracture.

Distal interphalangeal joint stiffness. Failure to flex the DIP joint approximately 30 degrees or impaling the lateral bands while passing the pull-out suture through the extensor mechanism on the dorsum of the middle phalanx may cause limitation of DIP flexion. Modifications in the technique help to decrease the risk of DIP stiffness. These include using two separate sutures for each side of the volar plate, tying the suture knots beneath the skin dorsally, or using small suture anchors in lieu of the pull-out suture. It is imperative to start DIP motion immediately postoperatively to regain the maximal motion possible.

Cerclage Wiring. A volar chevron incision is made from the MP joint to the DIP joint. The neurovascular bundles are mobilized away from the flexor sheath to avoid traction injury during the shotgun approach (previously). A dental pick is used to align and elevate fragments. Bone grafting of impacted subchondral bone is done as needed. Sharp dissection is used to clear the proximal 1 to 2 mm of the middle phalanx from the periosteum to allow the wire to be seated. A loop of 24-gauge wire is formed and twisted on itself, placed around the bone, and gently tightened (see Figure 8.6). The joint is gently distracted and reduced. The joint is placed through a range of motion to assess congruency and stability. A "V"-shaped wedge is removed from the volar plate and the lateral edges are repaired (Figure 8.18). This prevents hyperextension but eliminates bulk under the flexor apparatus. This also decreases tension on the repair, allowing for immediate full or nearly full extension in therapy.

Postoperative protocol. Therapy is initiated after 2 to 4 days to allow for edema control. Active and passive motion is allowed with interval gutter splinting. Dynamics are added at 2 weeks if motion is slow to progress.

❖ AUTHORS' PREFERRED TECHNIQUE FOR HEMIHAMATE RECONSTRUCTION

A midaxial incision is made centered on the PIP joint and extended obliquely across the proximal and middle phalanges (Figure 8.19). Sharp dissection passes superficial to the neurovascular bundle down to the flexor sheath, elevating the subcutaneous tissue off the sheath and including the neurovascular bundle on the hinge side of the retracted flap (see Figure 8.15). Incise the sheath between the A2 and A4 pulleys, and retract the flexor tendons. The accessory collateral insertion into the volar plate should be incised longitudinally from the volar plate. The volar plate is divided transversely at its distal insertion and elevated to its proximal insertion. Release the collateral ligaments from their proximal insertion as much as needed until the joint can be shotgunned open. In chronic cases, a Freer

elevator may be required to free dorsal capsular or extensor adhesions. Confirm on fluoroscopy that the dorsal residual intact articular base of the middle phalanx reduces anatomically with the head of the proximal phalanx. After exposing the articular base of the middle phalanx fracture, measurements are taken for the replacement graft with respect to the radioulnar width, anteroposterior height, and proximodistal length. It is best to harvest the hamate graft prior to final preparation of the recipient bed to preserve as much of the middle phalanx as possible and maximize the ability to properly position the graft.

Next a longitudinal incision is made over the bases of the fourth and fifth metacarpals, taking care to protect the ulnar sensory nerve branches. Retract the extensors to the fifth finger ulnarly and the fourth finger radially. Incise and elevate the capsule to expose the hamate and metacarpal articulation. Measure and mark the appropriate size for the donor graft, adding a few extra millimeters. The proximal end of the graft should be thicker than the articular portion to allow the graft to re-create the volar lip and appropriate buttress (Figure 8.20).

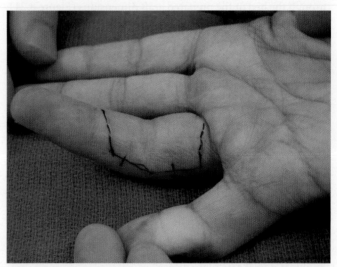

FIGURE 8.19 Incision for hemihamate arthroplasty extends obliquely proximally and distally, but continues along midaxial line at proximal interphalangeal joint to maximize exposure. (Courtesy Hill Hastings, MD.)

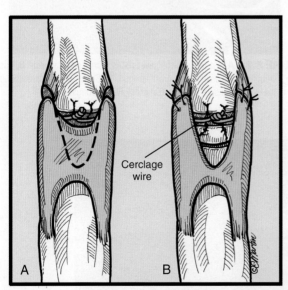

FIGURE 8.18 A, "V"-shaped segment is removed from volar plate. **B,** Edges are repaired to minimize bulk while allowing volar stabilization. (From Weiss AP: Cerclage fixation for fracture dislocation of the PIP joint, *Clin Orthop Relat Res* (327):21–28, 1996. Redrawn by Elizabeth Martin.)

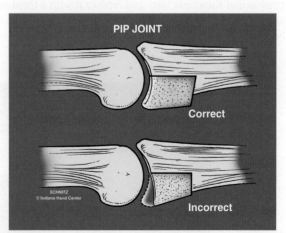

FIGURE 8.20 Graft is planned to be shaped such that when in place it tilts to re-create volar lip. *PIP,* Proximal interphalangeal. (From Strickland JW, Graham TJ, editors: *Master techniques in orthopaedic surgery: the hand,* 2nd ed, Philadelphia, Lippincott Williams & Wilkins, 2004.)

To harvest the hamate graft, mark the required dimensions on the dorsal surface of the hamate. Usually it will extend all the way to the ulnar border of the hamate. Place a Freer elevator in the fourth/fifth CMC joint to lever the joint open slightly. Use a thin sagittal saw blade to make sagittal cuts in the hamate radially and ulnarly, being sure that the depth of each cut is slightly greater than the needed anteroposterior thickness of the recipient defect. Be sure that the cuts extend distally though the articular surface of the hamate into the CMC joint. Make a similar transverse cut proximally at least 2 to 3 mm deeper than the axial cuts. The graft can be harvested in one of two ways. The goal is to create a coronal plane cut from the articular surface into the more proximal hamate in a direction that passes from distal into a more volar direction proximally. This will provide a graft that has a greater dorsal/volar depth or thickness proximally than distally. A curved osteotome is placed within the CMC joint to an appropriate depth that conservatively exceeds the required anteroposterior height of the desired graft. Once it is driven through the chondral and subchondral articular surfaces, a cleavage plane will usually propagate proximally through the bed of the prepared graft dimensions (Figure 8.21). The second, and perhaps safest, method is to make a coronal plane cut with a sagittal saw directed from the ulnar border of the hamate to the radial side. In most cases, in order to obtain a wide enough graft, harvest to the far ulnar side of the hamate will be required. This method provides the best control for ensuring that the plane of osteotomy is from a distal dorsal to a proximal volar direction. The shape of the graft obtained will ensure that the volar buttress of the articular base of the middle phalanx is properly restored (Figure 8.22).

Conservatively trim the recipient defect into a rectangularly shaped bed with a small oscillating saw (Figure 8.23). The graft should first be trimmed to re-create a proper "tip," such that the graft is slightly angled in the sagittal plane to re-create the volar lip buttress of the middle phalangeal base. Once a proper "tip" has been created, the graft is sequentially shortened or the recipient bed enlarged to align the articular surface of the graft with the intact dorsal articular surface.

Hold the graft in place with a provisional 0.028-inch Kirschner wire, and use two 1-mm screws in lag fashion to secure the graft on either side of the provisional Kirschner wire. Remove the provisional Kirschner wire and replace it with a third screw (Figure 8.24). In cases requiring replacement of more than 60% of the joint surface, consider adding a 1.3-mm buttress plate to

support the graft. Repair the medial and lateral edges of the volar plate back to the accessory collateral ligaments or proximal edge of the A4 pulley to prevent a swan neck deformity. Check the joint stability and the conformity in flexion and extension. At the surgeon flexion and the previously opened

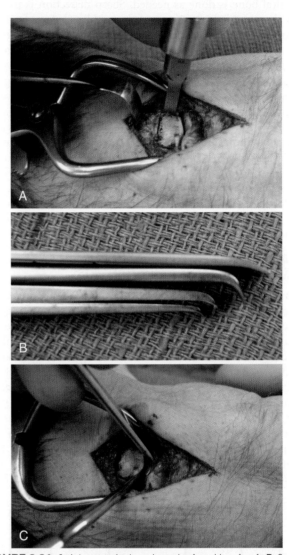

FIGURE 8.21 **A,** A 4-mm sagittal saw is used to free sides of graft. **B,** Custom-made osteotomes to assist with graft harvest. **C,** Small curved osteotomes are used to make coronal split in graft. (Courtesy Hill Hastings, MD.)

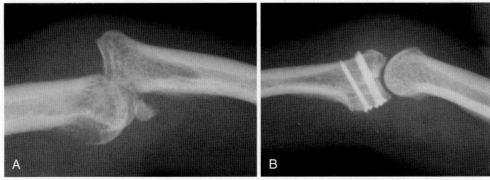

FIGURE 8-22 **A,** Preoperative lateral radiograph showing injury. **B,** Postoperative lateral radiograph showing reconstruction and congruent joint with volar buttress in place due to appropriate angling of graft. (Courtesy Hill Hastings, MD.)

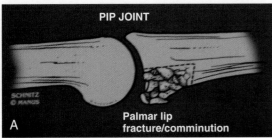

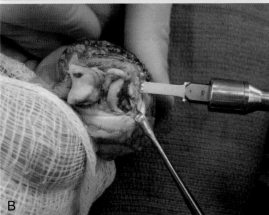

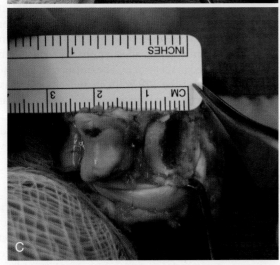

FIGURE 8.23 A, Diagram showing transverse and coronal cuts made to remove all comminuted fragments. **B,** Intraoperative photograph showing initial resection of fragments using 4-mm saw. **C,** This leaves a boxlike defect, where the remaining joint surface is structurally sound. *PIP,* Proximal interphalangeal. (**A,** From Strickland JW, Graham TJ, editors: *Master techniques in orthopaedic surgery: the hand,* 2nd ed, Philadelphia, Lippincott Williams & Wilkins, 2004. **B** and **C,** Courtesy Hill Hastings, MD.)

flexor sheath may be transposed beneath the flexor tendons to reinforce the volar plate and prevent adhesions (Figure 8.25).

Postoperative protocol. Patients are splinted with the PIP joint in 10 to 20 degrees of flexion and the MP joints in flexion. On postoperative days 2 to 4, a dorsal block splint for the PIP in 20 degrees of flexion is fitted and patients are instructed to perform full active and passive flexion exercises. A digital anesthetic block may be required to ensure that nearly full motion is established on this first therapy visit. The splint is removed at 4 weeks, and dynamic splints may be applied at 6 weeks as needed to address difficulties with flexion or extension. Radiographs are performed in the flexed and extended lateral posi-

tions to confirm joint congruency during the postoperative period (Case Study 8.1).

CRITICAL POINTS *Hemihamate Reconstruction*

Indications
- Acute or chronic unstable PIP fracture-dislocations with extensive joint impaction or comminution
- An option for previously failed external fixation, ORIF, or other treatments

Technical Points
- Preserve the flexor sheath between A2 and A4 on a hinge so that it can be transposed at the end of the procedure under the flexor tendon, to reinforce the repair site and minimize flexor tendon adhesions.
- Small comminuted fragments of volar bone are removed to make a precise box-shaped defect for reconstruction.
- The graft is harvested to be thicker proximally, in order to "tip" the chondral surface appropriately and reconstitute the natural joint curvature of the volar buttress.

Postoperative Plan
- The PIP joint is flexed 10 to 20 degrees for the first 4 weeks to allow volar plate healing.
- Patients should be advised to expect a mild flexion contracture at the final outcome.

Expected outcomes. All 22 patients in this study had unstable dorsal PIP fracture-dislocations of more than 50% of the middle phalangeal articular base that were not amenable to open reduction and fixation. At a mean follow-up of 4.5 years, active PIP motion averaged 70 degrees. The mean flexion contracture was 19 degrees (range, 0 degrees to 80 degrees). The mean VAS score for digit pain was 1.4 (acute, 0.7; chronic, 2.5). A mean DASH score of 5 (acute, 2; chronic, 9) and VAS functional score of 1.9 (acute, 1.4; chronic, 2.6) indicated little functional impairment (acute, 2; chronic, 9). Grip strength averaged 95% of the opposite hand. One dissatisfied patient required revision surgery.[15]

Chronic Proximal Interphalangeal Fracture-Dislocations

Occasionally, fracture-dislocations of the PIP joint remain untreated or the initial closed reduction is lost, resulting in a fixed dorsal subluxation with a malunited or nonunited volar buttress of the middle phalanx. Stiffness and progressive pain are inevitable.

Open reduction with a corrective osteotomy with or without bone graft of malunited fractures has been advocated.[125] Success of this technique is predicated on the accurate reduction of the joint and presence of reasonable chondral surfaces in chronic injuries, two conditions that may not be attainable. Resurfacing an IP joint with costal cartilage and perichondrium (perichondrial arthroplasty) has been used in a small number of chronic PIP joint fractures.[47,69] Free vascularized joint replacement with DIP joints or toe IP joints has also been reported.[51] The efficacy of these techniques for chronic fracture-dislocations has not been convincing to this author. Other treatment options include implant arthroplasty and arthrodesis, both of which are less than ideal in the relatively young patient population in whom this problem most often occurs.

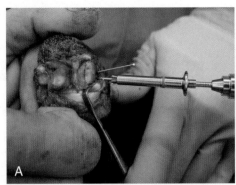 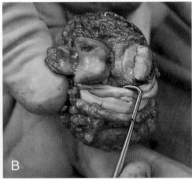

FIGURE 8.24 A, Graft is placed and held with provisional Kirschner wire while secured with 1-mm screws. **B,** Intraoperative photograph showing reconstructed joint. (Courtesy Hill Hastings, MD.)

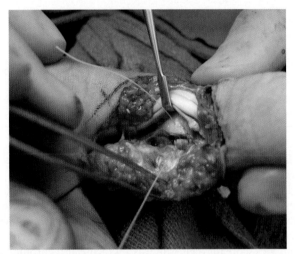

FIGURE 8.25   The flexor sheath between the A2 and A4 pulleys is transposed beneath the flexor tendons to prevent adherence at repair site. (Courtesy Hill Hastings, MD.)

Volar plate arthroplasty is a consideration for these injuries only when there is less than 40% volar articular involvement. The success of the procedure mainly depends on restoring proper reduction of the joint and less so on restoring the volar plate. Adequate advancement of the volar plate may require fractional lengthening of the proximal checkrein ligaments by making several 2- to 3-mm incisions in both lateral margins at intervals along their length. Complete *excision* of both PIP collateral ligaments is essential to achieve adequate exposure, a congruous joint reduction, and maximal postoperative motion.

❖ AUTHORS' PREFERRED METHOD OF TREATMENT

Hemihamate arthroplasty restores a smooth cartilaginous surface to the base of the middle phalanx and maintains a stable reduction. This technique can be used for PIP reconstruction provided there is enough intact articular surface on the dorsum of the base of the middle phalanx with which to form a congruous articulating facet and anchor the graft. In long-standing dislocations, a release of the dorsal capsule may be needed to regain flexion. Surgical technique and rehabilitation are the same as for acute fracture-dislocations. Surgical outcomes are less predictable for chronic injuries and in general less robust.[15]

Chronic Proximal Interphalangeal Subluxations (Hyperextension)

Untreated or underdiagnosed type I (hyperextension) injuries can result in PIP hyperextension or a swan neck deformity. It is important to compare the affected digit with neighboring digits and the opposite side, particularly for patients with ligamentous laxity. Patients may complain of pain from snapping lateral bands as they move to and from the hyperextended position. In swan neck deformities, the examiner must distinguish primary volar plate laxity from extensor mechanism imbalance, such as that after an untreated mallet finger. The distinction can usually be made by stabilizing the PIP joint in full extension as the patient attempts to actively extend the distal joint. A lag in active distal extension when the PIP joint is stabilized in neutral indicates incompetence of the extensor mechanism. If the distal joint extends normally, the problem is primarily with the volar support of the PIP joint.

Treatment

For minimally symptomatic PIP hyperextension deformity, custom or commercially available figure-of-eight splints provide a functional alternative to surgery. Splinting will not correct the problem and the splint must be worn full time to be effective. Surgical correction of these deformities involves either late reattachment/reconstruction of the volar plate or a tenodesis procedure.

Reattachment procedures include direct repair or advancement of the avulsed volar plate with sutures, a pull-out wire, or a bone anchor, following scarification of the base of the middle phalanx. Less severe deformities may be stabilized by advancement of the accessory collateral ligaments into the volar plate.[73]

Reconstruction of the volar plate by tenodesis can be achieved with one or both slips of the flexor digitorum superficialis[91] or by rerouting of one of the lateral bands. Use of both flexor digitorum superficialis slips is reserved for hyperextension deformities created by a severe chronic imbalance of forces, as in cerebral palsy, or in cases when the flexor digitorum superficialis slips may be quite thin. Lateral band tenodesis is a simple procedure that does not interfere with the flexor mechanism.

Technique of Lateral Band Tenodesis. A 2-cm ulnar-sided midlateral incision is made centered on the PIP joint. The Cleland ligament is incised to allow access to the neurovascular bundle and the flexor sheath. The neurovascular bundle is gently

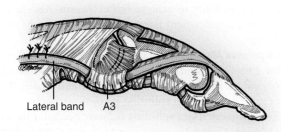

FIGURE 8.26 Treatment of flexible swan neck deformity by volar transposition of lateral band. (Copyright © Elizabeth Martin.)

retracted. The lateral band's relationship to the lumbrical is left undisturbed as it is incised from the extensor apparatus along its dorsal margin, keeping its distal attachment intact. It is mobilized palmar to the PIP joint. Several options exist for rerouting of the lateral band. I prefer to suture the intact lateral band to the lateral edge of the A3 pulley, taking care to avoid the flexor tendons. Another technique is to open the A3 pulley with a step-cut and sew it over the top of the lateral band, trapping it inside the pulley (Figure 8.26). Alternatively, one can release the ipsilateral flexor digitorum superficialis slip distally, interpose the lateral band between it and the volar plate, and reattach the flexor digitorum superficialis to the volar plate distally. The joint should rest in 20 to 30 degrees of flexion and on passive extension should still have a 5- to 10-degree flexion contracture. This allows for some stretching out of the soft tissue repair while still allowing for maintenance of the correction. Some prefer to approach the joint through a volar Bruner incision, divide the lateral band proximally, pass it beneath the Cleland ligament and the neurovascular bundle, and secure it to the A2 pulley on the opposite side of the finger.

Postoperative Management. On the first postoperative day a dorsal extension block splint is applied in 10 to 20 degrees of PIP flexion to allow immediate active flexion. After 3 weeks the extension block is reduced to 5 degrees. Unrestricted motion is permitted at 6 weeks, and unlimited sports activities are possible at 8 to 10 weeks with buddy taping until 3 months after the surgery.

Expected Outcomes. Patients seek treatment for PIP hyperextension deformities because of dysfunction in daily activities. We have found lateral band tenodesis to be reliable with generally good results. Immediate postoperative pain is mild, and recovery is brief with a rapid return to function. There are no published data for lateral band tenodesis that we know of to guide patient and surgeon expectations. Flexor digitorum superficialis tenodesis is another reliable option; in a series of 12 patients, 5 had excellent results, 5 had good results, and 2 had fair results, and all patients returned to their original occupations and recreational activities.[18] Two patients, both of whom were noncompliant with postoperative therapy, had flexion contractures of 30 and 60 degrees.

Complications. In spite of good-quality tissue and fixation, the final tenodesis position may not correspond to that which was set at surgery. There is more of a tendency toward a flexion contracture than residual hyperextension because the procedure weakens the extensor moment while providing a mechanical block to hyperextension. Therefore, it is important to set the tension on the tenodesis to no more than 5 or 10 degrees short of full extension and to monitor the patients carefully postoperatively.

Posttraumatic Fibrosis and Contracture of the Proximal Interphalangeal Joint

Flexion Contracture

When nonoperative treatment and dynamic splinting have failed, operative treatment options for flexion contractures run the gamut from soft tissue release to distraction external fixation.

Collateral ligament excision and, if necessary, a distal volar plate release have demonstrated good results.[1,24,82] Abbiati and associates recommended sparing the proper collateral ligaments while releasing the volar plate and accessory collateral ligaments.[1] Mansat and Delprat recommended a technique in which the volar plate and capsule are released and then the origins of the collateral ligaments are incised but not excised.[82] Diao and Eaton demonstrated no long-term collateral ligament insufficiency after complete excision of the collateral ligaments during joint release.[24] For severe contractures that may involve a postoperative skin deficiency, advancement flaps should be carefully planned to place skin graft over a defect in the palm rather than over the released joint; in cases with compromised volar tissue, a cross-finger flap may be useful.[35]

Concerns for PIP joint instability after collateral ligament excision are unfounded. A review of 16 patients who had total ligament excision and volar plate release for isolated posttraumatic PIP fibrosis showed an increase in total active motion from 38 degrees preoperatively to 78 degrees postoperatively at 1-year follow-up. In all patients, the joints were stable to lateral stress in all positions of flexion by 3 weeks.[24]

Preoperative Evaluation. The three requirements for successful treatment of a flexion contracture are absence of degenerative disease, a functional extensor mechanism, and a motivated and compliant patient. Conservative measures such as dynamic extension splints should be exhausted first. Radiographs should demonstrate a congruent, preserved joint space without mechanical block due to osteophytes. In that setting, release of the contracture, even if mild (<20 degrees), is quite reliable.

For more severe contractures, distraction external fixation achieved extension gains averaging 65 degrees in one series with a unilateral fixator and an average of 42 degrees with a compass hinge fixator.[56] Work by Houshian and Chikkamuniyappa also assessed different distraction rates and demonstrated equal results from an accelerated program with an average fixator time of only 17 days.[55]

An external device that uses extension torque was introduced in 2001 (Digit Widget, Hand Biomechanics Lab, Sacramento, CA).[4] This employs a dorsal bar fixed to the middle phalanx with two threaded pins and connected to a hand-based outrigger device with rubber bands (Figure 8.27). The device provides torque to progressively extend the PIP joint and is well tolerated because the patient can modulate the extension torque with different grades of rubber bands, as well as application times. It is important to control MP joint hyperextension when the device is being worn because this will limit gains in PIP extension (see Chapter 10).

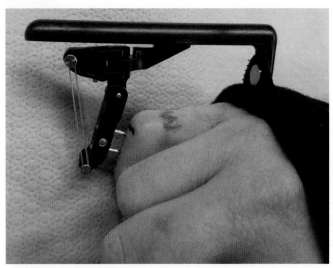

FIGURE 8.27 Digit Widget device (Hand Biomechanics Lab, Sacramento, CA) provides patient-controlled extension torque to a proximal interphalangeal contracture through dorsal rubber bands connected to a fixed dorsal outrigger. Metacarpophalangeal joint hyperextension can be controlled with an accessory strap. (Copyright © Scott W. Wolfe, MD.)

❖ AUTHORS' PREFERRED METHOD OF TREATMENT

The recent reports of external fixation PIP distraction are encouraging and worthy of further investigation.[4,55] At this time, we continue to achieve good results with open soft tissue release, although the time to return to full function may be longer than via a closed means of treatment. The PIP joint is approached through a Bruner style of volar incision. This is more expedient and safer because the bundles are easily identified, both the collaterals and the volar plate are easily accessed, and flexor tenolysis is accessible if needed. A midaxial incision has been shown in one series to produce better results and could be considered, although it is technically more demanding.[14] A tray with self-retaining ball-and-chain hooks facilitates retraction. The A3 pulley is released on one side, and this may be subsequently repaired or excised at the surgeon's discretion. The flexor tendons are gently retracted to allow exposure of the volar plate. Care is taken to protect the distal flexor digitorum superficialis insertion. The authors have never encountered a stiff PIP joint made unstable by full release of collaterals, accessory collaterals, and the volar plate. "Springy" PIP joints that have not had full release of all the aforementioned structures may not progress well postoperatively. A full release of all structures is typically necessary; however, one should proceed in a stepwise fashion, checking motion between steps. A Beaver blade is used to release the collaterals, starting in the joint and working proximally. The volar plate and checkrein ligaments are elevated off the proximal phalanx. There are often fibrotic bands from the volar plate that extend laterally upward dorsally under the neurovascular bundles, which also need to be removed. I have not found that excision of the collaterals is required; full release off the proximal condyles is all that is needed.

At this point in most cases, the digits achieve full extension with little flexor tone. If not, check the flexor tendons for adhesions and treat as needed. In long-standing severe contractures, one may have to consider the trade-offs of flexor digitorum superficialis release if it appears that tendon contractures contribute to an inability to achieve full extension. Also in severe contractures, advancement flaps or skin grafts may be needed for coverage.

Postoperative Management. The digit is splinted in full extension for 2 to 3 days and elevated. This allows for some edema control prior to initiating therapy for active and passive flexion exercises. Static extension splinting is continued between exercises. Dynamic extension splinting is rarely needed if the surgical release was complete. The patient is weaned from daytime extension splinting after a few weeks, but nighttime extension splinting is continued for 3 months.

Expected Outcomes. Ghidella and associates reported on 68 PIP joint contracture releases in 44 patients at minimal 2-year follow-up. Some results were sobering, with an average of only 8 degrees of improvement overall (range, 35-degree loss to 70-degree gain).[38] Younger patients, those with less severe contractures, those without a diagnosis of complex regional pain syndrome or crush injury, and those who had not had prior revascularization did better. Bruser and coworkers reported better overall results in 45 fingers, especially when the surgeon used a midlateral incision instead of a volar incision.[14] With a median contracture of 50 degrees, they achieved nearly 0 degrees of contracture at a 1.5-year follow-up. Careful patient selection is certainly important.

CRITICAL POINTS *Proximal Interphalangeal Contracture Release*

Indications
- Functional deficit secondary to a mature contracture in a compliant patient with no arthritic changes in the joint

Technical Points
- Midaxial incisions may produce better results but are technically more difficult.
- With full release of the collateral ligaments and proximal attachment of the volar plate and checkrein ligaments, instability will not be a problem.
- The joint should lay flat on the table at the end of the procedure and not be "springy."
- After sharp release of contracted structures, gently hyperextend the finger to release any remaining adhesions.

Postoperative Care
- Apply extension splinting between exercises.
- Initiate active and passive range-of-motion movements at postoperative day 2 to 3 to allow for some edema control initially.
- Apply dynamic splinting early if the patient is struggling to achieve full extension.

DISTAL INTERPHALANGEAL JOINTS OF THE FINGER AND INTERPHALANGEAL JOINTS OF THE THUMB

The ligamentous anatomy of the distal articulation of the finger and thumb is analogous to that of the PIP joint of the finger. However, due to the shorter lever arm of the distal phalanx and the enhanced stability provided by the adjacent insertions of the flexor and extensor tendons, dislocations are not as frequent.

Dislocations of the DIP joint are usually dorsal or lateral and often associated with an open wound because of the snug soft tissue envelope about the joint.

Treatment of these dislocations consists of closed reduction under digital or wrist block anesthesia. The reduction maneuver consists of longitudinal traction, direct pressure on the dorsum of the distal phalanx, and manipulation of the distal phalanx into flexion. If the dislocation is open, the joint is contaminated by definition, and treatment should include thorough irrigation and débridement in a controlled, sterile setting. After reduction, joint stability should be tested actively with range of motion by the patient and passively by the examiner to gently stress the collateral ligaments. Postreduction radiographs are mandatory to confirm congruous reduction. Instability after pure dislocations is rare, and the joint is immobilized in slight flexion using a dorsal splint for 2 to 3 weeks. After the first week, the patient should be encouraged to remove the distal tape or Velcro fixation of the splint and actively flex the DIP joint while avoiding the last 20 degrees of extension.

DIP and thumb IP dislocations are rarely irreducible. When they do occur, it is most commonly the result of proximal disruption of the volar plate, which then becomes interposed between the head of the digital middle or thumb proximal phalanx and the base of the distal phalanx, preventing reduction (Figure 8.28).[92] Interposition of the flexor tendon,[102] a fracture fragment,[113] digital nerves,[103] and a sesamoid bone[72] have also been reported, and the condyles of the middle phalanx can become entrapped in a longitudinal rent in the flexor digitorum profundus tendon.[39] Irreducible dislocations require surgical removal or manipulation of the offending anatomic structure(s) to facilitate reduction. It is sometimes possible to approach these cases with a small dorsal incision, thereby avoiding a larger volar dissection. A Freer elevator is introduced to push interposed structures out of the joint in an atraumatic manner and lever the joint back into position.

Rarely, a dorsal dislocation may be associated with a fracture of the volar lip of the distal phalanx, akin to a PIP joint dorsal fracture-dislocation.[54] If the volar fragment is not avulsed with the flexor digitorum profundus tendon, the goal of treatment remains a stable closed reduction. If the profundus tendon is avulsed, however, it must be reattached surgically. Even when the flexor digitorum profundus is intact, a volar fracture fragment may be large enough to render the joint unstable. If mild to moderate flexion of the DIP joint is insufficient to keep the joint reduced and especially if more than 40% of the articular surface has been fractured, a volar plate arthroplasty is indicated.

Volar plate arthroplasty can be an effective treatment for this problem. One series of 10 patients (4 thumb IP joints and 6 finger DIP joints) who underwent volar plate arthroplasty for chronic dorsal fracture-subluxation had an average of 51 degrees and 42 degrees, respectively, of stable active motion. All patients had a flexion contracture, which averaged 12 degrees. Patient satisfaction was high, and there were no complications.[99]

Dorsal dislocation of both IP joints of a single digit, most often the small finger, has also been reported.[6] The force required to cause this double dislocation implies more extensive soft tissue injury. Aggressive hand therapy is instituted soon after stable reduction to maximize the range of motion.

Pure volar dislocations of the DIP joint are rare and probably spontaneously reduce. These are essentially mallet injuries and require splinting in full extension for 6 weeks, followed by progressive mobilization. However, an irreducible volar dislocation of a DIP joint has been reported in which the extensor mechanism was longitudinally split and the terminal tendon interposed, preventing reduction.[62]

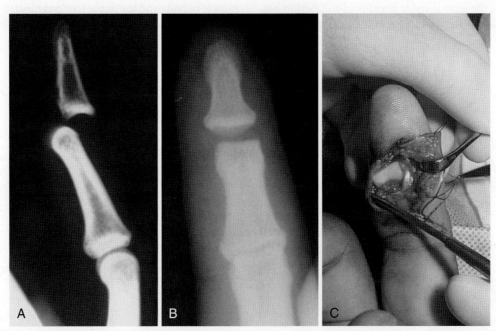

FIGURE 8.28 A, Irreducible dorsal dislocation of index distal interphalangeal joint. **B,** Posteroanterior view shows wide gap between middle and distal phalanges suggestive of soft tissue interposition. **C,** These injuries are commonly open, and, at exploration, the head of the middle phalanx was seen ulnar to the displaced flexor tendon. The volar plate was interposed between base of distal phalanx and head of middle phalanx.

METACARPOPHALANGEAL JOINT OF THE FINGER

ANATOMY

The MP joints of the fingers are relatively resistant to ligament injury and dislocation because of their intrinsic ligamentous structure, the surrounding tendons, and their protected position at the base of the fingers. They are most vulnerable to injury from forces directed ulnarly and dorsally. The articular surfaces form a condyloid joint. The metacarpal head is narrow dorsally, with a widened volar flare; this shape results in progressively more contact with the base of the proximal phalanx with increasing flexion.

The capsule of the MP joint extends from the metacarpal neck to the base of the proximal phalanx and is reinforced by specialized structures on all sides. The capsule is composed of areolar tissue dorsally and is reinforced by the loose insertion of the common extensor tendon. On the volar side, the joint is supported by the volar plate, which is continuous laterally with the deep transverse metacarpal (intervolar plate) ligament (Figure 8.29). The volar plate has a thick fibrocartilaginous distal portion and a thin membranous proximal portion. It does not have strong proximal checkrein ligaments comparable to those of the PIP joint. Lateral reinforcement for the volar plate is afforded by the collateral and intervolar plate ligaments, which insert into its lateral margins to produce linked support from one MP joint to the next.[85] The sagittal bands and the tendons of the intrinsic muscles provide additional, secondary support.[95] The collateral ligaments are more taut in flexion than in extension because of the cam effect created by the nonspherical shape of the metacarpal head, which has a longer dorsovolar axis than proximodistal axis (Figure 8.30). There is also broader and more stable articular contact between the metacarpal head and the base of the proximal phalanx beyond 70 degrees of flexion. Therefore, the joint is stable laterally in full flexion but allows some abduction and adduction in full extension.

Dorsal Metacarpophalangeal Dislocations

Dorsal dislocations of the MP joints of the fingers are relatively uncommon injuries. The most frequently involved digit is the index finger followed by the small finger. With exceptions,[90] dorsal dislocation of the central digits is usually seen only with concomitant dislocation of a border digit. Dorsal dislocation of a DIP joint and an MP joint in the same finger has been reported.[58]

The mechanism of injury is usually forced hyperextension of the digit as might occur from falling on an outstretched hand. The pathologic findings of complete dislocation of the index finger and the small finger are similar but not identical. In both instances, the volar plate ruptures in its membranous proximal portion and becomes interposed dorsally between the base of the proximal phalanx and the dorsal metacarpal head. If this were the only structure blocking reduction, reduction could be accomplished by using traction sufficient to draw the proximal edge of the volar plate over the metacarpal head. This is not possible, however, because the medial and lateral structures draw tightly around the narrow metacarpal neck and become even more taut with traction.

ANATOMY

Kaplan, in 1957, described the pathomechanics of the volar structures that block reduction of the dislocated MP joint.[66] The anatomic basis for complete, irreducible dislocation of the MP joint involves the following structures: the volar plate, the A1 pulley, the flexor tendons, the lumbricals, and, in the small finger, the abductor and flexor digiti quinti. As the volar plate is drawn distally over the metacarpal head by the dislocating proximal phalanx, the periarticular tendons are drawn dorsally past the metacarpal head. In this manner, a tendon noose forms around the metacarpal head and tightens further with traction. In the index finger, these structures include the lumbrical muscle radially and the flexor tendons ulnarly. The latter remain in the proximal flexor pulleys, which are attached to the dorsally

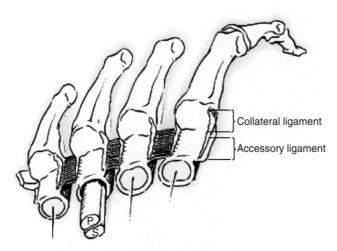

FIGURE 8.29 Intervolar plate ligaments that reinforce the ligament-box complex at each metacarpophalangeal joint. Because the volar plate is most securely attached to the proximal phalanx, this transverse ligament primarily supports the proximal phalanges. (From Eaton RG, Littler JW: Joint injuries and their sequelae, *Clin Plast Surg* 3:85–98, 1976.)

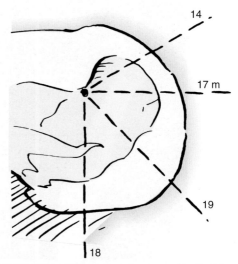

FIGURE 8.30 Diagram of cam effect of metacarpal head contour and relative length of collateral ligaments with increasing flexion. Shortening or loss of elasticity of collateral ligaments limits flexion. Metacarpophalangeal joint must be splinted in at least 50 degrees of flexion to maintain ligament length.

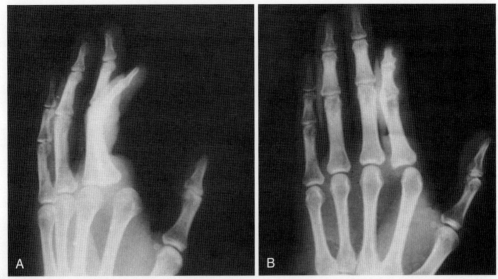

FIGURE 8.31 Radiographs of dorsal irreducible (complex) dislocation. **A,** Oblique view shows dorsal dislocation and a widened joint space caused by interposition of the volar plate. **B,** Ulnar shift of proximal phalanx suggests rupture of the radial collateral ligament.

displaced volar plate. In the small finger, the entrapping structures include the common tendon of the abductor digiti quinti and the flexor digiti minimi ulnarly and the lumbrical muscle and flexor tendons radially. The tendons are also drawn taut by the dorsally displaced volar plate and pulley.

Distinction must be made between subluxation (simple) and complete (complex) dorsal dislocations. Understanding this anatomic distinction is important in planning treatment, because the former is reducible by closed means whereas the latter is not. Similarly, an incomplete or simple dislocation can be converted into a complete or complex dislocation by an inappropriate attempt to reduce the finger by exaggerating the hyperextension deformity.

Simple Metacarpophalangeal Subluxation

Subluxation differs anatomically from complete dislocation because the volar plate is draped over the metacarpal head instead of entrapped within the joint, and the base of the proximal phalanx is postured in 60 to 80 degrees of hyperextension. If either hyperextension or traction is employed as part of the reduction maneuver of this incomplete lesion, it is possible to draw the entire volar plate dorsally, where it becomes folded between the base of the proximal phalanx and the metacarpal head, converting a subluxation into a complete or irreducible dislocation. The reduction maneuver for incomplete dislocations should therefore be performed by flexing the wrist to relax the flexor tendons and applying simple distally and volarly directed pressure to the dorsal base of the proximal phalanx. This *slides* the proximal phalanx and its attached volar plate over the metacarpal head into a reduced position. Early range of motion is encouraged, with a dorsal extension block splint to prevent extension beyond the neutral position.

Complete (Complex) Metacarpophalangeal Dislocation

Preoperative Evaluation. In contrast to the hyperextended proximal phalanx of a simple subluxation, patients with complete (complex) dislocations present with the MP joint of the digit held in slight extension; flexion is impossible. The distal joints are slightly flexed, and the digit itself is mildly deviated toward the adjacent, more central digit. A prominence is felt in the palm corresponding to the metacarpal head, and the adjacent skin may be puckered. Dorsally, a hollow can be palpated proximal to the base of the proximal phalanx.

Posteroanterior radiographs of complete dislocations show widening of the joint space (Figure 8.31). The identification of a sesamoid within the joint confirms the presence of an entrapped volar plate. In the lateral view, the dorsal dislocation is obvious and a large osteochondral shearing fracture from the metacarpal head may be identified. A Brewerton view may help demonstrate a fracture of the metacarpal head. This radiographic view is produced by placing the palm up and the dorsum of the MP joints against the radiograph plate. With the MP joints flexed approximately 65 degrees, the radiograph beam is tilted 15 degrees in an ulnar-to-radial direction. Be mindful on preoperative radiographs, as well as during surgical exploration, of the presence of osteochondral fragments that may need fixation or excision depending on size and location.

Surgical Techniques

MP dislocations can be approached either dorsally or volarly or in a combined approach. The dorsal technique popularized by Becton uses a straight dorsal incision to expose the extensor tendon and joint capsule, which are split longitudinally to gain access to the interposed volar plate.[9] After dividing the volar plate longitudinally in the midline, the two halves fall away as the proximal phalangeal base is gently reduced onto the metacarpal head.

The longer a dorsal dislocation remains unreduced, the more likely is the development of degenerative arthritis and the less satisfactory the result of surgery in terms of pain and ultimate range of motion. That notwithstanding, fair results have been reported after open reduction as long as 5 months after the original dislocation. This generally also requires a combined volar and dorsal approach to release the contracted collateral ligaments.

❖ AUTHORS' PREFERRED METHOD OF TREATMENT

A volar approach allows excellent visualization of any entrapped structures and the ability to extricate and repair them as needed. A regional brachial block is helpful to relax the extrinsic flexors. The index finger is exposed through an oblique volar incision running between the proximal and distal volar creases and extending as needed along the radial midaxial line of the affected proximal phalanx. A mirror image incision is used for the small finger, extending to the ulnar midaxial line. The radial neurovascular bundle is invariably tented over the protruding index metacarpal head and lies immediately beneath the skin. It may be easily damaged if the incision is not made with great care. Similarly, the ulnar neurovascular bundle is displaced in dislocations of the small finger MP joint. Once the skin is incised, the metacarpal head is immediately obvious in the subcutaneous tissue, herniated between the entrapping structures.

The main deterrent to reduction is the tension in the previously described muscle-tendon noose around the narrow metacarpal neck. This tension is maintained by the dorsal displacement of the flexor tendon that remains within the flexor sheath, which has been displaced dorsally with the volar plate. Reduction can be accomplished atraumatically by releasing the A1 pulley. This relaxes the tension of one tendon limb of the noose mechanism and allows the proximal phalanx and the attached volar plate to fall back or be gently manipulated into the normal anatomic position.

Postoperative Management

Immobilization of the joint in 30 degrees of flexion is continued for 2 weeks, after which active range of motion is begun using a removable 10-degree dorsal extension block splint. At 4 weeks the splint is used only for protection and at 6 weeks is discontinued. Unlimited activity is allowed at 12 weeks.

Complications

Complex dorsal MP joint dislocations are not uncommon in children. Closure of the metacarpal head physis has been reported as a rare sequela of this injury.[79] Therefore, the family should be warned of this possibility at the time of treatment.

Repeated attempts at closed reduction, traumatic open reduction (i.e., prying the proximal phalanx volarly), or late reduction may lead to degenerative arthritis and, occasionally, osteonecrosis of the metacarpal head.[40] Failure to recognize the very superficial position of the neurovascular bundle tented over the metacarpal head may lead to its division during surgical exposure of the joint. Prolonged immobilization, late reduction, or severe adjacent tissue injury may produce excessive fibrosis and reduce the final range of motion. However, motion may continue to improve for as long as 6 to 8 months.

Expected Outcomes

Timely open treatment of irreducible MP dislocations is the single most important factor in determining patient outcomes and will lead to good results in a majority of patients.

Volar Metacarpophalangeal Dislocations

Irreducible volar dislocations of the MP joints of the fingers have been reported but are extremely uncommon. Four different anatomic structures that may prevent reduction have been

---

> **CRITICAL POINTS** *Volar Approach to Complex Metacarpophalangeal Dislocations*
>
> **Preoperative Evaluation**
> - Document sensibility, because digital nerves are at risk in this approach.
> - Obtain standard radiographs as well as Brewerton views (see text).
>
> **Technical Points**
> - Make an oblique volar incision over the metacarpal head.
> - Incise *skin* only to avoid division of nearby digital nerves.
> - Use blunt dissection to identify and retract nerves.
> - Release the A1 pulley.
> - Inspect for osteochondral lesions and address as needed.
> - Use a blunt elevator or hemostat to leverage tendons away from the metacarpal head as the joint is reduced.
> - No soft tissue repair is necessary; close the skin.
>
> **Postoperative Care**
> - Immobilize the joint in 30 degrees of flexion for 2 weeks.
> - Begin active motion with an extension block splint at 10 degrees of MP flexion for 2 more weeks.
> - Buddy tape the digit to the adjacent digit at 8 weeks.
> - Unlimited use is allowed at 12 weeks.

---

reported. The dorsal capsule may be avulsed from the metacarpal proximally and become interposed between the base of the proximal phalanx and the metacarpal head. The distal insertion of the volar plate and/or collateral ligament can be avulsed and become lodged between the dislocated articular surfaces and prevent reduction.[87] In a border digit, a junctura tendinum may slip distal and volar to the metacarpal neck, also leading to an irreducible MP joint.[93] Successful closed reduction has been described and should be attempted under adequate anesthesia; failure necessitates an open reduction through a dorsal approach.

Isolated Radial Collateral Ligament Ruptures of the Metacarpophalangeal Joints

Although isolated MP ulnar collateral ligament (UCL) ruptures are extremely rare, isolated radial collateral ligament (RCL) ruptures of the MP joints of the fingers are not. The mechanism of injury is forced ulnar deviation with the MP joint flexed. Patients will often present late for evaluation and treatment owing to persistent swelling and pain in a "jammed finger" that is not improving. The clinician should first examine the contralateral digit to determine normal tension in the RCL with the MP joint in both extension and flexion. Differential tension in the two positions is normal due to the aforementioned cam effect of the metacarpal head. In the injured digit, there will be tenderness along the radial aspect of the joint at either the origin or the insertion of the ligament (in a series of 12 patients with complete tears, 7 were avulsed from the metacarpal and 5 from the proximal phalanx; none was a midsubstance rupture).[65] Passive MP flexion of the injured digit will usually cause pain; forced ulnar deviation of the proximal phalanx will demonstrate gross instability and exacerbate the pain. Radiographic evaluation should include a Brewerton view to look for avulsed bone fragments, which are not uncommon.[76] Magnetic resonance imaging (MRI) has been suggested to help identify the nature and location of the ligament disruption, although we have not found this necessary.

Like other ligament injuries, treatment depends entirely on the grade of injury. A grade I sprain is pain without laxity; a grade II injury demonstrates an endpoint to passive stress testing in 60 degrees of flexion; and a grade III injury represents avulsion with no endpoint to passive stress. Grades I and II injuries will heal with favorable outcomes when treated with splinting.[37] Grades III tears in two case series have worse outcomes with conservative treatment.[37,65] A digital block can be used to fully assess ligamentous integrity if the examination is too limited by pain.

Initial treatment for grades I and II injuries usually consists of immobilization of the joint in 30 degrees of flexion for 3 weeks for comfort. Alternatively, some physicians encourage immediate protected motion with a buddy strap to the ulnar adjacent digit. Clinical reassessment with gentle RCL stress is performed at 3 weeks, and if notable tightening or stability of the RCL is appreciated and the patient confirms a decrease in symptoms, primary healing of the ligament is likely. Further splinting or buddy taping is adjusted on an individual basis. Patients should be counseled that even with a stable MP joint, pain with maximal MP flexion and forceful gripping may continue for up to a year. If instability or pain is not markedly improved at 6 weeks, despite an endpoint, surgical repair or reconstruction may be considered and will give satisfactory results.

Grade III injuries or those with avulsion fragments and instability in the young and active patient should be repaired primarily. In these cases, there is no advantage to a trial of conservative care.[37,65] A dorsal radial incision is made over the joint. Sensory nerves are protected. The extensor hood is divided along the radial aspect of the tendon. The capsule is similarly divided. The injured ligament is identified and mobilized. The site of reattachment is cleared to bleeding bone and a minisuture anchor is placed, directed obliquely away from the joint. The ligament is tensioned with the MP joint in at least 45 degrees of flexion. The capsule and extensor hood are repaired separately with 4-0 suture. The joint is immobilized for 5 to 6 weeks in 45 degrees of flexion. A range of motion of 0 to 80 degrees without pain in acute repairs could be expected.[65]

Patients with grade I or II injuries do not tend to present late because most of these injuries eventually heal. If a patient presents with a subacute or chronic complete RCL injury, conservative treatment is not recommended. In one case series of nine chronic presentations (average, 28 weeks; maximum, 150 weeks), primary ligament repair was possible and all patients improved following surgery.[65] Some authors have preferred tendon graft reconstruction for chronic RCL injuries.[37]

Locked Metacarpophalangeal Joints

Locking of the MP joint of a finger is an unusual entity characterized by a moderate flexion deformity of the joint but normally functioning PIP and DIP joints. The locked MP joint must be differentiated from a locked trigger finger. This should not be difficult, because in a locked trigger finger, full active extension of the IP joints is not possible.

Although various causes have been reported, such as sesamoid entrapment or periarticular exostoses,[98] the usual cause of locking is the restriction of collateral or accessory collateral

ligament excursion by a prominent metacarpal head radial condyle or actual impalement on a marginal degenerative osteophyte.[96] The condition can be degenerative or idiopathic. In the former group, the patients tend to be older, and oblique or specialized radiographs will usually demonstrate degenerative changes and a marginal osteophyte. Although any finger may be involved, the long finger is the most frequently affected. In the idiopathic group, the patients are younger and have no degenerative disease. The index finger is usually involved, and the pathologic structure is a very prominent radial condylar margin of the metacarpal head that entraps the RCL.

Most cases can be resolved with the following technique.[124]

1. Inject 2 mL of normal saline dorsally into the MP joint. Lidocaine can be used, but it may increase the risk of fracture due to an anesthetic joint. The injection is hypothesized to distend the joint capsule and displace the ligament laterally enough to disengage it.
2. Flex the joint.
3. Perform radial deviation and external rotation of the joint, with the goal of disengaging a ligament that is still entrapped.
4. Gently extend the digit. The joint is kept in an extension splint for 1 week after which normal motion is allowed. Recurrence has been reported.[124]

If this maneuver is unsuccessful, or if there has been a previous episode of locking, it is necessary to explore the joint and remove the offending osteophyte or condylar margin. Occasionally, a patient will present with a chronically locked MP joint. Because the collateral ligaments are at full length in flexion, good to excellent motion is still usually achieved after surgery.

METACARPOPHALANGEAL JOINT OF THE THUMB

ANATOMY

The primary arc of motion of the thumb MP joint is in the flexion/extension plane, with secondary, minor arcs of abduction/adduction and pronation/supination. The radial condyle of the metacarpal head has greater dorsovolar height than the ulnar condyle, which allows an element of conjunct rotation in pronation with increasing flexion. The range of motion of the thumb MP joint is the most variable of any joint in the body, resulting from different radii of curvature of metacarpal heads. There is some evidence for an inverse relationship between the range of motion and the incidence of injury (i.e., limited range of motion is associated with an increased frequency of joint injury).[104]

Because of the relatively large radius of curvature of the base of the proximal phalanx, the MP joint of the thumb has little intrinsic stability and depends instead on a complex arrangement of capsular, ligamentous, and musculotendinous structures. It is supported laterally by the strong proper collateral ligaments, which arise from the lateral condyles of the metacarpal and pass obliquely to insert on the volar third of the proximal phalanx. The accessory collateral ligaments originate from a more volar site on the metacarpal head and insert on the volar plate and sesamoids on either side of the joint. The proper collateral ligaments are tight in flexion and loose in extension, and, conversely, the accessory collateral ligaments are tight in extension and loose in flexion. The floor of the joint is formed by the volar plate, creating a three-sided ligament-box configuration similar to that described previously at the PIP joint. However, it differs from the PIP complex because there is no flexor sheath proximal to the plate and, consequently, no strong checkrein ligaments are present. In addition to the fibrocartilaginous plate, volar support is provided by the thenar intrinsic muscles that insert into a pair of sesamoid bones, embedded in the thickened distal volar plate. The adductor pollicis inserts on the ulnar sesamoid, and the flexor pollicis brevis and abductor pollicis brevis insert on the radial sesamoid. Both muscles also have secondary insertions into the extensor mechanism via the adductor and abductor aponeuroses, which provide additional dynamic lateral stability.

The anatomy of the ulnar and RCL origins is important when considering surgical repair. Carlson and colleagues[17] demonstrated that the UCL origin is 4.2 mm from the dorsal edge and 5.3 mm from the joint. Its insertion is 2.8 mm from the volar lip and 3.4 mm from the joint. The RCL origin is 3.5 mm from the dorsal margin and 3.3 mm from the articular surface. The radial collateral insertion is 2.8 mm from the volar lip and 2.6 mm from the joint line. Because these are average measurements on a large cohort of male and female cadavers, it is important to know that the metacarpal origin of the ligaments is approximately a third of the distance volar from the dorsal cortex, and the proximal phalangeal insertions are approximately 25% dorsal to the volar cortex. These origin and insertion sites differ substantially from those in the published literature.[17]

Acute Ulnar Collateral Ligament Injuries (Skier's Thumb)

Preoperative Evaluation

Injuries to the ulnar collateral ligament (UCL) of the MP joint of the thumb are common, particularly among skiers and ball-handling athletes. Moberg and Stener[86] noted UCL injuries to be 10 times more common than RCL injuries. The mechanism of injury is sudden, forced radial deviation (abduction), often resulting from a fall on an outstretched hand with the thumb abducted. In skiing, if a person falls while gripping the ski pole, the handle abducts the thumb. Most modifications in ski pole design, including elimination of the strap, have not been shown to substantially reduce the incidence of thumb injuries.[36] Snowboarders also catch a thumb during falls and turns. Associated injuries include tears of the dorsal capsule and ulnar aspect of the volar plate and occasionally a rent in the adductor aponeurosis. Volar subluxation of the MP joint may result from concomitant tears of the dorsal capsule and UCL. Distal tears of the UCL at its insertion are more common than proximal tears. Ruptures within the substance of the ligament or avulsion of the ligament from the metacarpal head occasionally occur.

Smith[107] observed that not only do the collateral ligaments of the thumb MP joint afford lateral stability but they also resist volar subluxation. If one ligament is torn, the proximal phalanx tends to rotate volarly on the side of the tear, with the opposite intact ligament serving as the axis. In the case of an isolated UCL rupture, the proximal phalanx rotates in supination

around the intact RCL. Conversely, if the RCL is torn, the proximal phalanx pronates relative to the metacarpal.

Several fracture patterns may be associated with UCL injuries. An avulsion fracture of the ulnar base of the proximal phalanx at the insertion of the ligament is most common. Typically, the fracture fragment is small and includes little of the articular surface. Fractures involving more than 10% of the articular surface can occur and may require fixation if they are displaced 2 mm or more and associated with articular incongruity. Somewhat surprisingly, there is incomplete agreement about the optimal treatment for small, minimally displaced or nondisplaced avulsion fractures. Cast immobilization is generally believed to be adequate, but one series found that nine of nine patients with small avulsion fractures and displacement of less than 2 mm had persistent pain after immobilization, and all required secondary ORIF.[25] Avulsion fractures from the metacarpal head and intraarticular shearing fractures of the volar surface of the radial condyle of the metacarpal head have also been reported.[110] An interesting fracture pattern that is rare but potentially problematic is one in which there is an avulsion of the UCL with or without an avulsion fracture attached to the ligament and a simultaneous articular shear fracture of the proximal phalangeal base.[67] If attention is directed solely to the shear fracture, a complete tear of the UCL might be missed. In the skeletally immature individual, isolated rupture of the UCL without a Salter fracture of the proximal phalanx is rare but does occur.

Stener Lesion

In 1962, Stener[109] described the lesion that has come to bear his name, which he observed in 25 of 39 cases of complete rupture of the UCL of the thumb (Figure 8.32). At surgery he found the adductor aponeurosis interposed between the distally avulsed ligament and its insertion into the base of the proximal phalanx. He concluded that without contact at the site of rupture, ligament healing would be imperfect and would result in ulnar laxity regardless of the period of immobilization.

Adductor aponeurosis interposition does not occur in partial ruptures. Therefore, it is critical to distinguish between acute complete and partial ruptures of the UCL. That differentiation can usually be made clinically, although there is no absolute consensus in the literature concerning the criteria for making the diagnosis. Biomechanical modeling suggests the ligament is under maximum tension at 40 degrees of flexion, which would therefore be the best position for testing the proper collaterals.[46]

Patients with injuries to the UCL usually have tenderness, ecchymosis, and swelling along the ulnar border of the joint. Most authors use the criteria of 30 degrees of laxity of the ulnar side of the joint when stressed radially in MP extension and 40 degrees of flexion, as well as 15 degrees more laxity when compared with the contralateral thumb. The examination in flexion is far more relevant to the diagnosis of a complete tear because the volar plate will provide substantial lateral stability in full extension. It is hard to imagine that clinical testing is sufficiently precise to determine the difference between 30 and 35 degrees of laxity. I find it more helpful to assess instability by the presence or absence of an endpoint to valgus stress. If the ligament is completely torn, the joint can be manually opened without resistance and without a clear endpoint. A partially torn

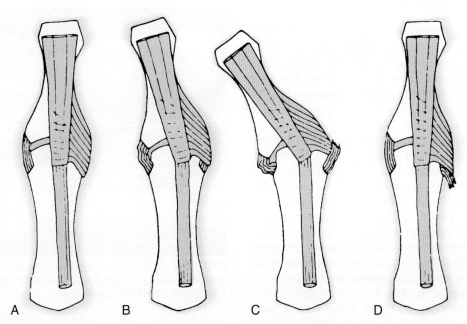

A B C D

FIGURE 8.32 Diagram of the displacement of the ulnar collateral ligament of a thumb metacarpophalangeal joint. **A,** Normal relationship with the ulnar ligament covered by the adductor aponeurosis. **B,** With slight radial angulation, proximal margin of the aponeurosis slides distally and leaves a portion of ligament uncovered. **C,** With major radial angulation, the ulnar collateral ligament ruptures at its distal insertion. In this degree of angulation, the aponeurosis has displaced distal to the rupture and permitted the ligament to escape from beneath it. **D,** As the joint is realigned, the proximal edge of the adductor aponeurosis sweeps free end of the ligament proximally and becomes interposed between the ligament and its insertion (Stener lesion). Unless surgically restored, the ulnar ligament does not heal properly and is unstable to lateral stress. (From Stener B: Skeletal injuries associated with rupture of the ulnar collateral ligament of the metacarpophalangeal joint of the thumb: a clinical and anatomic study, *Acta Chir Scand* 125:583–586, 1963.)

ligament (grade II sprain) has a discrete endpoint even if there is some laxity with stress. Rarely, patients have too much pain and guarding to allow an adequate assessment of stability. In that case, the MP joint can be anesthetized with a local nerve block before stressing the joint.

Standard posteroanterior, lateral, and oblique radiographs should be obtained in all patients with suspected UCL injury to identify an accompanying avulsion or condylar fracture. Radiographs should be done before stressing the joint. In the absence of a fracture, the posteroanterior view is usually normal. A rare exception is when the joint is so unstable that there is radial deviation of the proximal phalanx at rest. Volar subluxation of the proximal phalanx in the lateral view suggests an associated dorsal capsular tear or extensor insertion injury that may require repair. For some patients with generalized ligament laxity, a small degree of volar subluxation is normal. To be certain that the subluxation is pathologic, comparison should be made with radiographs of the contralateral thumb. We have not found stress radiographs helpful in the diagnosis or treatment algorithm. A diagnosis of a torn UCL remains primarily a clinical diagnosis. The use of diagnostic ultrasound and MRI has received considerable attention in recent years, particularly in the radiology literature. In one series, ultrasound accurately diagnosed the Stener lesion in 32 of 39 patients in whom there was operative confirmation of the findings. There were four false-positive results and three false-negative results.[52] MRI is slightly more accurate but considerably more expensive.[108]

Historical Review

Campbell[16] described the injury as a "gamekeeper's thumb," although the pathologic process that he was describing was chronic repetitive attenuation of the ligament by a radially directed force on the ulnar side of the thumb among Scottish gamekeepers who fractured the necks of rabbits between their thumbs and index fingers. The phrase *gamekeeper's thumb* describes chronic instability of the UCL, although it has been repeatedly misapplied in the literature when referring to any instability of the UCL, acute or chronic.

Treatment

There is general agreement that acute partial ruptures of the UCL can be effectively treated by a 4-week period of continuous immobilization in a thumb spica cast or splint to immobilize only the MP joint while leaving the IP joint free. This is followed by an additional 2-week period of splint immobilization, during which active range-of-motion exercise is begun. Because the injured ligament maintains its normal anatomic relationship, healing with full recovery can be expected. Strenuous activity with the thumb is avoided for 3 months after the injury. It is common for patients to have a degree of aching pain on the ulnar side of the MP joint for 6 or more months after the injury despite having no laxity on examination. Athletes with minor injuries to the UCL can be returned to play after 2 to 4 weeks of immobilization with a protective "playing splint."

Operative intervention is recommended for repair of complete tears as a more predictable and perhaps quicker path to recovery. Clinical diagnosis of a Stener lesion is difficult. Therefore if conservative treatment is even to be considered it is incumbent on the physician to rule out a Stener lesion, usually with advanced imaging. Conversely, if after clinical examination, a diagnosis of a complete tear requiring operative repair is made, MRI or ultrasound imaging is unnecessary.

Types of Operations

The technique used for repair of complete tears of the UCL depends, in part, on the location of the tear within the ligament. Intrasubstance tears are less common and can be fixed by direct suture of the ligament to itself or to the periosteum. The more common distal avulsion of the ligament necessitates reattachment of the ligament to its bony insertion using any of a number of techniques, including a pull-out suture or bone anchor.

Arthroscopic treatments have also been described. Ryu and Fagan monitored eight patients in whom complete tears of the UCL were treated successfully by arthroscopic reduction of Stener lesions without suture repair.[101] The results were good, but the series was small. Slade and Gutow[106] performed arthroscopic-assisted repair of the ligament using a bone anchor for bony reattachment or direct arthroscopic suture for midsubstance tears. The theoretical advantage of arthroscopic repair is the decreased manipulation of the adductor aponeurosis and capsule, which may result in less postoperative scarring and more rapid restoration of motion. A potential disadvantage includes the limited visualization of the dorsal sensory nerve branches, which are susceptible to injury. Introduction of arthroscopic instruments into a small joint by an inexperienced operator has the potential to traumatize the articular cartilage. There are no comparative studies to assess whether the technique is time efficient or clinically advantageous.

❖ AUTHORS' PREFERRED METHOD OF TREATMENT

In patients having less than 30 degrees of laxity of the UCL, less than a 15-degree differential in laxity compared with the contralateral side, and a discrete endpoint to joint opening, the assumption is that the tear is incomplete. Nonoperative treatment consists of immobilization of the MP joint for 4 weeks in neutral alignment and slight flexion. Adams and Muller have shown that excessive flexion and premature range of motion increase the strain on the healing ligament.[3] The IP joint is left free and IP range of motion is encouraged to avoid adherence of the extensor tendons to the injured MP joint capsule. The MP joint can be immobilized either with a custom-molded splint or a cast. The splint may be a short opponens splint that extends to a point just proximal to the thumb CMC joint or a shorter splint that leaves the CMC joint completely free. Take care when molding the spica cast to avoid the natural tendency to abduct the thumb ray and to be certain that no radial deviation occurs through the unstable MP joint. The functional results of splint and cast immobilization have been shown to be comparable, and most patients prefer splinting.[2]

Technique of Open Repair of the Thumb Metacarpophalangeal Ulnar Collateral Ligament. If clinical evaluation confirms that an acute complete rupture of the UCL is present, surgical repair is indicated. A lazy-"S"–shaped incision is used that parallels the ulnodorsal border of the thumb metacarpal to the MP joint, curving sharply in a volar direction to parallel the joint and extending distally along the ulnar midaxial line (Figure 8.33). The distal limb of the incision should be sufficiently volar to give easy access to the volar base of the proximal phalanx and the volar plate. Branches of the superficial radial nerve lying in the deep subcutaneous plane should be identified and protected. The proximal edge of the adductor aponeurosis is identified. When a Stener lesion is present, it appears as an edematous, rounded mass that may obscure this otherwise well-defined

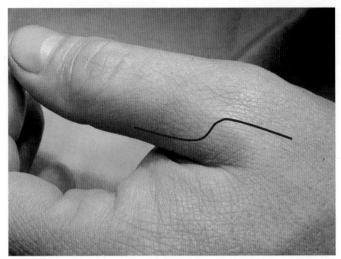

FIGURE 8.33 Incision for repair or reconstruction of ruptured ulnar collateral ligament of metacarpophalangeal joint of thumb. Exposure is excellent, and healing leaves almost imperceptible scar.

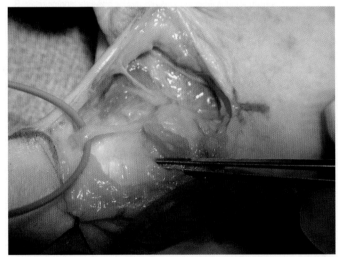

FIGURE 8.34 Displaced edematous end of ulnar collateral ligament lying proximal to edge of adductor aponeurosis, creating a palpable mass, which was noted preoperatively. Forceps is beneath the aponeurosis; the radial sensory nerve is protected with a loop. (Copyright © Scott Wolfe, MD.)

proximal border (Figure 8.34). A longitudinal incision is made at the dorsal margin of the sagittal bands incorporating 1 to 2 mm of the ulnar edge of the extensor pollicis longus tendon to facilitate repair of the sagittal bands at the end of the procedure. The aponeurosis is reflected to expose the ulnar aspect of the MP joint, including the volar base of the proximal phalanx. The joint should be examined to inspect the articular cartilage. A small cartilaginous shear fragment will occasionally be found and should be removed if loose.

Tears in the middle two thirds of the ligament can be reapproximated with interrupted figure-of-eight or horizontal mattress sutures using nonabsorbable 4-0 braided synthetic suture material. However, the ligament is usually avulsed distally and can be approximated to the distal stump or into the bone defect from which it was avulsed with a pull-through suture technique

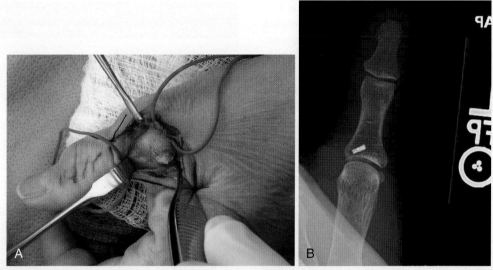

FIGURE 8.35 Ulnar collateral ligament (UCL) repair with bone anchor. **A,** Acute distal UCL disruption with Stener lesion. Vessel loop is around the dorsal sensory nerve branch. **B,** Postoperative posteroanterior radiograph demonstrating anchor in the ulnar base of the proximal phalanx and restoration of alignment and congruency of the metacarpophalangeal joint.

or a small bone anchor (Figure 8.35, *A* and *B*). In either case, the repair is performed with the joint flexed at 45 degrees to avoid overtightening.

Secure fixation of the ligament to bone can be achieved by a pull-through suture technique after scarifying the bone at the site of reattachment with a curet or rongeur. A 2-0 nonabsorbable suture is placed in the proximal stump of the UCL with a Krakow stitch. Keith needles are drilled using a Kirschner wire driver across the base of the proximal phalanx in an ulnoradial direction, exiting on the radial side with a small bone bridge between the needles. The ends of the suture in the UCL stump are threaded through the eye of the Keith needles, which are then pulled through the proximal phalanx. The ligament is pulled up to the shallow trough previously made in the ulnar base of the phalanx, and the ends of the suture are tied over the bone bridge through a small radial incision. The repair is robust and can be tensioned easily. The repair can be supplemented by suturing the proximal stump of the ligament to any remnants of the distal stump or periosteum. If I am concerned about the quality of the collateral ligament to hold a stitch, I find the Krakow stitch in this technique may work better than the simpler stitches used typically with a bone anchor repair.

When the collateral ligament tear extends volarly to also involve the accessory collateral ligament, sutures should be preplaced for accessory collateral ligament repair prior to reattachment of the proper collateral ligament.

Most ligament avulsions are repaired using a bone anchor. The pilot hole for the anchor is drilled in the ulnar base of the proximal phalanx after the reattachment site is cleared of soft tissue. The anatomic attachment site for a distal avulsion of the UCL is 25% dorsal from the volar surface of the proximal phalanx.[17] A single anchor is placed volar to the axis of the joint. The anchor is advanced into the drill hole, and one suture is securely locked into the proximal stump of the ligament. The second suture (the "post") glides through the eyelet in the anchor such that the tension will "dock" the ligament into

the repair site The second suture is passed through the ligament at its insertion point, separated as widely as possible from the first to spread out the ligament. A single simple throw may be placed in the suture and tightened down to check the range of motion and ensure satisfactory tension on the repair before completing the knots.

A few additional steps should be considered before closure. First, a suture should be placed between the distal volar portion of the repaired ligament and the volar plate to secure this vital three-dimensional complex. Second, if there is a large capsular tear and joint subluxation or rotation, the tear should be repaired. Third, gentle radial stress is applied to the joint to test the stability of the repair. A Kirschner wire across the MP joint can be used to secure the joint and can be placed dorsal to the repair site.

If a fragment of bone accompanies the avulsed ligament, the repair depends on the size of the fragment. If the fragment is small (>10% to 15% of the articular surface), it may be excised and the ligament inserted directly into the defect with a pull-out suture or anchor. If the fragment is large, it is reduced anatomically into the defect with a pull-out suture, Kirschner wires, one or more minifragment screws, or an interosseous wire.

The adductor aponeurosis is repaired with braided nylon suture, with care taken to avoid capturing the capsule with the repair. The skin is reapproximated with a running subcuticular suture of 4-0 monofilament suture. The thumb is immobilized in a thumb spica molded splint or cast with the IP joint left free to prevent adhesions of the extensor mechanism during healing. Immobilization is continued for 4 weeks, after which a hand-based thermoplastic splint is used to protect the repair. The splint is removed approximately four times per day for controlled active range-of-motion exercise, preferably under the supervision of a hand therapist. Some biomechanical studies suggest that the load during active motion is one third of the failure load of a suture anchor repair, so that active range of motion might be able to be initiated earlier than 4 weeks in compliant patients.[46] Splint protection is discontinued 6 to 8 weeks postoperatively. Activities that stress the UCL are avoided, and unrestricted use is not recommended for 3 to 4 months after surgery. Vague discomfort and some tenderness and thickening on the ulnar side of the joint can be expected to persist for as long as 1 year.

Postoperative Management and Expectations

We advise patients that when rehabilitation is begun 4 weeks postoperatively, they will be stiff and that it will take several weeks to work out that stiffness with therapy and exercise. Ultimately, they can expect range of motion of the MP joint averaging 80 to 90% of the uninjured thumb and nearly full range of motion of the IP joint. Pinch and grip strength are usually regained to within 5 to 10% of the contralateral side. Patients are often concerned about whether they will be able to return to preinjury sporting activities. In the majority of cases, full athletic participation, including contact sports, can be resumed by approximately 4 months postoperatively. Selective return to recreational activities can be considered sooner, but only if the thumb is protected with a splint and/or taped securely.

After 4 weeks of immobilization, MP and IP flexion and extension and full range of motion in the CMC joint and wrist are encouraged. Radially directed force on the tip of the thumb and resisted activities with the thumb are prohibited. The splint is worn full time except for during bathing and exercise.

During the ensuing 2 weeks (weeks 6 to 8) the patient gradually weans from the splint. During the first week, it is off primarily at mealtimes and during sedentary activity. In the second week, nonstrenuous activities at home and in an office are allowed and patients begin light resisted activities such as manipulating zippers and buttons. Flexion of the IP joint against slight resistance is begun with the therapist. By the seventh postoperative week, full active range of motion of the thumb is encouraged.

By 9 to 10 weeks postoperatively, the patient should have regained nearly full active range of motion. Focused exercises compensate for any deficit in that range. The patient is expected to have between 60 and 75% of normal pinch strength. The only activities that are restricted are forceful torque and radially directed pressure on the thumb tip. Full, unrestricted activity is allowed at 3 months, with the exception of contact sports, which can be played, if necessary, with taping or semirigid splinting of the MP joint.

The most common complication of UCL repair is neurapraxia of the crossing branches of the dorsal sensory branch of the radial nerve. Manipulation and traction on the nerve during the procedure can cause numbness and tingling on the dorsoulnar aspect of the thumb in 10 to 15% of patients, and they should be counseled about this possibility preoperatively. These symptoms are usually self-limited but can last from days to weeks and can be disconcerting, particularly if the patient is not forewarned. The likelihood of the problem arising can be diminished by fully mobilizing the nerve during the exposure and retracting it gently. If vessel loops are used for retraction, a suture should be used to secure the loop rather than an instrument. Another potential complication is stiffness, which can result from reattaching the ligament in a nonanatomic location, particularly one too dorsal relative to the axis of the joint (see previously).

CRITICAL POINTS *Repair of Complete Acute Ulnar Collateral Ligament Tears*

Preoperative Evaluation
- Physical examination is usually adequate for diagnosis; look for lack of a firm endpoint to valgus stress.
- Obtain posteroanterior, lateral, and oblique radiographs to assess for osteochondral lesions or fractures.
- Consider advanced imaging to assess for a Stener lesion if nonoperative treatment of a complete UCL tear is elected.

Technical Points
- Avoid injury to the dorsal sensory nerve branch that crosses the operative field.
- Intrasubstance tears are sutured with 3-0 or 4-0 braided synthetic suture, but consider a longer period of immobilization than with a repair to bone.
- Reattach the ligament avulsions at their anatomic insertion site[17] with a bone anchor or pull-out suture.
- Remember that avulsion fractures and ligament tears have been reported together, so if the fracture is repaired, check the ligament origin and insertion as well.
- Tie down sutures with the joint flexed at 45 degrees to avoid overtightening.
- Repair the accessory collateral component using additional sutures to the volar plate.
- Repair the adductor aponeurosis with 4-0 absorbable suture.
- Avoid stress on the repair when molding a splint or cast.

Postoperative Care
- The joint is immobilized for 4 weeks following operation.
- Apply a thermoplastic splint for 2 to 4 additional weeks.
- Begin range-of-motion exercises at 4 weeks.
- Avoid radially directed stress on the thumb tip for 12 weeks.

Chronic Ulnar Collateral Ligament Injuries (Gamekeeper's Thumb)

Preoperative Evaluation

Causes of chronic instability of the UCL include an untreated acute tear, failure to recognize a Stener lesion, or progressive attenuation of the ligament. Patients with chronic instability usually present with pain, swelling, and weakness of the involved thumb. The pain tends to be exacerbated by forceful pinch and activities requiring torsional motions of the hand, such as unscrewing jar tops. Holding large objects like a half-gallon container of milk may be painful and may cause a feeling of instability or lack of power because of the thumb's inability to resist counterpressure.

Preoperative evaluation of patients with chronic instability of the UCL is similar but less challenging than that of patients with acute instability. The resting posture of the thumb should be observed for volar subluxation or radial deviation of the MP joint. Chronic instability is manifested by gross instability to valgus stress with no endpoint. The presence of a Stener lesion in chronic instability is a moot point, because symptomatic chronic tears likely require repair or reconstruction. Crepitus with active motion suggests degenerative disease.

Radiographic assessment includes posteroanterior, lateral, and oblique views of the thumb. Specific attention should be paid to the presence of degenerative disease, as well as volar and/

or radial subluxation of the joint. Stress views occasionally help clarify the degree of laxity when clinical examination is not definitive. Advanced imaging studies are not indicated to define a Stener lesion.

In all but the most sedentary patients, in whom a splint may suffice, repair, reconstruction, or joint fusion will be necessary.

Types of Operations

Increased time from injury to treatment may decrease the likelihood of direct repair, and the patient and surgeon must be prepared preoperatively for either repair or reconstruction. In many cases, repair is still possible by mobilizing the retracted ligament from the surrounding and scarred soft tissue bed. If augmentation of a local tissue repair is required, the adductor tendon can be split longitudinally and left attached distally, and the volar half can be swung into place proximally to reconstitute or reinforce local tissue. If no local tissue is available, UCL reconstruction is most commonly performed with a free tendon graft. There are technical variations as to how grafts are passed through or attached to the metacarpal and proximal phalanx.

Smith[107] treated chronic UCL instability with reconstruction using a free tendon graft. The ulnar aspect of the MP joint is exposed with a midaxial incision. The adductor aponeurosis is incised longitudinally and mobilized from the underlying soft tissue, exposing the capsule. A 2.8-mm hole is drilled in the ulnar base of the proximal phalanx in the area of the anatomic insertion of the UCL[7,17] (Figure 8.36). A tendon graft is obtained (Smith preferred the palmaris longus), and a figure-of-eight suture is placed in the free end of the graft. The two ends of that suture are placed on needles and passed through the holes in the base of proximal phalanx and through the radial cortex, where the sutures are brought out through the skin and tied over a button; alternatively, the tendon graft can be woven through a channel in the base of the proximal phalanx (see Figure 8.36), The torn UCL is identified and dissected free of

surrounding scar tissue. If a proximal stump of ligament remains on the metacarpal head, the graft is woven into the ligament remnant through parallel longitudinal incisions. If there is no usable remnant of ligament, the tendon graft is fixed to the metacarpal through drill holes in the metacarpal head at its anatomic origin[7,17] (Figure 8.37, A and B). Graft positioning is essential because even small variations from the anatomic origin and insertion sites will limit motion (see previously). The abductor aponeurosis is repaired and the skin is reapproximated. A thumb spica cast is worn for 4 weeks postoperatively. Thereafter, the thumb is protected for an additional 5 weeks in a splint.

The only absolute contraindication to reconstruction is osteoarthritis of the MP joint, in which case arthrodesis is a dependable option, with rapid pain relief and recovery of function. A relative contraindication to ligament reconstruction is marked volar subluxation and/or supination of the MP joint,

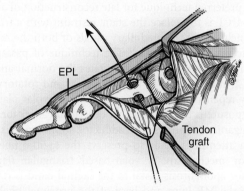

FIGURE 8.36 Method for reconstruction of the ulnar collateral ligament with a free tendon graft. Gouge holes are made at the 1 o'clock and 5 o'clock positions on the ulnar base of the proximal phalanx. A second gouge hole is made slightly obliquely across the metacarpal neck. *EPL,* Extensor pollicis longus. (Copyright © Elizabeth Martin.)

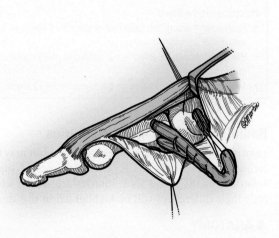

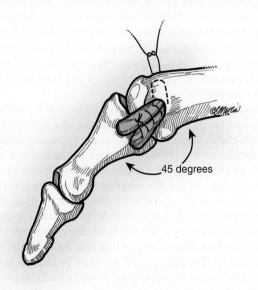

A   B

FIGURE 8.37 Free tendon graft tensioning. **A,** The ends of the free graft are whipstitched, and the suture ends are passed on straight needles through radial cortex. **B,** Graft is tensioned into the docking hole in the metacarpal head, and the suture is tied down over the radial cortex through a small counterincision. (Copyright © Elizabeth Martin.)

which may not be adequately addressed by these reconstructive procedures.

❖ AUTHORS' PREFERRED METHOD OF TREATMENT

The authors use 6 weeks as a general criterion for distinguishing between acute and chronic UCL injuries. It is certainly the case that local tissue can sometimes be used for repair of injuries that occurred more than 6 weeks earlier. The remnant of the torn ligament must be supple. Characteristically, the proximal stump of the ligament is shortened, retracted, and surrounded with a layer of fibrous tissue. To use the ligament for repair, that layer of fibrous tissue needs to be mobilized and the substance of the ligament brought out to its physiologic length. It is reattached to the base of the proximal phalanx with a bone anchor. If the local tissue is of questionable length or quality, a primary repair should not be done. This is typically the case in surgery performed more than 6 to 12 weeks after injury; this time frame is not absolute, however; it is the character of the tendon that should be the main guide for decision making.

My preferred technique for late reconstruction of an incompetent UCL is to replace the static restraint with a free tendon graft anchored in the medullary canals of both the metacarpal and the proximal phalanx.[41] The technique of passage of the tendon graft very nearly recapitulates the normal anatomy of the UCL and attempts to resist the volar and rotatory translation by repair of surrounding capsular and volar plate tissues. The exposure is the same as that described earlier for repair of acute ligament ruptures. The adductor aponeurosis is exposed, and an attempt is made to preserve the sagittal fibers of the extensor mechanism. A volar-based triangular flap of the adductor aponeurosis distal to the sagittal band is reflected to expose the MP joint and base of the proximal phalanx. The scarred, redundant UCL and capsule are resected from the concavity of the metacarpal head to the base of the proximal phalanx. A unicortical 2.5-mm hole is made in the proximal phalanx 3 mm from the joint and 3 mm from the volar cortex. Another unicortical hole is made in the metacarpal at the anatomic UCL origin. This hole is approximately 7 mm from the joint line and 5 mm from the dorsal cortex of the metacarpal.[17] A Kirschner wire is driven across the joint after joint reduction in 30 degrees of flexion, making sure to correct positioning in coronal and sagittal planes. The wire can be placed dorsal to the drill hole on the proximal phalanx and can run volar to the drill hole in the metacarpal.

A palmaris longus tendon graft is obtained if available. In the absence of the palmaris longus, a longitudinal strip of the flexor carpi radialis, extensor carpi radialis longus, long toe extensor, or abductor pollicis longus may be used. A 2-0 nonabsorbable stitch is placed in Krakow fashion in one end of the graft. Using Keith needles, the suture ends are passed through the radial cortex of the metacarpal head with a small bone bridge and tied over periosteum through a radial incision, drawing the graft down into the drill hole. The graft is measured and cut to length to allow it to pass just into the proximal phalangeal drill hole. The free end of the graft is stitched with a second Krakow suture; the sutures are passed with Keith needles through the drill hole in the proximal phalanx and out a bone bridge radially. This construct allows the surgeon to pull quite strongly on the graft to make sure it is tight and docked, and the suture strands are then tied radially over a bone bridge. It

is recommended that a small counterincision be made to avoid injuring the sensory nerve. Various anchors or tenodesis screws can also be used to avoid making a counterincision, although I like the tensioning effect of pulling a graft into a bone tunnel; it also obviates the risk of a tenodesis screw fracture.

Postoperative Management and Expectations. The MP joint is immobilized for 6 weeks, after which motion is started with protective interim splint wear. Full-time splinting is weaned at 8 weeks. Full activity, including contact sports, should be postponed for at least $4\frac{1}{2}$ months postoperatively.

Typically, the thumb is stabilized by the reconstruction; two thirds of patients have no pain postoperatively, and one third have mild, occasional pain. Approximately 80% of the motion of the MP joint and more than 90% of the motion of the IP joint are regained when compared with the contralateral side.[41] There is mild loss of key pinch strength and mild weakness with radially directed pressure on the ulnar aspect of the thumb tip. The overall satisfaction rate among patients who have had the procedure is high.

CRITICAL POINTS *Chronic Ulnar Collateral Ligament Repair*

Preoperative Evaluation
- Indicated for any complete tear (no endpoint) or partial symptomatic tear
- Rule out degenerative joint changes with radiographs.

Technical Points
- Avoid injury to the dorsal sensory branch of the radial nerve.
- Incise the adductor aponeurosis.
- Resect the remnant of the collateral ligament.
- Make a 2.5-mm hole in the base of the proximal phalanx 3 mm from the volar cortex and 3 mm from the joint.
- Make another 2.5-mm hole in the metacarpal head 7 mm from the joint and 5 mm from the dorsal cortex.
- Dock the tendon into the metacarpal drill hole with 2-0 nonabsorbable suture on Keith needles.
- Cut the tendon graft to length.
- Dock the tendon into the proximal phalanx hole by using Keith needles to pass the suture ends through the radial cortex.
- Tension and tie suture ends over bone using a small radial incision.
- Repair capsular tissue if possible and then the adductor.

Postoperative Care
- Apply a short-arm thumb spica cast or splint for 6 weeks of full-time wear with no MP motion.
- Use a thermoplastic splint for 2 additional weeks while starting MP exercises.
- Avoid radially directed stress on the thumb tip for 12 weeks.

Radial Collateral Ligament Injuries

Injuries to the RCL are much less common but may be as debilitating as tears of the UCL. The principles of diagnosis and treatment of RCL and UCL injuries are similar and therefore only their differences will be highlighted in this discussion.

⬛ ANATOMY

The principal difference between the anatomy on the radial and the ulnar sides of the thumb is that the abductor aponeurosis is broad and covers most of the radial side of the MP joint whereas the adductor aponeurosis is a narrower sheet of tissue that is easily interposed between the torn UCL and its insertion (i.e., the Stener lesion). There is little potential for an interposition lesion on the radial side comparable to the Stener lesion, although it has been reported.[21] The mechanism of RCL injuries is forced adduction or torsion on the flexed MP joint. The ligament is torn proximally or distally with about equal frequency and, somewhat more commonly than the UCL, is ruptured in its midsubstance.[27] The abductor aponeurosis may be torn as well. A tear in the RCL, as noted previously for the UCL, creates a rotatory deformity of the MP joint in which the proximal phalanx shifts volarly on the radial side and rotates around the intact UCL into pronation. This is responsible for dorsoradial prominence of the metacarpal head, a common physical finding seen with RCL rupture.

Preoperative Evaluation

Partial tears of the RCL are characterized by swelling, tenderness, and sometimes ecchymosis over the radial side of the joint and metacarpal head. There is little or no laxity with stress of the RCL, but if laxity is present there usually remains a clear end point to opening of the joint. Laxity of 30 degrees in flexion or extension or 15 degrees of increased laxity when compared with the contralateral thumb are guidelines indicating a complete tear. The most dependable diagnostic finding is the absence of a firm endpoint to varus stress.

Radiographic evaluation should include standard posteroanterior, lateral, and oblique views. Volar subluxation of the proximal phalanx, best detected on the lateral radiograph, usually accompanies the more extensive radial ligament tears and is strongly suggestive of an extension of the tear into the dorsal capsule. Volar subluxation is reported more frequently in RCL injuries than in UCL injuries, being seen in as many as 86% of complete tears.[21] The posteroanterior radiograph occasionally shows ulnar angulation of the proximal phalanx at rest and suggests gross instability. Avulsion fractures are best seen on the posteroanterior view. Stress radiographs, MRI studies, or ultrasound images offer little additional information for the guidance of diagnosis or treatment.

Treatment

Partial tears of the RCL can be treated the same as partial tears of the UCL, with a cast or splint. For complete acute tears, most authors advocate early surgical repair as a more predictable way of achieving good results.[19] For chronic instability without arthritic changes, surgical repair (when possible) or reconstruction (more likely) is necessary. For chronic instability with arthritic change, arthrodesis is preferable.

Types of Operations

Acute repairs typically involve the use of a suture anchor. Treatment options for reconstruction of chronic radial instability are either direct ligament repair (documented as late as 10 years from injury),[21] abductor advancement, or free tendon grafting.

The technique of abductor advancement is a mirror image of Neviaser adductor advancement, either alone or in combination with repair and/or reefing of the remnant of the RCL.[89] In these techniques, any ligament remnant that can be mobilized is repaired. This is reinforced by advancement of the extensor

pollicis brevis tendon into a drill hole in the proximal phalanx 1 cm from the articular surface and tied over bone on the ulnar side of the thumb.[27]

Two recent technique articles describe dorsal advancement of the abductor pollicis brevis origin on the metacarpal head with encouraging results.[53,59]

The abductor advancement procedures have the same potential shortcomings as the adductor advancement for UCL instability: it is a dynamic reconstruction that is used to replace a static restraint. The procedure involves ligamentous or capsular reefing, which may compensate for the dynamic component of the reconstruction.

❖ AUTHORS' PREFERRED METHOD OF TREATMENT

The principles of treatment are similar to those for the UCL. Partial tears of the RCL are best treated by immobilization of the MP joint full time for 4 to 5 weeks in either a thumb spica cast or splint. A splint is worn the majority of the time for an additional 2 weeks during which active range-of-motion movement in flexion and extension is begun. The literature does not resolve the question of whether all complete tears of the RCL need to be repaired, although I do routinely offer surgical repair when there is lack of a firm endpoint or significant laxity on examination. Complete tears with volar subluxation of the MP joint should be repaired. Patients with symptomatic chronic RCL instability are also offered surgery unless they are elderly or sedentary and are satisfied with a splint.

For acute repairs, the radial side of the MP joint is exposed, using a lazy-"S" incision in which the proximal limb is along the dorsoradial aspect of the thumb metacarpal and the central limb extends from dorsal to volar and parallel to the joint line. The distal limb parallels the radial volar base of the proximal phalanx in the midaxial line. A longitudinal incision is made in the abductor aponeurosis just radial to the extensor pollicis brevis. The aponeurosis is reflected volarly to expose the radial side of the joint. Midsubstance tears are repaired with figure-of-eight or mattress sutures using a 3-0 or 4-0 braided synthetic suture. Avulsions of the ligament from the metacarpal or proximal phalanx can be fixed with a bone anchor. Subluxation of the proximal phalanx must be reduced and the dorsal capsule accurately repaired without overtightening. If present, disruption of the insertions of the extensor pollicis brevis and the extensor mechanism at the base of the proximal phalanx must also be repaired. In the setting of marked volar subluxation of the joint, the repair can be supplemented with a 0.045-inch Kirschner wire to transfix the joint. The thumb MP joint is immobilized for 5 weeks in a splint or cast.

The treatment of chronic complete ruptures is similar to that for UCL ruptures. Unlike the UCL, the torn RCL almost always lies beneath the abductor aponeurosis. Consequently, it is more likely that the ends of the RCL can be mobilized and repaired in the chronic situation by using the same technique as described for acute tears. The joint should be immobilized for an additional week because healing of a chronically torn ligament is not as rapid or as strong as with a ligament repaired acutely. If the ruptured RCL is too fibrotic or shortened to be repaired, ligament reconstruction with a free tendon graft is performed (Figure 8.38). The technique of reconstruction is the mirror image of that described earlier for the ulnar side. The sagittal band is incised longitudinally along with the abductor

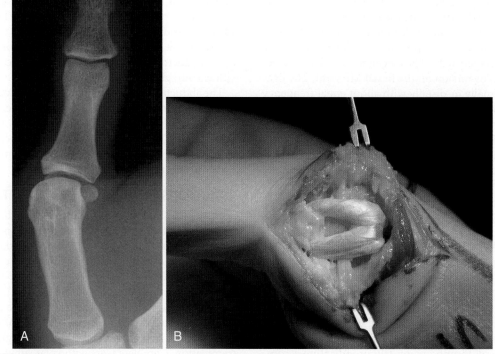

FIGURE 8.38 A, Typical radiographic appearance of chronic radial collateral ligament (RCL) instability demonstrates ulnar deviation of proximal phalanx even at rest. **B,** Chronic RCL instability may be reconstructed with a free tendon graft by using a mirror-image technique similar to that described for ulnar collateral ligament instability.

aponeurosis and repaired at the end of the procedure. The holes in the proximal phalanx and route of passage of the tendon are the same.

Postoperative Management and Expectations

The postoperative management of acute RCL repairs and RCL reconstructions is identical to that described previously for UCL repairs and reconstructions, with the single exception that the acute RCL repairs are immobilized for an additional week, beginning rehabilitation at 5 weeks postoperatively. Chronic UCL and RCL reconstructions are immobilized for 6 weeks before beginning the therapy protocol.

Postoperative expectations are also similar to those for UCL repair and reconstruction. Patients should be advised that they may have a persistent prominence of the radial side of the thumb metacarpal head postoperatively. This results from fibrosis of the soft tissue in the area of the repair or reconstruction. It may represent a mild degree of laxity of the ligament that, however, has not, in our experience, been a functional problem. Expectations for acute repairs can be guided by a report of long-term follow-up on 38 patients: 87% were symptom-free, 92% had normal pinch and grip strength, and 79% had full range of motion.[21] Although these results are encouraging, patients should be advised that some motion and strength will be lost.

Metacarpophalangeal Dislocations

Historical Perspective

Most dislocations of the thumb MP joint are dorsal, although volar dislocation has been reported and may be irreducible.[115] The mechanism of dorsal dislocation is hyperextension, with

---

CRITICAL POINTS *Chronic Radial Collateral Ligament Repair*

Preoperative Evaluation
- Physical examination usually adequate for diagnosis
- Posteroanterior, lateral, and oblique radiographs to rule out degenerative joint changes

Technical Points
- Avoid injury to the dorsal sensory branch of the radial nerve.
- Incise the abductor aponeurosis.
- Resect the remnant of collateral ligament.
- Make holes in the base of the proximal phalanx similar to the procedure for UCL reconstruction.
- Make a 4-mm hole in the metacarpal head.
- Pass a tendon graft through the distal holes.
- Whipstitch the tendon ends with nonabsorbable suture.
- Dock in the proximal hole using Keith needles to pass suture through the radial cortex.
- Set tension on the graft with the joint flexed 45 degrees.
- Tie down sutures on the ulnar side of the thumb over bone.
- Repair the abductor aponeurosis.
- Transfix the MP joint with a 0.045-inch Kirschner wire if needed.
- Avoid stress on the repair when molding a splint or cast.

Postoperative Care
- Apply a short-arm thumb spica cast for 6 weeks.
- Use a thermoplastic splint for 2 additional weeks.
- Begin range-of-motion exercises when the cast is removed.
- Avoid forceful pinch, torsional activities, and ulnarly directed stress on the thumb tip for 12 weeks.

complete rupture of the volar plate, capsule, and at least part of the collateral ligaments. Rupture of the volar plate usually occurs proximally but can be through or distal to the sesamoid bones. Most dorsal dislocations are reducible, although some are more complex injuries and are irreducible. Reduction is blocked typically by the volar plate and less commonly by the flexor pollicis longus. The flexor pollicis longus tendon more often remains within the flexor tendon sheath and displaces to the ulnar side of the metacarpal head, creating a "noose" around the metacarpal neck together with the radially displaced thenar intrinsic musculature. Volar dislocations have been described and in some cases can be reduced without surgery.[8]

Preoperative Evaluation

Diagnosis of an MP joint dislocation is generally not difficult. Clinically, the MP joint has an obvious hyperextension deformity and the metacarpal is adducted. There may be dimpling of the skin on the volar aspect of the MP joint that is suggestive of a complex dislocation. Radiographs typically show the MP joint to be hyperextended, with the proximal phalanx dorsal and sometimes lying in "bayonet" apposition to the metacarpal. There may be an increased space between the metacarpal head and the proximal phalanx suggestive of interposed soft tissue. Interposition of the sesamoids between the metacarpal head and the proximal phalanx is evidence of a complex, irreducible dislocation.

Treatment Options

The majority of dorsal dislocations can be easily reduced without surgery. Simple longitudinal traction as a reduction maneuver should be avoided because it might convert a simple dislocation into an irreducible complex one. The preferred reduction technique is hyperextension of the MP joint, followed by direct pressure on the dorsal base of the proximal phalanx to gently push it over the metacarpal head.

Less severe hyperextension injuries can cause dorsal subluxation of the MP joint rather than frank dislocation. This may present as a locked MP joint in which the joint cannot be flexed actively or passively. The pathoanatomy is thought to be entrapment of the radial condyle in a tear of the radial part of the volar plate, proximal to the sesamoid. Closed reduction may be attempted with regional anesthesia or a lidocaine block of the MP joint. The examiner applies volar-directed pressure on the proximal phalanx while twisting it on the metacarpal head.[74] If closed reduction fails, open reduction may be necessary and can be done through several approaches.

The surgical approach may be dorsal, volar, or lateral. Bohart and Gelberman and colleagues[11] prefer the dorsal approach because of its simplicity. A longitudinal skin incision exposes the extensor tendons. The interval between the extensor pollicis longus and extensor pollicis brevis tendons is developed. The dorsal capsule is incised. The tissue interposed in the joint is identified and mobilized using blunt instruments such as hooks, forceps, and periosteal elevators. The tissue is pushed over the metacarpal head and the joint is reduced. Occasionally, a dorsal MP dislocation will present with a volar laceration that necessitates débridement and extension of the volar wound. The proximal phalanx is hyperextended, and the interposed soft tissue is extricated from the joint. The advantage of the volar approach is that it allows the interposed structures to be pulled

from within the joint and affords an excellent view of the neurovascular bundles, tendons, and affected structures.[57] Once reduced, the joint is usually stable, but if not, ligament and volar plate repair can be performed.

❖ AUTHORS' PREFERRED METHOD OF TREATMENT

Closed reduction is usually successful with the following technique. Under radial and median nerve wrist block or Bier block anesthesia, distally directed pressure is applied to the base of the proximal phalanx with the metacarpal in a position of flexion and adduction. This maneuver relaxes the noose that the thenar muscles and flexor pollicis longus occasionally create around the metacarpal neck. If necessary, flexing the IP joint and the wrist will relax an entrapped flexor pollicis longus tendon that is blocking reduction. After reduction, collateral ligament stability is tested and a congruous reduction confirmed by radiographs. Stability is assessed by extending the joint to determine the point at which it starts to subluxate. The thumb should be fitted with a dorsal block splint in 10 degrees more of flexion than the point of instability. This can be extended 10 degrees per week. If there is significant collateral ligament instability, consideration should be given to immobilization of the MP joint for 4 weeks or open collateral ligament repair. Open reduction is required when closed reduction fails. If the case presents within 24 hours of injury, we make a small dorsal incision, insert a Freer elevator, and try to push interposed tissue from within the joint. If that fails or if the dislocation is more than 24 hours old, the joint is exposed through a volar zigzag incision. Interposed or entrapped structures are reduced with blunt instruments, avoiding injury to the metacarpal head. Stabilization of the joint in 25 degrees of flexion with a Kirschner wire should be done if the joint is unstable. If the volar plate is detached from the base of the proximal phalanx, surgical repair using bone anchors or repair of surrounding soft tissue is recommended after closed reduction.

Postoperative Management and Expectations

Patients are advised that they will most likely have a stable joint after closed or open reduction. However, stiffness is possible after any dislocation, and the chance of stiffness is greater if surgery is required. Recovery of motion can be slow and require several weeks of therapy. Patients should be counseled at the time of injury that stability is a more important consideration than full range of motion of the MP joint. The protocol for rehabilitation is similar to that for acute collateral ligament injury of the MP joint, with a focus on avoidance of forceful extension while the volar plate is healing during the initial 6 to 8 weeks after the injury.

Chronic Volar Instability of the Thumb Metacarpophalangeal Joint

Preoperative Assessment

Chronic laxity of the thumb MP joint occurs most commonly in the context of generalized ligament laxity and is rarely symptomatic. Symptomatic laxity may be a manifestation of systemic conditions such as collagen vascular disease, congenital or acquired paralytic disorders, collapse deformity secondary to basal joint arthritis, or trauma. Posttraumatic hyperextension of the MP joint is infrequent and may be the consequence of an unrecognized or undertreated volar plate injury or MP dislocation. Patients with instability caused by generalized ligament laxity are able to volitionally maintain the joint in flexion during pinch and grip, whereas those with posttraumatic laxity cannot, and the resultant collapse of the joint causes pain and weakness. Radiographs are usually normal but may show an avulsion fleck of bone at the site of the volar plate injury.

Types of Operations

If there has been a relatively recent hyperextension injury of the MP joint, it may be possible to reattach the volar plate to its metacarpal origin. A zigzag incision is used to expose the volar aspect of the MP joint. The volar plate is identified and mobilized. Its proximal end is minimally débrided and reattached to the volar aspect of the metacarpal neck with two bone anchors. The MP joint is immobilized in a cast for 1 month, after which range of motion with a 20-degree extension block splint is encouraged for an additional 2 weeks. The procedure is unlikely to be successful if the injury is chronic and the volar plate attenuated.

Several techniques have been described to treat chronic symptomatic hyperextension of the MP joint. Kessler[70] transected the extensor pollicis brevis proximally and reconstructed the volar plate with the distally attached segment. The graft was directed in a dorsovolar direction along the radial side of the MP joint and passed along the volar aspect of the joint in a radioulnar direction. The tendon was passed through a hole in the metacarpal neck from ulnar to radial and again passed across the volar aspect of the MP joint to the ulnar side, where it was sutured to the adductor tendon. The reconstruction creates a static restraint to hyperextension, while simultaneously removing the extensor pollicis brevis extension moment on the MP joint. Tonkin[117] reported good results with sesamoid arthrodesis to the metacarpal head for 42 thumbs in 37 patients with either cerebral palsy or osteoarthritis of the CMC joint. Eaton and Floyd[32] used a volar capsulodesis as an adjunct to basal joint arthroplasty for osteoarthritis in patients with MP hyperextension of 30 degrees or more.

The joint is approached through a volar Bruner incision and an interval between the volar plate and the RCL. The cortex of the retrocondylar fossa is decorticated, one or two suture anchors are placed, and the volar plate is advanced proximally. The RCL is sutured to the volar plate and the joint transfixed with a 0.045-inch Kirschner wire for 4 weeks, after which range-of-motion movement is begun. The joint is protected in a splint for 2 more weeks.

THUMB CARPOMETACARPAL JOINT

Carpometacarpal Joint Dislocations

▌ ANATOMY

The articular surfaces of the CMC joint of the thumb resemble two reciprocally opposed saddles with perpendicular transverse axes. The CMC joint has motion in three principal planes: flexion-extension, abduction-adduction, and pronation-supination (or opposition-retropulsion). There is an element of conjunct rotation in pronation that results from the asymmetric height of the radial and ulnar condyles of the trapezial articulating surface. These concavoconvex contours by themselves produce a degree of intrinsic stability, but the ligaments

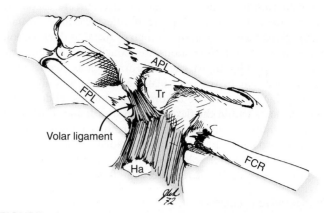

FIGURE 8.39 Essential anatomy of thumb carpometacarpal joint. A key structure is the volar oblique ligament, a short reflection of the transverse carpal ligament that maintains the thumb metacarpal within the biconcave contour of trapezium. *APL,* Abductor pollicis longus; *FCR,* flexor carpi radialis; *FPL,* flexor pollicis longus; *Ha,* hamate; *Tr,* trapezium. (From Eaton RG, Littler JW: Joint injuries and their sequelae, *Clin Plast Surg* 3:85–98, 1976.)

selves produce a degree of intrinsic stability, but the ligaments and joint capsule play the principal role in stabilization. There are four major ligaments: volar (anterior oblique), intermetacarpal, dorsoradial, and dorsal oblique (posterior oblique). The volar oblique ligament, which passes from the trapezium to the volar beak of the thumb metacarpal (Figure 8.39), has traditionally been considered to provide the primary restraint to dorsal subluxation force that is inherent with pinch. The dorsal ligament is thin but is reinforced by the expanded insertion of the abductor pollicis longus.

Historical Review

All reported CMC dislocations have been dorsal. It is generally believed that the mechanism of injury is axial compression on a flexed thumb metacarpal, driving the metacarpal base out dorsally. There is some disagreement concerning which ligaments must be injured to allow complete dislocation to occur. It has been suggested that the dorsoradial ligament has to be torn for a dorsal dislocation to occur but that the volar ligament is often sheared off its insertion on the metacarpal base as well. Strauch and colleagues[112] made observations using a ligament-cutting cadaver model and concluded that the dorsoradial ligament had to be disrupted for a complete dislocation to occur and that the volar ligament was insufficient to resist dislocation.

Preoperative Evaluation

Injuries to the ligaments of the thumb CMC joint may be complete or partial. Complete rupture permits the thumb metacarpal to dislocate dorsally (Figure 8.40). Partial rupture of the ligaments permits varying degrees of displacement. The more extensive the tear, the greater the displacement and, hence, the more obvious the diagnosis. Less severe tears are particularly difficult to diagnose because the contours of the joint tend to maintain gross alignment of the metacarpal base within the concavity of the trapezium. There may be minimal detectable dorsal translation of the metacarpal on clinical and radiographic examination. The difference between normal mobility and hypermobility is difficult to measure because these structures are at least partially enclosed within the thenar muscles.

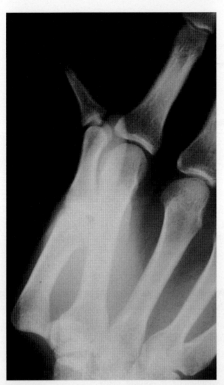

FIGURE 8.40 Dislocations of the thumb carpometacarpal joint are uncommon; they are invariably dorsal and usually unstable. The thumb is generally adducted.

Standard posteroanterior and true lateral radiographs must be taken to rule out existing joint pathologic developments and the relatively more frequent Bennett fracture-dislocation. Widening of the joint space or a slight dorsoradial shift of the metacarpal may be apparent on these routine radiographs. A useful diagnostic technique is the stress radiograph, which is a posteroanterior view of both thumbs positioned parallel to the radiograph plate with the distal phalanges pressed firmly together along their radial borders. This tends to lever the base of the metacarpal laterally, and in the presence of a capsular tear or laxity, radial shift of the metacarpal on the trapezium will occur. Because both thumbs are included on the film, a comparison with the uninjured joint is possible.

Treatment

Because acute complete dislocations are quite rare and partial tears of the CMC joint are rarely recognized, the relevant literature is composed largely of case reports with few specific recommendations about the management of these injuries. Simonian and Trumble[105] reported persistent instability in four of eight patients after closed reduction and percutaneous Kirschner wire fixation of acute CMC dislocations and significantly better results with early ligament reconstruction. The commonly used techniques for ligament reconstruction are those described by Eaton and Littler[29] and Brunelli and associates.[13]

❖ AUTHORS' PREFERRED METHOD OF TREATMENT

Patients with acute posttraumatic pain in the CMC joint of the thumb but without gross clinical instability or radiographic subluxation should be considered to have a partial volar ligament tear and immobilized in a long opponens or thumb spica splint with the metacarpal in palmar abduction and extension

for 4 to 6 weeks. The thumb should be positioned to prevent its tip from opposing the digits, which would create axial compression along the thumb ray.

Patients with a documented dislocation or with clinical instability and radiographic subluxation require special consideration. If postreduction radiographs show the metacarpal to be well reduced initially and maintained at 5 to 7 days, cast immobilization may be adequate treatment. However, if the metacarpal is not well seated radiographically or is clinically lax, surgical reduction is indicated. In light of the study by Simonian and Trumble,[105] the indications for closed reduction under anesthesia with percutaneous Kirschner wire fixation of the CMC joint should be narrow. A possible exception might be a patient in whom closed reduction resulted in a stable joint, suggesting that there is no interposed soft tissue. The joint may then be transfixed with a percutaneous 0.045-inch Kirschner wire down the medullary canal or obliquely across the base of the metacarpal. When the pin is driven across the joint, the metacarpal should be held in abduction and extension as the joint is held manually reduced. Pressure at its dorsoradial base seats the metacarpal and approximates the metacarpal beak to the volar ligament, to encourage ligament healing. If the metacarpal will not reduce congruously but remains dorsally or laterally translated, or if the joint continues to feel unstable, it must be assumed that soft tissue is interposed or that a small, undetected bony or chondral fragment is preventing reduction. Open reduction is indicated, and the volar ligament should be reconstructed with a tendon graft.

Technique of Volar Ligament Reconstruction of the Thumb Carpometacarpal Joint. The CMC joint of the thumb is exposed through a modified Wagner volar approach that curves ulnarly into the distal wrist flexion crease. Care is taken to avoid injury to the palmar cutaneous branch of the median nerve, the superficial radial artery, and branches of the lateral antebrachial cutaneous and radial nerves. The thenar muscles are elevated extraperiosteally. The intact volar and radial capsule is incised, and any interposed tissue is removed from the joint. The flexor carpi radialis tendon is identified at the wrist flexion crease and unroofed distally as far as the midportion of the trapezium.

Reconstruction of the volar ligament is begun by first creating a channel in the base of the metacarpal in a sagittal plane perpendicular to the thumbnail. A small incision is made in the dorsal periosteum through which a hole is made in the metacarpal base and enlarged with progressively larger handheld gouges. It emerges just distal to the volar beak, at the site of the volar ligament insertion. A 28-gauge stainless steel wire is placed through this channel for subsequent passage of the tendon graft used for ligament reconstruction (Figure 8.41).

The radial half of the flexor carpi radialis is mobilized, beginning 6 to 8 cm proximal to the wrist through one or more short transverse incisions. Alternatively, a looped monofilament suture or an arthroscopic suture passer can be passed from the incision at the wrist crease, beneath the skin bridge, to emerge through a proximal forearm incision and thereby avoid the need for multiple incisions on the forearm. The loop of the suture or the suture passer is placed through a split in the flexor carpi radialis tendon and firmly pulled distally into the distal wound to continue the split longitudinally. The distal end is left in continuity with the index metacarpal insertion, and the transected proximal end is passed through the channel in the volar

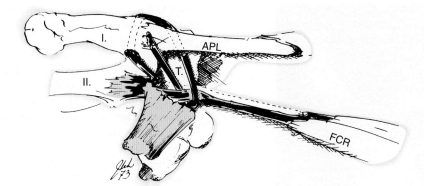

FIGURE 8.41 Schema for routing of the flexor carpi radialis tendon in a reconstruction of the volar ligament of carpometacarpal joint of the thumb. Volar, dorsal, and radial capsules are reinforced by this routing. *APL,* Abductor pollicis longus; *FCR,* flexor carpi radialis; *I,* thumb; *II,* index finger; *T,* trapezium. (From Eaton RG, Littler JW: Ligament reconstruction for the painful thumb carpometacarpal joint, *J Bone Joint Surg Am* 55:1655–1666, 1973.)

base of the metacarpal to emerge dorsally. The metacarpal is held reduced under direct vision as the tendon is drawn tight to remove any kinks along its passage, and then traction is relaxed slightly to keep the reconstruction from being too tight. The tendon is sutured to the dorsal periosteum to set proper tension in the new ligament, and its free end is passed deep to the insertion of the abductor pollicis longus on the metacarpal base. It is sutured at this point to reinforce the dorsal capsule. The free end is further passed volarly around the intact flexor carpi radialis tendon and finally reflected distally across the radial aspect of the joint, where it is sutured to a remnant of the capsule. Kirschner wire fixation of the trapeziometacarpal joint is optional. It is important that the new volar ligament not be sutured with excessive tension, which may restrict joint motion, particularly rotation. The thenar muscles are reattached. Immobilization is continued for 4 weeks, at which time the cast and Kirschner wire are removed and gentle progressive motion is begun.

Postoperative Management and Expectations

During the 4 weeks of immobilization after volar ligament reconstruction, patients are encouraged to move the digits and thumb IP joint within the limits of the cast. The cast and Kirschner wire are removed after 4 weeks, and patients are referred to a hand therapist. A custom-molded thermoplastic long opponens splint is worn for 2 weeks and removed for range-of-motion exercises. Patients are encouraged to oppose the tip of the thumb to the index and long fingers during the first 2 weeks. In the ensuing 2 weeks (beginning at 6 weeks postoperatively), they oppose the tip of the thumb to the ring and small fingers. Strengthening of the thenar musculature begins 2 months postoperatively and strengthening of pinch and grasp at 10 to 12 weeks postoperatively. It is important that the therapist not be overly aggressive with strengthening during the first 2 months postoperatively, because this may contribute to the reconstruction "stretching out." Patients are allowed essentially full use of the thumb at 3 months.

Patients are advised that volar ligament reconstruction predictably stabilizes the unstable basal joint, whether due to dislocation, subluxation, or atraumatic laxity of the basal joint, provided there is no degenerative disease. The vast majority of patients who have undergone CMC ligament reconstruction are

---

CRITICAL POINTS *Volar Ligament Reconstruction*

Indications
- Acute, irreducible dislocation of the thumb CMC joint
- Redislocation of the CMC joint after reduction
- Subacute or chronic posttraumatic instability
- Chronic symptomatic atraumatic laxity
- Persistent pain despite conservative treatment

Technical Points
- Use a modified Wagner incision.
- Avoid injury to the dorsal sensory branch of the radial nerve.
- Elevate the thenar musculature extraperiosteally.
- Inspect the CMC joint through a transverse arthrotomy.
- Make a dorsovolar hole in the metacarpal base perpendicular to the plane of the thumbnail. The hole should exit just distal to the volar beak at the insertion point of the volar oblique ligament.
- Place a 28-gauge stainless steel wire through the hole for later passage of the tendon graft.
- Harvest a distally based slip of the flexor carpi radialis tendon, starting ulnarly so that as it spirals it ends radially.
- Tie the volar end of a 28-gauge wire to the proximal end of the flexor carpi radialis tendon slip.
- Pull the tendon through the hole from volar to dorsal.
- Position the thumb in abduction and extension.
- Set tension on the flexor carpi radialis graft by pulling tightly and then relaxing 2 to 3 mm.
- Suture the graft to the periosteum adjacent to the dorsal hole with 3-0 braided polyester suture.
- Place the free end of the graft beneath the abductor pollicis longus to which it is sutured.
- Loop the graft around the intact flexor carpi radialis and then back dorsally.
- Reattach the thenar musculature.

Postoperative Care
- Apply a short-arm thumb spica cast for 4 weeks.
- Use a thermoplastic long opponens splint for 2 additional weeks.
- Begin range-of-motion exercises when the cast is removed.
- Begin gentle strengthening at 8 weeks.
- Avoid strenuous pinch and torsional motions for 3 months.

either pain free or have mild, intermittent pain postoperatively. It is very unlikely for laxity or pain to recur in the short and intermediate term, and patients should have essentially full function of their thumb and hand and be able to participate in all activities, including athletics. However, dislocation of the thumb CMC joint represents a significant injury not only to the ligaments but to the articular cartilage as well and raises the possibility of long-term degenerative arthritis. Postoperative mild limitation in range of motion of the basal joint is not uncommon, including the possibility the patient will not be able to fully flatten the palm on a countertop. This can usually be avoided by ensuring that the reconstruction is not overly tightened.

Patients commonly have some numbness on the dorsal radial aspect of the thumb after volar ligament reconstruction. It is most often due to traction on the branch of the dorsal sensory branch of the radial nerve that crosses the operative field. This complication can be avoided by being particularly attentive to identification and gentle retraction of the nerve throughout the procedure. Clamps attached to vessel loops around the nerve should be avoided. Occasionally, the nerve can become entrapped in scar tissue at the site of the fixation of the flexor carpi radialis tendon slip to the periosteum of the thumb metacarpal base. Neurapraxia resulting from traction almost invariably resolves completely over weeks to months. Rarely, entrapment of the nerve in scar tissue may require neurolysis and transposition of the nerve away from the previous point of fixation.

For Case Studies, Videos, and more, please visit ExpertConsult.com.

REFERENCES

1. Abbiati G, Delaria GE, Saporiti E, et al: The treatment of chronic flexion contractures of the proximal interphalangeal joint. *J Hand Surg [Br]* 20:385–389, 1995.
2. Abrahamsson SO, Sollerman C, Lundborg G, et al: Diagnosis of displaced ulnar collateral ligament of the metacarpophalangeal joint of the thumb. *J Hand Surg [Am]* 15:457–460, 1990.
3. Adams BD, Muller DL: Assessment of thumb positioning in the treatment of ulnar collateral ligament injuries: A laboratory study. *Am J Sports Med* 24:672–675, 1996.
4. Agee JM, Goss BC: The use of skeletal extension torque in reversing Dupuytren contractures of the proximal interphalangeal joint. *J Hand Surg [Am]* 37(7):1467–1474, 2012.
5. Aladin A, Davis TR: Dorsal fracture-dislocation of the proximal interphalangeal joint: a comparative study of percutaneous Kirschner wire fixation versus open reduction and internal fixation. *J Hand Surg [Br]* 30:120–128, 2005.
6. Andersen MB, Andersen-Ranberg F: Dislocation of the distal interphalangeal and the metacarpophalangeal joints in the same finger: A case report. *J Hand Surg [Am]* 20:574–575, 1995.
7. Bean CHG, Tencer AF, Trumble TE: The effect of thumb metacarpophalangeal ulnar collateral ligament attachment site on joint range of motion: An in vitro study. *J Hand Surg [Am]* 24:283–287, 1999.
8. Beck JD, Klena JC: Closed reduction and treatment of 2 volar thumb metacarpophalangeal dislocations: report of 2 cases. *J Hand Surg [Am]* 36(4):665–669, 2011.
9. Becton JL, Christian JD, Goodwin HN, et al: A simplified technique for treating the complex dislocation of the index metacarpophalangeal joint. *J Bone Joint Surg Am* 57:698–700, 1975.
10. Bilos ZJ, Vender MI, Bonavolonta M, et al: Fracture subluxation of proximal interphalangeal joint treated by volar plate advancement. *J Hand Surg [Am]* 19:189–196, 1994.
11. Bohart PG, Gelberman RH, Vandell RF, et al: Complex dislocations of the metacarpophalangeal joint. *Clin Orthop Relat Res* 164:208–210, 1982.
12. Bowers WH, Wolf JW, Jr, Nehil J, et al: The proximal interphalangeal joint volar plate: I. An anatomical and biomechanical study. *J Hand Surg [Am]* 5:79–88, 1980.
13. Brunelli G, Monini L, Brunelli F: Stabilisation of the trapeziometacarpal joint. *J Hand Surg [Br]* 14:209–212, 1989.
14. Bruser P, Poss T, Larkin G: Results of proximal interphalangeal joint release for flexion contractures: Midlateral versus volar incision. *J Hand Surg [Am]* 24:288–294, 1999.
15. Calfee RP, Kiefhaber TR, Sommerkamp TG, et al: Hemi-hamate arthroplasty provides functional reconstruction of acute and chronic proximal interphalangeal fracture-dislocations. *J Hand Surg [Am]* 34(7):1232–1241, 2009.
16. Campbell CS: Gamekeeper's thumb. *J Bone Joint Surg Br* 37:148–149, 1955.
17. Carlson MG, Warner KK, Meyers KN, et al: Anatomy of the thumb metacarpophalangeal ulnar and radial collateral ligaments. *J Hand Surg [Am]* 37(10):2021–2026, 2012.
18. Catalano LW, Skarparis AC, Glickel SZ, et al: Treatment of chronic traumatic hyperextension deformities of the proximal interphalangeal joint with flexor digitorum superficialis tenodesis. *J Hand Surg [Am]* 28:448–452, 2003.
19. Catalano LW, 3rd, Cardon L, Patenaude N, et al: Results of surgical treatment of acute and chronic grade III (corrected) tears of the radial collateral ligament of the thumb metacarpophalangeal joint. *J Hand Surg [Am]* 31:68–75, 2006.
20. Cheah AE, Tan DM, Chong AK, et al: Volar plating for unstable proximal interphalangeal joint dorsal fracture-dislocations. *J Hand Surg [Am]* 37(1):28–33, 2012.
21. Coyle MP, Jr: Grade III radial collateral ligament injuries of the thumb metacarpophalangeal joint: treatment by soft tissue advancement and bony reattachment. *J Hand Surg [Am]* 28:14–20, 2003.
22. Deitch MA, Kiefhaber TR, Comisar BR, et al: Dorsal fracture-dislocation of the proximal interphalangeal joint: Surgical complications and long-term results. *J Hand Surg [Am]* 24:914–923, 1994.
23. Deshmukh SC, Kumar D, Mathur K, et al: Complex fracture-dislocation of the proximal interphalangeal joint of the hand. Results of a modified pins and rubbers traction system. *J Bone Joint Surg Br* 86:406–412, 2004.
24. Diao E, Eaton RG: Total collateral ligament excision for contractures of the proximal interphalangeal joint. *J Hand Surg [Am]* 18:393–402, 1993.
25. Dinowitz M, Trumble T, Hanel D, et al: Failure of cast immobilization for thumb ulnar collateral ligament avulsion fractures. *J Hand Surg [Am]* 22:1057–1063, 1997.
26. Dionysian E, Eaton RG: The long-term outcome of volar plate arthroplasty of the proximal interphalangeal joint. *J Hand Surg [Am]* 25:429–437, 2000.
27. Durham JW, Khuri S, Kim MH: Acute and late radial collateral ligament injuries of the thumb metacarpophalangeal joint. *J Hand Surg [Am]* 18:232–237, 1993.
28. Durham-Smith G, McCarten GM: Volar plate arthroplasty for closed proximal interphalangeal joint injuries. *J Hand Surg [Br]* 17:422–428, 1992.
29. Eaton RG, Lane LB, Littler JW, et al: Ligament reconstruction for the painful thumb carpometacarpal joint: A long-term assessment. *J Hand Surg [Am]* 9:692–699, 1984.
30. Eaton RG, Littler JW: Joint injuries and their sequelae. *Clin Plast Surg* 3:85–98, 1976.
31. Eaton RG, Malerich MM: Volar plate arthroplasty for the proximal interphalangeal joint: A ten-year review. *J Hand Surg [Am]* 5:260–268, 1980.
32. Eaton RG, Floyd WE, III: Thumb metacarpophalangeal capsulodesis: An adjunct procedure to basal joint arthroplasty for collapse deformity of the first ray. *J Hand Surg [Am]* 13:461–465, 1988.
33. Ellis SJ, Cheng R, Prokopis P, et al: Treatment of proximal interphalangeal dorsal fracture-dislocation injuries with dynamic external fixation: a pins and rubber band system. *J Hand Surg [Am]* 32:1242–1250, 2007.
34. Failla JM: Extrusion of fracture fragment into flexor sheath following proximal interphalangeal joint fracture-dislocation: A case report. *J Hand Surg [Am]* 21:253–255, 1996.
35. Fei X, Feng S, Gao S: Microsurgery for severe flexion contracture of proximal interphalangeal joint. Article in Chinese. *Zhongguo Xiu Fu Chong Jian Wai Ke Za Zhi* 26(7):803–805, 2012.
36. Fricker R, Hintermann B: Skier's thumb. Treatment, prevention and recommendations. *Sports Med* 19:73–79, 1995.
37. Gaston RG, Lourie GM: Radial collateral ligament injury of the index metacarpophalangeal joint: an underreported but important injury. *J Hand Surg [Am]* 31:1355–1361, 2006.
38. Ghidella SD, Segalman KA, Murphy MS: Long-term results of surgical management of proximal interphalangeal joint contracture. *J Hand Surg [Am]* 27:799–805, 2002.
39. Ghobadi F, Anapolle DM: Irreducible distal interphalangeal joint dislocation of the finger: A new cause. *J Hand Surg [Am]* 19:196–198, 1994.
40. Gilsanz V, Cleveland RH, Wilkinson RH: Aseptic necrosis: A complication of dislocation of the metacarpophalangeal joint. *AJR Am J Roentgenol* 129:737–738, 1977.
41. Glickel SZ: Thumb metacarpophalangeal joint ulnar collateral ligament reconstruction using a tendon graft. *Tech Hand Up Extrem Surg* 6:133–139, 2002.
42. Grant I, Berger AC, Tham SK: Internal fixation of unstable fracture dislocations of the proximal interphalangeal joint. *J Hand Surg [Br]* 30:492–498, 2005.

43. Grant IR: Irreducible rotational anterior dislocation of the proximal interphalangeal joint: A spin drier injury. *J Hand Surg [Br]* 18:648–651, 1993.

44. Hamer DW, Quinton DN: Dorsal fracture subluxation of the proximal interphalangeal joints treated by extension block splintage. *J Hand Surg [Br]* 17:586–590, 1992.

45. Hamilton SC, Stern PJ, Fassler PR, et al: Mini-screw fixation for the treatment of proximal interphalangeal joint dorsal fracture-dislocations. *J Hand Surg [Am]* 31:1349–1354, 2006.

46. Harley BJ, Werner FW, Green JK: A biomechanical modeling of injury, repair, and rehabilitation of ulnar collateral ligament injuries of the thumb. *J Hand Surg [Am]* 29:915–920, 2004.

47. Hasegawa T, Yamano Y: Arthroplasty of the proximal interphalangeal joint using costal cartilage grafts. *J Hand Surg [Br]* 17:583–585, 1992.

48. Hastings H, Stern PJ, Capo JT, et al: *Hemicondylar hamate replacement arthroplasty (HHRA) for PIP fracture/dislocation.* Paper presented at 54th Annual Meeting of The American Society for Surgery of the Hand, September 2–4, 1999, Boston, MA.

49. Hastings J, III, Hamlet WP: *Critical assessment of PIP joint stability after palmar lip fracture dislocations.* Presented at the 56th Annual Meeting of The American Society for Surgery of the Hand, October 3–6, 2001, Baltimore, MD.

50. Henry M: Prosthetic hemiarthroplasty for posttraumatic articular cartilage loss in the proximal interphalangeal joint. *Hand (N Y)* 6(1):93–97, 2011.

51. Hierner R, Berger AK: Long-term results after vascularised joint transfer for finger joint reconstruction. *J Plast Reconstr Aesthet Surg* 61:1338–1346, 2008.

52. Hoglund M, Tordai P, Muren C: Diagnosis by ultrasound of dislocated ulnar collateral ligament of the thumb. *Acta Radiol* 36:620–625, 1995.

53. Horch RE, Dragu A, Polykandriotis E, et al: Radial collateral ligament repair of the thumb metacarpophalangeal joint using the abductor pollicis brevis tendon. *Plast Reconstr Surg* 117:491–496, 2006.

54. Horiuchi Y, Itoh Y, Sasaki T, et al: Dorsal dislocation of the D.I.P. joint with fracture of the volar base of the distal phalanx. *J Hand Surg [Br]* 14:177–182, 1989.

55. Houshian S, Chikkamuniyappa C: Distraction correction of chronic flexion contractures of PIP joint: comparison between two distraction rates. *J Hand Surg [Am]* 32:651–656, 2007.

56. Houshian S, Gynning B, Schroder HA: Chronic flexion contracture of proximal interphalangeal joint treated with the compass hinge external fixator: A consecutive series of 27 cases. *J Hand Surg [Br]* 27(4):356–358, 2002.

57. Hughes LA, Freiberg A: Irreducible MP joint dislocation due to entrapment of FPL. *J Hand Surg [Br]* 18:708–709, 1993.

58. Hutchison JD, Hooper G, Robb JE: Double dislocations of digits. *J Hand Surg [Br]* 16:114–115, 1991.

59. Iba K, Wada T, Hiraiwa T, et al: Reconstruction of chronic thumb metacarpophalangeal joint radial collateral ligament injuries with a half-slip of the abductor pollicis brevis tendon. *J Hand Surg [Am]* 38(10):1945–1950, 2013.

60. Ikeda M, Kobayashi Y, Saito I, et al: Open reduction and internal fixation for dorsal fracture dislocations of the proximal interphalangeal joint using a miniplate. *Tech Hand Up Extrem Surg* 15(4):219–224, 2011.

61. Inanami H, Ninomiya S, Okutsu I, et al: Dynamic external finger fixator for fracture dislocation of the proximal interphalangeal joint. *J Hand Surg [Am]* 18:160–164, 1993.

62. Inoue G, Maeda N: Irreducible volar dislocation of the distal interphalangeal joint of the finger. *J Hand Surg [Am]* 12:1077–1079, 1987.

63. Isani A: Small joint injuries requiring surgical treatment. *Orthop Clin North Am* 17:407–419, 1986.

64. Jespersen B, Nielsen SN, Bonnevie BEB, et al: Hyperextension injury to the PIP joint or to the MP joint of the thumb: A clinical study. *Scand J Plast Reconstr Hand Surg* 32:317–321, 1998.

65. Kang L, Rosen A, Potter HG, et al: Rupture of the radial collateral ligament of the index metacarpophalangeal joint: diagnosis and surgical treatment. *J Hand Surg [Am]* 32:789–794, 2007.

66. Kaplan EB: Dorsal dislocation of the metacarpophalangeal joint of the index finger. *J Bone Joint Surg Am* 39:1081–1086, 1957.

67. Kaplan SJ: The Stener lesion revisited: A case report. *J Hand Surg [Am]* 23:833–836, 1998.

68. Kato H, Minami A, Takahara M, et al: Surgical repair of acute collateral ligament injuries in digits with the Mitek bone suture anchor. *J Hand Surg [Br]* 24(1):70–75, 1999.

69. Katsaros J, Milner R, Marshall NJ: Perichondrial arthroplasty incorporating costal cartilage. *J Hand Surg [Br]* 20:137–142, 1995.

70. Kessler I: A simplified technique to correct hyperextension deformity of the metacarpophalangeal joint of the thumb. *J Bone Joint Surg Am* 61:903–905, 1979.

71. Kiefhaber TR, Stern PJ, Grood ES: Lateral stability of the proximal interphalangeal joint. *J Hand Surg [Am]* 11:661–669, 1986.

72. Kitagawa H, Kashimoto T: Locking of the thumb at the interphalangeal joint by one of the sesamoid bones: A case report. *J Bone Joint Surg Am* 66:1300–1301, 1984.

73. Kleinert HE, Kasden ML: Reconstruction of the chronically subluxated proximal interphalangeal finger joint. *J Bone Joint Surg Am* 47:958–964, 1965.

74. Kojima T, Nagano T, Kohno T: Causes of locking metacarpophalangeal joint of the thumb and its nonoperative treatment. *Hand* 11:256–262, 1979.

75. Krakauer JD, Stern PJ: Hinged device for fractures involving the proximal interphalangeal joint. *Clin Orthop Relat Res* 327:29–37, 1996.

76. Lane CS: Detecting occult fractures of the metacarpal head: the Brewerton view. *J Hand Surg [Am]* 2:131, 1977.

77. Lee JY, Teoh LC: Dorsal fracture dislocations of the proximal interphalangeal joint treated by open reduction and interfragmentary screw fixation: indications, approaches and results. *J Hand Surg [Br]* 31:138–146, 2006.

78. Leibovic SJ, Bowers WH: Anatomy of the proximal interphalangeal joint. *Hand Clin* 10:169–178, 1994.

79. Light TR, Ogden JA: Complex dislocation of the index metacarpophalangeal joint in children. *J Pediatr Orthop* 8:300–305, 1988.

80. Lutz M, Fritz D, Arora R, et al: Anatomical basis for functional treatment of dorsolateral dislocation of the proximal interphalangeal joint. *Clin Anat* 17:303–307, 2004.

81. Malerich MM, Eaton RG: The volar plate reconstruction for fracture-dislocation of the proximal interphalangeal joint. *Hand Clin* 10:251–260, 1994.

82. Mansat M, Delprat J: Contractures of the proximal interphalangeal joint. *Hand Clin* 8:777–786, 1992.

83. McCue FC, Honner R, Johnson MC, et al: Athletic injuries of the proximal interphalangeal joint requiring surgical treatment. *J Bone Joint Surg Am* 52:937–956, 1970.

84. McElfresh EC, Dobyns JH, O'Brien ET: Management of fracture-dislocation of the proximal interphalangeal joints by extension-block splinting. *J Bone Joint Surg Am* 54:1705–1711, 1972.

85. Minami A, An KN, Cooney WP, et al: Ligament stability of the metacarpophalangeal joint: A biomechanical study. *J Hand Surg [Am]* 10:255–260, 1985.

86. Moberg F, Stener B: Injuries to the ligaments of the thumb and fingers: Diagnosis, treatment and prognosis. *Acta Chir Scand* 106:166–186, 1953.

87. Moneim MS: Volar dislocation of the metacarpophalangeal joint: Pathologic anatomy and report of two cases. *Clin Orthop Relat Res* 176:186–189, 1983.

88. Morgan JP, Gordon DA, Klug MS, et al: Dynamic digital traction for unstable comminuted intraarticular fracture-dislocations of the proximal interphalangeal joint. *J Hand Surg [Am]* 20:565–573, 1995.

89. Neviaser RJ, Wilson JN, Lievano A: Rupture of the ulnar collateral ligament of the thumb (gamekeeper's thumb): Correction by dynamic repair. *J Bone Joint Surg Am* 53:1357–1364, 1971.

90. Nussbaum R, Sadler AH: An isolated, closed, complex dislocation of the metacarpophalangeal joint of the long finger: a unique case. *J Hand Surg [Am]* 11:558–561, 1986.

91. Palmer AK, Linscheid RL: Chronic recurrent dislocation of the proximal interphalangeal joint of the finger. *J Hand Surg [Am]* 3:95–97, 1978.

92. Palmer AK, Linscheid RL: Irreducible dorsal dislocation of the distal interphalangeal joint of the finger. *J Hand Surg* 2:406–408, 1977.

93. Patel MR, Bassini L: Irreducible volar metacarpophalangeal joint dislocation due to junctura tendinum interposition: A case report and review of the literature. *J Hand Surg* 25:166–172, 2000.

94. Peimer CA, Sullivan DJ, Wild DR: Volar dislocation of the proximal interphalangeal joint. *J Hand Surg [Am]* 9:39–48, 1984.

95. Posner MA, Langa V, Ambrose L: Intrinsic muscle advancement to treat chronic volar instability of the metacarpophalangeal joint of the thumb. *J Hand Surg [Am]* 13:110–115, 1988.

96. Posner MA, Langa V, Green SM: The locked metacarpophalangeal joint: diagnosis and treatment. *J Hand Surg [Am]* 11:249–253, 1986.

97. Posner MA, Wilenski M: Irreducible volar dislocation of the proximal interphalangeal joint of a finger caused by interposition of an intact central slip: a case report. *J Bone Joint Surg Am* 60:133–134, 1978.

98. Quinton DN: Dorsal locking of the metacarpophalangeal joint. *J Hand Surg [Br]* 12:62–63, 1987.

99. Rettig ME, Dassa G, Raskin KB: Volar plate arthroplasty of the distal interphalangeal joint. *J Hand Surg [Am]* 26:940–944, 2001.

100. Ruland RT, Hogan CJ, Cannon DL, et al: Use of dynamic distraction external fixation for unstable fracture-dislocations of the proximal interphalangeal joint. *J Hand Surg [Am]* 33:19–25, 2008.

101. Ryu J, Fagan R: Arthroscopic treatment of acute complete thumb metacarpophalangeal ulnar collateral ligament tears. *J Hand Surg [Am]* 20:1037–1042, 1995.

102. Salamon PB, Gelberman RH: Irreducible dislocation of the interphalangeal joint of the thumb: Report of three cases. *J Bone Joint Surg Am* 60:400–401, 1978.

103. Shah SR, Bindra R, Griffin JW: Irreducible dislocation of the thumb interphalangeal joint with digital nerve interposition: case report. *J Hand Surg [Am]* 35(3):422–424, 2010.

104. Shaw SJ, Morris MA: The range of motion of the metacarpophalangeal joint of the thumb and its relationship to injury. *J Hand Surg [Br]* 17:164–166, 1992.

105. Simonian PT, Trumble TE: Traumatic dislocation of the thumb carpometacarpal joint: early ligamentous reconstruction versus closed reduction and pinning. *J Hand Surg [Am]* 21:802–806, 1996.

106. Slade JF, Gutow AP: Arthroscopy of the metacarpophalangeal joint. *Hand Clin* 15:501–526, 1999.

107. Smith RJ: Post-traumatic instability of the metacarpophalangeal joint of the thumb. *J Bone Joint Surg Am* 59:14–21, 1977.

108. Spaeth HJ, Abrams RA, Bock GW, et al: Gamekeeper thumb: differentiation of nondisplaced and displaced tears of the ulnar collateral ligament with MR imaging. *Radiology* 188:553–556, 1993.

109. Stener B: Displacement of the ruptured ulnar collateral ligament of the metacarpophalangeal joint of the thumb: a clinical and anatomical study. *J Bone Joint Surg Br* 44:869–879, 1962.

110. Stener B: Hyperextension injuries to the metacarpophalangeal joint of the thumb: rupture of ligaments, fracture of sesamoid bones, rupture of the flexor pollicis brevis: An anatomical and clinical study. *Acta Chir Scand* 125:275–293, 1963.

111. Stern PJ: Stener lesion of the lateral dislocation of the proximal interphalangeal joint: indication for open reduction. *J Hand Surg [Am]* 6:602–604, 1981.

112. Strauch RJ, Behrman MJ, Rosenwasser MP: Acute dislocation of the carpometacarpal joint of the thumb: an anatomic and cadaver study. *J Hand Surg [Am]* 19:93–98, 1994.

113. Stripling WD: Displaced intraarticular osteochondral fracture: cause for irreducible dislocation of the distal interphalangeal joint. *J Hand Surg [Am]* 7:77–78, 1982.

114. Suzuki Y, Matsunaga T, Sato S, et al: The pins and rubbers traction system for treatment of comminuted intraarticular fractures and fracture-dislocations in the hand. *J Hand Surg [Br]* 19:98–107, 1994.

115. Tajima K, Sasaki T, Yamanaka K: Vertical locking of the metacarpophalangeal joint of the thumb. *Hand Surg* 10:279–284, 2005.

116. Tekkis PP, Kessaris N, Gavalas M, et al: The role of mini-fragment screw fixation in volar dislocations of the proximal interphalangeal joint. *Arch Orthop Trauma Surg* 121:121–122, 2001.

117. Tonkin MA, Beard AJ, Kemp SJ, et al: Sesamoid arthrodesis for hyperextension of the thumb metacarpophalangeal joint. *J Hand Surg [Am]* 20:334–338, 1995.

118. Viegas SF: Extension block pinning for proximal interphalangeal joint fracture dislocations: Preliminary report of a new technique. *J Hand Surg [Am]* 17:896–901, 1992.

119. Vitale MA, White NJ, Strauch RJ: A percutaneous technique to treat unstable dorsal fracture-dislocations of the proximal interphalangeal joint. *J Hand Surg [Am]* 36(9):1453–1459, 2011.

120. Waris E, Alanen V: Percutaneous, intramedullary fracture reduction and extension block pinning for dorsal proximal interphalangeal fracture-dislocations. *J Hand Surg [Am]* 35(12):2046–2052, 2010.

121. Weiss APC: Cerclage fixation for fracture dislocation of the proximal interphalangeal joint. *Clin Orthop Relat Res* 327:21–28, 1996.

122. Wiley AM: Instability of the proximal interphalangeal joint following dislocation and fracture dislocation: Surgical repair. *Hand* 2:185–194, 1970.

123. Wolfe SW, Katz LD: Intra-articular impaction fractures of the phalanges. *J Hand Surg [Am]* 20:327–333, 1995.

124. Yagi B, Yamanaka K, Yoshida K, et al: Successful manual reduction of locked metacarpophalangeal joints in fingers. *J Bone Joint Surg Am* 82:366–371, 2000.

125. Zemel NP, Stark HH, Ashworth CR, et al: Chronic fracture dislocation of the proximal interphalangeal joint: treatment by osteotomy and bone graft. *J Hand Surg [Am]* 6:447–455, 1981.

126. Zhang X, Yang L, Shao X, et al: Treatment of bony boutonniere deformity with a loop wire. *J Hand Surg [Am]* 36(6):1080–1085, 2011.

9

Perionychium

Nicole Z. Sommer

Acknowledgment: Thank you to Richard E. Brown and Elvin G. Zook for their past contributions to the creation of this chapter.

The fingernail serves many functions that are taken for granted in everyday use of the hand. The nail protects the fingertip, helps in regulation of peripheral circulation, and contributes to tactile sensation that assists us in picking up small objects. An abnormal nail is a functional and a cosmetic problem. Because of the prominence of the nail on the tip of the finger, the perionychium is the most frequently injured part of the hand.

ANATOMY

The anatomic landmarks of the nail are shown in Figure 9.1. The perionychium includes the nail bed, nail fold, eponychium, paronychium, and hyponychium. The nail bed, the soft tissue beneath the nail, includes the germinal matrix proximally and the sterile matrix distally. The nail fold, which is the most proximal extent of the perionychium, consists of a dorsal roof and a ventral floor. The ventral floor is the germinal matrix portion of the nail bed. Paronychium refers to the skin on each side of the nail, and hyponychium refers to the skin distal to the nail bed. The eponychium is the skin proximal to the nail that covers the nail fold. Extending distally from the eponychium onto the nail is the nail vest or cuticle. The white arc of the nail just distal to the eponychium, known as the lunula, is the distal extent of the germinal matrix.

The germinal matrix produces about 90% of the nail,[65] an important point in reconstruction of the nail bed. The sterile matrix adds a thin layer of cells to the undersurface of the nail, keeping the nail adherent to the nail bed.[12,29,53] Scarring of the germinal matrix leads to absence of the nail, whereas injury to the sterile matrix leads to nail deformity. The dorsal roof of the nail fold produces the shine on the nail.

The blood supply of the perionychium comes from the terminal branches of the radial and ulnar volar digital arteries and capillary loops (Figure 9.2).[47] The veins drain into the proximal nail bed and nail fold, then course randomly over the dorsum of the finger.[73,103] Sensation to the nail bed is supplied by dorsal branches of the volar radial and ulnar digital nerves and the most distal extent of the dorsal radial digital nerve branches.[99]

The numerous lymphatics of the nail bed roughly parallel the veins. The hyponychium contains the greatest density of lymphatics of any dermal area in the body,[93] which aids in deterring infection in this frequently exposed area.[102]

PREOPERATIVE EVALUATION

In the case of fingertip injuries, evaluation of the perionychium usually begins in the office or emergency department with the patient history. Evaluation of an injured perionychium includes assessment for associated injuries. We recommend a radiograph of the involved finger because of the 50% chance of fracture with a nail bed injury.

Doors are the most common source of trauma to the perionychium, followed by smashing the finger between two objects and lacerations from yard or workshop tools. Patients are most often older children or young adults. The long finger is most frequently injured because of its increased exposure distal to the other digits. Similarly, the most distal part of the nail bed is the most frequently injured part of the perionychium, and often the hyponychium is involved as well.

Most nail bed trauma falls into the classification of simple lacerations, stellate lacerations, severe crush, or avulsions (Figure 9.3).[44,104] These injuries occur in the same order of frequency. A fifth category of injury is subungual hematoma. Because of the inability to see the extent of the nail bed laceration, subungual hematomas can be the most challenging injury to treat.

TYPES OF OPERATIONS

Subungual Hematoma

Compression of the nail onto the underlying distal phalanx can lead to a laceration in the nail bed and bleeding beneath the nail, known as subungual hematoma. If the nail is intact, the pressure of the blood within this confined space frequently causes severe throbbing pain, and evacuation of the hematoma is indicated.

Before evacuation of the hematoma, the finger should be surgically prepared. Surgical preparation is essential to decrease the chance of bacterial inoculation of the subungual space on trephination of the nail. We prefer a povidone-iodine (Betadine) soap scrub. Trephination of the nail has been performed with drills, needles, and paperclips heated in an open flame until red hot. We prefer a battery-powered microcautery unit, available in most emergency departments (Figure 9.4). The heated tip is passed through the nail and is cooled by the hematoma, avoiding injury to the nail bed. The hole must be large enough to allow continued drainage; otherwise, the hematoma recurs if a clot seals the hole.

In the past, we recommended removal of the nail and repair of the nail bed if greater than 25% to 50% of the nail was undermined by blood.[97,107] However, a prospective 2-year study of 48 patients with hematomas showed no complications of nail deformity with drainage only, regardless of hematoma size or the presence of a distal phalangeal fracture.[88] Our cutoff for nail removal and repair subsequently became greater than 50%. At

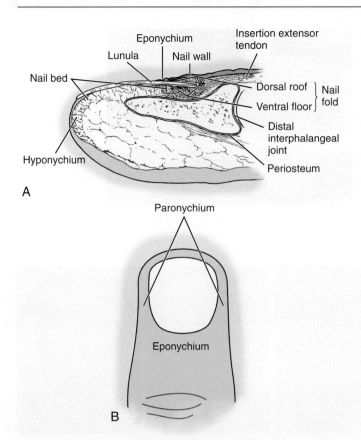

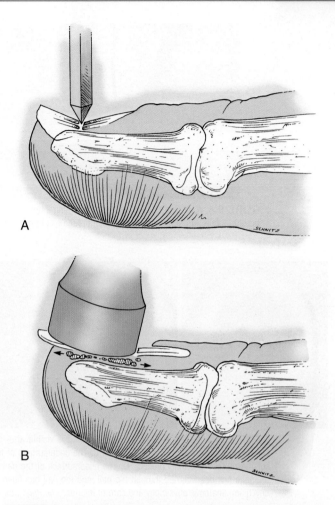

FIGURE 9.1 A, Anatomy of the nail bed shown in sagittal section. **B,** The perionychium includes the paronychium, eponychium, hyponychium, and nail bed.

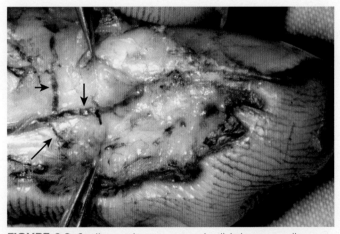

FIGURE 9.2 *Small arrow* shows common volar digital artery, *medium arrow* indicates dorsal branch to the nail fold, and *large arrow* shows artery that progresses along the perionychium and sends branches to the nail bed. The terminal branch to the pad of the finger is not shown.

the present time, the decision for removal of the nail is based primarily on evaluation of the nail edges, rather than the percentage of hematoma. Generally, if the nail edges are intact, we recommend drainage only. If the nail is broken or the edges are disrupted, we recommend removal of the nail with exploration and repair of the nail bed.

FIGURE 9.3 A, A relatively sharp object compressing the nail between the nail and bone causes a splitting laceration (simple). **B,** A wider area of compression of the nail bed between the nail and the bone causes an exploding-type injury that results in multiple fragments (stellate or crush).

Nail Bed Repair

This discussion on nail bed repair includes the various points pertinent for treatment of simple lacerations, crush injuries, and avulsion injuries. A finger block is performed with 1% plain lidocaine. Lidocaine with epinephrine (1:100,000) has also been shown to be safe for digital blocks.[25] The finger and often the entire hand are surgically prepared and draped. After exsanguination, a finger tourniquet is placed around the proximal phalanx to allow for hemostasis and adequate visualization of the nail bed. The nail is removed with a periosteal elevator or iris scissors. The scissors are inserted beneath the free edge of the nail and gently opened and closed working them proximally. If curved scissors are used, the tips are pointed superficially toward the nail to avoid injury to the nail bed. Caution must be used with an elevator because blunt force can tear the nail bed. We recommend a Kutz elevator because it is smaller than a Freer elevator and does less damage to the nail bed. The nail is cleaned by scraping the undersurface to remove the residual fibrinous tissue and soaked in povidone-iodine during the repair of the nail bed laceration.

The nail bed is examined under loupe magnification. Irregularities of the edges are trimmed if it is possible to do so without

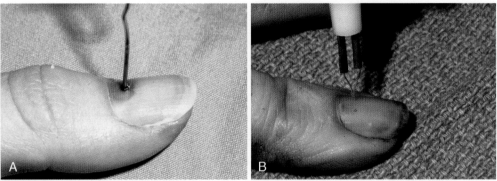

FIGURE 9.4 A, A time-honored method of burning a hole through the nail is with a heated paperclip. **B,** The authors' preferred method of burning a hole through the nail is with an ophthalmic battery-powered cautery.

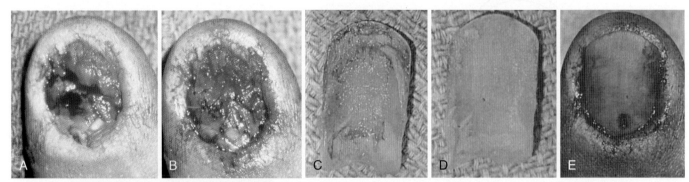

FIGURE 9.5 A, Stellate laceration of nail bed is visible after the nail is removed. **B,** The lacerations are approximated with fine 7-0 chromic sutures under loop magnification. **C,** The undersurface of the nail after it has been removed from the nail bed shows the residual soft tissue that is usually present. **D,** The undersurface of the nail after it has been cleaned and soaked. **E,** A hole large enough to allow drainage has been burned through the nail, and the nail has been inserted back into the nail fold. (**C** through **E,** From Zook EG: The perionychium: anatomy, physiology and care of injuries. *Clin Plast Surg* 8:21–31, 1981, with permission.)

compromising the repair. Débridement must remain conservative, however. The nail bed is adherent to the distal phalanx and difficult to mobilize. Undermining the edges approximately 1 mm allows for slight eversion, but minimal to no mobilization. It is better to leave contused edges in place if there is doubt of closure, rather than to leave a defect from aggressive débridement. The wound is copiously irrigated with normal saline. The nail bed is repaired with a 7-0 chromic suture on a micropoint spatula, double-arm, GS-9 ophthalmic needle (Ethicon). The curve of this needle allows easier passage through the nail bed, which is adherent to the periosteum. The double needle provides a spare in case one is bent or broken. Simple nonburied sutures are placed.

With stellate lacerations and especially with crush injuries, the nail is often fragmented. The nail is removed very cautiously to avoid injury to the small segments of adherent nail bed. With meticulous approximation of the multiple segments, stellate lacerations have a good outcome (Figure 9.5). Crush injuries have a poorer prognosis likely because of the presence of greater contusion along with the complicated laceration.

After repair of simple or complex lacerations (or placement of a nail bed graft, when needed), the nail bed must be protected. The best option is the native nail if this is available. The nail also acts as a perfect mold for the repaired nail bed.[85] The nail is removed from the povidone-iodine soak and irrigated with normal saline. A hole is cut in the nail with a pair of fine scissors or burned with a battery-operated cautery to allow

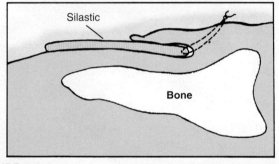

FIGURE 9.6 Horizontal mattress suture through the nail wall is used to hold a silicone sheet in the nail fold.

drainage of serum or hematoma from the subungual space. We prefer to place the hole away from the repair when possible. The nail is secured in place with a 5-0 nylon mattress suture through the nail and nail fold or a simple suture through the edge of the nail and hyponychium. The nail prevents scar formation between the ventral and dorsal surface of the nail fold. The nail stiffness prevents it from flipping out of the nail fold when the hyponychium suture is used. Dermal adhesives[45,94] have been advocated for nail adhesion, but we have no experience with this technique. If the nail is unavailable or is too badly damaged, a nail-shaped piece of 0.020-inch reinforced silicone sheeting may be substituted. Silicone is less stiff and requires a nail fold suture to hold it in place beneath the nail fold (Figure 9.6). We

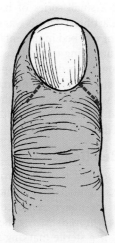

FIGURE 9.7 When incisions are made in the eponychium, they should be made at 90-degree angles from the eponychium to prevent deformity.

believe that the silicone is able to mold the edges of the repair more accurately than firmer prosthetic materials recommended by Ogunro.[78] If neither nail nor silicone is available, a single thickness of nail-shaped nonadherent gauze or suture packet material may be placed in the nail fold.

The finger is wrapped in nonadhesive gauze and small gauze bandages and wrapped with a small gauze roll. We recommend a four-prong or volar aluminum splint for protection of the repair and reduction of pain. The splint is worn for 2 to 3 weeks, or longer if a fracture is present. Immobilization of the distal interphalangeal (DIP) joint is necessary only if a significant distal phalanx fracture is present. Patients are instructed to keep the finger and dressing dry until follow-up and to keep the hand elevated. If a nail bed graft is taken, the donor site is treated in a similar fashion with replacement and stabilization of the nail and a protective dressing.

Avulsion

Nail bed avulsion often leaves a fragment of nail bed attached to the undersurface of the avulsed nail and often involves most of the nail bed. An avulsion commonly manifests as laceration of the nail bed within the nail fold with the nail bed attached distally. In a child, avulsion of the nail bed out of the nail fold suggests a Salter I fracture. Radiographic evaluation, especially in the lateral view, is recommended.

Adequate visualization and repair require an incision in the eponychium. The incision is made perpendicular to the lateral curved portion of the eponychial fold and may be necessary on both sides (Figure 9.7). The nail bed is repaired under direct visualization, and the eponychial incisions are closed with 6-0 nylon.

An attempt should be made to find the nail if it does not accompany the patient. The avulsed nail bed is replaced as a nail bed graft with the nail acting as an optimal graft bolster. If the fragment is large, the nail is trimmed back 1 to 2 mm from the outer edge of the nail bed to allow suturing of the nail bed (Figure 9.8). Small fragments of nail bed are removed from the nail and replaced as nail bed grafts. A graft 1 cm in diameter usually takes by inosculation and vascular ingrowth from the periphery. The distal phalanx is one of the few sites where a

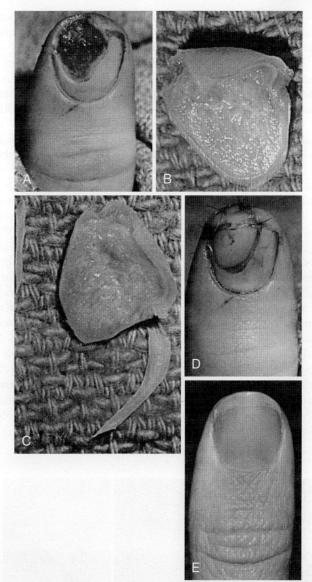

FIGURE 9.8 A, Avulsion of a small portion of the nail and nail bed. **B,** Undersurface of the nail fragment with attached nail bed. **C,** Only that portion of the nail that is overhanging the nail bed is removed. **D,** The nail with attached nail bed is accurately approximated and held in place with a few fine chromic sutures. **E,** Nail bed 12 months after injury.

graft can survive on bare cortex. Very small nail bed fragments may be more difficult to remove. Although rarely the case, if there is concern about further injury to the nail bed fragment on attempted removal, the entire nail is replaced without separation of the nail bed fragment from the nail or suturing of the nail bed.

Nail Bed Defect

A split-thickness injury of the nail bed regenerates and does not need closure. Small areas of full-thickness nail bed loss have been left to heal by secondary intention; however, this generally results in scarring and nail deformity. Johnson[52] advocated releasing incisions in the lateral paronychial folds with advancement of the germinal matrix toward the center of the nail. Favorable features that increase success of this lateral mobilization include a defect less than one third of the nail width, good condition of the matrix to be mobilized, and careful elevation and advancement of the matrix.[3] We have found this technique useful in the acute setting with a defect of 3 to 5 mm.

There are other options for closure of sterile matrix defects, including split-thickness or full-thickness nail bed grafts.[84] Use of a split-thickness nail bed graft[90] allows for harvest of nail bed from adjacent uninjured nail bed without altering nail growth at the donor site. It has been our experience that if there is inadequate undamaged area on the injured nail bed from which to harvest, such as a defect greater than 50% of the nail bed, the nail bed graft should be harvested from an adjacent finger or toe. Patients often choose to have a graft harvested from the toe rather than another finger. From a clinical standpoint, the toe is likely a better option, owing to the small risk of donor site nail deformity if the graft is harvested too deeply (Figure 9.9).

Full-thickness nail bed grafts are rarely used except when there are salvageable spare parts that would otherwise be discarded. Otherwise, a full-thickness graft would leave a deformity of the nail at the donor site. A full-thickness nail bed graft is necessary, however, when replacing lost germinal matrix. Another situation in which full-thickness grafts are chosen involves injury to the perionychium surrounding the nail bed. Zaias[100] determined that there are no living cells in split-thickness nail bed grafts, and the recipient site is resurfaced with cells from the surrounding hyponychium, eponychium, and paronychium. If the surrounding perionychium is also missing, a full-thickness nail bed graft, which possesses living cells, would yield superior results compared with a split-thickness graft.

Sugamata treated a small series of nail bed wounds with artificial dermis. The artificial dermis was placed as a substitute for the missing part of nail bed in patients without an available amputated piece or unwilling to sacrifice another digit for the nail bed graft. Although he does not specify if the nail bed wound involved the sterile versus germinal matrix, all patients regenerated nail and were satisfied with the result.[95] We suspect this technique would be less successful if the germinal matrix portion were involved.

Harvest of Nail Bed Graft

The finger or toe to be used as the donor is anesthetized with a digital block. After exsanguination, a digital tourniquet is placed for hemostasis, and the nail is removed. If possible, only a portion of the nail is removed, leaving the proximal nail intact within the nail fold. If a sterile marking pen is available, it is helpful to mark the area of graft needed on the donor site. A split-thickness nail bed graft (approximately 0.010 inch thick) is harvested with a No. 15 scalpel (see Figure 9.9, C). Harvesting must be done carefully and slowly. The scalpel is placed parallel to the nail bed, and a back-and-forth sawing motion is used. To ensure thinness of the graft, we recommend visualization of the blade through the graft. It is better for the graft to be too thin than too thick. If a thick graft results in full-thickness donor loss, donor site deformity is likely. A large graft is more difficult to harvest because of the curve of the nail bed and increases the chance of an accidental full-thickness harvest. To avoid this possibility, we use the tip of the blade while picking up the edge of the graft with fine forceps. The graft is sutured into the defect with 7-0 chromic sutures.

Fracture

An associated distal phalanx fracture occurs with 50% of nail bed injuries.[104] Nondisplaced fractures and distal tuft fractures are treated with repair of the nail bed and replacement of the nail as a splint. The curve of the nail and its close approximation to the underlying bone makes an excellent splint to maintain fracture reduction. A tension band suture over the replaced nail can provide further stability to the fracture (Figure 9.10).[15] If

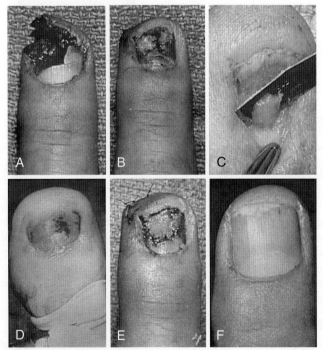

FIGURE 9.9 A, Nail bed and fingertip injury with avulsion of approximately 25% of the nail bed. **B,** Tip skin and nail bed surrounding the avulsion have been repaired. The white area at the distal left portion of the nail bed is bare cortical bone of the distal tuft. **C,** Technique of harvesting a small, split-thickness nail bed graft. **D,** Large toe after the nail has been removed and a split-thickness graft has been removed from the sterile matrix. The germinal matrix should not be included in a split-thickness graft. **E,** Split-thickness graft of sterile matrix is sutured in place on the nail bed. **F,** Fingernail 1 year later.

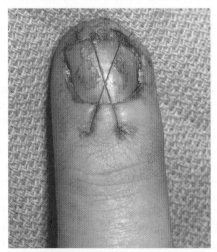

FIGURE 9.10 Figure-of-eight stitch holds nail in place and adds stability to fracture.

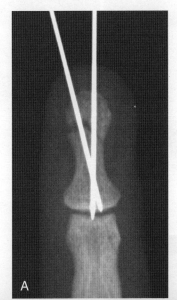

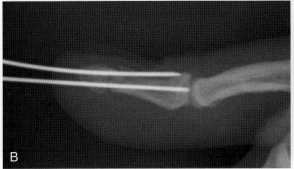

FIGURE 9.11 A and **B,** Distal phalanx fractures with Kirschner wire fixation. (From Brown RE: Acute nail bed injuries. *Hand Clin* 18:561–575, 2002.)

the nail is missing, the fracture may need to be pinned for better stabilization.

Displaced fractures, especially fractures proximal to the nail fold, are accurately reduced and fixed with 0.028-inch longitudinal or crossed Kirschner wires (Figure 9.11). The use of a single wire is not recommended. Although a single wire can reduce the fracture, it cannot eliminate axial rotation. If only a small nail bed laceration is present, wires are passed in a retrograde fashion. However, with large nail bed lacerations, the wires are passed antegrade through the distal fragment, then retrograde into the proximal fragment. Crossing the DIP joint should be avoided if possible. With crush injuries, the distal phalanx fracture is often comminuted with small fractured pieces adherent to the nail bed. In this case, the bony fragments are reduced with reapproximation of the nail bed using the nail as a splint. If the nail is unavailable for use as a splint, a piece of reinforced silicone is recommended. The goals of distal phalanx reduction are bony union and an even dorsal cortex. An uneven cortex would impair nail bed healing and lead to a nail deformity.

Salter I fractures are often reduced with repair of the nail bed alone. Pinning of the fracture should be avoided unless it is unstable. The patient and parents should be informed that growth of the distal phalanx may be affected, even with adequate reduction.

Amputation

Amputation can be treated in multiple ways, usually based on the remaining proximal tissue and the presence and quality of the amputated piece. Options include revision amputation, closure with flaps and grafts, or replantation. Our preference for treatment is discussed for a distal to proximal direction of injury.

On the rare occasion that the distal phalanx is covered by a layer of soft tissue, the amputated piece can be defatted and replaced as a skin or nail bed graft, or the area can be left to heal by secondary intention, especially if less than 1 to 1.5 cm in size. If the distal phalanx is exposed, the options consist of trimming back the bone to allow for primary closure or rotation of local or regional skin flaps to preserve length. In both cases, when suturing the fingertip skin to the distal nail bed, tension should be avoided. Tension at the closure causes volar curvature of the distal nail bed and plate, leading to a hook nail. If a portion of the distal phalanx is absent, the nail bed should be shortened to the end of the remaining distal phalanx before repair to avoid hooking of the nail from loss of bony support.

More proximal amputations involving the midportion of the nail bed can be managed with local and regional flaps.[20] We use local volar and lateral "V-Y" advancement flaps and regional cross-finger and thenar flaps to provide tip coverage (Figures 9.12 and 9.13).[18,5,39] "V-Y" advancement flaps cannot be advanced more than 5 to 10 mm.[18] These flaps can be used to close defects primarily involving the volar and distal fingertip or can be used with nail bed grafts to reconstruct the entire fingertip. Such flaps provide excellent coverage and can be deepithelialized to provide a vascularized bed for placement of the nail bed graft. Full-thickness nail bed grafts from the amputated part or a split-thickness nail bed graft from an adjacent finger or toe may be used. Eponychial advancement flaps or cutaneous translation flaps have been successfully used to advance the nail distally in reconstruction of amputation defects.[7] The eponychial flap is used in conjunction with a volar flap to preserve length of the digit.[35]

Amputations through the eponychium may be replanted, but success is variable. We tend to perform revision amputation at the level of the eponychium. If 25% or greater of the nail bed distal to the eponychium is present, the patient benefits from maintaining that nail. If less than 25% remains, however, we recommend resection of the remaining nail bed. This resection requires removal of the dorsal roof and ventral floor of the nail fold. The eponychial skin is left intact to use for coverage. Netscher and Meade[76] described success with the use of full-thickness graft of hyponychium, nail bed, and paronychium for amputations between the midportion of the nail and just proximal to the eponychium. In several cases, the distal phalanx was replaced as a graft and covered with regional flaps. The graft was placed onto the deepithelialized flaps. This would allow for preservation of length when successful.

Replantation is most successful when the amputation is proximal to the area of the paronychium through the proximal aspect of the distal phalanx. Amputations through the nail bed are less successful because of the size of the vessels.

In children, the tip of the finger is often avulsed with the nail bed. In these cases, we approximate the edges of the nail bed

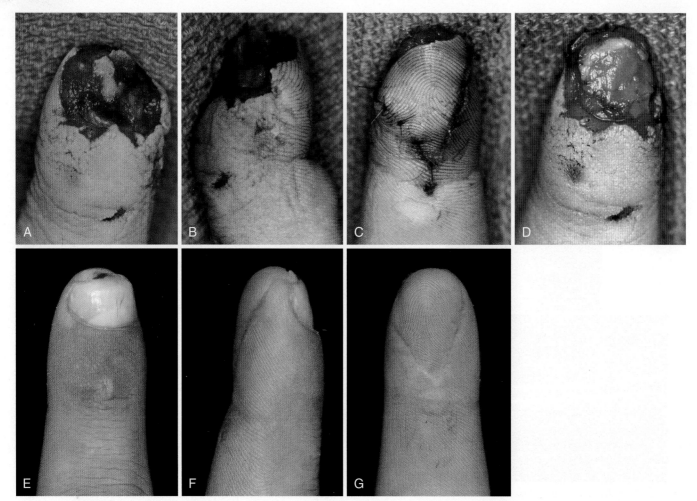

FIGURE 9.12 **A,** Fingertip injury with avulsion of nail bed. **B,** Dorsal tip defect with intact volar skin. **C,** "V-Y" volar advancement flap for coverage and nail bed support. **D,** Nail bed replaced as graft. **E** to **G,** Results after partial nail regrowth. (**D,** From Brown RE, Zook EG, Russell RC: Fingertip reconstruction with flaps and nail bed grafts. *J Hand Surg [Am]* 24:345–351, 1999.)

and fingertip skin as a composite graft. Débridement of this composite graft is minimal to allow for maximal inosculation effect. Longitudinal or crossed pins are used to hold the bone in place. With young children, we occasionally use hypodermic needles in place of Kirschner wires for the bony reduction. The younger the child, the better chances for "take" of a composite graft of skin and nail bed. Our greatest success rate is for children 3 years old and younger. Alternatively, in an older child, a "cap" graft[83] is likely to have greater success. This procedure includes removal of the bone fragment and defatting of the skin for use of the piece as a full-thickness skin or nail bed graft.

Delayed Treatment of Acute Injuries

Occasionally, a nail bed injury is seen hours or days after the injury, with or without previous treatment. The first decision must be whether the initial care was adequate and, if it was not, whether more should be done. If there is any question, the nail bed is explored and accurately approximated; this can usually be done 7 days after injury. Any untreated or maltreated distal phalangeal fractures should also be treated appropriately, and the patient should be placed on perioperative antibiotics. Although the chance of infection may be greater with delayed treatment, a nail deformity occurs if nothing is done. We believe the risk is worth taking.

POSTOPERATIVE MANAGEMENT

Patients are seen at 5 to 7 days after surgery. It is usually necessary to soak the finger with normal saline and peroxide to remove the dressing. The bandage is removed gently and slowly to protect the repair. This removal is especially difficult when nonadherent gauze alone is used for the nail fold because it adheres to the nail bed. If it does not loosen, we instruct the patient to perform warm soapy soaks at home several times a day. It generally separates as the nail grows.

The nail is checked for subungual seroma or hematoma. If either is present, the hole is reopened, or the nail is very gently raised at the edge to permit drainage. The suture used to hold the nail or silicone sheet in place within the nail fold should be removed 5 to 7 days after injury to avoid a sinus tract formation through the nail fold. Sutures placed through the hyponychium or the paronychium (lateral skin) may be left in longer and removed in 10 to 14 days as would be customary for sutures in the hand. The old nail is likely to adhere to the nail bed for 1 to 3 months until pushed off by the new nail. Silicone sheeting will fall off sooner.

The nail bed repair is protected, and distal phalangeal fractures are immobilized with a splint dressing for the first 3 to 4 weeks. After this time, a bandage is adequate for protection of

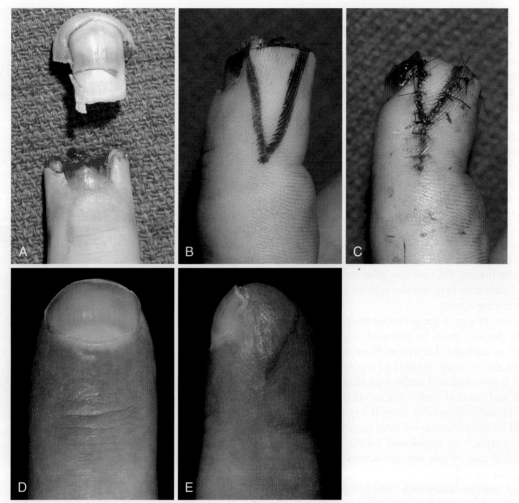

FIGURE 9.13 A, Fingertip amputation through the sterile matrix. **B,** Outline of bilateral "V-Y" advancement flaps for soft tissue coverage of fingertip. **C,** Flaps advanced and sutured together in midline. **D** and **E,** Appearance after regrowth of nail.

the repair and for assisting in retention of the old nail. Retention of the nail protects the nail bed and creates a much less tender fingertip while the new nail grows. Distal phalanx fractures are followed by x-ray evaluation at 3 to 4 weeks and clinical resolution of pain.

Scarring of the nail bed is reduced with surgical repair, and growth of a normal new nail is expected. Nail bed scarring and nail deformities do occur, however, and the patient should be reminded of this at the postoperative visit.

The nail grows at approximately 0.1 mm per day[6] or 2 to 3 mm per month. After removal of the nail for nail bed repair, there is a delay of new growth for 3 to 4 weeks.[6] If the proximal nail was uninjured and left in place during repair of a distal nail bed injury, growth of that nail occurs at a normal rate without delay. As the nail grows, there is a bulge on the leading edge. This distal end is expected to reach the distal finger at 6 to 9 months after injury. Toenail growth occurs four times more slowly than fingernail growth.[79]

COMPLICATIONS

Postoperative complications can be divided into problems at the site of nail growth (i.e., the germinal and sterile matrix and nail fold) and the site of nail support, the distal phalanx. Scar

within the sterile matrix results in various deformities, including notching, splitting, elevation, and nonadherence, because the nail does not grow over or adhere to a nail bed scar.[48] Scar within the germinal matrix may lead to absence of nail growth. Splitting or absence of the nail may also be caused from scarring of the nail fold dorsal roof to the ventral floor, which again emphasizes the importance of placing the nail or a silicone sheet under the nail fold after acute repair. All of these deformities can be functional and cosmetic. Bony complications include an uneven dorsal cortex and loss of bony support secondary to overdébridement of the distal phalanx, nonunion of the distal phalanx, or osteomyelitis.

Late reconstruction of the nail bed is commonly not as successful as the surgeon or the patient would desire. These less than satisfactory results have discouraged and hindered progress in reconstruction of the perionychium. Every reconstructive problem of the nail bed is different and must be approached individually. A thorough understanding of the anatomy and physiology of the nail bed of the fingers and toes is essential to devise and carry out a treatment plan.

Nail Ridges

Nail ridges are caused by an uneven dorsal cortex or scar beneath the nail bed. Because nail growth follows the shape of the nail bed, an uneven surface beneath the nail bed leads to an irregular nail bed and a subsequent nail ridge. A transverse nail ridge can raise the nail off of the nail bed preventing distal adherence. Ridging is typically a cosmetic problem except in the instance of nonadherence, where the free nail edge can catch on objects such as clothing, making this a functional problem as well. Correction requires elevation of the nail bed off of the distal phalanx and surgical excision of the scar or leveling of the uneven dorsal cortex to create a flat nail bed.[4,96]

We have noted minor transverse ridges of the nail after general hypoxic illness and local hypoxia from use of an arm tourniquet for upper extremity procedures. Hypoxia leads to temporary abnormality of germinal matrix cells; the ridges resolve as the nail grows.

Split Nail

A split nail may be caused by a longitudinal ridge or scar in the germinal or sterile matrix. Because scar does not produce nail cells, there is a blank area between the regions of normal nail production, producing a split.

If the split is due to scar in the germinal matrix with lack of nail production, the scar must be removed, and the nail bed must be repaired or replaced. The eponychium is elevated with incisions at right angles to the corners to expose the germinal matrix. The nail is removed, and under loop magnification, the scar is identified and resected. Rarely, the defect is small enough (<2 mm) to be closed primarily. If there is any tension, a nail bed graft should be used instead. We have found lateral mobilization of the matrix,[53] as mentioned earlier, to be mostly unsuccessful in the case of late reconstruction owing to scar interfering with flap rotation.

A larger defect must be closed with a nail bed graft. We prefer to use a germinal matrix graft from a toe that is similar in size and shape to the resected scar (Figure 9.14). The germinal matrix must be taken as a full-thickness graft for it to produce nail at the recipient site. Because a full-thickness graft frequently requires the elimination of nearly an entire toenail bed, the second toenail is more acceptable to most individuals, rather than having a significant deformity of the large toenail.[26] The third through fifth toes usually do not have enough germinal matrix available for a graft.

If the scar involves the sterile matrix, it can rarely be treated with resection and primary closure. In our experience, the scar is frequently too wide to approximate the edges without significant tension and recurrence of the scar and subsequent split. We recommend resection of the scar and replacement with a split-thickness nail bed graft. A defect in the sterile matrix does not require a full-thickness graft as does the germinal matrix. Harvest of the graft should cause no donor site deformity.[81,91] Donor site options include adjacent nail on the injured finger, an adjacent finger, or the first or second toe (Figure 9.15).

Nonadherence

The sterile matrix adds nail cells to the undersurface of the nail, resulting in adherence of the nail to the nail bed. Scars within the sterile matrix do not produce nail cells, allowing for loosening of the nail attachments. The nail is lifted off of the nail bed by transverse and diagonal scars and is unable to adhere distally. Resection of the scar is essential for correction. For replacement,

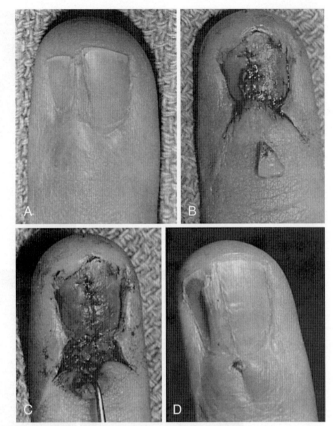

FIGURE 9.14 A, Split nail with a pterygium caused by scarring of the germinal matrix. **B,** Scar of the germinal matrix has been removed, and a fragment of germinal matrix from the second toe has been cut to shape to fit the defect. **C,** Germinal matrix graft sutured in place. **D,** Nail can be seen growing from the germinal matrix graft 6 months later.

we prefer a split-thickness sterile matrix graft from either an adjacent area of the nail bed or a toenail bed (Figure 9.16).[81,101,106]

Chronic nonadherence of the nail to the distal nail bed can also occur with repetitive trauma, such as using the fingernails to pry open objects. Cutting back or avoiding the activity is advised. If no improvement is seen, replacement of this distal nail bed segment with a split-thickness sterile matrix graft is recommended.

Absence

Absence of a nail may be congenital or may result from avulsion, severe crush, infection, or burn, and is a disconcerting deformity to the patient. Absence may be partial or complete. Absence of nail distal to the germinal matrix is treated with removal of the scar and replacement with a split-thickness sterile matrix nail bed graft. Lemperle and associates[64] reported success with serial excisions of 4-mm wide, crescent-shaped, full-thickness scars at 2-month intervals that resulted in distal migration of the nail bed by wound contraction. This technique seems to eliminate morbidity of a donor graft site, while increasing the number of procedures required in serial excision.

Complete absence of nail is more difficult to reconstruct, especially when the proximal nail fold is absent along with the germinal matrix. A simple but suboptimal treatment is resection of an area of skin in the shape of a slightly larger than normal nail.[46] A full-thickness or split-thickness skin graft is

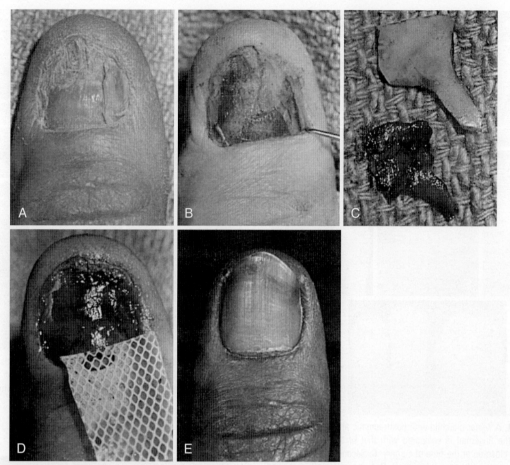

FIGURE 9.15 **A,** Preoperative view of a thumbnail after injury by a car door. The nail grows out and becomes nonadherent every 2 to 3 months. **B,** Nail remnant has been removed, and scar can be seen in the nail bed on the right side. **C,** An exact template in the configuration of the scar is used to shape a split-thickness nail bed graft from sterile matrix of the toe. **D,** Split-thickness nail bed graft has been sutured in place, and a silicone sheet has been placed over it and into the nail fold. **E,** The nail 11 months postoperatively with complete adherence of the nail.

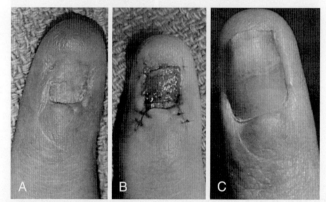

FIGURE 9.16 **A,** Finger with normal germinal matrix, but absent sterile matrix and nonadherence of the nail. The patient had had repeated infections beneath the nail. **B,** Scarred nail bed has been removed, and a full-thickness sterile matrix graft from the second toe has been used to replace it. **C,** Nail 1 year later adheres to the full-thickness toenail graft, but does not adhere to the distal scar. (From Zook EG: The perionychium: anatomy, physiology and care of injuries. *Clin Plast Surg* 8:21–31, 1981, with permission.)

used to mimic the appearance of a nail. Artificial nails applied with glue have been unsuccessful.[13] Buncke and Gonzalez[22] advocated reconstruction of a nail fold pouch to aid in artificial nail adherence. As time passes, the pouch becomes obliterated, however, and no longer holds the edge of the prosthetic nail.[13]

Baruchin and colleagues[12a] described the use of titanium implants inserted into the distal phalanx as a method of artificial nail fixation. A small patient series showed favorable results with this simple, cost effective and sustainable procedure.

Composite toenail grafts that include germinal and sterile matrix and the dorsal roof have been used for nail reconstruction (Figure 9.17). The few reported cases have produced unpredictable results. In our experience, the results do not seem to be directly related to patient age or size of the graft.[66] We inform the patients of the expected toenail deformity and the potentially suboptimal fingernail outcome. In selecting a donor site for composite grafts, we prefer to use the second toe because it is usually approximately the width of the fingernail. A toenail is not as long as a fingernail, however, and a split-thickness sterile matrix graft from another toe needs to be placed distal to the composite graft to lengthen the attachment area. The large toenail or a portion of it is necessary for thumbnail reconstruction with composite grafts.

The most reliable treatment to produce a growing nail is a free microvascular transfer of the dorsal tip of the toe, including the nail bed (Figure 9.18).[34,71,72,92,98] This procedure requires very skilled microvascular technique, has some risk of failure, and leaves significant scars on the foot, toe, and finger. Nakayama[75] and Iwasawa and coworkers[50] described microsurgical transfers of small toenail flaps that result in less donor and defect site

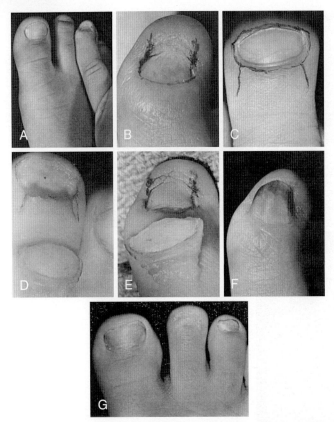

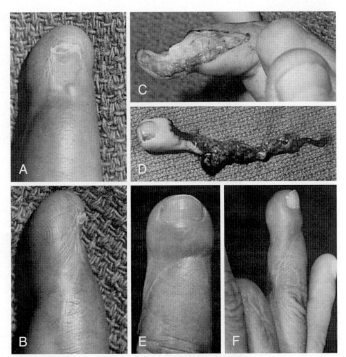

FIGURE 9.18 A and **B,** Minimal nail growth and soft tissue loss after oblique amputation of ring fingertip. **C,** Defect after excision of the scarred nail bed and tip. **D,** Partial second toe free flap. **E** and **F,** Postoperative appearance of ring finger.

FIGURE 9.17 A, A 7-year-old child with posttraumatic absence of the index nail; the width of the fingernail is compared with that of the second toenail. **B,** Nail bed is seen close-up at the time of surgery. **C,** Second toe is marked for removal of the composite nail and nail bed graft. **D,** Composite graft is excised. **E,** Composite graft is placed on the dorsum of the finger after the nail fold has been created. The toenail does not have as much length as a normal fingernail. The sterile matrix was advanced distally to create a recipient site for the graft. **F,** Nail 1 year postoperatively. **G,** Postoperative view of second toe. A split-thickness skin graft was applied to the periosteum.

morbidity than the larger wraparound flaps. Nakayama[75] successfully transferred a venous flap based on the venous system only, and Iwasawa and coworkers[50] reported a case of a venous flap anastomosed to a digital artery and vein. Nail flaps with short vascular pedicles have been reported for decreased scarring owing to less dissection at both sites, but these require expert microsurgical skill because of the small size of the vessels.[27,32,33,61]

Nail Spikes, Cysts, and Cornified Nail Bed

Nail cysts most commonly occur from failure to remove the entire germinal matrix from the nail fold during revision amputation. The skin is closed over the germinal matrix, producing a cyst wall, which continuously produces nail. They manifest as painful, enlarging masses at the site of the previous nail fold. Treatment consists of complete resection of the nail cyst and wall (Figure 9.19).

Nail spikes also result from incomplete removal of the germinal matrix. They are unenclosed and produce nail, which grows distally. They are a frequent occurrence after removal of the side of the nail and nail bed for an ingrown toenail. Treatment is complete removal of the spike and the residual germinal matrix.

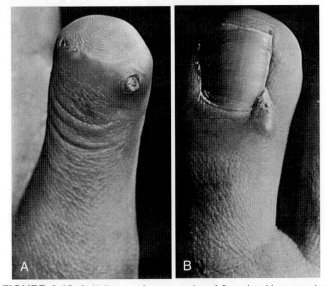

FIGURE 9.19 A, Nail cysts after amputation of fingertip without complete removal of the nail bed. **B,** Nail spike resulting from incomplete removal of nail bed after resection of an ingrown toenail.

A cornified nail bed occurs in patients whose germinal matrix has been removed to eliminate nail growth, but the sterile matrix has been left intact. The nail bed does not produce nail, but the sterile matrix continues to produce the keratinizing material, which in a normal nail bed maintains nail adherence. To relieve this, the sterile matrix is excised, and a split-thickness skin graft is applied.

Eponychial Deformities

Traumatic loss of the eponychium exposes the proximal nail and leads to loss of the nail shine, which is produced by the dorsal roof of the nail fold. This is commonly an aesthetic defect only because there is no abnormality in actual nail growth. Notching of the eponychium is often a primarily aesthetic concern, but can be functional if the free edge is frequently caught on objects. Notching is usually secondary to loss of part of the eponychium or failure to repair an eponychial laceration.

Scarring of the eponychium and nail fold to the nail bed, also known as pterygium, leads to functional and aesthetic deformities, such as absence of nail growth and splitting of the nail. This webbing between the eponychium and the nail bed most commonly occurs secondary to trauma, but has also been associated with ischemia and collagen vascular diseases. In trauma, scarring is minimized with precise repair of the nail bed within the fold and separation of the dorsal and ventral layers of the nail fold during healing, as previously mentioned. Scarring remains a possible complication, however. Absence or splitting of the nail occurs with scarring of the eponychium to the germinal matrix. The nail is unable to grow in the area of scar, leading to absence, or the nail grows around the scar, leading to splitting.

For a persistent pterygium of the eponychium, we recommend freeing the dorsal roof of the nail fold from the nail and inserting a small piece of silicone sheet into the nail fold with a horizontal mattress suture. The undersurface of the nail fold epithelializes preventing readherence. If this procedure is unsuccessful, it may be necessary to separate the dorsal roof from the nail and to place a thin split-thickness sterile matrix graft on the undersurface of the eponychium to prevent the adherence.[89] The nail bed must also be examined for scarring, especially in patients with absence of nail growth.

An eponychial defect may be reconstructed by a composite toe eponychial graft,[66] the helical rim of the ear,[82] or rotation flaps.[1] We recommend use of a composite eponychial graft from an appropriate toe to replace missing eponychium. A template of the eponychial defect is used to plan the composite graft of eponychium and underlying dorsal roof. With this graft, there is only a small area of raw surface on the proximal end for revascularization. To improve the chance of graft take, we harvest a larger area of dorsal skin with the graft that corresponds to a deepithelialized area on the finger, which lies just proximal to the defect. This leaves a slightly larger area on the toe that is left to heal secondarily. The resultant toe deformity has been minimal.

Eponychial deformities from burn injury result in contracture of soft tissue proximal to the eponychium. Donelan and Garcia have found a reliable treatment for this proximal retraction of the eponychium with a distally based bipedicle flap which unfurls the nail fold advancing the eponychium distally and replacing the resultant soft tissue defect with a skin graft.[30]

Hyponychial Deformities

Pterygia can also occur within the hyponychium secondary to trauma. Other sources of scarring within the hyponychium include denervation and ischemia. The tip of the finger may become painful and tender. We recommend removal of the

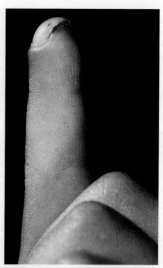

FIGURE 9.20 Hooked-nail deformity caused partially by loss of distal bony support but primarily from the nail bed being pulled over the tip to close the amputation.

distal 5 mm of nail from the nail bed and hyponychial area. A narrow strip of nail bed and hyponychium, 3 to 4 mm wide, is resected and replaced by a split-thickness skin graft. This procedure causes nonadherence in the hyponychial area and usually provides relief of pain.

Hooking of the nail occurs with tight closure of a fingertip amputation or loss of bony support under the nail bed, which leads to curving of the matrix in a volar direction (Figure 9.20). Because the growing nail follows the nail matrix, any alteration in the support of the distal finger would alter the direction of nail growth. To avoid this alteration in nail growth, the nail should not be pulled over the distal phalanx. Acutely, when the distal bone is absent, it must be replaced, or the nail bed must be trimmed back to the end of the bone so the nail bed does not curve over the end.

After a hooked nail has developed, a decision must be made whether to shorten the bone or attempt to add support to the nail bed. If the distal nail bed had been pulled over the end of the finger, a "V-Y" advancement flap, cross-finger flap, or full-thickness skin graft can be used to replace the soft tissue for the tip and allow replacement of the nail bed onto the dorsum of the bone.[63] This procedure usually improves the hook, although complete correction is uncommon. Correction of a hooked nail with maintenance of nail length requires replacement of the distal phalanx or tuft with a bone graft. Additional tip soft tissue before or at the time of bone grafting may be required. Initially, bone grafts support the nail bed satisfactorily, but as with most bone grafts that do not have bone apposition on both ends, in time they tend to resorb, and the correction is lost. A free vascularized transfer of second toe tip, including the distal phalanx and nail, is the best, although most complex, solution.[60] A prosthesis, rather than reconstruction, is a simple solution that may give very satisfactory results.[13]

Hyponychial nonadherence occurs with loss of the hyponychial barrier from exposure of the fingertips to acids or alkali or chronic exposure to liquid. Without the barrier, fungus, bacteria, and dirt have direct access to the subungual space, causing nonadherence of the nail. If removing the cause does not result

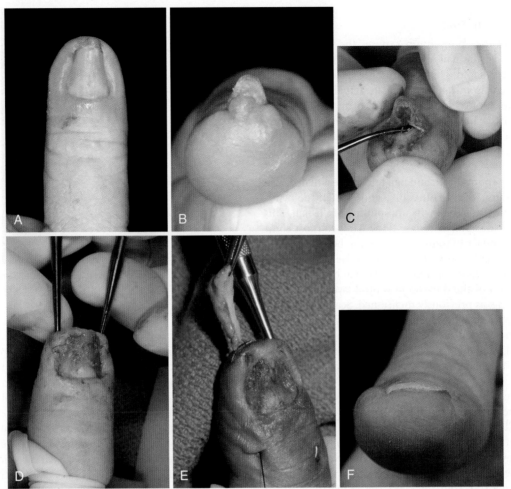

FIGURE 9.21 **A** and **B,** Pincer nail deformity with tubing of nail. **C,** Removal of nail. **D,** Elevation of sides of nail bed from underlying distal phalanx. **E,** Placement of dermal graft into created tunnel. **F,** Improvement of pincer nail 1 year after surgery.

in readherence, it is usually secondary to the presence of keratinous material. The nail is removed to a point just proximal to the nonadherence and the keratin is scraped from the nail bed to allow for adherence as the nail grows distally. The nail may need to be scraped multiple times as the nail grows to the desired length.

Dull Nail

A dull nail is another minor complication that is cosmetic in nature. The dorsal roof of the nail fold is responsible for the shiny surface to the nail. Scar within the dorsal roof may lead to a dull streak within the nail.[103] No treatment is necessary as long as there are no associated functional problems.

PINCER NAIL

Although the pincer or trumpet nail deformity has been attributed to several causes, the exact etiology of this deformity is uncertain. It consists of excess transverse curvature of the nail and progressive pinching off of the soft tissue of the distal fingertip with resultant pain and an unaesthetic deformity. Although partial or complete nail ablation may provide symptomatic relief, various nail-preserving methods have been

reported. Kosaka and Kamiishi[59] showed satisfactory success in treatment of severe pincer deformity with a contracted hyponychium. This method involves a fish-mouth incision near the nail margin, elevation of the nail bed, flattening of the distal phalanx dorsal surface, widening of the contracted hyponychium, and a "W"-plasty type of closure between the distal nail bed flap and hyponychium. Our preferred treatment consists of nail plate removal, elevation of the sides of the nail bed from the distal phalanx, and placement of autogenous dermal grafts[21] or AlloDerm under the lateral portions of the nail bed, between the nail bed and periosteum (Figure 9.21).[105]

ACUTE INFECTIONS

Fungal Infections

Perionychial infections of the subungual area are the most common infections in the hand. These are most frequently onychomycosis or chronic fungal infections (although superimposed bacterial infections may occur) and are usually treated medically by primary care physicians or dermatologists.[10] Treatment usually starts with topical therapy with nail lacquer placed over the nail. Systemic treatments are started if this is unsuccessful after 6 months. Options include terbinafine (250 mg/day

CRITICAL POINTS *Pincer Nail Treatment*

Indications
- Painful nail
- Disfigured nail

Technical Points
- Use a digital block and apply a tourniquet to finger.
- Remove the nail with an elevator or curved iris scissors.
- Perform stab incisions to the radial and ulnar hyponychium.
- Place a Kleinert-Kutz elevator into stab incisions.
- Carefully elevate the nail bed from the underlying periosteum.
- Harvest dermal graft or prepare AlloDerm.
- Cut graft or AlloDerm to length and tube.
- Perform a stab incision to the ulnar and radial proximal eponychium.
- Pass the dull end of a Keith needle proximal to distal beneath the nail bed, leaving the needle within the wound.
- Thread 5-0 nylon suture through the end of graft or AlloDerm.
- Thread suture into the Keith needle.
- Pull the needle proximally to pull the graft or AlloDerm into the space beneath the nail bed.
- Close stab incisions with superficial stitches.

Pitfall
- Tearing the radial or ulnar paronychium on nail bed elevation may occur.

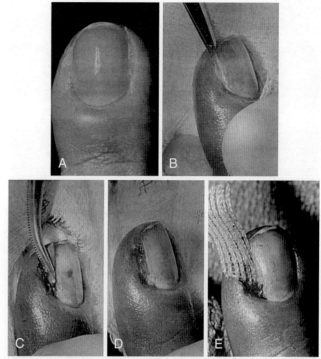

FIGURE 9.22 A, Paronychia is seen on the left side of this nail, with pus extending beneath the nail. **B,** Fine pair of iris scissors is used to elevate the side of the nail from the nail bed and the eponychium from the dorsum of the nail. **C,** Loosened fragment of nail is split longitudinally and removed from nail fold. **D,** Adequate drainage is performed after partial removal of the nail. **E,** Small wick of gauze is used to promote drainage.

for 6 weeks for fingernails and 12 weeks for toenails), itraconazole (200 mg twice a day for 1 week every month for 2 months for fingernails and 200 mg once daily for 12 weeks for toenails), or fluconazole (150 to 300 mg once a week for 3 to 6 months for fingernails and 6 to 12 months for toenails). Surgical intervention is required in 25% of patients who do not respond to systemic treatment.[10]

We most commonly see patients after these first lines of treatment have been unsuccessful. At this point, we recommend removal of the nail and application of 4% Mycolog-nystatin, triamcinolone acetonide cream twice a day to the nail bed until the nail has completely regrown. This approach allows for exposure of the subungual fungal infection and, if needed, debulking of the onychomycosis for improved penetration. Occasionally, we have performed total ablation of the nail for recurrent or persistent fungal infections.[103]

Recently, gentian violet solution has been found to be successful in treatment of chronic fungal infections without the need for removal of the nail (verbal correspondence, Wyndell Merritt, MD). This age-old drug has reemerged in the field of dermatology as well as a potentially simple option for a difficult problem.[68]

Bacterial Infections

Bacterial infections of the nail most commonly involve the paronychium. The dermal and epidermal layers of the paronychium are arranged in an overlapping fashion, similar to the shingles of a house. When one of these layers is pulled up, an open wound (hangnail) is created. Subsequent infection produces a paronychia. *Staphylococcus aureus* is the most frequent organism isolated.[69]

If the infection involves the paronychium, but is above the nail, it can be drained by lifting the paronychium away from the nail, followed by soaks to encourage adequate drainage. If the infection and purulence have progressed beneath the edge

of the nail, a portion of the nail must be removed to permit drainage (Figure 9.22). Local anesthesia is used, but commonly does not bring complete anesthesia because of the underlying infection. If a tourniquet is to be used for hemostasis, the finger should not be exsanguinated to avoid proximal spread of infection. The nail is dissected from the underlying nail bed and the overlying proximal eponychium with fine scissors or a periosteal elevator. The nail is split longitudinally, and the undermined portion is removed to allow drainage. Adequate open drainage is maintained by soaking the digit in warm soapy water three to four times per day. Antibiotics are indicated if tissue cellulitis is present. If the abscess dissects beneath the dorsal roof of the nail fold or beneath the nail in the nail fold, the proximal portion of the nail must be removed. The distal portion of the nail may be left in place to decrease discomfort. Incisions should not be made in the eponychium to drain the infection. Such incisions frequently do not heal primarily in the presence of infection, and a notch or square corner in the eponychium may result. We have never seen a paronychia or abscess that required incision in the eponychium for adequate drainage.

CHRONIC INFECTIONS

Chronic paronychia usually occurs between the nail and the dorsal roof of the nail fold and results in a tender, erythematous, and swollen fingertip. The infection is most commonly caused by gram-negative organisms and fungus, primarily *Candida*.[9] They are often seen in diabetic patients, immunocompromised patients, and patients whose jobs involve frequent hand soaking

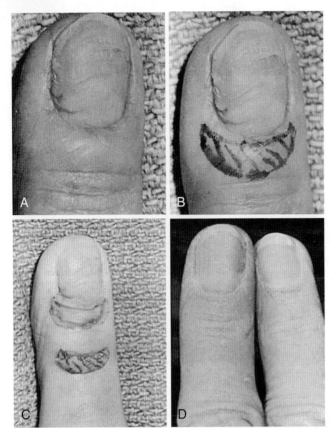

FIGURE 9.23 A, Chronic paronychia that has been present for 2 years. **B,** Area on the dorsal roof is marked for excision. **C,** Dorsal roof of nail fold has been removed down to the nail. **D,** Appearance 1 year after injury with no further infection.

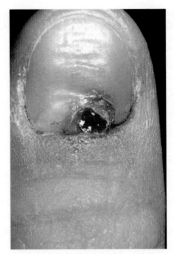

FIGURE 9.24 Pyogenic granuloma growing through the nail after perforation of nail with cuticle scissors.

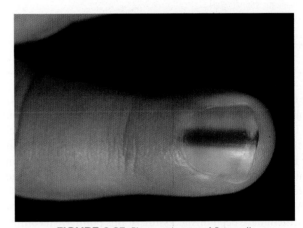

FIGURE 9.25 Pigmented nevus of fingernail.

in water. Treatment involves topical or oral antifungal agents and preventive measures such as avoidance of moisture, trauma from cuticle treatments, and irritants such as citrus fruits and cosmetic nail products.[100] For resistant cases, treatment is a Keyser-Eaton marsupialization of the nail fold.[1,14,54,55] A 3- to 4-mm–wide crescent is excised from the proximal nail fold, preserving the cuticle. The skin and dorsal roof of the nail fold are excised down to the nail, taking care not to injure the germinal matrix (Figure 9.23). The wound is allowed to heal secondarily. We have found this treatment generally successful (see Chapter 3).

TUMORS OF THE PERIONYCHIUM

Benign Tumors

Pyogenic Granuloma

Pyogenic granulomas manifest as rapidly growing lesions with a round, red, elevated area similar to granulation tissue, growing through the nail. They are usually the result of perforations of the nail by trauma or iatrogenic causes (Figure 9.24). The most common treatment is repeated silver nitrate cauterization, which may result in some nail deformity. Excision is also an option, but is likely to require a nail bed graft for closure. Differential diagnosis for these lesions includes squamous cell carcinoma and amelanotic melanoma. If the lesion is persistent or recurrent after cauterization, biopsy is needed.

Subungual Nevi

Nevi of the nail bed are common. The nail produced by a nail bed with a pigmented nevus is also pigmented because the nevus cells are added to the nail as it grows distally (Figure 9.25). Roughening of the nail surface usually does not occur, but elevation and ridging of the nail may. A nevus is frequently present at birth and first noticed in childhood. As years pass, it may become lighter or darker.

In the past, nevi of the nail bed were commonly observed owing to the potential deformity of the nail on nail bed biopsy. Because of a greater potential for malignant degeneration within the nail bed, we generally recommend incisional biopsy of the nevi. Watching the nevi for changes and delaying the biopsy until the child is older is also a reasonable option. We discuss the options with the patient and parents. On biopsy, if atypical cells are present, the involved portion of the nail bed is removed, and the nail bed is reconstructed as needed.[37]

It is important to remember the other causes of subungual pigmentation, including melanonychia striata and hematoma. Melanonychiae are benign longitudinal bands of pigmentation most often seen in African Americans and are usually present on multiple nails. They can be difficult to diagnose; Glat and colleagues[40] recommend biopsy in whites with any longitudinal

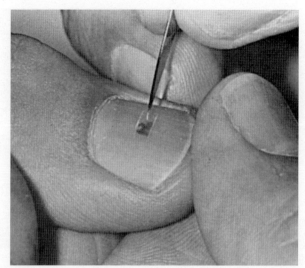

FIGURE 9.26 Marking the nail over a pigmented area to monitor pigment growth in relation to nail growth (see text Subungual Nevi in text).

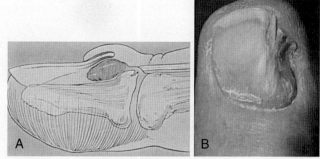

FIGURE 9.27 A, Dissection of a ganglion between the periosteum of the distal phalanx and the nail bed. **B,** Typical (but extreme) longitudinal groove deformity that results when the ganglion is located as shown in **A**.

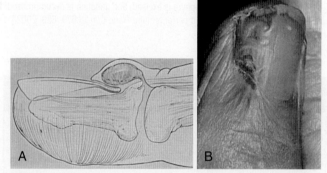

FIGURE 9.28 A, Dissection of ganglion into the dorsal roof of the nail fold compresses the nail bed volarly. **B,** Irregular breakup of the nail (or a longitudinal groove) is the deformity frequently caused by a ganglion.

pigmented band and in African Americans if only one digit is involved. A subungual hematoma is the most common cause of subungual pigmentation in an adult, even when there is no history of trauma. These areas of pigmentation should be monitored closely for resolution. We make a scratch into the surface of the nail at the proximal and distal borders of the pigmented area (Figure 9.26) and monitor the pigment in relation to the scratches for approximately 3 weeks. If the pigment is from a hematoma, it progresses toward the free edge of the nail with the scratches. If the pigment is nevus or melanoma in the nail bed, the scratches progress distally away from the area of pigmentation, necessitating a biopsy.

Verruca Vulgaris

Hand surgeons usually see patients with verruca vulgaris (viral warts) of the perionychium after they have been treated by their primary physician or dermatologist. We recommend laser therapy for patients with persistent warts. The keratin outer layer is shaved off to allow better penetration, and a pulsed dye laser is used to target the vessels within the wart. To avoid injury to the nail bed, laser treatment should remain superficial. Multiple treatments may be necessary. Our estimated success with this has been upwards of 75% resolution. Schellhaas and colleagues have seen a remission of 89% with the pulsed dye laser treatment, with only 4% failure.[87]

We also see patients with nail deformity that occurred from treatment of the wart. The resulting scar tissue in the nail bed prevents return of normal nail growth. Reconstruction consists of surgical excision of the nail bed scar and nail bed grafting, usually from the toes, as previously discussed.

Ganglion

Ganglions of the DIP joint, incorrectly known as mucous cysts, are the most common tumors that deform the nail bed. Kleinert and coworkers[58] reported a communication between these cysts and the DIP joint in the area of an arthritic spur (osteophyte). When the cystic expansion of the ganglion is between the floor of the nail and the periosteum, upward pressure on the nail bed causes a ridged, curved, or ragged nail (Figure 9.27). If the cyst

lies dorsal to the nail bed within the nail fold, the pressure is downward on the nail, causing grooving, thinning, or roughening of the nail (Figure 9.28).

If there is severe nail deformity, we believe that the best treatment is removal of the nail followed by débridement of the DIP osteophytes and drainage of the cyst through a "T"-shaped incision over the joint (Figure 9.29). A piece of 0.020-inch silicone sheet is placed into the nail fold to help mold the nail bed back into its normal position. For minor grooves or flattening, removal of the deformed nail is unnecessary. In our early experience, débridement of the osteophytes and removal of the cyst wall resulted in a residual minor nail deformity in 36% of cases.[19] Our more recent experience with only débridement of the osteophytes and drainage of the cyst through the incision resulted in minor nail deformity in 10% with no recurrence of the cyst.[38] We believe that osteophyte débridement is the key to preventing recurrence. Removal of the cyst wall is unnecessary and increases the risk of nail deformity owing to possible nail bed damage.

Ganglions occasionally rupture and drain through the nail fold of the overlying skin. If infection occurs, permanent nail deformity and limitation of joint motion may result. If the ganglion ruptures, the appropriate treatment is antibiotics until the skin is closed, followed by surgical removal of the osteophyte before the ganglion ruptures again. A ganglion should not be surgically treated while it is actively draining because of an increased risk of subsequent infection and deformity.

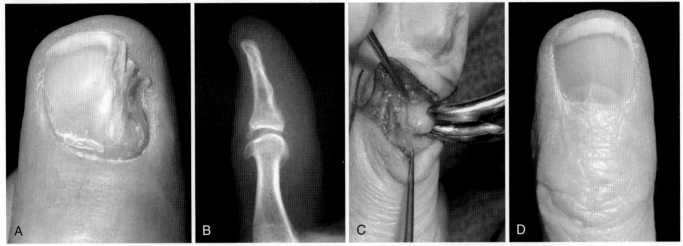

FIGURE 9.29 **A,** Distal interphalangeal (DIP) joint ganglion causing nail deformity. **B,** Radiographic evidence of osteophytes of DIP joint. **C,** Offending osteophyte is excised, and ganglion is decompressed. **D,** Normal nail growth at 1-year follow-up. (From Sommer N, Neumeister MW: Tumors of the perionychium. *Hand Clin* 18:673–689, 2002.)

CRITICAL POINTS *Treatment of Distal Interphalangeal Joint Ganglion*

Indications
- Pain
- Recurrent ganglion rupture or infection
- Significant nail deformity

Pearls
- Nail deformity resolves with removal of osteophyte and ganglion drainage.
- Chance of nail deformity is decreased with drainage rather than excision of ganglion.
- Infection of draining cyst must be resolved before definitive treatment.

Technical Points
- Use a "T"-shaped or "H"-shaped incision over dorsal DIP joint.
- Elevate and retract the extensor tendon without disrupting the insertion.
- Identify and drain the ganglion.
- Excise the osteophyte with a small rongeur.
- Irrigate the joint and wound with normal saline.
- Use superficial interrupted closure of skin.
- Apply a volar DIP joint digital splint for comfort.

Pitfalls
- Extensor lag may develop with extensor tendon elevation that is too aggressive.
- Patients must be willing to accept a lengthy recovery with a painful joint and swollen finger.
- Healing difficulties may occur at the "T" junction.

Postoperative Care
- Use a splint for 1 week if there is only minimal traction of the extensor tendon.
- Use a splint for 3 to 4 weeks if the extensor tendon is attenuated during retraction.
- Begin active range-of-motion exercises after the splint is removed.

Glomus Tumor

A glomus tumor arises from the glomus body that regulates blood flow and temperature in the finger.[11] Although not limited to the nail bed, 50% occur subungually. Proliferation of this angiomatous tissue within the confined space of the nail bed results in exquisite pain. On presentation, the patient may have a bluish discoloration beneath the nail. The nail may be exquisitely tender to pressure and sensitive to temperature changes, especially cold. An ice cube held over the nail bed may reproduce the pain. Ultrasound[24] and magnetic resonance imaging (MRI)[31] have been reported as highly successful in identifying subungual glomus tumors.

Treatment consists of removal of the nail, identification of the glomus tumor or tumors, and surgical excision. The entire nail bed should be carefully examined for multiple tumors after the nail is removed. A longitudinal incision is made over the glomus tumor, and the tumor is dissected out from the surrounding tissue. The tumor frequently "shells out," similar to a lipoma (Figure 9.30); this allows primary closure of the nail bed incision. Alternatively, the nail bed may be raised up as a flap from distal to proximal to provide exposure for tumor excision.

Malignant Tumors

Basal cell carcinoma is rare in the hand and even more so in the finger. Only 11 cases have been reported.[56] Basal cell carcinoma most frequently occurs after radiation exposure or other chronic trauma or exposure. Arsenic exposure is also thought to be a risk factor.[56] Complete resection of the tumor with frozen section examination of the margins is recommended to ensure complete removal. If the distal phalanx is involved, amputation at the DIP joint level is recommended. Repair consists of nail reconstruction with a split-thickness nail bed graft or skin graft closure.

Squamous cell carcinomas, although uncommon, are the most common malignant tumor of the perionychium[51] and can be secondary to radiation exposure (Figure 9.31).[2,23,67] In the past, dentists' hands were commonly affected, owing to chronic

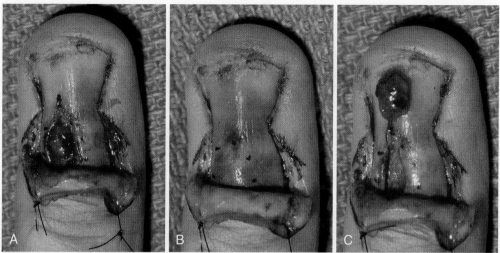

FIGURE 9.30 **A,** Perpendicular incisions at the eponychium expose a glomus tumor at the junction of the germinal and sterile matrices. **B,** Approach is through a longitudinal incision in the nail bed. **C,** Appearance after excision.

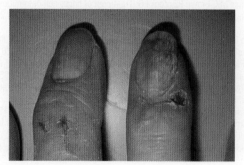

FIGURE 9.31 A veterinarian with many years of radiation exposure to his fingers contracted squamous cell carcinoma of the perionychium.

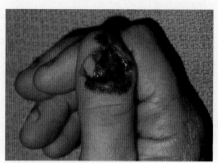

FIGURE 9.32 Malignant melanoma of the nail bed.

radiation exposure; this became much less common with the knowledge of radiation-induced tumor formation. Other predisposing factors include repeated trauma, infection, arsenic exposure, or presence of human papillomavirus.[23,74,86] In a retrospective review at the Cleveland Clinic of 12 patients in 10 years with squamous cell carcinoma of the nail, only two causes were clearly defined: human papillomavirus and radiation.[43]

Squamous cell carcinomas may manifest as a raised, red, sometimes ulcerated, bleeding lesion or as a simple nail deformity. They are slow growing and are frequently misdiagnosed as paronychia. Carroll[23] showed that the average length of time between appearance and treatment was 4 years. This tumor is seen more commonly in men and usually involves the thumb. A lesion without bony involvement requires resection of the entire lesion with adequate margins, frequently requiring a nail bed or skin graft. If the carcinoma has been present for a long time, is large, or involves the bone, amputation at the DIP joint or even more proximally is indicated. Node dissection is indicated only if the nodes do not disappear after amputation because most nodal enlargements are inflammatory.

Melanomas of the hands and feet have a poorer prognosis than melanomas elsewhere on the body.[28] They are almost always pigmented and may or may not have nail deformity (Figure 9.32). Fungal infection, paronychia, warts, pyogenic granuloma, foreign bodies, subungual hematoma, and melanonychiae striata may mimic a melanoma of the perionychium.

Consequently, the diagnosis is often missed initially and delayed 2 to 3 years.[62,70]

Any pigmented lesion that does not advance with nail growth, such as the case with subungual hematoma, should raise suspicion. If the lesion has not changed in 4 to 6 weeks, biopsy with permanent pathologic examination is recommended.[17] Margins of excision are based on thickness of the skin melanoma, but thickness is difficult to determine in cases of subungual melanoma.[36] We recommend complete excision with clear margins for lesions with dysplasia or atypia. Melanoma in situ requires excision with 5-mm margins. For invasive melanoma, early studies recommended metacarpal ray amputation for stage I (local) disease.[16,42] More recent recommendations include more conservative amputation[36] at the proximal interphalangeal joint[49] or at the joint just proximal to the nail bed melanoma[41] with preservation of as much function as possible.[77]

Evaluation for metastatic disease should include physical examination of the regional lymph nodes, a chest radiograph, and liver function tests. Opinions have varied regarding the advisability and timing of lymph node dissections in subungual melanoma. As in other areas of the body, elective lymph node dissection in the absence of palpable nodes is controversial and is still being evaluated, whereas therapeutic lymph node dissection is indicated for palpable nodes. Glat and colleagues[40] recommended lymph node dissection for lesions greater than

1 mm in thickness, which is in line with the recommendation for intermediate cutaneous melanomas (1 to 4 mm). The use of sentinel node biopsies has shown promising results for the detection of lymph node metastases, while potentially preventing unnecessary nodal dissections. With a negative sentinel node, the chance of regional lymph node metastasis was found to be less than 1%.[8]

Survival rates for subungual melanomas are varied. Park and colleagues[80] found a poorer 5-year survival for subungual melanomas (41%) versus cutaneous melanomas (72%). Klausner and coworkers[57] reported 5-year survival rates of 28% to 30% and 10-year survival rates of 0% to 13%.

REFERENCES

1. Achauer BM, Welk RA: One stage reconstruction of the postburn nailfold contracture. *Plast Reconstr Surg* 85:937–940, 1990.
2. Alport LI, Zak FG, Werthamer S: Subungual basal cell epithelioma. *Arch Dermatol* 106:599, 1972.
3. Antony AK, Anagnos DP: Matrix-periosteal flaps for reconstruction of nail deformity. *Plast Reconstr Surg* 109:1663–1666, 2002.
4. Ashbell TS, Kleinert HE, Putcha SM, et al: The deformed fingernail, a frequent result of failure to repair nail bed injuries. *J Trauma* 7:177–190, 1967.
5. Atasoy E, Iokamidis E, Kasdan ML, et al: Reconstruction of the amputated fingertip with a triangular volar flap: a new surgical procedure. *J Bone Joint Surg Am* 52:921–926, 1970.
6. Baden HP: Regeneration of the nail. *Arch Dermatol* 91:619–620, 1965.
7. Bakhach J, Demiri E, Guimerteau JC: Use of the eponychial flap to restore the length of a short nail: a review of 30 cases. *Plast Reconstr Surg* 116:478–483, 2005.
8. Balch CM: The role of elective lymph node dissection in melanoma: rationale, results and controversies. *J Clin Oncol* 6:163–169, 1988.
9. Baran R: Onychia and paronychia of mycotic, microbial and parasite origin. In Pierre M, editor: *The nail, GEM monograph series*, vol 5, New York, 1981, Churchill Livingstone.
10. Baran R: Nail fungal infections and treatment. *Hand Clin* 18:625–628, 2002.
11. Barre JA, Masson PV: Anatomy—clinical study of certain painful subungual tumors (tumors of the neuromyoarterial glomus of the extremities). *Bull Soc Fr Dermatol Syph* 31:148, 1924.
12. Barron JN: The structure and function of the skin of the hand. *Hand* 2:93–96, 1970.
12a. Baruchin AM, Nahlieli O, Vizethum F, et al: Harnessing the osseointegration principle for anchorage of fingernail prosthesis. *Hand Clinic* 18(4):647–654, 2002.
13. Beasley RW, deBeze GM: Prosthetic substitution for fingernails. *Hand Clin* 6:105–111, 1990.
14. Bednar MS, Lane LB: Eponychial marsupialization and nail removal for surgical treatment of chronic paronychia. *J Hand Surg [Am]* 16:314–317, 1991.
15. Bindra RR: Management of nail bed fracture-lacerations using a tension-band suture. *J Hand Surg [Br]* 21:1111–1113, 1996.
16. Booher RJ, Pack GT: Malignant melanoma of the feet and hands. *Surgery* 42:1084–1121, 1957.
17. Briggs JC: Subungual melanoma: a clinico-pathological study of 24 cases. *Br J Plast Surg* 38:174–176, 1985.
18. Brown RE: Acute nail bed injuries. *Hand Clin* 18:561–575, 2002.
19. Brown RE, Zook EG, Russell RC, et al: Fingernail deformities secondary to ganglions of the distal interphalangeal joint (mucous cysts). *Plast Reconstr Surg* 87:718–725, 1991.
20. Brown RE, Zook EG, Russell RC: Reconstruction of fingertips with combination of local flaps and nail bed grafts. *J Hand Surg [Am]* 24:345–351, 1999.
21. Brown RE, Zook EG, Williams J: Correction of pincer-nail deformities using dermal grafting. *Plast Reconstr Surg* 105:1658–1661, 2000.
22. Buncke HJ, Jr, Gonzalez RI: Fingernail reconstruction. *Plast Reconstr Surg* 30:452–461, 1962.
23. Carroll RE: Squamous cell carcinoma of the nail bed. *J Hand Surg* 1:92–97, 1976.
24. Chen SH, Chen Y, Cheng M, et al: The use of ultrasonography in preoperative localization of digital glomus tumors. *Plast Reconstr Surg* 112:115–120, 2003.
25. Chowdhry S, Seidenstricker L, Cooney DS, et al: Do not use epinephrine in digital blocks: myth or truth? Part II. A retrospective review of 1111 cases. *Plast Reconstr Surg* 126:2031–2034, 2010.
26. Clark WE, Buxton LHD: Studies in nail growth. *Br J Dermatol* 50:221–235, 1938.
27. Dautel G, Corcella D, Merle M: Reconstruction of fingertip amputations by partial composite toe transfer with short vascular pedicle. *J Hand Surg [Br]* 4:457–464, 1998.
28. Day CL, Jr, Lew RA, Mihm MC, Jr, et al: A multivariate analysis of prognostic factors for melanoma patients with lesions greater than or equal to 3.65 millimeters in thickness. *Ann Surg* 195:44–49, 1982.
29. DeBerker D, Mawhinney B, Sviland L: Quantification of regional matrix nail production. *Br J Dermatol* 134:1083–1086, 1996.
30. Donelan MB, Garcia JA: Nailfold reconstruction for correction of burn fingernail deformity. *Plast Reconstr Surg* 117:2303–2308, 2006.
31. Drape JL, Idy-Peretti I, Goettmann S, et al: Subungual glomus tumors: evaluation with MR imaging. *Radiology* 195:507–515, 1995.
32. Endo T, Nakayama Y: Short pedicle vascularized nail flap. *Plast Reconstr Surg* 97:656–661, 1996.
33. Endo T, Nakayama Y: Microtransfers for nail and fingertip replacement. *Hand Clin* 18:615–622, 2002.
34. Endo T, Nakayama Y, Soeda S: Nail transfer: evolution of the reconstructive procedure. *Plast Reconstr Surg* 100:907–913, 1997.
35. Fakin RM, Biraima A, Klein H, et al: Primary functional and aesthetic restoration of the fingernail in distal fingertip amputations with the eponychial flap. *J Hand Surg Eur Vol* 39(5):499–504, 2014.
36. Finley RK, Driscoll DL, Blumenson LE, et al: Subungual melanoma: an eighteen year review. *Surgery* 116:96–100, 1994.
37. Fleegler EJ, Zeinowicz RJ: Tumors of the perionychium. *Hand Clin* 6:113–136, 1990.
38. Gingrass MK, Brown RE, Zook EG: Treatment of finger nail deformities secondary to ganglions of the distal interphalangeal joint. *J Hand Surg [Am]* 20:502–505, 1995.
39. Gharb BB, Rampazzo A, Armijo BS, et al: Tranquilli-Leali or Atasoy flap: an anatomical cadaveric study. *J Plast Reconstr Aesth Surg* 63:681–685, 2010.
40. Glat PM, Shapiro RL, Roses DF, et al: Management considerations for melanonychia striata and melanoma of the hand. *Hand Clin* 2:183–189, 1995.
41. Glat PM, Spector JA, Roses DF, et al: The management of pigmented lesions of the nail bed. *Ann Plast Surg* 37:125–134, 1996.
42. Goldsmith HS: Melanoma: an overview. *CA Cancer J Clin* 29:194–215, 1979.
43. Guitart J, Bergfeld WA, Tuthill RJ, et al: Squamous cell carcinoma of the nail bed: a clinicopathological study of 12 cases. *Br J Dermatol* 123:215–222, 1990.
44. Guy RJ: The etiologies and mechanisms of the nail bed injuries. *Hand Clin* 6:9–21, 1990.
45. Hallock GG, Lutz DA: Octyl-2-cyanoacrylate adhesive for rapid nail plate restoration. *J Hand Surg [Am]* 25:979–981, 2000.
46. Hanraham EM: The split-thickness skin graft as a covering following removal of a fingernail. *Surgery* 20:398–400, 1946.
47. Hasegawa K, Pereira BP, Pho R: The microvasculature of the nail bed, nail matrix, and nail fold of a normal human fingertip. *J Hand Surg [Am]* 26:283–290, 2001.
48. Hashimoto H: Experimental study of histogenesis for the nail and its surrounding tissue. *Niigate Med J* 82:254, 1971.
49. Heaton KM, el-Naggar A, Ensign LG, et al: Surgical management and prognostic factors in patients with subungual melanoma. *Ann Surg* 219:197–204, 1994.
50. Iwasawa M, Furuta S, Noguchi M, et al: Reconstruction of fingertip deformities of the thumb using a venous flap. *Ann Plast Surg* 28:187–189, 1992.
51. John HG: Primary skin cancer of the fingers stimulating chronic infection. *Lancet* 1:662, 1956.
52. Johnson RK: Nailplasty. *Plast Reconstr Surg* 47:275, 1971.
53. Johnson M, Shuster S: Continuous formation of nail along the bed. *Br J Dermatol* 128:277–280, 1993.
54. Keyser JJ, Eaton RG: Surgical care of chronic paronychia by eponychial marsupialization. *Plast Reconstr Surg* 58:66–70, 1976.
55. Keyser JJ, Littler JW, Eaton RG: Surgical treatment of infections and lesions of the perionychium. *Hand Clin* 6:137–157, 1990.
56. Kim H, Kim Y, Suhr K, et al: Basal cell carcinoma of the nail bed in a Korean woman. *Int J Dermatol* 39:397–398, 2000.
57. Klausner JM, Inbar M, Gutman M, et al: Nail-bed melanoma. *J Surg Oncol* 34:208–210, 1987.
58. Kleinert HE, Kutz JE, Fishman JH, et al: Etiology and treatment of the so-called mucous cyst of the finger. *J Bone Joint Surg* 54:1455–1458, 1972.
59. Kosaka M, Kamiishi H: New strategy for the treatment and assessment of pincer nail. *Plast Reconstr Surg* 111:2014–2019, 2003.
60. Koshima I, Moriguchi T, Umeda N, et al: Trimmed second toetip transfer for reconstruction of claw nail deformity of the fingers. *Br J Plast Surg* 45:591–594, 1992.
61. Koshima I, Soeda S, Takase T, et al: Free vascularized nail grafts. *J Hand Surg [Am]* 13:29–32, 1988.
62. Krige JE, Hudson DA, Johnson CS, et al: Subungual melanoma. *S Afr J Surg* 33:10–14, 1995.

63. Kumar VP, Satku K: Treatment and prevention of "hook nail" deformity with anatomic correlation. *J Hand Surg [Am]* 18:617–620, 1993.

64. Lemperle G, Schwarz M, Lemperle SM: Nail regeneration by elongation of the partially destroyed nail bed. *Plast Reconstr Surg* 111:167–172, 2003.

65. Lewis BL: Microscopic studies of fetal and mature nail and surrounding soft tissue. *AMA Arch Dermatol* 70:732–747, 1954.

66. Lille S, Brown RE, Zook EG, et al: Free nonvascularized composite nail grafts: an institutional experience. *Plast Reconstr Surg* 105:2412–2415, 2000.

67. Lumpkin LR, Rosen T, Tschen JA, et al: Subungual squamous cell carcinoma. *J Am Acad Dermatol* 11:735–738, 1984.

68. Maley AM, Arbiser JL: Gentian violet: a 19th century drug re-emerges in the 21st century. *Exp Dermatol* 22:775–780, 2013.

69. McGinley KJ, Larson EL, Leyden JJ: Composition and density of microflora in the subungual space of the hand. *J Clin Microbiol* 26:950–953, 1988.

70. Metzger S, Ellwanger U, Stroebel W, et al: Extent and consequences of physician delay in the diagnosis of acral melanoma. *Melanoma Res* 8:181–186, 1998.

71. Morrison WA: Microvascular nail transfer. *Hand Clin* 6:69–76, 1990.

72. Morrison WA, O'Brien BM, McLeod AM: Thumb reconstruction with a free neurovascular wrap-around flap from the big toe. *J Hand Surg [Am]* 5:575–583, 1980.

73. Moss SH, Schwartz KS, von Drasek-Ascher G, et al: Digital venous anatomy. *J Hand Surg [Am]* 10:473–482, 1985.

74. Moy RL, Eliezri YO, Nuovo GJ, et al: Human papillomavirus type DNA in periungual squamous cell carcinomas. *JAMA* 261:2669–2673, 1989.

75. Nakayama Y: Vascularized free nail grafts nourished by arterial inflow from the venous system. *Plast Reconstr Surg* 85:239–245, 1990.

76. Netscher DT, Meade RA: Reconstruction of fingertip amputations with full-thickness perionychial grafts from the retained part and local flaps. *Plast Reconstr Surg* 104:1705–1712, 1999.

77. Nguyen JT, Bakri K, Nguyen EC, et al: Surgical management of subungual melanoma: Mayo Clinic experience of 124 cases. *Ann Plast Surg* 71:346–354, 2013.

78. Ogunro EO: External fixation of injured nail bed with the INRO surgical nail splint. *J Hand Surg [Am]* 14:236–241, 1989.

79. Pardo-Castello V: *Disease of the nail*, ed 3, Springfield, IL, 1960, Charles C Thomas.

80. Park KGM, Blessing K, Kernohan NM: Surgical aspects of subungual malignant melanomas. *Ann Surg* 216:692–695, 1992.

81. Pessa JE, Tsai T-M, Li Y, et al: The repair of nail deformities with the nonvascularized nail bed graft: indications and results. *J Hand Surg [Am]* 15:466–470, 1990.

82. Rose EH: Nailplasty utilizing a free composite graft from the helical rim of the ear. *Plast Reconstr Surg* 66:23–29, 1980.

83. Rose EH, Norris MS, Kowalski TA, et al: The "cap" technique: non-microsurgical reattachment of fingertip amputations. *J Hand Surg [Am]* 14:513–518, 1989.

84. Saito H, Suzuki Y, Fujino K, et al: Free nail bed graft for treatment of nail bed injuries of the hand. *J Hand Surg [Am]* 8:171–178, 1983.

85. Schiller C: Nail replacement in fingertip injuries. *Plast Reconstr Surg* 19:521–530, 1957.

86. Schwartz GB: Subungual squamous cell carcinoma of a nail bed. *Orthop Rev* 17:884–885, 1988.

87. Schellhaas U, Gerber W, Hammes S, et al: Pulsed dye laser treatment is effective in the treatment of recalcitrant viral warts. *Dermatol Surg* 34:67–72, 2008.

88. Seaberg DC, Angelos WJ, Paris PM: Treatment of subungual hematomas with nail trephination: a prospective study. *Am J Emerg Med* 9:209–210, 1991.

89. Shepard GH: Treatment of nail bed avulsions with split thickness nail bed grafts. *J Hand Surg [Am]* 8:49–54, 1983.

90. Shepard GH: Nail grafts for reconstruction. *Hand Clin* 6.79–102, 1990.

91. Shepard GH: Perionychial grafts in trauma and reconstruction. *Hand Clin* 18:595–614, 2002.

92. Shibata M, Seki T, Yoshizu T, et al: Microsurgical toenail transfer to the hand. *Plast Reconstr Surg* 88:102–109, 1991.

93. Smith DO, Oura C, Kimura C, et al: The distal venous anatomy of the finger. *J Hand Surg [Am]* 16:303–307, 1991.

94. Stanislas JM, Waldram MA: Keep the nail plate on with histoacryl. *Injury* 28:507–508, 1997.

95. Sugamata A: Regeneration of nails with artificial dermis. *J Plast Surg Hand Surg* 46:191–194, 2012.

96. Tajima T: Treatment of open crushing type industrial injuries of the hand and forearm: degloving, open circumferential, heat press and nail bed injuries. *J Trauma* 14:995–1011, 1974.

97. Wei FC, Epstein MD, Chen HC, et al: Microsurgical reconstruction of distal digits following mutilating hand injuries: results in 121 patients. *Br J Surg* 46:181–186, 1993.

98. Wilgis EF, Maxwell GP: Distal digital nerve graft: clinical and anatomical studies. *J Hand Surg [Am]* 4:439–443, 1979.

99. Yates YJ, Concannon MJ: Fungal infections of the perionychium. *Hand Clin* 18:631–642, 2002.

100. Zaias N: *The nail in health and disease*, ed 2, Norwalk, CT, 1990, Appleton & Lange.

101. Zook EG: The perionychium: anatomy, physiology and care of injuries. *Clin Plast Surg* 8:21–31, 1981.

102. Zook EG: Fingernail injuries. In Strickland JW, Steichen JB, editors: *Difficult problems in hand surgery*, St. Louis, 1982, Mosby.

103. Zook EG: Discussion of "nail fungal infections and treatment." *Hand Clin* 18:629, 2002.

104. Zook EG: Reconstruction of a functional and aesthetic nail. *Hand Clin* 18:577–594, 2002.

105. Zook EG, Chalekson CP, Brown RE, et al: Correction of pincer-nail deformities with autograft or homograft dermis: modified surgical technique. *J Hand Surg [Am]* 30:400–403, 2005.

106. Zook EG, Guy RJ, Russell RC: A study of nail bed injuries: causes, treatment and prognosis. *J Hand Surg [Am]* 9:247–252, 1984.

107. Zook EG, Van Beek AL, Russell RC, et al: Anatomy and physiology of the perionychium: a review of the literature and anatomic study. *J Hand Surg [Am]* 5:528–536, 1980.

10

Treatment of the Stiff Finger and Hand

Robert N. Hotchkiss

Acknowledgments: The author gratefully acknowledges the extensive analysis and expertise of previous authors of this chapter, including Peter Amadio, MD, Alex Shin, MD, and Richard J. Smith, MD.

This chapter is intended to provide guidance regarding the treatment of a stiff digit following trauma, primarily with a focus on the metacarpophalangeal (MP) and proximal interphalangeal (PIP) joints. There are numerous resources, including several sections in this book, dedicated to preventing stiffness and maximizing motion and mobility after specific injuries such as fractures, tendon lacerations, or burns. This chapter will not supplant or replace this specific guidance. Instead, this discussion is dedicated to the surgical treatment of a stiff digit caused by trauma, including the timing, methods, potential pitfalls, and expectations of operation.

Curtis's elegantly simple work from 1954[15] and Smith's[45] elucidation of intrinsic tightness cannot be improved upon. The detailed, granular record provided by Curtis is an accurate reflection of the complexity and variability of every patient. Reading this work removes any illusions about surgical formulas and reinforces the need for careful analysis and strategies that are designed for each individual. If the reader simply put down this volume and concentrated on those two masterpieces, little more would be required for a conceptual grasp of the digit's anatomy, pathologic findings, and reliable strategies for treatment.

You can learn more about the anatomy of the MP joint online at ExpertConsult.com.

PATHOPHYSIOLOGIC FINDINGS

The initial response to nearly any injury to the hand or finger is edema.[8,12,39] The injured hand and digit are bathed in a macrophage- and protein-rich fluid that not only encompasses the injured structure but surrounds and bathes adjacent uninjured structures. Accumulation of edema fluid or hematoma within the layers of tendons, sheaths, and capsular structures of the joint or within the synovial spaces physically limits mobility.[3,7,8,12] The swollen hand assumes a characteristic posture that maximizes the capacity of the joint and comfort of the hand; for the MP joint, this is full extension, and for the PIP joint, this is flexion[51] (Figure 10.1).

In contrast to the MP joint, the capacity of the interphalangeal joints is affected little by joint position and is minimally affected by the hydrostatic effect of edema, although skin tension does have some limiting effect. The posture of resting

MP extension following injury has a reciprocal influence on the PIP joint, by tipping the finely tuned balance between the extrinsic flexors and extensors in favor of a flexed position. Without intervention, this can become fixed and often does.

DIGIT FUNCTION AND MOBILITY

The functional demands of the hand obviously vary depending on activity, task, and occupation. However, the basic functions of pinch, grasp, and grip form the contextual basis for considering the need for motion, stability, and strength in the digits. For effective pinch, a stable, well-positioned thumb is crucial. Extremes of movement of the thumb interphalangeal or MP joint are less important for effective pinch than is stability in a functional position at these joints. Some movement of the carpometacarpal (CMC) joint of the thumb may be advantageous but is not crucial.[28] Meeting the thumb at the tip requires MP motion of the index and long fingers, with less motion needed at the PIP joints of these two radial digits. In contrast, power grip requires the composite motion of the MP and PIP joints, especially the ulnar three digits. Therefore before embarking on complex and challenging operative attempts to improve mobility of a given digit or joint, a full assessment of need and impact must be undertaken.

The highest priority of function combined with the highest probability of success is seen with attempts to improve *flexion* at the MP and PIP joints following trauma. Improvement of active and passive flexion of the joints is usually more likely than improvement of extension (e.g., patients with fixed contractures resulting from intrinsic tightness are excellent candidates for improvement following surgery).

Musicians present a unique and interesting challenge, because different instruments place vastly different demands on the fingers and hands and require an individualistic analysis. Pianists, who play with both hands, can adapt so that little PIP motion is needed. In contrast, musicians who play string instruments need both strength and mobility, especially of the fingering or fretting hand and even out to the DIP joint.

TREATMENT

Evaluation and Planning

Status of the Articular Surface of the Metacarpophalangeal and Proximal Interphalangeal Joints

If the joint shows signs of posttraumatic arthritis or articular malalignment, the likelihood of improvement with capsular release is quite poor. Although implant arthroplasty following

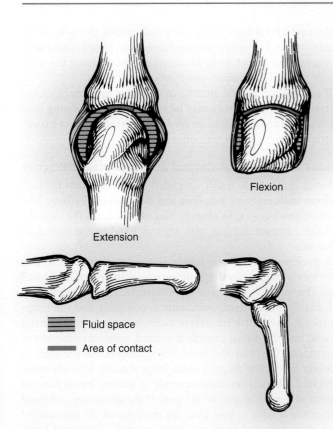

FIGURE 10.1 The anatomy of the extended metacarpophalangeal (MP) joint differs significantly from that of the fully flexed MP joint. In extension, the bone contact surface area is minimal. The collateral ligaments are loose, intracapsular fluid space is at a maximum, and the joint is relatively unstable. The proximal phalanx rotates, abducts, and adducts on the metacarpal. In full flexion, the metacarpal condylar surface is broad and the contact area is maximal between the metacarpal and proximal phalanx. The collateral ligaments are tight secondary to a cam effect and the necessity of the collaterals to pass around the metacarpal head prominences. The intracapsular fluid space is minimal, and the joint is highly stable because of the bone and ligament configurations in the flexed position. (Copyright © Elizabeth Martin.)

posttraumatic stiffness has been successful in the hip, knee, and elbow, this has not been the case for the MP or PIP joints. The reported motion gain is minimal, and implant failure is quite common.[20] Therefore if the joint is in poor condition, contracture release surgery should be avoided. Although some limited success has been reported for distraction arthroplasty, at this time a general recommendation regarding this procedure cannot be made.[30]

Capsular Contracture, Tendon Adherence, and Extrinsic and Intrinsic Assessment

The examination of the stiff joint requires a fundamental understanding of the interdependence and relative roles of the joint capsule, extrinsic tendon adherence, and intrinsic function (see Anatomy of the Intrinsics on ExpertConsult.com). It is vital to distinguish between active and passive motion and to determine the position of the adjacent joint in which these parameters are measured.

If the joint cannot be moved at all, it is difficult to tell whether the problem is due to joint incongruity, capsular

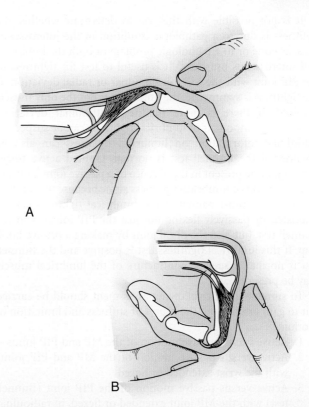

FIGURE 10.2 Intrinsic tightness test. In most cases of intrinsic tightness, there is less flexion of the proximal interphalangeal joint when the metacarpophalangeal (MP) joint is held extended **(A)** than when the MP joint is flexed **(B)**. (From Smith RJ: Intrinsic muscles of the fingers: function, dysfunction and surgical reconstruction. *Instr Course Lect* 24:200–220, 1975, with permission.)

contracture, or tendon adhesions or to some combination of factors. If active motion and passive motion are equal but diminished, the joint capsule or articular surface is likely to be a primary limiting factor. However, tendon adherence or dysfunction cannot be ruled until the joint is fully or maximally mobilized. If passive motion exceeds active motion, the musculotendinous unit is incompetent or adherent, or both. The adequacy of a motor unit or tendon can only be fully assessed once the joint contracture is resolved. Manual motor testing can identify any element of motor weakness.

After testing active and passive motion, a test of the extrinsic/intrinsic system is required. To test for extensor tendon tightness, the wrist and the MP joints are flexed, and passive flexion of the interphalangeal joints is assessed. In the normal state there is easy passive flexion of the interphalangeal joints. If extensor adhesions or tightness exists, flexion of the interphalangeal joints will be difficult. Similarly, if interphalangeal extension is less with the wrist and MP joints extended, extrinsic flexor tightness may be the problem.

Because the intrinsic system spans both the MP and PIP joints, testing requires fixing the position of the one joint when testing the other. The *Bunnell intrinsic tightness test* examines the effect of MP joint position on PIP joint flexion (Figure 10.2). The test is considered positive when there is less flexion of the PIP joint when the MP joint is held extended than when the MP joint is flexed. A positive intrinsic test indicates that there is some element of intrinsic muscle tightness contributing to the finger stiffness.

It is not possible with this test to determine whether the tightness is due to a pathologic condition of the interosseous muscle alone or to a pathologic problem of both the lumbrical and interosseous muscles.[14] It is useful to test for tightness of the PIP joint with the MP joint in ulnar or radial deviation. If the tightness is symmetric, the lumbrical is not the only muscle involved. If there is more tightness with ulnar deviation, however, a component of lumbrical tightness can be suspected. Additional information on lumbrical tightness can also be obtained if the Bunnell test is normal. Limited active finger flexion may be present in the absence of a passive joint contracture as a result of lumbrical tightness alone because the lumbrical fibers are most palmar. Thus, lumbrical tightness can be evaluated by passively flexing not just the PIP joint, as in the Bunnell test, but also the distal joint by making a passive hook grip. If this lumbrical tightness test is positive and the Bunnell test is normal, a specific contracture of the lumbrical muscle may be present.

To summarize, the following assessment should be carried out to gain insight into the causes of stiffness and limitation of motion:

1. Active versus passive motion of the MP and PIP joints
2. Active versus passive motion of the MP and PIP joints with the wrist extended or flexed
3. Active versus passive motion of the PIP joint (Bunnell test) with the MP joint extended or flexed, in radioulnar deviation

Nonoperative Intervention

Edema can often be diminished and mobilization promoted by applying low-load, prolonged stress during active exercise to encourage functional use of the hand in light and moderate activities. It has been estimated that 87% of MP and PIP joint contractures can be successfully managed nonoperatively.[52] As long as there is positive progress, nonoperative treatment should continue. Only when a plateau in active and passive range of motion has been reached and the result is functionally unacceptable should surgical options be considered.

For more information on nonoperative treatment of joint contractures, see ExpertConsult.com.

Operative Intervention

Before developing and implementing an operative approach to joint stiffness, it is essential to confirm that a compliant patient and competent therapist will be permitted to work together and that the postoperative therapy visits are indeed recognized by all concerned parties as being an essential part of the treatment plan. If all three conditions (willing patient, capable therapist, and third-party approval when required) are not met, the surgery should not be performed.

For more information on skin and soft tissue intervention, please see ExpertConsult.com.

Anesthesia

When possible, local anesthesia with intravenous sedation is optimal for contracture release and tenolysis. It permits the patient to have active motion without pain and allows the surgeon to assess active motion intraoperatively. If sedation is used, the anesthesiologist can often titrate the timing and degree of sedation, so that the patient is more sedated at the beginning

of the case and is later able to flex and extend the joint when asked to do so. The upper arm tourniquet can be alternated with a forearm tourniquet, both for comfort and to avoid the temporary palsy of tourniquet pressure.

If regional or general anesthesia is used, a proximal incision for traction on the flexors may be needed. It is surprising how much can be accomplished under local anesthesia using a combination of bupivacaine and lidocaine.

Release of Metacarpophalangeal Joint Extension Contracture

A dorsal approach to a stiff, extended MP joint is best because it allows both extensor tenolysis and dorsal capsulectomy. The extensor tendon is split sharply and elevated off the capsule, and the extensor tendon and sagittal band are reflected to either side.

A preliminary extensor tenolysis can be performed at this point by sliding an elevator both proximal and distal to the MP joint. The tenolysis may need to be extended further proximally and distally once the capsulectomy is complete and the range of motion is tested. A transverse incision is made in the dorsal capsule, and the dorsal capsule is excised, with inclusion of the most dorsal fibers of the collateral ligaments. As the joint is passively flexed, the surgeon must judge if more ligament must be incised. There is no absolute angle of flexion, but at least 70 degrees of flexion should be the goal. If the remaining collateral ligament is unable to pass over the condyles of the metacarpal head, it is detached from its origin on the metacarpal head. Although satisfactory flexion can be obtained by detaching the ulnar collateral ligament alone, it is often necessary to detach both collateral ligaments to prevent abnormal rotation as flexion occurs.

Once the collateral ligaments have been released, an elevator is used to free any adhesions between the volar plate and the volar capsule. It is best to keep testing passive motion, releasing more collateral ligament tissue as needed. Occasionally, the MP joint will jump or trigger as the joint reaches full extension. In such cases, any remaining accessory collateral ligament should be divided. Following release, the extensor tendons are again examined for excursion and any adhesions. The tourniquet is used sparingly to eliminate any degree of tourniquet palsy, and the patient is asked to actively move the affected finger. If a block or general anesthesia has been used, a second incision and proximal traction on the tendons will be necessary. In either case, if the extensor tendons do not glide freely, tenolysis may need to be extended.

Decisions Regarding When to Stop Excising and Releasing Tissue. In every one of these cases, one must decide when the "law of diminishing returns" should be invoked. For instance, there is no value in releasing the MP joint to the point of instability because immobilization or pin fixation of an unstable joint will defeat any gains in motion achieved. Instead, if one has achieved improvement in passive and active flexion from 0 to 60 degrees, excising more tissue may risk destabilizing the joint and the necessary smooth articulating movement.

The use of pin fixation is not necessarily a poor choice, especially in severe cases of global trauma, but if used, the timing of pin removal for activation of the mobilization program has to be carefully considered and individualized. Removal may take place as early as 5 to 7 days following the original procedure.

There is no substitute for experience in these cases, and consultation with colleagues is strongly encouraged, no matter the age or track record of the surgeon.

Closure and Postoperative Management. Once the release is complete, repair the extensor mechanism and skin in layers using 4-0 nonabsorbable sutures. The degree of flexion can be retested, being careful not to rupture the repaired extensor mechanism. The hand is placed in a bulky dressing, with dorsal and volar plaster splints holding the MP joints at 70 degrees of flexion and the PIP joints in extension.

The hand should be elevated for 24 to 36 hours and mobilization initiated in 2 to 3 days, if possible. The use of removable static splints and dynamic splints is dictated by individual circumstance and opportunity.

Methylprednisolone (Medrol Dosepak, Pfizer, New York) can effectively reduce swelling and pain in the immediate postoperative period in many cases and should be strongly considered if progress appears to have stalled.

Expectations and Complications. Most patients do not maintain the degree of improvement observed in the operating room, despite intensive and persistent rehabilitation programs; every patient needs to be fully informed of this difficulty. In general, patients with direct trauma and extensive local scarring do less well than patients with the sequelae of chronic regional pain syndrome.

Complications include wound separation and lack of skin pliability, especially in the first 2 weeks after release. It may be necessary to suspend rehabilitation for a few days until the skin and wound better tolerate flexion. At 10 to 12 days following operation the wounds can better tolerate mobilization and direct pressure. Diligent attention to the patient and rehabilitation program is an absolute necessity.

More information on this topic can be found online at ExpertConsult.com.

Release of Flexion Contractures of the Proximal Interphalangeal Joint

The primary challenge in the treatment of fixed flexion contracture of the PIP joint, after accounting for the health of the articular cartilage of the joint, is the integrity and function of the extensor mechanism. If there is attenuation of or injury to the extensor, release of the volar contracture tissue alone will not restore active extension. Instead, a plan to release the joint, including the volar collateral ligament, and reconstruction of the extensor mechanism must be considered.[1,23]

Surgical approaches to the PIP joint have been well described in the literature. All use either the volar zigzag Bruner incision or the midaxial approach. The use of local anesthesia with intravenous sedation is preferred to allow the patient to actively flex and extend the joint after release of contractures. This enables immediate evaluation of the effectiveness of the procedure, and any fine-tuning or additional releases can be performed if full extension is not achieved. If local anesthesia with sedation is not possible, an arm block or general anesthesia can be used, but in this case the effectiveness of the releases cannot be thoroughly evaluated intraoperatively without an additional proximal incision and applied traction to the affected motors.

For information on the volar surgical approach, please see ExperConsult.com.

❖ AUTHOR'S PREFERRED APPROACH: Proximal Interphalangeal Flexion Contractures

Under local anesthesia, a midlateral skin incision is made that extends from the midshaft of the proximal phalanx to the midshaft of the middle phalanx (Figure 10.3). The neurovascular bundle is identified and retracted palmarly. The transverse retinacular ligament is divided and the accessory collateral ligament and volar plate are visualized. Although a unilateral incision is preferred, a bilateral incision can be used if exposure of the contralateral collateral ligament is difficult. Once exposure is achieved, the checkrein ligament is released and the accessory collateral ligament is completely excised as necessary. The exposure can be extended to the dorsal side as needed for extensor tenolysis or central slip reconstruction. This situation is not substantially different from release and reconstruction of the chronic, fixed boutonnière reconstruction (see Chapter 5).

The dressing is removed at 3 days following operation and active motion is encouraged under the supervision of a hand therapy specialist. Two splints are made at that time, one for extension and one for flexion, and they are alternated as needed. Static splinting in extension is continued at night for up to 6 months.

For expectations and outcomes of PIP flexion contracture release, please see ExpertConsult.com.

External Fixation Devices for Proximal Interphalangeal Joint Contractures. External fixation provides a sustained forceful moment and exerts control through the bone, as opposed to pressure on the skin, thus offering a promising way of both stabilizing and mobilizing the PIP joint.[2,19,29,30]

Though several devices have been reported to have successful outcomes, the Digit Widget (Hand Biomechanics Laboratory, Sacramento, CA) is a unique device that uses extension torque rather than a distractive force, is controlled entirely by the patient, and has a reasonably low profile. This device allows a range of motion of the PIP joint during the application of extension torque on the contracted joint, via a series of rubber bands that are applied to the device (Figure 10.4, *A* to *E*). The device may be applied for a wide variety of reasons, is simple to apply and maintain, and "burns no bridges" should further reconstructive procedures be required (Case Study 10.1).

Release of Posttraumatic Proximal Interphalangeal Joint Extension Contractures

Surgery for extension contractures of the PIP joint is best performed under local anesthesia with sedation. This enables testing of the contracture release via the patient's voluntary control and allows fine-tuning. The operative approach for extension contractures can be from a dorsal or dorsolateral approach (Figure 10.5). The extensor mechanism is exposed, and the transverse fibers of the retinacular ligament are identified and longitudinally divided on either side of the central tendon. The extensor tendon is then elevated, with care taken to avoid injury to the central slip insertion. This provides exposure of the dorsal capsule and the collateral ligaments. Extensor tenolysis is performed, and the surgeon can continue as far proximally and distally as needed to free the tendon from underlying bone and overlying skin. The dorsal capsule is excised, and the range of motion of the joint is assessed. If full flexion is not possible, the dorsalmost fibers of the collateral

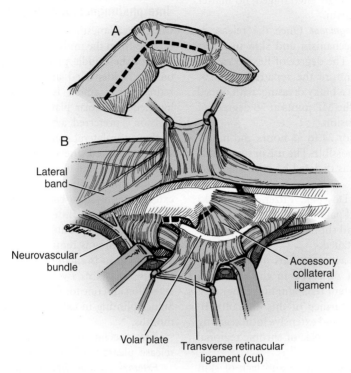

FIGURE 10.3 A, Flexion contracture release at the proximal interphalangeal joint as performed via a midlateral approach. Though technically easier, the results of a volar Bruner approach have been shown to result in less favorable outcomes. B, The transverse retinacular ligament is divided and the lateral aspect of the joint is visualized. The volar plate checkrein ligaments are released, as well as the accessory collateral ligament at its origin on both the radial and ulnar aspects of the joint. If motion is not improved, the proper collateral ligament is also released. (Copyright © Elizabeth Martin.)

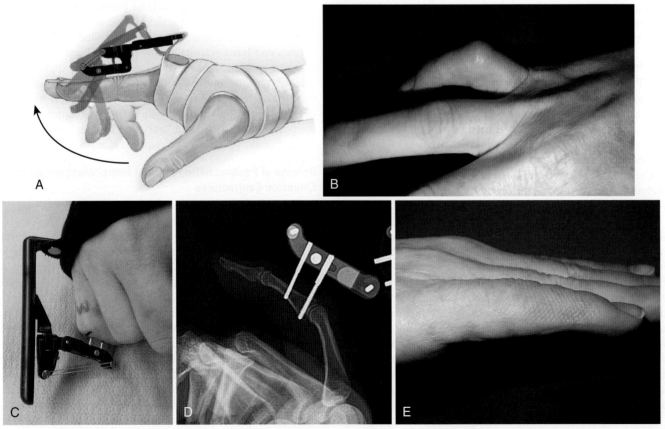

FIGURE 10.4 A, The Digit Widget, a device that uses extension torque rather than a distractive force, was introduced in 2001 (Hand Biomechanics Laboratory, Sacramento, CA). B, A 38-year-old woman 1 year after flexor tendon repair complicated by a 90-degree flexion contracture. C, The device allows range of motion while extension torque is applied via rubber bands with different grades of elasticity. D, Radiographs 4 weeks following application of device. E, Active extension 3 months following removal and vigorous splinting protocol.

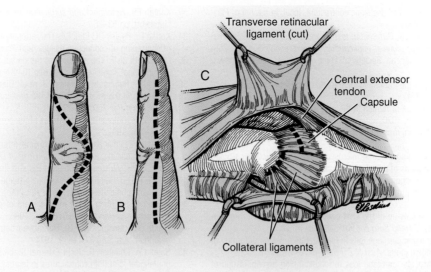

Transverse retinacular
ligament (cut)

Central extensor
tendon
Capsule

Collateral ligaments

FIGURE 10.5 A to C, Extension contracture release of the PIP joint can be performed through a dorsal curvilinear or midlateral approach. Once the skin is elevated and mobilized, the transverse retinacular ligament is divided to expose the joint. Extensor tenolysis is performed, and a dorsal capsulotomy is made. The collateral ligaments are then released at their insertion on the proximal phalanx. (Copyright © Elizabeth Martin.)

ligaments should be released. If full flexion is still not obtained, the rest of the collateral ligaments are released off the proximal phalanx origin. Once passive flexion is satisfactory, the patient is asked to voluntarily flex the digit to determine whether there are any extrinsic causes of blocked flexion. It is impossible to know whether flexor tenolysis will be needed in the presence of an extension contracture. Thus, active flexion always needs to be checked after release of the contracture, and the patient must be advised preoperatively of the possible need for flexor tenolysis. If the patient does not tolerate local anesthesia with sedation, the procedure can be done under regional or general anesthesia, and a proximal counterincision must be made in the distal part of the forearm to apply traction to the flexor tendons.

No discussion of PIP extension contractures is complete without mentioning the possibility of intrinsic contractures. After surgical release is completed, the Bunnell intrinsic tightness test is performed to determine whether there is residual contracture of the intrinsics. If the test is positive, release of the intrinsics should be performed as described by Dr. Richard J. Smith (see ExpertConsult.com). If the patient is awake, the active hook grip should be tested following release, to detect more subtle degrees of intrinsic tightness that will respond to stretching postoperatively.

An alternative to capsulotomy is release of the lateral bands on either side of the central slip, followed by the gentle passive flexion maneuver described by Inoue.[32] In this technique, the passive flexion breaks up adhesions of the extensor tendon and intraarticular adhesions. A dorsal extension block with a Kirschner wire prevents active extension beyond the desired flexed position, and active flexion exercises are initiated immediately postoperatively. The wire is removed at 2 weeks, and vigorous flexion exercises are initiated with a dynamic flexion splinting device. The results in 10 patients treated in this manner demonstrated an average gain of 47.5 degrees of flexion without complications.

The results of release of extension contractures have been reported by Mansat and Delprat.[37,38] In a multicenter study involving 10 institutions in France, 246 contracture releases of the PIP joint were performed, of which extension contractures accounted for 45% of cases. The average improvement in flexion was 28 degrees, with a preoperative range of motion of 19 to 34 degrees as compared with a postoperative range of motion of 8 to 62 degrees.

For Case Studies, Videos, and more, please visit ExpertConsult.com.

REFERENCES

1. Abbiati G, Delaria G, Saporiti E, et al: The treatment of chronic flexion contractures of the proximal interphalangeal joint. *J Hand Surg [Br]* 20(3):385–389, 1995.
2. Agee JM, Goss BC: The use of skeletal extension torque in reversing Dupuytren contractures of the proximal interphalangeal joint. *J Hand Surg [Am]* 37(7):1467–1474, 2012.
3. Akeson WH, Amiel D, Woo SLY: Immobility effects on synovial joints. The pathomechanics of joint contracture. (Third International Congress of Biorheology: Symposium on Soft Tissues Around a Diarthrodial Joint.) *Biorheology* 17:95–110, 1980.
4. Allieu Y, Ould Ouali A, Gomis R, et al: Simple arthrolysis for flexor rigidity of the proximal interphalangeal joint. *Ann Chir Main* 2:330–335, 1983.
5. Backhouse KM, Catton WT: An experimental study of the function of the lumbrical muscles in the human hand. *J Anat* 88:133–141, 1954.
6. Bain GI, Mehta JA, Hepinstall RJ, et al: Dynamic external fixation for injuries of the proximal interphalangeal joint. *J Bone Joint Surg Br* 80:1014–1019, 1998.
7. Brand PW: Drag. In *Clinical mechanics of the hand*, St. Louis, 1985, Mosby, pp 61–87.
8. Brand PW: Mechanical factors in joint stiffness and tissue growth. *J Hand Ther* 8:91–96, 1995.
9. Bruser P, Poss T, Larkin G: Results of proximal interphalangeal joint release for flexion contractures: midlateral versus palmar incision. *J Hand Surg [Am]* 24:288–294, 1999.
10. Buch VI: Clinical and functional assessment of the hand after metacarpophalangeal capsulotomy. *Plast Reconstr Surg* 53:452–457, 1974.
11. Bunnell S: Ischaemic contracture, local, in the hand. *J Bone Joint Surg Am* 35:88–101, 1953.
12. Bunnell S: *Surgery of the hand*, ed 3, Philadelphia, 1956, JB Lippincott.

13. Bunnell S, Doherty DW, Curtis RM: Ischemic contracture, local, in the hand. *Plast Reconstr Surg* 3:424–433, 1948.
14. Colditz JC, Erdmann D, Levin LS: *Differential testing and stretching of the interosseous and lumbrical muscles: clinical implications.* Paper presented at the 25th Annual Meeting of the American Society of Hand Therapists, 2002, Ottawa, Canada.
15. Curtis RM: Capsulectomy of the interphalangeal joints of the fingers. *J Bone Joint Surg Am* 36:1219–1232, 1954.
16. Curtis RM: Surgical restoration of motion in the stiff interphalangeal joints of the hand. *Bull Hosp Jt Dis* 31:1–6, 1970.
17. Eaton RG, Littler JW: Joint injuries and their sequelae. *Clin Plast Surg* 3:85–98, 1976.
18. Enna CD, Zimny M: A scanning electron microscopy study of articular cartilage obtained from contracted joints of denervated hands. *Hand* 6:65–69, 1974.
19. Feldscher SB, Blank JE: Management of a proximal interphalangeal joint fracture dislocation with a compass proximal interphalangeal joint hinge and therapy: a case report. *J Hand Ther* 15(3):266–273, 2002.
20. Field J: Two to five year follow-up of the LPM ceramic coated proximal interphalangeal joint arthroplasty. *J Hand Surg Eur Vol.* 33(1):38–44, 2008.
21. Field PL, Hueston JT: Articular cartilage loss in long-standing flexion deformity of the proximal interphalangeal joints. *Aust N Z J Surg* 40:70–74, 1970.
22. Field PL, Hueston JT: Articular cartilage loss in long-standing immobilization of interphalangeal joints. *Br J Plast Surg* 23:186–191, 1970.
23. Ghidella SD, Segalman KA, Murphey MS: Long-term results of surgical management of proximal interphalangeal joint contracture. *J Hand Surg [Am]* 27:799–805, 2002.
24. Gould JS, Nicholson BG: Capsulectomy of the metacarpophalangeal and proximal interphalangeal joints. *J Hand Surg [Am]* 4:482–486, 1979.
25. Harris C, Jr, Riordan DC: Intrinsic contracture in the hand and its surgical treatment. *J Bone Joint Surg Am* 36:10–20, 1954.
26. Harris C, Jr, Rutledge GL, Jr: The functional anatomy of the extensor mechanism of the finger. *J Bone Joint Surg Am* 54:713–726, 1972.
27. Harrison DH: The stiff proximal interphalangeal joint. *Hand* 9:102–108, 1977.
28. Hartigan BJ, Stern PJ, Kiefhaber TR: Thumb carpometacarpal osteoarthritis: arthrodesis compared with ligament reconstruction and tendon interposition. *J Bone Joint Surg Am* 83(10):1470–1478, 2001.
29. Houshian S, Chikkamuniyappa C: Distraction correction of chronic flexion contractures of PIP joint: comparison between two distraction rates. *J Hand Surg [Am]* 32(5):651–656, 2007.
30. Houshian S, Jing SS, Kazemian GH, et al: Distraction for proximal interphalangeal joint contractures: long-term results. *J Hand Surg [Am]* 38(10):1951–1956, 2013.
31. Hunter E, Laverty J, Pollack R, et al: Nonoperative treatment of fixed flexion deformity of the proximal interphalangeal joint. *J Hand Surg [Br]* 24:281–283, 1999.
32. Inoue G: Lateral band release for post-traumatic extension contracture of the proximal interphalangeal joint. *Arch Orthop Trauma Surg* 110:298–300, 1991.
33. Kaplan EB: *Functional and surgical anatomy of the hand*, Philadelphia, 1965, JB Lippincott, pp 53–86.
34. Kottke FJ, Pauley DL, Ptak RA: The rationale for prolonged stretching for correction of shortening of connective tissue. *Arch Phys Med Rehabil* 10:345–352, 1966.
35. Landsmeer JMF: The anatomy of the dorsal aponeurosis of the human finger and its functional significance. *Anat Rec* 104:31–44, 1949.
36. Lewis AR, Ralphs JR, Kneafsey B, et al: Distribution of collagens and glycosaminoglycans in the joint capsule of the proximal interphalangeal joint of the human finger. *Anat Rec* 250:281–291, 1998.
37. Mansat M, Delprat J: Contractures of the proximal interphalangeal joint. *Hand Clin* 8:777–786, 1992.
38. Mansat MF: Volar aspect of the proximal interphalangeal joint. An anatomical study and pathological correlations. *Bull Hosp Jt Dis Orthop Inst* 44:309–317, 1984.
39. Merritt WH: Written on behalf of the stiff finger. *J Hand Ther* 11:74–79, 1998.
40. Milz S, Putz R, Ralphs JR, et al: Fibrocartilage in the extensor tendons of the human metacarpophalangeal joints. *Anat Rec* 256:139–145, 1999.
41. Prosser R: Splinting in the management of proximal interphalangeal joint flexion contracture. *J Hand Ther* 9:378–386, 1996.
42. Rhode CM, Jennings WD, Jr: Operative treatment of the stiff proximal interphalangeal joint. *Am Surg* 37:44–59, 1971.
43. Salafia A, Chauhan G: Joshi External Stabilising System (JESS) in proximal interphalangeal joint (PIP) contractures in leprosy. *Indian J Lepr* 69:331–339, 1997.
44. Shrewsbury MM, Johnson RK: A systemic study of the oblique retinacular ligament of the human finger. Its structure and function. *J Hand Surg [Am]* 2:194–199, 1977.
45. Smith RJ: Balance and kinetics of the fingers under normal and pathological conditions. *Clin Orthop Relat Res* 104:92–111, 1974.
46. Sprague BL: Proximal interphalangeal joint injuries and their initial treatment. *J Trauma* 15:380–385, 1975.
47. Sprague BL: Proximal interphalangeal joint contractures and their treatment. *J Trauma* 16:259–265, 1976.
48. Stack HG: Muscle function in the fingers. *J Bone Joint Surg Br* 44:899–909, 1962.
49. Tubiana R, Valentin P: The anatomy of the extensor apparatus of the fingers. *Surg Clin North Am* 44:897–906, 1964.
50. Watson HK, Light TR, Johnson TR: Checkrein resection for flexion contracture of the middle joint. *J Hand Surg [Am]* 4:67–71, 1979.
51. Watson HK, Weinzweig J: Stiff joints. In Green DP, Hotchkiss RN, Pederson WC, editors: *Green's operative hand surgery*, Philadelphia, 1999, Churchill Livingstone, pp 552–562.
52. Weeks PM, Wray RC, Jr, Kuxhaus M: The results of non-operative management of stiff joints in the hand. *Plast Reconstr Surg* 61:58–63, 1978.
53. Weeks PM, Young VL, Wray RC, Jr: Operative mobilization of stiff metacarpophalangeal joints: dorsal versus volar approach. *Ann Plast Surg* 5:178–185, 1980.
54. Wynn Parry CB: Management of the stiff joint. *Hand* 3:169–171, 1971.
55. Young VL, Wray RC, Jr, Weeks PM: The surgical management of stiff joints in the hand. *Plast Reconstr Surg* 62:835–841, 1978.

Treatment of the Osteoarthritic Hand and Thumb

Peter M. Murray

▶ These videos may be found at
ExpertConsult.com:
11.1 Volar approach for proximal interphalangeal joint implant arthroplasty
11.2 Physical examination for osteoarthritis of the thumb

Osteoarthritis of the hand and thumb is one of the most common symptomatic conditions of the hand, particularly for people over the age of 75 years. Osteoarthritis of the thumb, for example, occurs in one of three females and in one of eight males.[5] Ring and colleagues have studied the prevalence of thumb carpometacarpal (CMC) arthritis in a consecutive series of patients and found the condition present in 91% of patients over the age of 80 years, with complete joint destruction present three times more often in females.[118] Osteoarthritis affects the small joint of the hand more commonly than any other location in the body and is among the leading conditions for which surgery of the hand is performed.[101]

Although the cause of osteoarthritis of the hand still engenders much debate, mechanical stress is supported by many. In a study of over 2500 individuals in China, Hunter and associates found that chopstick use accounted for 19% of thumb arthritis cases in men and 36% in women.[46] Interestingly and perhaps counterintuitively, handedness has not been shown to influence the development of osteoarthritis of the hand.

The indications for surgical reconstruction of the rheumatoid hand have declined over the last three decades, but the need for reconstruction of the osteoarthritic hand has remained constant, with reconstruction of the thumb CMC among the most commonly performed hand surgery procedures. A number of successful procedures have been employed for reconstruction of the arthritic thumb CMC joint. Traditionally, reconstruction for arthritis of the small joints of the hand has primarily involved arthrodesis. In recent decades, joint arthroplasty procedures have been used with increasing frequency and success.

OSTEOARTHRITIS OF THE SMALL JOINTS OF THE HAND

Preoperative Evaluation

Physical Examination

Physical examination of the hand begins with a careful inspection of the dorsal and palmar surfaces. Several distinguishing characteristics may be obvious in the osteoarthritic hand. At the metacarpophalangeal (MCP) joints, swelling and volar subluxation may be present, with an associated flexion contracture or extension lag. Likewise, the proximal interphalangeal (PIP) joints may display flexion contractures; a more common distinguishing characteristic is the Bouchard node. Similarly, inspection of the osteoarthritic distal interphalangeal (DIP) joint is heralded by the presence of Heberden nodes, which signifies swelling and periarticular osteophyte formation. Additionally, mucous cyst formation may occur in relation to an osteoarthritic DIP joint.

Palpation of the acutely inflamed osteoarthritic MCP, PIP, or DIP joint will elicit tenderness as well as a fullness about the joint and loss of the typical bony contour of the joint. While gently holding the joint between the dominant thumb and index finger, the examiner can carefully apply a small amount of pressure to detect tenderness and synovitis. The range of motion of each joint may be limited due to a superimposed flexion contracture. The digital range of motion is often expressed in terms of total active range of motion, approximately 250 degrees, but individual ranges are also often measured: The MCP joint has 0 to 90 degrees, the PIP joint 0 to 100 degrees, and the DIP joint 0 to 60 degrees.

Tendon integrity may be compromised in the osteoarthritic hand. Pathologic conditions of the flexor tendon may uncommonly occur, generally because chronic tenosynovitis of the flexor tendon sheath has caused a zone 2 flexor digitorum superficialis (FDS) or flexor digitorum profundus (FDP) tendon rupture. More commonly, the extensor tendons are involved, with ulnar subluxation of these tendons occurring at the level of the MCP joints owing to failure of the sagittal bands. The result is ulnar drift and flexion positioning of the digits at the level of the MCP joints. In the acute phase of this condition, extensor tendon subluxation and ulnar drift/MCP flexion may be passively correctable and amenable to individual digital splinting. In the more chronic situation, the only treatment option is surgical release of the sagittal bands, with or without intrinsic releases and extensor tendon realignment.

Erosive or inflammatory osteoarthritis is an uncommon variant of osteoarthritis first described in 1966 by Peter and coworkers.[101,104] Like primary osteoarthritis, it is more common in women and the symptoms appear abruptly and interestingly involve the joints on the radial aspect of the hand while sparing the joints on the ulnar side (Figure 11.1). The DIP joint is the most commonly affected joint, but the PIP joint is most

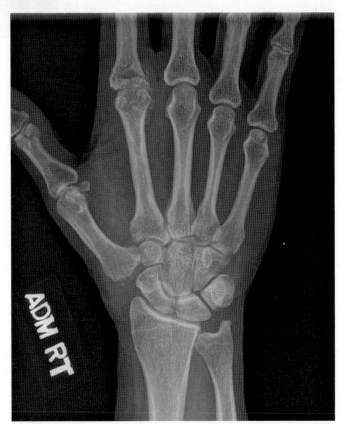

FIGURE 11.1 51-year-old right hand–dominant female with a 1-year history of right index finger pain located at the MCP joint.

commonly the symptomatic joint. In some patients, erosive osteoarthritis will seroconvert to rheumatoid arthritis at a later time.

Diagnostic Imaging

Plain PA, lateral, and oblique radiographic views can adequately image the osteoarthritic hand. Further detail can be obtained by directly imaging the individual digit, with an attempt made to center the radiograph beam over the joint in question (i.e., the MCP, PIP, or DIP joint). Further definition of the MCP joints can be obtained with a Brewerton view radiograph. Originally described for the rheumatoid hand, this view is obtained by placing the supinated hand on the cassette and flexing the MCP joints 45 to 60 degrees. This view may also be helpful in imaging the hand with osteoarthritis or erosive osteoarthritis. Advanced imaging such as computed tomography (CT) scanning and magnetic resonance imaging (MRI) is seldom necessary for osteoarthritis of the small joints of the hand; however, it may be helpful in the early stages of the condition, showing synovial changes in the joint along with effusion.

⬧ PERTINENT ANATOMY AND BIOMECHANICS

The PIP joint is a simple uniaxial hinge joint, stabilized by the extensor mechanism, the collateral and accessory collateral ligaments, the volar plate and articular contact between the bicondylar proximal phalangeal head, and the articular surface of the middle phalanx. The center of rotation of the PIP joint is within the condylar area of the proximal phalanx.[136] Minamikawa and coworkers[85] have shown that in the normal state, the PIP joint

may deviate 5 degrees in the radioulnar plane and supinate 9 degrees when subjected to lateral stress. This may increase to 20 degrees of deviation following complete sectioning of the collateral ligaments, with laxity greatly reduced when the PIP joint is in full extension and complete flexion. The primary stabilizer of the PIP joint is the lateral collateral ligament, and stability of the joint is maintained as long as half of this ligament remains intact.[85]

There are several unique characteristics of the MCP joints of the hand that can affect their surgical reconstruction and rehabilitation. In the sagittal plane, the metacarpal head has an elliptical shape that influences the arc of motion of the MCP joint such that a cam effect occurs during flexion and extension. The radial and ulnar collateral ligaments of the MCP joint originate along recesses of the metacarpal heads and course obliquely to insert along the base of the proximal phalanx. By virtue of the sagittal elliptical shape of the metacarpal head, the radial and ulnar collateral ligaments of the MCP joints are lax in extension and taut in full flexion. This integrity of the collateral ligament system has certain implications when it comes to joint immobilization, given the tendency for joint contracture of the MCP when immobilized in full extension.

Historical Review

Moberg and colleagues[87] and Carroll and Hill[19] reported on some early experiences with interphalangeal (IP) joint arthrodesis, citing a low pseudarthrosis rate. Since these early experiences, many authors have reported successful results using a variety of techniques (Table 11.1).

The first reported attempt at prosthetic replacement of the PIP joint was made by Burman using a Vitallium cap for arthroplasty in 1940.[12] In 1959, Brannon and Klein from Lackland Air Force Base, Texas, published the first series of digital total joint replacements. This was a hinged prosthesis initially indicated in PIP joint fractures and fracture-dislocations.[12] Flatt reported on a more rotationally stable device with two intermedullary prongs as opposed to the single-pronged Brannon prosthesis[36] (Figure 11.2). In 1979, Linscheid and Dobyns developed the surface replacement arthroplasty (SRA) for the PIP joint.[70] The development of these linked and unlinked metal arthroplasty designs were paralleled by the development of the Swanson silastic implant in the 1960s, which has been successful for management of osteoarthritis in both the MCP and PIP joints.[125] Carroll and Taber[20] reported on soft tissue interposition techniques for management of osteoarthritis of the IP joints of the hand.

Distal Interphalangeal Joint Arthrodesis
Indications and Contraindications

The main indication for DIP joint arthrodesis is primary osteoarthritis or posttraumatic arthritis. The patient should have pain referable to the DIP joint and static deformity or instability that interferes with activities of everyday living. The symptomatic digit may become less painful and the deformity less of an impairment with time, rendering the need for surgery less imperative. Therefore, it is advisable to treat the patient nonoperatively with analgesics, hand therapy modalities, a removable finger-based splint, and a period of prolonged observation prior to deciding to proceed with surgery. DIP joint arthrodesis may

TABLE 11.1 Studies of Interphalangeal Arthrodesis Fixation and Outcomes

Study	Fixation Technique	Time to Union (weeks)	Failure Rate (%)
McGlynn et al[79]	Cup and cone, Kirschner wire	~8	0
Lewis et al[66]	Tension and mortise, Kirschner wire	~8	2
Khuri[57]	Tension band wire	7	0
Hogh and Jensen[45]	Kirschner wire/cerclage	8	7-16
Granowitz and Vainio[42]	Crossed Kirschner wire	—	7
Carroll and Hill[19]	Cup and cone, Kirschner wire	6-8	10 (all cases)
Lister[72]	Intraosseous wire	10	13
Burton et al[17]	Kirschner wire	8	0
Buchler and Aikin[16]	Plate	—	8
Ayres et al[6]	Herbert screw	—	2
Moberg and Henrickson[87]	Bone peg	~6	6
Allende and Engelem[4]	Tension band wire	—	0
Wright and McMurtry[149]	Plate	—	0
Potenza[105]	Bone peg and Kirschner wire	7	—
Ijsselstein et al[47]	Kirschner wire	≈6	8
Ijsselstein et al[47]	Tension band wire	—	3
Stern and Fulton[121]	Kirschner wire	—	12
Stern and Fulton[121]	Interosseous wire	—	12
Stern and Fulton[121]	Herbert screw	—	11
Katzman et al[56]	Herbert screw	8	0
Stern et al[122]	Tension band wire	—	3
Braun and Rhoades[13]	External fixator	≈8	0
Seitz et al[117]	External fixator	6	9
Teoh et al[131]	Compression screw	8.2	4
Watson and Shaffer[145]	Kirschner wire	6	0
Leibovic and Strickland[64]	Kirschner wire	10	21
Leibovic and Strickland[64]	Tension band wire	11	5
Leibovic and Strickland[64]	Herbert screw	9	0
Leibovic and Strickland[64]	Plate	12	>50

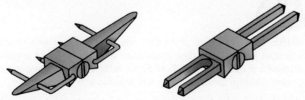

FIGURE 11.2 Drawing of the dual-pronged Flatt proximal interphalangeal (PIP) joint arthroplasty on the right and the single-prong Brannon PIP joint arthroplasty on the left.

be done following joint degeneration because of remote septic arthritis.

Contraindications for DIP arthrodesis include active infection of the finger, septic arthritis of the DIP joint, or an open wound in the proximity of the joint. Other potential contraindications include unhealthy atrophic skin over the joint, as may occur following long-term steroid usage. Patients with compromised blood flow or ischemic fingers should not undergo DIP joint arthrodesis.

Preoperative Planning

Critical to the preoperative assessment of the patient and planning for care are dedicated PA and lateral radiographs of the finger. It is important to identify the appropriate implant for arthrodesis based on the size of the distal phalanx. It is also important to identify any periarticular degenerative cyst formation or bone loss that may necessitate bone graft augmentation.

Technique

DIP joint arthrodesis can be performed under regional anesthesia or even digital block anesthesia using finger tourniquet control. The technique involves a dorsal exposure of the joint, followed by removal of all remaining articular cartilage. The natural contour of the head of the middle phalanx may be retained if it matches well with the resulting contour of the base of the distal phalanx following removal of articular cartilage. Typically, a reasonable fit is obtainable, but bone defect causing shortening may be encountered, which may require either allograft or autograft supplementation. Alternatively, the head of the middle phalanx and the base of the distal phalanx may be contoured into a cup and cone match.[19] Full extension to slight flexion is desirable for positioning of the joint and is limited due to fixation considerations. Fixation techniques for DIP joint arthrodesis include percutaneous pin fixation or low-profile, variable-pitch compression screw fixation.

Percutaneous pin fixation configurations include crossed pinning of the arthrodesis site or percutaneous longitudinal pinning with two parallel Kirschner wires. Longitudinal pinning is best done by advancing two 0.045-inch wires antegrade through the distal phalanx articular surface and exiting the tuft of the distal phalanx. The arthrodesis site is reduced. The wires are recovered beyond the skin of the fingertip and sequentially advanced in a retrograde manner such that the arthrodesis site is stabilized (Figure 11.3, *A* to *F*).

If a headless variable-pitch screw is chosen for fixation, attention must be paid to the dimension of the distal phalanx because the diameter of the bone in smaller individuals, particularly of the small finger, may not accommodate the caliber of the screw. This technique is detailed below.

❖ AUTHOR'S PREFERRED METHOD OF TREATMENT

DIP joint arthrodesis is accomplished through the extensile "H" incision (Figure 11.4). Full-thickness skin flaps are elevated and the terminal tendon is exposed. The terminal tendon is incised transversely, exposing the articular surfaces of the joint. Hyperflexion of the joint facilitates exposure of the articular surfaces. I avoid excessive shortening of the finger by using a 2-mm high speed bur to remove the remaining articular cartilage, preferably following the natural contours of the head of the middle

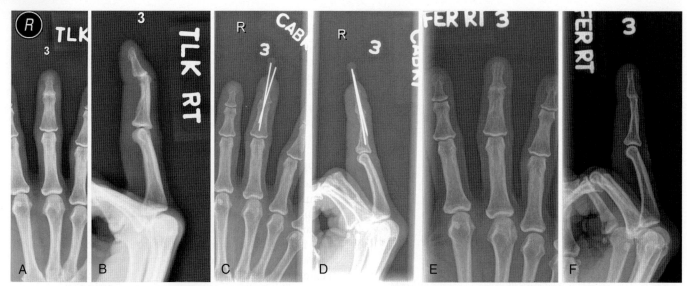

FIGURE 11.3 **A** and **B,** Preoperative radiographs of a 55-year-old female with distal interphalangeal (DIP) joint destruction following septic arthritis caused by an infected mucous cyst. **C** and **D,** Postoperative radiographs following DIP joint arthrodesis with K-wire stabilization. **E** and **F,** Final follow-up radiographs of healed DIP joint arthrodesis.

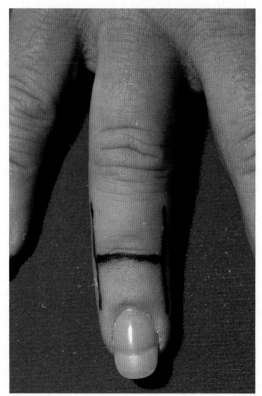

FIGURE 11.4 "H" incision for arthrodesis of the distal interphalangeal joint of the finger.

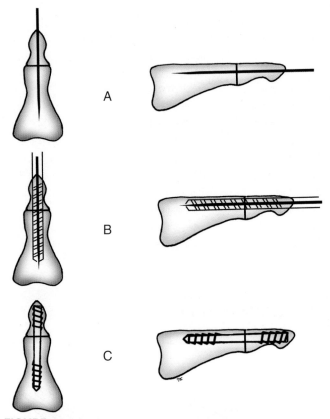

FIGURE 11.5 Arthrodesis of the distal interphalangeal joint with the use of a cannulated, low-profile headless compression screw. **A,** Guidewire placement. **B,** Placement of cannulated drill. **C,** Headless, variable-pitch compression screw placement. (© Mayo Clinic, Rochester, MN. Modified with permission.)

phalanx and the articular base of the distal phalanx. Though desirable, a tight, flush contact of surfaces is often not achieved; the arthrodesis site can be supplemented with a small portion of autograft or allograft material of choice. The position of full extension is generally preferred.

For fixation, I prefer a variable-pitch, headless compression screw no larger than 2.4 mm in diameter. This affords immediate, stable fixation and is available from a variety of different

manufacturers. Initially, a guidewire is driven retrograde to the level of the subchondral bone of the base of middle phalanx (Figure 11.5). A cannulated drill is advanced over the guidewire, and a screw of appropriate length is advanced across the arthrodesis. Care is taken to avoid inside-out contact with the nail bed. It is also important that the distal aspect of the compression screw be completely buried in the tuft of the distal phalanx so there is no screw prominence.

If inside-out contact with the nail bed occurs during placement of the compression screw, screw fixation is abandoned in favor of fixation with a 0.062-inch percutaneous pin placed longitudinally across the arthrodesis site in a retrograde fashion. To the extent possible, the drill track is packed with autograft or allograft bone substitute material. Placement of percutaneous pins or the cannulated drill bit and variable-pitch screw is done using biplanar fluoroscopy.

CRITICAL POINTS *Distal Interphalangeal Joint Arthrodesis*

Indications
- Osteoarthritis
- Posttraumatic arthritis
- Postseptic arthritis

Technique
- "H" incision
- Articular cartilage removed and joint surfaces matched (alternative is cup and cone technique)
- Fixation with headless screw or K-wires in extension or slight flexion
- Headless screws can cut out into nail bed if distal phalanx is of a small diameter.

Rehabilitation
- Immediate motion of the finger is permitted following headless screw fixation.

Outcomes
- High union rates can be anticipated with either head compression screw devices or K-wire fixation.
- Preoperative planning is important to avoid nail bed complications and prominent hardware.

Postoperative Management and Expectations

At 5 days following operation, the dressings are removed and the wound is inspected. Following DIP arthrodesis with a variable pitch, headless compression screw, a removable finger-based splint is fabricated by a hand therapist. The splint may be removed and immediate motion initiated. This should include active and passive range-of-motion exercises of the PIP, MCP, and wrist joints. Radiographs are obtained at 6- to 8-week intervals, and the splint is maintained until radiographic healing is evident.

If DIP arthrodesis is performed with percutaneous pin fixation, the wires are cut at the surface of the pulp of the finger and left in place for 8 weeks. The patient is treated with a nonremovable finger-based splint for 4 weeks, allowing active and passive MCP and wrist motion only. This is followed by fabrication of a removable finger-based splint allowing PIP motion at 4 weeks following operation. Radiographs are followed until solid fusion is achieved, at which time unrestricted activity is resumed.

Expected Outcomes. DIP joint arthrodesis is considered a reliable procedure. Accordingly, high rates of union and patient satisfaction can be expected.[144] Burton and coworkers reported

a 100% union rate using K-wire fixation,[17] and in 1984 Faithfull and Herbert originally reported on successful union using a headless compression screw.[33] More recently, Cox and colleagues and Matsumoto and associates have reported 94% and 97% union rates, respectively, for different compression screw devices at 12 months and 35 months of follow-up.[27,78] Alternatively, successful union has been reported using obliquely placed headless compression screws to avoid nail bed complications (96%)[48] as well as using fixation with a small plate placed laterally (100%).[75]

Complications. Mismatch between the caliber of the variable-pitch, headless compression screw and the diameter of the distal phalanx can result in inside-out damage of the nail bed, particularly in small individuals and particularly involving the small finger.[121] Furthermore, variable rates of nonunion, infection, and hardware prominence at the fingertip have been reported.[48,78] Stern and Fulton, for instance, in a study published in 1992, reported a nonunion rate of 12% and a complication rate of 21%.[121] Less common complications include malunion, cold intolerance, reflex sympathetic dystrophy, paresthesias, PIP joint stiffness, and skin necrosis.[121]

Proximal Interphalangeal Joint Arthrodesis
Indications and Contraindications

The principle indication for PIP joint arthrodesis is painful primary osteoarthritis or posttraumatic osteoarthritis that is refractory to nonoperative measures. Patients will often complain of diminishing motion of the joint in conjunction with aching pain with use. Other indications are unreconstructable fractures, fracture-dislocations, or chronic instability of the joint.

Contraindications for the procedure are recent infection or a poor soft tissue envelope. A relative indication for PIP joint arthrodesis is a history of septic arthritis. Patients with residual articular destruction following chronic septic arthritis may under certain circumstances be considered for arthrodesis, assuming that the level of pain and functional loss warrant the intervention. Bone loss is a relative indication for arthrodesis in that bone can often be reconstructed in such a way as to achieve arthrodesis when the appropriate fixation is used.

Preoperative Planning

Critical to preoperative assessment and planning are dedicated, high-quality PA and lateral radiographs of the finger. It is important to identify the appropriate implant for arthrodesis; surgeon preference is the deciding factor in most circumstances. In cases of trauma where bone loss has occurred, fixation must be planned in order to best accommodate the bone deficiency. It is also important to identify any periarticular degenerative cyst formation, which may necessitate bone graft augmentation and fixation modification.

Technique

Arthrodesis of the PIP joint is performed under regional anesthesia and upper arm or forearm tourniquet control. A dorsal longitudinal incision can be used in most patients. In patients with atrophic or compromised skin, a longitudinal incision can create insufficient skin margins for closure. A carefully designed serpentine incision over the dorsal aspect of the affected digit creates a flap well positioned to cover the hardware and arthrodesis site. The articular surfaces are exposed, and an osteotomy of the head of the proximal phalanx and the base of the middle phalanx is performed so that two flush bony surfaces are achieved. This requires the removal of the entire articular surface of the head of the proximal phalanx and the entire articular base of the middle phalanx. Positioning of the PIP joint arthrodesis is critical. The index finger PIP arthrodesis is positioned in 30 degrees of flexion, and the arthrodesis position of each successive finger should be in approximately 10 degrees more of flexion (Figure 11.6). Realistically, accuracy of arthrodesis positioning cannot often be scrutinized to the 10-degree level; an arthrodesis position of 30 to 40 degrees is preferred for the index and long fingers and 50 to 60 degrees for the ring and small fingers in most cases.

Several fixation techniques are available for stabilization of the arthrodesis. Options include K-wire fixation with or without tension band wiring; variable-pitch, headless compression screw fixation; or small joint plate fixation. Tension band wire fixation will be detailed in the following section. Variable-pitch, headless compression screw fixation requires adequate bone stock and accurate screw placement. A 2.4-mm cannulated screw is preferred. Plate fixation uses a 2-inch low-profile plate, bent to accommodate the bone contours and desired angle of the arthrodesed digit. In general, it is desirable to achieve six cortices of fixation on both sides of the arthrodesis. Immediate mobilization of the finger is possible following tension band wiring, screw fixation, and plate fixation. The compression screw has a low profile and usually does not cause irritation, as some hardware might. Plate fixation of an arthrodesis is generally reserved for situations in which trauma-related bone loss has occurred and a corticocancellous bone graft is needed to fill the defect.

❖ AUTHOR'S PREFERRED METHOD OF TREATMENT

The extensor mechanism is incised longitudinally and the articular surfaces exposed subperiosteally. The collateral ligaments are released, providing further PIP joint flexion and enabling correction of any joint contracture. Using a handheld oscillating saw, the articular surfaces of the PIP joint are removed just proximal to the condylar flares of the proximal phalanx and just distal to the articular surface of the middle phalanx. The angle of the arthrodesis is imparted on the bony cut of the proximal phalanx. Beginning with the index finger at 30 degrees, the long, ring, and small fingers are positioned at 40, 50, and 60 degrees, respectively. The oscillating saw is used to create the thin middle phalanx cut, just proximal to the articular base. It is important to make these cuts perpendicular to the longitudinal axis of the digit; otherwise, an angulated digit will result.

Once the bony surfaces are prepared, irrigated, and dried, the arthrodesis is stabilized. The author's preferred method is a K-wire tension band technique (Figure 11.7, *A* to *D*). Using fluoroscopic guidance, two parallel 0.035-inch K-wires are drilled in a retrograde fashion perpendicular to the osteotomy cut at the distal aspect of the proximal phalanx. This is necessary in order that the K-wires, when driven antegrade, migrate down the center of the middle phalanx. It is important that the tips of the K-wires stop about 5 mm shy of the distal articular aspect of the middle phalanx because they will be advanced further later to capture the figure-of-eight tension band. Once the articular surfaces are stabilized, another 0.035-inch K-wire is drilled transverse to the axis of the middle phalanx through the dorsal cortex at the junction of the proximal and middle thirds of the shaft. Through this transverse hole, the 22-gauge wire is passed and then passed in a figure-of-eight fashion beneath the K-wires, which are still exposed beyond the dorsal cortex of the proximal phalanx. The 22-gauge wire is twisted several times on the radial or ulnar aspect of the digit prior to cutting and burying the twist. Although sometimes difficult, the twist of the wire can be turned down around the side of the digit to prevent prominence of the material beneath the skin. Next, the exposed K-wires are cut approximately 1 cm superficial to the dorsal cortex of the proximal phalanx and are bent 90 degrees in order to capture and secure the figure-of-eight wires. The figure-of-eight wire is gently driven down over the middle phalanx with a small bone tamp and mallet with the aid of fluoroscopic imaging. Bone grafting is usually not necessary (see Figure 11.7, *A* to *D*). The extensor mechanism is closed over the hardware, and the skin reapproximated. The wounds are sterilely dressed and placed in a forearm-based resting hand splint.

Postoperative Management and Expectations

The wounds are inspected at postoperative day 5, and a rigid finger-based splint supporting the affected digits is created by a hand therapist. The patient is allowed to remove the hand from the fabricated splint and begin gentle active range of motion. At 4 weeks following operation, most activities of daily living are resumed. Radiographs are assessed at 6 weeks and 12 weeks for healing of the arthrodesis. Once healing has been achieved

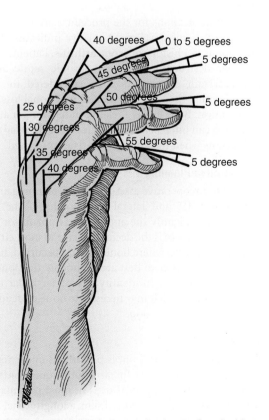

FIGURE 11.6 Drawing displaying the progressive degree of proximal interphalangeal joint arthrodesis flexion.

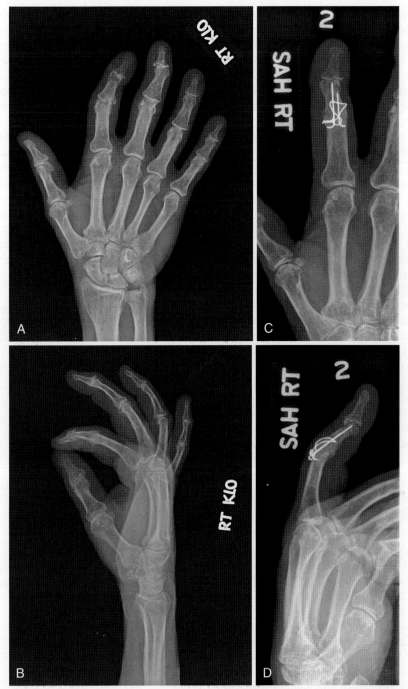

FIGURE 11.7 A and **B,** An 80-year-old male with gradual onset of index finger pain and limited mobility. **C** and **D,** Index finger with fresh interphalangeal joint arthrodesis.

CRITICAL POINTS *Proximal Interphalangeal Joint Arthrodesis*

Indications
- Osteoarthritis
- Inflammatory arthritis
- Posttraumatic arthritis
- Postseptic arthritis (relative)

Technique
- Dorsal midline incision
- Articular surfaces prepared so the angle of the arthrodesis is achieved on the proximal phalanx

- Angle of the arthrodesis for the index, long, ring, and small fingers is 30, 40, 50, and 60 degrees, respectively.
- Variety of fixation techniques available

Rehabilitation
- Immediate motion possible with most fixation techniques

Outcome
- High union rates can be expected using either K-wires and tension band wiring or headless compression screw fixation.
- Hardware removal is not unusual following fixation with K-wires and tension band wiring.

radiographically, the patient is released to full activity. The rationale behind tension band wiring of the PIP joint arthrodesis is that active flexion of the digit enhances compression of the arthrodesis surface.[62] Caution should be exercised in the patient with osteopenia or osteoporosis.

Expected Outcomes. High union rates have been reported using a number of fixation methods for PIP joint arthrodesis, including headless compression screws, K-wire fixation, and tension band wiring/K-wire techniques.[64,122] Carroll reported on 635 IP arthrodeses and found only a 5% nonunion rate.[19] Stern has reported a 97% fusion rate among 290 consecutive MCP and PIP joint arthrodeses using a tension band wiring technique.[122] A 98% union rate with the use of a headless compression screw has been reported by Ayres and colleagues.[6]

Throughout the arc of PIP joint flexion and extension, 5 degrees of adduction and 9 degrees of supination are anticipated.[85] Loss of this degree of freedom, as would be expected with PIP joint arthrodesis, has been shown to alter precision pinch in the index finger PIP joint.[31]

Complications. Nonunion, malunion, hardware prominence, fracture, infection, skin necrosis, and complex regional syndrome have been described as complications following arthrodesis of the PIP joint.[6,64,122] Ayres and associates reported fracture of the proximal phalanx following headless compression screw insertion.[6] Leibovic and Strickland reported on 3 of 224 PIP arthrodesis patients who ultimately required amputation, 1 for osteomyelitis and the other 2 for complications following the development of RSD.[64] Hardware removal can be anticipated in up to 9% of patients following PIP arthrodesis with K-wire and tension band wiring.[122]

Metacarpophalangeal Joint Arthrodesis
Indications and Contraindications

MCP joint arthrodesis is not typically recommended for osteoarthritis of the index, long, ring, and small fingers. It is, however, performed on the thumb MCP joint in cases of primary osteoarthritis or posttraumatic arthritis. Like the other arthrodeses, the procedure should not be performed in the setting of active or recent infection or in patients with a poor skin envelope. Reconstruction of chronic arthritis following a history of remote septic arthritis is considered a relative indication.

Preoperative Planning

Critical to the preoperative assessment and planning are dedicated PA and lateral radiographs of the thumb. An appropriate fixation technique is chosen based on surgeon preference. It is important to identify any periarticular degenerative cyst formation or bone loss that may necessitate bone graft augmentation of the arthrodesis or dictate the fixation technique.

Technique

Arthrodesis of the thumb MCP joint is accomplished through a dorsal longitudinal incision. The extensor mechanism is incised in line with the skin incision and the arthritic joint exposed. As in the PIP joint, the proximal phalanx and the metacarpal head are prepared with a handheld oscillating saw. The preferred position for arthrodesis is 20 degrees of flexion. As previously described for preparation of the PIP joint arthrodesis surfaces, a transverse osteotomy of the base of the middle

phalanx is accomplished just proximal to the subchondral bone of the proximal articular surface of the thumb proximal phalanx. Next, the flexion angle of the arthrodesis is accomplished by orienting the oscillating saw 20 degrees volar, just proximal to the metacarpal head. The two bony surfaces are approximated and secured by any of several fixation techniques, including the tension band technique described for arthrodesis of the PIP joint. Alternatively, two crossing percutaneous K-wires placed from distal to proximal can be used. The K-wires can be removed in 8 weeks but are preferably maintained, if possible, until bony union is achieved. Fixation can also be achieved with a 2.0 dorsal plate, obtaining six cortices proximal and six cortices distal to the arthrodesis site. Variable-pitch, cannulated headless screw fixation with one or two screws is another option. Alternatively, use of a standard cortical screw and washer has been described. The extensor mechanism is closed and the skin approximated. A sterile dressing is applied, followed by a thumb spica splint.

CRITICAL POINTS *Metacarpophalangeal Joint Arthrodesis*

Indications
- Osteoarthritis
- Inflammatory arthritis
- Posttraumatic arthritis
- Postseptic arthritis (relative)

Technique
- Dorsal midline incision
- Articular surfaces prepared so that the angle of arthrodesis is achieved on the proximal phalanx
- Desired angle of arthrodesis is 20 degrees.
- Fixation techniques available include tension band wiring, screw fixation, and plate fixation.
- Bone graft may be required in some posttraumatic situations.

Rehabilitation
- Immediate motion is possible with most fixation techniques.

Outcome
- A high union rate can be expected using either the K-wire and tension band technique or the headless compression screw technique.
- The need for hardware removal following the K-wire fixation and tension band technique is relatively common.

Postoperative Management and Expectations

At 5 days following operation, the dressing and splint are removed, a removable forearm-based thumb spica splint is fabricated, and gentle active motion is initiated. For reasons stated previously, active motion, including pinch, is encouraged for patients with stabilization using the tension band wire or headless compression screw technique. Protective splinting is maintained, however, until radiographic healing is seen, at which time activity without restriction may resume.

Expected Outcomes. High union rates can be expected with arthrodesis of the MCP joint of the thumb, irrespective of the form of fixation. Breyer and colleagues compared healing rates of thumb MCP arthrodesis using either a tension band wiring technique or a headless compression screw technique. The union rate among 28 patients with the tension band technique was 92.8%, whereas the union rate among the 28 patients treated with a headless compression screw was 85.7%. Overall, there was no significant difference in healing rates.[15]

Complications. Much like arthrodesis of the PIP joint, complications following arthrodesis of the thumb MCP joint can include nonunion, malunion, hardware prominence, infection, and fracture. Breyer and associates found no significant differences in the incidence of nonunion, delayed union, infection, or intraoperative fracture when comparing arthrodesis using tension band wiring or headless compression screw fixation. However, 25% of patients in the tension band wiring group (7/28) required hardware removal, compared with no patients in the headless compression screw group. This reached statistical significance.[15]

Proximal Interphalangeal Joint Arthroplasty
Indications and Contraindications

Indications for use of the PIP surface replacement arthroplasty (SRA) include primary degenerative osteoarthritis or posttraumatic arthritis in elderly patients. Ideally, this would include less active patients who desire to maintain PIP joint motion in deference to arthrodesis. Relative indications include severe fractures or fracture-dislocations of the PIP joint in older, less active patients. Contraindications for use of PIP arthroplasty include current or chronic infection, loss of extensor mechanism integrity such that the patient has a boutonnière deformity, with either PIP joint extension lag or fixed flexion contracture, or complete absence of extensor function. Additional contraindications include poor or absent flexor tendon function, a poor soft tissue envelope including atrophic skin on the dorsum of the digit, absent PIP collateral ligament function, and incompetence of the PIP joint volar plate rendering the PIP joint unstable or creating a swan neck deformity.

Preoperative Planning

The preoperative evaluation should include a thorough assessment of patient expectations and a clear articulation of the activity restriction imposed by this procedure. Documentation should include PIP range of motion, angular deformity, joint stability, and soft tissue integrity. Dedicated PA and lateral radiographs of the digit centered over the PIP joint are necessary for templating purposes. Seldom do radiographs of the entire hand suffice. Irrespective of the device chosen for implantation, template devices are available from the device manufacturer.

Success has been reported with a variety of PIP joint implant arthroplasties, including the silicone, pyrocarbon, and surface replacement implants. Choice of the implant is largely left to surgeon preference and experience; evidence suggests that a semiconstrained implant is advantageous in the index PIP joint for resisting enhanced forces encountered during thumb-index pinch maneuvers.[68,71,85,90]

Technique

PIP implant arthroplasty can be performed using one of three surgical approaches, each having advantages and disadvantages: dorsal, lateral and anterior.[21,68,116] With the dorsal approach, care is taken to preserve the extensor tendon insertion at the base of

the middle phalanx. Complications with this approach can include extensor tendon dysfunction and the development of a boutonnière deformity. The volar plate must be repaired following the volar or anterior approach. Failure to do so may result in PIP joint hyperextension instability and the development of a swan neck deformity (Video 11.1). With the lateral approach, the ulnar collateral ligament must be repaired in order to prevent PIP joint instability.

With the pyrocarbon and surface replacement arthroplasties, the proximal phalanx is prepared in such a way that the collateral ligaments of the PIP joint are preserved, although it has been shown that up to 50% of the radial or ulnar collateral ligament can be sacrificed without compromising stability of the joint.[85] With the silicone implant, a more generous phalangeal osteotomy is required, which sacrifices the radial and lateral collateral ligament origins. Merle and coworkers have reported on a lateral approach technique for silicone implant placement that advances, embrocates, and repairs the ulnar and radial collateral ligaments following initial sectioning for exposure.[82] Their study discusses 51 arthroplasties in 43 patients with a mean follow-up of 36 months, finding an average axial deviation of 17 degrees. The middle phalanx is prepared in order to accept the stem of either the middle phalanx component or the stem of the silicone implant. The canals are prepared with device-specific broaches and, not uncommonly, are further modified with a high-speed bur. Implantation of undersized components is a common mistake in implant arthroplasty of the digits and can result in limited motion because of subsidence and subsequent bony impedance to flexion.[89,90]

Most authors currently recommend fixation of the pyrocarbon implant using a press-fit technique.[21,60,96,126,120] Iagil and Geijer and colleagues reported subsidence of up to 8% of the prosthetic length of the proximal phalanx component and up to 7% of the prosthetic length of the middle phalanx component.[128] Sweets and Stern reported a 48% radiographic loosening rate in their series of 31 patients, followed up at a minimum of 2 years.[126] Silicone is implanted as a spacer and, therefore, is stabilized with neither a cement nor a press-fit technique.

Debate continues concerning the use of cement for implantation of the SRA of the PIP joint. Originally, the PIP surface replacement was designed for implantation using cement,[70,71] but more recently there have been reports about a cementless version of the prosthesis and a press-fit technique.[74,90] Jennings and Livingstone reported that the majority of loosening complications in their series of 43 arthroplasties in 25 patients with an average follow-up of 37 months were the result of inadequate cement technique.[49] At an average follow-up of 4 years, Johnstone and associates compared the results of 18 patients with 27 cemented PIP SRAs, with 18 patients having 21 joint replacements using the uncemented PIP surface replacement version of the prosthesis with an average length of follow-up of 4 years. They reported a very strong association between cementless implantation and prosthetic subsidence. However, there was no correlation with the use of cement and postoperative pain, range of motion, or joint failure.[51] In a study of 67 PIP SRAs in 47 patients with a follow-up averaging 8.8 years, Murray and colleagues[90] showed no correlation with cement use and overall implant survival. Implant subsidence and radiolucencies about the prosthesis bore no clinical association with the patients' final results in their series. A dorsal incision is

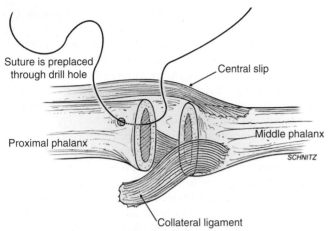

FIGURE 11.8 Dorsal approach for silastic implant arthroplasty of the proximal interphalangeal joint demonstrating the interval between the extensor mechanism and the ulnar collateral ligament. The ulnar collateral ligament is released and repaired in order to achieve the proper proximal phalanx cut. (From Bickel KD: The dorsal approach to silicone implant arthroplasty of the proximal interphalangeal joint. *J Hand Surg [Am]* 32(6):909–913, 2007.)

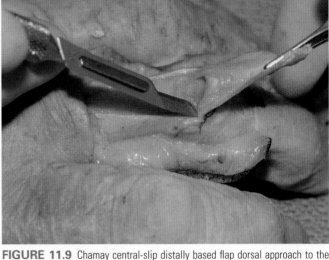

FIGURE 11.9 Chamay central-slip distally based flap dorsal approach to the proximal interphalangeal joint. (From Chamay A: A distally based dorsal and triangular tendinous flap for direct access to the proximal interphalangeal joint. *Ann Chir Main* 7(2):179–183, 1988.)

generally preferred for silicone spacer implantation of the PIP joint.[9] However, success has been reported with the use of the anterior approach as well as with the lateral approach as described by Segalman.[68,116] Merle and associates reported on 51 NeuFlex silicone spacers in 43 patients with a mean follow-up of 36 months. They found improvement in pain and function scores.[82] The primary technical distinction with silicone PIP arthroplasty is the more extensive proximal phalanx and middle phalanx bone resections required (Figure 11.8). The proximal phalanx cut is made just proximal to the articular head of the phalanx after the radial and collateral ligaments are released from the proximal phalanx (with either the anterior or dorsal approach) or the ulnar collateral ligament alone when using the lateral approach.

Whether approaching the joint laterally, where the ulnar collateral ligament only is taken down; anteriorly or dorsally, where both ligaments are taken down; or between the extensor mechanism and the ulnar collateral ligament, repair of the collateral ligaments is imperative. This is accomplished with the use of a 3-0 braided suture. Under most circumstances a cutting needle housing the suture can be used to penetrate the cortices of the proximal or middle phalanges. Alternatively, a free needle, a 2-mm drill bit, or a 0.045-inch K-wire can be used. The suture is first passed through the proximal phalanx and a Bunnell stitch is placed in the collateral ligament. Once the needle is passed back out of the ligament, it is again advanced through the proximal phalanx until it is taut and tied over the cortical bridge between the two holes in the cortex. If a drill or free needle is used to penetrate the cortex of the proximal phalanx, the needle is removed from the suture after it is passed through the ligament and the free ends are passed through the holes in the proximal phalangeal cortex and tied as before.

❖ AUTHOR'S PREFERRED METHOD OF TREATMENT

The bulk of my clinical experience with PIP joint arthroplasty has been with PIP SRA (Small Bone Innovations, New York,

NY). I prefer a dorsal, midline approach to the PIP. The extensor mechanism is incised and reflected according the technique described by Chamay[21] (Figure 11.9).

Remnants of the dorsal PIP joint capsule are identified and incised longitudinally.

As the joint is hyperflexed to expose the articular surfaces, it is imperative to protect the radial and ulnar collateral ligaments using small, narrow Hohmann retractors. Placement of the retractors will bring the articular surfaces of the proximal and middle phalanges into view, facilitating the bone cuts (Figure 11.10, A and B).

The proximal phalangeal head is prepared by accomplishing a perpendicular osteotomy just proximal to the most proximal extent of the articular surface. This cut is also perpendicular to the long axis of the proximal phalanx. Again, it is important to protect the proximal origin of the radial and ulnar collateral ligaments while using the handheld oscillating saw. At times, it may be necessary to release a small distal portion of the proximal phalangeal origin of the collateral ligaments to facilitate the proximal phalangeal osteotomy and subsequent prosthesis insertion. One biomechanical study has shown that up to 50% of the radial or ulnar collateral ligament may be undermined or released with little biomechanical consequence.[85] In some patients with heterotopic bone adjacent to the collateral ligaments, proximal release of the collateral ligament with repair back to the proximal phalanx may be necessary to facilitate prosthetic implantation. It has been, however, the author's experience that any release of the radial or ulnar collateral ligaments should be done cautiously and subsequently repaired.

A "chamfer" back cut of the proximal phalanx is necessary so the proximal phalanx can adequately accept the proximal phalangeal component (Figure 11.11). This important cut can be done with an oscillating saw, but the use of the saw may place the flexor tendons, volar plate, digital nerves, and arteries at risk. Alternatively, while protecting the volar plate with a small retractor, a high-speed 2-mm bur or a small rongeur can be used to make this cut.

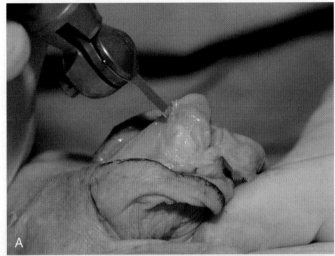

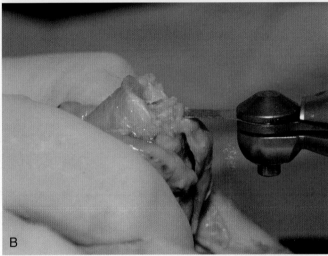

FIGURE 11.10 A and **B,** Proximal phalanx cut and middle phalanx articular "wafer" cut.

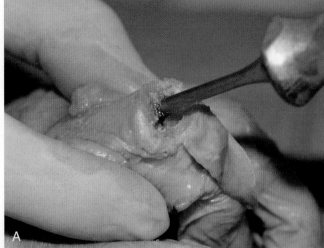

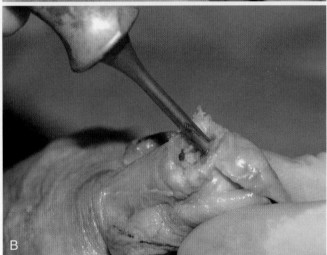

FIGURE 11.12 A and **B,** Broaching of the proximal phalanx and distal phalanx.

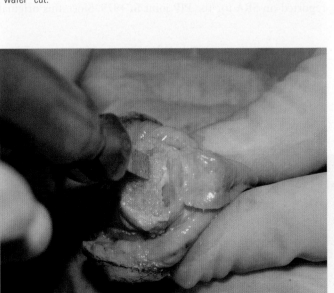

FIGURE 11.11 Chamfer back cut of proximal phalanx. This cut is necessary for placement of the proximal phalanx component.

After the proximal phalanx has been prepared, an oscillating saw is again used to make an osteotomy at the base of the middle phalanx, perpendicular to its long access. This is done while exercising caution not to violate the insertion of the central slip on the middle phalanx. Similar to the way in which the origin of the collateral ligaments on the proximal phalanx was protected, the collateral ligament insertions are protected with Hohmann retractors or simply by hyperflexion of the digit, bringing the base of the middle phalanx into full view. This osteotomy should be no more that 1 to 2 mm thick. Under circumstances of severe articular erosion or bone loss, adequate preparation of the bone surface may be accomplished with the use of a small rongeur, whereby the remaining articular cartilage is removed and subchondral bone exposed and an oscillating saw cut is not necessary.

Next, the proximal and middle phalanges are broached with the device-specific instrumentation. Specific proximal phalanx broaches and middle phalanx broaches are used (Figure 11.12, *A* and *B*). It is sometimes necessary to initially locate the intermedullary canal of the proximal or middle phalanx with a high-speed 2-mm bur. It is imperative to broach and then trial the proximal and middle phalanges to the largest size accepted by these bones. Failure to do so results in the implantation of undersized components, a common technical error.

Trial components are inserted next. Proximal and middle phalanx-specific impactors are available for trial component insertion. With the trial components in place, the digit is examined for range of motion and stability. If bony impingement occurs between the posterior cortices of the proximal and middle phalanges, the trial components are removed and their sizes reassessed or the canals are rebroached such that the largest trial components are accepted. Posterior osteophyte removal is sometimes necessary.

Once permanent components are chosen, they are delivered to the back table and kept in their protective packing. It remains my preference to insert the final components with a press-fit technique using clean gloves and the "no touch technique" whereby the implants are handled only with forceps. Using the proximal and middle phalanx component-specific impactors, the permanent components are seated. I reserve the use of cement for cases of osteoporosis or overly capacious canals. Patients who have substantial preoperative bone loss from degenerative cyst formation or following trauma may also require prosthesis implantation with cement. Alternatively, bone graft augmentation may be used in these patients. The extensor mechanism is repaired with a 3-0 nonabsorbable suture (Figure 11.13, *A* and *B*).

Postoperative Management and Expectations

Immediately following the operation, a volar plaster splint is placed with the MCP and PIP joints held in full extension. After 5 to 7 days, the initial dressing is removed and the patient is placed in a dynamic extension splint, affording active flexion and passive extension. During the first 6 weeks, the amount of active flexion is gradually increased every 2 weeks in the following progression: 30 degrees for the first 2 weeks, 60 degrees for the next 2 weeks, and 90 degrees for the next 2 weeks. At the end of 6 weeks, full digital flexion and extension are permitted

> ## CRITICAL POINTS *Proximal Interphalangeal Joint Surface Replacement Arthroplasty*
>
> ### Indications
> - Osteoarthritis
> - Posttraumatic arthritis
> - Inflammatory arthritis (relative)
>
> ### Technique
> - Dorsal, volar, or lateral incision
> - Preservation of the radial and ulnar collateral ligaments
> - Broach and trial components to the largest allowable size
> - Assess for bony impingement
> - Components press fit
> - Cement reserved for overly capacious canals or patients with osteoporosis
>
> ### Rehabilitation
> - Early motion allowed with constraints based on surgical approach
> - Extension outrigger for passive extension or flexion block is used following dorsal approach
> - Unrestricted range of motion is permitted at 6 weeks postoperative
> - Nighttime extension splinting may be necessary after 6 weeks if extension lag present
>
> ### Outcome
> - Good pain relief and modest improvement in range of motion and function expected
> - Similar results are found irrespective of surgical approach
> - Controversy exists regarding the use of cement
> - 16% failure rate at 15 to 25 years has been reported

without the splint. The dynamic outrigger device is continued for an additional 6 weeks if an extension lag is present.

Expected Outcomes

Surface Replacement Arthroplasty. Linscheid and Dobyns first reported on SRA for the PIP joint in 1979. Since this original

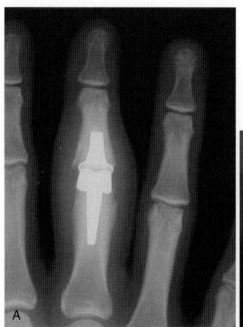
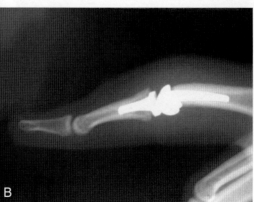

FIGURE 11.13 A and **B,** Postoperative radiographs showing proximal interphalangeal-surface replacement arthroplasty implanted with press-fit technique.

report, there has been general agreement that patient satisfaction is good and function is improved.[70] In 1997, Linscheid and Murray reported on 66 PIP joint SRA implants in 47 patients over a 14-year period, with a mean follow-up of 4.5 years. Results were good in 32 fingers, fair in 19, and poor in 15. Results in this study were better in patients with the dorsal approach. There was a 12-degree increase in range of motion in these patients.[71] Jennings and Livingstone reported on 43 SRA implants in 25 patients with an average follow-up of 37 months. They found a nominal increase in range of motion; 26 patients were very satisfied and 12 fairly satisfied; 5 were not satisfied. There were 11 failures, which were attributed to the lack of cement use in these joints.[49] Luther and colleagues reported on 24 PIP SRAs in 23 patients followed for an average of 27 months.

There was an average increase of range of motion of 21 degrees. Seventy percent of the patients were satisfied overall with the result of the operation; however, 58% of the patients needed a reoperation.[74]

Murray and associates[90] provided further follow-up on their original 1997 series from the Mayo Clinic with a report on 67 SRA PIP implants in 47 patients followed for a mean of 8.8 years. The mean range of motion was 40 degrees. The failure rate was found to increase from 3% at 1 year to 8% at 3 years, 11% at 5 years, and 16% at 15 to 25 years. Prostheses implanted through a volar approach failed more often than those implanted through a dorsal approach. Failure rates did not differ among patients with degenerative arthritis, rheumatoid arthritis, or posttraumatic arthritis. The use of cement also did not affect results.[90] Johnstone and coworkers[51] compared 18 patients who had 27 cemented PIP SRA implants with 18 patients who had 21 uncemented PIP SRA implants with a follow-up of 4 years and 6 years, respectively. Although functional results were not significantly different, there were 13 implants in the uncemented group with subsidence and loosening compared with 1 in the cemented group, leading the authors to favor the use of cement for the implantation of this prosthesis.

Other areas of controversy exist regarding the outcomes of the SRA implants. Despite earlier reports citing superior results with the dorsal approach, Stoecklein and coworkers have reported good results with significant improvements using the volar approach in six patients with an average follow-up of 35 months.[71,89,90,124] In another study that included 91 SRA implants, Pritsch and Rizzo reported that 26 reoperations were necessary; extensor mechanism dysfunction was identified as the most common reason for failure.[107] Daecke and colleagues[28] recently reported a prospective multicenter study involving 62 PIP SRAs among 43 patients followed up at 35 months. They noted comparable results among pyrocarbon, SRA, and silicone devices, with a tendency toward greater early range of motion in the pyrocarbon and SRA devices compared with the silicone devices. There were significantly more complications with the pyrocarbon and SRA devices compared with the silicone devices. Adams and associates published a metaanalysis finding that the dorsal approach produced the most successful result.[1]

Pyrocarbon Implant. Nunley and colleagues[96] reported disappointing results with the pyrocarbon PIP implant, with no real improvement postoperatively with respect to scores on the Disabilities of the Arm, Hand, and Shoulder (DASH) scale and

pain scale. The range of motion actually decreased at an average 17-month follow-up.[96] Subsequent studies have been more encouraging. Bravo and associates[14] reported on 50 implants in 35 patients at a minimum follow-up of 27 months, finding an overall patient satisfaction rate of 80% and a revision rate of 8%. Similarly, Mashhadi, McGuire, and Tagil and Geijer and their colleagues, each with midterm follow-up, reported improvements in pain and function as well as good patient satisfaction.[77,80,128] Osteolysis and implant subsidence in 40% of joints have been reported.[80,128] Wijk and associates have reported on 53 joints in 43 patients with an average follow-up of 24 months. On average, rates of pain at rest, pain with activity, patient satisfaction, and occupational performance as well as DASH scores all improved. There were seven reoperations, and the range of motion and grip strength did not improve.[147]

Sweets and Stern reported on their experience with pyrocarbon arthroplasty of the PIP joint in a series of 31 arthroplasties in 17 patients with an average follow-up of 55 months. They found a decrease in average range of motion postoperatively from 57 degrees to 31 degrees. Six joints required a reoperation, and implant migration was severe for seven proximal phalanx implants and three distal phalanx implants.[126] Although Ono and coworkers[97] reported improvement in pain on average and good patient satisfaction, they found a complication rate of 42.9% in their series of 21 implants in 13 patients. Presumably in an earlier report on the same cohort of patients, Chung and colleagues[24] noted implant squeaking in three patients and implant dislocation in three patients.

Silastic Implant. Success with the use of the silicone PIP joint spacer has been reported by many investigators. Swanson and colleagues[125] reported on 424 implants with a minimum of 1 year of follow-up. In this series, the majority of digits had at least 40 degrees of range of motion. Lin and associates analyzed 69 silicone PIP spacers at an average follow-up of 3.4 years. Pain was improved in 67 of the 69 digits. Range of motion was not improved following operation.[68] Takigawa and associates[130] reviewed 70 implants in 48 patients at an average follow-up of 6.5 years. They found no significant change in the active range of motion or correction of deformity, but pain had been relieved in 70% of patients.

Recently, several comparative studies involving the silicone spacer have been published. One study compared the NeuFlex implant (Small Bone Innovations, New York, NY) and Swanson implant, finding better objective results with the Swanson implant but better patient satisfaction with the NeuFlex implant at 34 months of follow-up.[120] Chan and coworkers[22] compared pyrocarbon arthroplasty with silicone implants in a systemic analysis. In this study, 35 citations were identified, and the authors found no clear superiority of pyrocarbon arthroplasty over silicone implants; they expressed concern over the number of identified complications in the pyrocarbon implants. Branam and colleagues[11] reviewed 41 arthroplasties in 22 patients, comparing results of silicone implants and pyrocarbon implants. At an average of 45 months of follow-up, the results were comparable, although 8 of the 19 pyrocarbon joints squeaked. Interestingly, Adams and associates[1] concluded in a recent metaanalysis that in general, the effectiveness of PIP joint arthroplasty has not been adequately established, citing short-term follow-up and insufficient data as limiting the value of current evidence.

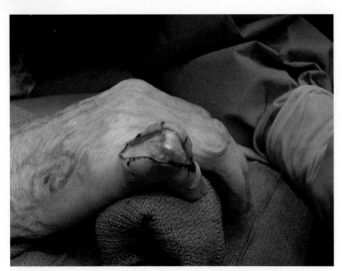

FIGURE 11.14 Proximal interphalangeal-surface replacement arthroplasty implant has failed because of extensor mechanism incompetence.

Complications. Complications from implant or spacer arthroplasty of the PIP joint are largely dependent on the surgical approach and device used. Extensor mechanism failure is a complication with the dorsal approach and in one study, accounted for the majority of indications for reoperation[107] potentially leading to the development of a boutonnière deformity (Figure 11.14). Alternatively, the anterior approach can lead to failure of the volar plate and the development of a swan neck deformity.

For the purpose of clarity, complications specific to the individual devices have been mentioned in the outcomes section above. Silicone spacer devices are known to fracture over time but may remain in service even if fractured. Stern and Ho have cautioned about the use of silicone spacer implants because of concerns about the development of instability with pinch.[123] Problems encountered with the pyrocarbon implant osteoplasty include squeaking, osteolysis, prosthesis migration, and dislocation.[24,80,97] Interestingly, infection has only rarely been reported among implant arthroplasty series of the hand, perhaps because the vasculature supply of the hand is robust.

Metacarpophalangeal Joint Arthroplasty
Indications and Contraindications

Most indications for MCP arthroplasty are in patients with rheumatoid arthritis, and the vast majority of published reports involve rheumatoid patients. Osteoarthritis of the MCP joint can be seen primarily in the index and long fingers as well as the thumb. Nonoperative measures such as splinting, medication with nonsteroidal antiinflammatory drugs (NSAIDs), activity modifications, and injections are often helpful in primary osteoarthritis or posttraumatic osteoarthritis. When nonoperative measures fail, arthroplasty may be indicated for the relief of pain but generally not for functional improvement. For MCP arthroplasty to be considered, adequate bone stock is necessary as well as a stable soft tissue envelope. For the nonconstrained pyrocarbon or metal-on-plastic surface replacement implants, this means preservation of the radial and ulnar collateral ligaments.

Contraindications to arthroplasty include compromised or atrophic skin as well as acute infection and a local open wound. A relative indication is a remote history of infection, but in certain well-controlled circumstances, replacement of a degenerative joint following a remote history of MCP joint septic arthritis may be indicated. Situations such as these should be scrutinized on a case-by-case basis.

The operative technique for MCP arthroplasty, including preoperative planning and postoperative management, will be discussed in Chapter 55.

Expected Outcomes

Pyrocarbon Implant. It is generally recognized that nonconstrained pyrocarbon implants have better material properties than silicone implants; however, limited follow-up data are available for the treatment of MCP joint osteoarthritis.[26,107] Parker and colleagues have reported on 21 MCP joints treated with pyrocarbon arthroplasty in the context of a study involving 142 total implants, with an average of 17 months of follow-up. Amid the osteoarthritis group, pain and function improved as did the arc of motion (from 44 degrees before operation to 58 degrees following operation), oppositional pinch (126% improvement), and grip (40% improvement).[100]

Silastic Implant. Silastic implant arthroplasty remains the standard for reconstruction of the MCP joints.[107,125] Rettig and Luca[109] reported on 13 MCP silicone implants in 12 patients, finding good or excellent overall improvement in all patients at an average of 40 months of follow-up. Increases in joint flexion were seen, but grip strength at follow-up was well below average. Neral and coworkers[93] reported on 30 patients with 38 MCP silicone implant arthroplasties at a follow-up of 56 months. They found improvement in range of motion and function and less pain. As with Rettig and Luca, no difference was found for grip strength. Overall, 73% were satisfied with the outcome of surgery. Namdari and Weiss have also reported good results with the use of a silicone implant for MCP joint osteoarthritis at 4 years of follow-up.[92]

Other Procedures. A surface replacement, metal-on-plastic MCP arthroplasty device has been developed as another option. The anatomic design of this implant (Small Bone Innovations, New York, NY) as well as its material properties are intriguing. To date, no series has reported on the clinical results of this implant, and currently its use is relegated to experimental protocols. Pain relief has been reported with the Tupper resection-interposition volar plate arthroplasty in one recent small series of patients, which included two patients with posttraumatic osteoarthritis of the MCP joint.[69]

Complications

Deformity and fracture of silicone implant arthroplasties following years of service are well recognized. Trail and coworkers found an implant fracture rate of 66% at 17 years among 1000 implants reviewed retrospectively.[135] Periprosthetic erosions have been reported, as have radiolucent lines surrounding pyrocarbon implants; the latter have been considered benign.[100] Ulnar drift with extensor tendon subluxation can complicate the use of either implant. Implant squeaking can occur with pyrocarbon implants.

OSTEOARTHRITIS OF THE CARPOMETACARPAL JOINT OF THE THUMB

Epidemiologic Findings

The prevalence of osteoarthritis of the thumb CMC joint is striking, with the condition affecting up to 10% of women in the middle years of life. Postmortem studies have found thumb CMC arthritis in 75% of cases.[98] In a study by Armstrong and colleagues, 143 postmenopausal women were found to have a 25% prevalence of thumb CMC osteoarthritis; 55% of patients with combined CMC and scaphotrapezial osteoarthritis of the thumb had pain.[5] The condition is regarded as a major cause of disability in the aging population.

Evaluation

Physical Examination

Patients with osteoarthritis of the thumb CMC joint may present with varied complaints of pain localized to the area or more vague complaints of throbbing or even burning in the radial aspect of the hand. A thorough physical examination of the joint begins with inspection. Patients with more advanced osteoarthritis will often display a thumb adduction contracture and a compensatory thumb MCP joint hyperextension deformity. Examination of the thumb MCP joint in these patients will show laxity of the joint in hyperextension. The degree of MCP joint instability can have implications for surgical management of the arthritic CMC joint when trapeziectomy procedures are indicated. This will be discussed in more detail later in this chapter.

After inspection, the CMC joint is evaluated using the grind test and joint subluxation test. To perform the CMC grind test, the examiner faces the patient, rests the patient's hand on a hand examining table, stabilizes the wrist with one hand, and applies an axial load to the thumb axis. Pain may be elicited as well as crepitus as the degenerative articular surfaces are compressed. The CMC subluxation test is done in a similar fashion, although the objective is to gently force the CMC joint to sublux; the examiner determines whether this elicits a pain response. Crepitus may also be apparent. Additionally, pinch strength testing, such as the two-point key pinch test or three-point chuck pinch test using a dynamometer, may be helpful when absolute values are compared with those of the contralateral side (Video 11.2). Pinch maneuvers such as the two-point or lateral pinch test may increase forces across the CMC joint by a factor of 12. The examiner should be aware that the association of carpal tunnel syndrome with CMC osteoarthritis approaches 30%.

Diagnostic Imaging

Radiographs to profile the thumb CMC joint include PA, lateral, and oblique views of the hand or, alternatively, PA and lateral views of the wrist. A Robert view of the thumb CMC joint is also helpful because it is a true PA view of the joint (Figure 11.15). The Robert view requires special positioning of the arm and hand that some patients may find difficult, particularly if they have limited or painful motion of the shoulder. The Robert view is obtained with the arm and hand in a combination of positions, including shoulder flexion, shoulder internal rota-

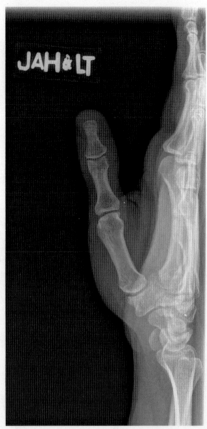

FIGURE 11.15 Robert's true PA radiograph of the thumb carpometacarpal (CMC) joint of a 52-year-old female with stage III CMC osteoarthritis.

tion, and wrist hyperpronation, so that the dorsal surface of the thumb can be placed directly on the radiograph cassette. Advanced imaging studies such as MRI or CT scanning are seldom necessary for operative procedures or surgical decision making about the thumb CMC joint.

Eaton and colleagues have described a widely accepted radiographic staging system for thumb CMC joint degenerative arthritis[32]:

Stage I: Normal or slight widening of the joint shadow due to synovitis

Stage II: Mild joint shadow narrowing with osteophyte formation of 2 mm or less

Stage III: Marked joint shadow narrowing with osteophyte formation of more than 2 mm

Stage IV: Stage III disease with scaphotrapezialtrapezoidal osteoarthritis

Although helpful for radiographic description and explanation, this staging system has never shown correlation with the intraoperative extent of disease or treatment outcome, irrespective of the treatment chosen.

ANATOMY AND BIOMECHANICS

The thumb CMC joint evolved as an unstable articulation providing prehension, opposition, and circumduction, which distinguished human hand function from that of the higher-order mammals. The joint is a biconcave, reciprocating saddle joint with little inherent stability. What stabilization it has is provided

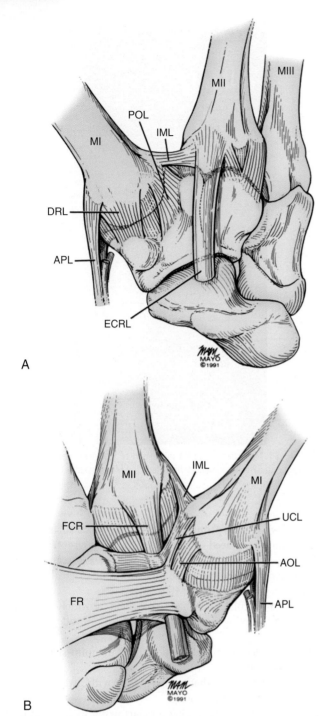

FIGURE 11.16 A, Posterior view and **B,** anterior view showing ligamentous anatomy of the thumb carpometacarpal joint. *APL,* Abductor pollici longus; *AOL,* anterior oblique ligament; *DRL,* dorsal radial ligament; *ECRL,* extensor carpi radialis longus; *FCR,* flexor carpi radialis; *FR,* flexor radialis; *IML,* intermetacarpal ligament; *MI,* metacarpal I; *MII,* metacarpal II; *MIII,* metacarpal III; *POL,* posterior oblique ligament; *UCL,* ulnar collateral ligament. (© Mayo Clinic, Rochester, MN. Modified with permission.)

by 16 ligaments, and it rests in pronation (Figure 11.16, *A* and *B*). There is a discrepancy in articular diameter; the thumb metacarpal articular surface is 34% smaller than the distal articular surface of the trapezium.

The primary stabilizer of the thumb CMC joint is the deep anterior oblique ligament, or palmar "beak" ligament. The deep anterior oblique ligament is an intracapsular ligament emanating from the volar tubercle of the trapezium and inserting on the ulnar volar aspect of the first metacarpal. The ligament tightens with pronation, abduction, and extension, preventing ulnar translation and dorsal translation of the first metacarpal relative to the trapezium. The ligament's obliquely oriented fibers serve to create a center of rotation about which the CMC joint may rotate. The superficial anterior oblique ligament tightens with pronation and extension of the thumb.

Other ligaments that contribute substantially to thumb CMC joint stability include the dorsoradial ligament and posterior oblique ligament, which stabilize and inhibit dorsal translation and ulnar translation of the joint, respectively. The dorsal intermetacarpal ligament of the thumb prevents radial translation of the thumb metacarpal as well as proximal migration of the thumb metacarpal following trapeziectomy.

Ultrastructurally, Mobargha and associates have noted in 11 patients with osteoarthritis that the deep anterior oblique ligament was composed of disorganized connective tissue, with little evidence of collagen fibers and few signs of innervation. Mechanoreceptors were identified in the dorsoradial ligament, and it was found to be innervated to a much greater extent than the anterior oblique ligament. In contrast, the collagen bundles of the dorsoradial ligament were found to be better organized. No association was noted with ligament innervation patterns and patient age.[86]

High compressive forces occur across the thumb CMC during pinch; they may reach in excess of 12 times the applied load and may approach 20 times the applied load during maximum grasp. Cantilever bending occurs with these applied forces such that shear forces are created that are highest at the volar half of the joint's articular surface. These forces are enhanced with CMC flexion, whereas the volar portion of the trapezial metacarpal joint is relatively unloaded.[88] Pellegrini has shown an association with degeneration of the volar half of the thumb CMC joint as the integrity of the deep anterior oblique ligament diminishes. Consequently, the dorsal cartilage is relatively spared, even in cases of advanced osteoarthritis.[102] In another study, Pellegrini showed that articular degeneration consistently involved a greater portion of the surface area of the trapezium compared with the metacarpal by a ratio of 3 : 1, and a decrease in this ratio was associated with more advanced disease.[103]

Treatment
Indications and Contraindications

Nonoperative Treatment. The first phase of management for patients with osteoarthritis of the thumb CMC joint is nonoperative treatment. This may include thumb spica splinting, which may be forearm or hand based but preferably leaves the thumb IP joint free for patient comfort. In addition to splinting, NSAIDs may be used orally or topically, depending on patient tolerance or physician preference. Outpatient hand therapy may consist of ultrasound, paraffin wax, heat, and deep tissue massage, along with activity modifications. The success of hand therapy protocols in these situations is variable. Sustained benefit from splinting and corticosteroid injections has been demonstrated by several authors[30,54]; however, one randomized, controlled, blinded trial has shown no difference in scores on the visual analog pain scale at 24 weeks when comparing a group treated with a thumb CMC joint steroid injection and another group treated with saline injection.[81]

First Metacarpal Osteotomy. Forces across the thumb CMC joint lead to cantilever bending and result in high concentrations of shear forces across the volar half of the joint. These forces are believed to be causative in the preferential development of osteoarthritis of this segment of the thumb CMC joint. Therefore, a 30-degree closing wedge, extension osteotomy of the thumb metacarpal has been theorized to unload the volar segment of the thumb CMC joint by redistributing the load through the more dorsal segment of the joint. The first metacarpal osteotomy is indicated for patients with stage I or II disease but contraindicated in patients with hypermobility, fixed subluxation, or hyperextension of the joint.

Tomaino[134] reported on 12 patients with stage I disease treated with extension osteotomy of the thumb metacarpal. All osteotomies healed within 7 weeks; 11 of the 12 were satisfied with the outcome, and all had increased grip and pinch strength at 2 years of follow-up. Parker and colleagues reviewed eight patients with stage I, II, or III disease at an average of 9 years of follow-up. They found that pinch and grip strength had improved and excellent functional outcomes were obtained in six of the eight patients.[99]

Ligament Reconstruction. For patients with stage I or II disease of the thumb CMC joint, ligament reconstruction alone may be preferred over other salvage techniques. Instability of the volar ligamentous complex of the joint, particularly the deep anterior oblique ligament, has been forwarded as a potential cause of osteoarthritis of the joint.[37] In a biomechanical study, Koff and coworkers have shown that ligament reconstruction improved stability of the joint.[60] It has generally been felt that ligament reconstruction be reserved for patients with very mild articular changes and that it is contraindicated in patients with stages III and IV disease.[98]

Resection Arthroplasty. The majority of reconstructive procedures for thumb CMC osteoarthritis involve resection arthroplasty of the trapezium, with removal of the articular base of the first metacarpal with or without ligament reconstruction and with or without interposition of autograft material. This procedure is typically reserved for patients with stage III or IV disease, although durability of this procedure has been reported in a younger population with stage I disease.[148] In 1984, Burton and Pellegrini described a technique for "advanced osteoarthritis of the thumb CMC joint," in part based on the procedure described by Eaton and Littler for reconstruction of the deep anterior oblique ligament.[18] This procedure involves resection of the trapezium and base of the first metacarpal, along with a stabilization procedure they termed the *flexor carpi radialis sling suspension interposition,* in which, similar to the Eaton and Littler procedure, a portion of the flexor carpi radialis (FCR) tendon is used to reconstruct the deep anterior oblique ligament (or perhaps more accurately, the intermetacarpal ligament) and to create an interposition arthroplasty, filling the void left by trapezium resection. Theoretically, this interposition and deep anterior oblique ligament reconstruction provides support and resists subsidence of the thumb metacarpal.

A number of different approaches to advanced thumb CMC arthritis have been described, centered on the concept of resection arthroplasty. Weilby has reported on a technique which involves passing half of the FCR tendon around the abductor pollicis longus (APL) tendon, making a suspension lattice in the void created by the trapezium resection.[142,143] Routing a slip of the APL tendon around the extensor carpi radialis longus (ECRL)[23] or passing half of the FCR around the ECRL has also been described to gain suspension and may be beneficial in revision procedures.

Kuhns and colleagues have described a procedure whereby no interposition material or ligament reconstruction was employed. Temporary K-wire stabilization is performed. They termed the procedure the *hematoma and distraction arthroplasty*.[35,43,63] Excision of the trapezium alone without stabilization of any kind has been reported by Gervis as well as others.[29,41]

Carpometacarpal Thumb Arthrodesis. Arthrodesis of the thumb CMC joint has historically been indicated for the young, high-demand laborer in whom stability and grip strength are considered a premium. More recently, the indications have been expanded to include older, less active patients, as an alternative to trapeziectomy with ligament reconstruction.[112] It is generally agreed that advanced osteoarthritis of the scaphotrapeziotrapezoidal (STT) joint is a contraindication to CMC joint arthrodesis, but there is less agreement about the relevance of mild or moderate osteoarthritis of the STT articulation. One challenge with CMC arthrodesis is the need for prolonged immobilization because notable nonunion rates have been reported.[112] Nevertheless, most continue to indicate this procedure in the young active individual.

Carpometacarpal Thumb Arthroplasty. Implant arthroplasty of the thumb CMC joint has met with varied, if not unpredictable, results. Several devices have been developed and used. These include the de la Caffinière prosthesis; Guepar implant; Elektra and Braun-Cutter implants and surface replacement arthroplasty (Small Bone Innovations, New York, NY); and Orthosphere implant (Wright Medical Technology, Memphis, TN). Among the most used and evaluated thumb CMC prostheses is the de la Caffinière prosthesis, which is a semiconstrained ball and socket design with both components cemented. The metacarpal component is made of cobalt chromium, and the trapezium component is a polyethylene cup. The Guepar prosthesis is also a cemented prosthesis with a cobalt chrome metacarpal component that snap-fits into a polyethylene trapezium component and functions in a constrained fashion. The Elektra prosthesis is a modular design made of cobalt chrome and threads into the trapezium. The Braun prosthesis is a cemented design that consists of a metallic metacarpal and a polyethylene socket. The Avanta SR TMC prosthesis is a cemented total joint surface replacement with matching sloped, saddle-shaped components approximating the natural contours of the base of the first metacarpal and the articular surface of the trapezium, with the trapezium component made of cobalt chrome and the first metacarpal component made of polyethylene.[7,65] Polycarbon has been used to develop replacement arthroplasties and hemiarthroplasties of the thumb CMC joint, including the pyrolytic carbon anatomic interposition arthroplasty, the pyrocarbon implant (BioProfile/Tornier, Montbonnot Saint Martin, France), the Pyrodisk (Integra Life Sciences, Plainsboro, NJ), and the pyrocarbon interposition implant (Pi2), which is a pyrolytic carbon interpositional disk (BioProfile/Tornier). The pyrolytic carbon hemiarthroplasty is a resurfacing implant with a stem that press-fits into the thumb metacarpal (NuGrip, Integra Life Sciences). This prosthesis has been used in patients with stage II or III disease. Confidence in many of these devices is hampered by its relatively recent use and high loosening rates.[44,108,139,140]

The most experience with implant arthroplasty of the thumb CMC joint is with silicone implants such as the Swanson implant (Wright Medical Technology) or Niebauer implant. In longer-term analysis of these implants, problems identified included breakage, subluxation/dislocation, bone erosion, and silicone synovitis; therefore, these implants are no longer available.[18,84,129] Regarding particulate debris synovitis, no clear best treatment alternative has been identified.[91] Interestingly, Umarji and colleagues[137] have recently reported their experience with 10 patients who had revision surgery with a silastic finger joint implant spacer following failure of simple trapeziectomy. At an average follow-up of 53 months, 9 of the 10 patients reported improvement in pain and were generally satisfied with their function.

Other Procedures and Devices

Artelon Implant. Porous polyurethane-urea (Artelon, Small Bone Innovations, Morrisville, PA) has been extensively trialed as an interpositional material following trapeziectomy. Multiple studies have called into question its efficacy, however. In a retrospective study, Blount and colleagues have reported that 37% of patients had their implants explanted, largely due to pain or extrusion of the implant.[10] Jorheim and associates, in a matched cohort study, were unable to show any advantage of the spacer over a tendon suspension procedure.[53] Similarly, Nilsson and coworkers could not show superior results with the implant compared with tendon interposition procedures.[94] Robinson and Muir, in a report of three cases, have described a histologic foreign body reaction that caused pain requiring removal of the implant.[113] Based on these recent series, use of this implant is generally not recommended.

Carpometacarpal Arthroscopy. Small joint arthroscopy procedures have been advocated by some for limited synovectomy and ligament stabilization through thermal shrinkage for stage I disease; however, outcome data are limited.[98] Arthroscopy has also been advocated for partial resection of the thumb CMC joint and the STT joint with reported success.[2,25]

Operative Techniques

First Metacarpal Osteotomy. The first metacarpal is approached through a dorsal longitudinal incision and exposed subperiosteally in the interval between the extensor pollicis longus (EPL) and extensor pollicis brevis (EPB) tendons. This requires elevation of the thenar muscles off of the radial aspect of the metacarpal. Care is taken to protect branches of the radial sensory nerve. In the ulnar proximal aspect of the wound, the deep branch of the radial artery is identified, along with two accompanying veins. These structures are retracted with the aid of a small vessel loop. Two curved Hohmann retractors are placed radially and ulnarly around the first metacarpal in order to fully expose the base of the first metacarpal. A location for the osteotomy is chosen approximately 1 cm distal to the trapezial metacarpal joint. The joint may be identified by making a small incision through the trapezium and first metacarpal joint capsule. A microsagittal saw is used to accomplish a transverse

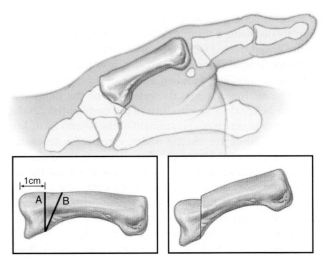

FIGURE 11.17 Wilson first metacarpal osteotomy for stage I and II carpometacarpal osteoarthritis. (© Mayo Clinic, Rochester, MN. Modified with permission.)

osteotomy, perpendicular to the axis of the first metacarpal and parallel to its base (Figure 11.17). The saw is stopped at the level of the volar cortex and removed, but the saw blade is left in place. A second saw blade is used to make a second cut approximately 2 mm distal to the first cut, and the two saw blades are converged at the level of the volar cortex. This will accomplish the desired 15-degree apex volar osteotomy.[99] A variety of different fixation options may be used to stabilize the first metacarpal, including crossed K-wires, crossed wires with a tension wire, or a small "T"-plate.

The author prefers to pass a 20-gauge surgical steel wire through drill holes made in the distal and proximal portions of the osteotomized metacarpal and then twist-tie the wires together, compressing the osteotomy surfaces. The wire twist is cut and bent beneath the thenar musculature on the radial aspect of the metacarpal. Drill holes through the metacarpal to accommodate the 20-gauge wire can be made with a 0.045-inch K-wire advanced perpendicular to the osteotomy sites in the proximal and distal portions of the metacarpal. Ideally the drill holes are made 5 mm proximal and distal to the osteotomy sites. The tension wire fixation is further augmented by a crossing 0.045-inch K-wire placed in a retrograde, oblique direction using fluoroscopy.

Following routine postsurgical wound inspection and management, a thumb spica cast is applied for 6 weeks; the percutaneous K-wire is removed when the cast is removed. The patient is transitioned to a removable forearm-based thumb spica splint and followed radiographically until healing occurs. At this time, the splint may be discontinued and full activity resumed.

Ligament Reconstruction. The standard volar (Wagner) approach is used. The thenar muscles are sharply dissected extraperiosteally from the underlying metacarpal, trapezium, and trapeziometacarpal (TMC) and scaphotrapezoid joints.

The deeper dissection begins at the transverse fascial fibers overlying the FCR tendon and continues distally along the overhanging ulnar border of the trapezium, from which the transverse carpal ligament attaches.

The proliferative synovium is débrided while preserving the joint capsule. The TMC joint is manually reduced to ensure that a concentric reduction is possible. The terminal branch of the superficial radial nerve courses along the dorsum of the metacarpal superficial and parallel to the EPB tendon. The nerve and EPB tendon are retracted, and the periosteum is incised parallel and volar to the EPB tendon 1 cm distal to the TMC joint. This is just distal to the abductor pollicis brevis insertion. The arthrotomies are closed with interrupted 3-0 braided nonabsorbable suture.

A volar-to-dorsal gouge tract of progressively larger diameters is created across the base of the metacarpal, parallel to the TMC joint and perpendicular to the metacarpal long axis. In harder bone, a 0.062-inch K-wire can be used to establish the initial tract orientation and facilitate gouge usage. The volar aspect of the gouge tract must be cleared of soft tissue and bone fragments to allow the smooth passage of the FCR tendon graft. A 28-gauge stainless steel wire is fed through the gouge tract, and the ends are clamped. Only half of the FCR tendon width is needed. The FCR tendon is identified at the proximal-ulnar extent of the primary incision.

The proximal tendon is isolated with blunt dissection and cleared of distal muscle fibers. A suture passer is gently bent at the tip and placed within the FCR sheath distally. As it is pushed proximally along the sheath, digital palpation ensures that the nylon loop remains volar to the tendon. The loop is delivered into the smaller proximal incision. A No. 2 monofilament suture is passed through the midportion of the tendon, and the needle is cut off. The two free ends of the suture are placed into the loop of the suture passer, which is drawn distally, bringing the monofilament suture limbs out of the distal end of the FCR sheath. The monofilament suture ends are grasped with a hemostat, and then with steady force the stitch is teased along the FCR tendon distally, splitting the tendon in half. The ulnar half of the tendon is used for the procedure; this ensures that the harvested tendon is in close apposition to the volar beak of the metacarpal. The ulnar portion of the FCR tendon is divided proximally, and the proximal free end of the FCR graft is delivered into the primary incision.

The FCR graft is held in a moist sponge and pulled distally just beyond the distal trapezium as it is separated from the intact tendon with a probe or fingertip. A loop is made in the previously placed 28-gauge wire and tightened around the last 2 mm of the tendon graft free end. The wire with tendon is drawn through the gouge tract from volar to dorsal. Using 3-0 braided nonabsorbable suture, a series of stay sutures are placed beginning with the periosteum of the dorsal metacarpal. During suturing, the joint is held reduced by an assistant. With the aid of a small hemostat, the free graft end is passed through and deep to the broad APL tendon insertion and across the volar capsule and sutured at both places. Finally, the FCR tendon graft is looped around the remaining FCR tendon and sutured to itself. It is important not to overtighten the graft. The thenar musculature is repaired anatomically with absorbable suture, beginning with the tagged slip of the APL tendon.

Gentle activities, including writing and typing, are allowed immediately as tolerated. The cast or splint is removed at 3 weeks, and progressive use and range-of-motion exercises are begun. Unlimited activities, including sports, are permitted at 6 weeks postoperatively.

Resection Arthroplasty. The trapeziectomy for thumb CMC osteoarthritis is essentially a resection arthroplasty procedure. In this procedure, a complete subperiosteal dissection is achieved so that the bone can be osteotomized with a small osteotome and removed in a piecemeal fashion. Next the base of the first metacarpal is prepared by removing the articular surface with a microsagittal saw. It should be noted that the osteotomy of the base of the first metacarpal requires removal of only a small wafer of bone of the first metacarpal should be removed. The trapeziectomy portion of this procedure has also been successfully performed with the small joint arthroscope; however, this technique generally involves resection of the distal half of the trapezium.[25]

Management of the CMC joint resection arthroplasty has been accomplished using a variety of methods:

1. *Hematoma:* The remaining capsule is closed over the defect and blood is allowed to fill the defect. A modification of this technique is to place thrombin-soaked Gelfoam in the defect.
2. *FCR sling suspensionplasty:* This classic method of reconstruction involves harvesting half or all of the FCR tendon, the base of which inserts on the base of the second metacarpal. The FCR is passed through the base of the first metacarpal, and the excess tendon is sutured together to create a ball, which in theory is used to provide a stable support for the thumb. It is important to understand that the FCR tendon may be absent, diminutive, or ruptured in some patients, and, in such cases, an alternative procedure would be necessary. Further details of this procedure are provided under Author's Preferred Technique.
3. *Weilby sling:* In this technique,[146] half of the FCR tendon is harvested and a lattice is created to support the thumb metacarpal by weaving the FCR back and forth in a figure-of-eight fashion between the APL and the remaining FCR (Figure 11.18).
4. *Thompson APL sling:* The entire APL is harvested at its musculotendinous junction, passed through a bone tunnel at the first metacarpal articular base, and passed through a transverse drill hole at the base of the second metacarpal. The remaining portion of the tendon is

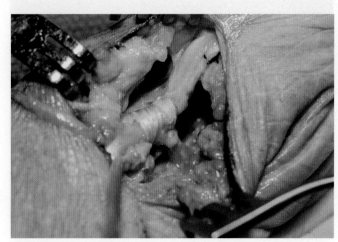

FIGURE 11.18 Weilby technique of flexor carpi radialis/abductor pollicis longus sling suspension.

woven around the ECRL tendon, in theory providing suspension to the first metacarpal. No interpositional material is placed into the void created by the trapeziectomy, according to Thompson's original description.[23] Chang and Chung have described a modification of the APL sling procedure whereby the most radial APL slip is released at the musculotendinous junction and advanced in a figure-of-eight fashion around the ECRL tendon, creating a sling for the first metacarpal of the thumb.

Carpometacarpal Arthrodesis. Exposure of the thumb CMC joint is gained through a dorsal longitudinal incision directly over the joint. Branches of the radial sensory nerve are identified and protected. The radial artery and accompanying veins are identified just proximal and ulnar to the thumb CMC joint and are retracted with a vessel loop. The interval between the EPB and the APL is used to expose the base of the first metacarpal and, subsequently, the trapezium in a subperiosteal fashion. The articular base of the first metacarpal and the distal articular surface of the trapezium are prepared by removing any remaining articular cartilage back to bleeding bone. The joint preparation is done in such a way that the contours of the opposing joint ends match and any voids are filled with autologous bone graft from the distal radius. The resultant fusion of the bone ends is stabilized by crossing 0.045-inch K-wires (Figure 11.19), which are placed percutaneously. Alternatively, a 2.4-mm low-profile "T"-plate can be used.

The thumb is placed in a thumb spica cast for 6 weeks, and the K-wires are removed at 6 weeks following operation. The patient is transitioned to a removable splint until radiographic arthrodesis can be determined. At that time, full activity may be resumed.

Carpometacarpal Arthroscopy. Thumb CMC arthroscopy involves the use of a 1.9-mm arthroscope inserted through either a 1R portal (positioned radial to the APL tendon) or a 1U portal (positioned ulnar to the EPB tendon).[3] The thumb may be suspended with a traction tower, with 5 to 10 pounds of traction applied. The 1R portal is helpful in visualizing the deep anterior oblique ligament insertion. A 25-gauge needle

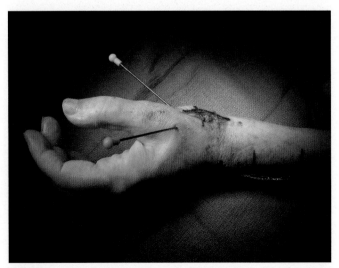

FIGURE 11.19 Carpometacarpal arthrodesis stabilized with cross K-wire technique.

with a small amount of saline may be used to inflate the thumb CMC joint through the 1U portal. With the scope through the 1R portal, the thumb CMC joint may be visualized. A 2.0-mm shaver may be inserted through the 1U portal for joint débridement. A 2.9-mm bur may also be inserted through the 1U portal to remove the distal articular surface of the trapezium. It is desirable to remove up to 4 mm of the distal trapezium in this fashion. Further details of small joint arthroscopy are described in Chapter 17. Once the partial trapeziectomy is complete, interpositional material such as autologous palmaris longus tendon or FCR tendon, Gelfoam, or GrafJacket (Wright Medical Technology, Memphis, TN) can be inserted.[3] Artelon has also been used in this manner, but recent studies question the predictability of its use.[10,53,94]

❖ AUTHOR'S PREFERRED METHOD OF TREATMENT

For patients with stage III or IV osteoarthritis of the thumb CMC joint, I prefer the trapeziectomy with the FCR sling suspension arthroplasty procedure. I have occasionally used the same procedure for older, less active patients with stage II disease, but in my experience, most patients with stage I and early stage II disease can be treated nonoperatively.

The patient is placed supine on the operating room table with the affected arm positioned comfortably on a hand table extension. After regional anesthesia is achieved, a well-padded upper arm tourniquet is applied and padding is also placed beneath the elbows, knees, and heels. The arm is prepped and draped, the limb exsanguinated, and the tourniquet inflated.

A longitudinal incision is made over the dorsum of the thumb CMC joint (alternatively, a volar radial or Wagner incision can be used) (Figure 11.20, *A* to *C*). The deep branch of the radial artery is identified and protected by placing a vessel loop around the artery and the accompanying veins. The dorsoradial sensory nerve branches to the thumb are also identified and protected. The dorsal capsule of the thumb CMC joint is incised in line with the skin incision. The trapezium is exposed in a subperiosteal fashion. Using a Hoke osteotome, the trapezium is osteotomized into four segments and removed piecemeal with a small rongeur, with care being taken to protect the FCR tendon at its insertion at the base of the second metacarpal. It is important to recognize that the FCR tendon is immediately deep to the trapezium and can be damaged with removal of the trapezium, particularly when overzealous attempts are made to remove osteophytes enshrouding the tendon. The trapezoid is also identified, as is the distal pole of the scaphoid. Care should be exercised not to violate the articular surface of these structures; however, they are carefully inspected for advanced osteoarthritis and treated accordingly. If there are advanced osteoarthritic changes at the scaphotrapezoidal articulation, resection of the proximal half of the trapezoid is performed with a one-quarter-inch osteotome and mallet. Interposition material is not used. With a 0.4-mm oscillating saw, the base of the first metacarpal is osteotomized, exposing subchondral bone. Next, using a curet and a 2-mm bur, an oval window is created over the dorsoradial aspect at the base of the first metacarpal, which communicates to the base of the first metacarpal and exits into the space previously occupied by the trapezium. During exposure of the base of the first metacarpal as well as during creation of the oval window, it is important to avoid the insertion of the APL tendon on the dorsal radial aspect of the

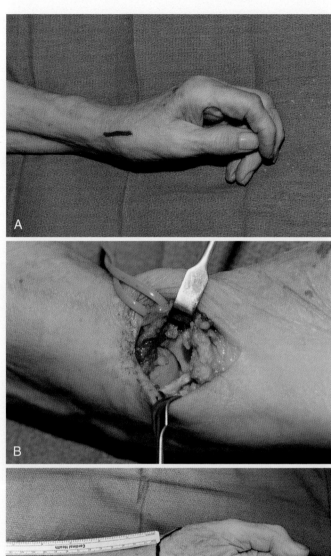

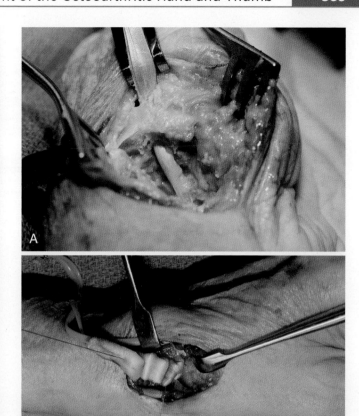

FIGURE 11.21 A, Flexor carpi radialis (FCR) tendon passed through osteoto-mized base of first metacarpal. **B,** FCR tendon anchovy achieved by placement of an alternating 2-0 nonabsorbable suture.

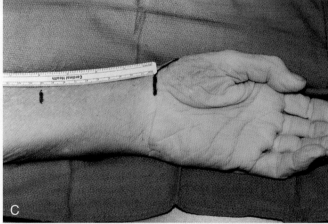

FIGURE 11.20 A, Dorsal approach with longitudinal incision for exposure of the thumb carpometacarpal joint. **B,** Following trapeziectomy. **C,** Wagner incision with transverse incision for flexor carpi radialis harvest positioned 10 cm proximal to the distal wrist flexion crease.

base of the first metacarpal. Using a 1-cm transverse incision in the forearm approximately 10 cm proximal to the wrist flexion crease, the myotendinous junction of the FCR tendon is identi-fied (see Figure 11.20, *C*). This is released sharply, and the FCR tendon is delivered into the distal wound. Thrombin-soaked Gelfoam can be placed in the base of the void created by the trapeziectomy. A 2-0 suture is placed in the proximal stump of the FCR tendon for the purpose of passing the tendon, and the FCR is delivered through the base of the first metacarpal and through the oval window with the aid of a small right angle. It

is tacked back upon itself using 2-0 nonabsorbable suture. A second nonabsorbable 2-0 suture is placed in the ulnar aspect of the capsule, deep in the wound. This 2-0 nonabsorbable suture is woven through the remaining FCR tendon so that it can be collapsed in accordion fashion into the void left by the trapeziectomy; the resulting FCR tendon "anchovy" is anchored into place, being secured with the limb of 2-0 nonabsorbable suture previously placed in the deep aspect of the void (Figure 11.21). The dorsal capsule of the thumb CMC joint is closed using a 4-0 absorbable suture.

At this point, the thumb MCP joint is assessed for stability. If more than 30 degrees of hyperextension instability is present, I favor some form of stabilization for the joint (Figure 11.22). This can include volar capsulodesis or MCP joint arthrodesis (described earlier in this chapter). Other described procedures include pinning of the MCP joint in flexion, sesamoid arthro-desis, or free palmaris longus tendon graft to the thumb MCP joint.[58]

The tourniquet is released prior to closure so hemostasis can be achieved. The wound is closed in layers using interrupted 4-0 absorbable suture for the CMC joint and subcutaneous tissue and 4-0 absorbable suture for the skin in a subcuticular fashion. A sterile dressing is applied. A thumb spica plaster splint is applied prior to leaving the operating room. See Case Studies 11.1 through 11.3.

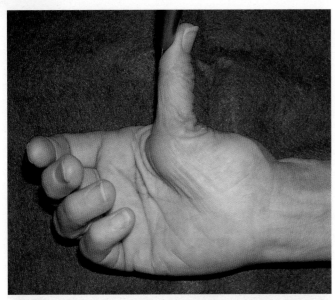

FIGURE 11.22 Hyperextension instability of the thumb MCP joint in the setting of advanced carpometacarpal osteoarthritis.

CRITICAL POINTS *Trapeziectomy and Flexor Carpi Radialis Sling Suspension Arthroplasty (LRTI)*

- A dorsal incision provides wide exposure to the trapezium.
- Identify the dorsal sensory nerve branches and the deep branch of the radial artery.
- Osteotomize the trapezium into pieces for removal with a rongeur.
- Using a 2-mm bur, create an oval window on the dorsal proximal aspect of the first metacarpal, avoiding the APL.
- Remove the articular surface of the base of the first metacarpal and a sliver of subchondral bone with a microsagittal saw.
- Carefully inspect the scaphotrapezoidal articulation for osteoarthritis and treat with resection of the proximal half of the trapezoid, if indicated.
- Protect the FCR tendon in the depths of the wound during extraction of the trapezium.
- Locate the FCR myotendinous junction 10 cm proximal to the wrist flexion crease.
- Harvest the entire FCR tendon and deliver the tendon into the trapeziectomy wound.
- Create an oval window and metacarpal base osteotomy of sufficient size to accommodate passage of the entire FCR tendon.
- Use the "anchovy procedure" for the remaining FCR tendon, securing it in the depths of the trapeziectomy wound with 2-0 nonabsorbable suture.

Postoperative Management and Expectations

Five to 7 days following surgery, provided the wound is in suitable condition, the patient is fitted for a removable custom forearm-based thumb spica splint with the thumb IP joint free. The splint is maintained for 6 weeks; it is removed daily for digital and wrist range-of-motion movements as well as hygienic care. This is followed by 6 weeks of strengthening, adaptation to activities of daily leaving, and occupational-related activities

as needed. Return to full activities is anticipated at 12 weeks following operation.

Expected Outcomes

First Metacarpal Osteotomy. Although studies are few and small in size, first metacarpal osteotomy is reliable in restoring thumb function and strength. Tomaino prospectively reported on 12 patients with stage I disease with follow-up at 2.1 years. All osteotomies had healed, and 11 of the 12 patients were satisfied with the outcome. Grip and pinch strength had both increased. Parker and colleagues,[99] in a longer-term follow-up, retrospectively reported on eight patients with a mean follow-up of 9 years. Excellent functional outcomes were reported in six of the eight patients, and the authors concluded that first metacarpal osteotomy is a durable procedure that has a predictable outcome in patients with early- to moderate-stage disease.

Resection Arthroplasty. Resection of the trapezium with or without ligament reconstruction and interposition has been shown by many authors to provide favorable results (Table 11.2), irrespective of the technique. More recently, different authors have published results comparing not only different technique modifications for traditional trapeziectomy and FCR sling suspension/interposition arthroplasty procedures but also suspension procedures using different tendons and, in some cases, synthetic material for the traditional trapeziectomy and FCR suspension/interposition procedure.

Davis and Pace compare in a prospective fashion the results of trapeziectomy and FCR ligament reconstruction and tendon interposition (LRTI) with or without K-wire stabilization and casting. At 1 year following surgery, clinical outcome measures did not differ among the two groups.[29] Field and Buchanan examined 65 patients randomized into two groups. One group had trapeziectomy alone and the other had FCR suspension-plasty. Patient satisfaction among the two groups was similar.[34] Gangopadhyay and associates[39] studied 174 thumbs in three groups: trapeziectomy alone, trapeziectomy with palmaris longus interposition, and trapeziectomy with suspensionplasty using half of the FCR tendon. At a minimum of 5 years of follow-up, they found no difference in pain relief, grip strength, pinch strength, and range of motion, causing them to conclude that there is no benefit from tendon interposition or ligament reconstruction following trapeziectomy for thumb CMC osteoarthritis.[39] In another study from the same group, Salem and Davis evaluated 114 thumbs in a randomized prospective series with a mean follow-up of 6.2 years, comparing trapeziectomy alone versus trapeziectomy and ligament reconstruction using FCR suspensionplasty and K-wire stabilization. Again, the authors found no difference in any subjective or objective outcome measures, causing them to conclude that evidence does not support the use of the LRTI procedure and K-wire stabilization following trapeziectomy.[114] Garcia-Mas and Sole Molins[40] compared the results of 94 thumbs that had been treated with partial trapeziectomy and FCR suspensionplasty with 18 thumbs treated with total trapeziectomy and FCR suspensionplasty and found no difference in outcome at a minimum of 3 years of follow-up.

It is worth noting that the partial trapeziectomy group included patients with stages II and III thumb CMC osteoarthritis, whereas all patients in the total trapeziectomy group had stage IV disease.[40] The approach to trapeziectomy was studied

TABLE 11.2 Studies of Carpometacarpal Arthroplasty

Technique	Study	Mean Follow-up Time (months)	Number of Procedures	Good to Excellent Outcome	Fair to Poor Outcome	Number of Complications	Male-to-Female Ratio	Level of Evidence
Double interposition	Barron, 1998[9]	34	21	95%	5%	4	8:12	IV
trapeziectomy, LRTI (FCR)	Burton, 1986[18]	24	25	92%	8%	2	3:21	IV
trapeziectomy, LRTI (APL)	Chang, 2008[23]	12	21	NA	NA	3	4:14	IV
trapeziectomy, LRTI (APL)	Kochevar, 2011[59]	66	25	94%	6%	0	1:17	IV
trapeziectomy, acellular matrix	Kokkalis, 2009[61]	30	82	NA	NA	6	15-67	IV
trapeziectomy	Kuhns, 2003[63]	24	26	96%	4%	2	7:19	II
trapeziectomy	Gray, 2007[43]	25	22	100%	0%	2	5:17	II
trapeziectomy, LRTI (APL-ECRL)	Sammer, 2009[115]	9	42	90%	10%	7	7:41	IV
trapeziectomy, LRTI (APL)	Soejima, 2006[119]	33.3	21	86%	14%	NA	2:16	IV
trapeziectomy, suture anchor/graft	Taghinia, 2008[127]	48	46	93%	7%	3	7:31	III
trapeziectomy, LRTI (FCR)	Tomaino, 1995[133]	108	24	95%	5%	3	3:19	IV
trapeziectomy, LRTI (Weilby)	Vadstrup, 2009[138]	12	106	83%	17%	18	18:87	II
trapeziectomy, LRTI (Weilby)	Vermeulen, 2009[143]	12	20	90%	10%	4	2:17	II
trapeziectomy	Wollstein, 2009[148]	86	8	100%	0%	NA	1:7	IV
trapeziectomy, FCR screw fixation	Wysocki, 2010[150]	19	29	NA	NA	1	5:24	IV
trapeziectomy, suture button suspension	Yao, 2013[152]	34	21	NA	NA	2	NA	IV
trapeziectomy, partial	Noland, 2012[95]	108	16	92%	7%	NA	4:9	IV

APL, Abductor pollicis longus; *ECRL,* extensor carpi radialis longus; *FCR,* flexor carpi radialis; *LRTI,* ligament reconstruction and tendon interposition.

by Ritchie and Belcher.[111] In this randomized study, they evaluated the results of trapeziectomy performed through either an anterior incision or a dorsal radial incision to the thumb CMC joint in 40 hands at a median follow-up of 33 months. They found that trapeziectomy performed through the anterior approach had better outcomes for power, scar tenderness, and overall patient satisfaction. The findings of these studies have been further amplified by Li and coworkers,[67] who published a systematic literature review that used electronic databases to identify previously published randomized controlled trials, including several of the previously mentioned studies, comparing trapeziectomy alone versus trapeziectomy with some form of FCR suspensionplasty and temporary K-wire stabilization. They concluded that neither procedure provided a clear benefit over the other.

Poulter and Davis[83,106] were unable to show any difference in outcome at 1 year for MCP joint hyperextension deformity of up to 30 degrees. For hyperextension beyond that, they showed that correction of the deformity was successful but were unable to draw definitive conclusions on how this affected outcomes. They did find value in volar plate advancement with suture anchors for correcting the MCP hyperextension deformity and

found little sustainable postoperative correction with simple, temporary K-wire fixation of the MCP joint.

In a follow-up questionnaire study comparing thumb CMC implant arthroplasty with trapeziectomy and FCR sling suspension arthroplasty, no significant difference could be demonstrated between the two. The device used was the de la Caffinière prosthesis (Stryker, Kalamazoo, MI) or Roseland prosthesis (DePuy Synthes, Warsaw, IN). Questionnaires regarding 89 CMC prosthetic implants were received, as well as questionnaires regarding 233 thumbs treated with trapeziectomy and the FCR sling suspension procedure. Given the cost of the implant and the fact that clear superiority of the implant could not be shown, the authors recommend trapeziectomy and FCR sling suspension as the preferred procedure for the treatment of thumb CMC osteoarthritis.[141]

In a randomized controlled study of 79 women over the age of 40 years with stage IV osteoarthritis of the thumb CMC joint, Vermeulen and colleagues[142] compared the clinical outcomes of trapeziectomy with the FCR sling suspension arthroplasty (Burton and Pellegrini technique) and the clinical outcomes of the FCR-APL suspension procedure (Weilby technique). At 3 months after surgery, the group treated with the Burton and

Pellegrini procedure demonstrated significant improvement in the Patient-Rated Wrist and Hand Function Evaluation, but by 12 months, no significant differences were seen in outcome scores or in rates of strength, return to work, patient satisfaction, or complications. The results led the authors to conclude that the trapeziectomy with the FCR suspension procedure using a bone tunnel offered a quicker initial recovery but by 1 year the results of the two procedures were similar.

A nuance of trapeziectomy with or without LRTI is the identification of scaphotrapezoidal involvement or the presence of stage IV disease. Tomaino and associates[134] have reported a sensitivity of radiographic diagnosis of 44% for scaphotrapezoidal disease and recommended visual inspection of the joint at the time of surgery. In the same study, the authors evaluated the results of proximal trapezoidal resection in 14 patients; they found no morbidity from the procedure and recommended its use in patients with trapezoidal osteoarthritis in the setting of thumb CMC osteoarthritis in order to prevent residual symptoms.

Carpometacarpal Arthrodesis. In a retrospective study of 59 trapezial metacarpal arthrodeses followed up at 7 years, Stern and Fulton[38] reported four nonunions following a technique that involved K-wire fixation and distal radius bone graft. Pain was assessed as an average of 1.5 on a scale of 10. In a more recent experience, the authors concluded that trapezial metacarpal arthrodesis in patients older than 40 years of age was successful for isolated trapezial metacarpal osteoarthritis. In a more recent, larger retrospective report, Rizzo and coworkers[112] reviewed 126 thumbs following trapezial metacarpal arthrodesis for osteoarthritis at an average follow-up of 11 years. Although they reported 17 nonunions, the oppositional pinch, grip strength, and pain scores of the entire group had significantly improved. Even though there was progression of osteoarthritis at the scaphotrapezoidal joint and MCP joint in 39 and 16 thumbs, respectively, over the study period, only 8 thumbs became symptomatic. The authors concluded that trapezial metacarpal arthrodesis improved functional results and resulted in excellent patient satisfaction despite the concomitant development of scaphotrapezoidal and first MCP osteoarthritis.

Carpometacarpal Arthroplasty. A number of implant arthroplasties have been designed for thumb CMC osteoarthritis. Perhaps the most widely used implant has been the de la Caffinière implant; however, it is no longer available. Johnston and colleagues[50] reported on 39 implants reviewed at 19 years. Survivorship was 73.9%, and patients continued to be satisfied with the implant arthroplasty. Lemoine and associates[65] reported on the Guepar prosthesis. In a retrospective review of 84 prostheses at 50 months, 92% of patients were satisfied with their results and more than 80% remained pain free. The authors concluded that use of this prosthesis for thumb metacarpal trapezial osteoarthritis is effective for improving strength and motion as well as providing a high degree of pain relief. However, it should be noted that less than half of patients had what would be typically considered advanced osteoarthritis of the thumb CMC joint. The authors go on to state that success with the use of this implant is dependent on compliance with the details of surgical technique. Badia and Sambandam[7] retrospectively reported on the results of the use of the Braun prosthesis in 26 thumbs with stages III and IV osteoarthritis of the thumb CMC joint. Ninety-six percent of patients reported complete pain

relief. The most widely used pyrolytic carbon device for the thumb CMC joint is the hemiarthroplasty. Martinez de Aragon and coworkers[76] have reported on 54 pyrolytic hemiarthroplasty implants; at 1.8 years, the survival rate was 80% and 71% of patients were pain free, but there was a high complication rate. Hansen and Snerum[44] reported on 17 Elecktra prostheses for the thumb CMC joint with a 35-month follow-up. Seven of the 10 prostheses had failed. Van Rijn and Gosens[140] reported on the results of the Avanta SR-TMC prosthesis (Small Bone Innovations, New York, NY) in 15 thumbs at a follow-up of 36 months. The range of motion and strength had not improved, but pain had subsided significantly.

Complications. The most common complication encountered with the first metacarpal osteotomy and the thumb CMC arthrodesis is nonunion. Fortunately, this complication is unusual, as is development of infection. Complications seen with implant joint replacement arthroplasty are loosening and subluxation. However, long-term studies for these implant arthroplasty procedures are not currently available. Implant subluxation is more often seen in the pyrocarbon hemiarthroplasty as reported by Martinez de Aragon and colleagues.[76] Kaszap and associates[55] have performed 15 secondary trapeziectomies following failure of trapeziometacarpal joint implant arthroplasty. Using subjective and objective evaluation measures, there was no difference in outcome when comparing secondary trapezium resection for revision surgery following failed CMC joint implant arthroplasty and primary trapeziectomy using a matched-pair analysis.

Following trapeziectomy, postoperative radiographic phenomena have been observed. Metacarpal subsidence has been demonstrated in excess of 30% with lateral pinch; however, this has not been shown to correlate with functional outcomes (Figure 11.23, A and B).[151] Yuan and coworkers[153] have reported on the development of carpal collapse following trapeziectomy. In a review of 33 wrists following surgery, they documented the increased presence of a dorsal intercalated segment instability deformity from 27% before operation to 50% following operation, noting an even greater tendency in patients with stage IV disease. Salem and Davis[114] have also shown the progression of degenerative changes in the pseudarthrosis site between the base of the first metacarpal and the scaphoid; however, these changes were not deemed clinically relevant in 25 thumbs at 6 years of follow-up.

Low and Hales[73] have reported a 25% incidence of FCR tendonitis 2 to 10 months following trapeziectomy and APL suspensionplasty, leading to persisting postoperative pain. Sixty percent of these patients required surgery, with some experiencing FCR rupture and pseudotendon formation. Jones and colleagues[52] have evaluated the consequences of and salvage options for complete FCR rupture during primary trapeziectomy and FCR sling suspensionplasty, including use of the partially ruptured FCR tendon or part of the ECRL tendon. Herniation of the tendon interposition material has been reported but can usually be treated with restabilization or excision of the material.[110]

Umarji and associates[137] have shown improvements in pain, pinch, activities of daily living, and overall satisfaction following silastic interposition finger arthroplasty treatment for failed trapeziectomy. This was a small series of 10 patients with an average follow-up of 53 months.

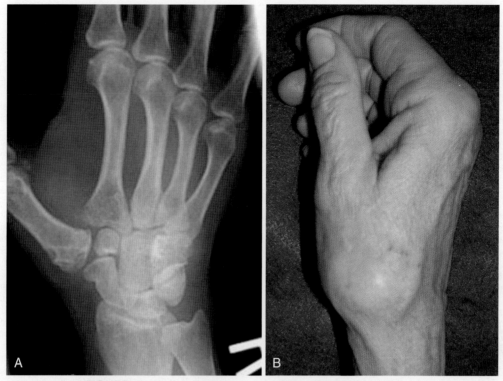

FIGURE 11.23 A and **B,** First metacarpal subsidence following trapeziectomy.

For Case Studies, Videos, and more, please visit ExpertConsult.com.

REFERENCES

1. Adams J, Ryall C, Pandyan A, et al: Proximal interphalangeal joint replacement in patients with arthritis of the hand: a meta-analysis. *J Bone Joint Surg Br* 94(10): 1305–1312, 2012.
2. Adams JE: Does arthroscopic debridement with or without interposition material address carpometacarpal arthritis? *Clin Orthop Relat Res* 472(4):1166–1172, 2014.
3. Adams JE, Steinmann SP, Culp RW: Bone-preserving arthroscopic options for treatment of thumb basilar joint arthritis. *Hand Clin* 27(3):355–359, 2011.
4. Allende BT, Engelem JC: Tension-band arthrodesis in the finger joints. *J Hand Surg [Am]* 5(3):269–271, 1980.
5. Armstrong AL, Hunter JB, Davis TR: The prevalence of degenerative arthritis of the base of the thumb in post-menopausal women. *J Hand Surg [Br]* 19(3):340–341, 1994.
6. Ayres JR, Goldstrohm GL, Miller GJ, et al: Proximal interphalangeal joint arthrodesis with the Herbert screw. *J Hand Surg [Am]* 13(4):600–603, 1988.
7. Badia A, Sambandam SN: Total joint arthroplasty in the treatment of advanced stages of thumb carpometacarpal joint osteoarthritis. *J Hand Surg [Am]* 31(10): 1605–1614, 2006.
8. Barron OA, Eaton RG: Save the trapezium: double interposition arthroplasty for the treatment of stage IV disease of the basal joint. *J Hand Surg [Am]* 23(2):196–204, 1998.
9. Bickel KD: The dorsal approach to silicone implant arthroplasty of the proximal interphalangeal joint. *J Hand Surg [Am]* 32(6):909–913, 2007.
10. Blount AL, Armstrong SD, Yuan F, et al: Porous polyurethaneurea (Artelon) joint spacer compared to trapezium resection and ligament reconstruction. *J Hand Surg [Am]* 38(9):1741–1745, 2013.
11. Branam BR, Tuttle HG, Stern PJ, et al: Resurfacing arthroplasty versus silicone arthroplasty for proximal interphalangeal joint osteoarthritis. *J Hand Surg [Am]* 32(6):775–788, 2007.
12. Brannon EW, Klein G: Experiences with a finger-joint prosthesis. *J Bone Joint Surg Am* 41(1):87–102, 1959.
13. Braun RM, Rhoades CE: Dynamic compression for small bone arthrodesis. *J Hand Surg [Am]* 10(3):340–343, 1985.
14. Bravo CJ, Rizzo M, Hormel KB, et al: Pyrolytic carbon proximal interphalangeal joint arthroplasty: results with minimum two-year follow-up evaluation. *J Hand Surg [Am]* 32(1):1–11, 2007.

15. Breyer JM, Vergara P, Parra L, et al: Metacarpophalangeal and interphalangeal joint arthrodesis: a comparative study between tension band and compression screw fixation. *J Hand Surg Eur Vol* 40(4):374–378, 2015.
16. Buchler U, Aiken MA: Arthrodesis of the proximal interphalangeal joint by solid bone grafting and plate fixation in extensive injuries to the dorsal aspect of the finger. *J Hand Surg [Am]* 13(4):589–594, 1988.
17. Burton RI, Margles SW, Lunseth PA: Small-joint arthrodesis in the hand. *J Hand Surg [Am]* 11(5):678–682, 1986.
18. Burton RI, Pellegrini VD, Jr: Surgical management of basal joint arthritis of the thumb. Part II. Ligament reconstruction with tendon interposition arthroplasty. *J Hand Surg [Am]* 11(3):324–332, 1986.
19. Carroll RE, Hill NA: Small joint arthrodesis in hand reconstruction. *J Bone Joint Surg Am* 51(6):1219–1221, 1969.
20. Carroll RE, Taber TH: Digital arthroplasty of the proximal interphlangeal joint. *J Bone Joint Surg Am* 36(5):912–920, 1954.
21. Chamay A: A distally based dorsal and triangular tendinous flap for direct access to the proximal interphalangeal joint. *Ann Chir Main* 7(2):179–183, 1988.
22. Chan K, Ayeni O, McKnight L, et al: Pyrocarbon versus silicone proximal interphalangeal joint arthroplasty: a systematic review. *Plast Reconstr Surg* 131(1):114–124, 2013.
23. Chang EY, Chung KC: Outcomes of trapeziectomy with a modified abductor pollicis longus suspension arthroplasty for the treatment of thumb carpometacarpal joint osteoarthritis. *Plast Reconstr Surg* 122(2):505–515, 2008.
24. Chung KC, Ram AN, Shauver MJ: Outcomes of pyrolytic carbon arthroplasty for the proximal interphalangeal joint. *Plast Reconstr Surg* 123(5):1521–1532, 2009.
25. Cobb T, Sterbank P, Lemke J: Arthroscopic resection arthroplasty for treatment of combined carpometacarpal and scaphotrapeziotrapezoid (pantrapezial) arthritis. *J Hand Surg [Am]* 36(3):413–419, 2011.
26. Cook SD, Beckenbaugh RD, Redondo J, et al: Long-term follow-up of pyrolytic carbon metacarpophalangeal implants. *J Bone Joint Surg Am* 81(5):635–648, 1999.
27. Cox C, Earp BE, Floyd WE, 4th, et al: Arthrodesis of the thumb interphalangeal joint and finger distal interphalangeal joints with a headless compression screw. *J Hand Surg [Am]* 39(1):24–28, 2014.
28. Daecke W, Kaszap B, Martini AK, et al: A prospective, randomized comparison of 3 types of proximal interphalangeal joint arthroplasty. *J Hand Surg [Am]* 37(9):1770–1779, 2012.
29. Davis TR, Pace A: Trapeziectomy for trapeziometacarpal joint osteoarthritis: is ligament reconstruction and temporary stabilisation of the pseudarthrosis with a Kirschner wire important? *J Hand Surg Eur Vol* 34(3):312–321, 2009.

30. Day CS, Gelberman R, Patel AA, et al: Basal joint osteoarthritis of the thumb: a prospective trial of steroid injection and splinting. *J Hand Surg [Am]* 29(2):247–251, 2004.

31. Domalain M, Evans PJ, Seitz WH, Jr, et al: Influence of index finger proximal interphalangeal joint arthrodesis on precision pinch kinematics. *J Hand Surg [Am]* 36(12):1944–1949, 2011.

32. Eaton RG, Lane LB, Littler JW, et al: Ligament reconstruction for the painful thumb carpometacarpal joint: a long-term assessment. *J Hand Surg [Am]* 9(5):692–699, 1984.

33. Faithfull DK, Herbert TJ: Small joint fusions of the hand using the Herbert Bone Screw. *J Hand Surg [Br]* 9(2):167–168, 1984.

34. Field J, Buchanan D: To suspend or not to suspend: a randomised single blind trial of simple trapeziectomy versus trapeziectomy and flexor carpi radialis suspension. *J Hand Surg Eur Vol* 32(4):462–466, 2007.

35. Fitzgerald BT, Hofmeister EP: Treatment of advanced carpometacarpal joint disease: trapeziectomy and hematoma arthroplasty. *Hand Clin* 24(3):271–276, vi, 2008.

36. Flatt A: Restoration of rheumatoid finger-joint function: interim report on trial of prosthetic replacement. *J Bone Joint Surg Am* 43:753–774, 1961.

37. Freedman DM, Eaton RG, Glickel SZ: Long-term results of volar ligament reconstruction for symptomatic basal joint laxity. *J Hand Surg [Am]* 25(2):297–304, 2000.

38. Fulton DB, Stern PJ: Trapeziometacarpal arthrodesis in primary osteoarthritis: a minimum two-year follow-up study. *J Hand Surg [Am]* 26(1):109–114, 2001.

39. Gangopadhyay S, McKenna H, Burke FD, et al: Five- to 18-year follow-up for treatment of trapeziometacarpal osteoarthritis: a prospective comparison of excision, tendon interposition, and ligament reconstruction and tendon interposition. *J Hand Surg [Am]* 37(3):411–417, 2012.

40. Garcia-Mas R, Sole Molins X: Partial trapeziectomy with ligament reconstruction: tendon interposition in thumb carpo-metacarpal osteoarthritis: a study of 112 cases. *Chir Main* 28(4):230–238, 2009.

41. Gervis WH, Wells T: A review of excision of the trapezium for osteoarthritis of the trapezio-metacarpal joint after twenty-five years. *J Bone Joint Surg Br* 55(1):56–57, 1973.

42. Granowitz S, Vainio K: Proximal interphalangeal joint arthrodesis in rheumatoid arthritis. A follow-up study of 122 operations. *Acta Orthop Scand* 37(3):301–310, 1966.

43. Gray KV, Meals RA: Hematoma and distraction arthroplasty for thumb basal joint osteoarthritis: minimum 6.5-year follow-up evaluation. *J Hand Surg [Am]* 32(1):23–29, 2007.

44. Hansen TB, Snerum L: Elektra trapeziometacarpal prosthesis for treatment of osteoarthrosis of the basal joint of the thumb. *Scand J Plast Reconstr Surg Hand Surg* 42(6):316–319, 2008.

45. Hogh J, Jensen PO: Compression-arthrodesis of finger joints using Kirschner wires and cerclage. *Hand* 14(2):149–152, 1982.

46. Hunter DJ, Zhang Y, Nevitt MC, et al: Chopstick arthropathy: the Beijing Osteoarthritis Study. *Arthritis Rheum* 50(5):1495–1500, 2004.

47. Ijsselstein CB, van Egmond DB, Hovius SE, et al: Results of small-joint arthrodesis: comparison of Kirschner wire fixation with tension band wire technique. *J Hand Surg [Am]* 17(5):952–956, 1992.

48. Iwamoto T, Matsumura N, Sato K, et al: An obliquely placed headless compression screw for distal interphalangeal joint arthrodesis. *J Hand Surg [Am]* 38(12):2360–2364, 2013.

49. Jennings CD, Livingstone DP: Surface replacement arthroplasty of the proximal interphalangeal joint using the PIP-SRA implant: results, complications, and revisions. *J Hand Surg [Am]* 33(9):1565, 2008.

50. Johnston P, Getgood A, Larson D, et al: De la Caffiniere thumb trapeziometacarpal joint arthroplasty: 16-26 year follow-up. *J Hand Surg Eur Vol* 37(7):621–624, 2012.

51. Johnstone BR, Fitzgerald M, Smith KR, et al: Cemented versus uncemented surface replacement arthroplasty of the proximal interphalangeal joint with a mean 5-year follow-up. *J Hand Surg [Am]* 33(5):726–732, 2008.

52. Jones DB, Jr, Rhee PC, Shin AY, et al: Salvage options for flexor carpi radialis tendon disruption during ligament reconstruction and tendon interposition or suspension arthroplasty of the trapeziometacarpal joint. *J Hand Surg [Am]* 38(9):1806–1811, 2013.

53. Jorheim M, Isaxon I, Flondell M, et al: Short-term outcomes of trapeziometacarpal Artelon implant compared with tendon suspension interposition arthroplasty for osteoarthritis: a matched cohort study. *J Hand Surg [Am]* 34(8):1381–1387, 2009.

54. Joshi R: Intraarticular corticosteroid injection for first carpometacarpal osteoarthritis. *J Rheumatol* 32(7):1305–1306, 2005.

55. Kaszap B, Daecke W, Jung M: Outcome comparison of primary trapeziectomy versus secondary trapeziectomy following failed total trapeziometacarpal joint replacement. *J Hand Surg [Am]* 38(5):863–871 e863, 2013.

56. Katzman SS, Gibeault JD, Dickson K, et al: Use of a Herbert screw for interphalangeal joint arthrodesis. *Clin Orthop Relat Res* (296):127–132, 1993.

57. Khuri SM: Tension band arthrodesis in the hand. *J Hand Surg [Am]* 11(1):41–45, 1986.

58. Klinefelter R: Metacarpophalangeal hyperextension deformity associated with trapezial-metacarpal arthritis. *J Hand Surg [Am]* 36(12):2041–2042, quiz 2043, 2011.

59. Kochevar AJ, Adham CN, Adham MN, et al: Thumb basal joint arthroplasty using adductor pollicis longus tendon: an average 5.5 year follow up. *J Hand Surgery [Am]* 36A:1326–1332, 2011.

60. Koff MF, Shrivastava N, Gardner TR, et al: An in vitro analysis of ligament reconstruction or extension osteotomy on trapeziometacarpal joint stability and contact area. *J Hand Surg [Am]* 31(3):429–439, 2006.

61. Kokkalis ZT, Zanaros G, Weiser RW, et al: Trapezium resection with suspension and interposition arthroplasty using acellular dermal allograft for thumb carpometacarpal arthritis. *J Hand Surg [Am]* 34(6):1029–1036, 2009.

62. Kovach JC, Werner FW, Palmer AK, et al: Biomechanical analysis of internal fixation techniques for proximal interphalangeal joint arthrodesis. *J Hand Surg [Am]* 11(4):562–566, 1986.

63. Kuhns CA, Emerson ET, Meals RA: Hematoma and distraction arthroplasty for thumb basal joint osteoarthritis: a prospective, single-surgeon study including outcomes measures. *J Hand Surg [Am]* 28(3):381–389, 2003.

64. Leibovic SJ, Strickland JW: Arthrodesis of the proximal interphalangeal joint of the finger: comparison of the use of the Herbert screw with other fixation methods. *J Hand Surg [Am]* 19(2):181–188, 1994.

65. Lemoine S, Wavreille G, Alnot JY, et al: Second generation GUEPAR total arthroplasty of the thumb basal joint: 50 months follow-up in 84 cases. *Orthop Traumatol Surg Res* 95(1):63–69, 2009.

66. Lewis AR, Ralphs JR, Kneafsey B, et al: Distribution of collagens and glycosaminoglycans in the joint capsule of the proximal interphalangeal joint of the human finger. *Anat Rec* 250(3):281–291, 1998.

67. Li YK, White C, Ignacy TA, et al: Comparison of trapeziectomy and trapeziectomy with ligament reconstruction and tendon interposition: a systematic literature review. *Plast Reconstr Surg* 128(1):199–207, 2011.

68. Lin HH, Wyrick JD, Stern PJ: Proximal interphalangeal joint silicone replacement arthroplasty: clinical results using an anterior approach. *J Hand Surg [Am]* 20(1):123–132, 1995.

69. Lin SY, Chuo CY, Lin GT, et al: Volar plate interposition arthroplasty for posttraumatic arthritis of the finger joints. *J Hand Surg [Am]* 33(1):35–39, 2008.

70. Linscheid RL, Dobyns JH: Total joint arthroplasty. The hand. *Mayo Clin Proc* 54(8):516–526, 1979.

71. Linscheid RL, Murray PM, Vidal MA, et al: Development of a surface replacement arthroplasty for proximal interphalangeal joints. *J Hand Surg [Am]* 22(2):286–298, 1997.

72. Lister G: Intraosseous wiring of the digital skeleton. *J Hand Surg [Am]* 3(5):427–435, 1978.

73. Low TH, Hales PF: High incidence and treatment of flexor carpi radialis tendinitis after trapeziectomy and abductor pollicis longus suspensionplasty for basal joint arthritis. *J Hand Surg Eur Vol* 39(8):838–844, 2014.

74. Luther C, Germann G, Sauerbier M: Proximal interphalangeal joint replacement with surface replacement arthroplasty (SR-PIP): functional results and complications. *Hand* 5(3):233–240, 2010.

75. Mantovani G, Fukushima WY, Cho AB, et al: Alternative to the distal interphalangeal joint arthrodesis: lateral approach and plate fixation. *J Hand Surg [Am]* 33(1):31–34, 2008.

76. Martinez de Aragon JS, Moran SL, Rizzo M, et al: Early outcomes of pyrolytic carbon hemiarthroplasty for the treatment of trapezial-metacarpal arthritis. *J Hand Surg [Am]* 34(2):205–212, 2009.

77. Mashhadi SA, Chandrasekharan L, Pickford MA: Pyrolytic carbon arthroplasty for the proximal interphalangeal joint: results after minimum 3 years of follow-up. *J Hand Surg Eur Vol* 37(6):501–505, 2012.

78. Matsumoto T, Nakamura I, Miura A, et al: Distal interphalangeal joint arthrodesis with the reverse fix nail. *J Hand Surg [Am]* 38(7):1301–1306, 2013.

79. McGlynn JT, Smith RA, Bogumill GP: Arthrodesis of small joint of the hand: a rapid and effective technique. *J Hand Surg [Am]* 13(4):595–599, 1988.

80. McGuire DT, White CD, Carter SL, et al: Pyrocarbon proximal interphalangeal joint arthroplasty: outcomes of a cohort study. *J Hand Surg Eur Vol* 37(6):490–496, 2012.

81. Meenagh GK, Patton J, Kynes C, et al: A randomised controlled trial of intra-articular corticosteroid injection of the carpometacarpal joint of the thumb in osteoarthritis. *Ann Rheum Dis* 63(10):1260–1263, 2004.

82. Merle M, Villani F, Lallemand B, et al: Proximal interphalangeal joint arthroplasty with silicone implants (NeuFlex) by a lateral approach: a series of 51 cases. *J Hand Surg Eur Vol* 37(1):50–55, 2012.

83. Miller NJ, Davis TR: Palmar plate capsulodesis for thumb metacarpophalangeal joint hyperextension in association with trapeziometacarpal osteoarthritis. *J Hand Surg Eur Vol* 39(3):272–275, 2014.

84. Minami A, Iwasaki N, Kutsumi K, et al: A long-term follow-up of silicone-rubber interposition arthroplasty for osteoarthritis of the thumb carpometacarpal joint. *Hand Surg* 10(1):77–82, 2005.

85. Minamikawa Y, Horii E, Amadio PC, et al: Stability and constraint of the proximal interphalangeal joint. *J Hand Surg [Am]* 18(2):198–204, 1993.

86. Mobargha N, Ludwig C, Ladd AL, et al: Ultrastructure and innervation of thumb carpometacarpal ligaments in surgical patients with osteoarthritis. *Clin Orthop Relat Res* 472(4):1146–1154, 2014.

87. Moberg E, Henrikson B: Technique for digital arthrodesis. A study of 150 cases. *Acta Chir Scand* 118:331–338, 1960.

88. Moulton MJ, Parentis MA, Kelly MJ, et al: Influence of metacarpophalangeal joint position on basal joint-loading in the thumb. *J Bone Joint Surg Am* 83(5):709–716, 2001.

89. Murray PM: New-generation implant arthroplasties of the finger joints. *J Am Acad Orthop Surg* 11(5):295–301, 2003.

90. Murray PM, Linscheid RL, Cooney WP, 3rd, et al: Long-term outcomes of proximal interphalangeal joint surface replacement arthroplasty. *J Bone Joint Surg Am* 94(12):1120–1128, 2012.

91. Murray PM, Wood MB: The results of treatment of synovitis of the wrist induced by particles of silicone debris. *J Bone Joint Surg Am* 80(3):397–406, 1998.

92. Namdari S, Weiss AP: Anatomically neutral silicone small joint arthroplasty for osteoarthritis. *J Hand Surg [Am]* 34(2):292–300, 2009.

93. Neral MK, Pittner DE, Spiess AM, et al: Silicone arthroplasty for nonrheumatic metacarpophalangeal joint arthritis. *J Hand Surg [Am]* 38(12):2412–2418, 2013.

94. Nilsson A, Wiig M, Alnehill H, et al: The Artelon CMC spacer compared with tendon interposition arthroplasty. *Acta Orthop* 81(2):237–244, 2010.

95. Noland SS, Saber S, Endress R, et al: The scaphotrapezial joint after partial trapeziectomy for trapeziometacarpal joint arthritis: long-term follow-up. *J Hand Surg [Am]* 37(6):1125–1129, 2012.

96. Nunley RM, Boyer MI, Goldfarb CA: Pyrolytic carbon arthroplasty for posttraumatic arthritis of the proximal interphalangeal joint. *J Hand Surg [Am]* 31(9):1468–1474, 2006.

97. Ono S, Shauver MJ, Chang KW, et al: Outcomes of pyrolytic carbon arthroplasty for the proximal interphalangeal joint at 44 months' mean follow-up. *Plast Reconstr Surg* 129(5):1139–1150, 2012.

98. Parker WL: Evidence-based medicine: thumb carpometacarpal arthroplasty. *Plast Reconstr Surg* 132(6):1706–1719, 2013.

99. Parker WL, Linscheid RL, Amadio PC: Long-term outcomes of first metacarpal extension osteotomy in the treatment of carpal-metacarpal osteoarthritis. *J Hand Surg [Am]* 33(10):1737–1743, 2008.

100. Parker WL, Rizzo M, Moran SL, et al: Preliminary results of nonconstrained pyrolytic carbon arthroplasty for metacarpophalangeal joint arthritis. *J Hand Surg [Am]* 32(10):1496–1505, 2007.

101. Pellegrini V: Hand osteoarthritis. In Glickel S, Bernstein S, editors: *Arthritis of the hand and upper extremity: a master skills publication*, Rosemount, IL, 2011, American Society for Surgery of the Hand, pp 167–176.

102. Pellegrini VD, Jr: Osteoarthritis of the trapeziometacarpal joint: the pathophysiology of articular cartilage degeneration. I. Anatomy and pathology of the aging joint. *J Hand Surg [Am]* 16(6):967–974, 1991.

103. Pelligrini VD, Jr: Osteoarthritis of the trapeziometacarpal joint: the pathophysiology of articular cartilage degeneration. II. Articular wear patterns in the osteoarthritic joint. *J Hand Surg [Am]* 16(6):975–982, 1991.

104. Peter JB, Pearson CM, Marmor L: Erosive osteoarthritis of the hands. *Arthritis Rheum* 9(3):365–388, 1966.

105. Potenza AD: Brief note. A technique for arthrodesis of finger joints. *J Bone Joint Surg Am* 55(7):1534–1536, 1973.

106. Poulter RJ, Davis TR: Management of hyperextension of the metacarpophalangeal joint in association with trapeziometacarpal joint osteoarthritis. *J Hand Surg Eur Vol* 36(4):280–284, 2011.

107. Pritsch T, Rizzo M: Reoperations following proximal interphalangeal joint nonconstrained arthroplasties. *J Hand Surg [Am]* 36(9):1460–1466, 2011.

108. Regnard PJ: Electra trapezio metacarpal prosthesis: results of the first 100 cases. *J Hand Surg [Br]* 31(6):621–628, 2006.

109. Rettig LA, Luca L, Murphy MS: Silicone implant arthroplasty in patients with idiopathic osteoarthritis of the metacarpophalangeal joint. *J Hand Surg [Am]* 30(4):667–672, 2005.

110. Rhee PC, Shin AY: Complications of trapeziectomy with or without suspension arthroplasty. *J Hand Surg [Am]* 39(4):781–783, quiz 784, 2014.

111. Ritchie JF, Belcher HJ: A comparison of trapeziectomy via anterior and posterior approaches. *J Hand Surg Eur Vol* 33(2):137–143, 2008.

112. Rizzo M, Moran SL, Shin AY: Long-term outcomes of trapeziometacarpal arthrodesis in the management of trapeziometacarpal arthritis. *J Hand Surg [Am]* 34(1):20–26, 2009.

113. Robinson PM, Muir LT: Foreign body reaction associated with Artelon: report of three cases. *J Hand Surg [Am]* 36(1):116–120, 2011.

114. Salem H, Davis TR: Six year outcome excision of the trapezium for trapeziometacarpal joint osteoarthritis: is it improved by ligament reconstruction and temporary Kirschner wire insertion? *J Hand Surg Eur Vol* 37(3):211–219, 2012.

115. Sammer D, Shah H, Shauver M, et al: The effect of ulnar styloid fractures on patient-related outcomes after volar locking plating of distal radius fractures. *J Hand Surg [Am]* 34:1595–1602, 2009.

116. Segalman KA: Lateral approach to proximal interphalangeal joint implant arthroplasty. *J Hand Surg [Am]* 32(6):905–908, 2007.

117. Seitz WH, Jr, Sellman DC, Scarcella JB, et al: Compression arthrodesis of the small joints of the hand. *Clin Orthop Relat Res* 304:116–121, 1994.

118. Sodha S, Ring D, Zurakowski D, et al: Prevalence of osteoarthrosis of the trapeziometacarpal joint. *J Bone Joint Surg Am* 87(12):2614–2618, 2005.

119. Soejima O, Hanamura T, Kikuta T, et al: Suspensionplasty with the abductor pollicis longus tendon for osteoarthritis of the thumb. *J Hand Surgery [Am]* 31A:425–428, 2006.

120. Stahlenbrecher A, Hoch J: [Proximal interphalangeal joint silicone arthroplasty: comparison of Swanson and NeuFlex implants using a new evaluation score]. *Handchir Mikrochir Plast Chir* 41(3):156–165, 2009.

121. Stern PJ, Fulton DB: Distal interphalangeal joint arthrodesis: an analysis of complications. *J Hand Surg [Am]* 17(6):1139–1145, 1992.

122. Stern PJ, Gates NT, Jones TB: Tension band arthrodesis of small joints in the hand. *J Hand Surg [Am]* 18(2):194–197, 1993.

123. Stern PJ, Ho S: Osteoarthritis of the proximal interphalangeal joint. *Hand Clin* 3(3):405–413, 1987.

124. Stoecklein HH, Garg R, Wolfe SW: Surface replacement arthroplasty of the proximal interphalangeal joint using a volar approach: case series. *J Hand Surg [Am]* 36(6):1015–1021, 2011.

125. Swanson AB: Silicone rubber implants for replacement of arthritis or destroyed joints in the hand. *Surg Clin North Am* 48(5):1113–1127, 1968.

126. Sweets TM, Stern PJ: Pyrolytic carbon resurfacing arthroplasty for osteoarthritis of the proximal interphalangeal joint of the finger. *J Bone Joint Surg Am* 93(15):1417–1425, 2011.

127. Taghinia AH, Al-Sheikh AA, Upton J: Suture anchor suspension and fascia lata interposition arthroplasty for basal joint arthritis of the thumb. *Plast Reconstr Surg* 122:497–504, 2008.

128. Tagil M, Geijer M, Abramo A, et al: Ten years' experience with a pyrocarbon prosthesis replacing the proximal interphalangeal joint. A prospective clinical and radiographic follow-up. *J Hand Surg Eur Vol* 39(6):587–595, 2013.

129. Tagil M, Kopylov P: Swanson versus APL arthroplasty in the treatment of osteoarthritis of the trapeziometacarpal joint: a prospective and randomized study in 26 patients. *J Hand Surg [Br]* 27(5):452–456, 2002.

130. Takigawa S, Meletiou S, Sauerbier M, et al: Long-term assessment of Swanson implant arthroplasty in the proximal interphalangeal joint of the hand. *J Hand Surg [Am]* 29(5):785–795, 2004.

131. Teoh LC, Yeo SJ, Singh I: Interphalangeal joint arthrodesis with oblique placement of an AO lag screw. *J Hand Surg [Br]* 19(2):208–211, 1994.

132. Thompson JS: Complications and salvage of trapeziometacarpal arthroplasties. *Instr Course Lect* 38:3–13, 1989.

133. Tomaino MM, Pellegrini VD, Jr, Burton RI: Arthroplasty of the basal joint of the thumb. Long-term follow-up after ligament reconstruction with tendon interposition. *J Bone Joint Surg Am* 77(3):346–355, 1995.

134. Tomaino MM, Vogt M, Weiser R: Scaphotrapezoid arthritis: prevalence in thumbs undergoing trapezium excision arthroplasty and efficacy of proximal trapezoid excision. *J Hand Surg [Am]* 24(6):1220–1224, 1999.

135. Trail IA, Martin JA, Nuttall D, et al: Seventeen-year survivorship analysis of silastic metacarpophalangeal joint replacement. *J Bone Joint Surg Br* 86(7):1002–1006, 2004.

136. Uchiyama S, Cooney WP, 3rd, Linscheid RL, et al: Kinematics of the proximal interphalangeal joint of the finger after surface replacement. *J Hand Surg [Am]* 25(2):305–312, 2000.

137. Umarji SI, Arnander MW, Evans DM: The use of Swanson silastic interposition arthroplasty in revision thumb-base surgery for failed trapeziectomy: a case series of 10 patients. *J Hand Surg Eur Vol* 37(7):632–636, 2012.

138. Vadstrup LS, Schou L, Boeckstyns ME: Basal joint osteoarthritis of the thumb treated with Weilby arthroplasty: a prospective study on the early postoperative course of 106 consecutive cases. *J Hand Surg Eur Vol* 34(4):503–505, 2009.

139. van Cappelle HG, Elzenga P, van Horn JR: Long-term results and loosening analysis of de la Caffiniere replacements of the trapeziometacarpal joint. *J Hand Surg [Am]* 24(3):476–482, 1999.

140. van Rijn J, Gosens T: A cemented surface replacement prosthesis in the basal thumb joint. *J Hand Surg [Am]* 35(4):572–579, 2010.

141. Vandenberghe L, Degreef I, Didden K, et al: Long term outcome of trapeziectomy with ligament reconstruction/tendon interposition versus thumb basal joint prosthesis. *J Hand Surg Eur Vol* 38(8):839–843, 2013.

142. Vermeulen GM, Brink SM, Slijper H, et al: Trapeziometacarpal arthrodesis or trapeziectomy with ligament reconstruction in primary trapeziometacarpal osteoarthritis: a randomized controlled trial. *J Bone Joint Surg Am* 96(9):726–733, 2014.

143. Vermeulen GM, Brink SM, Sluiter J, et al: Ligament reconstruction arthroplasty for primary thumb carpometacarpal osteoarthritis (Weilby technique): prospective cohort study. *J Hand Surg [Am]* 34(8):1393–1401, 2009.

144. Villani F, Uribe-Echevarria B, Vaienti L: Distal interphalangeal joint arthrodesis for degenerative osteoarthritis with compression screw: results in 102 digits. *J Hand Surg [Am]* 37(7):1330–1334, 2012.

145. Watson HK, Shaffer S: Concave-convex arthrodesis in joints of the hand. *Plast Reconstr Surg* 46(4):368–371, 1970.

146. Weilby A: Tendon interposition arthroplasty of the first carpo-metacarpal joint. *J Hand Surg [Br]* 13(4):421–425, 1988.

147. Wijk U, Wollmark M, Kopylov P, et al: Outcomes of proximal interphalangeal joint pyrocarbon implants. *J Hand Surg [Am]* 35(1):38–43, 2010.

148. Wollstein R, Watson HK, Martin RT, et al: Long-term durability of tendon arthroplasty with excision of the trapezium in stage 1 osteoarthritis of the thumb CMC joint. *Ann Plast Surg* 62(4):358–360, 2009.

149. Wright CS, McMurtry RY: AO arthrodesis in the hand. *J Hand Surg [Am]* 8(6):932–935, 1983.

150. Wysocki RW, Cohen MS, Shott S, et al: Thumb carpometacarpal suspension arthroplasty using interference screw fixation: surgical technique and clinical results. *J Hand Surg [Am]* 35(6):913–920, 2010.

151. Yang SS, Weiland AJ: First metacarpal subsidence during pinch after ligament reconstruction and tendon interposition basal joint arthroplasty of the thumb. *J Hand Surg [Am]* 23(5):879–883, 1998.

152. Yao J, Song Y: Suture-button suspensionplasty for thumb carpometacarpal arthritis: a minimum 2-year follow-up. *J Hand Surg [Am]* 38(6):1161–1165, 2013.

153. Yuan BJ, Moran SL, Tay SC, et al: Trapeziectomy and carpal collapse. *J Hand Surg [Am]* 34(2):219–227, 2009.

12

Wrist Arthrodesis and Arthroplasty

Marco Rizzo

Acknowledgment: The author and editors wish to acknowledge and thank John K. Stanley, MD, who contributed this chapter to the sixth edition. This work is built on his foundation.

> ▶ These videos may be found at
> *ExpertConsult.com:*
> **12.1** Re-motion total wrist arthroplasty
> **12.2** Radiolunate arthrodesis with ligament-sparing approach

A pain-free, stable wrist joint is essential for normal function of the hand. Pain arising from a traumatized, arthritic, or unstable wrist will, through the unconscious spinal reflex, inhibit the function of the forearm musculature and result in weakness. Intermittent pain and instability result in an unreliable grasp that can fail capriciously and without warning. In addition to pain and instability, the problems of restricted range of motion and deformity may be present and may have an added adverse impact on function.[33]

Primary osteoarthritis of the wrist is a relatively uncommon cause of pain and is exemplified by degenerative changes at the scaphotrapeziotrapezoid (STT) joint. More commonly, arthritis ensues after trauma, instability and dislocation, crystalline deposition, or inflammatory processes. Less common causes include cerebral palsy, penetrating wounds, hemophilia, infection, or chondrolysis. On occasion, bone lesions, such as giant cell tumors or distal radius or synovial chondromatosis of the wrist, can be a source of pain and may require excision and/or wrist reconstruction.

A variety of surgical procedures are available for the management of the painful, unstable, degenerate, or stiff wrist. The choice of treatment depends on the cause and the pattern of the effects of the causative pathology and is dependent on the integrity of the articular cartilage. There are some minimally invasive surgical options that try to maintain motion, including partial denervation or metaphyseal decompression. The more extensively performed surgical procedures may be grouped into two principal treatment options: partial or total wrist arthrodesis and wrist arthroplasty.

The aim of any treatment is to provide a pain-free, stable, and functional wrist, and each patient will have a pattern of problems that guide the surgeon toward the appropriate treatment for that individual. Some patients cannot tolerate the loss of range of motion engendered by total wrist arthrodesis and will press for a motion-preserving procedure.[116] Therefore, careful assessment of the patient's needs and requirements is important.

Because the normal wrist enjoys considerable range of motion, loss of any of that range is perceived as an impairment that may give rise to a disability. However, a number of studies have been performed to examine the requirements for wrist motion for a variety of normal activities, and it is clear that most of the activities of daily living can be performed with quite a restricted range of motion of the wrist.

Palmer and colleagues[78] suggested that the functional range of wrist motion is 30 degrees of extension, 5 degrees of flexion, 15 degrees of ulnar deviation, and 10 degrees of radial deviation; these values were derived from a study in which they evaluated 52 standardized tasks involving activities of daily living and some aspects of work. Brumfield and Champoux found that in performing 15 activities of daily living, 10 degrees of wrist flexion was required and 35 degrees of wrist extension was used.[12] A later study by Ryu and colleagues evaluated a smaller number of activities of daily living and identified an ideal range of motion that they described as 60 degrees of extension, 54 degrees of flexion, 17 degrees of radial deviation, and 40 degrees of ulnar deviation.[89] They went on to state that the majority of hand placement and range-of-motion tasks studied in their project could be accomplished with 70% of maximum range of wrist motion, that is, 40 degrees each of wrist flexion and extension and 40 degrees of combined radial and ulnar deviation. Nelson demonstrated with use of a splint to mimic stiffness that 123 activities of daily living could be performed successfully with limited motion consisting of 5 degrees of flexion, 6 degrees of extension, 7 degrees of radial deviation, and 6 degrees of ulnar deviation.[73] This probably represents considerable coping strategies, compensatory motion of the shoulder and elbow, and modification of activity by the individuals in the study. Their study concluded that although having a wide range of motion is of great value, only a small arc of motion in each direction is *required* to maintain independence of existence. However, life involves a combination of hobbies, pastimes, and work, each of which may require a specific range of motion, and these must be considered when assessing an individual patient for treatment. Franko and associates highlighted the issues surrounding the capacity of volunteers to adapt to and compromise limitations of wrist motion.[33] The authors found that severe restriction of wrist motion with the use of splints gave rise to only a modest impairment in function of the wrist in activities of daily living. However, when some motion was allowed, there was a significant improvement in the ease of performance of the same tasks and a significant improvement in the *range* of tasks that could be performed. This study highlights the general need of patients to have some movement at the wrist but the fact that individual requirements will differ. Therefore, when patients seek advice and treatment for a painful, unstable wrist, it is important to identify not only the wrist impairment but also the net effect of that impairment on functional ability. This will be unique to each patient and will have a great influence on the choice of surgical procedure. With a thorough history, one can determine which activities are inhibited by the painful or unstable wrist and choose the correct motion-preserving procedure, such as limited arthrodesis or arthroplasty, or motion-ablating procedure, such as arthrodesis. Other factors, such as the patient's age, ipsilateral shoulder and elbow pathologic findings, and occupation may well affect the choice between arthroplasty and arthrodesis.[71] Preoperative assessment must include a detailed physical examination and a full radiographic analysis to determine bone quality, residual bone stock, and the pattern of the disease. Additional investigations may be needed to identify the underlying pathologic condition (e.g., whether the condition is due to an inflammatory or degenerative disease process), as well as any comorbidity that might prejudice the outcome of a surgical procedure. Scoring of the function, disability, and pain will facilitate measurement of the outcome of the intervention. It is important to evaluate the patient's willingness and ability to comply with the postoperative instructions and therapy program; such evaluation is essential to a successful outcome for most surgical procedures involving the wrist.

PREOPERATIVE ASSESSMENT

The preoperative assessment consists of four discrete elements.
1. Identification of the impairment or loss of faculty. *Impairment* is defined as the parameters that can be measured and includes range of motion, grip strength, deformity, and stability.
2. Assessment of *pain*, which by definition is a symptom and therefore cannot be objectively measured. The most reliable assessment tool for pain is the visual analog scale. A visual analog chart should be scored for pain at rest and pain with activity.
3. Identification of the presence of a disability, which is a condition that limits a person's ability to perform normal tasks and may include pain. The term *disability* includes the effects of pain and the limitations generated by the loss of faculty on an individual. The assessment identifies the activities of daily living that are affected and the areas of significant difficulty within patients' lives that they wish to resolve.
4. Radiographic assessment to determine which procedures may be possible as indicated by the patient's residual bone stock and pattern of degenerative changes.

Physical Examination of the Wrist

Examination of the wrist is necessary to establish the baseline values of movement, strength, deformity, and stability.[99,107] In addition, visual inspection will allow the physician to observe local swelling, scars, evidence of current or previous infection, and the patient's reaction to movement or provocative stress testing of the joint or joints. The associated physical signs of inflammatory joint disease may well be apparent, including multiarticular involvement, deformity, swelling, and effusion. The presence or absence of scaly patches and nail changes must be noted to rule out psoriasis. A patient with psoriasis must be warned of the *Koebner phenomenon*,[117] in which acute psoriatic plaques may develop along the length of a scar engendered by surgery. The presence of vasculitis or active rheumatoid disease may be a contraindication to any surgery until the condition is controlled.

Radiographic Evaluation

X-rays, including the standard posteroanterior (PA), oblique, and lateral views, should be the basis for the initial radiographic examination. Gross changes can be seen on these three standard views with the shoulder held at 90 degrees of abduction, the elbow at 90 degrees of flexion, and the hand placed flat on the radiographic plate. This gives a reproducible PA view in neutral rotation with the beam centered over the capitate and including the distal radioulnar joint (DRUJ). Marked changes, as seen in the scapholunate advanced collapse (SLAC) pattern of arthritis, the scaphoid nonunion advanced collapse (SNAC) pattern, and carpal coalitions, are easily identified. STT arthrosis may be associated with deposition of calcium pyrophosphate (Figure 12.1, *A* and *B*), and in this condition the radiolunate joint may well be involved (see Figure 12.1, *C*). Less obvious and more difficult to assess is arthrosis between the capitate and the lunate and between the head of the hamate and the lunate. In these circumstances, the so-called six-shot series includes a PA view of the wrist in full radial and full ulnar deviation, which is valuable in identifying elements of instability in patients with scapholunate injury. An anteroposterior (AP) grip view completes the series and can magnify carpal collapse or scapholunate diastasis and show whether there is impingement between the hamate head and the hamate facet on the lunate (Figure 12.2, *A* to *C*).[97] The recently described "pencil-grip" PA view profiles both scapholunate joints simultaneously and demonstrates scapholunate diastasis favorably when compared with other radiographic stress views.[58]

Specific x-rays are indicated by the history and examination. They may include, for example, a pisotriquetral skyline view (a lateral view with the wrist in 10 degrees of supination) (Figure 12.3, *A*) to exclude osteoarthritis of this joint, which can coexist with other areas of arthritis in the wrist and, if not identified, can give rise to residual symptoms that may overshadow any improvement after other surgical procedures.

Computed tomography (CT) scans and magnetic resonance imaging (MRI) may also be helpful in evaluating patients with arthritis. CT scans will better discern the bone quality and joint disease when compared with plain films (see Figure 12.3, *B* and *C*). MRI will be most helpful in confirming the vascularity of the carpus, identifying bone marrow changes, and delineating pathologic conditions of the soft tissues such as synovitis and

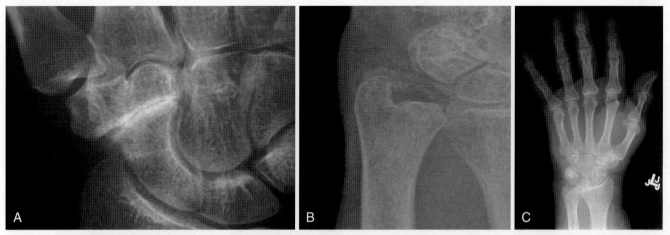

FIGURE 12.1 A, Scaphotrapeziotrapezoidal arthrosis may be localized to only one hand, although the majority of patients suffer from bilateral disease. **B,** The association with calcium pyrophosphate deposition disease (CPDD) is obvious in this patient with calcific changes in the triangular fibrocartilage complex. **C,** Figure demonstrates a posteroanterior view of a patient with known CPPD and obvious joint space narrowing at the radiolunate joint.

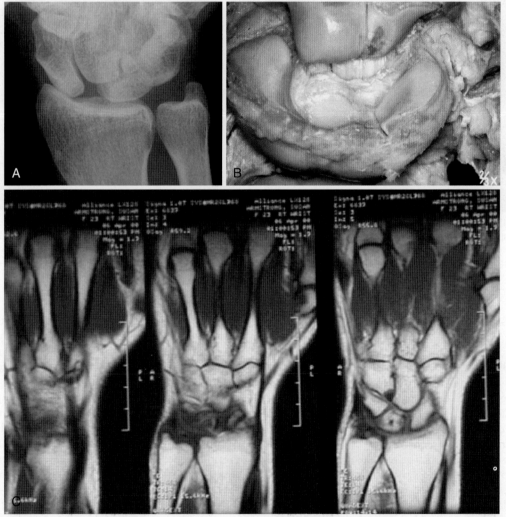

FIGURE 12.2 A, This radiograph of a wrist under axial load clearly demonstrates scapholunate dissociation but is also suggestive of hamolunate impingement. **B,** This cadaveric specimen demonstrates hamolunate impaction, which can occur and may compromise radiolunate and radioscapholunate arthrodesis. **C,** The most appropriate investigation is magnetic resonance imaging, which shows significant bone edema at the tip of the hamate.

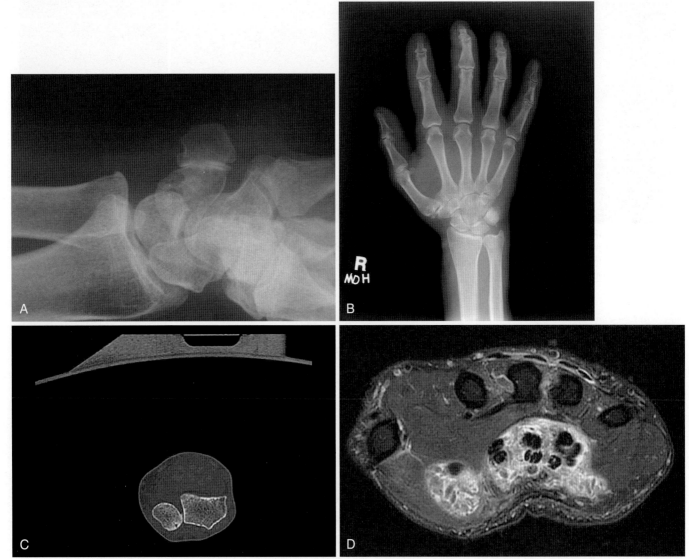

FIGURE 12.3 A, If not recognized preoperatively, pisotriquetral arthrosis can be painful, irritate the ulnar nerve in the canal of Guyon, and detract from an otherwise successful surgical wrist procedure. **B,** Posteroanterior radiograph of a patient with pain at the distal radioulnar joint and radiographic suspicion of arthritis. **C,** An axial computed tomographic scan of the same patient illustrates more clearly the arthritic process, demonstrating joint space narrowing; note also the subchondral cysts and volar osteophyte of the ulnar head. **D,** An axial T2-weighted image of a patient with inflammatory arthritis. Note the extensive flexor tendon tenosynovitis.

tenosynovitis associated with inflammatory diseases (see Figure 12.3, *D*).

Common Radiographic Patterns of Disease

Osteoarthritis. In osteoarthritis, a common pattern of the progression of degenerative change has been defined by Watson and Ballet as the SLAC pattern (Figure 12.4).[108] Vender and coworkers have described the SNAC pattern (Figure 12.5).[102]

Rheumatoid Arthritis. Because the variable picture seen in the inflammatory arthropathies such as rheumatoid arthritis does not lend itself to either of these classifications, treatment must be individualized. The following discussion is based on the Wrightington classification of rheumatoid wrist radiographs, which may be useful when considering surgical possibilities for various patterns of joint damage and residual bone stock.[47]

The Conservative Wrist. In general in the early stages of rheumatoid disease, x-rays show minor erosions but no significant bone loss or ligament injury and also show normal joint spaces. In these circumstances, simple synovectomy with disease-modifying drugs, splintage, and other measures may be all that is required. This would be called the conservative wrist (Figure 12.6, *A*).

The Restorative Wrist. As the disease progresses, localized loss of joint space becomes apparent in the radiocarpal joint (see Figure 12.6, *B*). There may be secondary changes consisting of translation and translocation of the carpus. Provided that the midcarpal joint is well preserved, patients at this stage are suitable candidates for radiolunate[17] or radioscapholunate fusion.[4,38,92]

The Reconstructive Wrist. Progression of the disease can lead to widespread loss of the joint surface, including the midcarpal joint, but if the bone stock is preserved, the surgical choices are total wrist replacement or total wrist arthrodesis (see Figure 12.6, *C*).

The Salvage Wrist. When the wrist has been so damaged by the disease process that a significant amount of bone stock has been lost, the only surgical procedure that is reasonably reliable is arthrodesis, and this is often the only practical course of action. Particular attention should be paid to the lateral x-ray of the wrist; it may show significant volar subluxation of the lunate, which will give rise to some difficulties in reducing the wrist and could precipitate carpal tunnel syndrome as the wrist is relocated and realigned (see Figure 12.6, *D*).

SURGICAL TECHNIQUES

Partial Wrist Fusions

History of Limited Wrist Arthrodesis

- Peterson and Lipscomb, 1967: Intercarpal arthrodesis[80]
- Chamay and colleagues, 1983: Radiolunate arthrodesis[17]
- Watson and Ballet, 1984: Surgical correction of the SLAC wrist[108]
- Pisano and associates, 1991: Scaphocapitate (SC) arthrodesis[81]
- Minamikawa and coworkers, 1992: The ideal sagittal scaphoid angle for STT and SC arthrodesis[67]
- Calandruccio and colleagues, 2000: Capitolunate fusion with excision of the scaphoid and triquetrum[14]

Much effort has gone into determining the most appropriate intercarpal arthrodesis for a given condition, and there is a wide range of opinions on the best options for particular patterns of disease and pathologic findings. The choices are described in the following sections.

Radiolunate Fusion

Indications

Localized degenerative change secondary to rheumatoid arthritis is the most common cause of isolated radiolunate arthritis. The indications for radiolunate fusion[10,17,94] are volar translation, ulnar carpal translocation (Figure 12.7, *A*), complex carpal instabilities, and localized radiolunate arthritis (see Figure 12.7, *B*), commonly seen in patients with rheumatoid arthritis but also noted in those with die punch fractures within the lunate fossa. This latter injury causes a disorder of normal mechanics, scapholunate dissociation, flexion of the scaphoid, and, ultimately, degenerative arthritis. Frequently, an ulnar abutment syndrome will accompany the situation because of subsidence of the lunate within the lunate fossa, and there may be associated damage to the DRUJ. This complex injury can be improved by radiolunate fusion, provided that carpal height is restored.

Technique for Radiolunate Fusion

Preparation of the bone surface is sometimes awkward and time-consuming because of the nature and shape of the lunate and the radial fossa, the presence of eburnation of subchondral bone in osteoarthritic patients, and the distortion of the anatomy as seen in rheumatoid disease (Figure 12.8). The lunate must be restored to its anatomic height, and this involves the use of iliac crest, distal radius, or ulnar head bone graft material if available and sufficient. Fixation can be accomplished with Kirschner wires, staples, miniature pin plates, blade plates, or screws. Headless cannulated or other compression screws passed through the dorsal horn of the lunate can also be used to achieve rigid fixation (Figure 12.9, *A* and *B*).

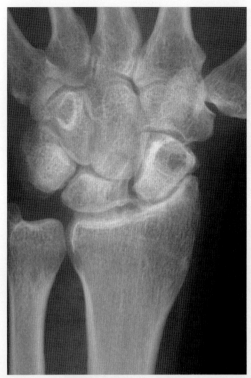

FIGURE 12.4 Scapholunate advanced collapse pattern of arthrosis of the wrist. Localized arthrosis of the scaphoid fossa begins at the styloid tip (stage I), proceeds to the proximal scaphoid fossa (stage II), and is followed by capitolunate arthrosis (stage III). The lunate may fall into dorsiflexion (dorsal intercalated segment instability [DISI]) and the scaphoid into flexion as seen here, but the integrity of the radiolunate articulation is preserved until late in the process.

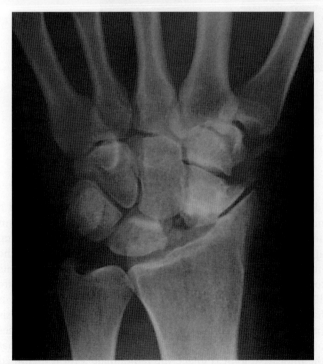

FIGURE 12.5 Scaphoid nonunion advanced collapse (SNAC) pattern of arthrosis of the wrist. Degenerative changes develop in the distal segment of the scaphoid (stage I), and the proximal segment is spared. As in this case, excision of the proximal pole of the nonunited scaphoid will precipitate a combination of instability and SNAC. The scaphocapitate joint deteriorates in stage II. (See Watson HK, Fink JS, Monacelli DM: Use of triscaphe fusion in the treatment of Kienbock's disease. *Hand Clin* 9(3):493–499, 1933.)

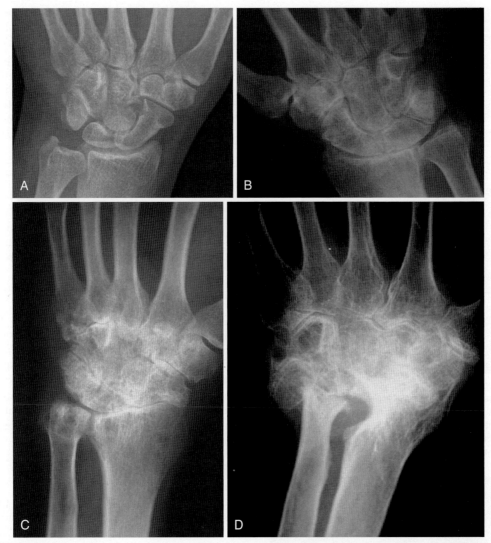

FIGURE 12.6 **A,** The conservative wrist. Integrity of the ligament and joint surfaces characterizes this phase of the disease, although erosions may be seen. **B,** The restorative wrist. The secondary arthrosis is principally confined to the lunate fossa and suggests that radiolunate fusion is an appropriate option. In this radiograph, the presence of translocation and radioscaphoid arthritis indicates that radioscapholunate fusion is the preferred option. **C,** The reconstructive wrist. Bony stock is well preserved, although all joints are significantly affected; wrist replacement may be considered as an option. **D,** The salvage wrist. Very poor bone stock remains, and with marked bone loss, arthrodesis remains the most likely choice, although each case must be taken on its merits.

❖ AUTHOR'S PREFERRED METHOD OF TREATMENT: Radiolunate Arthrodesis

The wrist is exposed through a standard longitudinal incision approximately 8 cm long in line with the third metacarpal and bisected by the radiocarpal joint line (Figure 12.10, *A* and *B*). The flaps are raised deep to the superficial fascia to preserve the vessels and cutaneous nerves while obtaining an excellent view of the extensor retinaculum. At this point, the Lister tubercle is identified by palpation and the extensor retinaculum is opened over the third compartment just to the ulnar side of the Lister tubercle while taking care not to damage the extensor pollicis longus (EPL). The digital extensor tendons contained within the fourth compartment are raised in the envelope created by the extensor retinaculum superficially and the capsule of the wrist on the deep surface. This prevents specific damage to the extensor tendons. The posterior interosseous nerve can be identified lying to the ulnar side of the Lister tubercle, and a neurectomy can be performed to help with postoperative pain and prevent scarring of the nerve.[60,114] A ligament-sparing approach to the wrist involves making an incision along the lines of the dorsal radiocarpal and dorsal intercarpal ligaments to expose the radiocarpal and midcarpal joints (see Figure 12.10, *C*). The capitolunate joint should be inspected; if it has degenerated, one would consider a full wrist arthrodesis (although some authors suggest that mild degenerative changes of the capitate head are acceptable).[96] Upon confirmation that the midcarpal joint is intact, the radiolunate joint is identified and the cartilage of the lunate fossa and the proximal lunate surface is denuded from the bone with curets, rongeurs, and limited use of a bur. A graft is taken from the area deep to the Lister tubercle if carpal height has been maintained. However, if carpal height needs to be restored, a corticocancellous bone graft is taken from the iliac crest with a trephine through a small

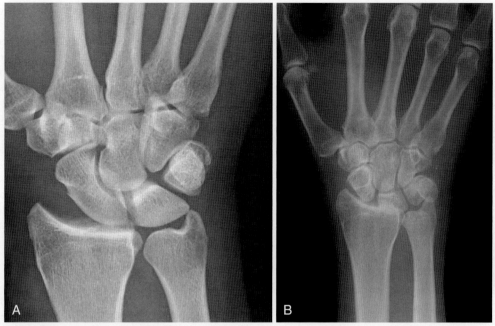

FIGURE 12.7 **A,** Posteroanterior (PA) view of the wrist demonstrating ulnar translocation of the lunate and carpus. **B,** PA view of the wrist illustrating significant radiolunate arthritis.

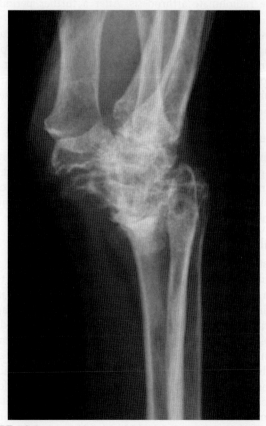

FIGURE 12.8 Volar subluxation of the lunate in a patient with inflammatory joint disease creates a new, more proximal pseudolunate fossa. This accentuates the supination deformity of the carpus and causes profound collapse of the scaphoid. Isolated radiolunate fusion in this patient would not be indicated.

incision. Care should be taken not to overcorrect the height of the proximal carpal row, because this has been associated with increased loading and progression of arthritis of the midcarpal joint.[24] If the ulnar head has been removed as part of the procedure, it may also be fashioned into a suitable graft (Figure 12.11, *A* and *B*). This yields a corticocancellous graft that may be shaped so that it can be inserted to restore carpal height, particularly if a die punch fracture has previously occurred (Figure 12.12).

In a patient with extension of the lunate, as seen in dorsal intercalated segment instability (DISI) deformity and SLAC/SNAC wrist or distal radius malunion with nondissociative carpal instability,[118] this must be corrected to achieve proper balance of the remaining carpus. Fixation of the lunate in extension during radiolunate arthrodesis will predictably result in impingement of the capitate with wrist flexion. To correct the extended lunate, one can fully flex the wrist and pass a 0.062-inch Kirschner wire through the dorsal aspect of the radius into the repositioned lunate. When the wrist is brought back to neutral flexion-extension, the lunate is in the correct position as seen in the sagittal view (Figure 12.13, *A* to *C*). Gentle manipulation of the wrist into extension stretches the anterior capsule, and this process can be repeated through two or three iterations. Extension of the wrist is then improved and arthrodesis can be completed. After preparation of the bone surface and grafting, fixation with Kirschner wires through the distal dorsal aspect of the radius into the lunate with the lunate in neutral rotation allows the position to be checked with intraoperative radiographs or fluoroscopy. The midcarpal joint should be carefully assessed to rule out hardware penetration. In patients with better bone quality, a cannulated headless bone screw or osseous staple can be inserted and the provisional wire removed. If the lunate does not lend itself readily to fixation with Kirschner wires through the dorsal horn, consideration can be given to

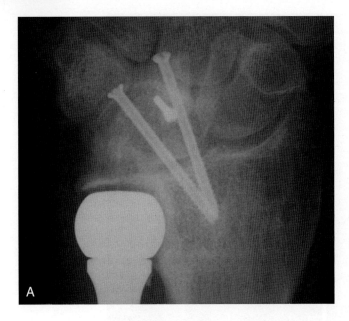

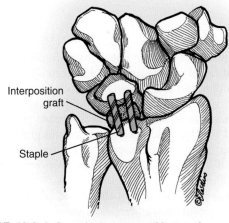

Interposition graft

Staple

B

FIGURE 12.9 A, Crossed screws are used here as the construct, the ulnar head has been replaced, and it is imperative that adequate clearance between the lunate graft and the implant be maintained to minimize the potential for the development of an ulnar abutment syndrome. **B,** Staples may provide a simpler method of fixation. (**B,** Copyright © Elizabeth Martin.)

removal of the proximal pole of the triquetrum. This maneuver reveals the ulnar aspect of the lunate and allows a Kirschner wire or headless bone screw to be inserted through the lunate into the radius from the ulnar side. This ensures better fixation, may increase the range of motion, and helps to prevent translocation.

Pitfalls

1. Failure to appreciate that the posterior interosseous nerve can be damaged or become scarred following surgery, resulting in traction pain or neuroma in continuity. A relatively straightforward solution is to simply excise 1 cm of the nerve proximal to the joint. This will prevent problems associated with scarring of the tethered posterior interosseous nerve.[60] In addition, performing a posterior interosseous neurectomy has been shown to relieve pain in many patients with arthritis. Thus, it is my preference to routinely perform a posterior interosseous neurectomy.[114]

2. Fusion of the lunate in an excessively dorsiflexed position (DISI). This restricts the range of motion in flexion considerably, and a neutral or 10-degree dorsiflexed position of the lunate in relation to the radius is essential.

3. Failure to restore carpal height, leading to a permanently flexed scaphoid and unnecessary restriction of the range of motion. However, overcorrection has been shown to increase loading of the midcarpal joint, and thus a proper balance needs to be achieved.

4. Problems related to hardware, such as violation of the capitolunate joint by wires or hardware extending from the radius into the lunate. In addition, dorsally prominent hardware can result in tendon or soft tissue irritation and pain.

Postoperative Management

Use of a bulky dressing with immobilization for 10 to 14 days with the hand elevated whenever possible allows the swelling to subside and the sutures to be removed. A short-arm cast immobilizes the wrist for a period of 5 to 6 weeks. At that point, early rehabilitation should be restricted to using the dart thrower's motion only, namely, radial deviation and extension to ulnar deviation and flexion. This prevents excessive forces from acting on the radiolunate arthrodesis. After a further period of 4 weeks, full mobilization can take place, provided that radiographs confirm the presence of union. Strengthening exercises for finger motion should start early. At 3 months it is appropriate to remove the splint entirely, but avoidance of contact sports for 2 to 3 additional months is recommended. Excessive attempts to mobilize the midcarpal joint can result in an increased risk for nonunion.

Net Analysis of the Literature

A nonunion rate of approximately 10%[56] and a 50% reduction in range of motion in flexion and extension are reported. Some authors have noted an increased risk of nonunion associated with staples and better union rates with the use of miniplates with oblique screws.[39,40]

Scaphocapitate Arthrodesis

Indications

Scaphocapitate (SC) fusion is considered an alternative to STT fusion for stabilization of the scaphoid.[68] Accordingly, indications include dynamic or rotatory subluxation of the scaphoid, nonunion of the scaphoid, Kienböck disease,[41,49] and midcarpal instability. It is particularly advantageous with chronic scaphoid nonunion to address the instability and to expand the area of bone healing from distal to proximal scaphoid to capitate.

Most authors believe that there are no significant loading differences between SC and STT fusion. Watson felt that better motion is achieved with STT fusion than with SC fusion. Two cadaveric laboratory studies found essentially no differences in motion between the two.[27,65] The authors noted that after both STT and SC fusion there is diminished joint reactive force at the radiolunate and capitolunate joints. The amount of restriction of motion very much depends on proper reduction of the scaphoid to an intermediate position of flexion with respect to the radius.

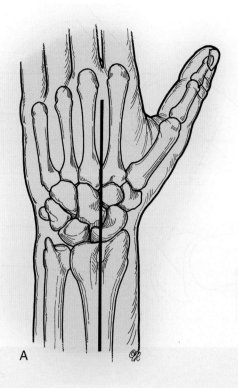

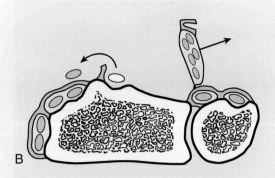

FIGURE 12.10 A single dorsal incision allows wide exposure of the dorsum of the wrist through the third dorsal compartment (**A**) and deep to the fourth extensor compartment (**B**), thereby maintaining the "extensor tube." See Video 12.2, demonstrating the ligament-sparing approach to the wrist, in line with the dorsal radiocarpal and dorsal intercarpal ligaments.

CRITICAL POINTS *Radiolunate Arthrodesis*

Indications
- Isolated cases of radiolunate arthritis, which usually arise as a result of localized die punch fractures or from rheumatoid arthritis
- Instability of the proximal row of the carpus in translation
- Severe nondissociative carpal instability with painful clunk[12,35,118]
- Failed soft tissue reconstruction of scapholunate dissociation[77,98,103]

Contraindications
- The presence of significant degenerative changes in the midcarpal joint or radioscaphoid joint

Radiographic Evaluation
- Assessment of the preoperative x-rays is essential to ensure that the midcarpal and radioscaphoid joints are free of any degenerative changes, there is no residual degenerative arthritis in the DRUJ or pisotriquetral joint, and the DRUJ is stable.

Pearls
- Maintain the fourth compartment "tube" intact to minimize the risk of tendon injury.
- Perform a posterior interosseous neurectomy to help with pain and avoid problems with scarring and traction pain of the nerve.
- Reduction of the lunate extension is very important; therefore, for reduction, fully flex the wrist, drive a Kirschner wire through the distal radius into the lunate, and extend the wrist to reduce the lunate to the remainder of the carpus.

- During the procedure, temporary fixation of the lunate to the radius followed by intraoperative radiographs helps identify whether adequate height has been achieved and whether the position of the lunate is not excessively extended with regard to the capitate and radius. In addition, the lunate must be placed so that it comes to lie underneath the capitate, not to the ulnar side of it.
- Excision of the proximal part of the triquetrum can provide easier access for screw fixation if there has been significant ulnar translocation of the lunate.
- Restoration of carpal height is important in injuries due to trauma and, to a lesser extent, in wrists affected by rheumatoid arthritis.
- When using a bur, care should be taken to irrigate to avoid overheating the bone and inviting osteonecrosis.

Expectations
- There will be permanent loss of some range of motion, usually 50% or slightly less than the range of a normal wrist.
- Full recovery may take 9 to 12 months; the patient will need to learn to adapt to the new situation, and coping strategies may be developed in conjunction with the hand therapist.
- Not all pain will be relieved, and aching may occur after heavy use.
- There is a risk for deterioration over time with the development of degenerative changes within the midcarpal joint. This may require further surgery in the future.

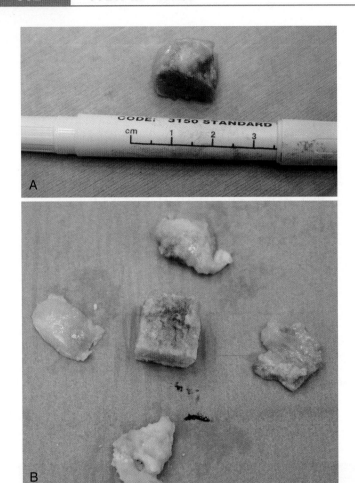

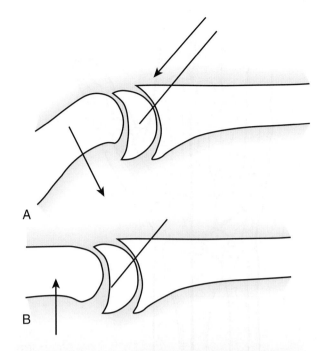

FIGURE 12.11 A, If the ulnar head is carefully excised as part of the procedure, it can, in many circumstances, be a sufficient graft to perform radiolunate or radioscapholunate arthrodesis. **B,** The head is held in a gauze sponge and the anterior, posterior, and medial surfaces are removed with an oscillating saw sequentially. The remaining cortical bone on the distal face provides a strong structural element for the graft.

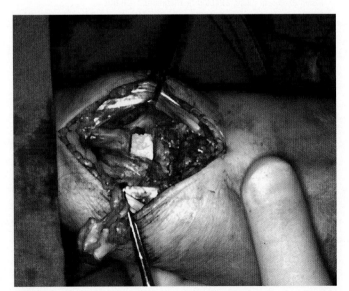

FIGURE 12.12 The size of the graft will often allow restoration of carpal height and is sufficiently robust to permit screw or staple fixation.

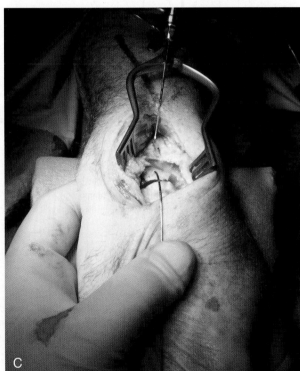

FIGURE 12.13 A, The wrist is fully flexed and a smooth 1.1-mm Kirschner wire is inserted into the distal radius to fix the lunate in neutral to slight flexion. If the wrist is moved into ulnar deviation and flexed before transfixion, the maneuver reduces both the translocation and flexion deformities. **B,** When the wrist is brought into neutral, the position of the lunate remains reduced and the capitate is in appropriate alignment with the lunate. **C,** A joystick in the lunate facilitates proper reduction of the lunate posture before transfixion.

Contraindications

Contraindications, as in STT fusion, include any abnormality of the radioscaphoid joint that would be susceptible to increased degeneration and symptoms because of the altered or increased loading through the radioscaphoid joint after SC fusion. Similarly, STT degenerative changes would be a contraindication to SC fusion.

Fixation

Fixation can be accomplished with Kirschner wires, staples, screws, or plates and screws (Figure 12.14). Safe hardware insertion requires identification and protection of the radial artery and the dorsal sensory radial nerve branches. Provided that normal intercarpal spacing is maintained by decorticating only the dorsal 75% of the articular surfaces and by packing the resultant space with bone graft, compression screws may be used between the scaphoid and capitate to hold the scaphoid in a 40- to 50-degree radioscaphoid angle.

❖ AUTHOR'S PREFERRED METHOD OF TREATMENT: Scaphocapitate Arthrodesis

The wrist is exposed through a longitudinal incision similar to that for a radiolunate fusion from the Lister tubercle to the base of the index metacarpal. The dorsal sensory radial nerve branches are identified and protected. The capsule is incised using a ligament-sparing approach within the fibers of the dorsal radiocarpal and dorsal intercarpal ligaments. When necessary for exposure, this approach can be extended radially along the radiocarpal joint to better expose the radioscaphoid interval. Both the radioscaphoid and capitolunate joints are inspected for healthy cartilage and protected. I prefer to use cannulated compression screws for fixation (Figure 12.15, *A*

and *B*). These can be placed in a radial to ulnar direction either percutaneously or directly within the exposure of the wound, depending on the visualization and access to the radial side of the scaphoid. Care is taken to ensure that the superficial branch of the radial nerve and dorsal branch of the radial artery are safely protected. The nerve can be visualized just deep to the

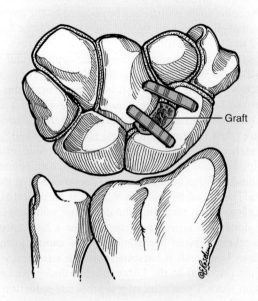

FIGURE 12.14 Scaphocapitate fusion with staples. Normal space between the scaphoid and capitate is maintained by preserving the volar 25% articulation of both bones. (Copyright © Elizabeth Martin.)

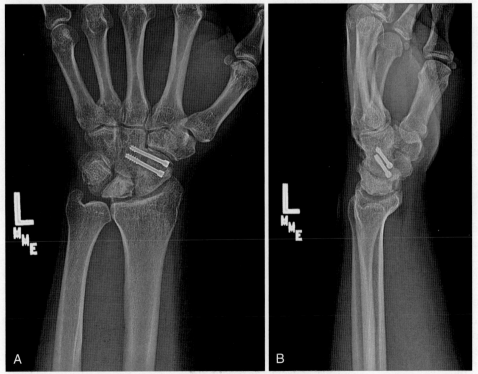

FIGURE 12.15 Figure shows (**A**) posteroanterior and (**B**) lateral views of a patient 5 years following scaphocapitate fusion using headless compression screws for the treatment of Kienböck disease.

skin to protect it from penetration or torsional damage by the guide pins. The artery will be deeper and needs to be seen to ensure it is safely out of the way. Reduction of a malrotated scaphoid is required. Similarly, if the lunate is tilted dorsally, this angulation must be corrected to ensure normal alignment of the fused capitate. For reduction, the proximal scaphoid pole is depressed and the distal pole of the scaphoid elevated with a 0.062-inch Kirschner wire "joystick," supplemented as needed with a large skin hook applied around the distal scaphoid. Correct capitolunate posture can be restored by the application of a palmar-directed load on the capitate until the lunate is restored to its normal tilt.

The guidewires are advanced into the capitate, and reduction to a 40- to 50-degree radioscaphoid angle is confirmed by fluoroscopy with the wrist in neutral alignment. If this is difficult to achieve within the wound, the guidewires can be placed through a small incision just distal to the radial styloid, with care taken to protect the dorsal radial artery and superficial branch of the radial nerve. Excessive scaphoid extension will impede radial deviation and extension. Any adjustments in scaphoid position are made before decortication of the joint surfaces. The dorsal 80% of the SC joint is decorticated down to cancellous bone, including the dorsal apposing edges. This can be done with curets, rongeurs, and/or a high-speed bur. Care is taken to avoid penetration of the capitolunate joint. Cancellous bone graft is harvested through a cortical window made just proximal to the Lister tubercle and is packed into the fusion space. Upon achieving appropriate reduction of the interval and bony preparation, the guide pins are inserted. Fluoroscopy is used to confirm the appropriate position of the proposed fusion and hardware placement. Drilling over the pins is then performed. I prefer to drill and place a screw in the first guide pin, prior to drilling over the second guide pin to maintain a point of fixation to resist rotation or loss of reduction. Take care not to overcompress the interval and not to overclose the normal intercarpal spacing with the compression screws. The provisional Kirschner wires are removed, and the capsule is closed with 3-0 braided absorbable suture. Alternatively, two staples 15 mm wide and 10 to 13 mm deep are inserted by power across the SC joint (see Figure 12.14). The skin is closed with a 4-0 polypropylene (Prolene) interrupted skin suture or subcuticular 3-0 polypropylene monofilament, followed by Steri-Strips. The hand and wrist are immobilized with a noncompressive short-arm bulky dressing and thumb spica splint.

Postoperative Management

At 10 days, the sutures are removed and a short-arm thumb spica cast is applied. At 6 to 8 weeks, radiographs are checked, and if satisfactory, a short-arm wrist splint is applied for intermittent protection. Active range of motion is initiated. Strengthening is usually deferred until 10 to 12 weeks postoperatively.

Postoperative Expectations

The range of motion should approximate 50% to 60% of the opposite side. Sennwald and Ufenast reported a flexion-extension arc of 62 degrees.[90] Viegas and associates reported a range of motion of 50% of the opposite side.[103] Grip strength will be approximately 80% of the opposite side; Pisano and coworkers reported 74% of the opposite side,[81] while Sennwald

and Ufenast documented 83% of the opposite side.[90] Nonunion rates of 6% to 28% can be expected, with a 95% confidence interval.[56]

CRITICAL POINTS *Scaphocapitate Arthrodesis*

Indications
- Dynamic or static rotatory subluxation of the scaphoid
- Chronic scaphoid nonunion
- Kienböck disease

Preoperative Evaluation
- Evaluate scaphoid stability with the scaphoid shift test (see Chapter 13)
- Obtain a supinated AP radiograph to evaluate the scapholunate joint for increased gap and to be sure that the radioscaphoid and STT joints are free of degenerative changes.
- Obtain a lateral radiograph to evaluate the scapholunate angle.
- Obtain a hyperpronated AP radiograph to evaluate the STT joint.

Pearls
- Preserve the volarmost cartilage surfaces between the scaphoid and lunate to maintain normal anatomic relationships.
- It is easier to reduce the scaphoid before decortication.
- When using a bur, irrigation should be done to avoid overheating the bone and inviting osteonecrosis.

Technical Points
- Protect the radial sensory nerve branches and radial artery by using a small drill guide during Kirschner wire placement.
- Confirm by fluoroscopy or radiographs proper reduction of the scaphoid to a 40- to 50-degree radioscaphoid angle. Separate lunate reduction is not required.

Pitfalls
- Avoid overreduction (extension > 50 degrees) of the scaphoid, which will limit motion, particularly radial deviation and extension.
- Avoid overcompression at the SC interval.

Postoperative Care
- The initial dressing should be bulky but noncompressive to avoid postoperative pain. Apply a short-arm thumb spica splint.
- At 10 days, apply a well-molded short-arm thumb spica cast.
- At 6 to 8 weeks, check radiographs and initiate active range-of-motion exercises.

Expectations
- Fifty percent to 60% range of motion in comparison to the opposite wrist
- Eighty percent grip strength
- Fifteen percent nonunion rate
- Minimum 4-month recovery time before sports participation

Athletic Participation

Athletic use of the involved extremity is precluded for at least 8 weeks. Nonloaded use is allowed at 8 weeks. Full use and any exposure to sudden force should be avoided for at least 10 to 13 weeks after surgery. Patients should not expect strong, relatively symptom-free wrist performance until at least 4 months after surgery.

What Patients Should Be Told

Patients are advised that pain relief is predictable and they will lose 40 to 50% of wrist motion but should still have a very

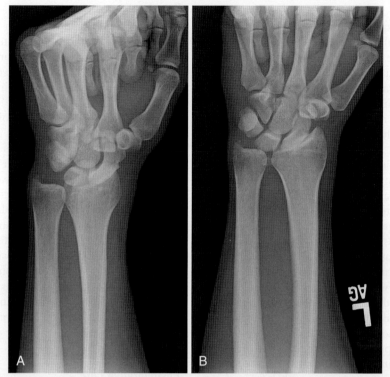

FIGURE 12.16 A, PA and **B,** oblique plain films of a patient who had prior trauma and now has degenerative changes in the radiocarpal joint as well as ulnar translation of the carpus.

functional arc. They may experience postoperative transient tingling over the dorsoradial aspect of the wrist or hand, which will resolve over time. Although the wrist will never feel "normal," almost all patients will feel improvement and regain 70 to 80% of grip strength. Patients who smoke are strongly advised to discontinue it preoperatively because smoking is associated with a higher likelihood of nonunion. Nonunion in other patients is unlikely but can occur in 15% of cases.

Radioscapholunate Arthrodesis

Indications and Contraindications

One indication for radioscapholunate arthrodesis is proximal row destruction, which is most commonly seen in posttraumatic patients (Figure 12.16, *A* and *B*) in whom there has been extensive intraarticular damage. It is also seen after chondrolysis, infection, or inflammatory arthritis (Figure 12.17). In fact, it is rare for patients with rheumatoid arthritis or osteoarthritis to have isolated radiolunate arthritis. Thus, in my experience it is more often necessary to perform a radioscapholunate arthrodesis.[4,38]

Preservation of midcarpal motion while dealing with painful radiocarpal motion is another indication for radioscapholunate arthrodesis. Contraindications include the presence of active infection or degenerative changes in the midcarpal joint.

❖ AUTHOR'S PREFERRED METHOD OF TREATMENT: Radioscapholunate Arthrodesis

Through a central longitudinal dorsal incision, full-thickness skin flaps are raised to identify the extensor retinaculum. The Lister tubercle is identified and an incision made in the extensor retinaculum in a line between the third and fourth compartments. The EPL tendon is dislocated from its groove. The Lister

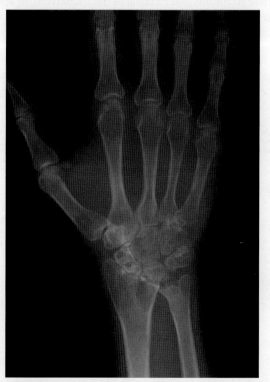

FIGURE 12.17 Patient with rheumatoid arthritis and severe articular destruction of the radiocarpal joint.

tubercle is removed with an osteotome. The retinaculum can be raised through the second compartment radially and (if necessary for exposure) the fifth compartment ulnarly. The extensor carpi radialis brevis (ECRB) and extensor carpi radialis longus (ECRL) are retracted to the radial side. Deep to the fourth compartment, a posterior interosseous neurectomy may be performed. The joint is exposed through a ligament-sparing approach, and the proximal radial exposure (if necessary) can be extended by elevating the capsule off the distal radius, leaving a cuff on the radius for reapproximation on closure.

Inspection of the midcarpal joint to ensure that there is adequate cartilage on the surface is the first prerequisite of this procedure. Any malalignment of the proximal row must be corrected by reduction of the lunate into the neutral position and reduction of the scaphoid into 45 degrees of radioscaphoid flexion, as determined by image intensification. The articular surfaces are excised down to cancellous bone. The space is filled with bone graft, which may be taken from the distal radius through a small defect created by removal of the Lister tubercle (Figure 12.18). Once the graft is in situ and the positions are satisfactory, memory staples can be used to maintain and compress the scaphoid-radial and lunate-radial interfaces (Figure 12.19, A to D). Alternative methods of fixation such as Kirschner wires, compressive screws, or plates can also be used. Once reduction and fixation of the arthrodesis have been achieved, the range of motion should be assessed. Because the scaphoid is fixed at 45 degrees of flexion, flexion-extension may be limited and radial deviation is particularly limited. The resultant motion is almost entirely in the dart thrower's plane of radial extension to ulnar flexion. When necessary or helpful, excision of the distal pole of the scaphoid can be performed to enable further radial deviation.[37,38,45] Separately, additional investigators have recommended removal of the triquetrum, in addition to the distal scaphoid, to enable a better ulnar-radial arc of motion of the wrist.[4,79]

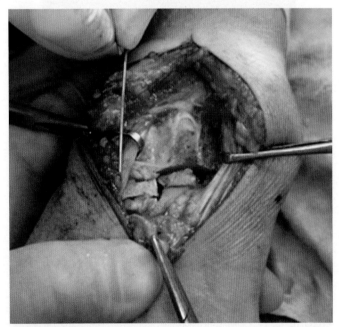

FIGURE 12.18 Example of radioscapholunate fusion. The diseased ulnar head has been excised and prepared in this case as the two grafts that are necessary to achieve restoration of carpal height and to ensure that the lunate is neutral in flexion and extension. Normally, it is our practice to excise the distal 20% of the scaphoid initially and then check during the dart thrower's range of motion that clearance is adequate. Further excision can be done until the surgeon is comfortable with the range of motion. Excision of the triquetrum follows the same principle.

Complications

Shin and Jupiter commented on the problems of nonunion after attempted radioscapholunate arthrodesis and the problems of using Kirschner wires or cannulated screws.[92] They reported successful use of 2.4-mm distal radial plates to provide locking plate stabilization of their radioscapholunate fusions. Nagy and Büchler identified two patients who exhibited secondary midcarpal degenerative joint disease.[72] Hamate-lunate impaction syndrome can occur in patients with a type II lunate and may be secondary to activities that require frequent flexion and ulnar deviation (see Figure 12.2, B).[97] Hamate-lunate impaction syndrome can be treated with amputation of 2 to 3 mm of the tip of the proximal hamate, which can be performed concurrently with radioscapholunate fusion. This causes no instability in the wrist and can ensure that impaction does not lead to pain and the late development of midcarpal degenerative joint disease. Arthrosis of the capitolunate joint is a contraindication to radioscapholunate arthrodesis, but Taleisnik suggested that mild arthrosis is acceptable and reported encouraging results with a motion-preserving adjunctive capitate interposition arthroplasty for patients with more severe capitolunate disease.[96]

Postoperative Care

As is standard for any fusion, initial immobilization in a bulky dressing for 10 to 14 days with the hand elevated whenever possible allows the swelling to subside. At 10 to 14 days a short-arm cast that allows finger and thumb motion is applied for 4 to 6 weeks. Once union is confirmed at 6 to 8 weeks, therapy is commenced with 1 to 2 weeks of dart thrower's motion, followed by 4 weeks of additional flexion-extension and radial-ulnar deviation exercises. Strengthening exercises with avoidance of heavy activities are then initiated for 4 to 6 weeks. Contact sports are not permitted for 4 to 5 months postoperatively.

What Patients Should Be Told

Provided union occurs (and even in select cases of pseudarthrosis), successful pain relief is predictable. There will be restricted range of motion, as identified by Garcia-Elias and colleagues.[36] The overall arc of flexion-extension and radioulnar deviation should be approximately half of the normal side, as one joint of a two-row system has been eliminated. Nagy and associates documented an average postoperative range of motion of 32 degrees of flexion, 35 degrees of extension, 14 degrees of radial deviation, and 19 degrees of ulnar deviation.[72] A metaanalysis from the mid 1990s documented a nonunion rate of 30%[56]; however, more recent investigations using more rigid fixation (e.g., compression screws, staples) and modification of technique to include distal scaphoid as well as triquetral excision have reported excellent union rates.[4,8,38,92] In addition, as previously mentioned, if it occurs, nonunion is not always painful (Figure 12.20). Recovery may require 9 to 12 months in some patients with poor bone stock, nonrigid fixation, or inflammatory disease. Patients should be warned that they are at some risk for midcarpal arthritis because of the altered wrist biomechanics and loads at that joint. Radioscapholunate fusion is an excellent motion-preserving procedure for radiocarpal arthrosis.

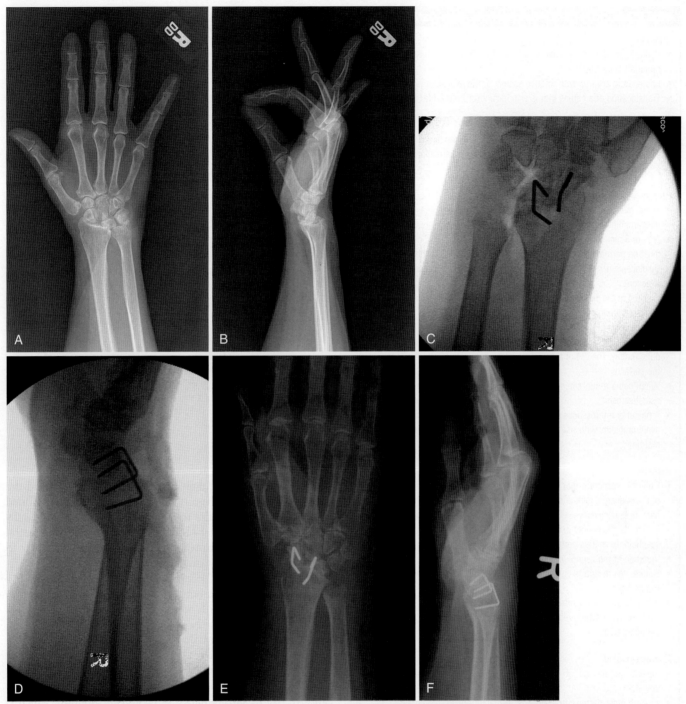

FIGURE 12.19 A, Posteroanterior (PA) and **B,** lateral x-rays of a 62-year-old female with significant radiocarpal arthritis. Note that the midcarpal joint has a fairly well maintained joint space. The patient underwent radioscapholunate (RSL) fusion using memory staples and intraoperative PA **(C)** and lateral **(D)** fluoroscopy images demonstrate the initial fixation. **E,** PA and lateral **(F)** radiographs 3 months after surgery show stable alignment and consolidation across the fusion mass.

Scapholunate Arthrodesis

Because motion of the scaphoid varies from individual to individual, the results of scapholunate arthrodesis[48] are unpredictable. In the hypermobile group of patients, the scaphoid will pronate and flex considerably with a small amount of translation. At the other extreme, the scaphoid does not flex or pronate in radial deviation.[23] In patients with hypermobile scaphoids, scapholunate arthrodesis is contraindicated. Nonunion rates

are high, the ability to achieve union is low, and the results are unpredictable. Because of nonunion rates of 50 to 85%,[48,56] this procedure has not proved to be a satisfactory treatment option for scapholunate dissociation.

Lunotriquetral Arthrodesis

Indications and Contraindications

Indications for lunotriquetral arthrodesis[51] include painful partial coalition of the lunotriquetral joint and symptomatic

CRITICAL POINTS *Radioscapholunate Arthrodesis*

Indications
- Radioscaphoid or radioscapholunate joint arthritic deformity after distal radial articular fractures
- Rheumatoid arthritis with relative sparing of the midcarpal joint
- Translocation of a carpus that is arthritic and/or irreducible

Preoperative Evaluation
- CT scanning or MRI can be helpful as an adjunct to standard x-rays to better delineate the nature of the midcarpal joint and, in particular, identify the presence or absence of a type II lunate facet.

Pearls
- There must be absent or minimal degenerative joint disease within the midcarpal joint.
- A 2- to 3-mm amputation of the impacting part of the head of the hamate must be performed if there is a significant type II joint on the lunate.
- Displacement of the ECRB and ECRL to the radial side gives adequate exposure.
- Excision of the distal pole of the scaphoid can be performed to allow better radial deviation of the wrist.
- Decortication of the posterior two thirds of the scaphoid, lunate, and radius preserves longitudinal alignment and length, and the area can be grafted quite readily. The use of a rongeur and/or a bur is most helpful in preparing the surfaces.
- When using a bur, copious irrigation is needed to avoid overheating and osteonecrosis.
- A posterior interosseous neurectomy can help with postoperative pain and avoid problems with scarring or tethering of the nerve with wrist range of motion.

Pitfalls
- Failure to recognize that a type II lunate is preventing full ulnar deviation of the midcarpal joint and therefore that excision of the proximal tip of the hamate is necessary
- Failure to adequately excise the distal pole of the scaphoid when distal scaphoid excision is performed
- Violation of the capitolunate joint
- Failure to recognize ulnar abutment between the ulnar head and triquetrum
- Irritation of a nerve, artery, or tendon caused by hardware. This is especially relevant when wires are placed from the radial side of the wrist percutaneously.

Expectations
- Seventy-degree arc of flexion-extension, 35-degree arc of radioulnar deviation
- As with other partial carpal fusions, incomplete relief of pain
- Prolonged recovery in some series
- Possible late-onset midcarpal degenerative changes

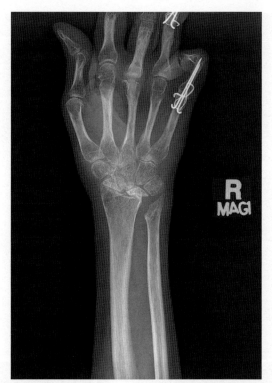

FIGURE 12.20 Posteroanterior x-ray at 9 months following surgery in a patient with rheumatoid arthritis who underwent attempted radioscapholunate fusion and developed nonunion. Despite nonunion, she remains symptom free with functional motion.

lunotriquetral dissociative instability. Contraindications include the presence of midcarpal arthritis, nondissociative ulnar midcarpal instability, or lunotriquetral dissociation with ulnocarpal impingement.

❖ AUTHOR'S PREFERRED METHOD OF TREATMENT: Lunotriquetral Arthrodesis

A longitudinal dorsal wrist incision is used. The lunotriquetral joint is approached through the fifth dorsal extensor compart-ment, and the extensor digiti minimi is dislocated toward the radial side. The triquetrum is identified through a longitudinal capsular incision, and the fourth compartment is raised subperiosteally off the distal radius to identify the lunotriquetral interval. Care is taken during this exposure to avoid injury to the dorsal radioulnar ligament origin on the radius. The triquetrolunate joint is decorticated with osteotomes and a rongeur. A distal radius bone graft is harvested as above. The fusion site is packed with bone graft while normal intercarpal spacing is maintained. Two 0.045-inch Kirschner wires are placed for fixation, and fluoroscopy is used to confirm the reduction and appropriate alignment. One Kirschner wire may be used to guide a cannulated drill or reamer and prepare for the insertion of a single cannulated headless bone screw; this can give rise to substantial compression of the joint, which is then usually stable. If there are any doubts about stability, the second Kirschner wire can be left in place and cut flush with the triquetrum.

Postoperative Management

Healing is somewhat less predictable and, in my experience, takes longer than with radiocarpal or four-corner arthrodesis. This is likely due to the small fusion area. Most patients require 6 to 10 weeks of immobilization. At this point the patient may be mobilized gently with flexion-extension and dart-throwing exercises. If the x-rays show satisfactory union, strengthening and more resistive activities can be started at 12 weeks. Heavy activities and contact sports should be avoided for 4 to 5 months.

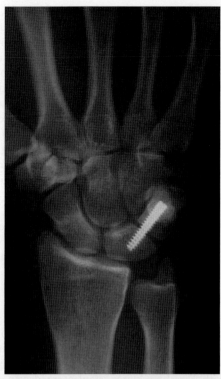

FIGURE 12.21 Headless bone screws are ideal for triquetrolunate (TL) fusion. A trial of TL fusion can be performed by percutaneous insertion of a TL screw.

Pearls

Because the effect of lunotriquetral fusion is unpredictable, temporary stabilization of the joint with a headless bone screw can be performed percutaneously through a small stab incision while taking care to avoid the dorsal branch of the ulnar nerve. After inserting a Kirschner wire and confirming its position with fluoroscopy, a cannulated drill and tap are used, followed by insertion of a headless bone screw across the joint (Figure 12.21). The patient can "try out" the fusion for the next 4 to 6 weeks; if successful, as a definite open procedure, the screw can be loosened, the joint prepared, the bone graft inserted, and the screw recompressed. Failure of the temporary fixation to improve the patient's symptoms indicates that the screw should be removed and the status quo should be reestablished. Further workup and consideration about management of the patient's condition are warranted.

Pitfalls

The dorsal branch of the ulnar nerve is highly vulnerable to percutaneous hardware insertion on the ulnar side of the wrist, and injury may give rise to a neuroma of this nerve and altered sensation on the dorsal-ulnar aspect of the hand. This complication causes considerable distress to patients and significantly detracts from any benefits of this procedure. To avoid this problem, a small skin incision should be made as is practiced in arthroscopy of the wrist, blunt dissection performed down to the triquetrum, and a drill sleeve used to protect the soft tissues.

Preoperative x-rays in full ulnar deviation and full axial compression of the forearm should identify whether there is abutment between the ulnar head and the triquetrum. Ulnar impaction is the leading cause of lunotriquetral disruption; it may also be a cause of significant pain. Treatment involves an isolated or combined wafer procedure[29] or ulnar-shortening osteotomy.

What Patients Should Be Told

There is a nonunion rate of 30%,[56] there will always be a loss of 30% to 40% of the range of motion, the results are somewhat unpredictable, and recovery takes 9 to 12 months. The pain may not be entirely relieved.

Triquetrohamate Fusion

Triquetrohamate fusion[85] is a less common intercarpal fusion; its primary indication is for treatment of painful midcarpal instability. Much like scapholunate arthrodesis, the complication rates are significant. Rao and Culver reported an almost 50% failure rate in providing relief of symptomatic midcarpal instability with triquetrohamate fusion[85]; therefore, this operation is not recommended. The author's experience mirrors that of these investigators.

Scaphotrapeziotrapezoidal Fusion

Indications

There are several indications for scaphotrapeziotrapezoidal fusion.[54,113] The presence of degenerative arthrosis localized to the STT joint is often associated with calcium pyrophosphate deposition disease. Primary osteoarthritis of this joint is not uncommon. Painful radial deviation and pain on gripping and when performing heavier tasks are the usual complaints of patients with scaphotrapeziotrapezoidal (STT) arthritis, and failure of conservative measures including corticosteroid injection is an indication for surgical intervention. STT arthrodesis (called triscaphe arthrodesis by Watson[109]) has also been used to treat selected cases of dynamic or static rotatory subluxation of the scaphoid, nonunion of the scaphoid, Kienböck disease,[41,109] scapholunate dissociation,[111] midcarpal instability, and congenital synchondrosis of the STT joint.

Contraindications

Contraindications primarily include radiographic narrowing or degenerative change of the radioscaphoid joint, which will become increasingly degenerative and symptomatic after the increased load transfer associated with STT fusion. The presence of thumb carpometacarpal (CMC) joint arthritis would also be considered a contraindication.

Preoperative evaluation should include radiography of the STT joint with full ulnar deviation views and full radial deviation views to identify whether the scaphoid moves. If the scaphoid is highly mobile, as characterized by considerable flexion and pronation during radial deviation, an STT fusion condemns patients to painful radioscaphoid subluxation each time they move into radial deviation. In this case, one should consider some form of interpositional arthroplasty or excisional arthroplasty rather than arthrodesis. Similarly, if there is substantial gap formation at the STT joint on full ulnar deviation that closes on radial deviation, there may be chronic bone loss involving the distal pole of the scaphoid. These patients have less satisfactory results with arthrodesis and in the author's experience are better served by excision of the distal pole of the scaphoid.[37]

❖ AUTHOR'S PREFERRED METHOD OF TREATMENT: Scaphotrapeziotrapezoid Fusion

The STT joint is approached through a dorsal radial curvilinear transverse wrist incision of 6 to 8 cm centered over the STT joint just distal to the radial styloid. The dorsal veins and branches of the superficial branch of the radial nerve are preserved. Care must be taken to identify and preserve the dorsal radial artery. The radial styloid is exposed through an incision in the capsule, and the distal 5 mm is removed with a rongeur. A transverse incision in the dorsal capsule is made, and the radioscaphoid joint is inspected. If significant degenerative disease is identified, the procedure of choice is proximal row carpectomy (if the capitate has a healthy articular surface) or scaphoid excision and four-corner fusion (if both the scaphoid fossa and head of the capitate show degenerative wear).

The distal aspect of the extensor retinaculum is opened along the EPL, and the STT joint is approached through a transverse capsular incision between the ECRL and ECRB tendons. The entire articular surfaces of the scaphoid, trapezium, and trapezoid are removed with a rongeur while taking care to remove the proximal half of the trapezium-trapezoid articulation only. It is mandatory that the subchondral hard cancellous bone also be removed and the softer cancellous surfaces exposed. The dorsal cortex of the trapezium and trapezoid is likewise removed to broaden the surface area for fusion. The volar lip of the scaphoid is decorticated by inserting a dental rongeur deep into the joint and levering the handle distally. Cancellous bone graft is then harvested from the distal radius at the Lister tubercle. Two 0.045-inch Kirschner wires are driven percutaneously from the distal aspect of the dorsal trapezoid proximally into the prepared space without crossing it. The first, radially positioned Kirschner wire is passed to the point of just touching the surface of the scaphoid. The second, ulnarly positioned Kirschner wire is passed proximally to the point of entering the scaphotrapezoid space. The wrist is placed in full radial deviation and 45 degrees of dorsiflexion while the scaphoid tuberosity is reduced by the surgeon's thumb to prevent overcorrection of the scaphoid (Figure 12.22, *A*). A 5-mm spacer, usually the handle of a small instrument, is placed into the scaphotrapezoid space to maintain the original external dimensions of the STT joint, and the radial Kirschner wire is driven into the scaphoid while avoiding placement into the radioscaphoid joint. The spacer is removed, and the ulnar Kirschner wire is similarly driven into the scaphoid (see Figure 12-22, *B*). After pinning, the scaphoid should lie at approximately 55 degrees of flexion relative to the long axis of the radius when seen from the lateral view. This ensures optimal radioscaphoid congruity and maximizes the postoperative range of motion. It is not necessary to correct any abnormal rotation of the lunate. Excessive extension of the scaphoid will limit the motion obtained after surgery. Cancellous bone is densely packed into the spaces between the scaphoid, trapezium, and trapezoid. The pins are cut beneath the skin level, and the wrist capsule and extensor retinaculum are simply realigned without suturing. The skin incisions are closed with a single-layer subcuticular monofilament suture. The postoperative dressing consists of a bulky noncompressive wrap incorporating a long-arm plaster splint. The hand is placed in a protected position with the wrist in slight extension and radial deviation, the forearm neutral, and the elbow at 90 degrees.

Postoperative Management

An above-elbow bulky dressing and splint including the thumb are applied for the first 2 to 3 weeks following surgery. Following suture removal, a long-arm thumb spica cast is applied. Following 4 additional weeks of above-elbow immobilization, a short-arm thumb spica cast can be added for an additional 2 to 3 weeks. If using Kirschner wire fixation, the proximal carpal row is easily immobilized by casting the forearm and arm, but it is difficult to adequately maintain the position of the distal carpal row. Therefore, Watson recommended casting the metacarpophalangeal (MP) joints of the index and middle fingers in 80 to 90 degrees of flexion (the so-called Groucho Marx cast) with the interphalangeal joints left free. When radiographic union is seen, the pins are removed in the office and the patient is referred to the hand therapy department for full wrist mobilization. A splint may occasionally be used for an additional 1 or 2 weeks if there is any doubt about the status of bone healing.

Alternative Techniques

Staple Fixation

Power-inserted staples can simplify the fixation process and prevent complications related to Kirschner wire irritation and potential infection. After provisional fixation in the appropriate position with Kirschner wires, staples are driven across the scaphotrapezial and scaphotrapezoid joints. The provisional Kirschner wires can then be removed. Postoperative care is as outlined earlier, although it is seldom necessary to include the index and middle digits in a cast when modern fixation techniques are employed.

Circular Plate Fixation

Small circular plates, commonly used in the management of four-corner fusions, may also be used for fixation of an STT arthrodesis. Most plate systems carry a smaller version that can be centered at the STT joint dorsally. The bone ends are prepared as in the above-mentioned technique and provisional Kirschner wires can be placed to hold the construct in reduction. Most systems use reamers to inset the plate into the fusion mass.

Screw Fixation

The STT joint should be reduced and provisionally held by two guidewires and checked by fluoroscopy. The length is measured, and an appropriate-length cannulated screw can be inserted over each wire.

What Patients Should Be Told

Watson has reported excellent functional results and pain-free, stable wrists after STT arthrodesis. In a review of over 800 STT fusions, the average range of motion has usually been 70 to 80% of that of the contralateral normal wrist and the grip strength has averaged 70 to 90% of that of the unaffected wrist.[113] Long-term radiographic follow-up has revealed only rare instances of progressive radioscaphoid or intercarpal degenerative changes, and they occurred only in patients who had some evidence of disease in these joints at the time of surgery. However, radial styloid-scaphoid impingement can occur and may be painful; styloidectomy is thus an important element of the procedure.[88] The nonunion rate is greater than 20% (Figure 12.23). Loss of

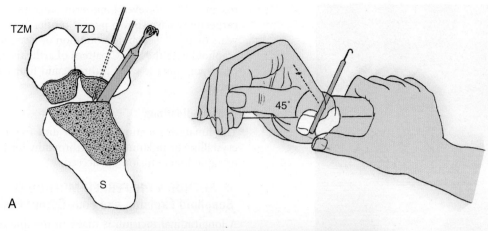

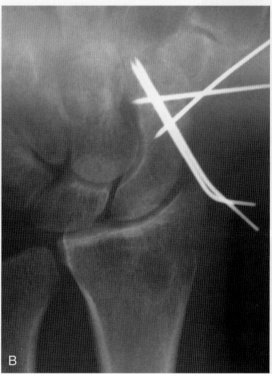

FIGURE 12.22 A, These diagrammatic representations of the preparation and positioning of the scaphoid highlight the requirement of ensuring that the scaphoid must lie in a flexed position at 45 to 55 degrees to the long axis of the radius before insertion of the Kirschner wires. **B,** Posteroanterior radiograph demonstrating scaphotrapezotrapezoidal arthrodesis with K-wire fixation. *S,* Scaphoid, *TZD,* trapezoid; *TZM,* trapezium.

wrist range of motion is unpredictable. Recovery takes 9 to 12 months, and pain relief may not be complete.

Few authors have reported results as successful as those reported by Watson and colleagues following STT arthrodesis. Kleinman and Carroll reported a 52% complication rate in 47 wrists monitored for 10 years and highlighted the need for precise positioning of the fused scaphoid.[54]

Reconstruction of Wrists With Scapholunate/Scaphoid Nonunion Advanced Collapse (Scaphoid Excision, Capitate-Lunate-Hamate-Triquetrum Fusion)

The SLAC and SNAC patterns of arthritis generally spare the radiolunate articulation, and therefore capitate-hamate-lunate-triquetrum arthrodesis (the four-corner fusion with scaphoid excision) has become the procedure of choice, particularly if the midcarpal joint is arthritic.[21,52,55,102,110,112] Excision of the scaphoid must include stabilization of the remaining carpus to prevent gross instability, and this is achieved effectively either through arthrodesis of the capitate, lunate, triquetrum, and hamate or by capitolunate fusion alone. Capitolunate arthrodesis reduces the area of cancellous bone exposed and may be less reliable than four-corner fusion.

Indications

The presence of degenerative changes in the radioscaphoid joint and the midcarpal joint identifies the pattern as SLAC wrist stage III (Figure 12.24). If the capitolunate joint is preserved, proximal row carpectomy is an alternative to four-corner

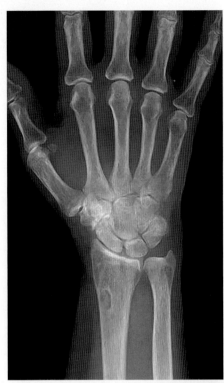

FIGURE 12.23 Posteroanterior view of the hand demonstrates a patient who had undergone attempted scaphotrapeziotrapezoid fusion 1 year earlier and now had a painful nonunion.

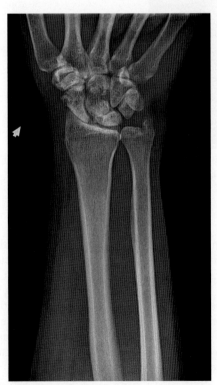

FIGURE 12.24 Stage III scapholunate advanced collapse wrist as seen on a radiograph. The prolonged scaphoid flexion and the deepening radial erosion force the lunate into extension, which becomes very difficult to reduce because of an associated anterior capsular contracture. Reduction, however, is essential to permit extension of the wrist, which after a four-corner fusion, occurs solely at the radiolunate articulation.

fusion.[21,25,105] However, long-term outcomes with proximal row carpectomy have shown poorer results in patients less than 40 years of age.[105] Scaphoid nonunion or avascular necrosis of the scaphoid with the SNAC pattern of arthritis may lead to significant symptomatic wrist arthritis, and four-corner fusion is an option.

Contraindications

The lunate fossa must be intact and free of disease such as crystalline or inflammatory arthropathy for four-corner fusion or capitolunate fusion to succeed.

❖ AUTHOR'S PREFERRED METHOD OF TREATMENT: Scaphoid Excision and Four-Corner Fusion

A longitudinal incision is made in the line of the third metacarpal. The extensor retinaculum is incised over the third compartment, and the fourth and second compartments are exposed over the carpus. Posterior interosseous neurectomy is performed by excising a 1-cm segment of the nerve proximal to the dorsal rim of the radius. The ligament-sparing capsulotomy is performed to expose the joint. Visual inspection of the lunate and the lunate fossa must confirm intact articular cartilage. On occasion, in more severe SLAC wrists and in wrists with extreme extension of the lunate, there may be some dorsal chondromalacia of the lunate and the dorsal rim of the lunate fossa. Because the lunate alignment will be corrected with the procedure, some of this is acceptable, but if it is too extensive, an alternative procedure, such as a complete wrist fusion, should be considered. The ECRL and ECRB are retracted to allow extension of the capsulotomy more radially for exposure of the scaphoid. The scaphoid is removed with a rongeur. The palmar radioscaphocapitate and long radiolunate ligaments are protected. The remaining cartilage and subchondral bone are removed from the surfaces of the capitate, distal lunate, hamate, and distal triquetrum until a broad cancellous surface is obtained. Bone graft is harvested from beneath the Lister tubercle. Next, 0.045-inch Kirschner wires are percutaneously preset through the capitate, hamate, and triquetrum so that they line up with the more proximal lunate. A fourth wire is passed into the triquetrum directed toward the capitate. Cancellous graft is packed into the deep interval between the capitate and lunate. The most important step in this procedure is to reduce the dorsiflexed position of the lunate in relation to the radius. A Kirschner wire inserted into the dorsal lunate is used as a joystick for reduction. With the lunate reduced into neutral alignment or very slight extension, the capitate is translated ulnarward to restore its normal position on the lunate in the coronal plane. It is important not to overcorrect the capitate position on the lunate, because the palmar extrinsic ligaments will tighten and limit ulnar deviation. The preset Kirschner wires are passed across the capitolunate, capitohamate, triquetrocapitate, and triquetrolunate joints under fluoroscopic guidance. The intervals between the bones are packed with cancellous bone harvested from the distal radius. Although I have no strong feelings about the hardware selection for fusion, I prefer a radiolucent circular plate (Figure 12.25, *A* and *B*). A reamer is used to inset the plate so that it will not impinge with extension of the wrist. Typically, I will try to place at least two screws into each bone; tightening the screws applies compression across the fusion mass. Each hole is drilled and the screw placed. I prefer to place subsequent

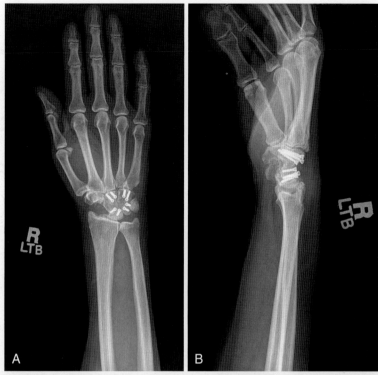

FIGURE 12.25   A, Posteroanterior view following a four-corner fusion using a radiolucent circular plate. Note the center of the plate is slightly distal to the four-bone center, which will minimize risk of plate impingement. **B,** Also, it is important to reduce the lunate from its extended position. Recessing the plate will also help to reduce the risk of impingement with extension, but care must be taken to avoid overrecessing because it will limit the strength of fixation.

screws opposite from the previous screw to maintain the balance of the plate and its position. I find that placing the center of the plate a bit distally from the center of the four bones provides a better position for the hardware (see Figure 12.25, *B*). Care should be taken to avoid penetration of the far cortex in the triquetrum and lunate as that would invite irritation of the pisotriquetral and radiolunate joints. Fluoroscopy should be used to confirm appropriate reduction of the lunate and carpus, as well as the hardware position and appropriate screw lengths. Upon completion of the construct, the wrist should be extended to confirm that there is no hardware impingement (Figure 12.26, *A* and *B*). The wires are removed after securing the plate. The capsule is closed, the retinaculum is repaired, the subcutaneous tissues are approximated, and the skin is closed with subcuticular sutures.

Postoperative Management

The extremity is immobilized in a bulky conforming dressing and splint in neutral to 20 degrees of extension. The fingers are left free for exercises. At 2 weeks the sutures are removed and a short-arm cast is applied. At 6 to 8 weeks after surgery, the patient is assessed clinically and radiographically, a lightweight removable splint is applied, and remedial exercises are commenced. In patients younger than 55 years, a more cautious approach consisting of the application of a long-arm cast for the first 5 weeks may be indicated. Some authors have allowed for earlier motion with the use of compression staples, circular plates, and compression screws. However, my preference is to protect the patient for approximately 6 weeks.

Alternative Methods of Fixation

In recent years a number of internal fixation devices have been designed and applied to limited wrist fusion in an attempt to provide more rigid fixation.

Kirschner Wire Fixation

Kirschner wires are a simpler method of fixation for maintaining the four-bone mass alignment and reduction (Figure 12.27). The pins are typically removed approximately 6 to 8 weeks following surgery. One can leave the pins out in the skin or bury the pins subcutaneously in case there is a need to leave them in longer. The pins have the advantage of being more forgiving in placement; also, there is no potential for problems with retained hardware.

Staple Fixation

Power fixation devices have facilitated placement of staples with both improved accuracy of placement and improved biomechanical properties.[7,91] The capitate, lunate, hamate, and triquetrum are prepared as described earlier and provisionally held with Kirschner wires. One staple is placed between the capitate and hamate, a second between the hamate and triquetrum, and a third between the lunate and capitate (Figure 12.28). Staples measuring 13 mm wide and 10 mm deep are normally chosen.

Screw Fixation

The development of headless compression screws has facilitated internal fixation of carpal bones by burying the screw within

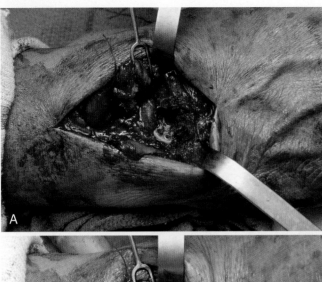

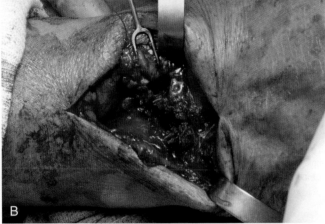

FIGURE 12.26 A, Intraoperative images following plate fixation and the use of a circular plate with the wrist in neutral. **B,** Note that in extension the plate glides without impingement on the dorsal lip of the radius.

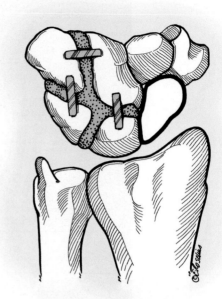

FIGURE 12.28 Diagram of staple fixation. (Copyright © Elizabeth Martin.)

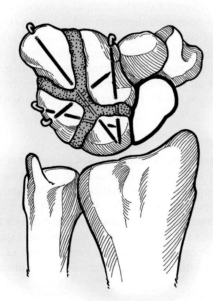

FIGURE 12.27 Kirschner wires fixing a four-corner fusion. (Copyright © Elizabeth Martin.)

the carpus. Several manufacturers have designed appropriate headless cannulated screws. Screw fixation affords the opportunity for initiation of earlier range of motion because a more reliable and rigid fixation can be achieved.

What Patients Should Be Told

When the procedure is successful, pain relief has been excellent. Neubrech and colleagues reviewed nearly 600 four-corner fusions, with over 100 followed for nearly 15 years.[74] Graduation to total wrist fusion was necessary in less than 7% of patients. The nonunion rate was 11%. Flexion-extension and radioulnar motions were 62% and 68%, respectively, of the motions of the contralateral sides. Grip strength was nearly 90% of that of the contralateral side. Subjective outcomes were generally excellent. Although some previous studies have shown that more rigid fixation methods were associated with earlier graduation to range of motion, these methods also had increased complication rates.[100] However, newer analyses have shown that with proper technique, success can be achieved with the newer-generation circular plates, headless compression screws, or staples.[3,5,76] I conclude again that the method of fixation is less important than the reduction of the fusion mass and appropriate bone preparation. In addition, I have found that with immobilization for 6 weeks following surgery, the rates of long-term motion are similar to those of the Neubrech and colleagues study.

Scaphoid Excision With Capitolunate Arthrodesis

Stabilization (fusion) of the midcarpal joint for reconstruction of a SLAC wrist can also be achieved by isolated capitolunate fusion (Figures 12.29 and 12.30).[2,14,50,52] Because there is no theoretical difference in motion between the two options, four-bone fusion has been recommended to enlarge the fusion surfaces and improve the rate of union. With the availability of more rigid methods of fixation, isolated capitolunate fusion has been used as a simpler procedure that requires only limited

CRITICAL POINTS *Scaphoid Excision and Four-Corner Fusion*

Indications
- SLAC or SNAC stage II or III
- Four-corner fusion is preferred over proximal row carpectomy in patients younger than 45 years of age

Preoperative Evaluation
- CT scanning or MRI can be helpful as an adjunct to standard x-rays to evaluate the cartilage of the radiolunate joint and confirm the SLAC stage.

Pearls
- There must be no degenerative joint disease at the radiolunate joint.
- A posterior interosseous neurectomy should be incorporated as part of the procedure.
- Protect the volar radial supporting ligaments and radioscaphocapitate ligament during the scaphoidectomy and scaphoid excision. This will minimize the risk of ulnar translation of the carpus.
- Proper bone preparation is critical to ensure a successful fusion. Decortication of the lunate-capitate-hamate-triquetral surfaces down to healthy cancellous bone is important. In patients with severe or long-standing SLAC III wrists, the lunate-capitate interval may be quite sclerotic, and denuding down to healthy cancellous bone may be challenging. A high-speed bur can be used to create "craters" on the surfaces that help to maintain the length of the fusion mass but also allow access to the healthy bleeding bone that helps facilitate fusion.
- When using a bur, copious irrigation is needed to avoid overheating and osteonecrosis.
- When choosing the fixation method, have fallback options or a plan B because the position of the four bones and their reduction may be somewhat different than originally expected.
- I feel strongly that the method of fixation is not as important as the application of meticulous carpentry in preparing the bone ends and bone grafting.

Pitfalls
- Avoid leaving prominent dorsal hardware because this may invite impingement with wrist extension.
- Do not overreduce the capitate in the coronal plane because this will tighten the extrinsic ligaments and reduce the ulnar deviation.
- Failure to adequately reduce the lunate from its extended position will invite impingement and result in limited wrist extension.
- With circular plates, avoid screws that penetrate the far cortex in the lunate and triquetrum. Inadequate bone preparation and denuding of cartilage down to cancellous bone will invite a higher risk of nonunion.

Expectations
- There will be 50 to 60% of contralateral flexion-extension and radioulnar deviation.
- The nonunion rate is 10 to 15%.
- Relief of pain is incomplete.
- The recovery time is 9 to 12 months.
- Late-onset radiolunate degenerative changes are possible.

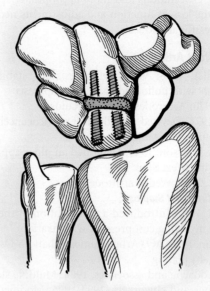

FIGURE 12.29 Excision of the scaphoid and localized capitolunate fusion fixed with headless bone screws. (Copyright © Elizabeth Martin.)

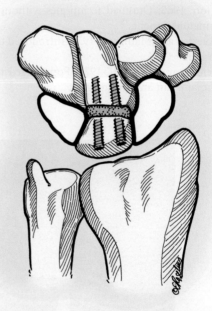

FIGURE 12.30 Excision of the scaphoid and triquetrum occasionally requires an additional capitohamate arthrodesis in the small group of patients with a mobile capitohamate joint. (Copyright © Elizabeth Martin.)

Total Wrist Arthrodesis

When the wrist has been so damaged by the disease process that significant bone stock has been lost, the only reliable surgical procedure is arthrodesis, and this is often the only practical course of action. Particular attention should be paid to the lateral x-ray of the wrist; it may show significant volar subluxation of the lunate, which will give rise to some difficulties in reducing the wrist and could precipitate carpal tunnel syndrome as the wrist is relocated and realigned. From a patient satisfaction perspective, I think it wise to have the patient wear

bone graft, which can be obtained from the excised scaphoid. Screw fixation permits earlier initiation of range of motion. Some authors recommend triquetral excision at the time of capitolunate fusion and have had results comparable to those of four-corner arthrodesis and improved motion in the radioulnar direction.[31]

a brace continuously in order to "simulate" a wrist fusion. It will help temper expectations and more appropriately prepare the patient for the loss of function and adjustments necessary following successful arthrodesis.

History of Wrist Arthrodesis

- Steindler, 1918: Wrist arthrodesis for stabilization in patients with polio and spastic hemiparesis
- Ely, 1920: Arthrodesis for tuberculosis
- Gill, 1923: Devised a method of corticocancellous grafting to provide stability
- Smith-Peterson, 1940: Described an ulnar approach with distal ulnar excision[93]
- Evans, 1955: Wedge arthrodesis[28]

Plates, Wires, and Staples

- Wood, 1987: Introduced a modification of the Gill technique involving compression wire fixation[119]
- Larsson, 1974: AO (Arbeitsgemeinschaft für Osteosynthesefragen) plating[57]
- Benkeddache and associates, 1984: Multiple staples[7]
- Hastings and coworkers, 1993/1996: Modified AO plate with compression[45]

Intramedullary Fixation

- Robinson and Kayfetz, 1952: Intramedullary rods in rheumatoid patients[87]
- Clayton, 1965: Outlined techniques without fixation in rheumatoid patients[18]
- Mannerfelt and Malmsten, 1971: Introduced the Rush pin technique[62]
- Millender and Nalebuff, 1973: Popularized the use of a Steinmann pin and sliding graft[66]

❖ AUTHOR'S PREFERRED METHOD OF TREATMENT: Total Wrist Arthrodesis

My preferred method of stabilizing the wrist for fusion is to use a dorsal wrist fusion plate applied using AO fixation principles.[45,116,120] Specially made plates that fix the radius with 3.5-mm screws and the metacarpal with 2.7-mm screws fit quite nicely and span the radiocarpal, intercarpal, and CMC joints nicely (Figure 12.31, A and B). Many fixation systems use precontoured plates that conveniently facilitate fixation and compression. Straight plates that one can customize are available for patients with severe disease or a shortened carpus resulting from a prior proximal row carpectomy. In addition, the newer-generation implants afford locking technology, which has been quite helpful in patients with weaker bone stock or bone deficits, such as those with severe rheumatoid arthritis or for whom arthroplasty has failed. As a result, I rarely use Steinmann pins or intramedullary fixation for total wrist fusion.

A standard longitudinal incision is begun in the midmetacarpal area and centered on the third metacarpal (Figure 12.32, A). The incision passes across the Lister tubercle and ends over the dorsum of the distal radius just proximal to the muscle belly of the adductor pollicis longus. The radial side of the incision is raised as a flap directly off the dorsal surface of the retinaculum and contains the superficial branch of the radial nerve. The dorsum of the retinaculum is opened by incising the third compartment (EPL) (see Figure 12.32, B and C) or through a Z-plasty of the fourth compartment retinaculum (see Figure 12.32, D). The EPL is mobilized from the compartment proximally and distally and transposed radially. The distal radius is exposed subperiosteally, and the longitudinal incision in the

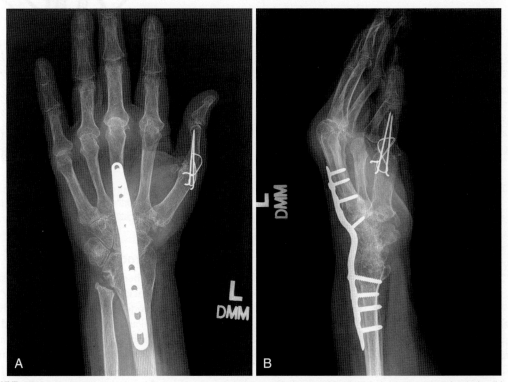

FIGURE 12.31 A, Posteroanterior and **B,** lateral x-rays of a patient with rheumatoid arthritis who underwent arthrodesis with a precontoured dorsal wrist fusion plate.

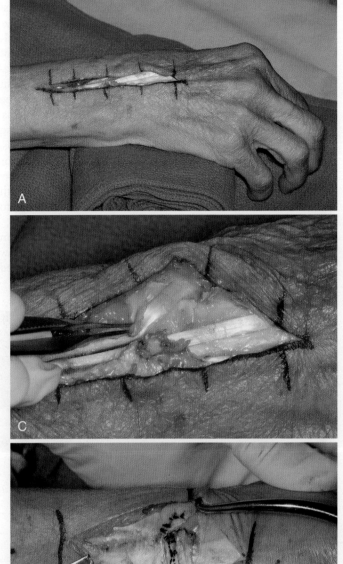

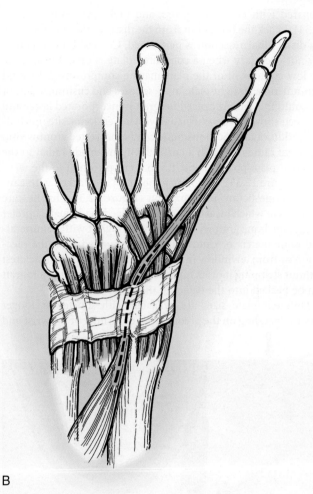

FIGURE 12.32 A, A dorsal approach to the wrist centered over the 3 to 4 compartments proximally and in line with the third metacarpal distally. **B** and **C,** A schematic drawing and an operative photo show the approach through the retinaculum in line with the EPL tendon. The obliquity of the retinacular exposure allows for adjustments in tension on closure. **D,** An alternative approach through the retinaculum is via a Z-plasty through the fourth compartment. I prefer to leave the extensor pollicis longus superficial to the retinaculum on closing. (**B,** Copyright © Elizabeth Martin.)

periosteum is extended distally through the capsule out to the radial base of the third metacarpal. A 1- to 2-cm portion of the posterior interosseous nerve is excised just proximal to the articular surface of the radius. The insertion of the ECRB is subperiosteally elevated by scalpel dissection and reflected radially. An incision is made in the interosseous fascia on the radial side of the third metacarpal. The dorsal surface of the third metacarpal is exposed without disturbing the intrinsic musculature on either side. A scalpel blade is used to elevate the two flaps of capsule from the carpus. The second dorsal compartment is elevated subperiosteally from the radius and reflected radially with its underlying capsule. If evaluation or resection of the DRUJ is necessary, the retinaculum should be elevated

through the fifth compartment; deep to that compartment, access to the distal radioulnar joint is afforded via an "L"-shaped capsular incision (Figure 12.33). The DRUJ is left undisturbed unless distal ulnar resection is needed for degenerative arthritis. To allow flat apposition of the plate on the radius, the Lister tubercle is removed with an osteotome. This also allows for access to a distal radius bone graft. The dorsal cortices of the base of the third metacarpal and the carpal bones are removed to give excellent visual access to all the joints to be included in the fusion.

Five articulations are generally necessary to facilitate a successful fusion: radiolunate, radioscaphoid, lunocapitate, scaphocapitate and the third CMC joints. The bone ends are prepared with curets, rongeurs, and high-speed burs (Figure 12.34). I pack the bone graft from the distal radius and the ulna, if a distal ulnar resection is performed. Cortical bone is generally not necessary when a contoured plate is used, but if used, the low-contour fit of the plate may be compromised. I would recommend a straight plate in these cases and customization of the contour. A purely cancellous graft is incorporated faster and has been shown to be associated with lower donor site morbidity.[45] Additional cancellous bone can be harvested from within the distal radius through a cortical window made radial to the intended plate position and 1.5 to 2 cm proximal to the wrist joint (Figure 12.35). All joints to be fused are packed with cancellous bone before plate fixation (Figure 12.36). In the rare instances in which local bone graft is judged inadequate, I prefer mixing the bone graft with cancellous allograft with demineralized bone matrix or cancellous bone harvested from the olecranon or from a window in the superior aspect of the iliac crest without stripping it of its musculature. Any remaining allograft can be packed into the defect of the distal radius.

Different plate sizes are available with shorter or longer bends depending on the preoperative deformity of the wrist and whether the proximal row is retained or excised. These plates do not typically require contouring and they position the wrist in slight extension. A straight version is used when large segmental carpal traumatic or tumor defects require corticocancellous intercalary graft replacement. When desired, a slight extension bend can easily be created with plate benders. If precontoured or 3.5/2.7-mm plates are not available, a straight 3.5-mm limited contact dynamic compression plate may be similarly contoured to follow the dorsal radius, carpal sulcus, and dorsal third metacarpal. One version has a distal taper so as to have a lower profile on the metacarpal. In small individuals, a nine-hole, 3.5-mm reconstruction plate is optimal. In persons with extremely small hands, a 2.7-mm reconstruction plate may be necessary. However, even in some of the smaller wrists with severe rheumatoid arthritis, it has generally been possible to secure the 3.5/2.7-mm plates (Figure 12.37, A and B).

The plate is affixed to the third metacarpal with 2.7-mm screws while taking care to ensure central drilling in its narrow isthmus. The distal metacarpal hole is drilled first and secured

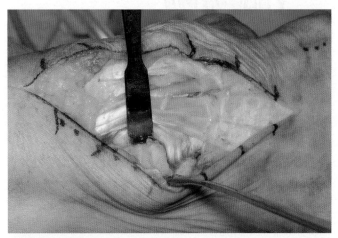

FIGURE 12.33 When necessary, exposure to the ulnar head is performed through the floor of the fifth compartment and the joint can be exposed via an "L"-shaped capsular incision.

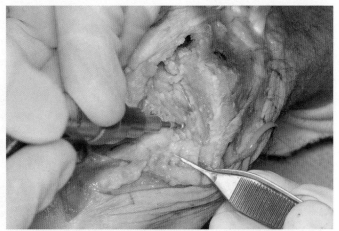

FIGURE 12.34 The use of curets, rongeurs, and, occasionally, burs, especially in hard sclerotic bony surfaces, is necessary to appropriately prepare the surfaces for bone grafting and fusion. This is arguably the most important aspect of surgery to help ensure fusion. When using a high-speed bur, liberal irrigation is needed to minimize heat-related damage to the bony surfaces.

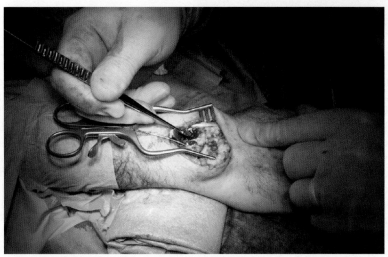

FIGURE 12.35 Cancellous graft is harvested from the distal radius through a window created by excision of the Lister tubercle.

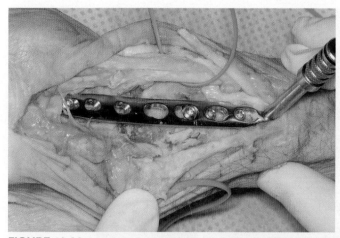

FIGURE 12.36 Placement of cancellous bone graft beneath the plate. Cortical screws help secure the plate to the bone and afford compression. In patients with severe rheumatoid arthritis and/or poor bone quality, locking screws can be added to enhance stability of the construct.

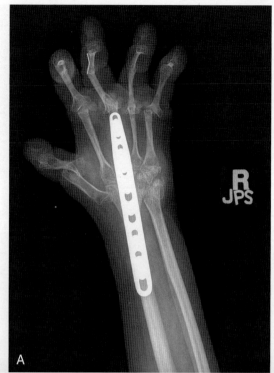

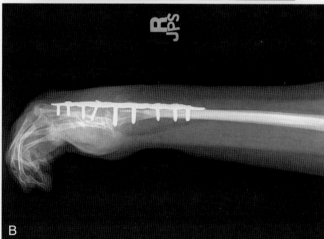

FIGURE 12.37 A, Posteroanterior and **B,** lateral radiographs of a 43-year-old female with juvenile rheumatoid arthritis and smaller bone structure who underwent arthrodesis for severe deformity and pain. Despite the smaller bone structure, fixation with the plate was feasible and fusion successful. Note that the most proximal screw was the smallest available and had to be cut so as not to be too prominent volarly.

with a cortical screw to enable fine-tuning of the position and compression of the plate to the bone. Accurate alignment of the plate in the dorsal midline of the metacarpal is essential to avoid malrotation and maximize grip strength potential.[82] Upon confirmation of adequate reduction and alignment of the wrist, a second screw may be placed in the metacarpal to ensure the plate will not rotate with compression prior to moving to the radius, or if I am comfortable with the bone quality and confident that the distal fixation is secure to the bone and will not rotate with compression, I will next fix the plate proximally in the radius with a 3.5-mm cortical screw in compression mode. Further compression at the fusion mass may be achieved with a second screw in the radius. After drilling the second compression screw, it is important to start the second screw; the tension from the first radial compression screw is released prior to securing the second screw, allowing for the further compression. The first radial screw can be retightened and secured. Because the radial screws are larger, better compression is achieved from them compared with the 2.7-mm metacarpal screws. The remaining screw holes in the metacarpal, capitate, and radius are filled in no-compression mode, or if the bone quality is poor, locking screws may be used to provide strength to the overall construct (Figure 12.38, *A* and *B*). The use of fluoroscopy will be most helpful during positioning for confirming appropriate plate/screw placement and screw lengths.

Closure

A small suction drain is routinely used and brought out proximally. The capsule is closed to the best extent possible to cover the plate with absorbable interrupted braided suture. The retained radial and ulnar flaps of the previously opened retinaculum are approximated, with the EPL left transposed radially out of the Lister canal to minimize potential irritation of the tendon (Figure 12.39).

Postoperative Management

A bulky short-arm dressing incorporating a volar plaster splint is applied. If a distal ulnar resection is performed, I will likely place a sugar-tong splint to prevent pronation and supination.

At week 2 the wrist is placed into a cast for an additional 2 to 4 weeks. If clinical healing is confirmed, the patient is graduated to a removable splint for support. Full active use of the hand and digits is allowed, but resistance or lifting is limited to 1 kg. The splint is discontinued at 8 to 10 weeks after surgery. Full use of the hand is allowed by the 10th week. Radiographic healing is to be expected by 8 to 10 weeks.

Complications

A union rate of nearly 100% can be expected when using a precontoured compression plate and local bone graft. Larsson reported a 0% nonunion rate in 23 cases,[57] and Weiss and

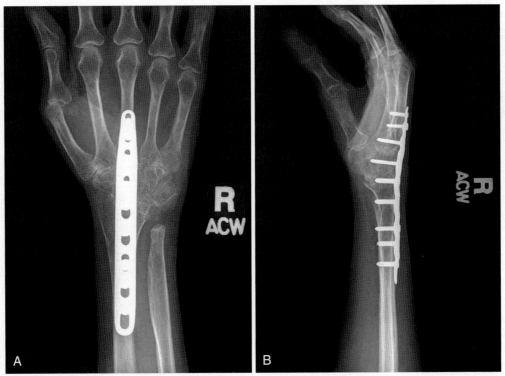

FIGURE 12.38 A, Posteroanterior and **B,** lateral x-rays of a 75-year-old female with severe rheumatoid arthritis and poor bone quality who underwent successful arthrodesis 1 year earlier. To enhance the rigidity and strength of the construct, the majority of screws placed were locking after securing the construct distally with a cortical screw and compressing it proximally with a 3.5-mm cortical screw.

CRITICAL POINTS *Plate Fixation for Wrist Arthrodesis*

Indications
- Pancarpal arthrosis of the radiocarpal and midcarpal joints
- Failed past limited arthrodesis
- Failed total joint or previous arthroplasty[86]
- Paralysis of the wrist or hand (with the potential for using functioning tendons for transfer)
- Reconstruction after segmental tumor resection, infection, or traumatic segmental bone loss of the distal radius and carpus[70]
- Inflammatory arthritis with healthy bone stock[45]

Pearls
- Decorticate the dorsal 80% of the third CMC joint.
- Remove the dorsal distal radius for improved plate fit.
- Harvest a distal radius metaphyseal bone graft and apply to the fusion site.
- In a patient with rheumatoid arthritis and ulnar translation, remove part of the radial styloid to facilitate realignment of the wrist.
- Fluoroscopy is helpful in ensuring that the plate position, wrist alignment, compression at the fusion mass, and screw lengths are appropriate.

Technical Points
- Transpose the EPL.
- Decorticate the third CMC joint, capitate, proximal hamate, and distal radius.
- Place graft in the third CMC joint.
- Fix the plate to the metacarpal first.
- Reduce the wrist and fix the plate to the radius in compression mode.
- Fill in any remaining screw holes in the metacarpal, capitate, and radius in neutral mode.
- In patients with poorer bone stock, locking screws will help strengthen the construct.

- Add additional graft from the dorsal distal aspect of the radius and excised carpal bones to the fusion area.
- The triquetrum can be removed if ulnocarpal impingement is of concern.

Pitfalls
- The drill hole through the metacarpal portion of the plate must be in the sagittal plane. If not, the plate will lie rotated on the metacarpal. Subsequent radius fixation will cause rotational deformity of the third metacarpal.
- If the capitate does not contact the undersurface of the plate and is lagged up to the plate, the screw may end up being too long and protrude into the carpal canal. Check screw length with fluoroscopy.
- If non–self-tapping screws are used, be careful to avoid excessive penetration of the tip through the metacarpal, which may injure the deep motor branch of the ulnar nerve as it crosses radially.
- If the ulna is not resected, failure to reduce the lunate to the lunate fossa may invite ulnocarpal impingement.

Postoperative Care
- Immobilize the hand and wrist in a bulky dressing and splint for 10 to 14 days.
- Apply a short-arm cast for 2 to 4 weeks longer.
- At 4 to 6 weeks, graduate to a removable splint.
- At 8 to 10 weeks, begin strengthening.
- Allow full use at 10 to 12 weeks.

Athletic Participation
- Patients are given a 5-lb weight limit for the first 8 weeks.
- Full use is allowed after 10 weeks as symptoms and radiographs permit.

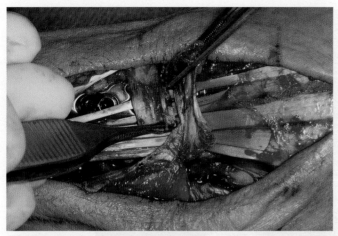

FIGURE 12.39 Repair of the retinaculum following fusion of the wrist. Even in cases of increased tension/volume due to hardware, bone graft, and/or correction of deformity, the Z-plasty affords reapproximation of a functional pulley. Note that the extensor pollicis longus in the most radial aspect of the wound is left superficial to the retinacular closure.

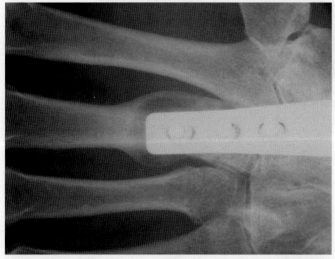

FIGURE 12.40 Failure to achieve sound arthrodesis at the third carpometacarpal joint in an active individual may give rise to loosening of the plate from the metacarpal as shown here, with subsequent painful swelling and diminished function.

Hastings also had a 0% nonunion rate in 28 patients with a plate and local bone graft.[116] When partial nonunion occurs, it most commonly occurs at the third CMC joint (Figure 12.40). With stabilization of the radiocarpal and midcarpal joints, stress may be concentrated distally, and micromotion can lead to fibrous union. Prevention depends on careful and complete decortication of the dorsal 80% of the third CMC joint down to cancellous bone. Although some authors have advised against attempts to formally include the third CMC joint in the fusion, subsequent plate removal is then mandatory to prevent hardware loosening or fatigue fracture. When not included in the fusion, the second and third CMC joints may be at risk for the later development of symptomatic degenerative changes. Standard 3.5-mm plates have been reported to have hardware complication rates of 19%, the majority at the metacarpal level. The incidence of plate removal for tenderness has been 12%.[45] The

lower-profile precontoured wrist fusion plate uses smaller 2.7-mm screws distally at the metacarpal level and has tapered edges, and the screws are recessed flush with the dorsal plate surface. With use of this lower-profile plate, symptoms requiring implant removal are rare. The incidence of carpal tunnel syndrome after AO plate fusion is as high as 10.5%, with approximately 67% requiring carpal tunnel release.[45] The surgeon must carefully assess for preoperative carpal tunnel symptoms that may become symptomatic postoperatively. Ideally, the three-dimensional architecture of the carpal canal should not be altered significantly by fusion. Although wrist fusion is generally predictable in providing pain relief, unexplained pain can persist despite successful fusion. This is most commonly seen in patients who have previously undergone multiple failed surgical procedures. When this is the case, selective wrist nerve blocks may be indicated to determine whether wrist denervation would be helpful.[13,114] DRUJ pain can occur after fusion in a small percentage of individuals.[19,115] In a series of 85 wrist fusions, new pain in the DRUJ was seen in just one case and resolved after injection of the joint with 1 mL of betamethasone. Plate fixation of the radius to the third metacarpal usually "radializes" the wrist and protects against impingement of the distal end of the ulna and carpus. Ulnocarpal abutment can occur when there is a discrepancy between the combined height of the radius and radial carpus and that of the ulna and ulnar part of the carpus.[34] When the surgeon chooses to maintain and incorporate the proximal row into the fusion, visual and radiographic means must be used to ensure that the triquetrum does not interfere with the distal end of the ulna. If insufficient space exists between the distal ulna and the triquetrum, the triquetrum should be excised (see Figure 12.30). Some surgeons first perform a proximal row carpectomy, fusing just the radial-capitate and third CMC intervals, simplifying the procedure and avoiding ulnocarpal impingement (Figure 12.41, A and B).[61]

Intramedullary Pin Fusion for Patients With Rheumatoid Arthritis

Intramedullary pin arthrodesis is an established technique for patients with rheumatoid arthritis and poor bone quality. This method of fusion was first described by Clayton[18] and further popularized by Millender and Nalebuff[66] uses a Steinmann pin, which is inserted down the third metacarpal shaft and into the radius (Figure 12.42). The technique is both technically simple and effective.

This technique is not without potential complications, because the third MP joint will have to be violated. In addition, because these patients have multijoint rheumatoid involvement, surgery will probably be needed to replace the third MP joint. The Steinmann pin may be difficult to countersink, and if there is a failure of union of the third CMC joint, continued motion at the joint may cause the pin to work loose and migrate distally. For these reasons, some surgeons prefer to place the pin retrogradely through the carpus and out the second intermetacarpal web space. The pin can then be redirected in an antegrade fashion down the shaft of the radius. The intermetacarpal pin position places the hand in a position of slight ulnar deviation, which is advantageous mechanically.

To counteract these problems and to improve the security of intramedullary fixation, the Wrightington unit developed a

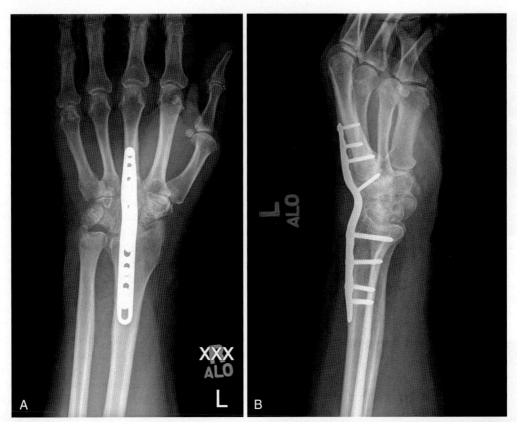

A

B

FIGURE 12.41 A, Posteroanterior and **B,** lateral x-rays of a patient following successful arthrodesis done with concomitant proximal row resection. This minimizes the risk of ulnocarpal impingement in this wrist with positive ulnar variance.

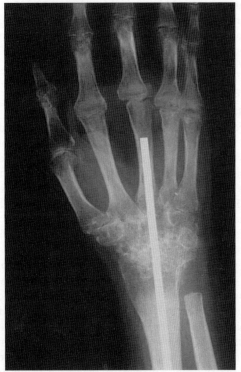

FIGURE 12.42 Introduction of intramedullary pins through the head of the third metacarpal is rapid and effective fixation for radiocarpal arthrodesis.

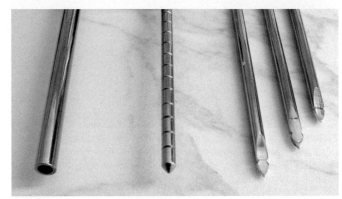

FIGURE 12.43 Three lengths of pins in two diameters for placement in the third metacarpal shaft are shown here. The introducer and countersink driver are also demonstrated.

specialized instrument kit consisting of modified pins, a driver, and a countersink driver (Osteotec Ltd, Christchurch, Dorset, UK). The tip of each pin has a flat cutting edge with a chip breaker so that it may be used as a drill when mounted on a hand drill piece. There are a variety of sizes and lengths (Figure 12.43). Preoperative radiographs must be assessed to identify the diameter of the third metacarpal so that the correct size and length of pin can be chosen. It is important that volar subluxation of the lunate be reduced, and any large anterior shelf of the distal radius should be excised when present to avoid postoperative median nerve compression (Figure 12.44).

In general, a single pin is all that is required unless there has been significant loss of bone, in which case two-pin fixation may be necessary (Figure 12.45, *B*). Rotational stability must be checked, and if there is any rotational movement, an additional 3-mm pin or a staple may be used to prevent rotation. Morselization of the carpus generates adequate bone stock to stimulate the healing process for fusion. If the ulnar head has been excised, it can be converted to a corticocancellous graft to lay on the surface of the radius and carpus (Figure 12.46, *A* and *B*).

What Patients Should Be Told

Most patients experience significant swelling requiring bed rest and strict hand elevation. Patients are told that they will be immobilized in a bulky dressing for 10 days followed by a removable splint until 6 weeks postoperatively and that they can expect a 98.5% union rate. Although full use is allowed at 10 weeks, they will not feel really adapted until 6 months after surgery. Complete pain relief cannot be guaranteed if the patient has undergone multiple previous surgeries. Grip strength will take a year to plateau and will approximate 72% of normal.[45] Bolano and Green found no significant difference in grip strength between fusion with retention of the proximal row and fusion with excision of the proximal row.[9] Patients should expect a 6-month period of learning and adaptation to the fusion. Ninety-two percent of tasks will be performed in a normal manner without undue delay. The greatest functional

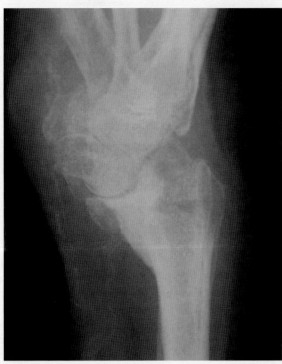

FIGURE 12.44 If the lunate is translated in the palmar direction, fusion in situ carries the risk of pin perforation into the flexor aspect of the forearm. Reducing the lunate to the radius without excision of the anterior shelf risks postoperative median nerve compression. The presence of marked arterial calcification indicates that excessive manipulation should be avoided.

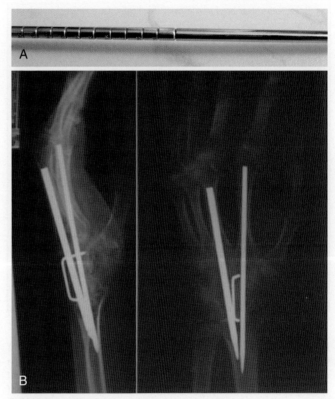

FIGURE 12.45 A, Once a stable construct is achieved, the driver is removed and the countersink tool is applied into the dimple at the base of the pin, which is driven into the metacarpal for a distance of approximately 1 inch. **B,** Two pins can be used if a single pin fails to prevent rotational stability.

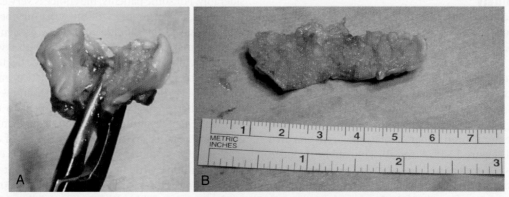

FIGURE 12.46 The extraperiosteal excised ulnar head can be used as a corticocancellous graft. **A,** The head is opened into a graft with a narrow bone rongeur. **B,** The softer bone of a rheumatoid patient is ideal for this technique. The periosteum holds the fragments together, and the graft remains a viable supplement to the main morselization of the carpus and distal radius.

CRITICAL POINTS *Wrist Arthrodesis With Intramedullary Pins*

Indications
- Pancarpal arthrosis of the radiocarpal and midcarpal joints
- Failed previous partial fusion
- Failed total joint or previous arthroplasty
- Significant bone loss of the distal radius and carpus[45]
- Other inflammatory arthritic disability or deformity[18,62]

Pearls
- Carefully assess preoperative carpal tunnel symptoms and perform a concomitant release, even for mild symptoms.
- Decorticate the dorsal 80% of the third CMC joint.
- Remove the ulnar head in one piece if indicated for additional source of graft.
- Morselize the dorsal two thirds of the scaphoid, lunate, and capitate and the entire radial articular surface, including the distal dorsal rim.
- When there is significant ulnar translation, remove part of the radial styloid to facilitate realignment of the wrist.
- Remove the anterior lunate fossa shelf if present.

Pitfalls
- Insufficient removal of the anterior shelf
- Acute carpal tunnel syndrome
- Pain from incomplete fusion of the third CMC joint
- Insufficient countersinking of the pin past the isthmus of the third metacarpal

Postoperative Care
- Immobilize the hand and wrist in a bulky dressing and splint for 10 days.
- Protect against excessive use with a removable short-arm splint until 6 weeks postoperatively.
- At 6 weeks, discontinue the splint.
- At 8 weeks, begin strengthening.

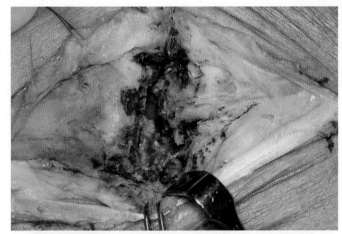

FIGURE 12.47 Patient following total wrist arthroplasty resection; note the metallosis and bony defect. Following debris removal and bone preparation, a sizable defect remained.

problems will be perineal care, lifting a glass or can from a low table, and horizontal use of a screwdriver. These potential concerns can be mitigated preoperatively by having the patient wear a splint day and night during all activities for a period of time. This will help the individual better understand the functional expectations following fusion. Further surgery for plate removal is unlikely with the low-profile precontoured plates.

Wrist Arthrodesis After Failed Total Wrist Arthroplasty

Fusion after failed total wrist arthroplasty can be challenging, and patients are often left with a sizable defect following implant resection (Figure 12.47, *A*), debris removal, and bone preparation. Although some investigators had encouraging union results with fusion following failed wrist arthroplasty,[15] others have had significantly higher nonunion rates ranging from 35% to 50%.[6,86] In these circumstances there is considerable loss of bone substance, and our preferred technique involves the use of morselized femoral head allograft that has been prepared with a bone mill (Figure 12.48, *A* and *B*). This can be included with an off-the-shelf graft as well as iliac crest (see Figure 12.48, *C*). The implants and cement, if present, are removed and the absence of infection confirmed. After three passages through the bone mill (to make the size of the fragments appropriate for the radius and carpus), the allograft femoral head is introduced

into the defect and impact grafted into the distal radius and into the defect within the carpus with bone tamps. Two pins are used for the second and third metacarpals to lock the carpus and hand in alignment with the radius. Any remaining gap may be filled with autologous bone from iliac crest if thought to be necessary. Structural bone graft may also be fashioned with tricortical iliac crest to maintain wrist length. An alternative to Steinmann pins is the use of locking wrist fusion plates (see Figure 12.48, *D* and *E*).

Total Wrist Replacement

Although total wrist arthrodesis yields significant pain relief, stability, and power grasp, immobility of the wrist requires compensatory motion of the elbow and shoulder to accurately place the hand in space and, more particularly, to allow the thumb, index finger, and middle finger to perform fine activities with precision. Therefore, loss of wrist motion can give rise to significant dysfunction in occupational, self-care, and recreational activities.[33,73] However, the individual patient's capacity to adapt, compromise, and develop coping strategies, coupled with support and assistance from family members, requires careful assessment and counseling to ensure the proper choice of surgical reconstruction. In individual patients, a decision has to be made whether to preserve motion at the expense of some residual pain or to remove motion and improve the pain considerably. For some patients, the choice is very easy and obvious; for others, loss of mobility of the wrist may be associated with difficulties with the shoulder and elbow, as seen in patients with inflammatory arthritis. Many patients with a wrist arthrodesis report significant impairment in fine dexterous activities, although they learn to cope. In our practice, patients who have undergone wrist arthrodesis on one side and wrist replacement on the other prefer the wrist replacement to the wrist fusion and state that they find preservation of some motion of considerable importance, particularly in activities of daily living.[69]

Normal wrist motion is accomplished by a complex interaction of multiple articulations involving the radius, ulna, and carpal bones. Total wrist arthroplasty cannot duplicate this intricate system, but it can potentially produce a stable, pain-free joint with a functional range of motion. Achieving a functional and durable outcome requires appropriate patient

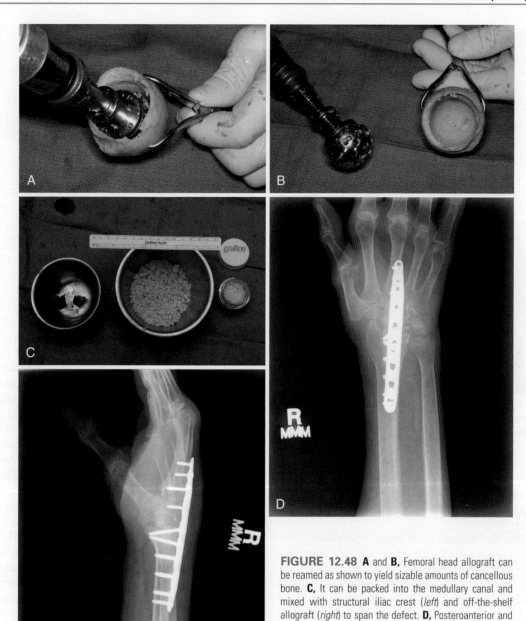

FIGURE 12.48 A and **B,** Femoral head allograft can be reamed as shown to yield sizable amounts of cancellous bone. **C,** It can be packed into the medullary canal and mixed with structural iliac crest (*left*) and off-the-shelf allograft (*right*) to span the defect. **D,** Posteroanterior and **E,** lateral radiographs of the patient shown in previous figures who underwent bone grafting and stabilization with a locking wrist fusion plate.

selection, preoperative planning, and accurate surgery. Because arthroplasty poses greater risks than arthrodesis does, low-demand patients with special needs or a desire for wrist motion are the best candidates. Recently, patients with degenerative arthritis are seeking to have replacement rather than fusion as they gain greater awareness of the surgical options. Careful patient selection is critical to a good outcome, and caution is advised when advising patients with high demands and perhaps unrealistic expectations.

History of Modern Total Wrist Arthroplasty

- Swanson, 1972: Flexible-hinge silicone arthroplasty[95]
- Volz, 1976: AMC/Volz prosthesis, a highly constrained implant[104]
- Meuli, 1980: The Meuli implant, a ball-and-socket design[64]
- Guepar, 1988: The first distal screw fixation device[1]
- Figgie and associates, 1988: Trispherical wrist[32]
- Ferlic and Clayton, 1995, The CFV wrist, a reverse-polarity implant[30]
- Cobb and Beckenbaugh, 1996: Biaxial wrist, ingrowth fixation into the radius and third metacarpal[20]
- Menon, 1998: Universal I, screw fixation of the distal component into the second metacarpal and hamate[63]
- Divelbiss, Sollerman, and Adams, 2002: Universal II (Integra Life Sciences, Plainsboro, NJ), change in design to reduce the risk for dislocation[26]
- Levadoux and Legré, 2003: Destot prosthesis[59]
- Radmer and colleagues, 2003: ATW/APH prosthesis[83]

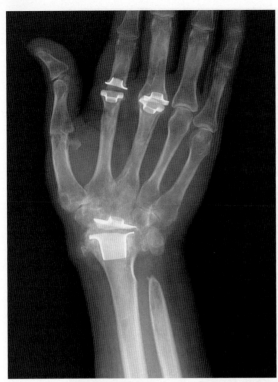

FIGURE 12.49 Imbalance of the wrist aggravated by ulnar translation of the common extensor tendons resulted in a high attrition rate of the silicone implant with consequent deterioration in function.

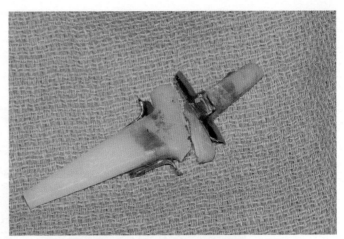

FIGURE 12.50 Excised fractured silicone wrist arthroplasty.

- Rahimtoola and Rozing, 2003: RWS implant[84]
- Palmer and associates, 2005: Maestro (Biomet Orthopaedics, Warsaw, IN), a design with alignment with the lunate fossa[75]
- Gupta, 2008: Re-Motion (Small Bone Innovations, Morrisville, PA), an implant with 10 degrees of pronation-supination of the components[43]

Swanson, in the late 1960s and early 1970s, developed a flexible-hinge silicone arthroplasty of the wrist,[95] similar to the successful MP joint implants. Patients initially had extremely good results, with a high level of pain relief and functional range of motion. Although the early results were encouraging, it became apparent over time that balance of the wrist was an important issue. Failure of the implant at its distal stem, when inserted into the carpus and third metacarpal, was a common feature, with loss of the ulnar shoulder (Figure 12.49) of the implant. This frequently occurred in association with ulnar deviation of the wrist and caused significant functional problems, and a number of implants fractured and/or had to be removed (Figure 12.50). The long-term results of Swanson arthroplasty showed that those that survived and were well balanced continued to give good pain relief, although with a gradually decreasing range of motion.[32] Even reports published within the last 10 years have concluded that for very low demand elderly patients with inflammatory arthritis, use of a Swanson flexible-hinge implant may still be considered.[53] However, the development of metal-on-plastic hip replacements encouraged many to attempt to reproduce this success at the wrist joint, and a number of implants were designed, including the early Volz,[104] Meuli,[64] and Guepar group implants.[1] Subsequently, the Mayo Clinic introduced the biaxial wrist.[20] All of these implants had

their particular foibles with difficulty in balancing the wrist. In 1998, Menon presented the first reports of the ellipsoid Universal I wrist design, which is composed of a metallic radial component and a polyethylene carpal component fixed to a metal carpal base plate.[63] The implant was a departure from the normal distal stem and cement fixation and instead relied on screw fixation in the second and fourth metacarpals and a central peg in the capitate. The particular design of this implant was attractive, and a number of these procedures were performed. The Universal I results as reported by Menon, however, identified a significant dislocation rate, and it became apparent that design modifications were required.[63] The Universal II implant restored the normal radial inclination of the distal radius and altered the shape and conformity of the implant with a subsequent reduction in the instability rate to 1% to 2%.[42] Short-term outcomes with the Universal II implant were encouraging.[26] Medium-term results focusing on rheumatoid patients have been published as well. Unfortunately, the authors noted a substantial loosening rate of the distal component necessitating revision surgery in 40%.[106] However, they went on to conclude that if the implant remained radiographically stable, the clinical results and patient satisfaction were generally excellent.

Further developments and designs have also been introduced and include the Re-Motion and Maestro designs. The Re-Motion design was introduced in 2003, and the design rationale, indications, and technique were described by Gupta with encouraging preliminary results.[43] It differs slightly from the Universal II device in that there is a 10-degree axial rotation of the carpal component allowing for some degree of intercarpal supination and pronation (Figure 12.51). In addition, the articular rims of the radius are preserved during preparation and placement of the Re-Motion implant so that the capsular attachments are preserved. The range of motion to be expected is 20 degrees of flexion, 30 to 40 degrees of extension, and an arc of motion of 25 degrees of radial and ulnar deviation. It is possible that marked distortion of the distal radius articular surface, as seen on occasion in rheumatoid arthritis, may make seating of the Re-Motion radial component more difficult.

Herzberg and coworkers prospectively reported their results in using the Re-Motion implant in over 200 wrists performed in a multicenter prospective trial.[46] Sixty percent of their patients

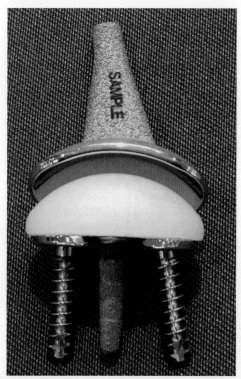

FIGURE 12.51 The Re-Motion total wrist replacement (Small Bone Innovations, Morrisville, PA).

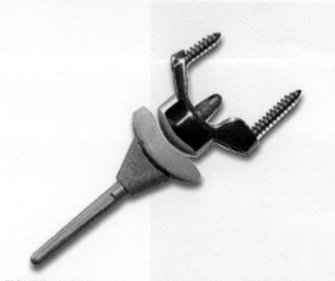

FIGURE 12.52 The Maestro total wrist replacement (Biomet Orthopaedics, Warsaw, IN).

had rheumatoid arthritis. Results at an average 4-year follow-up demonstrated improvement in subjective patient assessments such as pain scores and disability of shoulder arm and hand (DASH) scores. Although there was no significant difference in the range of motion postoperatively, grip strengths did improve. A total of 11 patients (6 in the group with rheumatoid arthritis and 5 in the group without rheumatoid arthritis) underwent revision to either fusion or revision total wrist arthroplasty (TWA).

The Maestro (Figure 12.52) implant is designed to mimic proximal row carpectomy and depends on replacement primarily of the capitate head; articulation is achieved with a polyeth-

ylene proximal component seated in the radius. Nydick and colleagues retrospectively published their results using the Maestro total wrist arthroplasty in 23 cases.[75] Short-term follow-up at an average of 28 months demonstrated excellent pain relief and patient-related outcomes (DASH and Mayo Wrist Scores). One wrist failed secondary to infection and was successfully revised to a fusion.

Cooney and associates described a retrospective review comparing the outcomes of the newer-generation (Universal II and Re-Motion) implants with the previous-generation biaxial design implants.[22] The authors found that both designs were associated with excellent pain relief and functional motion; however, lower rates of complications and reoperation were noted with the newer-generation designs.

Preoperative Evaluation

Clinical Examination. Examination must include an accurate range of active and passive motion, most particularly to determine whether there is subluxation or dislocation of the carpus and whether the DRUJ is stable. The status of the flexor and extensor tendons of the wrist and hand must be assessed. Functional assessment of the patient should be performed and a detailed history taken of the patient's activities, including home circumstances, hobbies, and pastimes. Patients who live alone have no one to assist them with important activities of daily living. Some patients with a sedentary occupation can have quite high-demand leisure activities that are a balance to their lives. Joint-preserving procedures should be considered in a patient who finds a trial period of splint immobilization unacceptable.

Surgical Technique (Universal II Implant)

Perioperative antibiotics are used, and fluoroscopy is an integral part of the procedure. The dorsal aspect of the wrist is exposed through a longitudinal central incision with reflection of the extensor retinaculum either through the fourth compartment Z-plasty or radially from the first compartment across through to the sixth compartment. The extensor tendons of the fourth compartment are retracted ulnarly and those of the third and second compartments to the radial side. A segment of the posterior interosseous nerve can be excised just proximal to the radiocarpal joint at the discretion of the surgeon. The distal radius is identified, and the dorsal capsule of the radiocarpal joint is defined and raised (Figure 12.53, *A* and *B*). Two methods can be used for this: (1) raising the capsule either in one or two distally based flaps with a "U" or an inverted "T" incision or (2) an ulnar-based flap by raising the dorsal radiolunotriquetral ligament from the rim of the radius, incising along the distal edge of the dorsal intercarpal ligament fibers, and detaching the fibers on the radial side and leaving them attached to the hamate and triquetrum on the ulnar side. The object of preserving the capsule is to provide cover for the implant and to place a layer of tissue between the implant and the extensor tendons. The proximal half of the scaphoid, the lunate, and the triquetrum is excised. During proximal scaphoid excision and sizing of the carpal component, it is helpful to temporarily pin the distal scaphoid to the distal carpal row. The distal radius is examined for bone loss, particularly in the lunate fossa. A central guide pin is introduced through the dorsal radial quadrant of the radius 5 mm below and in line with the Lister tubercle. This is

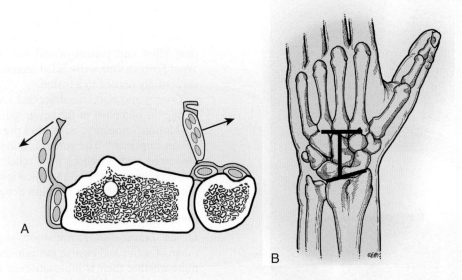

FIGURE 12.53 The incision is along the line of the third metacarpal and may be extended proximally and distally to facilitate exposure of the wrist. **A,** The fourth compartment is raised as for wrist fusion. The second compartment must be raised as shown. When the retinaculum has been raised in this manner, it can be passed deep to the extensor carpi radialis longus, extensor carpi radialis brevis, and extensor pollicis longus and, with a hemostat, can be used to maintain radial displacement of the radial-side tendons to facilitate the exposure. **B,** The dorsal capsule is raised as shown. (Copyright © Elizabeth Martin.)

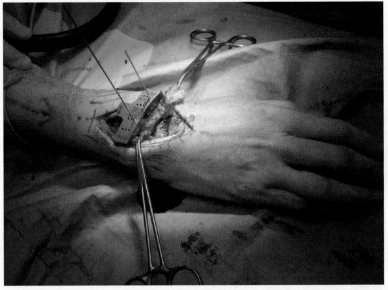

FIGURE 12.54 The cutting guide temporarily held in place by Kirschner wires after removal of the intramedullary guide rod. If a satisfactory position is achieved, as seen on intraoperative radiographs, the distal radial articular surface can be excised with an oscillating saw.

checked on the image intensifier to ensure that it is correctly located parallel to the cortices in both the sagittal and coronal planes. Introduction of a cutting guide along the central pin allows the radial cutting guide to be located and fixed with temporary Kirschner wires. Removal of the central pin allows the radial guide to be checked for position with intraoperative radiographs. The distal radius is cut and removed (Figure 12.54). Reinsertion of the medullary guide pin allows introduction of the cannulated reamers, and reaming of the shaft can proceed (Figure 12.55, *A* and *B*). A trial radial component of the appropriate size is inserted. Having completed preparation

of the radius, preparation of the distal component may be performed.

A Kirschner wire is introduced through the head of the capitate and into the third metacarpal with use of the wire guide. This again is checked on the intensifier to ensure that its placement within the third metacarpal and the capitate is, in fact, aligned in both the sagittal and coronal planes (Figure 12.56, *A* and *B*). A cannulated drill is introduced along the guidewire and drilled to the appropriate depth as marked on the drill. The wire and drill are removed and the distal alignment guide is placed in the drill hole. The cutting guide is placed on the

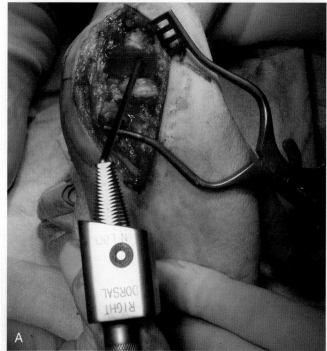

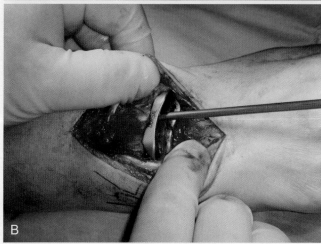

FIGURE 12.55 **A,** With the guide pin reinserted, the medullary canal can be reamed. **B,** The trial radial component is then inserted.

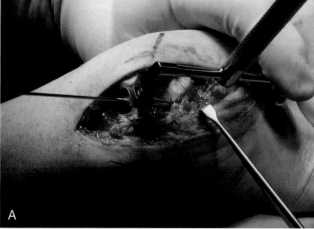

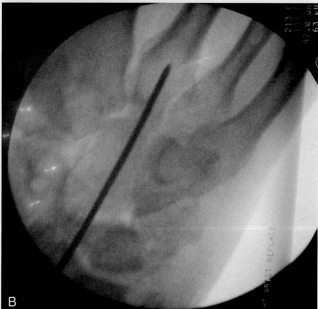

FIGURE 12.56 **A,** A Kirschner wire is inserted into the capitate and passed through to the third metacarpal. **B,** The position of the Kirschner wire must be assessed with intraoperative radiographs or fluoroscopy.

alignment guide, and temporary Kirschner wires are inserted through the cutting guide (Figure 12.57). The position is checked with a radiograph. With the cutting guide in place, the appropriate amount of capitate head, residual scaphoid, and, if necessary, part of the hamate is removed. The distal trial implant is inserted after removal of the guides (Figure 12.58). The metacarpal alignment guide is placed on the second metacarpal to guide introduction of the screws through the plate and into the second metacarpal. A similar process allows introduction of the screw into the hamate by alignment with the fourth metacarpal guides (Figure 12.59). The screw must be in the hamate but must not cross the fourth CMC joint (which is mobile). The polyethylene central component is attached (Figure 12.60, *A* and *B*), and the range of motion and stability are assessed. It is particularly important to assess axial distraction to ensure that there is no excessive laxity within the joint that would encourage dislocation. The distal component has modular sizes so that

appropriate tension can be attained. However, if the component is too large and prevents extension, a smaller component should be inserted. If this is not possible, 2 mm must be removed from the distal radius.

When satisfied with the sizing, the trial components can be removed and the final components implanted. The components may be inserted with or without cement. It is important to complete an intercarpal fusion of the distal row bones for support of the carpal component plate. After confirmation of adequate range of motion, particularly in extension, the wounds are closed, the capsule is closed, and the extensor tendons are examined. Provided that the common extensors are suitably centralized and aligned, closure of the superficial fascia and skin is all that is required. If there is a tendency for the tendons to lie to the ulnar side of the long axis of the implant, they should be centralized to properly balance the implant (see later).

The patient is immobilized in plaster for a period of 2 weeks for wound healing. The sutures are removed at 2 weeks, at

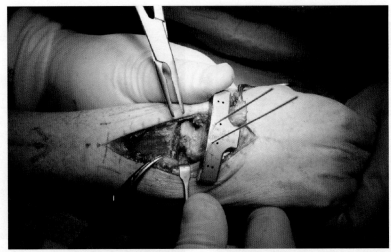

FIGURE 12.57 The distal cutting guide is held with two Kirschner wires and the position checked and adjusted if necessary.

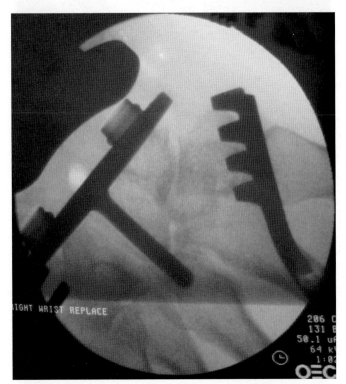

FIGURE 12.58 The distal implant must lie in contact with the cut surface of the capitate, scaphoid, and triquetrum, and the central stem of the implant should remain within the body of the capitate.

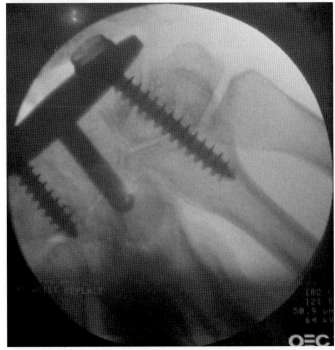

FIGURE 12.59 Seating of both components is followed by placing the trial screws into the second metacarpal and hamate.

which time early controlled motion in the form of flexion-extension and some radial-ulnar deviation is allowed. Over a period of 3 months, the wrist range of motion recovers and plateaus.

Surgical Technique (Re-Motion Implant) (Video 12.1)

The approach and exposure are similar to those for the Universal II implant, and differences or deviations from the above approach are mentioned below. The Re-Motion system has a carpal alignment guide that can be centered in the lunate fossa to allow for proper positioning in preparation for the carpal cut

at the level of the capitate head (Figure 12.61, *A* and *B*). In addition, it allows for a radial alignment guide to be attached to ensure proper positioning of the anticipated proximal component, and this can be confirmed radiographically (see Figure 12.61, *C*). A carpal bone resection guide is situated in line with the lunate (when reduced) and lines up with the third metacarpal distally (Figure 12.62). The anticipated carpal cut should be made at the level of the proximal capitate. Upon confirmation of appropriate alignment, the proximal carpal cut can be performed (Figure 12.63, *A* and *B*). A proximal radius alignment guide appropriately positioned, centered on the radius, will allow for preparation of the distal radius surface and properly align in the center of the medullary canal. The radial surface is

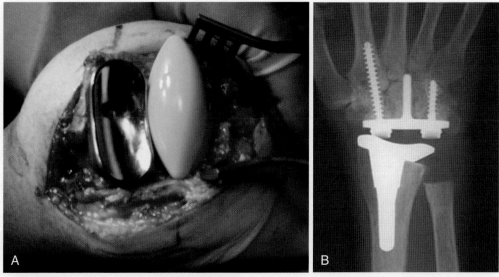

FIGURE 12.60 A, A trial central polyethylene bearing surface is placed. **B,** Verification with radiographs.

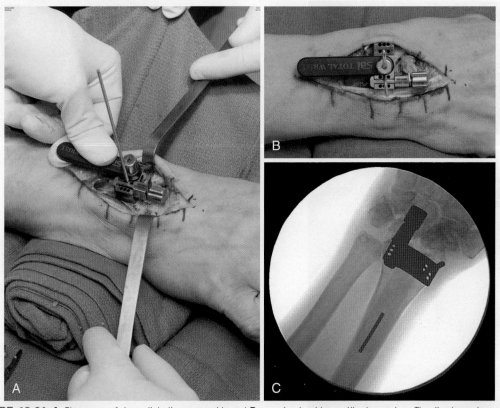

FIGURE 12.61 A, Placement of the radial alignment guide and **B,** securing it with two Kirschner wires. The distal attachment slides proximal to the lunate and sits on the lunate fossa. **C,** The black portion of the guide has a radiopaque rod to help confirm appropriate alignment. Fluoroscopy will help confirm alignment in the anteroposterior and lateral planes.

prepared using the appropriately sized high speed bur (Figure 12.64, *A*). The surgeon may also use the bur in a freehand position to fine-tune the preparation of the radial surface (see Figure 12.64, *B*). The next step involves placement of the intramedullary radial alignment guide and insertion of a medullary pin into the shaft of the radius (Figure 12.65). The Lister tubercle is a good landmark for the centering drill hole, and in the axial plane, it should sit in the middle-distal third junction

of the radius. Upon fluoroscopic confirmation that the guide pin is appropriately aligned, the radial canal can be reamed, broached, and trialed (Figure 12.66).

The carpal side can be prepared. The trial guide is based on the center of the capitate and a Kirschner wire is used to locate its center (Figure 12.67), followed by broaching to the correct size. The broach into the capitate has three slots on it corresponding to small, medium, and large, and much like the

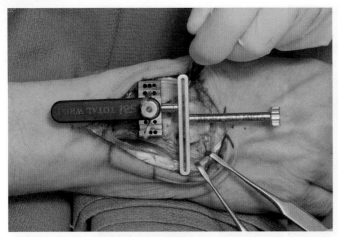

FIGURE 12.62 The carpal cutting guide attaches to the radial alignment guide as shown. It has three notches to correspond with the appropriate size.

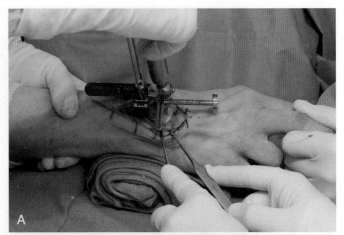

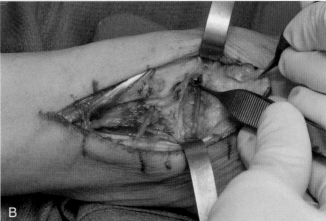

FIGURE 12.63 A, An oscillating saw is used to initiate the carpal cut. The cut should be made to remove only the tip of the capitate head. **B,** The cut should be perpendicular to the long axis of the capitate and long finger metacarpal.

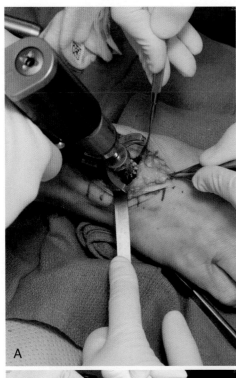

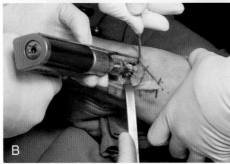

FIGURE 12.64 A, Another attachment with a large bur is used to prepare the radius. The aim is to smooth out the articular surface but preserve the subchondral bone. **B,** In my experience, freehand use of the bur is often necessary to appropriately prepare the radial surface.

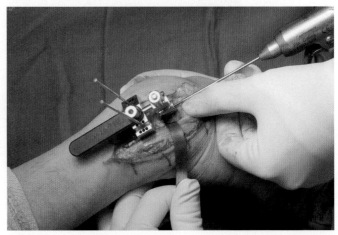

FIGURE 12.65 After preparing the radial surface, the intramedullary guide is placed into the radius. The Lister tubercle is a good marker for alignment in the coronal plane, and in the sagittal plane the guide pin should sit in the mid to distal third junction of the radial surface.

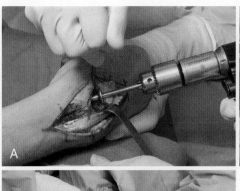

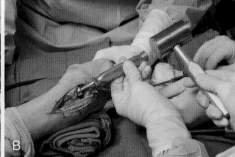

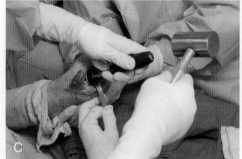

FIGURE 12.66 Upon confirmation of adequate alignment, the radius is drilled (**A**), broached (**B**), and trialed (**C**).

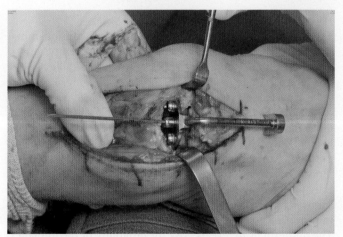

FIGURE 12.67 Attention turns to the carpal component. The drill guide is centered into the capitate and stabilized as shown.

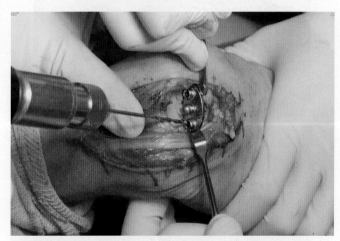

FIGURE 12.68 Drilling for the second metacarpal and hamate screws can be done with the alignment guide or after placement of the final component. It is acceptable to cross the carpometacarpal (CMC) joint with the radial screw, but if possible, the ulnar screw should not cross the fourth CMC joint.

Universal II, the distal trial has a peg for the capitate with holes for the 4.5-mm radial and ulnar carpal screws (Figure 12.68). The radial screw lines up with the second metacarpal distally, while the ulnar screw typically lies in line with the fourth meta-carpal. Use of a depth gauge will help ensure appropriate screw lengths. Upon completing the distal trial the proximal trial is inserted and the trial liner is secured (Figure 12.69). The wrist is assessed for stability, range of motion, and laxity. The wrist should be stable to 40 degrees of flexion and 40 degrees of extension, and the gap should be 2 to 3 mm with distraction. The radial and carpal components are placed, and the polyeth-ylene ball snaps on the carpal component. Radiographs confirm that the implant size and placement and the wrist alignment are appropriate (Figure 12.70, A and B).

Centralization of the Extensor Tendons

When the extensor tendons do not align in the midline of the wrist, they should be centralized to provide appropriate exten-sion moments across the implant. Centralization is achieved by

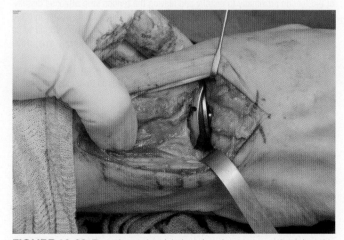

FIGURE 12.69 The wrist can be trialed one last time to ensure that it is stable to flexion and extension of 80 degrees and radial-ulnar deviation of 40 degrees. In addition, gapping of 2 to 3 mm with distraction should be appreciable.

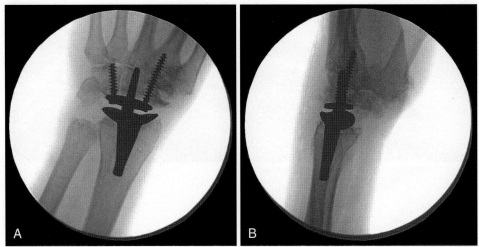

FIGURE 12.70 A, Posteroanterior and **B,** lateral fluoroscopy images show appropriate alignment of the wrist and screw lengths as well as implant position.

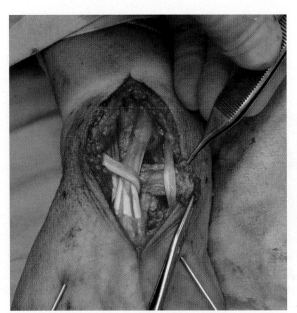

FIGURE 12.71 Use of half of the extensor carpi radialis longus (ECRL) tendon to align and stabilize the common extensor tendons is achieved by harvesting part of the tendon proximally to distally and leaving the tendon strip attached distally. The strip of tendon is taken deep to the common extensors and woven into the remaining ECRL to create an open loop. The tension in this loop is judged to be correct when the common extensors are aligned with the longitudinal axis of the implant. Similarly, the extensor carpi ulnaris (ECU) tendon is brought up to the dorsum by bringing the extensor retinaculum deep to the tendon. The free edge of the retinaculum is brought over the ECU tendon and sutured to itself under appropriate tension to realign the tendon dorsally.

performing a hemitransection of the ECRL proximally, raising a strip to its insertion on the base of the second metacarpal, and threading it deep to the ECRB and the common extensor tendons.[16] This should not include the extensor digiti minimi. The strip of ECRL is taken superficial to the common extensors and woven through the ECRB. The loop that has been generated maintains the extensor tendons in the proper alignment (Figure 12.71). This is very often necessary in a rheumatoid patient when preservation of the tube of the fourth compartment is not

always possible and when extensor tenosynovectomy may be necessary.

What Patients Should Be Told

The results of wrist replacement for a patient with inflammatory arthritis are very good for pain relief, but attempts at restoration of a normal range of motion are undesirable because this increases the risk of dislocation and loosening. The range to be expected is 25 to 35 degrees of extension, 30 to 40 degrees of flexion, 10 degrees of radial deviation, and 15 degrees of ulnar deviation; however, these ranges can be highly variable. For patients with severe rheumatoid disease, the outcome in terms of range of motion may be less predictable, but the motion obtained is of great value in improving the capacity for activities of daily living.[33] The recovery period after the acute surgical phase is 6 to 8 weeks, but the wrist will continue to improve for up to 1 year after implantation of the prosthesis. The midterm (1 to 5 years) risk for instability of the implant is reported to be 15%.[69] The loosening rate is dependent on time and the level of activity.

The early results are very encouraging, but as always with all implants, some failures are inevitable and the patient and treating physician should be aware of the potential risks associated with implant arthroplasty. The surgical technique should be meticulous and cutting guides used to ensure accuracy of bone preparation. Repeated intraoperative radiographs are important to ensure correct alignment to minimize the risk for early and midterm mechanical failure. Longer-term results will better help us understand the indications and limitations of these implants.

Wrist Hemiarthroplasty

One of the primary concerns regarding total wrist arthroplasty is distal component loosening; consequently, some investigators have proposed the concept of radial hemiarthroplasty as an alternative motion-preserving procedure for wrist disease.[11,24,44,101] The concept and rationale were introduced by Boyer and Adams in a case report whereby a proximal row carpectomy was performed with replacement of the proximal articulation with the radial component of the Universal II

CRITICAL POINTS *Total Wrist Arthroplasty*

Indications
- Pancarpal arthrosis of the radiocarpal and midcarpal joints in patients with low demand
- Failed past limited arthrodesis
- Rheumatoid wrist arthritis and other inflammatory arthritis or deformity with radiocarpal ulnar translocation instability
- SLAC pattern of arthritis in older low-demand patients
- Avascular necrosis of the carpal bones

Pearls and Technical Points
- Carefully assess for preoperative carpal tunnel symptoms, and perform a concomitant release, even for mild symptoms.
- Template the preoperative radiographs to guide selection of the appropriate implant size.
- In the event that it is difficult to raise a continuous capsuloperiosteal tube containing the fourth compartment tendons for adequate exposure (see Figure 12.10), the fourth compartment extensor retinaculum can be released and taken off the tendons and the tendons allowed to be retracted to the ulnar side.
- It is important to see the entire distal end of the radius when opening the capsule, and on occasion the extensor tendons can interfere with such visualization. Be generous with your exposure to minimize the risk of malpositioning the implant.
- Expose the distal radius and free the first compartment.
- Removal of the proximal row and the proximal half of the scaphoid and part of the triquetrum will expose both the distal radius and the distal row of the carpus.
- Check the alignment of the guide pin within the radius in the sagittal and coronal planes on intraoperative radiographs.
- Measure *three* times; cut *once*.
- In rheumatoid arthritis with ulnar translation, remove part of the radial styloid to facilitate realignment of the wrist.
- Check the insertion of the radial component with radiographs.
- Check the alignment of the carpal guide with radiographs.
- Preparation of the distal row includes very accurate placement of the central peg and accurate placement of the screws.
- The carpal screws may cross at the second CMC joint, but whenever possible, they should not cross the fourth CMC joint.

- Intercarpal arthrodesis is helpful to ensure stability of the distal component.
- Cement fixation is an option, but it is not commonly used.
- The range of motion to aim for is 40 degrees of extension, 20 degrees of flexion, 10 degrees of radial deviation, and 15 degrees of ulnar deviation.

Pitfalls
- Overstuffing the joint causes significantly restricted range of motion.
- Failure to remove and deal with the anterior lunate fossa lip can lead to acute carpal tunnel syndrome if the wrist is then relocated into its normal position.
- A very large lunate fossa defect gives rise to poor support of the implant of whatever type.
- Extreme palmar subluxation of the carpus on preoperative lateral radiographs and rupture of the radial and ulnar wrist extensor tendons are contraindications to total wrist arthroplasty.
- On completion of surgery, an x-ray must be taken before closure to ensure that there is no likelihood of ulnar abutment between the head of the ulna and the implant on the radius. If there is, a wafer type of procedure can be performed, and in a rheumatoid patient one may consider distal ulnar excision.

Postoperative Care
- Immobilize for 3 to 5 days in a bulky conforming dressing.
- Immobilize in a splint for 10 to 14 days.
- Begin an active supervised gentle exercise program for 4 to 6 weeks with a rest splint used between exercise periods for comfort.
- At 6 to 8 weeks, increase mobilization but permanently avoid repeated forceful activities (e.g., hammering) and avoid heavy manual work and contact sports.
- Further postoperative care includes encouraging patients to develop the appropriate range of motion for their lifestyle by encouraging them to perform tasks at an early stage in a planned, progressive, and purposeful fashion with a structured rehabilitation program of activities.

Joint Protection
- Advice regarding avoidance of stressful and staccato activity is crucial for long-term survival of the implants.

---

implant.[11] Culp and coworkers performed radial hemiarthroplasty in 10 patients, with an average 19-month follow-up, and reported a myriad of complications.[24] Unfortunately, there was a 30% rate of osteolysis and a significant incidence of wrist contracture and stiffness and diminished grip strength postoperatively. In addition, when polyethylene had been used, its erosion was a problem. The authors concluded that better materials and techniques were necessary. Wolfe introduced the first implant intended specifically for radial hemiarthroplasty (KinematX, Extremity Medical, Parsippany, NJ). The implant has a pronounced radial aspect to better emulate the distal carpal row. In addition, it maintains an anatomic center of motion while preserving the dart thrower's motion arc. Preliminary short-term results were published for nine patients with an average 31-week follow-up.[101] Most patients did not have rheumatoid arthritis, and both subjective and objective outcomes were excellent, with few or no complications.

The technique has the advantage of being simpler than a total wrist arthroplasty. A longitudinal incision is made, the proximal row of the carpus is removed, and the retinaculum is elevated between the third and fourth compartments. A posterior interosseous neurectomy is performed. The wrist can be exposed through a proximally based "U"-shaped flap and the proximal carpal row excised. The volar ligaments of the wrist can be preserved. The radial surface can be prepared or cut. An intramedullary alignment guide is used to confirm alignment within the radius. The distal radius is drilled, broached, and trialed. The final component is press-fit and the capsule closed with interrupted braided absorbable sutures. The retinaculum is reapproximated with the EPL translocated superficial to the retinaculum. The skin is closed over a drain, if necessary. Postoperatively, the recovery is similar to if not faster than that for a total wrist arthroplasty.

A hemiarthroplasty design that does not require proximal row carpectomy has been developed by Liverneaux (Prosthelast, Argomedical GmbH, Cham, Switzerland). The rationale and use have been to treat cases of irreparable distal radius fractures or lesions of the distal radius such as giant cell tumor of bone.[44] Although no reports have been published, carpal hemiarthroplasty designs are being developed.

The capitate component of the Maestro system has been suggested as a hemiarthroplasty in rheumatoid patients, but no formal reports have been published to date.

Longer-term studies and analysis will better help validate the use of hemiarthroplasty in the treatment of early arthritis of the wrist. Wrist hemiarthroplasty is not currently approved by the Food and Drug Administration for use in the United States.

For Case Studies, Videos, and more, please visit ExpertConsult.com.

REFERENCES

1. Alnot JY: [Guepar's total arthroplasty of the wrist in rheumatoid polyarthritis]. *Acta Orthop Belg* 54(2):178–184, 1988.
2. Alnot JY, Bruchou F, Couturier C: [Lunocapitate shortening arthrodesis after scaphoid and triquetrum resection: treatment of Watson stage III advanced scaphoid periarthrosis]. *Rev Chir Orthop Reparatrice Appar Mot* 88(2):125–129, 2002.
3. Bain GI, McGuire DT: Decision making for partial carpal fusions. *J Wrist Surg* 1(2):103–114, 2012.
4. Bain GI, Ondimu P, Hallam P, et al: Radioscapholunate arthrodesis: a prospective study. *Hand Surg* 14(2–3):73–82, 2009.
5. Bedford B, Yang SS: High fusion rates with circular plate fixation for four-corner arthrodesis of the wrist. *Clin Orthop Relat Res* 468(1):163–168, 2010.
6. Beer TA, Turner RH: Wrist arthrodesis for failed wrist implant arthroplasty. *J Hand Surg [Am]* 22(4):685–693, 1997.
7. Benkeddache Y, Gottesman H, Fourrier P: Multiple stapling for wrist arthrodesis in the nonrheumatoid patient. *J Hand Surg [Am]* 9(2):256–260, 1984.
8. Biswas D, Wysocki RW, Cohen MS, et al: Radioscapholunate arthrodesis with compression screws and local autograft. *J Hand Surg [Am]* 38(4):788–794, 2013.
9. Bolano LE, Green DP: Wrist arthrodesis in post-traumatic arthritis: a comparison of two methods. *J Hand Surg [Am]* 18:786–791, 1993.
10. Borisch N, Haussmann P: Radiolunate arthrodesis in the rheumatoid wrist: a retrospective clinical and radiological longterm follow-up. *J Hand Surg [Br]* 27(1):61–72, 2002.
11. Boyer JS, Adams B: Distal radius hemiarthroplasty combined with proximal row carpectomy: case report. *Iowa Orthop J* 30:168–173, 2010.
12. Brumfield RH, Champoux JA: A biomechanical study of normal functional wrist motion. *Clin Orthop Relat Res* (187):23–25, 1984.
13. Buck-Gramcko D: Denervation of the wrist joint. *J Hand Surg [Am]* 2(1):54–61, 1977.
14. Calandruccio JH, Gelberman RH, Duncan SF, et al: Capitolunate arthrodesis with scaphoid and triquetrum excision. *J Hand Surg [Am]* 25(5):824–832, 2000.
15. Carlson JR, Simmons BP: Wrist arthrodesis after failed wrist implant arthroplasty. *J Hand Surg [Am]* 23(5):893–898, 1998.
16. Cerovac S, Stanley JK: The centralization of extensor tendons during wrist surgery. *Tech Hand Up Extrem Surg* 12(3):188–190, 2008.
17. Chamay A, Della Santa D, Vilaseca A: Radiolunate arthrodesis. Factor of stability for the rheumatoid wrist. *Ann Chir Main* 2(1):5–17, 1983.
18. Clayton ML: Surgical treatment at the wrist in rheumatoid arthritis: a review of thirty-seven patients. *J Bone Joint Surg Am* 47:741–750, 1965.
19. Clendenin MB, Green DP: Arthrodesis of the wrist: complications and their management. *J Hand Surg [Am]* 6:253–257, 1981.
20. Cobb TK, Beckenbaugh RD: Biaxial total-wrist arthroplasty. *J Hand Surg [Am]* 21(6):1011–1021, 1996.
21. Cohen MS, Kozin SH: Degenerative arthritis of the wrist: proximal row carpectomy versus scaphoid excision and four-corner arthrodesis. *J Hand Surg [Am]* 26(1):94–104, 2001.
22. Cooney W, Manuel J, Froelich J, et al: Total wrist replacement: a retrospective comparative study. *J Wrist Surg* 1(2):165–172, 2012.
23. Craigen MA, Stanley JK: Wrist kinematics. Row, column or both? *J Hand Surg [Br]* 20(2):165–170, 1995.
24. Culp RW, Bachoura A, Gelman SE, et al: Proximal row carpectomy combined with wrist hemiarthroplasty. *J Wrist Surg* 1(1):39–46, 2012.
25. DiDonna ML, Kiefhaber TR, Stern PJ: Proximal row carpectomy: study with a minimum of ten years of follow-up. *J Bone Joint Surg Am* 86(11):2359–2365, 2004.
26. Divelbiss BJ, Sollerman C, Adams BD: Early results of the Universal total wrist arthroplasty in rheumatoid arthritis. *J Hand Surg [Am]* 27(2):195–204, 2002.
27. Douglas DP, Peimer CA, Koniuch MP: Motion of the wrist after simulated limited intercarpal arthrodeses. An experimental study. *J Bone Joint Surg Am* 69(9):1413–1418, 1987.
28. Evans DL: Wedge arthrodesis of the wrist. *J Bone Joint Surg Br* 37(1):126–134, 1955.
29. Feldon P, Terrono AL, Belsky MR: Wafer distal ulna resection for triangular fibrocartilage tears and/or ulna impaction syndrome. *J Hand Surg [Am]* 17(4):731–737, 1992.
30. Ferlic DC, Clayton ML: Results of CFV total wrist arthroplasty: review and early report. *Orthopedics* 18(12):1167–1171, 1995.
31. Ferreres A, Garcia-Elias M, Plaza R: Long-term results of lunocapitate arthrodesis with scaphoid excision for SLAC and SNAC wrists. *J Hand Surg Eur Vol* 34(5):603–608, 2009.
32. Figgie HE, 3rd, Ranawat CS, Inglis AE, et al: Preliminary results of total wrist arthroplasty in rheumatoid arthritis using the Trispherical total wrist arthroplasty. *J Arthroplasty* 3(1):9–15, 1988.
33. Franko OI, Zurakowski D, Day CS: Functional disability of the wrist: direct correlation with decreased wrist motion. *J Hand Surg [Am]* 33(4):485–492, 2008.
34. Friedman SL, Palmer AK: The ulnar impaction syndrome. *Hand Clin* 7(2):295–310, 1991.
35. Garcia-Elias M: The non-dissociative clunking wrist: a personal view. *J Hand Surg Eur Vol* 33(6):698–711, 2008.
36. Garcia-Elias M, Cooney WP, An KN, et al: Wrist kinematics after limited intercarpal arthrodesis. *J Hand Surg [Am]* 14(5):791–799, 1989.
37. Garcia-Elias M, Lluch A: Partial excision of scaphoid: is it ever indicated? *Hand Clin* 17(4):687–695, x, 2001.
38. Garcia-Elias M, Lluch A, Ferreres A, et al: Treatment of radiocarpal degenerative osteoarthritis by radioscapholunate arthrodesis and distal scaphoidectomy. *J Hand Surg [Am]* 30(1):8–15, 2005.
39. Gaulke R, O'Loughlin PF, Kendoff D, et al: Radiolunate fusion in the rheumatoid wrist via three point fixation with a mini-titanium-T-plate and oblique screw. *Technol Health Care* 17(4):345–351, 2009.
40. Gaulke R, Suppelna G, Hildebrand F, et al: Radiolunate fusion in the rheumatoid wrist with Shapiro staples: clinical and radiological results of 22 cases. *J Hand Surg Eur Vol* 35(4):289–295, 2010.
41. Graner O, Lopes EI, Carvalho BC, et al: Arthrodesis of the carpal bones in the treatment of Kienbock's disease, painful ununited fractures of the navicular and lunate bones with avascular necrosis, and old fracture-dislocations of carpal bones. *J Bone Joint Surg Am* 48(4):767–774, 1966.
42. Grosland NM, Rogge RD, Adams BD: Influence of articular geometry on prosthetic wrist stability. *Clin Orthop Relat Res* 421:134–142, 2004.
43. Gupta A: Total wrist arthroplasty. *Am J Orthop* 37(8 Suppl 1):12–16, 2008.
44. Hariri A, Facca S, Di Marco A, et al: Massive wrist prosthesis for giant cell tumour of the distal radius: a case report with a 3-year follow-up. *Orthop Traumatol Surg Res* 99(5):635–638, 2013.
45. Hastings H, 2nd, Weiss AP, Quenzer D, et al: Arthrodesis of the wrist for post-traumatic disorders. *J Bone Joint Surg Am* 78(6):897–902, 1996.
46. Herzberg G, Broekstyns M, Sorensen AI, et al: "Remotion" total wrist arthroplasty: preliminary results of a prospective international multicenter study of 215 cases. *J Wrist Surg* 1(1):17–22, 2012.
47. Hodgson SP, Stanley JK, Muirhead A: The Wrightington classification of rheumatoid wrist X-rays: a guide to surgical management. *J Hand Surg [Br]* 14(4):451–455, 1989.
48. Hom S, Ruby LK: Attempted scapholunate arthrodesis for chronic scapholunate dissociation. *J Hand Surg [Am]* 16(2):334–339, 1991.
49. Iwasaki N, Genda E, Barrance PJ, et al: Biomechanical analysis of limited intercarpal fusion for the treatment of Kienbock's disease: a three-dimensional theoretical study. *J Orthop Res* 16(2):256–263, 1998.
50. Kadji O, Duteille F, Dautel G, et al: [Four bone versus capito-lunate limited carpal fusion. Report of 40 cases]. *Chir Main* 21(1):5–12, 2002.
51. Kirschenbaum D, Coyle MP, Leddy JP: Chronic lunotriquetral instability: diagnosis and treatment. *J Hand Surg [Am]* 18(6):1107–1112, 1993.
52. Kirschenbaum D, Schneider LH, Kirkpatrick WH, et al: Scaphoid excision and capitolunate arthrodesis for radioscaphoid arthritis. *J Hand Surg [Am]* 18(5):780–785, 1993.
53. Kistler U, Weiss AP, Simmen BR, et al: Long-term results of silicone wrist arthroplasty in patients with rheumatoid arthritis. *J Hand Surg [Am]* 30(6):1282–1287, 2005.
54. Kleinman WB, Carroll CT: Scapho-trapezio-trapezoid arthrodesis for treatment of chronic static and dynamic scapho-lunate instability: a 10-year perspective on pitfalls and complications. *J Hand Surg [Am]* 15(3):408–414, 1990.
55. Krakauer JD, Bishop AT, Cooney WP: Surgical treatment of scapholunate advanced collapse. *J Hand Surg [Am]* 19(5):751–759, 1994.
56. Larsen CF, Jacoby RA, McCabe SJ: Nonunion rates of limited carpal arthrodesis: a meta-analysis of the literature. *J Hand Surg [Am]* 22(1):66–73, 1997.

57. Larsson SE: Compression arthrodesis of the wrist. A consecutive series of 23 cases. *Clin Orthop Relat Res* (99):146–153, 1974.

58. Lee SK, Desai H, Silver B, et al: Comparison of radiographic stress views for scapholunate dynamic instability in a cadaver model. *J Hand Surg [Am]* 36(7):1149–1157, 2011.

59. Levadoux M, Legré R: Total wrist arthroplasty with Destot prostheses in patients with posttraumatic arthritis. *J Hand Surg [Am]* 28(3):405–413, 2003.

60. Loh YC, Stanley JK, Jari S, et al: Neuroma of the distal posterior interosseous nerve. A cause of iatrogenic wrist pain. *J Bone Joint Surg Br* 80(4):629–630, 1998.

61. Louis DS, Hankin FM, Bowers WH: Capitate-radius arthrodesis: an alternative method of radiocarpal arthrodesis. *J Hand Surg [Am]* 9(3):365–369, 1984.

62. Mannerfelt L, Malmsten M: Arthrodesis of the wrist in rheumatoid arthritis: a technique without external fixation. *Scand J Plast Reconstr Surg* 5:124–130, 1971.

63. Menon J: Universal total wrist implant: experience with a carpal component fixed with three screws. *J Arthroplasty* 13(5):515–523, 1998.

64. Meuli HC: Arthroplasty of the wrist. *Clin Orthop Relat Res* 149:118–125, 1980.

65. Meyerdierks EM, Mosher JF, Werner FW: Limited wrist arthrodesis: a laboratory study. *J Hand Surg [Am]* 12(4):526–529, 1987.

66. Millender LH, Nalebuff EA: Arthrodesis of the rheumatoid wrist: an evaluation of sixty patients and a description of a different surgical technique. *J Bone Joint Surg Am* 55:1026–1034, 1973.

67. Minamikawa Y, Peimer CA, Yamaguchi T, et al: Ideal scaphoid angle for intercarpal arthrodesis. *J Hand Surg [Am]* 17(2):370–375, 1992.

68. Moy OJ, Peimer CA: Scaphocapitate fusion in the treatment of Kienbock's disease. *Hand Clin* 9(3):501–504, 1993.

69. Murphy DM, Khoury JG, Imbriglia JE, et al: Comparison of arthroplasty and arthrodesis for the rheumatoid wrist. *J Hand Surg [Am]* 28(4):570–576, 2003.

70. Murray JA, Schlafly B: Giant-cell tumors in the distal end of the radius. Treatment by resection and fibular autograft interpositional arthrodesis. *J Bone Joint Surg Am* 68(5):687–694, 1986.

71. Murray PM: Current status of wrist arthrodesis and wrist arthroplasty. *Clin Plast Surg* 23(3):385–394, 1996.

72. Nagy L, Buchler U: Long-term results of radioscapholunate fusion following fractures of the distal radius. *J Hand Surg [Br]* 22(6):705–710, 1997.

73. Nelson DL: Functional wrist motion. *Hand Clin* 13(1):83–92, 1997.

74. Neubrech F, Mühldorfer-Fodor M, Pillukat T, et al: Long-term results after midcarpal arthrodesis. *J Wrist Surg* 1(2):123–128, 2012.

75. Nydick JA, Greenberg SM, Stone JD, et al: Clinical outcomes of total wrist arthroplasty. *J Hand Surg [Am]* 37(8):1580–1584, 2012.

76. Ozyurekoglu T, Turker T: Results of a method of 4-corner arthrodesis using headless compression screws. *J Hand Surg [Am]* 37(3):486–492, 2012.

77. Palmer AK, Dobyns JH, Linscheid RL: Management of post-traumatic instability of the wrist secondary to ligament rupture. *J Hand Surg [Am]* 3(6):507–532, 1978.

78. Palmer AK, Werner FW, Murphy D, et al: Functional wrist motion: a biomechanical study. *J Hand Surg [Am]* 10(1):39–46, 1985.

79. Pervaiz K, Bowers WH, Isaacs JE, et al: Range of motion effects of distal pole scaphoid excision and triquetral excision after radioscapholunate fusion: a cadaver study. *J Hand Surg [Am]* 34(5):832–837, 2009.

80. Peterson HA, Lipscomb PR: Intercarpal arthrodesis. *Arch Surg* 95(1):127–134, 1967.

81. Pisano SM, Peimer CA, Wheeler DR, et al: Scaphocapitate intercarpal arthrodesis. *J Hand Surg [Am]* 16(2):328–333, 1991.

82. Pryce JC: The wrist position between neutral and ulnar deviation that facilitates the maximum power grip strength. *J Biomech* 13(6):505–511, 1980.

83. Radmer S, Andresen R, Sparmann M: Total wrist arthroplasty in patients with rheumatoid arthritis. *J Hand Surg [Am]* 28(5):789–794, 2003.

84. Rahimtoola ZO, Rozing PM: Preliminary results of total wrist arthroplasty using the RWS prosthesis. *J Hand Surg [Br]* 28(1):54–60, 2003.

85. Rao SB, Culver JE: Triquetrohamate arthrodesis for midcarpal instability. *J Hand Surg [Am]* 20(4):583–589, 1995.

86. Rizzo M, Ackerman DB, Rodrigues RL, et al: Wrist arthrodesis as a salvage procedure for failed implant arthroplasty. *J Hand Surg Eur Vol* 36(1):29–33, 2011.

87. Robinson RF, Kayfetz DO: Arthrodesis of the wrist; preliminary report of a new method. *J Bone Joint Surg Am* 34(1):64–70, 1952.

88. Rogers WD, Watson HK: Radial styloid impingement after triscaphe arthrodesis. *J Hand Surg [Am]* 14(2 Pt 1):297–301, 1989.

89. Ryu JY, Cooney WP, III, Askew LJ, et al: Functional ranges of motion of the wrist joint. *J Hand Surg [Am]* 16(3):409–419, 1991.

90. Sennwald GR, Ufenast H: Scaphocapitate arthrodesis for the treatment of Kienbock's disease. *J Hand Surg [Am]* 20(3):506–510, 1995.

91. Shapiro JS: Power staple fixation in hand and wrist surgery: new applications of an old fixation device. *J Hand Surg [Am]* 12(2):218–227, 1987.

92. Shin EK, Jupiter JB: Radioscapholunate arthrodesis for advanced degenerative radiocarpal osteoarthritis. *Tech Hand Up Extrem Surg* 11(3):180–183, 2007.

93. Smith-Petersen MN: A new approach to the wrist joint. *J Bone Joint Surg* 22:122–124, 1940.

94. Stanley JK, Boot DA: Radio-lunate arthrodesis. *J Hand Surg [Br]* 14(3):283–287, 1989.

95. Swanson AB: Flexible implant resection arthroplasty. *Hand* 4(2):119–134, 1972.

96. Taleisnik J: Combined radiocarpal arthrodesis and midcarpal (lunocapitate) arthroplasty for treatment of rheumatoid arthritis of the wrist. *J Hand Surg [Am]* 12(1):1–8, 1987.

97. Thurston AJ, Stanley JK: Hamato-lunate impingement: an uncommon cause of ulnar-sided wrist pain. *Arthroscopy* 16(5):540–544, 2000.

98. Trumble T, Bour C, Edwards GS, et al: [Partial arthrodesis of the wrist for internal instability of the wrist]. *Rev Chir Orthop Reparatrice Appar Mot* 74(Suppl 2):147–149, 1988.

99. Tubiana RT, Thomine JM, Mackin E: *Examination of the hand and wrist*, St. Louis, 1996, Mosby.

100. Vance MC, Hernandez JG, DiDonna ML, et al: Complications and outcome of four-corner arthrodesis: circular plate fixation versus traditional techniques. *J Hand Surg [Am]* 30(6):1122–1127, 2005.

101. Vance MC, Packer G, Tan D, et al: Midcarpal hemiarthroplasty for wrist arthritis: rationale and early results. *J Wrist Surg* 1(1):61–68, 2012.

102. Vender MI, Watson HK, Wiener BD, et al: Degenerative change in symptomatic scaphoid nonunion. *J Hand Surg [Am]* 12(4):514–519, 1987.

103. Viegas SF, Patterson RM, Peterson PD, et al: Evaluation of the biomechanical efficacy of limited intercarpal fusions for the treatment of scapho-lunate dissociation. *J Hand Surg [Am]* 15(1):120–128, 1990.

104. Volz RG: The development of a total wrist arthroplasty. *Clin Orthop Relat Res* 116:209–214, 1976.

105. Wall LB, DiDonna ML, Kiefhaber TR, et al: Proximal row carpectomy: minimum 20-year follow-up. *J Hand Surg [Am]* 38(8):1498–1504, 2013.

106. Ward CM, Kuhl T, Adams BD: Five- to ten-year outcomes of the Universal total wrist arthroplasty in patients with rheumatoid arthritis. *J Bone Joint Surg Am* 93(10):914–919, 2011.

107. Watson HK, Ashmead DT, Makhlouf MV: Examination of the scaphoid. *J Hand Surg [Am]* 13(5):657–660, 1988.

108. Watson HK, Ballet FL: The SLAC wrist: scapholunate advanced collapse pattern of degenerative arthritis. *J Hand Surg [Am]* 9(3):358–365, 1984.

109. Watson HK, Fink JA, Monacelli DM: Use of triscaphe fusion in the treatment of Kienbock's disease. *Hand Clin* 9(3):493–499, 1993.

110. Watson HK, Goodman ML, Johnson TR: Limited wrist arthrodesis. Part II: Intercarpal and radiocarpal combinations. *J Hand Surg [Am]* 6(3):223–233, 1981.

111. Watson HK, Ryu J, Akelman E: Limited triscaphoid intercarpal arthrodesis for rotatory subluxation of the scaphoid. *J Bone Joint Surg Am* 68(3):345–349, 1986.

112. Watson HK, Weinzweig J, Zeppieri J: The natural progression of scaphoid instability. *Hand Clin* 13(1):39–49, 1997.

113. Watson HK, Wollstein R, Joseph E, et al: Scaphotrapeziotrapezoid arthrodesis: a follow-up study. *J Hand Surg [Am]* 28(3):397–404, 2003.

114. Weinstein LP, Berger RA: Analgesic benefit, functional outcome, and patient satisfaction after partial wrist denervation. *J Hand Surg [Am]* 27(5):833–839, 2002.

115. Weiss AC, Wideman G, Jr, Quenzer D, et al: Upper extremity function after wrist arthrodesis. *J Hand Surg [Am]* 20(5):813–817, 1995.

116. Weiss AP, Hastings H, 2nd: Wrist arthrodesis for traumatic conditions: a study of plate and local bone graft application. *J Hand Surg [Am]* 20(1):50–56, 1995.

117. Weiss G, Shemer A, Trau H: The Koebner phenomenon: review of the literature. *J Eur Acad Dermatol Venereol* 16(3):241–248, 2002.

118. Wolfe SW, Garcia-Elias M, Kitay A: Carpal instability nondissociative. *J Am Acad Orthop Surg* 20(9):575–585, 2012.

119. Wood MB: Wrist arthrodesis using dorsal radial bone graft. *J Hand Surg [Am]* 12(2):208–212, 1987.

120. Wright CS, McMurtry RY: AO arthrodesis in the hand. *J Hand Surg [Am]* 8(6):932–935, 1983.

13

Wrist Instabilities, Misalignments, and Dislocations

Marc Garcia-Elias and Alberto L. Lluch

> ▶ These videos may be found at
> *ExpertConsult.com:*
>
> 13.1 Dorsal view of a dissected cadaveric wrist set in a jig that allows isometric loading of different tendons. The entire scapholunate (SL) ligament complex has been sectioned. When the extensor carpi ulnaris (ECU) tendon is loaded, the distal row pronates and pulls the scaphoid away from the lunate. By contrast, loading of the extensor carpi radialis longus (ECRL) and abductor pollicis longus closes the SL gap. Certainly, the latter, and not the ECU; are the muscles that need to be emphasized when performing proprioceptive exercises for SL dissociations. *(Courtesy of Marc Garcia-Elias and Alberto L. Lluch.)*
>
> 13.2 Dynamic 3D computed tomography (also known as 4D computed tomography) of a patient with a scapholunate dissociation while performing dart thrower's exercises. Note that the scaphoid no longer behaves as a proximal row bone. It moves as if it were an extension of the distal carpal row; thus, the formation of a large gap in ulnar-flexion. *(Courtesy of Marc Garcia-Elias and Alberto L. Lluch.)*
>
> 13.3 Clinical example of a catch-up clunk phenomenon in a patient with carpal instability nondissociative–volar intercalated segmental instability. *(Courtesy of Marc Garcia-Elias and Alberto L. Lluch.)*
>
> 13.4 Volar approach of a perilunate dislocation. The distal surface of the lunate bone may be seen before the dislocation is reduced. *(Courtesy of Marc Garcia-Elias and Alberto L. Lluch.)*

The wrist has often been described as an irrelevant articulation that can be fused without causing much functional impairment to the upper extremity. Undoubtedly, patients with a fused wrist may recover enough grip strength so as to return to their previous occupation; their hands, however, will never be completely normal.[77] A stiff wrist does not allow, for instance, washing one's own back, dusting a low surface, turning a steering wheel, or beating an egg without overloading the adjacent upper limb articulations. If the wrist is fused, the hand can reach distant objects, but it cannot be properly oriented to grasp, push, or manipulate them effectively. Certainly this is one of the most important roles of the wrist: to place the hand in the position that ensures its maximal efficiency with minimal energy cost.

If properly identified and treated, wrist injuries tend to heal without sequelae, with a very low complication rate. When there is a complication, the carpus may remain aligned or it may collapse in a variety of ways. The articular cartilage may deteriorate or remain normal and asymptomatic. Identifying which injuries will evolve into significant dysfunctions is not always easy. How does one prevent an injured wrist from becoming

unstable? How does one differentiate between carpal instability and carpal misalignment? There are no good answers to these questions; certainly, the more these subjects are analyzed, the more unknowns arise, leading to the realization that further research is needed.

Progress is being made, however, and the proof can be found in this chapter. Only 5 years have passed since the sixth edition of this book was published, yet most chapters have had to be extensively rewritten. The goals have been: (1) to incorporate new knowledge acquired during this period, (2) to propose changes to the classification of carpal disorders, (3) to question misleading terminology, and (4) to eliminate concepts that the test of time has proved obsolete. The book's title itself has been modified to emphasize the fact that not all carpal misalignments are necessarily unstable, and that normal alignment does not guarantee stability.[2]

Undeniably, there is a growing interest in the wrist. What follows is an earnest attempt to respond to that interest by offering an updated description of how to assess and treat the various disorders of the wrist, truly one of the most complex joints of the human body.

Terminology. Most terms used to describe carpal misalignment and wrist instability were introduced in the 1970s, when these subjects were discussed for the first time.[57] Some of them have passed the test of time and are still useful and widely utilized; others have been proven less effective, if not misleading or totally incorrect, and need to be revised. The following are some suggestions in this regard. The goal is to improve the clarity of what is taught and to avoid misinterpretation of the facts.

The term *rotary (or rotatory) instability of the scaphoid,*[116] used to describe the advanced stage of carpal collapse where the scaphoid has lost its oblique alignment relative to the radius, is not correct: The scaphoid not only undergoes flexion and pronation but also translates dorsolaterally. There is never a pure rotation as implied by the adjective "rotary" or "rotatory." Furthermore, such an advanced stage of misalignment involves not only a complex displacement of the scaphoid but also of the lunate, which should be mentioned as well.

The terms *dorsal intercalated segment instability* (DISI) and *volar intercalated segment instability* (VISI)[42] seem quite appropriate for cases where the entire proximal carpal row adopts a position of abnormal extension or flexion in relation to the long axis of the radius. However, its use to define deformities secondary to dissociative carpal instabilities may create some confusion: only the lunate is in DISI not the scaphoid, which goes into flexion and pronation. Both are intercalated bones, and the deformity of each should be defined separately to prevent confusion; the scaphoid flexes and pronates, while the lunate extends.

While reading the literature, it is not uncommon to find confounding descriptions of wrist pathology that are a sign of a limited understanding of the basic principles of its mechanics. A typical example would be the use of redundant expressions such as "rotation into flexion" or "rotation into extension"—"flexion" or "extension" is enough. Another example is the use of "dorsiflexion" or "palmar-flexion." The first is a contradiction and the second is another redundancy; "extension" and "flexion" need no embellishments.

Although radial and ulnar *deviation* are widely accepted expressions, following the recommendations of the Committee on Standardization of Nomenclature of the International Federation of Societies for Surgery of the Hand (IFSSH),[58] they should be replaced by radial and ulnar *inclination*. An inclination is a mathematical term used to define the angle between two lines or planes. The term deviation is to be used when something departs from an acceptable standard or norm, and this is not what happens when the wrist is moved.

The inclination of the distal articular surface of the radius in relation to its longitudinal axis is frequently referred to as *radial tilt*, an expression that could be misinterpreted as an inclination toward the radial side. We suggest using the term *ulnar tilt of the radius*; for the same reason, it is best to use the term *volar tilt* to refer to the anterior inclination of the radius.

By consensus, wrist joints are termed by juxtaposing the names of the bones that meet in that articulation in an orderly manner, from proximal to distal and from radial to ulnar. Ligaments are named in a similar way. Based on this, the central midcarpal articulation should not be called "capitolunate" but "lunocapitate," and the ligaments connecting the triquetrum to the lunate should not be called "triquetrolunate" but "lunotriquetral."

WRIST ANATOMY

Carpal disorders cannot be properly diagnosed without a first-rate understanding of what is normal and what is abnormal in a symptomatic wrist. This requires a thorough knowledge of both the anatomy and mechanics of the normal wrist. This section reviews the former. The terminology used from here on is in accordance with the recommendations made by the IFSSH,[58] as well as by the International Wrist Investigators' Workshop (IWIW).[42] A list of abbreviations used in this chapter is shown in Table 13.1.

Osseous Anatomy

The wrist is a complex, composite joint formed by 20 interdependent articulations binding 15 bones: radius, ulna, 8 carpal bones, and the bases of 5 metacarpals. In the frontal (coronal) plane, the carpus is arranged in two rows (proximal and distal). The distal carpal row consists of 4 tightly bound bones (i.e., trapezium, trapezoid, capitate, hamate) with little mobility between them. The proximal carpal row, by contrast, exhibits substantial intercarpal mobility. It consists of three bones (i.e., scaphoid, lunate, triquetrum), interconnected by two intercarpal joints: scapholunate (SL) and lunotriquetral (LTq) (Figure 13.1). The pisiform, usually considered a proximal row bone, is actually a sesamoid bone that increases the lever arm of the flexor carpi ulnaris (FCU) tendon.

The radiocarpal joint is an oval-shaped glenoid articulation that connects the proximal convexities of the scaphoid, lunate

TABLE 13.1	Abbreviations Used in This Chapter
Acronym	**Definition**
AAOS	American Academy of Orthopedic Surgeons
AIN	Anterior interosseous nerve
APL	Abductor pollicis longus
ASSH	American Society for Surgery of the Hand
CIC	Carpal instability complex
CID	Carpal instability dissociative
CIND	Carpal instability nondissociative
CMC	Carpometacarpal
DASH	Disabilities of the arm, shoulder, and hand
DISI	Dorsal intercalated segment instability
DRUJ	Distal radioulnar joint
DT	Dart thrower's
ECRB	Extensor carpi radialis brevis
ECRL	Extensor carpi radialis longus
ECU	Extensor carpi ulnaris
EPL	Extensor pollicis longus
FCR	Flexor carpi radialis
FCU	Flexor carpi ulnaris
FPB	Flexor pollicis brevis
FPL	Flexor pollicis longus
FR	Flexor retinaculum
L	Lunate
LC	Lunocapitate
LTq	Lunotriquetral
RASL	Reduction association scapholunate
RL	Radiolunate
RS	Radioscaphoid
RSC	Radioscaphocapitate
RSL	Radioscapholunate
S	Scaphoid
SC	Scaphocapitate
SL	Scapholunate
SLD	Scapholunate dissociation
SLIL	Scapholunate interosseus ligament
SNAC	Scaphoid nonunion advanced collapse
STT	Scaphotrapeziotrapezoid
TFCC	Triangular fibrocartilage complex
Tq	Triquetrum
TqC	Triquetrocapitate
TqH	Triquetrohamate
VAS	Visual analog scale
VISI	Volar intercalated segment instability

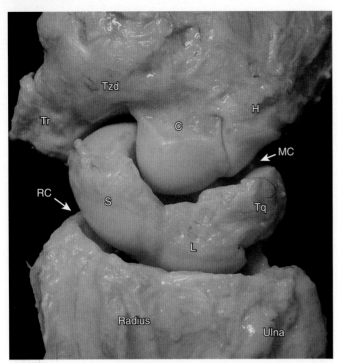

FIGURE 13.1 Dorsal view of a dissected cadaver specimen. The proximal row behaves as an intercalated segment between the radiocarpal (RC) and the midcarpal (MC) joints. *C,* Capitate; *H,* hamate; *L,* lunate; *S,* scaphoid; *Tq,* triquetrum; *Tr,* trapezium; *Tzd,* trapezoid.

and triquetrum—the so-called "carpal condyle"—with the antebrachial glenoid formed by the shallow concavities of the distal radius and triangular fibrocartilage complex (TFCC). The distal radius is tilted in two planes: the sagittal plane, where there is an average 10 degrees inclination toward the palm, and the frontal plane, where there is an average inclination toward the ulna of 24 degrees.[95] The proximal joint surface of the scaphoid is more curved than that of the lunate. To ensure articular congruency, the radius has two articular facets (i.e., scaphoid and lunate fossae), often separated by a cartilaginous sagittal ridge (i.e., interfacet prominence).

The midcarpal joint is a combination of three types of articulations. On the radial side, the convex distal surface of the scaphoid articulates with the concavity formed by the trapezium and the trapezoid—the scaphotrapeziotrapezoid (STT) joint. This is also known as the radial column. The central portion of the midcarpal joint is concave proximally and convex distally and has two sectors: the scaphocapitate (SC) and lunocapitate (LC) joints. The column formed by the lunate and capitate is also known as the central column. The lunate may have only one distal facet articulating with the capitate (lunate type I) or have two distal facets to articulate with the capitate and proximal pole of the hamate (lunate type II).[82,112] On the ulnar side, the triquetrum articulates with the hamate through the helicoidally shaped triquetrohamate (TqH) joint. This is known as the ulnar column.

The bones of the central column are collinear in the sagittal plane in only one-third of cases. In another 30%, the lunate is slightly flexed relative to the longitudinal axis of the forearm, while in the remaining 40% is slightly extended.[34] The scaphoid is placed obliquely in ~45 degrees of flexion in relation to the radius (range 30-60 degrees) to provide support to the thumb

metacarpal, which is located anteriorly to the plane of the capitate.[6]

In the axial (transverse) plane, the carpus forms the carpal tunnel, a palmar concavity, enclosed by the transverse carpal ligament (also known as the flexor retinaculum). The narrowest portion of the carpal tunnel is located at the level of the distal carpal row.

Ligamentous Anatomy

The bones of the wrist are interconnected by a complex arrangement of ligaments[7,23,81,86] (Figure 13.2, *A–C*). Some ligaments are mechanically important structures, formed by tightly packed collagen fibers with a minimal amount of sensory corpuscles. Others are sensorially important structures with a rich population of Ruffini, Pacini, or Golgi corpuscles embedded within a less dense structure of collagen fibers.[35,91] The former are static structures designed to hold the bones together. The latter provide the necessary proprioceptive information that the sensorimotor system uses to guarantee joint stability.[84]

The ligaments are extracapsular or intracapsular. Only three are extracapsular: the transverse carpal ligament, and the two ligaments that connect the pisiform to the hook of the hamate and to the base of the fifth metacarpal. All other ligaments are contained within the depth of the capsule, surrounded by sheaths of loose connective tissue.

Two categories of intracapsular ligaments exist: extrinsic and intrinsic. Extrinsic ligaments connect the forearm with the carpus, whereas intrinsic ligaments originate and insert within the carpus[23,86] (Figure 13.3, *A, B*). Histological and biomechanical differences exist between the two types. Extrinsic ligaments are mostly inserted onto bone, whereas intrinsic ligaments insert mostly onto cartilage. The extrinsic ligaments are more elastic and less resistant to traction (i.e., lower yield strength) than most intrinsic ligaments. Not surprisingly, the extrinsic ligaments tend to sustain midsubstance ruptures, whereas the intrinsic ligaments are more frequently avulsed than ruptured. The best way to assess the intracapsular ligaments is to use an arthroscope.[20,31,100] Inside the joint, most extrinsic ligaments can be identified under a thin synovial sheath.

Extrinsic Ligaments

There are four palmar radiocarpal ligaments: radioscaphoid (RS), radioscaphocapitate (RSC), long radiolunate, and short radiolunate ligaments (long RL and short RL).[7,23] The first three originate from the anterolateral margin of the distal radius and take an oblique course to insert onto the proximal edge of the scaphoid tuberosity (RS ligament), the palmar aspect of the capitate (RSC ligament), and the palmar surface of the lunate (long RL ligament). The short RL ligament originates from the anteromedial margin of the distal radius and has a vertical direction until merging with fibers of the long RL ligament. The RSC ligament courses around the palmar concavity of the scaphoid, forming a sling over which the scaphoid rotates. Between the two diverging RSC and long RL ligaments is the so-called "interligamentous sulcus" (i.e., space of Poirier), which represents a weak zone through which perilunate dislocations frequently occur.[45,94]

There are three palmar ulnocarpal ligaments: one superficial (ulnocapitate) and two deep (ulnotriquetral and ulnolunate).[7,23,69] The ulnocapitate ligament arises from a rough

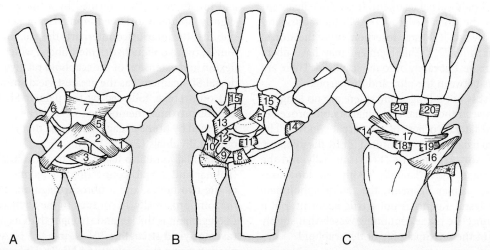

FIGURE 13.2 Schematic representation of wrist ligaments. These drawings do not replicate the exact shape and dimensions of the actual ligaments or their frequent anatomic variations. **A,** Palmar superficial ligaments: radioscaphoid (*1*), radioscaphocapitate (*2*), long radiolunate (*3*), ulnocapitate (*4*), scaphocapitate (*5*), pisohamate (*6*), and flexor retinaculum or transverse carpal ligament (*7*). **B,** Palmar deep ligaments: short radiolunate (*8*); ulnolunate (*9*); ulnotriquetral (*10*); palmar scapholunate (*11*); palmar lunotriquetral (*12*); triquetral–hamate–capitate, also known as the ulnar limb of the arcuate ligament (*13*); dorsolateral STT (*14*); and palmar transverse intercarpal ligaments of the distal row (*15*). **C,** Dorsal ligaments: radiotriquetral, also referred to as dorsal radiocarpal (*16*); triquetrum–scaphoid–trapeziotrapezoid, also known as the dorsal intercarpal ligament (*17*); dorsal scapholunate (*18*); dorsal lunotriquetral (*19*); and dorsal transverse intercarpal ligaments of the distal row (*20*). *Red asterisk,* triangular fibrocartilage complex.

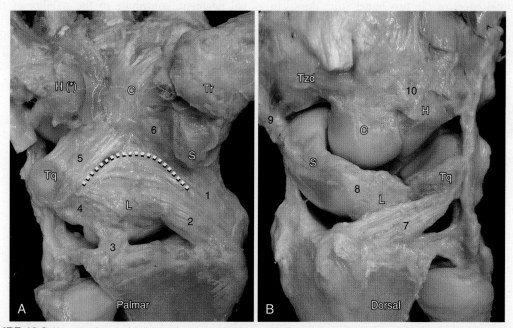

FIGURE 13.3 Human cadaver wrist dissected to show the relationship of some ligaments with the underlying joint surfaces. **A,** Palmar view: radioscaphocapitate (*1*); long radiolunate (*2*); short radiolunate (*3*); palmar lunotriquetral (*4*); triquetral–hamate–capitate (*5*); scaphocapitate (*6*). The so-called "space of Poirier" (*white dotted line*) is a relatively weak interligamentous sulcus through which most perilunate dislocations occur. **B,** Dorsal view: radiotriquetral (*7*); dorsal scapholunate (*8*); scaphoid–trapeziotrapezoid (*9*); dorsal transverse intercarpal ligaments (*10*). *Asterisk,* hook of the hamate. *C,* Capitate; *H,* hamate; *L,* lunate; *S,* scaphoid; *Tq,* triquetrum; *Tr,* trapezium; *Tzd,* trapezoid. (Not shown: dorsal intercarpal ligament.)

surface at the base of the ulnar styloid (i.e., the basistyloid fovea) and courses distally to attach onto the neck of the capitate. The ulnotriquetral and ulnolunate ligaments are deep fascicles that emerge from the palmar edge of the TFCC and run toward their distal insertions onto the anterior aspects of the lunate and triquetrum. The distal insertions of the ulnocapi-

tate ligament blend with those of the triquetrocapitate ligament before inserting onto the capitate. That combined ligament, together with the RSC ligament, form the "distal V" ligament, also known as arcuate ligament.

There is only one dorsal extrinsic ligament binding the radius to the carpus—the dorsal radiotriquetral ligament, also known as the dorsal radiocarpal ligament. It is a wide ligament that emerges from the dorsal edge of the distal radius and courses obliquely toward its distal insertion onto the dorsal ridge of the triquetrum.[76,86,100] This ligament may have fibers inserted onto the lunate, but rarely onto the scaphoid. There are no dorsal ligaments between the ulna and the carpus.

Because the wrist is not a hinge joint, there are no longitudinal ligaments between the radial and ulnar styloid processes and the medial and lateral corners of the carpal condyle. The absence of collateral ligaments is substituted for by the dynamic actions of the extensor carpi ulnaris (ECU) medially and the abductor pollicis longus (APL) laterally.[92] Although long considered an extrinsic palmar ligament, the radioscapholunate (RSL) ligament of Testut-Kuentz is not a true ligament, but a bundle of loose connective tissue containing vessels that supply the palmar corner of the proximal pole of the scaphoid.[7]

Intrinsic Ligaments

There are two types of intrinsic carpal ligaments: transverse intercarpal and midcarpal. The former interconnect bones from the same carpal row, while the latter link bones across the midcarpal joint.[7,11,23,81,86]

The SL joint is stabilized by two distinct transverse intercarpal ligaments (palmar and dorsal) and the proximal fibrocartilaginous membrane uniting both of them. The latter follows the arc of the proximal edges of the two bones from dorsal to palmar, separating the radiocarpal and midcarpal joint spaces. The dorsal SL ligament is located in the depth of the dorsal capsule and connects the dorsal–distal corners of the scaphoid and lunate bones. It is formed by a thick collection of fibers, slightly obliquely oriented, and plays a key role in scaphoid stability. Its anterior counterpart, the palmar SL ligament, has longer, more obliquely oriented fibers, which allow substantial flexion and extension of the scaphoid relative to the lunate. The dorsal SL ligament has the greatest yield strength, 260 newtons (N) on average, followed by the palmar SL ligament (118 N) and the proximal membrane (63 N).[7] The proximal membrane is formed by fibrocartilaginous tissue that is often perforated in older individuals (Figure 13.4).

The LTq joint also has two transverse intercarpal ligaments (palmar and dorsal) connecting the palmar and dorsal aspects of the two bones, and a fibrocartilaginous membrane closing the joint proximally. In contrast to the SL ligaments, the palmar LTq ligament is thicker and stronger than its dorsal counterpart (average yield strengths: 301 N and 121 N) with the proximal portion being the weakest (64 N).[54,87] Unless perforated by age or injury, this proximal membrane prevents communication between the radiocarpal and midcarpal joint spaces. The fibers of the two LTq ligaments are under greater tension through all ranges of motion than the fibers of the SL ligaments. The most distal fibers of palmar and dorsal LTq ligaments are often connected to the distal fibers of the SL ligaments, forming the palmar and dorsal scaphotriquetral ligaments.[113] These structures, as well as the interdigitating fibers of the dorsal intercarpal ligament, contribute to the stability of the LC joint by increasing the depth of the midcarpal fossa.[27,118]

The distal carpal row bones are strongly bound to each other by stout transverse intercarpal ligaments (i.e., dorsal, palmar,

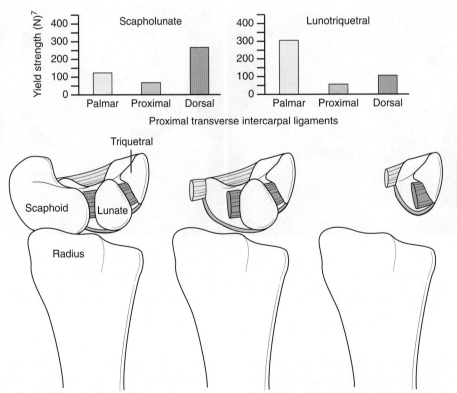

FIGURE 13.4 Schematic representations of the scapholunate (SL) and lunotriquetral (LTq) ligamentous complexes. At both levels there are one proximal fibrocartilaginous membrane (*in blue*) and two transverse intercarpal ligaments: palmar (*in yellow*) and dorsal (*in red*). The dorsal SL ligament has the greatest yield strength of the three components of the SL joint (*upper left bar chart*), whereas the palmar LTq ligament is stronger than it dorsal counterpart (*upper right bar chart*).[7]

intraarticular). They are essential to ensure the rigidity of the transverse carpal arch and to protect the carpal tunnel contents.[80]

The midcarpal joint is crossed by three palmar ligaments (i.e., triquetrohamate [TqH], triquetrocapitate [TqC], and scaphocapitate), one dorsolateral STT ligament, and one dorsal intercarpal ligament.[11,23,56] The TqH and TqC ligaments are thick structures, variable in size and shape, that play an important role in the stabilization of the midcarpal joint.[27,118] Their anatomy varies according to the type of lunate (I or II).[23,82,112] The TqC ligament is also known as the ulnar arm of the arcuate ligament.[56] Laterally, the scaphoid tuberosity is linked to the distal row by the anteromedial SC ligament and the dorsolateral STT ligament. These two ligaments behave as collateral ligaments for the STT joint.[70]

The only ligament crossing the dorsum of the midcarpal joint is the dorsal intercarpal ligament.[11,76,113] On the ulnar side, it arises from the dorsal ridge of the triquetrum and courses transversely along the dorsal edges of the proximal row bones, distal to the scaphotriquetral ligament. At the level of the scaphoid, this ligament fans out to insert onto the dorsal rim of the scaphoid, the trapezium, and the trapezoid. There are no ligaments, palmar or dorsal, between the lunate and capitate.

WRIST BIOMECHANICS

The wrist is a highly mobile, composite articulation that links the two forearm bones and the hand, characterized by its ability to sustain substantial amounts of load in all positions.[46,57] To achieve this, there must be appropriate interaction between wrist motor tendons, joint surfaces, and soft tissue con-

straints.[35,84] What follows is a brief description of how the wrist moves (i.e., kinematics) and how it withstands loads without yielding (i.e., kinetics).

Carpal Kinematics

The wrist can be moved passively by an external force, or actively by contracting muscles with a tendon crossing the joint. None of these tendons inserts onto the proximal carpal row; all of them insert distal to the midcarpal joint.[18,76,99] Consequently, when these muscles contract, the distal carpal row is the first to move. The bones of the proximal row do not start rotating until the midcarpal ligaments become taut and pull them into motion. In other words, around the neutral position, the only joint that moves is the midcarpal articulation.[18,29,67]

Flexion–Extension

In the sagittal plane, the scaphoid rotates more than the lunate, owing to differences in the shape of their proximal and distal articulating surfaces and surrounding ligamentous anatomy (Figure 13.5). From neutral-to-maximal wrist flexion, the scaphoid and lunate contribute 70% and 46%, respectively, to the total range. Similarly, during maximal wrist extension, the scaphoid and lunate contribute 72% and 42%, respectively.[67,76] The shape of the two bones also deserves a comment: the scaphoid is obliquely oriented relative to the longitudinal axis of the forearm; because of that, it is easier for it to flex than to extend.

The lunate, by contrast, has an inherent tendency to extend as it is narrower dorsally than palmarly. With this in mind, it is easy to understand why the contribution of the radiocarpal and midcarpal joints to the total range of wrist flexion–extension is different in the central column (55% of the total range takes

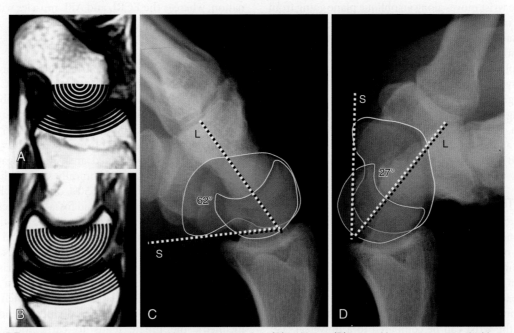

FIGURE 13.5 Sagittal computed tomography scans of the scaphoid **(A)** and lunate **(B)**, covered by a transparent card with concentric circle scale marks. Indeed, the radii of curvature of the lunate (L) is longer than that of the scaphoid (S). Because of this, the scaphoid needs to rotate more than the lunate to get to the limits of flexion–extension. Unlike the distal row, where the four bones form a fixed unit with little motion between them, the proximal row exhibits substantial SL and lunotriquetral (LTq) rotations. The proof of this may be found by comparing the SL angle in full flexion **(C)** and full extension **(D)**. In this particular case the scaphoid rotates 35 degrees more than the lunate.

place in the midcarpal joint) than in the radial column (70% of motion happens at the RS joint).[34]

Radioulnar Inclination

When the wrist moves along the frontal (i.e., coronal) plane, both the proximal and distal rows go into radial and ulnar inclination, but the proximal carpal row also flexes and extends. In radial inclination, the trapezium and trapezoid approximate to the radius and therefore the scaphoid has to flex because the space is reduced, and its longitudinal axis becomes almost perpendicular to that of the radius. The lunate and triquetrum also flex, although to a lesser degree.[67,105]

When the wrist goes into ulnar inclination the scaphoid extends, pulled by the trapezium and trapezoid, with its longitudinal axis becoming practically collinear to that of the radius. The lunate and triquetrum also extend during ulnar inclination, although to a lesser degree. For this reason, if the wrist is ulnarly inclined when a plain radiograph or a sagittal tomogram is obtained, one may erroneously think that the extended position of the lunate is secondary to misalignment.[59]

Dart-Thrower's Motion

The orthogonal (i.e., frontal and sagittal) planes of motion are seldom utilized in activities of daily living. The most commonly used plane of motion goes from extension and radial inclination to flexion and ulnar inclination.[9,18] Fisk described this plane as "when someone is casting a fly or throwing a dart"; thus, hand surgeons use the term "dart-thrower's" (DT) motion.[70]

When the wrist is in radial inclination, the scaphoid and lunate are flexed. If the wrist is then brought into extension, the lunate recovers its initial alignment, as when the wrist was in neutral. When the wrist goes into ulnar inclination, the scaphoid and lunate extend, but they regain that neutral position when the wrist is flexed while in ulnar inclination.[30] In other words, when the wrist moves along an oblique plane going from extension and radial inclination to neutral, and finally into flexion and ulnar inclination, the scaphoid and lunate remain in neutral position. Indeed, during DT motion, most wrist mobility takes place at the midcarpal joint.[18,30,70]

The obliquity of the DT plane of motion is unique to each individual, ranging from 37 to 59 degrees from the sagittal plane, according to various authors.[9,18,30,70] This oblique plane of wrist motion, generated by the pull of two wrist extensors—extensor carpi radialis longus (ECRL) and extensor carpi radialis brevis (ECRB)—and one wrist flexor, the FCU, is one of the most frequently used in activities of daily living.

Reversed Dart-Thrower's Motion

The opposite rotation, from extension–ulnar inclination to flexion–radial inclination has been referred to as the "reversed dart-thrower's" motion. It is a rotation mediated by the FCR on the volar side and the ECU on the dorsal side of the wrist. As opposed to what happens during DT rotation, the contribution of the midcarpal joint to the reversed dart-thrower's type of rotation is minimal: only the radiocarpal joint is mobilized. Based on this, the wrist can be compared to a universal (i.e., cardan) type of articulation with two axes of rotation: one for the midcarpal joint and another for the radiocarpal joint. The midcarpal dart-throwing axis and the radiocarpal reversed DT axis do not coincide in space: the first would be located at about

the center of the head of the capitate, while the second would be more proximally located at about the LC joint.[18]

Needless to say, this way of describing wrist motion is an oversimplification. In reality, each bone has its own center of rotation that changes in location and orientation as the wrist moves. There are substantial synergies between the bones of each row that make this simplified model useful for the clinician, however. In fact, this model is the first to provide a convincing explanation of how the wrist is able to transmit pronosupination torques, from distal-to-proximal or vice versa, in all wrist positions, without losing stability (Figure 13.6).

Intracarpal Pronosupination

Most axial rotation of the hand takes place in the forearm, with the radius rotating around a slightly oblique longitudinal axis running from the center of the head of the radius to the center of the head of the ulna. However, some pronation and supination also take place in the wrist, mainly at the midcarpal joint. Passive intracarpal pronation and supination are greater than active rotation.

The mechanism of active intracarpal pronosupination has recently been elucidated[91,92] and can be explained as follows. Distal to the extensor retinaculum, most wrist motor tendons change direction, taking an oblique path to their distal insertion. The ECU tendon, for instance, from a dorsal position at the level of the ulnar head, courses obliquely toward its distal insertion onto the volar–ulnar corner of the fifth metacarpal. The ECRL and the APL also have an oblique course but in the opposite direction, toward the lateral border of the wrist.

All of them are dorsal at the radiocarpal level but diverge distally toward their ulnar or radial insertions. If the wrist is in a neutral position, isolated isometric contraction of any of these muscles will generate a pronation or supination moment to the distal row: ECU muscle contraction will cause intracarpal pronation, whereas the ECRL and APL muscles will induce a supination moment to the distal row.[91,92]

Carpal Kinetics

Hand function generates a considerable amount of force that is transmitted across the carpometacarpal (CMC) joints into the carpus.[63,99,112] At the distal row, loads are distributed among the midcarpal joints with the SC and LC joints transmitting ~50%, the STT joint ~30%, and the TqH joint ~20%.[112] The fact that most synovial cysts emerge from the SL interval proves this to be a particularly overloaded area; indeed, ganglions tend to appear on the surface of chronically strained ligaments.

Once in the proximal row, 50% of the total load is transmitted across the RS joint (scaphoid fossa), 35% across the RL joint (lunate fossa), and 15% across the TFCC into the ulna.[63,112] The average pressure values within the radiocarpal joint may be as high as 5.6 MPa, which is approximately 0.5 N/mm^2 or 810 lb/in^2. These figures vary substantially with wrist position. The lunate fossa is increasingly loaded with ulnar inclination, the scaphoid fossa with radial inclination. When the wrist is in the "position of function" (i.e., slightly extended and radially inclined), the lunate tends to carry more load than the scaphoid.[63]

When axially loaded, the carpal bones become displaced following specific patterns.[2] The magnitude and direction of displacement depend on the shape of the articular surfaces, the

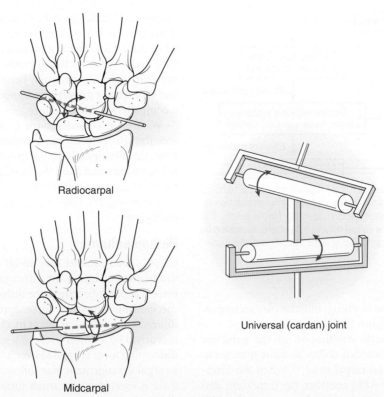

Radiocarpal

Midcarpal

Universal (cardan) joint

FIGURE 13.6 The wrist is a universal (cardan) type of articulation, able to transmit torques across the proximal row in all wrist positions without losing stability. Henle was the first to describe this phenomenon in 1871.[21]

orientation and point of application of the incoming loads, and the status of the various soft tissue constraints (i.e., capsule, ligaments, muscles).

A wrist is stable when it is able to sustain physiological loads in all positions without experiencing abnormal carpal displacement.[2] When a stable wrist is loaded, the carpal bones do not displace beyond normal limits. For this to happen, the articular surfaces must be normally oriented and congruous, the ligaments must be all present and active; and the forces generated by the muscles acting on the carpal bones must be balanced.

The Role of Ligaments in Carpal Stabilization

The proximal carpal row, truly an intercalated segment between the radius and distal carpal row, is inherently unstable. If not for the capsule, ligaments, and muscles, the three bones would collapse when compressed by the distal carpal row against the radius. The obliquely oriented scaphoid would rotate into flexion and pronation, while the wedge-shaped (thinner dorsally than palmarly) lunate and triquetrum would collapse into extension and supination[34] (Figure 13.7).

In theory, if the SL ligaments were all intact, the flexion tendency of the scaphoid would be counteracted by the opposite tendency of the loaded lunate and triquetrum to rotate into extension, and stability would be achieved. In practice, these ligaments cannot do that alone.[7] The tensile forces involved in most hand activities are far too high for these ligaments to be the only wrist stabilizers. To achieve stability, ligaments need to be protected by muscles.[35,91,92]

To ensure a timely and protective muscle response, the carpal ligaments contain mechanoreceptors providing the proprioceptive information required by the sensorimotor system to acti-

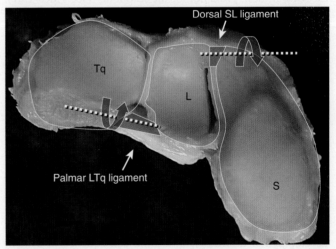

FIGURE 13.7 Human wrist dissected to show the distal articular surfaces of the proximal row and the transverse intercarpal ligaments. The main role of the dorsal scapholunate (SL) ligament is to avoid excessive flexion–pronation of the scaphoid (S; *blue curved arrows*), whereas the palmar lunotriquetral (LTq) ligament is responsible for the neutralization of the extension tendency of the triquetrum (Tq) under load. *L*, Lunate.

vate that response.[84] In other words, the ligaments provide the first line of defense against instability, but the muscles are the ultimate stabilizers.[35,91]

The Role of Muscles in Carpal Stabilization

Until recently, muscles were considered to have a negative influence on carpal stability. Instability was assumed to be a ligament insufficiency problem made worse by muscle contraction. Now

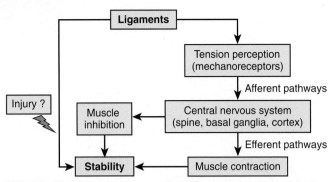

FIGURE 13.8 Schematic representation of the mechanism of carpal stabilization. Ligaments are the primary stabilizers. When one ligament is seriously injured, a secondary neuromuscular reflex develops to compensate for the defect. This entire mechanism is mediated by the central nervous system and, depending on which ligament is injured, involves contraction of some muscles, and inhibition of others muscles.

we know that the assumption is wrong: muscles play an important stabilizing role[35,91,92] (Figure 13.8).

The mechanisms of muscle stabilization of the wrist are based on the previously mentioned ability of some muscles to pronate or supinate the distal carpal row.[91,92] When the intracarpal supinators (ECRL or APL) contract, the trapezium displaces dorsally, thus tightening the STT ligament. If the STT ligament is taut, the scaphoid cannot collapse into flexion and pronation. The intracarpal supinators, therefore, protect against excessive flexion–pronation of the scaphoid[92] (see Video 13.1). In contrast, when the ECU contracts, the distal row pronates, tightening the TqH ligament and preventing the proximal row from collapsing into flexion.[54] Thus, the supinators are useful in the treatment of scaphoid instabilities, and the pronators in the treatment of most ulnarside carpal instabilities.[35] Again, muscles are the ultimate carpal stabilizers.[84]

WRIST DISORDERS

Wrist function may be altered in a variety of ways. A change in the shape of the articulating bones, a rupture or insufficiency of specific ligaments, and/or a loss of the stabilizing effect of specific muscles can explain most carpal disorders. The resulting malfunction may be present at birth (i.e., congenital disorders); may appear slowly as a result of abnormal growth (i.e., developmental disorders); or be the consequence of violent trauma, repetitive stress, or a joint damaging disease (i.e., acquired disorder). This chapter discusses the assessment and treatment of most acquired disorders of the wrist.

With time, most wrist disorders evolve into carpal misalignment. In theory, the most misaligned wrists should all be unstable. In practice, this is not always true. Instability is a multifactorial phenomenon that may or may not be associated with an alteration of the carpal alignment.[2] The misalignment of the so-called "adaptive wrists", for instance, is not a sign of ligament-related instability, but an adaptation of a normal carpus to compensate for an extracarpal bone deformity.[1] Another example is the constitutional hyperlax wrist: It may appear misaligned, yet it frequently remains asymptomatic, able to handle most activities of daily living, and seldom requires treatment. Chronic unreduced perilunate dislocations are also

examples of malaligned, but not unstable wrists. Certainly, if a dislocation is left unreduced, the joint will be unstable for a while until it undergoes a process of arthrofibrosis and becomes stiff, and stiffness is the opposite of being unstable. Indeed, a normally aligned carpus may behave as an unstable articulation; and vice versa, a grossly misaligned wrist may behave as if it was a completely stable structure.[1]

With these considerations in mind, this chapter differentiates the unstable carpus secondary to intracarpal pathology from the misaligned, yet normal carpus secondary to extracarpal pathology, and from the misaligned but stiff wrist secondary to posttraumatic arthrofibrosis. What follows is a review of some aspects that are common for these three clinical conditions.

Pathomechanics

Carpal derangements may result from a direct or an indirect mechanism of injury. In direct mechanisms, the destabilizing force is applied directly to the dislocating bone, whereas indirect mechanisms involve a force applied at a distance from the injured joint. A typical direct mechanism occurs when the wrist is crushed by a power press or a wringer-type machine.[80] If the dislocating force is applied over a large surface area of the hand, a carpal derangement may follow. In contrast, if the dislocating force is exerted over a small surface area, a localized fracture–dislocation may occur.

Wrist extension is the primary component of injuries causing distal radial fractures, scaphoid fractures, or perilunate dislocations. Differences in bone stock, the direction and magnitude of the deforming forces, and/or the position of the wrist at the time of incident may explain which type of injury occurs.

Perilunate dislocations are complex carpal derangements, usually the result of a combination of loaded hyperextension and intracarpal axial rotation.[43,64] A typical case would be a head-on motorbike collision, where the hand gets pinned to the handlebar while the body is violently projected forward. The wrist, in such instances, becomes the pivot point about which the body rotates. When this happens, carpal destabilization undergoes a quite consistent four-stage pattern called "progressive perilunar instability," described by Mayfield et al.[44,45,64] The stages shown in Figure 13.9 are described in the following subsections.

Stage I: SL Dissociation or Scaphoid Fracture

When the wrist is violently twisted into extension and intracarpal supination, if the STT and SC ligaments are intact, the scaphoid extends and supinates, dragged by the trapezium. The lunate, in contrast, stays behind, constrained by the two long and short RL ligaments. With this, an increasing SL torque is created. When this torque reaches a certain level, progressive tearing of the SL intercarpal membrane and ligaments tends to occur. Usually, this happens from palmar-to-dorsal.

The end stage would be a complete SL dissociation. If the same process happens when the wrist is radially inclined (i.e., when the proximal pole of the scaphoid is powerfully constrained by the RSC ligament), instead of SL dissociation, an scaphoid fracture is likely to occur. More rarely, the lunate may suffer a coronal fracture, the volar portion of it remaining attached to the radius while the dorsal fragment follows the scaphoid and distal row in their dorsal displacement.[5]

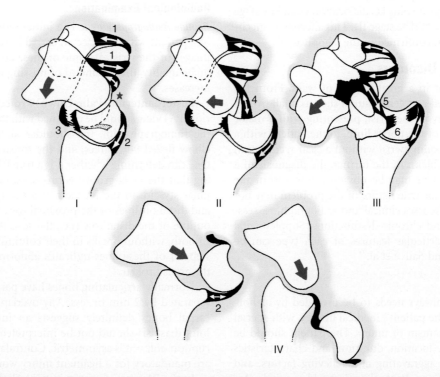

FIGURE 13.9 Schematic representation of the four stages of perilunate instability, viewed from the ulnar side. Stage I: As the distal carpal row is forced into hyperextension (*red arrows*), the scaphotrapezoid–capitate ligaments (*1*) pull the scaphoid (S) into extension, opening the space of Poirier (*asterisk*). The lunate (L) cannot extend as much as the scaphoid because it is directly constrained by the short RL ligament (*2*). When SL torque reaches a certain value, the SL ligaments may fail, usually from palmar to dorsal. A complete SL dissociation is defined by the rupture of the dorsal SL ligament (*3*). Stage II: When dissociated from the lunate, the scaphoid–distal row complex may dislocate dorsally relative to the lunate (*red arrow*). The limit of such dorsal translation is determined by the radioscaphocapitate (RSC) ligament (*4*). Stage III: If hyperextension persists, the ulnar limb of the arcuate ligament (*5*) may pull the triquetrum (Tq) dorsally, causing failure of the lunotriquetral (LTq) ligaments (*6*). Stage IV: Finally, the capitate may be forced by the still-intact RSC ligament (*4*) to edge into the radiocarpal space and push the lunate palmarward until it dislocates into the carpal canal in a rotary fashion. (Modified from Mayfield JK, Johnson RP, Kilcoyne RK: Carpal dislocations: pathomechanics and progressive perilunar instability. *J Hand Surg Am* 5:226–241, 1980.[64])

Stage II: Perilunate Dislocation

Once the SL joint is disrupted, if the destabilizing force continues, the capitate may leave the lunate concavity, leading to a dorsal perilunate dislocation. If instead of SL dissociation there is a scaphoid fracture, the wrist will suffer a transscaphoperilunate dislocation. Less commonly, the capitate may undergo a fracture. In such cases, only the body of the capitate dislocates dorsally with the rest of the distal row. The head of the capitate stays behind, sometimes completely rotated. In most instances, the displacement of the distal row is associated with a midsubstance stretching injury of the RSC ligament.

Stage III: LTq Disruption or Triquetrum Fracture

As the distal row dislocates dorsally, the TqH and TqC ligaments become extremely taut, generating an extension/dorsal translation vector to the triquetrum. This may result either in the separation of the triquetrum from the lunate, owing to tearing of the LTq ligaments, or a sagittal fracture of the triquetrum.

Stage IV: Lunate Dislocation

When all perilunate ligaments are torn, only the dorsal capsule and palmar RL ligaments can hold the lunate in place. In such circumstances, the dorsally displaced capitate, propelled by the forearm muscles, may enter the radiocarpal joint and push the lunate palmarly, out of the lunate fossa. This results in an anterior dislocation of the lunate. Such a dislocation is often associated with a variable degree of lunate flexion into the carpal tunnel.

Depending on the amount of lunate rotation, lunate dislocation has been subdivided into three categories: type I, in which the lunate exhibits greater than 90 degrees of flexion deformity; type II, in which the lunate is flexed >90 degrees around an intact, undisrupted, palmar RL capsule and ligament; and type III, which is a complete palmar enucleation of the lunate with rupture of the palmar capsule.[38]

There are cases where the carpal derangement starts at the ulnar side and proceeds radially around the lunate. Usually, this happens as a result of a backward fall on the outstretched hand with the upper limb externally rotated. In such circumstances, the disrupting load is applied to the hypothenar area, the triquetrum being forced by the pisiform to displace dorsally relative to the lunate. Since the lunate cannot displace in the same direction because it is constrained by the radius, an increasing shear stress develops between the two bones. In such cases, complete rupture of the LTq ligaments would be stage I of a reversed perilunate destabilization pattern of the wrist, ulnocarpal ligament rupture plus LC dislocation would be stage II, and SL dissociation would be stage III. This alternative mechanism has recently been confirmed in the laboratory.[71]

Diagnosis of Wrist Disorders

Wrist disorders present in a great variety of ways. From the patient who has suffered a violent trauma such as a fall from a height or a crush injury to the wrist, presenting with a major fracture or dislocation of the upper limb, to the patient with a symptomatic malfunctioning wrist without a clear recollection of what caused the problem. In the former, the diagnosis of a major carpal derangement may be obvious; however, in the latter, identification of the true nature of the problem may not be easy. This section discusses clinical and radiographic assessments of both acute and chronic dysfunctions. Supplemental information on the particular features of each type can be found in Rhee et al[83] and Sauvé et al.[93]

Clinical Examination

Physical examination always needs to be preceded by a thorough investigation of the patient's medical history, with special emphasis on the mechanism of injury. The patient should be asked details about the location, duration, and characteristics of any pain including aggravating and relieving factors, and previous treatments, if any. With chronic problems, it is also important to inquire about the patient's jobs and hobbies, and whether there has been exposure to repetitive stress, vibrating tools, or potentially dangerous instruments.

The next step is inspection. Except in cases with an open dislocation, the external appearance of most wrist dislocations may not be dramatic. Swelling is generally moderate, and bone displacements may be evident only if the patient is seen immediately after experiencing the trauma. If there has been a delay since the accident, swelling may have increased significantly, making visualization of the displaced bones more difficult. When present, skin abrasions, contusions, or ecchymosed areas may be helpful in determining the mechanism of injury and the potential areas of damage.

Palpation for areas of maximal tenderness is one of the most useful tools in the diagnosis of wrist pathology, especially in patients with chronic dysfunctions.[83,93] In acute dislocations, because of extensive soft tissue damage, tenderness is seldom elicited at specific points, but rather in a diffuse manner. Nonetheless, palpation should always be performed in a methodical way.

Acutely, range of motion is usually limited by pain, whereas it may be reduced or normal in more chronic cases. In the latter, passive mobilization of the joints is valuable not only in determining the presence of abnormal motion or crepitus but also in reproducing the patient's pain. Grip and pinch strength also need to be measured for chronic problems to uncover underlying pathology. Strength may be reduced due to muscle atrophy or by pain inhibition. A local injection of anesthetic within the affected joint may normalize the dynamometer readings in the latter.

A careful assessment of neurovascular status is imperative, with particular attention being paid to the median and ulnar nerves, which may be injured by direct contusion at the moment of impact, by compression from displaced bones, or by swelling in the carpal canal.

Radiological Examination

Routine Radiograph Views. The initial radiographic examination of a patient with a suspected carpal injury should include four images of the wrist. If some of these are omitted, or of inadequate quality, the likelihood of missing important information increases.[59,120]

Posteroanterior (Palm Down) Projection. The posteroanterior (PA) view should be obtained with the hand placed flat over the radiograph film, the shoulder abducted 90 degrees, the elbow flexed 90 degrees, and the forearm in neutral rotation. One can determine whether it is a true PA radiograph by checking that the ECU groove is projected radial to the axis of the ulnar styloid. In the PA view of a normal wrist, the proximal and distal outlines of the proximal row, as well as the proximal outline of the distal row (i.e., the so-called "Gilula's lines") are smooth, without breaks in their continuity (Figure 13.10). Any step-off of these lines indicates abnormality at the site where the arc is broken.[120]

Normally articulating bones have parallel opposing surfaces separated by 2 mm or less. Any overlap between well-profiled carpal bones definitely suggests an intercarpal abnormality. Joint diastasis should not be interpreted as a sign of joint disruption unless it is asymmetric. Contralateral wrist radiographs are mandatory for a ligament injury workup.

In the PA view of a wrist in neutral, the normal lunate has a trapezoidal configuration. It is possible to differentiate a flexed from an extended lunate based on the shape of its contour (Figure 13.11). To do so, it is important to remember that, in the transverse plane, the lunate is wider palmarly than dorsally. Therefore, when abnormally extended, the lunate has an ovoid configuration due to the distal displacement of the wider anterior horn. Conversely, when abnormally flexed the lunate is triangular shaped, often with a half moon-like configuration, with its concavity facing toward the scaphoid.[34,82]

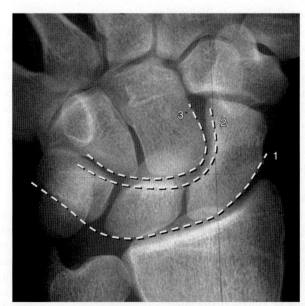

FIGURE 13.10 Gilula[120] defined three smooth, curved lines (*1, 2,* and *3*) joining the proximal and distal cortical surfaces of the carpal bones that help assess normal carpal relationships. A disruption or step-off in any one of these lines may indicate a major carpal derangement.

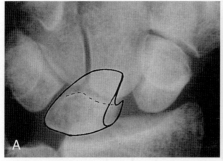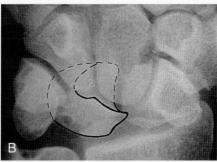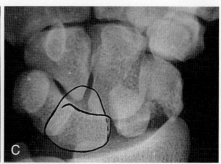

FIGURE 13.11 The shape of the lunate (L) on a posteroanterior view may help differentiate a dislocated from a malaligned lunate. **A,** The lunate in a dorsal intercalated segment instability (DISI) position tends to have an ovoid configuration, with a prominent ulnar corner pointing toward the medial aspect of the wrist. **B,** The lunate in volar intercalated segment instability (VISI) has a "C"-shaped or moonlike appearance. **C,** In dorsal perilunate dislocations, the subluxed lunate appears as an isosceles triangle pointing distally.

Lateral Projection. The lateral view must be taken with the arm adducted to the patient's side, and with both the forearm and the wrist in neutral rotation. For a lateral projection to be correct, the axis of the third metacarpal needs to be parallel to that of the radius, and the palmar outline of the pisiform needs to be located between (and equidistant to) the palmar surfaces of the scaphoid tuberosity and the capitate head.[120]

Scaphoid Projection. The best projection to confirm a scaphoid fracture is a PA view centered on it, with the wrist in ulnar inclination and the fingers fully flexed.

Semipronated (Oblique) Projection. A 45-degree semipronated oblique view profiling the anterolateral and posteromedial corners of the carpus is useful to investigate the presence of fractures of the dorsal ridge of the triquetrum and of the scaphoid tuberosity.

Additional Radiograph Views. When routine radiographs do not confirm the suspected diagnosis, obtaining additional views is recommended. The following are the most commonly used projections for the wrist.

- *Anteroposterior (palm up) view with a clenched fist:* Alternatively, get radiographs with a longitudinal compression force applied to the wrist by an assistant, which may accentuate the gap that often appears in SL dissociation (Figure 13.12). It is preferable to obtain this view without wrist extension or flexion. Correct positioning can be objectively evaluated by looking at the third CMC joint. When the wrist is in neutral, the joint's surfaces are parallel.
- *PA (palm down) view with 10 degrees of tube angulation from ulna toward radius:* This view is ideal to assess the SL interval. Measurement of its separation (SL gap) is made at the midportion of the joint where its anatomy is more consistent. The spacing should be compared with the opposite wrist and with the surrounding carpal articulations.
- *Clenched-pencil view:* This is one of the best ways to demonstrate SL dissociation because it optimally profiles the joint while it is being separated with some grip force. It consists of a PA view of both wrists while the two hands are gripping one pencil tightly, with the index fingers apposed and the thumb metacarpals lying flat on the radiographic cassette. The technique provides comparison of both wrists at the same time.[51a]
- *Oblique view at 20 degrees of pronation from the lateral position:* This view is used to visualize the dorsum of the triquetrum, where avulsion fractures frequently occur, and to

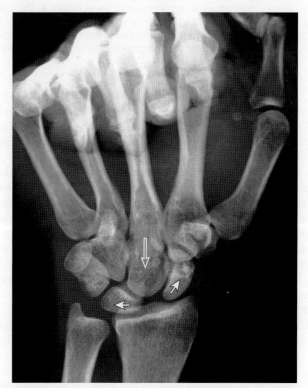

FIGURE 13.12 Compression of the carpus by having the patient make a fist (*large arrow*) may accentuate the gap in complete scapholunate dissociation (*small arrows*).

evaluate the distal tuberosity and waist of the scaphoid. It is ideal for fracture–subluxations of the fifth CMC joint.
- *Oblique view at 30 degrees of supination from the lateral position:* The pisotriquetral relationship is best seen with this view.
- *Lateral view with the wrist radially inclined:* The palmar outline of the hook of the hamate can be seen on a lateral view with the wrist radially inclined and the thumb in maximal anteposition. It places the hook of the hamate between the bases of the first and second metacarpals.
- *Carpal tunnel view:* By profiling the carpal concavity of the wrist, a clearer view of the hook of the hamate, the pisiform, and the palmar ridge of the triquetrum can be obtained. In patients with acute injuries, however, pain produced by extending the wrist may not allow the radiograph to be taken.

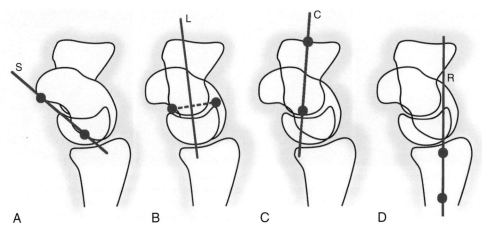

FIGURE 13.13 Carpal angle determination is based on tracing axes to the carpal bones on true lateral radiographs. The most reproducible methods of axis determination are as follows: **A,** The scaphoid (S) is represented by a tangential line that connects the two palmar convexities of the bone. **B,** The lunate (L)-axis is perpendicular to a line that joins the two distal horns of the bone. **C,** The capitate (C)-axis is determined by the center of the two proximal and distal articular surfaces. **D,** The axis of the radius (R) is obtained by tracing perpendicular lines to its distal third and connecting the center of these lines.

- *Static motion views:* For patients suspected of having carpal instability, a routine "motion" series may be needed. It should include PA and anteroposterior views in radial and ulnar inclination, in addition to lateral views in extension and flexion.

Carpal Bone Alignment Measurement. Carpal misalignment has traditionally been determined by measuring specific distances and angles on PA or lateral radiographs.[57,120] When interpreting these data, however, one must be aware that the normal ranges for these parameters are quite diverse. Also, reproducibility is low and small errors in rotational positioning of the hand at the time of radiograph exposure may result in substantial variation in angle determination. The following are the most frequently used measurements to define carpal bone alignment (Figure 13.13).

- *LC angle:* This is helpful to quantify midcarpal misalignment. The axis of the lunate is a line perpendicular to a line connecting the palmar and dorsal tips of it. The capitate axis is identified by connecting a point in the center of the convexity of its head to a point at the center of the third CMC joint. A normal LC angle should be 0 ± 15 degrees with the wrist in neutral.[120]
- *SL angle:* This angle, formed by a line tangential to the proximal and distal convexities of the scaphoid's palmar aspect and that of the lunate, has been quoted extensively in the literature as one of the major determinants of SL dissociation. Normal values range from 30 to 60 degrees (average, 47 degrees).[57,120] Although angles greater than 80 degrees indicate SL ligament disruption, lower readings do not rule out this pathology. Values less than 30 degrees are not unusual for patients with STT joint osteoarthritis.
- *RL angle:* This gives objective evidence of the dorsal or palmar tilt of the lunate. The normal RL angle should be 0 ± 15 degrees.[120]
- *Ulnar variance:* The relative lengths of the radius and ulna, or "ulnar variance," and the possible effects of this parameter on various carpal disorders have long been investigated.[95] Ulnar variance is usually measured on standard PA radiographs, although lateral radiographic projections also offer

very accurate readings. The usual way to assess ulnar variance is to measure the distance between two lines perpendicular to the longitudinal axis of the radius. One is tangential to the most distal point of the ulnar dome, and the other is tangential to the distal articular surface of the lunate fossa. When the ulna is shorter than the radius, the ulnar variance is negative, and when longer, it is positive.

- *Carpal height ratio:* This is another parameter in the evaluation of carpal collapse. The term *carpal height* refers to the distance between the base of the third metacarpal and the distal articular surface of the radius measured along the proximal projection of the axis of the third metacarpal. The ratio (carpal height ÷ length of third metacarpal) was found to be 0.54 ± 0.03 in normal wrists.[95] Because wrist radiographs often do not include the entire third metacarpal, some authors have proposed using the length of the capitate instead (i.e., carpal height ÷ capitate length), with a normal range of 1.57 ± 0.05[120] (Figure 13.14).
- *Ulnar translocation ratio:* In some instability conditions, there is an ulnar shift of the carpal bones. The amount of translocation can be quantified using a variety of techniques. The more commonly used one measures the perpendicular distance from the center of the head of the capitate to a line from the radial styloid, which extends distally and parallel to the longitudinal axis of the radius. The carpal translocation ratio (calculated as the ratio of this distance to the length of the third metacarpal) in normal wrists is 0.28 ± 0.03.[8] Other techniques use the axis of the ulna or the axis of the radius as a reference (Figure 13.15). However, they may not be as accurate as the ulnar translocation ratio.

Other Diagnostic Tests

Computed Tomography. Computed tomography (CT) scans are usually taken at 1- to 2-mm intervals along the axial, sagittal, and coronal planes, or any plane in which the structure of interest can be best visualized. CT scan images following the longitudinal axis of the scaphoid, at approximately 45 degrees to the long axis of the radius, are best at showing the amount of collapse in a "humpback" scaphoid deformity. CT is also useful in

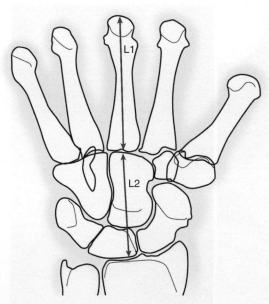

FIGURE 13.14 Carpal height ratio is calculated by dividing the carpal height (*L2*) by the length of the third metacarpal (*L1*). The normal ratio is 0.54 ± 0.03.117.

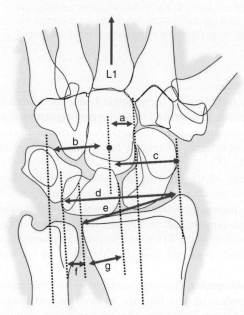

FIGURE 13.15 Ulnar translocation of the carpus can be quantified in different ways according to various authors. [8,64,78,95,120] McMurtry and colleagues[64] suggested using the axis of the ulna as a reference to determine whether there is an ulnar shift of the center of the capitate head. In normally positioned wrists, the distance *b* divided by the length of the third metacarpal (*L1*) should equal 0.3 ± 0.003. According to Chamay and coworkers, a vertical line extending distally from the radial styloid offers a more reliable reference to measure the ulnar shift of the capitate. Normal values for the distance *c* divided by L1 are 0.28 ± 0.03. A similar method was described by Di Benedetto and colleagues by using the longitudinal axis of the radius as a reference. The distance divided by L1 should be 0.015 ± 0.024. The so-called "lunate (L)-uncovering index" has been suggested by Linn and colleagues as another method to determine the relative position of the lunate with respect to the radius. According to Schuind and associates,[95] the ratio between the length of uncovered lunate (*f*) and the maximal transverse width of this bone (*f/g*) should equal 32.6 ± 11. To measure lunate translocation, Bouman and associates found it more reproducible to use the ratio *e/d*, which in normal wrists equals 0.87 ± 0.04. The last two methods are more likely to detect ulnar translocations of the lunate than the first three methods, at the expense of being strongly dependent on the wrist being precisely positioned in neutral. Even minor degrees of radial or ulnar inclination may significantly alter the results.

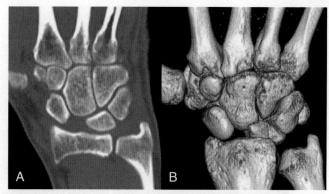

FIGURE 13.16 Computed tomography provides information about the amount and direction of carpal bone displacement **(A)**. For a better visualization of the deformity, a 3D rendering of bone surfaces is recommended **(B)**.

evaluating the union of fractures or arthrodeses, although in many instances the image can be altered by the presence of retained hardware.

CT has the added advantage of allowing computer manipulation to obtain three-dimensional (3D) images of the carpal bones, which help visualize the structure to be analyzed. When surgery is planned on a malunited scaphoid or a complex carpal dislocation, a 3D reconstruction provides excellent visual information about the amount and direction of the displacement (Figure 13.16). However, it is important to note that all the information provided by such a reconstruction is already present in the original CT image.[59,120]

The recent introduction of ultrafast CT scans has substantially reduced image-acquisition time to a fraction of a second.[30] By observing a sequence of 3D representations of the wrist, one can get the impression of seeing it in motion (see Video 13.2). This is called "dynamic 3D," also known as "four dimensions–computed tomography" (4D-CT scan). Although promising, this technology needs to be used with caution owing to the higher dose of radiation involved.[30]

Distraction Views. In patients with acute fracture–dislocations, the four routine views described earlier may be difficult to interpret because of the overlapping of displaced carpal bones. In such cases, obtaining anteroposterior and lateral radiographs with the hand suspended in finger traps is recommended. Distraction views may reveal intraarticular fracture fragments or joint dissociations in the form of a step-off that cannot be seen on routine films.

Stress Views. In some instances, obtaining radiographs while stressing the joints in various directions may help visualize the abnormality[120] (Figure 13.17). A commonly used technique consists of taking PA projections of the wrist while forcing it into maximal radial or ulnar inclination. Lateral views while applying a dorsal or palmar force to the distal carpal row ("drawer test") are also helpful to identify midcarpal instabilities.

Lateral radiographs, while extending a fully flexed wrist against resistance ("resisted extension test"), may reveal dynamic dorsal subluxation of the proximal scaphoid. In this case, if the SL ligaments are disrupted, the lunate will remain in a neutral or extended posture, substantially increasing the previously measured SL angle.

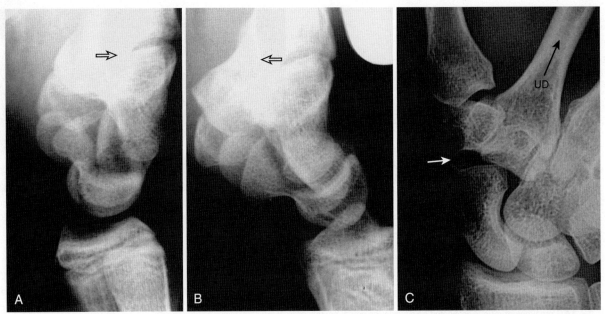

FIGURE 13.17 Stress views are particularly important to assess dynamic instabilities. **A,** In this 15-year-old girl with hyperlax wrists, dorsal stress (*white arrow*) shows the existence of a multilevel (radiocarpal and midcarpal) joint subluxation. **B,** A palmarly directed force (*white arrow*) in the same patient seems to be better tolerated, without any noticeable subluxation. **C,** In a 23-year-old patient, a combination of traction (*black arrow*) and ulnar inclination (UD) showed an increased scaphotrapezial gap (*white arrow*), which was not present on the contralateral side. Because this finding coincided with the location of major tenderness, a ligament injury was suspected and treated nonoperatively.

Cineradiography. Dynamic cineradiographic examination of the wrist provides considerable information for the evaluation of patients with altered kinematics ("clunking" wrists).[30,105] Cineradiography routinely includes observation of active motion from a radial-to-ulnar inclination in PA views; flexion and extension in lateral views, and radial and ulnar inclination in lateral views. If the patient has a painful clunk, the true nature of the subluxation can be identified by observing the moving wrist under an image intensifier. Provocative stress maneuvers may be of help to document the location of maximal dysfunction. In a recent study, cineradiography has been found to have a sensitivity of 90%, a specificity of 97%, and a diagnostic accuracy of 93% in detecting SL dissociation.[105]

Arthrography. Although long considered the gold standard in the assessment of intercarpal derangements, wrist arthrography is now rarely performed as an isolated procedure. The technique was originally introduced based on the assumption that any flow of dye from the radiocarpal to the midcarpal space or vice versa was pathologic. Since then, it has been proven that asymptomatic degenerative tears of the proximal SL or LTq membranes are not unusual, especially in older adults.

Nonetheless, arthrography still has some potential, particularly in association with high-resolution tomography (i.e., arthroscan), to assess cartilage defects and ligament injuries. When injecting the joint, it is important to watch the pattern of dye flow because this facilitates detection and estimation of the size of communicating defects.[12]

Magnetic Resonance Imaging. Compared with arthroscopy, traditional MRI without dedicated wrist coils shows reduced sensitivity and specificity (63% and 86%, respectively) in the diagnosis of SL ligament injury. When intravenous contrast medium is injected, these parameters may slightly improve,[12,88]

and this technique is increasingly being used. Technical improvements and advanced wrist imaging algorithms enable accurate measurement of the articular cartilage thickness, the length and integrity of specific ligaments, as well as injuries of the TFCC.[12,88]

Because of its superior soft tissue contrast, direct multiplanar acquisition, and lack of ionizing radiation, MRI is an effective means to evaluate the ligaments of the wrist. High-resolution noncontrast techniques have proven efficacious in the evaluation of the TFCC and intrinsic ligaments, but require a dedicated wrist coil and slice thickness of no more than 1 mm.[88]

Ultrasonography. This is gaining a well-deserved reputation in the assessment of both intrinsic and extrinsic wrist ligaments.[81] High-frequency linear transducers have been shown to have great potential. Ultrasonography is considerably less expensive than MRI, is real time (permitting dynamic evaluation of kinematic instabilities), and does not require intraarticular injection of a contrast medium or the use of ionizing radiation. No doubt, in the near future, ultrasonography will be incorporated into clinical practice as an inexpensive and safe method to get most of the information required to make accurate treatment decisions.

Arthroscopy. Wrist arthroscopy provides the technical capabilities to examine and treat intraarticular abnormalities without an arthrotomy.[17,20,31,100] As well as allowing direct visualization of the articular surfaces, synovial tissues, and intercarpal ligaments, arthroscopy has proved to be a useful adjunct in the management of various acute and chronic wrist lesions. Arthroscopy is an important wrist surgery tool; indications for its use are mentioned throughout this chapter and reviewed in detail in Chapter 17.

Carpal Instability

Definition

Injuries to the wrist that induce carpal misalignment have long been recognized in the medical literature. In 1968, Fisk was the first to use the term "carpal instability" to describe a zigzag pattern of carpal misalignment present in some fractured scaphoids.[21] In 1972, a landmark article by Linscheid and coworkers[57] helped define specific patterns of carpal malalignment secondary to carpal ligament injury. Unfortunately, an oversimplified interpretation of those publications propagated the incorrect view that all carpal misalignments are unstable. As emphasized earlier, the term *instability* cannot be used as a synonym for *misalignment*, and an alteration of carpal alignment is not always pathologically unstable.[1]

From a mechanical point of view, stability can be defined as the ability of a joint to avoid subluxations or dislocations under physiologic loads in all wrist positions.[2] Stability not only implies the capacity to transfer loads without yielding (i.e., kinetic stability) but also the ability to maintain smooth carpal rotations without sudden, unexpected changes in bone position and/or alignment (i.e., kinematic stability). However, it is important to emphasize from a mechanical point of view, that the presence of symptoms and carpal instability are not synonymous. In fact, asymptomatic instabilities are frequent and many do not require treatment.

Analysis of Carpal Instability

Carpal instability is a multifactorial phenomenon that is difficult to diagnose and treat unless there is a thorough understanding of all the factors contributing to each individual case. What follows is an analytical scheme developed by Larsen et al[50] to help the clinician in the assessment and interpretation of patients with carpal instability (Table 13.2). According to this scheme, any carpal instability can be characterized by investigating the following five features.

- *Chronicity:* Traditionally, ligament injuries have been classified depending on the time elapsed from injury to diagnosis into three categories: acute, subacute, and chronic. In acute injuries, diagnosed within a week, the ligament-healing potential is likely to be optimal. In subacute injuries, diagnosed between 1 and 6 weeks, the deformity is still easily reducible but the ligaments may have reduced healing potential because of retraction and/or necrosis. After 6 weeks, or in chronic cases, the possibility of achieving an acceptable reduction and primary ligament healing, although possible, is unlikely. The exception would be some ligament avulsions where the ligament is detached but not resorbed; it remains capable of being repaired with good healing potential beyond the time limit quoted for mid-substance ligament ruptures.

- *Severity:* Any carpal instability can be analyzed according to the severity of the resulting subluxation. If carpal misalignment appears only under high stress in specific wrist positions, the case is less severe than if it were permanently present. Based on this idea, three groups of instabilities exist: occult (partial ligament tears with no misalignment under stress), dynamic (complete ruptures exhibiting carpal misalignment only under certain loading conditions), and static (complete ruptures with permanent alteration of carpal alignment).[116]

- *Etiology:* Although most instability problems are caused by trauma, certain diseases (e.g., inflammatory arthritis) may also be responsible for a similar constellation of radiographic findings. In traumatic cases, especially if diagnosed early, effective repair of the ruptured ligaments is possible. If ligament rupture results from rheumatoid arthritis, strong remaining ligament tissue is unlikely.

- *Location:* It is important to investigate the location of the most important dysfunctions (e.g., subluxation or joint gapping), which may or may not coincide with the location of the primary lesion. This is especially important in the nondissociative instabilities in which treatment depends on which joint (i.e., radiocarpal or midcarpal) is more unstable under stress. It is also important to consider whether the pathology affects only one or several joints.

- *Direction:* When present, the direction of the carpal misalignment is an important factor to consider; several patterns have been recognized (Figure 13.18). The most common are: (1) DISI, when the lunate is regarded as an intercalated segment and appears abnormally extended relative to the radius and capitate; (2) VISI, when the lunate appears abnormally flexed; (3) ulnar translocation, when a portion of, or the entire proximal row, is (or can be) displaced ulnarly beyond normal limits; (4) radial translocation, when the proximal row can be passively displaced radially beyond normal, usually in the context of a radially malunited distal radius fracture; (5) dorsal translocation, when the carpal condyle, often as a result of a dorsally malunited fracture of the radius, is (or can be) displaced in a dorsal direction.[42]

TABLE 13.2 Analysis of Carpal Instability

Category I: Chronicity	Category II: Constancy	Category III: Etiology	Category IV: Location	Category V: Direction
Acute, >1 week (maximum primary healing potential)	Occult	Congenital	Radiocarpal	VISI rotation
	Dynamic	Traumatic	Proximal intercarpal	DISI rotation
Subacute, 1–6 weeks (some healing potential)	Static reducible	Inflammatory	Midcarpal	Ulnar translation
	Static irreducible	Neoplastic Iatrogenic	Distal intercarpal	Dorsal translation
		Miscellaneous	CMC	Other
Chronic, >6 weeks (little healing potential)			Specific bones	

CMC, Carpometacarpal; *DISI,* dorsal intercalated segmental instability; *VISI,* volar intercalated segmental instability.
Modified from Larsen et al.[50]

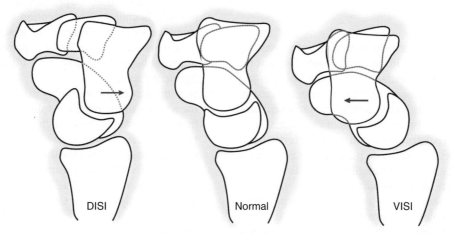

FIGURE 13.18 Views of the two major patterns of sagittal malalignment as described by Linscheid and coworkers.[57] In dorsal intercalated segment instability (DISI) and volar intercalated segment instability (VISI; also known as PISI, for palmar) the lunate (L) and triquetrum (Tq) rotate abnormally in a dorsal or volar direction, respectively (*red arrows*).

Classification of Carpal Instability

Classifying the great variety of conditions that can cause carpal instability depends in large part on the findings from the preceding analysis.[29] Many classification systems exist based on the location of the predominant disorder, the direction of the abnormal alignment, and the severity of the misalignment itself. However, none of these systems is exhaustive enough to allow categorization of all types of carpal instability or simple enough to be easily remembered and used clinically. Despite its limitations, the Mayo Clinic classification is the most commonly used by the majority of wrist specialists and therefore, it is recommended.[50]

Having clarified that neither adaptive misalignments nor all types of fracture–dislocations are necessarily unstable,[1] there are three major instability patterns of the wrist. The first group includes the so-called "dissociative carpal instabilities," also known as carpal instability dissociative (CID), in which the predominant dysfunction (i.e., ligament rupture or insufficiency) occurs between bones of the same carpal row.[29] Most CIDs occur between the scaphoid and lunate, and less often between the lunate and triquetrum.[48,87] Dissociative instabilities between the bones of the distal carpal row are rare, usually the result of a violent dorsopalmar crushing mechanism.[80]

The second group includes the nondissociative carpal instabilities, also known as carpal instability nondissociative (CIND).[28,56,118,119] This group includes radiocarpal, midcarpal, and combined radiocarpal–midcarpal instabilities. If the entire carpus is malaligned (translocated) with respect to the radius in any direction, this is radiocarpal instability.[8,78] If the proximal carpal row as a unit collapses and becomes unstable, either in flexion or extension, this is a combined radiocarpal–midcarpal instability, a condition that is also known as nondissociative instability of the proximal carpal row.[119] Less frequently, there are cases where there is only a dysfunction at the midcarpal level, the radiocarpal joint being normal. Only these cases can be called true midcarpal instabilities.[29]

The third group of instabilities is formed by the so-called "carpal instability complex" (CIC), where there are features of both CID and CIND types. Carpal dislocations, if treated inadequately, may generate complex (i.e., CIC) patterns of instability where the dysfunction affects both the radiocarpal and the proximal intercarpal joint. With time, however, the untreated or suboptimally reduced carpal derangement may evolve into a stiff misaligned joint. When this happens, the wrist may no longer be considered unstable, but stiff, and stiffness is the opposite of instability. This is why, in this edition, carpal dislocations are discussed in a section different from that of true carpal instabilities.

Dissociative Carpal Instability

In this group of instabilities, the misalignment occurs between two adjacent bones of the proximal carpal row, such as between the scaphoid and lunate or between the lunate and triquetrum.[29,48,50] Dissociative instabilities seldom occur between the bones of the distal carpal row, as there is little mobility between them.

Scapholunate Dissociation. Although this condition was recognized in the early 20th century,[21] it was not until 1972 that the clinical features of SL dissociation were described by Linscheid and associates.[57] SL dissociation is the most frequent carpal instability[48,88] and can appear either as an isolated injury or in association with other local injuries (e.g., distal radial fractures, perilunate injuries, or displaced scaphoid fractures).

Pathomechanics of SL Dissociation. A fall on the outstretched hand with the wrist in extension and ulnar inclination and associated with midcarpal supination may cause a wide spectrum of injuries, from minor SL sprains to complete perilunar dislocations. Although apparently different, these clinical conditions are stages of the same progressive perilunar destabilization process described earlier.[64]

Different authors have investigated the kinematic and kinetic consequences of having a complete SL dissociation.[30,72,99] In the cadaver, if only the palmar SL ligament and the proximal membrane are sectioned, minor kinematic alterations may appear. The SL joint, however, does not show an acutely detectable gap, not even under stress (occult instability). Scapholunate kinematics is altered, however, and heavy mechanical activity may cause symptoms. When painful, this may be due to the presence of joint synovitis and may improve with rest and anti-inflammatory agents.[88]

Complete sectioning of the SL ligaments results in substantial alterations of wrist kinematics and force transmission parameters, but acutely does not result in carpal misalignment. Immediate carpal misalignment only occurs if there is concomitant rupture of the secondary scaphoid stabilizers; that is, the palmar RSC, the palmar SC, and the anterolateral STT ligament.[99] These ligaments may gradually attenuate with time and lead to secondary malrotation and carpal collapse. In these cases, the dissociated lunate and triquetrum rotate into extension under load. The scaphoid and the lunate separate in the coronal plane and adopt opposite deformities. The scaphoid flexes around the RSC ligament, while pronating and translocating toward the radial side.[30] As a result of the scaphoid collapsing into flexion and pronation and the lunate and triquetrum into extension, the distal row is forced to rotate into pronation (Figure 13.19).

It seems evident that axial loads will increase the normal flexed stance of the scaphoid. However, there is controversy regarding the mechanisms causing the lunate to go into extension. According to Kauer,[46] the unconstrained lunate has a natural tendency toward displacing into extension owing to its configuration (with the dorsal horn being narrower than its palmar counterpart), but also to the fact that it is set onto a radial surface that is volarly inclined. Other authors believe that

the lunate, when free from the constraints of the scaphoid, tends to follow the triquetrum toward extension under the influence of the helicoid TqH joint surfaces.[21,107]

When the SL joint is completely dissociated, with the proximal pole of the scaphoid subluxed dorsoradially, the forces crossing the wrist cannot be distributed normally.[72,99] An increased compressive and shear stress appears on the dorsal and lateral aspect of the radioscaphoid fossa, a situation that Watson and associates[115,116] compared to two spoons sitting on top of each other with the handles out of alignment. Such peripheral contact may explain the frequent development of degenerative changes at the dorsolateral corner of the RS fossa. The lunate extends but remains stable with the radius because both opposing articular surfaces have the same radius of curvature. This explains why the RL joint is seldom affected by the degenerative process.

The term scaphoid–lunate advanced collapse (SLAC) has been proposed by Watson and associates[5,116] to define the progression of degenerative changes secondary to SL dissociation. Although only three stages were initially proposed, a recent investigation by Lluch[57a] identified five stages: stage I, radioscaphoid; stage II, scaphocapitate; stage III, lunocapitate; stage IV, triquetrohamate; and stage V, radiolunate.[57a] In stage I, the earliest osteoarthritic changes will differ among SLAC and scaphoid nonunion advanced collapse (SNAC) wrists. In SLAC wrists, osteoarthritis includes the proximal scaphoid and the dorsal rim of the radius. In SNAC wrists, osteoarthritis develops between the distal scaphoid and the radial styloid, while the proximal fragment of the scaphoid remains free of pathology.

Diagnosis of SL Dissociation. A history of a fall on an outstretched hand should warn the clinician about the possibility of an SL injury, sometimes masked by fractures of the scaphoid or the distal radius. SL dissociation is frequently missed at presentation, especially in isolated partial lesions, or when it is masked by other, more obvious injuries.[48] When SL dissociation is static or results from a perilunate dislocation, the diagnosis is more obvious. According to Geissler and colleagues,[31] up to 30% of distal radial fractures are associated with variable degrees of carpal ligament disruption. Aside from wrist trauma, iatrogenic SL injury can occur with excessive capsular excision when removing dorsal ganglions, or after ligament attenuation from rheumatoid, metabolic, or septic arthritis. Although SL dissociation is rare in children, diagnosis is more problematic because it is not easy to clearly identify bone axes in an immature skeleton and performing a careful clinical examination is difficult.

In both children and adults, a high index of suspicion is needed to avoid missing this injury. The symptoms of SL dissociation vary markedly depending on the magnitude of the ligament rupture, the extent of the associated injuries, and the time elapsed since the accident. Poor grip strength, limited mobility, dorsoradial swelling, and point tenderness over the dorsal aspect of the SL interval are the most common findings.[48,93] Pain is common and is usually aggravated by intense use of the hand. The patient may report a clunking sensation during wrist movement due to dislocation or reduction of a dorsally subluxed proximal scaphoid.

Physical examination. On inspection, there may be minimal or no changes in the appearance of the wrist with SL instability. Even in the acute phase, swelling may be moderate. Palpation

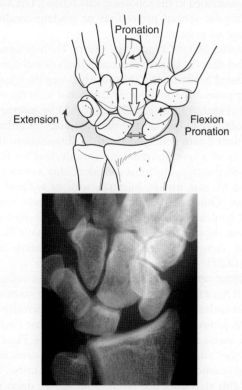

FIGURE 13.19 Schematic representation (*left*) and a case example (*right*) of the most frequent displacements (*red curved arrows*) exhibited by a static SL dissociation under axial load (*white arrow*): the scaphoid tends to rotate into flexion and slight pronation; the unconstrained triquetrum (Tq) and lunate (L) extend (dorsal intercalated segment instability [DISI] pattern of misalignment); the distal carpal row pronates and a gap appears between the scaphoid and lunate (*yellow double arrow*).

at the areas of maximal tenderness is useful in the diagnosis of wrist pathology, especially for patients with chronic SL instability. By flexing the wrist and palpating the dorsum of the capsule distal to the Lister tubercle, one can obtain important information about the SL joint. If sharp pain is elicited by pressing this area, the probability of either a recent injury or a chronic localized synovitis is high. Most of these patients also have tenderness in the anatomical snuffbox and over the palmar scaphoid tuberosity. In acute cases, range of motion is usually limited by pain, whereas it may be normal in chronic cases.

Scaphoid shift test. Passive mobilization of an unstable SL joint is valuable not only in determining the presence of abnormal scaphoid subluxation but also in reproducing the patient's pain. A positive scaphoid shift test, as described by Watson and colleagues,[115] is said to be diagnostic of SL dissociation. The examiner places four fingers behind the radius, and the thumb on the scaphoid tuberosity (distal pole). The other hand is used to move the wrist passively from ulnar-to-radial inclination. In ulnar inclination, the scaphoid is extended and assumes a position more in line with the forearm. In radial inclination, the scaphoid is flexed. Pressure on the tuberosity while the wrist is moved from ulnar-to-radial inclination prevents the scaphoid from flexing. If the SL ligaments are completely ruptured or elongated, the proximal pole subluxes dorsally out of the radius, inducing pain in the dorsoradial aspect of the wrist (Figure 13.20). When pressure is released, a typical clunking may occur, indicating self-reduction of the scaphoid over the dorsal rim of the radius.

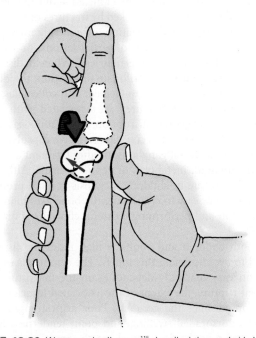

FIGURE 13.20 Watson and colleagues[115] described the scaphoid shift test. Firm pressure is applied to the palmar tuberosity of the scaphoid while the wrist is moved from ulnar-to-radial inclination (*curved arrow*). In normal wrists, the scaphoid cannot flex because of the external pressure by the examiner's thumb. This may produce pain on the dorsal aspect of the scapholunate (SL) interval owing to synovial irritation. A "positive" test is seen in a patient with an SL tear or in a patient with a lax wrist; the scaphoid is no longer constrained proximally and subluxes out of the scaphoid fossa (*straight arrow*). When pressure on the scaphoid is removed, it goes back into position and typically a clunk occurs.

When performing the scaphoid shift test, one should be aware of its low specificity. If the SL ligaments are intact, but there are other local problems inducing local synovitis (e.g., occult ganglion or dorsal RS impingement), this test may also provoke sharp pain, making it difficult to discern whether there is an abnormally subluxable proximal scaphoid. Alternatively, patients with generalized laxity may exhibit painless clunks during this maneuver, which most likely emanate from the midcarpal joint. Comparison of the two sides is important, although sometimes the opposite "asymptomatic" wrist has a painful scaphoid shift test as well.[74,115] Experience with this test is necessary before it can be interpreted with confidence.

Resisted finger extension test. The ability of the proximal pole of the scaphoid to carry a load without producing pain can be explored by asking the patient to extend the index and middle fingers fully against resistance with the wrist partially flexed.[115] In the presence of an injury or insufficiency of the dorsal SL ligament, a sharp pain is elicited in the SL area, probably due to the presence of synovitis at the RS joint. This maneuver is very sensitive but not specific for this pathology.

SL Ballottement Test. The lunate is firmly stabilized with the thumb and index finger of one hand, while the scaphoid, held with the other hand (i.e., thumb on the palmar tuberosity and index on the dorsal proximal pole) is displaced dorsally and palmarly. The test is positive when there is pain, crepitus, and excessive mobility of the scaphoid.

Radiological examination. On standard radiographs, SL dissociation is suspected in the presence of one or more of the features described in the following subsections. Dynamic instabilities require special projections or loading conditions for these features to be observed.

Increased SL joint space. The "Terry Thomas sign," named by Frankel after the English film comedian's dental diastema,[21,48] is considered positive when the space between the scaphoid and lunate appears abnormally wide compared with the contralateral side (Figure 13.21). The SL gap should be measured in the middle of the flat ulnar facet of the scaphoid.[120] A unilateral gap greater than 5 mm is diagnostic of SL dissociation. If there is no history of a specific traumatic episode, and yet there is an obvious SL diastasis, one must consider either a constitutionally increased SL gap, usually bilateral, with or without hyperlax ligaments. Other less common causes include rheumatoid arthritis, gout, and calcium pyrophosphate deposition disease.[48] To rule out the presence of an occult asymptomatic SL ligament injury, a comparative radiographic examination is critical (Figure 13.22).

Scaphoid ring sign. When the scaphoid has collapsed into flexion, it has a foreshortened appearance in the anteroposterior view.[93] In such circumstances, the scaphoid tuberosity is shown in the PA projection in the form of a radiodense circle or ring over the distal two-thirds of the scaphoid (see Figure 13.21). This is the "ring sign" and is present in all cases where the scaphoid is abnormally flexed, regardless of the cause. The presence of this sign does not always indicate SL dissociation, as both the scaphoid and lunate can be flexed with the SL ligaments remaining intact.

Increased SL angle. In the lateral view, if the scaphoid lies more perpendicular to the long axis of the radius and the lunate appears normally aligned or abnormally extended, SL dissociation should be suspected. In such circumstances, the

SL angle is greater than the usual 45 to 60 degrees (Figure 13.23). This angle will progressively increase as the lunate extends to accommodate the loss of height of the radial column, causing a dorsal subluxation of the capitate.

Palmar V sign. In the lateral view of a normal wrist, a wide "C"-shaped line can be drawn by joining the palmar margins of the scaphoid and radius. When the scaphoid is abnormally flexed, the palmar outline of it intersects the palmar margin of the radial styloid at an acute angle, forming a sharper, "V"-shaped pattern.[107]

Advanced imaging. When the patient's history, clinical examination, and radiographs are inconclusive, magnetic resonance imaging, computed arthrotomography,[12] or diagnostic arthroscopy[20,31,100,113] may be helpful to assess the degree of injury to the intercarpal ligaments, the secondary supporting ligaments, and the articular cartilage.

Treatment of SL Dissociation. Numerous factors may explain why the treatment of SL dissociation is difficult and not always predictable.[19,48,68,88,101,107] When the initial injury is a partial SL ligament derangement, radiographs are usually normal, and the injury is frequently missed at presentation. Even if diagnosed early, the ligament remnants are short and difficult to repair. Because the SL ligament is exposed to

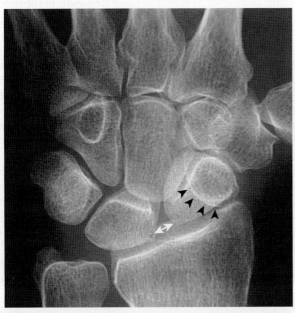

FIGURE 13.21 Posteroanterior view of the wrist of a 35-year-old man who sustained a hyperextension injury 4 months before seeking medical attention. Note the foreshortened scaphoid (S) with the ring sign (*arrowheads*), representing the frontal projection of the palmar tuberosity, and the increased scapholunate (SL) joint space (*white double arrow*), indicating the presence of SL dissociation with carpal malalignment.

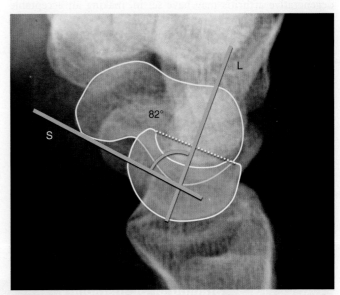

FIGURE 13.23 Lateral view of the same patient shown in Figure 13.22. The scapholunate (SL) angle is abnormally wide (82 degrees) as a result of an abnormally flexed scaphoid and a slightly extended lunate. *L*, Lunate axis; *S*, scaphoid axis.

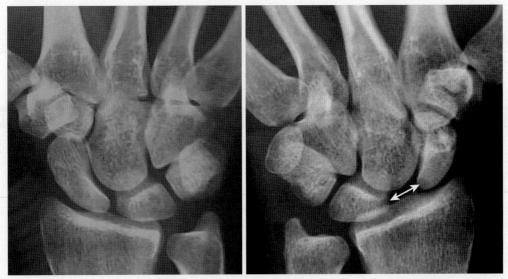

FIGURE 13.22 Bilateral radiographic scapholunate (SL) widening is not uncommon. True traumatic SL disruption is less common. To rule out this possibility, it is imperative to obtain comparative radiographs of both sides. In this case, a closed fist radiograph was obtained from both sides but only one had substantial widening of the SL joint (*white double arrow*), a finding known as the Terry Thomas sign.[21]

considerable tension and torsion, it is not unusual for successful repairs to deteriorate with time. There is no guarantee that a repaired SL ligament will retain good functional strength and adequate stabilizing capability, even with early diagnosis and proper treatment.

More commonly, SL dissociation is discovered in the subacute or chronic phase, when carpal malalignment is evident on plain radiographs. This occurs because abnormal SL kinematics gradually attenuate the secondary ligamentous stabilizers under load. At this stage, the underlying pathology no longer involves a single structure but consists of a complex multilevel ligament injury. Some ligament remnants are retracted, whereas others are attenuated and/or insufficient to stabilize the joint.[3] Furthermore, if substantial time has elapsed since the initial injury, degenerative arthritis may have set in, making an acceptable outcome from ligament repair less likely.[19,48,88]

For these reasons, treating the injury in the acute phase, when the healing potential is greatest, is generally more rewarding than trying to treat chronic or degenerative injuries. It is important to carefully consider the patient's age, occupation, recreational demands, and level of symptoms prior to embarking on a treatment plan.[88] To facilitate patient selection and appropriate treatment, Garcia-Elias[27,29] has recently modified a previously published algorithm for the treatment of SL dissociation, based on the six questions listed in the following Critical Points box.

The answers to these questions enable categorization of the SL dissociation into seven stages (Table 13.3). An increased number of negative answers indicates progression from a minor problem (Stage I) to a global dysfunction (Stage VII). In theory, all SL dissociations sharing similar features could be treated similarly. In practice, it is wise to tailor treatment to the specific peculiarities of each individual case. The following subsections describe all the stages in turn, including the most commonly used treatment for each.

Stage I: partial SL ligament injury. In stage I, the SL ligament is only stretched or partially disrupted. These patients still have an uninjured dorsal and/or volar SL ligament. Arthrography may suggest this diagnosis, but most commonly this is made arthroscopically or with high-resolution MRI. The degree of SL ligament incompetence varies from minimal distention (Geissler grade I; see Table 17.1) to a partial rupture of the proximal membrane without gross instability (Geissler grade II or III; see Table 17.1).[31] The European Wrist Arthroscopy Society (EWAS) suggested modifying Geissler's classification to include subtypes of SL ligament disruption, and the authors recommend this[66] (Table 13.4). At this stage, wrists do not exhibit misalignment or widening of the SL joint space on standard or stress radiographs. Based on this finding, some authors have suggested using the term predynamic or occult

---

CRITICAL POINTS *Six Questions to Consider When Evaluating an SL Injury*

- Is the dorsal SL ligament intact and functional?
- If the ligament has ruptured, does it have good integrity for repair?
- Is the scaphoid alignment normal?
- Is radiolunate alignment still retained?
- Are abnormal carpal alignments easily reducible?
- Is the articular cartilage normal?

TABLE 13.3   Staging of SL Instability

	Stage I	Stage II	Stage III	Stage IV	Stage V	Stage VI	Stage VII
Partial injury	Yes	No	No	No	No	No	No
Repairable	Yes	Yes	No	No	No	No	No
Normal RS angle	Yes	Yes	Yes	No	No	No	No
Lunate aligned	Yes	Yes	Yes	Yes	No	No	No
Reducible	Yes	Yes	Yes	Yes	Yes	No	No
Normal cartilage	Yes	Yes	Yes	Yes	Yes	Yes	No

Modified from Garcia-Elias.[29]

TABLE 13.4   Arthroscopic EWAS Staging of Scapholunate Interosseous Ligament Ruptures

Stage	Description	Arthroscopic Testing of Scapholunate Joint From the Radial Midcarpal Portal
I	Elongation	No passage of the probe
II	Rupture of the proximal SL membrane	Passage of the tip of the probe in the SL space without widening
IIIA	II + disruption of the volar SL ligament	Volar SL joint widening when tested with the probe (anterior laxity)
IIIB	II + disruption of the dorsal SL ligament	Dorsal SL joint widening when tested with the probe (posterior laxity)
IIIC	II + rupture of the volar and dorsal SL ligaments	Global widening of SL space, reducible with removal of probe
IV	IIIC + SL gap (no misalignment)	SL diastasis without radiographic abnormalities; arthroscope may enter the radiocarpal space
V	IV + carpal misalignment	Wide SL gap with radiographic anomalies

SL, Scapholunate.
Modified from Messina et al.[66]

instability to refer to such cases.[116] Dysfunction derives from increased motion between the two bones, generating abnormal cartilage loading and painful local synovitis.

If a subtotal ligament rupture (Geissler II or III; EWAS II or IIIA) is diagnosed in the acute phase, when the healing potential of the disrupted ligaments is greatest, a percutaneous or arthroscopically guided K-wire fixation is recommended.[31] For acute complete scapholunate interosseus ligament (SLIL) tears without carpal malalignment (Geissler grade III; EWAS Grades IIIB and IIIC), open repair should be considered in young patients. In chronic incomplete SLIL tears, three different approaches have been proposed: proprioception reeducation and strengthening of the intracarpal supination muscles, arthroscopic debridement of the torn ligament edges, and electrothermal ligament shrinkage. There are few data on the long-term clinical or radiographic outcomes of these techniques. Arthroscopic techniques for acute and chronic stage I instability are discussed in Chapter 17.

Percutaneous Kirschner wire fixation of the SL joint. Acute partial ruptures of the SL ligaments without carpal misalignment may benefit from pinning the joint with Kirschner (K) wires and a period of rigid joint immobilization to enable ligament healing. Obviously, the ligament remnants will only heal if there is no carpal malalignment (i.e., secondary stabilizers are intact), and there is close contact between the two edges of the injured ligament. To ensure this, K-wire insertion should be done under arthroscopy or fluoroscopy control.[31,100] However, open repair can also be done in these cases because it will provide more precise information on the degree and extent of the lesion.

Sometimes, a slight rotational displacement may keep the two ends of a disrupted ligament apart. To solve this, it is helpful to introduce two percutaneous K-wires into the dorsal aspects of the scaphoid and lunate to be used as "joysticks." If there is no soft tissue interposition, minimal displacement may be reduced by pulling the scaphoid wire proximally and ulnarly while the lunate wire is directed distally and radially.

To avoid injuring the dorsal sensory branches of the radial nerve, a small incision is made distal to the radial styloid. Blunt dissection of the subcutaneous tissue with a hemostat allows safe introduction of a soft tissue protector directly onto the scaphoid. Two or more 1.2-mm K-wires are inserted across the SL joint to keep the two bones together during the ligament-healing process. To ensure maximal stability, a third wire transfixing the SC joint can be used.

The wrist is immobilized in a below-elbow cast for 8 to 10 weeks, at which time the K-wires are removed. Physical therapy with range-of-motion exercises of the fingers is initiated immediately. The wrist is protected with a removable splint for an additional 4 weeks. Range-of-motion and grip-strength exercises of the wrist are begun at 3 months. Strenuous activities are discouraged for the first 6 months.

Reeducation of wrist proprioception. As stated previously, the muscles are the ultimate carpal stabilizers.[35,91] Without their protection, most wrist-stabilizing ligaments would not resist the amount of tension and torque generated in most accidents, and ligament ruptures would be even more common. To remain stable, the wrist does not need powerful muscles, but ones that are able to react quickly to protect the underlying ligaments. Even if some ligaments have failed, however, promptly reacting muscles may succeed in maintaining relatively normal kinematics of mildly unstable joints, avoiding the development of cartilage wear and reactive synovitis. Thus, the immediate goal of proprioception reeducation is not to increase grip strength but to optimize the "latency time" (i.e., the time taken by the stabilizing muscles to react to any potentially damaging force).[84]

Under axial load, the scaphoid tends to flex and pronate. That tendency can be counteracted by supinating the distal row. Indeed, if the STT capsule and ligaments are intact, a distal row supination will draw the trapezium dorsally, thus preventing the scaphoid from collapsing into flexion and pronation. Laboratory studies have shown ECRL and APL to be distal row supination muscles, while ECU is a pronation muscle.[54,92] If properly trained, the former may become effective dynamic scaphoid stabilizers. Isometric contraction of ECU, by contrast, increases scaphoid misalignment and widens the SL gap (see Video 13.1). A quick response of the intracarpal supinators (i.e., ECRL and APL), on one side, and avoidance of the ECU, on the other, may explain why many dynamic SL dissociations remain asymptomatic for a long time.

The FCR has also been said to have a positive effect on SL stability owing to its ability to close the SL gap by supinating the scaphoid. Indeed, if the dorsal SL ligament is not completely torn, the FCR also may be counted as a dynamic scaphoid stabilizer.[91,92]

As more research is being published, it appears that avoidance of the ECU's deleterious effects on SL stability, combined with adequate proprioception reeducation of FCR, APL, and ECRL will play an important role in the control of dynamic SL instabilities. What is not known is which of the many protocols being currently tested will prove to be the most useful, and in what circumstances.[35] In all cases, adequate evaluation of the extent of ligament damage is a prerequisite for this type of approach.

In recent years, special attention has been drawn to the fact that, during DT motion, the majority of carpal motion occurs at the midcarpal joint, the proximal row remaining relatively stationary. Based on these findings, it has been suggested that, after a SL ligament repair, early dart-throwing mobilization of the midcarpal joint could have a beneficial effect on stiffness, while avoiding tension on the repair. This is not entirely correct, and caution is warranted. Recent studies using dynamic 3D CT of patients with SL dissociations have shown that, once disconnected from the lunate, the scaphoid no longer behaves as a proximal row bone but follows the capitate as if it was a distal row element.[30] Certainly, unless the dorsal SL ligament is fully competent, or the repair is protected with additional fixation, DT exercises are not recommended, at least not in the early stages of healing.

Arthroscopic debridement of torn ligament edges and electrothermal ligament shrinkage. Debridement of the irregular edges of a torn SL proximal membrane has proved to be beneficial in the treatment of dynamic SL dissociation. Eliminating unstable flaps may help prevent joint synovitis and pain.[31,52,100] Another alternative is to shrink them with radiofrequency under arthroscopic control (see Chapter 17). Although one should not expect long-lasting results from the latter technique, acceptable results at an average follow-up of 53 months have been published by Lee et al.[52]

Stage II: complete SL ligament injury, repairable. This stage is characterized by complete disruption of the SL ligamentous complex, with good healing potential because of a repairable dorsal component.[28] The carpal bones are minimally displaced without cartilage degeneration. The distal–palmar connections of the scaphoid to the distal row (i.e., STT and SC ligaments) are still intact. The scaphoid is not abnormally flexed, the RS angle is normal, and there is little or no SL gap.

According to Andersson et al,[3] there are four major types of dorsal SL ligament ruptures: avulsion from the scaphoid (42% of all dorsal SL ligaments), avulsion from the lunate (18%), midsubstance rupture (20%), and partial rupture plus elongation (22%).[10] If the remnants and vascular supply of the disrupted SL ligament are preserved, one option is an arthroscopy-guided closed reduction and percutaneous fixation (Figure 13.24); another is a direct repair of the disrupted ligaments. In general, the second is recommended. If the ligament is avulsed, with or without a small piece of bone, successful reattachment of it can be expected beyond the time limits of what could be expected from a ligament rupture.

Proprioceptive reeducation of the intracarpal supinator muscles is no longer adequate in stage II as an isolated treatment. Indeed, if the dorsal SL ligament is disrupted, supination of the distal carpal row does not reduce the SL joint; however, it creates an unconstrained dorsally directed vector that promotes scaphoid dorsal subluxation of its proximal pole. Certainly, proprioceptive exercises of the intracarpal supinator muscles are only recommended in EWAS II and IIIA partial injuries, where the dorsal SL ligament is intact.

Open reduction, internal fixation, and dorsal SL ligament repair. This approach offers the same advantages as when treating acute ligament injuries in other joints, provided the subluxation is reduced. A direct, solid repair of torn ligaments should be carefully performed and all associated osteochondral injuries explored and repaired. Most failures may be explained by the excessive forces produced by the capitate trying to separate the SL joint, the poor healing potential of chronic or devascularized

ends of the disrupted ligaments, and the prolonged immobilization required after surgery. Despite these factors, we agree with authors who believe there is a place for acute primary repair in properly selected patients.[16,75]

Several biomechanical studies in cadaveric specimens concluded that only the dorsal SL ligament needs to be repaired to achieve relatively normal carpal kinematics.[99] Other authors claim better results by repairing both the palmar and dorsal SL ligaments, through a double palmar and dorsal approach, despite the obvious difficulty of getting access to the palmar component without damaging the palmar extrinsic ligaments. In this regard, the short-term results obtained after arthroscopic dorsal SL ligament repair and capsuloplasty by Wahegaonkar and Mathoulin[113] and the arthroscopic repair of the palmar SL ligament by Piñal[20] are truly encouraging. See arthroscopic techniques in Chapter 17.

Open dorsal ligament repair is performed as follows. The skin incision may be longitudinal, "Z"-shaped, or transverse, with the last two incisions resulting in a more aesthetic scar (Figure 13.25). The extensor retinaculum is divided longitudinally at the level of the Lister tubercle, being careful not to injure the extensor pollicis longus (EPL) tendon, running on its ulnar side. The author recommends visualizing the dorsal capsule by creating two retinacular flaps: one radial-based, uncovering the second extensor compartment; and the other ulnar-based, exposing the third, fourth, and fifth extensor compartments.

Next, the floor of the fourth compartment is explored, and if the posterior interosseous nerve is found to be normal, a proximally based capsular flap sparing the nerve is recommended. The incision starts at the dorsal rim of the lunate fossa. It takes a distal-oblique course following the fibers of the dorsal radiotriquetral ligament until its distal insertion on the dorsal ridge of the triquetrum. Another vertical incision is made from the tip of the radial styloid to the lateral corner of the STT joint. The distal ends of the two incisions are then connected by a third transverse incision that splits the fibers of the dorsal intercarpal ligament. This flap is carefully elevated by sectioning its

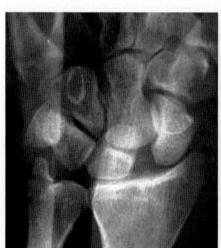
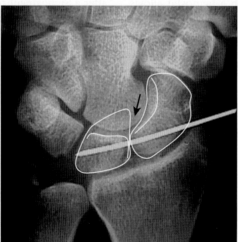
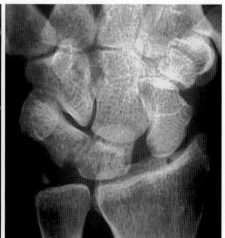

Closed reduction | 6 days post-fixation | 4 months follow up

FIGURE 13.24 Unless controlled arthroscopically, closed reduction and percutaneous Kirschner (K)-wire fixation cannot ensure that the two ends of the disrupted ligaments are in contact so that they can heal (*black arrow*). If there is no ligament healing, the intraarticular fibrosis that forms between the two bones is seldom enough to maintain stability. The case shown would not be an ideal indication for closed reduction and percutaneous K-wire fixation.

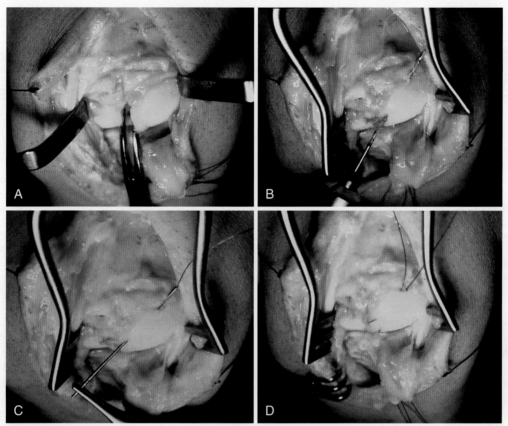

FIGURE 13.25 Open reduction and scapholunate (SL) ligament repair in a 27-year-old man who sustained SL dissociation 6 weeks before surgery. **A,** Through a dorsal approach and the wrist in flexion, the SL interval may be opened, allowing inspection of the anterior aspect of the joint. **B,** Fine drills are used to create tunnels connecting the dorsal edge of the scaphoid to the origin of the disrupted ligament. **C,** Transosseous sutures are passed through the perforations. **D,** Sutures are finally tied to bring the two ends of the ruptured ligament into contact. Previously, two Kirschner wires have been inserted to secure adequate immobilization of the reduced carpal bones.

connections to the dorsal edge of the three bones of the proximal row. Care is taken to leave enough dorsal radial triquetrum ligament attached to the triquetrum to facilitate capsular repair later.

If the posterior interosseous nerve is felt to be nonfunctional, damaged, or irregularly thick, a laterally based capsulotomy, following the "fiber-splitting" concept described by Berger[7] is recommended. This starts at the tip of the radial styloid and proceeds medially along the dorsal edge of the radius until it meets the center of the origin of the radiotriquetral ligament. From there it follows an oblique course toward the dorsal rim of the triquetrum and returns back to the lateral edge of the wrist, splitting the fibers of the dorsal intercarpal ligament. In these cases, the posterior interosseous nerve should be excised proximal to the joint; otherwise, a neuroma may develop leading to painful wrist flexion from traction on the nerve.

Frequently, when operating early on a torn dorsal SL ligament, there is sufficient ligamentous tissue to permit a reasonable repair. If the ligament is not ruptured but avulsed, the repair is more effective and consists of reattaching the avulsed ligament, with or without a bone fragment, to the freshened dorsal edge of the scaphoid or lunate. Transosseous sutures[16] or suture anchors[89] are used. The repair is protected by transfixing the SL and SC joints with K-wires. Several authors recommend reinforcing the repair with a dorsal capsulodesis, as will be described in the following.[48] The wires are maintained for 8 to

10 weeks with protection in a removable splint for an additional 4 weeks.

Several series of patients with SL dissociation treated by means of direct repair have been published.[16,25,75,88] By combining the data from 100 reported cases, with an average follow-up of 37 months, pain was absent or significantly reduced in 70% of patients, with more than 80% grip strength and 75% wrist motion compared with the normal contralateral side. Radiographs showed degenerative changes in one-third, but the condition had not progressed to an advanced collapse pattern except for those who had placed high demands on the wrist on a daily basis.[48,116]

Stage III: complete SL ligament injury, nonrepairable, normally aligned scaphoid and lunate. Stage III is characterized by complete rupture of the SL ligament, with poor healing capacity at its dorsal component.[28] When the dorsal SL ligament is disrupted through its mid-substance, the two ends tend to degenerate quite rapidly, thus diminishing the chance of a successful repair.[3] Carpal misalignment is not yet present because the scaphoid is constrained by the anterolateral STT ligament, volar capsule, and dorsal intercarpal ligaments.[11] No permanent misalignment exists at this stage, and an increased SL gap may appear only under specific loading conditions. However, the wrist may yield or give way when attempting tasks in certain wrist positions. From a radiologic point of view, stages II and III are "dynamic" instabilities.[116]

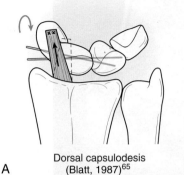
A Dorsal capsulodesis
(Blatt, 1987)[65]

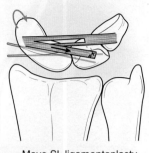
B Mayo SL ligamentoplasty
(Linscheid & Dobyns, 1992)[68]

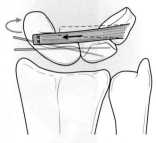
C DIL capsulodesis
(Szabo et al., 2002)[25]

FIGURE 13.26 Schematic representation of three capsulodeses described to stabilize the wrist with complete, but reducible, scapholunate (SL) dissociation: **(A)** proximally based dorsal capsulodesis described by Blatt[65] to prevent scaphoid flexion, **(B)** laterally based dorsal intercarpal ligamentoplasty (DIL) described by Linscheid and Dobyns,[68] and **(C)** medially based DIL described by Szabo et al.[106] Although similar in final results, they all aim to correct different aspects of carpal misalignment (*green curved arrows*): Blatt's procedure[65] aims at preventing scaphoid flexion; Szabo's technique prevents scaphoid pronation, whereas the Linscheid and Dobyns method attempts to correct both flexion and pronation using the lunate as a reference.

If the dorsal ligament cannot be repaired, one alternative is to reconstruct it, either by using local tissues from adjacent ligaments[11,68] or by using a bone–ligament–bone autograft.[37,101] Another commonly used method is to perform a capsulodesis.[25,106] Closed reduction and cast immobilization is not an acceptable treatment for complete SL disruption in active patients.

Dorsal capsulodesis. When detached from the lunate, the scaphoid has a natural tendency to collapse into flexion and pronation. To prevent this, several forms of dorsal capsulodesis have been recommended.[68,106] The most commonly used technique was popularized by Blatt[65,71a] and consists of tightening the RS capsule to prevent excessive palmar rotation of the scaphoid (Figure 13.26, *A*). A 1-cm-wide capsular flap is created, leaving its proximal edge attached to the dorsal rim of the radius. After the scaphoid is reduced by manipulation and stabilized with one or two K-wires passed obliquely from the distal pole of the scaphoid into the capitate, the flap is tightly inserted into a notch created on the dorsum of the neck of it, just distal to its axis of rotation. Sutures within the capsular flap are passed through the scaphoid using Keith needles and tied on a button over the thenar skin. Bone-anchored sutures are favored by some surgeons. A thumb spica cast should be worn for 2 months, followed by protected active range-of-motion exercises. The K-wires may be left in place for an additional month.

Various modifications of Blatt's technique have been published. The so-called "Mayo Clinic SL ligamentoplasty" was first suggested by Linscheid and Dobyns.[58] It uses one-half of the dorsal intercarpal ligament, released from the triquetrum and freed from the dorsal rim of the lunate (see Figure 13.26, *B*). This ligament flap is redirected and pulled on to the dorsum of the lunate, where it is securely anchored. Another option is "dorsal intercarpal ligamentoplasty," first described by Szabo and colleagues[25,106] (see Figure 13.26, *C*). It consists of advancing the scaphoid insertion of the dorsal intercarpal ligament from its dorsal ridge to a more radial position at the scaphoid neck to control the pronation component of SL instability.

According to the study of Megerle et al,[65] at an average of 8 years' follow-up, most of the 59 patients who underwent Blatt's dorsal capsulodesis for this condition had acceptable wrist function. The mean range of flexion–extension was 88 degrees, and the mean disabilities of the arm, shoulder, and hand (DASH) and Mayo wrist scores were 28 and 61, respectively. This technique could not prevent progressive carpal collapse. After significant postoperative improvement in the carpal alignment, the mean SL angle returned to the preoperative value of 70 degrees at final follow-up, with more than two-thirds of patients having radiological evidence of degenerative arthritis. Radiology aside, the overall results are satisfactory when used in dynamic instabilities.[25,65] Similar findings have been published for the other two capsulodesis options, none being superior to the other.[25,68,106] These methods can be done successfully in the skeletally immature carpus without adverse effects on growth.

Soft tissue reconstruction of the dorsal SL ligament. More recent publications have reported acceptable results in the treatment of dynamic SL instabilities by replacing the nonrepairable dorsal SL ligament with a strip of either the dorsal intercarpal ligament or the dorsal radiocarpal ligament.[25,61,68,106] Both methods involve using a portion of dense connective tissue, preserving its triquetral attachment. The free end of the ligament flap is tightly reinserted onto the dorsal and ulnar corner of the proximal scaphoid. Bone-anchored sutures should be used to facilitate incorporation of the ligament into the previously denuded dorsal and distal cortices of the scaphoid and lunate. Both techniques are very appealing in their simplicity and low local morbidity. Early results are said to be satisfactory, but they should be used with caution until further long-term results are available.[25,106]

Bone–ligament–bone grafts. Based on the proven success of replacing knee ligaments with bone–ligament–bone grafts, several investigators addressed the in vitro feasibility of using allografts to replace a dorsal SL ligament. Weiss[101] reported transferring a bone-retinaculum–bone autograft harvested from the region of the Lister tubercle. Harvey and associates[37] advocated the use of the third metacarpal–capitate dorsal ligament. The surgical approach is the same as used for a direct repair. After the scaphoid and lunate are reduced and transfixed by wires, a deep trough is carved on either side of the SL joint, and a bone–ligament–bone graft is impacted and fixed with miniature screws, small wires, or interference screws.

Theoretically, by providing tissue with similar elasticity and strength as the original ruptured ligament, there is a better chance of achieving an adequate SL linkage. However, the following three problems may arise. First, the proximal scaphoid is poorly vascularized and so healing of the bone graft may be delayed. Second, after a long period of postoperative immobilization, the mechanical properties of the ligament in the graft may deteriorate and fail from heavy use of the hand. Finally, reconstructing the dorsal SL ligament alone does not solve the palmar–distal ligament insufficiency present in complete SL ruptures. The early clinical results are encouraging in dynamic instabilities, when the secondary stabilizers are still preserved.[37,101] The reported failures of this technique, when used in static instabilities, makes this technique less desirable.

Dynadesis. First suggested by Seradge et al,[96] the so-called "dynadesis" (i.e., *dynamic ECRL tendon transfer to the distal scaphoid plus volar FCR tenodesis*) procedure consists of passing two-thirds of the ECRL tendon through a 3.5-mm tunnel drilled across the distal pole of the reduced scaphoid and anchoring the end to the FCR tendon (Figure 13.27). The portion of FCR distal to the scaphoid becomes a check-rein that tightens with contraction of the ECRL. In the 2014 meeting of the American Society for Surgery of the Hand (ASSH), Seradge et al[96] reported their experience with this procedure: out of 18 patients followed for an average of 20 years, complete relief of pain was obtained in 14 and 11 had excellent functional results according to Mayo wrist score. Whether such outstanding results can be replicated by other authors is not known.

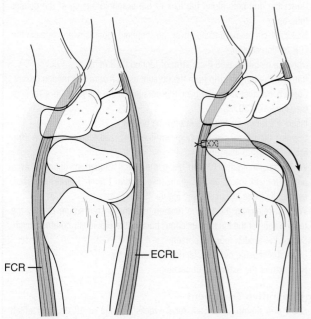

FIGURE 13.27 Schematic representation of the so-called "dynadesis" procedure described by Seradge et al.[96] A large anteroposterior tunnel across the distal scaphoid (S) is used to suture a strip of extensor carpi radialis longus (ECRL) to the flexor carpi radialis (FCR) tendon. In theory, the ECRL becomes a dynamic extensor of the scaphoid, whereas the FCR is converted into a static tether that inhibits scaphoid flexion. An average 20-year follow-up study presented recently by the authors demonstrates this method to be very efficient in dynamic scapholunate dissociations.

FCR —   — ECRL

Stage IV: complete SL ligament injury, nonrepairable, reducible flexion deformity of the scaphoid. Stage IV is characterized by complete loss of the proximal and distal scaphoid stabilizers. The scaphoid subluxates dorsally over the dorsolateral rim of the radius and increases its flexed position, showing an RS angle greater than 45 degrees. The lunate extends only slightly but does not translocate toward the ulnar side. For this to occur, there must be normal functioning of the long- and short-palmar RL ligaments.[29] The scaphoid misalignment is easily reduced, and there is no cartilage deterioration as yet. Because the misalignment is at rest, stage IV is categorized as a static instability. Clunking secondary to self-reduction of the subluxation is a common finding.

Two different treatments have been proposed for this stage: reconstruction of the disrupted ligaments with tendon grafts and reduction-association of the SL joint (i.e., RASL procedure).

SL ligamentoplasty using a tendon graft. The use of tendon grafts to reconstruct disrupted ligaments in the wrist has evolved considerably since their first description in 1972.[21,57,107] The initial technique was simple: anteroposterior bone tunnels were drilled across the lunate and proximal pole of the scaphoid along the margins of the joint, and a strip of tendon, usually the ECRL, was threaded through these tunnels to form a loop that closed the SL gap. These techniques involved large drill holes across poorly vascularized areas, so bone fractures and joint degeneration were not unusual. As such, the technique was abandoned in the early 1980s in favor of partial fusions.

In the 1990s, there was renewed interest in tendon reconstruction resulting in the publication of more complex and theoretically safer alternatives.[21] The technique described by Brunelli and Brunelli received great attention.[10] The goal was to provide sagittal stability to the scaphoid by reconstructing both the palmar–distal connections to the distal row and the dorsal–proximal connections to the radius. To achieve that, a strip of FCR tendon was obtained from the ipsilateral wrist, leaving its distal end attached to the second metacarpal. Through a separate dorsal incision, all fibrous tissue filling the STT joint was removed and the scaphoid reduced and neutralized with Kirschner wires (Figure 13.28). A 3.2-mm tunnel, perpendicular to the main axis of the scaphoid, was drilled from the center of the scaphoid tuberosity to the neck and the strip of FCR passed through it. Once at the dorsum, the split tendon was pulled taut proximally and anchored to the dorsal rim of the distal radius at the level of the origin of the dorsal radiocarpal ligament. This technique offered excellent stabilization of the scaphoid. Unfortunately, it resulted in a marked reduction in wrist flexion, and with time, an increased rate of RS osteoarthritis.

In 2005, Van den Abbeele and associates[110] proposed modifying the Brunelli technique in two ways to avoid this complication. First, the transscaphoid drill hole was placed slightly oblique rather than perpendicular to the axis of the scaphoid with its end coinciding with the insertion of the dorsal SL ligament; and second, the tendon did not cross the radiocarpal joint, but used the dorsal radiocarpal ligament as an anchor point for the tendon to be tensioned before being sutured onto itself. With further refinements, this technique was published with a new name: *three-ligament tenodesis*[27] (Figure 13.29).

According to its proponents, this procedure is indicated when the SL joint is easily reducible, the cartilage is undamaged,

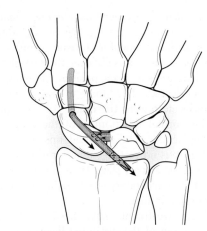

Scaphotrapezoid tenodesis
(Brunelli & Brunelli, 1995)[10]

FIGURE 13.28 Despite the initial discouraging results obtained after the first attempts to reconstruct the scapholunate (SL) linkage using tendons (*black arrows*),[21] the technique described by Brunelli and Brunelli[10] was the first to be successful in reducible SL dissociations for ligaments that cannot be optimally repaired (stage IV, SL dissociation). Unlike previous tendon reconstructions of the SL linkage, this technique was successful because it was based on the stabilization of both the proximal and the distal ends of the subluxating scaphoid, without creating bone holes in the vicinity of the vascularly compromised SL joint.

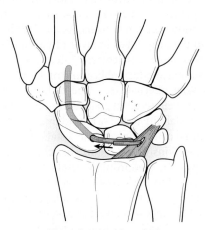

Three-ligament tenodesis
(Garcia-Elias et al., 2006)[27]

FIGURE 13.29 Schematic representation of "three-ligament tenodesis." This technique was designed to stabilize nonrepairable, easily reducible scapholunate (SL) dissociations.[27,110] A strip of flexor carpi radialis (FCR) tendon is passed obliquely from the palmar scaphoid (S) tuberosity to the dorsal ridge of the scaphoid where the dorsal SL ligament inserts. The tendon is buried in a trough created on the dorsum of the lunate by means of an anchor suture. To adjust the tension of the graft, a slit in the distal portion of the dorsal radial triquetrum ligament is made through which the tendon is looped around and sutured onto itself (*black arrow*).

and the lunate is stable relative to the radius (see the following Critical Points box). The series published by Garcia-Elias et al,[27] with an average follow-up of 46 months, indicated that 28 out of 38 patients had complete pain relief. Compared to the contralateral side, the operated wrist had a 24% reduction in global motion and a 35% reduction in grip strength. Recurrence of carpal collapse with an SL gap wider than 5 mm was frequently seen at follow-up (Figure 13.30). However, a recent publication by Sousa et al[103] has shown that in most cases this is asymptom-

atic. Indeed, the window of opportunity for this technique to be successful is quite narrow.[61] When the technique is used in poorly reducible subluxations, in cases with an ulnarly translocated lunate, or in cases with preexistant degenerative arthritis the results are consistently disappointing.[19]

CRITICAL POINTS *SL Stabilization With Three-Ligament Tenodesis*

Indications
- Dynamic SL dissociation, reducible, with normal cartilage (stage III)
- Static SL dissociation, reducible, with normal cartilage (stage IV)

Preoperative Evaluation
- Routine radiograph examination
- Clenched-fist view
- Fluoroscopic evaluation of abnormal carpal motion
- MRI to check integrity of FCR tendon if injury or discontinuity suspected
- Arthroscopy or MRI to rule out cartilage degeneration, LTq injury, or both

Technical Points
- Perform a dorsal (zigzag, lazy scaphoid, or longitudinal) approach centered at the Lister tubercle.
- Incise the extensor retinaculum along the third compartment.
- Open septa between II and III, III and IV, and IV and V; coagulate intraseptal arteries.
- If the posterior interosseous nerve is intact, perform a proximal-based, nerve-sparing capsulotomy[91]; if it is not intact, perform a dorsal capsulotomy with the fiber-splitting technique by Berger.[7]
- Reducibility is checked by traction or by direct manipulation with K-wires as joysticks.
- Enter the scaphoid with a 2.7-mm cannulated drill hole at the point of insertion of the dorsal SL ligament.
- Direct the drill hole along the axis of the scaphoid aiming at the palmar tuberosity.
- Make a 1-cm palmar incision over the scaphoid tuberosity and release the FCR tendon sheath.
- Obtain a distally based 8-cm strip of tendon (0~3 mm).
- Retrieve the tendon strip from the dorsum using a wire or a tendon passer.
- Carve a transverse trough over the dorsum of the lunate with a rongeur (see Figure 13.30, *C*).
- Insert a 1.8-mm anchor suture into the lunate.
- Localize the dorsal radial triquetrum ligament, and loop the tendon strip around its distal insertion.
- While tensioning the tendon using the radial triquetrum ligament as a pulley, transfix the SL and SC joints (usually two 1.5-mm K-wires are used; eventually three are used) (see Figure 13.30, *E*).
- Without releasing the tendon tension, use the anchor suture to bury the tendon against the lunate cancellous bone in the previously created trough.
- Suture the tendon loop onto itself.
- Close the capsule over the tendon strip carefully.
- Reconstruct the extensor retinaculum.

Postoperative Treatment
- Short arm thumb spica cast for 6 weeks; change at 10 days for stitch removal and radiographs
- Removal of wires at 6 weeks and protection in a removable splint for an additional 4 weeks
- Rehabilitation after cast removal to regain motion and grip strength
- Contact sports not allowed until 6 months postoperatively
- Probable outcome: a painless wrist with 20 degrees loss of flexion and 75% grip strength

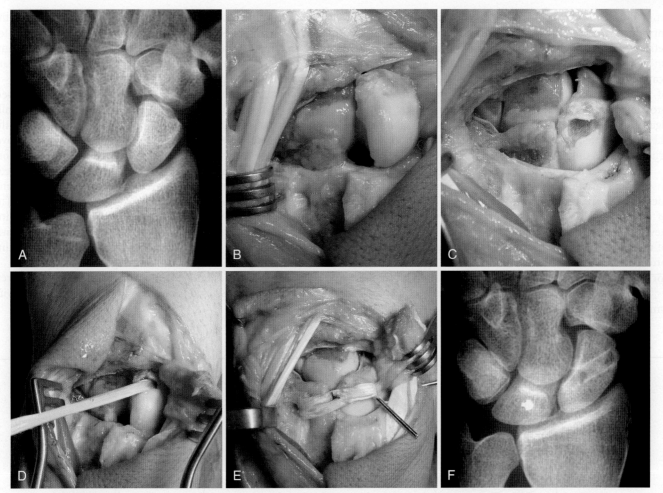

FIGURE 13.30 A 32-year-old lawyer sustained an injury to his left wrist while playing soccer 8 months ago. **A,** Posteroanterior (PA) radiograph showing relatively shortened scaphoid (S) with mildly increased scapholunate (SL) interval. **B,** The scaphoid viewed from the dorsum could easily sublux because the entire SL ligamentous complex was ruptured and could not be repaired (static reducible SL dissociation). **C,** A transverse trough was created on the dorsal aspect of the lunate (L). To ensure that the tendon would be permanently in contact with the lunate cancellous bone, an anchor suture was placed in the trough. **D,** A strip of flexor carpi radialis was harvested at the palmar side but left attached distally. Its proximal end was passed through a tunnel emerging at the distal–medial corner of the scaphoid. **E,** The tendon used the dorsal radial triquetrum ligament as an anchor point for adequate tension before being sutured onto itself. Two Kirschner wires were used to immobilize the reconstructed ligament for 6 weeks, with 4 more weeks in a removable splint. **F,** PA view obtained 8 months postoperatively. The patient had resumed his former sport activity at 6 months. At 18 months, the wrist remained stable and pain-free with 90% grip strength and 85% motion compared with the contralateral side.

To ensure better functional and radiographic results, several modifications to the technique have been proposed. In 2014, Ross et al[95] recommend drilling two tunnels: one across the scaphoid, as for the three-ligament tenodesis, and another across the lunate and triquetrum, from the lunate insertion site of the SL ligament to the medial corner of the triquetrum (Figure 13.31). The tendon strip is passed through these tunnels and secured using an interference screw in the triquetrum. The dorsal intercarpal ligament is then reinforced with the remnants of the tendon graft. A prospective series of 11 patients demonstrated good early radiological and clinical outcomes.

Corella et al[17] recommend a minimally invasive, arthroscopic, controlled technique to reconstruct both the dorsal and palmar SL ligaments (Figure 13.32). Two small incisions are placed at each end of the scaphoid, and a strip of FCR is passed through a tunnel similar to the one used for the three-ligament tenodesis. A second dorsopalmar tunnel is drilled across the lunate, again through a small incision, and the tendon graft is passed

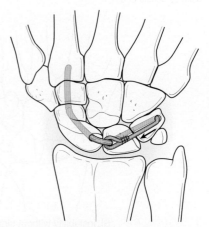

Scapholunotriquetral tenodesis
(Ross et al., 2014)[90]

FIGURE 13.31 Schematic representation of the scapholunotriquetral tenodesis suggested by Ross et al[90] to avoid recurrence of gap formation after tendon reconstruction of the dorsal scapholunate ligament (*black arrow*).

from dorsal-to-palmar. To facilitate this, a tendon passer is introduced between the FCR and the median nerve and used to retrieve the graft and tension it while it is being secured by two interference screws—one in the lunate and the other in the scaphoid. Once in the volar surface of the lunate, the remnant of the tendon graft is reattached to the volar surface of the proximal scaphoid to augment the volar component of the SL ligament. There have been no long-term results published for these recently described methods of SL stabilization, so their true efficacy is unknown.

It is important to emphasize that the use of a strip of tendon to stabilize unstable segments of the wrist is feasible but not ideal. The elastic properties of a tendon will never match those of a ligament. Also, the resultant neoligament probably will never contain mechanoreceptors, so will not participate in one of the most important functions of these ligaments—that is, to provide the necessary information required by the sensorimotor system to activate proper muscle stabilization of the joint.

Before deciding on one of the preceding techniques, it is imperative not to forget that stability cannot be built on an unstable foundation. If the lunate is unstable, reestablishing the SL ligament connections will not solve the problem. Indeed, for the techniques just discussed to be successful, the lunate must be stable. If it is not, the options described later for stage V are recommended (Figure 13.33).

Reduction-association of the SL joint. Based on the observation that failed SL fusions tend to do better clinically than successful fusions,[104] the "reduction-association of the scapholunate" (RASL) procedure was proposed as a novel approach to static SL instabilities[60,101a] (Figure 13.34). Before repairing the ligament remnants, the articular cartilage between the scaphoid and lunate is removed and the joint is reduced and transfixed with one headless screw for 12 months or more. The goal is to create a fibrous union of the SL joint and allow loading these bones without fear of recurrent joint widening. Early results have been encouraging, with most patients exhibiting excellent ranges of motion and a strong grip.[60]

Unfortunately, as reported by Larson and Stern,[51] the screw often becomes loose, and the outcomes tend to deteriorate with

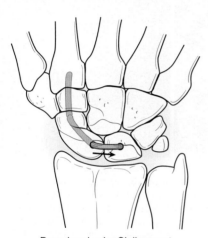

Dorsal and volar SL ligament
(Corella et al., 2013)[17]

FIGURE 13.32 Arthroscopically guided tendon reconstruction of both dorsal and volar scapholunate (SL) ligaments using a strip of flexor carpi radialis tendon (*arrow*), as described by Corella et al.[17]

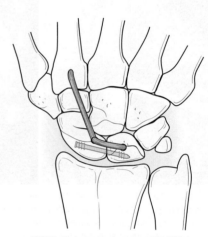

ECRL ligamentoplasty and RASL
(Fernandez DL, 2014)

FIGURE 13.34 Reduction-association of the scapholunate joint, the so-called "RASL procedure,"[60] has been suggested to avoid the problem of recurrent diastasis after an SL ligament repair. DL Fernandez has recently reported good results by combining the RASL procedure with an extensor carpi radialis tenodesis, as illustrated in this figure. *ERCL*, Extensor radialis carpi longus.

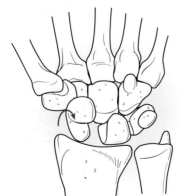

SL instability without ulnar translation
(Taleisnik type 1)

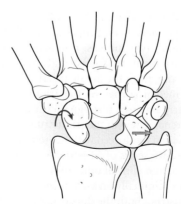

SL instability with ulnar translation
(Taleisnik type 2)

FIGURE 13.33 Tendon reconstructions of scapholunate (SL) dissociations can only be effective if the lunate is stable. An associated radiocarpal instability is the cause of most failures.[29] When evaluating an SL dissociation, therefore, it is imperative to rule out this problem, as emphasized by Taleisnik in 1988.[108] The *red arrows* indicate subluxation of the scaphoid and the *yellow arrows* indicate ulnar translocation of the lunate.

time, resulting in frequent recurrences of the misalignment once the screw is removed. To avoid these complications several alternatives have been proposed. One is to introduce a specially designed jointed screw into the SL interval that allows some rotation of the scaphoid about the lunate (SLIC screw, Acumed®, Hillsboro, OR). Another is to insert a tendon autograft along the axis of SL rotation that will act as a flexible biological link between the two bones (SL-axis method, Arthrex®, Naples, FL).[53] Yet another technique is to associate the RASL procedure with a more solid tendon reconstruction of the SL ligaments (Fernandez, DL, personal communication, 2014) (see Figure 13.34). Whether these alternatives will avoid the complications observed with current techniques is unknown, but that are certainly worth investigating.

Stage V: reducible carpal collapse due to chronic SL ligament injury, plus instability of radiolunate joint and normal joint cartilage. As stated earlier, rupture of both the primary and secondary ligament stabilizers of the scaphoid is frequently associated with distention or rupture of the RL ligaments. In such instances, both the scaphoid and lunate are unstable (see Figure 13.33). In general, it is accepted that an unstable segment cannot be stabilized using another unstable segment. If the lunate is unstable, most reconstructions of the SL ligaments are bound to fail. In those cases, stability is only possible if the reconstruction is based on the radius. This is the rationale for "spiral tenodesis"[13] (Figure 13.35).

Spiral Tenodesis. As described in the kinetic section of this chapter, under axial load the distal row tends to pronate, the scaphoid to flex and pronate, and the lunate to translocate ulnarly down the ulnar inclination of the radius. To constrain all these displacements, a number of ligaments need to be ruptured and/or attenuated, including: the long and short RL, the dorsal radiotriquetral (RTq), the palmar and dorsal LTq, the dorsal SL, the dorsal intercarpal, and the palmar SC ligaments. Except for the dorsal RTq ligament, all these structures spiral around the central column so as to prevent excessive pronation of the distal row under load. The so-called "antipronation spiral tenodesis," described by Chee et al,[13] was aimed at reconstructing this spiral arrangement of ligaments using one single strip of FCR (see Figure 13.35).

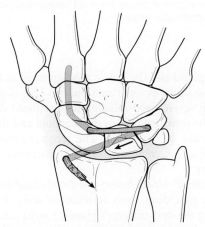

Antipronation spiral tenodesis
(Chee et al., 2012)[13]

FIGURE 13.35 Schematic representation of the so-called "antipronation spiral tenodesis" (*arrows*) described by Chee et al.[13] It is recommended for reducible scapholunate dissociation with instability of the radiolunate articulation.

The technique begins the same as for the three-ligament tenodesis. However, once on the dorsum of the triquetrum, the FCR is threaded through a dorsopalmar tunnel across it to exit at the floor of the carpal tunnel. From there, it is brought under the flexor digitorum profundus (FDP) to emerge in a separate incision over the radial styloid where it is inserted. This procedure is only indicated if the instability is easily reducible and there is no cartilage damage. The early results in the index patient obtained with this new alternative are encouraging (Figure 13.36).

Stage VI: irreducible carpal collapse due to chronic SL ligament injury, with normal joint cartilage. This stage is defined by the presence of carpal misalignment that cannot be reduced easily owing to deformation of the subluxed joint surfaces, fibrosis formation within the empty spaces left by the subluxing bones, and capsular retraction. If the joint cartilages are normal despite this, then the criteria for stage VI SL dissociation are fulfilled.

When cases are symptomatic, the most frequently recommended treatment is a partial carpal fusion. Compared to a total wrist fusion, the advantages of only arthrodesing the destroyed joint have long been recognized.[104] What follows is a brief description of the most commonly used partial fusions for the treatment of SL dissociation. Further details about these techniques and their results are provided in Chapter 12.

Scaphoid–trapezium–trapezoid arthrodesis. The goal of this procedure is to reduce the proximal pole of the scaphoid into the scaphoid fossa, restoring RS congruency and decreasing the chance of developing degenerative changes.[104,116] When planning, it is important that the external dimensions and alignment of the resultant fused block are the same as the external dimensions of the bones in the normal wrist. Underreduction (scaphoid flexed) fails to close the SL gap correctly, and overreduction (scaphoid extended) may result in more restricted motion and more severe RS impingement postoperatively.

As experience with STT joint fusion has increased, complications and long-term outcomes have been reported.[104] The average rate of nonunion among all the reported series is 14%. Postoperatively, range of motion and strength are frequently decreased, and the results in terms of pain relief are not uniformly predictable. Painful RS impingement is a frequent problem, owing to the fact that in radial inclination the distally fused scaphoid can no longer rotate into flexion, resulting in increased pressure on the scaphoid fossa. To solve this problem, Watson and coworkers[5,116] recommended incorporating a dorsolateral radial styloidectomy as part of the STT joint fusion. This is likely to prevent peripheral, but not central, RS impingement. Any preexisting cartilage degeneration between the scaphoid and radius is a formal contraindication to STT joint fusion.

SL arthrodesis. Previously believed to be the ideal method of treating SL dissociation, fusion of the SL joint has proved to be one of the least reliable treatments for this condition.[73,104] The small surface area of the articular surfaces coming into contact and the magnitude of forces transmitted by the capitate, tending to separate the two bones, make this fusion difficult to achieve. After this procedure, the mutual shifting that occurs between the two bones is no longer possible, resulting in increased demands on the arthrodesis, predisposing the fusion to refracture. Bony union occurs in only 50% of cases.[73,104] However, the nonunions may have created enough fibrosis between the scaphoid and lunate to decrease the patient's symptoms.[104]

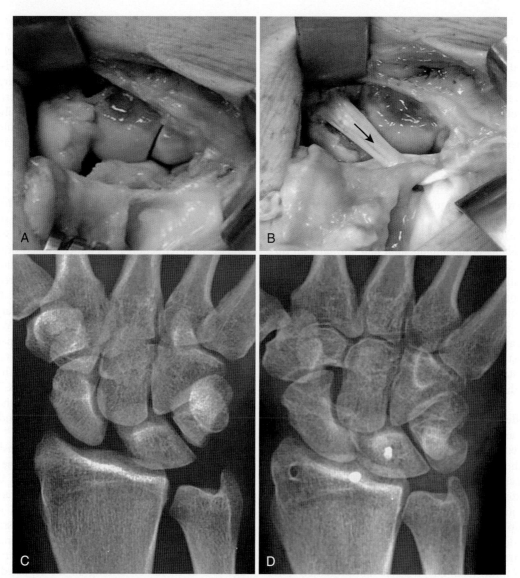

FIGURE 13.36 A 33-year-old male, after a motor vehicle accident, was diagnosed with scapholunate (SL) dissociation. A more detailed radiographic assessment under stress, however, showed the lunate to be excessively displaceable toward the ulna. Under the diagnosis of a combined radiocarpal–intracarpal derangement, he was scheduled for an antipronation spiral tenodesis, as described by Chee et al.[13] **A, B,** Photographs taken during surgery. Dorsal view of the SL dissociated joint, before and after the tendon graft (*arrow*) replaced the dorsal SL ligament. **C,** Posteroanterior radiograph before surgery. **D,** A radiograph obtained 8 months after surgery shows full restoration of the normal alignment. The patient was able to resume his occupation without limitations 4 months after surgery.

Scaphoid–capitate arthrodesis. Theoretically, SC fusion should have consequences similar to STT joint fusion. In the laboratory, the kinematic and kinetic carpal behavior after both types of fusion is similar—that is, both cause abnormal transfer of load and significant loss of midcarpal joint motion, especially in radial and ulnar inclinations. Watson and coworkers[104] found less of a reduction of motion after STT joint fusion than after SC fusion, probably because of increased rotation at the trapezoid–capitate joint. The long-term results of this procedure are quite acceptable, with more than two-thirds of patients satisfied, with minimal disability, although approximately 30% of patients develop degenerative changes at the RS joint.[62]

Scaphoid–lunate–capitate arthrodesis. Adding the lunate to the scaphoid–capitate fusion offers a method of controlling both the scaphoid and the lunate misalignment at the expense of a 50% reduction in wrist motion.[62,104] This is indicated in patients with severe fixed misalignment without degenerative changes of the proximal pole of the scaphoid and the opposing articular surface of the radius. The recommendation is that this procedure be combined with a generous dorsoradial styloidectomy.

Radioscaphoid–lunate fusion and distal scaphoidectomy. As stated in the preceding, most activities of daily living involve motion along the dart-thrower's plane-of-wrist rotation, going from extension and radial inclination to flexion and ulnar inclination. This motion occurs mainly at the midcarpal joint.[9,70] Consequently, if the cartilage of that joint is normal, and the fixed misalignment or degenerative arthritis of the scaphoid and lunate requires an arthrodesis, it is reasonable to fuse only

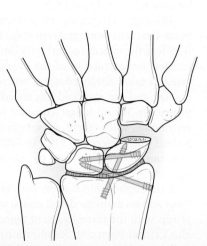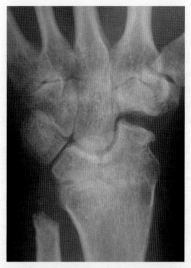

FIGURE 13.37 Schematic representation (*left*) and case example (*right*) of the technique that is preferred when a scapholunate dissociation is not easily reducible but the cartilage at the midcarpal joint is intact: radioscapholunate fusion plus distal scaphoidectomy to allow wider radial inclination.

the RSL joint. Fusing it eliminates pain induced by degenerative arthritis, while stabilizing the proximal component (i.e., SL acetabulum) of the midcarpal joint. After this fusion, the STT joint may degenerate with time and become painful due to the inability of the scaphoid to flex during wrist flexion and radial inclination, creating a local impingement.

To avoid this complication, and to increase the resultant motion, Garcia-Elias et al[26] suggested excision of the distal third of the scaphoid (Figure 13.37). Other authors have also recommended excising the triquetrum.[10a] With this modified technique, the midcarpal ball-and-socket articulation is freed from its lateral constraint, allowing more than 50% of overall wrist motion. Furthermore, the chances of achieving an RSL arthrodesis are improved due to the loss of distal scaphoid constraint.

Despite the published and encouraging early results, it is important to note that, by resecting the distal scaphoid, the area of contact between the proximal and distal rows is reduced substantially. If the joint is not misaligned, however, that reduction of contact should be well tolerated. Indeed, if the lunate is arthrodesed in a proper axial alignment, dorsal dislocation of the capitate will not occur, preserving full joint contact, thus preventing degenerative arthritis of the LC joint. Needless to say, the operation should not be performed if the LC cartilage is not normal.

Stage VII: complete SL ligament injury with irreducible misalignment and cartilage degeneration. Long-lasting carpal misalignment, with irreducible subluxation of the scaphoid, will cause joint cartilage destruction. This is secondary to decreased joint contact areas, which prevent successful ligament repair or reconstruction. Stage VII is the beginning of a pattern of progressive joint degeneration known as SLAC wrist.[5,116] The cartilage wear begins between the tip of the radial styloid and the adjacent surface of the scaphoid and progresses proximally until the entire RS joint is involved. At a later stage, the midcarpal joint may also degenerate, usually starting at the LC joint. In advanced cases, the rest of the carpus may be involved, with the exception of the RL joint, which is usually spared. The following subsections contain a brief review of the surgical alternatives that exist to tackle these conditions. Detailed information

about most of these procedures is provided in Chapters 12, 16, and 17.

Arthroscopy. Wrist arthroscopy plays a limited role in patients with SLAC wrist. It can be used to evaluate the degree and extent of articular degeneration to decide which salvage procedure is best. Wrist arthroscopy can be a valuable adjunct in determining the status of the radial and capitate articular cartilages, particularly in the decision-making process between a four-corner fusion or proximal row carpectomy.

Radial styloidectomy. This is one of the oldest procedures used to relieve wrist pain caused by an impingement between the tip of the radial styloid and a misaligned distal scaphoid. Despite removing the degenerated radial styloid process, the SLAC wrist sequence will continue to progress. When performing a radial styloidectomy through an open lateral approach, caution is required to protect the dorsolateral branches of the superficial radial nerve. At its palmar margin, it is important to avoid detaching the origin of the radiocarpal ligaments, which would lead to further instability.[7] For individuals who desire minimal surgical intervention, arthroscopic radial styloidectomy may be an option.

Scaphoidectomy and midcarpal fusion. Popularized by Watson and coworkers[116] the SLAC procedure (i.e., scaphoid excision plus capitate–lunate–triquetrum–hamate fusion; also known as four-corner fusion) has gained an excellent reputation for the treatment of chronic SL dissociation. For the operation to be successful, good articular cartilage at the RL level is required. A frequent complication is the development of dorsal impingement between the dorsal edge of the radius and the capitate. An important step to avoid this is to fully correct the extension deformity of the lunate before stabilizing the midcarpal joint. Several new implants, including circular or square plates, staples, and locking screws have been designed to be countersunk below the dorsal intersection of the four carpal bones so that radial impingement is avoided.

In selected cases, fusion is limited to the LC joint, and reported results have been comparable.[10a] In patients with ulnar-positive variance (in which an excessively rigid triquetrum could precipitate ulnocarpal abutment), or in cases with chronic combined SL and LTq instability, the scaphoid and triquetrum can be excised before fusing the LC joint.

Proximal row carpectomy. This is another salvage operation in which the scaphoid, lunate, and triquetrum are excised, creating a neoarticulation between the capitate and lunate fossa of the radius.[114] In most published series, this procedure is said to be good in terms of pain relief, restoration of functional wrist motion, and grip strength, with high overall patient satisfaction.

In mechanical terms, this operation converts a complex composite articulation into a single ball-and-socket joint with nonmatching articular surfaces. The wrist can adjust to such an incongruity only if there is a good articular cartilage on the proximal pole of the capitate and in the lunate fossa of the radius. Compared with midcarpal arthrodesis, this technique avoids long immobilization and the risk of nonunion. It has the added advantage of being able to be converted into a wrist arthrodesis or arthroplasty if at a later date it evolves into a painful osteoarthritis. Long-term radiocapitate degeneration, although often asymptomatic, is present in about one-third of patients with more than 10 years of follow-up. In one series, 6 out of 17 patients at 20 years follow-up had been reoperated on.[114] With a success rate (65%), Walls et al[114] recommends adequate preoperative counseling of this increased failure risk when this procedure is offered to patients younger than 35 years old.

Total wrist arthroplasty. Advances in total joint replacement of the wrist have made this option a reasonable treatment for patients who place low demands on the wrist. Most patients with late posttraumatic instability are young and active individuals or manual laborers, for whom a joint prosthesis is seldom an acceptable choice (see Chapter 12). If the cartilage of the proximal surface of the capitate is preserved, there is the option of replacing only the proximal row by a hemiarthroplasty.[48]

Total wrist arthrodesis. Although many surgeons believe that a total wrist arthrodesis should rarely be considered in patients with a posttraumatic unstable osteoarthritis, arthrodesis is still the procedure of choice for patients who perform heavy manual work. According to some sources, complete pain relief can be expected in 85% of patients with 65% of them returning to their former occupations.[77] As shown in many clinical series, most patients with total wrist fusion are able to accomplish all daily tasks by learning to compensate for the loss of wrist motion.

❖ AUTHORS' PREFERRED METHOD OF TREATMENT: SL Dissociation

Partial ruptures of the SL ligamentous complex (i.e., stage I, occult SL dissociation) may respond well to physiotherapy. Particularly promising are the results of proprioception reeducation of the wrist muscular stabilizers, promoting the combined action of the APL and ECRL muscles by asking them to extend and radially incline wrists against resistance. In more advanced partial injury, we believe in arthroscopic debridement of the unstable remnants of the disrupted membrane, plus percutaneous pinning of the SL joint with two or more Kirschner wires for 8 weeks. It is always important to check for the integrity of the dorsal SL ligament. If insufficient or torn, but repairable (stage II, SL dissociation), we prefer the open technique of joint reduction, ligament repair, and dorsal capsulodesis as proposed by Cohen[16] (see Figure 13.25).

Although recognizing its potential use, we no longer use bone–ligament–bone grafts in stage III SL dissociation because it stiffens the radiocarpal articulation too much. In our opinion, isolated reconstruction of the dorsal SL ligament is not indicated in more advanced stages where the secondary stabilizers are lost and the scaphoid has already yielded into flexion and pronation. We no longer consider SL ligament repair, even if repairable, when there is substantial lunate misalignment. Indeed, the presence of DISI indicates a more global problem that can hardly be solved by addressing only the dorsal SL ligament.

If the subluxation is easily correctable (stage IV, SL dissociation) and no cartilage defect exists, we have had very acceptable results with the three-ligament tenodesis (see Figure 13.29; see also Critical Points: SL Stabilization). However, in recent years, we have paid more attention to the level of RL instability than we have admitted in previous editions of this book. In our experience, one cannot build SL instability on an unstable lunate. If the lunate is ulnarly translocated, or if it exhibits substantial sagittal misalignment (stage V, SL dissociation), we look for reducibility. If it is easily reducible, we trust the recently described spiral tenodesis (see Figure 13.35).

When the misalignment is irreducible (stage VI, SL dissociation), but no cartilage damage is present, we have achieved good results by fusing the radiocarpal joint and excising the distal third of the scaphoid[26] (see Figure 13.37). In our experience, most midcarpal-crossing arthrodeses provide excellent short-term results but poor long-term outcomes. When the radioscaphoid and the midcarpal joints are involved by the arthritic process (stage VII, SL dissociation, SLAC wrist), we prefer to do a total scaphoidectomy plus a midcarpal fusion. Being skeptical of the long-term viability of a joint with mismatched articular surfaces, we perform proximal row carpectomies only occasionally.

Lunotriquetral Dissociation. Posttraumatic or degenerative LTq dissociations are not unusual. The literature may be scarce and often misleading, but disruptions of the LTq joint are not infrequent. The first case of a LTq dissociation was identified in the early 20th century,[21] but it was not until the 1970s, following the work of Reagan and associates,[79] that the problem became more widely recognized. Since then, this problem has become better understood and treatment results have improved. Yet, the chance that this condition is missed or confused with other ulnar-sided wrist problems (e.g., midcarpal instabilities or TFCC injuries) remains high.[15,83]

Pathomechanics of LTq Dissociation. Most isolated injuries to the LTq ligaments are secondary to a backward fall onto the outstretched hand, with the arm externally rotated, the forearm supinated, and the wrist extended and radially inclined. In such circumstances, the impact is concentrated on the hypothenar area, and particularly on the pisiform, which acts as a punch against the extended triquetrum.[71] Such a dorsally directed force to the triquetrum induces its dorsal displacement. The lunate does not follow the triquetrum because it is constrained by the radius and the volar long RL ligament. As a result of this, substantial shear stress is created at the LTq joint, causing progressive stretching and ultimately tearing of the three components of the LTq ligaments (i.e., volar, dorsal, and proximal).

If, aside from this, there is a violent rotation of the distal row into further pronation, the palmar TqHC ligament adds the extra destabilizing force required for the palmar LTq ligament to fail. Supporting this explanation is the fact that the two ligaments (i.e., palmar LTq and TqHC) are rarely disrupted simultaneously.

Injury to the LTq ligaments is often associated with peripheral tears of the TFCC and a distal avulsion of the ulnotriquetral ligament.[71] The mechanism of these combined injuries is similar to the mechanism discussed for the isolated LTq injury, except for the predominance of radial inclination and pronation as torque-inducing vectors. In this respect, any ligament avulsion of the palmar rim of the triquetrum should be interpreted as a sign of a combined ulnocarpal and LTq injury.

In other cases, a perilunate destabilization process, as postulated by Mayfield and colleagues,[64] may lead to LTq instability. In such instances, the wrist has undergone violent extension, ulnar inclination, and midcarpal supination, usually from motorcycle accidents or falls from a height. Rupture of the SL ligaments (stage I) occurs first, followed by LC dislocation (stage II), and finally rupture of the LTq ligaments (stage III). If the SL ligament lesion is successfully treated, but the LTq lesion remains, symptoms from LTq instability may require treatment.

The LTq joint may become progressively disrupted as the result of a long-standing ulnocarpal abutment. In the presence of an ulnar-plus variant, attritional degeneration of the proximal membranous portion of the LTq joint is frequent and should never be confused, or treated, as if it was the result of an isolated traumatic event.

In the laboratory, several attempts to ascertain the consequences of LTq ligament disruptions have been made.[87] When the LTq and dorsal radiotriquetral ligaments were experimentally sectioned in axially loaded cadaveric wrists, the flexion moment of the scaphoid became unconstrained, causing a conjoint flexion of the scaphoid and lunate, with secondary anterior subluxation of the capitate (Figure 13.38). This represents the more advanced stage of the disease, resulting in a static VISI pattern of instability. By contrast, when only the palmar and dorsal LTq ligaments were sectioned, increased mobility of the LTq joint was detected (dynamic instability), but not a complete destabilization of the carpus. These findings may explain the relatively low incidence of radiocarpal arthrosis in late static LTq dissociations. This is probably because the scaphoid and lunate maintain their normal alignment with the radius.

Diagnosis of LTq Dissociation. LTq dissociation manifests as a spectrum of clinical conditions, ranging from asymptomatic partial tears to a painful complete dissociation with static carpal collapse. Although the former does not deform the wrist, the latter may exhibit a reversed "fork-like" or "bayonet" deformity. This is similar to the deformity seen in volarly displaced distal radius fractures, except that the carpal sag is distal and not lateral to the prominent distal ulna.[81] Some patients describe painful crepitus as they incline the hand ulnarly.[57] Symptomatic injuries invariably exhibit point tenderness directly over the dorsal aspect of the joint. Pain is usually aggravated with ulnar inclination of the wrist and supination of the forearm. Wrist motion is seldom diminished except in the more advanced cases with carpal collapse. Patients frequently complain of weakness

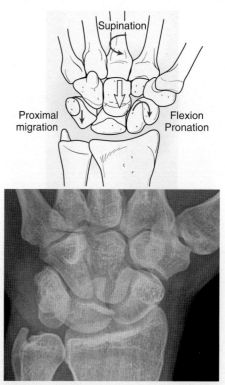

FIGURE 13.38 Schematic representation and radiograph of typical carpal bone displacements (*curved arrows*) that occur when the extrinsic and intrinsic lunotriquetral-supporting ligaments have failed. The scaphoid and lunate as a unit fall into flexion; the unconstrained triquetrum migrates proximally, especially in ulnar inclination (*straight arrows*); and the distal row supinates.

and a sensation of the wrist giving way, and some may also have ulnar nerve paresthesias.

Physical examination. A pathognomonic finding is a positive ballottement test, as described by Reagan and coworkers.[79] The lunate is firmly stabilized with the thumb and index finger of one hand, while the triquetrum and pisiform are displaced dorsally and palmarly with the other hand. A positive result elicits pain, crepitus, and abnormal displacement of the joint. The so-called "shear test" described by Kleinman[83] is a variation of the ballottement test that can be done with a single hand: By stabilizing the dorsal aspect of the lunate with the index finger, the pisiform is loaded by the thumb in a dorsal direction, creating a shear force at the LTq joint that causes pain (Figure 13.39).

The Derby test reported by Christodoulou and Bainbridge is also useful in the reducible LTq dissociation without a fixed VISI type of deformity.[83] This test starts by realigning the lunate and scaphoid relative to the radius. This is done by placing the wrist in extension and at a slight ulnar inclination. If, in that position, we reduce the LTq joint by pushing the pisiform dorsally, the feeling of instability disappears immediately, and grip strength increases as long as pressure over the pisiform is maintained.

Most of these provocative maneuvers are of reasonable sensitivity but poor specificity. Painful ulnar-sided conditions that may elicit a pain from these tests include: LTq synchondrosis, fracture of an incomplete congenital coalition; triquetrum–hamate impingement and degeneration; avulsion fractures of the dorsal triquetrum; pisotriquetral arthropathy; traumatic or degenerative TFCC tears; ulnocarpal impaction syndrome; ECU tenosynovitis; and entrapment of the dorsal branch of the

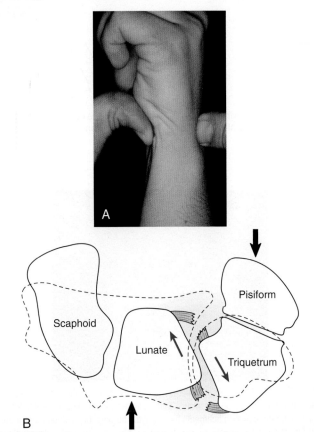

FIGURE 13.39 A, The "shear test" as described by Kleinman[83] is similar to the ballottement test described by Reagan and coworkers.[79] **B,** Opposite force (*black arrows*) is applied to induce abnormal displacement (*red arrows*) to a lunotriquetral (LTq) joint suspected of ligament injury. This test is painful for a patient with a sprain or instability in the LTq joint.

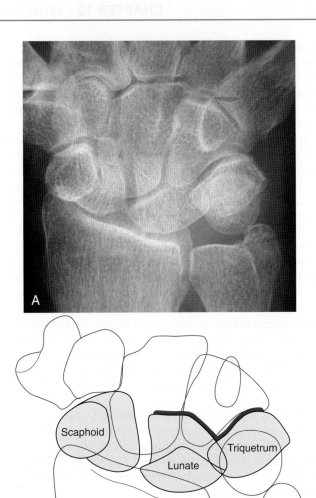

FIGURE 13.40 A, Posteroanterior view of a static lunotriquetral (LTq) dissociation in a 44-year-old lawyer who had suffered a fall from a height 2 years before, without apparent consequences. Six months after the accident, he complained of painful snapping during lateral inclinations. **B,** Note the moonlike configuration of the lunate in volar intercalated segmental instability and the "seagull"-appearing outline of the distal LTq border (*red line*). The scapholunate joint was slightly widened probably the result of the palmar fibers of this joint being longer than the dorsal ones.

ulnar nerve. Indeed, careful differential diagnosis is mandatory before deciding on a treatment for ulnar-sided pain.[12]

Radiographic examination. Standard wrist views appear normal in most patients with partial tears of the LTq interosseous membrane. Occasionally, in chronic dynamic instabilities, a slight narrowing of the LTq joint with subchondral cyst formation on the opposing sides of the joint may appear. This finding should not be confused with similar features seen in patients with a fracture of an incomplete LTq coalition.[120]

When there is a static VISI pattern of misalignment secondary to complete rupture of both intrinsic and extrinsic LTq supporting ligaments, radiographic diagnosis is obvious. Most characteristic is the disruption of the normal convex arc of the proximal carpal row (the Gilula line) in the PA radiograph projection. A "moon-like" lunate facing a foreshortened scaphoid is also typical of this condition (see Figures 13.15 and 13.40). In such cases, the lunate's dorsal pole is superimposed on the distal part of the capitate, implying an abnormal flexion of the bone. It is also pathognomonic of this problem, the so-called "seagull sign"—the distal outlines of the lunate and triquetrum adopt the form of a flying seagull (Figure 13.40). A widened SL joint is paradoxically common in LTq dissociations. It is important to note, however, that the gap does not represent a rupture of the SL ligaments, but is instead the result of an axial load being applied to the most palmar SL ligament fibers. These fibers are longer and obliquely oriented, allowing an

increased, but normal, separation of the two bones.[46] None of these radiographic findings changes with the wrist in ulnar inclination, except for an increased proximal displacement of the triquetrum relative to the rest of the proximal carpal row (Figure 13.41). In collapsed cases, the carpal height ratio may be diminished.

In the lateral projection, aside from the VISI pattern of misalignment, it is sometimes possible to find a decreased LTq angle. According to Reagan et al,[79] the average LTq angle is 14 degrees. Assessment of this angular measurement requires films of excellent quality and considerable practice taking them because the longitudinal axis of the triquetrum is difficult to identify. Yet, identifying the relative position of the triquetrum axis relative to the lunate axis may help to discriminate between a CIND–VISI and an LTq dissociation (Figure 13.42). Both in normal as in CIND–VISI wrists, the triquetrum-axis is palmar

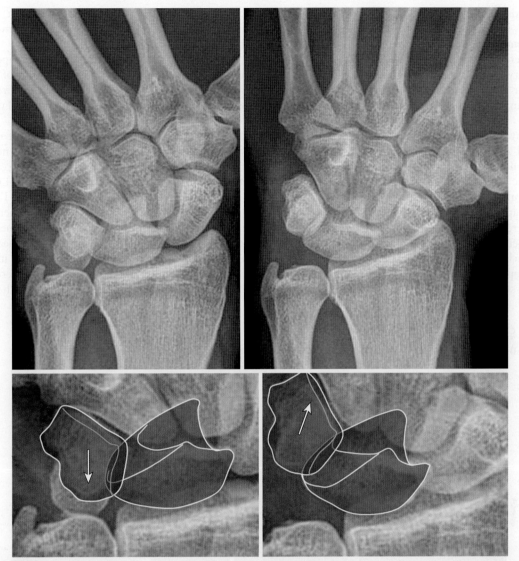

FIGURE 13.41 Dynamic radiographs of static lunotriquetral dissociation. During radial inclination (*right*), the scaphoid (S) and the lunate (L) are abnormally palmar flexed, but the triquetrum (Tq) is normally aligned relative to the lunate (*up arrow*). During ulnar inclination (*left*), there is a significant step-off between the lunate and the triquetrum (*down arrow*). Note the scaphoid and lunate remain in the flexed position, despite the ulnar inclination of the wrist.

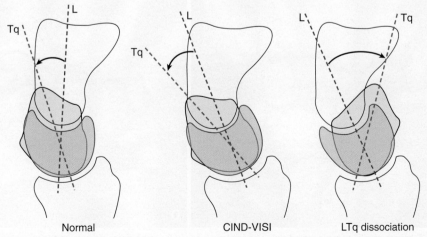

Normal   CIND-VISI   LTq dissociation

FIGURE 13.42 The lunotriquetral (LTq) angle is difficult to identify in a lateral radiograph, and its quantification difficult to reproduce. Yet, identifying the relative position of the triquetrum (Tq) axis relative to the lunate (L) axis may be of help to discriminate between a carpal instability nondissociative (CIND)–volar intercalated segmental instability (VISI) and an LTq dissociation. Both in normal wrists (*left*) and in CIND–VISI (*center*) wrists, the triquetrum-axis is palmar to the lunate-axis. In the LTq dissociated wrist (*right*), by contrast, the triquetrum-axis is always dorsal to the lunate-axis.

to the lunate-axis. In the LTq dissociated wrist, by contrast, the triquetrum-axis is always dorsal to the lunate-axis.

Other diagnostic tests. Advanced imaging is particularly useful when there is doubt about the etiology of a chronic LTq tear. If the injury is due to a chronic ulnocarpal impingement, a bone scan or MRI frequently shows an area of increased uptake in the lunate. In pure LTq instabilities, the scan is seldom positive.

Arthrography may show a communication of dye between the radiocarpal and midcarpal joints. An arthrographic communication is nonspecific and may result from a traumatic injury, a chronic age-related perforation, or ligament degeneration caused by ulnocarpal impaction syndrome.[12]

Cineradiography may be very helpful and is always recommended.[105] In relatively acute situations, the wrist may still exhibit a sudden reduction of the abnormally flexed lunate during ulnar inclination, manifesting as a clunk. However, such self-reducing capability is rapidly lost, and the VISI misalignment becomes static (Figure 13.43). In such instances, as the wrist moves from radial-to-ulnar inclination, the triquetral–hamate joint is always engaged, and the SL complex remains in the flexed position in ulnar inclination.

Arthroscopy has become an increasingly important diagnostic and therapeutic tool for the evaluation of lesions on the ulnar side of the carpus, and it may identify previously unrecognized types of ligamentous disruptions.[105] Further technical details are provided in Chapter 17.

LTq Dissociation Treatment. As with all other forms of carpal instability, treatment of LTq instability needs to be individualized according to the patient's age, occupation, recreational demands, and intensity of symptoms. LTq injuries may be acute or chronic. They may involve only the LTq interosseous ligaments and maintain normal bony alignment, or they may have a more global intrinsic and extrinsic ligament insufficiency resulting in carpal collapse. An injury may appear as an isolated ulnar-sided problem or be part of a perilunate instability. There are different clinical conditions in which there is substantial damage to the LTq supporting ligaments, each having its own

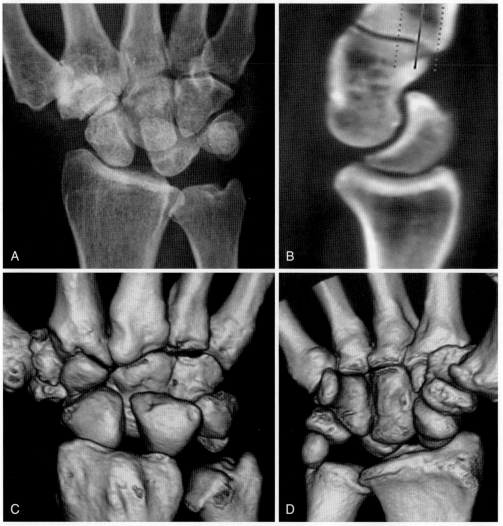

FIGURE 13.43 Images of a 56-year-old retired man who fell from a height 8 years before, without short-term consequences. Treated conservatively, he did well until 10 months ago when a mild sprain triggered an increasingly dysfunctional process characterized by wrist pain, progressive loss of motion, and increasing weakness. Plain radiographs **(A, B)** disclosed the presence of a static carpal collapse secondary to lunotriquetral dissociation, a diagnosis that was made fully evident by a 3D rendering of the bones' surfaces **(C, D)**.

prognosis and treatment. A description of the treatment of the five most common forms of LTq ligament injury seen in clinical practice follows. Cases in which there is degeneration of the lunotriquetral proximal membrane as a result of a chronic ulnocarpal abutment are not included in this section (see Chapter 14).

Acute LTq injury without carpal collapse. The so-called "dynamic or occult LTq instability" is usually diagnosed by arthroscopy. The degree of LTq ligament incompetence varies from a minimal disruption to complete rupture of the proximal membrane and both volar and dorsal LTq ligaments; yet, the wrist does not exhibit misalignment because the extrinsic ligaments are not injured. The condition may be painful as a result of increased motion between the two bones, generating shear stress and local synovitis.

In the past, most authors agreed that acute LTq injuries should be treated conservatively, with the wrist immobilized in a carefully molded cast or splint, with a pad beneath the pisiform and over the dorsum of the distal radius to maintain optimal alignment.[79] Failures using that approach, however, were not unusual. Unless pronosupination is blocked by including the elbow in the cast, the amount of motion that occurs in the LTq joint during forearm rotation is substantial, owing to the "pistonage" effect of the ulna against the carpus through the TFCC. Such micromotion prevents proper connective tissue formation at the repair site. Thus, should conservative treatment for an acute LTq ligament be chosen, an above-elbow cast is imperative.

The introduction of arthroscopy as a routine exploration in wrist trauma allowed earlier recognition of the extent of these lesions, and an increased awareness of their potential risk. To avoid an above-elbow cast, some authors recommend multiple percutaneous pinning of the acutely injured joint. The arthroscopic method of pinning the joint is discussed in Chapter 17. Postoperatively, it is important to remember the positive stabilizing effects of the ECU muscle in preventing VISI.[54] Thus, adequate proprioceptive reeducation of this muscle is recommended during rehabilitation.

Chronic LTq injury without carpal collapse. LTq instability is considered chronic when the two ends of the disrupted ligaments have degenerated, diminishing the chances for successful healing. If the extrinsic ligaments maintain their secondary stabilizing efficacy, carpal alignment may still be normal. In symptomatic cases, a more aggressive approach is necessary to reestablish the synchronicity of motion between the triquetrum and lunate.

A variety of strategies have been proposed including simple arthroscopic debridement, electrothermal shrinkage, ligament reconstruction using a strip of the ECU tendon, and LTq arthrodesis.[87,98] None of these methods has attained consistent success for chronic injuries.

The various arthroscopic techniques for the management of chronic tears of the lunotriquetral interosseous ligament are reviewed in Chapter 17. These include debridement of the frayed ends of the disrupted proximal membrane, capsular shrinkage, or closing the interval between the ulnolunate and ulnotriquetrum ligaments with sutures under arthroscopic control.[100]

Complete disruption of the LTq ligaments associated with reducible chronic instability is best treated by ligament reconstruction with a tendon graft (Figure 13.44). The technique recommended by Shin et al[98] consists of reconstructing the LTq linkage with a strip of ECU tendon, left attached distally and passed through holes in the lunate and triquetrum. By tightly looping the tendon graft around the LTq joint, immediate stability is achieved. The reconstruction is further secured by transfixing the joint with one or two Kirschner wires for 8 weeks, followed by 4 more weeks in a protective splint. A group of 8 patients treated with this technique showed encouraging results.[98]

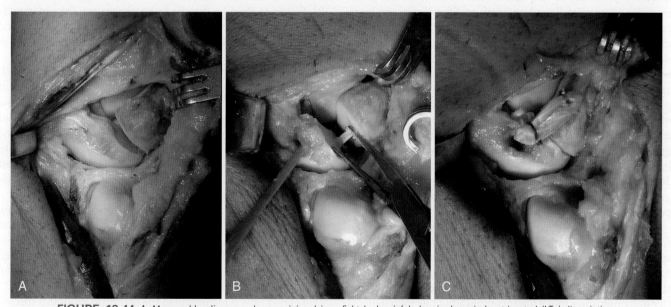

FIGURE 13.44 A 44-year-old policeman who was injured in a fight had painful chronic dynamic lunotriquetral (LTq) dissociation. A complete nonrepairable LTq injury was found arthroscopically **(A)**, so it was decided to perform an open tendon reconstruction of the palmar **(B)** and dorsal **(C)** LTq ligaments using a slip of the extensor carpi ulnaris tendon, according to Shin and colleagues.[98] The patient had regained normal hand function 6 months after surgery with 35% reduced flexion but a strong and painless grip.

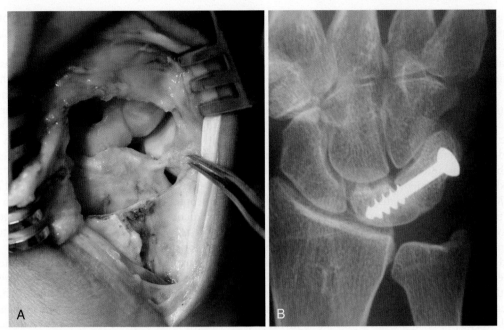

FIGURE 13.45 A 28-year-old woman, who could not recall any traumatic event, had chronic ulnar-side wrist pain. **A,** Increased hypermobility and complete rupture of the lunotriquetral intercarpal ligaments were shown at operation, so a local fusion was done. Following publication by Guidera and colleagues,[33] we tend to use compression screws to improve the chances of healing. **B,** The fusion was solid 15 months after surgery, but some tenderness persisted.

Shahane and coworkers[97] published a slightly different approach, also using a strip of ECU tendon, to tether the dorsal aspects of the triquetrum–hamate joint. This approach seems to control the abnormal triquetral motion and provides good pain relief and acceptable function in most patients with isolated chronic LTq dissociations.

Fusing the unstable LTq joint is another alternative. The procedure has met with variable success due to a relatively high nonunion rate[98,104] (Figure 13.45). According to Guidera et al,[33] most complications of LTq fusion result from technical problems. By using cancellous bone graft to fill a biconcave space created in the adjoining bones and stabilizing the joint with multiple Kirschner wires, these authors reported a 100% consolidation rate (see the following Critical Points box). In their series of 26 patient wrists, postoperative flexion–extension averaged 78% of the range measured on the contralateral side, with good or excellent pain relief in 83% of the cases and with 88% of patients returning to their previous occupations.[33] A meta-analysis of 143 LTq fusions, however, demonstrated that lunotriquetral fusions are not without problems, particularly if they have been incorrectly planned or executed. A nonunion rate of 26% and a complication rate of 43%, mostly in the form of persistent pain, were reported.[104] The procedure should not be performed in the presence of a VISI deformity.

The only study comparing ligament reconstruction with LTq fusion has been reported by Shin and colleagues.[98] They retrospectively reviewed 57 patients with an average postoperative follow-up of 9.5 years. Patients who underwent tendon reconstruction of the LTq ligaments had higher subjective and objective outcomes and a much lower complication rate than patients having an arthrodesis.

Chronic LTq dissociation with carpal collapse. LTq dissociation with carpal collapse is secondary to complete disruption of the intrinsic LTq ligaments and attenuation or disruption of the extrinsic stabilizing ligaments—dorsal and palmar radiocarpal ligaments. As a result of such a global ligament insufficiency, the carpus collapses into a dissociative VISI pattern of misalignment. The underlying pathology involves the intrinsic and extrinsic ligaments, so partial carpal fusion of the lunate and triquetrum is unsuccessful in controlling the misalignment. Neither an isolated fusion of the LTq joint nor any sort of tendon reconstruction is likely to reliably correct such a complex unstable condition. Halikis and associates[36] suggested adding an RL fusion to the LTq fusion. As an alternative, the ulnar midcarpal joint, between triquetrum and hamate, may be included in the fusion site. There is little guidance in the literature about this condition.

Acute perilunate instability (combined SL and LTq instability). Stage III perilunate instabilities involve a combination of injuries around the lunate, including complete rupture of the SL and LTq interosseous ligaments. If the LTq injury is not treated, carpal instability is more likely to result, and the outcome will be worse than that of an isolated injury. Owing to their inherent instability, all perilunate dislocations are best managed surgically. Treatment of perilunate dislocations is discussed in more detail later in this chapter.

Chronic perilunate instability (SL plus LTq instability). When not adequately addressed, most perilunate injuries evolve into a state of permanent misalignment (i.e., carpal collapse into either VISI or DISI) with reduced wrist motion, decreased grip strength, progressive joint degeneration, and painful synovitis.

There is little information in the literature about this specific problem. Generally, when the proximal row presents with a combined SL and LTq dissociation, most authors recommend a proximal row carpectomy.[114] Alternatively, excision of the

CRITICAL POINTS *LTq Arthrodesis*

Indications

- Dynamic LTq instability secondary to complete intrinsic ligament rupture in the absence of an ulnocarpal abutment syndrome (i.e., normal TFCC) and normal midcarpal joint
- Perilunar SL and LTq instability
- No radiographic evidence of VISI

Preoperative Evaluation

- Positive LTq ballottement test
- Fluoroscopic evaluation of abnormal proximal–distal shift of the triquetrum during radioulnar inclination
- Arthroscopy to rule out TFCC degeneration or triquetrum–hamate impingement

Technical Points

- Perform a dorsal (e.g., zigzag, lazy "S," or longitudinal) incision centered at the IV–V septum.
- Perform a longitudinal incision of the extensor retinaculum along the V compartment.
- Open the septum between IV–V; coagulate intraseptal artery.
- Perform a Z capsulotomy creating two flaps following the fiber-splitting concept.[10]
- Complete section of the remnants of LTq ligaments.
- Open the LTq as a book and remove the adjacent articular surfaces with a dental rongeur to expose cancellous bone. Do not excise the rim of the opposing cortical edges to preserve the normal intercarpal separation.
- Harvest cancellous bone from the radius through a window created under the infratendinous sheath at the floor of compartment IV.
- Two 1.5-mm nonparallel K-wires are preset in the ulnar aspect of the triquetrum. Bone graft is densely packed in the biconcave cavity.
- The joint is reduced, and two K-wires are driven into the lunate and their position verified.
- One wire is used to insert a headless cannulated compression screw. Beware of the dorsal branch of the ulnar nerve.
- Cut the second wire below the skin's surface.
- Perform standard capsular and retinacular closure.

Postoperative Regimen

- Short arm thumb spica cast for 6 weeks, changed at 10 days for stitch removal and radiographs
- At 6 weeks, cast removal, radiographs, and new cast applied
- Out-of-cast radiographs until healing is obvious, at which point wires are removed under local anesthesia
- Rehabilitation after cast removal to regain motion and grip strength
- Contact sports not allowed until 6 months postoperatively
- Probable outcome: 75% of patients have a painless wrist with 80% of global motion and 75% grip strength

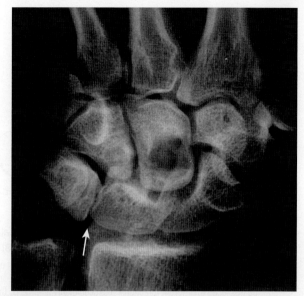

FIGURE 13.46 Late degenerative changes of static lunotriquetral (LTq) dissociation. Note the typical step-off in the LTq interval, a break in Gilula's line (*arrow*), and the midcarpal (hamate–lunate) articular deterioration involving cystic formation within the head of the capitate. Radioscaphoid–lunate joints are usually spared.

outweighs the minimal morbidity from pinning the joint. By ensuring complete immobilization of the joint with wires, the wrist can be mobilized earlier (at 4 weeks), which allows a much faster recovery of motion.

For chronic instability without carpal collapse, we have had very encouraging experience with the ECU tendon reconstruction suggested by Shin and colleagues[98] (see Figure 13.44). It is an anatomically sound solution for chronic, dynamic LTq dissociation because it replaces the most important stabilizer of the joint—the palmar LTq ligament.

We seldom perform LTq fusions, owing to the substantial rate of complications. When there is no other alternative than fusing the joint, we prefer the method described by Guidera et al,[33] in which the empty space left in the LTq joint, after resecting cartilage and subchondral bone from the central portion of the two articular surfaces, is filled with abundant, tightly packed cancellous bone graft from the distal radius. Thus, the joint is stabilized by multiple K-wires or a compression screw (see Figure 13.45). We believe it is important to check to see whether there is a relatively long ulna because, if there is an ulna-plus variant, lunate–triquetrum fusions tend to remain symptomatic. In such instances, it is better to add a "wafer" procedure or an ulnar shortening to the LTq fusion. We do not recommend an LT fusion if there is static carpal misalignment (i.e., VISI) or a chronic SL and LTq dissociation. Our first choice for the former would be fusion of the RL and LTq joints and, for the latter, an RSL fusion plus a distal scaphoidectomy.

Nondissociative Carpal Instability

As stated previously, a painful wrist is said to have a CIND pattern of instability when there is dysfunction of the radiocarpal and/or the midcarpal joints with complete integrity of the ligaments connecting the bones of the proximal and distal rows.[8,28,50,56,118,119] Depending on which joints are affected the most, CIND problems can be further subdivided into

scaphoid and triquetrum, while fusing the LC joint, may also give good results. The long-term comparative outcomes of these approaches are unknown. A less radical, motion-sparing solution for this problem is spiral tenodesis, described by Chee et al in 2012[13] (Figure 13.46).

❖ AUTHORS' PREFERRED METHOD OF TREATMENT: LTq Dissociation

We believe that acute tears of the LTq ligaments are best treated by percutaneous LTq joint fixation with Kirschner wires and cast immobilization. The good ligament healing obtained

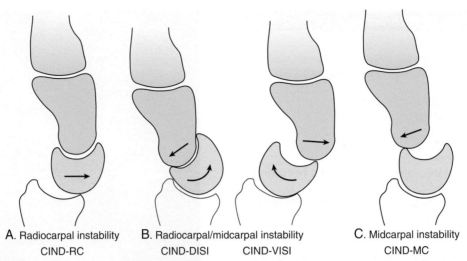

A. Radiocarpal instability
CIND-RC

B. Radiocarpal/midcarpal instability
CIND-DISI   CIND-VISI

C. Midcarpal instability
CIND-MC

FIGURE 13.47 Simplified representation of the four types of carpal instability nondissociative (CIND), and the most common displacements involved (*arrows*). **A,** Radiocarpal instability (CIND–RC), in which the entire carpus is dissociated from the radius and ulna and may be displaced in different directions, most commonly ulnarly. **B,** Combined radiocarpal and midcarpal, also known as proximal row instability, where there is instability at both levels: the proximal row rotating either volarly (CIND–VISI) or dorsally (CIND–DISI). **C,** Pure midcarpal instability (CIND–MC): this is an uncommon type in which only the midcarpal joint is unstable, the radiocarpal joint being normal, or following fusion to the radius.

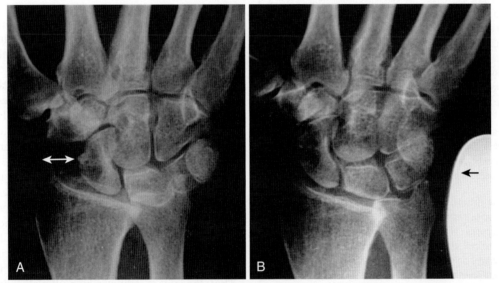

FIGURE 13.48 Ulnar translocation in a 50-year-old woman with rheumatoid arthritis. **A,** Widened radial styloid–scaphoid space (*white double arrow*). **B,** This unstable situation can be easily reduced by laterally directed pressure (*black arrow*).

radiocarpal, midcarpal, and combined radiocarpal–midcarpal (Figure 13.47). Combined radiocarpal–midcarpal instability is also known as "proximal row instability" and has two distinct varieties: CIND–VISI (i.e., flexion rotation of the proximal row with a tendency of the capitate to sublux volarly) and CIND–DISI (i.e., extension rotation of the proximal row with a dorsal capitate sublux tendency).

Radiocarpal Instability. Radiocarpal CINDs occur in patients with excessive laxity, insufficiency, or rupture of the radiocarpal ligaments. In these cases, the carpal condyle can be easily displaced beyond normal limits down the slope of the radius. With time, further stretching of the capsule may occur, and the carpus becomes permanently translocated.[8,78] This condition is

commonly seen in rheumatoid patients or in patients with developmental deformities such as the Madelung deformity (Figure 13.48). Posttraumatic radiocarpal instability is less frequent, most often associated with a distal radial malunion or the result of a pure radiocarpal dislocation.[22] In rheumatoid patients, the radiocarpal ligaments fail as a result of the attritional effects of synovitis. The displacement is not always anteromedial; if the instability is due to a malunion, the carpus may displace in a dorsal or dorsoradial direction, depending on the direction of the deformity. The most common form of radiocarpal CIND, however, is ulnar translocation.

The first traumatic ulnar translocation of the carpus caused by complete disruption of the extrinsic ligaments was described by Rayhack and associates.[78] There are two types of ulnar translocations. Type I involves displacement of the entire carpus, including the scaphoid, and the distance between the radial styloid process and the scaphoid is widened.[13,108] In type II, the relationship between the distal row, the scaphoid, and the radius remains normal. The SL space is widened and the LTq complex is ulnarly translocated.

The distinction between type I and type II is important for various reasons. Conceptually, type I is a true CIND instability, whereas type II is a combined SL and RL injury—a condition already discussed as stage V SL dissociation.[13] In practice, distinguishing between the two types is essential because different ligaments are involved that require differing treatment; type I injuries result from failure of all radiocarpal ligaments, including the RS and RSC. In type II injuries, neither the RSC ligament nor the RS ligament is ruptured; however, there is complete SL and RL ligament disruption. When presented with a widened SL joint, the possibility of an ulnar translation of the LTq complex (type II injury) must be kept in mind to avoid misdiagnosis. If a type II ulnar translocation is treated by stabilizing only the apparent SL dissociation, the underlying radiocarpal instability remains unresolved. If easily reducible, type II is an excellent choice for spiral tenodesis (see SL dissociation, stage V, and Figure 13.35).

As described in the discussion of the radiographic examination of carpal instabilities, a variety of methods for assessing ulnar translation have been reported. None is universally reliable. The indices using the center of the capitate head as a carpal reference should not be used in type II injuries because in those cases only the LTq complex is significantly displaced.[120] On the other hand, when using the lunate as a reference, if the wrist is slightly radially or ulnarly inclined, the measurements may be unreliable. Dynamic stress views under fluoroscopy are useful in the assessment of this type of instability. When the joint is axially loaded in radial inclination, the proximal row is brought into maximal flexion. If the dorsal radiocarpal ligament is disrupted or elongated, the axial load induces abnormal ulnar translation of the lunate beyond the sigmoid notch of the radius.

Rayhack and associates[78] reported a single series of eight patients with traumatic ulnar translocation of the carpus. Their experience indicates that this is a difficult problem to treat. They had disappointing results with delayed ligament repairs and suggested that probably a radiocarpal fusion is the only reliable alternative for such patients[28,36] (see Figure 13.37).

Isolated Midcarpal Instability. Strictly speaking, the term *midcarpal instability* should only be used to describe cases where the midcarpal joint is unstable but not the radiocarpal joint. In reality, most unstable midcarpal joints are associated to a variable degree of radiocarpal instability. One condition with potential for developing a pure midcarpal instability would be the wrist with incompetent midcarpal ligaments after radiocarpal fusion or a hemiimplant arthroplasty.[118] When loaded in full flexion, those wrists could exhibit capitate subluxations or even dislocations over the edge of the fixed proximal row. This is a theoretical possibility, however, that has not been published yet.

Volar Instability of the Proximal Row (CIND–VISI). Often referred to as "palmar (or anterior) midcarpal instability," this condition was first described in 1934 by Mouchet and Belot.[21] It is usually seen in patients with attenuation or rupture of the palmar

midcarpal ligaments associated with insufficiency of the dorsal radiocarpal ligament. The proximal row remains flexed (i.e., VISI) until near the end of ulnar inclination, where it suddenly rotates into extension. This phenomenon has been termed the "catch-up" clunk[27,56,118] (see Video 13.3).

Pathomechanics. As discussed previously, under axial compressive load, the proximal row tends to rotate into flexion and pronation, a tendency that is normally constrained by the palmar midcarpal crossing ligaments.[7,23] Especially important stabilizers are the palmar TqH ligament, the palmar TqC ligament, the dorsolateral STT ligament, and the SC ligament. These ligaments not only play a key kinetic role in preventing midcarpal collapse but also are essential to ensure a smooth, progressive transition of the proximal row from flexion to extension as the wrist inclines ulnarly. Consequently, any injury or condition resulting in increased laxity of the TqH, TqC, STT, and SC ligaments is likely to have two consequences: (1) a kinetic instability (i.e., loss of the ability to transfer loads adequately without collapsing); and (2) a kinematic problem in which the transition of the proximal row from flexion to extension is sudden and sometimes painful, rather than smooth and progressive, when the wrist reaches a certain amount of ulnar inclination (Figure 13.49). In the laboratory, several studies have addressed the intricate mechanism of stabilization of the proximal row. The consequences of sectioning the midcarpal crossing ligaments are better understood but, comparatively, little is known about what causes these ligaments to fail.

Diagnosis. Proximal row instability seldom results from injury of one specific ligament. Most have congenital laxity with poor neuromuscular control, plus some sort of repetitive stress initiating the symptoms. In these cases, there is an obvious sag

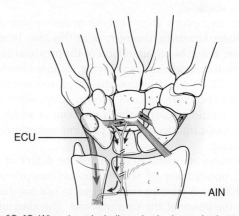

FIGURE 13.49 When the wrist inclines ulnarly, the proximal row undergoes a progressive extension. In some cases, however, that extension is not smooth and progressive—that is, the proximal row suddenly rotates at the end of ulnar inclination. What follows is a tentative explanation of why this happens. Because the wrist's center of rotation during radioulnar inclination lies around the center of the head of the capitate, all ligament fibers inserted proximal or radial to it are likely to increase in tension (*small arrow*) as the wrist inclines ulnarly. These fibers contain mechanoreceptors able to detect changes in tension. When taut, they send afferent messages (*red arrows*) through different nerves, here represented by the anterior interosseous nerve (AIN). These messages return in the form of efferent orders to those muscles (here represented by the extensor carpi ulnaris [ECU]) in which contraction (*blue arrow*) most effectively can realign with the proximal row. When this feedback mechanism fails, the proximal row does not extend until the hamate comes into contact with the lunate, forcing its sudden extension. It is the so-called "catch-up clunk."

of the wrist in the palmar direction, indicating a palmar translation plus supination of the distal row relative to the forearm—a misalignment that corrects itself in ulnar inclination.[28,118]

The role of arthroscopy in the diagnosis and grading of nondissociative instability is minimal. Under traction, the elongated palmar capsule allows greater joint separation than normal, but the palmar ligaments usually look normal.[52] In long-standing cases, recurrent subluxation may have caused degenerative changes at the proximal pole of the hamate, which can be assessed and often treated arthroscopically with debridement or drilling.

Physical examination. A useful maneuver to determine the amount of midcarpal joint laxity is the midcarpal shift test, described by Lichtman and colleagues.[56] It consists of reproducing the painful clunk by passive palmar translation and ulnar inclination of the wrist in pronation. Based on how much force is necessary to maintain the wrist palmarly subluxed in ulnar inclination, wrists are classified into five grades. In grade I, the palmar midcarpal ligaments are so tight that the distal row can hardly be displaced palmarly. Grades II and III can still be found in normal individuals and represent increasing levels of midcarpal laxity allowing the palmar sag to be obtained in ulnar inclination, although it reduces when the applied force is removed. In grade IV, subluxation is easily achieved, and the wrist remains subluxed after removal of the external force. Grade V instability occurs when the patient can actively reproduce and maintain the palmar sag in ulnar inclination without assistance from the examiner.

Radiographic examination. Radiographs usually show a VISI pattern of misalignment, especially on unsupported lateral views compared with the opposite wrist. In the frontal view, the scaphoid is foreshortened and exhibits the ring sign, whereas the lunate has a moon-like appearance, its concave surface facing the scaphoid.

Cineradiography is always helpful in cases where there is a predominant kinematic disorder, as in this one. In a normal wrist, there is synchronized motion of the proximal carpal row from flexion to extension as the wrist inclines ulnarly. In the wrist with CIND–VISI, the proximal carpal row remains flexed throughout the entire range of motion except when the wrist reaches a certain ulnarly inclined position, at which point it suddenly snaps into an extended position, sometimes with an audible clunk.

Stress views are useful to determine the degree of laxity or ligament insufficiency of the various radiocarpal–midcarpal joint stabilizers. A traction view is useful to rule out disruptions between the bones of the proximal row. The anterior drawer view[20] is recommended under fluoroscopic visualization. In this test, the distal row is translated palmarly, and the relationship between the scaphoid, lunate, and distal row is observed. If the STT joint widens palmarly (i.e., the so-called "yawning sign"), the STT and SC ligaments are probably stretched or excessively lax (see Figure 13.17). If there is also palmar LC subluxation, the ulnar midcarpal ligaments must be somehow incompetent. It is important to compare such findings with the contralateral normal side.

Differential diagnosis. When the radiographs of a clunking wrist reveal abnormal flexion of the proximal row (i.e., VISI), the differential diagnosis must include LTq instability. The diagnosis can be established by using the LTq ballottement and shear maneuvers.[79,82] Both tests are negative in nondissociative instabilities and induce pain and a typical grinding sensation when there is LTq dissociation. Radiographically, the SL and LTq angles are normal in nondissociative instabilities, whereas they may be altered in wrists with dissociative instability (see Figure 13.42). When the LTq ligaments are completely torn, the triquetrum appears proximally migrated relative to the lunate in the ulnar inclination stress test; this does not occur in a wrist with nondissociative instability. When in doubt, arthroscopy is recommended. Inspection with a probe shows a tightly closed LTq intercarpal space in nondissociative instabilities and a space easily opened up if there is substantial ligament damage of the LTq-stabilizing ligaments.[100]

Treatment. Several strategies have been recommended for the painful CIND–VISI. Patients should initially be treated by splint immobilization, antiinflammatory medication, and avoidance of activities that reproduce the painful clunk. In the initial inflammatory phase, the wrist should be protected by the so-called "pisiform boost splint," a gutter splint with padding to the volar surface of the pisiform that maintains the proximal row neutrally aligned (Figure 13.50). When symptoms have subsided, a supervised therapy program to reestablish adequate proprioceptive control of the wrist may help eliminate further symptoms.[35]

Excessive flexion of the proximal row can be dynamically controlled by the coupled action of the FCU and ECU muscles. Isometric contraction of the FCU muscle generates a dorsally directed force onto the triquetrum via the pisiform, which helps stabilize the proximal row in a neutral position.[54] Concomitant isometric contraction of the ECU pronates the distal row relative to the proximal row, further promoting reduction of the VISI misalignment. Poor proprioception and inadequate neuromuscular control are probably what differentiates symptomatic from asymptomatic wrists.[35,54,118]

When all conservative measures have failed to control the symptoms of patients with CIND–VISI, the following three options exist: capsular shrinkage, ligament reconstruction, and limited intercarpal arthrodesis.

- *Capsular shrinkage:* Based on experience with other joints, electrothermal shrinkage of insufficient or stretched ligaments has been proposed for the stabilization of CIND–VISI.[52] Local heat is applied to the loose palmar midcarpal and dorsal radiocarpal capsule to create areas of collagen damage.[100] Fibroblasts grow into the injured tissues, building a new structure simulating normal tissue. Despite some promising reports, the use of capsular shrinkage in this field is still considered experimental. See Chapter 17 for further details about this technique.

- *Soft tissue reconstruction of the midcarpal ligaments:* In the past, most attempts to resolve CIND–VISI through a soft tissue procedure were based on the assumption that the underlying pathology was an elongation of both TqH and TqC ligaments.[56,104,118] In most instances, surgery consisted of reefing or advancing the portion of capsule that contains these ligaments. Most attempts, however, failed and symptoms persisted.[56] Recreation of the palmar TqC and dorsal radiocarpal ligaments with a tendon graft was also proposed (Figure 13.51); however, no long-term results are ready to be published.[118] Again, it is implausible that a tendon graft can adequately simulate the mechanical properties of these

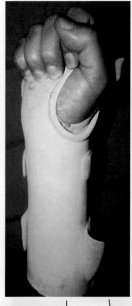

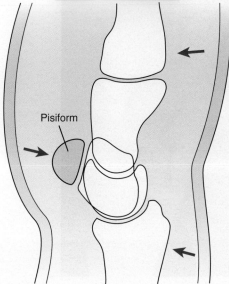

FIGURE 13.50 In the initial inflammatory phase, wrists with a painful carpal instability nondissociative–volar intercalated segmental instability should be protected by the so-called "pisiform boost splint"—a three point (*red arrows*) gutter splint (*left*) with padding on the volar surface of the pisiform that maintains the proximal row neutrally aligned (*right*).

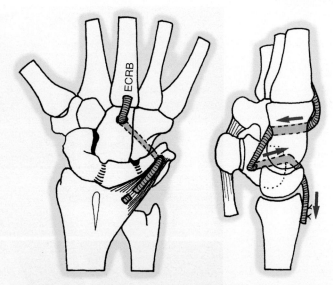

FIGURE 13.51 The author's preferred tenodesis procedure to reinforce the two major ligament problems in cases of a carpal instability nondissociative–volar intercalated segmental instability. A distally attached strip of the extensor carpi radialis brevis (ECRB) tendon is raised and passed through holes in the capitate and triquetrum (*red arrows*) to recreate the ulnar limb of the arcuate ligament (triquetrum–capitate fascicles) and the dorsal radial triquetrum ligament.

highly specialized and tensioned ligaments over a prolonged period and heavy use.

- *Limited intercarpal arthrodesis:* Limited midcarpal arthrodeses (mostly triquetrum–hamate fusions) have also been recommended for this type of instability[32,56] (Figure 13.52). In a study comparing the results of fusions with those of a variety of soft tissue reconstructions, Lichtman and colleagues[56] confirmed the advantage of the former in the treatment of patients with CIND–VISI. All of them were able to return to their normal level of activity with less than one-third loss of motion and no clunking. However, later publications have been less enthusiastic about such an approach.[32] Although this type of procedure is effective in eliminating the carpal clunking, this is achieved at the expense of creating a painful RS impingement. Furthermore, when the mid-

carpal joint is fused, DT motion is unnaturally performed by the radiocarpal joint[18,70]; this eventually results in either a dorsolateral overload of the scaphoid fossa or a progressive deterioration of the LTq.

More recently, it has been suggested that carpal clunking may also be eliminated by fusing the RL joint instead of the midcarpal joint.[28,36,118] By fixing the lunate to the radius, the cornerstone of the carpus is placed in a neutral position, allowing more stable midcarpal motion. The lunate is fused with crossed K-wires and a corticocancellous graft to preserve normal carpal height, allowing the scaphoid and triquetrum to move normally. Not only does the clunking disappear but also the wrist retains a substantial amount of motion, mostly along the dart-throwing plane. Certainly, RL fusion allows a more natural way of moving the wrist.[28]

Dorsal Instability of the Proximal Row. In dorsal instability of the proximal row (i.e., CIND–DISI), the wrist appears normally aligned except in ulnar inclination, where a dorsal subluxation of the capitate may appear, often with a clunk. These are often called "dorsal midcarpal instability" or "capitate-lunate instability pattern" (CLIP) wrists.[44] The posterior drawer test is useful to assess this type of condition.

If the capitate can be passively translocated beyond the dorsal edge of the lunate with manual dorsal translation of the hand while stabilizing the radius, the dorsal intercarpal ligament is attenuated, lax, or congenitally deficient. The RSC ligament is generally stretched in this condition as well. In ulnar inclination, slight subluxation of the capitate may occur. In normal wrists, the alignment should return to normal after the dorsally directed force is removed. When minimal force is necessary to dislocate the capitate in neutral position, a posterior midcarpal instability is likely.[28,56,118] The posterior drawer test is also useful to assess radiocarpal instability.[120] A dorsal tilt of the lunate causing anterior widening of the joint is indicative of a lax palmar RL ligament (see Figure 13.17).

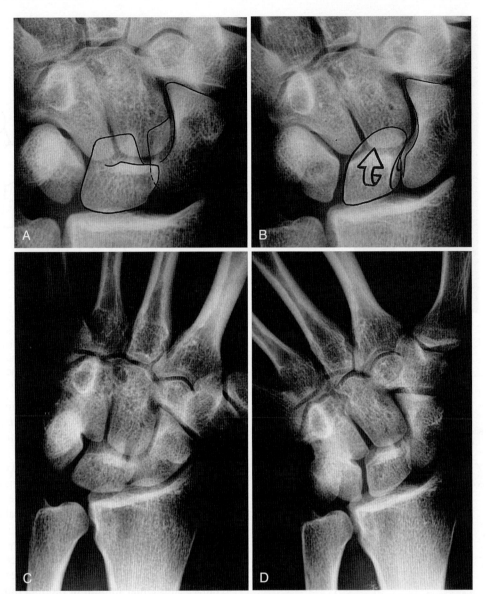

FIGURE 13.52 A 21-year-old man sustained a hyperextension injury to the right wrist 2 years earlier. Since then, there has been painful clunking during radioulnar inclinations. Dynamic radiographs showed a sudden shift (*arrow*) of the lunate and scaphoid from a flexed **(A)** to an extended **(B)** position as the wrist reached a certain degree of ulnar inclination. Conservative treatment did not succeed in relieving the patient's symptoms, and a triquetrum–hamate fusion was performed. Four months after surgery, the patient was back to his former occupation without any complaint. At 18 months of follow-up, the clunking had not recurred but an obviously altered carpal kinematics was evident. From radial **(C)** to ulnar **(D)** inclination, little midcarpal motion exists. Whether such increased radiocarpal shear will result in early degeneration is unknown, but it is a good possibility.

Patients with CIND–DISI should always undergo a dedicated program of physical rehabilitation. In this case, hand therapy should emphasize proprioceptive reeducation of the ECU, ECRL, and ECRB muscles. When these muscles contract, an extension moment to the distal row is generated that results in a shift of the midcarpal joint contact forces from a dorsal position to a more palmar one. Such compressive forces prevent excessive extension of the proximal row.

Failing proprioceptive reeducation, one option is the surgical procedure described by Johnson and Carrera.[44] Through an extended anterior approach to the carpal tunnel, the sulcus that exists between the long RL and RSC ligaments (i.e., space of Poirier) is obliterated with sutures to avoid dorsal translocation of the capitate. According to its proponents, most patients obtain good or excellent results with little loss of motion, especially in extension. Alternatively, a transverse dorsal midcarpal capsulodesis to reinforce the dorsal intercarpal ligament, similar to the one suggested by Gajendran and colleagues,[25,106] may be as effective.

❖ AUTHORS' PREFERRED METHOD OF TREATMENT: Nondissociative Instability

Our assessment of painful clunking wrists is mostly based on a thorough physical examination, plus cineradiography and stress views. The goal is to rule out CID and determine the location and characteristics of the predominant dysfunction. In case of doubt, occasionally arthroscopy is used. In our setting, most nondissociative disorders respond well to conservative treatment. This consists of splinting, avoidance of activities that produce the painful snapping, plus a controlled hand therapy program aimed at maximizing the stabilizing action of the ECU and FCU. Surgery is only indicated when the conservative protocol fails to control the patient's symptoms.

We are reluctant to recommend capsular shrinkage as an option in hyperlax individuals with CIND. By creating zones of stiff scarred tissue, radiofrequency may provide some static stability to the joint, but not a long-term solution. Indeed, by applying heat to the capsule, we neutralize the intracapsular mechanoreceptors that provide the proprioceptive information required by the sensorimotor system to ensure long-lasting stability. Without proprioception, a hypermobile wrist is bound to suffer continuous subluxations, cartilage damage, and synovitis, and the condition will ultimately deteriorate rather than improve. In the past at our institution, most patients with a clunking wrist were treated by fusing the triquetral–hamate joint. We have failed to reproduce the encouraging results reported by Lichtman and colleagues.[56] Some patients complained of RS impingement, whereas others disliked not being able to move the hand naturally because midcarpal fusion blocked the DT motion.

Some time ago, we designed a tenodesis procedure that is able to recreate the TqC ligament and augment the dorsal radiocarpal ligament (see Figure 13.51). Two longitudinal incisions (i.e., dorsal and palmar) are used. Two drill holes, 3.2 mm in diameter are made: (1) one from the dorsal aspect of the capitate into the carpal canal and (2) another from the palmar aspect of the triquetrum into its dorsal ridge. A strip of ECRB tendon is passed through the capitate hole, retrieved palmarly, and passed again through the triquetrum hole. The tendon is pulled taut, and sutures reinforcing the remnants of the palmar TqC and TqH ligaments are placed. On the dorsum, the tendon is tightly sutured to the origin of the dorsal–radiocarpal ligament. Generally, K-wires are used to stabilize the construct further.

The results obtained in seven patients have been promising, with minimal discomfort, excellent grip strength, and minimal loss of motion. All patients returned to their occupations without clunking. Nowadays, this option is used only when the dysfunction is easily reducible, with perfectly normal cartilages. In all other instances, we recommend an RL arthrodesis.

Our experience with the use of RL fusion for the treatment of combined radiocarpal and midcarpal instability, although limited in number, has been most satisfying. Not only were nearly all patients able to return to their previous activities but also the range of flexion–extension at follow-up was only slightly reduced, grip strength was normal, and no clunking recurred.[28] Indeed, patients are happy after an RL fusion because pain and instability disappear at the expense of losing only a moderate portion of wrist mobility.

When surgery is required for dorsal midcarpal instability, we no longer believe in obliterating the space of Poirier with nonabsorbable sutures; such an intervention would excessively decrease the midcarpal extension. In our experience, a dorsal reinforcement of the midcarpal capsule by using the capsulodesis technique[25,106] is less morbid, and it is as effective as other soft tissue procedures.

Carpal Misalignments

The introduction of this chapter emphasizes that ligament injury, wrist instability, and carpal misalignment, although frequently associated, are independent events—the presence of one does not necessarily imply the presence of the other two.[2] Indeed, not all wrists with a ligament injury develop carpal instability, and not all unstable wrists are misaligned. The previous section discussed carpal instabilities secondary to ligament injuries. This section reviews the "adaptive misalignments" (i.e., the carpal misalignment that is not caused by a ligament injury).

The concept of adaptive misalignment was introduced in 1984 by Allieu[1] to refer to those conditions where carpal misalignment is not a sign of instability but a way to preserve global joint congruity in the presence of a deformed bone. An adaptive carpus is a normal joint that adjusts its alignment to compensate for extracarpal defects. The adaptive misalignment is there to preserve joint coherence.[1,28] Usually, if the bone deformity is corrected, the misalignment disappears and no ligament reconstruction is needed. However, if the misalignment continues for a prolonged period of time, the taut ligaments may stretch and progress toward a true carpal instability problem. In other words, if the cause of an adaptive misalignment is not corrected early enough, the wrist may deteriorate and become unstable with time. Thus, early detection and correction of the deformity that is causing an adaptive misalignment are always recommended. What follows is a review of the most common adaptive misalignments of the carpus.

Carpal Misalignment Secondary to Deformity of the Distal Radius

If not properly reduced and immobilized, distal radial fractures may heal significantly misaligned. Of all possible deformities, the most frequent involves radial shortening plus extension, radial deviation, and supination misalignment of the distal fragment relative to the radial shaft. No matter how inclined the distal radial surface is, patients always try to realign the hand along the longitudinal axis of the forearm. Obviously, this implies forcing the wrist into considerable misalignment.

If the distal radial surface is for the most part tilted dorsally, the defect will be compensated for by flexion of the midcarpal joint. Prolonged flexion of that joint, however, tends to distend the dorsal capsule.[27,108] This, together with the lack of tension experienced by the volar midcarpal ligaments when the wrist is flexed, explains the frequent clunking that occurs during ulnar inclination.[108] Similar to the catch-up clunk of nondissociative instabilities, this clunking indicates the presence of a recurrent dorsal subluxation of the capitate over the dorsal edge of the midcarpal socket.

It is important to note that the primary cause of this type of kinematic dysfunction is not ligament insufficiency but radial deformity; there is no ligament repair that will correct this. The misalignment is an adaptive phenomenon that tends to disappear when the radial deformity is corrected. As stated earlier, if the normal alignment of the distal radius is not restored early enough, some ligaments may stretch out, and some portions of capsule may contract. In these circumstances, the wrist may become progressively unstable (i.e., CIND–DISI or CIND–VISI, depending on radius malunion direction), and a corrective osteotomy may not be enough to solve the dysfunction.

If the predominant deformity involves mostly the coronal plane, as when the frontal inclination of the radius is excessively steep or too shallow, a lateral (closing or opening) wedge osteotomy of the distal radius may be indicated. If, aside from radial misalignment, there is excessive radioulnar length discrepancy, a leveling procedure may be required as well. By doing so, the tendency of the carpal condyle to translate ulnarly will be inhibited as a result of the TFCC being pushed against the ulnar corner of the lunate.

When the deformity involves misalignment in more than one plane, as in the Madelung congenital deformity, a tailored corrective osteotomy addressing all rotations and translations is mandatory. Additional soft tissue procedures are seldom necessary. Aside from the clunking phenomenon, patients with distal radius malunion may also complain of pain in the dorsoradial corner of the wrist. This is typically due to midcarpal synovitis induced by the recurrent subluxation of the capitate. With time, if the misalignment is not corrected, permanent damage to the attenuated ligaments may occur, resulting in more pain and nondissociative radiocarpal instability.

In 1985, Taleisnik and Watson[108] reported on a series of 13 patients with a clunking wrist secondary to a distal–radial malunion. A distal–radial osteotomy was performed for 9, and all attained an excellent result. The only failure occurred in one patient who underwent a soft tissue stabilization of the midcarpal joint without correction of the radial deformity. Clearly, this patient was misdiagnosed as a CIND–VISI. Detailed information about the planning and execution of the corrective osteotomy is provided in Chapter 15 .

Carpal Misalignment Secondary to Deformity of the Scaphoid

When an unstable wrist is axially loaded, the scaphoid prevents what Fisk termed *concertina deformity* (i.e., carpal collapse).[21] Not only is scaphoid alignment important but also its own geometry needs to be normal so as not to create a global carpal destabilization. If the scaphoid has fractured into two or more unstable fragments, the distal portion has a tendency to follow the motion of the distal row, whereas the proximal fragment acts in concert with the proximal row.[6] Under such circumstances, the necessary coordinated motion of the two carpal rows is lost, resulting in an abnormal kinematics of the midcarpal joint. When fractured, the scaphoid cannot transfer load normally and acts as an imperfect kinetic linkage between the two rows. Under load, its proximal part tends to follow the unconstrained lunate and triquetrum by rotating into extension, whereas the distal fragment is forced into flexion by the axial force exerted by the trapezoid and trapezium.[6]

If not properly reduced and stabilized, the fractured scaphoid is likely to develop a pseudarthrosis. Stable nonunions rarely have global mechanical consequences. If the nonunion is unstable and motion occurs at the nonunion site, the scaphoid may undergo resorption of its palmar cortex at the fracture site. In these instances, a "humpback" deformity may appear—the distal scaphoid fragment becomes flexed and inclined ulnarward with respect to the proximal fragment. The resultant misalignment can be categorized as CID because the disruption occurs within the proximal row and typically progresses into a DISI pattern of carpal misalignment. In the presence of a scaphoid fracture, DISI should be regarded as an indirect sign of a fracture displacement.

If the scaphoid fracture finally heals, but in a deformed palmar-flexed posture, its external dimensions will not be normal, and the orientation and congruency of its articular facets will be inadequate to perform its important stabilizing role. Scaphoid malunions can be the source of painful instability, weakness, and reduced motion, especially wrist extension.

Surgery for an unstable scaphoid is technically demanding. The surgeon must be aware of the necessity of obtaining fracture consolidation and, most important, of reestablishing the normal length and shape of the scaphoid so that the anatomic relationship between the bone and the rest of the carpus is normalized. A thorough description of the techniques to achieve these goals is provided in Chapter 16.

Carpal Misalignment Secondary to STT Arthritis

Another rather frequent condition that causes scaphoid deformity, and secondarily carpal misalignment, is STT osteoarthritis.[59] For unknown reasons, it begins as an isolated degenerative phenomenon, often bilateral, and rapidly erodes the cartilage and subchondral bone of the distal scaphoid. In such circumstances, the shorter the scaphoid, the more the proximal row extends to compensate for the defect. In the early stages, the resultant misalignment should not be confounded with carpal instability: it is merely an adaptive phenomenon that can become asymptomatic when the normal length of the lateral column is restored, for instance, by means of an interposition implant.

Needless to say, if the misalignment continues long enough, the taut extrinsic volar radiocarpal ligaments may deteriorate and even disrupt, the dorsal RS capsule may contract, and the space of Poirier may become fibrotic. In such circumstances, restoring the scaphoid normal length may not restore the normal alignment. This would be an example of CIND–DISI.

Carpal Misalignment Secondary to Deformity of the Lunate.

Although Kienböck disease is discussed fully in Chapter 16, a brief comment here about the peculiar features of the carpal instability that appears when the diseased lunate collapses is pertinent. One of the prognostic factors of Kienböck disease is the absence (stage 3A) or presence (stage 3B) of abnormal flexion and pronation deformity of the scaphoid. In stage 3A, the carpus remains relatively stable, whereas in stage 3B, it has collapsed. Fragmentation of the lunate results not only in loss of the mechanical strength of the central column but also in a disruption of the kinematic linkage of the proximal row, secondary to slackening of the SL and LTq ligaments. In such circumstances, the loaded scaphoid is apt to follow its natural tendency and progressively collapse into flexion, whereas the triquetrum migrates proximally. Conceptually, the resultant misalignment would be categorized as a CID pattern. Depending on which part of the bone is most involved (i.e., palmar, dorsal, or global), the resultant lunate misalignment may range from neutral to VISI or DISI.

In the past few years, numerous limited intercarpal arthrodeses have been found to be beneficial in the treatment of late stage Kienböck disease. Some of them, especially procedures eliminating motion between the scaphoid and the distal carpal row (i.e., STT and SC joints), are said to be the most effective at unloading the lunate. Despite controversies about their effects on lunate load, these interventions have proved valuable in preserving carpal stability by preventing scaphoid rotary subluxation.

Wrist Dislocations and Fracture–Dislocations

Definition

According to the Mayo Clinic classification, when there is complete rupture of the ligaments binding bones of the same row, the resultant instability fulfills the criteria of a CID.[27,50] If the carpal derangement has preserved the ligaments that connect the bones of the same row, but not the ones that stabilize the radiocarpal and/or midcarpal ligaments, it fulfills the criteria of a CIND. When a carpal derangement shares features of both CID and CIND, the instability can be categorized as a "complex instability of the carpus" (CIC). Acute carpal fracture–dislocations are examples of CIC.

It is important to note that a dislocation is only unstable in the early stages of the injury, particularly if it has not been reduced. With time, the unreduced dislocation becomes stiff, and stiffness is the opposite of instability.[41,43,94,103] Indeed, chronic unreduced fracture–dislocations should not be classified as a carpal instability problem but as a more complex injury that tends to progress to stiffness and degenerative disease.

There are six types of wrist dislocations[94]: dorsal perilunate, lesser arc; dorsal perilunate fracture–dislocations, greater arc; palmar perilunate, lesser or greater arc; radiocarpal; axial; and isolated carpal bone. The first two groups have in common a carpal derangement occurring around the lunate; the first as a pure ligament disruption problem, the second involving one or more fractures of the adjacent bones. The third group, although perilunate, results from a different mechanism producing a palmar displacement of the distal row relative to the lunate. The fourth and fifth groups are nonperilunate dislocations, usually the result of high-energy trauma.

Dorsal Perilunate Dislocations (Lesser-Arc Injuries)

Under the diagnosis of dorsal perilunate dislocation, there are various forms of carpal injury, all confined to a relatively vulnerable area around the lunate (Figure 13.53). They can be pure ligamentous injuries or in combination with fractures of the bones around the lunate (see Chapter 16). Johnson[43] suggested using the term *lesser-arc injuries* to refer to pure perilunate dislocations, as opposed to *greater-arc injuries*, in which one or several bones around the lunate have a concomitant fracture.

Bain et al[5] have expanded this concept further by including the translunate arc, a particular type of wrist dislocation where the lunate has suffered a coronal fracture—the dorsal portion of it displaces together the distal row. This section focuses on lesser-arc injuries: dorsally displaced perilunate dislocations without an associated fracture.

Throughout the literature, there has been a tendency to consider dorsal perilunate dislocations and palmar–lunate dislocations as separate and distinct entities. In reality, as discussed in the pathomechanics section of this chapter, the two conditions represent different stages of the same injury—the so-called "progressive perilunate instability" pattern.[64] When one attempts to reduce a palmarly dislocated lunate, a dorsal perilunate dislocation can be easily reproduced. In other words, the position of the bones when the patient is seen in the emergency department does not reflect the degree of instability or the full extent of the ligamentous damage. Perilunate and lunate dislocations are pathogenically equivalent lesions, and their management is almost identical.

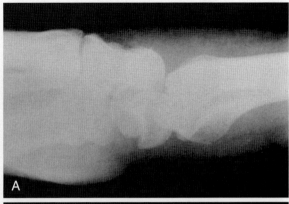
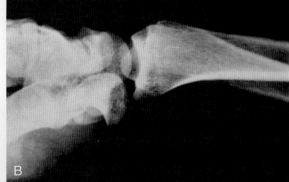
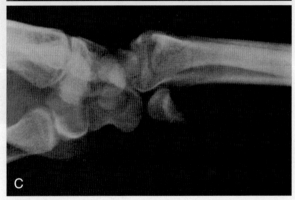

FIGURE 13.53 Carpal dislocations constitute a spectrum of injury, and the initial lateral radiograph in a patient with carpal dislocation may depict a configuration at any point on that spectrum. **A,** "Pure" dorsal perilunate dislocation. **B,** Intermediate stage. **C,** "Pure" volar lunate dislocation.

Another frequent misconception is that when the LC joint dislocates (i.e., the Mayfield stage II), the scaphoid has either fractured or torn its ligamentous attachments to the lunate, but not both. In the literature, perilunate dislocations with a simultaneous scaphoid fracture and SL dissociation have been reported, showing that the two lesions are not mutually exclusive.[14] Most experimentally produced scaphoid fractures have an associated partial SL intercarpal ligament failure. In a multicenter study of 166 perilunate dislocations, Herzberg and coworkers[38] found 6 cases (3.8%) with a concomitant scaphoid fracture and SL dissociation (Figure 13.54).

Treatment of Perilunate Dislocations. In the literature, three major methods of treating carpal dislocations have been suggested: closed reduction and cast immobilization, closed

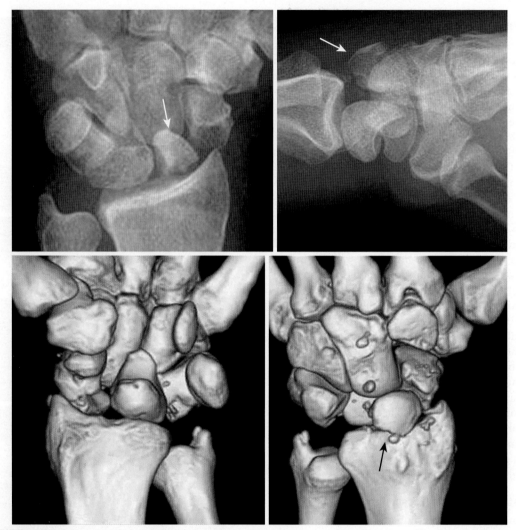

FIGURE 13.54 Posteroanterior (*upper left*) and lateral (*upper right*) radiographs, as well as 3D reconstruction of a computed tomography scan seen from both the volar (*lower left*) and dorsal (*lower right*) sides of the wrist of a patient who sustained a transscaphoid perilunate dislocation with dorsal enucleation of the proximal pole of the scaphoid.

reduction and percutaneous pinning under arthroscopy control, and open reduction and internal fixation.[39,94]

Closed Reduction and Cast Immobilization. Since the 1920s, when case reports of lunate dislocations began to appear, many methods have been suggested for closed reduction. Of importance is the contribution by Böhler, who emphasized the necessity of prolonged continuous traction before attempting to reduce the dislocation.[21] Some authors even considered the use of an external fixator spanning the wrist in old unreduced dislocations to neutralize muscle contraction and apply ligamentotaxis.[102]

Complete muscle relaxation is essential for an atraumatic reduction of a carpal dislocation. General anesthesia, axillary block, and intravenous regional anesthesia (i.e., Bier block) all provide satisfactory muscle relaxation. Local anesthesia or a "hematoma block" does not. An initial period of 10 minutes of uninterrupted traction with the elbow flexed 90 degrees is helpful before reduction begins. During traction, PA and lateral radiographs with the carpus distracted are obtained. These films are valuable in delineating the full extent of carpal damage. When the wrist has been distracted for 10 minutes, traction is

released, and the method of reduction described by Tavernier is attempted as follows[21,94] (Figure 13.55).

With one hand, the patient's wrist is extended (maintaining longitudinal traction), while the thumb of the other hand stabilizes the lunate on the palmar aspect of the wrist. Gradual flexion of the wrist allows the capitate to snap back into the lunate concavity. To facilitate this maneuver, the operator's thumb stabilizes the lunate to prevent it from being displaced forward by the capitate. When the LC joint is reduced, and without releasing traction, the wrist is extended gradually while the lunate is pushed dorsally with the thumb, and a full reduction is usually achieved. The sooner after injury this technique is performed, the easier it is to do the reduction.

Postreduction radiographs are taken. It is imperative to take enough different views and to assess "very critically" the relationship of the capitate and lunate and the position of the scaphoid. An SL angle greater than 80 degrees and an SL gap greater than 3 mm have been shown to indicate a poor prognosis if not corrected.[38,43] The wrist may be initially immobilized with a dorsal short arm and thumb spica plaster splint with the wrist in neutral. Unless operative treatment is medically contraindicated, surgery should be done expeditiously. In the few cases in which closed reduction alone is indicated, most authors recommend at least 12 weeks of immobilization, with weekly radiographic reassessment of the reduction for at least the first 3 weeks. Closed treatment should be continued only when medical reasons contraindicate surgical intervention.

Closed Reduction and Percutaneous Fixation Under Arthroscopic Control. Percutaneous pin fixation is acceptable only if the reduction achieved by closed manipulation of all the perilunate joints is completely anatomic. Minor degrees of

scaphoid malrotation would prevent the SL ligaments from being in contact for proper healing, leading to later SL or LTq instability, or both (Figure 13.56). The introduction of arthroscopy to ensure proper reduction of the carpal displacements has made this alternative more attractive. The technique of percutaneous fixation is as follows.

The hand is prepared with standard surgical preparation. The procedure starts by inserting from two K-wires dorsally, one into the lunate and one into the scaphoid; they are used as joysticks to manipulate and align the carpus into an anatomic reduction. Arthroscopy is performed in the radiocarpal and midcarpal joints to verify carpal bone alignment and carpal posture with the image intensifier.[117] While a knowledgeable assistant holds the lunate wire in the reduced position relative to the radius, a 1.2- or 1.5-mm oblique pin from the radial aspect of the radial metaphysis is inserted across the RL joint under fluoroscopy.

The scaphoid joystick wire is used to reduce the SL joint anatomically, and two slightly divergent pins are inserted transversely from the dorsoulnar corner of the lunate across the SL joint. These wires also can be introduced across the anatomical snuffbox; however, the wires should be placed through a small open incision using drill sleeves to minimize risk to the radial artery and radial sensory nerve branches. The wrist is then inclined somewhat radially to bring the triquetrum up into a reduced position relative to the lunate, and two more K-wires are inserted through a small incision from the anteromedial corner of the triquetrum across the LTq joint. Arthroscopy can be utilized to ensure that wires are intraosseous, and that the SL and LTq joints are anatomically coapted.

Lunocapitate joint mobility is inspected under fluoroscopy. If there is a tendency for the capitate to sublux dorsally in flexion, a further pin is passed across the SC joint. The K-wires are left protruding through the skin, bent at right angles, or cut just under the skin to facilitate later removal. A padded thumb

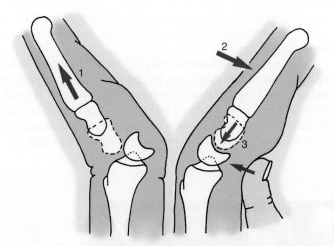

FIGURE 13.55 Schematic representation of Tavernier's method[21,94] of reduction of dorsal perilunate dislocations. With the wrist slightly extended, gentle manual traction is applied (*1*). Without releasing such traction, and while the lunate (L) is stabilized palmarly by the surgeon's thumb, the wrist is flexed until a snap occurs (*2*). This indicates that the proximal pole of the capitate has overcome the dorsal horn of the lunate. At this point, traction is released, and the wrist is brought back to neutral (*3*).

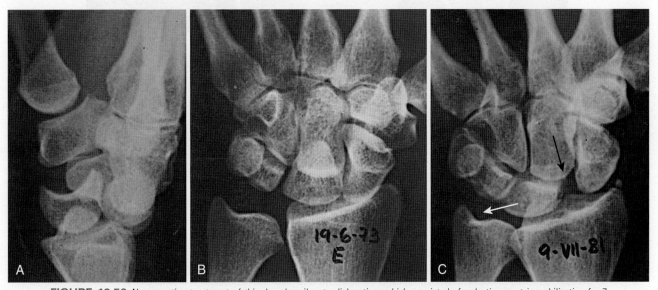

FIGURE 13.56 Nonoperative treatment of this dorsal perilunate dislocation, which consisted of reduction, cast immobilization for 7 weeks, and physical rehabilitation, was considered successful until the patient was assessed 8 years after the injury. **A-C,** Chronic scapholunate dissociation (*black arrow*) associated with ulnar translation of the lunate (*white arrow*) was the result of this suboptimal reduction. The wrist was not unstable, however, it continued to be stiff and painful.

spica splint is applied immediately after the final radiographs have been obtained. This is converted to a thumb spica cast at 7 to 10 days after swelling has subsided and assuming the pin tracts are free of infection. Radiographs are taken in the new cast to ensure proper maintenance of reduction.

The cast and pins are removed at 8 weeks, and immobilization in a dorsal splint is continued for an additional 4 weeks, for a total of 12 weeks after reduction. Until long-term results become available to critically appraise this procedure, a strictly percutaneous technique should be used with some caution. One can be sure though that the most significant drawback of this technique is the fact that it does not address the disruption of the critical dorsal component of the SL ligament, a factor that has been shown to lead to diminished long-term outcomes.[38,109]

Suboptimal reductions of perilunate dislocations will inevitably lead to poor long-term results[38] (see Figure 13.54). Even when an acceptable restoration of the anatomy has been obtained, one must consider the benefits of an open procedure to ensure adequate repair of the dorsal SL interosseous ligament, and to avoid missing osteochondral defects and loose intraarticular bone or cartilage fragments that may lead to poor outcomes.

Open Reduction and Internal Fixation. Generally, open surgery of a carpal dislocation is likely to achieve better results than closed treatment because it allows: (1) complete recognition of all bone and soft tissue damage, (2) removal of interposed soft tissue, (3) removal of unstable chondral fragments, (4) an accurate reduction of bone displacement, and (5) suture of repairable ligaments (Figure 13.57). Many long-term follow-up studies have shown the superiority of open reduction, ligament repair, and percutaneous K-wire fixation over any other alternative in the treatment of perilunate dislocations.[38,109,117] Although some authors still prefer using only a dorsal approach to treat perilunate dislocations,[94] the alternative of combining a dorsal and a palmar approach to allow repair of the palmar LTq ligament, while assessing the reduction and repair of the dorsal SL ligament from the dorsum, is gaining wider recognition.[109]

Some authors recommend using an external fixator to facilitate exposure while protecting the repair.[102] This is especially indicated in longstanding dislocations with extensive fibrosis. In these cases, several days of progressive joint stretching may facilitate surgery. A description of dual-approach treatment of a perilunate dislocation follows in the Critical Points box.

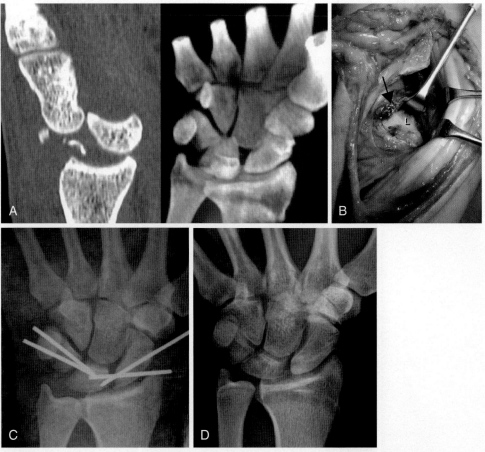

FIGURE 13.57 A 31-year-old male professional motorcycle racer fell during a race. **A,** Computed tomography scan and 3D reconstruction of unreduced perilunate dislocation obtained 3 days after the injury. The dislocation had been missed at presentation. **B,** Surgical approach using an extended carpal tunnel incision allows visualization of the distal surface of the lunate (L). After reduction, the disrupted palmar lunotriquetral (LTq) ligament (*arrow*) was repaired adding further stability to the proximal row. **C,** Placement of stabilizing Kirschner wires across the scapholunate and LTq joints. **D,** Posteroanterior view obtained 8 months after injury. The patient had resumed his racing activities with about a 25% reduction of wrist motion.

CRITICAL POINTS *Perilunate Dislocations: Technique for Open Reduction and K-wire Fixation (Combined Dorsal and Palmar Approach)*

Indication
- All perilunate dislocations, unless unstable medical condition contraindicates surgery

Preoperative Evaluation
- Under axillary block, the dislocation is reduced in the emergency department (Tavernier's maneuver) (Figure 13.55).
- During reduction, traction views are obtained.
- The forearm is elevated in a well-padded above-elbow cast until definitive surgery is possible.

Surgical Approach
- Perform a dorsal 6-cm straight incision centered on the Lister tubercle.
- Open the extensor retinaculum along the third compartment, and expose the second through fourth compartments. Elective neurectomy of the posterior intercarpal nerve may be performed.
- Perform a palmar carpal tunnel incision, extending proximally across the wrist in a zigzag fashion. Flexor tendons and the median nerve are retracted radially.

Usual Findings
- The dorsal capsule is generally found avulsed off the radius. If the dislocation has not been reduced, an obvious empty space between the capitate and radius appears.
- Exploration of the palmar capsule reveals a consistent arciform rent, coinciding with the space of Poirier, coursing along the sulcus between the radiocarpal and long RL ligaments, and ulnarly curving across the palmar LTq ligament (see Figure 13.58). If the dislocation is unreduced, one can see the distal articular surface of the lunate through this rent.

Reduction and Fixation
- The lunate can be easily reduced under direct vision by manually pushing it back in between the capitate and radius, while applying gentle longitudinal traction on the hand.
- The ulnar portion of the capsular rent (i.e., disrupted palmar LTq ligament) is repaired with 3-0 nonabsorbable sutures.

- The lateral portion of the palmar capsular derangement does not need to be repaired because it is an anatomic defect—the interligamentous sulcus between the long RL ligament and the RSC ligament.
- Through the dorsal approach, reduce the LTq joint, stabilize it with a K-wire, and repair the dorsal ligaments.
- Reduce, stabilize, and carefully repair the dorsal SL ligament.
- If the LC joint feels unstable, stabilize it with two crossed K-wires—one through the scaphoid and the other across the triquetrum.
- Obtain radiographs, and assess the quality of the reduction and the purchase of the pins.
- Except for the flexor retinaculum (FR), all anatomic planes are closed with sutures, leaving drains.

Important Tips
- Even if repair of the dorsal ligaments is impossible, their remnants should be tacked back into position; suboptimal repairs may still result in acceptable function.
- Make sure that no osteochondral fragments are left inside the articulation.
- If there is substantial damage of the lunate's cartilage, proximal row carpectomy may be an acceptable solution.
- When present, radial styloid fractures should be reduced anatomically and held with additional K-wire or screw fixation. If the fracture is comminuted, do not excise the unstable fragments so as not to destabilize the radiocarpal ligaments. Molding the fragments back into place as anatomically as possible is recommended.

Postoperative Regimen
- A short arm thumb spica cast is worn for 6 weeks; it is changed at 10 days for stitch removal and radiographs.
- At 8 weeks, cast and wires are removed and rehabilitation to regain range of motion and grip strength starts. A protective removable splint is used between sessions.
- Most patients have some permanent limitation of motion, and several months of rehabilitation are required to regain function. Return to heavy labor is rarely possible before 6 months and more commonly requires up to 12 months.

The dorsal capsule is exposed through a longitudinal incision centered on the Lister tubercle, dividing the extensor retinaculum between the second and third compartments. The fourth compartment is also opened by sectioning the septum between the third and fourth compartments. The capsule often is found disrupted or avulsed at its proximal insertion on the radius. This tear is extended medially following the fibers of the dorsal radiocarpal ligament, and a distally based capsular flap is elevated to uncover the radiocarpal and midcarpal joints.

The palmar approach consists of a carpal tunnel incision extended proximally in a zigzag fashion. The flexor tendons and median nerve are carefully elevated and protected. This allows inspection of the floor of the carpal tunnel, where an lunate-shaped transverse capsular rent along the sulcus between the RSC and long RL ligaments is identified. This capsular rent typically curves proximally across the palmar LTq ligament. Through this rent, the distal articular surface of the lunate can be easily inspected by carefully reproducing the dislocation (see Video 13.4). Before reducing the dislocation, all unstable rem-

nants of the capsule are removed, and the joints are freed from any interposed soft tissue. The lunate is reduced under direct vision by manually pushing it in a dorsal direction while gentle longitudinal traction is applied to the hand. The ulnar corner of the capsular rent, which contains the disrupted palmar LTq ligament, is repaired with nonabsorbable sutures (Figure 13.58).

The carpus is then inspected through the dorsum, and the SL and LTq joints are reduced and stabilized as described previously for the closed percutaneous fixation. Some authors use cerclage wire around the SL joint to provide further stability and allow earlier mobilization. Others insert a headless screw across the SL joint as described for the RASL joint.[60] When possible, direct repair of the dorsal SL and LTq intercarpal ligaments using nonabsorbable sutures is recommended.[39,61]

A reduction clamp to approximate the dissociated bones and facilitate a more reliable ligament repair may be useful. The two ends of all disrupted ligaments are intimately approximated to ensure healing. If there is an associated radial styloid fracture, the dorsal approach is used to reduce it anatomically and to fix

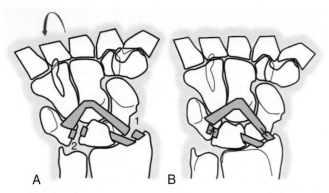

FIGURE 13.58 A, Schematic representation of the two levels of ligament disruption that need to be addressed when approaching a perilunate dislocation (*red arrow*) palmarly: the origin of the radioscaphocapitate (RSC) ligament may have avulsed off the radial styloid (1), and the palmar lunotriquetral ligament often is disrupted through its midsubstance (2). **B,** When properly reduced, the two ligament injuries need to be repaired to recreate or reinforce the distal portion of the ulnar limb of the arcuate ligament (triquetrum-capitate fascicles), and the dorsal radiotriquetral ligament. The apparent rent that exists between the avulsed RSC ligament and the long radiolunate ligament needs no repair because it is an anatomic sulcus (space of Poirier).

it with an additional screw. The postoperative regimen for open treatment of perilunate dislocations is identical to the closed method. If screws are used for fixation of the SL or LTq joints, they should be removed 3 to 5 months after insertion.

Frequently, during the first months after reduction, the lunate may show increased radiodensity. This finding should not be interpreted as posttraumatic Kienböck disease, however, because it tends to progress toward slow recovery without bone collapse in most cases.

According to a multicenter study by Herzberg and colleagues,[38] functional results of open reduction, ligament repair, and K-wire fixation are significantly better than the outcomes with other alternatives, with an average Green and O'Brien wrist functional score of 86 points in stages II and III and 79 points in stage IV (normal score = 100). Similar results have been published by others.[94,40a,109] Patients require a long period of rehabilitation to regain their maximal possible range of motion (~70% of their normal side) and grip strength. Less than one-third of patients are able to return to heavy manual work. With a minimum of 10 years' follow-up, only 8 out of 18 patients treated by Forli et al[24] exhibited a good or excellent clinical outcome; the main problems among the unsuccessful cases were wrist stiffness and articular degeneration.

❖ AUTHORS' PREFERRED METHOD OF TREATMENT: Perilunate Dislocations

All perilunate dislocations need to be reduced by closed means in the emergency department as soon as possible. The reason for such urgency is to decompress the median nerve and to release tension on the vascular supply to the displaced carpal bones. When the dislocation has been reduced, a well-padded bandage is applied, and the forearm is elevated until a definitive surgical treatment can be initiated. If the dislocation has been reduced, delaying the definitive treatment several hours or even a few days to get the right equipment and trained personnel is not a problem, as long as the patient is comfortable with proper analgesia.

We strongly recommend a double-approach open reduction—dorsal SL and palmar LTq ligament repair—and SL and LTq K-wire fixation. I have not used the alternative of reducing displacements anatomically under arthroscopic guidance and stabilizing the SL and LTq joints with temporary screw fixation, as is done in the RASL procedure for SL dissociation. We believe that surgery is always indicated, regardless of the quality of reduction obtained by closed means, unless an underlying medical condition contraindicates it. If the patient is reluctant to allow open surgical treatment, or if an unstable medical condition is likely to persist for more than a week, closed reduction and percutaneous fixation need to be considered. Operative treatment for dorsal perilunate (the Mayfield stage II or III) and palmar lunate (stage IV) dislocations is identical.

Dorsal Perilunate Fracture–Dislocations

Most perilunate fracture–dislocations (i.e., greater-arc injuries) combine ligament ruptures, bone avulsions, and fractures in various clinical forms. The most frequent is the dorsal transscaphoid perilunate dislocation.[38] Much less common, but interesting from a pathomechanic point of view, are dislocations involving a displaced fracture of the capitate[55,111] and dislocations with a displaced fracture of the triquetrum in the sagittal plane.

Transscaphoid Perilunate Fracture–Dislocations. According to most study series, approximately 60% of all perilunate dislocations are associated with a displaced scaphoid fracture, usually in the middle third.[38,94] Most often, the proximal fragment remains connected to the lunate, even if this has undergone a palmar dislocation. The exceptions are rare instances in which there is a concomitant SL dissociation, with the proximal scaphoid being extruded dorsally.[14]

The initial management of transscaphoid perilunate dislocations, including the need for adequate anesthesia and preliminary traction, is identical to the management described for dorsal perilunate dislocations. Radiographs taken with the hand suspended in finger traps are particularly helpful in the assessment of bone damage and should be obtained routinely. Rigid screw fixation of the scaphoid fracture simplifies treatment and rehabilitation because motion can begin before complete healing of the scaphoid fracture. Alternative methods of treatment are as follows.

Closed Reduction and Cast Immobilization. According to Herzberg and associates,[39] the average healing time reported for this injury is 16 weeks when treated with closed reduction and immobilization. The rate of nonunion after treatment approaches 50%.[38] Although not recommended as definitive treatment, the technique for closed reduction is the same regardless of whether the lunate is palmarly displaced or normally aligned, and it is almost identical to that described for lesser-arc injuries. While maintaining some longitudinal traction, the surgeon stabilizes the lunate by pressing the palmar aspect of the wrist with the thumb. From extension, the wrist is gradually flexed. Unless there is some soft tissue interposition, this maneuver brings the capitate back into the concavity of the lunate, sometimes with a snap. The wrist is held in slight flexion and radial inclination, and a padded thumb spica cast is applied.

At this point, it is important to take enough radiographic views to assess the scaphoid fracture reduction. Not only must the scaphoid be anatomically reduced but also the DISI deformity has to be corrected. If one of these two factors is not completely resolved (usually because of capsular interposition between the two scaphoid fragments), open treatment should be performed.

Closed Reduction and Percutaneous Fixation. If surgery is contraindicated, or the patient refuses open treatment, and provided that the dislocation has been acceptably reduced by closed means, percutaneous treatment is an alternative to avoid progressive loss of reduction. Two or more percutaneous K-wires are driven across the fracture, and two additional ones are used to stabilize the LTq joint. If available, arthroscopically guided percutaneous screw fixation may achieve improved results over those obtained using only the fluoroscope.[117] No long-term results have been published, however, to compare these techniques.

Open Reduction and Internal Fixation. Open reduction and internal fixation is the recommended treatment for achieving anatomic reduction of the many structures that need to be repaired (Figure 13.59). The dorsal approach that is used in lesser-arc injuries is utilized. Palmarly, the Russe approach, as described for grafting scaphoid nonunions, is adequate. This approach is mostly used to free the scaphoid fracture from interposed soft tissue, to apply bone graft if necessary, to address palmar comminution, and to repair the capsular tear that typically coincides with the scaphoid fracture.

The sequence of joint reduction is identical to that described earlier. Usually, bone reduction is better controlled from the dorsum by using K-wires as joysticks. If the fracture is to be stabilized with a headless compression screw, this can be done from either approach. Many surgeons prefer free-handed insertion of the screw from the dorsal aspect of the proximal pole aiming at the palmar–distal scaphoid tuberosity.

Different outcome studies using this open approach have been published.[38,94] According to Herzberg and Forissier,[39] the average Mayo wrist function score obtained at 8 years of follow-up in 14 transscaphoid perilunate dislocations treated with early surgery was 79 points, which is considered a good outcome. Most authors agree that this approach allows recovery of ~110 degrees of active flexion–extension and 75% of grip strength. Most reports emphasize, however, that fixation of the scaphoid alone is insufficient. Poor results may ensue from insufficient stabilization of the LTq joint or from an ulnar translation of the carpus. The worst outcomes are found among more severely displaced dislocations (stage IV), especially if the diagnosis was missed or treatment was delayed for any reason.

Transscaphoid–Transcapitate–Perilunate Fracture–Dislocations. The scaphocapitate syndrome consists of a variation of a greater-arc dislocation in which the scaphoid and the capitate are fractured, the latter being displaced with the proximal pole rotating 90 or 180 degrees.[4,111] Although not fully understood, the capitate fracture seems to be produced by direct impact of the bone against the dorsal lip of the radius when the wrist is hyperextended and ulnarly inclined (Figure 13.60). Rotation of the proximal fragment seems to occur secondarily, forced by the distal fragment as it returns to the neutral position.

Because radiographic interpretation of this injury may be confusing, films with the hand suspended in finger trap traction should be obtained routinely. The squared-off end of the proximal capitate is easily seen in this view. Many of these fractures are not recognized at presentation, however. Fenton[4] advocated excision of the proximal pole of the capitate as primary treatment because he believed that avascular necrosis and nonunion were inevitable. Rarely does the proximal capitate fragment heal in its malrotated position, but this is the distinct exception, and numerous necrotic nonunions have been reported in patients treated nonoperatively. By contrast, most cases treated by open reduction through a dorsal approach and internal fixation with K-wires or screws healed uneventfully 2 to 6 months after surgery.[111]

In comminuted cases, primary bone grafting may be indicated. Vance and coworkers[111] recognized six forms of displacement and recommended that the first step in the operative

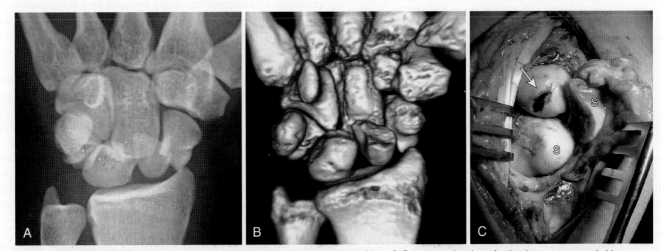

FIGURE 13.59 A 19-year-old man sustained trauma in a motorcycle accident. **A,** Posteroanterior view of wrist shows a transscaphoid perilunate dislocation. **B,** 3D reconstruction of computed tomography scan obtained soon after confirms the injury. **C,** Dorsal surgical approach provided excellent visualization of the structures involved. The two fragments of the scaphoid were completely displaced to each other. Cartilage injury to the proximal pole of the capitate (*arrow*) is quite frequent with this sort of injury, explaining why some patients rapidly develop midcarpal degenerative arthritis. *S,* Scaphoid.

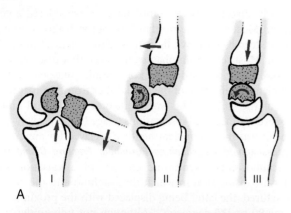

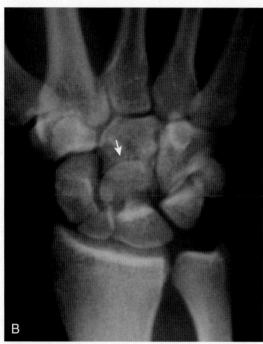

FIGURE 13.60 A, Probable mechanism of fracture–dislocation of the capitate as part of the scaphocapitate syndrome, popularized by Fenton.[21] Extreme wrist hyperextension can result in impaction of the neck of the capitate against the dorsal lip of the radius, causing its fracture (*I*). When the wrist is brought back into neutral position, the roughened surface of the fracture may contribute to further displacement of the unconstrained proximal pole of the capitate in a rotatory fashion (*II*). In some cases, the subsequent axial compression can displace the proximal fragment further, which now appears fully (180 degrees) rotated (*III*). **B,** Posteroanterior view of a wrist with scaphocapitate syndrome, with the proximal capitate fragment fully rotated, its articular portion facing distally (*arrow*).

treatment be reduction and fixation of the capitate fracture. The capitate is generally fixed with a headless screw. If capitate fixation is not done, the distal fragment of the scaphoid tends to migrate medially, making its reduction and stabilization difficult. It is equally important to achieve anatomic reduction and stabilization of the scaphoid and lunate using the techniques previously described. Transient avascular changes in the proximal pole of the capitate are common, but healing usually occurs. The overall long-term results after open reduction and internal fixation have been good.

Transtriquetrum–Perilunate Fracture–Dislocations. As previously explained, the third stage of the Mayfield "progressive perilunate instability" is defined by the occurrence of LTq

dissociation.[45,64] The lunate is constrained by the two strong RL ligaments (i.e., long and short), and a sudden extension moment is exerted by the dislocating distal row via the triquetrum–hamate–capitate ligaments. Such opposing forces usually result in rupture or avulsion, from palmar-to-dorsal, of the LTq ligaments. In about one-fourth of patients, instead of ligament derangement there is either a sagittal fracture of the body of the triquetrum or a proximal pole avulsion fracture, representing a ligament detachment (Figure 13.61). During the open procedure, this fragment should not be excised but replaced carefully in its original position to ensure correct LTq ligament stability. The triquetrum is a well-vascularized bone, and necrosis or nonunion reports have seldom been published after a wrist dislocation.

Late Treatment of Unreduced Fracture–Dislocations. Despite increased awareness of their clinical and radiological features, the diagnosis of perilunate dislocation is still frequently missed at presentation (in 16-25% of the cases, according to a different series), resulting in chronic wrist disorders and degenerative arthritis.[38] Delay in treatment has repeatedly been found to be an important factor influencing the long-term outcome for patients.

Even though it is unclear how late an open reduction can be accomplished, successful cases have been reported 35 weeks after injury[41] (Figure 13.62). This repair generally requires dorsal and palmar approaches. The use of wrist distraction with an external fixator for a week before surgery seems to facilitate open reduction of old dislocations.[102] If the bones can be reduced and fixed anatomically, satisfactory results can be expected. If reduction cannot be accomplished, or if there is significant cartilage damage, either a proximal row carpectomy or a total wrist arthrodesis is indicated. The results of isolated excision of only the lunate are uniformly poor.[41]

Palmar–Perilunate Dislocations

A palmar dislocation of the capitate relative to the lunate is a very rare injury, representing less than 3% of all wrist dislocations[94] (Figure 13.63). They may occur in association with a fracture of the lunate in the frontal plane,[5] or as a result of a progressive perilunate instability induced by a combination of forced hyperflexion and supination of the wrist relative to the radius.[45] In the former, the capitate subluxation is mild and the consequence of the dorsally displaced lunate fracture. In these circumstances, closed treatment is seldom effective, owing to the fracture's inherent instability. Open reduction using palmar and dorsal approaches and internal fixation of the lunate fracture with wires or screws is the method of choice.

In palmarly displaced perilunate dislocations without a lunate fracture, either SL dissociation or a scaphoid fracture is inevitably present. One or the other typically has a very unstable vertical orientation in the frontal plane, making recognition of it difficult on a standard PA view; a diagnosis is more readily apparent on the lateral view. Reported cases with concomitant rupture of extensor tendons suggest that the mechanism of injury is violent. In acute injuries, closed reduction using finger trap traction should be the initial step in management. Although successful treatment has been reported with closed reduction alone, these are exceedingly unstable injuries; in most cases, the only reliable way to realign and stabilize the scaphoid and perilunate injury is operative treatment.

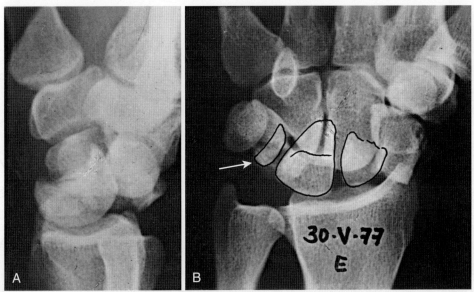

FIGURE 13.61 Lateral (**A**) and posteroanterior (**B**) radiographs of a transscaphoid, transtriquetrum, perilunate dislocation. In this case, there is a sagittal fracture of the triquetrum (*arrow*). The intercarpal lunotriquetral ligaments are probably intact.

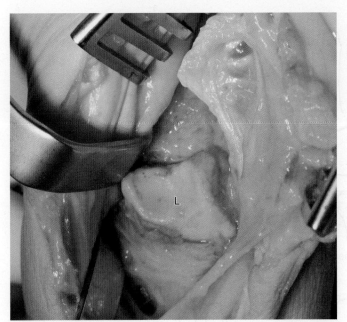

FIGURE 13.62 Volar lunate (L) dislocation was not diagnosed at presentation until median nerve symptoms forced reexamination of the initial radiographs. The wrist was explored at 8 weeks' postinjury with volar and dorsal approaches. The enucleated lunate, surrounded by scar tissue, is demonstrated in the carpal tunnel. The injury was treated with reduction, ligament repair, and Kirschner wire stabilization for 3 months. The final outcome was acceptable, with less than 25% loss of grip strength and 20% loss of range of motion.

Radiocarpal Dislocations

According to Dumontier and coworkers,[22] there are two types of radiocarpal dislocations. Type I includes patients with a pure radiocarpal dislocation, without an associated fracture of the distal radius. Type II involves a radiocarpal dislocation with an avulsion fracture of the radial styloid, which contains the origin of the palmar RS and RSC ligaments. This first type is exceedingly rare; no more than 20 cases have been reported; usually, they are the result of severe shear and rotational injury in young subjects. Associated neurovascular damage is not unusual. Reduction is easy by external manipulation, but maintenance of reduction is difficult because of the loss of radiocarpal ligament attachments. Type II radiocarpal dislocations, with an associated avulsion fracture of the radial styloid, have been reported more frequently. These have a much better prognosis provided that the styloid fracture, which contains the avulsed radiocarpal ligaments, is anatomically reduced and fixed.

Axial Fracture–Dislocations

When the palmar concavity of the carpus is involved in a high-energy dorsal–palmar compression (crush mechanism), a longitudinal disruption of the carpal arch may occur.[80] In most instances, the wrist splits into two axial columns, one remaining normally aligned with the radius and the other shifting in a radial or ulnar direction (Figure 13.64). The metacarpals usually follow the displacement of their corresponding carpal bones, causing an intermetacarpal derangement. As the carpal arch flattens, the FR may either disrupt or avulse from its lateral insertions. Because carpal derangement appears more or less parallel to the long axis of the forearm, Cooney and associates[21] coined the term "axial dislocation" to describe these injuries. Other descriptive terms, such as longitudinal disruption, sagittal splitting, or intercarpal diastasis, may also be appropriate.

Axial dislocations are common in developing countries, where safety measures for wringer-type machines, roller presses, and molding presses are not available. Because of the high energy involved, most patients present with severe associated soft tissue damage, including disruption of the FR with traumatic decompression of the carpal tunnel and subsequent nerve and vascular injuries.

Two major groups of dislocation injuries have been described: axial ulnar and axial radial. In the former, the carpus splits into two columns, with the radial column aligned and stable with respect to the radius, and the ulnar column unstable and displaced proximally and ulnarly (Figure 13.65). In the latter, the

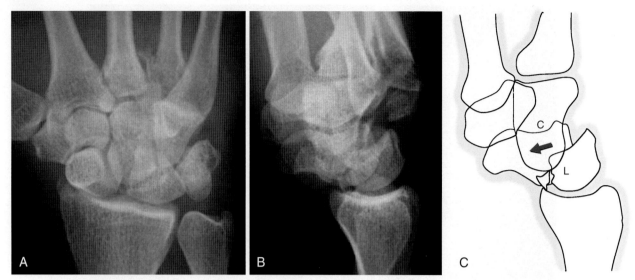

FIGURE 13.63 Example of a rare translunate anterior dislocation of the wrist. **A,** Initial posteroanterior view could be easily diagnosed as a static lunotriquetral dissociation because the lunate (L) shows the typical moonlike configuration. **B,** Careful assessment of the lateral view shows the presence of a fracture of the palmar lip of the lunate and an anterior dislocation of the distal row. **C,** Schematic representation of the sagittal view, demonstrating a capitate subluxation relative to the fractured lunate (*red arrow*).

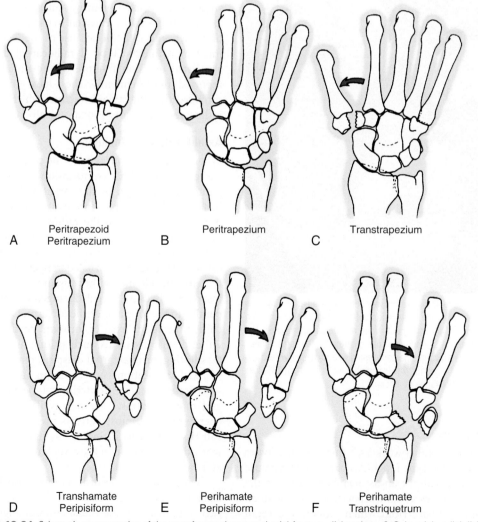

| A | Peritrapezoid Peritrapezium | B | Peritrapezium | C | Transtrapezium |

| D | Transhamate Peripisiform | E | Perihamate Peripisiform | F | Perihamate Transtriquetrum |

FIGURE 13.64 Schematic representation of the most frequently reported axial fracture–dislocations. **A-C,** In axial–radial dislocations, there is an unstable segment displaced in a radial direction. **D-F,** The opposite instability is seen among the axial–ulnar derangements. (From Garcia-Elias M, Dobyns JH, Cooney WP, III, et al: Traumatic axial dislocations of the carpus. *J Hand Surg [Am]* 14:446–457, 1989.[80])

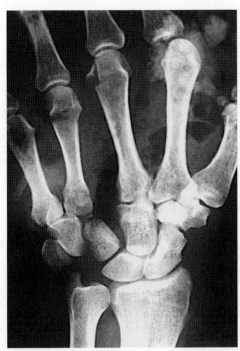

FIGURE 13.65 Perihamate, peripisiform axial–ulnar dislocation. Vertical disruption involves the distal carpal row and the base of the third and fourth metacarpals. The pisiform is ulnarly displaced because it remains attached to the flexor carpi ulnaris tendon complex.

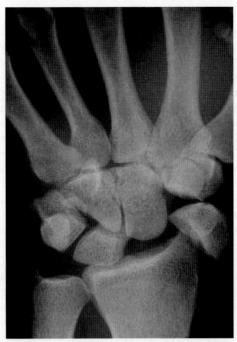

FIGURE 13.66 Anterolateral dislocation of the scaphoid, type I (without concomitant hamate-capitate axial–ulnar dislocation). (Courtesy of Dr. Fabio Urraza.)

ulnar part of the carpus remains normally aligned with the radius, and the radial aspect of the carpus is displaced and unstable.

The tendons within the carpal tunnel have divergent directions when they emerge into the palm. If their corresponding muscles contract, the flexor tendons of the little finger force the hook of the hamate toward the ulnar side. This force would be opposite in direction to the force generated when the FPL contracts against the inner surface of the triquetrum. Such opposing forces tend to open the palmar carpal concavity (i.e., trapezium toward the radial side, hamate toward the ulnar side) if it were not for the presence of the FR and the strong and taut transverse intercarpal ligaments of the distal carpal row. Their annular disposition maintains adequate transverse stability to the carpal arch. Catastrophic failure of these intrinsic carpal ligaments creates a particular type of carpal instability, termed *axial* or *longitudinal*, with the tunnel splitting into two or more unstable columns and moving in divergent directions.

When dealing with these complex fracture–dislocations, a careful assessment of the associated neurovascular and musculotendinous injury is necessary. A radical debridement of devitalized muscle, subcutaneous tissue, and skin is critical. Closed reduction and percutaneous fixation of the displaced bones may be successful, but open reduction and K-wire or screw fixation has yielded more reliable results. A dorsal approach to control bone reduction and an extended palmar approach to assess associated soft tissue injuries are usually required. Repair of the damaged intercarpal ligaments is seldom possible because of the high energy of the injury and ligamentous shredding. In many instances, decompression of the carpal tunnel is unnecessary because the FR has been disrupted or avulsed already by the trauma. In case of doubt, however, inspection of the carpal

tunnel is recommended. Immobilization in a cast for 6 to 8 weeks, depending on the extent of injury, is advisable. Early intensive physical and occupational therapy facilitate rehabilitation. The long-term results are not good, in the most part because of associated tendon and neurovascular involvement.

In less severe dorsal–palmar compressions of the carpal concavity, complete rupture of the transverse intercarpal ligaments between bones of the distal row may occur. If not properly healed, patients may complain of localized discomfort and lack of stability at the dissociated site.

Isolated Carpal Bone Dislocations

When a localized, direct or indirect force is concentrated over a single bone of the wrist, the resulting pressure may be sufficient to cause a localized fracture–dislocation.[47,49] Although the bones of the radial column appear to be more vulnerable to this type of aggression, each carpal bone has been reported to be dislocated. In contrast to axial disruptions, isolated carpal bone dislocations do not imply a global carpal derangement. Actually, except for the lunate and scaphoid, the carpal disorder created by removing the enucleated bone seems to be well tolerated.

Palmar dislocation of the scaphoid is a rare injury, with less than 40 cases reported in the literature.[47] Two clinical forms have been described: isolated anterolateral dislocation of the proximal pole of the scaphoid (type I) and scaphoid dislocation associated with an axial derangement of the capitate–hamate joint (type II) (Figure 13.66). The most probable mechanism of type I injuries involves a violent hyperpronation injury to an extended and ulnarly inclined wrist, causing SL dissociation first, followed by the enucleation of the proximal pole of the scaphoid around the RSC ligament. These injuries also may be the result of a self-reduced palmar–perilunate dislocation, the scaphoid having been left unreduced by capsular interposition.

Type II injuries are thought to involve a high-energy axial compressive load along the third and fourth metacarpals, creating enough shear stress to the capitate–hamate joint to disrupt its strong ligament attachments. None of these mechanisms has been established, however. Diagnosis of the condition is straightforward. An abnormal bony prominence adjacent to the radial styloid has been described frequently. In PA and lateral views, the proximal scaphoid appears enucleated forward and outward, whereas its distal end remains attached to the triquetrum. In type II dislocations, there is also a proximal migration of the capitate and an obvious derangement of the capitate–hamate joint. Closed reduction is easily accomplished by traction and direct manual pressure in most acute cases, all with good results. More recent publications have advocated an open reduction through a dorsal approach, however. Avascular necrosis of the scaphoid has not been reported.

Most reported cases of trapezium dislocation can be described as peritrapezium axial–radial dislocations; that is, the triquetrum appears displaced together with the first metacarpal. Complete enucleations with proximal and distal joint disruption are very rare[40]; usually they are the result of a blow to the dorsolateral aspect of the wrist or a consequence of a hyperextension–supination injury to the radial-inclined wrist. Although some reported cases were openly reduced, excision seems to be a reasonable solution, as shown by the many instances in which trapeziectomy alone has been done, with good patient satisfaction, for the treatment of trapeziometacarpal (TM) arthritis.

Most trapezoid dislocations described in publications manifested with a concomitant displacement of the second metacarpal. According to a literature review by Koenig and West,[49] dislocations of the trapezoid without other associated fractures or dislocations of adjacent bones are very rare. Palmar dislocations may cause attritional rupture of flexor tendons. There is no clear explanation as to how a wedge-shaped bone (wider dorsally) dislocates palmarly. It is plausible that a direct blow, associated with hyperextension of the midcarpal joint, is involved. Successful closed reduction of the dislocated bone has been achieved only in dorsal dislocations. Most volar dislocations of the trapezoid underwent bone excision and localized fusion with acceptable results.

For Case Studies, Videos, and more, please visit ExpertConsult.com.

REFERENCES

1. Allieu Y: Carpal instability—ligamentous instabilities and intracarpal malalignments—explication of the concept of carpal instability. *Ann Chir Main* 3:366–367, 1984.
2. Anatomy and Biomechanics Committee of the International Federation of Societies for Surgery of the Hand: Definition of carpal instability. *J Hand Surg [Am]* 24:866–867, 1999.
3. Andersson JK, Garcia-Elias M: Dorsal scapholunate ligament injury: a classification of clinical forms. *J Hand Surg Eur Vol* 38:165–169, 2013.
4. Apergis E: Scaphocapitate fracture-dislocation. In Garcia-Elias M, Mathoulin C, editors: *Articular injury of the wrist*, Stuttgart, 2014, Thieme, pp 61–65.
5. Bain GI, McGuire DT: Decision making for partial carpal fusions. *J Wrist Surg* 1:103–104, 2012.
6. Berdia S, Wolfe SW: Effects of scaphoid fractures on the biomechanics of the wrist. *Hand Clin* 17:533–540, 2001.
7. Berger RA: The ligaments of the wrist: a current overview of anatomy with considerations of their potential functions. *Hand Clin* 13:63–82, 1997.
8. Berschback JC, Kalainov DM, Husain SN, et al: Traumatic ulnar translocation of the carpus: early recognition and treatment. *J Hand Surg Eur Vol* 37:755–764, 2012.
9. Brigstocke GH, Hearnden A, Holt C, et al: In-vivo confirmation of the use of the dart thrower's motion during activities of daily living. *J Hand Surg Eur Vol* 39:373–378, 2014.
10. Brunelli GA, Brunelli GA: Carpal instability with SL dissociation treated using the flexor carpi radialis and scapho-trapezoid ligament repair: foundations, technique and results of preliminary series. *Rev Chir Orthop Reparatrice Appar Mot* 89:152–157, 2003.
10a. Calandruccio JH, Gelberman RH, Duncan SF, et al: Capitolunate arthrodesis with scaphoid and triquetrum excision. *J Hand Surg [Am]* 25(5):824–832, 2000.
11. Camus EJ, Van Overstraeten L: Dorsal scapholunate stabilization using Viegas' capsulodesis: 25 cases with 26 months follow-up. *Chir Main* 32:393–402, 2013.
12. Cerezal L, de Dios Berná-Mestre J, Canga A, et al: MR and CT arthrography of the wrist. *Semin Musculoskelet Radiol* 16:27–41, 2012.
13. Chee KG, Chin AY, Chew EM, et al: Antipronation spiral tenodesis—a surgical technique for the treatment of perilunate instability. *J Hand Surg [Am]* 37:2611–2618, 2012.
14. Cheng CY, Hsu KY, Tseng IC, et al: Concurrent scaphoid fracture with scapholunate ligament rupture. *Acta Orthop Belg* 70:485–491, 2004.
15. Christodoulou L, Bainbridge LC: Clinical diagnosis of triquetrolunate ligament injuries. *J Hand Surg [Br]* 24:598–600, 1999.
16. Cohen MS: Scapholunate acute repair techniques. In Shin AY, Day CS, editors: *Epub-Advances in scapholunate ligament treatment*, Chicago IL, 2014, American Society for Surgery of the Hand, pp 75–83.
17. Corella F, Del Cerro M, Ocampos M, et al: Arthroscopic ligamentoplasty of the dorsal and volar portions of the scapholunate ligament. *J Hand Surg [Am]* 38:2466–2477, 2013.
18. Crisco JJ, Heard WM, Rich RR, et al: The mechanical axes of the wrist are oriented obliquely to the anatomical axes. *J Bone Joint Surg Am* 93:169–177, 2011.
19. de Smet L, Goeminne S, Degreef I: Failures of the three-ligament tenodesis for chronic static scapholunate dissociation are due to insufficient reduction. *Acta Orthop Belg* 77:595–597, 2011.
20. del Piñal F: Arthroscopic volar capsuloligamentous repair. *J Wrist Surg* 2:126–128, 2013.
21. Dobyns JH, Linscheid RL: A short history of the wrist joint. *Hand Clin* 13:1–12, 1997.
22. Dumontier C, Meyer ZU, Reckendorf G, et al: Radiocarpal dislocations: classification and proposal for treatment: a review of twenty-seven cases. *J Bone Joint Surg Am* 83:212–218, 2001.
23. Feipel V, Rooze M: The capsular ligaments of the wrist: morphology, morphometry and clinical applications. *Surg Radiol Anat* 21:175–180, 1999.
24. Forli A, Courvoisier A, Wimsey S, et al: Perilunate dislocations and transscaphoid perilunate fracture-dislocations: a retrospective study with minimum ten-year follow-up. *J Hand Surg [Am]* 35:62–68, 2010.
25. Gajendran VK, Peterson B, Slater RR, Jr, et al: Long-term outcomes of dorsal intercarpal ligament capsulodesis for chronic SL dissociation. *J Hand Surg [Am]* 32:1323–1333, 2007.
26. Garcia-Elias M: Classification of scapholunate injuries. In Shin AY, Day CS, editors: *Epub-Advances in scapholunate ligament treatment*, Chicago IL, 2014, American Society for Surgery of the Hand, pp 52–62.
27. Garcia-Elias M: The non-dissociative clunking wrist: a personal view. *J Hand Surg Eur Vol* 33:698–711, 2008.
28. Garcia-Elias M, Alomar Serrallach X, Monill Serra J: Dart-throwing motion in patients with scapholunate instability: a dynamic four-dimensional computed tomography study. *J Hand Surg Eur Vol* 39:346–352, 2014.
29. Garcia-Elias M, Lluch L, Ferreres A, et al: Treatment of radiocarpal degenerative osteoarthritis by radioscapholunate arthrodesis and distal scaphoidectomy. *J Hand Surg [Am]* 30:8–15, 2005.
30. Garcia-Elias M, Lluch AL, Stanley JK: Three-ligament tenodesis for the treatment of SL dissociation: indications and surgical technique. *J Hand Surg [Am]* 31:125–134, 2006.
31. Geissler WB: Arthroscopic management of scapholunate instability. *J Wrist Surg* 2:129–135, 2013.
32. Goldfarb CA, Stern PJ, Kiefhaber TR: Palmar midcarpal instability: the results of treatment with 4-corner arthrodesis. *J Hand Surg [Am]* 29:258–263, 2004.
33. Guidera PM, Watson HK, Dwyer TA, et al: Lunotriquetral arthrodesis using cancellous bone graft. *J Hand Surg [Am]* 26:422–427, 2001.
34. Gupta A: Factors affecting the sagittal alignment of the lunate. *J Hand Surg Eur Vol* 32:155–159, 2007.
35. Hagert E: Proprioception of the wrist joint: a review of current concepts and possible implications on the rehabilitation of the wrist. *J Hand Ther* 23:2–16, 2010.
36. Halikis MN, Colello-Abraham K, Taleisnik J: RL fusion: the forgotten partial arthrodesis. *Clin Orthop Relat Res* 341:30–35, 1997.

37. Harvey EJ, Berger RA, Osterman AL, et al: Bone-tissue-bone repairs for SL dissociation. *J Hand Surg [Am]* 32:256–264, 2007.
38. Herzberg G, Comtet JJ, Linscheid RL, et al: Perilunate dislocations and fracture-dislocations: a multicenter study. *J Hand Surg [Am]* 18:768–769, 1993.
39. Herzberg G, Forissier D: Acute dorsal trans-scaphoid perilunate fracture-dislocations: medium-term results. *J Hand Surg [Br]* 27:498–502, 2002.
40. Ichikawa T, Inoue G: Complete dislocation of the trapezium: case report. *Scand J Plast Reconstr Surg Hand Surg* 33:335–337, 1999.
40a. Inoue G, Kuwahata Y: Management of acute perilunate dislocations without fracture of the scaphoid. *J Hand Surg [Br]* 22(5):647–652, 1997.
41. Inoue G, Shionoya K: Late treatment of unreduced perilunate dislocations. *J Hand Surg [Br]* 24:221–225, 1999.
42. International Wrist Investigators' Workshop (IWIW), Terminology Committee: Wrist: terminology and definitions. *J Bone Joint Surg Am* 84(Suppl 1):1–69, 2002.
43. Johnson RP, Carrera GF: Chronic capitolunate instability. *J Bone Joint Surg Am* 68:1164–1176, 1986.
44. Johnson RP: The acutely injured wrist and its residuals. *Clin Orthop Relat Res* 149:33–44, 1980.
45. Jones DB, Jr, Kakar S: Perilunate dislocations and fracture dislocations. *J Hand Surg [Am]* 37:2168–2173, 2012.
46. Kauer JM: Functional anatomy of the wrist. *Clin Orthop Relat Res* 149:9–20, 1980.
47. Kennedy JG, O'Connor P, Brunner J, et al: Isolated carpal scaphoid dislocation. *Acta Orthop Belg* 72:478–483, 2006.
48. Kitay A, Wolfe SW: Scapholunate instability: current concepts in diagnosis and management. *J Hand Surg [Am]* 37:2175–2196, 2012.
49. Koenig TR, West OC: Palmar dislocation of the trapezoid. *Skeletal Radiol* 32:95–98, 2003.
50. Larsen CF, Amadio PC, Gilula LA, et al: Analysis of carpal instability, I: description of the scheme. *J Hand Surg [Am]* 20:757–764, 1995.
51. Larson TB, Stern PJ: Reduction and association of the scaphoid and lunate procedure: Short-term clinical and radiographic outcomes. *J Hand Surg [Am]* 39:2168–2174, 2014.
51a. Lawand A, Foulkes GD: The "clenched pencil" view: a modified clenched fist scapholunate stress view. *J Hand Surg [Am]* 28(3):414–418, 2003.
52. Lee JI, Nha KW, Lee GY, et al: Long-term outcomes of arthroscopic debridement and thermal shrinkage for isolated partial intercarpal ligament tears. *Orthopedics* 35:e1204–e1209, 2012.
53. Lee SK, Zlotolow DA, Yao J: Scapholunate axis method. In Shin AY, Day CS, editors: *Epub-Advances in scapholunate ligament treatment*, Chicago IL, 2014, American Society for Surgery of the Hand, pp 124–135.
54. León-Lopez MM, Salvá-Coll G, Garcia-Elias M, et al: Role of the extensor carpi ulnaris in the stabilization of the lunotriquetral joint. An experimental study. *J Hand Ther* 26:312–317, 2013.
55. Leung YF, Ip SP, Wong A, et al: Transscaphoid transcapitate transtriquetral perilunate fracture-dislocation: a case report. *J Hand Surg [Am]* 31:608–610, 2006.
56. Lichtman DM, Wroten ES: Understanding midcarpal instability. *J Hand Surg [Am]* 31:491–498, 2006.
57. Linscheid RL, Dobyns JH, Beabout JW, et al: Traumatic instability of the wrist: diagnosis, classification, and pathomechanics. *J Bone Joint Surg Am* 54:1612–1632, 1972.
57a. Lluch A: Osteoarthritis of the wrist and DRUJ. In Trail IA, Fleming ANM, editors: *Disorders of the hand*, Volume 3: Inflammation, arthritis and contractures, London, 2015, Springer-Verlag, pp 41–69.
58. Lluch AL, Garcia-Elias M, Lluch AB: Arthroplasty of the scaphoid-trapezium-trapezoid and carpometacarpal joints. *Hand Clin* 29:57–68, 2013.
59. Lluch A, Hooper G, Kapandji A, et al: *Terminology for hand surgery*. Nomenclature Committee of the International Federation of Societies for Surgery of the Hand. London: Hartcourt Health Sciences, 2011.
60. Lombardi JM, Rodriguez RR, Rosenwasser MP: Reduction and association of scaphoid and lunate for scapholunate instability. In Shin AY, Day CS, editors: *Epub-Advances in scapholunate ligament treatment*, Chicago IL, 2014, American Society for Surgery of the Hand, pp 153–162.
61. Luchetti R, Atzei A, Cozzolino R, et al: Current role of open reconstruction of the scapholunate ligament. *J Wrist Surg* 2:116–125, 2013.
62. Luegmair M, Saffar P: Scaphocapitate arthrodesis for treatment of scapholunate instability in manual workers. *J Hand Surg [Am]* 38:878–886, 2013.
63. Majima M, Horii E, Matsuki H, et al: Load transmission through the wrist in the extended position. *J Hand Surg [Am]* 33:182–188, 2008.
64. Mayfield JK, Johnson RP, Kilcoyne RK: Carpal dislocations: pathomechanics and progressive perilunar instability. *J Hand Surg [Am]* 5:226–241, 1980.
65. Megerle K, Bertel D, Germann G, et al: Long-term results of dorsal intercarpal ligament capsulodesis for the treatment of chronic scapholunate instability. *J Bone Joint Surg Br* 94:1660–1665, 2012.
66. Messina JC, van Overstraeten L, Luchetti R, et al: The EWAS classification of scapholunate tears: An anatomical arthroscopy study. *J Wrist Surg* 2:105–109, 2013.
67. Moojen TM, Snel JG, Ritt MJPF, et al: In vivo analysis of carpal kinematics and comparative review of the literature. *J Hand Surg [Am]* 28:81–87, 2003.
68. Moran SL, Ford KS, Wulf CA, et al: Outcomes of dorsal capsulodesis and tenodesis of SL instability. *J Hand Surg [Am]* 31:1438–1446, 2006.
69. Moritomo H, Apergis EP, Garcia-Elias M, et al: International Federation of Societies for Surgery of the Hand 2013 Committee's report on wrist dart-throwing motion. *J Hand Surg [Am]* 39:1433–1439, 2014.
70. Moritomo H, Murase T, Arimitsu S, et al: Change in the length of the ulnocarpal ligaments during radiocarpal motion: possible impact on triangular fibrocartilage complex foveal tears. *J Hand Surg [Am]* 33:1278–1286, 2008.
71. Murray PM, Palmer CG, Shin AY: The mechanism of ulnar-sided perilunate instability of the wrist: a cadaveric study and 6 clinical cases. *J Hand Surg [Am]* 37:721–728, 2012.
71a. Nathan R, Blatt G: Rotatory subluxation of the scaphoid revisited. *Hand Clin* 16(3):417–431, 2000.
72. Omori S, Moritomo H, Omokawa S, et al: In vivo 3-dimensional analysis of dorsal intercalated segment instability deformity secondary to scapholunate dissociation: a preliminary report. *J Hand Surg [Am]* 38:1346–1355, 2013.
73. Petterson K, Wagnsjö P: Arthrodesis for chronic static SL dissociation: a prospective study in 12 patients. *Scand J Plast Reconstr Surg Hand Surg* 38:166–171, 2004.
74. Picha BM, Konstantakos EK, Gordon DA: Incidence of bilateral scapholunate dissociation in symptomatic and asymptomatic wrists. *J Hand Surg [Am]* 37:1130–1135, 2012.
75. Pomerance J: Outcome after repair of the SL Intercarpal ligament and dorsal capsulodesis for dynamic SL instability due to trauma. *J Hand Surg [Am]* 31:1380–1386, 2006.
76. Rainbow MJ, Crisco JJ, Moore DC, et al: Elongation of the dorsal carpal ligaments: a computational study of in vivo carpal kinematics. *J Hand Surg [Am]* 37:1393–1399, 2012.
77. Rauhaniemi J, Tiusanen H, Sipola E: Total wrist fusion: a study of 115 patients. *J Hand Surg [Br]* 30:217–219, 2005.
78. Rayhack JM, Linscheid RL, Dobyns JH, et al: Posttraumatic ulnar translation of the carpus. *J Hand Surg [Am]* 12:180–189, 1987.
79. Reagan DS, Linscheid RL, Dobyns JH: LTq sprains. *J Hand Surg [Am]* 9:502–514, 1984.
80. Reinsmith LE, Garcia-Elias M, Gilula LA: Traumatic axial dislocation injuries of the wrist. *Radiology* 267:680–689, 2013.
81. Renoux J, Zeitoun-Fiss D, Brasseur JL: Ultrasonographic study of wrist ligaments: review and new perspectives. *Semin Musculoskelet Radiol* 13:55–65, 2009.
82. Rhee PC, Moran SL, Shin AY: Association between lunate morphology and carpal collapse in cases of scapholunate dissociation. *J Hand Surg [Am]* 34:1633–1639, 2009.
83. Rhee PC, Sauvé PS, Lindau T, et al: Examination of the wrist: ulnar-sided wrist pain due to ligamentous injury. *J Hand Surg [Am]* 39:1859–1862, 2014.
84. Riemann BL, Lephart SM: The sensorimotor system, part I: the physiologic basis of functional joint stability. *J Athl Train* 37:71–79, 2002.
85. Rikli DA, Honigmann P, Babst R, et al: Intra-articular pressure measurement in the radioulnocarpal joint using a novel sensor: in vitro and in vivo results. *J Hand Surg [Am]* 32:67–75, 2007.
86. Ringler MD: MRI of wrist ligaments. *J Hand Surg [Am]* 38:2034–2046, 2013.
87. Ritt MJPF, Linscheid RL, Cooney WP, et al: The LTq joint: kinematic effects of sequential ligament sectioning, ligament repair, and arthrodesis. *J Hand Surg [Am]* 23:432–445, 1998.
88. Rohman EM, Agel J, Putnam MD, et al: Scapholunate interosseous ligament injuries: a retrospective review of treatment and outcomes in 82 wrists. *J Hand Surg [Am]* 39:2020–2026, 2014.
89. Rosati M, Parchi P, Cacianti M, et al: Treatment of acute scapholunate ligament injuries with bone anchor. *Musculoskelet Surg* 94:25–32, 2010.
90. Ross M, Peters SE, Couzens GB: Scapho-luno-triquetral tenodesis. In Shin AY, Day CS, editors: *Epub-Advances in scapholunate ligament treatment*, Chicago IL, 2014, American Society for Surgery of the Hand, pp 111–123.
91. Salva-Coll G, Garcia-Elias M, Hagert E: Scapholunate instability: proprioception and neuromuscular control. *J Wrist Surg* 2:136–140, 2013.
92. Salva-Coll G, Garcia-Elias M, Leon-Lopez MT, et al: Effects of forearm muscles on carpal stability. *J Hand Surg Eur Vol* 36:553–559, 2011.
93. Sauvé PS, Rhee PC, Shin AY, et al: Examination of the wrist: radial-sided wrist pain. *J Hand Surg [Am]* 39:2089–2092, 2014.
94. Scalcione LR, Gimber LH, Ho AM, et al: Spectrum of carpal dislocations and fracture-dislocations: imaging and management. *AJR Am J Roentgenol* 203:541–550, 2014.
95. Schuind FA, Linscheid RL, An KN, et al: A normal data base of PA roentgenographic measurements of the wrist. *J Bone Joint Surg Am* 74:1418–1429, 1992.
96. Seradge H, Baer C, Dalsimer D, et al: Treatment of dynamic scaphoid instability. *J Trauma* 56:1253–1269, 2004.

97. Shahane SA, Trail IA, Takwale VJ, et al: Tenodesis of the extensor carpi ulnaris for chronic, post-traumatic LTq instability. *J Bone Joint Surg Br* 87:1512–1515, 2005.

98. Shin AY, Weinstein LP, Berger RA, et al: Treatment of isolated injuries of the LTq ligament: a comparison of arthrodesis, ligament reconstruction and ligament repair. *J Bone Joint Surg Br* 83:1023–1028, 2001.

99. Short WH, Werner FW: The biomechanics of the scapholunate joint. In Shin AY, Day CS, editors: *Epub-Advances in scapholunate ligament treatment*, Chicago IL, 2014, American Society for Surgery of the Hand, pp 21–33.

100. Slutsky DJ: Current innovations in wrist arthroscopy. *J Hand Surg [Am]* 37:1932–1941, 2012.

101. Soong M, Merrell GA, Ortmann F, 4th, et al: Long-term results of bone-retinaculum-bone autograft for scapholunate instability. *J Hand Surg [Am]* 38:504–508, 2013.

101a. Souer JS, Rutgers M, Andermahr J, et al: Perilunate fracture-dislocations of the wrist: comparison of temporary screw versus K-wire fixation. *J Hand Surg [Am]* 32(3):318–325, 2007.

102. Sousa HP, Fernandes H, Botelheiro JC: Pre-operative progressive distraction in old transscapho-peri-lunate dislocations. *J Hand Surg [Br]* 20:603–605, 1995.

103. Sousa M, Aido R, Freitas D, et al: Scapholunate ligament reconstruction using a flexor carpi radialis tendon graft. *J Hand Surg [Am]* 39:1512–1516, 2014.

104. Stewart DT, Froelich JM, Shin AY: Intercarpal arthrodeses. *J Hand Surg [Am]* 39:373–377, 2014.

105. Sulkers GS, Schep NW, Maas M, et al: The diagnostic accuracy of wrist cineradiography in diagnosing scapholunate dissociation. *J Hand Surg Eur Vol* 39:263–271, 2014.

106. Szabo RM: Dorsal intercarpal ligament capsulodesis. In Shin AY, Day CS, editors: *Epub-Advances in scapholunate ligament treatment*, Chicago IL, 2014, American Society for Surgery of the Hand, pp 84–96.

107. Taleisnik J: Current concepts review. Carpal instability. *J Bone Joint Surg Am* 70:1262–1268, 1988.

108. Taleisnik J, Watson HK: Midcarpal instability caused by malunited fractures of the distal radius. *J Hand Surg [Am]* 9:350–357, 1984.

109. Trumble T, Verheyden J: Treatment of isolated perilunate and lunate dislocations with combined dorsal and volar approach and intraosseous cerclage wire. *J Hand Surg [Am]* 29:412–417, 2004.

110. Vance RM, Gelberman RH, Evans EF: Scaphocapitate fractures: patterns of dislocation, mechanisms of injury, and preliminary results of treatment. *J Bone Joint Surg Am* 62:271–276, 1980.

111. Van den Abbeele KLS, Loh YC, Stanley JK, et al: Early results of a modified Brunelli procedure for SL instability. *J Hand Surg [Br]* 23:258–261, 1998.

112. Viegas SF, Patterson RM, Todd PD, et al: Load mechanics of the midcarpal joint. *J Hand Surg [Am]* 18:14–18, 1993.

113. Wahegaonkar AL, Mathoulin CL: Arthroscopic dorsal capsulo-ligamentous repair in the treatment of chronic scapho-lunate ligament tears. *J Wrist Surg* 2:141–148, 2013.

114. Wall LB, Didonna ML, Kiefhaber TR, et al: Proximal row carpectomy: minimum 20-year follow-up. *J Hand Surg [Am]* 38:1498–1504, 2013.

115. Watson HK, Ashmead D, IV, Makhlouf MV: Examination of the scaphoid. *J Hand Surg [Am]* 13:657–660, 1988.

116. Watson HK, Weinzweig J, Zeppieri J: The natural progression of scaphoid instability. *Hand Clin* 13:39–49, 1997.

117. Weil WM, Slade JF, 3rd, Trumble TE: Open and arthroscopic treatment of perilunate injuries. *Clin Orthop Relat Res* 445:120–132, 2006.

118. Wolfe SW, Garcia-Elias M, Kitay A: Carpal instability nondissociative. *J Am Acad Orthop Surg* 20:575–585, 2012.

119. Wright TW, Dobyns JH, Linscheid RL, et al: Carpal instability non-dissociative. *J Hand Surg [Br]* 19:763–773, 1994.

120. Yin Y, Gilula LA: Imaging of the symptomatic wrist. In Watson HK, Weinzweig J, editors: *The wrist*, Philadelphia, 2001, Lippincott-Raven, pp 61–82.

Distal Radioulnar Joint

Brian D. Adams and Fraser J. Leversedge

> ▶ These videos may be found at
> *ExpertConsult.com:*
> **14.1** Dynamic ultrasound for tendinopathy. (Copyright © Scott W. Wolfe.)

The distal radioulnar joint (DRUJ) is a diarthrodial, synovial articulation that provides the distal link between the radius and the ulna and a pivot for pronation and supination (Figure 14.1). Because the radii of curvature of the articular surfaces of the radius and ulna are different, the soft tissues are critical for guiding and restraining the joint; pathologic alterations of the soft tissues can adversely influence joint motion or stability. During normal forearm motion, the DRUJ moves synchronously with the proximal radioulnar joint, and any injury or deformity involving the radius or ulna can alter the function of both joints.

The DRUJ and ulnocarpal joint are anatomically and functionally integrated, so both are affected by traumatic and arthritic conditions. Because of these interdependences, evaluation and treatment of the DRUJ are challenging. This chapter presents the relationships between anatomy, function, injury, and disease that affect the DRUJ and ulnocarpal joint and explains how these relationships influence the rationale for and technique of treatment options for these various conditions.

⬛ ANATOMY AND BIOMECHANICS

The sigmoid notch of the radius is a shallow concavity that articulates with the ulnar head. In anatomic studies, the radius of curvature of the sigmoid notch averaged 15 to 19 mm compared with only 10 mm for the ulnar head. The dorsal and palmar rims of the sigmoid notch contribute substantially to DRUJ stability. Typically, the dorsal bony rim is angled acutely, whereas the palmar rim is more rounded and is augmented by a fibrocartilaginous lip, which is prominent in 80% and more subtle in 18% (Figure 14.2). The importance of these rims has been shown clinically and in biomechanical investigations in which posttraumatic deficiencies substantially reduce joint stability.[1,156,162,171]

The articular contour of the DRUJ varies considerably among individuals in both the coronal and transverse planes. In the coronal plane, the slopes of the opposing articular surfaces of the notch and ulnar head may be parallel (55%), oblique (33%), or reverse oblique (33%) relative to the long axis of the radius and ulna.[162] Although slope has no proven impact on joint function in its natural state, acquired changes in length of the radius or ulna can alter peak DRUJ articular pressures. A shortening osteotomy through the ulnar shaft for the treatment of ulnar impaction syndrome in a patient with a reverse oblique slope of the DRUJ has the potential to increase articular pressures at the proximal edge of the notch and the opposing surface of the ulnar head.[135]

In the transverse plane, the average sigmoid notch subtends an arc of approximately 50 degrees (see Figure 14.2). Based on an anatomic study of 50 cadavers, four different sigmoid notch shapes were found: flat face (42%), ski slope (14%), "C" type (30%), and "S" type (14%) (Figure 14.3).[162] The shape has potential implications for risk of traumatic instability and its treatment alternatives. A flat sigmoid notch may be more prone to instability and less responsive to treatment by soft tissue repair alone.[162]

The ulna is the stable unit of the forearm and supports loads transmitted from the radius and carpus. The ulnar head serves as the articular seat around which the radius rotates via the sigmoid notch. The surface of the ulnar head that faces the sigmoid notch forms a slightly asymmetric, partial cylinder of about a 130-degree arc. The articular cartilage coverage of this arc ranges from 50 to 130 degrees and is located on the dorsal, lateral, palmar, and distal surfaces.[3] Due to a slight asymmetry in its curvature, there is a small cam effect at the DRUJ during forearm rotation. The articular surface is generally inclined and shaped to match the slope of the sigmoid notch, but a radiographic appearance of a mismatch is common.

In a radiographic study, the mean inclination of the sigmoid notch was found to be 8 degrees, ranging from −24 to 27 degrees, whereas the inclination of the opposing ulnar head surface averaged 21 degrees, ranging from −14 to 41 degrees.[135] These differences in inclination may partially explain why symptoms can develop after ulnar shortening or changes in radial length following distal radius fracture.[135]

The distal articular surface of the ulna (also called the "dome" or "pole" of the ulna[78]) that articulates with the articular disk of the triangular fibrocartilage complex (TFCC) varies in shape from a partial sphere to nearly flat. A semilunar distribution of cartilage covers much of the dome, which articulates with the articular disk of the TFCC. At the base of the styloid and encompassing the geometric center of the ulnar head is a shallow concavity called the "fovea" that is devoid of cartilage and replete with vascular foramina that supply vessels to the TFCC (Figure 14.4). The fovea is the primary attachment site for the radioulnar and ulnocarpal ligaments. The ulnar styloid is a continuation of the subcutaneous ridge of the ulna, projecting 2-6 mm distal to the dome of the distal ulna. It provides an increased area for soft tissue attachments, including the extensor carpi ulnaris (ECU) tendon sheath and the secondary attachments of the radioulnar ligaments. The dorsal (nonarticular) aspect of the head has a groove for the ECU tendon.

Ulnar variance is the term used to relate the difference in lengths of the radius and ulna. Ulna plus (or positive) and ulna minus (or negative) describe the ulna as longer or shorter than the radius, respectively. In a radiographic study of 120 normal Caucasian subjects, ulnar variance averaged −0.9 mm (range, −4.2-2.3 mm) with no differences between genders.[142]

The *TFCC*, named by Palmer and Werner,[120] is the term used most commonly to describe the interconnected soft tissues that span and support the DRUJ and ulnocarpal articulations. The TFCC is inclusive of other terms that have been used to emphasize either its fibrocartilage components (e.g., triangular cartilage, articular disk) or its ligament components (e.g., triangular ligament, ulnocarpal ligament complex). The TFCC is formed by the: (1) palmar and dorsal radioulnar ligaments; (2) triangular fibrocartilage proper, or articular disk; (3) floor of the ECU sheath; (4) ulnocarpal meniscal homologue; and (5) palmar ulnocarpal ligaments.[120] The primary functions of the TFCC are to (1) extend the smooth articular surface of the distal radius to cover the ulnar head; (2) transmit axial force across

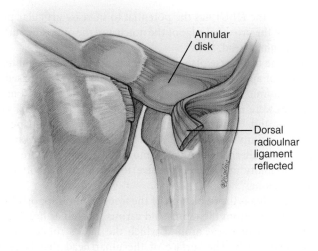

FIGURE 14.1 Distal radial ulnar joint with triangular fibrocartilage complex. (Copyright © Elizabeth Martin.)

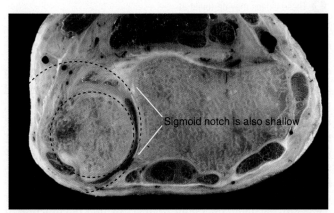

FIGURE 14.2 Cross section through distal radial ulnar joint in a cadaver. The rims of the sigmoid notch are augmented by fibrocartilaginous lips. The sigmoid notch is shallow, and its radius at curvature is substantially larger than at the ulnar head.

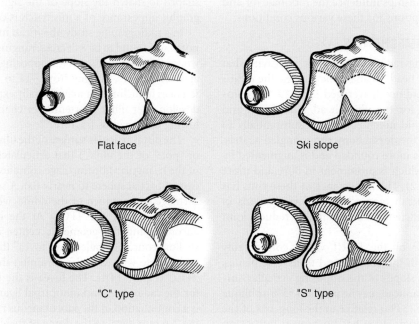

FIGURE 14.3 Various shapes of the articular surfaces of distal radial ulnar joint exist in the transverse plane. The shapes influence its stability. (Redrawn by Elizabeth Martin from Tolat AR, Stanley JK, Trail IA: A cadaveric study of the anatomy and stability of the distal radioulnar joint in the coronal and transverse planes. *J Hand Surg Br* 21:587–594, 1996.)

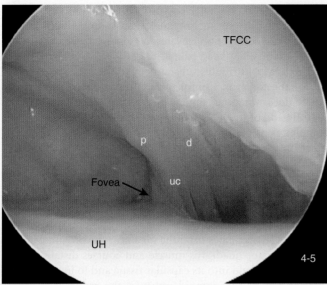

FIGURE 14.4 Arthroscopic evaluation of the ulnocarpal joint in the interval between the triangular fibrocartilage complex (TFCC) and ulnar head (UH). The inserting fibers of the deep limbs of the palmar (p) and dorsal (d) radioulnar ligaments converge as they insert into the foveal region of the distal ulna. The ulnar collateral ligament (uc) is considered a capsular condensation along the midsagittal aspect of the ulnocarpal joint. (Copyright David Slutsky. Reprinted with permission.)

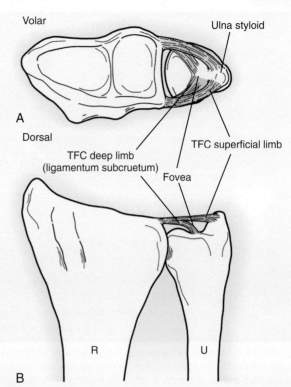

FIGURE 14.5 A, B, Normal division of dorsal and palmar radioulnar ligaments into superficial (distal) limbs that attach to the ulnar styloid and deep (proximal) limbs that attach at the fovea of the ulnar head. *R*, Radius; *TFC*, triangular fibrocartilage; *U*, ulna. (From Adams B: Distal radioulnar joint. In Trumble TE, editor: *Hand surgery update 3: Hand, elbow, and shoulder*, Rosemont, IL, 2003, American Society for Surgery of the Hand, pp 147–157.)

the ulnocarpal joint, while partially absorbing the load; (3) provide a strong but flexible connection between the distal radius and ulna that allows forearm rotation; and (4) support the ulnar portion of the carpus through connections to the ulna and the radius. Its anatomic complexity and multiple functions place the TFCC at substantial risk for injury and degeneration.

The radioulnar ligaments are the primary stabilizers of the DRUJ. The palmar and dorsal radioulnar ligaments are located at the common juncture of the articular disk, DRUJ capsule, and ulnocarpal capsule. These ligaments are composed of longitudinally oriented lamellar collagen to resist tensile loads and have a rich vascular supply to allow healing. The palmar and dorsal radioulnar ligaments extend from the palmar and dorsal distal margins of the sigmoid notch, respectively, and converge in a triangular configuration to attach to the ulna. As each radioulnar ligament courses ulnarly, it divides in the coronal plane into two limbs. The deep or proximal limbs attach to the fovea, just medial to the pole of the distal ulna, and are referred to as the *ligamentum subcruetum*.[77]

The superficial or distal limbs attach to the base and midportion of the ulnar styloid[9,77,110] (Figure 14.5). Stability of the DRUJ and treatment considerations, therefore, can be influenced by the location of an ulnar styloid fracture. A basilar styloid fracture imparts mechanical discontinuity to the superficial limbs and signifies potential disruption of the deep limbs because of its proximity to their foveal attachments.

The articular disk extends from the ulnar edge of the lunate fossa at the distal rim of the sigmoid notch and blends peripherally with the radioulnar ligaments. There is an inverse relationship between central disk thickness and ulnar variance.[118] The disk is composed of fibrocartilage, and its interweaving and obliquely oriented fibers are arranged to bear compressive loads

through its central portion.[21] In biomechanical cadaveric studies, approximately 20% of the load transmitted through the wrist passed through the ulna.[121] The transmitted force varied with wrist position and increased with ulnar deviation and pronation by up to 150%. Alterations in ulnar variance and the presence of the articular disk also affect load transmission. Shortening the ulna by 2.5 mm decreased ulnar load to 4%, whereas increasing ulnar length by 2.5 mm increased the load to 42%. Removal of two-thirds or more of the disk reduced ulnar load to 3%.[122]

Although the articular disk transmits and absorbs compressive forces, it provides minimal constraint to DRUJ translation.[2] The compression borne by the disk is converted partially to tensile forces that splay the TFCC.[141] These tensile forces are resisted by the radioulnar ligaments. The disk undergoes substantial deformation during forearm rotation. Increased strains are concentrated in its radial portion during axial loading of the wrist, especially in pronation.[2] This region corresponds to the junction of the radially oriented collagen fibers and the obliquely arranged fibers in the central region. These mechanical and histologic findings explain the frequency of traumatic tears near the disk's radial attachment.

The ECU sheath is a stout structure that extends from the dorsal groove in the ulnar head and the dorsal radioulnar ligament to the carpus. It augments the dorsal capsule and provides its own stabilizing effect separate from the ECU tendon.[110] There are three palmar ulnocarpal ligaments that are part of the TFCC. The ulnotriquetral and ulnolunate ligaments originate

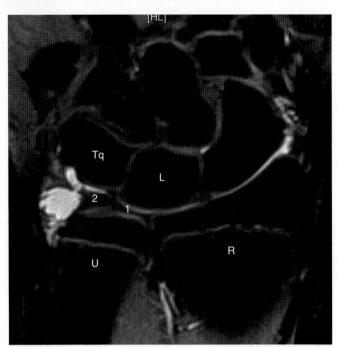

FIGURE 14.6 Meniscus homologue is an irregularly shaped soft tissue structure that variably fills the space between the ulnar capsule, disk, and proximal aspect of the triquetrum. *L*, Lunate; *R*, radius; *Tq*, triquetrum; *U*, ulna; *1*, articular disk of triangular fibrocartilage; *2*, meniscus homologue.

from the palmar radioulnar ligament and insert on their respective carpal bones. The ulnocapitate ligament, which lies just palmar to the other ulnocarpal ligaments, originates from the volar margin of the ulnar head and inserts on the capitate.[9,110] The contribution of the ulnocarpal ligaments to DRUJ stability is controversial. Because these ligaments have a common origin with the radioulnar ligaments, injuries or disease affecting soft tissue attachments at the fovea can affect DRUJ and ulnocarpal stability. This situation is seen commonly in inflammatory conditions, such as rheumatoid arthritis, in which synovitis around the fovea results in subluxation of the radioulnar joint and a supination deformity of the ulnocarpal joint.

The soft tissue structure between the ulnocarpal capsule, articular disk, and proximal aspect of the triquetrum has been referred to as the *meniscus homologue*[120] (Figure 14.6). Although its prevalence and function have not been defined precisely, it consists of well-vascularized loose connective tissue that is derived most likely from synovium. The size, shape, and distal insertion of the meniscus homologue can vary. There is a consistent insertion of the meniscal homologue into the triquetrum, but there is a broader insertion into the fifth metacarpal. In addition, occasionally there is an insertion into the articular surface of the triquetrum and/or into the lunotriquetral ligament that may obscure arthroscopic visualization of the lunotriquetral interosseous ligament.[111]

Several soft tissue structures are considered to be secondary stabilizers of the DRUJ, including the pronator quadratus, ECU, interosseous membrane (IOM), DRUJ capsule, and articular disk. The relative contributions of these structures to joint stability are controversial, but there is common agreement that gross instability requires disruption of multiple structures.[157] The pronator quadratus and ECU musculotendinous units provide dynamic stability. The pronator quadratus coapts the joint during active pronation and passive supination.[88] In pronation, ECU contraction elevates the ulnar carpus dorsally and depresses the ulnar head palmarly.[69,88]

The IOM contributes substantially to the mechanical integrity of the forearm. Complete radioulnar dissociation at the DRUJ does not occur unless the IOM is incompetent. The central band of the IOM that is part of the middle ligamentous complex runs proximally from the radius to its distal attachment on the ulna. The central band provides 71% of the soft tissue contribution to longitudinal forearm stiffness and is the main structure that resists proximal migration of the radius when the radial head is damaged or removed. The distal oblique bundle (DOB) was identified in all of a series of cadaver dissections, although its thickness varied widely among specimens.

The DOB originates from the ulna near the proximal border of the pronator quadratus muscle and courses distally toward the DRUJ to blend into its capsular tissue and to insert into the inferior rim of the sigmoid notch of the radius. Also, some fibers course farther distally to insert on the anterior and posterior ridges of the sigmoid notch and to become continuous with the dorsal and palmar radioulnar ligaments.[112] Based on a cadaver model, the presence of the DOB may confer increased dorsal–palmar translational stability on the DRUJ when evaluated in a cadaver model.[76] This stabilizing effect of the distal IOM appears to influence DRUJ stability following ulnar-shortening osteotomy; osteotomy performed proximal to the distal IOM improves DRUJ stability compared to one done distal to the distal IOM.[103] Also, alterations in the anatomic relationships of the distal radius and ulna, such as following a displaced distal radius fracture, may compromise the stabilizing effect of the DOB on the DRUJ.[35]

The TFCC has a lesser role in dorsoulnar forearm stability. Traditionally, the DRUJ capsule has been considered too redundant and weak to provide effective joint stabilization. Although biomechanical studies have not emphasized the contribution of the capsule,[172] histologic studies show a well-defined fiber orientation and suggest a potential stabilizing role of the capsule.[78] The palmar capsule has a prominent, redundant fold extending from the inferior radial aspect to the distal ulna border that forms a pocket for the ulnar head in supination and helps to limit translation. The dorsal capsule is thinner and homogeneous with a transverse orientation, indicating less potential to provide stability.

The precise roles of the radioulnar ligaments have been debated. There are two clinically relevant themes concerning their stabilizing functions.[140] First, the ligaments act together with the morphologic boundaries of the sigmoid notch to constrain the joint. Second, both ligaments are necessary for normal joint stability in both palmar and dorsal directions.[156,172] Ligament tension peaks at the extremes of translation and rotation as the ulnar head simultaneously compresses against a rim of the notch creating both a tether and a buttress to resist dislocation. In one view of the functions of these ligaments, the dorsal ligament restrains the ulna from dorsal displacement during pronation and the palmar ligament prevents palmar displacement during supination. Supporters of this theory tested the joint with a passive rotation force applied to the joint and measured strain within the ligaments. The major restraining ligament was deemed the one with the greatest strain.[2,140,172]

In the opposing view, the palmar ligament prevents dorsal displacement in pronation, and the dorsal ligament restrains palmar displacement in supination. These results were found by testing the joint with a passive translation force and observing bone displacements.[3,156] Both theories have merit in the clinical management of instability, and the discrepancy can be considered by appreciating the dual insertions of each ligament on the fovea and ulnar styloid. Despite one ligament possibly providing the dominant restraint under a specific condition, the other ligament provides a secondary restraint, and both must be injured to allow complete dislocation.[172] In patients with bidirectional or severe unidirectional instability, injury of both ligaments should be suspected. From a clinical perspective, the foveal attachments of the radioulnar ligaments are the critical stabilizers of the DRUJ.

Improved understanding of the neurovascular supply to the TFCC has been developed using modern imaging and immunohistochemical staining studies. The vascular supply to the articular disk is variable and plays a central role in its healing potential and treatment options. The TFCC vascular supply is primarily via the anterior interosseous and ulnar arteries.[8] The anterior interosseous artery provides palmar and dorsal branches to the DRUJ. The dorsal branch supplies most of the dorsal periphery, and the palmar branch supplies the volar periphery near the radius. Dorsal and palmar branches of the ulnar artery supply the styloid area and ulnar part of the volar periphery. Vascular penetration into the disk extends only to its outer 15%, leaving the central portion hypovascular, or essentially avascular[8,21] (Figure 14.7). The vascular supply of the peripheral articular disk decreases with age.[95]

Based on these findings, a central disk injury has little or no possibility to heal, whereas injuries at the periphery have good healing potential. The neural supply of the TFCC is concentrated in the dense and loose connective tissues deep in the prestyloid recess and has been traced from the dorsal sensory branch of the ulnar nerve and inconsistently from the medial antebrachial cutaneous nerve, posterior interosseous nerve, anterior interosseous nerve, superficial branch of the ulnar nerve, and the palmar cutaneous branch of the median nerve.[82,146] Selective denervation of the TFCC has been suggested based on an algorithm associated with sequential nerve blocks.[82]

The normal arc of pronation and supination ranges among individuals from 150 to 180 degrees. Additional rotation of up to 30 degrees occurs through the radiocarpal joint. The axis of forearm motion varies during rotation, especially under load, but generally passes near the cross-sectional centers of the radial head proximally and ulnar head distally. At the level of the DRUJ, the axis of motion shifts slightly dorsally with pronation and slightly palmarly with supination. During forearm rotation, translation occurs between the ulnar head and sigmoid notch, resulting in a combination of rolling and sliding movements at the articular surface. The radius slides palmarly with forearm pronation and dorsally with supination.

Total dorsal–palmar translation with the forearm in neutral rotation was measured at 8 to 9 mm in normal cadaveric joints subjected to externally applied forces, although in vivo studies suggest that the actual amount of translation may be considerably less. Nonetheless, when the unloaded forearm is in the neutral position, articular contact is maximal, reaching 60% of

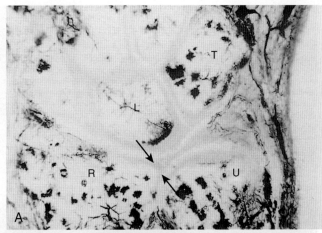

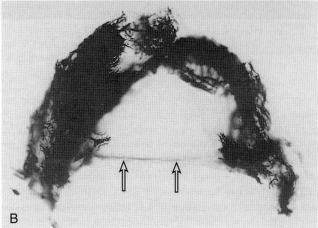

FIGURE 14.7 Triangular fibrocartilage complex (TFCC) is well vascularized in its periphery, whereas only the outer 15% of the disk has vascular penetration. *Arrows* in (**A**) and (**B**) identify avascular regions of TFCC at its attachment to radius. **A,** Coronal section through wrist. **B,** Axial view of TFCC. *L,* Lunate; *R,* radius; *T,* triquetrum; *U,* ulna. (From Bednar MS, Arnoczky SP, Weiland AJ: The microvasculature of the triangular fibrocartilage complex: its clinical significance. *J Hand Surg Am* 16:1101–1105, 1991.)

the available surface area. At the extremes of pronation and supination, there may be only 2 mm of articular contact at the margins of the sigmoid notch (<10% of the articular surface area).[3] Translation can occur because the sigmoid notch is shallow, and its radius of curvature is 50 to 100% greater than that of the ulnar head.

PHYSICAL EXAMINATION

A global examination of the involved upper extremity is warranted to evaluate for local and remote causes of wrist symptoms, and comparison with the contralateral limb is beneficial. The impact of elbow and forearm pathologic conditions, in particular those of the proximal radioulnar joint (PRUJ), on DRUJ function is necessary to avoid pitfalls and optimize treatment. Vascular or neurogenic causes, including cervical radiculopathy or ulnar neuropathy should be considered.

Inspect the upper limb for swelling and asymmetry with the other side. The evaluation progresses from a general inspection, to active and passive range of motion, strength, tenderness, and provocative maneuvers. Diagnostic injection can be useful in

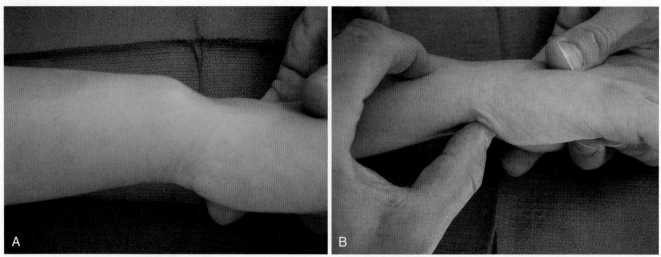

FIGURE 14.8 A, Appearance of the right distal ulnar forearm and wrist demonstrating the dorsal prominence of the ulnar head associated with volar subluxation of the distal radius and carpus. **B,** The examiner is able to reduce the wrist by placing the index and long fingers on the dorsal distal ulna and using the thumb to apply a dorsally directed force on the pisiform.

the evaluation. Evaluate for point tenderness using a single palpating fingertip at the distal radius and ulna, DRUJ, radiocarpal and ulnocarpal joints, ulnar styloid, proximal triquetrum, pisotriquetral joint, hook of the hamate, and the scapholunate and lunotriquetral intervals. Tenderness in the soft depression between the flexor carpi ulnaris (FCU) tendon, ulnar styloid, and triquetrum is suggestive of a TFCC injury.[160] Tenderness and or crepitus of the ECU and FCU tendons indicates possible tenosynovial hypertrophy or tendinopathy. A benign mass (e.g., lipoma or ganglion cyst) is not uncommon. An effusion at the ulnocarpal joint or radioulnar joint may indicate degenerative or inflammatory arthritis, especially when associated with dorsal prominence of the ulnar head. Symptoms elicited during provocation tests of the DRUJ may indicate instability, TFCC injury, or arthritic conditions of the DRUJ.

Active and passive motion of the wrist and forearm are measured and compared with the opposite side. Decreased motion and/or crepitus during pronation–supination are signs of DRUJ arthritis; pain may be heightened by manually compressing the joint. ECU tendinitis and lunotriquetral ligament tears can mimic DRUJ symptoms. ECU instability and subluxation is most apparent with forearm supination, flexion, and ulnar deviation of the wrist. The lunotriquetral joint is assessed with the shear or ballottement test. In this test, the examiner stabilizes the lunate between the thumb and index finger of one hand while manually shearing the triquetrum against the lunate articular surface in a dorsal–palmar direction with the thumb and index finger of the other hand. Distinguish between DRUJ conditions and pain associated with pisotriquetral arthritis by palpating the pisotriquetral interval and by pressing and manipulating the pisiform.

Several variations of ulnocarpal stress testing are useful when attempting to reproduce symptoms of ulnocarpal instability caused by disk tears or ulnocarpal degeneration. The patient's forearm is positioned vertically on the examination table and the examiner grasps the hand and applies an axial load through the wrist. The wrist is moved passively through radial and ulnar deviation while being moved through an arc of pronation and supination.[41,107] Alternatively, the wrist is moved

passively through a flexion and extension arc in different forearm positions while maintaining an ulnar deviation posture under axial load. Another maneuver involves placing the wrist in passive ulnar deviation while creating increased central loading of the disk and ulnar dome by simultaneously depressing the ulnar head volarly with the index and long fingers and pushing the pisiform dorsally (pisiform boost) with the thumb on its palmar surface. This maneuver is most effectively performed with the forearm in neutral rotation where the DRUJ is the most lax (Figure 14-8, A, B).

Increased anteroposterior translation of the radius on the ulna during passive manipulation is evidence of DRUJ instability. Because joint translation varies with forearm position and among individuals, the test should be done in all forearm positions and should be compared with the opposite side. A pianokey sign describes the relative hypermobility of the ulnar head with the forearm in full pronation and a positive test is defined by pain elicited following release of the ulnar head after transient palmar depression.[48] A DRUJ ballottement test, used to evaluate relative instability of the ulnar head with the forearm in neutral position, and the ulnocarpal stress test[107] are done with comparison to the contralateral side.

Clinical evaluation for DRUJ instability is challenging due to the subjective nature of the examination and the variability in "normal" DRUJ mobility, even with and without the influence of dynamic stabilizers. In a cadaveric model, one biomechanical study comparing these three clinical assessments suggested that the ballottement test was more accurate in detecting DRUJ instability following TFCC release at the fovea and base of the ulnar styloid.[105] Dynamic loading of the ulnocarpal joint by the patient can be done using the press test.[84] In this test, the patient grasps the arm of a chair and pushes up toward a standing position.

IMAGING

Radiography

Radiographic evaluation of the DRUJ should begin with standard posteroanterior, oblique, and lateral views. A standard posteroanterior radiograph (i.e., neutral forearm rotation) is taken with the shoulder abducted 90 degrees, the elbow flexed 90 degrees, the forearm and palm flat on the cassette, and the wrist in neutral flexion–extension and neutral radioulnar deviation. The position of the ECU groove can be used to determine whether the posteroanterior view is acceptable. When the cortical outline of the concavity of the groove is radial to the long axis of the ulnar styloid, the posteroanterior view is acceptable for measuring ulnar variance.[85]

A neutral rotation position has been recommended to standardize ulnar variance measurement, but a more recent study found minimal change in ulnar variance throughout the range of forearm rotation, differing only 0.6 mm between pronation and supination.[187] Although changes in variance can be subtle, a posteroanterior view with the forearm pronated,[38] or with the patient making a power grip,[42] or with combined pronation and grip can promote positive ulnar variance.[163]

Several techniques have been described to measure ulnar variance on the posteroanterior view.[117] In a study comparing three commonly used methods, differences were very small and not likely to be of clinical significance.[155] The method of perpendiculars is the most popular. In this method, a line is drawn through the volar sclerotic line of the distal radius perpendicular to its longitudinal axis. The distance between this line and the distal cortical rim of the ulnar dome is measured (Figure 14.9).

The standard lateral radiograph is taken with the shoulder at the patient's side (0 degrees abduction), the elbow flexed 90 degrees, and the wrist in a neutral position. An accurate lateral view is confirmed by the palmar surface of the pisiform visualized midway between the palmar surfaces of the distal pole of the scaphoid and the capitate (i.e., the so-called SPC lateral).[186] Other evidence of correct alignment includes superimpositions of the lesser four metacarpals, the proximal pole of the scaphoid on the lunate, and the radial styloid on the center of the lunate.

Despite attention to detail of positioning, the lateral view is imprecise for the diagnosis of DRUJ subluxation. Mino and associates showed that with 10 degrees of supination or pronation, subluxation appeared reduced and dislocation appeared subluxated.[101]

Several radiographic findings may support the diagnosis of DRUJ instability. Ulnar styloid fracture displacement greater than 2 mm associated with distal radius fractures may be consistent with DRUJ instability.[93] Arthroscopically confirmed foveal avulsions of the distal radioulnar ligaments in a group of 29 patients with displaced distal radius fractures were observed to have increased radial translation and radial shortening, decreased radial inclination, or 4 mm or greater ulnar styloid fracture displacement.[108] In the absence of bony abnormalities, however, DRUJ instability secondary to soft tissue deficiency may be highlighted through the use of radiographic stress views.

Several cadaveric studies have demonstrated DRUJ instability with dynamic stress testing following division of the dorsal and palmar distal radioulnar ligaments.[144,150] Clinically, Iida et al. demonstrated a significant increase in DRUJ gap compared to the uninjured side using a clenched-fist posteroanterior (PA) view with the forearm in pronation.[64] Evidence of DRUJ instability following Darrach excision can be accentuated in a lateral stress view in which the patient holds a 5-lb weight with the forearm in pronation and the x-ray beam is directed "cross-table"[138] (Figure 14.10). Semisupinated and semipronated radiographic views improve visualization of the palmar and dorsal rims of the sigmoid notch and the ulnar head and are useful to evaluate for fractures and arthritis. Osteophyte formation at the proximal margin of the ulnar head is an early sign of arthritis.

Ultrasonography

The reliability of ultrasound in the evaluation of DRUJ instability has not been demonstrated due to several confounding factors including its user-dependent nature, although recent work indicates the potential to assess DRUJ instability in a study comparing patients with and without TFCC injuries.[59] Ultrasound may also be helpful in the dynamic assessment of ECU instability.

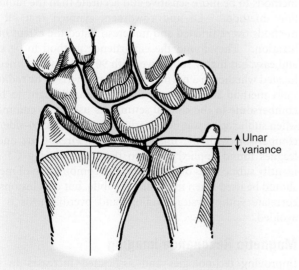

FIGURE 14.9 Ulnar variance is measured by drawing a line through the volar sclerotic line of the distal radius perpendicular to its longitudinal axis. Variance is the distance between this line and the distal cortical rim of the ulnar dome. (Copyright © Elizabeth Martin.)

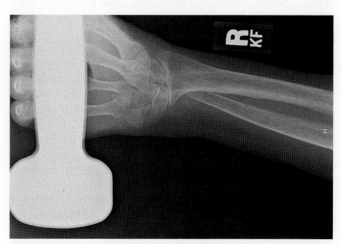

FIGURE 14.10 Weighted radiograph of the pronated forearm to demonstrate radioulnar convergence following distal ulna resection.

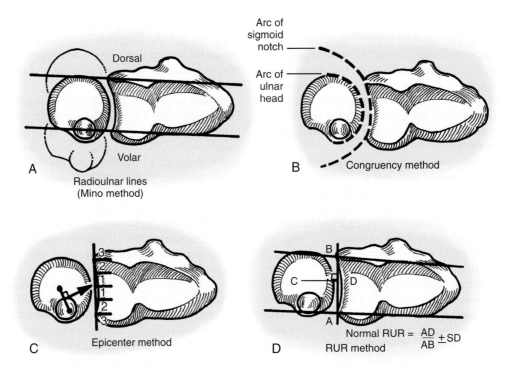

FIGURE 14.11 Measurement methods for assessing distal radial ulnar joint instability on axial computed tomography images. **A,** Radioulnar lines (Mino method). **B,** Congruency method. **C,** Epicenter method. **D,** Radioulnar ratio (RUR) method. (Redrawn by Elizabeth Martin from Adams BD: Distal radioulnar joint instability. In Berger RA, Weiss APC, editors: *Hand surgery* (vol 1). Philadelphia, 2004, Lippincott Williams & Williams, pp 337–354.)

Arthrography

Previously, wrist arthrography played an important role in assessing lesions of the TFCC[131] but was criticized subsequently because its findings showed poor clinical correlation and a low sensitivity compared with arthroscopy.[26] A high incidence of TFCC perforations is detected in asymptomatic wrists, including young adults. Generally, noninvasive magnetic resonance imaging (MRI) and arthroscopy have replaced arthrography. Despite these limitations, a negative arthrogram can be useful as a screening tool. In a retrospective study of patients with ulnar-sided wrist pain who had an inconclusive physical examination, normal standard radiographs, and a negative wrist arthrogram, most of the patients improved over time and few had persistent substantial disability.[67]

Computed Tomography

Computed tomography (CT) is a valuable tool for evaluating fractures, developmental deformities of the sigmoid notch and ulnar head, and degenerative arthritis. Rozental and associates evaluated a series of distal radius fractures with CT and identified displacement of sigmoid notch fractures that were not recognized on standard radiographs.[131] This radiographic study did not correlate radiographic results with patient outcome to determine the findings' clinical significance.

CT is a common method of imaging for DRUJ instability. To optimize its value, the forearms should be aligned with the axis of the gantry. When evaluating for DRUJ instability, it is important to image both wrists in identical forearm positions, including neutral, supination, and pronation. Several measurement

methods have been utilized, including use of dorsal and palmar radioulnar lines described by Mino and associates,[101] epicenter and congruency methods proposed by Wechsler and colleagues,[177] and radioulnar ratio described by Lo and coworkers[89] (Figure 14.11).

Wechsler and colleagues found the congruency and epicenter methods to be more sensitive and accurate than the radioulnar lines method.[177] Lo and coworkers claimed that all three methods overestimated and underestimated the extent of subluxation.[89] They found the congruency method to be simple and easy, but highly subjective, with 90% of cases deemed subluxated whether in a normal or abnormal wrist. The radioulnar ratio method was more reliable, but was thought to be too cumbersome in the clinical setting. Its use was recommended when subluxation was not clearly evident on side-to-side visual comparison with the unaffected wrist. Pirela-Cruz and colleagues found applied stress to the DRUJ during CT could identify subtle signs of instability.[126] A combination of methods should be used when instability is subtle, but conclusions must correlate with physical findings and overdiagnosis is to be avoided.

Magnetic Resonance Imaging

Improving technologies and associated increases in image resolution, as well as the use of adjuvant contrast-enhanced arthrography, have improved the sensitivity, specificity, and accuracy of MRI in the diagnosis of TFCC tears (Figure 14.12) (see Chapter 15). Similar to CT, MRI can be used to assess DRUJ instability through anatomic measurements.[37] Dynamic imaging may become an important tool to identify lesions and instability of the ulnocarpal joint and DRUJ.

Scintigraphy

Scintigraphy (bone scan) has a limited role in assessing the DRUJ but may be useful when the diagnosis is in question or concurrent problems are suspected. It is most useful in diagnosing ulnar impaction syndrome, in which the ulnar head, lunate, and triquetrum may show increased uptake consistent with chronic inflammation in the bone and soft tissues.

Arthroscopy

Arthroscopy is sensitive for identifying traumatic TFCC tears or degeneration in the central portion of the disk, chondromalacia, and ulnocarpal ligament injuries. In several studies, arthroscopy was more sensitive and more accurate than noninvasive imaging modalities.[26] Incomplete peripheral TFCC tears are more difficult to detect, however, and their severity is more complicated to judge. Scar and vascular invasion along the TFCC periphery and tears of the lunotriquetral interosseous ligament or ECU sheath are evidence of previous injury. A lax or hypermobile TFCC under direct probing—the so-called "trampoline effect"—is indicative of an unstable TFCC[58] although reduced tension in the TFCC does not establish the diagnosis of DRUJ instability.

In the assessment of DRUJ instability, arthroscopy can permit visualization of the foveal insertion of the deep fibers of the distal radioulnar ligaments[148] and guide arthroscopically assisted, transosseous repair techniques for foveal TFCC avulsion injuries.[147] Also, arthroscopy can facilitate the evaluation and treatment of secondary conditions that might contribute to the patient's symptoms, especially if these can be treated by arthroscopic debridement alone. A complete discussion of wrist arthroscopy is presented in Chapter 17.

TRIANGULAR FIBROCARTILAGE COMPLEX LESIONS

Palmer's classification divides TFCC lesions into two broad categories: traumatic and degenerative[116] (Table 14.1 and Figure 14.13). Traumatic TFCC injuries are classified further according to location of the tear. Most traumatic tears result from an acute rotational injury to the forearm, a combined axial load and distraction injury to the ulnar border of the forearm, or a fall on the pronated outstretched hand. Although Palmer's classification provides an accurate anatomic description of traumatic tears, it does not guide treatment or indicate prognosis. Additionally, the scheme implies that each type occurs in isolation, whereas clinical studies have found that multiple components of the TFCC may tear in the same injury.[94]

Most acute, isolated TFCC tears do not require early treatment. Although the incidence of TFCC injuries associated with distal radius fractures is estimated to be 13 to 60% using imaging methods or surgical inspection, the incidence of persistent problems related to these injuries is much less.[86,106,115,130] The necessity of treatment for TFCC tears depends on the presence of persistent joint pain from mechanical irritation or synovitis caused by the tear, associated fractures or malunions, or posttraumatic instability of the DRUJ. Diagnosis and treatment of isolated traumatic TFCC injuries are presented separately from associated injuries or DRUJ instability (see also Chapters 15 and 17).

A degenerative TFCC tear can result from chronic, excessive loading through the ulnocarpal joint and is a component of ulnar impaction syndrome. It is important to recognize, however, that natural degeneration of the ulnocarpal joint also occurs. In cadaveric examinations, TFCC perforations and chondromalacia of the ulnar head, lunate, and triquetrum were found in 30 to 70% of specimens.[95,120] Those with ulnar-negative

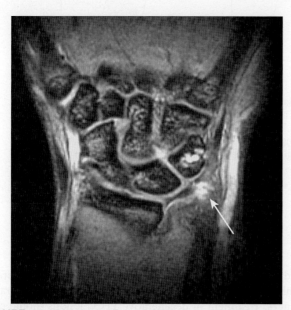

FIGURE 14.12 Magnetic resonance image of ulnar-peripheral tear of triangular fibrocartilage complex, shown by high-intensity signal on T2-weighted image (*arrow*). (From Adams B: Distal radioulnar joint. In Trumble TE, editor: *Hand surgery update 3: Hand, elbow, and shoulder*, Rosemont, IL, 2003, American Society for Surgery of the Hand, pp 147–157.)

TABLE 14.1 Palmer's Classifications of Triangular Fibrocartilage Complex Lesions	
Class	**Lesions**
1: Traumatic	A: Central perforation
	B: Ulnar avulsion
	With styloid fracture
	Without styloid fracture
	C: Distal avulsion (from carpus)
	D: Radial avulsion
	With sigmoid notch fracture
	Without sigmoid notch fracture
2: Degenerative (Ulnar Impaction Syndrome)	A: TFCC wear
	B: TFCC wear
	Plus lunate or ulnar head chondromalacia
	C: TFCC perforation
	Plus lunate or ulnar head chondromalacia
	D: TFCC perforation
	Plus lunate or ulnar head chondromalacia
	Plus lunotriquetral ligament perforation
	E: TFCC perforation
	Plus lunate or ulnar head chondromalacia
	Plus lunotriquetral ligament perforation
	Plus ulnocarpal arthritis

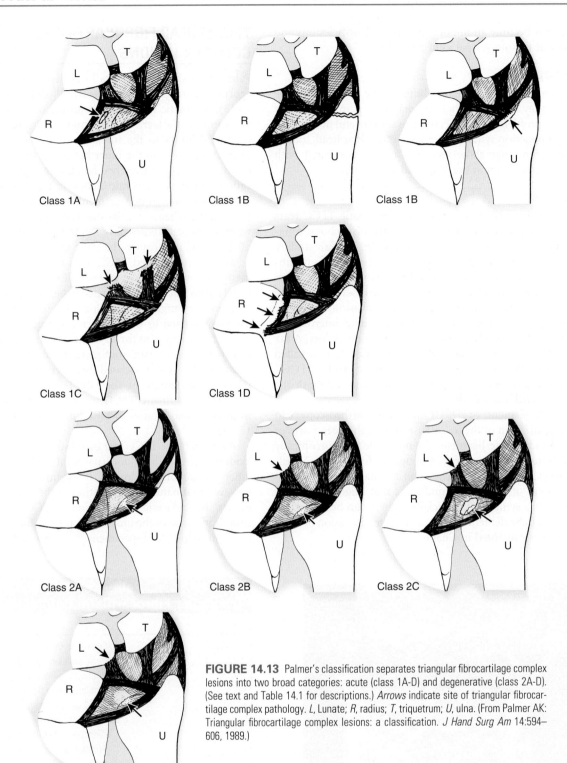

FIGURE 14.13 Palmer's classification separates triangular fibrocartilage complex lesions into two broad categories: acute (class 1A-D) and degenerative (class 2A-D). (See text and Table 14.1 for descriptions.) *Arrows* indicate site of triangular fibrocartilage complex pathology. *L*, Lunate; *R*, radius; *T*, triquetrum; *U*, ulna. (From Palmer AK: Triangular fibrocartilage complex lesions: a classification. *J Hand Surg Am* 14:594–606, 1989.)

variance had less severe degenerative changes.[120] Palmer classified degenerative lesions by the location and severity of degeneration involving the TFCC, ulnar head, and carpus.[116]

Although Palmer's classification implies a specific progression of degeneration among the structures, involvement and severity of degenerative changes in the articular disk, lunate, triquetrum, lunotriquetral interosseous ligament, and ulnar head vary widely in this condition, with any one structure or combination of structures having various stages of degenerative changes. Treatment of degenerative TFCC lesions should consider: (1) debridement of the joint, (2) reduction of load across the ulnocarpal joint, (3) DRUJ stability, (4) DRUJ articular congruity, and (5) presence of developmental or acquired skeletal deformities.

Palmer's Classification of TTFC Lesions

Class 1A Tear

A class 1A tear typically manifests as ulnar-sided wrist pain that is aggravated by power grip, especially with ulnar deviation or forearm rotation. It is a relatively common injury that can cause pain and mechanical symptoms, such as clicking, but does not cause DRUJ instability. Typically, this tear is confined to the disk, located 2 to 3 mm ulnar to its radial attachment, and oriented volar to dorsal. Initially, these injuries should be managed conservatively using rest; immobilization; antiinflammatory medications; and, occasionally, a corticosteroid injection. Patients with ulnar-positive wrists may be less likely to respond to conservative management.

When symptoms persist despite conservative management of traumatic TFCC tears, arthroscopic debridement is the preferred treatment and is discussed in Chapter 17. If a disk tear is identified during an open wrist procedure for another indication, the tear should be debrided to a clean and stable margin. It is important that the peripheral 1 to 2 mm of the articular disk be preserved to avoid injury to the radioulnar ligaments. Outcomes following debridement of the radial remnant of the disk and concomitant repair to the radius are controversial, particularly in light of the relatively good outcomes following arthroscopic debridement alone; this more complex technique is discussed later for the class 1D tear.

Class 1B Tear

A class 1B injury is a partial or complete avulsion of the TFCC from its ulnar attachments, with or without an ulnar styloid fracture. DRUJ instability may or may not be present. A fracture through the base of the styloid that can disrupt both the deep and superficial limbs of the TFCC is more predictive of DRUJ instability than the more common fracture through the shaft or tip.[57] However, most ulnar styloid fractures do not cause DRUJ instability, which is partially related to the dual ulnar attachments of the TFCC.[74,93,185] The ulnar styloid provides attachments for portions of the ulnocarpal ligaments,[9,104] ECU tendon sheath,[104] and superficial limbs of the radioulnar ligaments, whereas the deep limbs insert into the fovea of the ulnar head. The styloid tip is devoid of soft tissue attachments. In addition, a complete avulsion of the radioulnar ligaments and gross instability can occur without a styloid fracture.[94] Occasionally, a small fleck of bone is avulsed from the fovea indicating disruption of the deep limbs of the radioulnar ligaments. Recognition of these injury variations may prevent insufficient treatment.

Symptoms and physical findings associated with a class 1B tear are similar to those of a class 1A tear, although a click is usually absent and point tenderness is characteristically volar to the ulnar styloid. This localized tenderness coincides anatomically with the fovea and, appropriately, tenderness located here has been termed the *fovea sign*.[160] Evaluation of DRUJ stability, as described earlier, is likely to produce pain even if the DRUJ is stable.

Because these tears can progress to a destabilizing injury of the TFCC and DRUJ, initial treatment should restrict forces acting at the TFCC by protective above-elbow immobilization for 4 to 6 weeks with the forearm in neutral rotation. Subsequent treatment should be directed toward gradual recovery of motion and strength. Most of these injuries respond to conservative measures, with surgery indicated for persistent symptoms or evidence of DRUJ instability. Arthroscopic treatment of peripheral TFCC tears has evolved rapidly over the past few years. Symptomatic, complete tears can be repaired by arthroscopic-assisted techniques including transosseous or direct capsular suture repair[109,147,166,184] (see Chapter 17). An open repair is considered in grossly unstable or a chronic injury, provided there is good remaining ligamentous tissue. Chronic basistyloid nonunions associated with DRUJ instability can be addressed with surgical repair of the nonunion fragment (see section on acute DRUJ instability).

Class 1C Tear

A class 1C injury is a partial or complete tear of the ulnocarpal ligaments, either as an intrasubstance rupture or as an avulsion from their carpal insertion. These injuries can occur in combination with class 1B tears or lunotriquetral ligament tears, or both.[94] They are reported much less frequently than other TFCC injuries, probably because they are more difficult to diagnose. Contributions of the ulnocarpal ligaments to DRUJ stability are unclear. The most obvious sign of injury is a volar "sag" of the carpus relative to the ulnar head, analogous to the "caput ulnae" syndrome in rheumatoid arthritis (Figure 14.14). Generally, such injuries should be managed conservatively unless mechanical instability is present. Open repair has been reported in a few cases and arthroscopic-assisted techniques for suture repair or thermal capsular shrinkage have been described, but experience is limited (see Chapter 17).

Class 1D Tear

A class 1D tear is a partial or complete avulsion of the TFCC from the radius, with or without a bone fragment, and may involve one or both radioulnar ligaments. Some reports have confused class 1A and 1D repairs; it is important to reserve the class 1D designation for true radial detachments. Frequently, class 1D injuries are associated with a distal radius fracture and usually respond to accurate fracture reduction of the radius. In the absence of DRUJ instability, symptoms and physical findings are similar to other traumatic TFCC injury types.

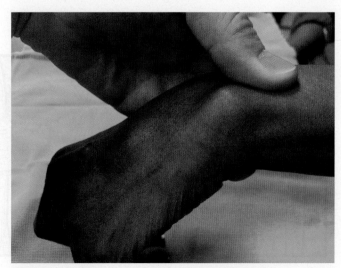

FIGURE 14.14 Example of the volar translation of the ulnar carpus and dorsal prominence of the ulnar head associated with rheumatoid arthritis.

Repair of the torn disk to the rim of the radius has been described[22] using open and arthroscopic techniques (Figure 14.15). A crucial concept underlying a successful repair is to provide a biologic environment conducive to healing by promoting vascular invasion from the bony rim. Various arthroscopic techniques have been described, including the use of specialized jigs.[7,22,166]

Open reduction and repair are indicated for large displaced avulsion fractures of the radius involving the rim of the sigmoid notch because the bony and ligament restraints are incompetent. Loss of the buttressing effect of the volar rim (e.g., with a displaced palmar lunate facet fracture) can be particularly destabilizing to the DRUJ. In most cases, these injuries are components of a more extensive distal radius fracture and are stabilized by fracture reduction and fixation (see Chapter 15). Special attention is warranted if DRUJ widening or substantial instability persists after reduction and stabilization of the radius.

❖ AUTHORS' PREFERRED METHOD OF TREATMENT: Open Triangular Fibrocartilage Complex Repair ± Ulnar-Shortening Osteotomy for Class 1B Tear

A 5-cm skin incision, centered over the ulnar head, is made between the fifth and sixth extensor compartments (Figure 14.16). The extensor digiti quinti (EDQ) sheath is opened, and the tendon is retracted. The DRUJ is exposed through an "L"-shaped capsulotomy. The longitudinal limb begins at the ulnar neck and extends to the distal edge of the sigmoid notch. Care should be taken to preserve the dorsal radioulnar ligament's origin at the sigmoid notch. The transverse limb is made by incising along the proximal edge of the dorsal radioulnar ligament and extends to the radial margin of the ECU sheath. The capsule is elevated and retracted proximally to expose the ulnar head and neck.

The proximal surface of the TFCC is inspected for injury, especially at its foveal attachment. If the dorsal and palmar radioulnar ligaments are suitable for repair, the distal surface of the articular disk is exposed through a transverse ulnocarpal capsulotomy made along the distal edge of the dorsal radioulnar ligament. A 0.045-in Kirschner wire is used to create 2 to 3 holes in the distal ulna extending from the dorsal aspect of the

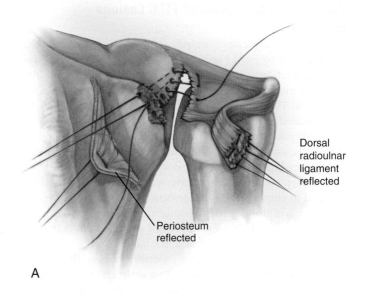

Dorsal radioulnar ligament reflected

Periosteum reflected

A

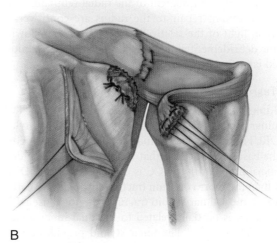

B

FIGURE 14.15 A, B, Class 1D injury involving dorsal radioulnar ligament can be repaired by an open technique using transosseous sutures. (Redrawn by Elizabeth Martin from Cooney WP, Linscheid RL, Dobyns JH: Triangular fibrocartilage tears. *J Hand Surg Am* 19:143–154, 1994.)

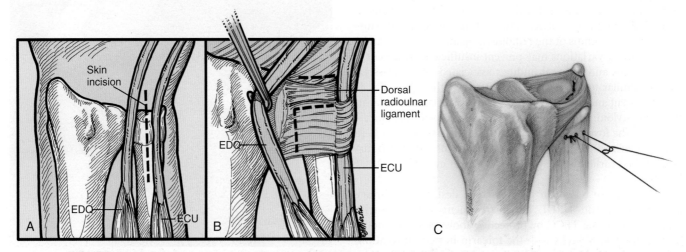

Skin incision

EDQ

ECU

Dorsal radioulnar ligament

ECU

EDQ

A

B

C

FIGURE 14.16 A-C, Open repair of class IB tear is performed through a dorsal approach, "L"-shaped capsulotomy, and horizontal transosseous mattress sutures through the ulnar neck. *ECU,* Extensor carpi ulnaris; *EDQ,* extensor digiti quinti. (Copyright © Elizabeth Martin.)

ulnar neck to the fovea. This site for the holes reduces irritation from suture knots compared with the subcutaneous ulnar border. Two horizontal mattress sutures (2-0 absorbable monofilament) are passed from distal to proximal through the ulnar periphery of the TFCC, which lies near the fovea, by entering through the ulnocarpal capsulotomy and exiting through the DRUJ capsulotomy. With the use of a straight needle or a small suture passer, they are passed through the bone holes. The sutures are tied over the ulnar neck with the joint reduced and the forearm in neutral rotation.

The dorsal DRUJ capsule and extensor retinaculum are either closed as separate layers or as a single layer together; the capsule should not be imbricated to avoid a potential loss of pronation. The EDQ is left superficial to the retinaculum to reduce the risk of peritendinous adhesions. A long-arm splint is applied with the forearm rotated 45 degrees toward the most stable joint position (e.g., supination for dorsal instability). At 2 weeks, the splint is converted to a long-arm cast for 4 weeks, followed by a well-molded short-arm cast for an additional 2 to 3 weeks. A removable splint is used for 4 weeks while motion is regained. Strengthening and resumption of activities are postponed until near-painless motion is possible. The surgical technique for ulnar-shortening osteotomy is described later in this chapter.

Outcomes

Hermansdorfer and Kleinman reported generally good results for open ulnar styloid nonunion excision with TFCC repair although patients with ulnocarpal joint arthritis responded less favorably.[58] For patients with instability and concomitant ulnar-positive variance, ulnar-shortening osteotomy should be considered. Trumble and colleagues reported satisfactory results after open TFCC repair, with some patients also undergoing simultaneous ulnar-shortening osteotomy.[166] The effectiveness of ulnar-shortening osteotomy alone for the treatment of class

1B tears was also reported with good results.[123] The role of ulnar-shortening osteotomy for patients with persisting symptoms following suture repair of a TFCC injury was demonstrated in selected patients.[182] This may be due to the tensioning effect of ulnar-shortening osteotomy on secondary stabilizers, including the DOB.[76] In selected pediatric patients with TFCC injuries, generally good results from repair were reported, although few studies are available.[6]

ACUTE DISTAL RADIOULNAR JOINT INSTABILITY

Although the radius and the carpus together make up the mobile unit of the DRUJ, by convention DRUJ dislocation or instability is described by the position of the ulnar head relative to the distal radius. A general classification of acute DRUJ instability can be considered based on anatomic sites of injury or deformity and is useful in guiding treatment.

Dorsal DRUJ dislocations are the most common and are caused by hyperpronation and wrist extension, as occurs in a fall on the outstretched hand. Conversely, volar dislocations occur with axial loading through a supinated forearm or from a direct blow to the ulnar aspect of the forearm (Figure 14.17). Although the most frequent cause for DRUJ instability is a distal radius fracture, instability after accurate reduction and fixation of the distal radius is uncommon. Initial radiographic findings of wide displacement of the DRUJ and severe radial shortening are the most important risk factors for persistent DRUJ instability. The radioulnar ligaments can tolerate no more than 5 to 7 mm of radial shortening before one or both ligaments tear. In the absence of a displaced sigmoid notch fracture, the TFCC typically tears at its ulnar attachments.[94]

In most cases, the integrity of the secondary stabilizers of the DRUJ, including the IOM, the DOB, the ECU subsheath, ulnocarpal ligaments, and lunotriquetral interosseous ligament,

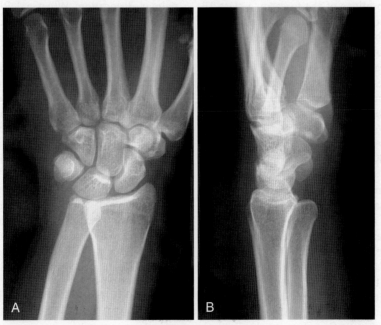

FIGURE 14.17 Radiograph of volar dislocation of distal radial ulnar joint shows overlap of ulnar head and sigmoid notch on posteroanterior view (**A**) and volar displacement of ulnar head on lateral view (**B**).

are preserved, thereby maintaining joint stability. However, as injury severity increases with progressive disruption of the secondary stabilizers, there is progressive instability of the DRUJ. Anatomic reduction of the radius is essential to facilitate DRUJ stability. In a series of articles evaluating young patients with distal radius fractures, unrepaired peripheral tears of the TFCC were a common cause of persistent symptomatic instability.[86,87]

It is important to evaluate DRUJ stability critically after treatment of a distal radius fracture. If instability persists after fracture repair, there are several options to promote a stable joint: (1) temporary immobilization of the forearm in the period of maximum stability using a sugar tong splint or long-arm cast and (2) percutaneous pinning of the ulna to the radius. Typically, the second option is done with one or two large pins (minimum of 0.062 in to resist breakage) driven proximal to the DRUJ from the palpable subcutaneous border of the ulna into the radius. When choosing this treatment, it is important to engage all four cortices of the radius and ulna, so that the pins are accessible should one or both break.

When treating open radius fractures with concomitant DRUJ instability, external fixation of the wrist, with an outrigger attached to the ulna in the position of maximum joint stability, may be considered.[133] When severe or bidirectional instability exists, ulnar styloid fixation or open TFCC repair, combined with radioulnar pinning, should be considered.

Ulnar head fractures and sigmoid notch fractures with or without a complex distal radius fracture pose additional challenges for restoring a congruous and stable DRUJ. Although distal radius fractures frequently involve the sigmoid notch, especially the dorsal rim, the extent of involvement is probably underestimated on standard radiographs and characterized more accurately by CT.[131,159] The clinical implication of residual incongruity of the sigmoid notch has not been studied sufficiently; however, anatomic and biomechanical studies and case reports[102,171] suggest that restoration of the sigmoid notch is essential for joint stability.

In Galeazzi fracture-dislocations of the forearm, a class 1B TFCC injury is present almost inevitably, although there may be a spectrum of DRUJ instability (Figure 14.18). Several studies demonstrated that the risk of DRUJ instability associated with a Galeazzi-type injury increases with a more distal fracture of the radial diaphysis; fractures in the distal one-third, or within 7.5 cm of the distal radius articular surface, have a higher risk of injury to the key soft tissue constraints of the DRUJ.[80,129]

Evaluation

An acute dislocation usually produces an obvious deformity with the ulnar head locked over a rim of the sigmoid notch. Local tenderness, swelling, and limited motion are the characteristic findings on presentation. Deep tenderness along the IOM and swelling or pain at the proximal radioulnar joint may indicate a concomitant Essex-Lopresti injury. Instability after reduction is marked by increased translation of the ulnar head in neutral forearm rotation and may be present in supination or pronation depending on the injured soft tissue stabilizers.

Accurate assessment of a DRUJ injury associated with a diaphyseal fracture of the radius or ulna is challenging and is usually impossible until the fracture is reduced and stabilized. Standard radiographs may show subluxation of the ulnar head

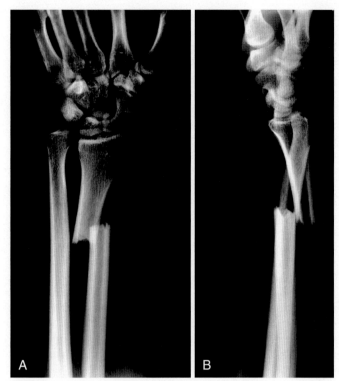

FIGURE 14.18 A, B, Galeazzi fracture disrupts distal radial ulnar joint (DRUJ) to varying degrees. After anatomic reduction of the radius, DRUJ stability is assessed and treated if necessary.

on the lateral view or partial overlap of the radius and ulna on the posteroanterior view. CT is useful to identify avulsion fractures of the rim of the sigmoid notch and to assess the adequacy of DRUJ reduction; postreduction images can be obtained through splinting or casting material.

Simple Dislocations

An isolated dorsal DRUJ dislocation is more common than a palmar dislocation. When a DRUJ dislocation is recognized acutely, reduction is accomplished easily, unless there is interposed soft tissue (e.g., ECU tendon). Under appropriate anesthesia, gentle pressure is applied over the ulnar head while the radius is rotated toward the prominent ulna. After reduction, joint stability should be evaluated over the full range of forearm rotation to determine the stable arc. Typically, joint reduction following a dorsal dislocation is most stable in supination and a palmar dislocation is most stable in pronation. If the joint is stable only in extreme pronation or supination, additional treatment, such as radioulnar pinning in the position of greatest stability or TFCC repair, should be considered. The TFCC is ruptured nearly always from the ulna.[58,94] If the joint is stable in an acceptable position of forearm rotation, it is treated with an above-elbow cast in this position for 3 to 4 weeks followed by use of a well-molded short-arm cast for 2 to 3 weeks. Interval evaluation with radiographs and/or fluoroscopy is recommended to ensure a stable reduction in the cast.

TFCC Repair (Class 1B Injury)

Peripheral TFCC tears can be diagnosed and sutured to the capsule using arthroscopic-assisted techniques; however, the indications for this technique in the treatment of acute dislocations of the DRUJ are not defined.[166] If the arthroscopic repair does not reconnect the TFCC to its anatomic attachments on the fovea or the ulnar styloid, it may not be as effective as an open repair in this situation. Ulnar-shortening osteotomy may be considered in conjunction with either an open or an arthroscopic TFCC repair to reduce the loads on the TFCC, especially in patients with positive ulnar variance (see later in the chapter for a description of ulnar-shortening osteotomy).[123,166,182]

Ulnar Styloid Fractures

In his classic article, Frykman reported that ulnar styloid fractures occurred in approximately 61% of distal radius fractures.[43] Most of these fractures are not associated with DRUJ instability or long-term symptoms. Fractures through the tip of the styloid do not require intervention because they do not cause DRUJ instability and are associated with a good prognosis.[18,29,46,81,152,180,188] Fractures through the styloid base, especially when displaced, are associated with a higher risk of DRUJ instability because of the increased potential for disruption of the inserting fibers of the deep limbs of the radioulnar ligaments.[57]

When the DRUJ remains unstable following anatomic fixation of the radius, fixation of an unstable basilar styloid fracture restores DRUJ stability through the restoration of radioulnar ligament integrity, provided that the TFCC is not otherwise damaged. Various methods have been described to fix fractures of the ulnar styloid, including the use of Kirschner wires, tension band wiring, compression screws, variable-pitch headless screws, mini-fragment plates, and suture anchors (Figure 14.19). The size of the ulnar styloid fragment influences fixation options. Soft tissue irritation associated with hardware prominence may require subsequent hardware removal.

Surgical exposure of the ulnar styloid can be accomplished by a dorsal approach if other procedures are being performed; however, the preferred approach is along the subcutaneous border just volar to the ECU tendon. The dorsal sensory branch of the ulnar nerve (DSBUN) is protected as it courses from volar to dorsal, typically crossing the midsagittal aspect of the wrist over the ulnocarpal joint. The ECU sheath is preserved. The ulnar styloid fracture is identified and cleared of any interposed soft tissue.

When using a tension band technique, one or two oblique Kirschner wires are passed through the tip of the ulnar styloid. A 24-gauge stainless-steel wire or heavy suture is passed around the tip of the wire and through a hole in the ulnar neck in a figure-of-eight fashion (see Figure 14.19, A). Multiple Kirschner wires or a screw can be used for larger fragments. Suture anchor fixation of the ulnar styloid is preferred by one author (B.D.A.) to minimize the potential to comminute the styloid and to reduce hardware irritation.

With this technique, a bone anchor is inserted into the fracture site and is seated well below the fracture line into the ulnar neck. The attached sutures are passed through drill holes in the styloid fragment if it is very large or passed around the fragment if smaller. The sutures are crossed over the subcutaneous surface of the ulna and one end is passed through a transverse drill hole made near the ulnar neck to create a figure-of-eight configuration. When the suture ends are tied, a combined interosseous compression and a tension band is created (see Figure 14.19, C).

Outcomes

The size and degree of displacement of the ulnar styloid fracture fragment are usually good predictors of DRUJ stability.[93] Although fracture union is not consistently achieved with any technique, sound fibrous healing in a good position is generally consistent with resolution of symptoms and DRUJ stability.[18,29,81,152,180,188] Independent of the presence and treatment of injuries of the ulna and TFCC, anatomic reduction and stability of the radius fracture and, in particular the sigmoid notch, are essential to achieve good DRUJ function.

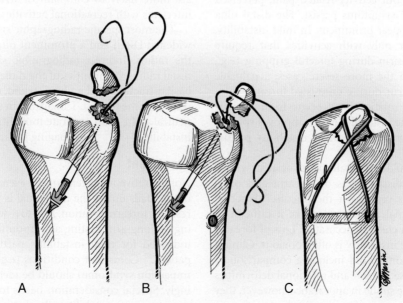

FIGURE 14.19 A-C, Several methods are available to fix a ulnar styloid fracture depending partially on the size of styloid fragment. Suture anchor technique is authors' preference (**C**). (Redrawn by Elizabeth Martin from Trumble TE, Culp R, Hanel DP, et al: Intra-articular fractures of the distal aspect of the radius. *J Bone Joint Surg Am* 80:595, 1998.)

CHRONIC DISTAL RADIOULNAR JOINT INSTABILITY

Symptomatic dysfunction of the DRUJ after wrist injury, especially after a distal radius malunion, is common. Residual dorsal angulation of the distal radius of greater than 20 to 30 degrees is associated with increased loading of the distal ulna, radioulnar incongruity, TFCC distortion, and palmar DRUJ instability.[4,28,62] In patients with a distal oblique bundle of the interosseous membrane, a coronal translation, or shift, of 2 mm or greater can also adversely influence DRUJ instability.[35]

DRUJ instability after a distal radius or forearm malunion usually manifests as loss of forearm rotation, prominence of the ulnar head, and ulnar-sided wrist pain. Symptoms are caused by a combination of effects of the malunion on the radiocarpal joint, ulnocarpal joint, and DRUJ. In isolation, loss of radial length is associated less frequently with a substantial loss of rotation or instability but causes a proportionate increase in ulnar load and symptoms of ulnar impaction.[17,127] Conversely, angular deformities of the distal radius or forearm are more likely to cause gross instability and unidirectional loss of motion.[127] Chronic length discrepancies caused by skeletal deficiencies in the proximal forearm (e.g., an Essex-Lopresti injury) are associated with IOM injuries and produce symptoms in the entire forearm axis.[145] Developmental skeletal deformities (e.g., Madelung deformity) behave similarly to their posttraumatic counterparts; however, the symptoms typically progress more slowly.[34]

Chronic posttraumatic DRUJ instability can occur in the absence of a distal radius fracture. A common history involves a fall on the outstretched hand or an unexpected forcible rotation of the wrist (e.g., a jammed power drill). Typically, the patient complains of intermittent ulnar-sided wrist swelling and pain that is aggravated by forearm and wrist motion, particularly with axial loading through an extended wrist or torsional activities against resistance. Untreated, pain at rest and swelling usually improve, but activity-related pain, perceived weakness, and mechanical symptoms persist. The distal ulna may remain tender and appear prominent. In mild instability, pain and weakness occur only with activities that require active rotation of the forearm during forceful gripping (e.g., turning a screwdriver). In the more severe cases, a palpable and painful clunk may occur during unresisted forearm rotation; a decreased arc of rotation may occur from chronic DRUJ subluxation. Chronic instability rarely improves spontaneously, and it is unknown whether DRUJ instability predisposes to arthritis.

DRUJ instability in children usually is associated with a previous fracture of the distal radius or forearm and often manifests later, sometimes years after the fracture.[4] Fracture remodeling and longitudinal growth can make it difficult to characterize a malunion in children accurately. Loss of forearm motion is variable, but the instability is often obvious. Clinical and radiographic evaluation should include a comparison to the noninjured side because angular and rotational deformities of the radius or ulna can be subtle in appearance; however, they can have a profound influence on function, leading to chronic ligament attenuation and associated DRUJ instability (Figure 14.20, A-D).

Evaluation

Chronic DRUJ instability can be demonstrated by reproducible clunking, both visible and palpable during active or passive forearm rotation as the ulnar head reduces into the sigmoid notch from a dislocated position. Passive manipulation of the joint is occasionally necessary to complete the dislocation, and compression across the joint may accentuate the clunk. Subtle DRUJ subluxation may be more difficult to detect. In palmar subluxation, a slight prominence of the ulnar head is seen on the palmar aspect of the wrist, and a depression of the soft tissues may be seen on the dorsal side (dimple sign). Tenderness is present diffusely around the distal ulna, but particularly over the fovea of the ulnar head, located in the natural depression between the FCU tendon and ulnar styloid.

Increased translation with passive force is nearly always present in at least one position of forearm rotation. Passive laxity should be assessed by holding the radius and carpus with one hand, while using gentle force with the examiner's opposite hand on the distal ulna with the forearm in neutral, supination, and pronation. Translation is normally greater in neutral compared to the extremes of pronation or supination. It is essential to compare findings with the contralateral extremity because the normal range of motion and laxity of the DRUJ vary considerably among individuals. Resisted forearm rotation, especially at the extremes of pronation and supination, is often painful.

A modification of the press test,[84] originally described to diagnose TFCC tears, is useful for evaluating suspected DRUJ instability.[1] In this modified test, the patient rises from a chair using the hands for assistance by pushing against a tabletop located to his or her front. Instability is shown by greater "depression" of the ulnar head on the affected side and is often coupled with pain. Tenderness over the ulnar styloid may signify an unstable nonunion. In a dorsally angulated malunion of the distal radius, the ulnar head is prominent volarly, especially with supination. Children are unlikely to have at rest pain and are more likely to complain of wrist pain and popping that interferes with recreational activities.

The most specific radiographic signs of instability include a widened DRUJ and a prominent ulnar head volar or dorsal to the radius. Indirect radiographic signs include a malunited distal radius, deformities of the radial or ulnar shafts, displaced basilar fracture of the ulnar styloid, and a displaced fleck fracture from the fovea. CT imaging in supination, pronation, and neutral is the most accurate modality to evaluate the DRUJ for instability.[89,126,177] (See Imaging section earlier in the chapter.)

Treatment

Nonoperative management of severe, chronic DRUJ instability usually fails unless the individual is willing to use a splint that restricts forearm rotation. A 4- to 6-week trial of forearm splinting or long-arm casting and antiinflammatory medications is indicated for mild instability, particularly in a low-demand patient.[97] Coexistent conditions (e.g., ECU tendinitis or ulnar impaction syndrome) should be identified and treated accordingly. Special consideration needs to be given to patients with symptoms of instability who have a flat sigmoid notch and bilateral DRUJ hypermobility because these patients respond less predictably to reconstructive surgery.

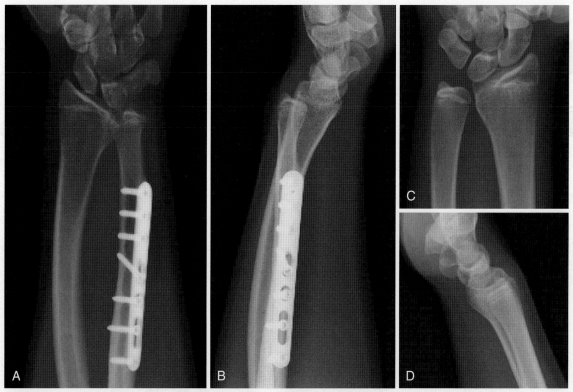

FIGURE 14.20 A 16-year-old female with a history of mild bilateral Madelung deformity and left forearm fracture treated with open reduction and internal fixation of the ulna and closed management of the radius. She complained of persistent instability and pain localized to the distal radial ulnar joint (DRUJ) and ulnocarpal joints. Posteroanterior (**A**) and lateral (**B**) radiographs of the left distal forearm demonstrate relative ulnar-positive variance and DRUJ subluxation. Comparison radiographs (**C, D**) of the contralateral extremity contrast the DRUJ alignment, despite mild morphologic changes of the distal radius.

To take advantage of dynamic DRUJ stabilizers, a strengthening program for the forearm and wrist, along with supportive soft bracing or taping during activities, can be considered. Recurrent dislocations may cause further attenuation of the soft tissue restraints and predispose to degeneration of the articular cartilage and the rims of the sigmoid notch. With young patients, it may be appropriate to accept intermittent dislocations and follow them regularly until skeletal maturity to avoid the potential for iatrogenic physeal injury with reconstructive surgery.

Restoration of stability and a full, painless arc of motion are the goals of surgical treatment for a posttraumatic unstable DRUJ. The anatomic derangements underlying the instability must be identified correctly, including bony deformity, ligament injury, and combinations. In established DRUJ instability without malunion or arthritis, late repair of a class 1B TFCC tear is an option if its radioulnar ligament components are otherwise robust, with the goal to restore their mechanical integrity.[58] Soft tissue repair or reconstruction in the presence of marked bony deformity, however, is likely to fail.

Symptomatic nonunion of the ulnar styloid is an uncommon problem that is usually best treated by simple subperiosteal excision. If the fragment is large, and the TFCC is unstable, it's repaired to the styloid base after fragment excision with transosseous sutures.[57] Alternatively, the nonunion can be repaired; although, fixation of a basilar ulnar styloid nonunion alone in chronic instability can be ineffective because the soft tissues may be attenuated.

A soft tissue reconstructive procedure is indicated when the TFCC is irreparable and the sigmoid notch is competent. Reconstructive techniques can be classified into three categories: (1) a direct radioulnar tether that is extrinsic to the joint, (2) an indirect radioulnar link via an ulnocarpal sling or a tenodesis,[16,60,168] or (3) reconstruction of the distal radioulnar ligaments.[1,70,138] The techniques in the first two categories may improve symptoms but are not anatomic; and in laboratory studies, they have not been shown to restore normal joint stability or mechanics.[124] Nonetheless, these reconstructions may be the only option in some cases and are occasionally used in conjunction with a Darrach excision of the distal ulna or to stabilize a previously resected distal ulna.[52]

An indirect radioulnar link is created using techniques described by Boyes and Bunnell[15] (Figure 14.21) and by Hui and Linscheid[60] (Figure 14.22) to reconstruct the volar ulnocarpal ligaments using a distally based strip of the FCU tendon. Such techniques are particularly applicable when ulnocarpal instability is the primary problem, and DRUJ instability is of a lesser concern.

Reconstruction of the distal radioulnar ligaments is the most anatomical approach and has the potential to restore stability without substantial loss of rotation or strength. The procedure is dependent on a mechanically competent sigmoid notch to provide a buttress effect for proper ligament function. If the notch is not competent, either an osteoplasty of the sigmoid notch (described later in this chapter) must be done concurrently, or another surgical option needs to be considered.

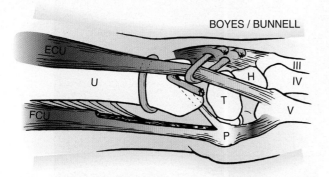

BOYES / BUNNELL

FIGURE 14.21 Technique described by Boyes and Bunnell for chronic distal radial ulnar joint instability reconstructs volar ulnocarpal ligaments and creates a tether between the distal radius and ulna. *ECU,* Extensor carpi ulnaris; *FCU,* flexor carpi ulnaris; *H,* hamate; *P,* pisiform; *T,* triquetrum; *U,* ulna; *III,* long finger metacarpal; *IV,* ring finger metacarpal; *V,* small finger metacarpal. (From Petersen MS, Adams BD: Biomechanical evaluation of distal radioulnar reconstructions. *J Hand Surg Am* 18:328–334, 1993.)

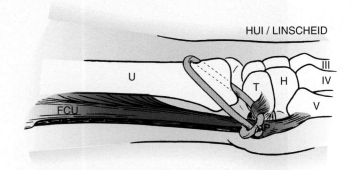

HUI / LINSCHEID

FIGURE 14.22 Hui and Linscheid procedure reconstructs volar ulnocarpal ligament using strip of flexor carpi ulnaris tendon. It is particularly useful for primary ulnocarpal instability and secondary distal radial ulnar joint instability. *FCU,* Flexor carpi ulnaris; *H,* hamate; *P,* pisiform; *T,* triquetrum; *U,* ulna; *III,* long finger metacarpal; *IV,* ring finger metacarpal; *V,* small finger metacarpal. (From Petersen MS, Adams BD: Biomechanical evaluation of distal radioulnar reconstructions. *J Hand Surg Am* 18:328–334, 1993.)

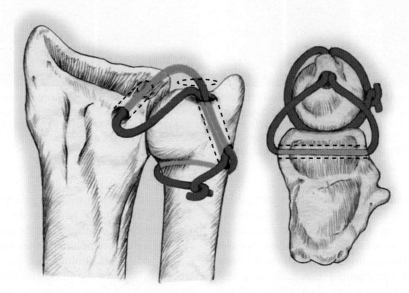

FIGURE 14.23 Method of reconstruction of both distal radioulnar ligaments that uses palmaris longus tendon graft passed through bone tunnels in distal radius and ulnar head is illustrated. Location of bone tunnels and route of tendon graft also are shown.

Scheker and associates described a technique for reconstruction of the dorsal radioulnar ligament using a tendon graft.[138] Three drill holes are placed in the distal radius and ulna, and the graft is woven and tied onto itself. Johnston Jones and Sanders described a technique for reconstruction of both radioulnar ligaments with a palmaris tendon graft.[70] A technique developed by the senior author reconstructs the anatomic origin and insertion of the palmar and dorsal radioulnar ligaments (Figure 14.23); it is presented next.[1]

❖ AUTHORS' PREFERRED METHOD OF TREATMENT: Distal Radioulnar Ligament Reconstruction

A 5-cm incision is made between the fifth and sixth extensor compartments over the DRUJ. Care is taken to preserve the dorsal sensory branch of the ulnar nerve and full-thickness soft tissue flaps are elevated off of the extensor retinaculum. The fifth extensor compartment is opened over the radioulnar joint, and the EDQ tendon is retracted (Figure 14.24, *A*). An

"L"-shaped DRUJ capsulotomy is made with the longitudinal limb along the dorsal rim of the sigmoid notch, leaving enough capsule attached to the rim for later repair, and the transverse limb just proximal to the dorsal radioulnar ligament (Figure 14.24, *B*).

The ECU sheath is not opened or dissected from the ulnar groove during the procedure. If the TFCC is irreparable, radioulnar ligament reconstruction is performed. Scar is debrided from the fovea, but the functioning remnants of the TFCC are retained. If an ulnar styloid nonunion is present, the fragment is resected subperiosteally through the same incision. A palmar exposure is made through a 3- to 4-cm longitudinal incision extending proximally from the proximal wrist crease in the interval between the ulnar neurovascular bundle and finger flexor tendons.

Although the palmaris longus is the easiest tendon graft to harvest, it is often too short and therefore the surgeon should be prepared to obtain an alternative graft (e.g., the plantaris, toe

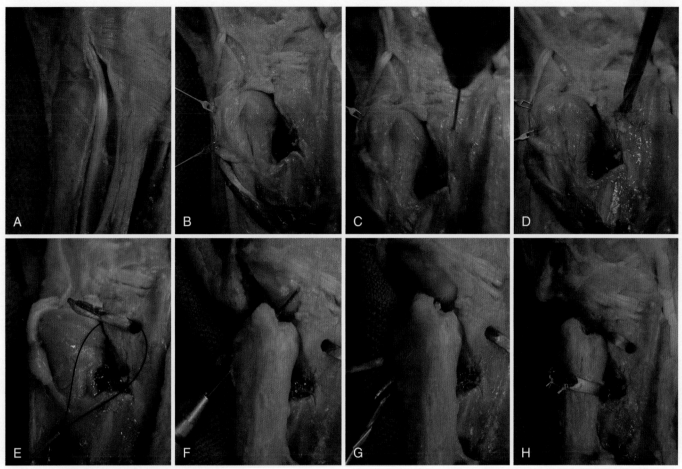

FIGURE 14.24 Surgical steps for the completion of a distal radioulnar ligament reconstruction demonstrated in a left wrist: **A,** Dorsal exposure and incision of the fifth extensor compartment. **B,** A dorsal capsulotomy using an L-shaped incision, preserving the dorsal radioulnar ligament. **C,** Dorsal-to-volar guide pin placement. **D,** Cannulated drilling of the osseous tunnel in the distal radius. **E,** Passage of the palmaris longus tendon graft using a Hewson tendon passer. **F,** The guide pin for the ulnar osseous tunnel may be placed from the ulnar neck with its trajectory toward the fovea, or from the fovea directed to the ulnar neck. **G,** Passage of the tendon graft from volar-to-dorsal within the distal radius before passing through distal ulnar osseous tunnel. **H,** The completed tendon graft passed through the distal radius and ulna, attempting to recreate the distal radioulnar ligaments. (**A–H:** Reprinted with permission: copyright © 2009, Leversedge FJ.)

extensor, or strip of the FCU or FCR)[66]; a narrow FCU strip is the authors' preferred choice because it can be harvested through the same palmar incision used for the reconstruction and a long graft can be obtained. The periosteum beneath the fourth dorsal extensor compartment is elevated sharply from the dorsal margin of the sigmoid notch. A guidewire for a 3.5-mm cannulated drill bit is driven through the radius several millimeters proximal to the lunate fossa and radial to the articular surface of the sigmoid notch. The wire is inserted parallel to the articular surfaces and located so that the tunnel can be made large enough to accommodate the graft without disrupting the subchondral bone of the lunate fossa or sigmoid notch (see Figure 14.24, *C*).

Fluoroscopic imaging is used to confirm proper guidewire position and the tunnel is made with a cannulated drill, exiting carefully through the palmar incision (see Figure 14.24, *D*). If a corrective osteotomy for a distal radius malunion is planned in conjunction with the ligament reconstruction, it is easier to create the tunnel before performing the osteotomy; however, tendon graft insertion and tensioning should not be done until the bony correction is completed. If a sigmoid notchplasty is

planned, the tunnel should be created prior to the notchplasty, but the tendon graft is not passed until the notchplasty is completed.

A second tunnel is created in the distal ulna between the fovea and ulnar neck. A 4- to 5-mm diameter drill hole is made in the ulnar neck at its subcutaneous border. A guidewire is inserted in the hole and driven through the fovea under direct visualization. Alternatively, the wrist is flexed, and the guidewire is driven through the fovea and out the ulnar neck. A 3.5-mm cannulated drill bit is used to create the tunnel. If necessary, it is enlarged further with larger drill bits or gouges to accommodate both limbs of the graft.

A suture retriever is passed through the tunnel in the radius from dorsal to palmar, and one end of the graft is pulled back through it (see Figures 14.24, *E-G*). Through the dorsal incision, a hemostat is passed over the ulnar head, adjacent to the ulnar styloid but proximal to the remaining TFCC, and pushed through the palmar DRUJ capsule. The other end of the graft is grasped with the hemostat and pulled back along this tract. Both graft limbs are passed through the ulnar tunnel to exit the ulnar neck. The limbs are passed in opposite directions around the ulnar neck, one passing radially and deep into the ECU sheath and the other passing palmarly. With the forearm in neutral rotation and the DRUJ manually compressed, the limbs are pulled taut, tied together, or passed through in a belt-loop fashion and secured with sutures (see Figure 14.24, *H*).

If the graft is too short to pass around the ulnar neck, alternative methods of graft fixation include making an additional hole in the neck dorsally and tying the graft over the bony bridge, or using a suture anchor or an interference screw. When the graft is too short, the senior author's preferred method is to tie the limbs around a broad, robust strip of elevated periosteum on the dorsum of the ulnar neck, typically located beneath the ECU tendon. The ECU sheath is opened at the level of the ulnar neck but not over the ulnar head, then one graft limb is passed under and then back over the periosteum through longitudinal splits but beneath the ECU tendon. The limbs are pulled taut around the periosteum and tied to each other.

The dorsal DRUJ capsule and extensor retinaculum are closed together as a single layer with 3-0 sutures, leaving the EDQ subcutaneous. The extremity is immobilized in a long-arm cast with the forearm in neutral rotation for 4 weeks, followed by use of a short-arm cast for 2 weeks. A wrist splint is used while motion and strength are gradually recovered. Near full activity is usually permitted after 4 months, but heavy lifting and impact loading are discouraged until 6 months postoperatively.

Outcomes

Scheker and associates reported complete resolution of pain in 12 of 14 patients at an average follow-up of 1.5 years with their technique.[138] Near full range of rotation and 76% increase in grip strength were achieved. Johnston Jones and Sanders reported 13 of 14 patients were satisfied at an average follow-up of 26 months.[70] Of these patients, 12 returned to their previous occupations and showed no evidence of recurrent instability; 2 patients had early failure of stability. No patient had loss of motion >10 degrees of supination or pronation.

Adams and Berger reported restoration of stability in 12 of 14 patients and resumption of previous work, sports, and avocations without limitations.[1] Recovery of strength and motion averaged 85%. Recurrent palmar instability occurred in one patient who had a posttraumatic defect in the palmar rim of the sigmoid notch and another patient had persistent ulnocarpal instability. The authors concluded that the procedure is effective for DRUJ instability but requires a competent sigmoid notch and does not fully correct ulnocarpal instability. If the notch is deficient, a sigmoid notch osteoplasty should be considered in conjunction with ligament reconstruction.

Osteoplasty of the Sigmoid Notch and Ulna

CT is helpful to evaluate the sigmoid notch in patients with a history of a fracture involving it, a suspected deformity of the DRUJ, or a developmentally flat notch. To improve the mechanical buttressing effect of the sigmoid notch's rim, an osteoplasty can be considered as an isolated procedure or to complement ligament reconstruction. In the procedure described by Wallwork and Bain, parallel osteotomies are made, with one just proximal to the lunate fossa and the other at the proximal margin of the sigmoid notch[171] (Figure 14.25).

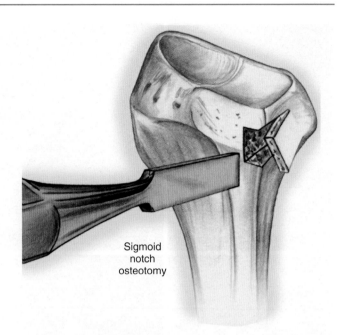

FIGURE 14.25 Sigmoid notch osteoplasty used for distal radial ulnar joint instability that is caused partially by deficiency of a rim of the notch. Bone graft is inserted beneath osteochondral flap. (From Adams B: Distal radioulnar joint. In Trumble TE, editor: *Hand surgery update 3: Hand, elbow, and shoulder*, Rosemont, IL, 2003, American Society for Surgery of the Hand, pp 147–157.)

A third osteotomy is made in the sagittal plane 5 mm from the articular surface of the notch and between the first two cuts; an osteotome placed in this longitudinal cut is carefully advanced, and at each increment it is levered in an ulnar direction to produce a thin, slightly curved osteocartilaginous flap. The wedge-shaped defect is filled with a bone graft harvested from the distal radius and fixed as necessary with Kirschner wires or sutures. When performed in conjunction with a ligament reconstruction, the tendon graft passes around the bone graft and the osteocartilaginous flap to stabilize the construct.

Published results about the procedure are limited, but the concept seems sound. It produced a good result when used as a sole procedure to treat palmar instability in a patient with a flat sigmoid notch.[171] The senior author uses it in conjunction with a radioulnar ligament reconstruction when the sigmoid notch is relatively flat and has been satisfied with the results.

An alternative osteoplasty is an angular osteotomy of the ulna. A closing wedge osteotomy is made in the distal third of the ulna to tilt the ulnar head toward the sigmoid notch with the forearm in the position of instability. The osteotomy is fixed with a compression plate. Preoperative planning, patient selection, and intraoperative assessment must be accurate to achieve a good result with this technique. It may be best utilized in patients with a preexisting ulnar deformity.

DISTAL RADIUS AND FOREARM MALUNIONS

In evaluating a patient with a distal radius malunion, both the radiocarpal joint and the DRUJ must be considered. Biomechanical studies have shown multiple effects of malunion on DRUJ function, with angulation and shortening of the radius more problematic than loss of radial inclination.[28] Isolated soft tissue reconstruction for instability fails when there is substantial radial deformity. Similarly, a Darrach resection of the distal ulna can result in instability of the residual ulnar stump if performed in the presence of a significant radial malunion.[47]

An osteotomy to correct angular deformity of the radius usually restores the sigmoid notch's orientation and DRUJ stability; however, radioulnar length discrepancy also must be addressed to improve carpal position and to prevent later development of an ulnar impaction syndrome. A trapezoidal graft to the radius can correct angulation and length discrepancy simultaneously. In malunions with severe length discrepancy, this

approach can be difficult because of the need for a large intercalated bone graft and the potential for delayed union.

As an alternative, leveling of the joint can be accomplished with concurrent ulnar-shortening osteotomy. If radial shortening is the only substantial deformity, and articular alignment of the radius and carpus is satisfactory, ulnar-shortening osteotomy is effective[154] (Figure 14.26). When bony realignment does not restore stability through a full arc of forearm rotation tested during surgery, TFCC repair or a soft tissue stabilization procedure is necessary (Figure 14.27). If DRUJ arthritis is present, one of the arthroplasty procedures described later in this

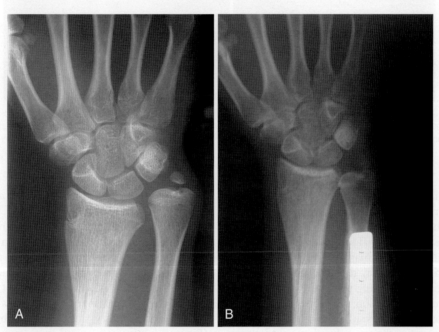

FIGURE 14.26 A, B, Radial shortening with disruption of distal radial ulnar joint can be effectively treated by ulnar shortening alone if joint widening is not present.

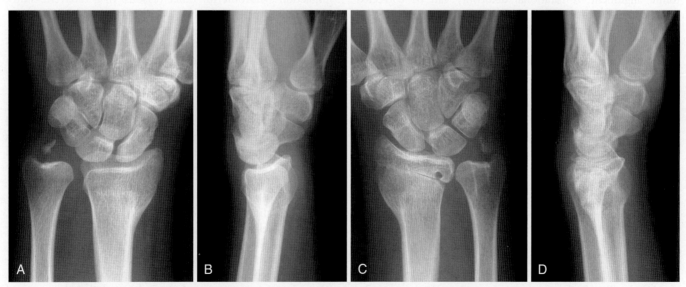

FIGURE 14.27 A, B, Views of distal radius malunion with distal radial ulnar joint (DRUJ) instability (i.e., angulation of the radius, DRUJ widening, and displaced fleck fracture from fovea). **C, D,** Treatment was by distal radius osteotomy and distal radioulnar ligament reconstruction as shown in Figure 14.20.

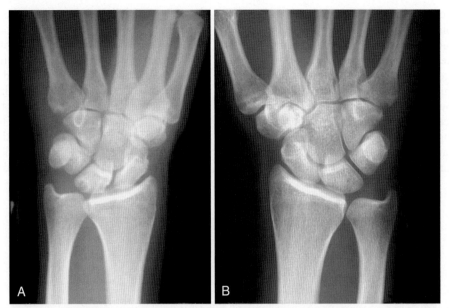

FIGURE 14.28 Comparison radiographs showing positive-ulnar variance with ulnar impaction syndrome (note cystic lesions in lunate) caused by premature physeal closure of distal radius (**A**) and opposite unaffected wrist (**B**). (From Adams B: Distal radioulnar joint. In Trumble TE, editor: *Hand surgery update 3: Hand, elbow, and shoulder,* Rosemont, IL, 2003, American Society for Surgery of the Hand, pp 147–157.)

chapter can be performed; however, radioulnar length discrepancy still needs to be corrected to prevent impingement between the ulnar styloid and the carpus.[14]

Forearm malunion can cause DRUJ instability in addition to loss of rotation. The deformity may manifest initially as limited forearm rotation, and instability may develop later as the soft tissues attenuate. Soft tissue stabilizing procedures alone fail in the presence of a forearm malunion. Conversely, corrective osteotomy with plate fixation often is sufficient to restore stability; TFCC repair or a reconstructive procedure is usually unnecessary.[165] The deformity may involve the radius and the ulna and require osteotomy of both bones. Angulation is corrected through the site of malunion whenever possible to attain anatomic alignment. A rotational deformity can be corrected simultaneously when an angular deformity is treated. Unless there is DRUJ arthritis, resection of the distal ulna should be avoided.

Preoperative planning is important to estimate the desired correction, but the final determination must be made intraoperatively. Temporary bony fixation can be used to assess the effect of the correction. If stability is not restored through a full arc of forearm rotation, a soft tissue stabilization procedure or DRUJ-salvage procedure may be combined with the corrective osteotomy. Operative techniques for correction of malunions are discussed in Chapter 15.

ULNAR IMPACTION SYNDROME

The ulnocarpal joint transmits a substantial load through a relatively small contact area and is at high risk for articular degeneration. This degenerative process is commonly called *ulnar impaction syndrome,* which implies that chronic compressive overloading is the primary cause. Shear forces over the articular surfaces and tensile forces through the soft tissues undoubtedly contribute to joint deterioration.

Acquired ulnar-positive variance is a known risk factor for ulnar impaction syndrome because of the associated increase in ulnocarpal loading. A 2.5-mm increase in ulnar variance increased ulnocarpal loading by 42% in a cadaveric study.[121] In a similar study, changing the tilt of the distal radius from normal to 40 degrees of dorsal tilt increased the ulnar load from 21 to 65%.[179a] Common causes of acquired positive variance include radial shortening from a distal radius fracture, Essex-Lopresti injury, and acute or chronic physeal injury[161] (Figure 14.28).

Although biomechanical studies have not shown increased load transmission through the ulnocarpal joint in developmentally ulnar-positive wrists, these wrists can still develop ulnar impaction syndrome for other reasons. In a cadaveric study, 73% of ulnar-neutral or ulnar-positive wrists had TFCC perforations, whereas only 17% of ulnar-negative wrists had perforations.[120] The thickness of the disk can play a role because there is an inverse relationship between ulnar variance and disk thickness; ulnar-positive wrists are associated with a thinner disk that may be more susceptible to perforation.[118] Also, physiologic increases in ulnar variance of 2 mm can occur during power grip, especially when the forearm is pronated. Palmer identified several additional structures at risk for degeneration in this process, including the ulnar head, lunate, triquetrum, and lunotriquetral interosseous ligament.[116]

Evaluation

Ulnar impaction syndrome is characterized by ulnar wrist pain, localized swelling, and occasional limitation of motion. The history and physical findings are similar to an acute TFCC tear. Pain is exacerbated by ulnar deviation during power grip, especially when combined with active pronation and supination. There is tenderness around the volar and dorsal aspects of the ulnar head and the triquetrum. Passive and active ulnar deviation produces pain, which is intensifed by the examiner simultaneously depressing the ulnar head and elevating the ulnar carpus (pisiform boost).

This maneuver better reproduces the joint reaction forces during power grip activities, which load the more central portions of the ulnar dome, TFCC disk, lunate, and triquetrum. While the wrist is loaded in this manner, the forearm can be rotated manually to add a shear force to the joint, which can increase pain and occasionally produces crepitus. The examiner should consider other diagnoses involving the ulnar side of the wrist that can manifest with similar findings or coexist, particularly arthritis of the DRUJ.

Standard wrist radiographs can be obtained to assess for arthritis involving the carpus and DRUJ and to measure ulnar variance. Because ulnar variance is dynamic, stress posteroanterior views can help. A pronated view,[38,117] a grip view,[42] or a view with combined pronation and grip[163] may reproduce dynamic increases in ulnar variance. In a study of 22 patients who presented with ulnar wrist pain, the pronated grip view resulted in statistically significant increases in ulnar variance with an average of 2.5 mm.[163]

Treatment

In treating ulnar-sided wrist pain, it is imperative to remember that degeneration is a common and natural occurrence in the ulnocarpal joint. Several months of conservative management are appropriate before proceeding to surgery. Options include modification of activities to avoid repetitive loading with the wrist in ulnar deviation, antiinflammatory medications, wrist splinting, and corticosteroid injections. Surgery is indicated for patients with clinical and radiographic evidence of ulnocarpal impaction without DRUJ arthritis whose symptoms do not resolve adequately despite conservative measures. The goal of surgery is to reduce ulnocarpal loading.

For a patient with negative or neutral ulnar variance, arthroscopic debridement of the articular disk, chondral surfaces, and lunotriquetral interosseous ligament can be effective. When static or dynamic ulnar-positive variance is present, decreased ulnar loading can be accomplished by a diaphyseal or metaphyseal[53,55] osteotomy, or a partial distal ulnar resection. Some surgeons prefer arthroscopic distal ulnar resection instead of open procedures because it avoids the potential for hardware irritation and the risk of nonunion (see Chapter 17). It is important to understand that distal ulnar-shortening osteotomies have no effect on tensioning of the secondary stabilizers of the DRUJ; consequently, when concern for subtle instability coexists with ulnar impaction syndrome, a diaphyseal osteotomy may be preferable.[76]

Partial Distal Ulnar Resection (Wafer Procedure)

Feldon and colleagues described the "wafer procedure" in which the distal 2 to 4 mm of the ulnar head is excised.[39] Although explained as an open procedure, it can be performed arthroscopically as well (see Chapter 17). The procedure is designed to retain the ulnar styloid and foveal attachments of the TFCC. It is not intended to disrupt the articular surfaces of the DRUJ, so no more than 3 to 4 mm of the distal ulna should be removed.

A dorsal approach to the DRUJ is used as described for distal radioulnar ligament reconstruction (see Figures 14.24, *A*, *B*). The distal 2 to 4 mm of the ulnar dome is resected with an osteotome or oscillating saw, taking care to preserve the TFCC's

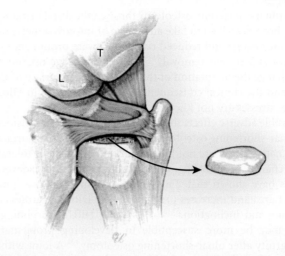

FIGURE 14.29 Resection of distal dome of ulnar head (wafer procedure) decompresses ulnocarpal joint for ulnar impaction syndrome. *L*, Lunate; *T*, triquetrum. (Copyright © Elizabeth Martin.)

ulnar attachments (Figure 14.29). If the TFCC becomes detached at the fovea, it is repaired using transosseous sutures as described for TFCC repair. The proximal surface of the disk is inspected and tears are debrided. The dorsal capsule is repaired, but not imbricated to avoid stiffness. A sugar tong splint is applied, with conversion to a removable wrist splint at the first postoperative visit. Digital, wrist, and forearm motion are started early, but full activity is not recommended for 8 to 12 weeks.

Outcomes. In a retrospective review of 13 cases by Feldon and associates, all achieved good or excellent results, and none required secondary procedures.[39] In a separate series of 26 patients, 23 were completely satisfied and obtained improved grip with this method. Two other smaller studies also reported positive results.[11,143] Despite such good final results, the procedure commonly requires a long recovery time. In comparison studies of ulnar-shortening osteotomy and the wafer procedure, outcomes were nearly identical, although reoperation, primarily for plate removal, was more frequent in the osteotomy group.[25,149]

Diaphyseal and Metaphyseal Ulnar-Shortening Osteotomy

Ulnar-shortening osteotomy (diaphyseal) has the advantage of preservation of the ulnar dome articular cartilage and does not violate the DRUJ or ulnocarpal joint. In cases of posttraumatic ulnar-positive variance, ulnar-shortening osteotomy may improve DRUJ congruity, improve forearm rotation, and reduce the risk of arthritis. The ulnocarpal ligaments are tightened by the procedure, and this may have a salutary effect on associated lunotriquetral or DRUJ instability.

An anatomical study of the interosseous membrane demonstrated the presence of a distal oblique bundle—a thickening of the IOM—in approximately 40% of specimens. The DOB originates from the distal 15% of the ulna diaphysis at approximately the proximal margin of the pronator quadratus, and it courses distally to insert into the capsular fibers of the DRUJ and the inferior rim of the sigmoid notch.[112] Based on its anatomic attachments, an ulnar-shortening osteotomy created proximal to the origin of the DOB may improve the stability of the DRUJ through its tensioning of the capsular structures.

An ulnar-shortening osteotomy through the distal metaphysis has been described to take advantage of improved metaphyseal bone healing and reduced risk of hardware prominence or need for subsequent removal.[55] The closing-wedge osteotomy does change the orientation of the distal articular surface of the ulna, and the clinical consequences of this alteration in DRUJ contact stresses are not known.[53]

Possible adverse effects should be recognized when considering ulnar-shortening osteotomy. Although the articular surfaces of the native DRUJ are not fully congruent and usually tolerate some change in joint alignment, radiographic and cadaveric studies have shown that 2 mm of shortening decreases joint contact area and increases pressures in the DRUJ regardless of its shape and inclination.[53,135,162,179] Some DRUJ morphologic types may be more susceptible to developing problematic incongruity after ulnar-shortening osteotomy.[135] A joint with a reverse oblique inclination in the coronal plane or a substantial articular mismatch between the sigmoid notch and ulnar head develops the greatest incongruity, with joint contact concentrated at the proximal margin of the notch. Similar changes occur in a joint with a deep sigmoid notch. Predicting the clinical outcome of surgically created DRUJ incongruity is difficult because it either may stimulate DRUJ remodeling or may cause arthritis.

Ulnar shortening was originally described by Milch in 1941 for the treatment of ulnar-positive variance after radial shortening from a Colles fracture.[96] Milch used a wire suture to fix the osteotomy. Although the principle remains the same, current methods include the use of an oblique osteotomy and techniques of osseous compression, with or without the use of special compression devices[20,178] or commercial plates designed specifically for this procedure.[128] An oblique osteotomy using a compression clamp and an interfragmentary screw increases compression and stability and may improve bone healing.[23,91]

❖ AUTHORS' PREFERRED METHOD OF TREATMENT: Ulnar-Shortening Osteotomy

The authors prefer the technique described by Chun and Palmer[23] (Figure 14.30). For patients with ulnar-positive variance, the amount of bone to be resected to obtain a final ulnar variance of 0 or −1 mm is determined on the posteroanterior radiograph. A 2- to 3-mm shortening is planned for patients with ulnar-neutral wrists. A skin incision is made along the subcutaneous border of the ulna extending proximally from its neck for 10 cm. The fascia is incised between the ECU and the FCU.

The dorsal sensory branch of the ulnar nerve typically lies volar and distal to the exposure and should be carefully protected. Minimal subperiosteal elevation is performed, so as not to strip the limited blood supply of the ulna. A 6- or 7-hole, 3.5-mm dynamic compression plate or specialty ulnar-shortening plate is contoured if necessary and applied to the ulna, with its distal edge about 1 cm proximal to the sigmoid notch. The two most distal screws are inserted in the neutral mode.

Electrocautery is used to make a mark on the ulna at the osteotomy site, which should lie opposite the third or fourth hole in the plate. A longitudinal mark is also made to ensure proper rotational alignment after osteotomy. When using the dynamic compression plate, the most distal screw is loosened and the other screw is removed to allow the plate to be swung away from the ulna. At 45 degrees to the coronal plane, an oblique cut is made through 75% of the ulna. A complete second cut is made parallel to the first. The kerf (i.e., width of bone it removes) of the saw blade is accounted for when making the second cut.

The first cut is completed and the resected bone is removed. The plate is swung back in place and the previously inserted screws are replaced and tightened. Axial compression is applied manually to the ulna to oppose the osteotomy, and the plate is clamped to the ulna proximally. In completing the plate fixation, one or two of the proximal screws are inserted eccentrically in the dynamic compression mode. At the osteotomy site, a compression screw is inserted through a gliding hole and across the oblique osteotomy using a standard interfragmentary compression technique.

In the senior author's experience, placement of the plate on the dorsal surface of the ulna reduces hardware irritation and the need for plate removal.[31] Commercially available systems incorporating a specialty plate and cutting jigs are commonly used for efficiency and accuracy; however, knowledge of the specific system is imperative to optimize its advantages. Postsurgery, an ulnar gutter splint is applied for 2 weeks. A removable splint is used with early forearm, wrist, and digital motion, but strenuous activity is restricted until bony union.

Outcomes. Several studies reported a high percentage of success with ulnar-shortening osteotomy. Combining the results using standard technique and equipment, 79 of 90 (88%) patients achieved good or excellent results with regard to pain relief and recovery of function with only one nonunion (1%).[20,23,30,178] Delayed union and symptomatic hardware prominence leading to plate removal are the most common

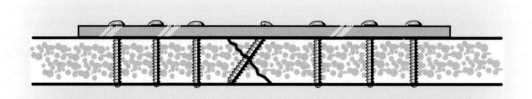

FIGURE 14.30 Ulnar-shortening osteotomy through the shaft is shown using oblique skeletal cut, compression plate, and interfragmentary screw. (Copyright © Elizabeth Martin.)

problems. Ulnar-shortening osteotomy has been used in conjunction with delayed repairs of traumatic TFCC injuries[166] and after failed arthroscopic debridement of central disk tears and incomplete avulsions of the TFCC.[61] The goal is to reduce the load on the injured TFCC. Ulnar shortening is reported as an effective treatment for Madelung deformity as well; remodeling of the joint may still occur even when performed in adolescents.[34]

DISTAL RADIOULNAR JOINT ARTHRITIS

Degeneration of the DRUJ can be caused by posttraumatic arthritis, inflammatory arthritis, osteoarthritis, but rarely by long-standing DRUJ instability. Differentiating between DRUJ arthritis and ulnocarpal impaction syndrome is important when treating degenerative conditions of the ulnar wrist. In some cases, both conditions are present and both require treatment to improve symptoms. Pain and swelling, decreased grip strength, and stiffness are the most common symptoms of DRUJ arthritis. Point tenderness is elicited directly over the DRUJ. Pain is exacerbated by forearm rotation, especially when the joint is manually compressed.

Early radiographic signs of degenerative arthritis of the DRUJ typically occur in the proximal portion of the joint. Osteophytes form along the proximal margin of the ulnar head, whereas the sigmoid notch often is spared. Based on these findings of localized articular involvement, nonablative procedures have been described. Ulnar shortening, which shifts the proximal margin of the ulnar head out of the sigmoid notch, was reported to relieve symptoms in early DRUJ posttraumatic arthritis.[139] Open surgical resection of the proximal one-third of the articular surface of the ulna around its entire circumference and 2- to 3-mm deep also has been employed. The procedure, called a modified arthroplasty, was reported to relieve pain and preserve motion and stability in 10 of 11 patients.[175] Although experience with these procedures is limited, similar approaches have been used successfully in other joints.

In more advanced arthritis, surgical treatments are designed to eliminate the articulation between the distal ulna and radius by resecting all or a portion of the distal ulna, fusing the joint, or replacing the distal ulna. Each of the many techniques described has advantages and disadvantages that should be considered when selecting treatment. Surgical options include the Darrach procedure, the Sauvé-Kapandji operation, hemiresection–interposition technique, implant arthroplasty, wide distal ulnar resection, and a one-bone forearm procedure. The last two options are reserved for ultimate salvage, particularly for a failed distal ulnar resection. Because these procedures do not restore normal anatomy, some compromised function and incomplete pain relief should be expected.

Operative Technique

Hemiresection–Interposition Arthroplasty

Because instability is occasionally associated with the Darrach procedure, Bowers designed a surgical procedure that removes the articular surface of the ulnar head and retains the critical ulnar attachments of the TFCC.[14] The procedure, which Bowers called the hemiresection–interposition technique, was derived from Dingman, who found the best clinical results of the Darrach procedure occurred in patients who had minimal distal

ulnar resection that was followed by regeneration within the retained periosteal sleeve.[33]

The primary indication for the hemiresection–interposition technique is posttraumatic or degenerative arthritis of the DRUJ. It may be useful also in patients with severe DRUJ contractures complicated by articular degeneration that may not be discovered until the surgical release. Caution should be observed before using this procedure for the treatment of combined DRUJ arthritis and instability because often the instability can be exacerbated.

Resection procedures in younger patients are less reliable because it may help to relieve pain but may result in loss of support for the ulnar carpus over time. Because some convergence of the radius and ulna occurs after partial resection of the ulnar head, ulnar-positive variance is a relative contraindication because it increases the likelihood of impingement between the ulnar styloid and triquetrum. Also, ulnar carpal translation is a contraindication to partial or complete excision of the ulnar head because the resection may exacerbate the translation. Irreparable damage to the TFCC is a relative contraindication because the hemiresection–interposition technique provides no theoretical benefit over a Darrach procedure.

In his original and modified techniques, Bowers created several retinacular flaps to reconstruct the capsule and to stabilize the ECU.[14] The arthroplasty can be augmented with a tendon or muscle interposition when local soft tissue is insufficient. The matched distal ulnar resection described by Watson and Gabuzda is a similar alternative.[174] Even though these authors do not stress preservation of the TFCC and ulnocarpal ligaments, it is advisable to do so. The concept is to remove all of the articular cartilage and subchondral bone on the radial and dorsal margins of the distal ulna so as to prevent radioulnar impingement during forearm rotation. An intact periosteal sleeve is preserved to maintain continuity with the ulnar carpus, and the exposed cancellous bone encourages very good healing of the surrounding soft tissue sleeve.

❖ AUTHORS' PREFERRED METHOD OF TREATMENT: Hemiresection-Interposition Technique Arthroplasty

The authors prefer a slight modification of Bowers' procedure, in which there is less resection of the ulnar head and the retinaculum and capsular flaps are secured within the resection site to create both interposition and stabilization (Figure 14.31). By resecting less ulnar head, the amount of radioulnar convergence that can occur is reduced. The seemingly increased risk of developing distal radioulnar bony contact is offset by the increased stability imparted from capturing a larger circumference of the distal ulna with a large capsular–retinacular flap, and it does not preclude adding free soft tissue for further interposition when desired.

The DRUJ is approached dorsally through the fifth extensor compartment in a manner similar to that described earlier for TFCC repair and distal radioulnar ligament reconstruction. An ulnar-based retinacular flap extending to the radial edge of the ECU sheath is elevated; its proximal margin is at the ulnar neck, and its distal margin is at the level of the ulnar styloid. The dorsal capsule is raised similarly as a large rectangular flap, with its base extending from the radial edge of the ECU sheath. (Note: The ECU sheath is not opened during this procedure.) The flap begins over the ulnar neck, continues along the rim of

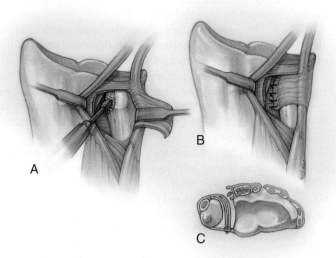

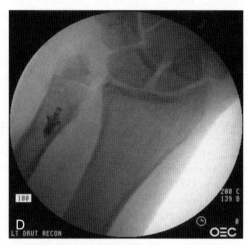

FIGURE 14.31 A–C, Hemiresection arthroplasty of distal ulna with soft tissue interposition for arthritis of distal radial ulnar joint (DRUJ). In this modification of the procedure described by Bowers, a single, broad dorsal flap composed of extensor retinaculum and dorsal DRUJ capsule is used for interposition and stabilization (see text). **D,** Concomitant interarticular ulnar-shortening osteotomy has been fixed with embedded suture anchor. (**A–C,** Copyright © Elizabeth Martin.)

the sigmoid notch, and courses ulnarly just proximal to the dorsal radioulnar ligament. Care should be taken not to cut the dorsal radioulnar ligament.

There is no need to expose the distal surface of the TFCC or carpus, unless symptomatic pathology is suspected. Small rongeurs and a bur are used to resect the surface of the ulnar head that articulates with the sigmoid notch to a depth of 3 to 7 mm; the depth of resection is guided by the size of the ulnar head. The head is shaped to resemble a dowel with approximately the same diameter as the ulnar neck. Slight distal tapering is done, but the fovea is not violated and the TFCC insertion is preserved. To reach the volar portion of the head, the radius and ulna are spread with strong retraction, or a laminar spreader is placed proximal to the DRUJ. The TFCC's proximal surface and the remaining ulnar dome are inspected for degeneration and debrided if necessary.

At this point, a decision about ulnar shortening is made. Usually, no more than 2 to 3 mm of ulnar-positive variance is accepted to avoid impingement between the triquetrum and the residual ulnar head or styloid. Similarly, in rare instances, an unusually long ulnar styloid may cause stylocarpal impingement.[164] An assessment for ulnar styloid impingement is done intraoperatively by compressing the radius and ulna while rotating the forearm with the wrist in ulnar deviation. If ulnar shortening is necessary, it can be done through the ulnar shaft, the base of the styloid, or the distal ulna. The goal is to create 1 to 2 mm of ulnar-negative variance. If styloid shortening is done, particular care is required not to cut the TFCC foveal attachment or release the TFCC from the styloid. A distal osteotomy can be repaired with wire or heavy nonabsorbable sutures using a figure-of-eight tension band or an interosseous compression loop.

We prefer to shorten the ulna through the midportion of the residual ulnar head because it can be done through the same incision, avoids the risk of injuring the TFCC foveal attachment, requires minimal fixation, and is in the metaphysis with good bone healing potential. With this technique, a slice is removed

with an oscillating saw at its midportion. The osteotomy can be fixed using a standard tension band technique with two parallel 0.045-in Kirschner wires passed obliquely across the osteotomy and a figure-of-eight wire suture. The Kirschner wires are bent over and tapped into the bone. Because the wires often create irritation and require removal, the authors prefer to fix the osteotomy using either a large suture anchor inserted deep into the ulnar neck as described earlier for fixation of ulnar styloid fractures or a headless cannulated screw (see Figure 14.31, *D*). To provide an interposition and to stabilize the joint, the ulnar edges of the retinacular and capsular flaps are sutured simultaneously to the volar DRUJ capsule. The EDQ tendon is left in a subcutaneous position.

Outcomes. Bowers reported on 38 patients, most of whom had rheumatoid arthritis.[14] Patient outcomes were generally good for pain relief and improved motion. Results were excellent in patients with degenerative or posttraumatic arthritis. Often, failures were related to residual ulnocarpal impaction. Bowers now recommends this procedure only in the early stages of rheumatoid arthritis when the stabilizing soft tissues are still effective. According to Bowers, the procedure is particularly valuable in posttraumatic arthritis and osteoarthritis if ulnocarpal impaction is avoided.[14] Fernandez found the procedure to be effective when used in conjunction with a radial osteotomy for malunited distal radius fractures.[40] It has been reported to also be successful in conjunction with repairs of the TFCC in patients with ulnar-positive variance.[99]

Sauvé-Kapandji Procedure

In 1936, Sauvé and, later, Kapandji described a procedure consisting of a radioulnar joint arthrodesis and creation of a pseudarthrosis proximal to the fusion (Figure 14.32). The procedure was developed as an alternative to resection of the distal ulna. Indications are similar to the Darrach procedure, including posttraumatic DRUJ arthritis, rheumatoid arthritis, and osteoarthritis. It has an advantage over a distal ulnar resection in patients with rheumatoid arthritis because it retains support for

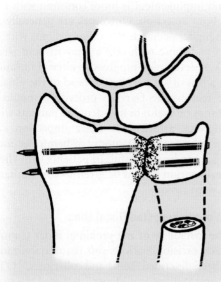

FIGURE 14.32 Sauvé-Kapandji procedure forms a fusion between ulnar head and sigmoid notch and creates a pseudarthrosis through ulnar neck. One or two cannulated screws are used instead of Kirschner wires if bone stock is adequate. (Copyright © Elizabeth Martin.)

the ulnar carpus and reduces the risk of ulnar translation. Some authors have suggested that the Sauvé-Kapandji procedure may be a better one for the treatment of posttraumatic arthritis in active young patients.[72] Potential complications include instability of the ulnar stump and regeneration of the resected segment resulting in loss of motion.

❖ AUTHORS' PREFERRED METHOD OF TREATMENT:
Sauvé-Kapandji Procedure

To improve visualization of the articular surfaces of the DRUJ and to avoid levering out the head fragment, we prefer a dorsal exposure. Some surgeons prefer an ulnar approach. A longitudinal incision is made over the sixth extensor compartment extending from the level of the ulnar styloid proximally for 5 to 6 cm. The fifth extensor compartment is opened and the EDQ tendon is retracted. The extensor retinaculum and DRUJ capsule are raised as an ulnar-based flap. The choice of fixation depends on the size and quality of the bone. If bone quality is sufficient, cannulated screw fixation is planned. Two parallel guidewires are inserted into the head just beneath the ECU sheath. The periosteum is excised around the ulnar neck, and 1 cm of the neck is resected with an oscillating saw. If there is ulnar-positive variance, a correspondingly greater segment of ulna is removed so that when the head is depressed to neutral variance the resulting gap is 1 cm. The opposing articular surfaces of the ulnar head and sigmoid notch are denuded to cancellous bone. The ulnar head is held against the sigmoid notch in neutral rotation and at the proper longitudinal position. The wires are driven into the radius, and acceptable alignment is confirmed with fluoroscopy.

Two 3.5-mm cannulated screws are inserted using a lag technique to gain compression, but tilting of the ulnar head must be avoided. If two screws cannot fit, one 3.5-mm and a smaller diameter screw, or one of the guidewires, can be used for

additional fixation. Prior to definitive fixation, a small portion of resected cancellous bone is placed into the arthrodesis site. The pronator quadratus muscle is detached from its ulnar insertion and advanced into the osteotomy site and sutured in place to the ECU sheath, followed by a layered wound closure.

To gain additional stability of the proximal ulnar stump in a young patient with posttraumatic arthritis, the FCU tenodesis technique described by Fernandez is used.[40] A distally based strip of FCU tendon is raised and passed into the exposed medullary canal of the ulnar stump and out through a drill hole in it. It is sutured back onto itself under tension. The pronator quadratus is brought into the gap and sutured in place. A long-arm splint is used for 2 to 4 weeks, followed by a short-arm cast until there is radiographic evidence of fusion.

A modified technique described by Fujita and colleagues is useful for patients with advanced rheumatoid disease and in whom the ulnar head is severely eroded. Therefore, a standard Sauvé-Kapandji procedure is not feasible.[44] In their modification, the ulnar osteotomy is made approximately 2 cm proximal to the head, the head–neck segment is rotated 90 degrees from its normal orientation; then, the neck is inserted into a large hole drilled in the sigmoid notch. A screw is inserted through the head, down the neck's medullary canal into the distal radius to stabilize the construct. Although the technique creates an articular surface with the nonarticular part of the ulna, it does construct a strong support for the ulnar carpus.

Outcomes. Goncalves reported on 22 patients whose results were "consistently better" than historical results with the Darrach procedure.[50] Taleisnik reported elimination of pain, restoration of forearm rotation, and few complications in 24 patients with a minimum 1-year follow-up.[158] Predictable complications of an unstable proximal ulnar stump were observed in only 3 of the 24 patients. Other authors have found instability of the ulnar stump more common, although not always symptomatic. A number of authors have expressed general satisfaction with the procedure.[40,51,72,98,100] Stern and colleagues reported unpredictable results in 12 patients—one underwent hardware removal and one underwent a Darrach procedure for persisting pain, with resolution of symptoms.[47]

Distal Ulnar Resection (Darrach Procedure)

Although Darrach's name has become synonymous with resection of the distal ulna, this technique was described by several others before him.[93] The general indication for a distal ulnar resection is any condition that causes incongruity or arthritis of the DRUJ, with resultant pain or stiffness. The procedure is particularly effective for a low-demand patient with an incongruous or degenerative sigmoid notch owing to the sequelae of an intraarticular fracture.

Probably more has been written about the Darrach procedure than any other operation concerning the DRUJ, with a wide variation of technical modifications, results, and opinions (Figure 14.33). Dingman[33] and, more recently, DiBenedetto and colleagues,[32] Nolan and Eaton,[113] and Tulipan and colleagues[169] reviewed the procedure with regard to the technical points of extraperiosteal or subperiosteal resection, the obliquity of the cut, whether to remove the styloid, and the amount of bone to be resected. Dingman's study suggested that none of these factors, other than the amount of bone resection, correlated with patient outcomes. He recommended that only the ulna

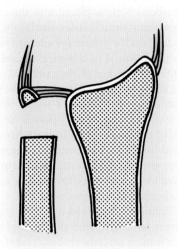

FIGURE 14.33 Darrach procedure resects distal ulna through ulnar neck. The ulnar styloid and its attachments can be retained. Various techniques have been described to help stabilize the ulnar stump. (Adapted from Dingman P: Resection of the distal end of the ulna (Darrach operation): an end result study of twenty-four cases. *J Bone Joint Surg Am* 34:893–900, 1952. Redrawn by Elizabeth Martin.)

adjacent to the sigmoid notch be resected and that subperiosteal resection was ideal because patients in whom regeneration had occurred seemed to have had better results. Dingman also preferred to retain the ulnar styloid. Although controversial, many surgeons would recommend that the procedure be combined with a soft tissue stabilization technique.

❖ AUTHORS' PREFERRED METHOD OF TREATMENT: Distal Ulnar Resection

An incision is extended 5- to 6-cm proximally from the ulnar styloid process along the midsagittal aspect of the distal ulna. The bone is approached just volar to the ECU sheath, with care taken to avoid the dorsal cutaneous branch of the ulnar nerve. The periosteum is incised and reflected from the distal 3 cm of the ulna, but the attachments to the ulnar styloid are retained. Fluoroscopy is used to confirm the preferred osteotomy site; a transverse ulnar osteotomy is made at the level corresponding to the proximal margin of the sigmoid notch. The distal fragment is dissected free, and the ulnar styloid process is osteotomized at its base and left in situ. The periosteal sleeve is closed to provide a firm attachment for the styloid and to help stabilize the ulnar stump.

We typically perform a soft tissue stabilization procedure as an adjunct to the resection (see next section). The wound is closed in layers. Darrach did not use a splint and allowed active motion within 24 h; however, the authors prefer to use a short-arm splint to support the wrist for 2 to 4 weeks to prevent full forearm rotation until the patient has recovered good digital motion and pain and swelling are minimal.

Outcomes. Regardless of the diagnosis, most patients achieve satisfactory pain relief and restoration of function.[52] Instability of the ulnar stump in the anteroposterior and coronal planes can develop and produce substantial weakness and pain. Convergence of the proximal ulnar stump can develop into radioulnar impingement and painful crepitus.[56] The amount of

instability and impingement is more common with increasing amounts of bony resection. Outcomes are generally worse in patients with higher demands.[14,56,174] For patients with rheumatoid arthritis and those with active synovitis and wrist laxity, there is a risk of developing progressive ulnar translation of the carpus from a loss of support by the head of the ulna.

For these reasons the Darrach procedure should be used selectively. It may be useful in low-demand patients with severe DRUJ incongruity, arthritis, or ulnar impaction syndrome when an ulnar-shortening osteotomy or hemiresection arthroplasty is unlikely to be successful. In patients with rheumatoid arthritis, consideration should be given to concomitant partial or complete wrist fusion.

Stabilization of the Resected Distal Ulna

To reduce the instability of the proximal ulnar stump created by the Darrach excision, various soft tissue stabilization techniques have been described. Leslie and colleagues,[83] O'Donovan and Ruby,[114] and Webber and Maser[176] tethered the stump with a distally based strip of ECU tendon. Spinner and Kaplan[153] transposed the ECU over the dorsum of the ulnar stump using a flap of retinaculum. Kessler and Hecht[73] created a dynamic sling for the ulnar stump by looping a strip of tendon around the distal ulnar stump and the ECU. Goldner and Hayes[49] passed a proximally based strip of the ECU through a drill hole in the ulnar stump with the forearm in supination. Breen and Jupiter used a combination of half FCU and half ECU, both threaded into the medullary canal of the stump.[16]

Tsai and coworkers used a distally based portion of the FCU tendon to stabilize the ulnar stump and looped this tendon over it also to stabilize the ECU.[167] Tsai and Stilwell[168] reported using the ECU in a similar manner. Hunter and Kirkpatrick[63] used Mersilene tape to bind the radius and ulna together. Watson and colleagues[173] lengthened the short ulnar stump to approximate the appearance of a successfully done partial ulnar resection. Advancement and dorsal redirection of the pronator quadratus was used by Johnson[68] as a soft tissue interposition and as a dynamic stabilizer for the proximal ulnar stump. Ruby and coworkers[132] described a similar use of the pronator quadratus. Blatt and Ashworth sutured a flap of volar capsule to the dorsal aspect of the ulnar stump, which is particularly useful in severe rheumatoid arthritis.[13] Insertion of soft tissue allograft with suture fixation to the ulna and radius was reported by Sotereanos and associates.[151]

❖ AUTHORS' PREFERRED METHOD OF TREATMENT: Stabilization of Resected Distal Ulna

In an elderly, low-demand, or rheumatoid patient, we prefer to stabilize the ulnar stump with a broad flap created from the palmar portion of the ulnocarpal capsule. The flap is transferred to the dorsum of the ulna and attached with sutures through drill holes in the dorsal cortex. The ECU tendon is positioned over the dorsum of the ulna using a sling made from the retinaculum, as described in the section on ECU tendon instability. In patients for whom the capsular tissue is attenuated or of poor quality, tenodesis using one-half of the ECU tendon or both the ECU and FCU tendons by Breen and Jupiter[16] is performed, as discussed next.

For patients with higher demands or patients presenting with an unstable previously resected distal ulna, we prefer to

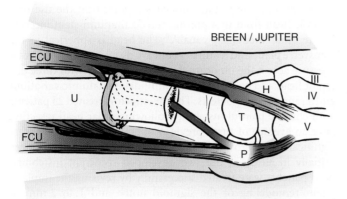

FIGURE 14.34 Tenodesis for stabilization of resected distal ulna using strips of flexor carpi ulnaris and extensor carpi ulnaris tendons as described by Breen and Jupiter. *ECU,* Extensor carpi ulnaris; *FCU,* flexor carpi ulnaris; *H,* hamate; *P,* pisiform; *T,* triquetrum; *U,* ulna; *III,* long finger metacarpal; *IV,* ring finger metacarpal; *V,* small finger metacarpal. (From Petersen MS, Adams BD: Biomechanical evaluation of distal radioulnar reconstructions. *J Hand Surg Am* 18:328–334, 1993.)

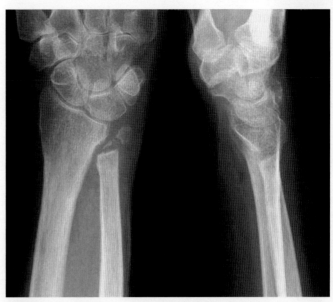

FIGURE 14.35 Radiograph showing excision and consequent radioulnar impingement after Darrach procedure. Note remodeling of radius at site of impingement.

stabilize the ulnar stump with a tenodesis using the technique described by Breen and Jupiter because it offers theoretical bidirectional control of the ulnar stump[16] (Figure 14.34). With this technique, a distally based strip of the FCU is passed into the canal of the ulna stump and out through a prepared bone hole in the ulnar shaft. A proximally based ECU strip is passed through the same hole, and both strips are wrapped around the shaft and sutured to each other. If the pronator quadratus has not been damaged previously, it is transferred to augment the stabilization and to provide soft tissue interposition to reduce radioulnar impingement. The muscle is detached from the palmar aspect of the ulna, routed through the radioulnar space, and attached to the dorsum of the distal ulna.[68] All of these procedures have been used successfully to reduce symptoms in small numbers of patients. Complete pain relief and restoration of full function are rare, however.

FAILED DISTAL ULNAR RESECTION

Instability of the distal ulna after a resection can develop early or late. Weakness and pain are associated with excessive dorsal–palmar translation and radioulnar convergence. Convergence can progress to impingement of the ulnar stump against the radius, producing crepitus and pain with forearm rotation (Figure 14.35). Although severe instability of the distal ulna is associated most commonly with the Darrach procedure, it also occurs after hemiresection or the Sauvé-Kapandji procedure. Typically, a history of painful crepitus around the distal ulna can be reproduced during the physical examination by manually compressing the radius against the ulna while passively rotating the forearm. A posteroanterior radiograph shows that the distal ulna touches the radius, which can be accentuated by having the patient hold a weight with the forearm in neutral rotation while the radiograph is taken in a "cross-table" direction (see Figure 14.10).

Treatment of radioulnar impingement is extremely difficult. Bieber and coworkers reported that patients failing a Darrach

procedure continued to do poorly despite undergoing up to seven additional operations.[10] Several of the ligament reconstructions described earlier have been used with varying success, but the techniques may need modification to produce a better mechanism to prevent recurrent impingement. If a tenodesis or soft tissue interposition was not used in the primary procedure, a revision using one, or a combination of the techniques, can be effective. A careful review of the patient's previous operation record provides important information regarding available tissues such as the volar DRUJ capsule, pronator quadratus, ECU, and FCU. Kleinman and Greenberg combined longitudinal intramedullary ECU tenodesis, dorsal transfer of the pronator quadratus, and temporary pinning of the distal radius and ulna.[79]

In a modestly active patient with adequate soft tissue and proper motivation for rehabilitation, the authors' preferred technique is ulnar head implant arthroplasty. This procedure is presented in the next section. When implant arthroplasty is contraindicated, we prefer to use the combined method of Breen and Jupiter[16] to stabilize the ulnar stump via tenodesis along with soft tissue interposition using the pronator quadratus when available or Achilles tendon interposition allograft.

In the challenging scenario where previous stabilization of the ulnar stump has failed, the allograft interposition arthroplasty described by Sotereanos and colleagues is a reasonable option because it has demonstrated favorable results for up to 10 years' follow-up.[151] Technically, it is important to secure the allograft tendon to the ulnar border of the distal one-third radius using multiple suture anchors and separate sutures fixing the allograft to the distal ulna using transosseous tunnels to reduce the risk of an ulnar stress fracture.

For patients who have had repeated failed surgeries, wide ulnar resection and creating a one-bone forearm are alternatives, but these procedures should be used with caution. Usually, extensive resection of the distal ulna is reserved for treatment of tumors,[27] but one study[183] reported generally favorable results in patients after failed DRUJ reconstruction. Range of motion and grip strength averaged 75 to 90%, but radioulnar instability and convergence led to failure in two cases. Radiocarpal instability and ulnar carpal translocation were rare. The surgical approach is straightforward; the ulna is exposed along its subcutaneous border, and subperiosteal resection of 25 to 30% of the ulnar length is recommended. Previous traumatic disruption of the interosseous membrane is an absolute contraindication to the procedure.[183]

The ultimate salvage for the dysfunctional forearm following attempts at surgical reconstruction of the radioulnar functional relationship is the creation of a one-bone forearm through a radioulnar fusion. A complete loss of forearm motion is what is sacrificed to reduce pain and to restore forearm stability. A preoperative test of immobilization in various positions of forearm rotation allows the patient to decide whether the procedure is appropriate and to determine the optimal position for fusion.

One study of 30 normal subjects determined that 63% of them preferred a neutral forearm position for activities of daily living. The procedure is indicated for end-stage radioulnar instability that is recalcitrant to surgical stabilization; paralytic instability; and, rarely, spastic contractures. The fusion can be accomplished by making osteotomies through the radial and ulnar shafts, discarding the proximal radius and the distal ulna, and transposition of the radius to the ulna with plate fixation. Alternatively, the radius and ulna can be collapsed against each other and fixed together with lag screws or a bridging plate. Iliac crest bone graft is recommended. Typically, the osteotomy is fixed with the forearm in neutral or slight pronation. Successful fusion was achieved in 60 of 65 cases in one study series with a distal radioulnar fusion fixed with dual lag screws. Complications are common, and the nonunion rate in one series was 32%.[125]

DISTAL ULNAR HEAD IMPLANT ARTHROPLASTY

Normal stability and function of the forearm rotation axis require an intact ulnar head, making implant arthroplasty an attractive concept for the treatment of ulnar head deficiencies and arthritis. Outcomes of soft tissue stabilization procedures for the treatment of the unstable, resected distal ulna are unpredictable. Successful ulnar head replacement arthroplasty would function to alleviate radioulnar impingement and replicate load transmission. Although a silicone implant, combined with soft tissue reconstruction, temporarily relieved symptoms and restored stability,[157] inevitable failure of the implant led to recurrence of symptoms and silicone synovitis. Silicone ulnar head implants therefore have been abandoned.

Various implant designs have become commercially available and can be divided into the following types: total ulnar head with or without an extended collar, partial ulnar head, unlinked total DRUJ arthroplasty, and linked DRUJ arthroplasty. None of these implants has had long-term clinical follow-up; however, biomechanical laboratory studies have shown excellent kinematic performance, and early clinical results are encouraging. Indications for ulnar head arthroplasty have expanded beyond the treatment of failed resection arthroplasty and include primary treatment of arthritis and irreparable ulnar head fractures.

van Schoonhoven and associates reported on the use of a ceramic head fixed to a porous-coated titanium stem inserted in the ulnar medullary canal.[170] The head is spherical in the transverse plane and features a concave distal surface to decrease pressure across the ulnocarpal joint. Modularity with three different head and collar sizes accommodates anatomic variations and a range of bony defects. The investigators treated 23 patients with chronic painful instability following ulnar head resection after an average of three previous operations. Symptoms were significantly improved in all patients. Stability was achieved initially in all cases, but two developed recurrent instability; both patients were treated successfully by revising the implant. Slight remodeling of the sigmoid notch and 1 to 2 mm of resorption beneath the collar occurred in all patients but was not progressive. These authors were cautiously optimistic with the short-term results.

A metallic ulnar head implant with a modular head and stem, including an extended collar for ulnar neck deficiencies has been developed.[92,181] The implant is indicated for use in acute ulnar head fractures, posttraumatic DRUJ arthritis, rheumatoid arthritis, and failed previous partial or complete resections of the distal ulna, including failed silicone implants. The implant head has a site for reattachment of the TFCC, ECU sheath, and ulnocarpal ligaments to help stabilize the DRUJ. Cement fixation of the stem is not typically necessary. In a prospective study of 19 implants in 17 patients treated for radioulnar convergence, impingement, or arthritis, results showed pain scores diminished by 50%, grip strength improved by 16%, and forearm rotation was unchanged. Many of these patients had multiple previous operations. Two failures occurred at 7 and 14 months postoperatively.[181]

A partial ulnar head replacement arthroplasty was designed for primary treatment of arthritis of the DRUJ, irreparable acute ulnar head fractures, and failed partial ulnar head resections. The concept is to replace only the articular surfaces of the ulnar head and to preserve the soft tissue restraints of the DRUJ. The implant is contraindicated for patients with substantial positive ulnar variance in which proper DRUJ congruity cannot be obtained or stylocarpal impingement would result, and for patients with a previous complete ulnar head resection. In a cadaveric study, the implant provided a close match to the native ulnar head and good joint stability.[24]

Scheker and associates designed a linked implant that replaces the ulnar head and the sigmoid notch, which they considered a total replacement of the DRUJ.[137] It is a ball-and-socket concept that allows some axial displacement of the radial component on the ulnar component to accommodate changes in ulnar variance during forearm rotation. The sigmoid notch component consists of a plate with a socket attached to its distal end and fixed to the distal radius by a peg and screws. The ulnar component is a polyethylene ball fitted on a peg that extends from a long stem fixed into the ulnar medullary canal. The ball can slide axially on the peg but cannot translate.

The purpose of this more complex implant is to stabilize the distal radioulnar relationship in cases with loss of skeletal and ligament support. The prosthesis was used in patients who had partial or complete destruction of the DRUJ, including loss from gunshot injuries, motor vehicle accidents, and excessive surgical resection of the distal ulna for posttraumatic arthritis. A dorsal surgical approach is used, and release of the distal IOM is occasionally performed to achieve proper motion. A long-arm splint is applied for 3 weeks for immobilization, after which active range-of-motion exercise is initiated.

Scheker and associates treated 23 patients who had at least one previous surgery with partial or complete distal ulna resection.[137] Mean follow-up was 15 months, with a maximum of 40 months. Complete pain relief was reported for all patients, and lifting capacity ranged from 2 to 50 lb with an average of 14 lb; however, a 25-lb lifting limit was recommended to reduce the risk of loosening. Normal pronation and supination were observed. The authors reported no complications; however, one prosthesis was removed for suspected infection.

Operative Technique for Ulnar Head Arthroplasty

A total ulnar head replacement is implanted through a dorsal approach. An ulnar-based flap, including the capsule and extensor retinaculum, is raised from the ulnar head with care to preserve the integrity of the ECU sheath. The amount of soft tissue release from the ulnar head and neck depends on the implant being used and the laxity of the joint. In the presence of a malunited radius, a corrective osteotomy is recommended before implant arthroplasty to achieve radioulnar stability. It is important to contour the sigmoid notch surgically when substantially misshapen by trauma or arthritis; however, breaching the subchondral bone can increase the risk of implant erosion into the radius.

The prosthetic head size is chosen to tension the soft tissues properly, but overstuffing the joint should be avoided. Typically, the implant is inserted without cement. The capsular and retinacular flaps are advanced on the radius as necessary during closure to create prosthetic stability. A long-arm splint is applied for 2 weeks, followed by a short-arm cast for 2 weeks, then a removable splint for another 4 weeks to allow sufficient soft tissue healing for joint stability and bone ongrowth for stem fixation. Strengthening and activities are advanced as wrist and forearm motion improves.

In previously operated cases, the senior author prefers an ulnar surgical approach between the FCU and ECU for ease of implantation and to preserve the capsule. The ECU sheath is elevated subperiosteally from the distal ulna along with the TFCC and ulnocarpal ligaments. The option exists to secure the confluence of the TFCC, ECU sheath, and ulnar wrist capsule with sutures placed through holes in the peripheral part of the implant head to gain joint stability. Rehabilitation is the same as described for the dorsal approach.

A partial ulnar head replacement can be implanted with less exposure than for a total head. A dorsal longitudinal skin incision is made over the ulnar head between the fifth and sixth extensor compartments. The fifth extensor compartment is opened from 2 cm proximal to the ulnar neck to 2 cm distal to the ulnar styloid. The EDQ tendon is retracted to expose the DRUJ dorsal capsule. A rectangular-shaped capsulotomy is made in the dorsal DRUJ capsule, with the longitudinal limb beginning at the ulnar neck and extending parallel to the attachment of the capsule at the sigmoid notch but stopping short of the dorsal radioulnar ligament.

The proximal transverse limb runs across the ulnar neck to the ECU tendon. The distal transverse limb runs parallel to the proximal edge of the dorsal radioulnar ligament and extends ulnarward to the ECU sheath. It is unnecessary to open the ECU sheath. To deliver the ulnar head dorsally, the foveal attachments of the TFCC are sharply released, but the remaining attachments are preserved. A small Hohmann retractor is placed beneath the ulnar head to lift it dorsally. The ulnar shaft is entered through the fovea with an awl. Serial reamers are used until there is cortical contact in the medullary canal. A cutting guide is applied to the reamer handle and properly aligned using the ulnar border of the ulna. The articular surfaces are resected using a small oscillating saw. The resected portion of the ulnar head is matched to the implant trials for proper size. The implant is inserted with a press-fit. The DRUJ capsule and retinaculum are closed in layers, with the EDQ tendon left subcutaneous over the DRUJ (Figure 14.36).

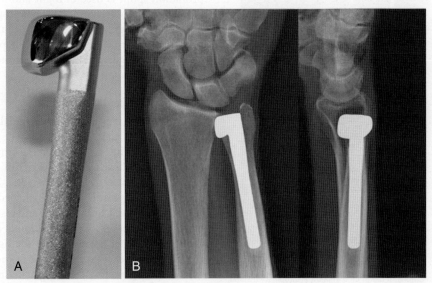

FIGURE 14.36 A, Partial ulnar head replacement prosthesis is designed to resurface only the articulating portion of distal ulna (Ascension Orthopedics, Austin, TX). **B,** Posteroanterior and lateral radiographs showing partial ulnar head replacement.

Outcomes

Experience with distal ulna implants is gradually increasing. Biomechanical testing shows that the implants restore DRUJ kinematics to near-normal.[92] The implants are particularly attractive for use for patients with radioulnar impingement after a failed partial or complete distal ulnar resection. In our experience, however, pain and instability are improved, with occasional minor pain and swelling being common after strenuous activities. Achieving a good, well-balanced soft tissue envelope around the implant can be challenging in a patient who has undergone multiple operations or poor-quality soft tissue constraints due to inflammatory arthritis. A substantial improvement in pain and range of motion in patients with rheumatoid arthritis was reported by Galvis et al.[45] Outcomes of ulnar head arthroplasty in patients with previous attempts at DRUJ reconstruction are worse than for primary arthroplasty.[134] Despite these concerns, implant arthroplasty results in less morbidity and appears to be more predictable in short-term follow-up than one-bone forearm or wide excision for radioulnar impingement (Figure 14.37).

In the absence of soft tissue constraints to support an implant arthroplasty, a linked total joint arthroplasty has been used. In this challenging condition, where a one-bone forearm reconstruction may otherwise be the only option, the linked prosthesis has shown promising early results. Several studies detailed good outcomes for decreased pain, forearm motion, and patient satisfaction, with no reported implant failures to date.[12,71,136] Kachooei et al. reported good outcomes for 14 prostheses with no implant failures and secondary procedures in only two patients for debridement of the radial screw tip at a mean follow-up of 60 months (range, 2-102 months).[71] Longer follow-up studies are needed to assess its full value.

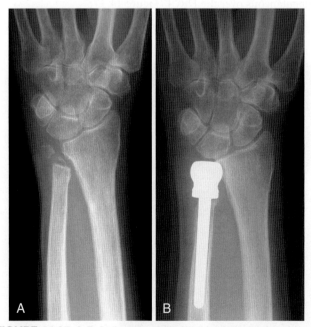

FIGURE 14.37 A, B, Radiographs of distal ulna implant arthroplasty (uHead; Avanta Orthopedics, San Diego) for treatment of radioulnar impingement. Note restoration of radioulnar alignment.

DISTAL RADIOULNAR JOINT CONTRACTURE

Acquired contractures of the DRUJ can be the result of trauma, arthritis, or spasticity. Conditions that mimic DRUJ contractures include forearm synostosis, radial head dislocation, and dysplastic congenital conditions. Posttraumatic contractures of the DRUJ capsule are common, especially loss of supination after a distal radius fracture. Physical therapy, including a splinting program, should be used for at least 4 to 6 months before considering surgery. Arthritis and DRUJ subluxation are contraindications to surgical release. CT should be performed if standard radiographs are inconclusive.

Posttraumatic DRUJ stiffness results from fibrosis and contracture of the capsule. The volar capsule normally has a redundant oblique fold that opens and forms a pocket to accept the ulnar head in supination.[78] Subsequent to trauma and immobilization in pronation, the capsular fold can become thickened, adherent, and shortened and can cause a restriction of supination. Contracture of the pronator quadratus from immobilization or injury can contribute to a pronation contracture. The dorsal capsule is normally much thinner and homogeneous, with transversely oriented fibers. It is much less likely to impede pronation after trauma or prolonged immobilization and is more likely to respond to therapy when contracted. Volar capsulectomy is performed for loss of supination, and dorsal capsulectomy is done for decreased pronation. Combined volar–dorsal capsulectomy is required for a severe bidirectional stiffness or fibrous ankylosis.

Operative Technique

Dorsal DRUJ Capsulectomy

A dorsal exposure of the DRUJ is made as described earlier for radioulnar ligament reconstruction. The entire dorsal capsule is excised to avoid damaging the dorsal radioulnar ligament or ECU sheath. The joint is inspected for injury or arthritis and carefully debrided if necessary. The forearm is gently manipulated into maximum allowable pronation. A long-arm or sugar tong plaster splint is applied with the forearm in full but not forced pronation and maintained for 2 to 3 weeks. A removable pronation splint is used at night and intermittently during the day for 1 month. Dynamic or static progressive splinting is used only if the original improvements in motion are not being sustained. Alternatively, if near full passive motion is easily achieved at surgery, immediate motion with night splinting is initiated.

Volar DRUJ Capsulectomy

A longitudinal incision is made radial to the FCU, extending proximal from the wrist crease. The pronator quadratus is exposed via the interval between the ulnar neurovascular bundle and the digital flexor tendons. The distal half of the pronator is raised subperiosteally from the ulna. The palmar radioulnar ligament is palpated, and an L-shaped capsulotomy is made, with the transverse limb parallel and just proximal to the palmar radioulnar ligament. The longitudinal limb is made parallel to the attachment of the capsule at the sigmoid notch. The entire volar capsule is excised with care so as not to damage the palmar radioulnar ligament. If the gain in supination is inadequate after gentle manipulation, the pronator quadratus is completely released or excised. A long-arm or sugar tong plaster splint is applied with the forearm in full but not forced supination and maintained for 2 weeks. A removable supination splint is used at night and intermittently during the day for 1 month. Dynamic or static progressive splinting is used only if the original gains in motion are lost.

Outcomes

In a report on a small series of patients, improvement in forearm motion was universal, with an average increase in supination of 51 degrees and in pronation of 28 degrees. There were no complications, including no iatrogenic cases of DRUJ instability.[78] In our experience, contracture release is a gratifying procedure for loss of supination after a distal radius fracture when the DRUJ is well aligned and not arthritic. A contracture release in the presence of a subluxated DRUJ or in the presence of DRUJ arthritis may result in a painful joint.

ECU TENOSYNOVITIS AND SUBLUXATION

The ECU tendon takes an angular path across the ulnar head to its insertion on the fifth metacarpal base when the forearm is supinated, which is accentuated further by ulnar deviation and flexion of the wrist (Figure 14.38). Normally, the ECU tendon is held within the groove of the ulnar head by a deep retinaculum, often referred to as the subsheath, which must resist the natural tendency for the tendon to subluxate.[119,153] The true extensor retinaculum passes over the subsheath without an attachment to the ulna and inserts on the pisiform, triquetrum, fifth metacarpal, and volar soft tissues. Repetitive stress on the subsheath can result in a stenosing tenosynovitis from fibrosis,[54,75] or the tendon can become unstable and dislocated from attenuation or tearing of its sheath.[19,36] Recurrent subluxation over the ulnar ridge of the groove can produce a partial tendon rupture. Variations in both the morphology of the ECU tendon and its groove and their relationship to one another have been described.[65] Such variation suggests that the diagnosis of ECU tenosynovitis and subluxation may be difficult to determine.[90]

Volar subluxation of the ECU is a common finding in rheumatoid arthritis and nearly always accompanies the caput ulna

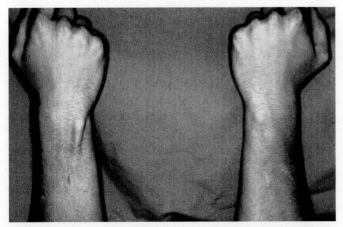

FIGURE 14.38 Subluxation of extensor carpi ulnaris tendon from groove in ulnar head is shown with wrist in supination.

syndrome, which is characterized by dorsal subluxation of the ulna and volar subluxation of the carpus.[5] Although ECU subluxation is rarely symptomatic in these patients, repositioning the tendon to the dorsal aspect of the ulna reduces its deforming force on the wrist and may help to stabilize the distal ulna; it should be considered whenever performing an isolated ECU tenosynovectomy, a complete extensor tenosynovectomy, DRUJ synovectomy, or distal ulnar resection (see Case Study 14.1).

Although ECU stenosing tenosynovitis and instability would seem to be different, their clinical presentations and treatments are quite similar. Typically, the patient can reproduce the pain or snapping by combined supination and ulnar deviation against resistance (see Video 5.1). Treatment of acute conditions include rest, immobilization with the forearm in pronation and the wrist in neutral, and antiinflammatory modalities. Even though snapping may not resolve, often pain is relieved. Stenosing tenosynovitis can be treated by corticosteroid injection into the sheath. Surgery is reserved for recalcitrant symptoms (see Case Study 5.6).

There are three general surgical categories for the ECU sheath: (1) release, (2) repair, and (3) reconstruction. Typically, we consider sheath release only for patients with low activity demands or for patients whose previous surgeries resulted in failure.

Operative Technique

Sixth Dorsal Compartment Release

A longitudinal incision is made over the sixth compartment, and the retinaculum and subsheath are divided. The tendon is inspected and debrided, as necessary, if tendinosis is present. A tenosynovectomy is performed when indicated. The groove is inspected for spurs and prominent ridges, which also should be debrided. The retinaculum can be left open or repaired beneath the tendon when degenerative changes are present within the ulnar groove. Ligament reconstruction (see next subsection) to stabilize the tendon is done only if there is audible snapping during passive forearm rotation.[75] The patient is immobilized with a plaster wrist splint for 2 weeks followed by return to activities over several weeks.

Extensor Carpi Ulnaris Tendon Stabilization

A longitudinal incision is made between the fifth and sixth extensor compartments. A volar skin flap is raised while protecting the dorsal sensory branch of the ulnar nerve. The extensor retinaculum is incised at the extreme volar margin of the sixth extensor compartment. The ECU subsheath is opened longitudinally at its midline. The tendon and groove are inspected, and any osteophytes are debrided. At this point, a decision is made regarding a subsheath imbrication versus a ligament reconstruction.

The decision depends on the quality of subsheath tissue and condition of the groove. In more acute cases (<6 months), a primary subsheath repair is preferred if the tendon has minimal fraying and the groove is smooth. The sheath should not be overtightened; placing a pediatric feeding tube next to the tendon during sheath suture repair reduces this risk. The extensor retinaculum is repaired anatomically. Alternatively, if the groove is excessively shallow, it can be deepened with a bur to increase tendon stability and to avoid tendon constriction. Care must be taken to ensure that the groove is smooth.

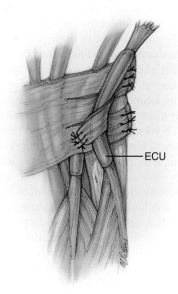

FIGURE 14.39 Extensor carpi ulnaris (ECU) stabilized by sling created from extensor retinaculum. (Copyright © Elizabeth Martin.)

When the groove is rough, when the subsheath is badly damaged, or in chronic cases, a ligament reconstruction to stabilize the tendon is preferred. Spinner and Kaplan employed a ½- to 1-in rectangular ulnar-based flap of retinaculum, using the septum between the fourth and fifth extensor compartments as its base.[153] The flap is raised to Lister's tubercle, folded back, and passed under the ECU tendon. The flap is brought back over the tendon and sutured to itself, which places the deep surface of the retinaculum against it. The previously released retinaculum over the sixth extensor compartment is repaired.

We prefer to create a flap from the retinaculum that had been raised previously for tendon exposure (Figure 14.39).[90] The central third of the retinaculum is raised using two parallel incisions extending from its divided ulnar edge to the septum between the fourth and fifth extensor compartments. The flap is passed under the ECU tendon and then is passed back over it. The flap is sutured to the more proximal portion of the retinaculum rather than to itself; this creates a loose sling rather than a tight noose. The remainder of the retinaculum is repaired anatomically. This method is easier and requires less exposure than that described by Spinner and Kaplan[153]; however, it places the superficial surface of the retinaculum against the tendon. The patient is immobilized for 3 weeks in a short-arm cast, followed by a wrist splint for 2 weeks. After this time, activities can be resumed as tolerated.

Outcomes

A few case reports and two larger series have reported good results for pain relief with conservative and surgical treatment for stenosing tenosynovitis.[54,75] These studies' authors reported no ECU instability by palpation or from passive or active wrist and forearm motion. Surgical failures were attributed to an incorrect diagnosis, with DRUJ arthritis being the most common. ECU tendon stabilization has been successful with good relief of pain and few recurrent subluxations.[19,32,56,60]

For Case Studies, Videos, and more, please visit ExpertConsult.com.

REFERENCES

1. Adams BD, Berger RA: An anatomic reconstruction of the distal radioulnar ligaments for posttraumatic distal radioulnar joint instability. *J Hand Surg [Am]* 27:243–251, 2002.
2. Adams BD, Holley KA: Strains in the articular disk of the triangular fibrocartilage complex: a biomechanical study. *J Hand Surg [Am]* 18:919–925, 1993.
3. af Ekenstam F, Hagert CG: Anatomical studies on the geometry and stability of the distal radioulnar joint. *Scand J Plast Reconstr Surg* 19:17–25, 1985.
4. Andersson JK, Lindau T, Karlsson J, et al: Distal radio-ulnar joint instability in children and adolescents after wrist trauma. *J Hand Surg Eur Vol* 39:653–661, 2014.
5. Backdahl M: The caput ulnae syndrome in rheumatoid arthritis: a study of the morphology, abnormal anatomy and clinical picture. *Acta Rheumatol Scand Suppl* 5:1–75, 1963.
6. Bae DS, Waters PM: Pediatric distal radius fractures and triangular fibrocartilage complex injuries. *Hand Clin* 22:43–53, 2006.
7. Bednar JM, Osterman AL: The role of arthroscopy in the treatment of traumatic triangular fibrocartilage injuries. *Hand Clin* 10:605–614, 1994.
8. Bednar MS, Arnoczky SP, et al: The microvasculature of the triangular fibrocartilage complex: its clinical significance. *J Hand Surg [Am]* 16:1101–1105, 1991.
9. Berger RA: The anatomy of the ligaments of the wrist and distal radioulnar joints. *Clin Orthop Relat Res* 383:32–40, 2001.
10. Bieber EJ, Linscheid RL, et al: Failed distal ulna resections. *J Hand Surg [Am]* 13(2):193–200, 1988.
11. Bilos ZJ, Chamberland D: Distal ulnar head shortening for treatment of triangular fibrocartilage complex tears with ulna positive variance. *J Hand Surg [Am]* 16:1116–1119, 1991.
12. Bizimungu RS, Dodds SD: Objective outcomes following semi-constrained total distal radioulnar joint arthroplasty. *J Wrist Surg* 2:319–323, 2013.
13. Blatt G, Ashworth C: Volar capsule transfer for stabilization following resection of the distal end of the ulna. *Orthop Trans* 3:13–14, 1979.
14. Bowers WH: Distal radioulnar joint arthroplasty: the hemiresection-interposition technique. *J Hand Surg [Am]* 10:169–178, 1985.
15. Boyes JH: Surgical repair of joints. In Bunnell S, editor: *Bunnell's surgery of the hand*, Philadelphia, 1970, Lippincott, pp 294–313.
16. Breen TF, Jupiter JB: Extensor carpi ulnaris and flexor carpi ulnaris tenodesis of the unstable distal ulna. *J Hand Surg [Am]* 14:612–617, 1989.
17. Bu J, Patterson RM, Morris R, et al: The effect of radial shortening on wrist joint mechanics in cadaver specimens with inherent differences in ulnar variance. *J Hand Surg [Am]* 31:1594–1600, 2006.
18. Buijze GA, Ring D: Clinical impact of united versus nonunited fractures of the proximal half of the ulnar styloid following volar plate fixation of the distal radius. *J Hand Surg [Am]* 35:223–227, 2010.
19. Burkhart SS, Wood MB, et al: Posttraumatic recurrent subluxation of the extensor carpi ulnaris tendon. *J Hand Surg [Am]* 7:1–3, 1982.
20. Chen NC, Wolfe SW: Ulna shortening osteotomy using a compression device. *J Hand Surg [Am]* 28:88–93, 2003.
21. Chidgey LK, Dell PC, et al: Histologic anatomy of the triangular fibrocartilage. *J Hand Surg [Am]* 16:1084–1100, 1991.
22. Cho CH, Lee YK, Sin HK: Arthroscopic direct repair for radial tear of the triangular fibrocartilage complex. *Hand Surg* 17:429–432, 2012.
23. Chun S, Palmer AK: The ulnar impaction syndrome: follow-up of ulnar shortening osteotomy. *J Hand Surg [Am]* 18:46–53, 1993.
24. Conaway DA, Kuhl TK, Adams BD: Comparison of the native ulnar head and a partial ulnar head resurfacing implant. *J Hand Surg [Am]* 34:1056–1062, 2009.
25. Constantine KJ, Tomaino MM, et al: Comparison of ulnar shortening osteotomy and the wafer resection procedure as treatment for ulnar impaction syndrome. *J Hand Surg [Am]* 25:55–60, 2000.
26. Cooney WP: Evaluation of chronic wrist pain by arthrography, arthroscopy, and arthrotomy. *J Hand Surg [Am]* 18:816–822, 1993.
27. Cooney WP, Damron TA, et al: En bloc resection of tumors of the distal end of the ulna. *J Bone Joint Surg Am* 79:406–412, 1997.
28. Crisco JJ, Moore DC, Marai GE, et al: Effects of distal radius malunion on distal radioulnar joint mechanics—an in vivo study. *J Orthop Res* 25:547–555, 2007.
29. Daneshvar P, Chan R, MacDermid J, et al: The effects of ulnar styloid fractures on patients sustaining distal radius fractures. *J Hand Surg [Am]* 39:1915–1920, 2014.
30. Darrow JC, Jr, Linscheid RL, et al: Distal ulnar recession for disorders of the distal radioulnar joint. *J Hand Surg [Am]* 10:482–491, 1985.
31. Das DS, Johnsen PH, Wolfe SW: Soft tissue complications of dorsal versus volar plating for ulnar shortening osteotomy. *J Hand Surg [Am]* 40(5):928–933, 2015.

32. DiBenedetto MR, Lubbers LM, et al: Long-term results of the minimal resection Darrach procedure. *J Hand Surg [Am]* 16:445–450, 1991.

33. Dingman P: Resection of the distal end of the ulnar (Darrach operation). An end result study of twenty-four cases. *J Bone Joint Surg Am* 34A:893–900, 1952.

34. dos Reis FB, Katchburian MV, Faloppa F, et al: Osteotomy of the radius and ulna for the Madelung deformity. *J Bone Joint Surg Br* 80:817–824, 1998.

35. Dy CJ, Jang E, Taylor SA, et al: The impact of coronal alignment on distal radioulnar joint stability following distal radius fracture. *J Hand Surg [Am]* 39:1264–1272, 2014.

36. Eckhardt WA, Palmer AK: Recurrent dislocation of extensor carpi ulnaris tendon. *J Hand Surg [Am]* 6:629–631, 1981.

37. Ehman EC, Hayes ML, Berger RA, et al: Subluxation of the distal radioulnar joint as a predictor of foveal triangular fibrocartilage complex tears. *J Hand Surg [Am]* 36:1780–1784, 2011.

38. Epner RA, Bowers WH, et al: Ulnar variance—the effect of wrist positioning and roentgen filming technique. *J Hand Surg [Am]* 7:298–305, 1982.

39. Feldon P, Terrono AL, et al: Wafer distal ulna resection for triangular fibrocartilage tears and/or ulna impaction syndrome. *J Hand Surg [Am]* 17:731–737, 1992.

40. Fernandez DL: Radial osteotomy and Bowers arthroplasty for malunited fractures of the distal end of the radius. *J Bone Joint Surg Am* 70:1538–1551, 1988.

41. Friedman SL, Palmer AK: The ulnar impaction syndrome. *Hand Clin* 7:295–310, 1991.

42. Friedman SL, Palmer AK, et al: The change in ulnar variance with grip. *J Hand Surg [Am]* 18:713–716, 1993.

43. Frykman G: Fracture of the distal radius including sequelae—shoulder-hand-finger syndrome, disturbance in the distal radio-ulnar joint and impairment of nerve function. A clinical and experimental study. *Acta Orthop Scand* (Suppl 108):3, 1967.

44. Fujita S, Masada K, et al: Modified Sauvé-Kapandji procedure for disorders of the distal radioulnar joint in patients with rheumatoid arthritis. *J Bone Joint Surg Am* 87:134–139, 2005.

45. Galvis EJ, Pessa J, Scheker LR: Total joint arthroplasty of the distal radioulnar joint for rheumatoid arthritis. *J Hand Surg [Am]* 39(9):1699–1704, 2014.

46. Geissler WB, Fernandez DL, et al: Distal radioulnar joint injuries associated with fractures of the distal radius. *Clin Orthop Relat Res* (327):135–146, 1996.

47. George MS, Kiefhaber TR, Stern PJ: The Sauvé-Kapandji procedure and the Darrach procedure for distal radio-ulnar joint dysfunction after Colles' fracture. *J Hand Surg [Br]* 29:608–613, 2004.

48. Glowacki KA, Shin LA: Stabilization of the unstable distal ulna: the Linscheid-Hui procedure. *Tech Hand Up Extrem Surg* 3(4):229–236, 1999.

49. Goldner J, Hayes M: Stabilization of the remaining ulna using one-half of the extensor carpi ulnaris tendon after resection of the distal ulna. *Orthop Trans* 3:330–331, 1979.

50. Goncalves D: Correction of disorders of the distal radio-ulnar joint by artificial pseudarthrosis of the ulna. *J Bone Joint Surg Br* 56B(3):462–464, 1974.

51. Gordon L, Levinsohn DG, et al: The Sauvé-Kapandji procedure for the treatment of posttraumatic distal radioulnar joint problems. *Hand Clin* 7:397–403, 1991.

52. Grawe B, Heincelman C, Stern P: Functional results of the Darrach procedure: a long-term outcome study. *J Hand Surg [Am]* 37:2475–2480, 2012.

53. Greenberg JA, Werner FW, Smith JM: Biomechanical analysis of the distal metaphyseal ulnar shortening osteotomy. *J Hand Surg [Am]* 38:1919–1924, 2013.

54. Hajj AA, Wood MB: Stenosing tenosynovitis of the extensor carpi ulnaris. *J Hand Surg [Am]* 11:519–520, 1986.

55. Hammert WC, Williams RB, Greenberg JA: Distal metaphyseal ulnar-shortening osteotomy: surgical technique. *J Hand Surg [Am]* 37:1071–1077, 2012.

56. Hartz CR, Beckenbaugh RD: Long-term results of resection of the distal ulna for post-traumatic conditions. *J Trauma* 19:219–226, 1979.

57. Hauck RM, Skahen J, 3rd, et al: Classification and treatment of ulnar styloid nonunion. *J Hand Surg [Am]* 21:418–422, 1996.

58. Hermansdorfer JD, Kleinman WB: Management of chronic peripheral tears of the triangular fibrocartilage complex. *J Hand Surg [Am]* 16:340–346, 1991.

59. Hess F, Farshad M, Sutter R, et al: A novel technique for detecting instability of the distal radioulnar joint in complete triangular fibrocartilage complex lesions. *J Wrist Surg* 1(2):153–158, 2012.

60. Hui FC, Linscheid RL: Ulnotriquetral augmentation tenodesis: a reconstructive procedure for dorsal subluxation of the distal radioulnar joint. *J Hand Surg [Am]* 7:230–236, 1982.

61. Hulsizer D, Weiss APC, et al: Ulnar-shortening osteotomy after failed arthroscopic débridement of the triangular fibrocartilage complex. *J Hand Surg [Am]* 22:694–698, 1997.

62. Hunt TR, Hastings H, 2nd, Graham TJ: A systematic approach to handling the distal radio-ulnar joint in cases of malunited distal radius fractures. *Hand Clin* 14:239–249, 1998.

63. Hunter JM, Kirkpatrick WH: Dacron stabilization of the distal ulna. *Hand Clin* 7(2):365–371, 1991.

64. Iida A, Omokawa S, Akahane M, et al: Distal radioulnar joint stress radiography for detecting radioulnar ligament injury. *J Hand Surg* 37A:968–974, 2012.

65. Iorio ML, Bayomy AF, Huang JI: Morphology of the extensor carpi ulnaris groove and tendon. *J Hand Surg [Am]* 39:2412–2416, 2014.

66. Jang E, Dy CJ, Wolfe SW: Selection of tendon grafts for distal radioulnar ligament reconstruction and report of a modified technique. *J Hand Surg [Am]* 39(10):2027–2032, 2014.

67. Jansen JC, Adams BD: Long-term outcome of nonsurgically treated patients with wrist pain and a normal arthrogram. *J Hand Surg [Am]* 27:26–30, 2002.

68. Johnson RK: Stabilization of the distal ulna by transfer of the pronator quadratus origin. *Clin Orthop Relat Res* 275:130–132, 1992.

69. Johnson RK, Shrewsbury MM: The pronator quadratus in motions and in stabilization of the radius and ulna at the distal radioulnar joint. *J Hand Surg* 1:205, 1976.

70. Johnston Jones K, Sanders WE: Posttraumatic radioulnar instability: treatment by anatomic reconstruction of the volar and radioulnar ligaments. *Orthop Trans* 19:832, 1995–1996.

71. Kachooei AR, Chase SM, Jupiter JB: Outcome assessment after aptis distal radioulnar joint (DRUJ) implant arthroplasty. *Arch Bone Jt Surg* 2:180–184, 2014.

72. Kapandji IA: The Kapandji-Sauvé procedure. *J Hand Surg [Br]* 17:125–126, 1992.

73. Kessler I, Hecht O: Present application of the Darrach procedure. *Clin Orthop* 72:254–260, 1970.

74. Kim JK, Koh YD, Do NH: Should an ulnar styloid fracture be fixed following volar plate fixation of a distal radial fracture? *J Bone Joint Surg Am* 92:1–6, 2010.

75. Kip PC, Peimer CA: Release of the sixth dorsal compartment. *J Hand Surg [Am]* 19:599–601, 1994.

76. Kitamura T1, Moritomo H, Arimitsu S, et al: The biomechanical effect of the distal interosseous membrane on distal radioulnar joint stability: a preliminary anatomic study. *J Hand Surg [Am]* 36:1626–1630, 2011.

77. Kleinman WB, Graham TJ: Distal ulnar injury and dysfunction. In Peimer CA, editor: *Surgery of the hand and upper extremity*, New York, 1996, McGraw-Hill, p 670.

78. Kleinman WB, Graham TJ: The distal radioulnar joint capsule: clinical anatomy and role in posttraumatic limitation of forearm rotation. *J Hand Surg [Am]* 23:588–599, 1998.

79. Kleinman WB, Greenberg JA: Salvage of the failed Darrach procedure. *J Hand Surg [Am]* 20(6):951–958, 1995.

80. Korompilias AV, Lykissas MG, Kostas-Agnantis IP, et al: Distal radioulnar joint instability (Galeazzi type injury) after internal fixation in relation to the radius fracture pattern. *J Hand Surg [Am]* 36:847–852, 2011.

81. Krämer S, Meyer H, O'Loughlin PF, et al: The incidence of ulnocarpal complaints after distal radial fracture in relation to the fracture of the ulnar styloid. *J Hand Surg Eur Vol* 38:710–717, 2013.

82. LaPorte DM, Hashemi SS, Dellon AL: Sensory innervation of the triangular fibrocartilage complex: a cadaveric study. *J Hand Surg [Am]* 39:1122–1124, 2014.

83. Leslie BM, Carlson G, et al: Results of extensor carpi ulnaris tenodesis in the rheumatoid wrist undergoing a distal ulnar excision. *J Hand Surg [Am]* 15:547–551, 1990.

84. Lester B, Halbrecht J, et al: "Press-test" for office diagnosis of triangular fibrocartilage complex tears of the wrist. *Ann Plast Surg* 35:41–45, 1995.

85. Levis CM, Yang Z, et al: Validation of the extensor carpi ulnaris groove as a predictor for the recognition of standard posteroanterior radiographs of the wrist. *J Hand Surg [Am]* 27:252–257, 2002.

86. Lindau T, Adlercreutz C, et al: Peripheral tears of the triangular fibrocartilage complex cause distal radioulnar joint instability after distal radial fractures. *J Hand Surg [Am]* 25:464–468, 2000.

87. Lindau T, Runnquist K, et al: Patients with laxity of the distal radioulnar joint after distal radial fractures have impaired function, but no loss of strength. *Acta Orthop Scand* 73:151–156, 2002.

88. Linscheid RL: Biomechanics of the distal radioulnar joint. *Clin Orthop* 275:46, 1992.

89. Lo IK, MacDermid JC, et al: The radioulnar ratio: a new method of quantifying distal radioulnar joint subluxation. *J Hand Surg [Am]* 26:236–243, 2001.

90. MacLennan AJ, Nemechek NM, Waitayawinyu T, et al: Diagnosis and anatomic reconstruction of extensor carpi ulnaris subluxation. *J Hand Surg [Am]* 33:59–64, 2008.

91. Martin DE, Zlotolow DA, Russo SA, et al: Comparison of compression screw and perpendicular clamp in ulnar shortening osteotomy. *J Hand Surg [Am]* 39:1558–1564, 2014.

92. Masaoka S, Longsworth SH, et al: Biomechanical analysis of two ulnar head prostheses. *J Hand Surg [Am]* 27:845–853, 2002.

93. May MM, Lawton JN, et al: Ulnar styloid fractures associated with distal radius fractures: incidence and implications for distal radioulnar joint instability. *J Hand Surg [Am]* 27:965–971, 2002.

94. Melone CP, Jr, Nathan R: Traumatic disruption of the triangular fibrocartilage complex: pathoanatomy. *Clin Orthop Relat Res* 275:65–73, 1992.

95. Mikic ZD: Age changes in the triangular fibrocartilage of the wrist joint. *J Anat* 126:367–384, 1978.

96. Milch H: Cuff resection of the ulna for malunited Colles fracture. *J Bone Joint Surg Am* 23:311–313, 1941.
97. Millard GM, Budoff JE, et al: Functional bracing for distal radioulnar joint instability. *J Hand Surg [Am]* 27:972–977, 2002.
98. Millroy P, Coleman S, et al: The Sauvé-Kapandji operation: technique and results. *J Hand Surg [Br]* 17:411–414, 1992.
99. Minami A, Kaneda K, et al: Hemiresection-interposition arthroplasty of the distal radioulnar joint associated with repair of triangular fibrocartilage complex lesions. *J Hand Surg [Am]* 16:1120–1125, 1991.
100. Minami A, Suzuki K, et al: The Sauvé-Kapandji procedure for osteoarthritis of the distal radioulnar joint. *J Hand Surg [Am]* 20:602–608, 1995.
101. Mino DE, Palmer AK, et al: Radiography and computerized tomography in the diagnosis of incongruity of the distal radio-ulnar joint: a prospective study. *J Bone Joint Surg Am* 67:247–252, 1985.
102. Morisawa Y, Nakamura T, Tazaki K: Dorsoradial avulsion of the triangular fibrocartilage complex with an avulsion fracture of the sigmoid notch of the radius. *J Hand Surg Eur Vol* 32:705–708, 2007.
103. Moritomo H: The distal interosseous membrane: current concepts in wrist anatomy and biomechanics. *J Hand Surg [Am]* 37:1501–1507, 2012.
104. Moritomo H: Anatomy and clinical relevance of the ulnocarpal ligament. *J Wrist Surg* 2:186–189, 2013.
105. Moriya T, Aoki M, Iba K, et al: Effect of triangular ligament tears on distal radioulnar joint instability and evaluation of three clinical tests: a biomechanical study. *J Hand Surg Eur* 34E:219–223, 2009.
106. Mrkonjic A, Geijer M, Lindau T, et al: The natural course of traumatic triangular fibrocartilage complex tears in distal radial fractures: a 13–15 year follow-up of arthroscopically diagnosed but untreated injuries. *J Hand Surg [Am]* 37:1555–1560, 2012.
107. Nakamura R, Horii E, et al: The ulnocarpal stress test in the diagnosis of ulnar-sided wrist pain. *J Hand Surg [Br]* 22:719–723, 1997.
108. Nakamura T, Iwamoto T, Matsumura N, et al: Radiographic and arthroscopic assessment of DRUJ instability due to foveal avulsion of the radioulnar ligament in distal radius fractures. *J Wrist Surg* 3:12–17, 2014.
109. Nakamura T, Sato K, Okazaki M, et al: Repair of foveal detachment of the triangular fibrocartilage complex: open and arthroscopic transosseous techniques. *Hand Clin* 27:281–290, 2011.
110. Nakamura T, Takayama S, Horiuchi Y, et al: Origins and insertions of the triangular fibrocartilage complex: a histological study. *J Hand Surg [Br]* 26(5):446–454, 2001.
111. Nishikawa S1, Toh S: Anatomical study of the carpal attachment of the triangular fibrocartilage complex. *J Bone Joint Surg Br* 84(7):1062–1065, 2002.
112. Noda K, Goto A, Murase T, et al: Interosseous membrane of the forearm: an anatomical study of ligament attachment locations. *J Hand Surg [Am]* 34:415–422, 2009.
113. Nolan WB, III, Eaton RG: A Darrach procedure for distal ulnar pathology derangements. *Clin Orthop* 275:85–89, 1992.
114. O'Donovan TM, Ruby LK: The distal radioulnar joint in rheumatoid arthritis. *Hand Clin* 5(2):249–256, 1989.
115. Ogawa T, Tanaka T, Yanai T, et al: Analysis of soft tissue injuries associated with distal radius fractures. *BMC Sports Sci Med Rehabil* 5:19, 2013.
116. Palmer AK: Triangular fibrocartilage complex lesions: a classification. *J Hand Surg [Am]* 14:594–606, 1989.
117. Palmer AK, Glisson RR, et al: Ulnar variance determination. *J Hand Surg [Am]* 7:376–379, 1982.
118. Palmer AK, Glisson RR, et al: Relationship between ulnar variance and triangular fibrocartilage complex thickness. *J Hand Surg [Am]* 9:681–682, 1984.
119. Palmer AK, Skahen FW, Glisson RR: The extensor retinaculum of the wrist: an anatomical and biomechanical study. *J Hand Surg [Br]* 10:11–16, 1985.
120. Palmer AK, Werner FW: The triangular fibrocartilage complex of the wrist—anatomy and function. *J Hand Surg [Am]* 6:153–162, 1981.
121. Palmer AK, Werner FW: Biomechanics of the distal radioulnar joint. *Clin Orthop Relat Res* (187):26–35, 1984.
122. Palmer AK, Werner FW, et al: Partial excision of the triangular fibrocartilage complex. *J Hand Surg [Am]* 13:391–394, 1988.
123. Papapetropoulos PA, Wartinbee DA, Richard MJ, et al: Management of peripheral triangular fibrocartilage complex tears in the ulnar positive patient: arthroscopic repair versus ulnar shortening osteotomy. *J Hand Surg [Am]* 35:1607–1613, 2010.
124. Petersen MS, Adams BD: Biomechanical evaluation of distal radioulnar reconstructions. *J Hand Surg [Am]* 18:328–334, 1993.
125. Peterson CA, 2nd, Maki S, et al: Clinical results of the one-bone forearm. *J Hand Surg [Am]* 20:609–618, 1995.
126. Pirela-Cruz MA, Goll SR, Klug M, et al: Stress computed tomography analysis of the distal radioulnar joint: a diagnostic tool for determining translational motion. *J Hand Surg [Am]* 16:75–82, 1991.
127. Pogue DJ, Viegas SF, Patterson RM, et al: Effects of distal radius fracture malunion on wrist joint mechanics. *J Hand Surg [Am]* 15:721–727, 1990.
128. Rayhack JM, Gasser SI, et al: Precision oblique osteotomy for shortening of the ulna. *J Hand Surg [Am]* 18:908–918, 1993.
129. Rettig ME, Raskin KB: Galeazzi fracture-dislocation: a new treatment-oriented classification. *J Hand Surg [Am]* 26:228–235, 2001.
130. Richards RS, Bennett JD, Roth JH, et al: Arthroscopic diagnosis of intra-articular soft tissue injuries associated with distal radial fractures. *J Hand Surg [Am]* 22:772–776, 1997.
131. Rozental TD, Bozentka DJ, et al: Evaluation of the sigmoid notch with computed tomography following intra-articular distal radius fracture. *J Hand Surg [Am]* 26:244–251, 2001.
132. Ruby LK, Ferenz CC, et al: The pronator quadratus interposition transfer: an adjunct to resection arthroplasty of the distal radioulnar joint. *J Hand Surg [Am]* 21:60–65, 1996.
133. Ruch DS, Lumsden BC, Papadonikolakis A: Distal radius fractures: a comparison of tension band wiring versus ulnar outrigger external fixation for the management of distal radioulnar instability. *J Hand Surg [Am]* 30(5):969–977, 2005.
134. Sabo MT, Talwalkar S, Hayton M, et al: Intermediate outcomes of ulnar head arthroplasty. *J Hand Surg [Am]* 39:2405–2411, 2014.
135. Sagerman SD, Zogby RG, et al: Relative articular inclination of the distal radioulnar joint: a radiographic study. *J Hand Surg [Am]* 20:597–601, 1995.
136. Savvidou C, Murphy E, Mailhot E, et al: Semiconstrained distal radioulnar joint prosthesis. *J Wrist Surg* 2:41–48, 2013.
137. Scheker LR, Babb BA, et al: Distal ulnar prosthetic replacement. *Orthop Clin North Am* 32:365–376, 2001.
138. Scheker LR, Belliappa PP, et al: Reconstruction of the dorsal ligament of the triangular fibrocartilage complex. *J Hand Surg [Br]* 19:310–318, 1994.
139. Scheker LR, Severo A: Ulnar shortening for the treatment of early post-traumatic osteoarthritis at the distal radioulnar joint. *J Hand Surg [Br]* 26:41–44, 2001.
140. Schuind F, An KN, Berglund L, et al: The distal radioulnar ligaments: a biomechanical study. *J Hand Surg [Am]* 16:1106–1114, 1991.
141. Schuind F, Linscheid RL, An KN, et al: Changes in wrist and forearm configuration with grasp and isometric contraction of elbow flexors. *J Hand Surg [Am]* 17:698–703, 1992.
142. Schuind FA, Linscheid RL, An KN, et al: A normal data base of posteroanterior roentgenographic measurements of the wrist. *J Bone Joint Surg Am* 74(9):1418–1429, 1992.
143. Schuurman AH, Bos KE: The ulno-carpal abutment syndrome: follow-up of the wafer procedure. *J Hand Surg [Br]* 20:171–177, 1995.
144. Shen J, Papadonikolakis A, Garrett JP, et al: Ulnar positive variance as a predictor of distal radioulnar joint ligament disruption. *J Hand Surg* 30A:1172–1177, 2005.
145. Shepard MF, Markolf KL, Dunbar AM: Effects of radial head excision and distal radial shortening on load-sharing in cadaver forearms. *J Bone Joint Surg Am* 83A:92–100, 2001.
146. Shigemitsu T, Tobe M, Mizutani K, et al: Innervation of the triangular fibrocartilage complex of the human wrist: quantitative immunohistochemical study. *Anat Sci Int* 82(3):127–132, 2007.
147. Shinohara T, Tatebe M, Okui N, et al: Arthroscopically assisted repair of triangular fibrocartilage complex foveal tears. *J Hand Surg [Am]* 38:271–277, 2013.
148. Slutsky DJ: Arthroscopic evaluation of the foveal attachment of the triangular fibrocartilage. *Hand Clin* 27:255–261, 2011.
149. Smet LD, Vandenberghe L, Degreef I: Ulnar impaction syndrome: ulnar shortening vs. arthroscopic wafer procedure. *J Wrist Surg* 3:98–100, 2014.
150. Smith AM, Urbanosky LR, Castle JA, et al: Radius pull test: predictor of longitudinal forearm instability. *J Bone Joint Surg* 84A:1970–1976, 2002.
151. Sotereanos DG, Gobel F, et al: An allograft salvage technique for failure of the Darrach procedure: a report of four cases. *J Hand Surg [Br]* 27:317–321, 2002.
152. Souer JS, Ring D, Matschke S, et al: AOCID Prospective ORIF Distal Radius Study Group. Effect of an unrepaired fracture of the ulnar styloid base on outcome after plate-and-screw fixation of a distal radial fracture. *J Bone Joint Surg Am* 91:830–838, 2009.
153. Spinner M, Kaplan EB: Extensor carpi ulnaris: its relationship to the stability of the distal radio-ulnar joint. *Clin Orthop Relat Res* 68:124–129, 1970.
154. Srinivasan RC, Jain D, Richard MJ, et al: Isolated ulnar shortening osteotomy for the treatment of extra-articular distal radius malunion. *J Hand Surg [Am]* 38:1106–1110, 2013.
155. Steyers CM, Blair WF: Measuring ulnar variance: a comparison of techniques. *J Hand Surg [Am]* 14:607–612, 1989.
156. Stuart PR, Berger RA, et al: The dorsopalmar stability of the distal radioulnar joint. *J Hand Surg [Am]* 25:689–699, 2000.
157. Swanson AB: Implant arthroplasty for disabilities of the distal radioulnar joint: use of a silicone rubber capping implant following resection of the ulnar head. *Orthop Clin North Am* 4:373–382, 1973.
158. Taleisnik J: The Sauvé-Kapandji procedure. *Clin Orthop* 275:110–123, 1992.
159. Tanabe K, Nakajima T, Sogo E, et al: Intra-articular fractures of the distal radius evaluated by computed tomography. *J Hand Surg [Am]* 36:1798–1803, 2011.

160. Tay SC, Tomita K, Berger RA: The "ulnar fovea sign" for defining ulnar wrist pain: an analysis of sensitivity and specificity. *J Hand Surg [Am]* 32(4):438–444, 2007.

161. Tolat AR, Sanderson PL, et al: The gymnast's wrist: acquired positive ulnar variance following chronic epiphyseal injury. *J Hand Surg [Br]* 17:678–681, 1992.

162. Tolat AR, Stanley JK, Trail IA: A cadaveric study of the anatomy and stability of the distal radioulnar joint in the coronal and transverse planes. *J Hand Surg [Br]* 21:587–594, 1996.

163. Tomaino MM: The importance of the pronated grip x-ray view in evaluating ulnar variance. *J Hand Surg [Am]* 25:352–357, 2000.

164. Tomaino MM, Gainer M, Towers JD: Carpal impaction with the ulnar styloid process: treatment with partial styloid resection. *J Hand Surg [Br]* 26:252–255, 2001.

165. Trousdale R, Linscheid RL: Operative treatment of malunited fractures of the forearm. *J Bone Joint Surg Am* 77:894–902, 1995.

166. Trumble TE, Gilbert M, et al: Ulnar shortening combined with arthroscopic repairs in the delayed management of triangular fibrocartilage complex tears. *J Hand Surg [Am]* 22:807–813, 1997.

167. Tsai T, Shimizu H, et al: A modified extensor carpi ulnaris tenodesis with the Darrach procedure. *J Hand Surg [Am]* 18(4):697–702, 1993.

168. Tsai TM, Stilwell JH: Repair of chronic subluxation of the distal radioulnar joint (ulnar dorsal) using flexor carpi ulnaris tendon. *J Hand Surg [Br]* 9:289–294, 1984.

169. Tulipan DJ, Eaton RG, et al: The Darrach procedure defended: technique redefined and long-term follow-up. *J Hand Surg [Am]* 16:438–441, 1991.

170. van Schoonhoven J, Fernandez DL, et al: Salvage of failed resection arthroplasties of the distal radioulnar joint using a new ulnar head prosthesis. *J Hand Surg [Am]* 25:438–446, 2000.

171. Wallwork NA, Bain GI: Sigmoid notch osteoplasty for chronic volar instability of the distal radioulnar joint: a case report. *J Hand Surg [Am]* 26:454–459, 2001.

172. Ward LD, Ambrose CG, et al: The role of the distal radioulnar ligaments, interosseous membrane, and joint capsule in distal radioulnar joint stability. *J Hand Surg [Am]* 25:341–351, 2000.

173. Watson HK, Brown RE: Ulnar impingement syndrome after Darrach procedure: treatment by advancement lengthening osteotomy of the ulna. *J Hand Surg [Am]* 14(2 Pt 1):302–306, 1989.

174. Watson HK, Gabuzda GM: Matched distal ulna resection for posttraumatic disorders of the distal radioulnar joint. *J Hand Surg [Am]* 17:724–730, 1992.

175. Watson HK, Manzo RL: Modified arthroplasty of the distal radio-ulnar joint. *J Hand Surg [Br]* 27:322–325, 2002.

176. Webber JB, Maser SA: Stabilization of the distal ulna. *Hand Clin* 7:345–353, 1991.

177. Wechsler RJ, Wehbe MA, Rifkin MD, et al: Computed tomography diagnosis of distal radioulnar subluxation. *Skeletal Radiol* 16(1):1–5, 1987.

178. Wehbe MA, Cautilli DA: Ulnar shortening using the AO small distractor. *J Hand Surg [Am]* 20:959–964, 1995.

179. Werner FW, Murphy DJ, Palmer AK: Pressures in the distal radioulnar joint: effect of surgical procedures used for Kienböck's disease. *J Orthop Res* 7:445–450, 1989.

179a. Werner FW, Palmer AK, Fortino MD, et al: Force transmission through the distal ulna: effect of ulnar variance, lunate fossa angulation, and radial and palmar tilt of the distal radius. *J Hand Surg* 17A:423–428, 1992.

180. Wijffels MM, Keizer J, Buijze GA, et al: Ulnar styloid process nonunion and outcome in patients with a distal radius fracture: a meta-analysis of comparative clinical trials. *Injury* 45:1889–1895, 2014.

181. Willis AA, Berger RA, Cooney WP, 3rd.: Arthroplasty of the distal radioulnar joint using a new ulnar head endoprosthesis: preliminary report. *J Hand Surg [Am]* 32(2):177–189, 2007.

182. Wolf MB, Kroeber MW, Reiter A, et al: Ulnar shortening after TFCC suture repair of Palmer type 1B lesions. *Arch Orthop Trauma Surg* 130:301–306, 2010.

183. Wolfe SW, Mih AD, et al: Wide excision of the distal ulna: a multicenter case study. *J Hand Surg [Am]* 23:222–228, 1998.

184. Wysocki RW, Richard MJ, Crowe MM, et al: Arthroscopic treatment of peripheral triangular fibrocartilage complex tears with the deep fibers intact. *J Hand Surg [Am]* 37:509–516, 2012.

185. Wysocki RW, Ruch DS: Ulnar styloid fracture with distal radius fracture. *J Hand Surg [Am]* 37:568–569, 2012.

186. Yang Z, Mann FA, Gilula LA, et al: Scaphopisocapitate alignment: criterion to establish a neutral lateral view of the wrist. *Radiology* 205(3):865–869, 1997.

187. Yeh GL, Beredjiklian PK, et al: Effects of forearm rotation on the clinical evaluation of ulnar variance. *J Hand Surg [Am]* 26:1042–1046, 2001.

188. Zenke Y, Sakai A, Oshige T, et al: The effect of an associated ulnar styloid fracture on the outcome after fixation of a fracture of the distal radius. *J Bone Joint Surg Br* 91:102–107, 2009.

15

Distal Radius Fractures

Scott W. Wolfe

Acknowledgments: I would like to acknowledge with sincere gratitude those giants who have written past editions of "Distal Radius Fractures," including Diego Fernandez and Andy Palmer. Their insightful perspectives, tricks, and techniques, as well as several of the original figures, tables, and parts of the text, have been an enormous asset to me in writing this chapter.

> ▶ These videos may be found at
> *ExpertConsult.com:*
> **15.1** Insertion of a novel intramedullary device for locked fixation of articular fractures. (© Scott W. Wolfe, MD)

With the wide array of options available, this is an exciting era for the treatment of fractures of the distal radius. An improved understanding of kinematics, bone quality, and muscle forces acting across the wrist has led to an increased awareness of a fracture's relative stability, as well as the development of innovative devices to counteract these forces and restore anatomy. Innovations have occurred in closed treatment; percutaneous or spanning fixation; and, in particular, internal fixation devices. However, new implants and techniques require careful assessment of efficacy, risk, and benefit as they are applied in practice, especially because the incidence of fractures is rising in our aging population.

Distal radius fractures are the most common ones seen in the emergency department; they represent approximately 3% of all upper extremity injuries, with an incidence of greater than 640,000 annually in the United States alone.[27] There is a bimodal distribution of these injuries, with a peak in the 5- to 24-year-old, predominantly male population—athletic and high-energy injuries—and a second peak in the elderly, predominantly female population—lower-energy or "fragility" fractures. US Census data indicate that the percentage of people older than 65 in the United States is expected to increase to 16.5% of the population by 2020 (50 million citizens). Osteoporosis is a leading cause of fractures in the elderly, and therefore improved attention to care for this condition may reduce the incidence of such fractures.[138]

The goals of this chapter are to provide the surgeon with a detailed understanding of fracture types, better knowledge of wrist and fracture mechanics, improved recognition of individual fracture fragments, and an understanding of the expectations of fracture treatment. Using a case-based approach, it is hoped that the reader will go away with a better appreciation of the factors influencing treatment results and that the information here will enable the surgeon to develop an effective approach to fracture injuries.

THE RATIONALE FOR MODERN TREATMENT

Beginning with Pouteau (1783), Colles (1814), and Dupuytren (1847), early reports of fractures of the distal radius considered them to be a group of injuries with a relatively good prognosis irrespective of treatment. Until the mid-1900s, nearly all fractures of the distal radius were treated in a closed fashion, with or without reduction of alignment. Patients' expectations were in line with the treatment tools available at the time, and certainly other public health issues surpassed the wrist in importance to a patient's long-term productivity. Since then, tens of thousands of clinical and basic science publications have contributed to an improved understanding of fractures' complexity, stability, and prognosis and have, consequently, driven the development of modern techniques and technology to optimize patient outcomes. A brief summary of the evolution of modern fracture fixation is shown in Table 15.1, with the sentinel publications and techniques that fundamentally changed treatment of these challenging injuries. See ExpertConsult.com for more information about this topic.

What is clear from an analysis of the evolution of wrist fracture treatment is that (1) there is both general consensus and scientific evidence that restoration of the anatomy of the distal radius is linked to restoration of function; and (2) no single technique or method will yield results superior to those of other treatment methods given the wide divergence in fracture subtypes, energy associated with the injury, age, activity level, and related injuries. The indiscriminate use of one method to treat all fractures of the distal radius predictably can lead to cases of fixation failure, soft tissue injury, and inability to achieve the goals of intervention.

FRACTURE EVALUATION

▌ PERTINENT ANATOMY

The distal radius functions as an articular plateau on which the carpus rests (Figures 15.1 and 15.2) and from which the radially based supporting ligaments of the wrist arise (Figure 15.3). The hand and radius, as a unit, articulate with and rotate about the ulnar head via the sigmoid notch of the radius (Figure 15.4). This latter relationship is maintained primarily by the ulnar-based supporting ligaments of the wrist—the TFCC.

The distal radius has three concave articular surfaces—the scaphoid fossa, the lunate fossa, and the sigmoid notch—for articulation with the scaphoid, lunate, and ulnar head, respectively (Figures 15.5 and 15.6). The sigmoid notch is concave, with a poorly defined proximal margin and well-defined dorsal, palmar, and distal margins (see Figure 15.6).

TABLE 15.1		Contributions to Understanding Distal Radius Fracture Treatment	
Author	**Year**	**Area of Contribution**	**Significance**
Colles	1814	Description of fracture and closed treatment	"[T]hat the limb will at some remote period again enjoy perfect freedom in all its motions."
Bohler	1929	Pins-and-plaster technique	Improvement over closed treatment for unstable fractures.
Anderson and O'Neil	1944	Principles and technique of external fixation	Reduction is easy to attain, maintenance is difficult. Advocated distraction by fixator, augmented with bone graft.
Gartland and Werley	1951	Outcome assessment	Of fractures treated with plaster, 60% collapse. A demerit point system is recommended; it has been in use for 7 decades.
DePalma et al.	1952	Closed-pin treatment	Outcomes linked to restoration of bony alignment.
Frykman	1967	Classification	Distinguished between radiocarpal and radioulnar articular involvement, and the importance of ulnar-sided injuries.
Vidal	1979	External fixation	Advanced the concept of "ligamentotaxis" to restore articular alignment in comminuted articular fractures.
Cooney et al.	1980s	Colles' fracture treatment	Treatment principles, complications of Colles' fractures, overdistraction, reflex sympathetic dystrophy, bone grafting.
Palmer et al.	1980s	Triangular fibrocartilage complex	Relationship of TFCC to radioulnar stability, malalignment to DRUJ dysfunction, and radial settling to ulnar impaction.
Fernandez	1982	Malunion	Established indications and technique for osteotomy of malunited distal radius fractures.
Taleisnik and Watson	1984	Carpal instability	Described relationship of dorsal malalignment to nondissociative carpal instability.
Knirk and Jupiter	1986	Articular congruency	Demonstrated relationship between articular incongruency and long-term arthritic change.
Axelrod and McMurty	1990	Internal-plate fixation	Recommended rigid internal fixation for comminuted articular fractures. Anatomically restored congruency, with higher complication rates.
Geissler	1990s	Percutaneous articular reduction	Percutaneous and arthroscopically assisted articular reduction.
Seitz	1991	Augmented external fixation	Advocated additional Kirschner wires and bone grafts to supplement external fixation so as to reduce dependency on traction.
Leung	1991	Bone graft external fixation	Bone graft reduces duration of external fixation, enables removal at 3-4 weeks postop.
Kaempffe et al.	1993	Complications of external fixation	Duration and degree of distraction related to RSD.
Gesensway et al.	1995	Dorsal fixed-angle plate fixation	Designed and demonstrated a fixed-angle blade plate that provided superior fixation strength to current ORIF designs.
Rikli and Regazzoni	1996	Columnar fixation	Defined radial, intermediate, and ulnar columns of wrist and advocated use of small implants with biplanar fixation.
Fitoussi et al.	1997	Dorsal and palmar plate fixation	Described ORIF with dual approaches for comminuted articular fractures.
Wolfe et al.	1998	External fixation	Fixation strength of augmented external fixation demonstrated to be comparable to ORIF.
Leslie and Medoff	2000	Fragment-specific fixation	Outlined principles and techniques of internal fixation using small "pin plate" and "wireform" implants.
Orbay	2000s	Palmar fixed-angle plate fixation	Proposed fixation and demonstrated outcomes of dorsally displaced fractures using palmar fixed-angle plates.
Kreder et al.	2005	Randomized trial ORIF vs. external fixation	Provided joint congruency can be attained; improved results demonstrated with percutaneous fixation vs. dorsal ORIF.
Goldfarb et al.	2006	Long-term evaluation of arthritis in ORIF patients	A 15-year follow-up with CT scans demonstrated arthrosis in 0.81% of ORIF patients. No correlation with upper extremity function.
Rozental and Blazar	2006	Complication of volar-plate fixation	Excellent functional outcomes with fixed-angle volar plate fixation, but high incidence of tendon and hardware complications.
Arora et al.	2011	Treatment of elderly	Unable to identify differences in outcomes of elderly patients with closed vs. ORIF of unstable radius fractures.
AAOS	2014	Appropriate use guidelines	Expert panels opine on appropriate treatment of 240 clinical scenarios of distal radius fracture fixation.

CT, Computed tomography; *DRUJ*, distal radioulnar joint; *ORIF*, open reduction internal fixation; *RSD*, reflex sympathetic dystrophy; *TFCC*, triangular fibrocartilage complex.

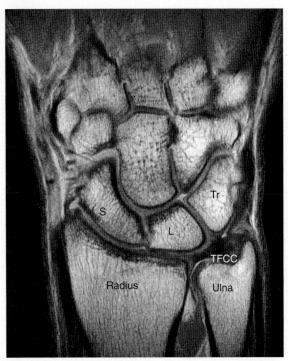

FIGURE 15.1 The scaphoid (S) and lunate (L) articulate with the distal articular surface of the radius, and the ulnar head articulates with the sigmoid notch. The triangular fibrocartilage complex (TFCC) is interposed between the ulnar carpus and the ulnar head. *Tq*, Triquetrum. (Magnetic resonance image, courtesy of Hollis Potter, MD, Department of Diagnostic Radiology, Hospital for Special Surgery.)

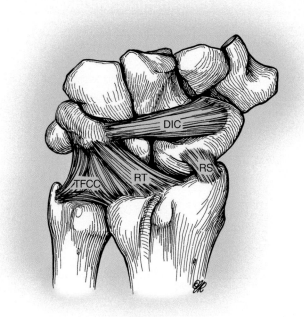

FIGURE 15.3 Dissection and illustration composite showing the dorsal ligaments of the wrist. *DIC*, Dorsal intercarpal ligament; *RS*, radioscaphoid; *RT*, radiotriquetral; *TFCC*, triangular fibrocartilage complex. (© Elizabeth Martin.)

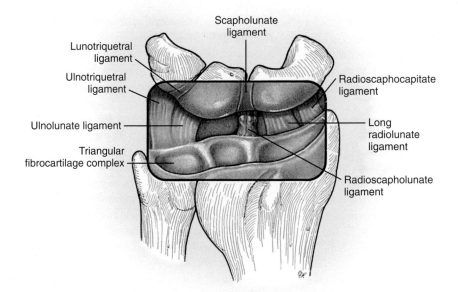

FIGURE 15.2 Arthroscopic anatomy of the radiocarpal joint. Pictured are the articular surfaces of the scaphoid, lunate, triquetrum, radius, and triangular fibrocartilage complex. The major extrinsic—radioscaphocapitate, long radiolunate, radioscapholunate, ulnolunate, and lunotriquetral—ligaments of the wrist are shown. The very important intrinsic ligaments of the wrist—the scapholunate ligament and lunotriquetral ligaments—are also shown. (© Elizabeth Martin.)

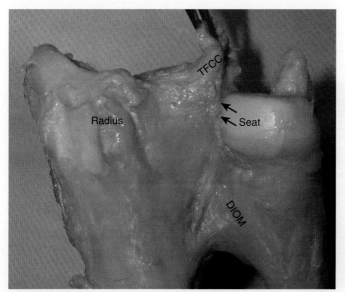

FIGURE 15.4 The ulnar head articulates with the sigmoid notch of the radius at the "seat" of the distal radioulnar joint (DRUJ). The triangular fibrocartilage complex (TFCC), detached to expose the ulnar head, is the primary restraint of the DRUJ, arising from the most ulnar border of the radius and inserts into the base and tip of the ulnar styloid process. The distal interosseous membrane (DIOM) is a secondary stabilizer, inserted on the radius at the base of the sigmoid notch.

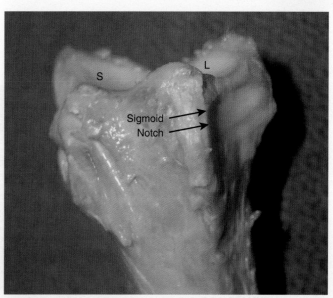

FIGURE 15.6 The sigmoid notch showing distinct dorsal, palmar, and distal borders and an indistinct proximal border. The scaphoid facet (S) and lunate facet (L) are also shown.

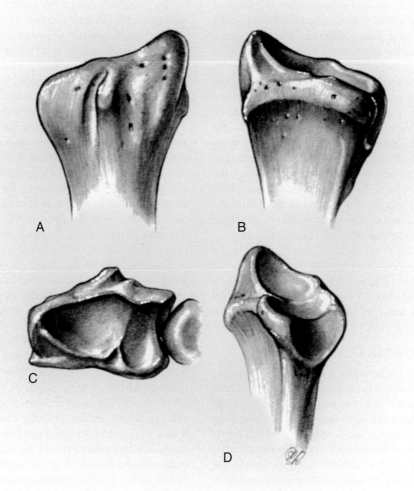

FIGURE 15.5 Artist's drawing of the distal radius. **A,** Dorsal view illustrating the Lister tubercle. **B,** Palmar view showing the scaphoid and lunate fossae distally, as well as the sigmoid notch ulnarly. Vascular foramina can be noted on the palmar and dorsal aspects of the distal radius. **C,** End-on view of the distal radius and radioulnar joint showing the scaphoid fossa, lunate fossa, and ulnar head resting in the sigmoid notch. **D,** View of the sigmoid notch from the ulnar aspect. (© Elizabeth Martin.)

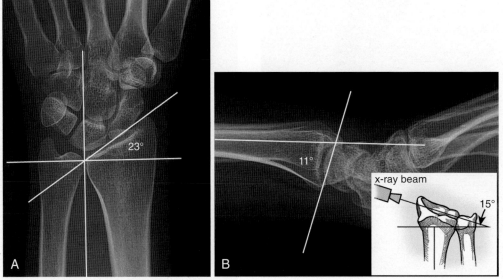

FIGURE 15.7 A, Posteroanterior radiograph of a wrist demonstrating radial inclination (23 degrees) and neutral ulnar variance. **B,** The "facet lateral" radiograph is performed by aligning the x-ray beam in a plane parallel to the lunate facet of the radius, approximately 15 degrees distal to proximal. (Drawing © Elizabeth Martin.)

The distal articular surface of the radius has a radial inclination, or slope, averaging 23 degrees and tilts palmarly an average of 11 degrees (Figure 15.7, A). Radial inclination is measured by the angle formed by a line drawn tangential to the distal radial articular surface on a posteroanterior (PA) radiograph and one perpendicular to the shaft of the radius. Palmar tilt is measured by the angle created by a line drawn between the dorsal and palmar lips of the lunate facet and the longitudinal axis of the radius. This angle is probably best appreciated on a *facet lateral* radiograph, performed with the beam inclined approximately 10 to 15 degrees distal-to-proximal, to profile the articular surface of the lunate facet and eliminate the bony overlap of the radial styloid (see Figure 15.7, B). Ulnar variance averages just under 1 mm negative[114] and ranges widely; variance is the axial difference between the subchondral bone of the lunate facet at the distal margin of the sigmoid notch and the most distal articular surface of the ulna, which is measured along the forearm's longitudinal axis (see Figure 15.7, A).

The dorsal aspect of the distal radius is convex and acts as a fulcrum for extensor tendon function (see Figure 15.5). The radial styloid area may have a groove for the tendon of the first dorsal compartment, and ulnar to this is a dorsal longitudinal prominence—the Lister tubercle, which acts as a fulcrum for the extensor pollicis longus (EPL) tendon.

RADIOGRAPHIC PATHOANATOMY

When evaluating fracture radiographs, it is important to understand several relationships and bony landmarks that may have subtle but important aberrations because of the malposition of fracture fragments. Perhaps the most important of these bony landmarks of the distal radius is the "teardrop,"[114] which represents the volar projection of the lunate facet of the distal radius and the mechanical buttress for subluxation of the lunate (see Figure 15.5, D). The teardrop projects 3-mm palmarward from the flat surface of the radial diaphysis, or 16% of the anterior-to-posterior height of the lunate facet.[3] A line drawn tangential

to the subchondral bone of the articular surface through the tip of the teardrop normally subtends an angle of 70 degrees with the longitudinal axis of the radius (Figure 15.8, A)[114]; consequently, subtle dorsal rotation of an extraarticular fractured radius alters this relationship and decreases the teardrop's angle. Similarly, an impaction injury that splits the lunate facet may drive the lunate into the metaphysis of the radius and rotate the teardrop relationship (see Figure 15.8, B, C). The teardrop measures just 5 mm at its greatest width, thus making it difficult to gain stable fixation with traditional volar implants.[3]

Another useful measurement on the facet lateral film is the anteroposterior (AP) distance, and it is measured between the distal apex of the dorsal and volar rims of the lunate facet (Figure 15.9, A, B). The average AP distance is 20 mm in males and 18 mm in females; however, for improved accuracy, the AP distance on the injured side should be compared with that on the uninjured side. An appreciably widened (or narrowed) AP distance, in relation to the opposite side, represents an alteration in the contour of the lunate facet secondary to impaction or articular split of the lunate facet (see Figure 15.9, B). In a group of 81 patients followed for an average of 9 years, increases in AP distance were correlated with increased radiographic evidence of osteoarthritis.[43] See ExpertConsult.com for more information on this topic.

Another useful parameter with which to evaluate the adequacy of reduction is articular cavity depth, which is measured by the perpendicular distance from the line measuring the AP distance to the greatest depth of the articular cavity (Figure 15.10, A, B). The measurement is compared to the uninjured side. Increases in the articular cavity depth of greater than 2 mm have been correlated mechanically with increased radiocarpal contact pressures and decreased contact area, and clinically with decreased range of flexion–extension and increased radiographic grade of radiocarpal osteoarthritis.[44]

On the normal PA view, the dorsal rim of the radius projects 3 to 5 mm beyond the dense subchondral bone of the volar rim

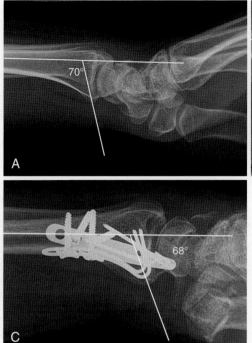
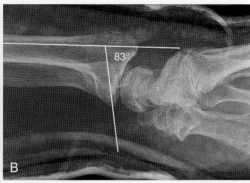
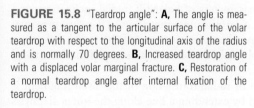

FIGURE 15.8 "Teardrop angle": **A,** The angle is measured as a tangent to the articular surface of the volar teardrop with respect to the longitudinal axis of the radius and is normally 70 degrees. **B,** Increased teardrop angle with a displaced volar marginal fracture. **C,** Restoration of a normal teardrop angle after internal fixation of the teardrop.

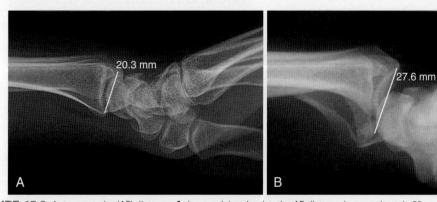

FIGURE 15.9 Anteroposterior (AP) distance: **A,** In an uninjured wrist, the AP distance is approximately 20 mm in males and 18 mm in females. **B,** In this lateral radiograph of an injured wrist, the AP diameter is grossly widened (~28 mm).

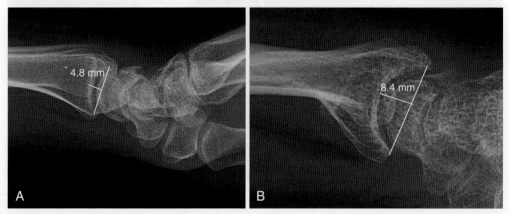

FIGURE 15.10 Articular cavity depth: **A,** Uninjured wrist's articular cavity depth as measured from anteroposterior distance is 4.8 mm. **B,** Healed comminuted impaction fracture with increased articular cavity depth of 8.4 mm. Increases in articular depth correlated with increased radiocarpal contact pressures, decreased range of motion and increased radiographic grade of arthritis.[44]

of the radius (Figure 15.11). Displaced fractures may increase, reduce, or invert this relationship, depending on the degree of sagittal plane rotation of the distal fragment. Breaks in the dense subchondral bone on the PA view can be recognized as step-offs or articular gaps, and impacted articular fragments can be identified as linear densities within the metaphyseal bone on either the PA or the lateral view.

Radial translation[134] or *coronal shift* of the distal radius describes abnormal radial translation of the distal fragment of the distal radius fracture in the coronal (PA) plane and has been shown to cause radioulnar instability through its slackening effect on the distal oblique bundle (DOB) of the interosseous membrane[38] (Figure 15.12, *A, B*). Coronal alignment should be carefully assessed as a useful parameter of reduction, alongside the traditional parameters of volar tilt, radial inclination, and ulnar variance. Loss of the ulnar metaphyseal flare just proximal to the sigmoid notch, or an overhang of the radial styloid on the radial metaphyseal flare, should raise suspicion of a coronal shift.

Measurement of radial translation of the distal fragment is easily performed by extending a line along the ulnar diaphysis of the radius distally across the carpus on a PA radiograph.[134] A transverse line is drawn across the lunate at its widest point on the PA film. The percentage of the lunate radial to the intersection point of the lines averages 45%. Patients in whom less than half of the lunate remains ulnar to this intersection point following distal radius reduction or internal fixation should be scrutinized for residual coronal shift of the articular fragment (see Figure 15.12, *A*).

Careful analysis of fracture radiographs, a thorough understanding of common fracture patterns, and an appreciation of

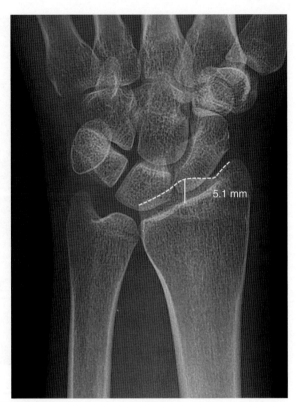

FIGURE 15.11 The dorsal rim of the radius normally projects 3 to 5 mm distal to the dense subchondral bone of the articular surface, and this relationship may be altered by posttraumatic changes in volar tilt or die-punch injuries.

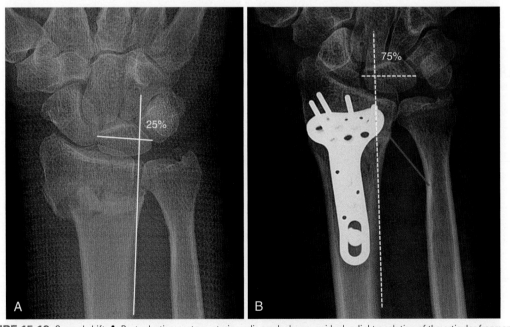

FIGURE 15.12 Coronal shift: **A,** Postreduction posteroanterior radiograph shows residual radial translation of the articular fragment and slackening the fibers of the distal interosseous membrane (DIOM). Less than 50% of the lunate (L) lies ulnar to a line drawn tangent to the ulnar diaphysis of the radius.[134] **B,** Following open reduction and internal fixation, the articular fragment is reduced, restoring the proper relationship of the L to the longitudinal line. Reduction restores tension to the DIOM, providing stability to the distal radioulnar joint by seating the ulnar head within the sigmoid notch.

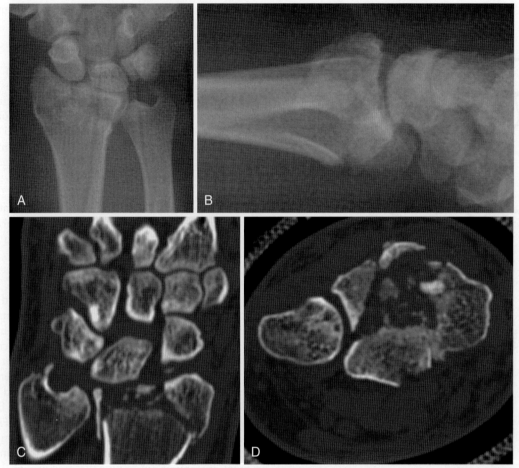

FIGURE 15.13 Use of computed tomography: **A, B,** Posteroanterior and lateral radiographs of a comminuted articular fracture after reduction that demonstrates what appears to be satisfactory reduction of the articular surface. **C, D,** Coronal and axial scans of the articular surface demonstrating multiple fragmentation, articular impaction, and incongruency. Note the separate volar lunate teardrop fragment that may not have been evident on the lateral radiograph.

the mechanism of the injury allows the examining physician to classify the fracture and begin to formulate a treatment plan. Generally, standard radiographic views (i.e., PA, facet lateral, oblique) are sufficient to understand a fracture's pathoanatomy. However, special imaging techniques (e.g., traction views after reduction, tomograms, CT scans) provide a more accurate diagnosis of the displacement pattern, the number of fragments, and the degree of joint involvement at both the radiocarpal and radioulnar levels (Figure 15.13, *A-D*). Three-dimensional reconstructions of CT scans of articular fractures more accurately define the number and presence of articular fragments and help guide the surgeon in the appropriate incision(s) and approach.[74] For unique injuries, modern software allows for the subtraction of the carpus with direct visualization of the articular surface of the radius in three dimensions.

RECOGNITION OF FRACTURE PATTERNS

There are few areas of skeletal trauma in which eponymic descriptions are so commonly used; contemporary authors have purposely avoided assigning their names to a particular fracture type and instead prefer to base newer classification systems on a variety of measurements, observations, and injury characteristics. As the common eponymous fractures are so

deeply engrained in the orthopedic literature, a brief illustrated review with images follows (Figures 15.14 through 15.16).

Fracture Classifications

Distal radius fractures tend to cluster in recognizable patterns, and it is important that the treating physician be familiar with the multiple fracture variants to recognize a fracture's "personality," as determined by the energy of injury, articular involvement, relative stability, associated soft tissue injuries, and radioulnar joint involvement. The ideal fracture classification should provide reproducible anatomic, diagnostic, and prognostic considerations; assess the associated soft tissue lesions; and infer appropriate treatment. Physicians dealing with distal radius fractures should adopt a classification scheme that fulfills their needs for clinical and scientific purposes. When reporting outcomes or designing a multicenter study, however, it is important to choose a system with a satisfactory degree of intraobserver and interobserver reproducibility.

Intraobserver and interobserver reliability and reproducibility of many of the distal radius fracture classifications has been analyzed repeatedly.[4,98] Agreement was considered adequate for the three main groups of the AO classification, but was suboptimal when analyzing subgroups. Interobserver agreement was rated moderate for the Mayo and fair for the Frykman, Melone,

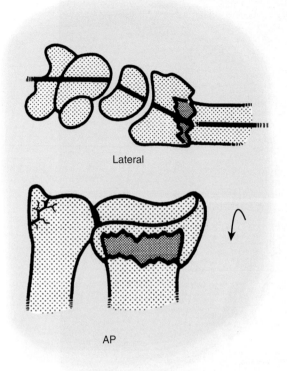

Lateral

AP

FIGURE 15.14 The typical features of a Colles' fracture, or a distal radius fracture with dorsal comminution, dorsal angulation, dorsal displacement, radial shortening, and an associated fracture of the ulnar styloid. (© Elizabeth Martin.)

and AO classifications. Most studies have concluded that these classifications lack the capacity for predicting outcome or comparing results among different studies. The AO system, while imperfect, is the most widely used when stratifying patients in a study protocol or registry. Three treatment-oriented classification systems are described as well.

Please see ExpertConsult.com for information on Frykman classification and Melone classification.

AO Classification

In 1986, the Swiss Association for the Study of Internal Fixation (ASIF) accepted a new classification of fractures that was further revised in 1990. In this system, applicable to all long bones, fractures are divided into three major types: type A (extraarticular), type B (partial articular), and type C (complete articular). This classification considers the severity of the fracture according to the extent of articular involvement and metaphyseal comminution. It is important to understand the distinction between type B fractures, in which some portion of the articular surface remains in continuity with the metaphysis, and type C fractures, in which no portion of the articular surface is in continuity with the metaphysis (Figure 15.17).

The three basic types are further subdivided into groups and subgroups to ultimately produce 27 different fracture patterns at the distal end of the forearm. Unfortunately, despite its ability to pigeonhole virtually every fracture variation, there is little interobserver agreement when the subdivisions are made; acceptable agreement is reached only when the three major subgroups have been chosen.[4]

Please see ExpertConsult.com for information on the Mayo Clinic classification.

"Fragment-Specific" Classification

Robert Medoff developed a simplified articular fracture classification by recognizing five major fragments—namely, the radial styloid, the dorsal wall, the impacted articular, the dorsal–ulnar corner (i.e., "die-punch"[115,141]), and the volar rim (Figure 15.18).[102] Articular fractures can be described by identifying their components, either alone or in combination. To more fully understand a fracture and to use this knowledge to plan treatment, the surgeon should also identify (1) the primary direction of the fracture angulation (dorsal–volar) and (2) the mechanism of the injury (see the Fernandez Classification later). The fragment-specific classification is treatment-oriented because fracture fixation is geared toward stabilization of each major fragment.

Columnar Classification

Daniel Rikli and Pietro Regazzoni introduced an important conceptual framework for the understanding and treatment of articular fractures by recognizing the three columns of the wrist (Figure 15.19).[133] The radial column, or *lateral* column, is composed of the radial styloid and scaphoid facet of the radius; restoration of this column reestablishes both length and alignment of the articular surface in the frontal and sagittal planes. The intermediate column includes the lunate facet and is the primary load-bearing column of the radius. Fractures of the intermediate column include the dorsal "die-punch" fragment, impacted articular fragments, and the volar–ulnar corner fragment. It is important to note that fractures of this column also disrupt the sigmoid notch of the radius and, consequently, the radioulnar joint.

The *medial* column constitutes the rotational column of the wrist and includes the distal ulna, the triangular fibrocartilage, and the radioulnar ligaments. To restore normal rotation of the forearm, it is critical that one assess and treat instability of this column when treating fractures of the radius. This, too, is a treatment-oriented classification system; Rikli and Regazzoni recommended orthogonally placed microplates to treat dual-column fractures of the radius and demonstrated the biomechanical and clinical efficacy of the concept.[132,133]

The Fernandez Classification

The author prefers the descriptive fracture classification developed by Diego Fernandez,[47] which is based on the *mechanism of injury* (Figure 15.20, A). In addition to the obvious bony injury to the radius, the associated ligamentous lesions, fractures of the neighboring carpal bones, and concomitant soft tissue damage are directly related to the direction and degree of trauma sustained. An understanding of the mechanism of the injury facilitates manual reduction through the application of a force opposite that produced by the injury and guides definitive treatment based on the direction and magnitude of impact, as well as the nature of associated soft tissue injuries (see Figure 15.20, A). Fractures of the distal radius can be divided into the following five types, recognizable on standard PA, facet lateral, and oblique radiographs:

Type I fractures are extraarticular *bending fractures of the metaphysis* in which one cortex fails with tensile stress and

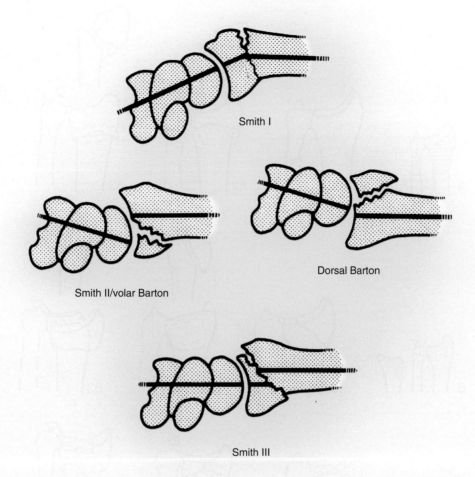

Smith I

Smith II/volar Barton

Dorsal Barton

Smith III

FIGURE 15.15 Thomas' classification (1957) of Smith fractures. A type I Smith fracture is an extraarticular one with palmar angulation and displacement of the distal fragment. A type II Smith fracture is an intraarticular one with volar and proximal displacement of the distal fragment along with the carpus. A Smith type II fracture is essentially a volar Barton fracture. A dorsal Barton fracture, illustrated for comparison, shows the dorsal and proximal displacement of the carpus and distal fragment on the radial shaft. A type III Smith fracture is an extraarticular one with volar displacement of the distal fragment and carpus. (In type III the fracture line is more oblique than in a type I fracture.) (© Elizabeth Martin.)

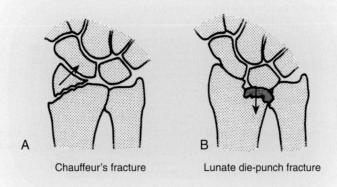

A   Chauffeur's fracture

B   Lunate die-punch fracture

FIGURE 15.16 A, A "chauffeur's" fracture is illustrated with the carpus translated ulnarly by the radial styloid fracture. The fracture earned its now antiquated name because of the propensity for the chauffeur to be struck by the backfire recoil of a starter crank on an early 1900s automobile engine. Despite its seemingly innocuous name, this fracture is notorious for concomitant injuries to the intercarpal and extrinsic radiocarpal ligaments. **B,** A lunate die-punch fracture is shown with a depression of the lunate fossa of the radius that allows proximal migration of the lunate or proximal carpal row (or both). (© Elizabeth Martin.)

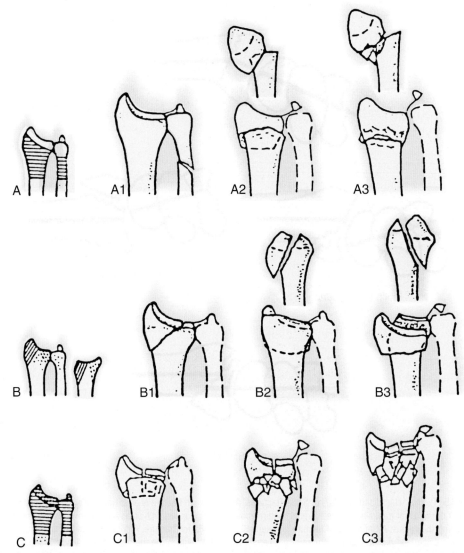

FIGURE 15.17 The comprehensive classification of fractures (AO): **A,** An extraarticular fracture affects neither the articular surface of the radiocarpal nor the radioulnar joints. **A1,** Extraarticular fracture of the ulna with the radius intact. **A2,** Extraarticular fracture of the radius, simple and impacted. **A3,** Extraarticular fracture of the radius, multifragmentary. **B,** A partial articular fracture affects a portion of the articular surface, but continuity of the metaphysis and epiphysis is intact. **B1,** Partial articular fracture of the radius, sagittal. **B2,** Partial articular fracture of the radius, dorsal rim (Barton). **B3,** Partial articular fracture of the radius, volar rim (reverse Barton; Goyrand-Smith II). **C,** A complete articular fracture affects the joint surfaces (i.e., radioulnar, radiocarpal, or both) and the metaphyseal area. **C1,** Complete articular fracture of the radius, articular simple and metaphyseal simple. **C2,** Complete articular fracture of the radius, articular simple and metaphyseal multifragmentary. **C3,** Complete articular fracture of the radius, multifragmentary.

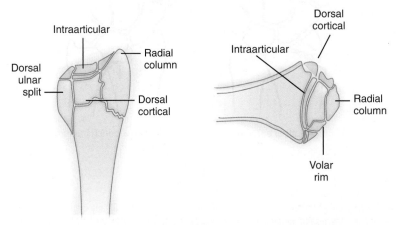

FIGURE 15.18 Fragment-specific classification.

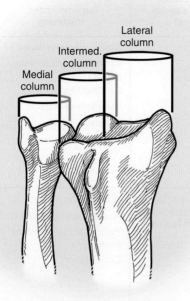

FIGURE 15.19 The columnar concept of the wrist. (© Elizabeth Martin.)

the opposite one undergoes a variable degree of comminution (Colles or Smith type I fractures; AO types A1–3).

Type II fractures are *shearing fractures of the joint surface* (the Barton, the reversed Barton, and chauffeur's fractures; AO types B1–3).

Type III fractures are *compression fractures of the joint surface* with impaction of subchondral and metaphyseal cancellous bone. These are generally high-energy injuries and usually involve disruption of both the radial and intermediate columns (Mayo type III, medial complex, die punch; AO types C1–2).

Type IV, or *avulsion fractures of ligament attachments*, includes dorsal rim and radial styloid fractures associated with radiocarpal fracture–dislocations.

Type V fractures are *high-velocity injuries* that involve combinations of bending, compression, shearing, and avulsion mechanisms or bone loss. Typically, there is diaphyseal as well as severe metaphyseal and articular disruption (AO type C3).

The treating physician should not lose sight of the purposes of fracture stratification when confronted by the multitude of eponyms and classifications that have been developed. The purpose of a classification should be to (1) catalog fracture types for subsequent reporting and comparison of outcomes and (2) understand fracture anatomy and guide treatment. The latter is perhaps best accomplished by describing the complexity, mechanism, and relative energy of the injury using the Fernandez system.

For extraarticular fractures, the primary determinant of treatment becomes the relative stability of the fracture. For articular fractures, in addition to an understanding of relative stability, the physician must obtain the necessary radiographs or advanced imaging studies (or both) to determine the location, number, and displacement of the articular fragments, as well as the integrity of the radial, intermediate, and ulnar columns. Careful consideration of these factors should enable

one to develop an appropriate treatment plan and, when indicated, the optimal surgical approach and fixation strategy.

Associated Injuries to the Distal Radioulnar Joint

Outcomes of treatment of distal radius fractures can adversely and seriously be affected by residual incongruity or instability of the distal radioulnar joint (DRUJ). Figure 15.20, *B*, illustrates a useful classification of concomitant ulnar injuries and guidelines for treatment. After satisfactory realignment of the radioulnar relationship is attained by restoring radial length and sagittal and coronal tilt, stability of the radioulnar joint depends on two factors:

- Restoration of the mechanical integrity of the sigmoid notch
- Continuity of the dorsal and volar radioulnar ligament components of the TFCC, which attach at the ulnar fovea (see Chapter 14)

Type I consists of stable DRUJ lesions, which means that adequate reduction of the radius will render the joint clinically stable without disruption of the articular surface. Such lesions include: (1) avulsion of the tip of the ulnar styloid and (2) stable fracture of the neck of the ulna. In both, the primary stabilizers of the joint (i.e., TFCC foveal attachment) are intact.

Type II consists of unstable DRUJ lesions. Despite satisfactory reduction of the radius, the ulna is unstable as a result of (1) a massive tear of the TFCC and (2) an avulsion fracture of the ulnar styloid through or below the fovea. These injuries may require supination casting, repair of the TFCC, fixation of the avulsed ulnar styloid, or temporary cross-pinning of the radius and ulna to restore stability.

Type III includes comminuted articular injuries of either the sigmoid notch or the ulnar head, and these injuries require reduction and stabilization to restore articular congruency and prevent degenerative changes.

Fracture Stability

Certain fractures are unstable by definition or require surgical management in healthy, active adults, including:

- Open fractures
- Displaced shear fractures (type II)
- Comminuted and displaced articular fractures with articular impaction (type III)
- Fracture–dislocations (type IV)
- Combined injuries with metaphyseal–diaphyseal comminution (type V)
- Fractures complicated by nerve compression, compartment syndrome, or multiple injuries

The majority of fractures, including extraarticular and simple articular ones, are not easily sorted into operative and nonoperative treatment regimens, and determination of fracture stability becomes a critical crossroad for fracture treatment.

Treatment of inherently unstable fractures with casting will fail and result in loss of radial length, carpal alignment, or articular incongruity. Unnecessary casting in this scenario may prolong overall treatment time and cost, may lead to digital stiffness and trophic changes, and may require subacute surgical intervention or corrective osteotomy to restore alignment and function, depending on the particular patient's needs. What is not immediately intuitive is how to identify stable and unstable fractures early to optimize patient outcome and minimize unnecessary surgery or ineffective cast immobilization.

Fracture type	Number of fragments	Associated injuries (nerve, tendon, ligament, skeletal trauma)	Recommended treatment
Type I Bending fracture of the metaphysis 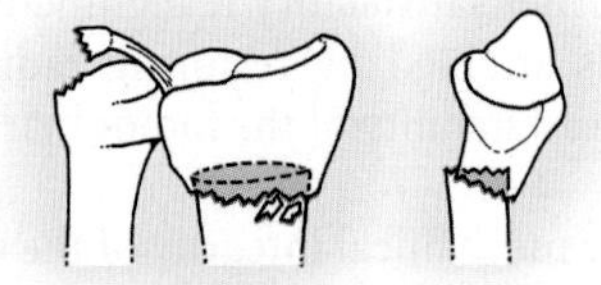 	Two-part ± metaphyseal comminution	Rare	Stable: Nonoperative Unstable: Percutaneous pinning External fixation Volar locked plate Intramedullary fixation
Type II Shear fracture of the articular surface 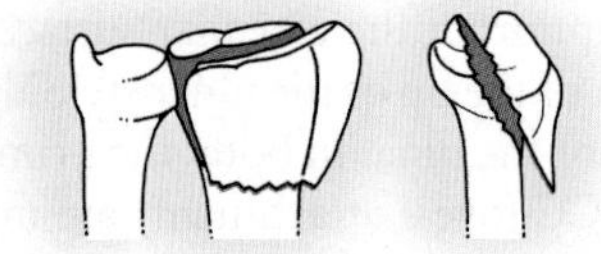 	Two-part Three-part Comminuted	Infrequent chauffeur: Suspect scapholunate interosseus ligament injury	Dorsal plate Radial columnar fixation Volar buttress or locked plate Combination
Type III Compression fracture of the articular surface 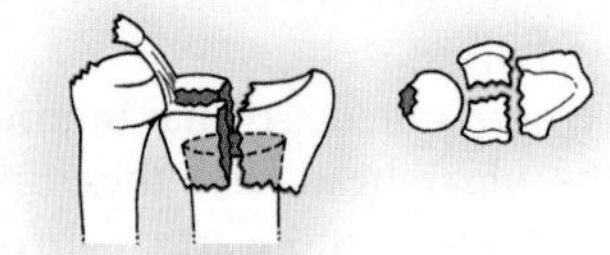 	Two-part Three-part Four-part Comminuted	Common	Open or arthroscopic reduction of articular surface, and dorsal, volar, or fragment-specific fixation ± bone graft Augmented external fixation ± bone graft Spanning plate fixation
Type IV Avulsion fracture, radiocarpal fracture-dislocation 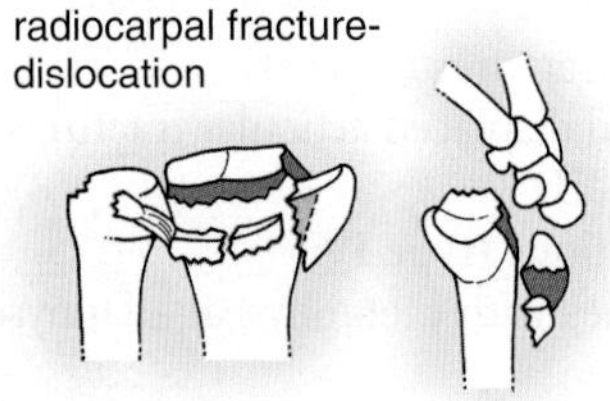 	Two-part: Radial styloid Three-part: Styloid plus volar or dorsal margin Comminuted	Frequent	Closed or open reduction and K-wire or tension band fixation Columnar fixation Fragment-specific fixation Spanning plate fixation Assess carpal translation, treat accordingly
Type V Combined fracture (I-II-III-IV) High energy injury 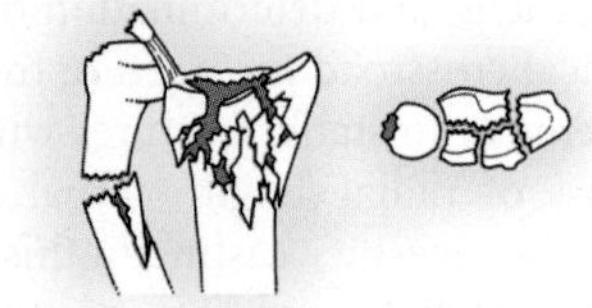 	Comminuted ± bone loss. Open injuries not uncommon.	Always	Angular stable fixation Fragment-specific fixation Spanning plate fixation Augmented external fixation Combination

A

FIGURE 15.20 A, B, The Fernandez classification of distal radius fractures and associated distal radioulnar joint (DRUJ) lesions.

	Pathoanatomy of the lesion		Joint surface involvement	Prognosis	Recommended treatment
Type I Stable (following reduction of the radius the distal radioulnar joint is congruous and stable)	A Fracture of the tip of the ulnar styloid	B Stable fracture of the ulnar neck	None	Good	Stable: Functional aftercare, early forearm rotation exercises Unstable: Assess and correct coronal shift. If still unstable, open reduction internal fixation ulnar neck or shaft.
Type II Unstable (subluxation or dislocation of the ulnar head present)	A Tear of the triangular fibrocartilage complex and/or palmar and dorsal capsular ligaments	B Avulsion fracture of the base of the ulnar styloid	None	• Possible chronic instability • Painful limitation of supination if left unreduced • Possible late arthritic changes	Anatomic reduction of radius and sigmoid notch, and *reduced coronal shift*. If still unstable: LAC for four weeks in position of stability, or dual 0.062-in K-wire fixation of radius and ulna, or ulnar styloid fixation, or open or arthroscopic triangular fibrocartilage complex foveal repair
Type III Potentially unstable (subluxation possible)	A Intraarticular fracture of the sigmoid notch	B Intraarticular fracture of the ulnar head	Present	• Dorsal subluxation possible together with dorsally displaced die punch or dorsoulnar fragment • Risk of early degenerative changes and severe limitation of forearm rotation if left unreduced	Anatomic reduction of radius and sigmoid notch, and *reduced coronal shift*. Open reduction internal fixation of ulnar head, immediate Darrach (sedentary), or early forearm rotation to enhance remodeling, and late ulnar head resection, arthroplasty, or Sauve-Kapandji if painful Open or arthroscopic triangular fibrocartilage complex repair if still unstable after anatomic fixation.

B

FIGURE 15.20, cont'd B, DRUJ injury classification. (© Elizabeth Martin.)

In a cohort of 32 patients treated nonoperatively for unstable Colles' fractures, Bickerstaff and Bell demonstrated that the two best predictors of poor functional, subjective, and objective outcomes were residual dorsal tilt of the radial articular surface and the associated nondissociative dorsal lunate instability.[15] In a group of patients who required operative treatment of unstable fractures that failed closed reduction, McQueen and colleagues also demonstrated that failure to restore carpal alignment in the sagittal plane, as demonstrated on lateral radiographs at one year, was the single most predictive factor in deterioration of functional outcomes and objective measures of strength.[112] Failure to restore radial length was significantly associated with a reduction in grip and pinch strength. These authors delineated a useful parameter of carpal malalignment on neutral-positioned lateral radiographs by defining intersecting lines of the capitate axis and the longitudinal axis of the radius.

Carpal malalignment is defined when the two lines intersect outside the boundaries of the carpus (Figure 15.21). On a perfect lateral radiograph, however, these two lines may be parallel, thus this method may not be accurate. The author considers the carpus malaligned if the center of the capitate proximal pole does not lie within a "radial box" defined by the dorsal or volar cortical confines of the radius (Figure 15.22).

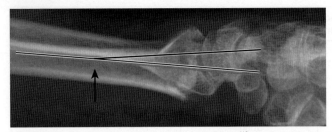

FIGURE 15.21 According to McQueen and colleagues,[112] carpal malalignment is defined when the longitudinal axis of the capitate and the radius intersect outside the boundaries of the carpus (*arrow*).

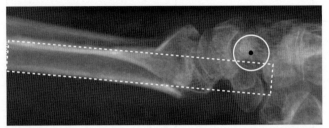

FIGURE 15.22 Alternative and rapid assessment of carpal malalignment using the "radial box" (*dashed lines*). The center of the capitate (*circle with black dot*) proximal pole should fall within a box generated along the dorsal and palmar cortical outlines of the radius on a true lateral radiograph.

Numerous authors have attempted to determine parameters that are predictive of radial instability in the acute setting. Lafontaine and colleagues defined five "instability parameters" and demonstrated a linear relationship between the number of instability parameters present on displaced fracture films and ultimate fracture collapse with closed treatment,[100] as follows:

- Dorsal angulation greater than 20 degrees
- Dorsal comminution
- Articular radiocarpal fracture
- Ulnar fracture
- Age of more than 60 years

Lafontaine et al recommended that patients with three or more of the five parameters be considered for surgical intervention at an early stage of management. Although inclusion of all the factors is the subject of some controversy, subsequent authors have confirmed that age, loss of radial length, and initial dorsal angulation are the most important predictors of collapse with cast treatment.

MacKenney and colleagues produced a quantitative, weighted formulaic approach for determination of fracture instability in a prospective study of 3559 patients with displaced and nondisplaced extraarticular fractures. They demonstrated a 60% malunion rate had all displaced fractures been treated by closed reduction.[107] Advanced age was the most predictive factor of instability, and the nature of the fracture on the initial films was also predictive of malalignment at healing. Specifically, in addition to a "relentless" association of instability and malalignment with *age, dorsal comminution,* and *increased ulnar variance* (≥ 3 mm) were important predictors of subsequent loss of reduction in plaster. Initial dorsal angulation was not predictive because it was confounded by the presence of dorsal comminution in the multivariate analysis. It is interesting to note from a historical perspective that 60 years ago Gartland and Werley

also demonstrated that 60% of reduced and casted fractures returned to their original position in plaster.[50]

Taken together, though not infallible, evidence shows that patient age and the position and comminution of the fracture on initial trauma films can be vital predictive tools for assessment and formulation of treatment plans. Patients with a constellation of instability factors should be advised of the relative probability of loss of reduction, and physiologically young or active patients should be counseled concerning the option of early operative intervention. Patients with initial radial shortening and dorsal comminution, who elect to forego surgical stabilization, particularly if older than 60, should be observed weekly for radiographic evidence of fracture settling. Understanding that malunion[20,61] and carpal malalignment are important predictors of diminished strength and function in otherwise healthy adults should enable the physician to tailor the treatment expeditiously.

TREATMENT OPTIONS AND TECHNIQUES

Closed Reduction

The greatest challenge of closed treatment of a dorsally angulated fracture is to reduce the fracture and maintain the position without excessive flexion of the wrist joint. Inherently unstable fractures with initially acceptable closed-reduction alignment often become displaced again and shorten secondary to the resting muscular tension, occasional involuntary contraction, and the load transmitted from normal digital motion. Although *extreme* palmar flexion and ulnar deviation (the so-called Cotton-Loder position[30]) may be mechanically effective in restoring volar tilt, this position should not be maintained because a fully flexed wrist may cause compression of the median nerve and is a mechanical disadvantage to the digital flexor tendons.

Closed Reduction Technique

In preparation for closed reduction, the first step is gentle surgical preparation of the dorsal surface of the wrist. The hematoma associated with the fracture is then sterilely infiltrated with 1% lidocaine without epinephrine, and the anesthetic is allowed to diffuse around the fracture site for approximately 5 minutes. If the fracture is seen belatedly, and there is significant soft tissue swelling, a regional nerve block (axillary) or general anesthesia may be necessary. The arm is gently suspended with finger traps attached to the thumb and the index and long fingers (Figure 15.23) and 5 to 10 lb of countertraction across the upper part of the arm.

Once the patient is comfortable, the arm is allowed to hang from the finger traps for 5 to 10 minutes, pressure is applied by the treating physician's thumb to the distal fracture fragment in a direction that will reduce the displacement (see Figure 15.23, D). For a dorsally displaced fracture, the distal fragment is rotated with the physician's thumb into a slightly flexed position with a palmarly directed force. Care should be taken to avoid overpronation of the fracture fragment on the radial shaft. When the distal fragment is translated dorsally as well as angulated, it is helpful to simultaneously distract and hyperextend the fracture to decrease the impact of the fragments before subsequently reducing the deformity with a traction–flexion maneuver. A stable reduction generally holds its position with fractures are generally unstable, the flexion–pronation deformity of them can be reduced and occasionally stabilized effectively in extension and supination (45-60 degrees) with a sugar tong splint.

Depending on the fracture type and stability, patients should be examined weekly with cast checks and serial radiographs. Patients with stable fractures can be changed to a well-molded short-arm cast at 2 or 3 weeks. The principles of three-point bending should be used to help maintain reduction; dorsal molds are applied over the metacarpals and the mid-diaphysis of the radius, and a third palmar countermold is placed over the apex of the fracture. "Six-pack" digital exercises are begun immediately to reduce edema and prevent contractures and disuse atrophy (Figure 15.26). If displacement in the cast occurs, skeletal fixation should definitely be considered for young or physiologically active patients.

Percutaneous Pin Fixation

Percutaneous pinning, supplemented by an external fiberglass cast, is a relatively simple and effective fixation method that is applicable for reducible extraarticular fractures and simple articular fractures without metaphyseal comminution but with good bone quality.

A variety of techniques have been described; the most commonly used methods are shown in Figure 15.27. These include pins placed through the radial styloid alone, crossed radial styloid and dorsal–ulnar corner pins, intrafocal pinning *within* the fracture site, transulnar oblique pinning without transfixation of the DRUJ, one radial styloid pin and a second across the DRUJ, and multiple transulnar-to-radius pins, including the DRUJ.[131]

The procedure is done in the operating room, usually under regional block anesthesia with fluoroscopic guidance. The hand is prepared and suspended in finger traps with 5 to 10 lb of countertraction applied across the upper part of the arm. A closed reduction is performed and the adequacy of reduction confirmed fluoroscopically. Pinning of the fracture may be done while traction is maintained, or the hand may be removed for ease of manipulation, with 0.0625-in Kirschner wires (K-wires) being preferred. The pins can be inserted with a minidriver by using only one hand so that the surgeon's other hand is free to manipulate and stabilize the fracture.

Care must be taken to avoid injury to the dorsal sensory nerves, particularly when transfixing the radial styloid. The styloid pin is inserted first to simultaneously restore length and inclination of the distal fragment. At the tip of the styloid, the surgeon brackets the tendons of the first dorsal compartment with his fingers and identifies the starting point of the styloid pin immediately dorsal to the tendons. A 0.062-in K-wire is placed by hand through the skin to engage the tip of the styloid and the position is checked with fluoroscopy. The pin is directed obliquely to engage the stout diaphyseal bone of the opposing cortex at the metaphyseal flare. Position of the fracture is assessed, and a few additional degrees of volar tilt can be "dialed in" by rotating the fragment around the styloid wire. The second 0.062-in K-wire is placed at the dorsal–ulnar corner of the radius, just radial to the sigmoid notch and between the fourth and fifth extensor compartment tendons.

The easiest way is to place a free K-wire percutaneously and check its position before engaging the wire driver. The ideal

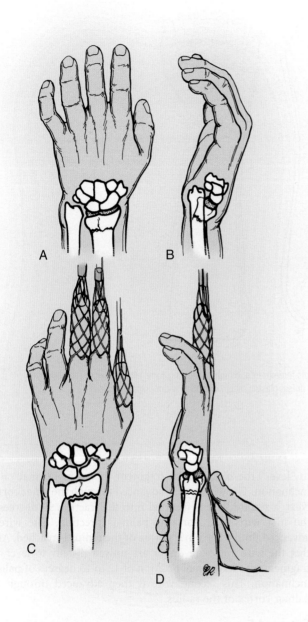

FIGURE 15.23 A, B, Distal radius (Colles') fracture. **C, D,** The author recommends reduction of this fracture. After suspending the arm from finger traps and allowing disimpaction of the fracture, apply pressure with the thumb over the distal fragment. (© Elizabeth Martin.)

the wrist only slightly flexed and ulnarly deviated. A sugar tong splint is applied to maintain the position (some prefer to apply it while still suspended in finger traps), and the fracture reduction can be fine-tuned as necessary with the splint in place (Figure 15.24).

Molding over the index metacarpal, with a countermold over the palmar apex of the fracture site, is helpful to maintain fracture position. The recommended position of immobilization for a dorsally angulated metaphyseal fracture is neutral to slight flexion, 20 to 30 degrees of ulnar deviation with neutral forearm rotation (Figure 15.25). Radiographs are obtained to confirm reduction. Although palmarly displaced, extraarticular Smith

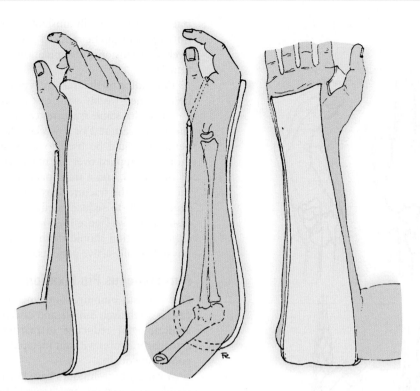

FIGURE 15.24 Sugar tong splint for a distal radius fracture. It controls forearm rotation while allowing some elbow flexion. The palmar crease should be free to allow full metacarpophalangeal flexion and the dorsal plaster should extend to the metacarpal heads.

starting position is just ulnar to the fourth dorsal compartment tendon in the "soft spot" of the 4-5 arthroscopy portal. The wire is gently navigated through subcutaneous tissues to engage the bone and its position is confirmed with fluoroscopy. The K-wire is then drilled at a 45- to 60-degree angle to the frontal and sagittal planes to engage the opposing stout volar bone well *proximal* to the fracture line. After confirmation of reduction, a second styloid wire increases the stability of the construct. For simple articular fractures, a fourth wire can be placed as necessary between the third and fourth dorsal compartments to stabilize the scaphoid facet fragment, but this is rarely necessary.

Before completion of the procedure, the extensor tendons are checked by passive flexion of the digits and wrist flexion tenodesis to be certain that they have not been tethered. Any skin tethering needs to be relieved with a No. 11 scalpel blade. The pins are bent and cut off 1 cm above the skin, and pin caps or petroleum gauze is applied. Alternatively, they can be cut beneath the skin. A well-padded sugar tong splint in supination is applied for 3 weeks, followed by a short-arm cast for an additional 3 weeks. Full forearm rotation is allowed after 2 weeks. The cast and pins are removed 5 to 6 weeks after reduction (Figure 15.28).

Kapandji popularized the technique of "double intrafocal wire fixation" to both reduce and maintain distal radial fractures (Figure 15.29).[85] This technique is best reserved for simple extraarticular fractures and is not without complications. Under fluoroscopic guidance, one K-wire is inserted into the fracture site in a radial-to-ulnar direction until the ulnar cortex of the radius is felt. The wire driver and wire are then moved distally

to "lever" the distal radial fragment to regain normal radial inclination. The wire is then advanced through the ulnar cortex. Next, a second wire is inserted into the fracture 90 degrees to the first wire in a dorsal-to-palmar direction. The wire is advanced until the palmar cortex of the radius is reached. After that the wire and wire driver are moved distally to lever the fragment into its normal position of 12 to 15 degrees of palmar inclination. This second wire is then advanced through the palmar cortex of the radius.

External Fixation

Since the original idea of Roger Anderson of applying skeletal traction with a "portable" external-fixation device for the treatment of comminuted distal radial fractures,[5] there has been a constant evolution in both technique and design technology. One of the two most important developments has been the recognition that excessive distraction was harmful and associated with multiple complications and poor outcomes.[82] The second development was that distraction alone (i.e., ligamentotaxis) could not reduce displaced and impacted articular fragments.

Modern techniques include limited open or arthroscopic reduction of the articular surface, subchondral support with bone graft or a bone graft substitute, and "augmentation" with supplemental pin fixation. Augmentation of fixation allows the fixator to be placed in a neutralization mode with only minimal distraction, thereby enabling immediate use of the fingers for light activity. Early controlled motion of the wrist is sometimes possible between 4 and 6 weeks after the injury by removing the

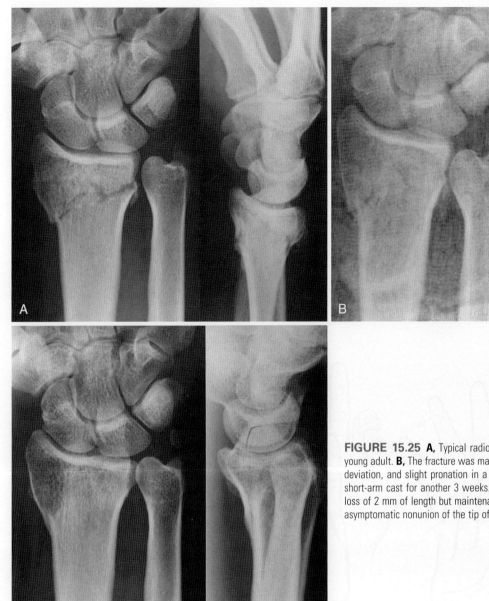

FIGURE 15.25 A, Typical radiographic appearance of a Colles' fracture in a young adult. **B,** The fracture was manually reduced and held in slight flexion, ulnar deviation, and slight pronation in a sugar tong splint for 3 weeks, followed by a short-arm cast for another 3 weeks. **C,** Follow-up radiographs at 1 year revealed loss of 2 mm of length but maintenance of normal volar and ulnar tilt. Notice the asymptomatic nonunion of the tip of the ulnar styloid.

fixator and leaving the pins in place for several additional weeks (Figure 15.30).

External-Fixation Technique

Under brachial block or general anesthesia, the anesthetized upper extremity is prepared and draped from the fingertips to the lower part of the arm, just below a pneumatic tourniquet. Sterile finger traps and a traction device can be used if preferred. Manual reduction is performed to grossly align the fracture fragments and approximate normal length, alignment, and tilt (see Figure 15.23).

A 2- to 3-cm-long incision is made over the dorsal radial aspect of the index metacarpal base. Blunt dissection with scissors exposes the metacarpal while carefully preserving and reflecting branches of the dorsal radial sensory nerve. A soft

tissue protector is then placed on the metacarpal, and 3-mm self-tapping half-pins are inserted at a 30- to 45-degree angle dorsal to the frontal plane of the hand and forearm. Pin position and length are confirmed with portable fluoroscopy. Next, a 4-cm skin incision is made 8 to 10 cm proximal to the wrist joint and just dorsal to the midline.

Blunt dissection exposes superficial branches of the lateral antebrachial cutaneous nerve, the brachioradialis (BR), the two radial wrist extensors, and the radial sensory nerve, which exits in the mid-forearm from the investing fascia between the BR and the extensor carpi radialis longus (ECRL) (Figure 15.31). Two 3-mm half-pins (1.5 cm apart) are then introduced through a soft tissue protector between the radial wrist extensors at a 30-degree angle dorsal to the frontal plane of the forearm. The pins should just perforate the medial cortex of the radius and

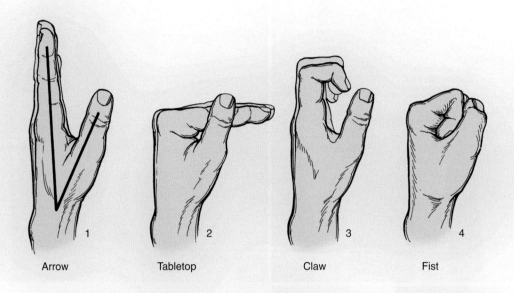

Arrow   Tabletop   Claw   Fist

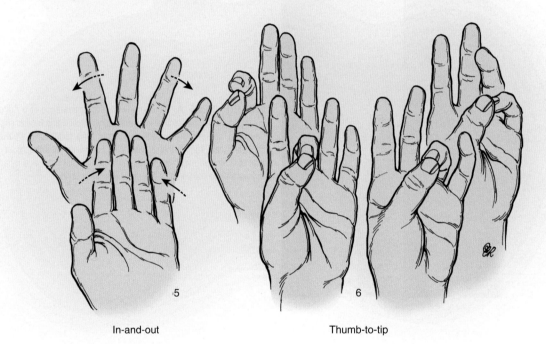

In-and-out   Thumb-to-tip

FIGURE 15.26 "Six-pack" exercises: Drawings 1 through 6 illustrate the position that the patient's hand should assume when performing these exercises. It is helpful to show the patient that full metacarpophalangeal (MP) extension makes the hand look like an arrow, full MP flexion makes the hand look like a tabletop; full MP extension combined with proximal and distal interphalangeal flexion, creates a claw; complete finger flexion creates a fist; and abduction and adduction of the fingers create an in-and-out motion. Finally, to complete the exercises, the individual touches the tip of the thumb to the tip of each finger. (© Elizabeth Martin.)

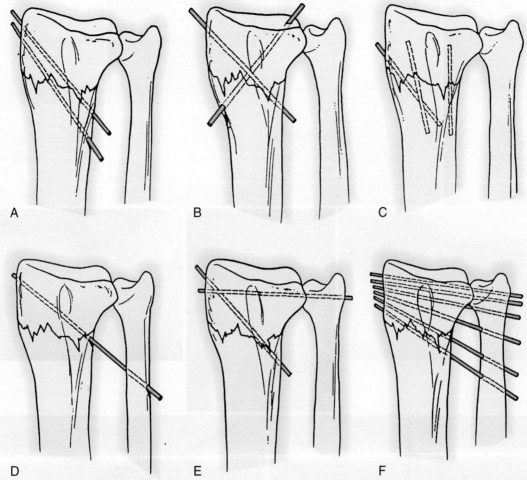

FIGURE 15.27 Several different techniques of percutaneous pinning of unstable bending fractures have been described. **A,** Pins placed primarily through the radial styloid. **B,** Crossing pins from the radial and ulnar sides of the distal fragment into the distal shaft. **C,** The intrafocal technique advocated by Kapandji. **D,** Ulnar-to-radius pinning without transfixation of the distal radioulnar joint (DRUJ). **E,** A radial styloid pin and one across the DRUJ. **F,** Multiple pins from the ulna to the radius, including transfixation of the DRUJ.

should be confirmed fluoroscopically. Both wounds are irrigated and closed with 4-0 nylon sutures before applying the frame.

For relatively stable fractures, and when performing augmented fixation with K-wires or a graft (or both), a simple single-bar external-fixation frame is ideal. The particular design or strength of the frame is less important from a mechanical perspective than the degree of stability attained by the supplemental K-wires (see Figure 15.30).[170]

If nonbridging external fixation is selected for a minimally comminuted extraarticular or simple articular fracture with good bone stock, proximal pin insertion is identical but the distal pins are introduced exclusively into the distal fragment. A radial-sided pin is placed through a small dorsal radial incision between the wrist extensors in the radial half of the distal fragment. Its direction is dorsal-to-palmar, parallel to the joint surface in the sagittal plane. A second pin is placed in the ulnar aspect of the distal fragment through a limited incision between the fourth and fifth extensor compartments. Its direction is also dorsal-to-palmar but aimed slightly obliquely from the ulnar-to-radial side to engage the palmar–ulnar cortex of the distal fragment.

Having securely fixed the distal pins, closed reduction is performed by using them as "joysticks" to restore volar tilt.[60,110] The pins are assembled with separate clamps and rods to create a triangular frame (Figure 15.32). An alternative design of nonbridging "crossed-pin" fixation is shown in Figure 15.33.

Augmented External Fixation

For all but minimally comminuted extraarticular fractures, augmented external fixation is recommended so as to provide additional support to individual fracture fragments and increase construct stability.[172] For unstable fractures without depressed articular fragments, 0.045- or 0.0625-in K-wires are introduced into the fragments in a crossed configuration according to the technique described earlier. One or two pins driven through the radial styloid fragment, and one through the dorsal–ulnar fragment into the radial shaft, combine to produce maximum additional stability.[172] The pins should pierce the ulnar cortex of the radius but not penetrate the ulnar shaft. The pins should be bent at an acute angle and cut off 1-cm external to the skin (eFigure 15.5).

Impacted and severely displaced fragments that do not respond to ligamentotaxis or external-reduction maneuvers

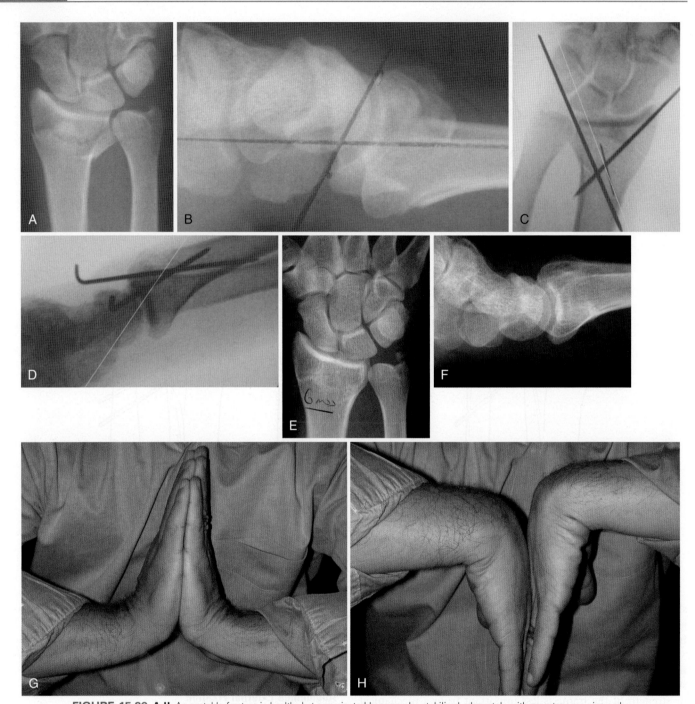

FIGURE 15.28 A-H, An unstable fracture in healthy but comminuted bone can be stabilized adequately with percutaneous pins and a cast for 6 weeks with the expectation of restoration of alignment and function.

require additional limited open reduction. This concept is defined as: selective surgical exposure of articular fragments that still remain displaced after the application of traction, closed manipulation, or percutaneous manipulation. The main objective of this technique is to achieve anatomic reduction with limited exposure and to minimize the use of implants in an effort to preserve ligament attachments, thereby minimizing iatrogenic soft tissue disruption and preserving the vascular supply of the fragments.

Limited open reduction is particularly useful for articular four-part fractures of the distal radius without metaphyseal comminution. Articular tilt, radial length, and reduction of the radial styloid fragments usually can be achieved with classic closed-reduction maneuvers alone or combined with longitudinal traction. However, the dorsal–ulnar and volar–ulnar fragments that disrupt the lunate fossa and the sigmoid notch may remain displaced because of either impaction or soft tissue interposition. The limited open reduction technique addresses the anatomic restoration of such fragments after percutaneous fixation of the radial styloid fragment.

After grossly aligning the fracture fragments, the external fixator is applied in slight distraction (see earlier), and the radial

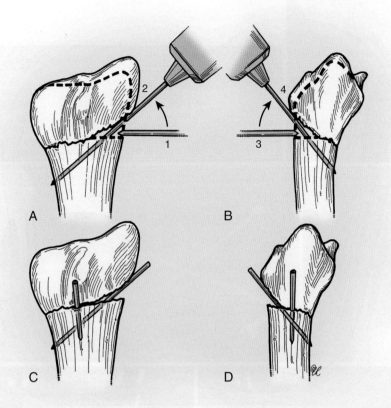

FIGURE 15.29 A-D, The Kapandji technique of "double intrafocal wire fixation" to reduce and maintain distal radial fractures. A 0.045- or 0.0625-in Kirschner wire is introduced into the fracture in a radial-to-ulnar direction. When the wire reaches the ulnar cortex of the radius, it is used to elevate the radial fragment and re-create the radial inclination. This wire is then introduced into the proximal ulnar cortex of the radius for stability. A second wire is introduced at 90 degrees to the first in a similar manner to restore and maintain volar tilt. (© Elizabeth Martin.)

articular surface is approached through a 3- to 4-cm dorsal longitudinal midline incision (Figure 15.34, A, B). The extensor retinaculum is opened over the Lister tubercle and the EPL transposed radially. The fourth compartment is opened, and a 2-cm section of the posterior interosseous nerve can be excised at the discretion of the surgeon. The EPL and wrist extensor tendons are retracted to the radial side and the finger extensors to the ulnar side. The wrist capsule is left intact; rarely is it necessary (or helpful) to perform an open inspection of the articular surface when using modern portable fluoroscopy.

If examination of the joint is deemed necessary, the surgeon is afforded a more complete view of all articular surfaces and associated soft tissues with the arthroscope (see next section). The radial styloid fragment is then reduced anatomically and stabilized with a single 0.062-in K-wire (or cannulated screw) as mentioned previously. Any traction that has been applied at this point is reduced, and the impacted articular fragments are elevated en bloc with a Freer elevator (Figure 15.35) or a pointed awl by using the opposing articular surfaces of the lunate and scaphoid as a template. The congruency of the reduction is checked with fluoroscopy, and the resultant metaphyseal void beneath the reduced subchondral bone is then packed with an autogenous bone graft or a structural bone graft substitute (see Figure 15.35, B).

Most advocates of augmented external fixation routinely graft all subchondral bone defects regardless of their size if the articular surface has been elevated. The bone graft provides mechanical buttressing of small cartilage-bearing fragments and may accelerate fracture healing by providing additional osteogenic potential. A second 0.045- or 0.062-in K-wire is then directed from the radial styloid transversely across the radius immediately beneath and tangent to the articular surface to engage the cortical bone of the sigmoid notch. Care should be taken to avoid protrusion of the wire into the DRUJ.

If there is joint incongruity involving the sigmoid notch of the radius, every attempt needs to be made to achieve an anatomic reduction. Usually, this can be accomplished with percutaneous manipulation of the fragment with a K-wire and K-wire fixation of the fragment to the stout volar metaphyseal bone (see earlier). If not reducible by percutaneous means, there may be soft tissue interposition; thus limited open reduction is required.

To gain access to the fragment, the fourth dorsal compartment tendons are retracted radially, and the extensor digiti minimi (EDM), which lies directly over the DRUJ, is exposed and retracted to the ulnar side. Great care needs to be taken to avoid disruption of the dorsal radioulnar ligament when exposing and realigning this fragment, and the periosteum is left intact to avoid vascular stripping. A 0.045-in K-wire can be passed at a 45-degree angle to the frontal and sagittal planes to engage the distal and ulnar margin of the dorsal–ulnar fragment and to secure it to the opposing palmar cortical bone. Reduction and fixation are confirmed with fluoroscopy.

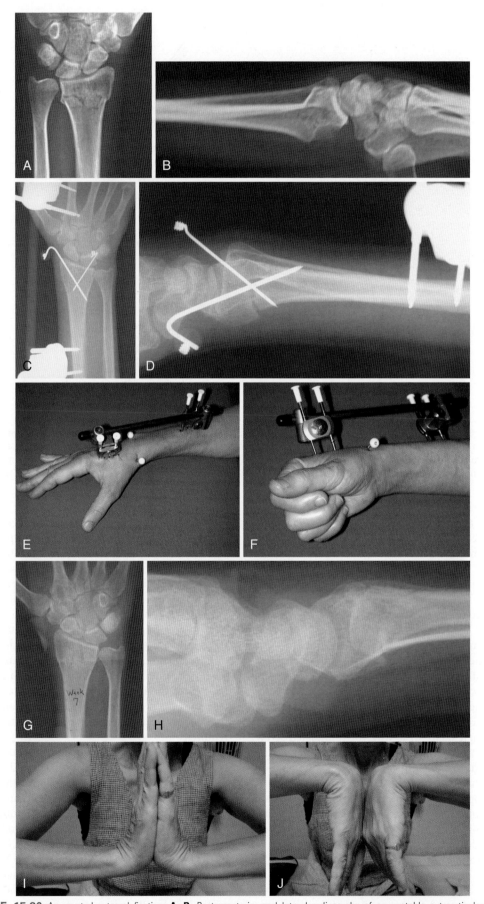

FIGURE 15.30 Augmented external fixation: **A, B,** Posteroanterior and lateral radiographs of an unstable extraarticular fracture. **C, D,** Crossed pin augmentation of external fixation yields optimal construct strength. **E, F,** Photos of the fixator shows it in a neutral position to allow full flexion and extension of the digits postoperatively. **G, H,** Healed fracture in satisfactory alignment. **I, J,** Photos showing symmetric range of motion postoperatively.

To help prevent pin-track infection, it is recommended that the patient clean the skin–pin interface with saline once or twice daily until the wounds have sealed. Active- and passive-finger motion can be begun as soon as the anesthetic wears off and is encouraged for the entire time that the frame is in place. Supination–pronation of the forearm is started at the first postoperative visit and its importance is reemphasized throughout the postoperative period. Supervised hand therapy is begun for patients who are unwilling, uncomfortable, or unable to mobilize their fingers and forearms independently.

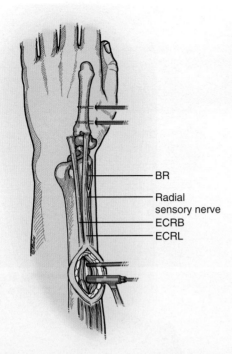

FIGURE 15.31 An external-fixation device being applied after two 3-mm half-pins have already been introduced into the base of the second metacarpal. Two 3-mm half-pins are then introduced into the distal radius via direct exposure of the radius between the extensor carpi radialis brevis (ECRB) and extensor carpi radialis longus (ECRL) at an angle 30 degrees dorsal to the coronal plane. The lateral antebrachial cutaneous and radial nerves are protected by directly identifying them and then inserting the half-pins through a tissue protector that is placed directly on the radius. *BR,* Brachioradialis. (© Elizabeth Martin.)

BR
Radial sensory nerve
ECRB
ECRL

If an unstable volar–ulnar fragment is identified, reduction and hybrid fixation (see eFigure 15.6) through a limited volar approach must be performed to prevent subsequent volar displacement of the carpus. Percutaneous fixation of the volar–ulnar fragment is not recommended because of the density of neural, vascular, and tendinous structures overlying it. A variety of small internal-fixation devices are available, including fixed-angle 2.4-mm plates, tension bands, wireforms, and pin plates.

The fixator is then adjusted to a neutral position in the frontal and sagittal planes, and any excess traction is removed. Full passive flexion and extension of the digits and thumb are ensured at this time to be certain that there is neither residual distraction nor tethering. The wound is closed by reapproximating the extensor retinaculum while leaving the extensor pollicis transposed. DRUJ stability is assessed with a manual "shuck" test of the radioulnar joint. Gross instability must be treated to avoid long-term sequelae.

The external fixator pin clusters are dressed with a compressive wrap to prevent skin shear, the wounds are covered, and the wrist is immobilized in a light compression bandage with a supportive splint. It is preferable to immobilize the wrist in a supinated position with a sugar tong splint for 10 days until pain and swelling have subsided in order to promote DRUJ stability and facilitate resumption of full supination postoperatively. The frame is usually removed at 6 weeks and the supplemental pins may be kept in place for an additional 2 weeks.

CRITICAL POINTS *Augmented External Fixation*

Indications
- Unstable extraarticular fractures of the distal radius (type I bending)
- Impacted articular fractures (type III compression)
- Comminuted unstable fractures with articular and metaphyseal involvement

Contraindications
- Severe osteoporosis
- Volar shear fractures (type II; Smith type II; volar Barton type)
- Patient preference, compliance concerns, or inability to care for the external fixation and pins

Technical Points
- Closed reduction with traction, finger traps, or both
- Mini-open placement of proximal- and distal-fixation pins to the index metacarpal and radius
- Placement of fixator pins in a plane 45 degrees oblique to the sagittal and frontal planes
- Closure of pin cluster incisions before assembly of the fixator
- Gross alignment of the fragments by fixation in moderate traction, flexion, and ulnar deviation
- Mini-open dorsal incision over the third dorsal compartment and transposition of the EPL
- Reduction of traction and elevation of impacted articular fragments with an elevator against the carpus
- Fluoroscopic check of reduction and support of fragments with graft or substitute
- Percutaneous 0.062- or 0.045-in K-wire or screw fixation through the radial styloid
- Percutaneous 0.045-in K-wire fixation transversely below the reduced subchondral bone
- Crossed percutaneous 0.062-in K-wire through the dorsal–ulnar corner
- Assessment of the volar ulnar fragment and performance of limited open reduction and fixation if needed
- Revision of the fixation posture to a neutral wrist angle to facilitate digital mobility and function
- Assessment of the DRUJ for stability and augmentation as needed

Postoperative Care
- Apply a sugar tong splint in supination for 5 to 10 days until suture removal.
- Begin digital range-of-motion exercises immediately.
- Use peroxide or dry pin care and apply compressive wraps until wounds are sealed.
- Begin forearm rotation and gentle active wrist motion exercises at the initial postoperative visit.
- Evaluate with radiographs at the initial postoperative visit and at 2 and 6 weeks postoperatively.
- Remove the fixator at 6 weeks while leaving the K-wires in place for 2 additional weeks.

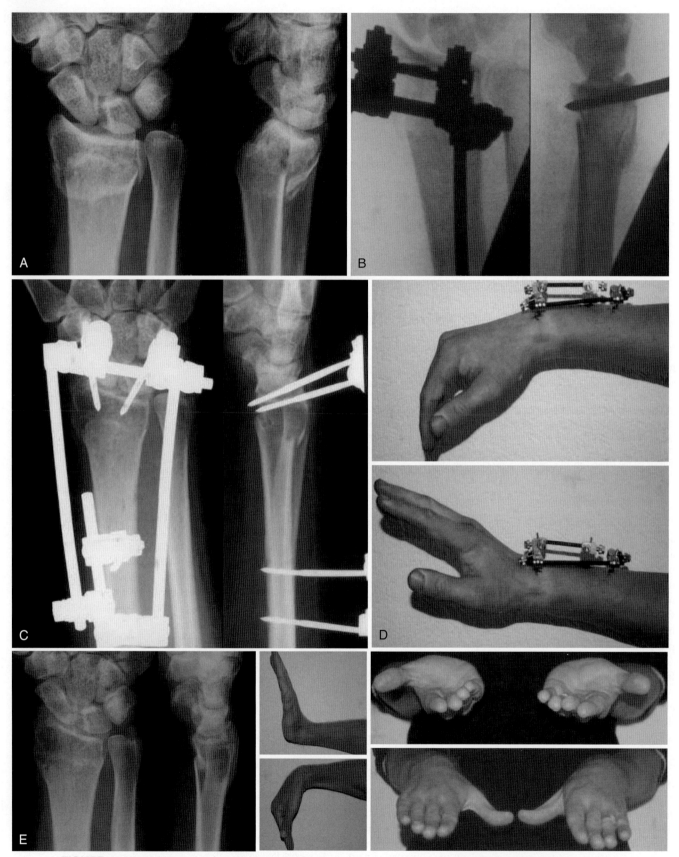

FIGURE 15.32 A, Radiographs of an unstable dorsally displaced extraarticular fracture of the distal radius. **B,** Fluoroscopic control of the nonbridging fixator. Notice the converging position of the distal pins in the frontal plane and parallel to the joint surface in the sagittal plane. **C,** Control radiographs 10 days after injury with well-maintained reduction. **D,** Early motion of the wrist is allowed as soon as the swelling has subsided. **E,** Radiographs at 3 months. The fracture has healed without displacement and correlates with free wrist motion and restoration of complete forearm rotation.

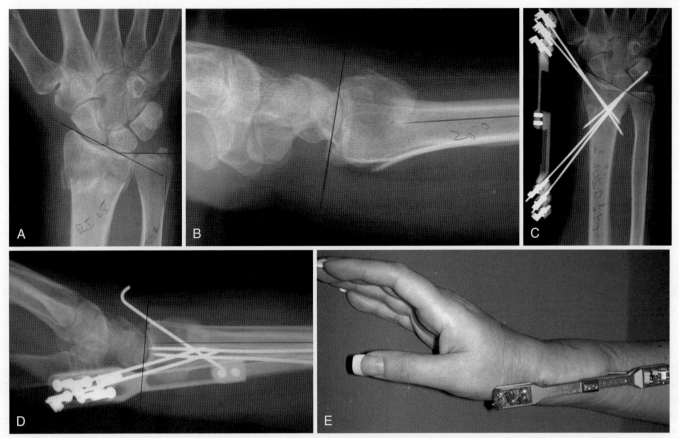

FIGURE 15.33 A-E, Cross-pinned nonbridging external fixation of the distal radius (CPX, AM Surgical, Smithtown, NY). For selected unstable fractures with large articular fragments and healthy bone, nonbridging fixation enables early wrist motion and compares favorably with bridging external fixation.

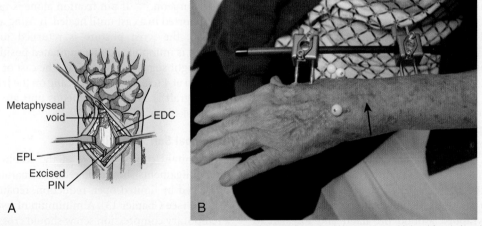

FIGURE 15.34 Limited open reduction: **A,** Limited exposure of the radial metaphyseal void between the third and fourth dorsal compartments enables percutaneous elevation of the articular surface and bone graft augmentation. **B,** Photo of healed 3-cm dorsal incision (*arrow*) for articular reduction and placement of bone graft. *EDC,* Extensor digitorum communis; *EPL,* extensor pollicis longus; *PIN,* posterior interosseous nerve. (**A,** © Elizabeth Martin.)

Arthroscopic Reduction and Percutaneous Fixation

Diagnostic and therapeutic wrist arthroscopy is widely used by many practicing hand surgeons. Its use in conjunction with a percutaneous means of fracture fixation offers several advantages in the management of articular fractures of the distal radius.[36,54] Arthroscopy is a minimally invasive means of monitoring articular reduction without the additional ligamentous and capsular damage that is inherent with open inspection of the articular surface. In addition, the arthroscope affords an unparalleled diagnostic view of the interosseous carpal ligaments, the carpal articular surfaces, and the TFCC. If indicated, arthroscopic or limited open management of concomitant soft

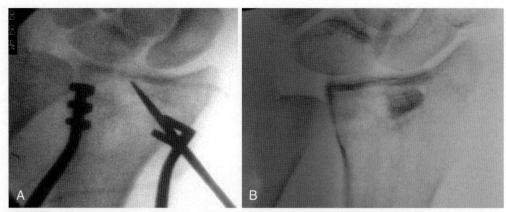

FIGURE 15.35 A, Limited open reduction of an impacted articular surface can be performed by inserting a Freer elevator into the metaphyseal defect through an area of comminution. Gentle pressure disimpacts and elevates articular fragments using the carpal bones as a template. **B,** Bone graft or graft substitute inserted into the metaphyseal defect supports the elevated articular surface.

tissue injuries of the carpus or DRUJ can be undertaken simultaneously.

Although the addition of arthroscopic inspection and reduction means additional operating room time and equipment, there is evidence to suggest that outcomes are improved. Doi and associates demonstrated improvements in range of motion and fracture reduction in a prospective cohort of patients treated by arthroscopically assisted percutaneous fixation when compared with a group treated by conventional open reduction and internal fixation (ORIF) for displaced articular fractures of the distal radius.[36]

Arthroscopic Reduction and Percutaneous Fixation Technique

When considering arthroscopically assisted reduction and fixation of an articular distal radius fracture, it is wise to reduce and stabilize the fracture in a splint for 3 to 7 days before surgery. Treatment of fractures acutely by arthroscopic means may limit visibility secondary to bleeding and may risk the development of compartment syndrome because of extravasation of fluid into the soft tissues. After 7 days, however, it becomes difficult to elevate impacted articular fragments without a formal open reduction.

The arm is prepared sterilely, draped in the usual manner, and suspended from sterile finger traps attached to the index and long fingers (Figure 15.36). The forearm may be exsanguinated with an Esmarch bandage that can be left in place from just proximal to the wrist up to the elbow to prevent fluid extravasation into the soft tissues. Alternatively, an elastic bandage can be wrapped around the hand and forearm to reduce soft tissue swelling. It is preferable to perform the arthroscopic portion of the procedure without a tourniquet, saving its use for any open reduction that may be required. The fracture is then evaluated under fluoroscopic guidance, and the fragments are manually manipulated into position. As an alternative to finger trap or tower traction, an external-fixation device can be applied before arthroscopy of the wrist to prevent the need for suspension traction.[171]

The arthroscope is inserted through the 3-4 portal, and an outflow portal is established in either the 4-5 or 6U position. Immediate and copious irrigation is critical to clear clot and debris and to improve visualization. Once this is done, con-

tinuous irrigation is maintained through the 6U portal, and working portals can be established in the 1-2 or 4-5 positions (or both). Doi and associates demonstrated the utility of an additional volar–radial portal created by means of a limited open incision over the flexor carpi radialis (FCR) tendon.[36] K-wires (0.0625 in) are useful as percutaneous joysticks when placed in the radial styloid and other large articular fragments.

Reduction of the fragment is then accomplished with the joysticks under fluoroscopic control, and it is stabilized as mentioned previously with either 0.045- or 0.0625-in K-wires (see Figure 15.36, D, E). Impacted articular fragments can be elevated through a mini-open dorsal approach (see earlier) and supported with a bone graft or substitute (see Figure 15.35, B). Pins can be replaced with cannulated screws at the discretion of the surgeon.[72,97] If pin fixation alone is used, the wrist must be supported in a cast until healed. If using augmented external fixation, the wrist posture is returned to neutral, and the forearm is immobilized in a supinated position for 7 to 10 days with a light sugar tong dressing. The cast or fixator is generally removed at 4 to 6 weeks, depending on the fracture and whether a bone graft is used; percutaneous pins are usually removed 2 to 3 weeks later.

Additional Soft Tissue Injuries

Concomitant complete tears of the scapholunate or lunotriquetral ligaments should be reduced anatomically and pinned or treated by limited open reduction, repair, and pin or screw fixation (see Chapter 13). A minimum of two divergent pins or a temporary compression screw should cross the affected intercarpal articulation, and one or two additional pins should be placed to temporarily stabilize the proximal row to the distal carpal row across the midcarpal joint. Intercarpal pins are left in place for at least 8 weeks and a graduated program of range-of-motion and resistive exercises is begun slowly thereafter. If using a temporary scapholunate screw, the device can be left in place while gentle midcarpal motion is begun with a dart-thrower's rehabilitation protocol[31] (see Chapter 13); the screw can be removed 4 to 6 months postoperatively. Complete peripheral detachment of the articular disk of the TFCC can also be treated by arthroscopically guided suture placement at the time of fracture reduction (see Chapter 14).

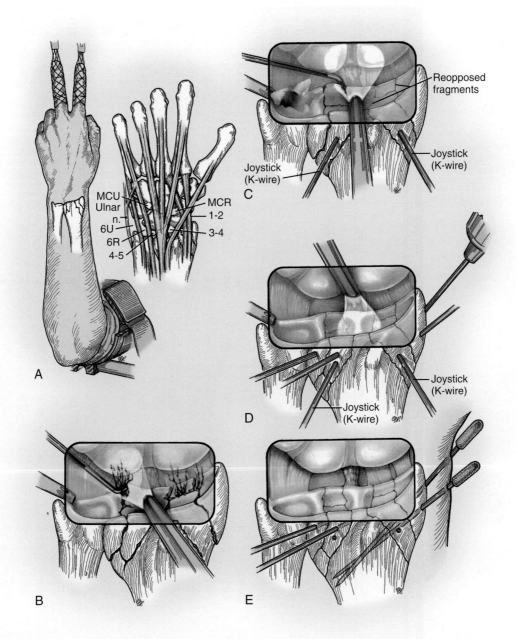

FIGURE 15.36 Operative technique for arthroscopic reduction and pinning of distal radial fractures: **A,** The arm is suspended from finger traps on the index and long fingers. The following anatomic landmarks are identified: arthroscopic portals 1-2, 3-4, 4-5, 6R (radial), 6U (ulnar), MCR (midcarpal radial), and MCU (midcarpal ulnar). The dorsal sensory branch of the ulnar nerve is noted. **B,** The arthroscope is introduced through the 3-4 or 4-5 portal, and with a probe through the 6R portal, the comminuted distal radial fracture is visualized. Clot and hemorrhage extrude from the fracture fragments. **C,** Joysticks (0.0625-in Kirschner wires [K-wires]) are introduced into the major fragments percutaneously to elevate the fracture fragments into an anatomic position. **D,** Additional K-wires are then introduced percutaneously into the fracture. **E,** The joysticks are then removed, the fixation pins are cut off outside the skin, and caps are applied. (© Elizabeth Martin.)

Bone Graft and Bone Graft Substitutes

A recent Cochrane systematic review of 10 trials involving 847 adult patients identified improvements in radiographic alignment among patients whose external or percutaneous fixation was supplemented by bone graft or bone graft substitutes; however, no differences in functional outcomes were identified.[70] The use of a bone graft to supplement internal or external fixation (see eFigure 15.7) has dramatically decreased during the last 5 years, in large part as a result of the seismic shift toward the use of angular stable implants[95,108] (Table 15.2).

Supplemental bone graft is now most often used in subacute or *nascent malunions* requiring osteoclasis[81]; malunited fractures; and, less frequently, in the acute situation to buttress the reduction of small articular fragments (see Case Study 15.1).

Iliac Bone Graft Harvesting Technique

After a rolled towel has been placed under the ipsilateral sacro-iliac joint, the iliac crest region is sterilely prepared and draped. A 5-cm-long incision is made over the iliac crest beginning 2-cm posterior to the anterior superior iliac spine and coursing

TABLE 15.2   Outcomes of Percutaneous and Single- and Multiple-Plate Fixation of Distal Radius Fractures

Year	Author	Number of Patients	Age	Female	C Type	C3	Follow-up Time (Months)	Grafted	Compl	Loss Redux	GE	PRWE	DASH	F/E	Grip
Volar-plate fixation															
2002	Orbay	31	54	55%	45%	10%	12	10%	3%	0%	100%			82%	77%
2004	Orbay	24	79	71%	10%	4%	12	38%	17%	13%				82%	79%
2005	Musgrave	32	57	91%	66%	0%	13	0%	34%	0%				80%	
2005	Kamano	40	57	70%	15%	3%	12	10%	5%	0%	100%			85%	78%
2006	Ruch	14	46	50%	100%	71%	22	14%	29%	0%	86%			85%	78%
2006	Rozental	41	53	63%	46%	12%	17	7%	22%	10%	100%			70%	94%
2007	Rein	15	54	47%	100%	100%	48	0%	13%	7%	47%			80%	90%
2008	Egol	38	52	57%	38%		12	0%	21%	0%			13	85%	85%
2009	Wei	12	61	75%	75%		12	33%	17%	0%			4	91%	94%
2009	Rozental	23	51	70%	57%		12	0%	9%	0%			4	88%	85%
2011	Yu	47	56	62%	68%		38	0%	28%	2%					
2011	Wilcke	33	55	76%	21%		12	0%	21%	0%		11	7	92%	94%
2012	Jakubietz	22	68	86%	100%	23%	12	0%	41%	0%	94%		11	87%	95%
2013	Williksen	52	54	80%	69%	2%	12	0%	29%	2%			9	88%	86%
2014	Karantana	66			3%	0%	12	0%	27%	2%			9	91%	95%
AVERAGE		**33**	**57**	**68%**	**54%**	**23%**	**17**	**7%**	**21%**	**2%**	**88%**		**8**	**85%**	**87%**
Dorsal-plate fixation															
2005	Grewel	29	46	62%	100%	100%	18	86%	72%	0%				60%	86%
2006	Kamath	30	59	53%	70%	13%	18	33%	13%	3%	93%			85%	78%
2006	Ruch	20	49	55%	100%	75%	21	45%	20%	25%	75%			75%	74%
2006	Simic	51	55	59%	16%	0%	24	0%	12%	0%	78%			81%	92%
2007	Rein	14	45	71%	100%	100%	48	0%	50%	14%	36%			70%	85%
2011	Yu	57	51	62%	58%		49	0%	18%	2%					
2012	Jakubietz	20	68	85%	100%	30%	12	0%	55%	15%	64%		14	68%	75%
AVERAGE		**32**	**53**	**64%**	**78%**	**53%**	**27**	**23%**	**34%**	**8%**	**69%**		**14**	**73%**	**82%**

Fragment-specific fixation													
2000	Jakob	74	60	70%	66%	41%	12	51%	22%	6%	97%			84%	90%
2002	Konrath	25	53	44%	70%	33%	29	0%	28%	4%	92%			82%	83%
2006	Benson	85	50	68%	89%	21%	32	76%	20%	0%	100%		9	88%	92%
2009	Jupiter	150	51	59%	71%		24	12%	16%	3%	96%		7	86%	90%
2009	Abramo	26	48	67%	85%		12	8%	31%	4%			9	86%	90%
2012	Gavaskar	105	43	41%	100%	31%	12	4%	21%	5%		10	8	87%	78%
AVERAGE		**78**	**51**	**58%**	**80%**	**32%**	**20**	**25%**	**23%**	**4%**	**96%**	**10**	**8**	**86%**	**87%**
External fixation													
2001	Sakano	25	49	40%	76%	8%	30	100%	0%	0%	100%			88%	89%
2003	Werber	50	58	70%	60%	0%	6	0%	14%	0%	90%			65%	60%
2004	Harley	25	43	52%	80%	44%	12	12%	56%	0%	48%			81%	79%
2005	Grewal	33	45	36%	100%	85%	18	45%	24%					65%	97%
2005	Kreder	88	40	43%	83%		24	13%	11%	0%				94%	90%
2005	Gradl	25	60	12%	44%	20%	24	0%	16%	4%	96%			92%	
2008	Leung	74	42	38%	100%	39%	24	22%	13%	0%	94%				
2008	Egol	39	50	100%	59%		12	0%	18%				17	87%	100%
2009	Abramo	24	48	71%	83%		12	8%	58%	21%			14	86%	78%
2009	Wei	22	55	73%	55%		12	18%	17%	0%			18	90%	94%
2011	Grewel	24	54	75%	42%		12	0%	46%	4%		15		84%	86%
2011	Wilcke	30	56	77%	27%		12	0%	43%	10%		15	11	84%	85%
2013	Williksen	59	54	80%	76%	3%	12	0%	30%	5%			11	83%	81%
AVERAGE		**40**	**50**	**59%**	**68%**	**28%**	**16**	**17%**	**27%**	**4%**	**86%**	**15**	**14**	**83%**	**85%**

Compl, Complications; *DASH*, disabilities of the arm, shoulder and hand; *F/E*, flexion/extensior; *GE*, good-to-excellent; *PRWE*, patient rated wrist evaluation.

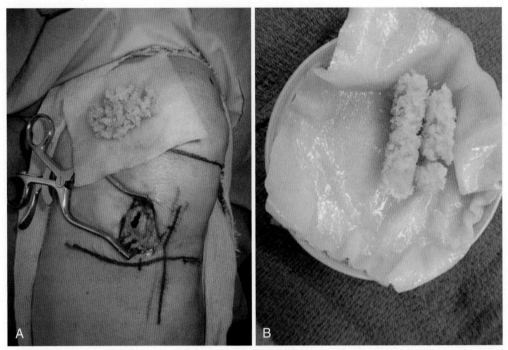

FIGURE 15.37 A, B, Approximately 25 cc of cancellous graft may be harvested rapidly with minimal morbidity from a small cortical window medial to the insertion of the patellar tendon on the tibia. The 2-cm oblique incision begins at a point 1 cm medial and 1 cm superior to the midpoint of the patellar tubercle.[76] (Redrawn with permission, Herford AS et al: Medial approach for tibial bone graft: anatomic study and clinical technique. *J Oral Maxillofac Surg* 61:358–363, 2003.)

posteriorly. With straight and curved 1-cm osteotomes, a section of the iliac crest 3 cm long and 1 cm thick is reflected cephalad on its medial periosteum and is still attached to the external oblique musculature. This exposes an abundant area of cancellous bone between the two cortical wings.

Cancellous bone is harvested and preserved in a moist saline-soaked sponge. The iliac crest flap is then turned back down into its bed and sutured in place. (This technique leaves virtually no cosmetic defect to either the eye or touch along the iliac crest.) The wound is then closed in layers over a suction catheter drain. Alternatively, a bone trephine set can be used to harvest one or more bicortical 10- to 12-mm plugs from the iliac wing through a 1- to 2-cm incision. Each harvest site is filled with thrombin-soaked Gelfoam® for hemostasis, and the area is infiltrated with a long-acting anesthetic. This procedure reduces the pain and local morbidity of iliac crest graft harvest, can be performed under local anesthesia with sedation, and generally obviates the need for an overnight stay or ambulatory assistance postoperatively.

Tibial Bone Graft Harvesting Technique

Up to 25 cc of cancellous graft can be harvested from the tibia, just medial to the tibial tubercle, without ambulatory aids or additional morbidity of an iliac crest graft.[76] The technique is rapid and straightforward and is adopted from work done by our maxilla-facial colleagues. The leg is prepared and draped from just below a sterile thigh tourniquet. A towel or sandbag is placed under the knee and the apex of the tibial tubercle is marked. Two perpendicular lines are marked, intersecting at this point: the first along the axis of the tibia and the second parallel to the joint line. The leg is exsanguinated and the tourniquet inflated.

A 2- to 3-cm oblique incision is made, centered on a point 1.5 cm proximal and 1.5 cm medial, at the tubercle apex (Figure 15.37) (see Case Study 15.1). Periosteum is incised and reflected, and a 15-mm oval or round defect is created with a K-wire driver and osteotomes. The cortical piece is lifted and saved for later replacement and an abundant cancellous graft is harvested. Thrombin-soaked Gelfoam is placed in the cavity, the cortical piece returned, and the periosteum and skin closed. A local compression dressing is applied, and the patient is allowed to bear weight immediately.

Bone graft substitutes may be used as an alternative to the harvesting of autogenous bone. With acute fractures, the need for structural support of the elevated articular surface generally outweighs the need for osteogenic stimulation of healing (see Figure 15.35, *B*). The intact radial metaphysis is normally an potent source of osteogenic cells, growth factors, and osteoinductive cancellous bone, and fractures through this area have a strikingly low rate of delayed union or nonunion.

The ability to expedite fracture healing by the addition of biologic products has not been demonstrated, except in situations in which healing potential has been compromised by disease or tobacco use.[99] Thus, bone graft substitutes that demonstrate compressive properties equal to or greater than cancellous bone are of greater utility in the management of comminuted articular fractures than are purely osteogenic or combined osteogenic-moldable putty formulations (see Case Study 15.2). The use of methyl methacrylate and other bone cements to support the articular surface has largely been abandoned because of their unfavorable mechanical properties.

The specific advantages and disadvantages of several common bone graft alternative categories are presented in eTable 15.1 (see ExpertConsult.com).

Open Reduction and Internal Fixation

Open reduction of distal radius fractures is indicated in active patients when satisfactory reduction cannot be achieved or maintained by closed manipulation and casting, and as an alternative to percutaneous fixation at the preference of the patient or surgeon. There is increasing evidence to support equivalent functional, clinical, and radiographic outcomes of fixed-angle internal fixation when compared with percutaneous and indirect fixation,[105,174] and it is an attractive alternative to the bulkiness and pin care issues of external fixation. Open reduction has also been demonstrated to yield improved radiographic alignment when compared with percutaneous pins and repeat closed reduction for fractures that have lost the original reduction after a trial of closed reduction and casting.[112]

Articular fractures in elderly, inactive patients, and in those with considerable osteoporosis, have traditionally been considered a contraindication to open reduction because in these patients there is a risk for complications, including fixation failure, nonunion, and reflex sympathetic dystrophy. However, since the introduction of fixed-angle internal-fixation devices, both unstable extraarticular and simple articular fractures in the elderly, active osteoporotic patients have had increasingly satisfactory outcomes with ORIF.[126] Subchondral buttressing with locking pins or screws secured to the plate greatly reduces the incidence of settling or secondary articular displacement, as well as the need for a supplemental bone graft (Figure 15.38).

The choice of surgical approach depends largely on the location and direction of displacement of the fracture fragments. Thus, dorsally or radially displaced fractures have been classically approached through dorsal incisions, whereas volarly displaced fractures (e.g., the Smith and reversed Barton) are classically approached through palmar exposures. There has been increased interest in the management of dorsally displaced nonarticular and articular fractures with volar fixed-angle plate fixation in an attempt to decrease the incidence of extensor tendon irritation associated with dorsal implants. When using multiple plates or fragment-specific fixation, dorsal, radial palmar, ulnar–volar, and ulnar incisions are used in combination, as dictated by the particular fracture's configuration.

General factors limiting surgical reconstruction of the articular surface include the number of fragments, their size, the amount of cancellous bone impaction, and associated traumatic lesions of the articular cartilage. Alternatives to open anatomic restoration, including percutaneous fixation and bridge plating, should be considered in cases of extreme articular comminution. In these cases, efforts should be directed at restoring the anatomic relationships of the radius and ulna and to ensuring normal alignment of the hand and carpus with the long axis of the forearm by percutaneous and indirect means. If radiocarpal arthritic changes subsequently occur, the restoration of normal length and alignment will greatly facilitate the performance of secondary reconstructive procedures.

Dorsal Plate Fixation

Although satisfactory outcomes have been reported with dorsal plating systems, the incidence of extensor tendon complications, including irritation, synovitis, attrition, and tendon rupture, is not negligible.[9,23,83] A dorsal approach is preferred by many surgeons in the more comminuted C3 type fractures because of improved visualization and ease of reduction of the impacted articular surface, or when the use of a bone graft is needed. Low-profile and stainless steel plates have a decreased incidence of dorsal tendinopathy when compared to traditional 3.5-mm implants[177]; however, with increased versatility, mechanical strength, and ease of application of fixed-angle volar devices, isolated dorsal-plate fixation for distal radius fractures is less commonly performed.

"Universal" Dorsal Approach to the Distal Radius. A 3- to 10-cm straight dorsal incision is made just ulnar to the Lister tubercle, centered over the radial metaphysis. Full-thickness skin flaps are raised at the retinacular level, including the dorsal sensory branches of the radial and ulnar nerves. An ulnar-based retinacular flap is begun just ulnar to the Lister tubercle and elevated to expose the EPL and the tendons of the fourth compartment. Some surgeons prefer to elevate the fourth dorsal compartment subperiosteally without exposing the tendons themselves. A 2-cm segment of the posterior interosseous nerve can be removed at the discretion of the surgeon. Subperiosteal exposure yields direct visualization of the fracture fragments, so rarely is it necessary to violate the wrist capsule. Additional exposure of the dorsal–radial styloid can be performed by undermining the second and first dorsal compartments.

Direct and indirect reduction of the fracture fragments is performed and confirmed with fluoroscopy, and temporary fixation is done with K-wires through the styloid and dorsal–ulnar corner of the radius. Articular reduction is facilitated by using a Freer elevator and subchondral elevation (see Figure 15.35), with the carpus being used as a template for reduction. Placement of the plate may be facilitated by removal of the Lister tubercle. The plate is contoured and fitted to the dorsal surface and conventional screws, or 2.4-mm fixed-angle pegs and screws, are inserted to support the subchondral bone. The tendons of the second and fourth compartments are put back over the plate, and a portion of the retinaculum can be used as an interposition flap between the tendons and the distal plate. The EPL tendon is primarily transposed to a subcutaneous position when closing the dorsal retinaculum (Figure 15.39).

If using older implants without angular stable fixation, the use of an autogenous iliac bone graft, or an appropriate structural bone graft substitute, to support comminuted or impacted articular fragments is important. If fixed-angle devices with subchondral buttressing are used, the need for bone grafting is reduced because the chance of secondary displacement of

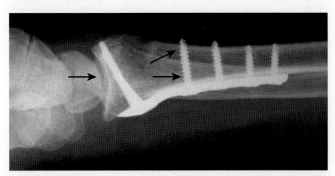

FIGURE 15.38 Ideal positioning of a volar fixed-angle plate. Notice the subchondral positioning of the distal fixed-angle pegs, by virtue of which axial loading is transmitted to the pegs and the volar plate and to the radial shaft. The dorsal comminuted area has not been grafted in this case.

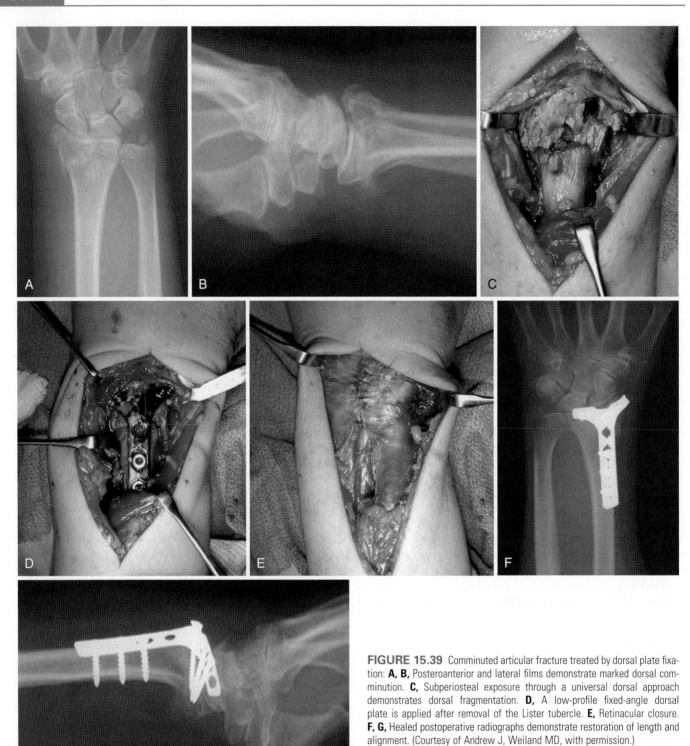

FIGURE 15.39 Comminuted articular fracture treated by dorsal plate fixation: **A, B,** Posteroanterior and lateral films demonstrate marked dorsal comminution. **C,** Subperiosteal exposure through a universal dorsal approach demonstrates dorsal fragmentation. **D,** A low-profile fixed-angle dorsal plate is applied after removal of the Lister tubercle. **E,** Retinacular closure. **F, G,** Healed postoperative radiographs demonstrate restoration of length and alignment. (Courtesy of Andrew J, Weiland MD, with permission.)

articular fragments is diminished by the increased structural properties of the fixed-angle plate. A compilation of published studies about internal fixation from 2000 to 2014 demonstrates that bone grafts were employed in 23% of cases in which single dorsal plates were used, in 25% of cases in which multiple fragment-specific plates were used, and in 7% of procedures that used volar fixed-angle plates (see Table 15.2). With the technologic improvements in angular stable plate design over the past 5 years, supplemental bone graft use has dropped to 8% or less for all types of internal fixations.

Volar Plate Fixation Technique. Regardless of the displacement of the distal fragment (i.e., dorsal, volar, radial), volar plating of both articular and nonarticular fractures is an effective fixation method that may reduce some of the soft tissue complications associated with dorsal plating. Advantages of palmar exposure and volar plating include the following:

- Minimal volar comminution facilitates reduction of dorsally displaced fractures.
- Anatomic reduction of the volar cortex facilitates restoration of radial length, inclination, and volar tilt.
- Avoidance of additional dorsal dissection helps preserve the vascular supply of comminuted dorsal fragments.
- Because the wrist's volar compartment has a larger cross-sectional space and the implant is separated from the flexor tendons by the pronator quadratus, the incidence of flexor tendon complications is minimized.
- The use of fixed-angle volar plate designs avoids screw "toggling" in the distal fragment and thus reduces the danger of secondary displacement.
- When stabilized with a fixed-angle, internal-fixation device that uses subchondral pegs or screws, control of shortening and late displacement of articular fragments are improved and the need for bone grafting is reduced (see Figure 15.38).

Fractures are exposed through the distal part of the Henry approach between the FCR and radial artery via an 8- to 9-cm longitudinal incision that courses proximally from the wrist crease. It is not generally necessary to cross the wrist crease, but an oblique "hockey-stick" extension can be made toward the scaphoid tubercle if additional exposure is required. The subsheath of the FCR is opened along its radial border to avoid inadvertent injury to the nearby palmar cutaneous branch of the median nerve. The virtual space beneath the flexor tendons is developed and the FCR and flexor tendons are retracted to the ulnar side, thus protecting the median nerve and its palmar branch.

The radial vascular bundle is retracted radially to expose the flexor pollicis longus (FPL) and the pronator quadratus, then transverse radial artery branches are cauterized. The distal fibers of the FPL muscle belly may require partial release from the radius for adequate radial shaft exposure. The brachioradialis tendon is sharply separated from overlying soft tissues and split longitudinally at the level of the pronator quadratus for 5 to 8 cm to its insertion on the radial styloid. It is not necessary to completely transect the BR tendon in most acute cases, though many surgeons do this routinely; there are no reported adverse consequences of BR release.

The first dorsal compartment is easily released to improve visualization of the radial styloid. Elevation of the pronator in continuity with the volar half of the split BR tendon facilitates anatomic suture repair and ensures plate coverage at the conclusion of the procedure (Figure 15.40; see also Figure 15.42 later). The distal border of the pronator is sharply incised at the volar lip of the radius and the muscle sharply reflected ulnarly from the radius and volar fragments. A manual reduction is performed, usually aided by traction and manipulation of the fragments against the surgeon's thumb that is held as a buttress on the metaphyseal flare of the radius. If anatomic reduction is confirmed clinically and with fluoroscopy, it is preferable to fix the fracture temporarily with an oblique 0.062-in K-wire inserted percutaneously through the radial styloid. Any degree of coronal shift of the articular fragment should be corrected at this juncture.[38,134]

I prefer to deliver a radial-directed moment via a small Bennett retractor, placed strategically on the ulnar metaphyseal flare of the radial shaft fragment. A clamp on the radial shaft proximal to the fracture is also useful in this regard. Counterpressure on the articular fragment in an ulnar direction is performed to reduce the fragment (Figure 15.41, A, B). Reduction

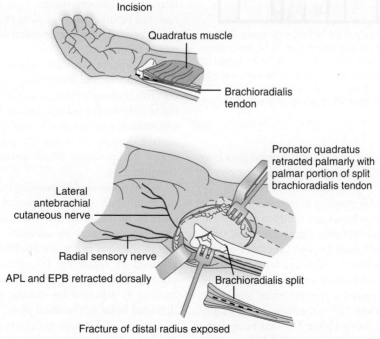

Incision

Quadratus muscle

Brachioradialis tendon

Lateral antebrachial cutaneous nerve

Pronator quadratus retracted palmarly with palmar portion of split brachioradialis tendon

Radial sensory nerve

APL and EPB retracted dorsally

Brachioradialis split

Fracture of distal radius exposed

FIGURE 15.40 Volar–radial approach to the distal radius. The brachioradialis tendon may be split and elevated subperiosteally to expose the radial and intermediate columns and the volar aspect of the distal radius. *APL,* Abductor pollicis longus; *EPB,* extensor pollicis brevis. (© 2001, Virginia Ferrante.)

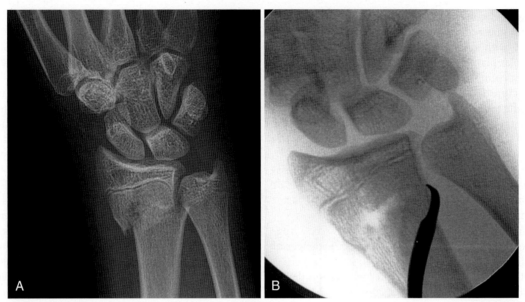

FIGURE 15.41 Reduction of radial translation (coronal shift): **A,** Prereduction fluoroscopy indicating a 4-mm radial coronal shift of the articular fragment in a 16-year-old golfer. **B,** A Hohmann retractor is placed on the ulnar border of the radial metaphyseal flare, proximal to the fracture line. Firm radial directed force is applied while the fracture fragment is pushed ulnarward to seat the ulna in the sigmoid notch.

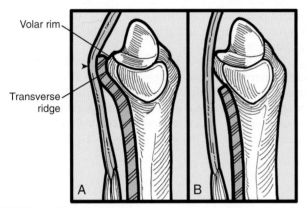

Volar rim

Transverse ridge

FIGURE 15.42 A, Incorrect placement of a volar fixed-angle device. A Soong grade 2 plate placement,[147] characterized by prominence of the hardware above the critical line, and within 2 mm of the tip of the volar rim. Without coverage by the pronator, the flexor tendons are in direct contact with the plate and may rupture. **B,** Correct placement of the implant, recessed proximally and with sufficient soft tissue coverage to prevent flexor irritation and rupture. (© Elizabeth Martin.)

of the coronal shift and anatomic seating of the distal ulna into the sigmoid notch of the radius is confirmed fluoroscopically on the frontal view.

A volar plate is chosen and contoured as necessary to fit the volar metaphyseal flare of the radius. Care needs to be taken to avoid placement of the plate distal to the transverse radial ridge (i.e., the so-called "watershed" line) because implants on the volar lip of the radius are in direct continuity with the flexor tendons, and there is a risk of tendon irritation and rupture (Figure 15.42).[33] Hardware placed 2 mm or more above the volar critical line (Soong Grade 1)[147] or within 3 mm of the distal edge of the volar rim (Soong Grade 2)[147] has been demonstrated to have a high rate of tendon rupture.[90] If fixation of the plate distal to this ridge is deemed necessary to stabilize small marginal or volar ulnar fragments, I recommend consid-

eration of a tension-band fixation[25] or a low-profile miniplate or a wireform construct as alternative solutions to avoid the serious complication of flexor tendon rupture. If a decision is made to use a volar plate in this position, scheduled hardware removal should be discussed with the patient.

When optimal plate position is confirmed, the plate is provisionally fixed with K-wires or with a single screw in the oval hole of the plate at the diaphyseal level. Distal or proximal fine-tuning of plate position can be performed, as determined with fluoroscopy, to align the projected angles of the distal screws or pegs immediately beneath the subchondral bone on the facet lateral fluoroscopic image. It is important that volar tilt be restored before finalizing plate position to optimize peg placement beneath the subchondral bone and minimize articular penetration.

This is particularly important for patients with osteoporotic bone; subchondral buttressing with the locked pegs effectively controls fracture settling or dorsal displacement. It is also essential to contour the plate to match the patient's normal metaphyseal volar flare; undercontouring it can translate the articular surface dorsally or rotate the fragment into an unacceptable dorsal tilt position when associated with extensive dorsal comminution.

When optimal plate position is realized, the remainder of the proximal shaft screws are placed. It is important to have six cortices proximal to the fracture site for adequate fixation, although four may be adequate with locking screws. Longer metadiaphyseal plates are available in most sets to span comminuted or segmental fracture varieties. With the proximal plate fixed, fine-tuning of the reduction is performed and distal fixation is achieved by locking smooth pegs or screws into threaded holes in the distal plate.

Dozens of different plates are available, and several feature "multiaxial" screw projection to enable alteration of screw or peg angle to suit a particular fracture anatomy. Precise drilling with custom drill guides that are screwed or snapped into the

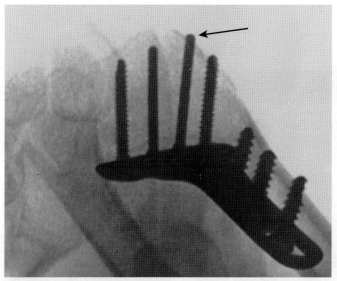

FIGURE 15.43 Tangential fluoroscopic or "horizon" views of the radius are essential to avoid protrusion of locking screws dorsally (*arrow*), risking delayed tendon rupture.

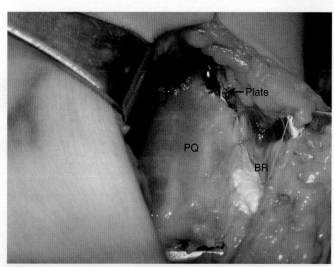

FIGURE 15.44 Splitting the brachioradialis (BR) longitudinally and leaving its volar tendinous portion attached to the pronator quadratus (PQ) allows a stout repair over the volar plate on closure.

distal holes is necessary when using fixed-angle devices to ensure engagement of the threaded heads on the plate. While most plates feature double rows of screw holes, inserting half of the pegs or screws achieves comparable mechanical strength,[120] especially if staggered between proximal and distal rows.[32] Use of screws or pegs is largely the surgeon's preference; there is no mechanical advantage to either, and the ease of insertion of smooth pegs may be offset by the increased difficulty of removal at a later date.[64]

Careful fluoroscopic assessment of screw length is mandatory to prevent its prominence dorsally and to detect articular protrusion. Several specialized views have been recommended to detect dorsal protrusion, and it is sensible to thoroughly evaluate final screw placement with a combination of lateral, supination, pronation, and dorsal tangential[127] or "horizon" views[78] (Figure 15.43). With locked screws or pegs, there is no mechanical advantage to penetration or purchase of the dorsal cortical bone; thus, it is recommended that screws 2 mm shorter than the measured length be routinely employed distally.

Although there is no demonstrated advantage to closure of the pronator quadratus, the implant can be easily covered with the pronator by restoring the split portion of the BR to the remaining tendon on the radius (Figure 15.44). The wound is closed in layers, and drainage is rarely necessary. The stability of the radioulnar joint is assessed and addressed as necessary. I routinely utilize a plaster sugar tong splint in full supination until suture removal 10 to 14 days postoperatively, followed by use of a removable wrist brace for comfort. Patients are encouraged to mobilize the digits immediately after surgery. Light functional use of the hand and wrist (e.g., eating, dressing, writing, typing) is permitted after suture removal (Figure 15.45). For elderly patients with an osteoporotic bone, the postoperative regimen can be modified as needed; if insufficient fixation is suspected, a light forearm cast is applied for 4 to 5 weeks after suture removal.

If anatomic reduction of the articular surface and dorsal marginal fragments cannot be achieved with manual reduction through the volar Henry incision, Orbay and Fernandez recommend an extended Henry approach to enable direct articular reduction.[125] To gain this degree of exposure, the entire proximal radius is pronated away from the fractured articular components by performing an extensive soft tissue release. It is theorized that complete subperiosteal elevation from the metaphyseal diaphyseal portion of the radius is tolerated because of a rich endosteal blood supply.

The first step in the exposure is release of the radial septum (insertion of the BR and the palmar sheath of the first extensor compartment) to facilitate reduction of the radial styloid fragment. Next, the surgeon performs a subperiosteal exposure of the distal third of the radial diaphysis. Finally, to visualize the dorsal die-punch and centrally impacted fragments through the fracture plane, the proximal shaft fragment is fully pronated with a bone clamp. Using direct visualization, the fragments can be manipulated into a reduced position against the proximal carpal row (Figure 15.46). Thereafter, the proximal fragment is supinated back into place and a volar fixed-angle plate is applied. An attempt is made to fix large dorsal–ulnar fragments with locking screws through the plate. Orbay and Fernandez cite preservation of the extensor tendon sleeve and a reduced incidence of extensor tendinopathy as advantages of this exposure.

Alternatively, displaced fragments of the dorsal rim or intermediate column can be reduced and fixed by direct exposure through a limited dorsal incision with the application of additional 2.0- or 2.4-mm implants (or by reduction and stabilization with distal screws from the volar plate). Similarly, if complete capture of a large or comminuted radial styloid fragment cannot be attained with one or two of the locked pegs, the surgeon should definitely consider the addition of a radial column plate to complement volar fixation and prevent undesirable settling and consequent incongruity of the styloid and its scaphoid facet (Figure 15.47). Finally, volar fixed-angle plate fixation is not ideal for a small volar–ulnar corner or "teardrop" lunate facet fragments.[39] Failure to adequately capture this fragment with plate coverage and one or two locked pegs may

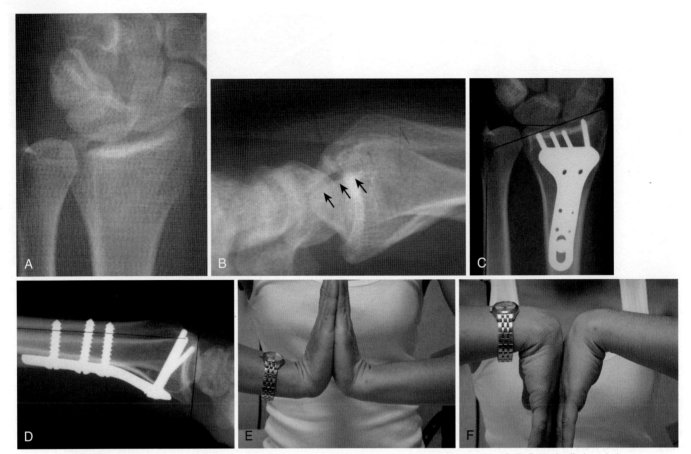

FIGURE 15.45 Coronal split Smith type II fracture fixed with a volar locked-plate and immediate motion: **A, B,** Coronal split through the articular surface (*arrows*). **C, D,** Volar locked-plate fixation. **E, F,** Photos of range of flexion and extension 12 weeks postoperatively.

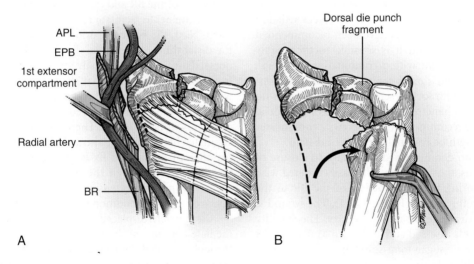

FIGURE 15.46 A, B, The extended volar approach enables direct disimpaction of articular fragments by subperiosteal exposure of the distal third of the radius and pronation of the proximal fragment. *APL,* Abductor pollicis longus; *BR,* brachioradialis; *EPB,* extensor pollicis brevis. (Adapted from Orbay JL, Fernandez DL: Volar fixation for dorsally displaced fractures of the distal radius: a preliminary report. *J Hand Surg [Am]* 27:205–215, 2002. Redrawn and © by Elizabeth Martin.)

result in loss of fixation[12] and palmar translation of the entire carpus during the postoperative period (Figure 15.48). Additional fixation of this fragment may be achieved with K-wires, a tension band, a 2.0-mm miniplate, a spring wire,[117] or a volar buttress pin.

Fragment-Specific Fixation

In an attempt to minimize the morbidity of extensive surgical dissections associated with conventional dorsal plate fixation of distal radius fractures, Robert Medoff devised a hybrid technique of percutaneous wire and plate fixation designed

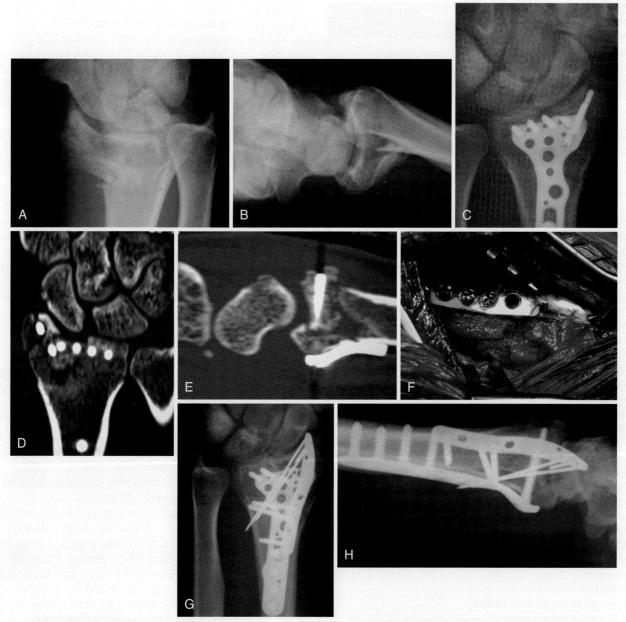

FIGURE 15.47 Hybrid fixation of the radial styloid: **A, B,** Posteroanterior (PA) and lateral radiographs demonstrating a comminuted articular fracture with palmar displacement and a large radial styloid fragment. **C,** PA radiograph 3 weeks postoperatively demonstrating incomplete fixation of the radial styloid. **D, E,** Computed tomography confirms insufficient styloid fixation with articular incongruency. **F,** Photo of revision stabilization of the radial column with a radial column plate and bone graft. **G, H,** PA and lateral radiographs of the healed construct.

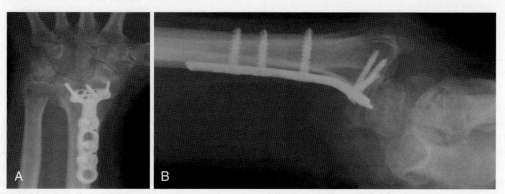

FIGURE 15.48 A, B, Palmar subluxation of the carpus after volar plate fixation. Note the palmar and proximal translation of the carpus as a result of loss of fixation of the volar ulnar fragment on the lateral radiograph.

CRITICAL POINTS *Volar Fixed-Angle Plate Fixation*

Indications

- Unstable nonarticular fractures of the distal radius (including osteoporotic bone)
- Nascent and established distal radius malunion
- Articular fractures

Contraindications

- Marginal shear fractures; very distal fracture–dislocations
- Small volar–ulnar corner fragment

Technical Points

- Make a longitudinal incision along the FCR tendon.
- Expose the pronator quadratus between the FCR and the radial artery.
- Release the first dorsal compartment tendons to expose the radial styloid.
- Detach the pronator quadratus with an "L"-shaped incision and leave a portion of the split BR attached to the pronator for subsequent closure.
- Reduce the fracture by restoring the volar cortex.
- Reduce any residual coronal shift of the distal fragment.
- Provide temporary fracture fixation with an oblique K-wire through the radial styloid.
- Apply the plate volarly and fix it to the shaft through an oval hole.
- Determine the ideal plate position with fluoroscopy, then place the remaining shaft screws.
- Avoid placement of plate on distal transverse ridge of the radius to prevent tendon rupture.
- Insert fixed-angle pegs or screws in a subchondral position.
- Insert screws 2 mm shorter than the measured length.
- Use a facet lateral fluoroscopic view to prevent articular protrusion.
- Use multiple fluoroscopic views, including a dorsal tangential one, to prevent dorsal screw prominence.
- Assess the adequacy of dorsal–ulnar fragment and radial styloid reduction and fixation and augment, as necessary, with columnar plates.
- Consider alternative or additional fixation of the volar lunate facet fragment if not adequately captured by the volar plate.
- Assess stability of the distal radioulnar joint, and treat as necessary.
- For articular fractures that are not reducible, an extended FCR approach is an option:
  - Perform a tenotomy of the BR tendon.
  - Release the first dorsal compartment.
  - Pronate the proximal fragment to expose the articular surface.

Postoperative Care

- Apply a sugar tong splint in supination for 10 to 12 days until suture removal.
- Begin digital range-of-motion exercises immediately.
- Begin forearm rotation and gentle active wrist motion exercises at the first postoperative visit.
- Evaluate with radiographs at the initial postoperative visit and at 6 weeks postoperatively.

---

to fix individual fracture fragments through several small incisions.[10,102] His "fragment-specific" classification (see Figure 15.18) defines articular fractures of the radius by recognition of five elemental fragments present alone or in combination in every fracture. The technique involves the use of ultrathin modular implants that can be shaped to customize fixation for various fragment configurations; the Medoff technique builds on the work of Rikli and Regazzoni[133] by placing these implants strategically along the radial and intermediate columns (see Figure 15.19) to maximize construct rigidity.[77]

The key component of the implant system is the so-called *pin plate* (TriMed, Inc., Valencia, CA), which combines the versatility of a K-wire with the rigidity of plate-and-screw fixation. The bending stiffness of conventional K-wire fixation is dramatically increased by passing the wire through the free end of a miniature 2.0-mm plate, secured proximally to the radial shaft, to create a pin plate hybrid with a three-point fixation. Mechanical studies using an unstable metaphyseal fracture model have demonstrated that dual 2.0-mm plates, when placed at 50- to 90-degree angles to each other in the axial plane, provide fixation that is statistically superior to that of either K-wire–augmented external fixation or to a traditional 3.5-mm dorsal "T"-plate.[35,129] Thus, the use of the term "fragment-specific fixation" in this text does not refer to a particular implant type but to the concept of the use of two or more low-profile implants placed strategically along the columns of the distal radius to fix individual fracture fragments.

Five recent single-cohort clinical series and one randomized trial totaling more than 450 patients, and using a variety of bicolumnar low-profile miniplate or wireform fixations, documented good-to-excellent results in 96% of patients at an average follow-up of 20 months (see Table 15.2).[13,77,94] The fractures were predominantly AO C-type (80%), and a supplemental bone graft was used for 25% of them. Grip strength was restored to 87% of the opposite side and flexion–extension to 86%. Average disabilities of arm, shoulder and hand (DASH) scores on 366 of the patients measured 8 on a 100-point scale. Fragment-specific fixation is indicated for most unstable and high-energy articular fractures of the distal radius and is generally contraindicated for fractures with substantial metaphyseal–diaphyseal extension or severe osteoporosis.

The radial styloid fragment is regarded as the cornerstone for reduction and stability of articular distal radius fractures and is therefore addressed first in the sequence of multifragment reduction and fixation. The other key fragments to be considered include the volar lip, the dorsal wall, the dorsal and volar components of the lunate facet, and the impacted articular (see Figure 15.18). Traction of 5 to 10 lb, applied via finger traps on the index and long fingers or through the use of a formal traction table, is helpful to grossly align fragments. Fluoroscopic images in traction are a valuable adjunct to assess the nature of the fracture and its key components.

The radial styloid is approached through a 4- to 5-cm incision on the volar–radial aspect of the metaphyseal flare, just radial to the radial artery and palmar to the tendons of the first dorsal compartment. Superficial branches of the radial sensory and antebrachial cutaneous nerves are retracted in the skin flaps, and the first dorsal compartment is opened to expose and retract its tendons. The BR tendon is split longitudinally and the tendon and periosteum are elevated in a dorsal and palmar plane to expose the radius (see Figure 15.40).

Complete palmar exposure of the radius is accomplished by elevating the pronator quadratus in continuity with the palmar margin of the BR. If necessary, the entire radial styloid can be exposed by dorsal elevation beneath the second dorsal compartment. The styloid fragment is reduced anatomically and fixed provisionally with a 0.045-in K-wire. At this time, attention is directed to the intermediate column of the radius for reduction and fixation of the lunate facet and impacted articular fragments.

Dorsal intermediate column fragments are most commonly approached through a 4- to 5-cm universal dorsal incision over the third dorsal compartment, where the dorsal wall, articular fragments, and the dorsal–ulnar corner can be simultaneously addressed. The EPL is isolated and primarily transposed out of its compartment, and the radial metaphysis can be widely exposed by elevating the second or fourth (or both) compartments in a subperiosteal fashion. The comminuted dorsal cortical wall can be lifted to expose the radial metaphysis and a Freer elevator used to disimpact the articular fragments and elevate the articular surface en bloc against the template of the proximal carpal row bones (see Figure 15.35).

It is not generally necessary to open the dorsal capsule to directly inspect the articular surface because fluoroscopy is used to document reduction of the fracture fragments and the articular surface. An autogenous bone graft or a suitable structural bone graft substitute can be utilized at the surgeon's discretion to augment the reduction of the impacted articular fragments (see Figure 15.35, B). The dorsal intermediate column fragments are then directly reduced and fixed in position with any of a series of modular wireform implants, 2.4-mm angular stable plates[80] that capture and hold the small periarticular fragments (Figure 15.49; see also Case Study 15.2).

An isolated dorsal–ulnar fragment may be accessed and reduced using a limited approach through the fifth dorsal compartment. It is important to note that this incision is not extensile and cannot be readily enlarged to gain access to larger metaphyseal and impacted articular fragments; thus, if multiple dorsal fragments require reduction and fixation, a standard dorsal approach is preferred. A 3- to 4-cm incision is made directly over the radioulnar joint. The EDM is identified and transposed out of its compartment after dividing the extensor retinaculum of the fifth dorsal compartment. Great care needs to be taken to avoid iatrogenic disruption of the dorsal radioulnar ligament as the dorsal–ulnar fragment is exposed and reduced. Reduction is facilitated by the use of a dental pick to anatomically align the fragment's proximal cortical margins.

A 0.045-in K-wire is placed obliquely from the dorsal and ulnar margin of the fragment into the stout volar metaphyseal bone. A three-hole ulnar pin plate or a 2.0- to 2.4-mm low-profile locked plate is contoured and applied so it fits over the fragment with care taken to not overlap the radioulnar joint. The pin plate is secured proximally with two bicortical screws. A second wire is driven through one of the distal holes and the two wires are sequentially measured, cut, and bent 180 degrees at their tips before being impacted back into a free hole in the plate (Figure 15.50).

A frequently overlooked, but critically destabilizing intermediate column fragment, is the volar–ulnar or teardrop fragment. It constitutes the volar half of the lunate facet and is thus the primary restraint to volar subluxation of the carpus. It also represents the volar rim of the sigmoid notch and contains the origin of the volar radioulnar ligament—a prime stabilizer of the distal radioulnar joint. Failure to recognize or adequately stabilize this fragment can result in dramatic palmar subluxation of the carpus, articular incongruency, radioulnar instability, and ulnocarpal impaction (see Figure 15.48). The fragment is often too small, too distal, and/or too ulnar to be adequately captured by the pegs or screws of a fixed-angle palmar plate and, consequently, can complicate volar-plate fixation by the delayed development of carpal subluxation.[73]

Surgical Approach to the Volar–Ulnar Fragment. Because only the volar aspect of the DRUJ and the ulnar corner of the radius need to be visualized, a limited incision that parallels the FCU tendon just proximal to the transverse wrist crease provides sufficient exposure. Surgical release of that ligament can be performed if necessary by extending the incision in a zigzag fashion across the wrist crease and into the palm (i.e., extended carpal tunnel incision). The interval between the flexor tendons and the ulnar artery and nerve is easily developed by blunt dissection, through which the pronator quadratus and volar wrist capsule are exposed. Usually, the distal border of the pronator quadratus has been disrupted by the fracture; this allows visualization of the metaphyseal fracture line and displaced volar–ulnar fragment with minimal soft tissue dissection. The pronator quadratus is partially released from its ulnar insertion and

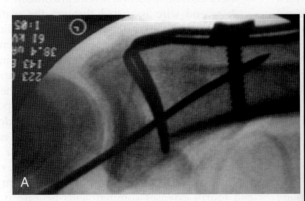
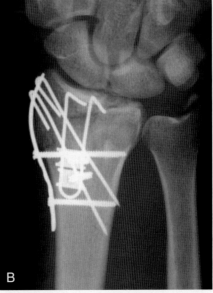

FIGURE 15.49 A, Intraoperative fluoroscopy demonstrating subchondral support for the articular surface and fixation of the comminuted dorsal cortex with a dorsal wireform implant. **B,** Posteroanterior view of a wireform implant used to secure a shear-type fracture of the articular surface.

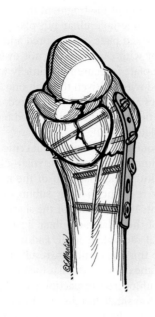

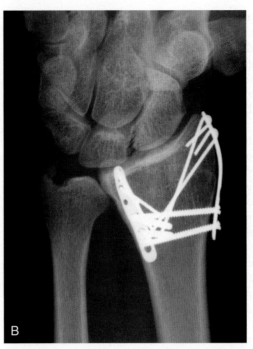

FIGURE 15.50 A, An ulnar "pin plate" or 2.0-mm miniplate can be used to fix unstable dorsal intermediate column fragments. **B,** The ulnar pin plate uses 0.045-in Kirschner wires and 2.0-mm screws and can be placed through a limited fifth dorsal compartment incision. It is important for most fractures that fixation of the intermediate column be supplemented with orthogonal (90–90) fixation of the radial column. (**A,** © Elizabeth Martin.)

retracted radially and proximally to expose the fracture site. Extreme care must be taken to avoid injury to the volar arm of the radioulnar ligamentous complex.

The volar–ulnar fracture fragment is then carefully reduced to restore continuity of the palmar cortex at the metaphyseal area by applying a dorsally directed force with an awl or periosteal elevator. Although not in rigid fixation, the fragment may be fixed by introducing a K-wire obliquely in a volar-to-dorsal direction. The wire is retrieved through the dorsal skin while making sure that its palmar end lies flush with the cortical level of the fragment to avoid impingement of the flexor tendons. For more stable fixation, the wire should be augmented with a suture or figure-of-eight wire placed through the proximal metaphyseal cortex in a tension band configuration.[25] Alternatively, if using a volar locked plate, the wire can be bent to match the curvature of the volar metaphyseal flare and captured beneath the volar plate as a "spring wire." Moore and Dennison reported maintenance of reduction in 9 of 9 patients treated in this fashion.[117]

I find that a volar buttress pin provides the most stable fixation for this fracture fragment and prevents carpal subluxation (Figure 15.51). The two prongs of the implant serve as a fixed-angle support for the subchondral bone, and the proximal implant is rigidly secured to the intact diaphyseal bone with washers and 2.3-mm screws. This restores the palmar stability of the fracture and provides a solid base on which the overlying dorsal–ulnar or die-punch fragment can be reduced. Additional volar rim fragments of the scaphoid facet can be stabilized with a volar buttress pin or a fixed-angle volar plate, at the surgeon's discretion.

The construct is completed by returning to the radial styloid to finish fixation with a radial columnar plate and screws (see Figure 15.51). To maximize stability of the fixation construct, it is important to place the radial styloid implant in a plane 50 to 90 degrees counter to the intermediate column's plane of fixation. The ideal position for a radial column implant lies directly beneath and oblique to the first dorsal compartment tendons, such that the distal tip of the plate is dorsal to the tendons and the plate's proximal end is palmar to them. If the previously placed provisional styloid K-wire is in an optimal position, a 3-, 5-, or 7-hole radial column pin plate is slid over the wire and positioned beneath the first dorsal compartment tendons. The plate is fixed to the intact metaphyseal–diaphyseal flare with two or more 2.3-mm bicortical screws proximally.

A second wire is passed through the plate distally and obliquely across the styloid to engage the opposing cortex. Each K-wire is sequentially measured, cut, and bent 180 degrees before being inserted into a neighboring hole in the pin plate. Final reduction and position of the implants are checked with fluoroscopy, and the BR tendon is closed over the radial column plate with a single running suture to interpose soft tissue between the implant and the overlying first dorsal compartment's tendons. By closing the BR tendon, the attached pronator quadratus simultaneously covers the volar implants. The dorsal wound is closed by transposing the EPL out of its compartment and closing the extensor retinaculum of the second and fourth extensor compartments beneath it. The DRUJ is then carefully assessed for stability, and appropriate treatment is rendered for residual instability. The wrist and forearm are temporarily immobilized in supination with a sugar tong splint for 5 to 10 days to allow soft tissue healing.

Rehabilitation is predicated on the strength of fracture fixation, but generally patients can be started on a program of active, unresisted motion exercises within a week of

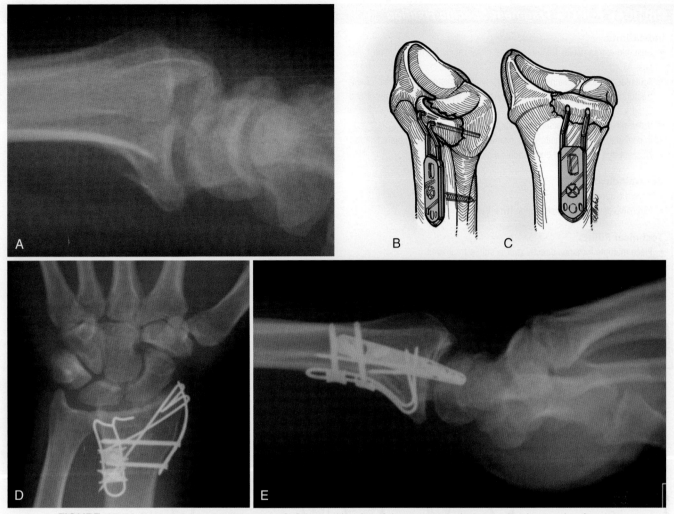

FIGURE 15.51 Fixation of the volar ulnar corner: **A,** Palmar subluxation of the carpus secondary to a volar ulnar teardrop fracture. **B, C,** A volar buttress pin is contoured to support the articular surface and can be placed immediately atop the palmar ridge of the radius and secured proximally beneath the pronator quadratus. **D, E,** Posteroanterior and lateral radiographs of the healed fracture at 1 year. (**B** and **C,** © Elizabeth Martin.)

surgery. Strengthening exercises are begun after radiographic evidence of fracture consolidation, generally at 6 to 8 weeks postoperatively.

Other Fixation Methods

Virtually all fractures of the distal radius can be managed with the previously detailed fixation strategies—namely, percutaneous/external, low-profile dorsal plate, angular stable volar plate, and fragment-specific. A surgeon versed in each of these techniques can apply them in isolation or in combination to effectively reduce a distal radius fracture and maintain fragment stability until healing. Conversely, failure to understand the indications and contraindications, or an inability to execute a difficult technique when necessary, can lead the surgeon to use an inappropriate application of a more familiar technique to a complicated fracture, with potential consequences of instability or loss of reduction.

On occasion, a highly comminuted distal radius fracture, if not amenable to complex periarticular reconstruction as detailed earlier or when associated with multiple extremity trauma, will need rapid, stable, and durable fixation to grossly restore radial alignment and length. In selected cases, the technique of distraction plating with an internal bridge plate, as initially described by Burke and Singer,[22] can provide highly satisfactory results. Hanel and colleagues recently published outcomes and complications of the treatment of 144 fractures in 140 patients treated with this technique over a 6-year period; the study demonstrated highly satisfactory results, with a 12.3% complication rate, for a very difficult injury cohort.[71]

Distraction Plating Technique. Incisions 4-cm long are centered over the long metacarpal and the dorsal–radial aspect of the radial midshaft, and a third 2-cm incision is done over the radiocarpal joint at the Lister tubercle.[56] A 3.5-mm low-contact compression plate that will span the fracture from the metacarpal shaft to a point at least three screw holes proximal to the most proximal fracture line is chosen. The plate is passed bluntly beneath the extensor tendons and across the fracture site to lie in the floor of the fourth dorsal compartment. To facilitate its passage, the EPL is freed from the retinaculum and an elevator is used to develop a plane below the fourth dorsal compartment tendons, through which the plate is tunneled proximally into the most proximal wound (Figure 15.52).

CRITICAL POINTS *Fragment-Specific Fixation*

Indications

- Unstable extraarticular fractures of the distal radius (Fernandez' type I; AO type A)
- Articular fractures, simple-to-complex, multifragmentary fractures, shear fractures, fracture–dislocations (the Fernandez types II–IV; AO types B and C, all subtypes)
- Volar–ulnar teardrop fracture with carpal subluxation
- In combination with percutaneous fixation or volar fixed-angle plate fixation
- Nascent and established distal radius malunion

Contraindications

- Severe osteoporosis
- Extensive diaphyseal comminution (type V)

Technical Points

- Place multiple incisions directly over unstable fragments.
- Make a volar–radial incision to the radial column, and split the brachioradialis.
- Elevate the pronator quadratus with a portion of the split BR as needed to expose the volar surface.
- Reduce the fracture with traction and direct manipulation of the fragment.
- Provide temporary fracture fixation with an oblique K-wire through the radial styloid.

- Expose the intermediate column fracture via dorsal, volar, or both approaches and reduce it.
- Elevate impacted articular fragments through a dorsal 3- to 4-cm incision under fluoroscopic guidance.
- Support impacted articular fragments with a graft or substitute.
- Choose a dorsal wireform, 2.4-mm plate, or a pin plate to secure the intermediate column.
- Complete fixation of the volar rim or teardrop as needed with a 2.4-mm fixed-angle implant or a volar buttress pin.
- Apply a radial columnar plate or radial pin plate along the reduced styloid and fix proximally with a minimum of 2 to 3 screws.
- Assess distal radioulnar stability manually and repair or use internal fixation as needed.

Postoperative Care

- Apply a sugar tong splint in supination for 10 to 12 days until suture removal.
- Begin digital range-of-motion exercises immediately.
- Begin forearm rotation and gentle active wrist motion exercises at the initial postoperative visit.
- Evaluate with radiographs at the initial postoperative visit and at 2 and 6 weeks postoperatively.

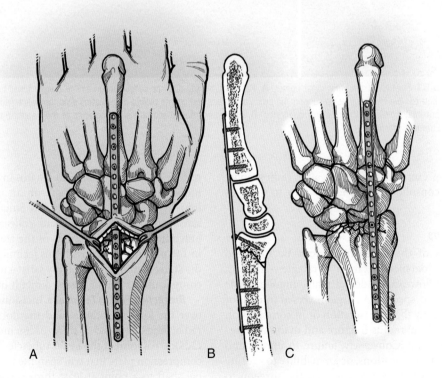

FIGURE 15.52 A, Distraction plating is performed through a limited dorsal incision with tunneling of the plate beneath the fourth dorsal compartment. Screws are placed proximally and distally to span the fracture site. **B,** Additional screw or wire fixation of the articular fragments may be performed through or outside the plate. **C,** Alternative positioning of a low-profile 2.4-mm plate below the second dorsal compartment and affixed to the index metacarpal. (© Elizabeth Martin.)

The plate is fixed to the third metacarpal with a single screw, ideally in the midshaft of it to enable fine-tuning of fracture reduction. The hand and forearm are supinated approximately 60 degrees to avoid fixing the fracture in pronation, and a provisional fracture-reduction clamp is applied to hold the plate to the radius proximally. The forearm is taken through a full range of rotation and gross alignment is assessed with fluoroscopy. Care needs to be taken to prevent excess radiocarpal or midcarpal distraction when setting the final position, and the author recommends a maximum radiocarpal gap of 5 mm. Proximal and distal fixation is finalized with a minimum of three bicortical screws.

Attention is directed to the radiocarpal joint, where articular congruency is restored by subchondral elevation of the impacted fracture fragments, generous subchondral support with allograft, and percutaneous fixation of the periarticular fragments with K-wires or screws (see Mini-Open Fixation earlier). It is helpful to place one screw through the plate and immediately beneath the subchondral bone of the intermediate column.

Contraindications to bone grafting include grade III open fractures, prior contamination, or insufficient soft tissue coverage. After assessing the radioulnar joint for stability and treating as necessary (see earlier), the wounds are closed and splint immobilization is applied. Within 3 days of surgery, the splint is removed (except in cases of radioulnar instability), and patients can begin forearm supination–pronation and digital range-of-motion exercises. A 5-lb weightlifting limit is advised. The percutaneous wires are generally removed at 6 weeks and the plate at 4 to 6 months when healing should be complete.

Hanel and colleagues recommend placement of a smaller, 2.7-mm stainless steel custom locking plate on the index metacarpal, beneath the second dorsal compartment tendons at the radiocarpal level and fixed to the dorsal radial surface of the midshaft of the radius beneath the tendons of the two radial wrist extensors (see Figure 15.52, C). This is a rapid and simple approach that minimizes interference with extensor tendon function postoperatively, and the internal position of the low-profile device allows it to be used for an extended period if necessary[71] (Figure 15.53).

Intramedullary Implants. Recently, novel intramedullary (IM) methods have been developed to achieve rapid restoration of radial length, alignment, and tilt; they are designated low-profile, minimal-incision alternatives to locked volar–dorsal plate, fragment-specific, or bridging external fixation. These techniques are indicated primarily for unstable, nonarticular, or simple articular fractures and combine the stability and early mobility of internal fixation with minimal additional surgical intervention of percutaneous fixation. The techniques are deficient in long-term outcome or prospective comparative data and are offered as alternative fixation methods for predominantly lower-energy injuries.

The first is an IM device that uses locked, diverging screws distally to support the articular surface and interlocking screws proximally to provide stability across the fracture. The implant is inserted percutaneously in a retrograde manner at the radial styloid "bare spot" between the first and second dorsal compartments. Care must be taken to prevent injury to branches of the radial sensory nerve during the procedure. In the setting of acute fractures, indications for this IM implant include unstable

extraarticular fractures, the reduction of which cannot be maintained by closed treatment (AO types A2 and A3), and simple articular fractures with large articular fragments that can be reduced percutaneously (AO types C1 and C2).

Other relative indications include AO type B fracture patterns (i.e., provided that the distal fragment can be captured with at least two screws), potentially unstable fractures in active patients who desire wrist motion during the healing period, and individuals requiring early return to work for whom cast immobilization is impractical. In a recent prospective study, 29 patients treated with IM fixation were followed for one year and were demonstrated to have excellent radiographic, clinical, and patient-rated outcomes; complications included two cases of lost reduction.[121] Complex articular fractures with multiple small articular fragments (AO type C3) are relative contraindications to fixation with this device (Figure 15.54).

A second IM device uses an expandable nitinol cage inserted into a prepared cavity within the metaphyseal flare of the radius, augmented by percutaneous fragment-specific cannulated screws that engage the rigid nitinol cage (Figure 15.55). The implant is inserted through a small diaphyseal incision proximal to the fracture, and the locking screws are inserted in a percutaneous or open approach through the radial styloid, dorsal, and volar–ulnar corner fragments (see Video 15.1). Biomechanical data support the stiffness of the device as being comparable to locked-plate fixation in axial bending and compression.[155] The device is novel in its low profile and high strength, intended for use in A-, B-, and C-type fractures, but there are no comparative clinical data at the time of this writing (see Case Study 15.3).

The Ulnar Column

The most frequent complaints of residual disability and functional loss following healed fractures of the distal radius emanate from the ulnar column. Therefore, it deserves as thorough an evaluation in the acute stage as the distal–radial fracture itself to address these injuries and prevent long-term dysfunction.

Some element of DRUJ involvement is present in every displaced distal radius fracture. The acute pathoanatomy of the ulnar column can be reduced to several discrete entities: articular incongruity (e.g., sigmoid notch, ulnar head), disruption of the TFCC, and changes in radioulnar alignment. Fernandez classified DRUJ injuries into a simple and useful three-group system that is helpful in defining treatment (see Figure 15.20, B). The key to a successful result depends on precise restoration of the anatomic relationships of the radius and the ulna; correction of articular incongruity at the sigmoid notch; identification of residual DRUJ instability through manual assessment; repair, or reconstruction as necessary; and maintenance of stability throughout the first 4 to 6 weeks after injury.

Ulnar Styloid Fixation

When fractured, realignment and fixation of the ulnar head, neck, or shaft may be necessary to restore the integrity and alignment of the ulnar column. There is considerable controversy, however, concerning the need to repair fractures of the ulnar styloid, including the so-called *basilar styloid (basistyloid) fracture.* It is of particular concern because of the attachment of the dorsal and volar radioulnar ligaments at its base (the fovea). A number of studies in the last decade have questioned

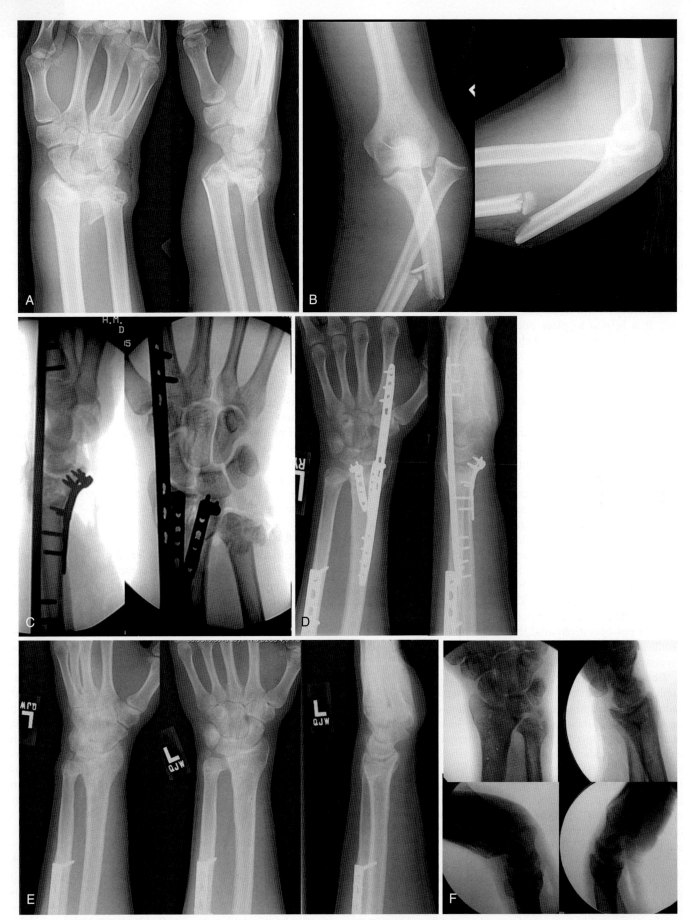

FIGURE 15.53 Bridge plate fixation: A 20-year-old man sustained life-threatening polytrauma in a fall from a height, including bilateral distal radius fractures (**A**) and a Monteggia fracture–dislocation on the left (**B**). **C,** The ulnar fracture was stabilized with a plate, the volar rim of the left radius was reconstructed with volar 2.5-mm implants, the impacted subchondral bone was elevated and supported with allograft cancellous bone, and the severely comminuted dorsal metaphyseal bone was stabilized with a spanning plate in the second dorsal compartment. **D,** Healed fracture at the time of removal of the spanning plate at 4 months postoperatively. **E,** The volar plates were removed at 1 year. **F,** Radiographs at 1 year demonstrating active range of motion. (Courtesy of Douglas P. Hanel, MD, University of Washington, Seattle.)

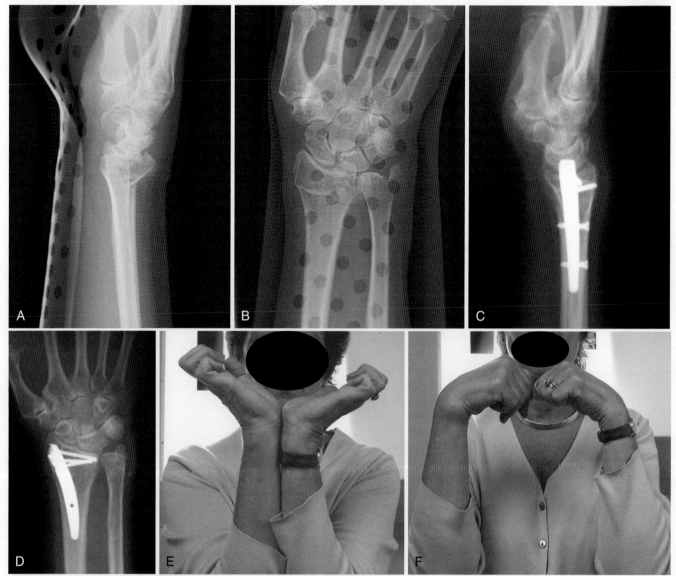

FIGURE 15.54 A, B, Posteroanterior and lateral radiograph of an intraarticular distal radius and ulnar styloid base fracture. **C, D,** A locked intramedullary nail (Micronail, Wright Medical, Arlington, TN) was used to stabilize the distal radius fracture, and suture fixation of the ulnar styloid was performed. **E, F,** Photos of range of motion 2 months postop; no immobilization was used postoperatively. (Courtesy of Virak Tan, MD, with permission.)

the importance of an ulnar styloid fracture to radioulnar stability. To summarize these findings, among operatively treated fractures without identifiable evidence of radioulnar instability, the presence or absence of an ulnar styloid fracture,[140] styloid fracture displacement,[148] or ulnar styloid nonunion[166] had no bearing on the radiographic or functional outcome of the distal radius fracture.

Even though underpowered, in the only prospective level II trial of nonrepaired ulnar styloid fractures, Kim et al demonstrated no influence of the size or displacement of ulnar styloid fractures on fracture outcome or on DRUJ stability as assessed manually.[89] However, it is important to note that all patients with intraoperative DRUJ stability in this study were treated with 4 weeks of long-arm casting. A study of the efficacy of internal fixation of the ulnar styloid for patients with manually identified DRUJ instability has not been performed.

The Coronal Shift (Radial Translation)

Anatomic reduction of the radius generally results in relocation of the ulnar head within the sigmoid notch, as occurs after reduction of Galeazzi-type fractures of the radial shaft. Recent attention has been given to the importance of anatomic reduction of the radius in the coronal plane to restore tension of the interosseous membrane and "seat" the ulna into the sigmoid notch (see Figures 15.12 and 15.41).[134,124] Investigators have identified the distal interosseous membrane (DIOM) and, in particular, the distal oblique bundle as the "major restraining structures" of dorsal and volar laxity of the distal radius relative to the ulnar head[161] when the TFCC is disrupted. The DIOM is tense in all positions of forearm rotation.[161] A recent anatomic study defined the ligament to insert distally and dorsally on the radius, coursing to insert palmar and proximal on the ulna, confirming its primary role in resisting dorsal translation of the

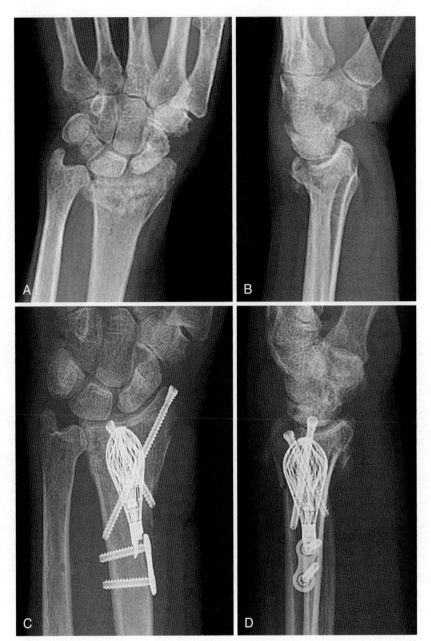

FIGURE 15.55 A-D, A novel intramedullary implant using an expandable nitinol cage and crossed locked screws (Conventus Orthopaedics, Maple Grove, MN) inserted percutaneously. Mechanical data demonstrate comparable rigidity to volar plate fixation.

radius on the ulna in supination.[118] As reviewed earlier, studies have demonstrated the lack of correlation between ununited or unrepaired basilar ulnar styloid fractures and DRUJ instability,[140,148] and this author and others[134] have noticed residual DRUJ instability despite isolated ulnar styloid repair when the anatomic spacing between the radius and ulna was not restored and the radius was translated radialward. Orbay noted that, when the DIOM is not torn, anatomic restoration of radial position in the coronal plane tensions the DIOM and stabilizes the radioulnar joint without need for TFCC reattachment.[124]

Nakamura and colleagues[119] demonstrated that radial translation, loss of radial inclination, ulnar shortening, and 4-mm radial translation of the ulnar styloid were all predictive of a foveal avulsion of the DRUJ ligaments; however, *radial translation was the only independent predictive variable.* Previously, this phenomenon had been referred to as ulnar transla-

tion of the proximal fragment[65,130]; by convention, it is probably more precise to describe position of the distal component of the fracture—that is, the articular fragment.[134] Failure to correct the coronal shift leads to laxity of the interosseous membrane, the pronator quadratus, and the distal interosseous membrane.[122,161]

Conversely, reduction of this deformity tensions the distal interosseous membrane and increases contact pressures by tensioning the surrounding soft tissue sleeve.[38,66,79,118,124] Dy et al, in a mechanical simulation of distal radius fractures in 10 cadaveric wrists, demonstrated that DRUJ instability was produced by a 2-mm coronal shift of the radius in forearms with an intact DOB.[38]

Reduction of the coronal shift is easily performed through any approach used for distal radius fracture fixation. Application of a radial reduction moment by a curved Hohmann retractor placed in the interosseous space on the ulnar metaphyseal flare, while counterpressure is applied on the radial styloid, will translate the fragment back to normal alignment (see Figure 15.41). Rapley et al described the insertion of an "Army-Navy" retractor in the interosseous space and rotating it 90 degrees until the radius and ulna were restored to their normal relationship.[130] Alternatively, a Gelpi retractor can be used to spread the radius and ulna apart until the proper tension is restored.

The deformity can also be corrected after preliminary application of a volar plate using the technique of Moritomo et al.[118] With the most proximal screw in place (but not fully tightened), several distal locked screws are applied to the distal fragment. A lion jaw clamp is applied between the ulnar cortex of the radius just proximal to the fracture site and the distal radial edge of the plate. Compression of the clamp reduces the distal fragment and seats it onto the ulnar head, restoring tension in the DIOM.

Distal Radioulnar Joint Injury Treatment Options

As outlined earlier in Figure 15.20, *B*, three treatment options are possible: (1) early mobilization, (2) closed treatment and cast immobilization with or without radioulnar pinning, and (3) operative management, including open and arthroscopic techniques.

To assess radioulnar stability following completion of radial fixation, a manual "shuck" test of the ulna is performed by grasping the ulnar head between the examiner's thumb and index finger and translating it dorsally and palmarly within the sigmoid notch. Gross instability is manifested by frank dislocation, but more subtle instability can be appreciated by the loss of a firm endpoint to translation and by increased subluxation of the ulna relative to the uninjured wrist. I find it helpful to have assessed the contralateral wrist's DRUJ stability before preparing and draping the injured wrist. It is important that the shuck test be performed in all rotation positions to specifically test both the palmar and the dorsal radioulnar ligaments (see DRUJ section).

For type I stable injuries, *functional aftercare* with early active forearm rotation exercises and minimal external support is recommended. Early motion is likewise recommended for patients with fractures of the distal ulna or ulnar styloid in which radioulnar stability has been restored with stable internal fixation, and for type III comminuted fractures of the ulnar head that are not amenable to internal fixation to allow fracture remodeling.

Type II subluxation can be treated successfully in a number of ways. Many prefer 4 weeks of cast immobilization with the forearm in the most stable rotation position; most often this is partial to complete supination.[153] Grossly unstable DRUJ dislocations may require percutaneous transfixion of the ulna to the radial shaft in the position of greatest stability with dual 0.062-in K-wires. The wires are placed just proximal to the joint, and it is helpful to leave their tips protruding through both the radial and ulnar cortices in the unlikely event that wire breakage occurs in the interosseous space. The wires may be removed at 4 weeks postoperatively and rotation exercises begun (Figure 15.56).

For type II *unstable* DRUJ lesions with a large ulnar basistyloid fragment, fracture fixation should be considered. The styloid is exposed with a 3- to 4-cm incision midway between the extensor carpi ulnaris (ECU) and the flexor carpi ulnaris (FCU). Care is taken to identify and preserve the dorsal sensory branch of the ulnar nerve, which courses through the ulnar "snuffbox" just distal to the styloid tip. A 24-gauge wire or nonabsorbable suture can be passed either around or preferably through the styloid fragment and then through the ulna at the axilla of the shaft and the articular surface. The suture/wire is tensioned and tied with the forearm in neutral rotation. Alternatively, the fragment can be stabilized with two 0.035-in K-wires and a tension band wire passed proximally through the ulnar shaft. The forearm is immobilized in neutral rotation for 4 to 6 weeks, depending on the degree of stability attained.

Large fracture fragments also can be fixed with a compression screw or a cannulated headless screw. With the advent of ultrathin pin plates, basilar styloid fractures can be rigidly fixed with two K-wires and an ulnar pin plate contoured to the ulnar shaft (Figure 15.57). The stability of the DRUJ is then assessed manually again; if stable, gentle forearm rotation can be initiated within 7 to 10 days of surgery. Implants on the ulnar side of the wrist can, on occasion, cause irritation (of the ECU tendon) and discomfort when patients rest their hands on a tabletop; consequently, ulnar styloid hardware may need to be removed in 10 to 20% of patients.

For patients who have residual manual DRUJ instability in all rotation positions following anatomic reduction of the distal radius and without a basistyloid fracture, open or arthroscopic reattachment of the foveal attachment of the distal radioulnar ligaments may be considered (see Chapter 14). Repairs must be protected by cast immobilization in the position of maximum stability in an above-elbow cast for 4 to 8 weeks to allow the TFCC to heal.

When type III DRUJ instability is associated with a dorsally displaced dorsal–ulnar fragment of the sigmoid notch or a displaced ulnar head fracture, precise anatomic reduction and fixation are imperative to restore stability. Associated TFCC lesions should be addressed simultaneously as described previously.

❖ AUTHOR'S PREFERRED METHOD OF TREATMENT: Ulnar Column Instability

Anatomic restoration of length, inclination, tilt, and coronal alignment of the fractured radius is performed with internal or percutaneous fixation at the surgeon's discretion. Unstable fractures of the dorsal and volar margins of the sigmoid notch are rigidly stabilized because unstable fragments have been demonstrated to mechanically lead to radioulnar subluxation.[28] Neck or head fractures of the ulna are anatomically reduced and fixed with 2.4-mm or 2.7-mm plates, interfragmentary screws, cerclage wiring, or a tension band, depending on the nature of the fracture and the degree of comminution.

Residual instability of the DRUJ, as determined by a dorsal and volar shuck test in neutral, pronation, and supination, is treated aggressively. If a basilar styloid fracture is present, I prefer open reduction and fixation followed by early range of motion (see Figure 15.57). If no fracture is present and stability can be restored in full or partial supination, simple immobilization in a sugar tong splint is performed in the operating room and converted to a long-arm cast at 10 days. The cast is removed 4 weeks postoperatively and supination–pronation exercises begun. If stability cannot be restored with positioning,

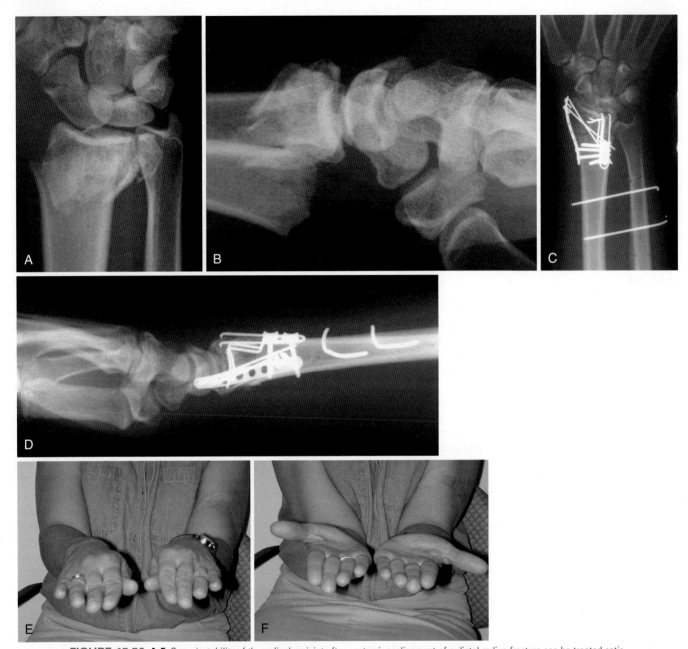

FIGURE 15.56 A-F, Gross instability of the radioulnar joint after anatomic realignment of a distal radius fracture can be treated satisfactorily with 4 weeks of cross-pinning of the ulnar and the radius. Dual 0.062-in Kirschner wires are recommended, and perforation of all four cortices is important.

augmentation with parallel 0.062-in transfixion wires is performed and maintained for 4 weeks (see Figure 15.56). I have not found open or arthroscopic repair of the TFCC to add appreciably to this algorithm.

EVIDENCE-BASED DECISION MAKING

Is there sufficient "evidence" in the literature in the form of randomized, prospective clinical trials to derive individual treatment decisions for distal radius fractures? Outcomes of treatment for such fractures have been the subject of several large Cochrane metaanalyses performed by Handoll and colleagues over the last decade.[67–69] Not surprisingly, the heterogeneity of the injuries, variations in reporting outcomes, and

differences in operative techniques and patient populations have made the extrapolation of any firm conclusions difficult. These authors made a plea for future investigators to use a common classification system and standardized validated outcome measurements so that data for distal radius fractures can be compared and contrasted.

A plethora of randomized studies have been performed since the Handoll et al attempt to identify a "best" treatment for distal radius fractures based on 1- and 2-year outcomes. The 2008 Cochrane review demonstrated that there was insufficient evidence to support the use of one mode of treatment over another for distal radius fractures.[68] The American Academy of Orthopedic Surgeons (AAOS) subsequently convened three expert panels to examine the best-available evidence and to develop

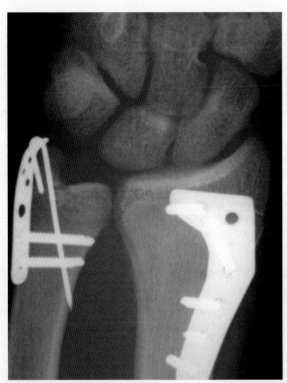

FIGURE 15.57 A 2.0-mm ulnar pin plate can be applied over a percutaneous Kirschner wire to rigidly fix unstable basilar ulnar styloid fractures with two proximal screws.

TABLE 15.3   Summary of Available Evidence

I.	Nondisplaced fractures, no reduction required	• Dorsal splint leads to improved motion and strength vs. short-arm cast[123]
II.	Nonoperative treatment, closed reduction, simple articular, healthy bone	• Sugar tong, short-arm cast, three-point brace: NMD[17,154]
III.	Loss of reduction in cast	• Operative treatment leads to improved radiographic alignment vs. another reduction and cast[112]
IV.	Simple bending (AO A) or simple articular (AO C1) fractures in healthy bone; anatomically reduced and maintained	• Casting, percutaneous fixation or ORIF: NMD[62,96,106,176]
V.	*Unstable* bending and articular fractures in healthy bone	• External fixation improvement over cast treatment[86,96] • Augmented external fixation vs. percutaneous pin fixation: NMD[72] • Nonbridging external fixation improved radiographic parameters over bridging EF[8,75] • Subtle early[40,42,109,137] and sustained[45,159,168] improvements of volar locked-plate vs. percutaneous fixation
VI.	Highly comminuted fractures	• No available evidence

EF, External fixation; *NMD,* no measureable difference; *ORIF,* open reduction internal fixation.

"appropriate use criteria" for treatment of distal radius fractures by voting on 240 different clinical scenarios.[164] Even though the panel was unable to identify "evidence-based conclusion[s] for the optimal operative treatment of distal radius fractures," the exhaustive report is a valuable resource that summarizes the conclusions of the many level II operative trials performed over the past two decades, along with consensus opinions of appropriate treatment.

A comparison of the randomized trials done during the past 8 years versus those done in the preceding decade reveals clear advances in the reporting of outcomes for distal radius fractures; specifically, the use of validated patient-rated functional outcome tools such as the DASH, quick-DASH, patient-rated wrist evaluation (PRWE), and Michigan Hand Outcomes Questionnaire (MHQ). By most modern functional outcome criteria, percutaneous fixation and open reduction with internal fixation led to similar outcomes for unstable distal radius fractures in several level II randomized trials,[62,87,137] calling into question the benefit of the increased cost of internal fixation.[40] Yet, several short studies in the literature argue against the immediate adoption of a treatment parity.

No standards for measurement of outcomes for distal radius fracture treatment have been universally adopted, making comparison of various series results difficult if not impossible.[59] Remarkably, pain is not consistently assessed as an outcome parameter in randomized trials of distal radius fracture treatment. In one study, only 37% of the variability of the patient assessments using the MHQ could be explained by measurable outcomes of wrist motion or grip strength.[144]

Another study demonstrated that it was only by inclusion of a pain-assessment visual analog scale (VAS), along with "objective" measurement of supination and grip strength, that the investigators could account for more than half of the variability of the DASH.[151] Perception of pain and, specifically, the *interference of pain on function* and activities, was the most significant predictor of patient-assessed arm disability as measured by quick-DASH scores in a third study.[116] Finally, no measures of activity level have been used to stratify distal radius fracture patients, despite the increasing use of activity level as an outcome measure in other orthopedic fields (e.g., hip, knee, shoulder, ankle).[21]

These data suggest that a battery of patient-rated and physician-rated outcome measures are critical to a complete assessment of outcomes. Comparisons across academic centers, states, countries, and continents could be facilitated by the use of accepted patient-rated functional scales, the VAS pain assessment, activity level and health stratification, physician-rated outcome parameters, complication analysis, and the return to activities or "life roles."[59]

With all its inherent limitations, what practical treatment recommendations can be assembled from the evidence? A concise summary of evidence-based recommendations is presented in Table 15.3, and the reader is referred to the complete AAOS report for an inclusive analysis of the available evidence.[164]

It is difficult to distill firm treatment recommendations from current "evidence" given the specific exclusion criteria of each study. All would agree that the restoration of pain-free hand and wrist function is the overarching goal of treatment for distal radius fractures. In studies where more patients are excluded than included,[42,137,169] and weighted heavily toward relatively noncomminuted dorsally displaced fractures,[87,109] the evidence supports intuition; for straightforward fractures, several fixation types are essentially interchangeable and will result in nearly equal outcomes at "some remote period [of time]."

Decisions must be made in part by the patient and in part by the surgeon's expertise and preference, and customized based on the patient's systemic factors and activity level. Patient preference for an internal implant rather than an external device because of the perceived benefit of early wrist motion and the avoidance of pin care and pin-tract infections may sway individual surgical decisions in favor of open reduction. However, bridging and nonbridging external-fixation techniques continue to demonstrate excellent outcomes in properly selected cases and should not be abandoned.

Treatment of the Elderly

Remarkable interest has been focused on the treatment of distal radius fractures in older individuals over the past 5 years, perhaps in part due to the recent focus on cost containment in medical care. Several prospective studies demonstrate a lack of significant functional outcome differences among elderly patients, and imply that treatment options for unstable distal radius fractures in this cohort are interchangeable.[1,6,41,57,173] However, several consistent findings of these studies, as well as notable shortcomings, should prompt considerable caution when interpreting the data.

The elderly cohort as a group takes longer to return of functional status,[26] has lower DASH functional scores, and has an inferior global health-related quality of life than their younger counterparts[2]; thus, the lack of differences within this group may be related to nonorthopedic factors. Conventional wisdom ascribes the lack of differences to the older cohort's "low functional demands."[1,175] In fact, up to 30% of US elderly patients describe themselves as "very active" and nearly 90% report no disability at all.[81] Notably, no study stratifies outcomes by activity level in the senior population; in actuality, only one validated elderly activity stratification exists.[160] To date, no prospective studies have utilized the physical activity scale for the elderly (PASE) to differentiate patients.

The AAOS appropriate use panel concluded that firm conclusions for distal radius fracture treatment in the elderly were confounded by the lack of studies that "distinguished patients based on infirmity, *functional demands*, bone quality, or energy of injury."[164] While Grewal et al identified no significant risk relationship between fracture alignment and outcome in their entire older cohort, their relative risk data suggest that their *active* elderly patients achieved better outcomes when the parameters of radial reduction were met.[61] It has been demonstrated that demented or infirm patients receive no benefit from anatomic reduction.[14]

Differences in perceived physiologic and actual age must be identified and considered when treating elderly patients.[2] Because malunion of the distal radius is associated with worse outcomes in women whose age is older than 55[18]; in all age cohorts,[51,61] patients with higher activity levels prior to injury will be disproportionately impaired. Second, in virtually all studies, early improvements in functional outcomes were noted in the operative cohorts; the importance of a 5-week earlier removal of immobilization and a 4-week earlier return to activities may be difficult to quantify; however, it is likely to be very important to a subset of active elderly individuals, especially those who live alone.

Shauver et al performed a cost–utility analysis with a group of seniors and identified a preference for internal fixation over other types of distal radius fracture treatments because of its more rapid return of function and a demonstrable improvement in quality-adjusted life years.[145] Although not consistently counted as a complication, the effect of a *100% loss of reduction* and deformity in the nonoperative cohort cannot be estimated using current functional scales.[6] Finally, the impact of a significant increase in arthritis[6,41] at *1 year* cannot be estimated for patients' future lifetime. Before we adopt a nihilistic approach to treatment of elderly patients and respond with more "cost-effective" solutions, further long-term studies need be performed.

❖ AUTHOR'S PREFERRED METHOD OF TREATMENT: The Elderly

Even though restoration of mobility, lack of pain, and return of function is the universal goal of treatment for the elderly, consideration must be given to the physiologic age and functional activity level so as to provide customized care. For the relatively inactive or sedentary patient, a treatment combining minimal morbidity with emphasis on maintenance of digital and forearm mobility is preferable; nonsurgical treatment is likely to result in very acceptable outcomes despite imperfect radiographic outcomes, and deficits in grip strength and range of motion are likely to be well tolerated.

For the highly active patients who place high functional demands on the wrist, deformity, pain, and loss of strength are not likely to be compatible with their lifestyle. In these individuals, efforts should be made to restore articular congruency, radial alignment, and a normal radioulnar relationship. Although several methods can achieve these goals, active elderly patients are quite conscious of quality of life and prefer a treatment that will return them to normal function earlier with minimal risk of complications.[145] Percutaneous methods have an increased risk of pin-tract infection and loss of reduction in osteopenic bone, while internal fixation has been noted to increase the risk of nerve or tendon complications.

My preference for the active elderly group is stable internal fixation with a fixed-angle volar plate, adding or substituting columnar fixation in the more comminuted or unstable fractures as needed. For those patients in the intermediate activity group, a customized decision is made after careful discussion with the patients, based on their needs, expectations, systemic issues, and fracture type. Those who prefer an earlier return to function may opt for internal fixation, with the assumption of additional risk and the knowledge that the long-term outcome may not be measurably different with any type of treatment.

❖ AUTHOR'S PREFERRED METHOD OF TREATMENT: A Case-Based Approach to Operative Management

…[It] is neither the fixation nor the implant [that] dictates the outcome but the ability of the surgeon to meet the goal of satisfactory reduction and vascular preservation with the least invasive procedure possible.

—Kreder et al, 2006

It is no surprise that randomized trials fail to show convincing evidence of the superiority of one treatment technique over another for the entire spectrum of distal radius fractures. The variety and complexity of fracture patterns, associated injuries to the distal radioulnar and intercarpal ligaments, and widely divergent patient factors (e.g., osteoporosis, activity level, systemic illness) mitigate against a single treatment modality for all types of injuries. Instead, a treatment strategy must be developed to customize the treatment to the injury, with the overarching principle that the least additional surgical disruption of the soft tissue sleeve that is necessary to gain fracture stability and articular congruency will generally impart the best functional outcome.

To paraphrase Lee Trevino, "It's the archer, not the arrow." Although the literature is replete with a bewildering array of techniques and implants, it is important to understand that it is the judgment and skill of the surgeon in reaching the operative goals that will be the most important determinant of success. The goals of operative treatment (i.e., ARMS) are the following:

1. **A**rticular congruity (to prevent shear on articular cartilage and degenerative changes)
2. **R**adial alignment and length (to enable normal kinetics and kinematics of the carpus and radioulnar joint)
3. **M**otion (of digits, wrist, and forearm to optimize return to function and activities)
4. **S**tability (to preserve length, alignment, and congruency until the fracture heals)

My approach is built around three fundamentally different categories of fixation that, when matched to the particular fracture pattern, enable the surgeon to plan and execute successful wrist fracture repair for nearly all of its variations:

- Percutaneous/indirect fixation
- Fragment-specific fixation
- Volar or dorsal fixed-angle plating

For treatment purposes, I present an algorithm based on the Fernandez mechanism–based classification of distal radius fractures. Treatment recommendations are based on fractures in a physiologically young and active patient cohort; treatment can be tempered according to the patient's age, activity level, functional impairments, and general medical condition.

Treatment of Nondisplaced Distal Radius Fractures

For all injuries, the patient's history and physical examination should include age, handedness, occupation, aerobic activity level, sports and leisure activities, an extensive medical record, and a list of medications. Particular attention must be paid to conditions that might affect bone mass or bone quality, including endocrine disorders, inflammatory diseases, renal disease, steroid use, and other factors. The wrist should be inspected for wounds and tendon and nerve function, paying special attention to function of the median nerve.

Nondisplaced distal radius fractures in the physiologically young and active cohort can be treated with either a splint or short-arm cast at the surgeon's discretion while leaving the elbow, fingers, and thumb free to avoid stiffness. Patients should be advised of the possibility of an EPL rupture that, although rare, can complicate treatment of nondisplaced fractures. Interval radiographs are not generally necessary for truly nondisplaced fractures; a single follow-up examination with radio-

graphs to determine union at 6 weeks is recommended.[136] Closer scrutiny should be given to elderly and osteoporotic patients as well as to any person's fracture that has an intraarticular component.

Type I—Bending Fractures

The prime determinant in dorsally displaced, nonarticular bending (Colles') fractures is the predicted stability of the fracture (see earlier). In younger patients with minimal comminution of the dorsal cortex and less than a 3-mm loss of radial length, an adequate closed reduction will be predictably quite stable. For active patients with a stable fracture type and excellent reduction, I prefer a sugar tong splint, which permits acute swelling for the first 2 to 3 weeks; then switch to a short-arm cast for 3 weeks until the fracture is healed both clinically and radiographically. Radiographs should be taken at 1, 2, or 3, and 6 weeks to ensure maintenance of the reduction.

A simple removable splint may be needed for comfort and support for an additional 2 weeks after cast removal. By providing patients with a removable splint that they can wean themselves from as they regain wrist motion and upper extremity confidence, much of their anxiety about possible reinjury is relieved and their rehabilitation process is shortened.

Minimizing Hand and Shoulder Stiffness

During the period of immobilization and weaning from the splint, all patients are instructed to keep their fingers, elbow, forearm, and shoulder mobile. The six-pack of hand exercises is illustrated earlier in Figure 15.26. Passive and active shoulder, elbow, and forearm motion should also be addressed as priorities as soon as the injury's pain subsides and specific immobilization requirements permit. In general, motion should be encouraged at least three times a day. Some patients benefit from supervised therapy, as well as a home program under the guidance of a hand therapist.

Unstable dorsal bending fractures are suspected in patients with comminution of greater than 50% of the lateral width of the radial diaphysis at the fracture site and initial radial shortening of greater than 3 mm. As MacKenney, Lafontaine, and others have demonstrated, advancing age is the most important predictor of instability, and a patient older than 60 years should be considered unstable when these two factors are present.[100,107]

Volar extraarticular bending fractures are decidedly less common than their dorsal counterparts and usually involve comminution of the important stout metaphyseal flare; consequently, these fractures are implicitly unstable and generally require operative stabilization. Patient education is extremely important for this group of injuries because she or he is likely to want to take an active role in the treatment decision. In healthy and active individuals, regardless of age, the patient should be counseled concerning the nature of the injury, its inherent instability, and the additional treatment time that may be required should the fracture demonstrate late instability and collapse in a cast.

If the patient elects nonoperative treatment, close observation of unstable fractures with weekly visits is necessary for the first 3 to 4 weeks, along with cast changes as necessary to maintain optimal three-point fixation. The surgeon should be vigilant for early signs of collapse and avoid the "slippery slope" of accepting a few degrees of additional dorsal tilt or loss of radial length on successive radiographs (see Case Study 15.4). The patient should be attuned to the potential need for relatively urgent operative intervention if the fracture collapses because a second attempt at closed reduction and casting is ineffective.[112] The author is not as aggressive in the treatment of unstable extraarticular fractures in elderly, sedentary patients because of the mitigating effect of advanced age (≥80 years) on hand dysfunction.[51]

Because the articular surface is intact, this group of injuries enjoys a high rate of functional return and patient satisfaction after several types of treatments, provided that anatomic indices of reduction are reasonably restored. Treatment possibilities include, but are not limited to, closed reduction and pinning, augmented bridging external fixation, nonbridging external fixation, low-profile columnar fixation, IM fixation, and volar locked plating (see Case Study 15.5). The surgeon should discuss the limitations and advantages of various techniques with the patient and tailor treatment to his or her preference and individual needs; each of these fixation techniques is used with some frequency. If a sizable metaphyseal bone void is anticipated because of the extremes of dorsal displacement or osteoporosis, the balance is tipped in favor of volar locked plating (see Case Study 15.6), augmented by bone graft or a substitute if necessary.

Similarly, if the fracture is several weeks old and a realignment of a "nascent" malunion is anticipated, volar locked plating is the preferred treatment (see Case Studies 15.7 and 15.8). For elderly and active patients who need or request operative fixation, especially those with decreased bone mass, the increased rigidity of volar locked-plate fixation is preferable. More and more frequently, active patients express the desire to avoid a 6-week period of casting when presented with a viable alternative; likewise, when given an option, most patients in the urban setting in which this author practices choose internal-fixation over external-fixation devices because of ease of care and avoidance of pin care. After surgery, immobilizing patients in a sugar tong splint in supination is necessary for 7 to 10 days and begin range of motion of the digits and shoulder immediately. Wrist and forearm motion is begun in a removable splint at the time of dressing change, and return to activity is initiated at 6 to 8 weeks, as permitted by radiographic evidence of healing.

Algorithm for Management of Articular Distal Radius Fractures

Type II—Shear Fractures

The basic feature common to *shearing marginal fractures of the joint surface* is that a portion of the metaphysis of the distal radius is intact and in continuity with the unaffected area of the joint surface. These fractures are inherently unstable because of the high deforming forces, and they fare poorly with nonoperative treatment. The ultimate prognosis of these fractures is generally good because the displaced articular fragment or fragments can be precisely reduced and solidly fixed to the intact radius. Furthermore, fractures with a distinct shearing component usually occur in young adults, whose firm cancellous bone offers ideal holding power for internal fixation.

Volarly displaced shear fractures (AO type C2) are not generally amenable to percutaneous fixation because of gross instability, the strong deforming forces of the flexor tendons, and the vulnerability of major nerves and vessels to percutaneous implant insertion. The obliquity of the fracture line and loss of palmar support of the carpus make these fractures inherently unstable. Shortening and palmar displacement of the fragment are always associated with volar subluxation of the carpus. This fracture may affect only the most radial aspect of the palmar articular surface, or it may extend ulnarly into the sigmoid notch. Depending on the quality of the bone and the severity of the impact, a variable amount of comminution of the volar fragment may be present.

Particular attention must be given to rule out the presence of a separate volar–ulnar or teardrop fragment (see earlier); its presence demands that the implant or implants rigidly capture and maintain reduction of this fragment to prevent postoperative carpal subluxation (see Figure 15.48 and Case Study 15.9). An increase in the AP distance on the lateral film (see earlier) suggests that a sagittal split in the articular surface is present and is of concern for a lunate facet or teardrop fragment. If there is any question about whether a separate lunate facet fragment is present, getting a CT scan is indicated.

For volarly displaced shear fractures with a single fragment, a volar fixed-angle plate is preferable, although a traditional 3.5-mm volar buttress plate or low-profile plate fixation is also appropriate (see Case Study 15.10). The standard FCR approach is performed, and provisional fixation of the fragment with one or more 0.062-in K-wires is helpful to maintain reduction before the application of a permanent fixation (see earlier). For injuries with a separate teardrop fragment, the author prefers fixing this lunate facet fragment with a volar buttress pin placed through a volar FCU approach (see earlier), followed by support of the radial column fragment with a 2.0-mm plate.

I am not impressed by the ability of most volar plates to adequately capture a small lunate facet teardrop fragment (see Figure 15.48), and advancement of the plate distally to cover the volar rim is not recommended because of concern for flexor tendon rupture (see Figure 15.42 and Figure 15.58).[33] In the event of primary median nerve signs and symptoms associated with a volar shear fracture, it is preferable to release the carpal tunnel through a separate 3-cm incision in the palm. Extension of the volar–radial approach into the palm risks injury to the palmar cutaneous branch of the median nerve.

A sugar tong splint in supination is worn for 7 to 10 days, followed by a removable wrist splint for 4 to 5 weeks until healing is complete. The patient is encouraged to use the hand for activities of daily living, but heavy manual work or sports are not allowed for 5 to 6 weeks after surgery, at which time the fracture should be healed.

Isolated dorsal shearing fractures (i.e., *dorsal Barton fractures*) are rare. As a group, dorsal marginal shear fractures represent less than 2% of all distal radius fractures and share the defining characteristic of (1) a fracture of the dorsal articular rim and (2) dorsal radiocarpal subluxation. This is a high-energy injury that occurs in a predominantly young male cohort. The injury is characterized by an intact volar metaphyseal rim in most cases.

Lozano-Calderón and colleagues identified four discrete subtypes of shearing fractures based on the degree of articular surface involvement (Figure 15.59).[104] The least common subtype is characterized by extension of the fracture line across the volar cortex with a relatively large and dorsally rotated volar lip component and no appreciable articular impaction. Fractures of this subtype often can be indirectly reduced and stabilized using a volar approach and a fixed-angle plate. For the remainder of these fractures, however, adequate articular disimpaction and support cannot be achieved without direct visualization, carpal reduction, and stabilization through a dorsal or combined approach.

I prefer to approach these fractures through dual incisions: a volar–radial columnar approach and a universal dorsal approach through the third extensor compartment. First, the radial styloid fragment is carefully reduced through the radial column incision, checked for proper realignment at the metaphyseal level, and pinned provisionally to the proximal–radial shaft with an oblique 0.45-in K-wire. Then, the dorsal rim fragment is reduced against the scaphoid and lunate, and dorsal subluxation of the carpus is corrected. The fragments are provisionally pinned, and articular congruity is confirmed with fluoroscopy.

Depending on the extent of metaphyseal comminution, an autogenous bone graft or a structural bone graft substitute (see earlier) may be required to support the reduced articular surface (see Figure 15.35, *B*). The dorsal rim fragment can then be secured to the intact radius with a dorsal wireform—typically a dorsal buttress pin or small-fragment buttress pin combination (Figure 15.60). As an alternative, use of 2.0- to 2.4-mm fixed-angle dorsal plates may provide sufficient stability to obviate the need for a structural bone graft.[104] A 3- or 5-hole radial column pin plate or a 2.4-mm fixed-angle radial column plate is then applied directly on the radial column to maintain reduction of the styloid fragment; this should also provide the increased mechanical stability of orthogonal fixation, with the implants placed in two planes at least 50 to 70 degrees apart (see Figure 15.60).[10,77] Fixation should be sufficiently stable to begin wrist and forearm range-of-motion exercises after removal of the sutures and the postoperative splint at 7 to 10 days.

Shear fractures of the radial styloid (chauffeur's fracture) are not uncommon and can be associated with intercarpal bony and soft tissue injuries. Scaphoid fractures and perilunate injuries, ranging from partial or complete scapholunate ligament disruption to lunate dislocation, on occasion may be associated with this injury (Figure 15.61, *A*). If the radial styloid fragment shows substantial proximal and radial displacement and the fracture line enters the joint at the level of the interfacet ridge between the scaphoid and lunate fossae, there is a distinct possibility of disruption of the scapholunate ligament. The scaphoid displaces proximally with the radial fragment, whereas the

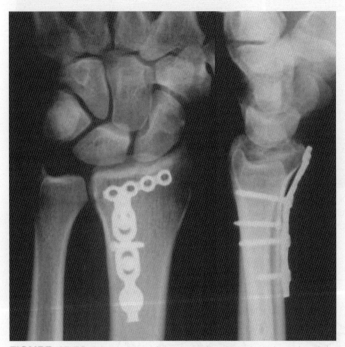

FIGURE 15.58 Advancement of a palmar plate onto the palmar rim of the radius should be avoided because there is no soft tissue buffer between the plate and the overlying flexor tendons.

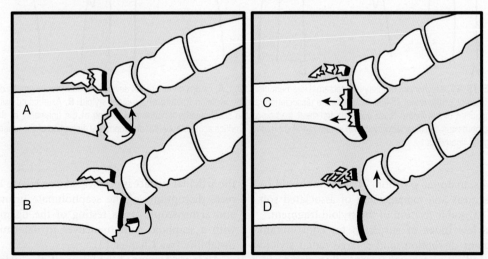

FIGURE 15.59 Four discrete types of dorsal shear fractures have been described by Lozano-Calderón and colleagues.[104] **A,** A relatively common variant has a large rotated volar fracture fragment that constitutes the majority of the articular surface. **B,** The most common subtype demonstrates a small volar lip (teardrop) fragment, from which the important short and long radiolunate ligaments originate. **C,** The central impaction pattern, associated with the shear fracture of the dorsal margin, is relatively uncommon, as is the true radiocarpal fracture–dislocation **(D),** which constitutes a serious combined ligamentous and bony injury. (© Elizabeth Martin.)

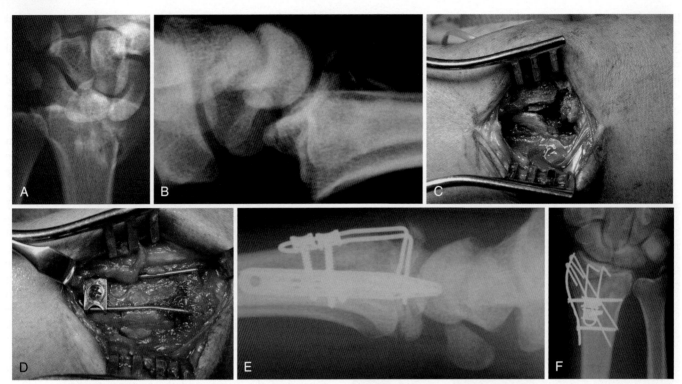

FIGURE 15.60 Type A dorsal shear fracture: **A, B,** Posteroanterior and lateral radiographs demonstrating shear of the entire articular surface with little attached subchondral bone. **C,** Dorsal view of the highly comminuted dorsal surface after closed reduction. **D,** Fixation of the thin dorsal rim and articular surface fragment with a dorsal wireform implant. **E, F,** Postoperative radiographs demonstrating restitution of articular alignment and length.

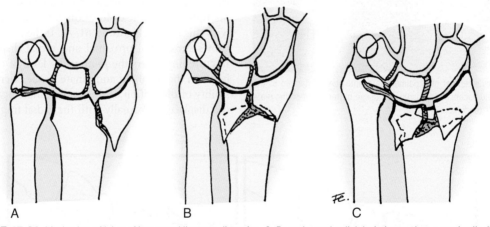

FIGURE 15.61 Mechanism of injury of intercarpal ligament disruption: **A,** Extension and radial deviation produce a proximally displaced shearing fracture of the radial styloid, scapholunate dissociation, and an avulsion fracture of the ulnar styloid. **B,** Axial compression with severe impaction of the lunate fossa accounts for shear loading of the scapholunate junction and tearing of the ligaments at this level. **C,** Axial compression and ulnar deviation with severe radial shortening produce acute ulnocarpal abutment and disruption of the lunotriquetral and triangular ligaments.

lunate remains in its anatomic position. Treatment should be directed at (1) diagnosis and management of associated soft tissue injuries and (2) stable fixation of the styloid fragment.

I recommend a low index of suspicion for concomitant scapholunate ligament disruption, and a large radial styloid fracture is a prime indication for arthroscopically assisted percutaneous reduction and fixation (see earlier).[52,171] In this procedure, irrigation of the articular hematoma, direct inspection of the scapholunate ligament from both the radiocarpal and midcarpal portals, and arthroscopic–fluoroscopic reduction of

the articular surface is performed (see Figure 15.36). For incomplete disruptions of the scapholunate ligament, fluoroscopic and arthroscopic stress testing of the ligament is performed with a scaphoid shift maneuver to determine the degree of instability (see Chapter 13).

After assessment of the ligament, the cartilage-bearing fragment is manipulated with an awl or a periosteal elevator through a small skin incision under fluoroscopic and arthroscopic guidance, with a minimum of soft tissue dissection. Most of these cases can be stabilized with percutaneously inserted implants (e.g., cannulated screws, K-wires, external fixation, bridging or nonbridging, or any combination of these) provided there is good bone quality (Figure 15.62). Care should be taken to protect the superficial radial nerve, the radial artery, and the extensor tendons at the anatomic snuffbox level. For larger or more unstable fragments, I prefer the rigidity of a radial column plate applied through a 3- to 4-cm volar–radial approach (see earlier) (see Case Study 15.2). A bone graft or bone graft substitute may be required if there is a subchondral–metaphyseal void after fragment reduction.

I repair *complete* ruptures of the dorsal component of the scapholunate ligament through a limited dorsal approach that involves the use of a bone anchor in the scaphoid and a double row of sutures.[84] Although there are limited data available, it is best to immobilize the reduced scapholunate joint with a temporary cannulated screw inserted just distal to the radial styloid. The advantage of a temporary screw over wires is that it may be left in place while radiocarpal wrist motion is initiated.

For incomplete tears with fluoroscopic or arthroscopic evidence of scapholunate instability during a scaphoid shift examination (e.g., Geissler grade 2), I perform percutaneous temporary pin or screw fixation without open ligament repair. If radial styloid fixation alone is performed, wrist and forearm range-of-motion exercise is begun at the first postoperative dressing change. If the scapholunate ligament was repaired and fixed with pins or a temporary screw, gentle wrist range of motion is begun 6 to 8 weeks postoperatively, and the screw is removed 4 months after surgery.

Type III—Joint Surface Compression Fractures

Compression fractures have a variety of configurations, but all variants share comminution of the articular surface of the intermediate column,[77,133] the so-called die-punch fracture (see Figure 15.16, *B*).[115] These fractures occur most commonly in young and active individuals, so accurate reduction and maintenance of reduction are essential for an optimal outcome. Critical to their treatment is a thorough understanding of the fracture anatomy, and I recommend the fragment-specific classification (see Figure 15.18) to identify critical fracture components and guide treatment options. The surgeon should have a low threshold for advanced imaging studies (i.e., CT with or without three-dimensional reconstruction) of these challenging injuries to better understand the fracture anatomy and plan the operative approaches.

Intermediate Column Single-Fragment Fractures. If an intermediate column fracture is characterized by a simple nondisplaced or minimally displaced articular fragment (and is without significant metaphyseal comminution), closed reduction and cast application may be all that is necessary. In many cases, however, the higher energy of this fracture group displaces the intermediate column fragment, so operative reduction and stabilization are required. Joint distraction with horizontal finger-trap traction is not generally capable of disimpaction and realignment of small cartilage-bearing fragments, nor can it accomplish reduction of rotated volar lip and dorsal–ulnar corner fragments.

Isolated and displaced fractures of the dorsal or volar–ulnar corner are rare, but they are potentially serious injuries (see Case Study 15.11). It is important to recognize these fractures and treat them aggressively to avoid late subluxation of the carpus. More commonly, the combination of a *radial column or dorsal-bending fracture and a dorsal or volar intermediate column fragment* is seen. They may be misdiagnosed as Colles' fractures because the small (but critically important) ulnar corner fragment may be overlooked. An unreduced intermediate column fragment can lead to carpal subluxation, distal radioulnar incongruency, or both. If closed manipulation fails to provide anatomic congruity and stability of the joint surface, open reduction with direct fragment fixation is my preference (see Case Study 15.11), although mini-open reduction with percutaneous–external fixation is a suitable alternative for many fractures with a dorsal–ulnar corner component and good bone quality.

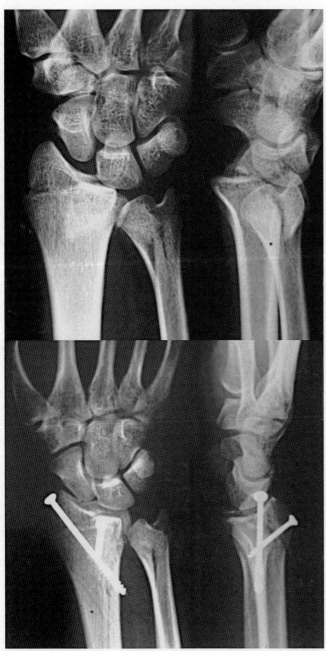

FIGURE 15.62 Combined radial styloid and dorsal shearing fracture (dorsal Barton) in a 23-year-old woman. Notice the intact volar–ulnar portion of the joint surface in the lateral view. Both fragments were securely stabilized with lag screws, which permitted early wrist motion after suture removal.

I begin with closed reduction under fluoroscopy and use finger-trap traction as necessary to maintain the reduction during the surgical exposure. The radial column is approached first through the volar–radial column method (see Case Study 15.11), and after reflection of the first dorsal compartment tendons, fixed provisionally to the proximal–radial shaft with an oblique 0.045-in K-wire. I expose dorsal–ulnar corner fractures that are not associated with an impacted articular or dorsal wall component with a limited, nonextensile incision over the fifth dorsal compartment (see earlier). A provisional 0.045-in K-wire is directed across the fragment at a 45-degree angle to both the coronal and sagittal planes and secured to the proximal–radial shaft. A three-hole ulnar pin plate or a 2.0- to 2.4-mm fixed-angle plate is affixed to the proximal metaphysis to stabilize the fragment (see Figure 15.50).

A radial pin plate or a 2.4-mm radial column plate is used to stabilize the radial styloid fragment. The wrist is taken through a full range of motion under fluoroscopy to confirm a stable reduction. Stable fractures are mobilized with early hand therapy beginning 7 to 10 days postoperatively.

Volar intermediate column fractures (e.g., volar–ulnar corner, teardrop) are exposed through a limited volar–ulnar approach, as well as the radial column approach, and radial columnar fixation is performed as described previously. Fixation of the volar teardrop fragment is performed as described earlier, with a volar buttress pin or a tension band fixation, followed by fixation of the radial column plate. Alternatively, a volar-locked plate and spring wire combination can be employed.[117] Patients with stable fracture reductions are started on an early mobilization protocol (see Case Study 15.12).

Three- and Four-Part Injuries. Further fragmentation of the intermediate column produces more complex diagnostic and treatment challenges. Delineation of the location, relative stability, and number of fragments is essential in planning the operative approach and fixation strategy. A CT scan in such cases is vital and has been demonstrated to alter not only the decision to operate but also the surgical approach in nearly 50% of cases.[74]

In general, these fracture types will require a combination of (1) longitudinal traction or reduction of the metaphyseal fracture, (2) open reduction for restoration of joint congruity, (3) possible bone grafting of the metaphyseal defect, and (4) augmented external or internal fixation. Angular stable plates and miniplate–wireform techniques have enabled stable internal fixation of complex injuries and have reduced the need for combined internal and external fixation. Subchondral placement of pegs to buttress the small articular fragments and simultaneously control shortening and angular displacement are particularly helpful in osteoporotic bones.[126]

Although fixed-angle volar plating is straightforward and provides outstanding fixation strength for the less comminuted fracture variants, it may be difficult to adequately reduce and stabilize small or unstable dorsal rims, central articulars, and dorsal–ulnar corner fragments with a volar fixed-angle device unless an "extended Henry approach" is used (see Figure 15.46). I avoid this particular approach for the more comminuted fractures because of the extensive subperiosteal exposure required and the potential for fragment devascularization.

Management of complex articular fractures through a traditional dorsal approach and dorsal single- or double-plate fixation enables reduction of the dorsal–carpal subluxation, the radial styloid, a central articular impaction fragment, the dorsal rim, and the dorsal–ulnar fragment (see Figure 15.50). Although it may be used with a nondisplaced volar–ulnar fragment, the risk for iatrogenic displacement of this fragment is relatively high. The major disadvantage of dorsal exposure is its inability to permit direct control and manipulation of the volar–ulnar teardrop fragment, which is the *cornerstone* of the distal–radial articular surface. Failure to restore the anatomy of the volar–ulnar corner, the correct depth and concavity of the lunate fossa, and the corresponding area of the sigmoid notch gravely compromises both the radiocarpal joint and the DRUJ.

I prefer fragment-specific fixation for the more highly comminuted fracture patterns because it allows me the greatest latitude for multifragmentary fixation. A combination of radial, dorsal, and volar incisions is used, depending on the number and displacement of the fracture fragments, as determined by preoperative radiographs and the CT scan. Through a volar–radial approach, the radial column can be reduced anatomically and provisionally pinned in position. Elevation of the pronator gives access to the volar rim through the same incision (see Figure 15.40), and manual reduction can be readily performed. A large scaphoid facet or volar rim fragments can be stabilized with a buttress plate or volar fixed-angle device as needed.

If there is a separate volar–ulnar fragment, it is next reduced and stabilized with a volar buttress pin through a volar–ulnar incision parallel to the FCU. The forearm is pronated and a universal dorsal approach (see earlier) is used to gain access to the dorsal rim, dorsal–ulnar corner, and impacted articular fragments. It is often helpful to make all incisions before final fixation of any particular fracture fragment to ensure simultaneous and optimal reduction in all planes. Elevation of one of the larger dorsal metaphyseal fragments (i.e., the "trapdoor") enables access to the subchondral impaction zone, where the articular fragments are elevated en bloc against the template of the scaphoid and lunate. Bone graft or a structural graft substitute may be packed into the resultant defect as necessary (see Figure 15.35, *B*), and the dorsal rim and dorsal–ulnar corner fragments are reassembled (see Case Study 15.3).

Dorsal fixed-angle wireforms and pin plates are contoured to support the elevated articular surface and simultaneously secure the articular and metaphyseal cortical fragments to an intact volar bone. The articular surface reduction and fixation are checked with fluoroscopy. The radial styloid fragment is fixed with a 3-, 5-, or 7-hole radial pin plate along the radial column. Stability of the ulnar column is checked manually before closure and treated as necessary. The wrist is immobilized in neutral and the forearm in supination for 10 days in a sugar tong splint. Digital and shoulder motion exercises are initiated immediately, and the operative splint and sutures are removed when the edema and swelling have subsided, at which point wrist and forearm range-of-motion exercises are begun.

Type IV—Radiocarpal Fracture–Dislocation

These are high-energy injuries in a young patient cohort that combine bony and soft tissue components and have the potential for significant wrist dysfunction. Dumontier and colleagues describe two distinct variants of radiocarpal fracture–dislocation, with important treatment implications (see eFigure 15.8).[37] Even though distinctly uncommon, a radiocarpal

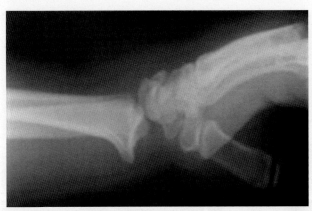

FIGURE 15.63 Radiocarpal fracture–dislocation with minimal bony avulsion. Treatment must be directed at the necessary subtotal ligamentous disruption with the use of multiple Kirschner wires. Alternatively, a temporary bridge plate could be considered. (Reprinted with permission from Dumontier C, Meyer zu Reckendorf G, Sautet A, et al: Radiocarpal dislocations: classification and proposal for treatment. A review of twenty-seven cases. *J Bone Joint Surg [Am]* 83:212–218, 2001.)

dislocation with only a small fleck of attached bone has by necessity disrupted each of the volar and dorsal extrinsic ligamentous stabilizers of the carpus and will predictably progress to an ulnar translational deformity unless meticulous repair of the volar ligaments is performed through an extended volar–carpal tunnel incision (Figure 15.63). Multiple K-wire or temporary dorsal distraction plating placement (see Figures 15.52 and 15.53) should be done to stabilize this injury during ligament healing.

More commonly, a large fragment of the radial styloid, with or without a portion of the articular surface and its attached dorsal–radial rim, is avulsed at the time of injury. Treatment consists of anatomic reduction and stable fixation of the styloid and dorsal rim fragments. Fragments that comprise at least a third of the scaphoid facet of the radius preserve the radioscapho-capitate and long radiolunate ligaments in continuity with the carpus such that anatomic reduction and healing restore stability to the carpus.[37] It is preferable to use a rigid columnar fixation of the styloid piece with a radial pin plate or a 2.4-mm radial column plate through a volar–radial incision (see earlier), combined with dorsal rim fixation using a dorsal wireform (see Case Study 15.13) or a 2.4-mm dorsal plate.[80] Fixation stability is tested in the operating room under fluoroscopy, and postoperative immobilization is customized. Cannulated screw fixation, isolated K-wires, or a tension band can also be used, depending on the size of the styloid fragment and surgeon's preference.

Type V—Combined/Complex Injury

Finally, for more *complex fracture patterns*, such as type V or C3-3 high-energy fractures (e.g., combined articular, metaphyseal, diaphyseal), no single implant or treatment paradigm is appropriate to solve all components of the fracture and the soft tissue injuries. If the fracture has a relatively simple articular component and extensive metaphyseal–diaphyseal comminution with large butterfly fragments, internal fixation with interfragmentary screws and a metadiaphyseal fixed-angle device is the method of choice to simultaneously restore radial alignment and length and to bridge the bony comminution. Initial

application of a bridging external fixator to gain length and alignment may be helpful, and it may be left in place at the surgeon's discretion for additional stability (see Case Study 15.14). For more comminuted articular fractures, a combined dorsal–volar exposure with compartment and median nerve release, autologous cancellous bone grafting of the metaphyseal defect, and a combination of external, internal, or fragment-specific fixation may be required (Figure 15.64).

For cases with extensive articular and metaphyseal–diaphyseal disruption, particularly for patients who present with multiple traumas, or those who require load bearing on their injured wrist in the immediate postoperative period, bridge (distraction) plating is a comparably rapid and effective solution that preserves radial length during the healing process. I prefer the use of the smaller 2.7-mm stainless steel bridge plate that spans the second extensor compartment and can be affixed to the index metacarpal distally (see Figures 15.52 and 15.53).

ASSOCIATED INJURIES

Distal radius fractures may be the result of significant trauma to the entire upper extremity. Whether evaluating a patient with an acute or chronic distal radius fracture, a complete examination of the entire upper extremity should always be undertaken to identify and treat associated musculoskeletal and neurovascular injuries. Conversely, on occasion, serious associated injuries (e.g., shoulder dislocation or scapulothoracic dissociation, elbow fracture–dislocation, plexus injury, or vascular injury) can overshadow a concomitant distal radius fracture. The associated injuries, particularly those to a peripheral nerve, often lead to more problems than the distal radius fracture itself.

Open Fractures

Most fractures of the distal radius are closed injuries, but I consider any fracture that communicates with the external environment to be an open fracture. The associated skin injury may be massive, or it may be a pinpoint, with the only real indication that it communicates to the fracture being a small amount of fatty fluid that exudes from the wound. All open fractures should be treated as surgical emergencies. My treatment plan for open distal radius fractures calls for clinical and radiologic evaluation in the emergency department followed by local cleansing, wound irrigation, and temporary stabilization in a splint. Specimens should be obtained from the wound for culture after initial cleansing, and intravenous broad-spectrum cephalosporin antibiotics need to be initiated before transport to the operating room.

Injuries that occur on a farm, or grossly contaminated wounds, should receive additional anaerobic and aminoglyco-side coverage. The patient should be transported to the operating room expeditiously, where the wound is enlarged, the skin and fracture margins are debrided, and the wound is irrigated with abundant quantities of saline. Restoration of stability is paramount to control infection; thus, if the fracture is unstable, there is adequate soft tissue coverage, and the wound has been suitably cleaned, I prefer to stabilize the fracture with internal or percutaneous fixation, depending on the fracture's particular characteristics. If the fracture is stable, the wound extensions can be closed primarily, while leaving the traumatic wound open, and the fracture immobilized in a cast. If the wound

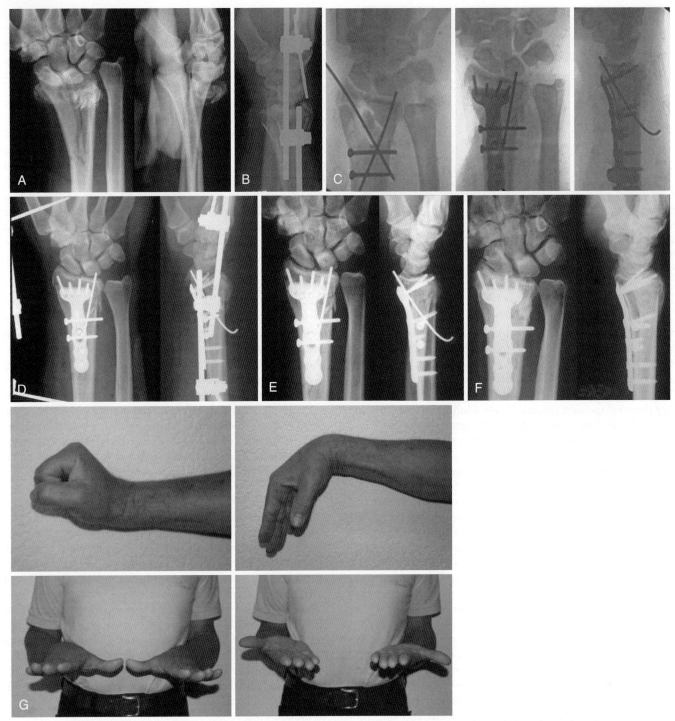

FIGURE 15.64 A, Radiographs of a severely displaced type V complex distal radial fracture with intraarticular and metaphyseal comminution. **B,** Partial insufficient reduction obtained with the application of an external fixator. **C,** Intraoperative fluoroscopic views showing reconstruction of the metaphyseal fracture with two transverse lag screws, provisional fixation of the radial and ulnar fragments with Kirschner wires (K-wires), and application of a volar fixed-angle device. An oblique K-wire inserted palmarly to dorsally has been applied to the volar–ulnar fragment. **D,** Postoperative radiographs showing acceptable reduction and restoration of radial length. The fixator was maintained for 3 weeks. **E,** Fracture was healed 6 weeks after surgery. Notice healing of the dorsal and ulnar comminuted area. At this time the additional K-wire was removed. **F,** Radiographs at 1 year show good restoration of the joint surface and a well-remodeled distal radius. **G,** Photos of adequate arc of flexion and with extension and free forearm rotation restored.

cannot be suitably cleaned or if it has been open for more than 12 h, the fracture should be stabilized with an external fixator, the wound left open, and the patient returned to the operating room at 48 h for definitive treatment and wound closure as possible.

Associated Median Nerve Injury

Varying levels of median nerve compromise, usually caused by blunt contusion or stretching of the nerve over the angulated distal radius, commonly accompany acute distal radius fractures. A fracture hematoma also can compromise the nerve within the carpal tunnel, particularly in patients who may have mild or nocturnal symptoms preceding the injury. It is essential to record the degree of nerve involvement with careful measurements of two-point discrimination and, if possible, thenar motor function before treatment. Closed reduction is performed under adequate local or regional anesthesia, and, if satisfactory reduction is obtained, observation plus careful follow-up is all that is necessary in most instances. If the reduction can be maintained, the nerve compression syndrome generally improves substantially over the subsequent 24 to 48 h. If neurologic symptoms get worse or show no improvement during that period, or if the reduction cannot be obtained or maintained in the presence of median nerve compression, early closed reduction under anesthesia, carpal tunnel release, and operative stabilization of the fracture is preferable. There are no data to support routine release of the carpal tunnel at the time of operative fixation in patients without preoperative evidence of median nerve compromise.

Associated Carpal Ligament Injuries

Carpal ligament disruption can occur with both intraarticular and extraarticular fractures of the distal radius and exacerbate the fracture's prognosis. Certain fracture patterns (e.g., radiocarpal fracture–dislocations and severely displaced radial styloid fractures entering the ridge between the scaphoid and lunate fossae) are particularly at risk for associated carpal ligament injury (see earlier). The incidence of associated carpal ligament disruption with fractures of the distal radius has been documented with arthroscopy by several authors, and an approximate incidence of 30% for partial or complete scapholunate tears and 15% for lunotriquetral tears has been demonstrated.[55] There is no clear association between fracture type and location or the extent of interosseous ligament injury.

Arthroscopic assessment is recommended when injury to the interosseous scapholunate or lunotriquetral ligament is suspected. Complete interosseous ligament injuries in young and active individuals require aggressive operative treatment. Open repair of scapholunate disruptions is recommended after reduction and fixation of the distal radial fracture (see Chapter 13). Arthroscopic pinning or cannulated screw fixation is appropriate for partial scapholunate lesions with instability and for unstable or complete lunotriquetral injuries.

OUTCOME AND PATIENT EXPECTATIONS

Table 15.2 summarizes a compilation of data from single-cohort studies published since 2000, broken down into broad fixation categories. One can generalize from these data that the use of modern fixation techniques generates highly successful

physician-rated outcomes in the vast majority of patients, with restoration of grip strength to 80 to 90% of preinjury values, restoration of range of wrist flexion–extension to 80 to 85%, and nonvalidated outcome measures indicating 85 to 95% good to excellent results. The more recent use of patient-rated validated functional outcome tools enables somewhat easier comparisons between series studies. The patient cohorts are largely comparable, with a trend toward less comminuted fractures in the fixed-angle volar plate group and lower use of bone graft in the fixed-angle plate cohorts.

It is difficult to draw definitive outcome inferences from the combined data considering differences in fracture types, patient age, and surgeon expertise, in particular because of the convergence of outcomes toward excellent anatomic and functional restoration in all cohorts. Whether improvement in outcomes is because of an intense concentration on the principles and techniques of operative indications, fracture fixation, technologic improvements, or some combination can only be speculated.

Factors that lead to a patient's perception of a successful outcome after any surgical intervention are inadequately understood and abundantly illustrated by the lack of consensus on primary outcome measures for management of distal radius fractures (see above). After an exhaustive review of 3371 comparisons in 48 randomized trials for treatment of distal radius fractures, Handoll and colleagues were unable to definitively identify particular surgical interventions that produced consistently improved long-term patient outcomes when compared with nonsurgical treatment. Their 2003 review was hampered by inconsistencies in reporting and the paucity of validated outcome tools in most publications. These authors made a plea for a validated "standard core dataset" for classification and uniform reporting of *objective* and *patient-derived* outcomes.[68]

More recently, Goldhahn et al presented a consensus document calling for the establishment of a core set of specific modules addressing both symptoms and function as separate domains.[59] Going forward, it will be increasingly important for wrist investigators to use common classification and outcome parameters if we are to successfully collect data with which to compare and contrast treatment interventions for wrist injuries. At a minimum, it would seem prudent to collect a standard core dataset that includes the following:

- AO classification of wrist fracture type
- Activity level stratification pre- and postop (PASE)
- Functional assessment (PRWE)
- Pain assessment (VAS)
- ROM of the digits, wrist, and forearm
- Grip strength (bilateral)
- Radiographic parameters
  - Congruence
  - Tilt
  - Variance
  - Inclination
  - Radial translation

COMPLICATIONS

Although it was once believed that all patients with distal radius fractures did relatively well regardless of treatment, it is now well recognized that treatment of these fractures is associated with a high complication rate. As can be seen earlier in Table 15.2, surgical complications with modern fixation techniques, particularly after articular or high-energy injuries (or both), are still reported for nearly 25% of patients and as many as 72% of them in some series.

The complications that continue to plague treatment of distal radius fractures include persistent neuropathy, tendinopathy or tendon rupture, radiocarpal or radioulnar arthrosis, malunion, nonunion, chronic regional pain syndrome (CRPS), ulnar impaction, loss of rotation, finger stiffness, and compartment syndrome, though rarely. An understanding of these complications should lead us to be more aggressive in the original care of such fractures.

Chronic Regional Pain Syndrome

Although full-blown reflex sympathetic dystrophy is a relatively infrequent problem, milder variants are surprisingly common in conjunction with distal radius fractures. Early recognition and attention to patients with an inordinate amount of pain, finger stiffness, swelling, allodynia, or paresthesias may prevent many of the problems of this serious complication. Removal or splitting of a dressing or cast to relieve pressure, elevation of an edematous hand, and intensive hand therapy are frequently very helpful in preventing the development of full-blown CRPS.

A short course of tapered prednisone is often a valuable means of intervention and may allow a patient to turn the corner and avoid escalation of symptoms. More often than not, an irritated or entrapped peripheral nerve underlies most cases of early dystrophy, and the surgeon should have a low threshold for performing electrodiagnostic studies or surgical decompression (or both) for suspected nerve entrapment. For patients who do not respond to early local measures, sympathetic blocks, even with a cast in place, should be considered (see Chapter 53).

Zollinger et al, in a well-controlled randomized trial, confirmed that a daily dose of 500 mg of vitamin C for 50 days reduced the incidence of symptoms associated with CRPS (e.g., swelling, pain, digital stiffness, elevated skin temperature, color changes) in patients treated for distal radius fractures.[178] Although independent confirmation of these findings is pending, the practice is endorsed by the AAOS guidelines and the risks and cost of treatment are decidedly low. For patients who have a previous history of CRPS, there may be value in preemptive treatment with a long-acting sympathetic block or indwelling catheter for a regional nerve blockade for any proposed surgical procedure.

Tendon Rupture

Cast treatment of nondisplaced or minimally displaced distal radius fractures is complicated by rupture of the extensor pollicis brevis (EPB) in up to 5% of cases, a number higher than previously reported in the literature.[135] Patients with painful thumb extension, especially if radiographs demonstrate an irregularity in the region of the Lister tubercle, should be examined by dynamic ultrasound for signs of tendon irritation or fraying. On occasion, decompression and/or internal fixation is warranted to prevent this complication; however, so far strict clinical guidelines are lacking.

The incidence of EPL tendinopathy and rupture appears to have risen following the introduction of locked fixed-angle volar plating. The best treatment of this complication is

prevention whenever possible. As mentioned earlier, precise placement of locked screws or pegs, deliberate downsizing of screw length to avoid dorsal protrusion, and careful assessment of screw placement through the use of specialized radiographic views is necessary to prevent this serious complication.[78]

Similarly, flexor tendon rupture complications following volar plating have been reported with increasing frequency. A systematic review of 21 studies that report flexor tendon ruptures documented the highest incidence in the FPL (57% of reported cases), followed by the index of flexor digitorum profundus (FDP) (15%).[7] The average time to rupture was 9 months postoperatively, but ruptures have been reported as late as 10 years following surgery. Guidelines for prevention of this complication is (1) careful placement of the implant proximal to the transverse ridge of the radial metaphyseal flare (i.e., the watershed line) and (2) avoiding plate prominence either above the volar critical line or within 3 mm of the articular rim of the radius[90] (see Soong guidelines).

Patients may present with volar swelling, tenderness, crepitus, or pain with finger or thumb motion months or years following surgery. I find ultrasound useful to identify flexor tendon proximity to the plate, tendinopathy, fraying, or tenosynovitis. If radiographs demonstrate Soong grade 1 or 2 positioning, I recommend plate removal if the fracture is fully healed to prevent rupture. Ruptured tendons require hardware removal and reconstruction with direct repair, a tendon graft, or a tendon transfer, as indicated by patient impairment (see Chapter 31).

Nonunion

Nonunion of distal radius fractures is rare but presents unique treatment challenges because of the associated pain, joint contractures, tendon imbalance or rupture, and occasional severe bone deformity. Treatment must be individualized, but generally involves workup for subclinical infection, removal of existing hardware, anatomic realignment of the radiocarpal and radioulnar joints, and stable fixation with a bone graft. In contrast, nonunion of ulnar styloid process fractures in conjunction with distal radius fractures is quite common and yet is rarely symptomatic.[166] Treatment of ulnar styloid nonunion must be individualized and based on the patient's symptoms and functional deficits.

Symptomatic nonunion of the ulnar styloid is best treated by excision of the styloid unless the ulnar styloid fragment is large enough for rigid internal fixation. It is essential, however, for the examiner to distinguish between radioulnar instability secondary to foveal avulsion of the TFCC and ulnar styloid nonunion or impingement. If DRUJ instability is suspected clinically, magnetic resonance imaging (MRI) of the radioulnar ligaments, or CT of both wrists in full supination and pronation (or both) can help differentiate between the various conditions (see Chapter 14). If a styloid nonunion is accompanied by distal–ulnar instability, the TFCC should be reattached to the fovea at the time of fragment excision or fixation.

Malunion

Malunion of distal radius fractures may result in wrist pain, decreased range of motion, midcarpal instability, or any combination of these complications. Two studies that examined threshold criteria for an acceptable reduction demonstrated a significant correlation between outcome and adverse radiographic parameters across all age groups, but mitigated to a great deal in patients older than 65.[20,61] Factors most closely correlated with outcome included ulnar variance,[19,61,93] radial inclination,[61] and volar tilt.[19,93] Greater disability was identified when two factors were present in combination,[19] and this effect was sustained at 2 years' follow-up.[20] In general, ulnar-sided wrist pain is the factor that leads most patients with malunited distal radius fractures to seek treatment because of the effect of changes in variance, congruency, or alignment of the sigmoid notch.

Recognition of associated carpal malalignment and DRUJ derangement is mandatory to decide whether additional procedures, together with radial osteotomy, are necessary to help ensure a good result. Assessment of carpal malalignment with malunited distal radius fractures includes determination of the presence of (1) dorsal subluxation of the carpus, (2) a type I (*adaptive*) dorsal intercalated segment instability (DISI) that is *reducible* by radial osteotomy, or (3) a type II (*fixed*) DISI pattern that does not improve after radial osteotomy. A reducible deformity is usually characterized by a mobile lunate on flexion and extension lateral radiographs. A fixed DISI is generally associated with a more chronic deformity and may be associated with an unrecognized disruption of the scapholunate or radiocarpal ligaments.

Correction of posttraumatic wrist deformity must be tailored to the specific site of the deformity and depends on whether the malunion is extraarticular, involves the radiocarpal or radioulnar joints (or both), or is complex (i.e., metaphyseal and articular deformity). The decision to perform a simultaneous procedure at the DRUJ depends on the amount of radial shortening and the presence of osteoarthritic changes or instability of the joint. Instability or ulnocarpal impingement that results from radial shortening, angulation, or malrotation without associated degenerative changes can generally be corrected by restoration of radial anatomy alone.

My indications for corrective osteotomy in a young, symptomatic, and active individual include articular step-off with or without carpal subluxation, 15 degrees or more of dorsal tilt, ulnar-positive variance with impaction, or marked loss of radial inclination. Less commonly, increased volar tilt results in carpal subluxation and manifests as a painful deformity and loss of extension, supination, or both. If an impending malunion is recognized in the subacute stage (i.e., before complete bony healing) and the patient is medically stable, early intervention provides easier realignment because of the absence of soft tissue and capsular contractures, and shortens the overall recovery–disability time. In patients with swollen and dystrophic changes, it may be prudent to wait until the soft tissues have stabilized and the patient has plateaued in wrist, digital, and forearm motion before osteotomy and fixation.

Extraarticular Radial Osteotomy Technique

The aims of radial osteotomy are to restore function and improve the appearance of the wrist by correcting the deformity at the level of the fracture site. The osteotomy should reorient the joint surface to restore normal load distribution, reestablish the mechanical balance of the midcarpal joint, and improve the anatomic relationships of the DRUJ. Because radial shortening is a constant component of the deformity in both volar and

dorsal malunions, an opening wedge osteotomy that is transverse in the frontal plane and oblique (i.e., parallel to the joint surface) in the sagittal plane is used to permit radial lengthening. Such an osteotomy allows for the following:

- Radial lengthening of up to 10 to 12 mm
- Correction of volar tilt in the sagittal plane
- Correction of radial inclination in the frontal plane
- Correction of rotational deformity in the axial plane

A 2011 comparative study showed improved correction of ulnar variance and better Mayo scores with closing wedge osteotomy and a simultaneous ulnar-shortening osteotomy.[158] Regardless of technique, it is important that the osteotomy be parallel to the articular surface, as close as possible to the site of the original fracture, so as to restore the relationship between the center of rotation of the carpus and the long axis of the radius (Figure 15.65).

With large defects created by an opening wedge osteotomy, a cancellous or corticocancellous bone graft (see earlier) can be used to fill the bone defect and to induce more rapid consolidation. Angular–stable plate fixation is ideal for corrective osteotomies in osteopenic bone and nascent malunions and when using nonstructural bone grafts. If partial or complete resection of the distal end of the ulna is performed simultaneously, the resected ulnar head can be sculpted and used to fill the radial defect. Preoperative planning and the use of K-wires to mark the angle of deformity help to facilitate accurate angular correction, simplify the procedure, and reduce the degree of exposure to fluoroscopy.[46] Radiographs of the uninjured wrist should be performed to determine the physiologic ulnar variance and calculate restoration of radial length (Figure 15.66).

Dorsal Approach for Osteotomy of Malunited Distal Radius Fractures

Dorsal malunions may be exposed through a universal dorsal incision between the third and fourth extensor compartments (see earlier). For severe deformities, this has the benefit of a single approach through which soft tissue release, bone grafting, and internal fixation can be performed. The healed fracture site is identified with fluoroscopy. If dorsal plate fixation of the osteotomy is planned, the Lister tubercle should be removed with a rongeur to provide a flat surface on which to apply the plate. If K-wire or low-profile columnar fixation of the osteotomy is planned, the Lister tubercle may be left undisturbed.

To be sure that the osteotomy, as seen in the sagittal plane, is parallel to the joint surface, a 25-gauge needle is introduced through the dorsal part of the capsule into the radiocarpal joint and along the articular surface of the radius. In accordance with the preoperative plan,[46] two 2.5-mm K-wires with threaded tips are inserted so that the angle of correction in the sagittal plane is subtended on both sides of the future osteotomy (see Figure 15.66). These wires not only control intraoperative angular correction but also help manipulate and maintain the distal fragment in the corrected position with a small external fixator bar until the graft is inserted in the defect.

The osteotomy is performed with an oscillating saw, with care taken to not osteotomize the volar cortex completely. It is then opened dorsally and radially by manipulating the wrist into flexion, by applying a laminar spreader dorsally, or by using 2.5-mm Schanz screws as joysticks. The osteotomy is opened until both wires are parallel in the sagittal plane. Opening up

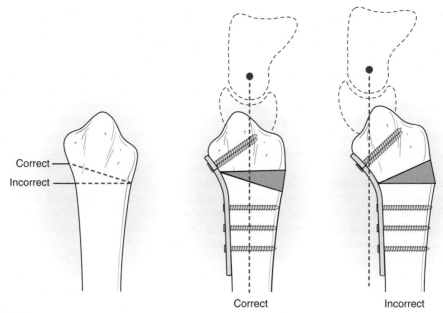

Correct
Incorrect

Correct   Incorrect

FIGURE 15.65 It is imperative that the osteotomy be parallel to the articular surface to avoid creating a secondary deformity. (© Elizabeth Martin.)

the osteotomy on the radial side can be difficult, and complete tenotomy of the BR tendon is recommended to facilitate realignment.

A small external fixator bar with two clamps can be attached between both Schanz screws to maintain reduction of the distal fragment. With the elbow in 90 degrees of flexion, intraoperative forearm rotation and wrist motion are checked. Radiographic control with the image intensifier may be advisable at this point to assess the quality of correction and radial lengthening before definitive internal fixation of the osteotomy is undertaken.

Depending on the rigidity of fixation planned, corticocancellous or cancellous bone graft can be inserted into the defect. At this point, a 1.6- or 2.0-mm K-wire is driven obliquely from the radial styloid across the graft and into the proximal fragment, after which the threaded screws and the external fixator bar can be removed. The osteotomy can be stabilized by a variety of methods. In young adults with good bone quality and, especially when the volar cortex is not disrupted, simple K-wire fixation (one through the radial styloid and one through the Lister tubercle in an oblique dorsal–palmar direction) offers adequate stability. However, this method requires casting and prolonged immobilization.

As an alternative, stable plate fixation can be used with the advantage of early wrist rehabilitation. The use of low-profile fixed-angle implants (2.4-mm condylar plates or any of a number of dorsal fixed-angle devices) has helped diminish extensor tendon irritation. For dorsal fixation, I prefer to use a radial column plate and a fixed-angle wireform implant that spans the opening wedge osteotomy and provides rigid fixation when combined with a corticocancellous graft (Figure 15.67).

Volar Approach for Osteotomy of a Malunited Distal Radius Fracture

Alternatively, malunited dorsally angulated fractures can be corrected through a volar approach to avoid extensor tendon

---

CRITICAL POINTS *Radial Osteotomy for Malunited Extraarticular Fracture*

Indications
- Symptomatic malunion (e.g., pain, weakness, cosmetic disturbance)
- Limited palmar flexion
- DRUJ incongruency, limited forearm rotation
- Adaptive carpal instability

Technical Points
- Use a 6- to 7-cm dorsal approach with the incision centered on the Lister tubercle.
- Expose the distal radius between the third and fourth compartments.
- Mobilize the EPL tendon.
- Mark the osteotomy at the previous fracture line.
- Use 2.5-mm K-wires (also can be used as joysticks) to determine the angle of correction.
- Perform an osteotomy parallel to the joint surface in the sagittal plane and transverse in the frontal plane.
- Open the osteotomy dorsally until the K-wires are parallel (use a laminar spreader or temporary external fixator).
- Fill the defect with corticocancellous bone graft.
- Use temporary K-wire fixation and fluoroscopic control (i.e., for position of the distal fragment and DRUJ congruency).
- Perform internal fixation of the osteotomy (low-profile fixed-angle plates).
- Morcellized cancellous grafts or bone substitutes can alternatively be used depending on rigidity of fixation.

Postoperative Care
- Apply a dorsal and palmar splint until suture removal. Use a sugar tong cast in supination for 2 weeks when concomitant distal–ulna excision is performed.
- Apply a short-arm cast for 4 to 6 weeks, when using pin fixation, until radiograph shows healing.
- Apply a palmar splint and initiate gentle range-of-motion exercises if fixed-angle fixation is used.

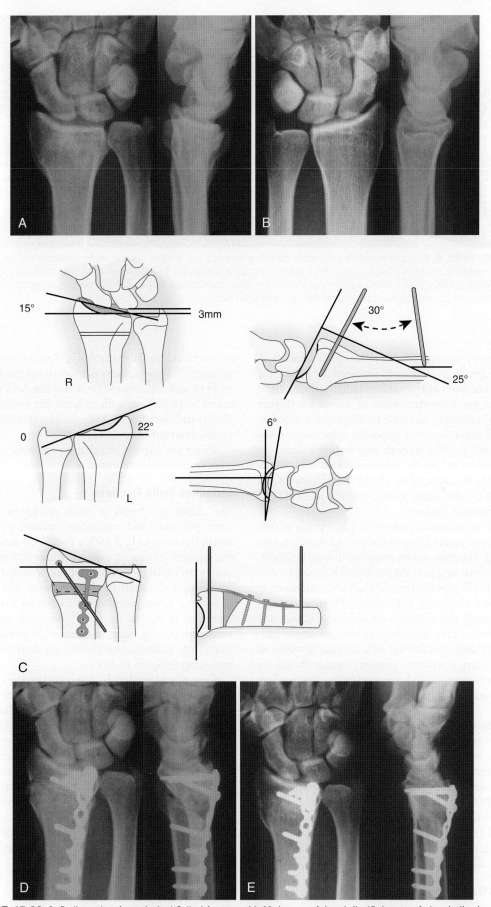

FIGURE 15.66 A, Radiographs of a malunited Colles' fracture with 30 degrees of dorsal tilt, 15 degrees of ulnar inclination, and an ulnar-plus variance of 3 mm. **B,** Comparative radiographs for preoperative planning. **C,** Preoperative planning for the opening wedge dorsal osteotomy and fixation with the minicondylar plate. **D,** Immediate postoperative radiographs. **E,** Radiographs 1.5 years after osteotomy with anatomic restoration of wrist anatomy and carpal alignment.

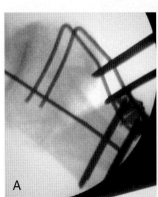
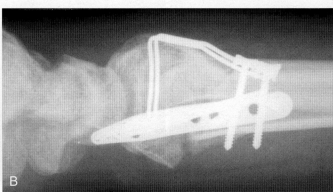
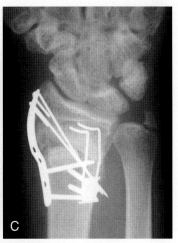

FIGURE 15.67 A, A dorsally malunited distal radius fracture is corrected with a dorsal opening wedge osteotomy and the use of a laminar spreader to correct volar tilt. A prebent dorsal wireform implant is in place, but final screw tightening has not yet been performed. **B,** Radiograph 2 weeks postoperatively demonstrates correction of volar tilt and biplane fixation. **C,** Posteroanterior radiograph at 2 weeks demonstrating an iliac crest graft and reduction of the radial inclination and length.

irritation that may be associated with dorsal plate fixation. A fixed-angle volar device anatomically designed to match the normal anatomic contours of the palmar–radial surface can be used as a guide for precision restoration of palmar tilt (Figure 15.68). The author prefers to calculate the degree of correction in the sagittal and coronal planes, apply the volar plate to the distal fragment with parallel smooth pegs before osteotomy, then remove the plate to cut the osteotomy (see Case Study 15.15). Care should be taken to finish the ostetotomy of the dorsal cortex with an osteotome to decrease the possibility of an injury to the extensor tendons.

The EPL and wrist extensor tendons are particularly at risk, and a small counterincision to isolate and protect these tendons may be considered. The plate is then reapplied distally by inserting the parallel smooth pegs into the predrilled holes and rotating into position on the proximal–radial shaft to simultaneously realign the articular surface in both planes. Fixation is completed both proximally and distally with additional screws and pegs. Large deformities may require a concomitant dorsal incision, periosteal division, and the use of a laminar spreader to gain length. If making a separate incision, I generally fill the resultant defect with a cancellous bone graft to expedite healing, although some surgeons rely on the rigidity of locked-plate fixation alone.

If the length discrepancy between the ulna and the radius is more than 10 mm, or if performing a closing wedge osteotomy, a combined radial osteotomy and simultaneous ulnar shortening can be performed.[158] Stable fixation of both the radius and the ulna is necessary. The presence of severe degenerative changes in the DRUJ mandates resection of the distal ulna or prosthetic replacement of the joint. If the radial shortening is greater than 2 to 3 cm, progressive lengthening with the distraction osteogenesis technique may be necessary to prevent nerve or tendon dysfunction, or both.

Ulnar-Shortening Osteotomy

Ruch and colleagues advocate isolated ulnar shortening osteotomy for patients with up to 20 degrees of symptomatic dorsal

extraarticular radial malunion and simultaneous ulnar-positive variance.[149] These authors demonstrated marked improvements in wrist and forearm range of motion, VAS scores, and DASH scores in 18 patients with isolated ulnar-shortening osteotomy (USO) and recommend it as a simpler treatment for a uniplanar radius deformity (see Chapter 14).

Please see ExpertConsult.com for information about Watson's trapezoidal osteotomy.

Malunited Smith Fractures

The classic symptoms of volar malunion include decreased wrist extension and supination because of the tendency for Smith fractures to heal with a pronation deformity. Symptomatic malunions can be exposed through a standard FCR incision, with radial detachment of the pronator quadratus muscle and partial elevation of the FPL from the radial shaft. Two K-wires or a two-pin external fixator are inserted on the volar aspect to mark the angle of correction and manually hold reduction during plate application. A palmar opening wedge osteotomy, grafting, and plating are then carried out as in the preceding (eFigure 15.10).

Care must be taken to not translate the entire distal radius fragment dorsally and, in so doing, shift the center of rotation of the carpus dorsally. Temporary K-wire fixation through the radial styloid and a second wire placed volar-to-dorsal from the radial rim helps stabilize the correction, which is verified with fluoroscopy. Application of a fixed-angle volar plate automatically derotates the pronation deformity of the distal fragment by virtue of the contoured surface of the plate. Dorsiflexion of the distal fragment and derotation, as well as lengthening, reorient the sigmoid notch of the radius with respect to the ulnar head. Degenerative arthritis of the DRUJ may necessitate simultaneous distal–ulnar excision or ulnar head replacement.

Articular Osteotomies

The role of an osteotomy in correcting an articular malunion of the radiocarpal joint after a distal–radius fracture is limited

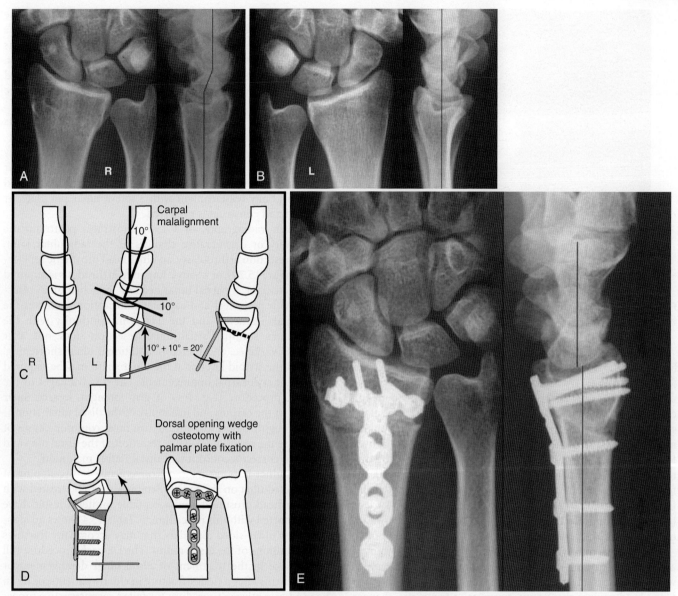

FIGURE 15.68 A, Dynamic midcarpal instability in a malunited Colles' fracture with 10 degrees of dorsal tilt. The patient has painful clicking on ulnar deviation of right wrist. **B,** Comparative radiographs of the left wrist showing normal carpal alignment. **C, D,** Preoperative radiographs and planning: An opening wedge osteotomy was performed through a volar approach and fixed with a fixed-angle plate and morcellized cancellous bone. Preapplication of the fixed-angle plate to the distal fragment at the anticipated angle of correction with two parallel pegs allows the surgeon to subsequently remove the plate, make the osteotomy, and then reattach the plate to precisely rotate the distal fragment into position. **E,** Realignment of the distal radius with restoration of a 10-degree volar tilt, improved carpal alignment, and controlled instability. Notice the subchondral positioning of the central fixed-angle pegs. (**D,** © Elizabeth Martin.)

by both chronology and the type of injury. The osteotomy should be done as early as possible after fracture, and the fracture plane can be readily identified upward of 8 to 12 weeks after injury (see Case Study 15.16). A high-resolution CT with multiplanar reformatting is particularly helpful in identifying the fracture plane and planning the osteotomy (see Case Study 15.1). Custom sterile cutting guides can be created to ensure precision correction of articular and combined defects[150] (see Case Study 15.16). MRI with cartilage-sensitive sequences or concomitant wrist arthroscopy may play a useful role in evaluating the amount of cartilage damage and articular incongruence. The presence of areas that lack subchondral bone represents a formal contraindication to osteotomy.

It is preferable to reserve such a procedure for malunited fractures that have a relatively simple articular component (Figure 15.69). Such fractures include malunited radial styloid, volar or dorsal shearing (i.e., a Barton fracture), dorsal die-punch, and palmar carpal subluxation due to a displaced palmar–lunate facet fragment.[139] The choice of surgical approach is as indicated for the fracture scenario in the acute stage. Stable fixation of the osteotomized fragment enables early rehabilitation of the radiocarpal and radioulnar joints.

Distal Radioulnar Joint Procedures

The most common cause of residual wrist disability after fracture of the distal radius involves the wrist's ulnar side. The three

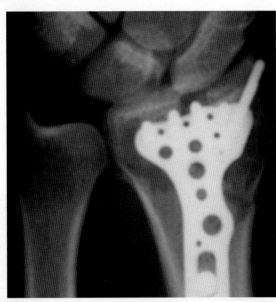

FIGURE 15.69 Relatively simple articular malunion involving articular depression of the scaphoid facet.

strated by CT, a shortening osteotomy of the ulna is the procedure of choice. Ulnar shortening decompresses the wrist's ulnar compartment, reestablishes DRUJ congruity, and tightens the TFCC, which exerts a stabilizing effect on the distal ulna. An oblique osteotomy with resection of a bony segment and rigid fixation with a compression plate is recommended (see Chapter 14).[24]

If associated instability of the DRUJ is present and persists following correction of the radial malunion, transosseous reattachment of the dorsal and palmar radioulnar ligaments may be required. If the DRUJ is unstable and the dorsal and palmar radioulnar ligaments are in continuity with a large ulnar styloid fragment, bony reattachment with a screw, ulnar pin plate, or tension band construct is preferred.

If plain radiographs or CT demonstrates posttraumatic incongruity or degenerative changes of the radioulnar joint, either a resection arthroplasty, an ulnar head prosthetic replacement (Figure 15.70), or a Sauvé-Kapandji arthrodesis is required to alleviate pain. A partial ulnar head or "matched ulna" resection[163] with periosteal and capsular imbrication preserves the ulnocarpal ligaments and the TFCC in continuity with the distal ulnar stump. Partial ulnar resection does not alter the ulnar variance, and therefore additional ulnar shortening, either at the styloid level or at the ulnar shaft, may be required to prevent stylocarpal impingement. The disadvantages of the Darrach procedure (e.g., loss of grip strength, loss of ulnar support of the carpus, and instability of the distal ulnar stump) are thoroughly described, but the two most common causes of failure are the result of excessive resection of the distal ulna and failure to correct a concomitant distal radius malunion.

Radioulnar impingement, or convergence and scalloping of the resected ulna on the radial metaphysis, can be treated with an ulnar head prosthesis, and acceptable midterm results have been reported with this procedure.[156] Table 15.4 shows an algorithm for ulnar-sided disorders that may accompany fractures and malunions of the distal radius. The Darrach procedure still has a place in the treatment of distal ulnar derangement or osteoarthritis after a Colles' fracture in elderly patients, or it can be used as a salvage procedure for failed reconstructive procedures of the radioulnar joint (see Chapter 14).

DRUJ arthrodesis with the creation of a proximal pseudarthrosis (i.e., Sauvé-Kapandji procedure) preserves both the ulnocarpal ligaments and the bony support of the carpus. This operation is useful for younger, active patients because it improves forearm rotation in those with fixed DRUJ subluxation after articular fractures of the distal radius and severe destruction of the joint (Figure 15.71). The author recommends primary stabilization of the remaining distal ulna with distally based tendon weaves using slips of both the FCU and the ECU, as described by Lamey and Fernandez.[101]

Distal Radioulnar Joint Contracture

Capsular contraction of the DRUJ may be responsible for limitation of forearm rotation after distal radius fractures. Having ruled out joint incongruity, subluxation, radioulnar synchondrosis, interosseous membrane contracture, or derangement of the proximal radioulnar joint as other possible causes of limited forearm rotation, surgical release is helpful if the condition does not improve after a trial of physiotherapy.

basic conditions responsible for pain associated with limited forearm rotation are sigmoid notch incongruency, positive ulnar variance, and instability of the joint. Less frequent (or concomitant) findings are painful nonunion of the ulnar styloid, capsular contracture of the joint, and radioulnar impingement (i.e., after distal ulnar resections or Sauvé-Kapandji procedures). Incongruency of the DRUJ may be due to (1) extraarticular deformity of the radius or ulna, which leads to an abnormal orientation of joint surfaces (sigmoid notch and ulnar head) in space; (2) disruption of the articular joint surface by a fracture line affecting the sigmoid notch or the ulnar head, or both; and (3) extraarticular and articular factors combined.

Ulnar impaction syndrome occurs at the ulnocarpal joint as a result of posttraumatic radial shortening and is synonymous with ulnocarpal abutment. With continuing impaction of the ulnar head against the carpus, progressive traumatic changes follow in a predictable sequence, including attenuation and tears of the TFCC; chondromalacia of the ulnar head, lunate, and triquetrum (Tq); attenuation and tears of the triquetrolunate ligament; and finally, ulnocarpal degenerative changes. Instability is the result of loss of ligament support, generally due to avulsion of the palmar and dorsal radioulnar ligaments from their foveal insertion. Additional injuries to the secondary joint stabilizers (e.g., capsular ligaments, sheath of the ECU, interosseous membrane, pronator quadratus) or disruption of the joint surface may aggravate the degree of laxity.

If the patient's main complaints are localized to the DRUJ (i.e., pain associated with limited forearm rotation) and the angulation of the radial articular surface in the sagittal and frontal planes is less than 20 degrees,[149] a reconstructive procedure at the distal radioulnar level is indicated, without a corrective radial osteotomy. However, if significant radial deformity is clearly associated with identifiable DRUJ problems, radial osteotomy and the appropriate DRUJ procedure can be performed simultaneously.

For radial shortening and ulnocarpal impaction with acceptable congruency of the sigmoid notch and ulna, as demonstrated by CT, a

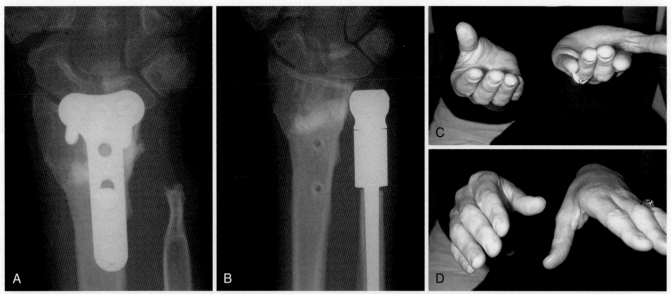

FIGURE 15.70 A 42-year-old with a chronically painful and unstable ulna after multiple procedures for distal radial malunion. **A,** Radically shortened ulna. **B,** Stability of the distal radioulnar joint was restored with a custom ulnar head replacement. **C, D,** Photos of functional and pain-free supination and pronation at 2 years postoperatively.

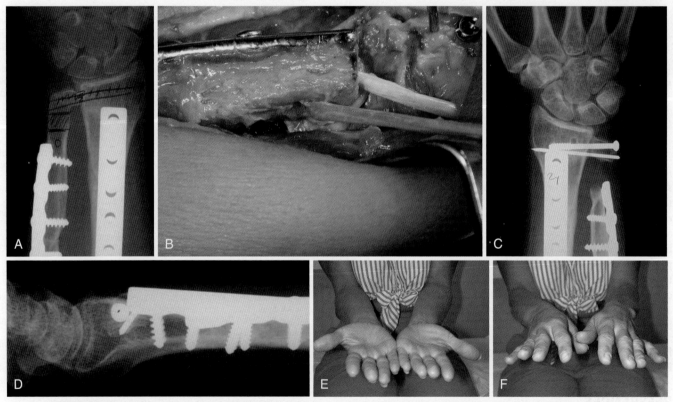

FIGURE 15.71 Suavé-Kapandji procedure: **A,** A 28-year-old emergency medical technician with a chronically unstable and degenerative distal radioulnar joint after multiple procedures for a malunited distal both-bones fracture. **B,** Intraoperative photograph of the flexor carpi ulnaris tendon woven through the proximal stump of the Sauvé-Kapandji reconstruction. **C, D,** Radiographs at 4 years postoperatively. **E, F,** Photos of pain-free functional rotation enabled return to all activities.

The volar aspect of the joint is exposed through a longitudinal incision just ulnar to the FCU tendon. Having exposed and protected the dorsal cutaneous branch of the ulnar nerve, the tendon and the ulnar neurovascular bundle are retracted radially. Next, the pronator quadratus is sectioned longitudinally 5 mm radial to its ulnar insertion. The contracted palmar capsule is exposed to retract the pronator quadratus radially. It is useful to place a 25-gauge needle between the TFCC and the ulnar head and confirm placement under fluoroscopy before resection of the palmar capsule. A longitudinal capsulotomy

TABLE 15.4 Algorithm for Management of DRUJ Disorders After Distal Radius Fracture

Disorder	Management
DRUJ incongruity	
Extraarticular	Reorient the sigmoid notch with a radial osteotomy
Articular	Depending on the severity of degenerative changes, age, dominance, and occupation, resection arthroplasty, Sauvé-Kapandji procedure, or prosthetic replacement
Combined	Radial osteotomy and DRUJ procedure as for an articular disorder
DRUJ instability	Reattachment of the dorsal and palmar radioulnar ligaments ORIF of an ulnar styloid nonunion Shortening osteotomy of the ulna
Ulnocarpal impaction	Restore the radioulnar index or ulnar variance to normal Ulna-shortening osteotomy Wafer procedure Combined radius–ulna osteotomies
Symptomatic (painful) nonunion of the ulnar styloid	Excision
Capsular contracture	Dorsal and/or palmar capsulotomy[91]
Radioulnar impingement	Ulnar head prosthesis

Note: If these conditions occur in association, two or more procedures may need to be combined. A classic example is a malunited Colles fracture and degenerative changes in the DRUJ.
DRUJ, Distal radioulnar joint; *ORIF,* open reduction internal fixation.

just proximal to the volar radioulnar ligament close to the sigmoid notch is performed and then continued proximally to the neck of the ulna. The entire palmar capsule is excised to expose the articular surface of the ulnar head.

A more radial approach between the ulnar neurovascular bundle and the digital flexor tendons can also be used for this purpose. A "silhouette" capsulotomy[91] of the dorsal capsule is then performed with a counterincision through the fifth dorsal compartment. Postoperatively, it is important to begin immediate mobilization of the forearm and use dynamic supination bracing if necessary.

For Case Studies, Videos, and more, please visit ExpertConsult.com.

REFERENCES

1. Aktekin CN, Altay M, Gursoy Z, et al: Comparison between external fixation and cast treatment in the management of distal radius fractures in patients aged 65 years and older. *J Hand Surg [Am]* 35(5):736–742, 2010.
2. Amorosa LF, Vitale MA, Brown S, et al: A functional outcomes survey of elderly patients who sustained distal radius fractures. *Hand (NY)* 6(3):260–267, 2011.
3. Andermahr J, Lozano-Calderón S, Trafton T, et al: The volar extension of the lunate facet of the distal radius: a quantitative anatomic study. *J Hand Surg [Am]* 31(6):892–895, 2006.
4. Andersen DJ, Blair WF, Steyers CM, Jr, et al: Classification of distal radius fractures: an analysis of interobserver reliability and intraobserver reproducibility. *J Hand Surg [Am]* 21(4):574–582, 1996.
5. Anderson R, O'Neil G: Comminuted fractures of the distal end of the radius. *Surg Gyn Obstet* 78:434–442, 1944.
6. Arora R, Lutz M, Deml C, et al: A prospective randomized trial comparing nonoperative treatment with volar locking plate fixation for displaced and unstable distal radial fractures in patients sixty-five years of age and older. *J Bone Joint Surg Am* 93(23):2146–2153, 2011.
7. Asadollahi S, Keith PP: Flexor tendon injuries following plate fixation of distal radius fractures: a systematic review of the literature. *J Orthop Traumatol* 14(4): 227–234, 2013.
8. Atroshi I, Brogren E, Larsson GU, et al: Wrist-bridging versus non-bridging external fixation for displaced distal radius fractures: a randomized assessor-blind clinical trial of 38 patients followed for 1 year. *Acta Orthop* 77(3):445–453, 2006.
9. Axelrod TS, McMurtry RY: Open reduction and internal fixation of comminuted, intraarticular fractures of the distal radius. *J Hand Surg [Am]* 15(1):1–11, 1990.
10. Barrie KA, Wolfe SW: Internal fixation for intraarticular distal radius fractures. *Tech Hand Up Extrem Surg* 6(1):10–20, 2002.
11. Bass RL, Blair WF, Hubbard PP: Results of combined internal and external fixation for the treatment of severe AO-C3 fractures of the distal radius. *J Hand Surg [Am]* 20(3):373–381, 1995.
12. Beck JD, Harness NG, Spencer HT: Volar plate fixation failure for volar shearing distal radius fractures with small lunate facet fragments. *J Hand Surg [Am]* 39(4):670–678, 2014.
13. Benson LS, Minihame KP, Stern LD, et al: The outcome of intra-articular distal radius fractures treated with fragment-specific fixation. *J Hand Surg [Am]* 31A:1333–1339, 2006.
14. Beumer A, McQueen MM: Fractures of the distal radius in low-demand elderly patients: closed reduction of no value in 53 of 60 wrists. *Acta Orthop Scand* 74(1):98–100, 2003.
15. Bickerstaff DR, Bell MJ: Carpal malalignment in Colles' fractures. *J Hand Surg [Br]* 14(2):155–160, 1989.
16. Bohler L: *The treatment of fractures,* New York, 1929, Grune and Stratton, p 420.
17. Bong MR, Egol KA, Leibman M, et al: A comparison of immediate postreduction splinting constructs for controlling initial displacement of fractures of the distal radius: a prospective randomized study of long-arm versus short-arm splinting. *J Hand Surg [Am]* 31(5):766–770, 2006.
18. Brogren E, Hofer M, Petranek M, et al: Fractures of the distal radius in women aged 50 to 75 years: natural course of patient-reported outcome, wrist motion and grip strength between 1 year and 2 to 4 years after fracture. *J Hand Surg Eur Vol* 36(7):568–576, 2011.
19. Brogren E, Hofer M, Petranek M, et al: Relationship between distal radius fracture malunion and arm-related disability: a prospective population-based cohort study with 1-year follow-up. *BMC Musculoskelet Disord* 12:9, 2011.
20. Brogren E, Wagner P, Petranek M, et al: Distal radius malunion increases risk of persistent disability 2 years after fracture: a prospective cohort study. *Clin Orthop Relat Res* 471(5):1691–1697, 2013.
21. Brophy RH, Lin K, Smith MV: The role of activity level in orthopaedics: an important prognostic and outcome variable. *J Am Acad Orthop Surg* 22(7):430–436, 2014.
22. Burke EF, Singer RM: Treatment of comminuted distal radius with the use of an internal distraction plate. *Tech Hand Up Extrem Surg* 2(4):248–252, 1998.
23. Carter PR, Frederick HA, Laseter GF: Open reduction and internal fixation of unstable distal radius fractures with a low-profile plate: a multicenter study of 73 fractures. *J Hand Surg [Am]* 23(2):300–307, 1998.
24. Chen NC, Wolfe SW: Ulna shortening osteotomy using a compression device. *J Hand Surg [Am]* 28(1):88–93, 2003.
25. Chin KR, Jupiter JB: Wireloop fixation of volar displaced osteochondral fractures of the distal radius. *J Hand Surg [Am]* 24(3):523–533, 1999.
26. Chung KC, Kotsis SV, Kim HM: Predictors of functional outcomes after surgical treatment of distal radius fractures. *J Hand Surg [Am]* 32(1):76–83, 2007.
27. Chung KC, Spilson SV: The frequency and epidemiology of hand and forearm fractures in the United States. *J Hand Surg [Am]* 26(5):908–915, 2001.
28. Cole DW, Elsaidi GA, Kuzma KR, et al: Distal radioulnar joint instability in distal radius fractures: the role of sigmoid notch and triangular fibrocartilage complex revisited. *Injury* 37(3):252–258, 2006.
29. Cooney WP, III, Dobyns JH, Linscheid RL: Complications of Colles' fractures. *J Bone Joint Surg* 62A:613–619, 1980.
30. Cotton FJ: *Dislocations and joint fractures.* 1-1-0024. Philadelphia, 1924, W.B. Saunders, pp 348–358.
31. Crisco JJ, Coburn JC, Moore DC, et al: In vivo radiocarpal kinematics and the dart thrower's motion. *J Bone Joint Surg Am* 87(12):2729–2740, 2005.
32. Crosby SN, Fletcher ND, Yap ER, et al: The mechanical stability of extra-articular distal radius fractures with respect to the number of screws securing the distal fragment. *J Hand Surg [Am]* 38(6):1097–1105, 2013.
33. Cross AW, Schmidt CC: Flexor tendon injuries following locked volar plating of distal radius fractures. *J Hand Surg [Am]* 33(2):164–167, 2008.
34. DePalma AF: Comminuted fractures of the distal end of the radius treated by ulnar pinning. *J Bone Joint Surg* 34A(3):651–662, 1952.

35. Dodds SD, Cornelissen S, Jossan S, et al: A biomechanical comparison of fragment-specific fixation and augmented external fixation for intra-articular distal radius fractures. *J Hand Surg [Am]* 27(6):953–964, 2002.
36. Doi K, Hattori Y, Otsuka K, et al: Intra-articular fractures of the distal aspect of the radius: arthroscopically assisted reduction compared with open reduction and internal fixation. *J Bone Joint Surg Am* 81(8):1093–1110, 1999.
37. Dumontier C, Meyer ZU, Reckendorf G, et al: Radiocarpal dislocations: classification and proposal for treatment. A review of twenty-seven cases. *J Bone Joint Surg Am* 83-A(2):212–218, 2001.
38. Dy CJ, Jang E, Taylor SA, et al: The impact of coronal alignment on distal radioulnar stability following distal radius fracture. *J Hand Surg Am* 39:1045–1052, 2014.
39. Dy CJ, Wolfe SW, Jupiter JB, et al: Distal radius fractures: strategic alternatives to volar plate fixation. *Instr Course Lect* 63:27–37, 2014.
40. Dzaja I, MacDermid JC, Roth J, et al: Functional outcomes and cost estimation for extra-articular and simple intra-articular distal radius fractures treated with open reduction and internal fixation versus closed reduction and percutaneous Kirschner wire fixation. *Can J Surg* 56(6):378–384, 2013.
41. Egol KA, Walsh M, Romo-Cardoso S, et al: Distal radial fractures in the elderly: operative compared with nonoperative treatment. *J Bone Joint Surg Am* 92(9):1851–1857, 2010.
42. Egol K, Walsh M, Tejwani N, et al: Bridging external fixation and supplementary Kirschner-wire fixation versus volar locked plating for unstable fractures of the distal radius: a randomised, prospective trial. *J Bone Joint Surg Br* 90(9):1214–1221, 2008.
43. Erhart S, Schmoelz W, Arora R, et al: The biomechanical effects of a deepened articular cavity during dynamic motion of the wrist joint. *Clin Biomech (Bristol, Avon)* 27(6):557–561, 2012.
44. Erhart S, Schmoelz W, Lutz M: Clinical and biomechanical investigation of an increased articular cavity depth after distal radius fractures: effect on range of motion, osteoarthrosis and loading patterns. *Arch Orthop Trauma Surg* 133(9):1249–1255, 2013.
45. Esposito J, Schemitsch EH, Saccone M, et al: External fixation versus open reduction with plate fixation for distal radius fractures: a meta-analysis of randomised controlled trials. *Injury* 44(4):409–416, 2013.
46. Fernandez DL: Correction of post-traumatic wrist deformity in adults by osteotomy, bone-grafting, and internal fixation. *J Bone Joint Surg Am* 64(8):1164–1178, 1982.
47. Fernandez DL: Fractures of the distal radius: operative treatment. *Instr Course Lect* 42:73–88, 1993.
48. Fitoussi F, Ip WY, Chow SP: Treatment of displaced intra-articular fractures of the distal end of the radius with plates. *J Bone Joint Surg Am* 79(9):1303–1312, 1997.
49. Frykman GK: Fracture of the distal radius including sequelae-shoulder-hand-finger syndrome, disturbance in the distal radioulnar joint and impairment of nerve function. A clinical and experimental study. *Acta Orthop Scand* 108:1–25, 1967.
50. Gartland JJ, Werley CW: Evaluation of healed Colles' fractures. *J Bone Joint Surg Am* 33A(4):895–907, 1951.
51. Gehrmann SV, Windolf J, Kaufmann RA: Distal radius fracture management in elderly patients: a literature review. *J Hand Surg [Am]* 33(3):421–429, 2008.
52. Geissler WB: Arthroscopically assisted reduction of intra-articular fractures of the distal radius. *Hand Clin* 11(1):19–29, 1995.
53. Geissler WB, Fernandez DL: Percutaneous and limited open reduction of the articular surface of the distal radius. *J Orthop Trauma* 5(3):255–264, 1991.
54. Geissler WB, Freeland AE: Arthroscopic management of intra-articular distal radius fractures. *Hand Clin* 15(3):455–465, viii, 1999.
55. Geissler WB, Freeland AE, Savoie FH, et al: Intracarpal soft-tissue lesions associated with an intra-articular fracture of the distal end of the radius. *J Bone Joint Surg Am* 78(3):357–365, 1996.
56. Ginn TA, Ruch DS, Yang CC, et al: Use of a distraction plate for distal radial fractures with metaphyseal and diaphyseal comminution. Surgical technique. *J Bone Joint Surg Am* 88(Suppl 1 Pt 1):29–36, 2006.
57. Goehre F, Otto W, Schwan S, et al: Comparison of palmar fixed-angle plate fixation with K-wire fixation of distal radius fractures (AO A2, A3, C1) in elderly patients. *J Hand Surg Eur Vol* 39(3):249–257, 2014.
58. Goldfarb CA, Rudzki JR, Catalano LW, et al: Fifteen-year outcome of displaced intra-articular fractures of the distal radius. *J Hand Surg [Am]* 31(4):633–639, 2006.
59. Goldhahn J, Beaton D, Ladd A, et al: Recommendation for measuring clinical outcome in distal radius fractures: a core set of domains for standardized reporting in clinical practice and research. *Arch Orthop Trauma Surg* 134(2):197–205, 2014.
60. Gradl G, Jupiter JB, Gierer P, et al: Fractures of the distal radius treated with a nonbridging external fixation technique using multiplanar k-wires. *J Hand Surg [Am]* 30(5):960–968, 2005.
61. Grewal R, MacDermid JC: The risk of adverse outcomes in extra-articular distal radius fractures is increased with malalignment in patients of all ages but mitigated in older patients. *J Hand Surg [Am]* 32(7):962–970, 2007.
62. Grewal R, MacDermid JC, King GJ, et al: Open reduction internal fixation versus percutaneous pinning with external fixation of distal radius fractures: a prospective, randomized clinical trial. *J Hand Surg [Am]* 36(12):1899–1906, 2011.
63. Grewel R, Perey B, Wilmink M, et al: A randomized trial on the treatment of intra-articular distal radius fractures: open reduction internal fixation with dorsal plating versus mini open reduction, percutaneous pinning and external fixation. *J Hand Surg [Am]* 30A:764–772, 2005.
64. Gyuricza C, Carlson MG, Weiland AJ, et al: Removal of locked volar plates after distal radius fractures. *J Hand Surg [Am]* 36(6):982–985, 2011.
65. Hagert CG: Distal radius fracture and the distal radioulnar joint—anatomical considerations. *Handchir Mikrochir Plast Chir* 26(1):22–26, 1994.
66. Hagert E, Hagert CG: Understanding stability of the distal radioulnar joint by understanding its anatomy. *Hand Clin* 26:459–466, 2010.
67. Handoll HH, Huntley JS, Madhok R: External fixation versus conservative treatment for distal radial fractures in adults. *Cochrane Database Syst Rev* (3):CD006194, 2007.
68. Handoll HH, Madhok R: Surgical interventions for treating distal radial fractures in adults. *Cochrane Database Syst Rev* (3):CD003209, 2003.
69. Handoll HH, Vaghela MV, Madhok R: Percutaneous pinning for treating distal radial fractures in adults. *Cochrane Database Syst Rev* (3):CD006080, 2007.
70. Handoll HH, Watts AC: Bone grafts and bone substitutes for treating distal radial fractures in adults. *Cochrane Database Syst Rev* (2):CD006836, 2008.
71. Hanel DP, Ruhlman SD, Katolik LI, et al: Complications associated with distraction plate fixation of wrist fractures. *Hand Clin* 26(2):237–243, 2010.
72. Harley BJ, Scharfenberger A, Beaupre LA, et al: Augmented external fixation versus percutaneous pinning and casting for unstable fractures of the distal radius—a prospective randomized trial. *J Hand Surg [Am]* 29(5):815–824, 2004.
73. Harness N, Ring D, Jupiter JB: Volar Barton's fractures with concomitant dorsal fracture in older patients. *J Hand Surg [Am]* 29(3):439–445, 2004.
74. Harness NG, Ring D, Zurakowski D, et al: The influence of three-dimensional computed tomography reconstructions on the characterization and treatment of distal radial fractures. *J Bone Joint Surg Am* 88(6):1315–1323, 2006.
75. Hayes AJ, Duffy PJ, McQueen MM: Bridging and non-bridging external fixation in the treatment of unstable fractures of the distal radius: a retrospective study of 588 patients. *Acta Orthop* 79(4):540–547, 2008.
76. Herford AS, King BJ, Audia F, et al: Medial approach for tibial bone graft: anatomic study and clinical technique. *J Oral Maxillofac Surg* 61(3):358–363, 2003.
77. Jakob M, Rikli DA, Regazzoni P: Fractures of the distal radius treated by internal fixation and early function. A prospective study of 73 consecutive patients. *J Bone Joint Surg Br* 82B(3):340–344, 2000.
78. Joseph SJ, Harvey JN: The dorsal horizon view: detecting screw protrusion at the distal radius. *J Hand Surg [Am]* 36(10):1691–1693, 2011.
79. Jupiter JB: Commentary: the effect of ulnar styloid fractures on patient-rated outcomes after volar locking plating of distal radius fractures. *J Hand Surg [Am]* 34(9):1603–1604, 2009.
80. Jupiter JB, Marent-Huber M: Operative management of distal radial fractures with 2.4-millimeter locking plates. A multicenter prospective case series. *J Bone Joint Surg Am* 91(1):55–65, 2009.
81. Jupiter JB, Ring D, Weitzel PP: Surgical treatment of redisplaced fractures of the distal radius in patients older than 60 years. *J Hand Surg [Am]* 27(4):714–723, 2002.
82. Kaempffe FA, Wheeler DR, Peimer CA, et al: Severe fractures of the distal radius: effect of amount and duration of external fixator distraction on outcome. *J Hand Surg [Am]* 18(1):33–41, 1993.
83. Kambouroglou GK, Axelrod TS: Complications of the AO/ASIF titanium distal radius plate system (pin plate) in internal fixation of the distal radius: a brief report. *J Hand Surg [Am]* 23(4):737–741, 1998.
84. Kang L, Ek E, et al: Biomechanical analysis of scapholunate ligament repair techniques. *JHS* 2015 epub ahead of print.
85. Kapandji AI, Epinette JA: Colles' fractures: Treatment by double intrafocal wire fixation. In Razemon JP, Fisk GR, editors: *The wrist*, New York, 1988, Churchill Livingstone, pp 65–73.
86. Kapoor H, Agarwal A, Dhaon BK: Displaced intra-articular fractures of distal radius: a comparative evaluation of results following closed reduction, external fixation and open reduction with internal fixation. *Injury* 31(2):75–79, 2000.
87. Karantana A, Downing ND, Forward DP, et al: Surgical treatment of distal radial fractures with a volar locking plate versus conventional percutaneous methods: a randomized controlled trial. *J Bone Joint Surg Am* 95(19):1737–1744, 2013.
88. Karnezis IA, Panagiotopoulos E, Tyllianakis M, et al: Correlation between radiological parameters and patient-rated wrist dysfunction following fractures of the distal radius. *Injury* 36(12):1435–1439, 2005.
89. Kim JK, Koh YD, Do NH: Should an ulnar styloid fracture be fixed following volar plate fixation of a distal radial fracture? *J Bone Joint Surg Am* 92(1):1–6, 2010.
90. Kitay A, Swanstrom M, Schreiber JJ, et al: Volar plate position and flexor tendon rupture following distal radius fracture fixation. *J Hand Surg [Am]* 38(6):1091–1096, 2013.

91. Kleinman WB, Graham TJ: The distal radioulnar joint capsule: clinical anatomy and role in posttraumatic limitation of forearm rotation. *J Hand Surg [Am]* 23(4):588–599, 1998.

92. Knirk JL, Jupiter JB: Intra-articular fractures of the distal end of the radius in young adults. *J Bone Joint Surg Am* 68(5):647–659, 1986.

93. Kodama N, Takemura Y, Ueba H, et al: Acceptable parameters for alignment of distal radius fracture with conservative treatment in elderly patients. *J Orthop Sci* 19(2):292–297, 2014.

94. Konrath GA, Bahler S: Open reduction and internal fixation of unstable distal radius fractures: results using the trimed fixation system. *J Orthop Trauma* 16(8):578–585, 2002.

95. Koval KJ, Harrast JJ, Anglen JO, et al: Fractures of the distal part of the radius. The evolution of practice over time. Where's the evidence? *J Bone Joint Surg Am* 90(9):1855–1861, 2008.

96. Kreder HJ, Agel J, McKee MD, et al: A randomized, controlled trial of distal radius fractures with metaphyseal displacement but without joint incongruity: closed reduction and casting versus closed reduction, spanning external fixation, and optional percutaneous K-wires. *J Orthop Trauma* 20(2):115–121, 2006.

97. Kreder HJ, Hanel DP, Agel J, et al: Indirect reduction and percutaneous fixation versus open reduction and internal fixation for displaced intra-articular fractures of the distal radius. *J Bone Joint Surg Br* 87-B:829–836, 2005.

98. Kreder HJ, Hanel DP, McKee M, et al: Consistency of AO fracture classification for the distal radius. *J Bone Joint Surg Br* 78(5):726–731, 1996.

99. Ladd AL, Pliam NB: The role of bone graft and alternatives in unstable distal radius fracture treatment. *Orthop Clin North Am* 30(2):337–351, 2001.

100. Lafontaine M, Hardy D, Delince PH: Stability assessment of distal radius fractures. *Injury* 20(4):208–210, 1989.

101. Lamey DM, Fernandez DL: Results of the modified Sauvé-Kapandji procedure in the treatment of chronic posttraumatic derangement of the distal radioulnar joint. *J Bone Joint Surg Am* 80(12):1758–1769, 1998.

102. Leslie BM, Medoff RJ: Fracture specific fixation of distal radius fractures. *Tech Orthop* 15(4):336–352, 2000.

103. Leung KS, So WS, Chiu VD, et al: Ligamentotaxis for comminuted distal radial fractures modified by primary cancellous grafting and functional bracing: long-term results. *J Orthop Trauma* 5(3):265–271, 1991.

104. Lozano-Calderón SA, Doornberg J, Ring D: Fractures of the dorsal articular margin of the distal part of the radius with dorsal radiocarpal subluxation. *J Bone Joint Surg Am* 88(7):1486–1493, 2006.

105. Lozano-Calderón SA, Doornberg JN, Ring D: Retrospective comparison of percutaneous fixation and volar internal fixation of distal radius fractures. *Hand (NY)* 3(2):102–110, 2008.

106. Ludvigsen TC, Johansen S, Svenningsen S, et al: External fixation versus percutaneous pinning for unstable Colles' fracture. Equal outcome in a randomized study of 60 patients. *Acta Orthop Scand* 68(3):255–258, 1997.

107. MacKenney PJ, McQueen MM, Elton R: Prediction of instability in distal radius fractures. *J Bone Joint Surg Am* 88:1944–1951, 2006.

108. Mattila VM, Huttunen TT, Sillanpaa P, et al: Significant change in the surgical treatment of distal radius fractures: a nationwide study between 1998 and 2008 in Finland. *J Trauma* 71(4):939–942, 2011.

109. McFadyen I, Field J, McCann P, et al: Should unstable extra-articular distal radial fractures be treated with fixed-angle volar-locked plates or percutaneous Kirschner wires? A prospective randomised controlled trial. *Injury* 42(2):162–166, 2011.

110. McQueen MM: Redisplaced unstable fractures of the distal radius. A randomised, prospective study of bridging versus non-bridging external fixation. *J Bone Joint Surg Br* 80(4):665–669, 1998.

111. McQueen MM, Caspers J: Colles' fracture: does the anatomical result affect the final function? *J Bone Joint Surg Am* 34A(3):649–651, 1988.

112. McQueen MM, Hajducka C, Court-Brown CM: Redisplaced unstable fractures of the distal radius: a prospective randomised comparison of four methods of treatment. *J Bone Joint Surg Br* 78(3):404–409, 1996.

113. McQueen MM, Michie M, Court-Brown CM: Hand and wrist function after external fixation of unstable distal radial fractures. *Clin Orthop* 285:200–204, 1992.

114. Medoff RJ: Essential radiographic evaluation for distal radius fractures. *Hand Clin* 21:279–288, 2005.

115. Melone CP, Jr: Articular fractures of the distal radius. *Orthop Clin North Am* 15(2):217–236, 1984.

116. Menendez ME, Bot AG, Hageman MG, et al: Computerized adaptive testing of psychological factors: relation to upper-extremity disability. *J Bone Joint Surg Am* 95(20):e149, 2013.

117. Moore AM, Dennison DG: Distal radius fractures and the volar lunate facet fragment: Kirschner wire fixation in addition to volar-locked plating. *Hand (NY)* 9(2):230–236, 2014.

118. Moritomo H, Omori S: Influence of ulnar translation of the radial shaft in distal radius fracture on distal radioulnar joint instability. *J Wrist Surg* 3(1):18–21, 2014.

119. Nakamura T, Iwamoto T, Matsumura N, et al: Radiographic and arthroscopic assessment of DRUJ instability due to foveal avulsion of the radioulnar ligament in distal radius fractures. *J Wrist Surg* 3(1):12–17, 2014.

120. Neuhaus V, Badri O, Ferree S, et al: Radiographic alignment of unstable distal radius fractures fixed with 1 or 2 rows of screws in volar locking plates. *J Hand Surg [Am]* 38(2):297–301, 2013.

121. Nishiwaki M, Tazaki K, Shimizu H, et al: Prospective study of distal radial fractures treated with an intramedullary nail. *J Bone Joint Surg Am* 93(15):1436–1441, 2011.

122. Noda K, Goto A, Murase T, et al: Interosseous membrane of the forearm: an anatomical study of ligament attachment locations. *J Hand Surg [Am]* 34(3):415–422, 2009.

123. O'Connor D, Mullett H, Doyle M, et al: Minimally displaced Colles' fractures: a prospective randomized trial of treatment with a wrist splint or a plaster cast. *J Hand Surg [Br]* 28(1):50–53, 2003.

124. Orbay JL: Ulnar head and styloid fractures. In Slutsky DJ, editor: *Principles and practice of wrist surgery*, Philadelphia, 2010, WB Saunders, pp 198–204.

125. Orbay JL, Fernandez DL: Volar fixation for dorsally displaced fractures of the distal radius: a preliminary report. *J Hand Surg [Am]* 27(2):205–215, 2002.

126. Orbay JL, Fernandez DL: Volar fixed-angle plate fixation for unstable distal radius fractures in the elderly patient. *J Hand Surg [Am]* 29(1):96–102, 2004.

127. Ozer K, Wolf JM, Watkins B, et al: Comparison of 4 fluoroscopic views for dorsal cortex screw penetration after volar plating of the distal radius. *J Hand Surg [Am]* 37(5):963–967, 2012.

128. Palmer AK, Werner FW: Biomechanics of the distal radioulnar joint. *Clin Orthop* 187:26–35, 1984.

129. Peine R, Rikli DA, Hoffmann R, et al: Comparison of three different plating techniques for the dorsum of the distal radius: A biomechanical study. *J Hand Surg [Am]* 25A(1):29–33, 2000.

130. Rapley JH, Kearny JP, Schrayer A, et al: Ulnar translation, a commonly overlooked, unrecognized deformity of distal radius fractures: techniques to correct the malalignment. *Tech Hand Up Extrem Surg* 12(3):166–169, 2008.

131. Rayhack JM, Langworthy JN, Belsole RJ: Transulnar percutaneous pinning of displaced distal radial fractures: a preliminary report. *J Orthop Trauma* 3(2):107–114, 1989.

132. Rikli DA, Kupfer K, Bodoky A: Long-term results of the external fixation of distal radius fractures. *J Trauma* 44(6):970–976, 1998.

133. Rikli DA, Regazzoni P: Fractures of the distal end of the radius treated by internal fixation and early function. A preliminary report of 20 cases. *J Bone Joint Surg Br* 78(4):588–592, 1996.

134. Ross M, Di ML, Peters S, et al: Defining residual radial translation of distal radius fractures: a potential cause of distal radioulnar joint instability. *J Wrist Surg* 3(1):22–29, 2014.

135. Roth KM, Blazar PE, Earp BE, et al: Incidence of extensor pollicis longus tendon rupture after nondisplaced distal radius fractures. *J Hand Surg [Am]* 37(5):942–947, 2012.

136. Roth KM, Blazar PE, Earp BE, et al: Incidence of displacement after nondisplaced distal radial fractures in adults. *J Bone Joint Surg Am* 95(15):1398–1402, 2013.

137. Rozental TD, Blazar PE, Franko OI, et al: Functional outcomes for unstable distal radial fractures treated with open reduction and internal fixation or closed reduction and percutaneous fixation. A prospective randomized trial. *J Bone Joint Surg Am* 91(8):1837–1846, 2009.

138. Rozental TD, Makhni EC, Day CS, et al: Improving evaluation and treatment for osteoporosis following distal radial fractures. A prospective randomized intervention. *J Bone Joint Surg Am* 90(5):953–961, 2008.

139. Ruch DS, Wray WH, III, Papadonikolakis A, et al: Corrective osteotomy for isolated malunion of the palmar lunate facet in distal radius fractures. *J Hand Surg [Am]* 35(11):1779–1786, 2010.

140. Sammer DM, Shah HM, Shauver MJ, et al: The effect of ulnar styloid fractures on patient-rated outcomes after volar locking plating of distal radius fractures. *J Hand Surg [Am]* 34(9):1595–1602, 2009.

141. Scheck M: Long-term follow-up of treatment of comminuted fractures of the distal end of the radius by transfixation with Kirshner wires and cast. *J Bone Joint Surg* 44A:337–351, 1962.

142. Seitz WH, Jr, Froimson AI, Leb R, et al: Augmented external fixation of unstable distal radius fractures. *J Hand Surg [Am]* 16(6):1010–1016, 1991.

143. Seitz WH, Jr, Putnam MD, Dick HM: Limited open surgical approach for external fixation of distal radius fractures. *J Hand Surg Am* 15A:288–293, 1990.

144. Shauver MJ, Chang KW, Chung KC: Contribution of functional parameters to patient-rated outcomes after surgical treatment of distal radius fractures. *J Hand Surg [Am]* 39(3):436–442, 2014.

145. Shauver MJ, Clapham PJ, Chung KC: An economic analysis of outcomes and complications of treating distal radius fractures in the elderly. *J Hand Surg [Am]* 36(12):1912–1918, 2011.

146. Short WH, Palmer AK, Werner FW, et al: A biomechanical study of distal radial fractures. *J Hand Surg [Am]* 12(4):529–534, 1987.

147. Soong M, Earp BE, Bishop G, et al: Volar locking plate implant prominence and flexor tendon rupture. *J Bone Joint Surg Am* 93(4):328–335, 2011.

148. Souer JS, Ring D, Matschke S, et al: Effect of an unrepaired fracture of the ulnar styloid base on outcome after plate-and-screw fixation of a distal radial fracture. *J Bone Joint Surg Am* 91(4):830–838, 2009.

149. Srinivasan RC, Jain D, Richard MJ, et al: Isolated ulnar shortening osteotomy for the treatment of extra-articular distal radius malunion. *J Hand Surg [Am]* 38(6):1106–1110, 2013.

150. Stockmans F, Dezillie M, Vanhaecke J: Accuracy of 3D virtual planning of corrective osteotomies of the distal radius. *J Wrist Surg* 2(4):306–314, 2013.

151. Swart E, Nellans K, Rosenwasser M: The effects of pain, supination, and grip strength on patient-rated disability after operatively treated distal radius fractures. *J Hand Surg [Am]* 37(5):957–962, 2012.

152. Taleisnik J, Watson HK: Midcarpal instability caused by malunited fractures of the distal radius. *J Hand Surg [Am]* 9(3):350–357, 1984.

153. Trousdale RT, Amadio PC, Cooney WP, et al: Radio-ulnar dissociation. A review of twenty cases. *J Bone Joint Surg Am* 74(10):1486–1497, 1992.

154. Tumia N, Wardlaw D, Hallett J, et al: Aberdeen Colles' fracture brace as a treatment for Colles' fracture. A multicentre, prospective, randomised, controlled trial. *J Bone Joint Surg Br* 85(1):78–82, 2003.

155. van Kampen RJ, Thoreson AR, Knutson NJ, et al: Comparison of a new intramedullary scaffold to volar plating for treatment of distal radius fractures. *J Orthop Trauma* 27(9):535–541, 2013.

156. van Schoonhoven J, Fernandez DL, Bowers WH, et al: Salvage of failed resection arthroplasties of the distal radioulnar joint using a new ulnar head prosthesis. *J Hand Surg [Am]* 25(3):438–446, 2000.

157. Vidal J, Adrey J, Connes H, et al: A biomechanical study and clinical application of the use of Hoffman's external fixator. In Brooker AF, Edwards CC, editors: *External fixation: current state of the art*, Baltimore, 1979, Williams & Wilkins, pp 327–343.

158. Wada T, Tatebe M, Ozasa Y, et al: Clinical outcomes of corrective osteotomy for distal radial malunion: a review of opening and closing-wedge techniques. *J Bone Joint Surg Am* 93(17):1619–1626, 2011.

159. Wang J, Yang Y, Ma J, et al: Open reduction and internal fixation versus external fixation for unstable distal radial fractures: a meta-analysis. *Orthop Traumatol Surg Res* 99(3):321–331, 2013.

160. Washburn RA, Smith KW, Jette AM, et al: The physical activity scale for the elderly (PASE): development and evaluation. *J Clin Epidemiol* 46(2):153–162, 1993.

161. Watanabe H, Berger RA, Berglund LJ, et al: Contribution of the interosseous membrane to distal radioulnar joint constraint. *J Hand Surg [Am]* 30(6):1164–1171, 2005.

162. Watson HK, Castle TH, Jr: Trapezoidal osteotomy of the distal radius for unacceptable articular angulation after Colles' fracture [see comments]. *J Hand Surg [Am]* 13(6):837–843, 1988.

163. Watson HK, Gabuzda GM: Matched distal ulna resection for posttraumatic disorders of the distal radioulnar joint. *J Hand Surg [Am]* 17(4):724–730, 1992.

164. Watters WC, Sanders JO, Murray J, et al: The American Academy of Orthopaedic Surgeons Appropriate Use Criteria on the treatment of distal radius fractures. *J Bone Joint Surg Am* 96(2):160–161, 2014.

165. Weber SC, Szabo RM: Severely comminuted distal radial fracture as an unsolved problem: complications associated with external fixation and pins and plaster techniques. *J Hand Surg [Am]* 11(2):157–165, 1986.

166. Wijffels M, Ring D: The influence of non-union of the ulnar styloid on pain, wrist function and instability after distal radius fracture. *J Hand Microsurg* 3(1):11–14, 2011.

167. Wilcke MK, Abbaszadegan H, Adolphson PY: Patient-perceived outcome after displaced distal radius fractures. A comparison between radiological parameters, objective physical variables, and the DASH score. *J Hand Ther* 20(4):290–298, 2007.

168. Wilcke MK, Abbaszadegan H, Adolphson PY: Wrist function recovers more rapidly after volar locked plating than after external fixation but the outcomes are similar after 1 year. *Acta Orthop* 82(1):76–81, 2011.

169. Williksen JH, Frihagen F, Hellund JC, et al: Volar locking plates versus external fixation and adjuvant pin fixation in unstable distal radius fractures: a randomized, controlled study. *J Hand Surg [Am]* 38(8):1469–1476, 2013.

170. Wolfe SW, Austin G, Lorenze MD, et al: Comparative stability of external fixation: a biomechanical study. *J Hand Surg [Am]* 24A:516–524, 1999.

171. Wolfe SW, Easterling KE, Yoo H: Arthroscopic-assisted reduction of distal radius fractures. *Arthroscopy* 11(6):706–714, 1995.

172. Wolfe SW, Swigart CR, Grauer J, et al: Augmented external fixation of distal radius fractures: A biomechanical analysis. *J Hand Surg [Am]* 23A(1):127–134, 1998.

173. Wong TC, Chiu Y, Tsang WL, et al: Casting versus percutaneous pinning for extra-articular fractures of the distal radius in an elderly Chinese population: a prospective randomised controlled trial. *J Hand Surg Eur Vol* 35(3):202–208, 2010.

174. Wright TW, Horodyski M, Smith DW: Functional outcome of unstable distal radius fractures: ORIF with a volar fixed-angle tine plate versus external fixation. *J Hand Surg [Am]* 30(2):289–299, 2005.

175. Young BT, Rayan GM: Outcome following nonoperative treatment of displaced distal radius fractures in low-demand patients older than 60 years. *J Hand Surg [Am]* 25(1):19–28, 2000.

176. Young CF, Nanu AM, Checketts RG: Seven-year outcome following Colles' type distal radial fracture. A comparison of two treatment methods. *J Hand Surg [Br]* 28(5):422–426, 2003.

177. Yu YR, Makhni MC, Tabrizi S, et al: Complications of low-profile dorsal versus volar locking plates in the distal radius: a comparative study. *J Hand Surg [Am]* 36(7):1135–1141, 2011.

178. Zollinger PE, Tuinebreijer WE, Breederveld RS, et al: Can vitamin C prevent complex regional pain syndrome in patients with wrist fractures? A randomized, controlled, multicenter dose-response study. *J Bone Joint Surg Am* 89(7):1424–1431, 2007.

16

Fractures of the Carpal Bones

Steve K. Lee

Acknowledgments: I would like to give full acknowledgment to the authors of the previous version of this chapter, Dr. William B. Geissler and the late Dr. Joseph F. Slade. Their chapter was the foundation of the current chapter; I have maintained many of their principles but have updated the chapter with my own thoughts, influenced by prime mentors of mine, Drs. Martin Posner, Scott Wolfe, and Michael Hausman. Dr. Slade was one of my mentors and teachers from residency. Most know of his contributions to hand and upper extremity surgery and his continual willingness to teach and instruct worldwide. His dedication and enthusiasm for hand surgery are legendary and are an inspiration to us all. Thank you also to Dr. Geissler, who continues to be a pioneer in our specialty. Acknowledgments to Dr. Dean G. Sotereanos and Dr. James P. Higgins, who authored two of the Case Studies for this chapter available on ExpertConsult.com. I also wish to acknowledge Zina Model, BA, for editorial assistance.

> ▶ These videos may be found at
> *ExpertConsult.com:*
> **16.1** Arthroscopic fixation scaphoid of nonunion

SCAPHOID FRACTURES AND NONUNION

The treatment of scaphoid fractures requires knowledge of the blood supply, surgical approaches, and effects that fractures and nonunions of the scaphoid have on carpal kinematics, stability, and arthritis.[211] Vigilant care of these fractures can usually lead to a functional result for the patient. However, incorrect fracture healing can potentially lead to a relentless downward spiral of wear and cartilage damage. Chronic pain and dysfunction of the wrist results, which affects both hand function and the entire upper extremity.

Within the past two decades, methods of scaphoid repair have been developed to minimize additional surgical trauma and optimize stabilization until healing. Minimally invasive fixation has been demonstrated to have a higher union rate than cast treatment and has relatively few complications. This approach allows the patient or athlete to return to work or sports within weeks or months, whereas a failed attempt at healing with cast immobilization can result in months of lost time, compounded by the increased complexity, cost, and complications of nonunion repair. This chapter will explore the mechanics, biologic factors, and modern treatment regimens for fractures of the scaphoid and neighboring carpal bones.

General Considerations in Fractures and Nonunion of the Scaphoid
Incidence and Cause of Scaphoid Fractures

The scaphoid bone garners more interest in upper extremity surgery for its weight and size than any other bone because it is the "keystone" of the carpus. In architecture, the keystone is the central stone at the summit of an arch, locking the whole together. Likewise, the scaphoid links the carpus together. Pathologic conditions of the scaphoid can affect the entire wrist.

The scaphoid is not only important but it is the most commonly fractured carpal bone. Scaphoid fractures account for 60% to 70% of all carpal fractures and are second in frequency of wrist fractures only to distal radius fractures. The majority of injuries are low-energy injuries, either from a sporting event (59%) or from a fall onto an outstretched wrist (35%); the remainder result from high-energy trauma such as a fall from a height or a motor vehicle injury. Howe documented that 82% of the scaphoid fractures in Norway occur in males, with an average age of 25 years (range, 11 to 79 years).[100] The age-specific incidence in males remained significantly higher than that in females until age 60 years, at which point the incidences were similar. The annual incidence was 43 per 100,000 people.[2] The statistics were similar in Larsen's series; the mechanism for scaphoid fracture was a fall in 69% of cases and a blow to the wrist in 28% of cases.[126]

More recently, Wolf studied a large U.S. military population and found a greater incidence of scaphoid fracture than the previous data had shown, 121 per 100,000 person-years.[224] Males and the 20- to 24-year-old age group were associated with higher rates of scaphoid injury.[224] The more active nature of the occupations of this population may explain this higher incidence. Van Tassel and colleagues[209a] showed a peak incidence in scaphoid fractures in the second decade, and few after age 50 years (Figure 16.1).

⬥ PERTINENT ANATOMY OF THE SCAPHOID

Bony and Ligamentous Anatomy. The shape of the scaphoid bone has been described with several terms: as a boat ("skaphos" in Greek), as a twisted peanut, and as bean shaped. The complex shape of the bone can present challenges to reconstruction and fixation. Approximately 80% of the scaphoid is covered by cartilage, limiting ligamentous attachment and vascular supply (Figure 16.2).[7,17] The scaphoid is divided into three regions: proximal pole, waist, and distal pole (tubercle). The proximal pole articulates with the scaphoid fossa of the distal radius and the lunate. The scaphoid is oriented in the carpus with an intrascaphoid angle averaging 40 ± 3 degrees in the coronal plane and 32 ± 5 degrees in the sagittal plane.[7,17]

The scaphoid is the only carpal bone that bridges the proximal and distal carpal rows and acts as a tie-rod. The carpal rows are supported by stout intrinsic ligaments and reinforced by a complex system of volar and dorsal extrinsic ligaments (Figure 16.3). The scapholunate interosseous ligament (SLIL) is a stout ligament connecting the scaphoid to the lunate and is the primary stabilizer. The dorsal aspect of this ligament is composed of transverse collagen fibers, whereas the palmar ligament is composed of oblique collagen fibers inserting to the volar capsular ligaments. The dorsal portion is twice as strong as the anterior portion. Only 20 to 30 degrees of motion is possible at an intact scapholunate interval.[2] The dorsal and palmar regions are critical in maintaining normal carpal kinematics and function of the scapholunate interval. The dorsal region resists palmar-dorsal translation and gap, whereas the volar portion resists rotation. The proximal fibrocartilaginous region is the weakest mechanically and is well suited to accept the compression and shear loads at the radiocarpal joint. The radioscaphocapitate (RSC) ligament originates from the volar radial aspect of the radius, crosses the volar concavity of the scaphoid waist, and proceeds ulnarly toward the capitate, acting as a fulcrum around which the scaphoid rotates. The scaphoid can also fracture around this fulcrum at the waist. The scaphocapitate ligament originates from the distal scaphoid at the border between the trapezoid facet and the capitate facet. It inserts into the volar

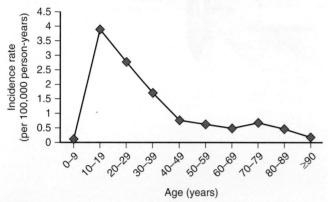

FIGURE 16.1 Incidence of scaphoid fracture by age decade. (See Van Tassel Reprinted, with permission, from Elsevier.)

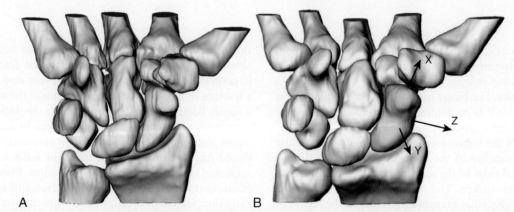

FIGURE 16.2 A, A three-dimensional reconstruction of the scaphoid from CT images of 25 normal wrists. Note the scaphoid's position spanning the proximal and distal carpal rows and acting as a "tie-rod" to coordinate smooth carpal motion. **B,** Eighty percent of the normal scaphoid surface is covered by articular cartilage. The scaphoid derives its name from its peculiar boat- or skiff-shaped contour. *X*, rotation (pronation/supination); *Y*, sagittal (flexion/extension); *Z*, coronal (radial/ulnar). (**A,** From Joseph J. Crisco, PhD, Department of Orthopaedics, The Alpert Medical School of Brown University and Rhode Island Hospital.)

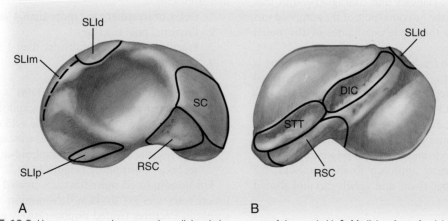

FIGURE 16.3 Ligamentous attachments to the radial and ulnar aspects of the scaphoid. **A,** Medial surface of a right scaphoid demonstrating the attachment zones of the scaphocapitate ligament (*SC*), the radioscaphocapitate ligament (*RSC*), and the dorsal (*SLId*), membranous (*SLIm*), and palmar (*SLIp*) regions of the scapholunate interosseous ligament. **B,** Right scaphoid from a dorsal radial perspective demonstrating the attachment zones of the scaphotrapeziotrapezoidal ligament (*STT*), RSC, dorsal intercarpal ligament (*DIC*), and SLId. (Copyright Elizabeth Martin.)

VOLAR   DORSAL

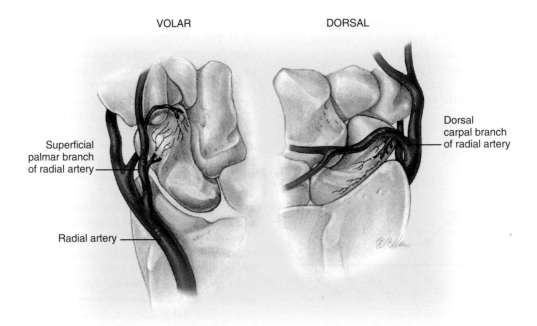

Superficial
palmar branch
of radial artery

Dorsal
carpal branch
of radial artery

Radial artery

FIGURE 16.4 Schematic representation of the blood supply of the scaphoid. (Copyright Elizabeth Martin.)

waist of the capitate distal to the RSC ligament. This ligament, along with the scaphotrapezial ligament, functions as a primary restraint of the distal pole.

Vascular Anatomy. The blood supply of the scaphoid bone is not robust, because it is predominantly retrograde. The major blood supply to the scaphoid is via the radial artery: Seventy percent to 80% of the intraosseous and proximal pole vascular supply is from branches of the radial artery entering distally through the dorsal ridge of the scaphoid between the proximal and distal articular surfaces. The radial artery or the superficial palmar arch also give volar branches that enter in the region of the tubercle and provide the blood supply to 20% to 30% of the bone in the region of the distal pole (Figure 16.4).[73] The proximal pole also gets blood supply from the radioscapholunate ligament (ligament of Testut, a neurovascular conduit) and directs scapholunate branches from the palmar and dorsal transverse carpal arches.[29] Handley and colleagues found that the venous drainage from the proximal pole of the scaphoid was via the dorsal ridge into the venae comitantes of the radial artery.[86]

The more proximal the fracture, the more likely the bone is to be dysvascular and the higher the risk of nonunion. Proximal pole fractures have been reported to have an incidence of avascular necrosis (AVN) of 13% to 50%.[194] Knowledge of the vascular anatomy has implications for sensible approaches to the scaphoid. Combined palmar and dorsal approaches taking off the soft tissue at the tubercle *and* the dorsal ridge would not be advisable. During the dorsal approach to the scaphoid, the majority of the dorsal ridge tissue and vessels can and should be left intact.

Biomechanics of Scaphoid Fractures and Implications of Nonunion

Although the exact mechanism of fracture is not completely understood, hyperextension past 95 degrees[219] is the usual posi-

tion of injury, but other mechanisms such as axial loading have also been postulated to produce scaphoid fractures,[99] as has hyperflexion of the wrist. With the hyperextension mechanism, a fracture of the scaphoid usually begins at the volar waist with a tensile failure; the forces propagate to the dorsal surface with compression loading, until failure occurs. In a cadaveric study, wrists placed in extreme dorsiflexion and ulnar deviation produced fractures through the scaphoid waist as the scaphoid impinged on the dorsal rim of the radius. Proximal scaphoid fractures resulted from dorsal subluxation during forced hyperextension. Carpal dislocations and scapholunate ligament tears were reproduced with wrist extension and ulnar deviation, combined with intercarpal supination.[138]

As with any fracture, the potential for healing relies on the fracture's location, vascularity, and stability. Nonunion occurs in 10% to 15% of all scaphoid fractures. The risk of nonunion increases with:

1. Delay of treatment for more than 4 weeks
2. Proximal pole fractures
3. Fracture displacement greater than 1 mm
4. Osteonecrosis
5. Tobacco use
6. Associated carpal instability (DISI = dorsal intercalated segmental instability with a scapholunate angle > 60 degrees and a capitolunate angle > 15 degrees) secondary to humpback (flexed with intrascaphoid angle > 45 degrees; the normal intrascaphoid angle is 24 degrees) scaphoid positioning (Figure 16.5).[40,125,199]

For nondisplaced waist fractures treated with casting, nonunion rates are 5% to 12%.[39] Nonunion rates for displaced scaphoid fractures treated nonoperatively are higher, reaching 50%.[199]

Untreated displaced fractures of the waist are subject to varying degrees of these forces and will usually angulate as the volar bone is reabsorbed, yielding a "humpback" of flexion

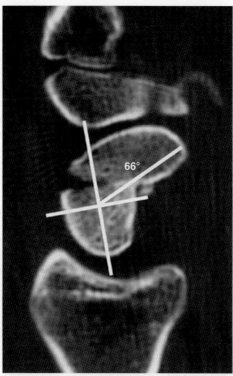

FIGURE 16.5 Example of intrascaphoid angle of 66 degrees. (From Trumble TE, Gilbert M, Murray LW, et al: Displaced scaphoid fractures treated with open reduction and internal fixation with a cannulated screw. *J Bone Joint Surg Am* 82(5):633–641, 2000.)

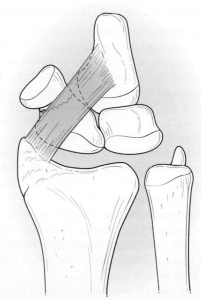

FIGURE 16.6 The radioscaphocapitate ligament crosses the scaphoid waist and acts as a fulcrum over which the scaphoid fractures.

deformity of the scaphoid. Simultaneous extension of the lunate through its attachment to the triquetrum results in a DISI deformity. Ultimate treatment of a humpback scaphoid non-union with DISI requires both restitution of scaphoid anatomy and reversal of the secondary changes in carpal kinematics.

Untreated scaphoid nonunion will predictably progress to arthritic change, in what has been termed scaphoid nonunion advanced collapse (SNAC).[211] Arthritic change arises at the radial styloid articulation with the distal scaphoid pole and is followed by degeneration of the midcarpal joint and ultimately by pancarpal arthritis. Arthritic changes have been found in 97% of the patients assessed at least 5 years after injury, with the degree of arthritic changes being proportionate to the duration of nonunion.[133] Patients generally present with escalating mechanical pain, with limitations in range of motion. Duppe[55] reviewed 30-year follow-up results of scaphoid fractures treated with thumb spica short-arm casts. Ten percent of the patients developed nonunion; 60% of these demonstrated radiographic evidence of radiocarpal osteoarthrosis, while only 2% of the healed group demonstrated degenerative change.

Examination and Imaging of the Scaphoid
Clinical Presentation

The patient usually presents with pain on the radial side of the wrist. There may be swelling on the radial side, as well. There is usually a history of trauma, such as falling on an outstretched hand, collision of the wrist against a person or heavy obstacle, or possibly a direct blow against an object. There may be limited

range of motion and pain when applying extended wrist loading or positioning the wrist in extreme positions of flexion or extension.

Physical Examination

Physical examination starts with visual inspection. Wrists with acute fractures may have swelling and bruising in the radial aspect of the wrist. There may be limited range of motion. Wrists with chronic injury may have swelling in the dorsoradial wrist. "Snuffbox tenderness" has become synonymous with scaphoid fracture, but this applies predominantly to waist fractures, which represent 70% of scaphoid fractures. The second most common type of scaphoid fracture is proximal pole fracture, at 20%. The least common is distal pole fracture, at 10%.[122] Fractures tend to occur at the waist partly because the RSC ligament acts as a fulcrum over which the scaphoid waist fractures (Figure 16.6).[35]

The full physical examination of the scaphoid bone should include all of its parts: the waist, distal pole, and proximal pole. To palpate the anatomic snuffbox for the waist examination, palpate just distal to the radial styloid in the "soft spot." The distal pole should be palpated at the scaphoid tubercle on the palmar aspect of the wrist. To do this, place the index finger in the anatomic snuffbox and place the thumb on the palmar aspect just distal to the anatomic snuffbox. The prominent bone palpated is the distal pole of the scaphoid. With radial deviation of the wrist, this prominence should move palmarly toward the examiner's thumb. This distal pole should be checked for tenderness. The proximal pole is palpated dorsally in line with the second ray just distal to the dorsal radius lip. The scapholunate ligament is in line between the second and third rays just distal to the dorsal radius lip and corresponds to the 3-4 wrist arthroscopy portal. The proximal pole is just radial to this scapholunate ligament/3-4 portal area. In diagnosing scaphoid fracture, physical examination is sensitive but its specificity is low, ranging from 74% to 80%.[82,158]

Diagnostic Imaging of Scaphoid Fractures and Nonunion

Computed Tomography. Computed tomography (CT) scanning helps elucidate scaphoid fracture displacement, bony morphologic findings, gapping, sclerosis, cysts, and evidence of healing. CT is particularly helpful in addressing nonunions. It is important that CT scans are taken with overlapping 1-mm cuts along the long axis of the scaphoid and with coronal and sagittal reconstructions. CT scans have particular utility in evaluating for healing after scaphoid surgery, especially because radiographs are often indeterminate.[94] CT scanning has also demonstrated some utility in evaluating the vascularity of the proximal pole of the scaphoid. Increased radiodensity of the proximal pole is a sign of dysvascularity.[186]

Magnetic Resonance Imaging. Magnetic resonance imaging (MRI) is best to determine whether there is occult scaphoid fracture. Specificity is 90% and sensitivity is between 90% and 100%,[164] as opposed to bone scintigraphy, which is 92% to 95% sensitive and 60% to 95% specific.[16]

Use of MRI to assess bony vascularity is controversial. Some authors advocate its use,[8] whereas others present cogent arguments questioning its efficacy and utility.[84,149,223] MRI findings of hypointense areas of bone on both T1-weighted and T2-weighted sequences have been suggested to be correlated with AVN.[8] However, subsequent studies have shown poor correlation,[54] and almost no data exist correlating MRI findings with operative or nonoperative healing rates.

In a study of 88 patients for which imaging results were compared with findings of intraoperative bleeding, Schmitt and colleagues[176] concluded that viability of the proximal fragment in scaphoid nonunion can be significantly better assessed with contrast-enhanced MRI than with nonenhanced MRI. Contrast-enhanced MRI has demonstrated significantly improved sensitivity (77% vs. 6%; $p < .001$) in detecting scaphoid AVN compared with nonenhanced MRI. However, this study suggests that, even with contrast enhancement, MRI might fail to detect proximal pole AVN in nearly a quarter of cases. This might be due to ingrowth of nonspecific inflammatory tissue into the proximal pole from the nonunion site, resulting in contrast enhancement despite the necrotic bone. Additional techniques for improving the sensitivity of MRI, such as dynamic gadolinium enhancement, are being developed and investigated,[153] but they are still currently inferior to standard gadolinium-enhanced MRI.[54] Therefore, MRI with or without contrast enhancement might be helpful in assessing the vascularity of the bone, but the entire picture must be taken into account using the patient history and CT imaging. Even though MRI with gadolinium was thought to have a better correlation with intraoperative scaphoid bleeding assessment,[33] MRI with gadolinium still could not predict fracture healing in a paper by Dawson and colleagues.[44]

One of the strongest arguments against MRI was presented by Willems and colleagues,[223] who studied vascularized bone grafting in a canine carpal AVN model. AVN was induced in carpal bones by excising bones, deep freezing, and coating in cyanoacrylate and then reimplanting them. A vascularized bone graft from the radius was implanted in the avascular carpal bone. The contralateral side served as an untreated ischemic control. Bone blood flow, bone volume, radiography, histomorphometry, histology, and MRI were analyzed at 4 weeks. T1 and T2 signals on MRI did not correlate with quantitative bone blood flow measurements. Necrotic bones with no blood flow had normal T1 and T2 signals, whereas revascularized bones had signal changes when compared with adjacent carpal bones. A major point of this work is that MRI did not necessarily correlate with known blood flow to the carpal bone in an animal model.[84]

Controversy about MRI is complicated by differences in techniques and image quality, which depend on programming of the image acquisition parameters and reading of the images and on the MRI machines, magnet power, and specialized wrist coils used; all of these factors influence the quality of information presented.

Preferred Modes of Diagnostic Imaging. I prefer to take five radiographic views for the assessment of scaphoid fractures: wrist posteroanterior (PA), lateral, and oblique views; scaphoid view; and clenched pencil view.[128] It is important to take a true scaphoid pisiform capitate (SPC) lateral radiograph of the wrist, wherein the palmar cortex of the pisiform bone overlays the interval between the palmar cortex of the distal scaphoid pole and the palmar cortex of the capitate. This allows true assessment of the carpal alignment.

A predictable scaphoid view is taken where a fist is made, with the thumb covering the dorsum of the middle phalanges of the index and middle fingers. The pronated forearm and hand are placed on the radiography table. The wrist is placed in ulnar deviation (Figure 16.7). The rationale behind this position is to take the scaphoid out of its usual position of flexion and pronation. With the thumb in the above position, the wrist is extended and supinated slightly. Ulnar deviation and wrist extension extend the proximal carpal row. This view allows a full view of the scaphoid bone with minimal overlap from neighboring bones.

A clenched pencil view is also taken.[127,128] This is the best view to assess associated dynamic scapholunate widening[128] (Figure 16.8, *A* and *B*) and in my experience also shows SNAC and SLAC (scapholunate advanced collapse) wrist changes better than standard PA views.

For better detail of bony anatomy, especially in patients with small proximal poles, comminution, or nonunion, I obtain a CT scan without contrast at 1-mm cuts, along the long axis of the scaphoid with coronal and sagittal reconstructions. If the status of the cartilage is in question, I obtain an MRI without contrast with cartilage-sensitive sequencing.

Scaphoid healing cannot be reliably determined by standard radiographs at 3 months;[49] consequently, CT provides enhanced resolution and definitive information regarding healing. Most acutely treated scaphoid fractures require approximately 10 to 12 weeks to heal. I obtain a CT scan at 3 months to determine healing and before allowing full return to heavy occupational demands, sports, or recreational pursuits.

Scaphoid Fracture Classification and Implications for Treatment

Scaphoid fractures have been classified by fracture location (proximal, waist, or distal), plane (transverse or oblique), and stability (stable or unstable). The goal of a fracture classification is to guide management of injuries, in order to enable rapid healing with minimal complications and allow return to activities of daily living, work, and sports or hobbies. The consequences of failed healing include wrist pain, loss of wrist

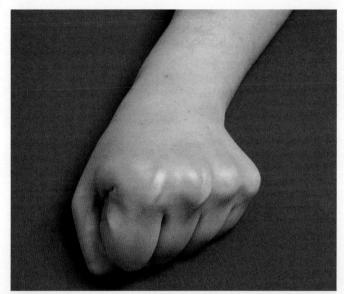

FIGURE 16.7 Scaphoid view. The subject makes a fist and places the forearm and fist pronated palm side down with the wrist in ulnar deviation. (Courtesy of Steve K. Lee, MD.)

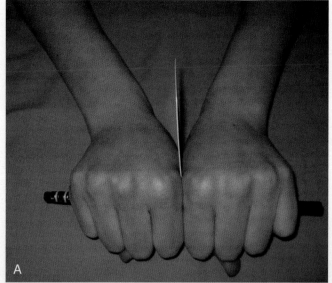

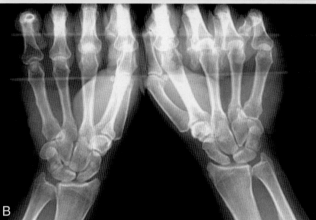

FIGURE 16.8 Clenched pencil views. **A,** The subject gently presses a card between the first dorsal interosseous muscles while gripping a pencil. **B,** Postero-anterior radiograph showing asymmetric scapholunate widening. (**A** and **B,** From Lee SK, Desai H, Silver B, et al: Comparison of radiographic stress views for scapholunate dynamic instability in a cadaver model. *J Hand Surg [Am]* 36:1149–1157, 2011.)

motion, loss of grip strength, loss of productivity, and premature articular degeneration. Of particular importance is identifying which scaphoid fractures require surgical intervention to heal. A failure to identify an unstable scaphoid fracture and treat it accordingly will predictably result in 6 months or more of additional treatment and restricted activities.

One of the earliest efforts to identify unstable fractures was to examine the scaphoid fracture plane. Russe recognized that oblique fractures were unstable and difficult to control with immobilization and that they resulted in an increased rate of nonunion.[172] Herbert and Fisher classified scaphoid fractures according to their stability.[91] Stable fractures, classified as type A, included incomplete fractures or fractures of the scaphoid tubercle. The authors stated that these fractures could be safely treated with immobilization with expectation of a high rate of union. All other fractures were considered potentially unstable and merited rigid fixation, a point of some controversy. Despite the assertions of these authors, however, Desai and colleagues were unable to predict fracture union with closed treatment using either the Russe or the Herbert classification system.[46]

Cooney and colleagues attempted to further define unstable injuries.[39] These included fractures with more than 1 mm of displacement, a lateral intrascaphoid angle of more than 35 degrees, bone loss or comminution, perilunate fracture-dislocation, DISI alignment, and proximal pole fractures. He advocated open surgical fixation for all unstable injuries.

Preferred Method of Classification

I prefer to use a classification method that mimics actual cases that present to the surgeon. It borrows from some elements of the Herbert and Fisher classification and from Cooney's definition of an unstable injury. It also includes a classification of scaphoid nonunions.

Stable Acute Fractures
  Distal pole fracture, nondisplaced
  Incomplete fracture through waist
  Negative radiographs, positive MRI

Unstable Acute Fractures
  Waist fracture, visible on radiographs
  Proximal pole fracture
  Displaced fracture
  (displacement is defined as DISI malalignment of 1 mm
    [DISI = dorsal intercalated instability with scapholunate
    angle > 60 degrees and capitolunate angle >15 degrees])
  Scaphoid fracture as part of perilunate fracture-dislocation
Nonunion
  Nonunion of waist fracture, no arthritis, acceptable alignment, stable
  Nonunion of waist fracture, no to minimal (only SNAC I) arthritis, humpback deformity
  Nonunion of proximal pole fracture, no arthritis
  Nonunion of waist fracture, arthritis, SNAC II to III, nonreconstructable, distal pole grossly deformed
  Nonunion of proximal pole fracture, no arthritis, not salvageable (proximal pole <5 mm)

For completeness, two other classification schemes of scaphoid nonunion are shown in Tables 16.1 and 16.2.

TABLE 16.1 Slade and Geissler Classification of Scaphoid Fracture Nonunion

Type	Description
Type 1	Delayed presentation for 4 to 12 weeks
Type 2	Fibrous union, minimal fracture line
Type 3	Minimal sclerosis of less than 1 mm
Type 4	Cystic formation of 1 to 5 mm
Type 5	Humpback deformity with cystic change of more than 5 mm
Type 6	Wrist arthrosis

From Geissler WB: Arthroscopic management of scaphoid fractures in athletes. *Hand Clin* 25(3):359–369, 2009.

TABLE 16.2 Alnot Classification of Scaphoid Fracture Nonunion

Grade	Description
I	Linear nonunion without altered scaphoid form, instability, or intracarpal malalignment
IIA	Stable nonunion with incipient bone resorption at fracture line, without instability or malalignment
IIB	More or less mobile nonunion with anterior defect and proximal pole flexion on distal tubercle inducing DISI
III	More or less mobile displacement nonunion with instability or reducible malalignment with IIIA: isolated styloscaphoid arthritis IIIB: radial and/or intracarpal arthritis
IV	Proximal fragment necrosis with IVA: malalignment IVB: radioscaphoid and/or intracarpal arthritis

DISI, Dorsal intercalated segmental instability.
From Gras M, Mathoulin C: Vascularized bone graft pedicled on the volar carpal artery from the volar distal radius as primary procedure for scaphoid non-union. *Orthop Traumatol Surg Res* 97(8):800–806, 2011.

TABLE 16.3 Algorithm for Acute Scaphoid Fracture Management

Type of Fracture	Treatment
Stable Fractures, Nondisplaced (Obtain CT Scan to Ensure the Fracture Is Completely Nondisplaced, Especially on Sagittal View)	
Tubercle fracture	Short-arm cast for 6 to 8 weeks
Distal third fracture or incomplete fracture	Short-arm cast for 6 to 8 weeks
Waist fracture	Short-arm thumb spica cast until healed, especially for pediatric patients and sedentary or low-demand patients, preference for nonoperative treatment Mini-open internal fixation (APM: dorsal approach), especially for active, young, manual worker, athlete, or worker in high-demand occupation, preference for early range of motion
Proximal pole fracture, nondisplaced	Mini-open internal fixation, dorsal approach
Unstable Fractures	
Displacement of more than 1 mm Lateral intrascaphoid angle of more than 35 degrees Bone loss or comminution Perilunate fracture-dislocation Dorsal intercalated segmental instability alignment (DISI = dorsal intercalated instability with scapholunate angle > 60 degrees and capitolunate angle > 15 degrees)	Mini-open internal fixation (APM: dorsal approach)

APM, Author's preferred method.

Management of Scaphoid Fractures

Up to 25% of scaphoid fractures are not visible on initial radiographs (see Preferred Modes of Diagnostic Imaging, above). Unless the x-ray beam lies in the same plane as the fracture, the fracture line may be missed. Because failure to treat a stable scaphoid fracture within 4 weeks increases the nonunion rate, all clinically suspected scaphoid fractures are treated as fractures with short-arm thumb spica cast immobilization until the cause of the symptoms is clarified (Table 16.3). Follow-up radiographs and clinical examination without the cast are performed at 10 to 14 days. If a fracture is clinically suspected in the presence of negative follow-up radiographs, we prefer MRI. At our institution, MRI is the most reliable imaging modality for the diagnosis of acute and occult fractures and is generally diagnostic within 24 hours of injury.

The obvious goal is to attain healing of the scaphoid fracture in an anatomic position while maintaining carpal alignment. Patients with union have better functional results.[40,109,165,192] Table 16.3 summarizes treatment options.

Stable Acute Fractures

Distal Pole Fractures. Distal pole and tubercle fractures of the scaphoid are generally treated nonoperatively. The distal pole of the scaphoid is well vascularized, and distal scaphoid pole fractures have a high rate of union after 6 to 8 weeks of plaster immobilization in a short-arm cast. The two predominant distal fracture types treated in plaster immobilization are (1) avulsion fractures from the radiopalmar lip of the scaphoid tuberosity and (2) impaction fractures of the radial half of the distal scaphoid articular surface. However, malunion of impacted radial-sided compression fractures may result in symptomatic degenerative arthritis. When in doubt, CT can delineate the articular surface, and operative fixation can be implemented if deemed necessary to try to reduce the risk of late degenerative arthritis of the scaphotrapezial joint.

Incomplete Fracture Through the Waist, Negative Radiographs, Positive MRI Studies. Incomplete fractures through the waist and injuries that have negative radiographs but positive MRI views for signal change probably need even less strict immobilization. Depending on the patient, a short-arm thumb spica cast or, in particularly compliant patients, a thumb spica splint has been used. Other authors recommend internal percutaneous fixation for these fractures (see the following).

Unstable Acute Fractures

Waist Fracture, "Nondisplaced." Even if a scaphoid fracture is visible but is "nondisplaced" on radiographs, it is arguably displaced and may be seen as a flexion deformity in the sagittal plane via CT scan. Therefore, an argument can be made for fixing all scaphoid fractures where a fracture line is seen on plain radiographs. In addition, there is evidence that fixing nondisplaced fractures allows for faster healing and earlier return to work. Bond and colleagues demonstrated that in a prospective study of 25 patients randomized to cast or screw treatment, union rates (time to healing) were significantly faster for the group who had surgery (7 vs. 12 weeks) and the return to work time was also significantly faster for this group (8 vs. 15 weeks).[23]

The choice of operative or nonoperative treatment must be individualized based on the discussion of pros and cons of treatment with the patient. If a cast is chosen, there are controversies about what type of cast to use. There is no agreement in the literature as to the optimum position of immobilization (extension, ulnar deviation, neutral) or type of cast (thumb spica, interphalangeal [IP] free, IP included, long arm, short arm), suggesting that many waist fractures can be treated in a variety of positions and casts.

Controversies include short-arm versus long-arm casting and whether to include the thumb. In a prospective, randomized trial of long-arm versus short-arm thumb spica casting, there was significantly faster healing with long-arm casting (9.5 vs. 12.7 weeks). The nonunion rate was not different, with numbers tested at 0 with long-arm casting and 2 with short-arm casting. The authors recommended long-arm thumb spica casting for the first 6 weeks, followed by short-arm casting until healing.[75] Immobilization of the elbow produced no long-term disability. Displaced fractures were excluded from this study, and the minimum follow-up was 6 months. This carefully conducted study is probably the best evidence in favor of the long-arm cast for the initial immobilization period.

In a cadaveric study, there was motion of 1 to 4 mm in simulated scaphoid fractures treated with a short-arm thumb spica cast. Therefore, the authors recommended a long-arm thumb spica cast.[116] Other indirect evidence that short-arm cast immobilization with the thumb free is inadequate is that in a series by Dias and colleagues; with this method of immobilization, 23% did not unite at 12 weeks.[50]

In the most recent literature, Symes and Stothard[198] performed a systematic review of cast versus surgery for acute scaphoid fractures. The rate of nonunion was three times less for surgery, and recovery was quicker. However, there were more complications with surgery. In the end, there was no difference in pain, cost, functional outcome, or patient satisfaction, though the secondary costs and morbidity of nonunion treatment were not taken into account. In two trials that compared long-arm casts versus short-arm casts and thumb spica casts versus short-arm cast, there was no difference in outcome.[198] Alshryda and associates performed a metaanalysis of 13 level I studies (randomized controlled trial [RCT]) and concluded that for closed treatment there is no difference between short-arm and long-arm casting or between thumb spica and short-arm casting. Union rates are the same for surgical and nonoperative treatment for undisplaced fractures. Surgery is recommended for displaced fractures.[6]

Taking all the above factors into account, I obtain a CT scan to ensure that a "nondisplaced" fracture on a radiograph is truly nondisplaced. I not uncommonly see fractures that seem to be nondisplaced on radiographs but are shown as displaced on CT scans, especially on sagittal views where the fracture is flexed at the waist. If the fracture is truly nondisplaced, I discuss with the patient the pros and cons of operative and nonoperative care. If the patient opts for nonoperative care, I prefer to treat with short-arm thumb spica casting until the fracture is healed. If healing has not occurred by 3 months and/or there are no longer interval changes, I consider operative intervention. If the fracture is displaced on CT scanning, I recommend operative intervention.

Proximal Pole Fracture. Proximal pole nonunion may be attributed to impaired vascularity or instability of the proximal fragment. Proximal pole fractures are considered unstable, whether or not they are displaced, because of their small size, their tenuous blood supply, their interarticular location, and the relatively large moment arms across the fracture site. Rettig and Raskin reported 100% healing of 17 proximal pole fractures treated acutely with operative screw fixation through a dorsal approach.[167] There is consensus that proximal pole fractures cannot be reliably treated nonoperatively. Consequently, I believe that any proximal pole fracture, whether nondisplaced or displaced, should be fixed operatively. The nonunion rate is higher for proximal pole fractures if treated closed. Because of the position of the fracture in that the proximal pole is dorsal, proximal pole fractures are best fixed from the dorsal approach.

Mechanics of Fracture Fixation

Bone healing requires viable bone cells, an adequate blood supply, and stabilization of the fracture site. For a fixation device to be successful in providing rigid fixation of scaphoid fractures, it must be able to resist complex bending, shearing, and translational forces during normal functional loading. Because the majority of the scaphoid is covered with cartilage, fracture callus is not produced, so primary bone healing is entirely dependent on rigid stabilization of the fracture fragments until healing.

The mechanical effectiveness of internal fixation is determined by the bone quality, fracture geometry, fracture reduction, choice of implant, and implant placement. While all five of these independent variables are important, bone quality and fracture geometry are intrinsic to the patient. Fracture reduction, choice of implant, and implant placement are all under the surgeon's control. Fracture reduction and placement of the implant in the biomechanically ideal position are the most important of the five variables. Trumble and colleagues observed that screws placed in the central third of the scaphoid were associated with significantly shorter healing times than screws placed outside of the central third axis ($p < .05$).[205] To explain this observation, McAdams and colleagues simulated scaphoid waist fractures and compared screws placed in the central axis with screws placed eccentrically.[140] This study demonstrated that screws centrally placed in the proximal fragment of the scaphoid had superior results compared with screws placed in an eccentric position. Fixation with central placement of the screw demonstrated 43% greater stiffness, 113% greater load at 2 mm of displacement, and 39% greater load at failure.[140]

Biomechanically, the longer the screw, the more rigid the fixation, because longer screws reduce forces at the fracture site and bending forces are spread along the screws.[51] In a cadaveric study by Slade and colleagues, short or long screws were placed along the central scaphoid axis after an osteotomy was simulated at the waist.[51] Scaphoids that were repaired with longer screws were significantly stiffer than those repaired with short screws. When rigid fixation cannot be provided by a central screw placement alone (as in extreme proximal pole fractures and nonunions), augmentation may be necessary to prevent micromotion at the fracture site. Supplemental fixation can be applied from the distal scaphoid to the capitate using a 0.045-inch or 0.062-inch Kirschner wire or a mini–headless screw. If a Kirschner wire is placed, it should be buried, because it usually has to stay in place for 3 months until the bone is healed.

Techniques for Rigid Fixation
Implants for Rigid Fixation of Scaphoid Fractures

Implants used included Kirschner wires, AO compression screws, headless compression screws, plates, and bioabsorbable implants. Solid and cannulated screws are available from several manufacturers. Any implant used must reduce bending, shearing, and translational forces acting at a fracture site.

Kirschner Wires

Although Kirschner wires are easy to insert, they have a narrow role for scaphoid fixation today, given the relatively insecure fixation and minimal compression afforded by these implants.[35] Kirschner wire fixation must be supplemented with a cast until healing, and a separate procedure for Kirschner wire removal is required. In multitrauma situations or open fractures, rapid stabilization of an unstable scaphoid fracture may be expedient.

Screws

In 1954, McLaughlin described fractures of the scaphoid as "an unsolved problem."[143] His main interest was returning a "breadwinner" to work with a treatment that would "hold bone fragments in apposition" until healing. He reported on the fixation of scaphoid fractures using solid lag screws. The operative procedure was technically challenging, the optimal screw position was not always achieved, and the incidence of nonunion in unstable fractures was not substantially reduced over that obtained by casting alone.

Herbert and Fisher in 1984 presented the results of the first headless screw used to treat 158 patients from 1977 to 1981. The rate of union was 100% for acute fractures and 83% overall.[91] This screw revolutionized bone fixation because it permitted compression of a fracture with two heads of differential pitches (Figure 16.9). The embedded threaded heads of headless screws are placed in the densest bone of both poles for maximum bony purchase. This paper also demonstrated that screws placed perpendicular to an acute fracture plane using compression and rigid fixation could successfully heal an acute fracture. The implant, however, is not technically easy to insert, and other centers reported lower rates of union with screw fixation of acute scaphoid fractures secondary to technical problems.[1]

The next major development in headless screw design was the cannulated compression screw. This device greatly simpli-

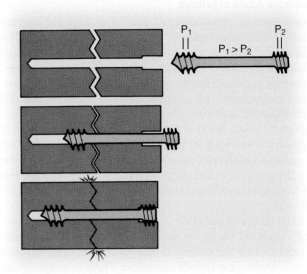

FIGURE 16.9 The difference in pitch between the leading thread (P_1) and the trailing thread (P_2) of the Herbert screw governs the rate of "take-up," or drawing together, of the two bone fragments to produce compression. (Redrawn, by Elizabeth Martin, from Herbert TJ, Fisher WE: Management of the fractured scaphoid using a new bone screw. *J Bone Joint Surg Br* 66:114–123, 1984.)

fied accurate placement of the screw within the scaphoid bone by using a thin guidewire placed under fluoroscopic control. A fully threaded, variable-pitch implant, the Acutrak screw (AcuMed, Hillsboro, OR), demonstrated compression comparable to that of a standard 4-mm compression screw and greater compression when compared with the Herbert screw in biomechanical testing.[222] Several manufacturers have developed cannulated compression screws with unique advantages and disadvantages. There have been a number of recent biomechanical studies comparing headless compression screws.[13,81,83,88,159] Most second-generation headless compression screws achieve adequate compression, the compression decreases by 50% 12 hours after placement, and the compression does not necessarily correlate with the feel of torque on the screwdriver.

What is unknown is how much compression is necessary for bone healing. Few clinical studies exist with which to compare implants, and which screw to use is still largely a matter of surgeon preference.

Other Implants. Bailey reported on the mechanics of a bioresorbable cannulated screw composed of poly-L-lactic acid and hydroxyapatite that was developed for small bone fracture fixation.[14] The bioresorbable screw has been shown to have good compressive properties compared with commonly used small bone fragment compression screws, but no clinical data have been presented.

Staple Fixation. The use of staples has had its proponents as a means of achieving stable fixation. Early studies demonstrated simple application and satisfactory healing rates among patients with scaphoid nonunions and acute fractures but long-term degenerative changes secondary to hardware impingement.[120] New staples with memory achieve compression after insertion as they warm to body temperature. These staples might be indicated for fractures or nonunions requiring open reduction through a palmar approach, and clinical data are lacking at this time.

Plate Fixation. Plate fixation has also been used to stabilize scaphoid fractures.[27] Huene and Huene reported their experience in 1991.[101] The Ender blade plate is suitable for adding stability in scaphoid nonunions with AVN, cystic degeneration, and osseous size discrepancy or compromise. Plate fixation can be used with scaphoid nonunion humpback deformity. Dodds and colleagues presented a combination of volar buttress plating and a vascularized volar distal radius wedge autograft pedicled on the volar carpal artery for salvage treatment of chronic scaphoid nonunion.[52] Ghoneim reported on healing of 13 of 14 scaphoid nonunions with an iliac crest wedge graft and a volar miniplate of 1.5 or 2 mm.[77]

Surgical Treatment Methods

❖ AUTHOR'S PREFERRED TREATMENT METHOD:
Dorsal Approach (Figure 16.10)

Scaphoid Open Reduction and Internal Fixation From the Dorsal Approach/Mini-Open Approach. The tourniquet is placed proximally on the arm and draped to allow full motion of the extremity. A small (≈2-3 cm) longitudinal or transverse incision should be made over the proximal pole at the position of the scapholunate ligament. A miniincision is safer than the purely percutaneous method when approaching from the dorsal wrist.

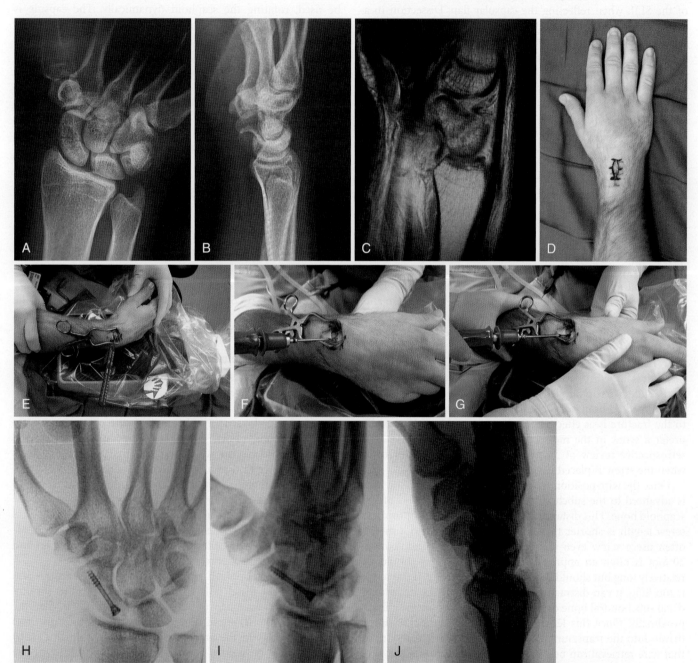

FIGURE 16.10 Acute scaphoid fracture at waist showing open reduction and internal fixation with a dorsally placed headless compression screw. Preoperative radiograph of scaphoid **(A)** and preoperative lateral radiograph **(B)** of wrist. **C,** Preoperative sagittal magnetic resonance imaging of wrist. **D,** Dorsal incision for drilling and screw placement. **E,** Measuring screw length. **F,** Countersinking to avoid hoop stresses. **G,** Screw placement. **H,** Intraoperative fluoroscopic view of scaphoid showing optimal screw position. **I,** Intraoperative fluoroscopic oblique view of wrist. **J,** Intraoperative fluoroscopic lateral view of wrist.

Weinberg and colleagues have shown that there is a 13% chance of tendon injury with a purely percutaneous technique.[220]

The incision is just radial to the area that corresponds with the 3-4 arthroscopic portal. This area is also in line between the second and third metacarpal interspaces, and just distal to the dorsal lip of the radius. The extensor pollicis longus (EPL) is carefully identified and the second and third dorsal compartment tendons are retracted radially. For the mini-open approach, the capsule is opened with a mini inverted-"T" incision. If more exposure is necessary, a ligament-sparing approach can be used[18] (see Chapter 13).

Extreme care is taken to avoid disruption of the dorsal fibers of the SLIL when reflecting the capsular flap. Dissection in a plane tangential to the dorsal surfaces of the scaphoid and the lunate can be performed with a scalpel or Beaver blade. The distal boundaries of dissection of the scaphoid are determined by the vascular supply along the dorsal ridge. Care is taken not to disrupt the blood vessels entering the waist of the scaphoid. Retractors are placed deeper to retract the capsule. If the scaphoid is displaced, the hematoma should be evacuated and the scaphoid reduced, possibly with the aid of smooth Kirschner-wire joysticks, if necessary. The wrist is flexed and the entrance point on the scaphoid is identified 1 to 2 mm radial to the membranous portion of the scapholunate ligament and in the midportion of the scaphoid in the sagittal plane. The guidewire for the headless compression screw is started there; the surgeon should aim the wire for the articular base of the thumb metacarpal (because the scaphoid distal pole, trapezium, and metacarpal base are collinear). Once this wire is placed, the surgeon must not extend the wrist, because this will bend the wire at the radiocarpal joint and not allow overdrilling and screw placement. Fluoroscopic images are taken to assess the fracture and wire position. Posteroanterior (PA), lateral, and oblique images are taken. It is important to take several oblique views to ensure that there is no screw penetration out of the scaphoid in any view. In order to obtain the PA images while keeping the wrist flexed, it is imperative to flex the elbow. A center-center position of the guidewire in all views (PA, lateral, and oblique) should be obtained. Although a screw that is shorter and perpendicular to the fracture is as effective as a long-axis screw,[58] I generally prefer a screw in the most central portion of the bone. In a retrospective review of 34 patients, time to union is shorter when the screw is placed in the central third.[205]

Once the wire position is determined to be optimal, the wire is advanced to the subchondral bone on the distal end of the scaphoid bone. This distance is then measured. The appropriate screw length is shorter than this distance by at least 4 mm; I often use a screw even shorter than this. For an adult man, 20 mm is often an appropriate length. The screw should be relatively long but should *definitely* not be too long. If the screw is too long, it can distract the fracture if it hits the unyielding distal subchondral bone or protrude out of the bone distally or proximally. Once this length is determined, the guidewire is driven into the trapezium bone and out of the thenar skin, so that wire retrieval can be easily accomplished should the wire break during drilling or screw insertion. A second, antirotation wire may be placed. The wire is overdrilled with a cannulated drill. Although some of the systems tout a "self-drilling" screw, my preference is to overdrill to the subchondral bone on the far end of the scaphoid bone as determined by fluoroscopy. After drilling, I believe it to be imperative to countersink the proximal

hole. Most systems come with a countersink. This is to decrease the hoop stresses placed on the proximal bone which can cause a fracture in the proximal bone. After countersinking, a screw of the appropriate size is placed, making sure that it is well seated below the cartilage and into the proximal subchondral bone. A study by Hart and colleagues showed that the torque of the screw turns felt by the surgeon does not correlate with fracture compression.[88] After the screw is placed, it is important to remove the guidewire and check all fluoroscopic views (PA, lateral, supinated and pronated oblique views) to ensure an excellent position of fracture reduction and hardware placement. If unsure about screw position, live fluoroscopy should be used, rotating the scaphoid dynamically. The capsule is closed with absorbable braided suture. The tourniquet is released and hemostasis achieved. The skin is closed and a well-padded short-arm splint is placed. Depending on fracture stability and patient compliance, a postoperative short-arm thermoplastic splint or short-arm cast may be placed at 2 weeks until the bone is healed; this may take 6 to 10 weeks following operation. Fracture healing is determined clinically by lack of tenderness and by imaging with radiographs and with CT scanning if there is any radiographic ambiguity.

Dorsal Percutaneous Slade Technique

The main difference in the Slade technique[76] is that it is a percutaneous technique; as such the entrance point is identified by flexing the wrist and identifying the superimposed rings on fluoroscopy of the proximal and distal poles. The guidewire is placed down the center of the superimposed rings. The wire is advanced out of the radial aspect of the thumb so the wrist can be extended for standard wrist radiographs. When satisfactory wire placement is confirmed, the wrist is again flexed and the wire driven dorsally for the remainder of the procedure, which is identical to the author's preferred method above.

Unstable Acute Fractures: Waist Fracture, Displaced

Acute waist fractures can be approached dorsally or palmarly. There are advantages and disadvantages to both approaches. The main advantage of the dorsal approach is that the fixation can get down the true axis better than the palmar approach. Many surgeons prefer dorsal percutaneous screw fixation because of the ease of access and the ability to place a screw closer to the central axis.[28,127] The disadvantages of the dorsal approach are that it either (1) requires a miniopen approach to retract extensor tendons or (2) risks injury or rupture of the extensor tendons with a percutaneous approach. The dorsal approach also requires flexion of the wrist, which may theoretically displace an unstable fracture. The dorsal miniopen and Slade percutaneous approaches are described above.

The palmar approach may be used for waist fractures and the infrequent distal pole fracture that may require surgical fixation. An advantage of the palmar approach is that the entrance of the scaphoid tubercle is subcutaneous; thus there are no tendons in the path of the approach. A small (1-cm) incision may be used if needed to allow overdrilling of the guidewire and placement of the screw. Another advantage of the palmar approach is that the wrist is extended, theoretically helping to reduce the fracture. A disadvantage is that it is not possible to place the screw down the true axis of the bone because the trapezium blocks the entrance of the center of the distal scaphoid (Figure 16.11, *A*).

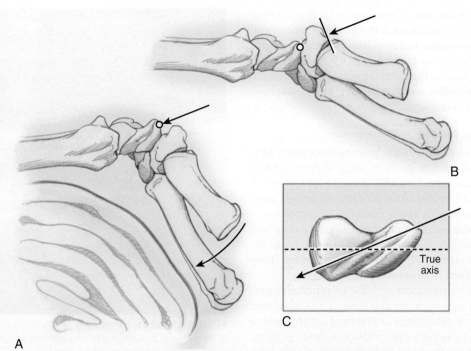

FIGURE 16.11 A, With the wrist in neutral position, the trapezium blocks the scaphoid bone. **B,** With the wrist in the hyperextended position, the trapezium moves dorsally out of the way for access to the starting point on the scaphoid bone. **C,** Even with the wrist extended, it is not possible to get down the true axis from the volar approach, because the trapezium is in the way.

The placement of the screw is always oblique; the more proximal the fracture, the higher the chance of not engaging enough screw threads in the proximal fragment. Another concern is penetration of the dorsal surface of the bone by the screw. The optimal radiographic views for determining screw prominence are the oblique views as reported by Kim and colleagues (Figure 16.12).[119]

Like the dorsal approach, the percutaneous approach can be extended if necessary to openly reduce the fracture or treat a nonunion.

Scaphoid Open Reduction and Internal Fixation From the Palmar Approach

In the open volar approach, a hockey-stick incision is made beginning between the flexor carpi radialis (FCR) tendon and the radial artery in the distal forearm and angled across the distal wrist crease toward the base of the thumb. The FCR tendon is retracted ulnarly and the radial artery radially. The wrist capsule is entered through a longitudinal incision from the volar lip of the radius to the proximal tubercle of the trapezium. The capsule and intracapsular ligaments are carefully divided and reflected sharply off of the scaphoid with a scalpel. The capsule needs to be preserved, as it contains the RSC ligament and will be repaired at the close of the procedure. Some surgeons prefer to tag the ligaments at this stage with nonabsorbable sutures for later repair. The entire volar scaphoid is exposed. Reduction is performed by manipulation or with joysticks, and Kirschner wires are used to provide provisional fixation. Bone grafting can be performed as required for volar comminution or in subacute fractures, with the grafts harvested from the volar radius beneath the pronator quadratus by extending the incision an additional 2 to 3 cm. The scaphotrapezial joint is opened to place a central guidewire in preparation for final fixation. If necessary, a small amount of the proximal

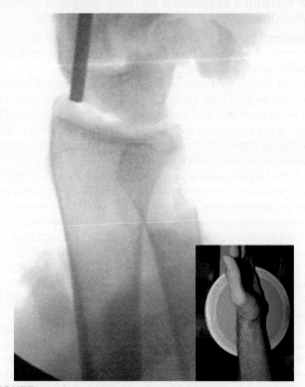

FIGURE 16.12 Supinated oblique view for assessment of proximal scaphoid articular cannulated screw penetration. (From Kim RY, Lijten EC, Strauch RJ: Pronated oblique view in assessing proximal scaphoid articular cannulated screw penetration. *J Hand Surg [Am]* 33(8):1274–1277, 2008.)

trapezium can be excised with a rongeur to clear an unobstructed path for the implant. Rigid internal fixation can be performed with the implant of choice.

With the volar approach, it is important to know that it is impossible to put the screw down the long axis of the scaphoid without violating the trapezium. Verstreken and colleagues have popularized a transtrapezial approach that enables more central screw position.[76,144] Leventhal and associates performed a computational analysis to identify the ideal starting point (1.7 mm dorsal and 0.2 mm radial to the tip of the scaphoid tubercle) to enable the longest possible screw trajectory in the scaphoid without violating the trapezium.[129]

Palmar Percutaneous Method

Streli[81] was the first to describe volar percutaneous screw fixation of the scaphoid fracture in 1970 using traction applied through the thumb and a standard ASIF screw. In 1991, Wozasek and Moser reported on an adaptation of Streli's technique using cannulated 2.9-mm screws via a volar percutaneous approach.[225] Later, Bond and colleagues demonstrated faster healing and return to work with percutaneous screw fixation from the palmar approach compared with cast immobilization. They used modern cannulated headless compression screws.[23]

Fractures suitable for treatment with the volar percutaneous (distal to proximal) approach are fractures at the waist and distal pole. Humpback deformities or scaphoid collapse with a DISI deformity usually require open reduction, bone grafting, and fixation. Unsuitable fractures include proximal pole fractures, which are best treated via a dorsal (proximal to distal) approach.

❖ AUTHOR'S PREFERRED METHOD: Scaphoid Mini-Open Screw From the Palmar Approach

The tourniquet is placed proximally on the arm and the upper extremity draped to allow for full motion of the extremity and enable adequate visualization with fluoroscopy. A tourniquet is used at the surgeon's discretion. A small longitudinal incision (≈1 cm, or just long enough to accommodate the drill bit/screw) is made over and just distal to the scaphoid tubercle. The wrist is hyperextended and ulnarly deviated over a bump. This moves the trapezium dorsally away from the entrance point on the scaphoid bone (see Figure 16.11, *B*).

If the trapezium has a particularly palmar location, a rongeur may be needed to remove a small amount of bone to gain access to the entrance point. The guidewire is started as dorsally as possible on the scaphoid in the sagittal plane without impinging on the trapezium. On the coronal plane, a good landmark for the starting point is a third of the distance from the radial side of the distal pole of the scaphoid (Figure 16.13). The surgeon should attempt to drop the hand to get as close as possible to the axis of the scaphoid (Figure 16.14). Fluoroscopy is used to optimize guidewire placement.

Once the guidewire is placed, multiple minifluoroscopic views are taken, including anteroposterior (AP), lateral, and oblique views. It is imperative to take 45-degree oblique views in supination and pronation to ensure that the wire is within the bone in all planes.[119] The wire should be advanced to the subchondral bone on the proximal side and measured.

The appropriate screw length is shorter than this distance by at least 4 mm; I often use a screw even shorter; a 20-mm screw is often an appropriate length for an adult male. The screw should be relatively long but should *definitely* not be too long. If it is too long, it can distract the fracture or protrude out of the bone distally or proximally. Once this length is determined, the guidewire is driven into the radius or out of the dorsal skin

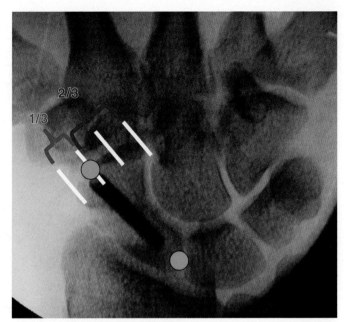

FIGURE 16.13 On the coronal plane, a good landmark for the starting point of the guidewire is one third of the distance from the radial side of the distal pole of the scaphoid. (Courtesy of Steve K. Lee, MD.)

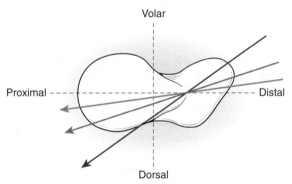

FIGURE 16.14 The surgeon should attempt to be closer to the *green line* and not the *red line* for wire placement from the volar approach. If the fracture is at the proximal waist, using the *red line* trajectory risks having minimal proximal bone purchase.

and clamped so that the wire will not come out during drilling. A second antirotation wire may be placed. The wire is overdrilled with a cannulated drill that is common to most headless compression screw systems. Although some of the systems tout a "self-drilling" screw, my preference is to overdrill up to the subchondral bone on the far end of the scaphoid as determined by fluoroscopy. After drilling, I believe it to be imperative to countersink the entrance hole. This is to decrease hoop stresses when tightening the screw, which can crack the distal fragment. After countersinking, a screw of appropriate size is placed, making sure that it is seated below the cartilage and flush with the subchondral bone. After the screw is placed and the guidewire removed, it is important to check all fluoroscopic views (AP, lateral, supinated and pronated oblique views) to ensure an excellent position of fracture reduction and hardware placement. If a tourniquet is used, it is deflated at this time. If an incision is used, it is closed with sutures or Steri-Strips. A well-padded short-arm splint is placed. Depending on fracture stability and patient compliance, a thermoplastic splint or short-arm cast is placed at 2 weeks until the bone is healed.

Some surgeons allow light activities as tolerated and early range-of-motion exercises to restore wrist mobility prior to complete healing. Fracture healing at 6 to 10 weeks postoperatively is assessed clinically by lack of tenderness and by imaging with radiographs and/or CT scans.

CRITICAL POINTS Pearls and Pitfalls for Surgical Treatment

- Place the guidewire as centrally as possible in the scaphoid.
- Consider using an antirotation wire.
- Common error is using a screw that is too long.
- Subtract at least 4 mm from the measured distance.
- A common screw length for an adult male is 20 mm.
- Do not ream past the far cortex.
- If feeling a lot of resistance (especially when reaming over wire), *stop* and look. The wire may be bent and break or the drill bit may break (Figure 16.15).[121]
- Beware of hoop stresses. Use countersinking to avoid excessive hoop stresses that can fracture the near fragment.
- Consider the use of joysticks to gain reduction.
- If needed, reduce and pin the lunate in neutral (out of DISI) (Figure 16.16, *A* to *C*).
- Consider supplemental fixation for more stability (Figure 16.17).

Palmar Percutaneous Method of Scaphoid Fixation (Alternate Method)

In the palmar percutaneous method of scaphoid fixation,[76] the patient is placed supine on an operating table and the hand is suspended vertically by the thumb using a finger trap (Figure 16.18).[85] This position extends the scaphoid and ulnarly deviates the wrist to improve access to the distal pole of the scaphoid. A fluoroscopic imaging unit is rotated parallel to the floor

and positioned so that the wrist is in its central axis. Traction from a tower permits full rotation of the scaphoid in the imaging beam. In the majority of cases, longitudinal traction is enough to reduce the scaphoid fracture. If the fracture is not reduced, Kirschner wires can be inserted and used as joysticks to manipulate the fragments into position. The quality of the reduction can then be checked radiographically.

Having achieved an acceptable reduction, the most important step is to establish the entry point of the guidewire. The ulnar deviation of the wrist extends the scaphoid to make the tubercle more accessible. The entry point, the scaphoid tuberosity, is located using a 12- or 14-gauge intravenous needle introduced on the anteroradial aspect of the wrist, just radial and

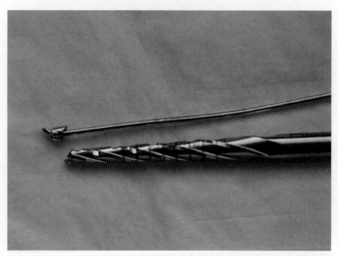

FIGURE 16.15 Broken drill bit from attempting to drill over a bent guidewire. (From Kosy JD, Standley DM: Retrieval of broken Acutrak drill bit. *J Hand Surg Eur* 35(8):683, 2010.)

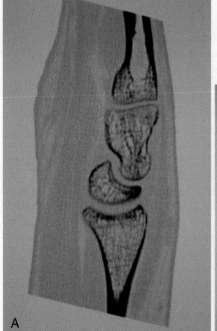
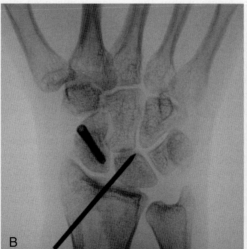
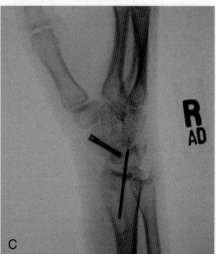

A B C

FIGURE 16.16 A, Preoperative computed tomographic scan showing dorsal intercalated segmental instability (DISI). Postoperative posteroanterior view **(B)** and lateral view **(C)** after reduction of DISI and Kirschner wire placement from radius to lunate. (Courtesy of Scott W. Wolfe, MD.)

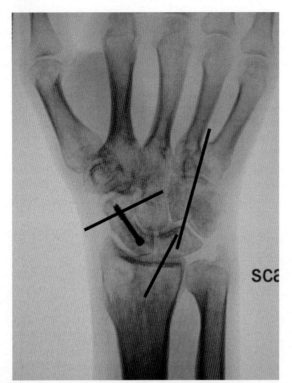

FIGURE 16.17 Example of supplemental fixation for stability. (Courtesy of Steve K. Lee, MD.)

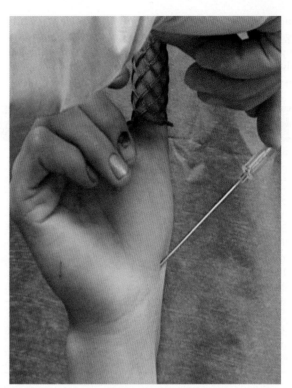

FIGURE 16.18 In 1998, Haddad and Goddard reported on a simplified volar percutaneous technique using traction and a cannulated screw to stabilize waist fractures. The thumb is suspended by a single finger trap. It permits free rotation of the hand throughout the operation, and the scaphoid remains in the center of an imaging unit. The C-arm is turned to a horizontal position surrounding the wrist. The most important step is to establish the entry point of the guidewire and the position of the screw. The ulnar deviation of the wrist is provided by thumb traction and allows the distal half of the scaphoid to slide out from under the radial styloid. The scaphoid tuberosity is easily palpable and is the key to the insertion point. The entry point is located using a 12- or 14-gauge intravenous needle, which is introduced radial and distal to the scaphoid tuberosity. (Haddad FS, Goddard NJ: Acute percutaneous scaphoid fixation: a pilot study. *J Bone Joint Surg Br* 80(1):95–99, 1998.)

distal to the scaphoid tuberosity. The needle serves as a trocar to guide the wire and establish a central path along the scaphoid. The needle is inserted into the scaphotrapezial joint and tilted into a vertical position. The needle is levered on the trapezium, which brings the distal pole of the scaphoid more radially and facilitates screw insertion. The wrist is rotated in the fluoroscopic beam to confirm that the needle is aligned along the axis of the scaphoid in all planes, with the intent of directing the guidewire into the proximal pole to a point just radial to the scapholunate ligament. Leventhal and colleagues identified the ideal starting point to be approximately 2 mm dorsal and just radial to the apex of the scaphoid tubercle, in order to achieve maximum guidewire length within the scaphoid.[129]

Once the entry point and the direction of the guidewire are confirmed, the needle is impacted into the soft articular cartilage over the distal pole of the scaphoid so that the tip does not slip during insertion of the guidewire. The guidewire is passed down through the needle and drilled across the fracture; its direction is continually checked on the image intensifier and adjusted as necessary, with the goal of entering the radial aspect of the proximal pole. The position is checked in multiple fluoroscopy planes, and, if satisfactory, a longitudinal incision of 0.5 cm is made at the entry point of the wire and deepened down to the distal pole of the scaphoid using a small hemostat and blunt dissection. This is a relatively safe zone, with minimal risk to the adjacent neurovascular structures.

The length of the screw is determined using a depth gauge or by advancing a second guidewire of the same length up the distal cortex of the scaphoid and subtracting the difference between the two. The correct screw size is 4 to 5 mm shorter than the measured length, which will ensure that the screw head

is fully buried below the cartilage and the subchondral bone on each end. In rare cases a second antirotation wire may be inserted parallel to the first prior to drilling and reaming. The wire is advanced into the radius or out of the dorsal skin and clamped, so as to avoid loss of wire position with drilling. The 12-gauge needle is removed and the cannulated drill is passed over the wire and advanced under imaging guidance, stopping 1 to 2 mm short of the far articular surface. At this point the hand is taken out of traction so that the screw will adequately compress the scaphoid. A countersink or a trailing drill is used, depending on the particular set. A self-tapping screw is advanced over the guidewire. The final position is checked with multiple fluoroscopic views to confirm complete containment within the scaphoid. A hyperpronated PA view profiles the dorsal-radial cortical margin of the scaphoid, where a perforation of the proximal cortical bone can occur. Compression of the fracture site is confirmed radiographically on the image intensifier. The wire is removed, the skin closed with a suture or Steri-Strips, and the wound covered with a sterile compressive dressing.

Postoperative Care. A volar plaster splint is removed at 10 to 14 days postoperatively. The sutures are removed at this stage, and wrist radiographs are taken to confirm that screw position is satisfactory. Depending on the bone quality, fixation, and assumed patient compliance, a short-arm thumb spica cast or well-molded Orthoplast short-arm thumb spica splint is used for 4 additional weeks or until the wrist has healed. Hand therapy may be useful to regain hand motion; no heavy carrying or weight-bearing activity is permitted. A return to sedentary work is allowed as soon as the patient feels ready or when 75% of the contralateral range of movement is achieved. When radiographic and clinical union have been achieved, the splint is discontinued and all previous activities are resumed as tolerated. CT is used to confirm healing before return to heavy lifting or competitive athletics.

Potential complications include malposition of the screw, violation of the cortical surface, and hardware protrusion within the radioscaphoid or scaphocapitate joint proximally, breakage of a guidewire, and fracture of the scaphoid during screw placement. Another potential problem is a failure to completely bury the head of the screw within the scaphoid, which can lead to scaphotrapeziotrapezoidal (STT) arthrosis. This problem is avoided by selecting a screw length approximately 4 to 5 mm shorter than measured with the depth gauge. Fracture displacement can occur with guidewire malposition or in proximal pole or oblique fractures. Other risks include transient dysesthesia just distal to the scar. This is secondary to a neurapraxia of a sensory branch of the median nerve and usually resolves within 4 to 6 weeks. Volar fixation of a small proximal scaphoid fragment is contraindicated because of tenuous fixation and minimal compression. Nonunions or delayed unions using the volar approach have occurred with proximal pole fractures, and small proximal pole fractures should be treated using a dorsal approach.

Arthroscopy-Assisted Percutaneous Scaphoid Fixation

The goals of arthroscopy-assisted stabilization of scaphoid fractures[76] are to reduce displaced fractures without an open incision and provide secure fixation that will permit early motion until solid union has been achieved.[71] The early results of arthroscopy-assisted percutaneous screw fixation of displaced fractures of the scaphoid suggest that minimally invasive reduction and fracture union can be predictably obtained with good to excellent functional results in the correctly selected patient.[184] Avoidance of open exposure limits the potential for wrist ligament injury, may help to preserve the blood supply, and minimizes postoperative stiffness. However, many scaphoid fractures are now treated with percutaneous or mini-open techniques that create little scarring and do not adversely affect postoperative motion.

Slade reviewed his results in arthroscopy-assisted fixation from a dorsal approach in 27 consecutive patients.[182] There were 18 waist fractures and 9 fractures of the proximal pole. Seventeen patients were treated within 1 month of injury, and 10 patients were treated late. All fractures healed, as documented by CT.

Arthroscopy-assisted fixation of scaphoid fractures also allows for simultaneous detection of associated intracarpal soft tissue injuries. Braithwaite originally reported on four patients with a fracture of the scaphoid with complete scapholunate dissociation.[26] As in fractures of the distal radius, associated soft tissue lesions may occur with scaphoid fractures, and arthroscopic evaluation allows detection and management. It is not known whether early arthroscopic detection and management of the associated injuries improve the final outcome. For operative details of arthroscopic-assisted percutaneous treatment of scaphoid fractures and scaphoid nonunions, the reader is referred to Chapter 17.

Delayed (Subacute) Presentation of Waist Fracture

Surgery is generally indicated for delayed presentation of a scaphoid fracture 4 to 6 weeks or more following injury. Patients with delayed presentation of scaphoid fractures have a higher likelihood of nonunion with closed treatment and require 4 to 6 months to heal in plaster.[134]

Managing Scaphoid Fractures in Athletes

Scaphoid fractures are common in competitive and recreational athletes, and such patients are reluctant to submit to the long period of immobilization and restricted activity that plaster requires. These factors may influence our treatment decisions. The treating physician may permit participation in athletic activity with a playing cast. Some organizations permit casts that are protected with foam padding. Whether the forces generated by firm gripping are detrimental to healing probably depends on the fracture's inherent stability. One study reported a faster return to play with internal fixation compared with a playing cast alone.[166] A potential problem with plaster immobilization is compliance. Young people often will modify or remove the cast and are increasingly noncompliant with follow-up over time. The pressure to return to sports may lead the patient and coach to seek ways of shortening the period off of the field. The player's ability to return to sports before the fracture is healed depends on the sport and its requirements. Options to be weighed will be surgery, a playing cast, and playing restrictions. The goal will be the successful union of the scaphoid fracture regardless of the patient's athletic responsibilities. Clearly, educating the patient, family, trainer, and coach is essential.

Complex Scaphoid Injuries
Combined Fractures of the Scaphoid and Distal Radius

Combined fractures of the distal radius and scaphoid are uncommon but present a challenging treatment dilemma. Scaphoid fractures may not be recognized when associated with a comminuted distal radius fracture and when untreated can result in carpal collapse, cystic degeneration, and eventual carpal degenerative arthritis. Although an isolated stable scaphoid fracture might be safely managed with plaster immobilization, the 12 to 16 weeks of immobilization required for healing are not appropriate for the treatment of the distal radius fracture. Prolonged immobilization may result in arthrofibrosis and atrophy of the forearm and hand, making the recovery of full hand function difficult.

A review of the published reports on combined scaphoid and distal radius fractures demonstrates that treatments have evolved over the past decade. Trumble and colleagues reported on six patients treated with internal fixation for ipsilateral combined fractures of the scaphoid and radius.[204] All patients sustained a high-energy injury from a fall from a substantial height. All of the fractures united, with the radial fractures healing in an average of 6 weeks and the scaphoid fractures healing in an average of 13 weeks. Internal fixation of the scaphoid in these combined injuries allowed for earlier and more aggressive therapy to maximize wrist and forearm motion. Treatment in my hands is usually open reduction and internal fixation (ORIF) of the distal radius fracture and the mini-open approach and fixation of the scaphoid fracture.

Transscaphoid Perilunate Fracture-Dislocations

Open and Arthroscopic Treatment. Acute fracture-dislocations of the carpus are uncommon. Perilunate fracture-dislocations represent approximately 5% of wrist fractures and are about twice as common as pure ligamentous dislocations. Transscaphoid perilunate fracture-dislocation is the most common type of complex carpal dislocation.

Treatment of these injuries can be challenging owing to the extensive soft tissue, cartilaginous, and bony damage. Furthermore, obtaining universally excellent long-term results can be elusive.[92] Various operative treatment options have been recommended, including dorsal, volar, percutaneous, and arthroscopic approaches.[189]

These injuries are usually due to a high-energy impact, as may occur in motor vehicle accidents, a fall from a height, or contact sports. The mechanism of injury characteristically involves forceful wrist extension, ulnar deviation, and intercarpal supination. The injuries have been classified as greater and lesser arc injuries. Greater arc injuries have associated fractures and lesser arc injuries do not; lesser arc injuries are purely ligamentous. Bone or ligament failure usually begins with the radial styloid and or scaphoid fracture or palmar capsuloligamentous disruption starting radially and propagating ulnarly. In the greater arc injury, the energy takes a transosseous route through the scaphoid, with usual disruption of the lunotriquetral interosseous (LTIO) ligament and fracture of the ulnar styloid. The proximal fragment of the scaphoid and the lunate remain with the radius, while the distal fragment of the scaphoid dislocates dorsal to the lunate with the attached distal carpal row. In 10% of dislocations, the distal scaphoid fragment and the distal carpal row dislocate palmarly to the lunate. Variations of perilunate fracture-dislocations include fractures of the capitate, triquetrum, radial styloid, and ulnar styloid. A specific variation of the perilunate fracture-dislocation is *scaphocapitate syndrome.* In this injury, the injury force passes through the neck of the capitate, fracturing both the scaphoid and the capitate. The proximal portion of the capitate may rotate 90 to 180 degrees, with the articular surface of the head of the capitate directed distally. The injury to the capitate can be missed on plain radiographs. If scaphocapitate syndrome is suspected, a CT scan will better elucidate the pathoanatomic situation. ORIF is indicated in scaphocapitate syndrome through a dorsal approach. Both the capitate and scaphoid should be reduced and fixed with proximal to distal headless compression screws. Briseno and Yao reported on a lunate fracture along with perilunate injury and stressed the importance of looking for this injury and treating it appropriately. Even with treatment, the simultaneous lunate fracture portends a worse prognosis.[28]

Herzberg and Forissier investigated the medium-term results (mean follow-up, 8 years) of a series of 14 transscaphoid dorsal perilunate fracture-dislocations treated operatively at an average of 6 days following injury.[92] Eleven underwent ORIF through a dorsal approach. Combined palmar and dorsal approaches were used in three cases: in two cases, ORIF, and in one case, proximal row carpectomy. All internally fixed scaphoids healed, and no carpal AVN or collapse was observed. Carpal alignment was satisfactory in most cases. Posttraumatic radiologic midcarpal arthritis or radiocarpal arthritis, or both, was almost always observed.

Nearly every combination of radiocarpal and intercarpal dislocation has been described, but few fit neatly into a particular pattern or classification scheme. These injuries may be subtle, and diagnosis is still frequently delayed; the dislocation is missed by primary providers in up to 25% of cases.[117] Prompt recognition, accurate reduction, and stable internal fixation all contribute to improved outcomes. Internal fixation techniques depend on the pathologic condition of the carpus. Although arthroscopic techniques and fluoroscopically aided percutaneous techniques have been described,[68] my preference for treatment is an open procedure. The wrist is approached dorsally primarily for treatment of the scaphoid fracture or the scapholunate tear if it is a lesser arc injury. In 3% of cases, a complete SLIL tear accompanies a scaphoid fracture-dislocation.[92] An extended carpal tunnel approach is added if one of two situations is present: (1) The preoperative history and examination are consistent with acute carpal tunnel syndrome. If left untreated, median nerve compression can lead to long-term nerve deficits, hand stiffness, and, potentially, a complex regional pain syndrome. (2) A perilunate fracture-dislocation is irreducible from the dorsal approach. The lunate is visualized in the space of Poirier between the RSC ligament and long radiolunate ligament. Using a Freer elevator or similar instrument from the volar approach and manual wrist manipulation, the lunate can be negotiated into reduction.

For associated lunotriquetral ligament injury, the lunotriquetral joint is reduced and held with two Kirschner wires. One technique that is very valuable and surgically efficient is to place one or two double-ended Kirschner wires from within the lunotriquetral joint out the ulnar side of the wrist through the triquetrum before the lunate is reduced. A similar technique can be used in the scaphoid when the SLIL is torn. It is important to protect the soft tissues (radial artery, superficial radial nerve, tendons, veins) on the radial side of the wrist. The lunate is reduced and the wires are driven back into the lunate from inside the triquetrum and scaphoid, respectively. If extended carpal tunnel release has been performed, the stronger palmar component of the lunotriquetral ligament can be sutured with nonabsorbable braided suture from the palmar side.

Occasionally the dorsal radioulnar ligament origin is avulsed off of the dorsal ulnar corner of the radius. The distal radioulnar joint will be unstable and the dorsal ulnar corner of the radius will be devoid of soft tissue during the exposure. It is

---

CRITICAL POINTS *Perilunate Dislocation*

1. It is imperative during reduction to restore Gilula's lines in coronal plane and attain neutral radiolunate and capitolunate alignment in the sagittal plane.
2. Consider starting K wires from within the scapholunate joint and going out radially and ulnarly. Reduce the joint, then drive wires back in to fix the scapholunate joint and lunotriquetral joints, respectively.
3. Bury K wires because they should stay for approximately 10 to 12 weeks.
4. Beware of concomitant wrist injuries, such as dorsal radioulnar ligament injury.

important to repair the ligament with bone suture anchor. Repairs are generally protected with cast immobilization for 8 to 12 weeks, followed by removal of Kirschner wires and then gentle active mobilization of the wrist over the next 4 to 8 weeks (Figure 16.19, *A* to *H*).

Complications of Scaphoid Fracture Treatment

The most common complications reported in the literature are delayed union, nonunion, arthritis, reduced wrist motion, and loss of strength. Prolonged cast immobilization leads to muscle atrophy, possible joint contracture, disuse osteopenia, and potential financial hardship. Closed treatment of scaphoid waist fractures may require cast immobilization for 3 months or longer, and fractures of the proximal third of the scaphoid in particular may take 6 months or longer to heal. Surgical repair of scaphoid nonunion is successful in 50% to 95% of patients, depending on the vascular status and presence of arthritis or carpal collapse; successfully repaired scaphoid nonunions may require up to 6 additional months for healing and rehabilitation.

Other complications are reported. Filan and Herbert in 1996 reported on 431 patients treated with ORIF using the Herbert bone screw.[63] They reported that 56 patients had hypertrophic scarring and 20 patients complained of postoperative pain and swelling at the donor site of a bone graft. Four superficial infections and one deep wound infection resolved satisfactorily with conservative treatment. Four patients had early signs of reflex sympathetic dystrophy after surgery. In two patients these signs resolved spontaneously, but two patients developed carpal tunnel syndrome, which required surgical decompression. Only two wrists showed instability of the scaphoid after surgery. One had sustained a tear of the scapholunate ligament at the time of injury; the other appeared to have a late rupture of this ligament. AVN developed after surgery in 20 scaphoids, all of which required further operations. In one case, a very small necrotic fragment of the proximal pole was excised and the scaphoid stabilized by dorsal capsulorrhaphy. Five wrists had a midcarpal fusion. The necrotic proximal pole was excised in 14 cases and was replaced with a stabilized silicone implant in 13 and an osteochondral autograft in one.

In another early report of headless screw fixation, Dias and colleagues investigated 88 patients with minimally displaced or nondisplaced bicortical fractures of the waist of the scaphoid in a prospective, randomized controlled study comparing plaster immobilization in a below-elbow plaster cast with early internal fixation with use of a Herbert or Herbert-Whipple screw.[50] Complications occurred in 13 patients (30%) who had been managed operatively, and nonunion occurred in 10 of 44 patients (23%) of those treated in a cast. Most operative complications were minor, and included superficial wound infection (in one patient), sensitive scar (in three patients), hypertrophic scar (in four patients), sensitive and hypertrophic scar (in three patients), hypoesthesia in the region of the palmar cutaneous branch of the median nerve (in one patient), and mild early complex regional pain syndrome (in one patient). Technical difficulty was experienced in seven patients (16%) during surgery. In four of them, there was initial misplacement of either the drill or the screw. In one patient, the scaphoid tuberosity split during screw insertion.

Bushnell reported his complications with repair of scaphoid fractures using a dorsal percutaneous approach and cannulated headless screw fixation in 24 cases performed over 5 years.[30] All cases involved nondisplaced (<1 mm) fractures of the scaphoid waist. The overall complication rate was 29%; there were five major complications (21%) and two minor complications (8%). Major complications consisted of one case of nonunion, three cases of hardware problems, and one case of postoperative fracture of the proximal pole of the scaphoid. Minor complications included intraoperative equipment breakage, with one case involving a screw and one case involving a guidewire.

Complications of internal fixation are usually due to screw placement and length.[146] Controversy exists as to whether the screw should be placed centrally in the scaphoid[141] or perpendicular to the fracture.[108,140] Eccentric screws decrease fixation strength and risk penetration out of the scaphoid.[141]

Use of Fluoroscopy and Surgical Navigation to Reduce Screw Malposition

The development of small cannulated screws has permitted minimally invasive percutaneous fixation of acute scaphoid fractures. There are known mechanical advantages to increased screw length and central screw placement. As cited above, there are potential deleterious effects of eccentric screw placement, including articular protrusion, proximal pole fracture, and nonunion. Tumilty and Squire reported that the curvilinear surface of the proximal pole of the scaphoid may lead to errors in calculation of screw length and penetration into the joint.[207] In this cadaveric study of six specimens, two screws were found to be penetrating subchondral bone. The plain x-ray films were accurate in only five of the six specimens, while 360-degree fluoroscopic views were accurate in all six. Fluoroscopy during placement of a scaphoid screw may decrease the rate of subchondral penetration.

Recently, investigators have evaluated CT-generated models to assist in the development of a targeting system for implantation of screws into a reduced scaphoid fracture. Several investigative teams have demonstrated that a computer-assisted navigation of volar percutaneous scaphoid screw placement improved accuracy and required less time, less use of fluoroscopy, and diminished radiation exposure when compared with traditional percutaneous techniques.[70,96,115,129,214] Hoffman and colleagues showed in a cadaveric model that compared with the standard fluoroscopic technique, an electromagnetic navigation technique had a higher accuracy rate and lower rates of complications and required less operative time and radiation exposure time.[96]

Cost of Surgical or Nonsurgical Treatment

The treatment of stable scaphoid waist fractures by surgery has raised the issue of cost. Would the health care system be better served by plaster immobilization of these stable fractures, not considering the costs of re-treating fractures that failed to heal (6% to 23% nonunion rate)? Arora and colleagues compared two groups of stable scaphoid fractures, one treated with plaster immobilization and the other with internal screw fixation.[11] They concluded that internal screw fixation of nondisplaced scaphoid fractures had a shorter time to bony union and that the patients returned to work an average of 7 weeks earlier than patients with cast immobilization. Although it is assumed that operative treatment is more expensive, in this study the overall cost was not found to be higher.[11]

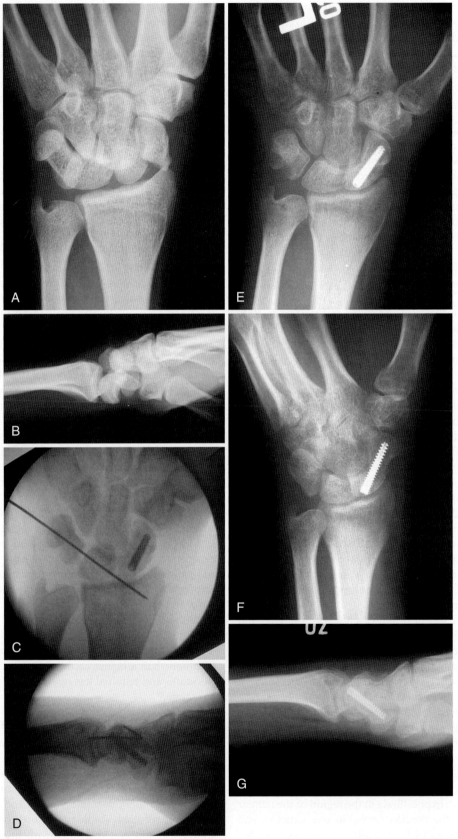

FIGURE 16.19 Transscaphoid perilunate fracture-dislocation. Preoperative posteroanterior (PA) **(A)** and lateral **(B)** radiographs of wrist. Intraoperative PA **(C)** and lateral **(D)** fluoroscopic images of wrist. At 3 months following operation, PA **(E)**, oblique **(F)**, and lateral **(G)** radiographs of wrist.

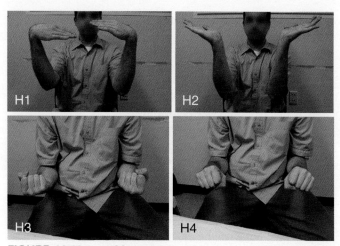

FIGURE 16.19, cont'd H, Postoperative range of motion at 6 months following operation.

Davis and colleagues conducted a cost/utility analysis to weigh ORIF against cast immobilization in the treatment of acute nondisplaced midwaist scaphoid fractures.[43] The authors used a model to calculate the outcomes and costs of ORIF and of cast immobilization, assuming the societal perspective. Medical costs were estimated using Medicare reimbursement rates, and costs of lost productivity were estimated by average wages obtained from the U.S. Bureau of Labor Statistics. ORIF offered greater quality-adjusted life-years than casting. ORIF was less costly than casting ($7940 versus $13,851 per patient) because of a longer period of lost productivity with casting. When considering only direct costs, the incremental cost/utility ratio for ORIF ranged from $5438 per quality-adjusted life-year for the 25- to 34-year-old age group to $11,420 for the 55- to 64-year-old age group, and $29,850 for the age group 65 years and older. They concluded that, unlike casting, ORIF is more cost-effective relative to other widely accepted interventions.[43]

Bone Growth Stimulators

The currently used bone stimulators that have been discussed in the context of scaphoid fractures fall into two major categories: external stimulation of ultrasound or pulsed electromagnetic field (PEMF) therapy. The external stimulators mimic stress to the bones, augmenting bone formation. Ultrasound (Exogen, Bioventus, Durham, NC) is used for only 20 minutes per day and PEMF for 8 to 12 hours per day; understandably, patient compliance with PEMF use is difficult to achieve. Randomized controlled data for ultrasound treatment in acute scaphoid fractures support its use. Mayr reported on 30 patients in a randomized study who had a cast with or without ultrasound for 20 minutes per day.[139] His results showed that fractures that underwent ultrasound treatment healed in 43.2 ± 10.9 days, versus 62 ± 19.2 days in the control group ($p < .01$). Using criteria of trabecular bridging as evidence of healing, 81.2% ± 10.4% of the ultrasound-stimulated fractures were healed at 6 weeks, versus 54.6% ± 29% in the control group ($p < .05$).[139] PEMF has been used to attempt to accelerate scaphoid healing. However, there are no reliable randomized controlled data for PEMF in scaphoid fractures. My preference is to use ultrasound for difficult scaphoid fractures.

Biologic Stimulation of Scaphoid Nonunions

Bone morphogenetic proteins play critical roles in both bone development and fracture healing. Urist first showed that extracts from demineralized bone matrix were capable of inducing new bone formation when implanted in an intramuscular site.[208] The osteoinductive properties of bone morphogenetic proteins for inducing bone formation in ectopic sites and producing healing of critical-sized segmental bone defects in experimental animal studies are attributable to their ability to stimulate the chemotaxis and differentiation of mesenchymal stem cells into chondroblasts or osteoblasts, or both. With the difficulty in treating proximal pole scaphoid nonunions, it is natural that these biologic enhancements would be investigated.

In a case reported by Jones and colleagues, a chronic nonunion of a proximal pole fracture of the scaphoid was treated by curettage of the nonunion, single Kirschner wire fixation, and implantation of 50 mg of human bone morphogenetic protein followed by 12 weeks of cast immobilization without any conventional corticocancellous bone grafting or rigid screw fixation.[111] Radiographs showed signs of bony healing by 12 weeks, and an MRI 6 years after surgery showed no signs of AVN. The authors discussed the potential future applications of human bone morphogenetic protein in hand surgery.[111]

Bilic and colleagues reported on 17 patients with scaphoid nonunion at the proximal pole treated with and without bone graft osteogenic protein-1 (OP-1) or bone morphogenetic protein 7 (BMP-7).[21] OP-1 improved the performance of both autologous and allograft bone implants and reduced radiographic healing time to 4 weeks compared with 9 weeks without OP-1. CT scans and scintigraphy showed that in patients treated with OP-1, sclerotic bone was replaced by well-vascularized bone. Allograft and autologous grafts treated with OP-1 healed at a similar rate.[21] At present, there is insufficient evidence to derive recommendations concerning the role of biologics in scaphoid fracture or nonunion treatment, and their use is not common.

Scaphoid Fracture in Children

Fractures of the immature scaphoid are uncommon and can be challenging to diagnose. These fractures most commonly involve the distal scaphoid and are effectively treated with cast immobilization. Fortunately most acute pediatric scaphoid fractures heal with nonoperative treatment, and surgery in children is indicated only if there is nonunion.[10]

The diagnosis of acute scaphoid fracture may be missed or delayed because of minimal symptoms. This is particularly true in athletic adolescents, who may return to sports prematurely after a seemingly minor injury to the wrist. The presentation of scaphoid fractures in adolescents has changed over the years and today more closely resembles the adult pattern. Malunion or nonunion may occur in patients with a missed diagnosis or delayed presentation and occasionally in patients treated promptly with immobilization. Surgical intervention should be considered for fracture nonunions in patients who are at or near skeletal maturity or in those in whom nonsurgical treatment has failed. Mintzer and Waters presented the outcome of 13 pediatric scaphoid fracture nonunions in 12 children treated over an 18-year period.[148] The average elapsed time between fracture and surgery was 16.7 months. Four of the nonunions were treated with inlay bone graft from a palmar approach, and nine were treated with Herbert screw fixation and iliac crest bone grafting. The average time of follow-up was 6.9 years (range, 2 to 19 years). All cases went on to clinical and radiographic union. Patients had no statistically significant difference in range of motion or strength between the operative and nonoperative wrists. The length of time for postoperative immobilization in the Herbert screw group was significantly less than that in the inlay bone graft group. Though scaphoid nonunions in children can heal with prolonged cast immobilization, the authors recommended that the treatment of scaphoid fracture nonunions in the skeletally immature patient be rigid fixation with a compression screw and iliac crest bone graft.

Masquijo and Willis presented their series of 23 pediatric (average age, 15 years) scaphoid nonunions fixed with iliac crest bone graft and screws, with a 95.6% union rate.[136]

Weber reported on six children with nonunited scaphoid fractures treated conservatively.[218] The mean age was 12.8 years (range, 9.7 to 16.3 years), and the mean follow-up time was 67 months. Five had no previous treatment, and the time to diagnosis averaged 4.6 months (range, 3 to 7 months) after injury. Treatment consisted of cast immobilization until clinical and radiologic union. Fractures united in all six children after a mean period of immobilization of 5 months (range, 3 to 7 months). All patients returned to regular activities. Although prolonged treatment with cast immobilization resulted in union of the fracture and an excellent subjective wrist score in all patients, this delay may not be well tolerated by the child or family.

Management of Scaphoid Nonunion

The ability to successfully treat scaphoid nonunions in part defines the abilities of a hand/upper extremity surgeon. Unfortunately, missed scaphoid fractures are relatively common, because oftentimes the patient, trainer, or urgent care personnel will dismiss a wrist injury as a "sprain." The traditional definition of scaphoid nonunion is failure of union following cast immobilization or surgical treatment of 6 months' duration. When most patients with scaphoid nonunion present, however, they have not had any form of treatment, months to years have elapsed since the injury, and secondary deformities and carpal collapse have occurred. If scaphoid nonunion is left untreated, the natural history is carpal collapse and degenerative arthritis.[133] In a long-term follow-up study of more than 30 years of scaphoid fractures treated with short-arm thumb spica casts, 10% had nonunion. Osteoarthritis with associated pain and weakness was present in 56% of patients. Only 2% of the healed group had osteoarthritis.[55]

To minimize the incidence of arthritis, the goal of treatment is to attain a healed scaphoid with anatomic alignment. Advanced imaging, including CT and MRI, aids in the evaluation of scaphoid alignment, bone loss, scaphoid humpback deformity, carpal collapse, and osteonecrosis. Generally, scaphoid nonunions from waist fractures with severe collapse and humpback deformity must be approached volarly with interposition of bone graft and internal fixation. For proximal pole nonunions, a dorsal approach allows access for curetting the nonunion site, bone grafting, and internal fixation of headless compression screw(s) from proximal to distal. The indications and best method of vascularized bone grafting are controversial.

Evaluation of Scaphoid Nonunion

When evaluating patients with scaphoid nonunion, the following issues regarding the fracture must be considered:

1. Where is the nonunion? At the waist or at the proximal pole?
2. Is the nonunion displaced?
3. Is there a humpback deformity?
4. Is there comminution, cyst formation, or cavitation?
5. Is DISI present?
6. Was there previous surgery?
7. Does the proximal pole look dysvascular?
8. Is there arthritis (SNAC wrist)? If so, at what stage?
9. Is the scaphoid deformed or salvageable?

Fracture Site. The more proximal the fracture, the more likely the proximal bone will be dysvascular. This may have implications for the choice of bone graft or other treatment.

Amount of Scaphoid Deformity and Carpal Malalignment. If there is humpback deformity and carpal malalignment, they may have to be corrected at the time of bone grafting and fixation.

Stability of Nonunion; Amount of Bone Loss. If the nonunion is stable and well aligned and bone loss is minimal, limited opening in the nonunion site, curetting as necessary, and cancellous bone grafting may be appropriate, followed by internal fixation by a headless compression screw. Slade and colleagues had previously reported on successful percutaneous bone grafting and fixation for nonunions.[182,183] I have not performed this and prefer an open technique, which also allows for confirmation of stability of the fracture and an intact cartilaginous envelope. Imaging, even CT scanning, does not necessarily predict the stability well (Mark Cohen, MD, personal communication).

Previous Treatment. Any previous surgical or other treatments should be taken into account because they would make further treatment more complex. We have had success with removal of the screw from the original surgery (usually, a volarly placed screw), cavitation of sclerotic or dysvascular bone, hybrid corticocancellous Russe autogenous bone grafting, and placement of a new screw from the opposite pole, usually from proximal to distal because the distal fragment has a hole from the previous screw.

Vascularity of Fragments. There is general agreement that vascularity is important. Green showed that 92% of scaphoid fractures with good vascularity healed when treated by Russe bone grafting. Union took place in 71% of patients when there was diminished vascularity in the scaphoid, but healing did not take place in any patients when the proximal pole was avascular.[80]

There is a lack of agreement on how to best determine vascularity. X-rays are not adequate to assess AVN,[177] and MRI and intraoperative punctate bleeding do not always correlate[84,112] (see previous section on Magnetic Resonance Imaging).

According to Green, vascularity was best determined by punctate bleeding. The use of punctate bleeding intraoperatively to determine AVN has recently been challenged. Even if the fragment is deemed to be dysvascular, there is lack of agreement about the optimal and necessary treatment, as will be discussed.

Possibly to better determine vascularity, curettings of the proximal and distal poles of the scaphoid should be evaluated by a pathologist who is experienced in bone histologic findings.

Salvageability of the Fragment. The fragment must not be collapsed or deformed beyond repair. In some cases the proximal pole has fragmented and collapsed and is not usable; this may occasionally happen with the distal pole, as well.

Presence and Location of Arthritis. If there is arthritis of the radiocarpal, midcarpal, or distal radioulnar joint, the treatment may have to be tailored accordingly For instance, if early arthritis (SNAC I) is confined to the radial styloid, radial styloidectomy and scaphoid bone grafting could be considered. With advanced arthritis, nonoperative management is considered if symptoms are not severe. With increasing pain, other options may include partial denervation or salvage procedures such as scaphoid excision and four-bone fusion, proximal row carpectomy, total wrist fusion, hemiwrist arthroplasty, and total wrist arthroplasty.

Patient parameters to consider when evaluating scaphoid nonunions include:

1. Length of time nonunion has been present
2. Age of patient
3. Amount of pain or dysfunction
4. Activity level
5. Systemic comorbidities present

Length of Time Nonunion Has Been Present. The longer the nonunion has been present, the more likely it is that there will be secondary issues such as arthritis, scaphoid deformity, and carpal instability. In a study by Mack and colleagues, older nonunion was associated with more severe arthritis.[133]

Age of the Patient. Although scaphoid fractures are usually a problem of young males, in the case of nonunion in an older patient, treatment might be tailored depending on individual needs and activity levels.

Amount of Pain or Dysfunction. In the case of nonunion with arthritis where a salvage procedure of scaphoid excision and four-bone fusion or proximal carpectomy might be an option, if the level of pain and dysfunction is tolerable, nonoperative treatment might be employed; the patient should be told that a salvage procedure may be needed later.

Activity Level. Elderly, inactive, or infirm patients may choose to accept the pain and limited range of motion of a scaphoid nonunion. There is no mandate for operative repair because salvage operations may always be considered if escalating arthritic pain causes increasing impairment.

Presence of Comorbidities. Scaphoid nonunion surgery can be complex and complicated, and the best efforts may be thwarted by heavy tobacco use, poor compliance, uncontrolled diabetes or inflammatory arthritis, steroid dependency, or other factors.

Operative Treatment of Scaphoid Nonunion (Table 16.4)

Type I: Delayed or Fibrous Union, No Deformity. Scaphoid nonunions without substantial bone loss require only rigid fixation to heal if there is adequate perfusion. These include fractures with a delayed presentation, fibrous unions, and nonunions with minimal sclerosis (<1 mm). Stable scaphoid fractures presenting for treatment after 1 month have already developed bone resorption at the fracture site from shearing. Early bony resorption is not typically detected by standard radiographs. Scaphoid fractures with delayed presentation (>4 weeks) have a poorer union rate with casting alone. Selected stable scaphoid delayed unions without deformity or substantial bone loss can

TABLE 16.4 Algorithm for Scaphoid Nonunion Management

Type of Fracture	Treatment
I. Delayed union	Mini-open rigid fixation with headless compression screw
II. Established waist nonunion, no deformity Fibrous nonunion, waist Sclerotic nonunion, waist	Open repair and autogenous bone grafting Dorsal or volar
Humpback nonunion	Volar approach Russe or Matti-Russe corticocancellous autograft Intercalated wedge autograft Hybrid Russe autograft
III. Proximal pole nonunion, viable	Dorsal approach Open bone grafting and fixation with headless screw Percutaneous bone grafting with headless screw Lock midcarpal joint with Kirscher wire(s) or miniscrew(s)
IV. Dysvascular nonunion, waist or proximal pole	Nonvascularized vs. vascularized bone graft: dorsal or palmar approach Osteoarticular graft

be successfully treated with reduction and internal rigid fixation without bone grafting using techniques described for acute fractures above.

Similarly, established fibrous nonunions stabilized with a compression screw and without a bone graft typically heal. Shah and Jones examined 50 scaphoid nonunions treated with open Herbert screw fixation and noted that the scaphoid nonunions that had an intact cartilaginous envelope or a stable fibrous union healed with screw fixation alone without bone grafting.[178]

Scaphoid nonunions that have minimal bone resorption of the anterior cortical bone and minimal fracture sclerosis (<2 mm confirmed by CT scan) still have the potential for healing in the early stages with screw fixation alone. Slade and coworkers successfully treated aligned nonunions without bone loss using headless screw fixation alone. All 15 patients in this case series healed at an average of 14 weeks and showed bridging cortical bone on CT scans.[182]

Type II: Scaphoid Waist Nonunion, Without Arthritis. The most common type of nonunion faced by the surgeon will be a midwaist fracture nonunion with fracture site resorption and varying degrees of deformity and bone loss. For this type, nonvascularized bone grafting either from the distal radius or iliac crest will generally suffice for healing of the bone as long as certain technical aspects are followed. A point of controversy is whether deformity must be corrected to provide an optimal outcome. In a long-term follow-up study of healed scaphoid nonunions, Jiranek and colleagues identified a higher percentage of arthritic changes in malunited scaphoid fractures.[109] The degree of arthritis did not correlate with the activity level, satisfaction, or return to work, however. Although anatomic alignment is intuitively preferable for restoration of normal

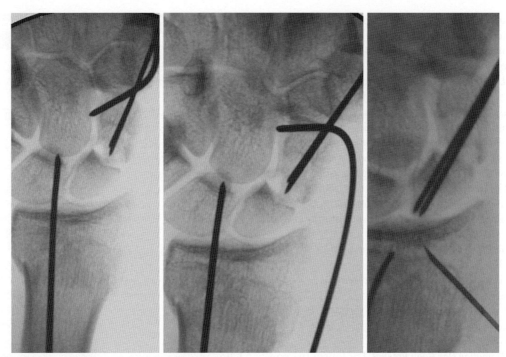

FIGURE 16.20 Once fracture reduction has been accomplished using the joysticks, the central axis guidewire in the distal scaphoid fragment is driven from volar to dorsal, capturing and holding the fracture reduction. Very unstable fractures may require two central axis wires to resist bending and fracture rotation.

kinematics, some degree of malunion seems to be tolerable.[37,50,64] I make every attempt to correct intercarpal malalignment and DISI at the time of nonunion surgery, especially in young and active patients, to avoid the otherwise inevitable progression of arthritis.

Surgical Fixation With Nonvascularized Bone Graft (Local). The procedure can be done from a volar or dorsal approach. Adequate preparation of the bone surfaces with care taken not to cause thermal necrosis with a bur or saw is imperative. Curetting to bleeding bone is necessary on both proximal and distal poles. The scaphoid is reduced and abundant autogenous bone graft packed into the proximal and distal poles. Fixation with a headless compression screw is optimal and is generally performed from distal to proximal in waist nonunions, as detailed in the section, Hybrid Russe Procedure. If the lunate is malrotated into dorsiflexion, reduction and temporary fixation of the lunate with a 0.062-inch radiolunate Kirschner wire will facilitate accurate alignment of the scaphoid proximal pole prior to scaphoid grafting and fixation (Figure 16.20). Supplemental fixation across the scaphocapitate joint may further stabilize the construct, especially if there is concern about the rigidity of fixation.

For nonvascularized bone graft, there is no difference in outcomes between distal radius and iliac crest bone grafts.[35,145] A systematic review of the literature showed the superiority of screw over Kirschner wires for fixation of the scaphoid.[145] Cohen and colleagues reported on 12 patients who all healed with cancellous bone graft from the distal radius and a distal to proximal headless compression screw. The average lateral intrascaphoid angles were improved from 49 degrees to 32 degrees.[37]

Matti Technique, Matti-Russe Technique, and Green's Modification of the Russe Technique. In the original Matti technique, only cancellous bone was used, and this is optimum

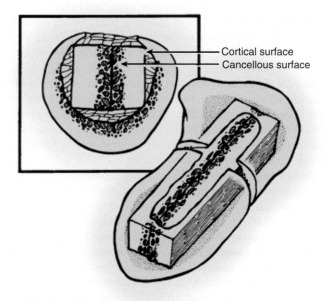

FIGURE 16.21 Russe technique using two corticocancellous bone grafts. (From Green DP: The effect of a vascular necrosis on Russe bone grafting for scaphoid nonunion. *J Hand Surg [Am]* 10:597–605, 1985.)

for scaphoid waist nonunions without humpback deformity and carpal collapse. The Matti-Russe technique and Green's modification of the Russe technique have a high percentage of cortical to cancellous bone (Figure 16.21). In the current author's preferred method of the hybrid Russe technique, the cortical strut volume is much smaller yet still "props open" the scaphoid, and it can be performed for both well-aligned and humpback scaphoid nonunions. The rest of the scaphoid is filled with cancellous bone, and a headless compression screw is used for both axial and centripetal compression.

Barton had less success in long-term evaluation of Russe bone grafting, especially in proximal pole nonunions, which demonstrated a success rate of only 54%.[15]

❖ AUTHOR'S PREFERRED METHOD:
Hybrid Russe Procedure

The hybrid Russe procedure is advantageous because it is effective for humpback scaphoid nonunions with DISI. The procedure exposes healthy bleeding cancellous bone in both scaphoid poles, uses a strut to maintain reduction of the humpback deformity, and resists collapse during screw compression. The technique incorporates abundant cancellous bone with optimal healing potential, which provides earlier healing than the standard Russe procedure.[80] It also avoids graft extrusion and uses local bone grafts.

In a series of hybrid Russe corticocancellous grafting procedures for scaphoid nonunion, we reported union in 16 of 16 patients at an average of 13 weeks. Compared with the contralateral side, the mean ipsilateral grip strength was 91% ($p = .029$). The mean postoperative scapholunate angle was significantly reduced when compared with the preoperative angle (47 degrees postoperatively from 70 degrees preoperatively, $p < .001$). The mean postoperative intrascaphoid angle was also reduced with surgery (32 degrees vs. 62 degrees, $p < .001$). Similarly, the mean radiolunate angle was reduced postoperatively by 30 degrees (−4 degrees vs. 26 degrees, $p = .031$). The median visual analog pain scale score postoperatively was 1, with a highest frequency of 0. There were no reported complications.[170]

Hybrid Russe Procedure. The patient is placed in the supine position under general or regional anesthesia with a pneumatic tourniquet on the injured extremity. The arm is cleansed with antimicrobial solution and draped using sterile technique. Exsanguination is performed with an Esmarch bandage, and an arm tourniquet is inflated to 250 mm Hg. A volar incision is made along the course of the FCR tendon and extended distally along the border of the glabrous skin of the thenar eminence. The distal incision is limited to the level of the scaphotrapezial joint in preparation for screw fixation starting in the distal pole of the scaphoid. Splitting the sheath of the FCR allows the FCR to be retracted ulnarly. The floor of the FCR sheath is incised longitudinally to expose the distal and proximal poles of the scaphoid. The superficial branch of the radial artery to the superficial arch is retracted radially or divided between sutures. The nonunion is exposed with the aid of skin hooks (Figure 16.22). All fibrous tissue at the nonunion site is removed and bone is curetted to remove sclerotic bone and fibrous tissue down to bleeding cancellous bone. In cases of humpback deformity and DISI, the lunate is reduced with a wrist flexion maneuver and a percutaneous radiolunate 0.062-inch Kirschner wire is placed dorsally or radially for temporary fixation and to correct proximal scaphoid pole alignment. Proximal dissection is carried out, incising and reflecting the pronator quadratus off the metaphysis of the radius toward the ulnar side. A cortical window of 20 × 5 mm is made on the volar cortex of the distal radius, and the cortical fragment is set aside for later use (Figure 16.23). Abundant cancellous bone graft is harvested from the radius. A "matchstick" is fabricated from the volar cortical window of the radius and sized to act as a cortical strut (to extend and reduce the humpback deformity and restore the

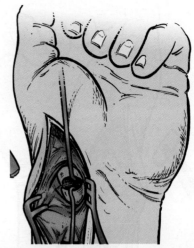

FIGURE 16.22 Volar incision over flexor carpi radialis. Nonunion site is exposed with aid of skin hooks, and fibrous tissue is resected. (Courtesy of Steve K. Lee, MD.)

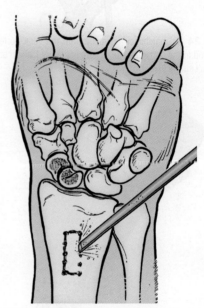

FIGURE 16.23 A cortical window is made on the volar cortex of the distal radius. Cancellous bone graft is harvested. (Courtesy of Steve K. Lee, MD.)

length of the scaphoid) (Figure 16.24). Using bone hooks to extend the prepared proximal and distal poles, the cortical strut is inserted in intramedullary fashion and tamped into position. Cancellous bone graft is packed into the remainder of the nonunion site (Figure 16.25), and this is followed with fixation with a headless screw (Figures 16.26 and 16.27). Intraoperative fluoroscopy is used as needed to confirm adequate reduction and fixation. The volar capsule and radiocarpal ligaments are repaired with interrupted nonabsorbable sutures, and the subcutaneous layer and skin are closed in layers. A splint is kept in place for 2 weeks following the operation. For patients with a radiolunate wire, above-elbow immobilization is critical to prevent wire breakage. The wire is removed in the office at 4 weeks, and a short-arm cast is applied until healing occurs. A CT scan is performed to confirm union at 10 to 14 weeks following operation, and immobilization is converted to a custom-molded removable splint.

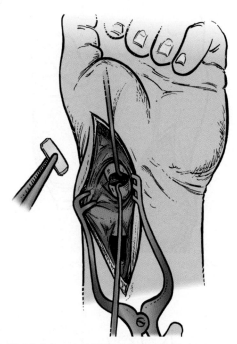

FIGURE 16.24 A "matchstick" is made from the volar cortex of the distal radius and placed in the nonunion site in intramedullary fashion as a strut. (Courtesy of Steve K. Lee, MD.)

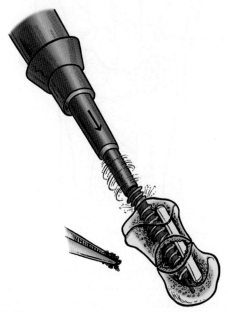

FIGURE 16.25 Cancellous bone graft is packed in the remainder of the nonunion site, followed by fixation with a headless compression screw. (Courtesy of Steve K. Lee, MD.)

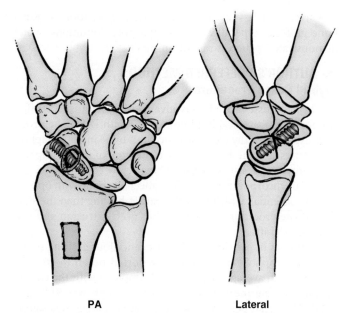

PA   Lateral

FIGURE 16.26 Posteroanterior (*PA*) and lateral line drawings showing the scaphoid after hybrid Russe procedure. The humpback deformity has been corrected and the length of the scaphoid has been restored. Headless screw provides additional fixation to the construct. (Courtesy of Steve K. Lee, MD.)

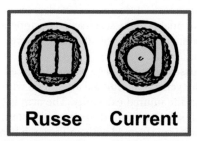

Russe   Current

FIGURE 16.27 Drawing showing axial cut through the scaphoid comparing the Green's modified Russe procedure *(left)* and the hybrid procedure *(right)*, showing the position of the screw as well as the graft.

If surgery has been performed previously, this technique may still be used, but the new screw should be placed from the opposite direction (Figure 16.28, *A* to *F*). The cortical strut may be inserted down the previous screw tract.

Surgical Fixation of Scaphoid Nonunion With Nonvascularized Bone Graft (Distant) Wedge Graft

Fernandez-Fisk wedge graft. In 1984, Fernandez presented his modification of the Fisk procedure to treat scaphoid nonunions associated with carpal instability.[60] His article described the

following modifications: (1) preoperative calculation of the exact scaphoid length and form based on comparative radiographs of the opposite wrist, (2) the use of a palmar approach, (3) the insertion of a wedge-shaped corticocancellous graft from the iliac crest after resection of the pseudarthrosis, and (4) the use of internal fixation (Figure 16.29, *A* to *D*).

Preoperative planning is considered essential to restore the anatomic length, analyze the angular deformity, evaluate the pathologic scapholunate angle, and calculate the resection and size of the graft needed. The palmar approach reduces the danger of iatrogenic damage of the vascular supply of the scaphoid and accidental lesions of the superficial branches of the radial nerve. Iliac bone is preferred to the radial styloid graft, as proposed by Fisk, because of its better ability to resist compression forces. Internal fixation adds rotational stability so that continued postoperative plaster immobilization can be reduced to a minimum of 8 weeks.

In 1990, Fernandez reported union of 19 of 20 established nonunions repaired with this technique, with an average time off work of 8.9 weeks.[61] In a review of the pertinent literature, he determined that the most common reasons for recalcitrant

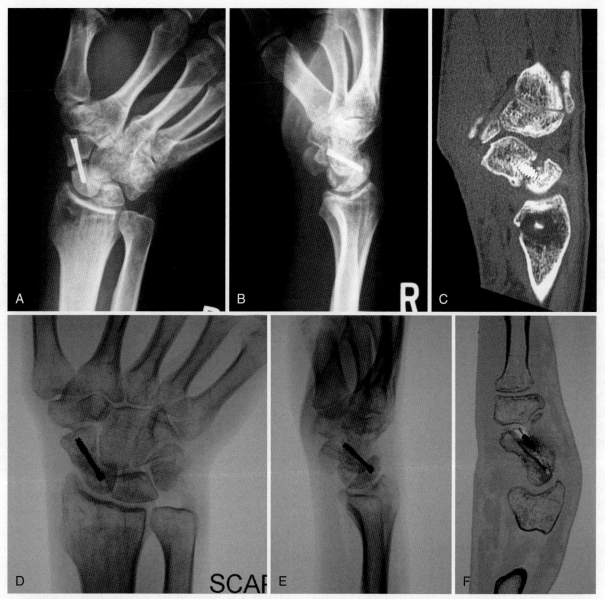

FIGURE 16.28 A, Oblique radiograph of wrist showing scaphoid nonunion after attempted open reduction and internal fixation. **B,** Lateral wrist radiograph. **C,** Computed tomography (CT) scan, sagittal view. At 12 weeks following operation, healing is evident on scaphoid **(D)** and lateral **(E)** radiographs and sagittal CT scan **(F)**. (Courtesy of Scott W. Wolfe, MD.)

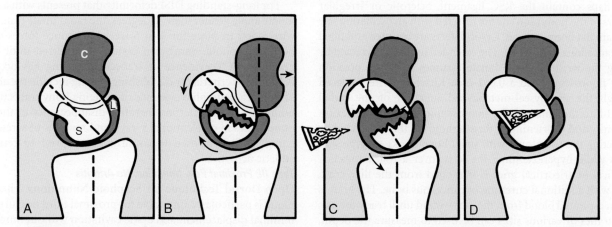

FIGURE 16.29 A, Schematic representation of normal alignment of the scaphoid (*S*), lunate (*L*), and capitate (*C*). **B,** Nonunion of a fracture of the scaphoid with palmar flexion of the distal fragment and a dorsal intercalated segmental instability pattern. **C,** The scaphoid alignment is corrected. **D,** It is maintained by the insertion of a palmar wedge-shaped bone graft. (From Taleisnik J: *The Wrist,* New York, 1985, Churchill Livingstone. Redrawn by Elizabeth Martin.)

nonunion were improper internal fixation techniques or the absence of bone grafting, or both.

Eggli reported on a retrospective review of 37 patients with scaphoid fracture nonunions treated by interpositional bone grafting and internal fixation at an average follow-up of 5.7 years.[56] Solid radiographic union was achieved in 35 cases. Pre-existing AVN was a major adverse factor for achievement of union and satisfactory outcome. Patients with preexisting degenerative changes had a significantly worse clinical outcome. The vast majority of the patients had satisfactory correction of scaphoid length and the associated DISI. Although 30 patients showed radiographic evidence of mild or moderate degenerative changes at their latest follow-up, there was no significant progression of arthrosis, and carpal collapse deformity did not progress after healing of the fracture nonunion.[56]

Arguments against the wedge graft. The wedge graft technique as described does not routinely incorporate curettage of the proximal and distal poles to bleeding cancellous bone. I would advise removing sclerotic, fibrotic, or cystic bone in the proximal and distal poles prior to insertion of the wedge graft and packing with additional cancellous graft. Volar wedge bone grafting may require 3 to 6 months to heal and may result in reduced wrist motion.[68] In documented avascular cases without punctate bleeding, volar wedge grafting with an autologous iliac crest graft is associated with union rates of only 30%.[168] Finally, the technique is exacting, and it may be challenging to simultaneously attain excellent compression, anatomic restitution of normal scaphoid anatomy, and rigid fixation.

Technique of anterior wedge grafting. Preoperative PA, lateral, and ulnar deviation PA radiographs of the injured wrist and the opposite normal wrist are used to determine the amount of resection and size of the graft needed. The surgeon must determine the amount of scaphoid flexion deformity, the extent of carpal collapse, and the scapholunate and lunocapitate angles (Figure 16.30, *A* to *C*). The humpback deformity can be evaluated more exactly using CT scans taken along the long axis of the scaphoid.

Nonunions of the distal third and waist are approached through a palmar hockey-stick incision along the FCR, extended obliquely toward the thenar eminence. The anterior capsule is incised from the distal radius to the scaphotrapezoidal joint to expose the most palmar-radial corner of the scaphoid. The capsular flaps contain the RSC ligament. Sclerotic or irregular borders of the nonunion site are resected with an oscillating saw to obtain flat bony surfaces. Cystic defects are curetted and filled with cancellous bone chips. The extended lunate is corrected by flexing the wrist until the lunate assumes a neutral position under fluoroscopy, and a 0.062-inch Kirschner wire is placed through the diaphyseal-metaphyseal junction of the radial styloid into the lunate under fluoroscopic control. The flexion deformity and shortening of the scaphoid are then corrected by distracting the osteotomy with small bone hooks or large skin hooks while hyperextending the wrist over a rolled towel. A bicortical or tricortical graft is harvested from the iliac crest, along with additional curetting of cancellous bone. The graft is kept in aspirated blood from the iliac wound until ready for use. Osteotomes of various sizes can be used to measure the depth, width, and length of the trapezoidal defect of the scaphoid,[168] and the graft is sculpted to the correct dimensions using a saw and osteotomes. The bone graft is impacted into the defect, and

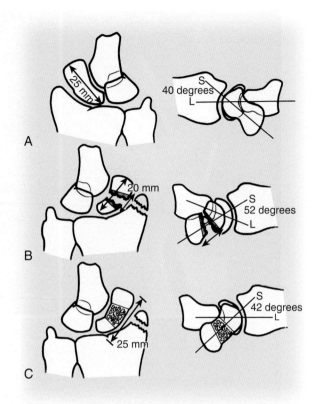

FIGURE 16.30 A, Preoperative planning for insertion of a wedge-shaped graft. Tracing of the opposite uninjured wrist and measurement of scaphoid length and scapholunate angle. **B,** Calculation of size, resection area, and form of graft. **C,** Definitive diagram of the operation. *L,* Lunate; *S,* scaphoid. (Redrawn from Fernandez DL: A technique for anterior wedge-shaped grafts for scaphoid nonunions with carpal instability. *J Hand Surg [Am]* 9:733–737, 1984. Redrawn by Elizabeth Martin.)

scaphoid alignment and posture are checked with fluoroscopy. A guidewire is advanced from distal to proximal across the scaphoid and intercalated graft. Finally, compression screw fixation of the scaphoid is performed. Careful closure of the palmar capsule and repair of the RSC ligament is done. A long-arm thumb spica postoperative splint is applied. Sutures are removed at 10 to 12 days, and the above-elbow immobilization is continued until the radiolunate pin is removed.

For long-standing DISI deformity that presents with a radiolunate angle greater than 20 degrees, the radiolunate transfixion wire is left in place for 4 to 6 weeks to reduce forces on the healing scaphoid. Short-arm casting is preferred until radiographic or CT evidence of trabecular healing has occurred. Fernandez's criteria for establishing healing include the absence of pain, radiographic evidence of bridging bony trabeculae on both sides of the interposed graft, a disappearance of the osteotomy lines in conventional x-rays, and no signs of screw loosening.[60] CT is advised to confirm union prior to return to athletic activities.

Type III: Proximal Pole Nonunion, No Arthritis

Open Dorsal Technique for Scaphoid Nonunions. This technique is particularly applicable for proximal third fractures with minimal displacement and cystic cavitation without humpback deformity. The technique is similar to that described above in the acute treatment of scaphoid fractures from the dorsal approach.

The tourniquet is placed proximally on the arm and draped to allow full motion of the extremity. A small (≈2-3 cm) longitudinal incision is made just radial to the 3-4 arthroscopic portal. This area is also in line between the second and third metacarpal interspaces and extends proximally just radial to the Lister tubercle, crossing the dorsal lip of the radius. The EPL is carefully identified by opening the third dorsal compartment and may be transposed external to the retinaculum at the conclusion of the case. The second and fourth dorsal compartments are retracted and protected with Penrose drains. The capsule is incised along the dorsal rim of the radius, splitting the dorsal radiotriquetral ligament in the line of its fibers. If more exposure is necessary, a full ligament-sparing approach can be used (see Chapter 13), reflecting a radially based capsular flap by splitting the dorsal intercarpal ligament in line with its fibers.[18]

Extreme care is taken to avoid disruption of the dorsal fibers of the SLIL when reflecting the capsular flap. Dissection in a plane tangential to the dorsal surfaces of the scaphoid and the lunate can be performed with a scalpel or Beaver blade. The distal boundaries of dissection of the scaphoid are determined by the vascular supply along the dorsal ridge. Care is taken not to disrupt the blood vessels entering the waist of the scaphoid. Retractors may be placed deeper to retract the capsule. The proximal pole nonunion site may not be immediately evident, and a 25-g needle can be inserted under fluoroscopy to confirm the location. A small dorsal window is created to expose the nonunion site, and curets are used to excavate cystic areas. The proximal and distal poles are débrided to bleeding cancellous bone, and if the nonunion is adherent and has a smooth cartilaginous shell, no attempt is made to disrupt the two poles. If displaced, the scaphoid is aligned using Kirschner wire joysticks.

The Lister tubercle is removed with an osteotome and saved for re-placement in the graft cavity. A large amount of cancellous bone can be harvested. The harvested cancellous bone graft can be compacted using a 3-mL syringe and its plunger and cut to size for impaction into the nonunion. Thrombin-soaked Gelfoam may be inserted into the radial defect, and the tubercle can be replaced or inverted as a lid. The nonunion site is packed with cancellous bone graft. Screw fixation is performed as is described in the section on Author's Preferred Treatment Method: Dorsal Approach. Use of two microheaded screws (1.2-1.7 mm) can also be considered, but it is important to countersink and bury these small noncannulated headed screws. The capsule is closed with a running suture, and the retinaculum is closed with 2-0 absorbable suture.

Additional maneuvers to augment stability of the construct are to place a 0.045- or 0.062-inch Kirschner wire or headless compression screw from the distal scaphoid to the capitate[68] and to reduce the lunate to be collinear with the radius and pin from the radius to the lunate. If used, the radiolunate pin is stabilized with an above-elbow cast and the pin removed after 4 weeks. Scaphocapitate fixation is retained until healing, which may take 10 to 12 weeks. Inoue reported a successful union rate of 80% with cancellous bone grafting and Herbert screw placement through a dorsal approach.[105]

Percutaneous Bone Graft or Bone Graft Substitute, Arthroscopic Technique (Video 16.1). Geissler and Slade are proponents of percutaneous bone grafting of proximal pole nonunions.[68] Slade and Gillon reviewed their experience with percutaneous bone grafting in a series of 234 scaphoid fractures.[183] Successful percutaneous treatment of scaphoid nonunions requires careful planning and the use of a number of imaging tools, including standard radiography, minifluoroscopy, CT or MRI, and arthroscopy. Chu and Shih reported that 14 of 15 (93%) scaphoid nonunions healed with arthroscopic-assisted use of injected bone graft substitute (Genex, Biocomposites, Keele, England). Herbert Whipple screw fixation was used.[36]

Percutaneous Bone Grafting of Scaphoid Nonunions. Selected minimally displaced or nondisplaced scaphoid fracture nonunions can be treated with percutaneous bone grafting and internal fixation. This may be particularly helpful for the small proximal pole fragment with cystic resorption at the fracture site but an intact cartilage shell. The technique for dorsal wire placement is the same as for acute fractures. The starting position for the guidewire is the proximal pole of the scaphoid. The wire is introduced into the proximal scaphoid pole using fluoroscopic imaging and is guided down the scaphoid central axis toward the thumb. The wrist is moderately flexed to avoid bending the guidewire. The wire is advanced toward the thumb base from a dorsal to volar position until the dorsal trailing end of the wire clears the radiocarpal joint, permitting full extension of the wrist. Once the dorsal trailing end of the guidewire has been buried into the proximal scaphoid pole, the wrist can be extended for imaging to confirm scaphoid alignment and correct positioning of the guidewire. If percutaneous wire placement is not possible, a mini-incision can be made over the 3-4 portal. The EPL tendon is located and retracted radially and the capsule is incised, exposing the proximal scaphoid pole. A drill guide is placed on the scaphoid proximal pole and a 0.045-inch double-cut guidewire is driven in a radial and distal direction toward the thumb base. Fluoroscopic imaging is used to confirm the correct course of the wire in the scaphoid.

Displaced nonunions may be percutaneously manipulated and reduced with the use of dorsally placed 0.062-inch joystick Kirschner wires in each fragment and a percutaneously placed hemostat, using the previously described techniques for acute fractures. Following accurate fracture reduction, placement of the guidewire, and measurement of the screw length, the wire is driven distally and out of the skin of the thenar eminence and clamped.

The scaphoid is reamed from the proximal scaphoid pole, crossing the nonunion site to the distal scaphoid 2 mm from the far cortex. The reaming of the distal scaphoid reestablishes a fresh blood supply and removes the devitalized bone at the nonunion site. The scaphoid wire is withdrawn distally across the nonunion site and into the distal fragment. A curet is placed through the proximal scaphoid portal to the nonunion site. This is done using real-time imaging. The outer cortex, which often has fibrous tissue, must not be violated, because this tissue acts as a net holding the percutaneously introduced bone graft. The wire is reintroduced across the fracture and out of the dorsal wound.

Percutaneous harvesting of bone graft. Bone graft can be percutaneously harvested from the distal radius or iliac crest using one of several bone-coring devices that are commercially available. We prefer a 4-inch 8-gauge bone biopsy needle (Baxter Jamshidi, Deerfield, IL) to percutaneously harvest cancellous bone graft. A guidewire is percutaneously inserted into the dorsal distal radius near or at the Lister tubercle. A small incision and blunt dissection expose the bone cortex. A hand reamer is used to penetrate the cortex. The bone biopsy cannula is introduced over the Kirschner wire, the Kirschner wire is removed, and cancellous bone plugs are harvested.

Attention is directed back to the scaphoid, and the biopsy cannula is inserted over the guidewire into the prepared nonunion site. The guidewire is withdrawn into the distal scaphoid pole. Guided by imaging, autogenous bone plugs are implanted through the cannula into the nonunion site using the plunger, and the graft is impacted. The guidewire is driven back across the proximal pole and out of the dorsal wound. Rigid fixation is obtained with percutaneous cannulated headless screw fixation along the guidewire axis. Additional implants may be inserted to further stabilize the fracture site and prevent bone shearing until bone healing has occurred as needed, including a screw or wire to temporarily lock the midcarpal joint and a radiolunate wire as needed. In some cases, extreme proximal scaphoid pole nonunions have been treated with bone grafting and compression by sandwiching a compression screw from the midscaphoid to the lunate in addition to the midcarpal locking screw.

Postoperative care. Immediate postoperative care includes a bulky compressive hand dressing and a volar splint. The patient is encouraged to initiate early finger exercises to reduce swelling. The therapist fashions a removable volar splint that holds the wrist and hand in a functional position at the first postoperative visit, and the patient is started on an immediate gentle strengthening program the purpose of which is to axially load the fracture site now secured with an intramedullary screw to stimulate healing. This early digital motion program decreases swelling and permits an early return of hand function. Patients with eccentric fractures, particularly proximal pole fractures, are restricted from wrist motion until CT scan confirms bridging bone at the fracture site at 6 weeks following operation. Although postoperative radiographs are obtained at the first postoperative visit and at 6-week intervals, a CT scan is used to confirm trabecular bridging.

Dysvascular Nonunion, Waist or Proximal Pole Fracture. When vascularized bone grafting was first introduced, the healing rate was reported to be 100%.[195,228] With time, the original enthusiasm has waned because more reports have shown much lower healing percentages. Hirche and colleagues reported a healing rate of only 75% with the 1,2 intercompartmental suprareticnacular artery bone graft.[94] Chang and associates reported a union rate of 50% with the same graft if AVN was present,[34] and Straw and coworkers reported a union rate of only 12% if AVN was present.[196] No distinct guidelines exist as to which cases would most benefit from vascularized bone grafting.

Previous papers reported low healing rates with the Russe technique[80] (0% union) or volar iliac crest wedge grafting[168] (30% union) when ischemic bone was diagnosed by the absence of punctate bleeding. Many of these patients were treated with Kirschner wire fixation, before the advent of headless screw fixation. Modern methods of rigid internal fixation have called into question the relative importance of ischemia versus fixation strength as the key parameter influencing healing of scaphoid nonunions. Whether removal of necrotic or dysvascular bone and replacement with healthy autogenous bone and rigid fixation is preferable to retention of ischemic bone and implantation of a vascular graft to encourage creeping substitution has not been answered by the current scientific evidence. In fact, few papers report the histologic findings of surgically treated nonunions, making comparative studies impossible. There is controversy as to how to best assess vascularity of the proximal pole, whether by preoperative MRI with or without contrast or by the presence or absence of bleeding bone intraoperatively. Given all of these unanswered questions, the role of vascular grafting for scaphoid nonunion cannot be stated with certainty; the various options available and current best evidence will be reviewed.

In 1979, Hori and colleagues performed elegant canine studies to demonstrate the efficacy of an implanted arteriovenous pedicle to treat osteonecrosis.[97] Sunagawa and colleagues, in a subsequent canine study, compared nonvascularized (conventional) grafts with arteriovenous pedicle graft implantation and quantitatively assessed bone blood flow, fracture healing, and bone remodeling.[197] They found that 73% of the vascularized grafts and none of the conventional grafts healed. At 6 weeks, bone blood flow in the proximal pole was significantly higher on the side of the vascularized graft. Quantitative histomorphometry of the avascular proximal segment demonstrated significantly higher levels of fluorochrome-labeled osteoid- and osteoblast-covered trabecular surfaces on the vascularized graft side. These data supported the clinical application of pedicled vascularized bundle implantation in the treatment of carpal osteonecrosis including proximal pole scaphoid nonunions (Figure 16.31).[62]

Vascularized Bone Grafting. Since 1986 there has been great interest in vascularized bone grafting to treat bony nonunion

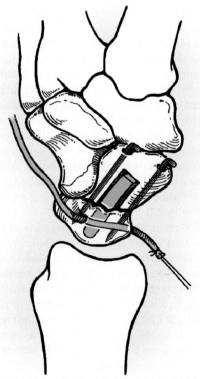

FIGURE 16.31 Second intermetacarpal vascular bundle implantation. (From Fernandez DL, Eggli S: Nonunion of the scaphoid: revascularization of the proximal pole with implantation of a vascular bundle and bone grafting. *J Bone Joint Surg [Am]* 6:883–893, 1995. Redrawn by Elizabeth Martin.)

including the scaphoid. Shi reported on an experimental study and clinical uses of the fasciosteal flap for bone healing.[180] In 1991, Zaidemberg and colleagues demonstrated a consistent vascularized bone graft source from the distal dorsal radial radius for the treatment of scaphoid nonunions using latex injection techniques.[228] In a preliminary series of 11 patients, these authors reported 100% success.[228]

Although when to use vascularized bone grafting is controversial, many authors discuss using it for AVN when there is lack of punctate bleeding witnessed intraoperatively. Another indication may be persistent nonunion following previously attempted surgical treatment. Some of the more common vascularized bone graft choices are:

1. 1,2 intercompartmental supraretinacular artery (ICSRA) pedicle (Zaidemberg)
2. Pedicled on the volar carpal artery (Mathoulin)
3. Dorsal capsular pedicle (Sotereanos)
4. Free medial femoral condyle graft (Doi, Bishop and Shin, Higgins)

1,2 Intercompartmental Supraretinacular Artery Pedicle

Vascular anatomy of dorsal radius grafts. The vessels supplying the nutrient arteries to the dorsal radius are best described by their relationship to the extensor compartments of the wrist and the extensor retinaculum. The 1,2 intercompartmental supraretinacular artery (1,2 ICSRA) is superficial to the extensor retinaculum and lies between the first and second compartments. The 2,3 intercompartmental supraretinacular artery (2,3 ICSRA) lies superficial between the second and third compartments. Both arteries are at areas where the extensor retinaculum is firmly attached to bone, allowing nutrient arteries to penetrate the cortex. In addition to the superficial vessels, two vessels are deep to the extensor tendons on the floor of the fourth and fifth dorsal compartments. These are the fourth and fifth extensor compartment arteries (ECAs). The 1,2 ICSRA branches from the radial artery 5 cm proximal to the radiocarpal joint and rises dorsally to lie on the extensor retinaculum between the first and second compartments.

Technique for surgical preparation of the 1,2 ICSRA graft. The 1,2 ICSRA graft for scaphoid nonunion described by Zaidemberg and colleagues[228] (Figure 16.32) is most useful for scaphoid nonunion, but it has a relatively short pedicle. A dorsal radial incision is centered over the radiocarpal joint between the first and second compartments. This allows good exposure of the dorsal radial scaphoid. Branches of the superficial radial

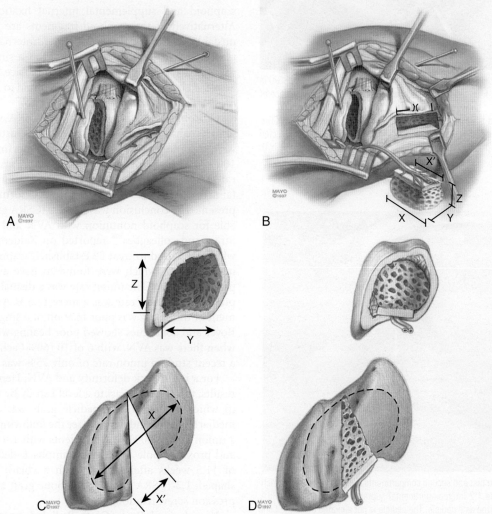

FIGURE 16.32 Use of a dorsal radius vascularized graft in cases of malunion or humpback deformity. **A,** The scaphoid is prepared before graft elevation. **B,** A large graft is harvested that can be shaped into a wedge. **C** and **D,** The graft is trimmed to fit the defect dimensions and used as a volar strut. *X,* length of intramedullary defect; *X′,* length of cortical gap; *Y,* width; *Z,* height. (By permission of Mayo Foundation for Medical Education and Research. All rights reserved.)

nerve need to be identified and protected. The 1,2 ICSRA is found coursing up dorsally from the radial artery to lie superficially on the surface of the extensor retinaculum between the first and second compartments (Figure 16.33). The first and second compartments are incised at their attachments to bone near the 1,2 ICSRA. The 1,2 ICSRA is carefully mobilized as a pedicle (Figure 16.34). Care is taken not to elevate the pedicle off the bone more than 10 to 15 mm proximal to the joint line, because this is the area where the nutrient vessels begin to penetrate the cortex. The pedicle is freed almost to the radial artery at the level of the first compartment.

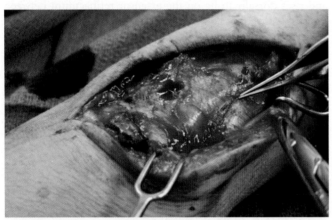

FIGURE 16.33 1,2 intercompartmental supraretinacular artery (1,2 ICSRA) is found coursing dorsally from the radial artery to lie superficially on the surface of the extensor retinaculum between the first and second extensor tendon compartments. The vascularized bone graft is harvested on a pedicle from the 1,2 ICSRA. Branches of the superficial radial nerve need to be identified and protected during the isolation of this pedicle. (Figure used with permission from Seth D. Dodds, MD.)

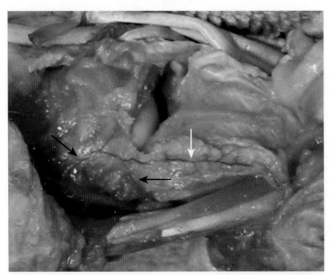

FIGURE 16.34 The first and second compartments are incised at their attachments to bone near the 1,2 intercompartmental supraretinacular artery (IC)SRA. The 1,2 ICSRA is mobilized as a pedicle. The pedicle is not elevated off the bone more than 10 to 15 mm proximal to the joint line, because this is the area where the nutrient vessels begin to penetrate the cortex (*arrows*). The pedicle is freed up almost to the radial artery at the level of the first compartment. (Figure used with permission from Seth D. Dodds, MD.)

After elevation of the pedicle, the scaphoid nonunion is approached through a radial longitudinal incision at the capsule. The nonunion site is identified and exposed. Ideally, a rectangular slot is created, bridging the fracture site in the scaphoid that will receive the bone graft. If the fracture is in the proximal pole, a slot can be created in the distal fragment, and the proximal pole can be curetted or burred out of avascular bone. In such a case, the graft would slide into the concavity of the proximal pole and fit into the slot in the distal fragment. A small, limited radiostyloidectomy can improve visualization but is often not needed. If the scaphoid is foreshortened with a humpback deformity, a vascularized graft may be placed as a volar wedge graft. This requires a wider exposure, which is accomplished by radial styloidectomy.

Once the nonunion site is prepared, the pedicled graft is carefully lifted from the radial metaphysis using small osteotomes. The 1,2 ICSRA is ligated proximal to the graft, and the graft is checked for flow by deflating the tourniquet. The graft is passed under the radial wrist extensors and impacted gently into place. If a significant concavity exists in either the proximal or distal fragment, additional cancellous bone is harvested from the distal radius to fill out the deep area of concavity in the scaphoid. Once the graft is in place, a screw is placed down the scaphoid and supplemental internal fixation may be used. Alternatively, if the scaphoid fragments are loose and grossly unstable with respect to each other, internal fixation can be placed first to stabilize the scaphoid as a single unit, and the vascularized graft can be impacted into place. The screw should be placed in the volar third of the scaphoid to reduce the chance of dislodging the graft.

Outcomes. Outcomes of the 1,2 ICSRA vascularized bone graft have had an interesting and evolving history. Initial reports were incredible, with some authors reporting union rates of 100%.[195,228] Later investigations were more critical, with healing rates of only 71%, and, if AVN was present, only 50%. Moreover, failures occurred in 64% if humpback deformity and DISI were present. The conclusion was that 1,2 ICSRA grafting is not suitable for scaphoid nonunion with AVN and carpal collapse.[34] Straw and colleagues[196] reported on Zaidemberg's technique, which they used to treat 22 established scaphoid fracture nonunions, 16 of which were found to have avascular proximal poles at surgery. The union rate was a dismal 27%. If AVN was present, the union rate was a mere 12.5%. A confounding element of this study was poor fixation of a single Kirschner wire. Boyer and colleagues showed poor healing with the 1,2 ICSRA when there was AVN, with 6 of 10 (60%) achieving union.[25] In a recent study, a union rate of only 75% was achieved.[94]

For a humpback deformity and AVN, Henry[90] showed good results; this is in contrast to a level I study by the Mayo group[110] in which a distal radial pedicle graft was compared with a medial femoral condyle graft (see the following). Henry reported a union rate of 100% in 15 patients with a scaphoid nonunion and proximal pole AVN with humpback deformity at a mean of 11.5 weeks after surgery with a volarly inserted, wedge-shaped, 1,2-ICSRA vascularized bone graft and headless compression screw fixation.[90]

Vascularized Bone Graft Pedicled on the Volar Carpal Artery. Kuhlmann and colleagues were the first to describe the vascularized bone graft pedicled on the volar carpal artery,[124] which lies between the palmar periosteum of the radius and the distal part of the superficial aponeurosis of the pronator quadratus. It is harvested from the distal radius along with a 5-mm-wide strip of fascia and periosteum, using a volar approach. A trapezoidal graft can be harvested and placed palmarly in the case of humpback deformity.

Dailiana reported its use in nine patients with scaphoid nonunion; union was achieved in 100% of cases. However, there was no preoperative carpal collapse and only one patient had AVN.[42] Gras and Mathoulin reported on the use of this vascularized bone graft in 111 patients, 47 of whom had DISI. None had AVN. The union rate was 96% for primary nonunions and 90% for secondary nonunions (Figure 16.35).[79]

Other Pedicled Bone Grafts

Surgical fixation of scaphoid nonunion with vascularized bone graft; dorsal capsular pedicle. Sotereanos and colleagues[188] described a dorsal capsular-based vascularized distal radius graft. This graft is harvested from the dorsal distal radius, just ulnar and distal to the Lister tubercle, and is based on a wide distally based strip of the dorsal wrist capsule, which is supplied by the artery of the fourth extensor compartment. The graft is placed as a dorsal inlay graft. Their series had 13 patients, 10 of whom had AVN and two of whom had DISI (Case Study 16.1). The rate of union was 10 of 13 (77%).[188]

Surgical fixation of scaphoid nonunion with vascularized bone graft; thumb metacarpal based on first dorsal metacarpal artery. Bertelli and colleagues[20] reported on the use of a bone graft from the thumb metacarpal pedicle on the first dorsal metacarpal artery used as a volar interposition graft to treat persistent scaphoid nonunions. They achieved a 90% union rate in 10 patients. Mathoulin and Brunelli presented the transfer of the index metacarpal pedicle (based on the dorsal intermetacarpal artery) for failed scaphoid surgery. Healing occurred in 14 of 15 patients, but only 10 patients had good function; previously unrecognized arthritis prevented good function in the other patients.[137]

Free Vascularized Bone Grafts

Iliac crest vascularized bone graft. The iliac crest vascularized bone graft is based on the deep circumflex iliac vascular pedicle. The vascular anastomosis is performed end-to-side to the radial artery and end-to-end to the venae comitantes. Gabl reported on its use in 15 patients with AVN and achieved union in 12 of 15 cases (80%).[65] Arora and colleagues reported on 21 patients in whom this technique was used for failed previous surgery with AVN; 76% achieved union.[12]

Surgical fixation of scaphoid nonunion with vascularized bone graft; free medial femoral condyle graft. In 1991 Doi and colleagues described the medial femoral condyle as a vascularized bone graft based on the articular branch of the descending genicular artery and vein or the superomedial genicular vessels.[173] Doi subsequently reported achieving union in 100% of 10 patients with scaphoid nonunion.[53]

Jones and colleagues[110] compared the medial femoral condyle vascularized bone graft with the 1,2 ICSRA graft. Twenty-two patients with scaphoid waist nonunions associated with an avascular proximal pole and carpal collapse were treated. Four of the 10 nonunions treated with the distal radial pedicle graft healed (40%) at a median of 19 weeks, and all 12 nonunions treated with the free medial femoral condyle graft healed (100%) at a median of 13 weeks. The rate of union was higher ($p = .005$) and the median time to healing was significantly shorter ($p < .001$) for the nonunions treated with the medial femoral condyle graft (Figure 16.36, *A* to *F* and Case Study 46.1).

Clinical use has spurred anatomic studies to further define the vascular anatomy. The descending genicular artery was present in 89% of specimens, originating at an average distance proximal to the articular surface of 13.7 cm, and the superior medial genicular artery was present in 100%, at 5.2 cm from the joint line. The average number of perforating vessels was greatest in the posterior distal quadrant condyle.[226]

Vascularized medial femoral trochlea osteocartilaginous flap reconstruction. Higgins and Burger published their series of vascularized medial femoral trochlea osteocartilaginous flap reconstruction of proximal pole nonunion and had healing in 15 of 16 patients. Similar to the rib osteochondral autograft, indications are unreconstructable or completely necrotic proximal poles without arthritis[93] (Case Study 16.2).

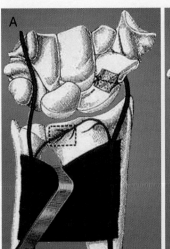
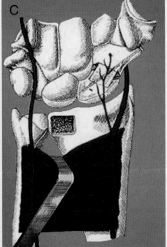
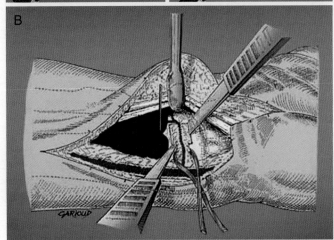

FIGURE 16.35 Harvest and inset of the volar distal radius vascularized bone graft based on the radial contribution to the volar carpal artery. Donor site (**A**), graft elevation with small osteotomes (**B**), and inset (**C**) are noted. A small pyramid-shaped graft is harvested, and a small rim of fascia is taken around the pedicle during its subperiosteal dissection from the distal radius. (Adapted, with permission, from Mathoulin C: Treatment of scaphoid nonunion with a vascularized bone graft harvested from the volar aspect of the radius, Maîtrise Orthopédique no. 105, June 2001. Reprint is in Derby BM, Murray PM, Shin AY, Bueno RA, Mathoulin CL, Ade T, Neumeister MW: Vascularized bone grafts for the treatment of carpal bone pathology. *Hand* 8(1):27-40, 2013.)

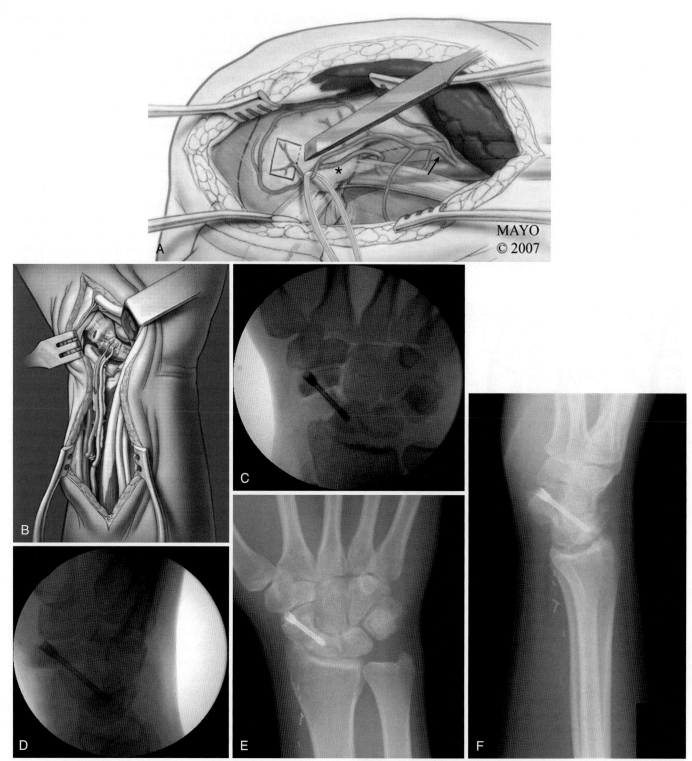

FIGURE 16.36 A, Raising the medial femoral condyle graft. **B,** The graft transferred to the scaphoid nonunion. **C** and **D,** Posteroanterior and lateral fluoroscopic intraoperative views after graft and screw placement. **E** and **F,** Posteroanterior and lateral radiographic views after healing. (From Jones DB Jr, Burger H, Bishop AT, et al: Treatment of scaphoid waist nonunions with an avascular proximal pole and carpal collapse: a comparison of 2 vascularized bone grafts. *J Bone Joint Surg Am* 90:2616–2625, 2008.)

Prognosis for Healing of Scaphoid Nonunion

Merrell and colleagues performed a systematic quantitative metareview of the literature to provide evidenced-based suggestions for the treatment of scaphoid nonunion.[145] This search identified 1121 articles, of which 36 met eligibility require-ments. In unstable nonunions, screw fixation with corticocan-cellous wedge grafting, which resulted in union in 94% of cases, was superior to Kirschner wires and wedge grafting, which resulted in union in 77% of cases. Immediate mobiliza-tion was compared with 6 weeks or more of casting, and they demonstrated comparable healing rates of 74%. For patients with reported AVN of the proximal fragment, union was achieved in 88% of patients with a vascularized graft versus 47% with screw and intercalated corticocancellous graft.

Shah and Jones reported on 50 scaphoid nonunions treated with Herbert screw fixation.[178] Success rates fell off as the duration of nonunion increased. The authors felt that this may have been related to the increased incidence of AVN with time. In their series, the major adverse determinants for outcome were AVN and a history of previous surgery for nonunion.

Inoue and colleagues retrospectively reviewed 160 cases of scaphoid nonunion treated by internal fixation using a Herbert screw with bone grafting at an average follow-up of 24 months.[104] Radiographic union was achieved in 90% of cases. Failure of union was related to the existence of avascular changes of the proximal fragment, instability of the fracture fragment, the prolonged delay in surgery, and the location of the fracture site. Persistent flexion deformity of the scaphoid adversely affected outcomes.

Schuind and colleagues reported on a multicenter study of 138 patients following scaphoid nonunion surgery.[177] Definitive healing occurred in only 74% of cases. Duration of nonunion longer than 5 years was associated with nonunion following the operation.

❖ AUTHOR'S PREFERRED METHOD:
Scaphoid Nonunion (Table 16.5)

Unsalvageable Scaphoid Proximal Pole Nonunion
Rib osteochondral autograft reconstruction of the proximal pole. Yao and colleagues[227] reported success in three cases with more than 2 years of follow-up of rib osteochondral autograft reconstruction of the proximal pole of the scaphoid. Indications are unreconstructable or completely necrotic proximal poles in the absence of arthritis. They all healed and had good function. Sandow reported on 47 cases, none going to revision surgery.[174] Veitch reported on success on 13 of 14 cases.[210]

1. For delayed union, use rigid fixation with headless compression screw. Nonvascularized bone graft should be used if CT shows bone loss. Dorsal versus palmar approach is dependent on the location of the fracture. For waist or proximal, use the dorsal approach. The palmar approach should be used if the fracture is distal to the waist.
2. For waist nonunion with humpback, use the Hybrid Russe procedure.
3. For proximal pole nonunion, dorsal approach, use nonvascularized bone graft and screw fixation. Consider supplemental K wire fixation of distal scaphoid to capitate to neutralize long lever arm.
4. If nonsalvageable proximal pole (fragmented), then use osteochondral medial femoral condyle free flap.

CRITICAL POINTS *Scaphoid Nonunion*

1. Preoperative CT is imperative to understand three dimensional pathoanatomy and plan surgical approach and appropriate hardware placement.
2. Carpal alignment should be corrected; use of joysticks (K wires in two poles) may be necessary.
3. Scaphoid nonunion site must be prepared adequately; use curettes to remove all nonunion fibrous tissue and callus to cancellous bone.
4. If the scaphoid has deformity, use cortical bone graft to strut open scaphoid and use cancellous bone to pack nonunion site tightly.
5. A central headless compression screw should be placed.
6. Supplemental K wire fixation, such as radiolunate wire and scaphocapitate wire, should be considered for unstable nonunions.
7. CT scan should be used postoperatively to confirm healing.

TABLE 16.5 Author's Preferred Treatment: Scaphoid Nonunion

Nonunion waist, no arthritis to minimal arthritis, with humpback deformity
- Hybrid Russe bone graft technique
- Headless compression screw
- Possible radial styloidectomy if SNAC I
- If surgery had been performed previously, the screw is removed and a new screw is placed from the opposite pole
- Consider radiolunate wire after lunate reduction if DISI is present

Nonunion proximal pole, no arthritis, with or without ischemia
- Nonvascularized bone graft, headless compression screw from dorsal approach
- Controversial to use vascularized bone graft during first surgery
- Consider scaphocapitate and, possibly, radiolunate temporary Kirschner wire or screw

Nonunion waist, no arthritis, acceptable alignment, stable
- In situ nonvascularized cancellous bone graft
- Headless compression screw

Nonunion waist, arthritis, SNAC II. nonreconstructable, distal pole grossly deformed
- Scaphoid excision with four-bone fusion
- Proximal row carpectomy
- Consider distal scaphoid pole excision if proximal scaphoid fossa is preserved and capitolunate arthritis is not present

Nonunion proximal pole, no arthritis, not salvageable (proximal pole < 5 mm)
- Scaphoid excision with four-corner fusion
- Proximal row carpectomy
- Osteoarticular autograft vascularized[93] or nonvascularized[227]

Treatment of Scaphoid Malunion

There are insufficient data to justify routine corrective osteotomy in patients with malunited scaphoids. The literature is mixed as to whether scaphoid deformity and associated lunate dorsal rotation influence the long-term outcome, provided the scaphoid is healed. In a recent study, Forward, Davis, and colleagues studied 42 patients with malunion and found no correlation between malunion measurements and functional outcome. They concluded that the goal of scaphoid treatment is to heal the scaphoid.[64]

Similarly, Jiranek and colleagues studied the effect of malunion on patients who had bone grafting for scaphoid nonunion.[109] Although there were significant objective differences and increased degenerative changes when patients with malunited and normally aligned scaphoids were compared, there were no subjective differences in satisfaction, pain relief, and return to work or sporting activities.

Amadio and colleagues reported on 45 patients with 46 scaphoid fractures that were studied more than 6 months after union by clinical examination and trispiral tomography.[7] Twenty fractures healed with normal scaphoid alignment as defined by lateral intrascaphoid angles of less than 35 degrees. There were satisfactory clinical outcomes in 83% and posttraumatic arthritis in only 22% of those with normal scaphoid anatomy. Worsening results were associated with increasing lateral scaphoid angulation and humpback deformity. In patients with more than 45 degrees of lateral intrascaphoid angulation present at the time of union, there was a satisfactory clinical outcome in 27% and posttraumatic arthritis in 54%. The authors felt that union alone is an insufficient criterion for measuring success in treating scaphoid fractures.

Similarly, Nakamura reported on 10 patients with symptomatic malunion of a carpal scaphoid fracture. All had displacement with DISI and suffered from pain, restricted range of movement at the wrist, and decreased grip strength. The restriction of flexion-extension and the decreased grip strength correlated with the severity of the DISI deformity. Seven patients had a corrective osteotomy using an anterior wedge-shaped bone graft with internal fixation by Herbert screw, and all had satisfactory results.[154]

Fernandez and colleagues presented a small series of three patients with painful rotational malalignment of the scaphoid and significant loss of active wrist extension who were treated with an opening wedge multiplanar osteotomy that corrected flexion, ulnar deviation, and pronation rotational malalignment of the distal fragment.[62] After a minimum follow-up of 4 years, all three patients were satisfied with the procedure and were pain free. The preoperative range of wrist motion had improved, and they had returned to their preoperative occupations.

Lynch and Linscheid reported on a long-term follow-up of five patients with DISI who underwent corrective osteotomy for symptomatic scaphoid malunion.[132] At an average of 9 years after the procedure (range, 1.5 to 19 years), all patients had healed and demonstrated an improvement in range of motion and grip strength. The preoperative intrascaphoid and carpal malalignments were reduced as demonstrated by trispiral tomography.

While firm evidence cannot be cited to justify routine osteotomy and correction of scaphoid malunion, clinical and laboratory studies support an attempt to restore correct alignment and length of the scaphoid and carpus when addressing scaphoid nonunion, particularly in active patients without degenerative change.

Nonunion of Distal Pole Scaphoid Fractures

Nonunion of distal pole scaphoid fractures is decidedly uncommon. Oron and colleagues[156] reported an incidence of 4.1% of 193 scaphoid nonunions at their institution. All were type IIC fractures of Prosser,[163] which are comminuted with a "Y"-split configuration at the scaphotrapeziotrapezoidal (STT) joint, and all had DISI deformity.[156]

Salvage Procedures for Scaphoid Nonunion Advanced Collapse

Radial Styloidectomy. Radial styloidectomy may be performed subperiosteally through the anatomic snuffbox. Care must be taken to avoid injury to the superficial radial nerve and potentially lateral antebrachial cutaneous nerves. It is important to preserve the important volar RSC ligament attachments; if more than 1 cm of styloid is removed, the RSC ligament origin will be significantly compromised, which could lead to instability.[181] Styloidectomies have been unsatisfactory as isolated procedures for SNAC arthritis, but they have enjoyed success for

stage I SNAC arthritis when combined with procedures to heal scaphoid nonunions. Although some surgeons have not considered styloidectomy to be an essential part of the treatment of nonunions, the procedure does consistently improve on the results of bone grafting alone.

Distal Scaphoid Resection Arthroplasty. Malerich, Eaton, Littler, and colleagues reported on 19 patients with chronic scaphoid nonunion and stage I (radioscaphoid) SNAC arthritis who were treated with distal scaphoid fragment excision.[135] The original series of 19 patients has been followed for 25 years. Grip improved from 36% of the unaffected side to 83% (range, 45% to 111%, $p < .001$). The range-of-motion arc improved from 72 degrees preoperatively to 139 degrees postoperatively ($p < .0001$). There has been minimal change in the radiolunate angle (from −28 to −33 degrees). There were two failures requiring revision surgery to proximal row carpectomy and scaphoid excision and four-bone fusion. Only one patient, other than the two failures, had pain that required nonsteroidal antiinflammatory drugs. More than half of the patients developed asymptomatic midcarpal arthritis. The authors recommended the procedure in selected cases because of its technical simplicity and high satisfaction rate and stated that it does not preclude later salvage procedures. Ruch and colleagues reported satisfactory results in a cohort of 13 patients treated for SNAC arthritis with scaphoid distal pole excision at 4 years postoperatively.[171] They documented significant increases in wrist range of motion but noted significant increases in DISI posture in six patients.

Current indications for the Malerich procedure are a waist fracture nonunion with SNAC I styloscaphoid arthritis with significant loss of wrist dorsiflexion and radial deviation and pain on wrist loading, gripping, and range of motion. Chronicity is a favorable indication. Contraindications are DISI of 60 degrees or greater, midcarpal subluxation, or scapholunate ligament incompetence with gapping (personal communication, Matthew Malerich, MD).

Surgical Technique for Distal Scaphoid Resection. A dorsal midline incision is made in line with the third ray. The sensory branches of the radial nerve are identified and protected. The third extensor compartment is released and the EPL tendon retracted radially. The second and fourth compartment tendons are mobilized and an inverted-"T" capsulotomy is made. The radial artery is identified and protected. The dorsal branch of the radial artery is vulnerable at the distal pole area. A 2-cm segment of the posterior interosseous nerve is resected. There are occasionally dorsal osteophytes around the dorsal radiocarpal joint that should be excised with a rongeur. The distal scaphoid fragment is excised while protecting the RSC ligament. To remove the distal fragment, negotiate a key elevator in the STT joint and use the trapezium and trapezoid as a fulcrum to elevate and remove the fragment. Some surgeons prefer to remove the distal scaphoid from a palmar approach.

When the distal scaphoid has been removed, it is essential to test the stability of the distal row relative to the proximal scapholunate socket. Should the capitate subluxate, a salvage procedure, such as scaphoid excision and four-bone fusion or proximal row carpectomy, should be considered instead. If stable, the capsule is closed and a bulky dressing applied. The wrist is splinted until suture removal and wrist motion exercises are initiated with therapy. Aggressive strengthening exercises are postponed until 3 months after surgery; heavy wrist loading in flexion would promote an excessive compressive load of the capitate against the dorsal lip of the lunate, thus inducing the appearance of further DISI malalignment and dorsal midcarpal subluxation. These patients are advised to avoid contact sports for the first 6 months after surgery.

Proximal Row Carpectomy. Proximal row carpectomy for advanced SNAC arthritis is a motion-preserving salvage operation. Compared with intercarpal arthrodesis, it is simple to perform, avoids the risk of nonunion, requires a short period of immobilization, and requires little rehabilitation. Several long-term studies have shown it to be a durable procedure with predictable results.[41,103] Patients can expect to achieve grip strength of 70% to 80% and a wrist arc range of motion of 50% to 60% of their contralateral extremity. Although the majority of patients develop radiographic degenerative change at the radiocapitate articulation, most are asymptomatic. In a recent review of patients with a minimum of 20 years of follow-up, Wall and colleagues[187] found that proximal row carpectomy provides satisfaction, with a survival rate of 65%; the 35% with failure went on to radiocarpal arthrodesis at an average time of 11 years after proximal row carpectomy. The majority of the 65% were satisfied, with a total arc of motion of 68 degrees and grip strength of 72% of the contralateral side. There was no correlation between radiographs and satisfaction. Patients who were younger than 40 years had a higher probability of failure; such patients should be counseled about this possibility.

Indications and Contraindications. The ideal candidate is a relatively low-demand patient older than 40 years with stage II or III SNAC with no to minimal capitolunate degenerative disease (may have scaphocapitate changes). Heavy laborers are usually excluded.

Surgical Technique. A dorsal incision about 8 cm long is centered over the Lister tubercle. The EPL tendon is identified distal to the extensor retinaculum. The third dorsal compartment is opened and the EPL is retracted radially. The second and fourth compartments are opened and the tendons retracted. A posterior interosseous neurectomy may be performed. An inverted-"T" capsulotomy is performed. The longitudinal portion is made in line with the third ray and the transverse limb is made off of the dorsal lip of the distal radius. The wrist is flexed to expose the proximal carpal row, and the capitate and the lunate fossa of the distal radius are inspected for degenerative change. If there is full-thickness cartilage loss, an intracarpal fusion or total wrist arthrodesis should be considered.

The removal of the proximal row begins with the resection of the scaphoid. Care must be taken to avoid injury to the RSC ligament that lies at the volar midportion of the scaphoid extending from the volar radial styloid to the volar capitate. The RSC ligament prevents postoperative ulnar translocation of the carpus because the other major palmar extrinsic wrist ligament will be taken during the proximal row carpectomy (the long radiolunate = radiolunotriquetral). The lunate and triquetrum are removed next, with care taken not to damage the articular surface of the head of the capitate. It may be helpful to use a threaded Steinmann pin or 3.5-mm threaded Schanz screw to drill into the carpal bones for assistance with manipulation and excision. If there is minimal wear in the capitate head, capsular interposition may be performed. A distally based flap

of the capsule is sutured to the volar capsule. The wrist capsule is closed. The EPL tendon is left transposed out of its compartment, and the extensor retinaculum is also closed. A short-arm wrist splint is applied and a PA fluoroscopic image is taken to confirm the location of the capitate within the lunate fossa of the radius while the splint is drying. Axial compression and slight ulnar deviation are often necessary to seat the capitate head in the lunate fossa. I do not place temporary fixation across the new radiocarpal articulation. A thermoplastic splint is applied at 2 weeks following operation to be worn full time. Gradual increased motion is permitted 6 weeks postoperatively. Patients are counseled that it can take 4 to 6 months or more to realize the benefit of surgery.

Intercarpal Fusion. The purpose of intercarpal fusion is to stabilize the midcarpal joint after the scaphoid is resected. Four-bone (capitate-lunate-hamate-triquetrum) fusion with scaphoid excision satisfactorily treats degenerative SNAC arthritis affecting the radioscaphoid and midcarpal joints while preserving an anatomically congruous radiolunate joint.

The priorities in properly executing four-bone fusion and scaphoid excision include (1) adequate decortication of joints, (2) correction of DISI deformity, (3) bone apposition, (4) rigid internal fixation, with options including headless compression screws, Kirschner wires, plates, or staples, and (5) appropriate postoperative immobilization. If the lunate is not derotated into neutral from its extended position and the capitate is fused in a dorsally subluxated position, as is often present in the SNAC wrist, radiocapitate abutment will prevent necessary wrist extension and cause pain.

Technique. A dorsal incision about 8 cm long is centered over the Lister tubercle. The EPL tendon is identified distal to the extensor retinaculum. The third dorsal compartment is opened and the EPL is retracted radially. The second and fourth compartments are opened and the tendons retracted. A posterior interosseous neurectomy may be performed. An inverted-"T" capsulotomy is performed. The longitudinal portion is made in line with the third ray and the transverse limb is made off of the dorsal lip of the distal radius. If more exposure is necessary to expose the proximal triquetrum for screw placement, the fifth compartment with the extensor digitorum quinti may need to be opened as well and the extensor digitorum quinti tendon retracted. The wrist is flexed to expose the proximal and midcarpal rows and scaphoid and lunate fossae of the distal radius to confirm degenerative changes.

The scaphoid is excised, with care taken to preserve the critical volar carpal ligaments (RSC and long radiolunate [LRL] ligaments). A threaded Steinmann pin or 3.5-mm Schanz screw may be inserted down the axis of the scaphoid as a joystick to manipulate and excise the bone. The midcarpal joint surfaces of the distal lunate and triquetrum and proximal capitate and hamate are decorticated to spongy cancellous bone. A combination of a rongeur, curets, and a 3-mm round bur may be used. Constant irrigation of the bur is important to avoid thermal necrosis of the bone, which may impede healing and bony fusion. I prefer to use a bur to create two to three channels, or "oil wells," in the articulation between the bones that will later be filled with bone graft. The primary joints to be fused are between the proximal row of the lunotriquetral complex and the capitohamate complex. The lunotriquetral and capitohamate joints are inherently very stable and are not formally taken down (two-column, or "bicolumnar," fusion). This method is much more surgically efficient than taking down all joints; in the latter situation, the presence of four independent and unstable bones makes the remainder of the procedure more difficult without appreciable clinical gain.

Bone graft is harvested from the excised scaphoid and/or a small window at the Lister tubercle and packed tightly into all intercarpal spaces. The lunate is derotated out of DISI to a neutral position. If there is difficulty in rotating the lunate out of DISI, the attachments of the dorsal radiocarpal ligament on the triquetrum may be released in the coronal plane, which will release both the lunate and triquetrum to allow them to palmarly flex back to anatomic position. The capitate is reduced to its anatomic position on the lunate. In the coronal plane, the lunate should be restored to its anatomic position, covering approximately two thirds of the capitate rather than the entire bone. The carpal bones are held reduced and axially compressed while one to three temporary 0.062-inch Kirschner wires are placed from distal to proximal (capitate to lunate and hamate to triquetrum).

My preference for fixation is staples, but Kirschner wires, plates, staples, or other techniques may be used. The wrist is placed in a volar/dorsal splint, and the splint is converted to a short-arm cast until union, which generally occurs 6 weeks postoperatively. Digital motion exercises are encouraged immediately following surgery, and wrist motion rehabilitation and strengthening are initiated at healing.

CRITICAL POINTS *Scaphoid Excision, Partial (Midcarpal) Wrist Fusion*

1. The joints to be fused need to prepared adequately to cancellous bone and packed with bone graft.
2. The midcarpal joint should reduced out of DISI. The dorsal radiocarpal ligament may need to be released in the coronal plane off of the lunate and triquetral bones.
3. The capitolunate joint should be fused in the anatomic position (the lunate usually covers approximately two thirds of the capitate).
4. Stable fixation must be achieved.

FRACTURES OF CARPAL BONES OTHER THAN THE SCAPHOID

Whereas fractures of the scaphoid are relatively common, fractures of the remaining carpal bones are relatively rare.[24] Larsen and colleagues reported that the relative incidence of carpal fractures excluding the scaphoid was 1.1% of all fractures.[126] They estimated the annual incidence to be 36 fractures per 100,000 people. In a review of 1000 consecutive hand injuries, only 18% involved fractures of the carpus, with the scaphoid being the most commonly injured carpal bone (58%).[126] Fractures of the carpus occur in three general groups: perilunate pattern injuries, axial pattern injuries, and local avulsion/impaction injuries.

Most carpal fractures are the consequence of a fall onto an outstretched hand. The energy from the fall may be focused on the distal carpal row. If the mechanism of injury continues, it produces an extension moment across the proximal carpal row

transmitted through the volar carpal ligaments. These ligaments may be disrupted or result in shear stress around the area of the lunate. This results in perilunate-pattern or "lesser arc" injuries. Carpal fractures or ligamentous injuries may occur in an arc around the lunate. Carpal fractures may occur on the volar aspect of the wrist from tensile stress, or dorsal cortical comminution may occur from compression shear stress. Fractures of the scaphoid, capitate, triquetrum, or radial styloid, or all four, in conjunction with perilunate instability, are known as "greater arc" injuries.

Strong anterior to posterior compression injuries may result in axial-pattern disruption of the carpus. The forced injury propagates both radially and ulnarly, separating the carpus on both sides of the capitate. Frequently, this may result in an open fracture associated with variable soft tissue injury. These injuries are usually unstable and require surgical stabilization.

Lastly, avulsions may occur owing to localized forced concentration. These forces commonly cause avulsion injuries at the volar/dorsal aspect of the triquetrum secondary to ligament insertions, but trapezial ridge, hamate hook, and pisiform fractures may occur as well.

Garcia-Elias noted several characteristics common to carpal fractures.[67] First, these injuries generally occur in young individuals with high functional demands; second, these injuries are frequently missed at initial presentation; third, the small size of the fractured carpal bone complicates surgical reduction and potentially compromises its vascular supply; fourth, the displaced carpal fracture may significantly affect the congruency of the articular surface to the wrist, resulting in posttraumatic degenerative changes; fifth, unstable carpal fractures frequently are associated with adjacent ligamentous injury, as previously described; and sixth, because of the close relationship of the carpus to the tendon and neurovascular structures, secondary entrapment neuropathies or tendon ruptures can occur by friction of nonreduced bone fragments.

The relative frequency of each carpal bone fracture is controversial (Table 16.6).[67] Many authors report that the triquetrum is second only to the scaphoid as the most commonly fractured carpal bone, with 3% to 5% of all carpal fractures.[3] Garcia-Elias reviewed 10,400 consecutive wrist injuries over a 10-year period and reported on 249 carpal fractures.[67] In his series, there were 153 scaphoid fractures, 64 triquetrum fractures, 15 trapezoid fractures, 5 capitate fractures, 5 hamate fractures, and 2 lunate fractures.

Fractures of the Triquetrum

In most authors' series, fractures of the triquetrum are reported to represent the second or third most common carpal bone fracture.[67,130] Three primary patterns are usually observed: dorsal cortical fracture, triquetral body fracture, and palmar cortical fracture (Box 16.1).

Triquetral Fracture Patterns

Dorsal Cortical Fracture. The dorsal cortical fracture is by far the most common (Figure 16.37).[66,95,130] Its frequency is often reported to be as high as 93% of all triquetral fractures.[130] Different mechanisms of injury have been proposed for dorsal triquetral fractures.[66,95,130] These include avulsion, shear forces, or impaction. Extreme palmar flexion with radial deviation would be a primary cause for a dorsal avulsion fracture due to

TABLE 16.6 Relative Incidence of Carpal Bone Fractures

Source	Total Number of Fractures	BONE FRACTURED							
		Scaphoid	Lunate	Triquetrum	Pisiform	Trapezium	Trapezoid	Capitate	Hamate
Garcia-Elias	249	153	2	64	5	15	1	5	4
Auffray	245	144	10	72	1	10	—	4	4
Snodgrass	170	144	11	7	1	3	1	2	1
Borgeskov	143	102	2	29	1	5	1	2	1
Franz	122	81	13	6	4	8	1	6	3
Dunn	72	59	1	5	1	2	—	—	4

Data from Garcia-Elias M: Carpal bone fractures (excluding scaphoid fractures). In Watson H, Weinberg J, editors: *The wrist*, Philadelphia, 2001, Lippincott Williams & Wilkins, pp 174–181.

BOX 16.1 Fractures of the Triquetrum

Incidence
Second most common carpal bone fracture; approximately 15% of all carpal fractures

Classification
Type 1 Dorsal cortical fracture (Figure 16.41), most common
Type 2 Triquetral body fracture
 Medial tuberosity fracture
 Sagittal plane fracture
 Transverse proximal pole fracture
 Transverse body fracture
 Comminuted fracture
Type 3 Palmar cortical fracture

Mechanisms
Type 1 Dorsal cortical fracture
Mechanism 1: Extreme palmar flexion/twist with avulsion by dorsal ligaments: radiotriquetral (dorsal radiocarpal) and triquetroscaphoid (dorsal intercarpal) ligaments
Mechanism 2: Hyperextension and ulnar deviation during fall with impaction by ulnar styloid or hamate
Type 2 Triquetral body fracture
Medial tuberosity fracture (caused by direct blow)
Sagittal plane fracture (anterior-posterior crush injury or axial dislocation)
Transverse proximal pole fracture (perilunate injury)
Transverse body fracture (perilunate injury)
Comminuted fracture (due to high-energy trauma)
Type 3 Palmar cortical fracture
Avulsion of palmar ligaments (palmar ulnar triquetral or lunotriquetral ligament)
Shear from pisiform

Special Imaging
CT scanning still often necessary
Oblique, 45-degree pronated view for dorsal cortical fracture

Palmar cortical fracture may be a harbinger of carpal instability, and MRI may be helpful in further assessment

Treatment
Type 1 Dorsal cortical fracture
Small fragment, no instability: short-arm cast for 3 to 4 weeks; then wrist splint for comfort. Progressive range of motion and strengthening. Excision if symptomatic after 6 to 9 months
Signs of carpal instability: ORIF
Type 2 Triquetral body fracture
Nondisplaced body fracture: short-arm cast for 4 to 6 weeks
Displaced body fracture: CRIF vs. ORIF with compression screws and/or Kirschner wires
Beware of associated lunotriquetral ligament injury. If lunotriquetral ligament is disrupted, pin across the joint
Type 3 palmar cortical fracture
Small fragment, no instability: Wrist splint vs. short-arm cast for 4 to 6 weeks
Ligamentous avulsion with carpal instability: ORIF
Shear from pisiform: short-arm cast for 4 to 6 weeks; excision of fragment and pisiform if injury remains symptomatic

Associated Injury
Perilunate fracture-dislocation
Axial pattern fracture-dislocations
Radius or ulna fractures

Complications
Nonunion
Persistent carpal instability
Pisotriquetral arthritis

CRIF, Closed reduction and internal fixation; *ORIF,* open reduction and internal fixation.

the attachment of the dorsal radiotriquetral and triquetroscaphoid ligaments. The most common mechanism is a fall onto a wrist in dorsiflexion and ulnar deviation. The ulnar styloid may act as a chisel and is driven into the dorsal cortex of the triquetrum. Garcia-Elias, in a study of 76 patients with triquetral fractures as compared with 100 uninjured patients, noted that the mean size of the ulnar styloid was significantly (p = .001)

longer in the fracture patients.[66] Lastly, the shear force applied by the proximal edge of the hamate against the distal dorsal triquetrum during wrist extension has also been shown as a potential mechanism of injury for dorsal triquetrum chip fractures.[95]

Triquetral Body Fracture. Triquetral body fractures are the second most common type of triquetral fractures. These

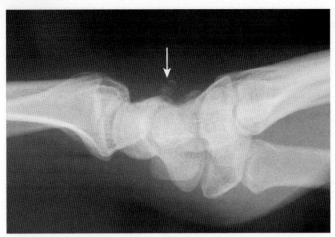

FIGURE 16.37 Wrist radiograph, lateral view. Dorsal cortical fracture of the triquetrum. (Courtesy of Steve K. Lee, MD.)

fractures generally require a high amount of injury to the wrist. Fractures of the body of the triquetrum are occasionally seen with perilunate fracture-dislocations. Perilunate fracture-dislocations are seen in 12% to 25% of triquetral injuries. A fracture of the body of the triquetrum should alert the physician to look for associated ligamentous injuries.

Fractures of the body of the triquetrum may be divided into five categories. These include sagittal fractures, fractures in the medial tuberosity, transverse fractures of the proximal pole, transverse fractures of the body, and comminuted fractures. A direct blow to the ulnar border of the wrist may cause a medial tuberosity fracture and occasionally involves the palmar articular surface of the triquetrum. Sagittal fractures are commonly associated with axial dislocations, with flattening of the transverse carpal arch. Small fractures of the proximal pole are frequently associated with perilunate dislocations. Small avulsion fractures to the volar aspect of the triquetrum may be the result of avulsion of the palmar LTIO ligaments and carry a much worse prognosis than isolated dorsal tip fractures, as noted by Smith and Murray.[185]

Palmar Cortical Fracture. Lastly, palmar cortical fractures have been described in the triquetrum. These fractures usually represent an avulsion of the palmar ulnar triquetral ligament and the LTIO ligament.

Clinical and Radiographic Features

Patients with a fracture of the triquetrum complain of point tenderness to palpation directly over the triquetrum. A patient who has a dorsal avulsion fracture is usually symptomatic with wrist flexion and extension.

Most triquetral fractures can be identified with anteroposterior (AP), lateral, and 45-degree pronated oblique radiographs of the wrist. The lateral and oblique views most often reveal the dorsal cortical fragments. Radial deviation views are helpful to diagnose a palmar cortical fragment that may be hidden behind the hamate or remaining triquetrum. Occasionally, CT scans are helpful in identifying occult triquetral fractures.

Treatment

Management of triquetral fractures depends on the fracture pattern. Most fractures are dorsal cortical fractures and are treated nonoperatively with immobilization for approximately

4 to 6 weeks. Immobilization is generally used in treating the underlying soft tissue injury. MRI is occasionally obtained to identify extrinsic intercarpal ligament injuries or occult fractures. It is important for the patient to understand that despite immobilization, fibrous nonunion of the fracture may occur. Patients generally complain of mild discomfort over the dorsum of the wrist for several months. Hocker reviewed his results in these injuries and showed excellent return of motion and function of the wrist.[95] In symptomatic nonunions, excision of the painful dorsal fragment may be performed.

Guidelines for treatment of triquetral body fractures are less clear. Isolated triquetral body fractures can generally be treated successfully by casting and immobilization for 4 to 6 weeks. Nonunion of a triquetral body fracture is very rare. Most fractures of the body of the triquetrum are associated with severe trauma and may be associated with a perilunate fracture-dislocation. Usually, treatment is directed toward managing the LTIO ligament by pinning the joint, ignoring the fracture of the body of the triquetrum. However, in cases of displaced triquetral body fractures, ORIF has been described (Figure 16.38).[162] A patient with an isolated triquetral body fracture in which the proximal row initially looks intact should receive close follow-up with radiographs looking for instability, particularly of the scapholunate interval, or further MRI. Fractures of the body of the triquetrum associated with scapholunate instability are best managed by early primary repair of the ligamentous disruption and fixation of the triquetral fracture with a compression screw.

Palmar cortical fractures of the triquetrum are rare. MRI to evaluate the fracture pattern and involvement of potential carpal instability is recommended. Treatment should be directed toward restoring carpal stability rather than treating the small avulsion fragment.

Fractures of the Trapezium

The trapezium forms a set articulation for the base of the thumb metacarpal. Fractures of the trapezium constitute approximately 1% to 5% of all carpal bone fractures, making the trapezium the third most commonly fractured carpal bone in most authors' series (Box 16.2).[161,209] The largest series of fractures of the trapezium was described by Pointu and colleagues, who reviewed 34 cases.[161] Fractures of the trapezium are usually associated with fractures of other bones, usually the distal radius or metacarpal. Isolated fractures occur rarely. Fractures of the trapezium typically involve the body or the ridge. The palmar ridge of the trapezium projects in a palmar direction and serves as an attachment for the transverse carpal ligament. The tendon of the FCR passes along a groove formed by the trapezial ridge. Fractures of the body are more common. Walker and colleagues described five different fracture patterns of the trapezium (Figure 16.39).[213] A vertical intraarticular fracture pattern is the most common, followed by fractures of the dorsoradial tuberosity.

Mechanism of Injury

The position of the trapezium below the thumb metacarpal generally protects it from a direct blow, making this an uncommon cause of trapezial fracture. Several mechanisms of injury have been described for fractures of the trapezium. These fractures are incurred from a fall onto an outstretched thumb,

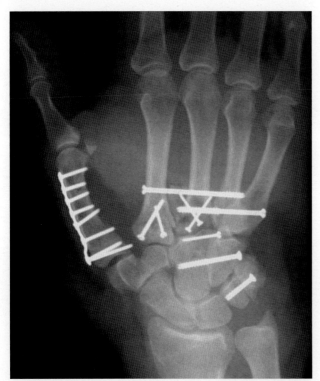

FIGURE 16.38 Posterioranterior radiograph of a patient following stabilization of multiple carpal fractures and instability, including stabilization of the fracture of the body of the triquetrum.

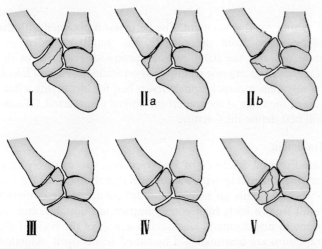

FIGURE 16.39 Classification of trapezial body fractures by Walker and colleagues: I, horizontal fractures; IIA, fractures of the radial tuberosity through the carpometacarpal joint; IIB, fractures of the radial tuberosity through the scaphotrapezial joint; III, fractures of the ulnar tuberosity; IV, fractures of the carpometacarpal joint (two-part); and V, fractures of the scaphotrapezial joint (comminuted). (From Walker JL, Greene TL, Lunseth PA: Fractures of the body of the trapezium. *J Orthop Trauma* 2:22–28, 1988.)

BOX 16.2   Fractures of the Trapezium

Incidence
Third most commonly fractured carpal bone; 1% to 5% of all carpal fractures

Classification (see Figure 16.40)
Type 1 Vertical intraarticular fracture, most common, frequently accompanies Bennett fracture
Type 2 Horizontal fracture (rare)
Type 3 Dorsoradial tuberosity fracture
Type 4 Palmar trapezial ridge fracture
    4A Fracture of base
    4B Fracture of tip
Type 5 Comminuted fracture

Mechanism
Type 1 Axial compression from first metacarpal
Type 2 Horizontal shear
Type 3 Vertical shear between radial styloid and first metacarpal
Type 4 Direct blow or avulsion of transverse carpal ligament
Type 5 High-energy injuries

Special Radiographs
CT scanning still often necessary
Bett view (see Imaging section)
Pronated AP view
Carpal tunnel view (for palmar trapezial ridge fractures)

Treatment
Fracture of body
    Nondisplaced: Short-arm thumb spica cast for 4 to 6 weeks
    Displaced: ORIF (palmar Wagnor approach, headless compression screws and/or Kirschner wires)
    Comminuted: ORIF combined with traction pin (first to second metacarpal) or external fixator
Palmar trapezial ridge fracture
    Type 4A (base of ridge): Short-arm thumb spica cast for 4 to 6 weeks (usually heals)
    Type 4B (tip avulsion): Short-arm thumb spica cast for 4 to 6 weeks (often does not heal; excise if symptomatic)

Associated Injury
Bennett fracture
Fracture-dislocations with fractures of scaphoid, trapezoid, capitate, metacarpals, distal radius

Complications
Basal joint posttraumatic arthritis
Contracture of first web space
Nonunion
Carpal tunnel syndrome
FCR tendinopathy and late rupture

ORIF, Open reduction and internal fixation.

causing the base of the thumb metacarpal to be driven axially into the trapezium. This results in a vertical intraarticular shear fracture on the radial aspect of the trapezial body (Figure 16.40). The body of the trapezium is split and displaced proximally with the attached metacarpal, resulting in subluxation or dislocation of the joint. Depending on the angle of compression, a fracture of the trapezium or a Bennett fracture of the

thumb metacarpal, or occasionally both, may occur. Dorsoradial trapezial fractures may be the result of vertical shear when the trapezium is being trapped between the metacarpal and the tip of the radial styloid. Most fractures of the trapezium have a vertical orientation consistent with a vertical shear force.

The ridge of the trapezium is superficial. It can be palpated just distal to the scaphoid tubercle at the base of the thenar

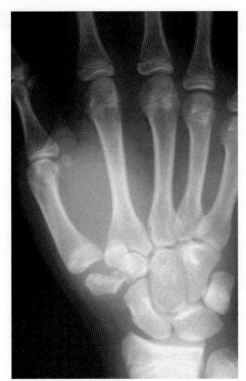

FIGURE 16.40 Posteroanterior radiograph demonstrating a fracture of the body of the trapezium that is split into volar and dorsal fragments. This was secondary to the thumb metacarpal being driven proximally into the body of the trapezium.

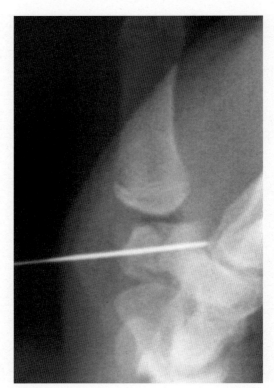

FIGURE 16.42 The fracture from Figure 16.41 was approached volarly, elevating the thenar musculature. The fracture was anatomically reduced and provisionally stabilized with Kirschner wire fixation.

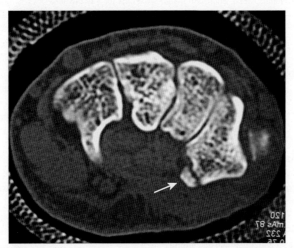

FIGURE 16.41 Computed tomography showing avulsion of the transverse carpal ligament produced by an anteroposterior crush. (Courtesy of Steve K. Lee, MD.)

eminence. Because the ridge is superficial, fractures of this structure are generally caused by direct trauma such as a fall onto an outstretched hand or being struck by a pitched ball. Other mechanisms include avulsion of the transverse carpal ligament produced by an AP crush (Figure 16.41).

Imaging

Fractures of the body of the trapezium can usually be identified on standard PA and lateral radiographic wrist views. A pronated AP view further defines the articular surface and is helpful for detecting any displacement. The Bett view is obtained with the elbow raised from the cassette, the thumb extended and abducted, and the hand partially pronated. Fractures of the trapezial ridge are not readily seen on standard PA and lateral radiographs. A carpal tunnel view is best for identifying a fracture of the ridge of the trapezium when it is suspected. CT scan will best define the fracture.

Treatment

Nondisplaced fractures of the trapezium are relatively rare; treatment would be with a short-arm thumb spica cast for 4 to 6 weeks. Patients do require close follow-up, as these injuries result from a fairly high-energy impact, are unstable, and are prone to displacement. Displaced fractures of the body of the trapezium are best managed by closed versus open reduction and internal fixation.[178] Fractures of the trapezium are best addressed through a volar approach. The thenar muscle is elevated, exposing the fracture site. The radial artery is at risk during the exposure and should be identified and protected during the procedure. The fracture may be stabilized by compression screws or Kirschner wires, or a combination of both (Figures 16.42 and 16.43). Frequently, because of the compressive forces involved in producing the fracture, bone grafts may be needed to support the articular surface. Allograft cancellous bone may be used because it has structural integrity or autologous cancellous bone graft may be obtained from the volar aspect of the distal radius or from the olecranon. Various bone substitutes may also be used.

Fractures of the ridge of the trapezium may be easily missed. Patients present with pain at the base of the thumb and pain

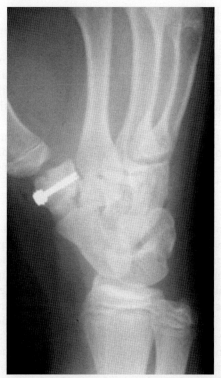

FIGURE 16.43 Following anatomic reduction of the fracture from Figure 16.41, a cannulated screw was placed over the guidewire, anatomically reducing the intraarticular fracture to the trapezium.

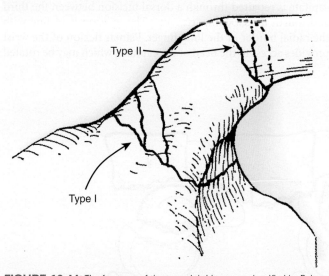

FIGURE 16.44 The fractures of the trapezial ridge were classified by Palmer. Type I fractures involve the base, and type II fractures involve the tip.

with wrist flexion. According to Palmer, two types of trapezial ridge fractures exist (Figure 16.44).[157] Type I fractures occur at the base of the ridge, and type II fractures are avulsion fractures at the tip of the ridge. The main aspect of these fractures is recognizing them by clinical suspicion via the patient's area of pain and tenderness, but CT scanning is frequently required for confirmation. Types I and II fractures may be treated in a short-arm thumb spica cast for 4 to 6 weeks. If the fracture does not heal and ends up in painful nonunion, excision of the fracture

---

BOX 16.3 Fractures of the Capitate

Incidence
Fourth most common carpal fracture; 1% to 2%

Classification
Type 1 Transverse body fracture; most common, associated with perilunate injuries, with or without fracture of scaphoid and/or radial styloid
Type 2 Transverse proximal pole (waist) fracture
Type 3 Coronal oblique fracture
Type 4 Parasagittal fracture

Blood Supply
Retrograde

Special Imaging
CT scan may be needed to confirm

Mechanisms
Most commonly, fall on outstretched hand; hyperextension with capitate striking distal radius
Axial load down the third metacarpal
Direct blow

Treatment
Nondisplaced fracture: Short-arm thumb spica cast for 6 to 8 weeks
Displaced fracture: ORIF (headless compression screws)
Beware of scaphocapitate syndrome (proximal capitate fragment rotates 180 degrees; ORIF is necessary for treatment)

Associated Injury
Perilunate injury

Complications
Most common is nonunion, which is often related to delay in diagnosis
Avascular necrosis of capitate
Posttraumatic arthritis
Malunion of capitate

ORIF, Open reduction and internal fixation.

fragments may be required. Padded gloves are used to help the patient return to activities as the scar may be tender for several months.

Fracture of the trapezium may result in chronic conditions such as carpal tunnel syndrome, tendinitis, or potential rupture of the FCR tendon as it passes by the trapezium. Excision of fracture fragments and bony osteophytes is recommended in chronic injuries that are symptomatic. The fragment is removed through a volar approach and the thenar musculature is elevated off of the capsule. The FCR tendon must be identified and carefully protected as it is easily injured during excision of fragments.

Fractures of the Capitate

Similar to the trapezoid, the capitate is centered within the carpus and is well protected from injury. Fractures of the capitate account for 1% to 2% of all carpal fractures (Box 16.3). Adler and Shaftan found 72 previously published cases in their review of the literature and published 12 additional cases of their own.[2] However, isolated fractures of the capitate are being diagnosed with increased frequency, and a heightened awareness of these injuries is important. The capitate articulates with the scaphoid and lunate proximally and is well attached along the metacarpal distally to form the central column of the hand and wrist. Fractures of the capitate are incurred as an isolated injury or more frequently are part of a transscaphoid perilunate fracture-dislocation. This was described by Fenton as a scaphocapitate fracture syndrome.[59]

Four major patterns of fractures have been observed in the capitate. These include transverse fracture of the body of the capitate, transverse fracture of the proximal pole of the capitate, coronal oblique fracture, and a parasagittal fracture pattern. Transverse fractures of the capitate occur most frequently and are usually associated with a transscaphoid, transcapitate perilunate fracture-dislocation.[59]

Mechanism of Injury

Stein and Siegel investigated the mechanism of injury for fractures of the capitate that can result from up to 180 degrees of rotation of the proximal fragment (Figure 16.45, *A* to *C*).[193] In the scaphocapitate perilunate fracture-dislocation, the mechanism of injury is a high-energy fall with the wrist hyperextended. The force is initially transmitted through the scaphoid, which fractures at the waist. As the wrist continues to extend, the neck of the capitate impacts on the dorsal ridge of the radius and fractures as a result of tensile forces on the palmar aspect.

When the wrist returns to neutral, shortening of the carpus prevents reduction of the proximal fragment. As the wrist continues to go into flexion, the fractured distal portion of the capitate exerts a flexion moment to the proximal pole, which may result in complete rotation, causing the articular surface of the capitate proximal pole to face distally into the capitate fracture site. Other possible mechanisms of capitate fracture include an axial load down the third metacarpal or a direct blow.

Radiographic Features

Routine PA, lateral, and oblique radiographs are usually sufficient to diagnose a capitate fracture (Figure 16.46, *A* and *B*). Occasionally, however, initial radiographs of a nondisplaced capitate fracture may appear normal. Close evaluation of the radiographs is important. A patient may present with a typical transscaphoid perilunate fracture-dislocation, and the capitate fracture may be overlooked. A patient's continued wrist pain following trauma may require serial radiographs and temporary immobilization until the pain resolves or a diagnosis is made. The fracture is subsequently recognized when resorption of the fracture site is noted.

Treatment

The head of the capitate is nearly completely covered with articular cartilage, similar to the proximal pole of the scaphoid. Like proximal pole scaphoid fractures, fractures of the head and neck of the capitate are subject to major vascular disruption and, hence, prolonged healing and poor outcome because the blood supply is retrograde. These fractures are inherently unstable and frequently lead to delayed union or nonunion. These factors need to be considered if casting and immobilization are recommended, because the several months of cast immobilization required for healing may result in additional morbidity. MRI has helped to evaluate the vascular supply of the proximal pole of the capitate and the healing capacity of the capitate head.

Displaced fractures of the capitate, delayed diagnosis of nondisplaced capitate fractures, and transscaphoid, transcapitate perilunate fracture-dislocations are best managed by ORIF. The capitate is repaired through a dorsal incision between the third and fourth dorsal compartments. The incision is in line with the radial border of the long finger. Palmar flexion of the wrist provides access to the head of the capitate, which may be rotated

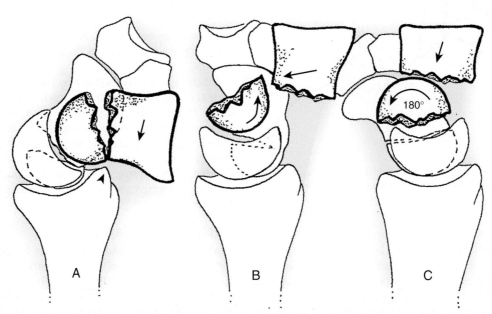

FIGURE 16.45 The mechanism of injury to fractures of the capitate. **A,** The neck of the capitate may impact on the dorsal ridge of the radius once the scaphoid has fractured. **B,** As the wrist recovers to its neutral position, shortening of the carpus prevents reduction of the proximal fragment. **C,** As the capitate regains its normal alignment in relation to the radius, it exerts a flexion moment to the proximal fragment that may result in a 180-degree rotation, with the fracture site facing the distal aspect of the lunate.

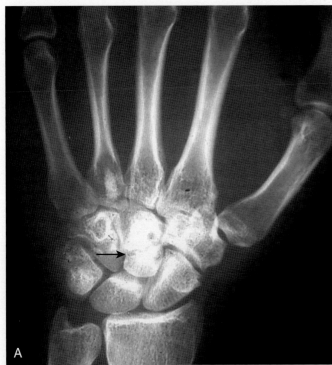

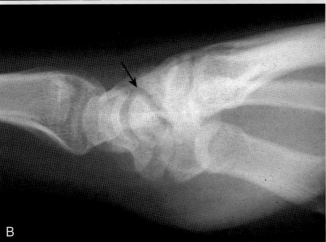

FIGURE 16.46 Capitate neck fracture. **A,** Posteroanterior radiographic view of the wrist. **B,** Lateral radiographic view of the wrist. (Courtesy of Martin A. Posner, MD.)

180 degrees. One or two headless compression screws may be placed from proximal to distal in the capitate to provide adequate stability (Figure 16.47, *A* and *B*).[69] The scaphoid may be stabilized from the same dorsal approach or through a separate volar approach if it is fractured.

It is important to reestablish the carpal height of the capitate when managing an established capitate nonunion. Corticocancellous interposition bone grafts are usually necessary to reestablish the carpal height to prevent carpal collapse and overloading to the scaphotrapezialtrapezoidal and triquetral hamate joints.

A coronal fracture is caused by transmission of an axial load along the shaft of the third metacarpal, resulting in a joint compressive force on the dorsal aspect of the capitate articular surface. This fracture is not well seen in typical AP radiographs but is seen on a lateral view. These fractures are managed by ORIF if displaced.

Fractures of the Hamate

It has been reported that hamate fractures make up approximately 2% of all carpal fractures (Box 16.4).[1,147] These fractures are probably underreported if carpometacarpal fracture-dislocations are taken into account where there are dorsal avulsion fractures related to the metacarpal bases. Also, hook fractures may be more common but may not be symptomatic enough for treatment by a hand surgeon. The unique anatomy of the hamate hook places it at risk: It protrudes from the base of the hamate into the hypothenar eminence. The hook of the hamate is the site of origin for the flexor digiti minimi muscles, opponens digiti minimi muscles, hypothenar muscles, pisohamate ligaments, and distal attachment of the transverse carpal ligament. Fractures of the hamate may be divided into two groups: those affecting the hook of the hamate and those involving the body.

Fractures of the Hook of the Hamate

Fractures of the hook of the hamate are relatively rare in the general population but more common in athletes.[69] The hook of the hamate is at risk for a fracture in any athlete who swings a racket, club, or bat (Figure 16.48).

Direct compression of the handle of the club against the protruding hook is the primary cause of fracture. In addition, shear forces from the adjacent flexor tendons or contraction of the attached hypothenar muscles may contribute to the fracture or displacement. The wrist nearest the handle is at risk for fracture. The nondominant hand is usually involved in golfers and baseball players, whereas the dominant hand is more likely involved in tennis and racketball players.

Clinical and Radiographic Presentation. Fractures of the hook of the hamate frequently present late as chronic pain at the base of the hypothenar eminence. Patients may complain of ulnar nerve paresthesia into the ring and small fingers and weakened grip strength. Tenderness to palpation is felt over the hamate hook approximately 2 cm distal and radial to the pisiform. Patients complain of pain aggravated by active grasping. Pain with resistance of ring- and small-finger flexion that is worst with the wrist in ulnar deviation and lessened by radial deviation can help further document a fracture of the hook of the hamate, which irritates the flexor tendons at the ring and small fingers. A chronic unrecognized hamate hook fracture may present with a rupture of the small or ring finger deep or superficial flexor tendon.

Fractures of the hamate hook are difficult to recognize on standard anterior, posterior, and lateral radiographs. Clues on the PA radiograph include absence of the hook or cortical ring or sclerosis in the region of the hook. The hamate hook can be visualized with radiographs taken with the wrist in 45 degrees of supination or with the carpal tunnel view. The carpal tunnel view is typically used to profile the hook of the hamate but may be difficult to obtain in patients with acute pain from a fracture precluding sufficient extension (Figure 16.49). A CT scan may be used to define the fracture. The superiority of CT scan over conventional radiographs was demonstrated by Andresen and colleagues.[9] CT was found to have a sensitivity of 100%, a speci-

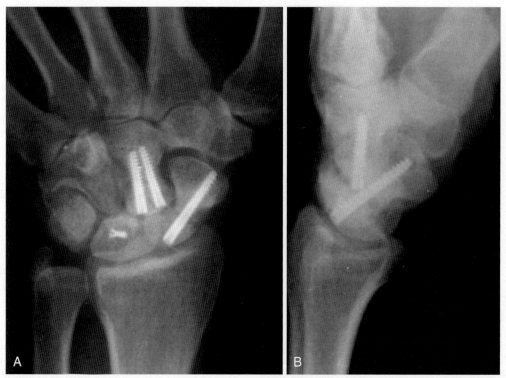

FIGURE 16.47 A, Transscaphoid, transcapitate perilunate fracture-dislocations are best stabilized through a dorsal approach. The capitate was stabilized with two headless cannulated screws, and the fracture of the scaphoid was stabilized with a single screw inserted in a proximal-distal direction. The patient had a complete tear of the lunotriquetral interosseous ligament; it was primarily repaired and provisionally stabilized with Kirschner wires, which were eventually removed. **B,** Lateral radiograph following open reduction and internal fixation of a transscaphoid, transcapitate perilunate fracture-dislocation. The radiograph confirms normal restoration of the scapholunate angle.

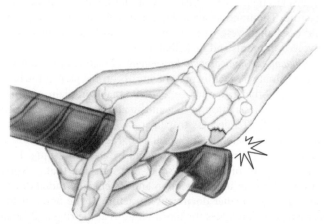

FIGURE 16.48 Mechanism of hook of hamate fracture. (From Sennwald GR: Carpal bone fractures other than the scaphoid. In Berger RA, Weiss AP, editors: *Hand Surgery*, Philadelphia, 2004, Lippincott Williams & Wilkins, p 418; with permission.)

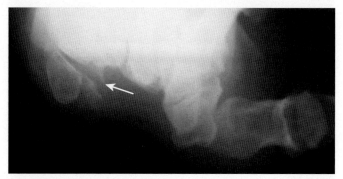

FIGURE 16.49 Hook of hamate fracture *(arrow)*. Carpal tunnel radiograph view. (Courtesy of Martin A. Posner, MD.)

ficity of 94%, and an accuracy of 97.2% in defining hook fractures, as compared with radiographs, which had a 72% sensitivity, an 88% specificity, and an 80.5% accuracy.

Blood Supply. The blood supply to the hamate has been studied extensively.[57] The hamate has three vascular pedicles. Palmar and dorsal vascular pedicles enter the hamate along the midcarpal capsular attachments and from the interosseous network that supplies the body of the hamate in a retrograde fashion. One group of small and nutrient arteries arising from the ulnar artery at the level of the Guyon canal supplies the hook of the hamate. Few anastomoses exist between the two systems. Failla described a vascular supply of the hamate as a variable pattern.[57] He described all hamates as having a nutrient vessel that enters the radial base of the hamate. However, only 71% have a nutrient vessel entering at its tip. Therefore, approximately 29% of the population is at risk for osteonecrosis of the hamate hook with a fracture distal to the basal nutrient artery. This poorly vascularized area adjacent to the base of the hook (watershed area) has a greater risk of nonunion if the fracture is not acutely immobilized.

Treatment. According to Milch, there are three different types of fractures of the hook of the hamate.[147] These have been classified as avulsion fractures of the tip of the hook, fractures through the base of the hamate hook, and fractures through the waist.

BOX 16.4 Fracture of the Hamate

Incidence

2%, probably more due to underreporting

Classification

Type 1 Hook fracture
  Fracture of tip (avulsion)
  Fracture of waist
  Fracture of base
Type 2 Body fracture
  Proximal pole fracture
  Medial tuberosity fracture
  Sagittal oblique fracture (usually radial to hook)
  Dorsal coronal fracture (usually with 4,5 carpometacarpal fracture-dislocation)

Blood Supply

Hook: Watershed region at waist
Body: Retrograde; distal hamate with volar and dorsal blood supply

Mechanisms

Type 1 Hook fracture
  Repeated trauma (golf, tennis, baseball) or direct blow
Type 2 Body fracture
  Wrist fracture-dislocation, shear
  Direct blow
  AP crush, high-energy trauma
  Axial load of fourth and fifth metacarpals

Special Radiographs

CT scanning still often necessary
Carpal tunnel view
Oblique (45-degree supinated) view

Treatment

Type 1 Hook fracture
Acute nondisplaced fracture: Ulnar gutter cast (IPs free) for 3 weeks, short-arm cast for 3 weeks (counsel that healing rate is 50% and future surgery is possible if symptomatic)
Acute displaced fracture: Early excision of bony fragment vs treatment as in acute nondisplaced hook of hamate fractures
  Chronic, symptomatic nonunion: excision of bony fragment
  Ulnar nerve/artery or tendon symptoms with displaced hook: decompression, excision. (This is controversial; some authors recommend ORIF; the author prefers excision because studies show no adverse sequelae of wrist range of motion or grip strength with hook of hamate excision.*)
It is important to identify and protect the ulnar nerve [especially the ulnar motor branch] and artery prior to hook of hamate excision).
Type 2 Body fracture
  Nondisplaced body fracture: Ulnar gutter cast (IPs free) for 3 weeks, short-arm cast for 3 weeks
  Displaced body fracture: ORIF with headless compression screws or low-profile plates and/or Kirschner wires

Associated Injuries

Ulnar artery/nerve injury in hook fractures
Fourth and fifth metacarpal fracture-dislocations in coronal body fractures
Greater arc perilunate fracture-dislocations in oblique body fractures
Axial carpal instability

Complications

Avascular necrosis in proximal wedge (pole) body fractures
Ulnar nerve compression in Guyon canal
Carpal tunnel syndrome
Flexor digitorum profundus tendon rupture
Ulnar artery thrombosis (hypothenar hammer syndrome)
Nonunion
Carpometacarpal posttraumatic arthritis

*See Devers BN, Douglas KC, Naik RD, et al: Outcomes of hook of hamate fracture excision in high-level amateur athletes. *J Hand Surg [Am]* 38(1):72–76, 2013; Stark HH, Chao EK, Zemel NP, et al: Fracture of the hook of the hamate. *J Bone Joint Surg Am* 71(8):1202–1207, 1989.

Acute nondisplaced fractures of the hook of the hamate may heal with casting and immobilization. With displaced hamate hook fractures or chronic injuries, most authors advise excision of the hook of the hamate fragment. One study noted less favorable results if hamate hook fractures are treated after the first week.[32] The unrecognized or untreated hamate hook fracture may lead to partial or complete rupture of the ring and small finger deep or superficial flexor tendons.

The reported results of hook of the hamate excision have generally been favorable.[187] Some pain and weakness may persist, but most patients will be able to return to full athletic and occupational activities. Occasionally, padded gloves are useful to allow the athlete to return to competition earlier following hook of the hamate excision. Watson and Rogers, however, noted that the hook of the hamate constitutes the medial wall of the carpal concavity, acting as an important pulley that enhances the action of the flexor tendons of the small finger by increasing its moment arm.[216] Excising the hamate may affect the function of the small finger. Because of this, some authors have recommended ORIF for hamate hook fractures.[216] There is little available literature reporting the results of ORIF.[216]

Most authors recommend excision of symptomatic fractures of the hook of the hamate,[187] and this is my preference. Studies show no adverse sequelae on wrist range of motion or grip strength with hook of hamate excision.[47,191] Excision is accomplished through a curvilinear incision centered over the hook of the hamate. If exposure requires crossing the flexor wrist crease, it is important to zigzag across the crease to avoid a flexion contracture. The ulnar nerve and artery are identified proximally in the incision and traced out distally through the Guyon canal past the hook of the hamate and protected. The distal portion of the transverse carpal ligament surrounding the tip of the hook of the hamate is released. The ulnar nerve and artery are traced along the ulnar border of the hook of the hamate. The motor branch exits from the ulnar nerve along the dorsal ulnar aspect of the nerve, passes deep to the remaining ulnar nerve, and dives beneath the flexor digiti minimi. This motor branch almost always lies at the fracture site at the base of the hamate (Figure 16.50). This nerve must be clearly identified and mobilized and retracted before the hook of the hamate fracture is excised. The hook of the hamate is a fairly long bone in the palmar-dorsal dimension. Close subperiosteal dissection is performed from palmar to dorsal to expose the base of the

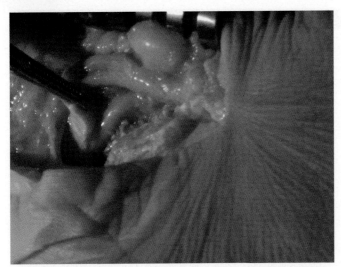

FIGURE 16.50 The motor branch of the ulnar nerve runs very near the base of the hook of the hamate. It should be identified prior to excision of the hook.

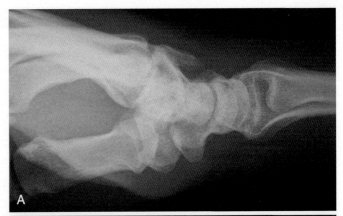

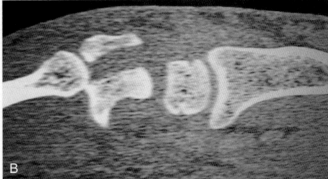

FIGURE 16.51 A lateral wrist radiograph **(A)** and computed tomography scan **(B)** to identify dorsal coronal hamate fractures. (Courtesy of Steve K. Lee, MD.)

hamate at the fracture site clearly while protecting the motor branch of the ulnar nerve. Once the fracture site has been clearly dissected and protected, the hook of the hamate fragment is removed. Any sharp bony edges are smoothed with a rongeur and/or rasp. The remaining periosteum is then closed over the base of the hamate body to decrease irritation from the remaining fracture surfaces to the ulnar nerve and flexor tendons.

Postoperative Care. Following removal of the hook of the hamate, patients can return to sports relatively quickly. Scar sensitivity is the primary factor limiting a return to sports. Physical therapy modalities, including scar massage, a silicone patch, and padded gloves, help with early return to activities. A 3% complication rate has been reported in association with excision of hamate hook fractures. Injury to the motor branch of the ulnar nerve was the most common complication.[188]

Fractures of the Body of the Hamate

Body of the hamate fractures have been divided into four major groups: proximal pole fractures, fractures of the medial tuberosity, sagittal oblique fractures, and dorsal coronal fractures. Proximal pole fractures usually are the result of shear forces in fracture-dislocations of the wrist. They are usually small intraarticular osteochondral fractures. Fractures of the medial tuberosity are usually the result of a direct blow to the ulnar side of the wrist. Sagittal oblique fractures are the result of high-energy trauma causing severe flattening of the transverse carpal arch. The ulnar nerve is at risk with this mechanism of injury. Dorsal coronal fractures are often the result of axial forces transmitted through the metacarpal. These fractures are best identified in lateral and 45-degree pronated oblique radiographs, and can be further defined with CT scan (Figure 16.51, *A* and *B*).

The small- and ring-finger hamate carpometacarpal joints are important for gripping and normally allow for approximately 30 degrees of motion. Isolated nondisplaced fractures of the body are generally stable and may be treated with casting and immobilization. Displaced fractures of the hamate that involve the carpometacarpal joint are best managed by ORIF. The fracture is exposed through a dorsal approach between the fourth and fifth extensor digitorum communis tendons. The

carpometacarpal joints are usually unstable and require reduction and fixation with Kirschner wires that are driven from involved metacarpals to carpal bones. The hamate fracture may be stabilized by small compression screws or by a small "H"-plate (Figure 16.52, *A* and *B*). Care must be taken when drilling dorsal to the palmar aspect of the hamate because of the close association of the motor branch of the ulnar nerve.

Injuries associated with fractures of the hamate body include ulnar artery or nerve injury in hook fractures, fourth and fifth metacarpal fracture-dislocations in coronal body fractures, greater arc perilunate fracture-dislocations in oblique body fractures, and axial carpal instability.

Fractures of the Pisiform

The pisiform is a sesamoid contained within the flexor carpi ulnaris (FCU) tendon. It articulates with a concave facet of the triquetrum. The pisiform serves as an attachment of the origin of the pisohamate and pisotriquetral ligaments, transcarpal ligament, and abductor digiti minimi muscle. Fracture of the pisiform accounts for approximately 2% of all fractures of the carpal bones (Box 16.5).[142] Approximately 200 reports of fractures of the pisiform have been published in the literature.[142]

Pisiform fractures occur in sports secondary to a direct blow, such as being struck by a baseball or a fall onto an outstretched hand. Occasionally, pisiform fractures are seen in marksmen from the force transmitted through a handgun, similar to the fracture of the hook of the hamate seen in players using a racket, club, or bat. Because of the pisiform's multiple soft tissue attachments, a fracture of the pisiform can also result from an avulsion mechanism. Fracture of the pisiform is frequently associated

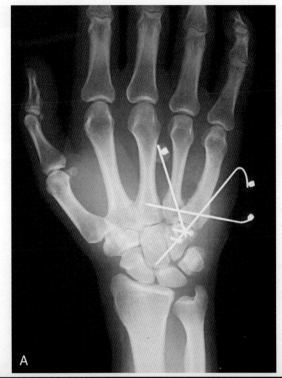

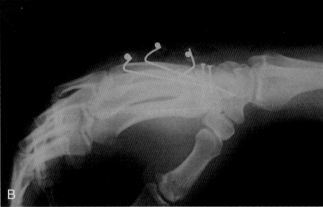

FIGURE 16.52 Postoperative radiographs after open reduction and internal fixation of hamate body fracture. Posteroanterior view **(A)** and lateral view **(B)** of wrist. (Courtesy of Steve K. Lee, MD.)

BOX 16.5 Fractures of the Pisiform

Incidence
2%

Classification
Type 1 Transverse fracture (most common)
Type 2 Parasagittal fracture
Type 3 Comminuted fracture
Type 4 Pisotriquetral impaction

Blood Supply
Robust (however, avascular necrosis has been reported)

Mechanisms
Direct blow, commonly in sports
Eccentric load of the FCU tendon
Repetitive trauma

Special Radiographs
CT scanning still often necessary
Reverse oblique view (45-degree supination with wrist extended)
Carpal tunnel view

Treatment
Acute treatment
    Nondisplaced to minimally displaced parasagittal fracture (in line with FCU) or transverse fracture: short-arm cast for 4 to 6 weeks
    Widely displaced fracture with loss of FCU continuity: comminuted: pisiform excision and FCU repair
Chronic, symptomatic nonunion or arthritic pisotriquetral joint: pisiform excision (it is important to identify and protect the ulnar nerve and artery prior to pisiform excision)

Associated Injury
50% with other upper extremity injury
Ulnar nerve injury

Complications
Posttraumatic pisotriquetral arthritis
    Nonunion

with digital, carpal, or ligamentous injuries. A high index of suspicion is warranted, as there is a high chance of an associated injury to the distal radius or carpus when a fracture of the pisiform is identified. With pisiform fractures involving the body of the triquetrum, there is a high incidence of additional injuries, and close follow-up is needed.

Four different types of pisiform fractures have been described: transverse fractures, parasagittal fractures, comminuted fractures, and pisiform-triquetral impaction fractures. Transverse fractures are most commonly associated with a sudden contracture of the FCU while the pisiform is locked between the triquetrum and the floor during a fall onto an outstretched palm. These fractures may represent discontinuity of the FCU tendon when they are severely displaced. Parasagittal fractures usually involve the ulnar rim of the pisiform and do not involve disruption of the FCU tendon. These fractures

have a better prognosis. Comminuted fractures usually result from a direct blow of the base in the hypothenar area and are associated with additional soft tissue injuries, particularly of the ulnar neurovascular bundle.

The pisiform is difficult to visualize on standard PA and lateral radiographs. It is best visualized on oblique radiographs taken with the wrist supinated 45 degrees from the lateral position in slight extension. A carpal tunnel view can be helpful (Figure 16.53). CT scan is usually obtained to clarify the injury.

Acute nondisplaced pisiform fractures are managed by casting and immobilization for 4 to 6 weeks. Most heal by bony or fibrous union. Comminuted fractures, widely displaced transverse fractures, and symptomatic nonunions are best managed with excision of the pisiform. Incongruence of the pisotriquetral joint can cause persistent pain, particularly with gripping and radioulnar motion. Athletes will continue to complain of pain while swinging a bat or golf club.

The pisiform is approached through a volar zigzag approach. The point of a zig or transverse limb is centered over the distal

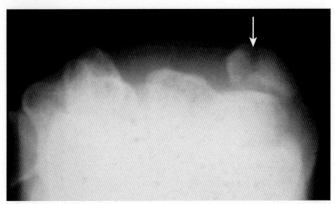

FIGURE 16.53 A radiograph with a carpal tunnel view indicating a pisiform fracture *(arrow)*. (Courtesy of Martin A. Posner, MD.)

BOX 16.6 Fractures of the Trapezoid

Incidence
Trapezoidal fractures are the rarest carpal fractures, at less than 1%

Classification
Type 1 Dorsal rim fracture
Type 2 Fracture of the body, often with proximal dorsal subluxation of the second metacarpal

Blood Supply
70% dorsal, 30% palmar

Mechanism
Axial load of index metacarpal
Extreme index metacarpal palmar flexion
High-energy trauma

Special Radiographs
CT scanning still often necessary
Standard radiographs; CT particularly helpful
MRI may be helpful for occult fractures

Treatment
Nondisplaced fracture: Short-arm thumb spica cast for 4 to 6 weeks
Displaced: ORIF with headless compression screws or Kirschner wires; excision of fragments is contraindicated because of risk of second metacarpal subluxation
Severe comminution with unreconstructable trapezoid: Primary carpometacarpal arthrodesis with possible bone grafting
Chronic fracture with arthritic changes: Carpometacarpal arthrodesis

Associated Injury
Dorsal or palmar dislocation of trapezoid or index metacarpal
Multiple injuries of carpal and metacarpal bones, other extremities, and systems due to high-energy trauma

Complications
Delayed union or nonunion
Posttraumatic arthritis
Possible avascular necrosis if dorsal fracture-dislocation has occurred

---

palmar crease. The ulnar neurovascular bundle is identified throughout the field and protected prior to excision of the pisiform. The pisiform is then carefully shelled out from the FCU tendon. The tendon fibers must be left intact to preserve function of the FCU. The FCU is repaired side-to-side with nonabsorbable braided suture.

Carroll and Coyle reviewed their results with excision of the pisiform.[31] They found little or no functional impairment with pisiform excision. Pisiform excision appears to have little effect on wrist flexion strength. Patients are returned to activities as tolerated.

Ulnar nerve injuries that occur at the same time as the pisiform fracture are usually neurapraxias. These usually resolve with observation. Nerve exploration is recommended with excision of the pisiform if symptoms persist or worsen after 12 weeks of observation. Immediate exploration of the ulnar nerve is recommended if ulnar nerve dysfunction occurs following pisiformectomy during which the nerve was not identified.

Fractures of the Trapezoid

The trapezoid is a wedge-shaped bone widest at its dorsal surface with strong ligament attachments that bind it to the adjacent bones. The dorsal surface is twice as wide as the volar surface. The trapezoid is well positioned between the trapezium, scaphoid, capitate, and index metacarpal. In its well-protected position, the trapezoid is the least commonly fractured carpal bone (<1% of all carpal fractures) (Box 16.6). Isolated fractures of the trapezoid are very rare. When the trapezoid is fractured, the mechanism of injury is usually a high-energy axial or bending mechanism transmitted through the index metacarpal proximally. This can result in a shear fracture, dorsal avulsion of the trapezoid, and dorsal dislocation of the index metacarpal or trapezoid.

Palmar dislocations and fracture-dislocations have also been reported. Fewer than 20 isolated fractures of the trapezoid have been reported.[67]

A fracture-dislocation of the trapezoid is usually evident on standard PA, lateral, and oblique radiographic views. Fracture-dislocations of the trapezoid–index metacarpal joint are usually better visualized on the PA view than on the lateral view. A dislocated trapezoid allows proximal migration and overlap of the index metacarpal. Patients present with tenderness at the base of the index metacarpal. Pain can be elicited with motion

of the index metacarpal. CT scans may help clarify the injury, and MRI may be helpful for occult fractures.

Isolated fractures of the trapezoid without displacement are usually treated nonoperatively. Displaced fractures are managed by ORIF. If the fragment is small, occasionally closed reduction with cast protection may provide satisfactory results. However, if the fragments are larger, ORIF is recommended. Fractures are stabilized with pin or screw fixation. Excision of the trapezoid is contraindicated secondary to potential proximal migration of the index metacarpal. The trapezoid receives approximately 70% of its interosseous blood supply through dorsal branches.[143] Dorsal dislocations have been complicated by AVN. Severe comminution with unreconstructable trapezoid and chronic injuries with arthritis are best managed by carpometacarpal arthrodesis owing to the minimal motion that occurs at the index carpometacarpal joint.

Fractures of the Lunate

The lunate is well enclosed within the large lunate fossa of the distal radius. Hence, isolated fractures of the lunate body are

BOX 16.7   Fractures of the Lunate

Incidence
1%
Controversy exists regarding relative frequency because Kienböck disease and congenital bipartite lunates confound diagnosis

Classification
Type I Palmar pole fracture
Type II Osteochondral chip
Type III Dorsal pole fracture
Type IV Sagittal body fracture
Type V Transverse body fracture
Type VI Comminuted fracture

Blood Supply
Most lunates have palmar and dorsal blood supply; 20% have palmar supply only

Mechanism
Usually, axial compression from capitate being driven into lunate with wrist in dorsiflexion and ulnar deviation; slight differences in position may lead to different fracture patterns
Type I Hyperextension, possible ligamentous avulsion fracture
Type II Shear
Type III Shear from capitate or ligamentous (scapholunate) avulsion fracture
Type IV Shear during radiocarpal fracture-dislocation
Type V
    Hyperextension with capitate forcing dorsal half of lunate into extension and short radiolunate ligament forcing palmar half into flexion; fracture in midsection results
    Shear with palmar displacement of capitate in palmar perilunate injury
Type VI Axial compression between radius and capitate

Special Radiographs
CT scanning still often necessary
Oblique wrist views

Treatment
First step is to determine if the pathologic process is Kienböck disease, congenital bipartite lunate, or acute traumatic fracture

If fracture fragments are too small but there is concern about instability, Kirschner wire to adjacent carpal bones may be needed
Carefully assess scapholunate and lunotriquetral ligaments for injury, and evaluate for carpal instability if small avulsion fractures appear benign on radiographs or CT scans because there may be extensive ligamentous disruption
Type I
    Nondisplaced and small, no instability: Short-arm cast for 4 to 6 weeks
    Large and/or displaced, or signs of carpal instability (usually VISI as lunate is unlinked from triquetrum): ORIF with headless compression screws or Kirschner wires; may need carpal reduction and Kirschner wire stabilization to adjacent bones if signs of carpal instability
Type II Short-arm cast for 4 to 6 weeks; arthroscopic débridement or excision if remains symptomatic
Type III
    Nondisplaced and small, no instability: Short-arm cast for 4 to 6 weeks
    Large and/or displaced, or signs of carpal instability (usually DISI as lunate is unlinked from scaphoid): ORIF with headless compression screws or Kirschner wires; may need carpal reduction and Kirschner wire stabilization to adjacent bones if signs of carpal instability
Type IV ORIF with headless compression screws or Kirschner wires *if displaced*
Type V ORIF with headless compression screws or Kirschner wires *if displaced or carpal instability*
Type VI Severe comminution or chronic (without capitate/lunate fossa arthrosis): Proximal row carpectomy

Associated Injury
Distal radius
Carpus
Metacarpals

Complications
Nonunion
Avascular necrosis
Carpal instability
Posttraumatic arthritis

DISI, Dorsal intercalated segmental instability; *ORIF*, open reduction and internal fixation; *VISI*, volar intercalated segmental instability.

rare (Box 16.7). Acute traumatic fractures of the lunate account for 1% of all carpal fractures.[202] However, fractures of the lunate are controversial. It is difficult to determine whether a fracture of the lunate is acute or whether the fracture is pathologic and the result of repetitive trauma on a weakened osteonecrotic bone resulting from Kienböck disease.[202]

Mechanism of Injury and Radiographic Presentation

Fractures of the body of the lunate usually occur from direct axial compression as the head of the capitate is driven proximally into the lunate. Differences in wrist position may lead to different fracture patterns. The dorsal lip of the lunate may be fractured as the head of the capitate impacts on it and on the dorsal distal edge of the radius in a severe hyperextension and ulnar deviation injury. If the capitate appears volarly subluxated on a lateral radiograph, a fracture of the volar lip of the lunate is suspected.

Teisen and Hjarbaek proposed a classification of fresh lunate fractures into five groups based on a review of 17 cases collected over 31 years.[202] These groups are palmar pole fractures with involvement of the palmar nutrient arteries, osteochondral chip fractures of the proximal articular surface without substantial damage to the nutrient vessels, dorsal pole fractures, sagittal fracture through the body of the lunate, and transverse fractures of the body (Figure 16.54). Fractures may also be comminuted.

Patients present with pain on the dorsum of the wrist and generalized swelling. Fractures of the lunate may be difficult to visualize on standard radiographs because of the overlapping adjacent carpal bones. CT is extremely helpful to visualize the fracture fragments and particularly to evaluate for any displacement. MRI may be helpful to evaluate for associated ligamentous injury. Signs of carpal instability should be evaluated, such as DISI, volar intercalated segmental instability (VISI), loss of Gilula lines, and asymmetric carpal bone gapping.

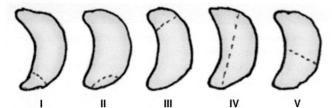

FIGURE 16.54 Lateral view line drawings of the five patterns of lunate fractures: palmar pole (I), osteochondral chip (II), dorsal pole (III), sagittal (IV), and transverse (V). (Courtesy of Steve K. Lee, MD.)

Fractures involving separation of the proximal articular surface from the body of the lunate are usually the result of Kienböck disease. A crescent line parallel to the proximal outline of the lunate is usually seen. Distinguishing fracture of a normal lunate from pathologic fracture of a lunate with AVN (as in Kienböck disease) must be done.

Treatment

Fractures of the lunate must be diagnosed and managed promptly. Careful assessment for carpal instability is imperative because a finding of small lunate fragments either dorsally or palmarly may seem benign by their size but may actually be a sign of major ligamentous disruptions. Imaging should be scrutinized for DISI or VISI deformity, loss of Gilula lines, and carpal gapping. Nondisplaced fractures of the lunate with no signs of carpal instability are treated by casting and immobilization, with close follow-up for any displacement.

Displaced fractures of the lunate require ORIF, particularly if there are signs of carpal instability. The carpus should be reduced and pinned. Lunate fragments are fixed. If open reduction is required, dorsal and body fractures are approached dorsally, palmar fragments palmarly, and osteochondral fragments either arthroscopically or dorsally.

Dorsal ridge fractures occur by shear force transmitted by the capitate. Most dorsal pole fractures are relatively benign. Treatment is determined according to the clinical findings (pain and swelling) and radiographic findings. Small dorsal chip fractures are treated with a short course of immobilization with close imaging follow-up.

Avulsions of the dorsal portion of the SLIL need to be repaired primarily. Malalignment of the capitate over the lunate (DISI) or scapholunate diastasis is consistent with carpal instability. This portion of the SLIL contains the stout transverse fibers important for stability across the scapholunate interval. The carpus needs to be reduced and pinned and the scapholunate ligament needs to be repaired primarily to the lunate with one or two micro-bone suture anchors.

Fractures of the body of the lunate and dorsal chip fractures are approached through a standard dorsal approach via the third dorsal compartment. The EPL is released, the second and fourth dorsal compartments are elevated, and the capsule is opened by the ligament-sparing technique of Berger and colleagues, exposing the carpus.[19] When the joint surface in a fracture of the body is involved, it is best seen through the dorsal approach. Body fractures may be fixed with headless compression screws and/or Kirschner wires. Comminuted fractures may require a cancellous bone graft harvested from the distal radius. Scaphocapitate pinning during slight distraction of

the wrist may take pressure off the healing lunate when internal fixation is performed. If there is severe comminution with an unreconstructable lunate or chronic injury with arthritis, proximal row carpectomy or scaphocapitate fusion may be indicated.

VISI deformity may be seen with palmar chip fractures. Palmar lunate fractures are probably the result of a wrist extension injury, with the proximal pole being avulsed by the short radiolunate ligament. The hyperextended capitate continues to load the dorsal portion of the lunate. The dorsal portion of the lunate shifts dorsally as it is no longer constrained by the palmar ligaments, and the capitate acts as a proximal wedge. This causes a separation and a high rate of nonunion, and there is a chance of palmar subluxation of the capitate and eventual degenerative disease.

Volar fragments are reduced through an extended carpal tunnel approach exposing the volar lunate. Because the incision crosses the palmar wrist crease, it is important that the incision be made in a zigzag fashion to avoid flexion contracture from the scar. The incision crosses ulnar to the palmaris longus tendon proximally so as not to affect the palmar cutaneous branch of the median nerve. Volar pole fractures are often small and may not tolerate screw fixation. In these cases, the fragment may be secured with a bone suture anchor that captures bone and palmar ligaments. Carpal reduction and stabilization by pinning the scapholunate and lunotriquetral ligaments may be needed. A pin from the scaphoid into the capitate is placed to hold the capitate reduced and to decrease compressive loads across the lunate (Figures 16.55, A to C and 16.56).

Blood Supply

The vascular supply of the lunate has been studied extensively (Figure 16.57).[57,72,74] Both a palmar and a dorsal blood supply are present in 74% to 100% of bones.[57,72,74] These studies have demonstrated a single vascular blood supply in approximately 7% of lunates. Of those lunates with a dual blood supply, 33% have a single palmar and dorsal vessel for anastomosis, 66% have a three-vessel anastomosis, and 10% have a four-vessel anastomosis.[57,72,74] In those lunates with a single nutrient vessel, interruption may lead to necrosis of the entire bone; similarly, a coronal fracture in these lunates can lead to avascularity of the opposite pole.

Injection studies of the anterior interosseous vascular lunate have demonstrated a consistent palmar blood supply but frequently an inconsistent dorsal blood supply. On the palmar aspect, the radial, ulnar, and palmar branches of the anterior interosseous artery combine to form three transverse arches to supply the lunate. Dorsally, the radial, ulnar, and dorsal branches of the anterior interosseous artery combine to form three arches. The dorsal blood supply to the lunate is drawn from the proximal two transverse arches over the radiocarpal and intercarpal joints.

Because of internal anastomoses, both dorsal and palmar flow must be interrupted for the lunate to lose circulation. Fractures that split the lunate into dorsal and palmar halves or dislocations that leave a dorsal hinge should not be expected to result in AVN. However, 20% of lunates have only a palmar nutrient artery supply in the bone. Displaced volar fragments left untreated may place predisposed lunates at risk for AVN. These fractures may be anatomically reduced and fixed.

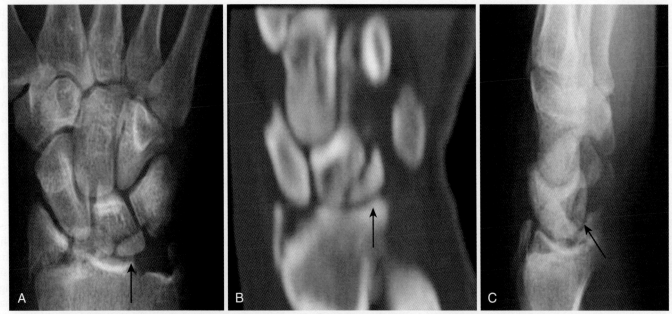

FIGURE 16.55 Lunate fracture *(arrows).* Plain radiographic **(A)** and tomographic (**B** and **C**) evaluations demonstrating a fracture to the body and volar lip of the lunate. Radial styloid fracture is also present.

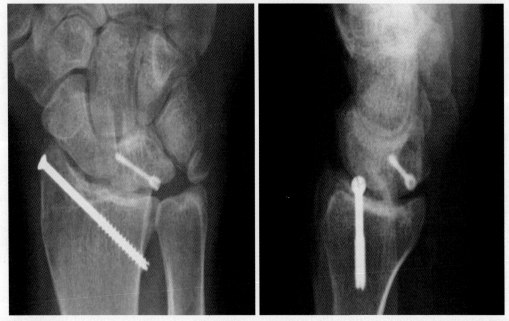

FIGURE 16.56 The lunate fracture in Figure 16.55 was approached through an extended carpal tunnel incision crossing in oblique fashion across the superficial wrist crease between the wrist flexor tendons and the ulnar nerve vascular bundle. The fracture was stabilized with a headless screw.

Osteonecrosis

Kienböck Disease

AVN of the lunate was first described in 1843 by Peste, who noted a collapsed lunate in certain cadaver dissections.[160] Robert Kienböck, a radiologist, described the x-ray changes associated with lunatomalacia that is now associated with his name.

Etiologic Findings

There is no consensus about the relationship between acute lunate fractures and Kienböck disease. Uncertainty exists as to whether some lunate fractures are actually pathologic fractures in patients with preexisting Kienböck disease. Teisen and Hjarbaek noted in a long-term follow-up series that lunate fractures had failed to show AVN even though half of the patients studied had ulnar-negative variance.[202] Persistent pain following a lunate fracture can be evaluated by MRI to see whether Kienböck disease is present.[202] However, radiographic findings of AVN in a patient with a fracture can be difficult to define. AVN of the lunate should be considered when there is homogeneous signal loss of the entire lunate rather than signal loss of a portion secondary to fracture.

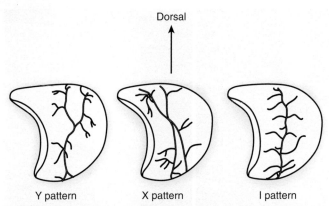

Dorsal

Y pattern   X pattern   I pattern

FIGURE 16.57 The vascular supply of the lunate has been thoroughly studied, and three major vascular patterns have been identified. These have been previously described as the Y, X, and I patterns. The I pattern is the only one with a single vessel to the lunate and is considered to be most at risk for development of avascular necrosis.

Despite years of clinical experience, the origin and natural history of Kienböck disease remain unclear. The loss of blood supply to the lunate has been attributed to primary circulatory problems, traumatic interference, poor circulation, ligament injury with collapse, and single or multiple fractures resulting in secondary vascular impairment. Although fracture-dislocation of the carpus may result in transient radial density of the lunate, the avascular changes of Kienböck disease are progressive. Kienböck disease has been associated with various medical conditions, including scleroderma, sickle cell anemia, systemic lupus erythematosus, and corticosteroid use. However, no consistent correlation with any specific disease process has been demonstrated. Most likely, the cause of Kienböck disease is multifactorial.

The relationship of ulnar variance and Kienböck disease is controversial. Gelberman and colleagues described a significant relationship between ulnar-negative variance and Kienböck disease.[72] However, D'Hoore and colleagues reviewed 125 normal wrists in 52 patients with Kienböck disease and found no significant statistical relationship between ulnar variance and Kienböck disease.[48] It was also noted that if Kienböck disease were related to ulnar-negative variance, the incidence of Kienböck disease would be higher, particularly in patients who had undergone Darrach procedures or ulnar shortenings. Nakamura and colleagues reviewed Kienböck disease in the Japanese population.[155] They found that ulnar-negative variance occurs with equal frequency in the general population and in the population with Kienböck disease.

Schiltenwolf and colleagues studied the interosseous pressure of the lunate with wrist motion.[175] In their study, they found that the interosseous pressure of the lunate is greater than its axial neighboring capitate by 40 mm Hg in wrist extension than in neutral. This rise in interosseous pressure may explain the lunate's predisposition to osteonecrosis.

The slope of the distal radius has been studied as a potential cause of Kienböck disease. Tsuge and Nakamura found that the radial inclination was lower in patients with Kienböck disease.[206] Other investigators found that the radial slope in the AP projection has a significant effect on both the forces transmitted to the lunate and the patient's age at the onset of Kienböck disease.

Clinical and Radiographic Presentation. The diagnosis of Kienböck disease is suspected particularly in young males with pain and stiffness in the dominant wrist. Tenderness is centered over the dorsal lunate, and patients experience decreased grip strength. The lunate lies just distal to the distal radius dorsal lip in line with the third ray. Patients frequently describe an insidious onset of dull pain centered over the radiolunate joint; however, some will provide a history of recent hyperextension injury. Patients complain of pain aggravated by activity and relieved with rest and immobilization.

On physical examination, patients may demonstrate a radiocarpal effusion with boggy synovitis of the radiocarpal joint. Range of motion of the wrist is limited, and grip strength is decreased compared with the opposite side.

Standard PA and lateral radiographs of the wrist are obtained with the wrist in neutral rotation. Increased bone density of the lunate is the early sign of avascularity on plain radiographs. MRI is the most sensitive imaging study for Kienböck disease. It is important not to confuse Kienböck disease with findings limited to the ulnar side of the lunate consistent with ulnar impaction (=abutment). Frequently, radiologists will diagnose ulnar impaction changes as Kienböck disease; the entire lunate must show signal loss on MRI to warrant the diagnosis of Kienböck disease, however.

Bone scintigraphy may also show increased uptake in the early stage of Kienböck disease. This technique is less commonly used today and has mostly been supplanted by MRI. Radiographic findings depend on the stage of the disease. Typical radiographic findings include lunate sclerosis, progressive loss of lunate height, fragmentation of the lunate, especially in the sagittal plane, progressive loss of carpal height as the capitate migrates proximally, and eventual degenerative joint changes related to rotation of the scaphoid and carpal collapse.

MRI will demonstrate a uniform decrease in signal intensity on T1 radial images due to the decreased vascularity. To make the diagnosis of Kienböck disease, a signal change must be seen throughout the entire lunate (*black lunate sign*). Ulnar impaction syndrome, fractures, interosseous ganglions, and enchondromas will cause MRI changes within the lunate, but these conditions will cause a focal change rather than a magnetic imaging change in the entire bone.

Staging. The most common method for staging Kienböck disease was first described by Stahl in 1947.[190] Lichtman and colleagues' 1977 modification of the system is widely used.[131] This classification system is based on plain radiographs and MRI findings. Treatment is based on the stage of disease (Table 16.7).

In stage I disease, plain radiographs may be normal or may show a linear compression fracture. Lunate collapse has not occurred. Diagnosis at this stage is usually made by MRI evaluation. A decreased signal on both T1- and T2-weighted images suggests AVN. Patients have intermittent dorsal wrist pain.

In stage II disease, there is sclerosis and fracture of the lunate but no change in the size or shape of the bone. There may also be multiple fracture lines, but the lunate is not collapsed. I find CT scan with sagittal and coronal reconstructions very helpful to assess for collapse and reconstructability of the lunate bone. Clinically, affected patients complain of pain, persistent swelling, and stiffness of the wrist.

TABLE 16.7 Lichtman Classification for Kienböck Disease

Stage	Description
I	Plain radiographs are generally normal, but a linear fracture through the lunate may be noted. MRI demonstrates diffuse T1 signal decrease in lunate. Bone scan is positive.
II	Sclerosis of the lunate is seen on plain radiographs. Multiple fracture lines may be seen, though collapse of the lunate has not occurred.
IIIA	Lunate collapse has occurred, but the carpal height alignments have been maintained.
IIIB	Lunate collapse has occurred, and the capitate has migrated proximally. The scaphoid assumes a hyperflexed position.
IV	This is a continuation of stage IIIB disease, with the addition of carpal (radiocarpal and/or midcarpal) arthritis.

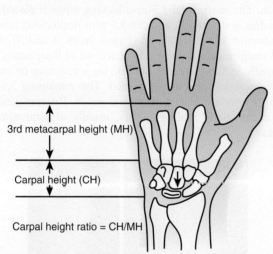

3rd metacarpal height (MH)

Carpal height (CH)

Carpal height ratio = CH/MH

FIGURE 16.58 The carpal height index is measured on the posteroanterior radiograph. The carpal height ratio is defined as the carpal height divided by the height of the third metacarpal.

From the Lichtman-Stahl classification, stage III disease is divided into stages A and B. In stage IIIA, the lunate has collapsed but the carpus remains unchanged, with normal alignment and height. Lateral radiographs show that the lunate is wider in its AP dimension. In stage IIIB, the capitate has migrated proximally and the scaphoid has assumed a flexed position. As the carpal height ratio decreases, the lunate collapses and the capitate migrates proximally (Figure 16.58). Scaphoid rotation produces a DISI pattern of carpal instability. Patients complain of progressive stiffness with diminished grip strength. Clunking with radial and ulnar deviation of the wrist may be found.

Using radiographs, Goldfarb and colleagues found that interobserver reliability for differentiating between stages IIIA and IIIB of the Lichtman classification was poor. With the additional criterion that the radioscaphoid angle must be greater than 60 degrees to qualify for stage IIIB, interobserver reliability increased to a Kappa value of 0.75.[78] Using radiographs, Jensen and colleagues reported a reliability Kappa value of between 0.45 and 0.52 and a reproducible Kappa coefficient of between 0.26 and 0.63, which is fair to moderate.[107] Jafarnia and colleagues reported an average paired weighted Kappa coefficient of 0.71 for interobserver reliability of the Lichtman classification among four observers who reviewed radiographs from 64 patients and 10 control subjects.[106] The coefficient for interobserver reliability was noted to be 0.77. Condit and colleagues found that the preoperative radioscaphoid angle correlated best with clinical outcomes.[38] Specifically, wrists with preoperative radioscaphoid angles of greater than 60 degrees tend to do poorly with any procedure aimed at salvaging the lunate.

In stage IV disease, continued carpal collapse is related to arthritic changes in the radiocarpal and midcarpal joints. Radiographs show subchondral sclerosis with joint space narrowing, osteophyte formation, and degenerative cysts. Patients complain of decreased range of motion of the wrist with constant pain and swelling.

Imaging. I currently use radiographs, MRI, and CT scans to assess Kienböck disease. MRI is best for the assessment of vascularity of the lunate, specifically documenting the absence of vascularity on *all* imaging sequences. On occasion, an abnormal signal in a portion of the lunate will be interpreted on MRI to represent Kienböck disease, when in fact clinical and radiographic signs point more toward ulnar impaction syndrome. MRI with cartilage-sensitive sequencing also aids in knowledge of the state of cartilage and arthritic change. I believe that the usefulness of staging classic IIIA and IIIB disease in guiding treatment is uncertain. I use CT scans to determine the morphologic condition of the lunate and the probability that it can be salvaged.

Treatment. Treatment algorithms for Kienböck disease have primarily been determined by the stage of the disease according to the Lichtman classification. There are many treatment options, but they basically fall into three main groups: procedures to unload the lunate, procedures to promote revascularization of the necrotic lunate, and salvage procedures used when the lunate is not reconstructable or arthritic conditions exist.

Stahl recommended prolonged immobilization for Kienböck disease.[190] Tajima reviewed 80 patients with Kienböck disease with a follow-up of 42 years and found no appreciable difference in the end results of nonoperative or surgical treatment.[200]

Kristensen and colleagues followed 46 patients with Kienböck disease treated nonoperatively for a minimum of 5 years, with a mean of 20 years.[123] Although 66% of the patients had arthritic changes of the wrist at follow-up, only 25% had significant pain. Taniguchi and colleagues found that although radiographic findings worsened in 70% of 20 patients followed for 35 years, only 20% had significant symptoms limiting their activities.[201] However, a recent study by Keith and colleagues reviewed 33 patients treated nonoperatively for Kienböck disease.[118] They found a predictable pattern of deterioration of motion, grip strength, and Disabilities of the Arm, Shoulder, and Hand (DASH) scores.

Stage I, II, or IIIA Kienböck Disease with Ulnar-Negative Variance. In stage I, II, or IIA Kienböck disease with ulnar-negative variance, carpal collapse into an instability pattern has not occurred (radioscaphoid angle < 60 degrees). Salvage of the lunate may be possible to maintain normal carpal kinematics. In a symptomatic patient with stage I, II, or IIIA disease with ulnar-negative variance, a joint-leveling procedure should be considered. Some authors have found that unloading the joint can be useful even in patients with stage IIIB pathologic changes.[5,221] The most common procedure for unloading the lunate in patients with ulnar-negative variance is radial-shortening osteotomy. This can be done through either a volar or dorsal approach, although the volar approach is more commonly performed. Specialized jigs and forearm-shortening plates have been designed to simplify the procedure. The goal is to leave the patient with ulnar-neutral or slightly ulnar-positive variance. Some authors have described lengthening of the ulna; however, this technique requires two osteotomy sites and a bone graft, unlike radial shortening, and is not commonly performed.

Joint-leveling procedures. Radial-shortening osteotomy is considered for patients with Kienböck disease who have an ulnar-negative variance, a salvageable lunate, no carpal collapse (radioscaphoid angle < 60 degrees), and no arthritic changes around the adjacent intercarpal or radiocarpal joints. Patients who are ulnar neutral or ulnar positive are at risk for developing ulnar impaction syndrome after ulnar shortening. Several biomechanical studies have compared the changes of force distribution across the carpus. Trumble and colleagues reviewed the force distribution across the carpus with various procedures for Kienböck disease.[203] In this study, capitate-hamate fusion did not significantly decrease lunate strain. However, ulnar lengthening, radial shortening, and STT fusion all produced a 70% decrease in lunate strain. The advantage of joint-leveling procedures such as radial shortening is that it does not affect the final range of motion of the wrist, unlike intraarticular procedures such as STT fusion, which limits wrist radial deviation and extension. Trumble and colleagues noted that 90% of the reduction in lunate strain following radial shortening or ulnar lengthening occurred in the first 2 mm of length alteration, although strain reduction increased in both procedures with up to 3 mm of length alteration.[203] Length alteration of more than 4 mm produced no further changes in the lunate load; in addition, shortening of more than 4 mm runs the risk of incongruence to the distal radioulnar joint. Based on the biomechanical studies, the object of radial shortening is to shorten the radius approximately 2 to 3 mm and not merely to obtain ulnar-neutral variance.

Similarly, Horii and colleagues used a mathematical model to evaluate joint-leveling procedures.[98] Ulnar lengthening and radial shortening were equivalent in this mathematical model, leading to a 45% decrease in the force transmitted through the radiolunate joint. This decrease was mostly borne by the ulnar lunate and ulnar triquetral joints, where force increased by 50% and 78%, respectively. The force transmitted to the radioscaphoid joint increased by 6%, and in the midcarpal region there was an increase in the lunatocapitate joint force of 13%. Scaphocapitate fusion led to a decrease in the radiolunate joint force of 12%, capitate hamate fusion had no change, and capitate shortening combined with carpal hamate fusion led to a 66% force decrease.

Radial-shortening osteotomy. Radial shortening may be performed through either a volar or a dorsal approach. In the volar approach, an incision is centered over the radial border of the FCR tendon. The tendon sheath is released, and the FCR is retracted ulnarly to protect the median nerve. The pronator quadratus is released from the radial border of the radius and retracted ulnarly. There are a few radial shortening plate systems on the market, or a freehand technique may be used with a dynamic compression plate and dynamic compression/distraction device using a screw placed outside of the plate.

A plate is placed on the volar aspect of the radius. It may be slightly prebent distally to fit the volar curvature to the distal radius. A locking screw is placed in the most distal screw hole, and a 3.5-mm nonlocking screw is placed in the oval reduction slot. The osteotomy will be performed over the oblique lag screw hole. This area is marked on the radius with the plate in place. The plate is removed. A transverse or oblique osteotomy to the distal radius is performed. If an oblique cut is made, a 2-mm wafer is removed because of the geometry of compression. If a transverse cut is made, a wafer of bone of approximately 3 mm is removed. The forearm osteotomy plate is replaced and fixed to the radius. An articulated distraction-compression device with which to gain increased compression at the osteotomy site may be used at the discretion of the surgeon. The most distal 3.5-mm locking screw is placed first. The radius is shortened, and the 3.5-mm nonlocking screw in the reduction slot is tightened (Figure 16.59. *A* and *B*). Additional compression is gained by a second oblique screw hole proximally in the plate. An oblique lag screw may be used if an oblique osteotomy is performed. The remaining 3.5-mm locking screws are placed in neutral mode. Patients generally wear a cast until healing occurs, usually at approximately 6 weeks.

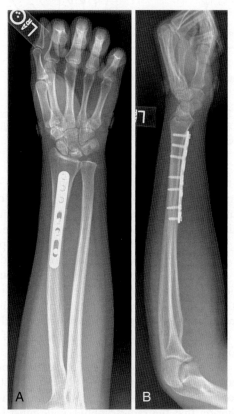

FIGURE 16.59 A, PA radiograph following radial-shortening osteotomy. A forearm-shortening osteotomy plate (AcuMed, Hillsboro, OR) was placed on the volar surface of the radius. The patient now is ulnar neutral. **B,** Lateral radiograph showing the anatomically contoured plate along the volar aspect of the radius following radial-shortening osteotomy.

Alternatively, an osteotomy can be performed more distally in the metaphyseal bone. In this incidence, a long distal radius plate may be used. The plate is initially placed with distal screws, and a proximal screw is inserted. The plate is removed, a transverse osteotomy is performed in the metaphysis of the distal radius, the radius is shortened, the distal plate is replaced, and the radius is compressed. This technique has a potentially better incidence of healing because the osteotomy is made in the metaphyseal bone. However, compression is more difficult to obtain at the osteotomy site as compared with a formal forearm osteotomy plate.

Alternatively, a plate may be placed dorsally. However, a dorsal plate may be symptomatic because of its more superficial location and may need to be removed in the future.

Most authors report good results after a radial-shortening osteotomy.[5,169,221] Weiss and colleagues reviewed the results of 29 patients who underwent the procedure for stages I through IIIB disease.[221] At a minimum follow-up of 2 years, they reported that 87% of the patients had decreased pain and that the wrist range of motion had increased by an average of 32%. There was no progressive evidence of carpal collapse. It is important to note there was no improvement in the radiographic appearance of the lunate. Rock and colleagues reviewed 16 patients who underwent radial-shortening osteotomy.[169] Six patients were classified as stage III and four were classified as stage IV. At an average follow-up of 4.5 years, 13 of 16 patients were pain free, and the range of motion improved in the AP plane by 15 degrees. Grip strength increased by 20% to 30%. Almquist and Burns reported pain relief in 11 of 12 patients, although no patient was pain free in their series at 5 to 10 years' follow-up.[5] Wrist range of motion increased by an average of 40 degrees, and grip strength improved.

Vascularized bone grafting. Vascularized bone grafting is another useful technique for patients with stage I, II, or IIIA disease; however, precise indications are not clear. The dorsal distal radius vascular anatomy is constant and demonstrates a consistent special relationship to anatomic landmarks. An anatomic network for the intercompartmental and compartmental arteries is provided by a series of arterial arches across the dorsum of the hand and wrist. These include the dorsum of the carpal arch, the dorsal radiocarpal arch, and the dorsal supraretinacular arch. Dorsal arterial arches are the source of the vascularized bone graft from the base of the second and third metacarpals. The vessels supplying nutrient branches directly to the dorsal radius and ulna are described at those locations with respect to the extensor compartments of the wrist and extensor retinaculum. *Intercompartmental vessels* are located between compartments, and *compartmental vessels* lie within an extensor compartment. Vessels lying superficial to the retinaculum are further described as *supraretinacular.*

Technique based on the fourth and fifth extensor compartment arteries. The most useful vessels for vascularized bone grafting for the treatment of Kienböck disease are the fourth and fifth ECAs. A vascularized bone graft using the fifth ECA's connection to the fourth ECA by way of their common origin is preferred because of the large diameter of the fifth ECA. The ECA pedicle provides an ideal pedicle length that can reach anywhere in the carpus.

A longitudinal incision is made to expose the lunate and distal radius. The fifth ECA is exposed by opening the fifth

dorsal extensor compartment. The fifth ECA is visualized on the radial floor of the compartment adjacent to or partially in the septum separating the fourth and fifth extensor compartments. The fifth ECA is traced proximally to its origin at the anterior osseous artery while the fourth ECA is identified and distally traced, opening the fourth compartment (Figure 16.60). A bone graft centered 11 mm proximal to the radiocarpal joint and overlying the fourth ECA to include the nutrient vessels is outlined (Figure 16.61). Ligation of the anterior osseous artery proximally to the fourth and fifth ECA is

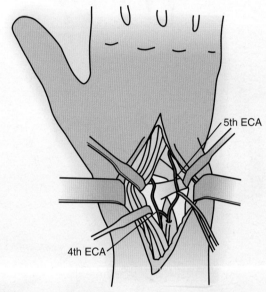

5th ECA

4th ECA

FIGURE 16.60 The fifth extensor compartment artery is identified by incising the fifth dorsal extensor compartment. It is visualized on the radial aspect of the compartment by an adjacent septum separating the fourth and fifth dorsal compartments. (By permission of Mayo Foundation for Medical Education and Research. All rights reserved.)

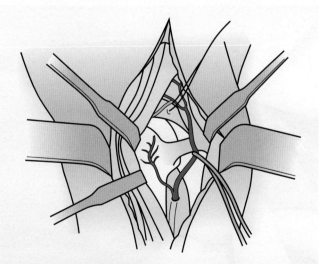

FIGURE 16.61 The fifth extensor compartment artery is identified and traced proximally to its origin from the anterior interosseous artery. The fourth extensor compartment artery is identified and traced distally to the distal radius. A bone graft is centered approximately 11 mm from the radiocarpal joint overlying the fourth extensor compartment artery. (By permission of Mayo Foundation for Medical Education and Research. All rights reserved.)

performed. Graft elevation is completed with the use of osteotomes (Figure 16.62). The tourniquet is deflated to verify blood flow to the graft. Cancellous bone graft can be additionally obtained from the donor site. While protecting the bone graft and its pedicle, the lunate is exposed via a dorsal ligament–sparing capsulotomy. A dorsal cortical window is made in the lunate, and the necrotic bone is removed (Figure 16.63). With

the wrist distracted, a scaphocapitate Kirschner wire is placed to unload the lunate. If partially collapsed, the lunate is reduced by a hemostat so that the morphologic condition is uncompressed. Cancellous bone graft is packed in the defect, leaving room for the vascularized bone graft. The 4,5 ECA vascularized bone graft is rotated and transferred into the lunate (Figure 16.64). Moran and colleagues reported on 26 patients with Kienböck disease who had the 4,5 ECA graft. Although they had a short follow-up of 3 months, 92% of patients had significant improvement in their pain. Grip strength improved from 50% to 89% of the unaffected side. Satisfactory results were seen in 85% of patients based on the Lichtman outcome score. Of patients who had a postoperative MRI, 71% showed evidence of revascularization.[151]

Other graft options include the 2,3 ICSRA graft based on antegrade flow through the fifth ECA. The 2,3 ICSRA has a proximal origin from the anterior interosseous artery or its posterior division. It lies superficial to the extensor retinaculum directly over the Lister tubercle and anastomoses with the dorsal intercarpal arch, the dorsal radiocarpal arch, and occasionally the fourth ECA. It is easily harvested and has an arc of rotation that reaches the entire proximal row.[179]

Technique based on the second or third metacarpal. This technique takes advantage of the distal vascular arcade to use the vascularized bone graft through a single midline incision. Releasing the distal portion of the fourth dorsal compartment exposes the distal vascular arcade. The pedicle may be mobilized in either an ulnar or a radial direction to a length sufficient to reach the lunate. The bone graft is harvested from the base of the second or third metacarpal, depending on where the artery has the greatest area of contact. The vascularized bone graft is harvested and is inserted into the lunate, as in the previously described technique using the fourth and fifth ECAs (Figure 16.65).

Technique for vascularized bundle implantation. Hori and colleagues described a technique for vascular bundle implantation using the second dorsal intermetacarpal artery.[97] Indications for this technique include patients who maintain a

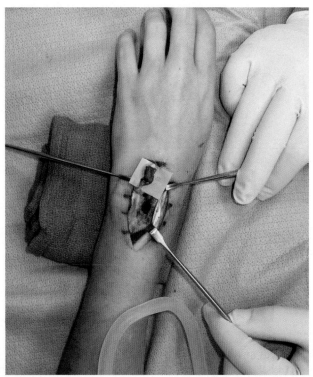

FIGURE 16.62 Graft elevation is completed with the use of osteotomes. (Courtesy of Steve K. Lee, MD.)

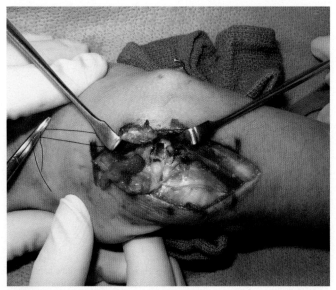

FIGURE 16.63 While protecting the bone graft and its pedicle, the lunate is exposed via a dorsal ligament–sparing capsulotomy. A dorsal cortical window is made in the lunate, and the necrotic bone is removed. (Courtesy of Steve K. Lee, MD.)

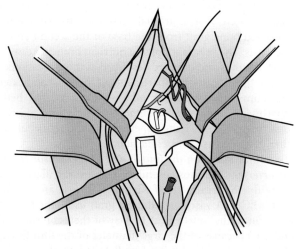

FIGURE 16.64 The vascularized bone graft is inserted into the lunate. The pedicle is oriented vertically with the cortical surface and arranged in proximal-distal orientation to maintain lunate height. (By permission of Mayo Foundation for Medical Education and Research. All rights reserved.)

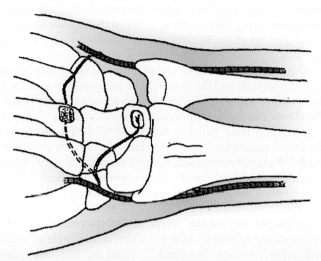

FIGURE 16.65 An optional source of vascularized bone graft may be obtained from the base of the second or third metacarpal based on the dorsal metacarpal arcade.

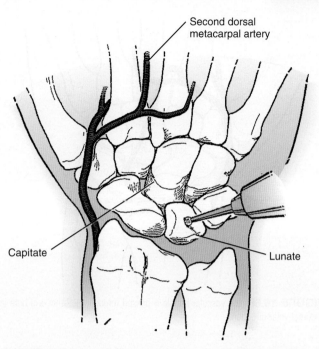

FIGURE 16.66 The dorsal second intermittent carpal artery lies just beneath the aponeurosis and covers the interosseous muscles. The fascia is divided to expose the intermittent carpal artery.

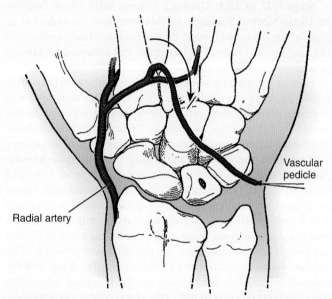

FIGURE 16.67 The distalmost extent of the artery is ligated with a 5-0 monofilament suture. This provides a 5- to 6-cm length of vessel.

relatively normal arch of the carpus. The second dorsal metacarpal artery is a branch of the dorsal metacarpal artery to the index and long fingers. It travels between the index and long metacarpals. If this vessel is damaged or cannot be found, the third dorsal metacarpal artery may be used. A dorsal incision is made starting proximal to the second metacarpophalangeal joint; it is continued proximally and curves around the Lister tubercle. Dissection is continued between the second and third extensor compartments, which are released, and the extensor carpi radialis longus and brevis are retracted radially. The extensor digiti communis tendon is retracted ulnarly so that the capsule of the carpus is visualized. A proximally based flap is made to visualize the lunate. In the nonarticular portion of the lunate a dorsal window is made in the bone using 0.035-inch Kirschner wires and a sharp osteotome to remove the outer layer of bone. Sclerotic bone is removed. The second dorsal intermetacarpal artery lies underneath the aponeurosis that covers the interosseous muscles (Figure 16.66). This fascial layer is divided from proximal to distal to the level of the second web space. The artery and venae comitantes are elevated with a thin layer of surrounding perivascular tissue. At the distalmost extent of the artery, the vessels are ligated with a 5-0 monofilament suture (Figure 16.67). This should provide a 5- to 6-cm length of vessel. The lunate should be unloaded by any number of procedures (such as external fixation, capitate shortening, or temporary scaphocapitate pinning). Devascularized and necrotic bone is removed from the lunate. Cancellous bone chips are packed into the defect. A 2.7-mm drill is used to create a hole in the proximal avascular portion of the lunate. The vascular bundle is passed through this hole in a dorsal to volar direction (Figure 16.68). This may be performed by attaching a fine resorbable suture on a straight needle to the 5-0 monofilament suture. The needle exits through the palmar skin just ulnar to the FCR tendon. A small skin incision is made, and the suture is tied over the palmar antebrachial fascia.

Hori and colleagues reported their experience with implantation of the dorsal metacarpal arteriovenous pedicle.[97] Nine cases of Kienböck disease were reviewed, with improvement

described in eight patients. Several authors have described their experience with transfer of the vascularized pisiform into the necrotic lunate. Bochud and Buchler reported on 32 patients with a follow-up of 2 years.[22] Initial restoration of the lunate anatomy was observed in 95% of the patients. However, only 33% retained a correction, and nearly half of the long-term results were only fair or poor. Moran and colleagues reviewed the results of vascularized bone grafting in 48 patients with follow-up over a 10-year period.[150] Ninety-eight percent of patients experienced significant pain relief. Grip strength

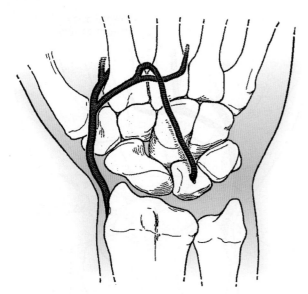

FIGURE 16.68 The vascular bundle is passed through a 2.7-mm drill hole in a dorsal-volar direction.

improved, although range of motion did not. Postoperative MRI showed evidence of vascularization in 60% of the patients in their series.

Stage I, II, or IIIA Kienböck Disease With Ulnar-Positive or Ulnar-Neutral Variance. In this situation, the radius is as short as the ulna, and further shortening is not likely to decrease the load on the lunate. The lunate has not collapsed, so salvage procedures are not warranted.

Capitate shortening alone or combined with capitate-hamate fusion has been reported in the literature.[5] This technique was first described by Almquist in 1993, and he reported lunate revascularization rates as high as 83%.[4] Stage IV Kienböck disease would be a contraindication to this surgical technique.

Technique for capitate shortening with capitate-hamate fusion. A dorsal incision is made from the base of the third metacarpal to the Lister tubercle. The fifth dorsal compartment is released, and the extensor digiti quinti tendon is retracted. The fourth dorsal compartment tendons are retracted radially, and the dorsal capsule is opened. Care is taken not to elevate the fourth compartment and disrupt the vascular supply. The capitate-hamate joint is incised from proximal to distal, and the waist of the capitate is identified for the proposed osteotomy. This level should correspond to the distal pole of the scaphoid. Almquist, in his technique, described using a sharp, thin osteotome to make the bone cut to avoid disruption of the volar capsule blood supply. A small curved elevator is inserted carefully into the capitolunate joint, avoiding injury into the articular surface. The elevator is used to compress the capitate head against the distal segment, and two crossed 0.062-inch Kirschner wires are used to stabilize the osteotomy site. Alternatively, headless compression screws can be used. If a capitate-hamate fusion is performed, all cartilage and subchondral bone at the capitate-hamate interface is removed, and bone harvested from the osteotomy or from a separate distal radius graft site is packed into the space. Kirschner wires or headless cannulated screws are placed percutaneously from the hamate into each of the capitate fragments. Viola noted that when performing this procedure, the tip of the hamate becomes prominent proximally, preventing the unloading effect of the capitate shortening.[212] The tip of the hamate may be removed to correct this problem.

Alternatively, the surgeon can perform the osteotomy across both the capitate and the hamate. The composite osteotomy is then reduced and secured with Kirschner wires or buried headless screws inserted from proximal to distal.

Hanel and Hunt noted in the review of their patients that the initial results in 1 year were remarkable with this technique.[87] Range of motion and strength plateaued between 8 and 12 months. Almquist noted grip strength of the affected hand to be 80% of the opposite side, and he reported an 83% satisfaction rate in his series.[4]

Technique for closing wedge radial osteotomy. Radial-closing radial osteotomy with reduction in the angle of radial inclination has been described.[215] Watanabe and colleagues' rigid body spring model showed that the axial load through the radiolunate joint is redistributed to the radioscaphoid joint without increasing the ulnar carpal load.[215] Radial osteotomy does not violate the intraarticular space of the wrist, so the range of motion is maintained. The technique is technically demanding. Radial osteotomy is not indicated in advanced Kienböck disease with collapse.

In this technique, a standard volar approach is made to the distal radius. The FCR is released and retracted ulnarly to protect the median nerve. The pronator quadratus is released along the radial surface. A trapezoidal wedge-shaped segment of bone may be removed from the distal quarter of the radius or metaphysis. The osteotomy would be wider radially than ulnarly to decrease the radial inclination (Figure 16.69, *A* to *C*).

Core decompression. Illarramendi and colleagues described their technique of coring out the metaphyseal region of the distal radius and ulna for treating Kienböck disease.[102] The idea for this technique arose from the authors' observation that complete resolution of Kienböck disease occurred in patients who sustained a distal radius fracture. By coring out the distal radius, they felt they would be able to create a scenario similar to that of a distal radius fracture. Twenty-two patients were followed for an average of 10 years. Sixteen patients were pain free and four patients had occasional pain. No patient required further surgery. This technique is used mainly to increase venous outflow, which is similar to cord decompression, and to decrease interosseous congestion.

Stage IIIB Kienböck Disease. If the disease has progressed to stage IIIB, the various salvage procedures should be considered.[155] Various intercarpal fusions have been described, including STT and scaphocapitate arthrodesis. Proximal row carpectomy has also been reported for stage IIIB disease. Watson and colleagues reported their results in 69 patients who underwent 71 triscaphe scaphotrapezial arthrodesis procedures for Kienböck disease.[217] (Two patients in the series had bilateral disease.) Initially, in the authors' series, the lunate was excised and Silastic lunate arthroplasty was performed. The prevalence of Silastic particulate synovitis led to the discontinuation of the Silastic prosthesis. In their series, 46% of the patients had excellent subjective results and 32% had good results. The carpal height index remained essentially unchanged in 35 of 36 patients. Eighty-two percent returned to their preoperative

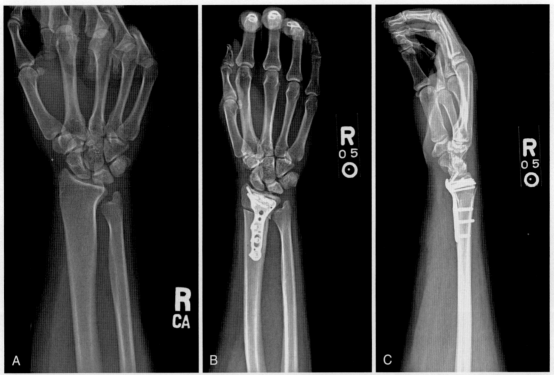

FIGURE 16.69 Closing wedge osteotomy. **A,** Posteroanterior wrist radiograph of a 23-year-old female with a congenital abnormality with increased radial tilt and Kienböck disease. **B,** Because of the increased tilt, a trapezoidal wedge osteotomy was performed. The osteotomy is stabilized by an AcuLoc (AcuMed, Hillsboro, OR) volar distal radial plate. **C,** Lateral wrist radiograph following trapezial wedge osteotomy.

work or avocational activities. Further wrist salvage procedures were needed in 5.6% of patients, including proximal carpectomy in two patients and total wrist arthrodesis in two patients. Scaphocapitate fusion is thought to be technically easier to perform than STT fusion. It is important to maintain the normal distance between the scaphoid and capitate.

De Smet and colleagues reported on their results for 21 patients who underwent proximal row carpectomy for advanced lunate AVN.[45] In their series, 13 patients had no pain to mild pain, 3 patients reported moderate pain, and 5 patients had severe pain. Nakamura and colleagues reported better results with proximal row carpectomy than with limited wrist arthrodesis for advanced Kienböck disease.[155] Based on their experience, they recommended proximal carpectomy over STT fusion, although the difference was not statistically significant (Figure 16.70, *A* to *F*).

Recently, pyrocarbon arthroplasty has become an option in patients with late-stage Kienböck disease. The pyrocarbon lunate may be stabilized by either suture or tendon. There are no long-term studies with this technique.

Stage IV Disease. In stage IV disease, there is significant collapse of the lunate in addition to perilunate arthritis. Generalized degenerative changes are noted at the radiocarpal and midcarpal joints. Proximal row carpectomy may be a possibility, but it is important to determine that the head of the capitate and the lunate fossa are relatively well preserved. Potentially, a dorsal capsule interposition or soft tissue graft may be placed on the lunate fossa.

In most instances with end-stage Kienböck disease and arthritic radiocarpal and midcarpal joints, total wrist fusion is recommended. Patients frequently achieve pain relief, but wrist fusion is not without potential complications and residual symptoms.

❖ AUTHOR'S PREFERRED METHOD

I prefer to think of Kienböck disease in two stages: (1) the lunate is salvageable and (2) the lunate is not salvageable. I base this decision on radiographs, MRIs, and CT scans and believe all three add to the decision-making process. MRI is best for specific evaluation of complete avascularity of the lunate on all sequences. MRI with cartilage-sensitive sequencing also provides knowledge of cartilage and arthritic changes. CT scans are used to assess the lunate morphologic conditions of collapse and carpal alignment. If the lunate is salvageable and there is ulnar-negative variance, I shorten the radius to 2 to 3 mm and perform a posterior interosseous nerve neurectomy. If the lunate is salvageable and there is ulnar-neutral or ulnar-positive variance, I perform vascularized bone grafting from the 4,5 ECA and posterior interosseous nerve neurectomy. If the lunate is not salvageable and the lunate fossa and capitate head cartilage are preserved, I perform proximal row carpectomy and posterior interosseous nerve neurectomy. If the lunate is not salvageable and the lunate fossa and capitate head cartilage are not preserved, I perform proximal row carpectomy and capsular interposition versus total wrist fusion, depending on a preoperative discussion with the patient regarding the possibility

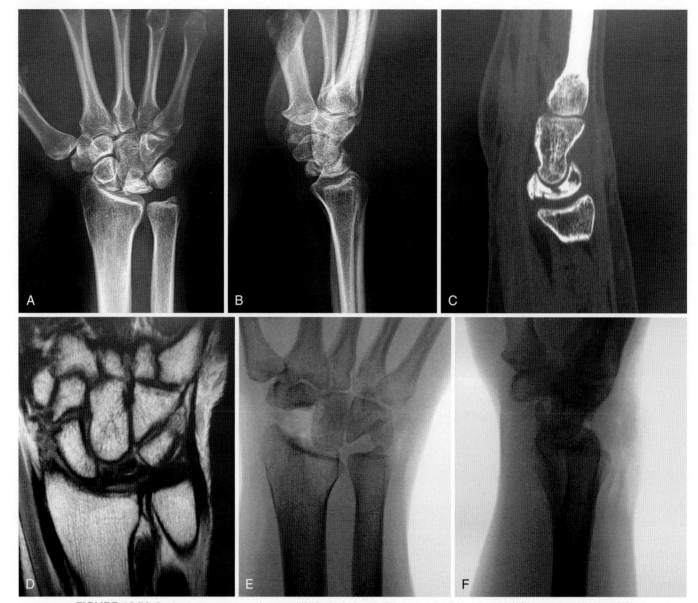

FIGURE 16.70 Proximal row carpectomy for stage IIIB Kienböck disease. Posteroanterior (PA) radiograph **(A)** and lateral radiograph **(B)** of the wrist. **C,** Computed tomography scan, sagittal view. **D,** Magnetic resonance image, coronal view. PA fluoroscopic image **(E)** and and lateral fluoroscopic image **(F)** of wrist following proximal row carpectomy. (Courtesy of Steve K. Lee, MD.)

that total wrist fusion may be needed later if proximal row carpectomy is first attempted.

Preiser Disease

In 1910, Preiser described a rarefying osteitis of the scaphoid that he distinguished from a scaphoid fracture. He compared the condition with Kienböck disease and thought that the causes were similar. However, recently Kallen and Strackee[114] have called into question Georg Preiser's original observations. They recovered the images of the five cases he described and showed that they all had fractures but did not have AVN. Kalainov and colleagues[113] described type 1, whole bone, and type 2, partial bone, patterns of Preiser disease. Type I has the propensity to fragmentation and collapse, no matter the treatment. Type 2 patterns usually maintain their architecture, with the same types of treatment. The cause has been related to

collagen vascular disease, steroid therapy, repetitive trauma, or idiopathic conditions. Clinical findings are related to local pain and tenderness. Radiographically, involved areas are typically sclerotic, and there is often fragmentation of the proximal articular surfaces. CT and MRI may be helpful to define the changes. This condition can present in children.

Treatment of Preiser disease has not been standardized. Nonoperative symptomatic management, joint débridement, silicone replacement arthroplasty, and electrical stimulation have all been tried, with mixed results. Reversed-flow vascularized bundle implantation has been performed in a limited number of cases with variable success. Vascularized bone grafting may also be considered, but results have been variable and revascularization has been incomplete.[152] Hayashi and associates reported on decreased but continued pain after closing wedge radial osteotomy.[89] The success of scaphoid-preserving procedures may be compromised by chronic degenerative changes that are often present in the carpus at the time of reconstruction, particularly at the radial styloid and radioscaphoid articulation; this makes pain-free motion following successful salvage difficult. Furthermore, there is often insufficient satisfactory cortical bone into which a graft can be inserted, as the surface is too fragmented. Therefore, if revascularization is to be considered, the patient should also consent to scaphoid excision and midcarpal arthrodesis or proximal row carpectomy should vascularized grafting prove technically impossible. If revascularization is attempted and proves unsuccessful, scaphoid excision combined with either midcarpal arthrodesis or proximal row carpectomy may be appropriate for persistently symptomatic cases. Given the lack of reliable treatment options, in the absence of severe pain and disability a conservative approach is probably warranted and should be discussed with the patient.

Avascular Necrosis of the Capitate

The capitate is at risk for AVN because the proximal pole is essentially an intraarticular structure. The retrograde intraosseous blood flow to the capitate is similar to that in the scaphoid, which makes the proximal pole of the capitate prone to AVN at its waist.[171] Dorsal and palmar vessels are present but vary considerably. Additional causes of AVN include vibration exposure, steroid use, repetitive wrist extension, and ligamentous laxity.[209]

Attempts to promote revascularization with bone grafting have had mixed results.[209] There are no long-term follow-up reports on AVN. AVN has been reported infrequently in isolated capitate fractures but is more common in higher-energy fractures, particularly when the capitate is rotated.

For Case Studies, Videos, and more, please visit ExpertConsult.com.

REFERENCES

1. Adams BD, Blair WF, Reagan DS, et al: Technical factors related to Herbert screw fixation. *J Hand Surg [Am]* 13(6):893–899, 1988.
2. Adler JB, Shaftan GW: Fractures of the capitate. *J Bone Joint Surg Am* 44:1537–1547, 1962.
3. Adolfsson L, Lindau T, Arner M: Acutrak screw fixation versus cast immobilisation for undisplaced scaphoid waist fractures. *J Hand Surg [Br]* 26(3):192–195, 2001.
4. Almquist EE: Capitate shortening in the treatment of Kienbock's disease. *Hand Clin* 9(3):505–512, 1993.
5. Almquist EE, Burns JF, Jr: Radial shortening for the treatment of Kienbock's disease: a 5- to 10-year follow-up. *J Hand Surg [Am]* 7(4):348–352, 1982.
6. Alshryda S, Shah A, Odak S, et al: Acute fractures of the scaphoid bone: systematic review and meta-analysis. *Surgeon* 10(4):218–229, 2012.
7. Amadio PC, Berquist TH, Smith DK, et al: Scaphoid malunion. *J Hand Surg [Am]* 14(4):679–687, 1989.
8. Anderson SE, Steinbach LS, Tschering-Vogel D, et al: MR imaging of avascular scaphoid nonunion before and after vascularized bone grafting. *Skeletal Radiol* 34(6):314–320, 2005.
9. Andresen R, Radmer S, Sparmann M, et al: Imaging of hamate bone fractures in conventional X-rays and high-resolution computed tomography: an in vitro study. *Invest Radiol* 34(1):46–50, 1999.
10. Anz AW, Bushnell BD, Bynum DK, et al: Pediatric scaphoid fractures. *J Am Acad Orthop Surg* 17(2):77–87, 2009.
11. Arora R, Gschwentner M, Krappinger D, et al: Fixation of nondisplaced scaphoid fractures: making treatment cost-effective: prospective controlled trial. *Arch Orthop Trauma Surg* 127(1):39–46, 2007.
12. Arora R, Lutz M, Zimmermann R, et al: Free vascularised iliac bone graft for recalcitrant avascular nonunion of the scaphoid. *J Bone Joint Surg Br* 92(2):224–229, 2010.
13. Assari S, Darvish K, Ilyas AM: Biomechanical analysis of second-generation headless compression screws. *Injury* 43(7):1159–1165, 2012.
14. Bailey CA, Kuiper JH, Kelly CP: Biomechanical evaluation of a new composite bioresorbable screw. *J Hand Surg [Br]* 31(2):208–212, 2006.
15. Barton NJ: Experience with scaphoid grafting. *J Hand Surg [Br]* 22(2):153–160, 1997.
16. Beeres FJ, Hogervorst M, Rhemrev SJ, et al: A prospective comparison for suspected scaphoid fractures: bone scintigraphy versus clinical outcome. *Injury* 38(7):769–774, 2007.
17. Berger RA: The anatomy of the scaphoid. *Hand Clin* 17(4):525–532, 2001.
18. Berger RA: A method of defining palpable landmarks for the ligament-splitting dorsal wrist capsulotomy. *J Hand Surg [Am]* 32(8):1291–1295, 2007.
19. Berger RA, Bishop AT, Bettinger PC: New dorsal capsulotomy for the surgical exposure of the wrist. *Ann Plast Surg* 35(1):54–59, 1995.
20. Bertelli JA, Peruchi FM, Rost JR, et al: Treatment of scaphoid non-unions by a palmar approach with vascularised bone graft harvested from the thumb. *J Hand Surg Eur Vol* 32(2):217–223, 2007.
21. Bilic R, Simic P, Jelic M, et al: Osteogenic protein-1 (BMP-7) accelerates healing of scaphoid non-union with proximal pole sclerosis. *Int Orthop* 30(2):128–134, 2006.
22. Bochud RC, Buchler U: Kienbock's disease, early stage 3: height reconstruction and core revascularization of the lunate. *J Hand Surg [Br]* 19(4):466–478, 1994.
23. Bond CD, Shin AY, McBride MT, et al: Percutaneous screw fixation or cast immobilization for nondisplaced scaphoid fractures. *J Bone Joint Surg Am* 83(4):483–488, 2001.
24. Botte MJ, Gelberman RH: Fractures of the carpus, excluding the scaphoid. *Hand Clin* 3(1):149–161, 1987.
25. Boyer MI, von Schroeder HP, Axelrod TS: Scaphoid nonunion with avascular necrosis of the proximal pole: treatment with a vascularized bone graft from the dorsum of the distal radius. *J Hand Surg [Br]* 23(5):686–690, 1998.
26. Braithwaite IJ, Jones WA: Scapho-lunate dissociation occurring with scaphoid fracture. *J Hand Surg [Br]* 17(3):286–288, 1992.
27. Braun C, Gross G, Buhren V: Osteosynthesis using a buttress plate: a new principle for stabilizing scaphoid pseudarthroses. *Unfallchirurg* 96(1):9–11, 1993.
28. Briseno MR, Yao J: Lunate fractures in the face of a perilunate injury: an uncommon and easily missed injury pattern. *J Hand Surg [Am]* 37(1):63–67, 2012.
29. Buchler U, Nagy L: The issue of vascularity in fractures and non-union of the scaphoid. *J Hand Surg [Br]* 20(6):726–735, 1995.
30. Bushnell BD, McWilliams AD, Messer TM: Complications in dorsal percutaneous cannulated screw fixation of nondisplaced scaphoid waist fractures. *J Hand Surg [Am]* 32(6):827–833, 2007.
31. Carroll RE, Coyle MP, Jr: Dysfunction of the pisotriquetral joint: treatment by excision of the pisiform. *J Hand Surg [Am]* 10(5):703–707, 1985.
32. Carroll RE, Lakin JF: Fracture of the hook of the hamate: acute treatment. *J Trauma* 34(6):803–805, 1993.
33. Cerezal L, Abascal F, Canga A, et al: Usefulness of gadolinium-enhanced MR imaging in the evaluation of the vascularity of scaphoid nonunions. *AJR Am J Roentgenol* 174(1):141–149, 2000.
34. Chang MA, Bishop AT, Moran SL, et al: The outcomes and complications of 1,2-intercompartmental supraretinacular artery pedicled vascularized bone grafting of scaphoid nonunions. *J Hand Surg [Am]* 31(3):387–396, 2006.
35. Christodoulou LS, Kitsis CK, Chamberlain ST: Internal fixation of scaphoid nonunion: a comparative study of three methods. *Injury* 32(8):625–630, 2001.
36. Chu PJ, Shih JT: Arthroscopically assisted use of injectable bone graft substitutes for management of scaphoid nonunions. *Arthroscopy* 27(1):31–37, 2011.
37. Cohen MS, Jupiter JB, Fallahi K, et al: Scaphoid waist nonunion with humpback deformity treated without structural bone graft. *J Hand Surg [Am]* 38(4):701–705, 2013.
38. Condit DP, Idler RS, Fischer TJ, et al: Preoperative factors and outcome after lunate decompression for Kienbock's disease. *J Hand Surg [Am]* 18(4):691–696, 1993.
39. Cooney WP, Dobyns JH, Linscheid RL: Fractures of the scaphoid: a rational approach to management. *Clin Orthop Relat Res* 149:90–97, 1980.
40. Cooney WP, 3rd, Dobyns JH, Linscheid RL: Nonunion of the scaphoid: analysis of the results from bone grafting. *J Hand Surg [Am]* 5(4):343–354, 1980.
41. Croog AS, Stern PJ: Proximal row carpectomy for advanced Kienbock's disease: average 10-year follow-up. *J Hand Surg [Am]* 33(7):1122–1130, 2008.
42. Dailiana ZH, Malizos KN, Zachos V, et al: Vascularized bone grafts from the palmar radius for the treatment of waist nonunions of the scaphoid. *J Hand Surg [Am]* 31(3):397–404, 2006.
43. Davis EN, Chung KC, Kotsis SV, et al: A cost/utility analysis of open reduction and internal fixation versus cast immobilization for acute nondisplaced mid-waist scaphoid fractures. *Plast Reconstr Surg* 117(4):1223–1235, discussion 1236–1238, 2006.

44. Dawson JS, Martel AL, Davis TR: Scaphoid blood flow and acute fracture healing. A dynamic MRI study with enhancement with gadolinium. *J Bone Joint Surg Br* 83(6):809–814, 2001.

45. De Smet L, Robijns P, Degreef I: Proximal row carpectomy in advanced Kienbock's disease. *J Hand Surg [Br]* 30(6):585–587, 2005.

46. Desai VV, Davis TR, Barton NJ: The prognostic value and reproducibility of the radiological features of the fractured scaphoid. *J Hand Surg [Br]* 24(5):586–590, 1999.

47. Devers BN, Douglas KC, Naik RD, et al: Outcomes of hook of hamate fracture excision in high-level amateur athletes. *J Hand Surg [Am]* 38(1):72–76, 2013.

48. D'Hoore K, De Smet L, Verellen K, et al: Negative ulnar variance is not a risk factor for Kienbock's disease. *J Hand Surg [Am]* 19(2):229–231, 1994.

49. Dias JJ, Taylor M, Thompson J, et al: Radiographic signs of union of scaphoid fractures: an analysis of inter-observer agreement and reproducibility. *J Bone Joint Surg Br* 70(2):299–301, 1988.

50. Dias JJ, Wildin CJ, Bhowal B, et al: Should acute scaphoid fractures be fixed? A randomized controlled trial. *J Bone Joint Surg Am* 87(10):2160–2168, 2005.

51. Dodds SD, Panjabi MM, Slade JF, 3rd: Screw fixation of scaphoid fractures: a biomechanical assessment of screw length and screw augmentation. *J Hand Surg [Am]* 31(3):405–413, 2006.

52. Dodds SD, Patterson JT, Halim A: Volar plate fixation of recalcitrant scaphoid nonunions with volar carpal artery vascularized bone graft. *Tech Hand Up Extrem Surg* 18(1):2–7, 2014.

53. Doi K, Oda T, Soo-Heong T, et al: Free vascularized bone graft for nonunion of the scaphoid. *J Hand Surg [Am]* 25(3):507–519, 2000.

54. Donati OF, Zanetti M, Nagy L, et al: Is dynamic gadolinium enhancement needed in MR imaging for the preoperative assessment of scaphoidal viability in patients with scaphoid nonunion? *Radiology* 260(3):808–816, 2011.

55. Duppe H, Johnell O, Lundborg G, et al: Long-term results of fracture of the scaphoid. A follow-up study of more than thirty years. *J Bone Joint Surg Am* 76(2):249–252, 1994.

56. Eggli S, Fernandez DL, Beck T: Unstable scaphoid fracture nonunion: a medium-term study of anterior wedge grafting procedures. *J Hand Surg [Br]* 27(1):36–41, 2002.

57. Failla JM: Hook of hamate vascularity: vulnerability to osteonecrosis and nonunion. *J Hand Surg [Am]* 18(6):1075–1079, 1993.

58. Faucher GK, Golden ML, 3rd, Sweeney KR, et al: Comparison of screw trajectory on stability of oblique scaphoid fractures: a mechanical study. *J Hand Surg [Am]* 39(3):430–435, 2014.

59. Fenton RL: The naviculo-capitate fracture syndrome. *J Bone Joint Surg Am* 38(3):681–684, 1956.

60. Fernandez DL: A technique for anterior wedge-shaped grafts for scaphoid nonunions with carpal instability. *J Hand Surg [Am]* 9(5):733–737, 1984.

61. Fernandez DL: Anterior bone grafting and conventional lag screw fixation to treat scaphoid nonunions. *J Hand Surg [Am]* 15(1):140–147, 1990.

62. Fernandez DL, Eggli S: Non-union of the scaphoid: revascularization of the proximal pole with implantation of a vascular bundle and bone-grafting. *J Bone Joint Surg Am* 77(6):883–893, 1995.

63. Filan SL, Herbert TJ: Herbert screw fixation of scaphoid fractures. *J Bone Joint Surg Br* 78(4):519–529, 1996.

64. Forward DP, Singh HP, Dawson S, et al: The clinical outcome of scaphoid fracture malunion at 1 year. *J Hand Surg Eur Vol* 34(1):40–46, 2009.

65. Gabl M, Reinhart C, Lutz M, et al: Vascularized bone graft from the iliac crest for the treatment of nonunion of the proximal part of the scaphoid with an avascular fragment. *J Bone Joint Surg Am* 81(10):1414–1428, 1999.

66. Garcia-Elias M: Dorsal fractures of the triquetrum: avulsion or compression fractures? *J Hand Surg [Am]* 12(2):266–268, 1987.

67. Garcia-Elias M: Carpal bone fractures (excluding scaphoid fractures). In Watson H, Weinberg J, editors: *The wrist*, Philadelphia, 2001, Lippincott Williams & Wilkins, pp 174–181.

68. Geissler W, Slade JF: Fractures of the carpal bones. In Wolfe SW, Hotchkiss RN, Pederson WC, et al, editors: *Green's operative hand surgery*, ed 6, Philadelphia, 2011, Elsevier/Churchill Livingstone.

69. Geissler WB: Carpal fractures in athletes. *Clin Sports Med* 20(1):167–188, 2001.

70. Geissler WB: Arthroscopic management of scaphoid fractures in athletes. *Hand Clin* 25(3):359–369, 2009.

71. Geissler WB, Hammit MD: Arthroscopic aided fixation of scaphoid fractures. *Hand Clin* 17(4):575–588, viii, 2001.

72. Gelberman RH, Bauman TD, Menon J, et al: The vascularity of the lunate bone and Kienbock's disease. *J Hand Surg [Am]* 5(3):272–278, 1980.

73. Gelberman RH, Menon J: The vascularity of the scaphoid bone. *J Hand Surg [Am]* 5(5):508–513, 1980.

74. Gelberman RH, Panagis JS, Taleisnik J, et al: The arterial anatomy of the human carpus. Part I: The extraosseous vascularity. *J Hand Surg [Am]* 8(4):367–375, 1983.

75. Gellman H, Caputo RJ, Carter V, et al: Comparison of short and long thumb-spica casts for non-displaced fractures of the carpal scaphoid. *J Bone Joint Surg Am* 71(3):354–357, 1989.

76. Geurts GF, Van Riet RP, Meermans G, et al: Volar percutaneous transtrapezial fixation of scaphoid waist fractures: surgical technique. *Acta Orthop Belg* 78(1):121–125, 2012.

77. Ghoneim A: The unstable nonunited scaphoid waist fracture: results of treatment by open reduction, anterior wedge grafting, and internal fixation by volar buttress plate. *J Hand Surg [Am]* 36(1):17–24, 2011.

78. Goldfarb CA, Hsu J, Gelberman RH, et al: The Lichtman classification for Kienbock's disease: an assessment of reliability. *J Hand Surg [Am]* 28(1):74–80, 2003.

79. Gras M, Mathoulin C: Vascularized bone graft pedicled on the volar carpal artery from the volar distal radius as primary procedure for scaphoid non-union. *Orthop Traumatol Surg Res* 97(8):800–806, 2011.

80. Green DP: The effect of avascular necrosis on Russe bone grafting for scaphoid nonunion. *J Hand Surg [Am]* 10(5):597–605, 1985.

81. Grewal R, Assini J, Sauder D, et al: A comparison of two headless compression screws for operative treatment of scaphoid fractures. *J Orthop Surg Res* 6:27, 2011.

82. Grover R: Clinical assessment of scaphoid injuries and the detection of fractures. *J Hand Surg [Br]* 21(3):341–343, 1996.

83. Gruszka DS, Burkhart KJ, Nowak TE, et al: The durability of the intrascaphoid compression of headless compression screws: in vitro study. *J Hand Surg [Am]* 37(6):1142–1150, 2012.

84. Gunal I, Ozcelik A, Gokturk E, et al: Correlation of magnetic resonance imaging and intraoperative punctate bleeding to assess the vascularity of scaphoid non-union. *Arch Orthop Trauma Surg* 119(5–6):285–287, 1999.

85. Haddad FS, Goddard NJ: Acute percutaneous scaphoid fixation. A pilot study. *J Bone Joint Surg Br* 80(1):95–99, 1998.

86. Handley RC, Pooley J: The venous anatomy of the scaphoid. *J Anat* 178:115–118, 1991.

87. Hanel DP, Hunt TR: Capitate shortening osteotomy: Kienbock's disease. *Atlas Hand Clin* 4:45–58, 1999.

88. Hart A, Harvey EJ, Lefebvre LP, et al: Insertion profiles of 4 headless compression screws. *J Hand Surg [Am]* 38(9):1728–1734, 2013.

89. Hayashi O, Sawaizumi T, Ito H: Closed radial wedge osteotomy for Preiser's disease: a report of four cases. *Hand Surg* 16(3):347–352, 2011.

90. Henry M: Collapsed scaphoid non-union with dorsal intercalated segment instability and avascular necrosis treated by vascularised wedge-shaped bone graft and fixation. *J Hand Surg Eur Vol* 32(2):148–154, 2007.

91. Herbert TJ, Fisher WE: Management of the fractured scaphoid using a new bone screw. *J Bone Joint Surg Br* 66(1):114–123, 1984.

92. Herzberg G, Forissier D: Acute dorsal trans-scaphoid perilunate fracture-dislocations: medium-term results. *J Hand Surg [Br]* 27(6):498–502, 2002.

93. Higgins JP, Burger HK: Proximal scaphoid arthroplasty using the medial femoral trochlea flap. *J Wrist Surg* 2(3):228–233, 2013.

94. Hirche C, Heffinger C, Xiong L, et al: The 1,2-intercompartmental supraretinacular artery vascularized bone graft for scaphoid nonunion: management and clinical outcome. *J Hand Surg [Am]* 39(3):423–429, 2014.

95. Hocker K, Menschik A: Chip fractures of the triquetrum: mechanism, classification and results. *J Hand Surg [Br]* 19(5):584–588, 1994.

96. Hoffmann M, Reinsch OD, Petersen JP, et al: Percutaneous antegrade scaphoid screw placement: a feasibility and accuracy analysis of a novel electromagnetic navigation technique versus a standard fluoroscopic method. *Int J Med Robot* 11(1):52–57, 2015.

97. Hori Y, Tamai S, Okuda H, et al: Blood vessel transplantation to bone. *J Hand Surg [Am]* 4(1):23–33, 1979.

98. Horii E, Garcia-Elias M, Bishop AT, et al: Effect on force transmission across the carpus in procedures used to treat Kienbock's disease. *J Hand Surg [Am]* 15(3):393–400, 1990.

99. Horii E, Nakamura R, Watanabe K, et al: Scaphoid fracture as a "puncher's fracture." *J Orthop Trauma* 8(2):107–110, 1994.

100. Howe LM: Epidemiology of scaphoid fractures in Bergen, Norway. *Scand J Plast Reconstr Surg Hand Surg* 33:423–426, 1999.

101. Huene DR, Huene DS: Treatment of nonunions of the scaphoid with the Ender compression blade plate system. *J Hand Surg [Am]* 16(5):913–922, 1991.

102. Illarramendi AA, Schulz C, De Carli P: The surgical treatment of Kienbock's disease by radius and ulna metaphyseal core decompression. *J Hand Surg [Am]* 26(2):252–260, 2001.

103. Imbriglia JE, Broudy AS, Hagberg WC, et al: Proximal row carpectomy: clinical evaluation. *J Hand Surg [Am]* 15(3):426–430, 1990.

104. Inoue G, Shionoya K: Herbert screw fixation by limited access for acute fractures of the scaphoid. *J Bone Joint Surg Br* 79(3):418–421, 1997.

105. Inoue G, Shionoya K, Kuwahata Y: Ununited proximal pole scaphoid fractures: treatment with a Herbert screw in 16 cases followed for 0.5-8 years. *Acta Orthop Scand* 68(2):124–127, 1997.

106. Jafarnia K, Collins ED, Kohl HW, 3rd, et al: Reliability of the Lichtman classification of Kienbock's disease. *J Hand Surg [Am]* 25(3):529–534, 2000.

107. Jensen CH, Thomsen K, Holst-Nielsen F: Radiographic staging of Kienbock's disease: poor reproducibility of Stahl's and Lichtman's staging systems. *Acta Orthop Scand* 67(3):274–276, 1996.

108. Jeon IH, Micic ID, Oh CW, et al: Percutaneous screw fixation for scaphoid fracture: a comparison between the dorsal and the volar approaches. *J Hand Surg [Am]* 34(2):228–236, e1, 2009.

109. Jiranek WA, Ruby LK, Millender LB, et al: Long-term results after Russe bone-grafting: the effect of malunion of the scaphoid. *J Bone Joint Surg Am* 74(8):1217–1228, 1992.

110. Jones DB, Jr, Burger H, Bishop AT, et al: Treatment of scaphoid waist nonunions with an avascular proximal pole and carpal collapse. A comparison of two vascularized bone grafts. *J Bone Joint Surg Am* 90(12):2616–2625, 2008.

111. Jones NF, Brown EE, Mostofi A, et al: Healing of a scaphoid nonunion using human bone morphogenetic protein. *J Hand Surg [Am]* 30(3):528–533, 2005.

112. Kakar S, Bishop AT, Shin AY: Role of vascularized bone grafts in the treatment of scaphoid nonunions associated with proximal pole avascular necrosis and carpal collapse. *J Hand Surg [Am]* 36(4):722–725, quiz 725, 2011.

113. Kalainov DM, Cohen MS, Hendrix RW, et al: Preiser's disease: identification of two patterns. *J Hand Surg [Am]* 28(5):767–778, 2003.

114. Kallen AM, Strackee SD: On the history and definition of Preiser's disease. *J Hand Surg Eur Vol* 39(7):770–776, 2014.

115. Kam CC, Greenberg JA: Computer-assisted navigation for dorsal percutaneous scaphoid screw placement: a cadaveric study. *J Hand Surg [Am]* 39(4):613–620, 2014.

116. Kaneshiro SA, Failla JM, Tashman S: Scaphoid fracture displacement with forearm rotation in a short-arm thumb spica cast. *J Hand Surg [Am]* 24(5):984–991, 1999.

117. Kardashian G, Christoforou DC, Lee SK: Perilunate dislocations. *Bull NYU Hosp Jt Dis* 69(1):87–96, 2011.

118. Keith PP, Nuttall D, Trail I: Long-term outcome of nonsurgically managed Kienbock's disease. *J Hand Surg [Am]* 29(1):63–67, 2004.

119. Kim RY, Lijten EC, Strauch RJ: Pronated oblique view in assessing proximal scaphoid articular cannulated screw penetration. *J Hand Surg [Am]* 33(8):1274–1277, 2008.

120. Korkala OL, Kuokkanen HO, Eerola MS: Compression-staple fixation for fractures, non-unions, and delayed unions of the carpal scaphoid. *J Bone Joint Surg Am* 74(3):423–426, 1992.

121. Kosy JD, Standley DM: Retrieval of broken Acutrak drill bit. *J Hand Surg Eur Vol* 35(8):683, 2010.

122. Kozin SH: Incidence, mechanism, and natural history of scaphoid fractures. *Hand Clin* 17(4):515–524, 2001.

123. Kristensen SS, Thomassen E, Christensen F: Ulnar variance in Kienbock's disease. *J Hand Surg [Br]* 11(2):258–260, 1986.

124. Kuhlmann JN, Mimoun M, Boabighi A, et al: Vascularized bone graft pedicled on the volar carpal artery for non-union of the scaphoid. *J Hand Surg [Br]* 12(2):203–210, 1987.

125. Langhoff O, Andersen JL: Consequences of late immobilization of scaphoid fractures. *J Hand Surg [Br]* 13(1):77–79, 1988.

126. Larsen CF, Brondum V, Skov O: Epidemiology of scaphoid fractures in Odense, Denmark. *Acta Orthop Scand* 63(2):216–218, 1992.

127. Lawand A, Foulkes GD: The "clenched pencil" view: a modified clenched fist scapholunate stress view. *J Hand Surg [Am]* 28(3):414–418, discussion 419–420, 2003.

128. Lee SK, Desai H, Silver B, et al: Comparison of radiographic stress views for scapholunate dynamic instability in a cadaver model. *J Hand Surg [Am]* 36(7):1149–1157, 2011.

129. Leventhal EL, Wolfe SW, Walsh EF, et al: A computational approach to the "optimal" screw axis location and orientation in the scaphoid bone. *J Hand Surg [Am]* 34(4):677–684, 2009.

130. Levy M, Fischel RE, Stern GM, et al: Chip fractures of the os triquetrum: the mechanism of injury. *J Bone Joint Surg Br* 61(3):355–357, 1979.

131. Lichtman DM, Mack GR, MacDonald RI, et al: Kienbock's disease: the role of silicone replacement arthroplasty. *J Bone Joint Surg Am* 59(7):899–908, 1977.

132. Lynch NM, Linscheid RL: Corrective osteotomy for scaphoid malunion: technique and long-term follow-up evaluation. *J Hand Surg [Am]* 22(1):35–43, 1997.

133. Mack GR, Bosse MJ, Gelberman RH, et al: The natural history of scaphoid non-union. *J Bone Joint Surg Am* 66(4):504–509, 1984.

134. Mack GR, Wilckens JH, McPherson SA: Subacute scaphoid fractures. A closer look at closed treatment. *Am J Sports Med* 26(1):56–58, 1998.

135. Malerich MM, Clifford J, Eaton B, et al: Distal scaphoid resection arthroplasty for the treatment of degenerative arthritis secondary to scaphoid nonunion. *J Hand Surg [Am]* 24(6):1196–1205, 1999.

136. Masquijo JJ, Willis BR: Scaphoid nonunions in children and adolescents: surgical treatment with bone grafting and internal fixation. *J Pediatr Orthop* 30(2):119–124, 2010.

137. Mathoulin C, Brunelli F: Further experience with the index metacarpal vascularized bone graft. *J Hand Surg [Br]* 23(3):311–317, 1998.

138. Mayfield JK, Johnson RP, Kilcoyne RK: Carpal dislocations: pathomechanics and progressive perilunar instability. *J Hand Surg [Am]* 5(3):226–241, 1980.

139. Mayr E, Rudzki MM, Rudzki M, et al: Does low intensity, pulsed ultrasound speed healing of scaphoid fractures? *Handchir Mikrochir Plast Chir* 32(2):115–122, 2000.

140. McAdams TR, Spisak S, Beaulieu CF, et al: The effect of pronation and supination on the minimally displaced scaphoid fracture. *Clin Orthop Relat Res* 411:255–259, 2003.

141. McCallister WV, Knight J, Kaliappan R, et al: Central placement of the screw in simulated fractures of the scaphoid waist: a biomechanical study. *J Bone Joint Surg Am* 85(1):72–77, 2003.

142. McCarty V, Farber H: Isolated fracture of the pisiform bone. *J Bone Joint Surg Am* 28:390, 1946.

143. McLaughlin HL: Fracture of the carpal navicular (scaphoid) bone: some observations based on treatment by open reduction and internal fixation. *J Bone Joint Surg Am* 36(4):765–774, 1954.

144. Meermans G, Verstreken F: Percutaneous transtrapezial fixation of acute scaphoid fractures. *J Hand Surg Eur Vol* 33(6):791–796, 2008.

145. Merrell GA, Wolfe SW, Slade JF, 3rd: Treatment of scaphoid nonunions: quantitative meta-analysis of the literature. *J Hand Surg [Am]* 27(4):685–691, 2002.

146. Meyer C, Chang J, Stern P, et al: Complications of distal radial and scaphoid fracture treatment. *J Bone Joint Surg Am* 95(16):1517–1526, 2013.

147. Milch H: Fracture of the hamate bone. *J Bone Joint Surg Am* 16:459–462, 1934.

148. Mintzer CM, Waters PM: Surgical treatment of pediatric scaphoid fracture nonunions. *J Pediatr Orthop* 19(2):236–239, 1999.

149. Moon ES, Dy CJ, Derman P, et al: Management of nonunion following surgical management of scaphoid fractures: current concepts. *J Am Acad Orthop Surg* 21(9):548–557, 2013.

150. Deleted in review.

151. Moran SL, Cooney WP, Berger RA, et al: The use of the 4 + 5 extensor compartmental vascularized bone graft for the treatment of Kienbock's disease. *J Hand Surg [Am]* 30(1):50–58, 2005.

152. Moran SL, Cooney WP, Shin AY: The use of vascularized grafts from the distal radius for the treatment of Preiser's disease. *J Hand Surg [Am]* 31(5):705–710, 2006.

153. Muller GM, Mansson S, Muller MF, et al: Assessment of perfusion in normal carpal bones with dynamic gadolinium-enhanced MRI at 3 tesla. *J Magn Reson Imaging* 38(1):168–172, 2013.

154. Nakamura P, Imaeda T, Miura T: Scaphoid malunion. *J Bone Joint Surg Br* 73(1):134–137, 1991.

155. Nakamura R, Horii E, Watanabe K, et al: Proximal row carpectomy versus limited wrist arthrodesis for advanced Kienbock's disease. *J Hand Surg [Br]* 23(6):741–745, 1998.

156. Oron A, Gupta A, Thirkannad S: Nonunion of the scaphoid distal pole. *Hand Surg* 18(1):35–39, 2013.

157. Palmer AK: Trapezial ridge fractures. *J Hand Surg [Am]* 6(6):561–564, 1981.

158. Parvizi J, Wayman J, Kelly P, et al: Combining the clinical signs improves diagnosis of scaphoid fractures. A prospective study with follow-up. *J Hand Surg [Br]* 23(3):324–327, 1998.

159. Pensy RA, Richards AM, Belkoff SM, et al: Biomechanical comparison of two headless compression screws for scaphoid fixation. *J Surg Orthop Adv* 18(4):182–188, 2009.

160. Peste JL: Discussion. *Bull Soc Anat* 18:169, 1843.

161. Pointu J, Schwenck JP, Destree G, et al: Fractures of the trapezium: Mechanisms: anatomo-pathology and therapeutic indications. *Rev Chir Orthop Reparatrice Appar Mot* 74(5):454–465, 1988.

162. Porter ML, Seehra K: Fracture-dislocation of the triquetrum treated with a Herbert screw. *J Bone Joint Surg Br* 73(2):347–348, 1991.

163. Prosser AJ, Brenkel IJ, Irvine GB: Articular fractures of the distal scaphoid. *J Hand Surg [Br]* 13(1):87–91, 1988.

164. Raby N: Magnetic resonance imaging of suspected scaphoid fractures using a low field dedicated extremity MR system. *Clin Radiol* 56(4):316–320, 2001.

165. Reigstad O, Grimsgaard C, Thorkildsen R, et al: Long-term results of scaphoid nonunion surgery: 50 patients reviewed after 8 to 18 years. *J Orthop Trauma* 26(4):241–245, 2012.

166. Rettig AC, Weidenbener EJ: Gloyeske R. Alternative management of midthird scaphoid fractures in the athlete. *Am J Sports Med* 22(5):711–714, 1994.

167. Rettig ME, Raskin KB: Retrograde compression screw fixation of acute proximal pole scaphoid fractures. *J Hand Surg [Am]* 24(6):1206–1210, 1999.

168. Robbins RR, Ridge O, Carter PR: Iliac crest bone grafting and Herbert screw fixation of nonunions of the scaphoid with avascular proximal poles. *J Hand Surg [Am]* 20(5):818–831, 1995.

169. Rock MG, Roth JH, Martin L: Radial shortening osteotomy for treatment of Kienbock's disease. *J Hand Surg [Am]* 16(3):454–460, 1991.

170. Roman J, Lockyer P, Paksima N, et al: *The modified Russe procedure for scaphoid waist fracture non-union with deformity.* Feb 7, 2012, AAOS.

171. Ruch DS, Papadonikolakis A: Resection of the scaphoid distal pole for symptomatic scaphoid nonunion after failed previous surgical treatment. *J Hand Surg [Am]* 31(4):588–593, 2006.

172. Russe O: Fracture of the carpal navicular: diagnosis, non-operative treatment, and operative treatment. *J Bone Joint Surg Am* 42:759–768, 1960.

173. Sakai K, Doi K, Kawai S: Free vascularized thin corticoperiosteal graft. *Plast Reconstr Surg* 87(2):290–298, 1991.

174. Sandow MJ: Costo-osteochondral grafts in the wrist. *Tech Hand Up Extrem Surg* 5(3):165–172, 2001.

175. Schiltenwolf M, Martini AK, Mau HC, et al: Further investigations of the intraosseous pressure characteristics in necrotic lunates (Kienbock's disease). *J Hand Surg [Am]* 21(5):754–758, 1996.

176. Schmitt R, Christopoulos G, Wagner M, et al: Avascular necrosis (AVN) of the proximal fragment in scaphoid nonunion: is intravenous contrast agent necessary in MRI? *Eur J Radiol* 77(2):222–227, 2011.

177. Schuind F, Haentjens P, Van Innis F, et al: Prognostic factors in the treatment of carpal scaphoid nonunions. *J Hand Surg [Am]* 24(4):761–776, 1999.

178. Shah J, Jones WA: Factors affecting the outcome in 50 cases of scaphoid nonunion treated with Herbert screw fixation. *J Hand Surg [Br]* 23(5):680–685, 1998.

179. Sheetz KK, Bishop AT, Berger RA: The arterial blood supply of the distal radius and ulna and its potential use in vascularized pedicled bone grafts. *J Hand Surg [Am]* 20(6):902–914, 1995.

180. Shi ZM, Xu ZG: Experimental study and clinical use of the fasciosteal flap. *Plast Reconstr Surg* 78(2):201–210, 1986.

181. Siegel DB, Gelberman RH: Radial styloidectomy: an anatomic study with special reference to radiocarpal intracapsular ligamentous morphology. *J Hand Surg [Am]* 16(1):40–44, 1991.

182. Slade JF, 3rd, Geissler WB, Gutow AP, et al: Percutaneous internal fixation of selected scaphoid nonunions with an arthroscopically assisted dorsal approach. *J Bone Joint Surg Am* 85(Suppl 4):20–32, 2003.

183. Slade JF, 3rd, Gillon T: Retrospective review of 234 scaphoid fractures and nonunions treated with arthroscopy for union and complications. *Scand J Surg* 97(4):280–289, 2008.

184. Slade JF, 3rd, Grauer JN, Mahoney JD: Arthroscopic reduction and percutaneous fixation of scaphoid fractures with a novel dorsal technique. *Orthop Clin North Am* 32(2):247–261, 2001.

185. Smith DK, Murray PM: Avulsion fractures of the volar aspect of triquetral bone of the wrist: a subtle sign of carpal ligament injury. *AJR Am J Roentgenol* 166(3):609–614, 1996.

186. Smith ML, Bain GI, Chabrel N, et al: Using computed tomography to assist with diagnosis of avascular necrosis complicating chronic scaphoid nonunion. *J Hand Surg [Am]* 34(6):1037–1043, 2009.

187. Smith P, 3rd, Wright TW, Wallace PF, et al: Excision of the hook of the hamate: a retrospective survey and review of the literature. *J Hand Surg [Am]* 13(4):612–615, 1988.

188. Sotereanos DG, Darlis NA, Dailiana ZH, et al: A capsular-based vascularized distal radius graft for proximal pole scaphoid pseudarthrosis. *J Hand Surg [Am]* 31(4):580–587, 2006.

189. Sotereanos DG, Mitsionis GJ, Giannakopoulos PN, et al: Perilunate dislocation and fracture dislocation: a critical analysis of the volar-dorsal approach. *J Hand Surg [Am]* 22(1):49–56, 1997.

190. Stahl F: On lunatomalacia (Kienbock's disease): a clinical and roentgenological study, especially on its pathogenesis and the late results of immobilization treatment. *Acta Chir Scand* 126(Suppl):1–133, 1947.

191. Stark HH, Chao EK, Zemel NP, et al: Fracture of the hook of the hamate. *J Bone Joint Surg Am* 71(8):1202–1207, 1989.

192. Stark HH, Rickard TA, Zemel NP, et al: Treatment of ununited fractures of the scaphoid by iliac bone grafts and Kirschner-wire fixation. *J Bone Joint Surg Am* 70(7):982–991, 1988.

193. Stein F, Siegel MW: Naviculocapitate fracture syndrome: a case report: new thoughts on the mechanism of injury. *J Bone Joint Surg Am* 51(2):391–395, 1969.

194. Steinmann SP, Adams JE: Scaphoid fractures and nonunions: diagnosis and treatment. *J Orthop Sci* 11(4):424–431, 2006.

195. Steinmann SP, Bishop AT, Berger RA: Use of the 1,2 intercompartmental supraretinacular artery as a vascularized pedicle bone graft for difficult scaphoid nonunion. *J Hand Surg [Am]* 27(3):391–401, 2002.

196. Straw RG, Davis TR, Dias JJ: Scaphoid nonunion: treatment with a pedicled vascularized bone graft based on the 1,2 intercompartmental supraretinacular branch of the radial artery. *J Hand Surg [Br]* 27(5):413, 2002.

197. Sunagawa T, Bishop AT, Muramatsu K: Role of conventional and vascularized bone grafts in scaphoid nonunion with avascular necrosis: a canine experimental study. *J Hand Surg [Am]* 25(5):849–859, 2000.

198. Symes TH, Stothard J: A systematic review of the treatment of acute fractures of the scaphoid. *J Hand Surg Eur Vol* 36(9):802–810, 2011.

199. Szabo RM, Manske D: Displaced fractures of the scaphoid. *Clin Orthop Relat Res* 230:30–38, 1988.

200. Tajima T: An investigation of the treatment of Kienbock's disease (abstract). *J Bone Joint Surg Am* 48:1649, 1966.

201. Taniguchi Y, Tamaki T, Nakatan N: Long-term results of non-surgical treatment in Kienbock's disease. *J Jpn Soc Surg Hand* (9):962–968, 1993.

202. Teisen H, Hjarbaek J: Classification of fresh fractures of the lunate. *J Hand Surg [Br]* 13(4):458–462, 1988.

203. Trumble T, Glisson RR, Seaber AV, et al: A biomechanical comparison of the methods for treating Kienbock's disease. *J Hand Surg [Am]* 11(1):88–93, 1986.

204. Trumble TE, Benirschke SK, Vedder NB: Ipsilateral fractures of the scaphoid and radius. *J Hand Surg [Am]* 18(1):8–14, 1993.

205. Trumble TE, Clarke T, Kreder HJ: Non-union of the scaphoid: treatment with cannulated screws compared with treatment with Herbert screws. *J Bone Joint Surg Am* 78(12):1829–1837, 1996.

206. Tsuge S, Nakamura R: Anatomical risk factors for Kienbock's disease. *J Hand Surg [Br]* 18(1):70–75, 1993.

207. Tumilty JA, Squire DS: Unrecognized chondral penetration by a Herbert screw in the scaphoid. *J Hand Surg [Am]* 21(1):66–68, 1996.

208. Urist MR, Strates BS: Bone formation in implants of partially and wholly demineralized bone matrix. including observations on acetone-fixed intra and extracellular proteins. *Clin Orthop Relat Res* 71:271–278, 1970.

209. Vander Grend R, Dell PC, Glowczewskie F, et al: Intraosseous blood supply of the capitate and its correlation with aseptic necrosis. *J Hand Surg [Am]* 9(5):677–683, 1984.

209a. Van Tassel DC, Owens BD, Wolf JM: Incidence estimates and demographics of scaphoid fracture in the U.S. population. *J Hand Surg [Am]* 35(8):1242–1245, 2010.

210. Veitch S, Blake SM, David H: Proximal scaphoid rib graft arthroplasty. *J Bone Joint Surg Br* 89(2):196–201, 2007.

211. Vender MI, Watson HK, Wiener BD, et al: Degenerative change in symptomatic scaphoid nonunion. *J Hand Surg [Am]* 12(4):514–519, 1987.

212. Viola RW, Kiser PK, Bach AW, et al: Biomechanical analysis of capitate shortening with capitate hamate fusion in the treatment of Kienbock's disease. *J Hand Surg [Am]* 23(3):395–401, 1998.

213. Walker JL, Greene TL, Lunseth PA: Fractures of the body of the trapezium. *J Orthop Trauma* 2(1):22–28, 1988.

214. Walsh E, Crisco JJ, Wolfe SW: Computer-assisted navigation of volar percutaneous scaphoid placement. *J Hand Surg [Am]* 34(9):1722–1728, 2009.

215. Watanabe K, Nakamura R, Horii E, et al: Biomechanical analysis of radial wedge osteotomy for the treatment of Kienbock's disease. *J Hand Surg [Am]* 18(4):686–690, 1993.

216. Watson HK, Rogers WD: Nonunion of the hook of the hamate: an argument for bone grafting the nonunion. *J Hand Surg [Am]* 14(3):486–490, 1989.

217. Watson HK, Ryu J, DiBella A: An approach to Kienbock's disease: triscaphe arthrodesis. *J Hand Surg [Am]* 10(2):179–187, 1985.

218. Weber DM, Fricker R, Ramseier LE: Conservative treatment of scaphoid nonunion in children and adolescents. *J Bone Joint Surg Br* 91(9):1213–1216, 2009.

219. Weber ER, Chao EY: An experimental approach to the mechanism of scaphoid waist fractures. *J Hand Surg [Am]* 3(2):142–148, 1978.

220. Weinberg AM, Pichler W, Grechenig S, et al: The percutaneous antegrade scaphoid fracture fixation: a safe method? *Injury* 40(6):642–644, 2009.

221. Weiss AP, Weiland AJ, Moore JR, et al: Radial shortening for Kienbock disease. *J Bone Joint Surg Am* 73(3):384–391, 1991.

222. Wheeler DL, McLoughlin SW: Biomechanical assessment of compression screws. *Clin Orthop Relat Res* 350:237–245, 1998.

223. Willems WF, Alberton GM, Bishop AT, et al: Vascularized bone grafting in a canine carpal avascular necrosis model. *Clin Orthop Relat Res* 469(10):2831–2837, 2011.

224. Wolf JM, Dawson L, Mountcastle SB, et al: The incidence of scaphoid fracture in a military population. *Injury* 40(12):1316–1319, 2009.

225. Wozasek GE, Moser KD: Percutaneous screw fixation for fractures of the scaphoid. *J Bone Joint Surg Br* 73(1):138–142, 1991.

226. Yamamoto H, Jones DB, Jr, Moran SL, et al: The arterial anatomy of the medial femoral condyle and its clinical implications. *J Hand Surg Eur Vol* 35(7):569–574, 2010.

227. Yao J, Read B, Hentz VR: The fragmented proximal pole scaphoid nonunion treated with rib autograft: case series and review of the literature. *J Hand Surg [Am]* 38(11):2188–2192, 2013.

228. Zaidemberg C, Siebert JW, Angrigiani C: A new vascularized bone graft for scaphoid nonunion. *J Hand Surg [Am]* 16(3):474–478, 1991.

Wrist Arthroscopy

William B. Geissler

> ▶ These videos may be found at
> *ExpertConsult.com:*
> **17.1** Diagnostic arthroscopy. *(Copyright © 2015, Scott W. Wolfe.)*

INTRODUCTION

Arthroscopy has revolutionized the practice of orthopedics by providing the technical capacity to examine and treat intraarticular abnormalities under magnified and bright conditions. The development of wrist arthroscopy was a natural progression in the successful application of it to larger joints. The wrist itself is a labyrinth of eight carpal bones, multiple articular surfaces with intrinsic and extrinsic ligaments, and a triangular fibrocartilage complex all within a 5-cm interval. Wrist arthroscopy has continued to see considerable growth since Whipple et al. reported on the original description of the techniques they developed.[130] The complex wrist joint continues to challenge clinicians with an array of potential diagnoses, pathology, and treatment options.

Indications for wrist arthroscopy continue to expand as new techniques and instrumentation are developed and improved. Diagnostic indications include assessment of the spectrum of interosseous ligament injuries, and an array of pathology that can occur on the ulnar side of the wrist, including injuries of the triangular fibrocartilage complex.[48,71,89,92,97] The use of wrist arthroscopy in fracture evaluation continues to grow with management of both radius and scaphoid fractures.[19,25] Wrist arthroscopy is extremely sensitive for detecting chondral defects of both the radial carpal and midcarpal joint, which frequently are difficult to evaluate by imaging studies alone.[25,27,67,70,87,93,96,126] These can be a source of chronic wrist pain of unknown etiology.[1] Arthroscopy of the thumb carpometacarpal joint (and the other small joints) continues to grow in popularity. Finally, the advantage of dry wrist arthroscopy and its indications are expanding.[69]

The purpose of this chapter is to present the indications for, techniques, and expected outcomes of wrist arthroscopy and how the techniques can be applied to an array of wrist pathology.

GENERAL SETUP FOR WRIST ARTHROSCOPY

Small joint instrumentation is absolutely essential for wrist arthroscopy.[129] Large joint instrumentation is not appropriate for the small joint of the wrist. In general, a small joint arthroscope (2.7 mm or less) is used with either a 30- or 70-degree visualization angle. Small joint punches and graspers are uti-

lized particularly for management of tears to the articular disk of the triangular fibrocartilage complex. A small joint shaver of 3.5 mm or less with varied tips is available for joint débridement.

Traction is essential for visualization.[39] This can be accomplished with the use of a commercial traction tower that stabilizes the forearm while traction is applied to two or more of the digits with finger traps. The amount of traction can be adjusted by means of a gear mechanism. Recent traction towers are now made with the traction bar at the side of the forearm rather than the middle, which makes the tower much more fluoroscopy friendly and expands the indication of wrist arthroscopy for management of carpal instability and fracture management (Figures 17.1 and 17.2). The traction tower has the advantage of applying constant traction to the wrist while it is slightly flexed; this wrist position makes it easier to insert the arthroscope and instruments. The improved visualization and increased ability to equip the wrist with newer traction towers continue to expand the possibility for treating various wrist pathologies.

If a traction tower is not available, a shoulder holder can be used to provide overhead support of the wrist. A countertraction band is placed around the arm. The wrist can be aligned in a horizontal manner on a hand table, which allows it to be stabilized by a pulley attached to the table, with weights hanging over the end (see Figure 17.2). Some surgeons prefer the horizontal position for wrist arthroscopy. In general, approximately 7 to 10 pounds (4.5 kilograms) is used for traction, depending on the intrinsic laxity of the individual.

PORTAL PLACEMENT

Radiocarpal Portals

Accurate portal placement in wrist arthroscopy is vital because of the small space available in the wrist joint.[19,21] eTable 17.1 reviews most of the common wrist arthroscopy portals and the articular structures that can be identified in their field of view. Appropriate portal placement begins with palpation and marking the base of the index, long, and ring metacarpals. Next the radial and ulnar borders of the extensor carpi ulnaris tendon are identified and marked (Figure 17.3). The radiocarpal space can be palpated and marked by rolling the surgeon's thumb over the dorsal rim of the distal radius and making an impression with the fingernail. The tendons of the extensor pollicis longus and extensor digitorum communis tendons can be palpated and marked unless obscured by swelling from an acute injury.

All portals should be drawn on the skin prior to making the incision, and after traction has been applied (Figure 17.4). The

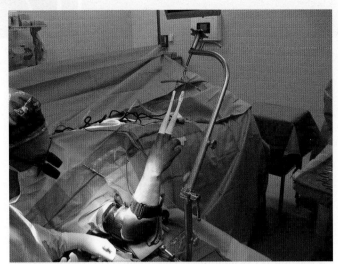

FIGURE 17.1 A traction tower is very helpful to support and distract the wrist during arthroscopic evaluation. They provide support of the forearm and allow the wrist to be slightly flexed to make it easier to initially insert the arthroscope, compared to overhead traction to keep the wrist straight.

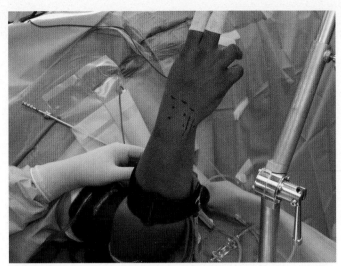

FIGURE 17.3 The bony landmarks can always be palpable even in swollen wrists. The base of the metacarpals and the tendon sheath of the extensor carpi ulnaris are identified. The standard 3-4 portal, 6-R portal, radial and ulnar midcarpal portals, and 6-U portal are marked.

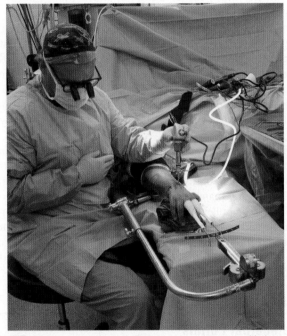

FIGURE 17.2 Some surgeons prefer to use the arthroscope with the wrist in a horizontal position. This may be more helpful particularly in addressing arthroscopic management of wrist fractures. Another option is to employ finger traps connected to weights that hang over the edge of the table with towels underneath the wrist so it is in a slightly flexed position.

portals are named by the position relative to the dorsal extensor tendons. The 3-4 portal is the most common viewing portal and is located between the third and fourth compartments on the dorsal aspect of the wrist. The 3-4 portal is identified by palpating Lister's tubercle and moving the finger approximately 1 cm distally until a soft spot is reached between the third and fourth compartments. The 3-4 portal also is in line with the radial border of the long finger. The 4-5 portal, which is located

between the fourth and fifth dorsal compartments, is the primary working portal. It is made by having the surgeon roll his or her finger ulnarward over the palpable fourth compartment and identifying a second soft spot immediately ulnar to the fourth compartment tendons. As a general rule, the 4-5 portal lies slightly more proximal than the 3-4 portal because of the normal radial inclination of the distal radius. The 4-5 portal also is in line with the midaxis of the ring finger.

The 1-2 portal is situated between the first extensor compartment containing the abductor pollicis longus (APL) tendon and the extensor pollicis brevis (EPB) tendon and the second dorsal compartment. It is important to remember that branches of the dorsal sensory branch of the radial nerve travel through the portal zone, as does the radial artery. One study showed that the radial artery is located at an average of 3 mm radial to the portal and the branches of the dorsal sensory branch of the radial nerve were within 3 mm radial and 5 mm ulnar to the portal. A separate study noted the mean distance of the superficial branch of the radial nerve was only 1.8 mm. It is generally recommended that, if this portal is utilized, it be as close as possible to the extensor pollicis longus (EPL) tendon (on its radial border) and just distal to the radial styloid to avoid injury to the radial artery. This portal is helpful for arthroscopic radial styloidectomy, as well as for peripheral triangular fibrocartilage (TFC) repair, using the Tuohy needle technique.[98]

The 6-R and 6-U portals are named according to their position relative to the extensor carpi ulnaris tendon, with the 6-R portal being radial and 6-U portal being ulnar to it. The 6-R portal is generally a working portal while the 6-U portal is frequently used for inflow of fluid. Normally, 3 to 5 mm of irrigation fluid is injected into the wrist at the radial carpal space through the inflow cannula at the 6-U portal. As the wrist joint is inflated with irrigation fluid, the dorsal aspect of the 3-4 portal bulges. This further helps to localize the proper position of the 3-4 portal. A pressurized pump can provide a feedback mechanism to maintain a constant pressure flow of irrigation into the joint.

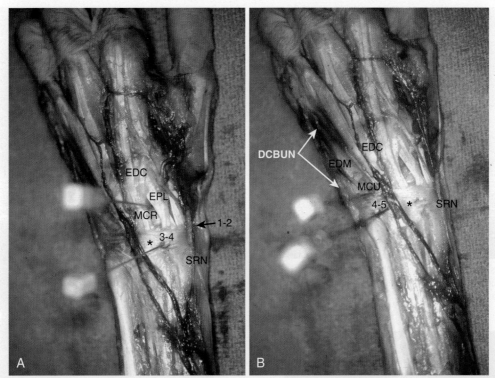

FIGURE 17.4 Dorsal portal anatomy. **A,** Cadaver dissection of the dorsal aspect of a left wrist demonstrating the relative positions of the dorsoradial portals. **B,** Relative positions of the dorsoulnar portals. *DCBUN,* Dorsal cutaneous branch of the ulnar nerve; *EDC,* extensor digitorum communis; *EDM,* extensor digiti minimi; *EPL,* extensor pollicis longus; *MCR,* midcarpal radial; *MCU,* midcarpal ulnar; *SRN,* superficial radial nerve; *,* the Lister tubercle.

The wrist is suspended in the traction tower in slight flexion, which makes it easier to insert the arthroscope and instrumentation. Prior to committing to a portal, a needle is placed in the proposed location to ensure that it passes easily into the joint without injuring the distal radius, ulna, or carpus. Portal incisions may be longitudinal or transverse. Transverse portals may be more cosmetic but potentially pose a slightly higher risk of injury to the underlying sensory branches of the radial and ulnar nerves. To avoid injury to the underlying sensory branches and extensor tendons, the surgeon uses his or her thumb to pull the skin against the tip of a number 11 scalpel blade, avoiding a deep plunge (Figures 17.5 and 17.6). Blunt dissection is continued down with the hemostat to the level of the joint capsule. The arthroscopic cannula with a blunt or semiblunt trocar is placed at approximately a 10-degree angle relative to the forearm to allow the cannula to enter the joint in line with the normal volar slope of the distal radius (Figures 17.7 and 17.8).

Two volar portals have been described to view the dorsal structures and the volar aspect of the radiocarpal interosseous ligaments.[109,110] The volar radial (VR) portal is made between the interval of the radioscaphocapitate ligament and the long radial lunate ligament. This portal is most easily made by placing the arthroscope directly through that interligamentous interval with the scope in the 3-4 portal. The scope is removed from the cannula, and a blunt trocar or switching stick is then inserted into the cannula and gently passed through the volar capsule, tenting the skin on the volar aspect of the wrist near the radial artery. A small incision is then made in the skin, and the switching stick is bluntly eased through the skin incision.

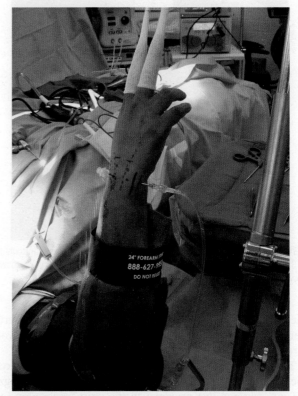

FIGURE 17.5 An 18-gauge needle is used to identify the precise location of the 3-4 portal prior to committing the skin incision. If the portal is located too far proximal or distal, it can damage the articular cartilage of the distal radius or carpus.

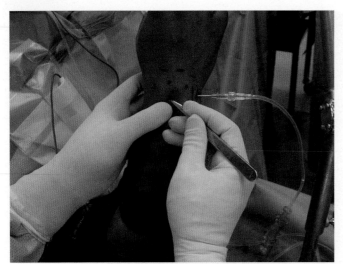

FIGURE 17.6 The skin is pulled with the thumb against the tip of the 11 blade to incise it to create the portal. In this manner, it decreases the risk of injury to the cutaneous nerves and tendons about the wrist.

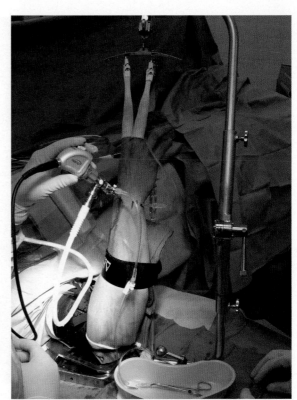

FIGURE 17.8 View of the arthroscope in the 3-4 portal. Note the approximately 10-degree tilt of the arthroscope to match the slope of the distal radius. It is the author's preference to have a separate inflow through the 6-U portal and outflow through the arthroscopic sheath, which drains into a basin. Because of the small diameter of the sheath, it is difficult to get much flow with the inflow attached directly to the arthroscopic sheath.

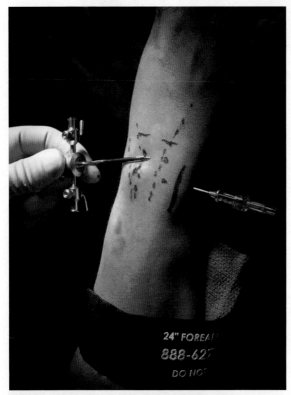

FIGURE 17.7 The arthroscope with a blunt trocar is introduced initially into the 3-4 portal. It is important to use a blunt trocar rather than a sharp one to avoid injury to the articular cartilage of the wrist.

Just distal to the pronator quadratus, the radiocarpal joint space is identified and pierced with a 22-gauge needle. Blunt tenotomy scissors are used to pierce the volar capsule, followed by insertion of the trocar/cannula, then the arthroscope. The ulnar nerve is protected by use of the cannula. The median nerve is protected by the adjacent flexor tendons. This portal penetrates between the ulnolunate and ulnotriquetral ligaments adjacent to the radial insertion of the TFC complex. The palmar region of the lunotriquetral interosseous ligament can usually be seen slightly distal and radial to the portal.

Alternatively, the VU portal can be made by an inside-out technique with the arthroscope in the 3-4 portal. A blunt trocar is inserted through the 6-U portal and pushed anteriorly through the ulnar carpal joint complex between the ulnolunate and triquetrum ligaments exiting the floor of the flexor tendons. It is important to remember that the ulnar artery and nerve have generally been found approximately 5 mm ulnar to the trocar, and the median nerve is protected by the flexor tendons. This portal provides a view of the dorsal articular surface of the radius and the dorsal extrinsic ligaments.

The cannula is removed from the dorsal portal and reinserted around the switching stick into the joint through the volar portal.

The volar ulna (VU) portal has been described by Slutsky.[109] The VU portal is established via a 2-cm longitudinal or zigzag incision centered just proximal to the wrist crease along the ulnar edge of the finger flexor tendons. Those tendons are retracted to the radial side and the flexor carpi ulnaris (FCU) and ulnar neurovascular bundle is retracted to the ulnar side.

MIDCARPAL PORTALS

The midcarpal portals are made approximately 1 cm distal to the 3-4 and 4-5 portals.[46] The radial midcarpal portal is in line with the radial margin of the long metacarpal. Radially, the extensor carpi radialis brevis tendon will pass and ulnarly the fourth dorsal extensor tendons. The midcarpal space is somewhat tighter than the radial carpal space, and care should be taken when entering with a blunt trocar. A needle is always used first to identify the precise position of the midcarpal portals prior to cutting the skin. The radial midcarpal portal has slightly less room compared to the ulnar midcarpal portal.

If the surgeon has difficulty entering the radial midcarpal portal, it is suggested that the arthroscope be placed in the ulnar midcarpal space first where there is more room to enter the joint. The ulnar midcarpal portal is situated in the soft depression of the four-corner intersection of the lunate, triquetrum, capitate, and hamate. It is in line with the midaxis of the ring metacarpal. This portal is situated approximately 1 to 1.5 cm distal to the 4-5 portal. It is bound radially by the extensor digitorum communis tendons, and ulnarly by the extensor digiti minimi tendon. Inflow is provided through the arthroscopic cannula, and a needle is used to provide outflow in the radial midcarpal space to improve visualization.

Four other midcarpal portals are described: the volar midcarpal (VM),[106] the scaphotrapeziotrapezoid (STT), the radial STT (STT-R), and the triquetral-hamate (TH).[22,106,120] To make the VM portal, a skin incision is made similar to the outside-in technique for the VR portal. The volar aspect of the midcarpal joint is identified with a needle at an average of 11 mm distal to the entry of the volar radial portal. The joint is enlarged with a hemostat and blunt trocar. This portal may be useful for assessing the palmar aspect of the capitate and hamate.

The scaphotrapezoid portal is found at the level of the STT joint in line with the radial margin of the index metacarpal just ulnar to the EPL tendon. The portal is bordered on its ulnar aspect by the extensor carpi radialis longus tendon and proximally by the distal pole of the scaphoid. The proposed portal site is located with an 18-gauge needle piercing the joint as viewed with the arthroscope in the radiomidcarpal space. This portal is used primarily for arthroscopic resection of the distal pole of the scaphoid in STT arthritis. Branches of the radial sensory nerve are in close proximity to this portal. The STT-R portal is located at the same level as the STT joint but radial to the APL tendon. This portal may be made in conjunction with the standard STT portal for resection of the distal portion of the scaphoid.

The TH portal is an infrequently used midcarpal portal, but it can help to define the ulnar aspect of the midcarpal joint. It is located between the extensor carpi ulnaris and FCU tendons and is bordered proximally by the triquetrum and distally by the base of the fifth metacarpal and hamate. This portal is more frequently used for instrumentation rather than viewing and can also be used for inflow or outflow. The dorsal ulnar sensory nerve crosses the midline just proximal to the portal site.

DISTAL RADIOULNAR JOINT PORTALS

Four portals for the distal radioulnar joint (DRUJ) have been described, including two dorsal, one volar, and a direct fovea.[8,20,107] The two standard portals are the distal DRUJ (D-DRUJ) and the proximal (P-DRUJ) portals for evaluation of the foveal insertion of the deep fibers of the radioulnar ligaments. A 1.9-mm small joint arthroscope is generally used at the outset since access to the DRUJ can be difficult; however, a standard 2.7-mm scope provides a better field of view.

The D-DRUJ portal is located in line with the 6-R portal approximately 5 to 8 mm proximal and just under the triangular fibrocartilage. This portal is bordered radially by the extensor digitorum minimi tendon and ulnarly by the ECU, tendon. Proximal to the portal is the ulnar head and distal is the articular disk. The portal is located with a needle prior to making a skin incision. For patients who are ulnar positive, this portal is of limited use. The proximal DRUJ (P-DRUJ) portal is useful for evaluating the articular surface of the ulnar head proximally and the undersurface of the articular disk distally. The P-DRUJ portal is situated approximately 1 cm proximal to the D-DRUJ portal. This portal is located in the axilla of the joint just proximal to the sigmoid notch of the radius in the flare of the ulnar metaphysis. This portal is useful to evaluate the articular cartilage of the sigmoid notch of the radius and the articular surface of the neck of the ulna.

The volar distal radial ulnar joint (V-DRUJ) uses the same landmarks as previously described for the VU portal. After a skin incision has been made, the flexor tendons are retracted radially and the flexor carpi ulnaris tendon and ulnar neurovascular bundle are retracted ulnarly to expose the joint capsule. The portal is located with a needle and then enlarged.

Finally, the direct fovea (DF) portal, as described by Atzei et al, is located 1 cm proximal to the standard 6-U portal.[8] To make the portal, the forearm is held in full supination. This portal is bound by the ECU tendon volarly and the FCU tendon volarly. Care should be taken to dissect and protect the dorsal sensory branch of the ulnar nerve. It may be helpful to encircle it with a vessiloop for additional protection. This portal is generally used as a working portal for possible repair of the articular disk to the ulnar fovea or débridement.

Trapeziometacarpal Arthroscopy

The portals for thumb basal joint arthroscopy are defined as the 1-R and 1-U portals.[15] The 1-R portal is just radial to the APL tendon. The 1-U portal is located just ulnar to the EPB tendon. The 1-R portal is best for viewing the dorsoradial ligament (DRL), posterior oblique ligament (POL), and the ulnar collateral ligament (UCL). The 1-U portal provides views of the anterior oblique ligament (AOL) and the ulnar collateral ligament (UCL). There is no true internervous plane because branches of the superficial radial nerve surround the field and are at risk for injury. The radial artery courses immediately posterior and ulnar to the arthroscopic field.

Accessory Thumb Carpometacarpal Portals

Accessory portals have been described by Orellana and Chow.[88] They discuss a modified radial portal (RP) for improving the radial view of the trapeziometacarpal joint. This portal is established by placing the scope in the 1-U portal and directed just radial to the AOL. A percutaneous 22-gauge needle is placed just distal to the ridge of the trapezium and visualized arthroscopically before finalizing the portal. Walsh et al. described a thenar portal, which is made by illuminating the thenar eminence with the arthroscope in the 1-U portal and inserting a 18-gauge needle through the bulk of the thenar muscles at the level of the carpometacarpal (CMC) joint.[125] This portal is approximately 90 degrees from the 1-U portal.

Slutsky developed a distal dorsal (D-2) accessory portal that allows one to look down the trapezium as opposed to across it,

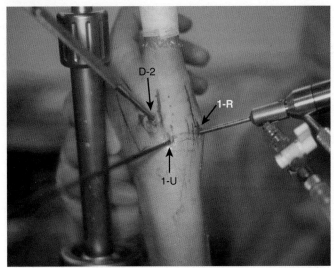

FIGURE 17.9 Trapeziometacarpal arthroscopy with use of the D-2 portal. The scope is in the 1-R portal, with a probe in the 1-U portal and a Freer elevator in the D-2 portal.

which he feels is safer for resection of medial osteophytes.[108] This portal is situated in the dorsal aspect of the first web space ulnar to the EPL tendon and 1 cm distal to the V-shaped soft spot at the junction of the index and thumb metacarpal bases. A 22-gauge needle is inserted 1 cm distal to the index–thumb metacarpal junction and angulated in a proximal, radial, and palmar direction while hugging the thumb metacarpal. Confirmation of joint access is performed from either the 1-R or 1-U portal. A small skin incision is made, and tenotomy scissors are used to spread the soft tissue and pierce the joint capsule followed by the arthroscope or instrumentation. There is no true safe zone for the D-2 portal, so a careful wound-spread technique is of paramount importance (Figure 17.9).

DRY ARTHROSCOPY

Dry arthroscopy has recently been increasing in popularity because of improved visualization, avoidance of normal tissue plane disruption by pressurized fluid, and the ability to use larger portals.[35,68] Dry arthroscopy avoids potential complications of extravasation of irrigation fluid into the soft tissues and the potential risk of compartment syndrome. An initial washing of the joint with 10 to 20 mm of fluid through a syringe attached to the side valve of the arthroscope sheath may be useful for evacuating hematoma or debris, especially if the procedure is indicated for the evaluation and reduction of articular fractures. The wrist arthroscope can be dried with small surgical padding inserted through a separate portal. *Tip:* To improve visualization immerse the tip of the arthroscope in warm water to prevent condensation. It is important to keep the side valve on the cannula open to air so that suction does not collapse the joint capsule. Suction should be used sparingly.

ARTHROSCOPIC ANATOMY

Arthroscopic evaluation of the radiocarpal space is started with the arthroscope in the 3-4 portal and progresses from a radial-to-ulnar direction. The radial styloid process articulates with

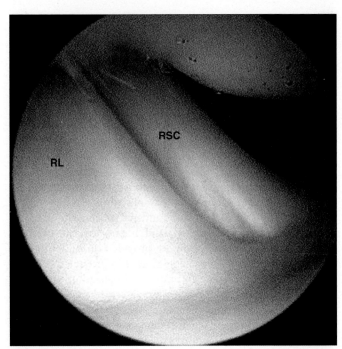

FIGURE 17.10 Arthroscopic view of the radioscaphocapitate (RSC) and long radial lunate (RL) ligaments with the arthroscope in the 3-4 portal. The RSC ligament is the most radial ligament and the long RL ligament is wider and lies just ulnar.

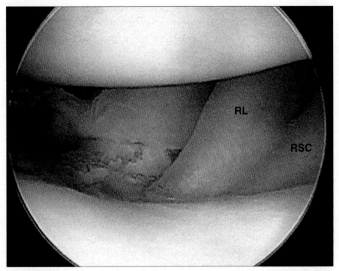

FIGURE 17.11 Arthroscopic view of the short radial lunate (RL) ligament and the well-vascularized ligament of Testut from the 3-4 portal. *RSC,* Radioscaphocapitate.

the proximal pole of the scaphoid and is examined for any signs of chondromalacia or synovitis, which can be seen in SLAC wrists. The volar extrinsic ligaments are then evaluated. The radial scaphocapitate ligament is the most radial extrinsic ligament that can be easily viewed.[18] The long radial lunate ligament is just ulnar to the radial scaphocapitate ligament and may be 2 to 3 times the width of the radial scaphocapitate ligament (Figure 17.10).[19,86]

Ulnar to the long radial lunate ligament is the short radial lunate ligament, which is a vascularized structure immediately volar to the scapholunate interval (Figure 17.11). The scapholunate interosseous ligament is then identified between the scaphoid and the lunate (Figure 17.12). It should have a normal concave appearance between the two carpal bones. As one continues to move ulnarward, the lunate facet of the distal radius is seen and the origin of the articular disk of the TFC complex is identified on the ulnar aspect of the radius.

The normal thickening of the volar and dorsal radial ulnar ligaments is also easily viewed. A probe may be inserted in either the 4-5 or 6-R portal to palpate the articular disk, which should be taut similar to a trampoline and can be balloted. The prestyloid recess is located dorsal to the ulnar carpal ligaments (Figure 17.13). This is a normal anatomic finding not to be confused with a peripheral tear of the articular disk of the TFC complex (Figure 17.14). The 6-U inflow cannula is traditionally

placed in this recess (Figure 17.15). The lunotriquetral interosseous and the ulnar carpal ligaments are best visualized with the arthroscope in either the 4-5 or 6-R portal. The ulnolunate and ulnotriquetral ligaments are capsular thickenings on the volar aspect of the ulnar capsule. The lunotriquetral interosseous ligament should have a normal concave appearance between the lunate and triquetrum that is very similar to the scapholunate interosseous ligament (Figure 17.16)

The midcarpal space is then examined after appropriate evaluation of the radial carpal space.[118] All six midcarpal portals can be used as needed for the particular pathology suspected.

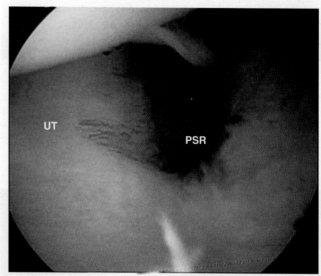

FIGURE 17.14 Arthroscopic view of the ulnotriquetral (UT) ligament with the arthroscope in the 6-R portal. Note the prestyloid recess (PSR) just dorsal and ulnar to this structure. It is important to note that this is a normal open space and not to mistake it for a peripheral tear of the articular disk, which is usually seen dorsal to the prestyloid recess.

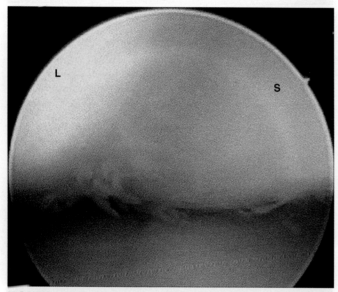

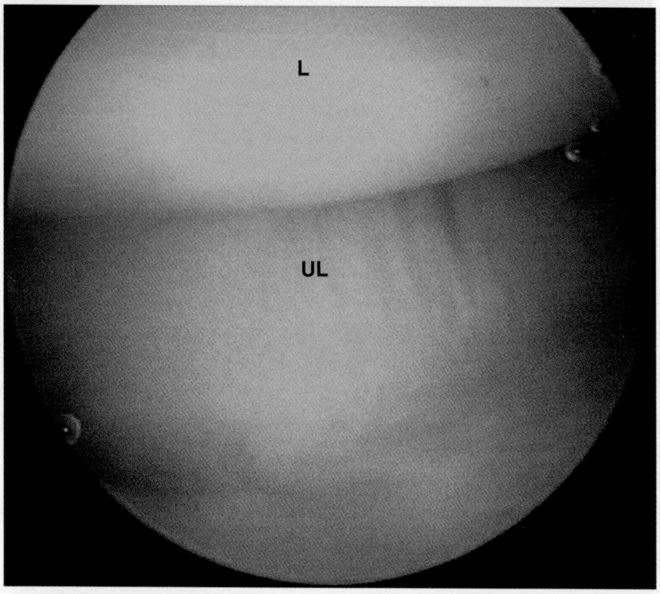

FIGURE 17.12 Arthroscopic view of the normal concave appearance of the scapholunate interosseous ligament between the scaphoid (S) and the lunate (L).

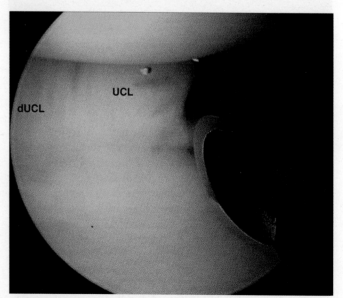

FIGURE 17.15 Arthroscopic view of the inflow needle being placed through the prestyloid recess. It is important to place the inflow distal to the articular disk so as not to injure this structure. *dUCL*, Distal ulnar collateral ligament; *UCL*, ulnar collateral ligament.

FIGURE 17.13 Arthroscopic view of the ulnolunate (UL) ligament with the arthroscope in the 3-4 portal. The lunate (L) is seen superiorly.

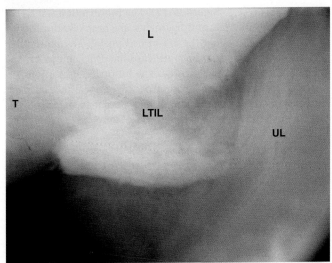

FIGURE 17.16 Arthroscopic view of a partial tear of the lunotriquetral interosseous ligament (LTIL) as seen with the arthroscope in the 6-R portal. It is important to note that this cannot be seen very well with the arthroscope in the 3-4 portal due to the more distal position of the triquetrum (T) in relation to the lunate (L). To thoroughly evaluate the lunotriquetral interval, the arthroscope needs to be placed on the ulnar side of the wrist, either in the 4-5 or 6-R portal. *UL,* Ulnar lunate.

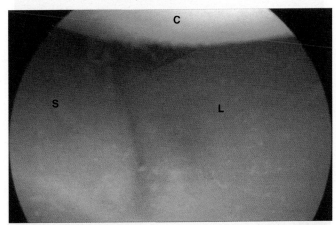

FIGURE 17.17 Arthroscopic view of the normal tight congruent articulation of the scaphoid (S) and lunate (L) as seen from the radial midcarpal portal. Note there is no step-off or gap between the scaphoid and lunate. The capitate (C) is seen distally.

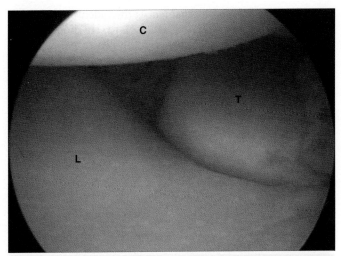

FIGURE 17.18 Arthroscopic view of the lunate (L) and triquetrum (T) as seen with the arthroscope in the radial midcarpal portal. Note that the triquetrum has about 1 mm of play or is positioned slightly distal to the lunate. This is a normal arthroscopic finding. *C,* Capitate.

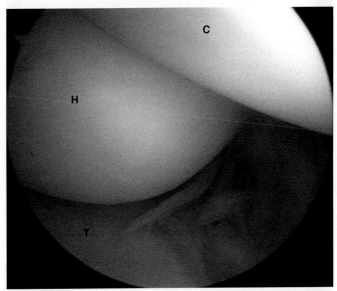

FIGURE 17.19 Arthroscopic view of the capitate (C), hamate (H), and triquetrum (T) as seen with the arthroscope in the ulnar midcarpal portal. This articulation can be a common location for symptomatic focal chondral defects, especially the proximal hamate, that can be difficult to image accurately.

The arthroscope is usually placed in the radial midcarpal portal, although in smaller wrists, it may be easier to start the examination with the arthroscope in the ulnar midcarpal portal.

The scapholunate interval proximally and the head of the capitate distally are initially identified as the arthroscope is placed in the radial midcarpal portal (Figure 17.17). This portal is useful for evaluating carpal instability, scaphoid fractures, articular cartilage defects to the midcarpal space, and the pathology of the STT joint. The lunotriquetral interval was seen as well as the proximal aspect of the hamate as the arthroscope is translated ulnarly (Figures 17.18 and 17.19). The arthroscope can then be translated radially and distally between the scaphoid and the capitate to visualize the STT joint. The trapezoid would be the carpal bone in the foreground and the trapezium in the background (Figure 17.20).

Two additional STT portals are established as in the preceding for arthroscopic treatment of the STT joint. The ulnar midcarpal portal is established, and the arthroscope can be moved back and forth between the two portals to evaluate and treat the appropriate conditions. Ulnar midcarpal viewing is helpful for suspected lunotriquetral tears, midcarpal instability, and to evaluate the type II lunate and any associated hamate impaction or degenerative disease.

DRUJ ARTHROSCOPY

The DRUJ is a very small space to arthroscopically evaluate and into which to insert instrumentation. Distal radioulnar joint

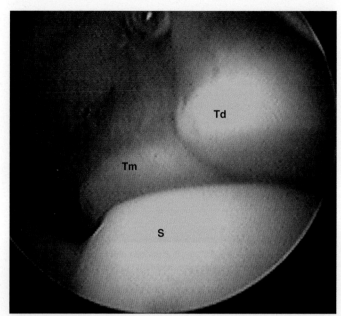

FIGURE 17.20 Arthroscopic view of the scaphotrapeziotrapezoid joint with the arthroscope in the radial midcarpal portal. The trapezium (Tm) is seen volar in relation to the trapezoid (Td). The scaphoid (S) is seen inferiorly.

TABLE 17.1	**Carpal Instability Chart**	
Grade	**Description**	**Management**
I	Attenuation or hemorrhage of interosseous ligament as seen from the radiocarpal space. No incongruency of carpal alignment in midcarpal space.	Cast immobilization
II	Attenuation or hemorrhage of interosseous ligament as seen from radiocarpal space. Incongruency or step-off seen in midcarpal space. There may be a slight gap (less than width of probe) between carpal bones.	Arthroscopic pinning
III	Incongruency or step-off of carpal alignment as seen from both radiocarpal and midcarpal space. Probe may be passed through gap between carpal bones.	Arthroscopic pinning/open repair
IV	Incongruency or step-off of carpal alignments as seen from both radiocarpal and midcarpal space. There is gross instability with manipulation. A 2.7-mm arthroscope may be passed through gap between carpal bones.	Open repair

arthroscopy is useful for evaluation of the articular cartilage of the ulnar head or sigmoid notch and assessment of soft tissue disorders that cannot be seen from the radiocarpal space. Indications include débridement of undersurface flap tears of the articular disk, removal of loose bodies, diagnosis and evaluation of sigmoid notch arthritis, capsulorraphy for arthrofibrosis, and débridement/resection of the ulnar head for class II degenerative lesions of the triangular fibrocartilage complex (TFCC). Four portals have been described: two dorsal, one volar, and one foveal. It is generally recommended that a 1.9-mm arthroscope be used and traction decreased to help reduce tension on the capsule so as to improve visualization. As the view improves with débridement and, particularly in larger joints, ultimately a 2.9-mm arthroscope can be inserted to improve visualization.

CARPAL INSTABILITY

The radiocarpal and midcarpal space both should be evaluated arthroscopically when carpal instability is suspected. The key to arthroscopic management of carpal instability is the recognition of what is normal and what is pathologic when viewing the interosseous ligaments and the alignment of the carpal bones. Wrist arthroscopy is not complete until the midcarpal space is examined when carpal instability is suspected. The interosseous ligaments are unusual in that they can stretch and attenuate substantially before they avulse. This can allow bulging of the interosseous ligament and rotation of the carpal bones even without complete tearing.

The mechanics of carpal instability are quite complex involving not only the interosseous ligaments but also the extrinsic ligaments.[16] This combination of both intrinsic and extrinsic pathology allows for malrotation of the carpal bones and clinical instability. As the interosseous ligament tears, it hangs down, blocking visualization with the arthroscope in the radial carpal space. Rotation of the carpal bones is best accomplished with the unobstructed view available with the arthroscope in the midcarpal space.

The scapholunate and lunotriquetral interosseous ligaments should have a normal concave appearance as seen from the radial carpal space. The scapholunate interosseous ligament is best seen with the arthroscope in the 3-4 portal and the lunotriquetral interosseous ligament is best seen with the arthroscope in either the 4-5 or 6-R portal because of its oblique distal relationship to the proximal carpal row. In the midcarpal space, the scapholunate interval should be tightly congruent without any step-off. The lunotriquetral interval should be congruent, but frequently a 1 mm distal step-off of the triquetrum to the lunate is seen; this is normal. When the triquetrum is palpated, there is generally slight motion between the lunate and the triquetrum.

A limited type of intraoperative arthrogram (poor person's arthrogram) may be performed for the evaluation of carpal instability. A needle is placed in either the radial or ulnar midcarpal portal, and a tear of the interosseous ligament is strongly suspected when there is free flow of irrigation fluid from one carpal space to the other.

A spectrum of injury can be seen in both the scapholunate and lunotriquetral interosseous ligaments when they are injured. The interosseous ligament appears to attenuate and then tear from a volar-to-dorsal direction. Geissler et al. devised an arthroscopic classification of carpal instability based on observations of injury to the scapholunate and lunotriquetral interosseous ligaments when associated with fractures of the distal radius (Table 17.1).[48]

In grade I injuries, there is loss of the normal concave appearance between the carpal bones. The interosseous ligament bulges with a convex appearance as seen with the arthroscope in the radial carpal space (Figure 17.21). Evaluation of the midcarpal space shows the carpal bones to be congruent

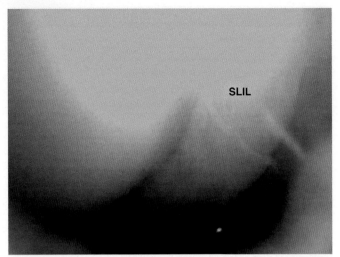

FIGURE 17.21 Arthroscopic view of a Geissler grade I injury to the scapholunate interosseous ligament (SLIL) as seen with the arthroscope in the 3-4 portal. Note the loss of the normal concave appearance of the interosseous ligament. The convex and stretched ligament bulges into the radiocarpal joint. In the midcarpal space, arthroscopic evaluation will show no step-off or congruency of the scapholunate interval in a grade I injury.

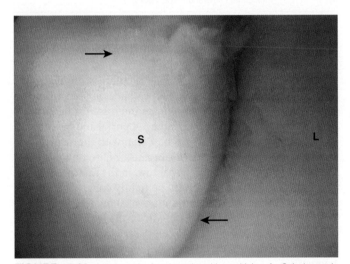

FIGURE 17.22 Arthroscopic view from the midcarpal joint of a Geissler grade II injury to the scapholunate interosseous ligament. Similar to a grade I injury, there is bulging of the ligament as seen in the radiocarpal space. In the midcarpal space as seen here, now there is joint incongruency and palmar flexion of the scaphoid in relation to the lunate as demonstrated by the *arrows*. *L*, Lunate; *S*, scaphoid.

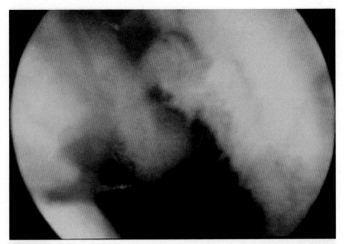

FIGURE 17.23 Arthroscopic view of a Geissler grade III injury to the scapholunate ligament as seen with the arthroscope in the radiocarpal space. Note a gap is seen between the scaphoid on the left and the lunate on the right. Normally, the ligament tears in a volar-to-dorsal direction.

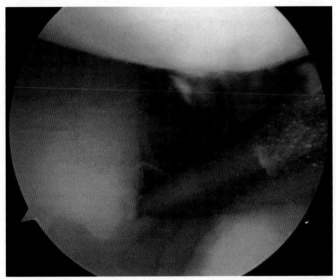

FIGURE 17.24 Arthroscopic view of a Geissler grade III injury as seen with the arthroscope in the radial midcarpal space. Note the separation between the scaphoid and lunate when palpated with a probe.

with no step-off. In grade II injuries, the interosseous ligament is again convex as seen with the arthroscope in the radial carpal space. In the midcarpal space, the carpal bones are no longer congruent (Figure 17.22). With scapholunate instability, the scaphoid is observed with a slight palmar flexion because the dorsal edge is distal compared to the lunate. However, there is no gap between the scaphoid and the lunate. In injuries to the lunotriquetral interosseous ligament, there is increased motion as seen in the lunate and triquetrum when palpated with a probe inserted through the ulnar midcarpal portal.

With grade III injuries, the interosseous ligament begins to tear and a gap is seen from the carpal bones of both the radial carpal and midcarpal spaces. A probe may be inserted between the scaphoid and lunate and gapping can be observed from the radiocarpal and midcarpal space (Figures 17.23 and 17.24). In grade IV injuries, the interosseous ligament is completely detached and the arthroscope can be passed freely from the radial carpal to the midcarpal space to the interval of the carpal bones. This is a so-called "drive-through sign." This corresponds to a widening scapholunate gap as seen on the radiographs of patients with a complete scapholunate disassociation (Figure 17.25).

Acute tears of the scapholunate or lunotriquetral interosseous ligaments that result in incongruency from the midcarpal space may be arthroscopically reduced and temporarily pinned. It is felt that in patients who have a grade I injury, typically the wrist sprain will resolve with immobilization alone as there is no incongruency.

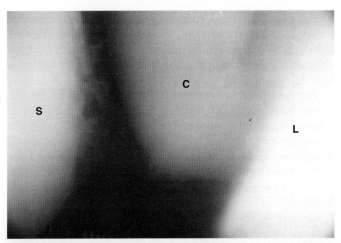

FIGURE 17.25 Arthroscopic view of a Geissler grade IV injury with the so-called "drive through sign." The arthroscope can freely be passed through the gap between the scaphoid (S) and lunate (L) and between the radiocarpal and midcarpal spaces. The capitate (C) is easily seen distally.

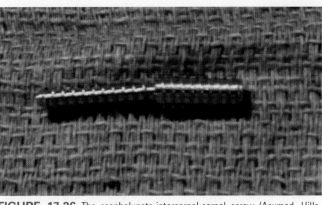

FIGURE 17.26 The scapholunate-intercarpal-carpal screw (Acumed, Hillsboro, OR). This screw rotates between the threaded portions on either end to allow rotation between the scaphoid and the lunate. It also has approximately 20 degrees of toggle at the two ends. This screw is designed to remain in place for a prolonged period of time while the repair of the interosseous ligament heals and matures.

Two or three guidewires are placed just distal to the radial styloid into the scaphoid under fluoroscopy. It is important to place the guidewire either through a cannula or in oscillation mode to avoid injury to the dorsal sensory branch of the radial nerve. The Kirschner wires are placed into the scaphoid aiming toward the lunate under fluoroscopic control. The wrist is suspended in the traction tower. The arthroscope is placed in the ulnar midcarpal portal. It is most effective arthroscopically to look across the wrist. A joystick may be placed into the lunate to help control rotation as well. The scapholunate interval is anatomically reduced as viewed from the midcarpal space. The Kirschner wires have been driven across the scapholunate interval.

Frequently, droplets of fat are seen exiting the interval between the scapholunate as Kirschner wires are being driven across the carpal bones. Three or four wires are placed and left in position for approximately 8 weeks. The Kirschner wires can be buried or left exposed for easier removal based on the surgeon's preference. The wrist is immobilized in a below-elbow cast and the wire tracks are evaluated every 2 to 3 weeks. Digital range of motion is encouraged. The wires are removed at 8 weeks and the wrist is immobilized an additional 4 weeks. Physical therapy for wrist range of motion and grip strength is initiated after a 3-month interval.

Management of acute tears to the lunotriquetral interosseous ligament is essentially the same except the arthroscope is placed in the radial midcarpal space as the pins are driven across the lunotriquetral interval. The Kirschner wires are placed through a catheter or in oscillation mode to avoid injury to the dorsal sensory branch of the ulnar nerve. Frequently, reduction of the lunotriquetral interval is not as difficult compared to the scapholunate interval.

There is a complete tear of the interosseous ligament in grade IV injuries to the wrist. It is felt that direct primary repair of a complete tear of the interosseous ligament is the best option; it is performed through a small arthrotomy rather than pinning alone. While Kirschner wires are effective for stabilization, they can only be left in for a short period of time (6-8 weeks). These wires have been associated with pin tract infec-

tions and potentially can limit rehabilitation. The concern is that the interosseous ligaments may take a long time to heal, and a period of 6 to 8 weeks may not be enough for them to heal when the pins are pulled.

An alternative is placement of a screw specially designed by Acumed (Hillsboro, OR) for carpal instability—the scapholunate-intercarpal-carpal (SLIC). A SLIC screw rotates in its midsection and has approximately 20 degrees of toggle (Figure 17.26). The theory with an SLIC screw is that it can be left in for a prolonged period of time (6-9 months) and allows rotation of the scaphoid and lunate in the sagittal plane while the ligament heals. The cannulated screw can be removed in the future. Using a screw to temporarily augment scapholunate repair has advantages over Kirschner wires, which are mechanically less secure and have problems of pin irritation and pin tract infection.

Whipple reviewed the results of arthroscopic treatment of scapholunate instability in patients who were followed for a duration of 1 to 3 years.[132] Patients were classified in two distinct groups of 40 patients each according to the duration of symptoms and the side-to-side scapholunate gap. Eighty-three percent of patients who had scapholunate instability of 3 months or less, and a gap of 3 mm or less, had symptomatic relief compared to only 21 patients (63%) who had symptoms greater than 3 months and more than a 3-mm side-to-side difference. The conclusion from the study was that arthroscopic pinning should be reserved for patients with an acute injury rather than a chronic, complete tear.

Osterman and Seidman reviewed their study's results of arthroscopic treatment of acute lunotriquetral instability in 20 patients who did not have volar intercalated segment instability.[91] Follow-up was done at an average of 32 months, and 16 patients had good-to-excellent relief of pain. Grip strength improved in 18 patients.

Weiss et al. reviewed results of arthroscopic débridement of interosseous ligament tears alone at an average of 27 months following the procedure.[127] In the study, 31 of 36 patients who had a partial tear of the scapholunate interosseous ligament had complete resolution or a decrease in their symptoms compared to 19 to 21 patients who had a complete tear of the scapholunate interosseous ligament. All 42 patients who had a partial tear of the lunotriquetral interosseous ligament and 26 of 33 patients who had a complete tear of the lunotriquetral interosseous ligament had complete resolution or a decrease in their symptoms. Grip strength improved in an average of 23% in study participants. Weiss et al. concluded that débridement of lunotriquetral interosseous ligament tears had a better result compared to injury to the scapholunate interosseous ligament. In addition, débridement of partial tears to the interosseous ligament had better results compared to complete tears.

Although electrothermal shrinkage of ligaments in other joints of the body, primarily the shoulder, has not been shown to be effective, electrothermal shrinkage may play a role in the management of chronic partial tears of the interosseous ligaments. This is because the wrist may be immobilized for a prolonged period of time, allowing the contracted collagen to mature. Electrothermal shrinkage is based on heating and denaturing of collagen, which results in shrinkage. This technique is best indicated for chronic grade I or grade II partial tears of the interosseous ligament. The monopolar or bipolar probe can be used. The monopolar probe is shown to lead to deeper penetration of heat to contract the interosseous ligament compared to a bipolar probe. In addition, a bipolar probe yields higher surface temperatures that can further increase the temperature of the irrigation fluid in the wrist due to its small volume.

An electrothermal probe is used to shrink the remaining portion of the interosseous ligament following mechanical débridement of the tear. It is important not to paint the tissue but to spot weld and to leave viable tissue in between the contracted areas (Figure 17.27). The probe addresses primarily the membranous portion of the interosseous ligament but also the dorsal and volar capsule may be shrunk. In addition, the probe can be placed in the midcarpal space to shrink the volar capsule. It is extremely important to increase the flow of irrigation fluid into the wrist joint during thermal shrinkage. Increasing the fluid's flow helps to disseminate the heat from the wrist probe. The volume of flow to the wrist joint is quite small and can be

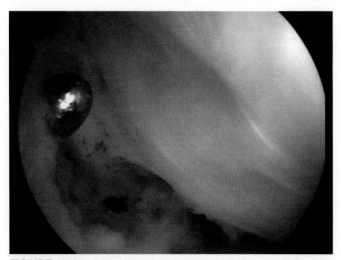

FIGURE 17.27 View with the arthroscope in the 6-R portal following electrothermal shrinkage of the scapholunate interosseous ligament. The thermal probe is inserted through the 3-4 portal. Note the caramel colorization following shrinkage of the scapholunate interosseous ligament and restoration of the normal concave appearance to the ligament.

rapidly heated up with a thermal probe. The temperature of the irrigation fluid as it leaves the wrist should be monitored as well to help prevent burns to the patient. It is recommended that a separate inflow through the 6-U portal be used to maintain a high volume of fluid in and out of the joint.

Postoperative management of thermal shrinkage for chronic partial tears of the interosseous ligament is controversial as minimal protocols are available. Some authors believe that immobilization alone is sufficient while others recommend temporary Kirschner wire stabilization. Patients' wrists are immobilized for approximately 8 weeks then for an additional 4 weeks in a removable brace after physical therapy exercises are initiated.

Geissler reviewed the results of 19 patients with chronic isolated interosseous ligament tears.[46] A chronic injury was defined as symptoms greater than 6 months. Geissler noted that grade II tears of the scapholunate and lunotriquetral interosseous ligaments had significantly better results compared to grade III tears. There is no real difference in the study between scapholunate and lunotriquetral interosseous ligament tears. The lunate was neutral in those patients with partial interosseous ligament injuries.

Darlis et al. performed arthroscopic débridement and capsular shrinkage on 16 patients with 14 reporting good-to-excellent results. In their series, eight of those patients were pain-free; there were two failures.[33] In a similar study, Hirsh et al. performed his study with 10 patients who were 90% pain-free on an average follow-up of 10 months.[61]

Mathoulin et al. described a unique arthroscopic dorsal capsule ligament repair for chronic reducible scapholunate interosseous ligament tears.[77,124] Their hypothesis is that the dorsal intercarpal ligament is avulsed from the intact dorsal scapholunate interosseous ligament (dSLI). In this technique, a 3.0 PDS suture is placed through a needle as visualized arthroscopically and passed through the dorsal intercarpal ligament (DICL) and the dorsal scapholunate ligament, tied to form a capsuloplasty. No pins are used. In their study series of 36 patients with a 13-month follow-up, results were generally excellent. Patients regained 96% of grip strength compared to the contralateral side and reported that seven of the patients involved in sports were able to return to the same level of activity postoperatively. The advantage of this technique is in the reduction of postoperative stiffness by minimizing the dorsal capsule dissection compared to traditional open surgery.

del Pinal et al. described an all-inside technique for arthroscopic suturing of the volar scapholunate interosseous ligament.[36] With this technique, sutures are placed volarly through a Tuohy needle to plicate the volar ligament remnants and the long radial lunate ligament. He described using this technique in four patients.

Van Kampen and Moran reported on a new technique for capsulodesis based on cadaver study.[118] With this technique, a volar capsulodesis is used to reconstruct the volar scapholunate interosseous ligament using a portion of the long radial lunate ligament; they included a detailed description.

As can be seen, more and more investigative work is being performed to address the difficult problem of scapholunate instability. More attention is being placed, in particular, on addressing the volar aspect of instability instead of concentrating on the dorsal aspects. Chronic isolated lunotriquetral interosseous ligament injuries have been treated with various techniques including ligament repair, ligament reconstruction, and lunotriquetral fusion.

Moskal and Savoie described a ligament plication of the ulnotriquetral-ulnolunate ligaments.[82] Contraindication to this technique would be a VISI deformity. In this technique, the standard 3-4, 6-R, and 6-U arthroscopic portals are made. A volar 6-U (v6-U) portal is established. The v6-U portal, similar to the normal 6-U portal, is placed just dorsal to the disk carpal ligaments. Through the v6-U portal an 18-gauge needle is passed just volar to the disk triquetral, ulnar capitate, and disk lunate in the radial carpal joint at the radial edge of the ulnolunate ligament just distal to the articular surface of the radius. A 2.0-PDS suture is placed through the needle into the joint. The suture is retrieved either sequentially through the 6-R and through the v6-U or directly through v6-U using a wire loop suture retriever. The suture is then tagged as the first plicating suture.

In a likewise fashion, a second plicating suture is placed approximately 5 mm distal to the first suture parallel to the lunate and triquetrum. Finally, through the v6-U a spinal needle is passed through the volar aspect of the capsule at the pre-styloid recess and then through the periphery of the articular disk of the TFCC. The retriever is introduced through the ulnar capsule, and the suture is brought out of the v6-U portal through the ulnar capsule. The three sutures are then tied after the lunotriquetral joint has been congruently reduced and stabilized with Kirschner wires. In their study series, 19 out of 21 patients had an excellent or good result with two fair.

Various authors have cast light on the importance of the dorsal radiocarpal ligament pertaining to carpal instability.[79,99,103,122] It is felt that tears of the dorsal radiocarpal ligament (DRCL) have been linked to the development of both volar and dorsal intercalated segmental instabilities. It also has been implicated as a cause of midcarpal instability.[66,81,121] It is generally felt that DRCL is commonly overlooked with the general arthroscopic examination of the wrist. The dorsal radiocarpal ligament may be seen through either the 1-2 or 6-R portals. Visualization may be difficult in a smaller, tight wrist. Wrist arthroscopy through a volar radial portal is the most ideal way to access the DRCL due to straight access of the site.

Slutsky described his technique for arthroscopic repair of a lesion to DRCL.[106] Using his technique, the VR portal is made as previously described. He feels that while the procedure may be done dry, it is easier to see the torn edges of the DRCL with fluid irrigation. The DRCL is seen just radial to the standard 3-4 portal underneath the lunate. He notes that the dorsal capsule may often appear redundant and can protrude into the joint; however, when a DRCL tear is present, the frayed ligamentous fibers can be seen. It is often helpful to insert a 3-mm hook probe through the 3-4 portal for orientation. The torn DRCL then may be pulled into the joint with a probe that differentiates it from the redundant dorsal capsule.

A repair of a DRCL is performed by inserting a 22-gauge spinal needle through the 3-4 or 4-5 portals (Figure 17.28). A 2.0 absorbable suture is threaded through the spinal needle and retrieved with a grasper or suture retriever and passed through the opposite portal. A curved hemostat is then used to pull either end of the suture underneath the dorsal extensor tendons. A suture knot is tied either at the 3-4 or 4-5 portal. Slutsky notes that usually one suture is sufficient but additional ones may be added. In this technique, the patient is placed in a cast for approximately 4 weeks followed by wrist mobilization.

Slutsky reviewed a retrospective series of 22 patients. There were 6 men and 16 women in his study.[105] A dorsal capsulodesis was performed with 7 patients as a primary treatment and 13 underwent DRCL repair with thermal shrinkage. It was noted that 5 patients who underwent an isolated DRCL repair were satisfied with the surgery's outcome and would repeat it because of the improvement. All 5 described their pain as none or mild, and all returned to their previous occupations without restrictions.

Wrist arthroscopy also can serve as a valuable adjunct in the management of chronic injuries to the interosseous ligaments beyond thermal shrinkage. Wrist arthroscopy can be used to evaluate the degree and extent of articular cartilage degeneration in patients with chronic scapholunate advanced collapsed (SLAC) wrist. Arthroscopic evaluation of the status of the articular cartilage to the head of the capitate is extremely useful to help determine the indications for four-corner fusion versus proximal row carpectomy, and it may be used as an alternative or an adjunct to magnetic resonance imaging.

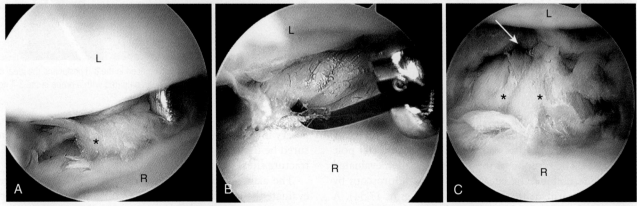

FIGURE 17.28 Dorsal radiocarpal ligament repair. **A,** View from the volar radial portal demonstrating the torn edge of the dorsal radiocarpal ligament (DRCL) (*) protruding into the joint space. **B,** The suture is entering from the 4-5 portal and being retrieved by a grasper in the 3-4 portal. **C,** Note how the suture (*arrow*) pulls the DRCL (*) up against the dorsal capsule. *L,* Lunate; *R,* radius.

FRACTURE MANAGEMENT

Scaphoid Fractures

Cast immobilization has shown a successful healing rate of 85 to 95% of acute nondisplaced scaphoid fractures.[54] While cast immobilization may be successful, it comes with a price: muscle atrophy, osteopenia, and potential wrist stiffness. An athlete may lose his scholarship, and an employee his job, should a prolonged period of immobilization and ultimately surgery for scaphoid nonunion be required. Arora et al. compared cast and operative fixation for stable scaphoid fractures.[7] They noted the operative group had a shorter time to union, decreased overall costs, and a 7-week earlier return to sports and/or work. Several minimal incision techniques have been developed, including a volar percutaneous approach, a percutaneous dorsal approach, mini-open, and all-arthroscopic fixation. The reader is referred to Chapter 16 for a complete description of operative techniques.

❖ AUTHOR'S PREFERRED TREATMENT: Arthroscopic Reduction and Internal Fixation of Scaphoid Fractures

Geissler Technique

This technique can be used for both acute fractures and selected scaphoid fracture nonunions.[53] The advantage of this technique is that the starting point is viewed directly arthroscopically and there is no guesswork concerning the insertion point of the guidewire and the headless cannulated screw. It is also felt that this technique may have a technical advantage over the dorsal percutaneous approach because the wrist is not hyperflexed during wire insertion, which could create a flexion/humpback deformity in the scaphoid. It is important to note that this technique is indicated for patients with acute fractures of the scaphoid and for nonunions without a humpback deformity or dorsal intercalated segment instability (DISI).

The wrist is placed in the traction tower and the arthroscope is inserted in the 3-4 portal to evaluate any associated soft tissue injuries that may be associated with the fracture. It is helpful to place the forearm baseplate on the dorsal aspect of the forearm to make it easier to flex the wrist (Figures 17.29 and 17.30). The arthroscope is then transferred into the 6-R portal and the wrist is flexed approximately 30 degrees. A 14-gauge needle is inserted through the 3-4 portal to align the ideal starting point for the guidewire in the scaphoid proximal pole. The needle should pass easily and care be taken to avoid puncture or injury to an extensor tendon.

Viewing from the 6-R portal, the needle is pushed by hand into the scaphoid proximal pole at its junction with the membranous portion of the scapholunate interosseous ligament at the approximate volar-dorsal midpoint (Figure 17.31). The flexed wrist is then evaluated under fluoroscopy in the PA plane and the starting point of the needle is confirmed and adjusted as necessary (Figure 17.32). The needle is next aimed toward the thumb and a guidewire is advanced under fluoroscopy down the central axis of the scaphoid to abut the distal pole (Figure 17.33). The position of the guidewire is then evaluated in the PA plane, oblique, and lateral views under fluoroscopy by rotating the forearm in the traction tower (Figure 17.34). A second guidewire is then inserted percutaneously to abut the proximal pole of the scaphoid, and the length of the screw is determined by the difference in the length of the two wires. It

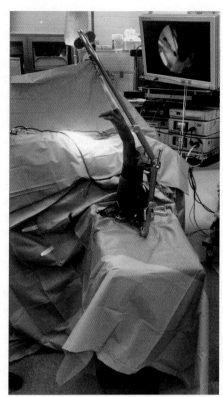

FIGURE 17.29 It is helpful with arthroscopic fixation of the scaphoid to place the forearm base plate of the traction tower on the dorsal aspect of the forearm. In this manner, it is easier to flex the forearm when evaluating the position of the needle and guidewire under fluoroscopy.

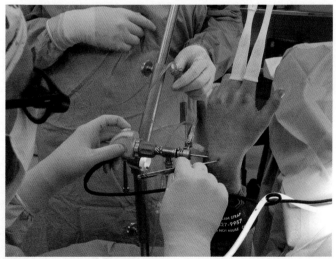

FIGURE 17.30 The arthroscope is placed in the 6-R portal and the ideal starting position for the scaphoid guidewire is palpated with a probe in the 3-4 portal.

is very important that a screw at least 4 mm shorter than measured be used to avoid screw prominence or distraction of the fracture site.

The arthroscope is then placed in the midcarpal space to evaluate the fracture reduction. Fractures of the proximal pole are best seen with the arthroscope in the ulnar midcarpal portal, and fractures of the waist are best visualized with the arthroscope in the radial midcarpal portal. The guidewire is then

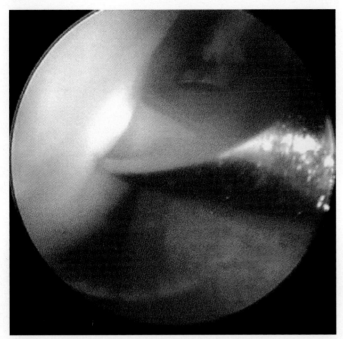

FIGURE 17.31 A 14-gauge needle is then brought in through the 3-4 portal and the proximal pole of the scaphoid is impaled just radial to the junction of the interosseous ligament. It is important as one passes the needle through the 3-4 portal that it easily goes through the portal so as not to injure an extensor tendon.

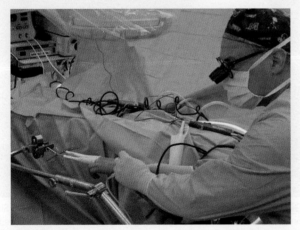

FIGURE 17.32 The traction tower is then flexed to horizontal to check position of the needle under fluoroscopy to be exactly at the proximal pole of the scaphoid.

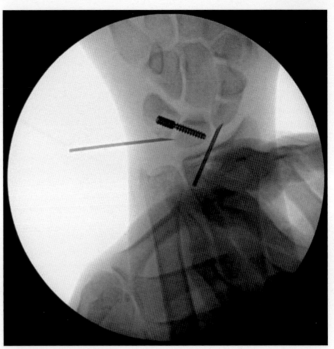

FIGURE 17.33 Fluoroscopic view showing ideal position of the 14-gauge needle on the proximal pole of the scaphoid so that the guidewire will pass perpendicular to the scaphoid fracture.

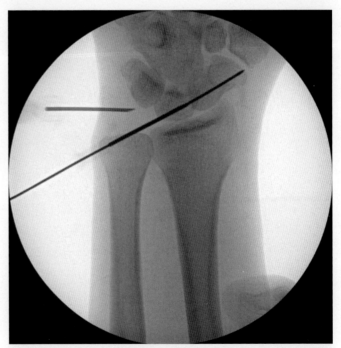

FIGURE 17.34 Fluoroscopic view showing the guidewire inserted through the 14-gauge needle and down the central axis of the scaphoid.

advanced out the volar aspect of the wrist, generally through the thenar eminence. This is an important step because if the guidewire breaks at any point during the procedure, the two ends can be retrieved from dorsal and palmar. If the reduction is not considered satisfactory, the wire is further withdrawn distally until it is in the distal fragment alone, and a joystick is inserted into the proximal pole to help manipulate the fracture to an anatomic reduction. Frequently, flexion and extension and radial and ulnar deviation of the wrist in the traction tower help facilitate the reduction. Once the fracture is felt to be anatomic, as viewed directly with the arthroscope in the midcarpal space, the guidewire is advanced proximally into the proximal pole of the scaphoid and out the initial 3-4 portal.

At this point, the guidewire should be exiting the volar and dorsal aspects of the wrist. The scaphoid is then reamed through a trocar to protect the extensor tendons and cutaneous nerves. A cannulated screw is then placed over the guidewire (Figure 17.35). The position of the screw is evaluated under fluoroscopy in the PA, oblique, and lateral planes (Figure 17.36). The wrist

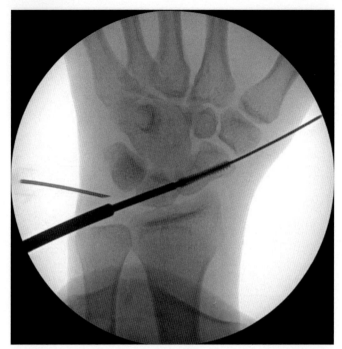

FIGURE 17.35 Fluoroscopic view showing the headless cannulated screw placed over the guidewire down the axis of the scaphoid. Note the wire exits the volar aspect of the wrist so it is easily accessible if there is any breakage or bending of the guide wire.

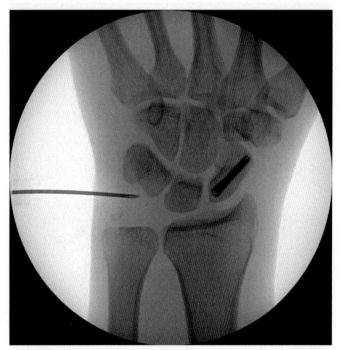

FIGURE 17.36 Fluoroscopic view showing ideal placement of the headless cannulated screw across the scaphoid fracture.

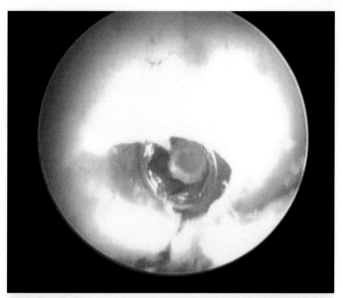

FIGURE 17.37 Arthroscopic view showing the headless cannulated screw buried beneath the articular cartilage to the level of the subchondral bone.

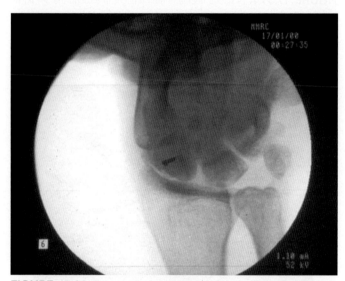

FIGURE 17.38 Fluoroscopic view of the guidewire in place using the Slade technique. The proximal and distal poles of the scaphoid have been aligned by hyperflexion to form the "ring sign." The guidewire is passed parallel to the fluoroscopic beam.

is then evaluated arthroscopically both from the midcarpal and radial carpal spaces. From the midcarpal space, the reduction and compression of the scaphoid are evaluated.

In the radiocarpal space, it is imperative to evaluate that the headless cannulated screw has been advanced below the articular cartilage (Figure 17.37). Occasionally, the screw may look to

be buried under fluoroscopy, but arthroscopic evaluation shows the screw remains slightly prominent, which could injure the articular cartilage of the distal radius. If this is the case, the screw is further advanced into the scaphoid.

Slade Technique

Slade et al. described the dorsal arthroscopic assisted technique.[104] In this technique, the wrist is flexed and pronated until the proximal and distal poles of the scaphoid are aligned into a cylinder. This forms a ring sign (Figure 17.38). Once the ring sign is achieved, a guidewire is placed down the center of the ring in line with the axis of the x-ray beam. The wire is advanced out the volar aspect of the wrist until it is flush with the dorsal pole of the scaphoid. In this manner, now the wrist can be extended to verify the precise position of the guidewire and the posterior, anterior, oblique, and lateral planes. The position of the guidewire in the proximal pole of the scaphoid can be verified with the arthroscope in the radiocarpal space. The arthroscope can be placed in the midcarpal space to evaluate reduction of the scaphoid fracture.

Fractures of the waist of the scaphoid are best seen with the arthroscope in the radial midcarpal portal, and proximal pole fractures are best seen with the arthroscope in the ulnar midcarpal portal. If reduction is not satisfactory, the guidewire can be advanced out the thenar eminence and withdrawn until it is only within the distal pole. Separate joysticks are placed in the proximal and distal poles to manipulate the fracture fragments; extension and radial deviation of the wrist in the traction tower also help to align the fracture anatomically. The wire can then be advanced back proximally across the fracture site. Once ideal reduction of the scaphoid is confirmed arthroscopically, the wrist is flexed and the guidewire is brought out dorsally through the 3-4 portal until it abuts the subchondral bone of the distal pole and is measured. It is imperative that a screw at least 4 mm shorter than the measured length be used to avoid prominence or fracture distraction. The scaphoid is then reamed and a headless cannulated screw is placed.

Herbert–Whipple Technique

Another arthroscopic-assisted technique using the Herbert-Whipple jig (Zimmer, Warsaw, IN) has been described. With the arthroscope in the 6-R portal, the jig is inserted into the 1-2 portal and the spike of the jig is placed at the junction of the scapholunate interosseous ligament and the proximal pole of the scaphoid, identical to the starting point of the Geissler technique (Figure 17.39). An incision is then made over the distal pole of the scaphoid and the barrel of the jig is advanced to the scaphoid tubercle to provide provisional compression of the fracture. The reduction of the scaphoid may be arthroscopically assessed by placing the arthroscope in the radial midcarpal portal (Figure 17.40).

If the fracture is not anatomically reduced, the barrel of the jig is released and with manipulation or joysticks, the scaphoid fracture is anatomically reduced (Figure 17.41). Once anatomic reduction of the scaphoid fracture is confirmed arthroscopically, the barrel of the jig is then compressed to provide provisional fixation (Figure 17.42). A guidewire is then

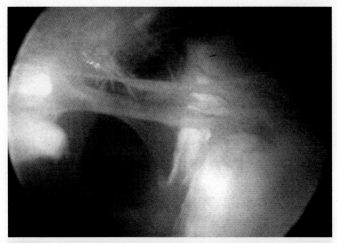

FIGURE 17.40 Arthroscopic view of the scaphoid fracture from the radial midcarpal space with the Herbert–Whipple jig applied but not tensioned. The fracture gap remains open.

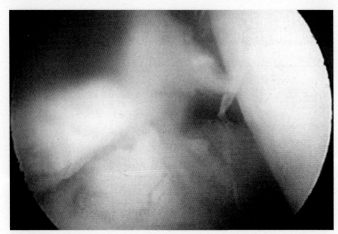

FIGURE 17.41 Arthroscopic view of the reduced fracture gap. In most incidences, with extension and radial deviation, the fracture can be manipulated in the tower to be anatomically reduced, and the jig is compressed to provide provisional stabilization.

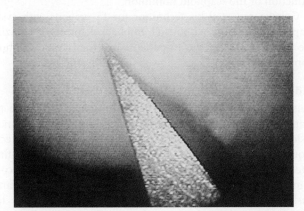

FIGURE 17.39 Arthroscopic view of the Herbert–Whipple jig being inserted through the 1-2 portal. The spike of the guide is placed at the junction of the scapholunate interosseous ligament and the proximal pole of the scaphoid.

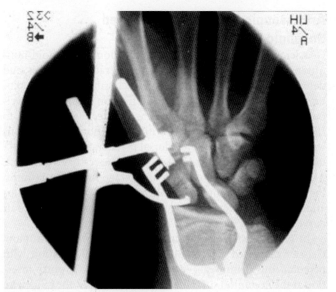

FIGURE 17.42 Fluoroscopic view showing ideal alignment of the scaphoid fracture with the Herbert–Whipple jig (Zimmer, Warsaw, IN) in place.

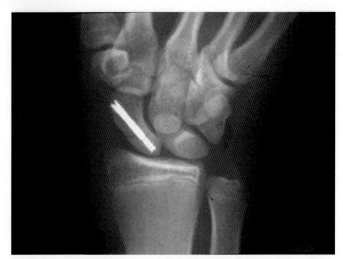

FIGURE 17.43 Fluoroscopic view showing the Herbert–Whipple screw (Zimmer, Warsaw, IN) placed across the fracture site.

TABLE 17.2   Scaphoid Nonunion Classifications of Slade and Geissler

Type	Description
I	Delayed presentation at 4-12 weeks
II	Fibrous union, minimal fracture line
III	Minimal sclerosis <1 mm
IV	Cystic formation, 1-5 mm
V	Humpback deformity, >5 mm cystic change
VI	Wrist arthrosis

From Geissler WB, Slade JF: Fractures of the carpal bones. In Wolfe SW, Hotchkiss RN, Peterson WC, et al, editors: *Green's operative hand surgery*, vol 1, ed 6, Philadelphia, 2010, Elsevier, pp 639–707.

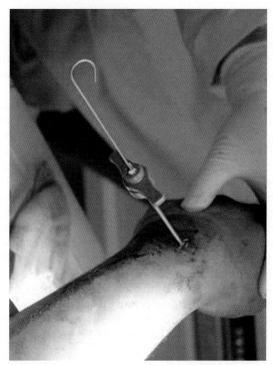

FIGURE 17.44 In cases of scaphoid nonunion without a humpback deformity, the nonunion can be addressed either with percutaneous bone grafting or injection of putty (DBM) into the nonunion site. Here a bone biopsy needle is filled with putty and inserted over a guidewire directly into the scaphoid nonunion site.

placed down the jig into the long axis of the scaphoid. It is then drilled from distal to proximal, measured, and the appropriate length Herbert–Whipple headless compression screw is placed (Zimmer, Warsaw, IN) (Figure 17.43).

Arthroscopic Reduction of Selected Scaphoid Nonunions

Geissler and Slade developed a classification of scaphoid nonunions based on the chronicity, degree of fracture sclerosis, and deformity (Table 17.2).[54] Utilizing this classification, the percutaneous arthroscopic-assisted dorsal fixation techniques developed for acute scaphoid fractures were effective in types I to III.[52] In addition, 15 patients with stable fibrous nonunions were treated with Slade et al's dorsal percutaneous technique[104] using a headless cannulated screw and no accessory bone graft. All patients' fractures healed in an average time of 3 months. Eight of the 15 patients had confirmed healing with CT evaluation. This technique avoided the morbidity of bone graft harvest from the iliac crest or distal radius.

In patients who have a type IV cystic scaphoid nonunion, Geissler described a technique for arthroscopic fixation with percutaneous demineralized bone matrix (DBM) putty insertion at the nonunion site. Utilizing this technique, the guidewire is placed arthroscopically as previously described. The scaphoid is then reamed with a cannulated reamer. A bone biopsy needle

is filled with DBM putty and placed directly over the wire into the cystic nonunion site of the scaphoid (Figure 17.44). The guidewire is then retracted distally but still remains in the distal pole of the scaphoid. The DBM putty is then injected through the bone biopsy needle directly into the central aspect of the scaphoid at the nonunion site that has been previously reamed. The guidewire is then advanced back through the bone biopsy needle from a volar-to-dorsal direction out the dorsum of the wrist following putty injection. In this manner, the guidewire passes through the original path of the proximal pole of the scaphoid and out the soft tissues. A headless cannulated screw is inserted over the wire across the scaphoid nonunion site. As before, both the radial carpal and midcarpal spaces are reevaluated arthroscopically to confirm position of the screw and reduction of the scaphoid nonunion.

Geissler reported his technique for 15 patients with cystic scaphoid nonunions without a humpback deformity.[53] Utilizing the technique, 14 of the 15 patients had their cystic scaphoid nonunions healed.

Transscaphoid Perilunate Fracture-Dislocations

Geissler recently described an all-arthroscopic technique for management of seven patients with transscaphoid perilunate dislocations (unpublished data) (Figure 17.45). With this technique, the wrist is initially arthroscopically evaluated to confirm a tear to the lunotriquetral interosseous ligament. Once confirmed, a SLIC screw (Acumed, Hillsboro, OR) is percutaneously inserted over a guidewire and stabilized across the lunotriquetral interval (Figure 17.46). The wrist is then suspended in a traction tower. The scaphoid is arthroscopically stabilized as previously described (Figures 17.47 through 17.50).

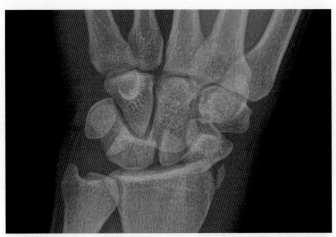

FIGURE 17.45 Radiographic view of a transscaphoid perilunate dislocation.

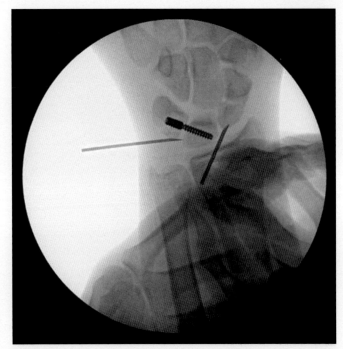

FIGURE 17.47 Fluoroscopic view following stabilization of the lunotriquetral interval. The wrist is arthroscopically evaluated and the exact location of the guidewire needle in the proximal pole of the scaphoid has been identified.

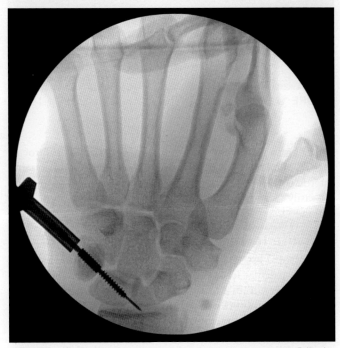

FIGURE 17.46 The dislocation has been anatomically reduced. Following arthroscopic confirmation of a complete tear to the lunotriquetral interosseous ligament, a scapholunate-intercarpal-carpal screw (Acumed, Hillsboro, OR) is percutaneously placed across the lunotriquetral interval.

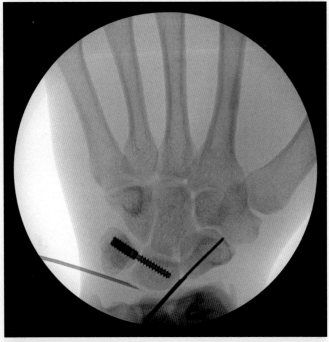

FIGURE 17.48 Fluoroscopic view showing ideal placement of the guidewire down the axis of the scaphoid.

At 3 months, all fractures had healed and the wrist flexion–extension arc ranged from 70 to 120 degrees. Five of the seven patients had no pain. Stabilization of perilunate dislocations without Kirschner wires allowed patients to participate in physical therapy at an earlier stage and resulted in a very functional range of motion at 3 months postoperatively.[55]

Fractures of the Distal Radius

Articular fractures of the distal radius are a unique subset of distal fractures.[70] The prognosis for these injuries depends on restoration of original length, articular inclination, and articular reduction both of the radial carpal and distal radial ulnar joint.[4,12,45,70,72,75,114,117,123] Arthroscopic-assisted fixation of intra-articular fractures allows for reduction of the joint surface

under bright light and magnified conditions.[74,131] It allows for lavage of hematoma and multiple-joint debris and management of associated soft tissue injuries that may occur with these fractures.[43,83,97]

Arthroscopic-assisted fixation can be used for simple articular fractures that have large, well-defined fragments, including the radial styloid, volar and dorsal die punch, volar and dorsal

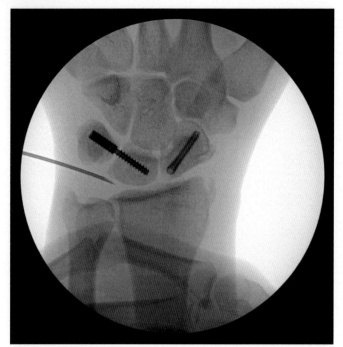

FIGURE 17.49 Fluoroscopic view showing screw stabilization of the lunotriquetral interval and the scaphoid fracture with a headless cannulated screw. The transscaphoid perilunate dislocation has been completely stabilized by percutaneous and arthroscopic fixation. Without a buried or protruding Kirschner wire earlier range of motion can be initiated.

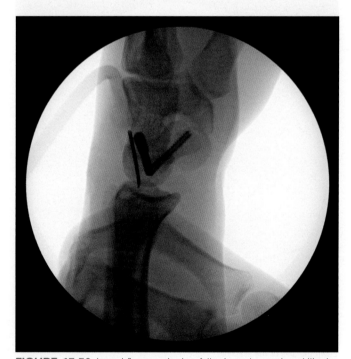

FIGURE 17.50 Lateral fluoroscopic view following arthroscopic stabilization of the transscaphoid perilunate dislocation.

Barton, and as an adjunct in the management of three- and four-part articular fractures with metaphyseal comminution.[49,134] It is well known that a fracture of the distal radius is a true wrist injury rather than a fracture alone and is associated with additional soft tissue injuries.[56,62,65,80,89] Both articular and nonarticular fractures of the distal radius have a high preva-

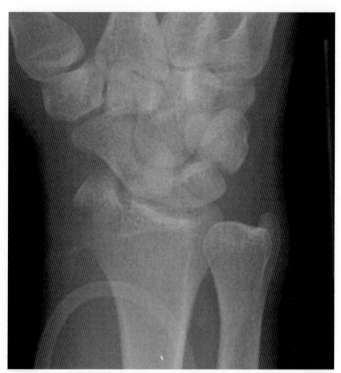

FIGURE 17.51 Fluoroscopic view of a displaced fracture of the radial styloid.

lence of associated soft tissue injuries of the triangular fibrocartilage complex as well as scapholunate and lunotriquetral interosseous ligaments.[50] These associated soft tissue injuries are easily seen arthroscopically and can be managed at the same sitting.

Operative Technique

Arthroscopic-assisted reduction and fixation of displaced unstable articular fractures of the distal radius should generally have surgery within 2 to 10 days from injury. A delay of at least 48 h helps to minimize bleeding from the fracture during the arthroscopy.[47] For fractures that are 10 days or older, it may sometimes be difficult to manipulate the fragments due to early healing. The operating room is set up so that both fluoroscopy and arthroscopy can be used simultaneously. The wrist is suspended with 10 lb of traction in a standard traction tower. The standard 3-4, 6-R, and 6-U portals are made. It is helpful to lavage the joint of fracture debris and hematoma prior to introduction of the arthroscope. This is done by placing the inflow through the 6-U portal and the arthroscopic cannula in the 3-4 portal. A shaver is brought in through the 6-R portal to remove any further fracture debris. A traditional diagnostic wrist arthroscopy is then performed (see Video 17.1).

Fractures of the radial styloid are ideal for arthroscopic management. Rotation is best judged by looking across the wrist from an ulnar portal. Under fluoroscopy, one or two guidewires are placed using oscillation mode into the tip of the radial styloid but not across the fracture site (Figures 17.51 and 17.52). Using the guidewires in the radial styloid fragment and a trocar placed in the 3-4 portal, the radial styloid fragment can be manipulated and anatomically reduced back to the radius (Figures 17.53 and 17.54). The guidewire is then advanced across the fracture site for provisional stabilization. Once the

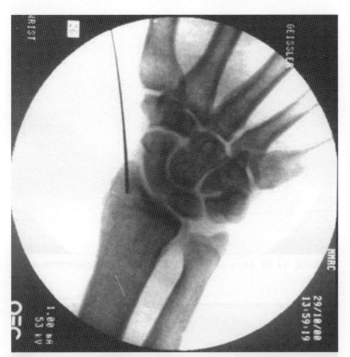

FIGURE 17.52 Fluoroscopic view of a guidewire placed into the radial styloid fragment. This can be used as a joystick to help reduce the fracture; it is not placed across the fracture site.

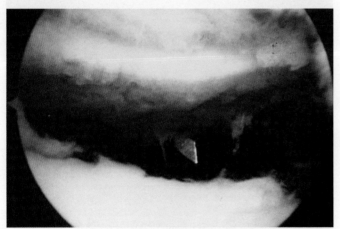

FIGURE 17.53 Arthroscopic view showing the guidewire in the radial styloid fragment. It is best to place the arthroscope in the 6-R portal to look across the wrist to judge rotation of the radial styloid fragment.

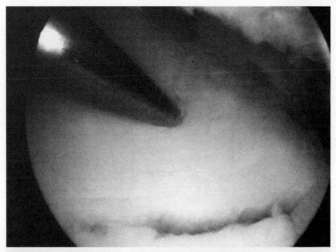

FIGURE 17.54 Arthroscopic view showing reduction of the radial styloid fragment with a combination of the guidewire joystick and a trocar inserted through the 3-4 portal to help control rotation and position of the fracture fragment.

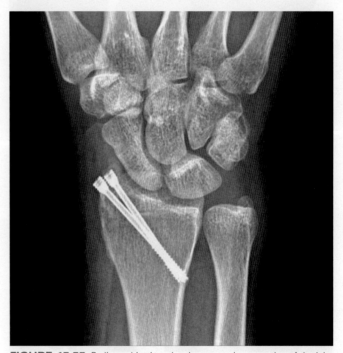

FIGURE 17.55 Radiographic view showing anatomic restoration of the joint surface with stabilization of the radial styloid fracture with two headless cannulated screws.

fracture is judged to be anatomically reduced by arthroscopic and fluoroscopic confirmation, additional wires are placed across the fracture site. One or two headless cannulated screws are then placed into the radial styloid fragment (Figure 17.55). By utilizing headless screws, the implant is contained within the bone, which decreases soft tissue irritation and enables early mobilization.

In three-part articular fractures without metaphyseal comminution, the radial styloid fragment may be closed, reduced, and provisionally pinned under fluoroscopy (Figure 17.56). This will serve as a landmark to elevate the lunate facet. The wrist is then suspended in a traction tower and the articular surface is evaluated. A headless cannulated screw is placed in

the radial styloid fragment as previously described. The lunate facet fragment is identified and a needle is placed over the fragment percutaneously. This is used as a fluoroscopic landmark. A Steinmann pin is placed approximately 2 cm proximal to the needle to percutaneously elevate the die punch fragment (Figure 17.57). The previously reduced radial styloid fragment is used as an arthroscopic landmark to ensure the lunate facet fragment is correctly reduced (Figure 17.58).

Once the fragment is elevated and judged to be anatomic, a guidewire is placed subchondrally transversely beneath the bone surface to stabilize the fragment, which is usually best seen

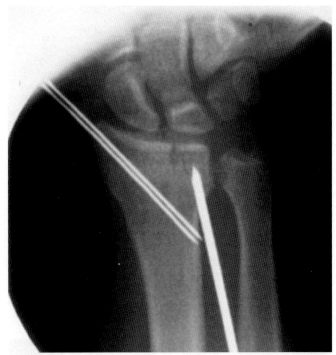

FIGURE 17.56 In three-part fractures, the radial styloid is provisionally pinned and reduced. This can then be used as a landmark to help reduce the impacted lunate facet fragment.

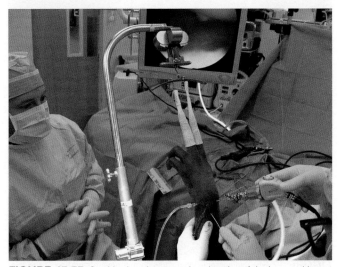

FIGURE 17.57 Outside view demonstrating elevation of the impacted lunate facet with a large Steinmann pin as viewed with the arthroscope in the 3-4 portal.

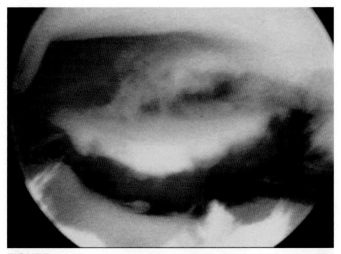

FIGURE 17.58 Arthroscopic view of a displaced three-part fracture to the distal radius.

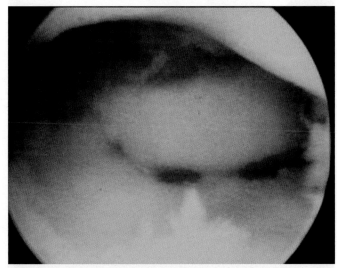

FIGURE 17.59 Arthroscopic view following reduction of the impacted lunate facet fragment with the arthroscope in the 3-4 portal.

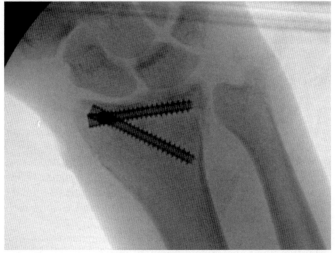

FIGURE 17.60 Fluoroscopic view showing anatomic restoration of the joint surface with two headless cannulated screws. One screw is placed perpendicular to the radial styloid fragment, and the second is placed transversely beneath the subchondral bone. Following placement of the screw, rotation of the forearm is performed to evaluate for any potential crepitus from a prominent screw.

with the arthroscope in the 3-4 portal (Figure 17.59). It is important to pronate and supinate the wrist to ensure the transverse guide pin does not violate the distal radial ulnar joint. An additional headless cannulated screw is then placed transversely over the guidewire to support the lunate facet fragment (Figure 17.60).

Usually the guidewire is aimed slightly dorsally because the fragment is generally a dorsal fragment. Following placement of the headless cannulated screw, the wrist is again pronated and supinated to make sure there is no violation of any hardware into the distal radial ulnar joint. Arthroscopic management of transradial perilunate fractures may be performed.

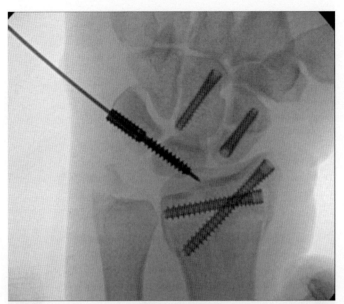

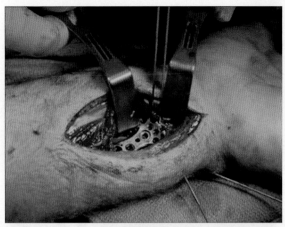

FIGURE 17.63 An Acu-loc (Acumed, Hillsboro, OR) is placed through a standard volar incision to stabilize the displaced fracture. Under fluoroscopic visualization, the articular reduction is provisionally stabilized.

FIGURE 17.61 Fluoroscopic view demonstrating arthroscopic and percutaneous fixation of a greater arc transscaphoid perilunate dislocation. The displaced fracture of the distal radius and scaphoid are arthroscopically reduced. The fracture of the capitate was percutaneously reduced and stabilized with a headless cannulated screw, and a scapholunate-intercarpal-carpal screw (Acumed, Hillsboro, OR) was placed percutaneously across the lunotriquetral interval to stabilize a complete tear of the lunotriquetral interosseous ligament.

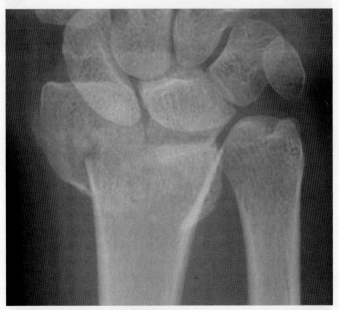

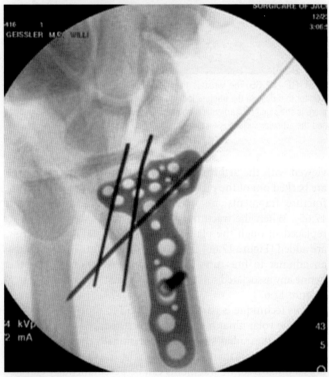

FIGURE 17.64 Fluoroscopic view following volar placement of the distal radius plate with reduction to the articular surface. Under fluoroscopy, the articular reduction looks satisfactory.

FIGURE 17.62 Radiographic view of a displaced articular fracture of the distal radius with metaphyseal comminution.

In this example, all fractures were treated percutaneously or arthroscopically, thereby enabling early range of motion (Figure 17.61).

For patients who have metaphyseal comminution, simple cannulated screw fixation alone may not sufficiently stabilize the fracture (Figure 17.62). Wrist arthroscopy is used as an adjunct in the management of such fractures. A standard volar approach is made over the flexor carpi radialis tendon to the wrist if a volar plate is being used. The flexor carpi radialis

tendon is retracted radially, the flexor pollicis longus is retracted ulnarly, and the pronator quadratus is released to expose the fracture site. The fracture is reduced under fluoroscopy and a volar plate is placed and attached proximally to the shaft. The plate is provisionally pinned distally to the fracture site (Figures 17.63 and 17.64). Following this, the wrist is suspended in a traction tower and the arthroscope is placed in the 3-4 portal. The joint is lavaged as before with inflow through the 6-U portal.

The fracture line is identified, and the distal screws are then placed in the plate if the fracture is anatomically reduced as

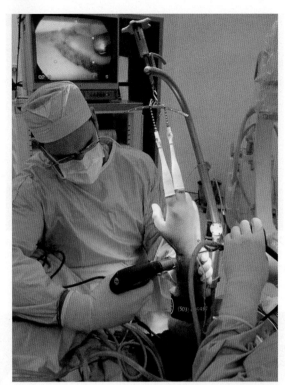

FIGURE 17.65 The wrist is then arthroscopically evaluated. Note at the monitor that despite the fracture looking anatomically reduced under fluoroscopy, there is still significant articular step-off. The pins are then backed off the fracture and the articular surface is anatomically reduced as viewed arthroscopically.

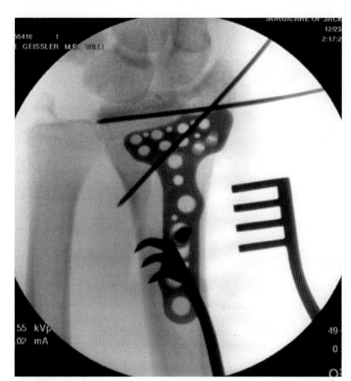

FIGURE 17.66 Fluoroscopic view showing anatomic restoration of the joint surface after being anatomically reduced as viewed arthroscopically.

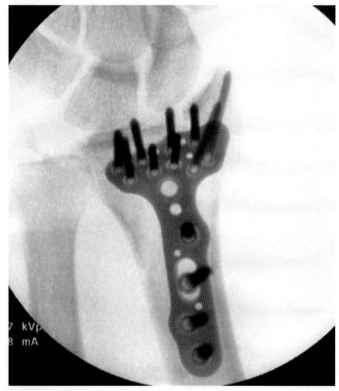

FIGURE 17.67 Fluoroscopic view showing anatomic restoration of the joint surface with the volar plate in place.

viewed with the arthroscope. The provisional Kirschner wires are backed out of the plate if the fracture is not reduced and the fracture fragments are manipulated percutaneously (Figure 17.65). When the fracture is reduced, the Kirschner wires are replaced through the plate and then the distal locking screws are added (Figure 17.66). In this manner, arthroscopy is used as an adjunct to fine-tune the anatomic reduction and further define any associated soft tissue injuries that occur in these areas (Figure 17.67).

This technique is particularly helpful in four-part fractures, where the volar ulnar fragments are first reduced with the radial styloid to the radial shaft and provisionally stabilized by the plate. The wrist is then suspended in the traction tower and the dorsal ulnar fracture fragments can be percutaneously elevated and reduced to the volar fragment. Once anatomic reduction has been achieved, the distal locking screws are placed.

del Pinal et al. have recently advocated the advantages of dry arthroscopy in the management of distal radius fractures. They described the technique that was used for seven patients.[35]

TREATMENT OF TRIANGULAR FIBROCARTILAGE COMPLEX INJURIES

Injuries to the triangular fibrocartilage complex (TFCC) typically occur with extension and pronation of the axial loaded wrist. The most common mechanism of injury is a fall on an outstretched hand. Peripheral tears of the articular disk are common athletic injuries that involve racket sports or golf that requires rapid twisting and loading to the ulnar side of the wrist. Peripheral ulnar-sided tears of the articular disk are also common work injuries. Patients often describe a mechanism of traction or torqueing of the forearm that occurred when a motorized drill bit suddenly binds. The reader is referred to Chapter 14 for a complete discussion of the anatomy, kinematics, and classification of injuries of the TFCC.

Patients with peripheral tears of the TFCC complain of deep diffuse pain across the ulnar side of the wrist. Frequently, they complain of weakness when gripping as well as a clicking sensation with rotation of the forearm. They complain particularly of pain with twisting of the wrist such as turning a doorknob or twisting the lid off a jar. Patients with a peripheral tear are point tender in the prestyloid recess. Patients who have a central tear of the articular disk frequently complain of pain over the distal aspect of the ulna. This pain can be accentuated by hyperpronation and supination of the wrist. Dorsal subluxation of the ulnar head in relation to the radius can be seen in foveal detachments.

Indications for surgical intervention include specific ulnar-sided wrist pain not relieved by conservative management for 3 months. An additional indication is for patients with symptomatic instability of the distal radial ulnar joint that is not relieved by immobilization.[60]

ARTHROSCOPIC MANAGEMENT OF TRAUMATIC INJURIES

Palmer Class IA tears (see Chapter 14) are perforations of the articular disk that are usually 1 to 2 mm wide and located approximately 2 to 3 mm just ulnar to its radial attachment to the sigmoid notch (Figure 17.68).[92] Arthroscopic débridement of the unstable flap of the tear is a preferred treatment in those patients whose symptoms do not resolve with temporary splinting and are ulnar neutral or minus. The arthroscope is placed in the 3-4 portal and a small banana blade is inserted through the 6-R portal. The unstable flap is outlined with a banana blade and a grasper is used to remove the fragment. The arthroscope is then transferred to the 6-R portal and a small punch is inserted through the 3-4 portal to débride the most ulnar aspect of the tear (Figure 17.69). A small joint shaver is then used to

smooth the remaining portion of the articular disk. Approximately two-thirds of the articular disk can be excised without causing instability. An approximately 2-mm rim should be left intact to protect the volar and dorsal radial ulnar ligaments, which are important stabilizers of the distal radial ulnar joint (Figure 17.70).

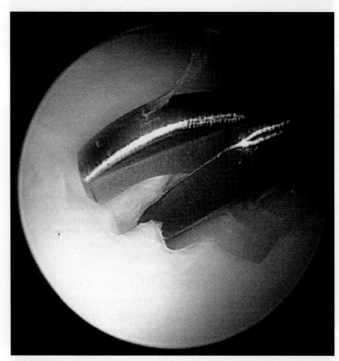

FIGURE 17.69 View with the arthroscope in the 3-4 portal and a wrist arthroscopic punch in the 6-R portal débriding the unstable tear back to a stable surface.

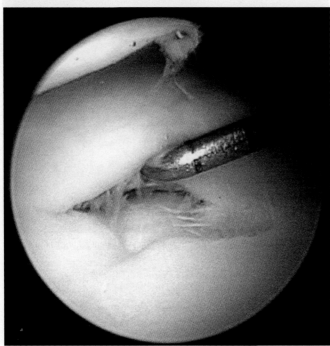

FIGURE 17.68 View with the arthroscope in the 3-4 portal demonstrating a Palmer type IA tear of the articular disk of the triangular fibrocartilage complex.

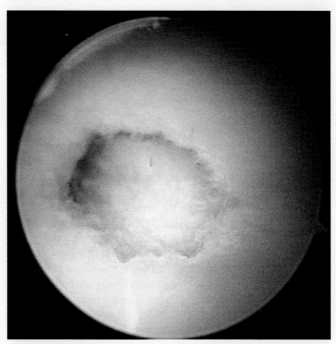

FIGURE 17.70 Arthroscopic view following débridement of the tear of the articular disk back to a stable surface. The ulnar head can be seen through the defect of the articular disk.

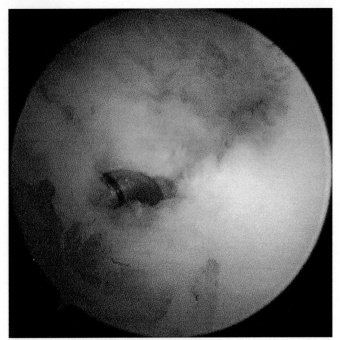

FIGURE 17.71 View with the arthroscope in the 3-4 portal demonstrating a peripheral tear of the articular disk (Palmer type IB).

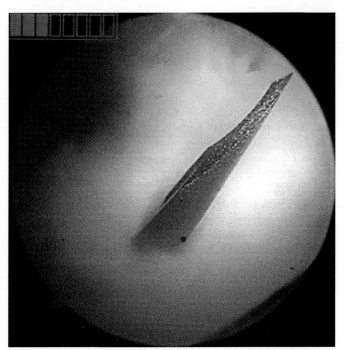

FIGURE 17.72 Arthroscopic view showing an 18-gauge needle being inserted through the floor of the extensor carpi ulnaris tendon sheath and perpendicular to the articular disk. It is imperative that the needle be placed as vertically as possible so that, as the suture is being inserted and tensioned, it will not shred through the articular disk.

Class IB injuries are traumatic avulsions of the triangular fibrocartilage complex from its insertion onto the distal ulna. These injuries usually are associated to some degree with instability to the distal radial ulnar joint. Several techniques for repair have been described in the literature.[3] These injuries are potentially reparable due to the blood supply.[13,112]

Whipple described an outside-in technique, wherein sutures are placed longitudinally to reattach the articular disk back to the floor of the tendon sheath of the extensor carpi ulnaris.[130] In this technique, the arthroscope is placed in the 3-4 portal and a peripheral tear is débrided with a small motorized shaver through the 6-R portal to help delineate the site of the tear and to facilitate revascularization (Figure 17.71). The 6-R portal is then elongated for approximately 1.5 cm and the retinaculum of the extensor carpi ulnaris tendon sheath is opened. The tendon is retracted ulnarly to expose the floor of the sheath of the ECU. An 18-gauge needle is then placed as vertically as possible to the floor of the sheath of the extensor carpi ulnaris to perforate the articular disk as viewed arthroscopically (Figure 17.72).

A 2.0-PDS suture is advanced through the needle into the radial carpal space (Figure 17.73). A suture retriever is then passed through the floor of the sheath of the extensor carpi ulnaris distal to the articular disk to retrieve the suture (Figures 17.74 and 17.75). Usually three sutures are placed, as described in the preceding, to close the tear (Figures 17.76 and 17.77). The wrist is taken out of traction and placed in slight supination and the sutures are tied. A sliding knot is very useful to tension the repair of the disk through such a small incision. It is vital to close the retinaculum of the ECU following the procedure. Corso et al. reported a high percentage of good-to-excellent results with this technique in a multicenter study.[29]

Ekman and Poehling described a Tuohy needle technique for repair of peripheral ulnar-sided tears to the articular disk.[39]

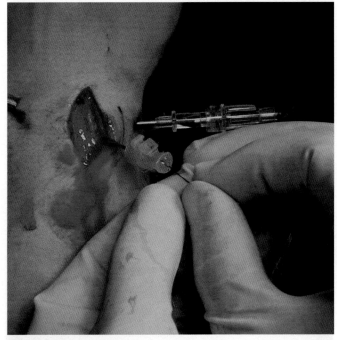

FIGURE 17.73 Outside view showing a monofilament suture being inserted through the needle.

With this technique, a 20-gauge anesthetic Tuohy needle is placed into the radial carpal space through either the 1-2 or 3-4 portal. The arthroscope is placed in the 4-5 portal. The Tuohy needle is passed across the wrist to the torn edge of the articular disk above the ulnar styloid process and advanced out of the

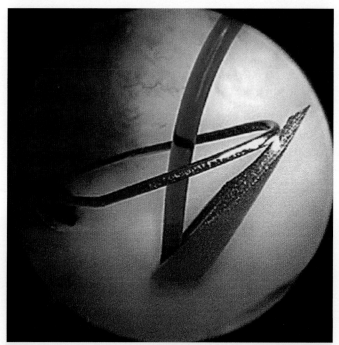

FIGURE 17.74 Arthroscopic view showing a suture grasper being inserted distal to the articular disk to grasp the monofilament suture as it is being inserted through the 18-gauge needle.

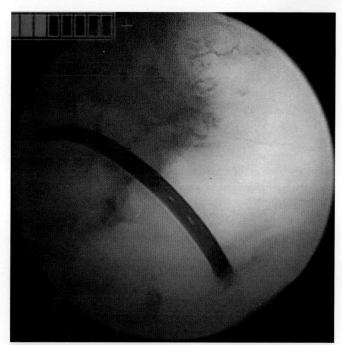

FIGURE 17.76 Arthroscopic view showing a monofilament suture placed across the peripheral tear in a vertical mattress suture.

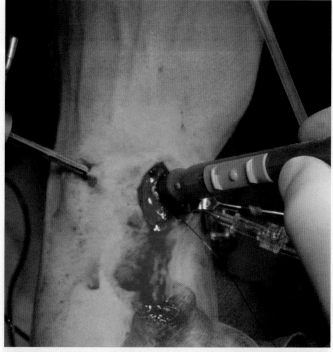

FIGURE 17.75 Outside view demonstrating the suture grasper pulling the suture out of the joint to be tied on the floor of the sheath of the extensor carpi ulnaris tendon.

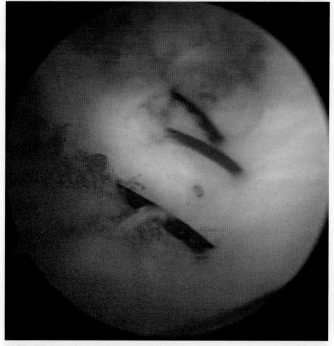

FIGURE 17.77 Arthroscopic view following placement of three monofilament sutures across the peripheral tear after being tied. Note the tensioning of the articular disk.

skin. A grasper may be helpful to direct the needle across the wrist and help perforate the articular disk.

A 2.0 absorbable suture is threaded through the entire needle and exits the skin. A hemostat is placed on the suture exiting the skin. The needle is retrieved back into the radial carpal space and repassed through the edge of the articular disk and advanced out the skin so a whole mattress suture is placed. The loop of

suture that is exiting the needle is then pulled out the ulnar side of the wrist. This process may be repeated two or three times to form a horizontal mattress suture. Blunt dissection is then carried out where the sutures are tied onto the joint capsule. It is very important to ensure that branches of the dorsal sensory branch of the ulnar nerve are not entrapped beneath the sutures as they are tied down to the capsule.

Geissler described an all-arthroscopic knotless technique for repair of peripheral ulnar-sided tears back to the ulna.[52] In this technique, the standard 3-4 and 6-R portals are made. An accessory 6-R portal is made approximately 1.5 cm distal to and in line with the 6-R portal. The accessory 6-R portal is made by using an 18-gauge needle inserted through the skin into the fovea at the base of the ulnar styloid (Figure 17.78). It is helpful if the wrist is flexed 20 to 30 degrees for easier access to the fovea. The accessory 6-R portal is enlarged with an 11 blade and blunt dissection is carried down with a hemostat to the capsule. A suture lasso is then inserted through the accessory 6-R portal into the radial carpal space. The curved suture lasso is then passed through the articular disk in a proximal-to-distal direction (Figures 17.79 and 17.80). It is helpful to gently twist the lasso with the thumb and index finger as it passes through the tough fibers of the articular disk.

The suture wire is then inserted through the lasso and retrieved through the 6-R portal with a crochet hook (Figure 17.81). A 2.0-fiber wire suture is then passed through the wire retriever and pulled out of the suture lasso distally through the handle (Figures 17.82 and 17.83). The suture lasso is then backed out of the articular disk and reinserted either anterior or posterior to the original perforation so that a horizontal mattress suture results (Figures 17.84 and 17.85). As the suture lasso passes through the articular disk for the second time, a loop of suture is formed; it will be retrieved through the 6-R portal with a suture retriever. At this stage, neither suture limb is exiting the 6-R portal (Figure 17.86).

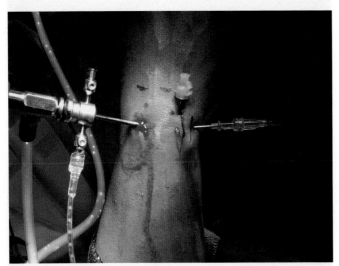

FIGURE 17.78 Outside view demonstrating the accessory 6-R portal. Note that this portal is approximately 1.5 cm distal and in line with the standard 6-R portal.

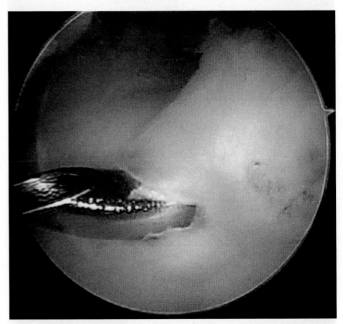

FIGURE 17.80 The suture lasso is then passed through the articular disk. It is helpful to gently twist the lasso between the thumb and index finger to allow it to penetrate through the articular disk.

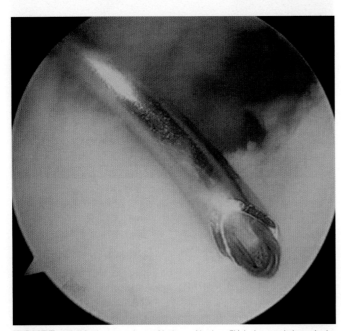

FIGURE 17.79 A suture lasso (Arthrex, Naples, FL) is inserted through the accessory 6-R portal.

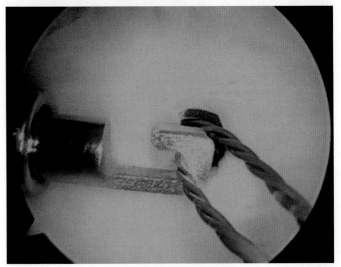

FIGURE 17.81 A crochet hook (Arthrex, Naples, FL) is inserted through the standard 6-R portal to grab the lasso suture wire.

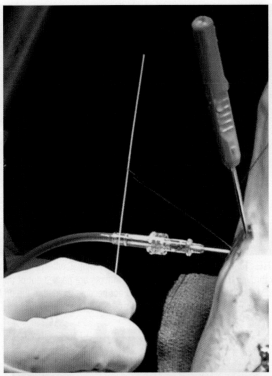

FIGURE 17.82 The suture wire is then pulled out of the standard 6-R portal. A 2.0-fiber wire suture (Arthrex, Naples, FL) is passed through the suture wire.

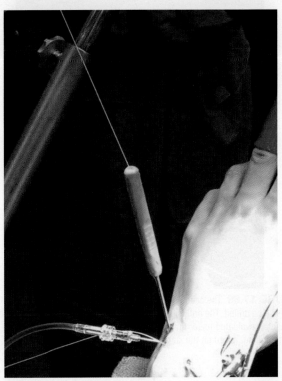

FIGURE 17.83 The suture wire is then used to pull the fiber wire suture out distally through the handle of the suture lasso.

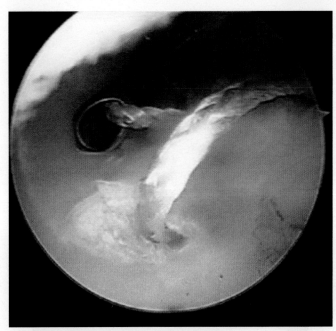

FIGURE 17.84 Arthroscopic view showing the suture lasso as it is about to be passed for the second time through the articular disk. It is important not to pull the suture lasso out of the joint following placement of the first suture to help eliminate any soft tissue bridge on the fiber wire suture.

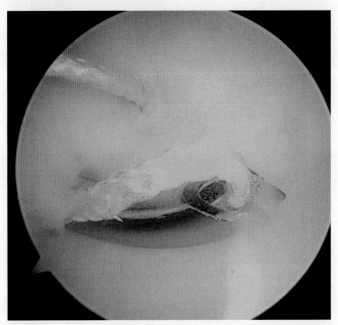

FIGURE 17.85 Arthroscopic view showing the suture lasso (Arthrex, Naples, FL) piercing through the articular disk for the second time.

A slotted cannula is then inserted through the accessory 6-R portal into the radial carpal space. Then a crochet hook is used to retrieve both sutures distally through the cannula in the accessory 6-R portal (Figure 17.87). The cannula is then advanced down directly onto the bone at the ulnar fovea and held in position. The two suture limbs are pulled out of the slot in the cannula so that they will not be twisted as the ulna is drilled (Figure 17.88). The drill is inserted through the cannula and the base of the ulna is drilled as the cannula is held firmly against the ulna bone (Figure 17.89). The two suture limbs are threaded through a suture anchor, and they are inserted down the cannula into the drill hole (Figure 17.90). The sutures are tensioned as the PushLock® is advanced into the ulnar head (Figures 17.91 and 17.92).

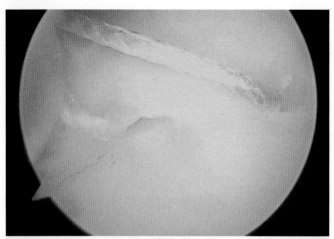

FIGURE 17.86 Arthroscopic view from the 3-4 portal showing a horizontal mattress suture of 2.0-fiber wire (Arthrex, Naples, FL) through the articular disk.

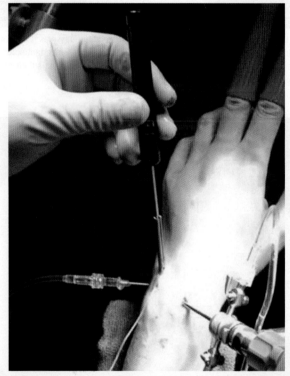

FIGURE 17.87 An outside view of a slotted cannula being passed through the accessory 6-R portal. A crochet hook is then used to pull the 2.0-fiber wire suture out through the cannula.

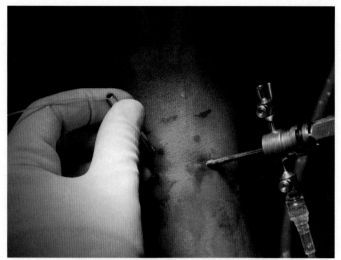

FIGURE 17.88 Outside view showing the 2.0-fiber wire being passed out distally through the slot of the cannula. The sutures are passed out of the slot so as the distal ulna is being drilled, they will not become twisted in the drill.

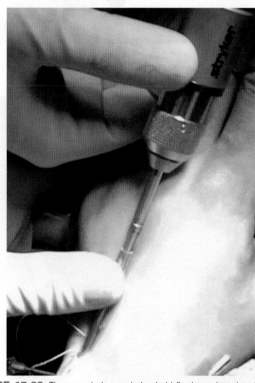

FIGURE 17.89 The cannula is now being held firmly against the ulnar fovea as it is being drilled. The drill is cannulated so that a guidewire can be placed and its position evaluated under fluoroscopy to confirm its location in the ulna fovea prior to drilling, based on the surgeon's preference.

After the anchor has been seated, moderate tension is applied to the handle to make sure the anchor and sutures cannot be pulled out. If there is resistance, the anchor has been inserted correctly into the bone. The tendency is for the anchor to slide off the volar aspect of the ulnar. If this occurs, the anchor will easily pull out with minimal tension on the handle and may be simply reinserted. When the correct anchor tension is confirmed, the suture ends are cut with a small up-biter and removed through the 6-R portal.

Postoperatively, the patient is immobilized in an above-elbow splint for approximately 4 weeks and then at week 3 a removable wrist brace is used. General wrist flexion–extension range-of-motion exercises start immediately. General pronation and supination exercises are initiated at week 4. At 7 weeks postoperatively, the patient is referred for a physical therapy program for grip strengthening and improved range of motion.

Class IC tears are rare and involve the distal attachment of the articular disk to the lunate and lunotriquetral ligaments (Figure 17.93). Complete tears of the ulnocarpal ligaments can result in ulnar carpal instability and/or translocation of the

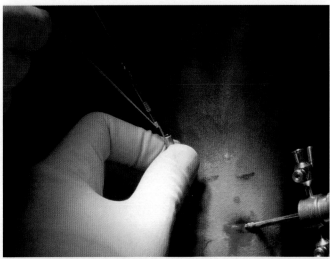

FIGURE 17.90 The suture is now being loaded into the mini-PushLock® anchor (Arthrex, Naples, FL) and then passed down the cannula.

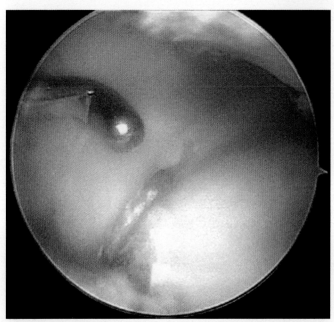

FIGURE 17.92 Arthroscopic view with the arthroscope in the 6-R portal showing repair of the peripheral tear of the articular disk back down to bone in an all arthroscopic knotless technique.

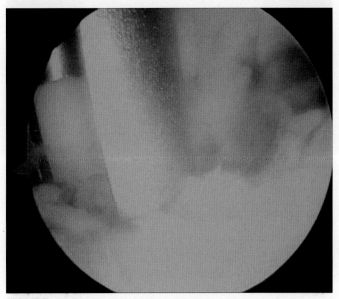

FIGURE 17.91 Arthroscopic view with the arthroscope in the 3-4 portal showing placement of the anchor down the cannula into the drilled hole.

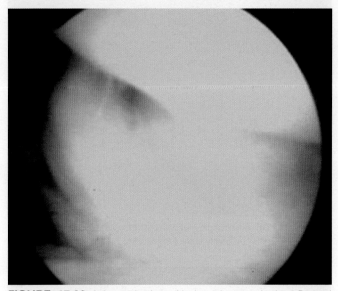

FIGURE 17.93 Arthroscopic view with the arthroscope in the 6-R portal demonstrating a distal tear of the ulnocarpal ligaments (Palmer type 1C).

ulnar carpus in relation to the radius. Patients complain of tenderness over the pisiform bone with locking and pain with grip exercises. Treatment recommendations include arthroscopic suture placement, as noted by Trumble, with good results (Figure 17.94).[115] Other options include simple débridement or electrothermal shrinkage which may restore tension back to the ulnar carpal ligaments (Figures 17.95 through 17.99).

Class ID lesions of the TFCC involve a traumatic avulsion of the articular disk from the attachment of the sigmoid notch of the distal radius and the volar and/or dorsal radial ulnar ligaments (see Figure 17-99). An ID tear may or may not be associated with a fracture of the distal radius involving the sigmoid notch. Patients may complain of diffuse tenderness along the ulnar side of the wrist.

In patients who have a traumatic avulsion, these fragments can be arthroscopically reduced and pinned.[41] Sagerman and

Short suggested suture repair if the patient does not have an avulsion.[101] In this technique, a cannula is placed in the 6-U portal and the arthroscope is placed in the 3-4 portal (Figures 17.100 and 17.101). A 0.062 Kirschner wire is put through the cannula in the 6-U portal and pushed from the sigmoid notch across the radius to exit the midaxial radial border near the diaphyseal–metaphyseal flare. Care must be taken to avoid injury to the radial sensory nerve; it is advisable to make a counterincision at the exit point of the K-wire and retract/protect the nerve. Three parallel drill holes are created. Long meniscus repair needles are then inserted at the 6-U portal through the articular disk and into the drill holes

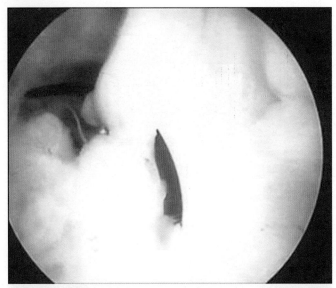

FIGURE 17.94 Arthroscopic view with the arthroscope in the 6-R portal showing placement of a suture through the articular disk and distally through the ulnocarpal ligament repairing the tear and restoring tension.

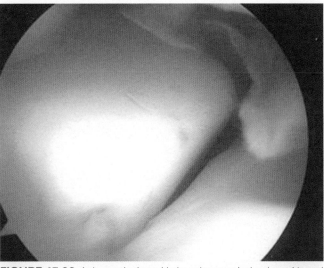

FIGURE 17.96 Arthroscopic view with the arthroscope in the ulnar midcarpal portal demonstrating instability to the lunotriquetral interval.

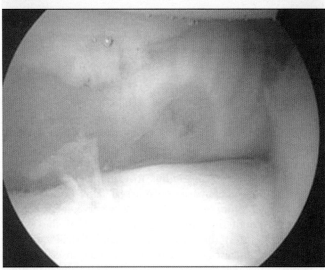

FIGURE 17.98 Arthroscopic view with the arthroscope in the 6-R portal following shrinkage of the ulnocarpal ligaments. Note the change in the apparent tension of the ligaments.

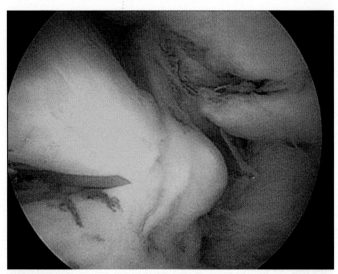

FIGURE 17.95 Arthroscopic view with the arthroscope in the 6-R portal demonstrating a tear and lack of tension to the ulnocarpal ligaments in a chronic Palmer type IC injury.

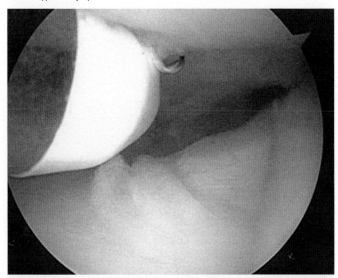

FIGURE 17.97 Arthroscopic view with the arthroscope in the 3-4 portal during thermal shrinkage to the ulnocarpal ligament.

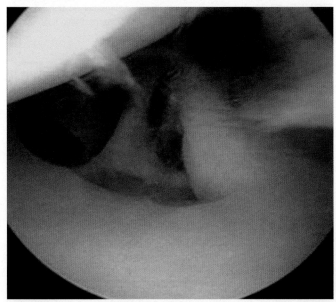

FIGURE 17.99 Arthroscopic view with the arthroscope in the 3-4 portal demonstrating a Palmer type 1D tear of the articular disk. This tear involved the volar radioulnar ligament.

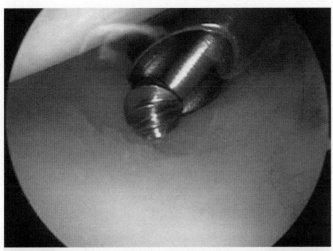

FIGURE 17.100 Arthroscopic burring of the sigmoid notch of the distal radius. Similar to a rotator cuff tear, the distal radius is lightly burred to subchondral bone to facilitate revascularization for the articular disk repair.

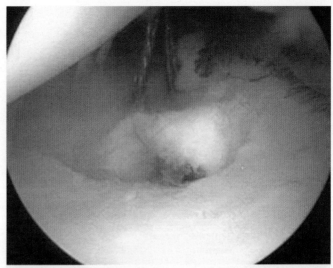

FIGURE 17.102 Arthroscopic view with the arthroscope in the 3-4 portal showing placement of a braided horizontal mattress suture through the articular disk for repair to the radius. Long meniscus needles have been placed through the articular disk and through transradial drill holes.

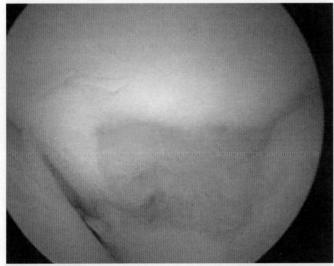

FIGURE 17.101 Arthroscopic view with the arthroscope in the 6-R portal following burring of the S notch. Note that just a minimal amount of bone is removed with this technique. If too much bone is taken, then the articular disk will not stretch to bone.

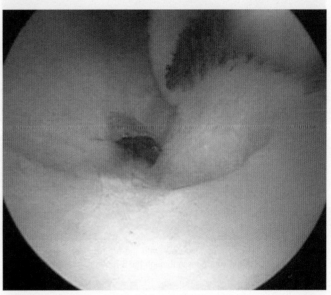

FIGURE 17.103 Arthroscopic view following placement of the meniscus needles through the distal radius as the suture is being tied. Note restoration of the tension of the volar radioulnar ligament.

(Figure 17.102). A grasper is helpful in terms of the 6-R portal to invert the disk to help with passage of the meniscus repair needle. Two stitches of a 2.0 Ethibond suture are placed horizontally in mattress fashion (Figures 17.103 and 17.104). Sutures are retrieved and tied to bone through the radial incision.

Recently, Corrella et al described a technique for all-arthroscopic knotless repair of radial-sided TFCC tears (Figure 17.105).[28] It requires use of the 3-4, 4-5, and 6-R portals. This technique requires one visualization portal (3-4) and two working portals (4-5 and 6-R). The 70-degree TFC suture lasso (Arthrex, Naples, FL) is inserted through the 6-R portal (Figure 17.106). The tip is situated just above the articular disk, and it penetrates from distally to proximally, coming out underneath the tear. It is sometimes helpful to insert a probe through the 3-4 portal to make counterpressure from the inferior side. The suture lasso is then loaded with a fiber stick suture (Arthrex,

Naples, FL), which is a 2.0-fiber wire suture with a more rigid end to facilitate insertion in the passer. It is recovered with a minisuture hook (Arthrex, Naples, FL) or with a grasper through the 4-5 portal (Figure 17.107). The suture is retrieved through the 4-5 portal.

Following this, the suture lasso is withdrawn and is reinserted a few millimeters from the first point in a distal-to-proximal direction. The loop of the suture from the suture lasso is then retrieved through the 4-5 portal, leaving a vertical mattress-type suture (Figure 17.108). The suture lasso is withdrawn and a slotted cannula with an operator (TFC instrument kit, Arthrex, Naples, FL) is inserted through the 6-R portal (Figure 17.109). The operator is withdrawn from the cannula

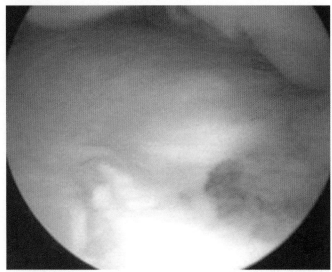

FIGURE 17.104 Arthroscopic view 2 years following repair of the articular disk. This demonstrates healing of the articular disk back to bone. In this case, the patient complained of pain over the screw where the suture was tied, so the screw was removed. This gave the opportunity to arthroscopically review the repair.

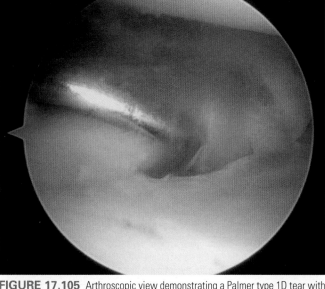

FIGURE 17.105 Arthroscopic view demonstrating a Palmer type 1D tear with instability of the distal radioulnar joint.

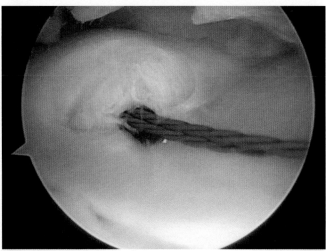

FIGURE 17.106 Arthroscopic view with the arthroscope in the 3-4 portal showing passage of the suture lasso through the 6-R portal.

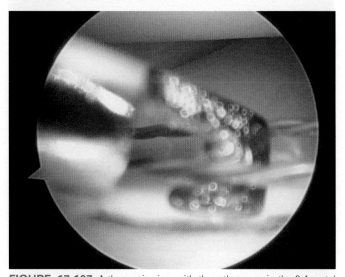

FIGURE 17.107 Arthroscopic view with the arthroscope in the 3-4 portal showing grasping of the suture wire with a crochet hook in the 4-5 portal.

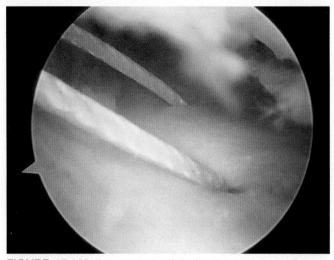

FIGURE 17.108 Arthroscopic view following placement of a 2.0-fiber wire (Arthrex, Naples, FL) stitch passed through the articular disk.

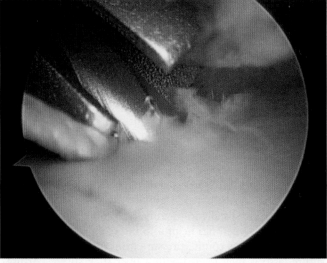

FIGURE 17.109 Arthroscopic view with the arthroscope in the 3-4 portal showing drilling of the distal radius with the cannula inserted through the 6-R portal.

and a minisuture hook is used to transfer the two sutures from the 4-5 portal to the 6-R portal. The sutures are passed outside the cannula through the slot so that drilling will not affect the sutures.

Through the obturator in the cannula, a guidewire can be placed to help confirm the ideal position of the eventual anchor. A cannulated drill is then used over the guidewire to drill the hole for the suture anchor (Figure 17.110). The 2.0-fiber wire suture is then inserted into a 2.5-mm PushLock anchor (Arthrex, Naples, FL), and the anchor is then inserted through the drill hole. Tension on the sutures can be performed by pulling the suture and holding the PushLock anchor in place. The anchor should be advanced until flush with the bone, locking the anchor and suture into the predrilled hole. The suture is cut and tension on repair of the articular disk is verified with a probe (Figure 17.111).

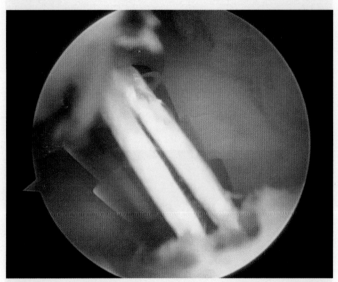

FIGURE 17.110 Arthroscopic view showing the mini-PushLock anchor (Arthrex, Naples, FL) being inserted through the 6-R portal repairing the articular disk back to the distal radius.

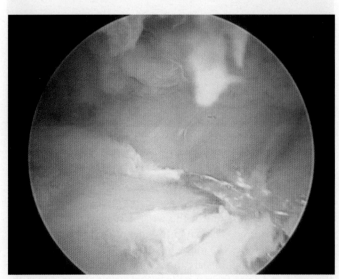

FIGURE 17.111 Arthroscopic view with the arthroscope in the 3-4 portal demonstrating repair of the Palmer type 1D tear back to the distal radius with an all-arthroscopic knotless technique.

DEGENERATIVE LESIONS CLASS II

Palmer class II lesions are degenerative lesions on the ulnar side of the wrist involving the TFCC (see Chapter 14). If a tear of the articular disk is present, it is usually circular as opposed to the typical traumatic longitudinal tear of an acute injury. The patient may also have chondromalacia of both the lunate and the ulna. The final stage includes disruption of the lunotriquetral interosseous ligaments. It is important to remember that in class II lesions, the prominent pathology is not the articular disk but the relatively long ulna, and ulna-shortening osteotomy is usually recommended. For patients who have a class IIA or IIB lesion when there is no perforation of the articular disk, an ulnar-shortening osteotomy is performed.[67,89,116] For patients who have a class IIC lesion, a perforation of the articular disk is present. In this instance, the surgeon has the option of an arthroscopic débridement of the ulnar head by working through the central tear of the articular disk.

Arthroscopic Wafer Resection of the Ulnar Head

The arthroscope is inserted in the 3-4 portal and a bur is placed in the 6-R portal. The head of the ulna is resected through the defect in the articular disk (Figure 17.112). The wrist is pronated and supinated to gain access to the peripheral margins of the ulnar head. In addition, the bur can be placed in a separate portal proximal to the articular disk to improve access to the ulnar head. Under normal conditions, approximately 3 to 4 mm of bone is resected. Fluoroscopy is strongly encouraged to monitor the amount of resection because arthroscopic magnification makes it difficult to judge the amount of bone that has been removed. Care should be taken not to take too much articular cartilage from the distal radial ulnar joint. When this happens, patients may have prolonged pain with forearm rotation.

The wafer procedure was first presented as an alternative to ulnar-shortening osteotomy by Feldon et al.[40] The wafer procedure was intended to resect the distalmost aspect of the ulnar head, while still preserving the attachments of the ulnar carpal

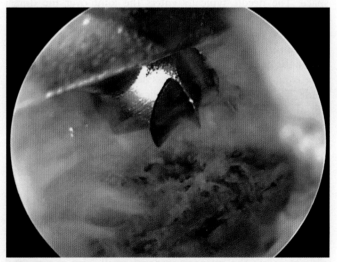

FIGURE 17.112 Arthroscopic wafer resection. The adequacy of the wafer resection of the ulnar head is viewed from the 6-U portal with the bur in the 4-5 portal.

ligaments in the TFCC's horizontal portion. By limiting the resection to 2 to 4 mm, the DRUJ is left relatively undisturbed. It has been shown that by shortening the ulnar head by 3 mm, the force transmitted across the ulna is decreased by 50%.[34,133]

Bernstein et al., in a retrospective comparative study, found that combined arthroscopic TFCC débridement and the arthroscopic wafer procedure provided similar pain relief and restorative function with fewer procedures compared to arthroscopic débridement of a torn TFC and ulnar-shortening osteotomy.[17] However, in this author's opinion, patients who have an arthroscopic wafer procedure have lingering discomfort with pronation and supination compared to open ulnar-shortening osteotomy.

In class IID lesions, there is instability to the lunotriquetral interval. An open ulnar-shortening osteotomy is recommended because traction on the ulnar carpal ligaments helps reduce instability to the lunotriquetral interval. In class IIE lesions, there are frank arthritic changes involving the distal radial ulnar joint, and treatment must address the arthritis in addition to any component of ulnar impaction.

ARTHROSCOPIC GANGLIONECTOMY

Arthroscopic excision of dorsal ganglions was popularized by Osterman and Rafael, who reported excellent initial results.[90] Open excision of dorsal ganglions is not a benign procedure, and patients occasionally complain of wrist stiffness during flexion. The arthroscopic procedure can be performed with less scarring and more rapid return of wrist flexion, compared to an open procedure.[51] Rate of recurrence is low and comparable to open procedures.[5]

Surgical Technique: Arthroscopic Ganglion Excision

The arthroscope is initially placed in the 4-5 or 6-R portal with inflow provided through a needle in the 6-U portal. A needle is then placed through the sac of the ganglion, usually located distal to the site of the 3-4 portal, into the radial carpal space. Because of this, the needle must be placed more obliquely into the joint to pass through the ganglion and into the radial carpal space. The needle typically enters the joint over the dorsal capsule at the level of the scapholunate interosseous ligament. A skin portal is made once ideal placement of the needle has been confirmed arthroscopically. A small joint shaver is then placed through the portal and into the joint (Figure 17.113). An approximately 1-cm full thickness defect in the capsule is then made. The capsular defect is typically at the junction of the dorsal capsule with the scapholunate interosseous ligament. Sometimes the stalk of the ganglion cyst can be identified and removed with débridement. A dorsal extensor tendon must be seen following removal of the capsule to ensure a full thickness defect and débridement of the capsule has been performed (Figure 17.114).

Palpation of the ganglion cyst as the capsule is being resected usually demonstrates a sudden blush because the cyst and stock have been débrided. A small joint punch can also be used to further débride the joint capsule. It is difficult but not impossible to injure the extensor tendons; small joint shavers and punches are minimally aggressive. The technique is particularly useful when a single-lobed ganglion is centered in the typical

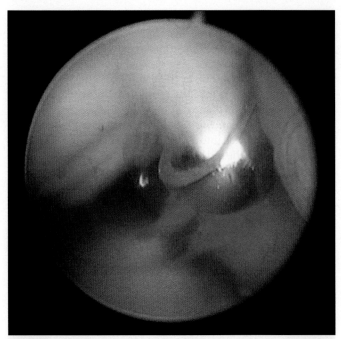

FIGURE 17.113 Arthroscopic view with the arthroscope in the 6-R portal demonstrating the shaver inserted through the sac of the ganglion with resection of the dorsal capsule.

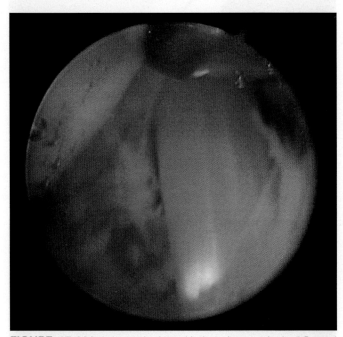

FIGURE 17.114 Arthroscopic view with the arthroscope in the 6-R portal demonstrating a full thickness defect of the capsule and exposure of the extensor tendons.

location on the dorsum of the wrist. Usually minimal formal therapy is required. The patient is encouraged to begin range-of-motion exercises the following day.

Volar wrist ganglions are the second most common mass in the wrist and arise from a pedicle that originates in either the volar scapholunate joint, the scaphotrapezial joint, or the trapeziometacarpal joint. They usually appear between the flexor

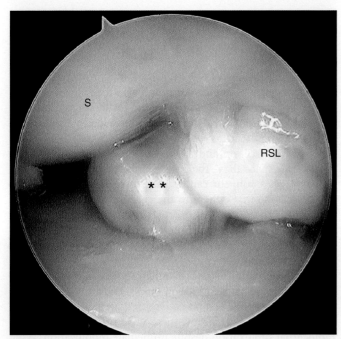

FIGURE 17.115 View of a volar ganglion (*asterisks*) from the 3-4 portal. *RSL*, Radioscapholunate ligament; *S*, scaphoid.

carpi radialis tendon and the flexor pollicis longus tendon. Arthroscopic excision of a volar ganglion has the advantage of avoiding extensive dissection, scarring, and potential damage to the surrounding structures. With this technique, the 3-4, 4-5, and 1-2 portals are used. The arthroscope is initially placed in the 3-4 portal. Synovial capsular abnormalities may be seen between the interval of the radioscaphocapite (RSC) and long radiolunate ligament (LRL) or between the LRL and short radiolunate ligament (SRL) (Figure 17.115).

It is helpful to manually compress the ganglion externally so that capsular bulging can be seen arthroscopically at the involved volar capsular sites. A 2.0–2.9 arthroscopic shaver is then introduced into the 1-2 portal to débride the region. Care needs to be taken to avoid injury to dorsal radial sensory nerves during establishment of this portal. Shaving is performed until a capsular defect of approximately 1 cm is created. It is important not to advance the shaver too far anteriorly to avoid injury to the volar structures. No attempt should be made to remove the ganglion wall as a separate structure.

Fernandez et al described their experience with 31 arthroscopic volar ganglionectomies.[42] It was their experience that the 4-5 portal is the ideal one for visualization, while instrumentation is best placed through the 1-2 portal. The authors noted one case of superficial radial neuritis, two hematomas, and one recurrence.

For those ganglions that arise from the scaphotrapeziotrapezoidal (STT) joint or another component of the midcarpal joint, a different approach is used. In these situations, finger-trap traction is applied to the thumb. A standard radial midcarpal portal is made, and an STT portal is established as previously described. A third portal is then made in the volar aspect of the trapeziometacarpal joint. The excision of a ganglion arising from the STT interval is more difficult compared to the standard volar ganglion.

WRIST ARTHRITIS

The arthroscope can play an important role in diagnosis and treatment of a wide array of arthritic conditions in the wrist. From palliative procedures, such as débridement of osteophytes or radial styloidectomy in an early SLAC wrist, to wrist synovectomy in inflammatory arthritis, to the more advanced procedures of carpectomy and partial arthrodesis, arthroscopic techniques have evolved to play a vital role in management of these common and disabling conditions.

Wrist Synovectomy

Adolfsson established the protocol for arthroscopic synovectomy in patients with rheumatoid arthritis.[2] Indications include persistent joint symptoms following a 6-month course of pharmacological treatment and only early radiographic degeneration or erosions as defined by Larsen et al.[73] The arthroscopic technique for synovectomy is straightforward. The standard 3-4, 4-5, and/or 6-R portals are established. A relatively rapid and efficient procedure is important to minimize wrist swelling and preserve visualization. With the arthroscope in the 3-4 portal, a synovectomy is performed in an ulnar-to-radial direction using instruments in the 4-5 and 6-R portals. The portals are then switched and with the arthroscope in the 6-R portal, the remaining synovitis on the radial side of the wrist is resected. Adolfsson et al. reported improved wrist arc of motion from 70 to 90 degrees and an 87% increase in grip strength in 18 patients 6 months following synovectomy.[3] In their longer-term follow-up study, the authors demonstrated continued improvements in pain for the majority of patients at 3.8 years after surgery.[2]

Chung et al. reviewed their series of 21 patients with rheumatoid arthritis following arthroscopic synovectomy.[24] At 3 months' follow-up, the authors noted arthroscopic synovectomy resulted in decreased pain, improved joint motion, and lower disability scores. It was felt that arthroscopic synovectomy should be considered an option for patients with mild-to-moderate stages of inflammatory arthritis.

Focal chondral defects are a common source of wrist pain. Proximal pole hamate arthrosis has been associated with the (bifacet) type II lunate morphology, and it can be a common cause of ulnar-sided wrist pain, particularly when sports or occupational demands require extremes of ulnar deviation (Figure 17.116). It has been noted that type II lunate can lead to chondral defects in approximately 44% of specimens but only 2% in type I lunates.[57,85,135] Arthroscopic or open resection of the proximal pole of the hamate has yielded good results, as noted by Yao et al.[136]

Patients with early SLAC disease and focal radioscaphoid arthritis may be candidates for arthroscopic radial styloidectomy. Patients with point tenderness directly over the tip of the radial styloid may attain improved function with a palliative procedure to remove the degenerated areas, provided they understand that the procedure will not restore normal joint kinematics and will not reverse the underlying condition. Arthroscopic radial styloidectomy ensures preservation of the critical RSC ligament, thus preventing iatrogenic ulnar translation of the wrist. In this technique, the arthroscope is placed in the standard 3-4 portal, and a 3.5-mm bur is inserted through the 1-2 portal. The chondromalacia noted on the scaphoid facet

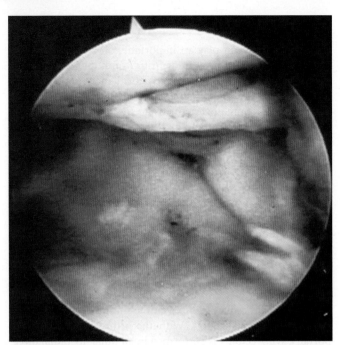

FIGURE 17.116 Arthroscopic view of a chondral defect of the hamate with the arthroscope in the radial midcarpal portal. This defect was débrided to relieve pain.

of the distal radius marks the area of resection. Approximately 4 mm of bone may be arthroscopically removed. Fluoroscopy is strongly encouraged to monitor the amount of resection.

Arthroscopic proximal carpectomy is a reproducible and effective arthroscopic technique that compares favorably to the established open technique.[30,32,128] Although there is a steep learning curve, arthroscopic proximal carpectomy can be accomplished in a reasonable amount of surgical time with routine small- and large-joint instrumentation. Arthroscopic proximal row carpectomy avoids disruption of the dorsal capsule allowing for immediate postoperative range of motion and improved wrist stability. Indications for arthroscopic proximal carpectomy are identical to the open procedure. The procedure is reserved for those patients with debilitating wrist pain and intact articular cartilage of the lunate fossa and capitate head.

To perform the procedure, the routine radiocarpal portals (i.e., 3-4, 4-5, 6-R, and 6-U) and midcarpal portals (i.e., midcarpal radial, midcarpal ulnar, and STT) are established. In the technique as described by Weiss et al, the arthroscope is placed in the ulnar midcarpal portal and a small joint arthroscopic bur is introduced through the radial midcarpal portal.[128] It is important at all times to avoid any injury to the articular cartilage of the capitate head. The hood of the shaver should always face the head of the capitate to avoid cartilage injury. Utilizing the small joint bur, the distal ulnar corner of the scaphoid is resected.

Once adequate resection of the ulnar corner of the scaphoid has been performed, a large joint shaver and, subsequently, a 4.0-mm bur can be introduced into the radial midcarpal portal. The larger bur obviously facilitates more rapid removal of bone. The scaphoid is then excised with the bur moving from ulnar-to-radial and distal-to-proximal. To complete resec-

tion of the most distal pole of the scaphoid, the bur can be placed through the STT portal. A small joint rongeur is helpful to remove small fragments that wind up in the joint capsule.

Following excision of the scaphoid, the arthroscope is moved to the STT portal. With the 4.0-mm bur in the radial midcarpal portal, the lunate is excised in a radial-to-ulnar and distal-to-proximal direction. Great care should be taken to avoid injury to the capitate head as well as the lunate facet of the distal radius. Wrist traction and adequate fluid flow are essential to create a safe space above the distal radius and protect the articular cartilage. A rongeur can be used to remove the final fragments of bone that adhere to the capsule. The arthroscope is then moved to the radial midcarpal portal and the bur is placed in the ulnar midcarpal portal to remove the triquetrum. Fluoroscopic views are made to confirm complete excision of the proximal row of the carpus.

Weiss and coauthors reviewed their series of 35 patients with an average of 33-months' follow-up.[128] The authors noted no major complications and no patients required conversion to an open procedure. Specifically, there were no complications of radiocarpal subluxation despite immediate mobilization. What is impressive is that the average length of surgery was 61 minutes. Patients retained an average 78% of the flexion–extension arc of the wrist and 70% of radial and ulnar deviation. Grip strength averaged 83% compared to the opposite wrist. The authors reported a 94% rate of patient satisfaction with the arthroscopic procedure.

Partial wrist fusion is a widely accepted technique for a patient with an arthritic wrist who still desires preservation of some motion and additional pain relief. Conventionally, these procedures are performed through an open approach. Ho described his case series of arthroscopic partial wrist fusion.[63] He notes an arthroscopic approach provides an excellent view of the wrist and is a viable adjunct for various techniques of partial wrist fusion. Ho combines an arthroscopic débridement of the cartilaginous surfaces with strong percutaneous fixation and feels that he can generate better functional outcomes by avoiding wrist arthrotomy.

Ho reported outcomes of 23 partial wrist fusions for patients with an average age of 42,[63] as follows: STT fusion in 3, scaphoidectomy and four-corner fusion in 5, scaphoidectomy and lunocapitate fusion in 4, lunate excision and scaphocapitate fusion in 3, radioscapholunate fusion in 4, radial lunate fusion in 2, and lunotriquetral fusion in 2. Surgical complications included superficial pin tract infections and a skin burn.[63] Radiographic fusion was completed in 19 cases, 3 cases were reported as having stable and asymptomatic fibrous union, and 1 case required revision of a nonunion.

Intercarpal Arthrodesis

Through the radial midcarpal portal, the corresponding articular surfaces are removed with an arthroscopic bur and curet. Carpal bones are provisionally transfixed with Kirschner wires and alignment confirmed under fluoroscopic control. A cancellous bone graft or bone substitute is inserted at the fusion site through a cannula under arthroscopic and fluoroscopic visualization. Final fixation was achieved with multiple Kirschner wire fixation or cannulated screws. Rigid fixation enabled early mobilization in most patients.

Arthroscopic Arthrolysis

Wrist stiffness is a debilitating condition that may be secondary to trauma or prolonged immobilization and may have intraarticular and extraarticular etiologies. Arthrofibrosis may involve the radiocarpal, radioulnar, and ulnocarpal joints. Arthroscopic arthrolysis is an effective treatment for restoring range of motion and reducing pain.

Contraindications

Carpal instability is a contraindication for capsular release, since release of the volar and/or dorsal extrinsic ligaments would likely exacerbate the condition. Similarly, the presence of posttraumatic arthritis or osteoarthritis would limit any potential gains. Patients who cannot comply with postoperative dynamic–static progressive splinting are not appropriate candidates.

Technique

The traditional radiocarpal portals are used for arthroscopic arthrolysis, and the volar radioulnar portals may be utilized as necessary. Although less common, if the midcarpal joint is involved, traditional midcarpal portals may be used. In a technique by Luchetti et al, dry arthroscopy is used more frequently and avoids fluid extravasation into the soft tissues.[76] Luchetti notes that arthroscopic arthrolysis always starts from the radial side of the radiocarpal joint. The traditional 3-4 viewing portal is used and 1-2 is a working portal. The portals are used interchangeably under triangulation. Once fibrosis is completely removed from the radial side of the wrist, the arthroscope is transferred to the 3-4 portal and the shaver through the 6-R portal.

It is noted that, frequently, a fibrotic band is identified between the scapholunate ligament and the interfacet ridge of the distal radius.[58] This fibrotic band can be partial or complete and is incised using a small dissector through the 6-R portal. Depending on the range of motion obtained from arthroscopic débridement of intraarticular adhesions, the volar and/or dorsal capsule may need to be released. Volar capsulectomy is usually easier than dorsal because the structures are immediately in the field of vision when viewing from the standard dorsal arthroscopy portals. A mini-banana blade can be inserted through the 1-2 portal with the arthroscope in the standard 3-4 portal. The radioscaphocapitate ligament is incised at its base and the procedure continues to the ulnar aspect of the wrist. The ulnar side of the volar capsule is released with a banana blade in the 6-R portal using the arthroscope in the 3-4 portal. The LRL should be preserved to minimize the risk of ulnocarpal translation. Following release of the volar capsule, manipulation can be performed.

To release the dorsal capsule, the arthroscope is placed through the 1-2 portal and the banana blade through the 6-R portal. The dorsal central portion of the capsule is resected first. The arthroscope is then transferred to the 6-R portal and the remaining radial side of the dorsal capsule is released with a banana blade inserted through the 1-2 portal. Small open incisions can be used as needed to protect the extensor tendons. Resection of a portion of the dorsal rim of the distal radius may be helpful when wrist extension is restricted secondary to a malunion of the distal radius. After dorsal capsule release has been performed, the dorsal rim is resected with a bur alternating between the 6-R and 1-2 portals. Following capsular release the wrist is taken out of traction and gently manipulated. The procedure is complete when a functional passive range of motion has been achieved as previously described. Postoperatively the patient is placed in a bulky splint for 2 to 3 days to reduce hematoma formation, followed by aggressive wrist mobilization.

Luchetti et al. published their results of five cases with a 10-month follow-up.[76] The patients' average flexion improved from 44 degrees to 54 degrees postoperatively. Similarly, wrist extension improved from 40 degrees preoperatively to 60 degrees postoperatively. Hattori et al. reported an improvement of 20 degrees in the flexion–extension arc of nine males and two females after arthroscopic capsular release for a variety of posttraumatic arthrofibrotic conditions.[2]

KIENBÖCK'S DISEASE

In 1999, Menth-Chiari et al first described the use of wrist arthroscopy in the treatment of Kienböck's disease.[78] The authors used arthroscopy in seven patients with late-stage disease (Lichtman stage IIIA or IIIB) to assess the articular surfaces, to débride the lunate, and to perform a synovectomy. At 19 months' follow-up all patients experienced relief of pain and improvement in mechanical symptoms; three of the seven experienced radiographic progression of the disease.

Bain and Begg described their arthroscopic classification in 2006 (Table 17.3).[10] The classification system is based on the number of nonfunctional articular surfaces. A normal articular surface was defined as having a glistening appearance or minor fibrillation with normal hard subchondral bone with probing. A nonfunctional articular surface is defined as having extensive fibrillation, fissuring, localized or extensive articular loss, floating articular surface, or fracture (Figures 17.117 and 17.118).

The number of nonfunctional articular surfaces determines the grade. In the Bain and Begg study series, they found a consistent pattern of changes within the lunate and that the changes always occurred initially on the proximal articular surface of the lunate. The more severe cases would develop a subchondral fracture and subsequently secondary chondral changes in the apposing lunate facet of the radius. They noted

TABLE 17.3 Bain and Begg Arthroscopic Classification

Grade	Description
0	All functional surfaces are working
I	One nonfunctional articular surface—usually the proximal articular surface of the lunate
II	Two nonfunctional articular surfaces divided into types A and B
IIa	Proximal lunate facet of the radius
IIb	Proximal surface of the lunate and distal articular surface of the lunate
III	Three nonfunctional articular surfaces—lunate facet of the radius, proximal and distal articular surfaces of the lunate with a preserved head of the capitate
IV	All functional surfaces are nonfunctional

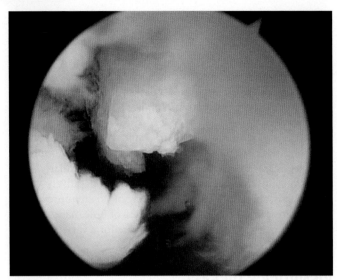

FIGURE 17.117 Arthroscopic view from the 3-4 portal demonstrating a necrotic lunate in Kienböck's disease.

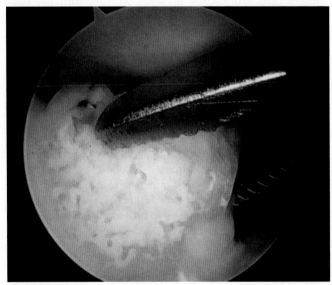

FIGURE 17.118 Arthroscopic view showing débridement and the removal of the necrotic fragments of the lunate.

that involvement of the distal articular surface of the lunate was rare; exceptions included a coronal fracture extending to the distal articular surface for chronic cases.

The authors found that the degree of synovitis correlated with the degree of articular damage. The severity of articular cartilage as seen on plain radiographs was underestimated when seen arthroscopically. They found that findings of arthroscopy commonly changed the initial treatment plan. More important, Bain and Begg identified cases where the articular cartilage envelope remained intact while the underlying subchondral bone had collapsed. The authors postulated that this subgroup may have undergone spontaneous lunate revascularization.

Bain and Durrant developed a treatment algorithm based on their arthroscopic grading.[11] The principles of the algorithm were to remove only the nonfunctional surfaces while maintaining range of motion. In grade 0, all the articular surfaces are

functional. Arthroscopic synovectomy is performed. Further treatment may include an unloading procedure, revascularization, arthroscopic or open core decompression, or bone grafting. Arthroscopic core decompression is recommended only for patients with a neutral or positive ulnar variance.[11]

Pegoli et al. described arthroscopic bone grafting for the necrotic lunate; it is drilled at a site near the dorsal insertion of the lunotriquetral interosseous ligament. The necrotic lunate is then débrided with a motorized shaver and osteoscopy is then performed by inserting a scope into the lunate to confirm adequate débridement. Cancellous bone graft is then harvested from the volar aspect of the distal radius and inserted into the lunate through a trocar.[94]

Grade I Kienböck's disease is defined by a nonfunctioning proximal lunate articular surface. Treatment options include proximal row carpectomy or radioscapholunate fusion. In grade IIa, both the proximal articular surface of the lunate and the lunate fossa are nonfunctional. In this case, radioscapholunate fusion removes the nonfunctional articular surface while maintaining normal midcarpal kinematics. In grade IIb, the proximal and distal articular surfaces of the lunate are nonfunctional. Bain and Begg feel a proximal carpectomy is the treatment of choice, provided the lunate articular facet of the radius is intact.

In grade III Kienböck's, three articular surfaces are nonfunctional although the capitate articular surface usually remains functional. In this instance, Bain and Begg recommend a salvage procedure such as a total wrist fusion or arthroplasty. A third option is a resurfacing hemiarthroplasty of the distal radius that articulates with the head of the capitate. In grade IV Kienböck's, all four articular surfaces are nonfunctional and a total wrist fusion or arthroplasty is recommended.

Tatebe et al. performed arthroscopic inspection of 57 patients who underwent radial osteotomy for Kienböck's disease.[111] All patients were classified using the Bain and Begg classification. They noted the number of articular surfaces involved did not correlate with the Lichtman radiographic stage or the duration from onset to surgery. The authors noted that all but two patients had cartilage lesions in the proximal articular surface of the lunate and that loss of additional articular surfaces correlated with patient age. For workup, staging, and a complete review of treatment options for Kienböck's disease, the reader is referred to Chapter 16.

THUMB CARPOMETACARPAL ARTHROSCOPY

The thumb carpometacarpal joint is the most common one in the hand to develop degenerative arthritis. While there has been considerable attention paid to the treatment of advanced disease, much less attention has focused on early intervention to prevent or delay the need for a salvage procedure.[37] Recent advances in small joint arthroscopy allow for treatment of symptomatic basal joint laxity in a minimally invasive fashion without joint destabilization.

Badia defined an arthroscopic classification of thumb carpometacarpal arthritis.[9] In stage 1, there is diffuse synovitis but the articular cartilage is intact and volar capsule laxity is demonstrated. In stage 2, there is central fovea articular cartilage loss of the trapezium, deep metacarpal base loss, and resulting synovitis. In stage 3, there is widespread articular cartilage loss and deep osteophyte on trapezium. The staging system was gradually developed as a result of more than 20 years performing arthroscopic assessment of recalcitrant basal joint arthritis, which did not improve after conservative management.

Thermal stabilization of the capsule ligamentous structures has been used with some success in hand and wrist surgery compared to its use in other joints. It is thought that prolonged immobilization allows for capsular shrinkage to mature.[6,59,84] Thermal stabilization exploits the heat liable intramolecular bonds that maintain the triple helix structure in type I collagen. Ideal temperatures for thermal stabilization have been described as between 60°C to 67°C. Thermal shrinkage occurs until a plateau is reached beyond which thermal shrinkage will not occur. As the tissue cools, it has been shown that up to 10% of initial shrinkage may be lost and some of the bonds renature. This technology has been most recently applied to the thumb carpometacarpal joint.

Indications

As a general rule, any patient who has isolated and refractory degenerative disease of the trapeziometacarpal joint is a candidate for an arthroscopic treatment. This form of treatment does not preclude an open trapeziectomy and/or ligament reconstruction at a later date as a salvage procedure.

Contraindications

This would include any general contraindication to thumb arthroscopy including distortion of the anatomy due to swelling, unstable or friable skin that would preclude the use of traction, and recent infection. The presence of pantrapezial degenerative disease is a relative contraindication, although simultaneous arthroscopic TM and STT arthroplasty has been reported. Because of excessive ligamentous laxity, patients with Ehlers-Danlos syndrome or lupus arthritis are not ideal candidates for this procedure although a successful arthroscopic tendon arthroplasty has been reported.[108] If present, MP joint hyperextension must be carefully considered and addressed separately (see Chapter 11).

Technique: Arthroscopic Capsular Shrinkage

Five to ten pounds of sterile finger trap traction is applied to the thumb so that the wrist is in slight ulnar deviation. The elbow is flexed 90 degrees, nearly parallel to the long axis of the traction tower. It is helpful to wrap Coban™ around the forearm and the tower itself to help stabilize the wrist. It is often helpful to have fluoroscopy in the room to verify correct placement of the portals for the thumb's carpometacarpal joint.

It is important to confirm each portal location using a 22-gauge needle inserted under fluoroscopy before committing to a skin incision. The 1-R and 1-U portals may be used interchangeably to inspect the joint, and visualization is markedly improved by the use of a synovial resector. Some authors prefer a standard 2.7-mm arthroscope for the thumb carpometacarpal joint. Others prefer a 1.9-mm scope.

For thermal capsular shrinkage, the arthroscope is initially placed in the 1-U portal and a thermal probe is introduced into the 1-R portal.[31] The probe is passed repeatedly over the capsule ligamentous structures in a controlled, systemic manner. It is important not to pass the probe too rapidly, which will result in insufficient shrinkage. Remember that the CMC joint is a very small space, and the fluid can heat up rapidly. If the probe is passed too slowly, this may result in excessive thermal damage. It is also important not to paint the capsular structures but rather to make precise stripes. The anterior oblique ligament is initially shrunk and progress is made toward the ulnar collateral ligament.

At this point, the portals are switched and the remaining ulnar collateral ligament and posterior oblique ligament, as well as the dorsal radial ligament, can be treated with the thermal probe. A pin should be placed across the thumb CMC joint or between the thumb and index metacarpals following the procedure to stabilize the joint. The pin is removed in 3 to 4 weeks and range-of-motion exercises begun. Strengthening exercises are started 6 weeks postoperatively.

With more severe degenerative disease of the thumb carpometacarpal joint, either arthroscopic hemitrapeziectomy or complete trapeziectomy are indicated.

Technique: Arthroscopic Hemitrapeziectomy

The arthroscope is inserted in the standard 1-U portal. A full-radius resector is placed through a thenar working portal to débride the synovitis and degenerative articular cartilage. The advantage of a thenar portal is that it is located further from the dorsal sensory branch of the radial nerve and is perpendicular to the 1-U portal to allow for easier triangulation. A 2.9-mm arthroscopic bur is then placed through the thenar portal to complete the hemitrapeziectomy. Approximately 3 to 5 mm of the distal aspect of the trapezium should be removed. The shaver and arthroscope are switched between the two portals for optimal visualization and débridement. It is vital to confirm the degree of trapezial resection under fluoroscopy.

A ballottement test can be performed by alternately applying traction and compression to the thumb metacarpal while visualizing the amount of translation. The thumb metacarpal should temporarily be pinned for 3 to 4 weeks to maintain the resection space. Alternatively, to decrease the amount of postoperative immobilization while still maintaining support to the thumb metacarpal, a mini-tightrope suture device (Arthrex, Naples, FL) can be placed between the thumb and the index metacarpal (see Chapter 11). A short explanation of the tight-rope device can be found in this chapter online at ExpertConsult.com.

Arthroscopic trapeziectomy has been described by Cobb et al.[26] In this technique, the standard 1-R and 1-U portals are made for thumb carpometacarpal arthroscopy. STT arthroscopy portals are made by using 1-R and 1-U portals placed approximately 1 cm proximal to the standard 1-R and 1-U portals as described earlier. These portals are ideally localized using fluoroscopy with 22-gauge needles. Initially, a 3.5-mm full resector is used to clean out debris within the joint. Cobb and coauthors recommend electrothermal shrinkage to tighten the capsule and create an articular denervation. It is critical to maintain high fluid flow to minimize overheating and potential burns with the use of radio frequency probes. A 3.0- or 4-mm bur is then used to resect 2 to 3 mm of bone from the distal aspect of the trapezium and the proximal aspect of the thumb metacarpal.

The STT resection arthroplasty is performed by removing 2 to 3 mm of bone from the distal aspect of the scaphoid and from the proximal aspect of the trapezium and trapezoid. Once space is more readily available, a 4-mm barrel bur can be used.

When an interposition material is to be utilized, Cobb et al recommend the graft jacket (Wright Medical Technology, Inc., Memphis, TN). They feel that this material tends to adhere effectively and has a decreased inflammatory response.[26] In Cobb and coauthors' earlier experience, no fixation methods were used to secure the interposition material.

To prevent extrusion, the interposition material is now secured with sutures tied over buttons external to the skin on the volar and dorsal aspect of the joint. Fixation is performed by passing absorbable sutures into the volar portal, across the joint and out the dorsum of the hand. The suture can be used to pull the graft into the prepared joint. A second suture is placed on the opposite side of the interposition material so that the interposition material can be manipulated to lie in the center of the joint as viewed arthroscopically. The sutures are then tied over buttons on the dorsal and volar sides of the joint. Postoperatively, the patients are immobilized in a thumb spica splint that is converted to a thermoplastic splint after 5 to 7 days. The pull-out suture is removed at approximately 2 weeks. It is felt that early range of motion provides for a better overall outcome.

Cobb et al reviewed their results in 35 patients with arthroscopic resection arthroplasty of the thumb carpometacarpal joint performed in 35 patients for thumb arthrosis.[26] The average pain level improved from 7 preoperatively to 1 postoperatively at 1-year follow-up. DASH scores improved from 46 preoperatively to 19 at 1-year follow-up. Grip strength improved 4.3 kg and key pinch improved 1.3 kg. There were four reoperations in his series. As Cobb et al noted, the indications for interposition are not well established. Good results have been reported with resection arthroplasty without interposition.[38,64]

SMALL JOINT ARTHROSCOPY

Please see www.expertconsult.com.

COMPLICATIONS

Complications of wrist arthroscopy are relatively rare.[44] Beredjiklian et al. reported 11 complications in 211 patients who underwent wrist arthroscopy.[14] There were two major complications in his studies: one case of severe arthrofibrosis and one case of a ganglion that developed at the 3-4 portal. Nine patients developed minor complications including transient ulnar neurapraxia, transient wrist and finger stiffness, skin burn, portal site infection, and extensor carpi ulnaris tendonitis. All complications had resolved at the last follow-up visit.[14] Pell and Uhl noted three tendon ruptures in their series of 47 patients treated with thermal ablation during wrist arthroscopy.[95] One patient had a full-thickness skin burn after the use of thermal shrinkage.

To prevent complications of wrist arthroscopy, careful portal planning is essential. A few millimeters difference with regard to placement of the portals can make a big difference in proximity to vital structures and ease of joint access. A needle should always be used, prior to cutting the skin, to determine precise portal placement. The needle should pass easily into the joint without impaling tendons, carpal bones, or the distal radius.

It is important to always use blunt trocars to prevent iatrogenic damage of the articular cartilage during introduction of the arthroscopic cannulae. Separate inflow and outflow portals limit fluid extravasation into the soft tissues. Use of physiological solutions (e.g., lactated Ringer) allows reabsorption of extravasated fluid and minimizes the risk of compartment syndrome. Kirschner wires should always be inserted with the use of a soft tissue protector or the oscillation mode to limit any potential damage to the numerous sensory branches surrounding the wrist.

CONCLUSION

In summary, arthroscopy continues to grow in popularity as a valuable diagnostic and therapeutic adjunct for complex disorders of the wrist. It allows for the evaluation of articular structures under bright light and magnified conditions with minimal morbidity. Continued improvement in the techniques will occur as more surgeons are exposed to wrist arthroscopy and better instrumentation is developed.

For Case Studies, Videos, and more, please visit ExpertConsult.com.

REFERENCES

1. Adolfsson L: Arthroscopic diagnosis of ligament lesions of the wrist. *J Hand Surg* 19B:505–512, 1994.
2. Adolfsson L: Arthroscopic synovectomy in wrist arthritis. *Hand Clin* 21:527–530, 2005.
3. Adolfsson L, Nylander G: Arthroscopic synovectomy of the rheumatoid wrist. *J Hand Surg [Br]* 18:92–96, 1993.
4. Anderson DD, Bell AL, Gaffney MB, et al: Contact stress distributions in malreduced intraarticular distal radius fractures. *J Orthop Trauma* 10:331–337, 1996.
5. Angelides AC, Wallace F: The dorsal ganglion of the wrist: its pathogenesis, gross and microscopic anatomy, and surgical treatment. *J Hand Surg* 1:228–235, 1976.
6. Arnoczky SP, Aksan A: Thermal modification of connective tissues: basic science consideration and clinical implications. *J Am Acad Orthop Surg* 8:305–313, 2000.
7. Arora R, Gschwentner M, Krappinger D, et al: Fixation of nondisplaced scaphoid fractures: making treatment cost effective. Prospective controlled trial. *Arch Orthop Trauma Surg* 127:39–46, 2007.
8. Atzei A, Rizzo A, Luchetti R, et al: Arthroscopic foveal repair of triangular fibrocartilage complex peripheral lesion with distal radioulnar joint instability. *Tech Hand Up Extrem Surg* 12:226–235, 2008.
9. Badia A: Trapeziometacarpal arthroscopy: A classification and treatment algorithm. *Hand Clin* 22:153–163, 2006.
10. Bain GI, Begg M: Arthroscopic assessment and classification of Kienbock's disease. *Tech Hand Up Extrem Surg* 10:8–13, 2006.
11. Bain GI, Durrant A: An articular-based approach to Kienbock avascular necrosis of the lunate. *Tech Hand Up Extrem Surg* 15(1):41–47, 2011.
12. Baratz ME, Des Jardins JD, Anderson DD, et al: Displaced intra-articular fractures of the distal radius: the effect of fracture displacement on contact stresses in a cadaver model. *J Hand Surg* 21A:183–188, 1996.
13. Bednar MS, Arnoczky SP, Weiland AJ: The microvasculature of the triangular fibrocartilage complex: its clinical significance. *J Hand Surg [Am]* 16(6):1101–1105, 1991.
14. Beredjiklian PK, Bozentka DJ, Leung L, et al: Complications of wrist arthroscopy. *J Hand Surg [Am]* 29:406–411, 2004.
15. Berger RA: A technique for arthroscopic evaluation of the first carpometacarpal joint. *J Hand Surg [Am]* 22:1077–1080, 1997.
16. Berger RA, Landsmeer JMF: The palmar radiocarpal ligaments: a study of adult and fetal human wrist joints. *J Hand Surg* 15A:847–854, 1990.
17. Bernstein MA, Nagel DJ, Martinez A, et al: A comparison of combined arthroscopic triangular fibrocartilage complex debridement and arthroscopic wafer distal ulna resection versus arthroscopic triangular fibrocartilage complex debridement and ulnar shortening osteotomy for ulnocarpal abutment syndrome. *Arthroscopy* 20(4):392–401, 2004.
18. Bettinger PC, Cooney WP, III, Berger RA: Arthroscopic anatomy of the wrist. *Orthop Clin North Am* 26:707–719, 1995.
19. Botte MJ, Cooney WP, Linscheid RL: Arthroscopy of the wrist: anatomy and technique. *J Hand Surg* 14A:313–316, 1989.

20. Bowers WHWT: Arthroscopic anatomy of the wrist. In McGinty J, editor: *Operative arthroscopy*, New York, 1991, Raven Press, pp 613–623.

21. Buterbaugh GA: Radiocarpal arthroscopy portals and normal anatomy. *Hand Clin* 10:567–576, 1994.

22. Carro LP, Golano P, Farinas O, et al: The radial portal for scaphotrapeziotrapezoid arthroscopy. *Arthroscopy* 19:547–553, 2003.

23. Chen YC: Arthroscopy of the wrist and finger joints. *Orthop Clin North Am* 10(3):723–733, 1979.

24. Chung CY, Yen CH, Yip ML, et al: Arthroscopic synovectomy for rheumatoid wrists and elbows. *J Orthop Surg (Hong Kong)* 20:219–223, 2012.

25. Chung KC, Zimmerman NB, Travis MT: Wrist arthrography versus arthroscopy: a comparative study of 150 cases. *J Hand Surg* 21A:591–594, 1996.

26. Cobb T, Sterbank P, Lemke J: Arthroscopic resection arthroplasty for the treatment of combined carpometacarpal and scaphotrapeziotrapezoid (pantrapezial) arthritis. *J Hand Surg [Am]* 36:413–419, 2011.

27. Cooney WP: Evaluation of chronic wrist pain by arthrography, arthroscopy, and arthrotomy. *J Hand Surg* 18A:815–822, 1993.

28. Corella F, Ocampos M, Del Cerro M: Are extensor tendons safe on your first wrist arthroscopy? *J Hand Surg Eur* 36(9):817–818, 2011.

29. Corso SJ, Savoie FH, Geissler WB, et al: Arthroscopic repair of peripheral avulsions of the triangular fibrocartilage complex of the wrist: a multicenter study. *Arthroscopy* 13:78–84, 1997.

30. Culp RW, McGuigan FX, Turner MA, et al: Proximal row carpectomy: a multicenter study. *J Hand Surg* 18A:19–25, 1993.

31. Culp RW, Rekant MS: The role of arthroscopy in evaluating and treating trapeziometacarpal disease. *Hand Clin* 17(2):315–319, 2001.

32. Culp RW, Osterman AL, Kaufmann RA: Wrist arthroscopy: operative procedures. In Green DP, Hotchkiss RN, Pederson WC, et al, editors: *Green's operative hand surgery*, ed 5, Philadelphia, 2005, Elsevier, pp 781–803.

33. Darlis NA, Weiser RW, Sotereanos DG: Partial scapholunate ligament injuries treated with arthroscopic debridement and thermal shrinkage. *J Hand Surg [Am]* 30:908–914, 2005.

34. Deitch MA, Stern SJ: Ulnocarpal abutment: treatment options. *Hand Clin* 14(2):251–263, 1998.

35. del Pinal F, Garcia-Gernal FJ, Pisani D, et al: Dry arthroscopy of the wrist: surgical technique. *J Hand Surg [Am]* 32:119–123, 2007.

36. del Pinal F, Studer A, Thams C, et al: An all-inside technique for arthroscopic suturing of the volar scapholunate ligament. *J Hand Surg [Am]* 36:2044–2046, 2011.

37. Eaton RG, Lane LB, Littler JW, et al: Ligament reconstruction for the painful thumb carpometacarpal joint: a long-term assessment. *J Hand Surg [Am]* 9:692–699, 1984.

38. Edwards SG, Ramsey PN: Prospective outcomes of stage 3 thumb CMC arthritis. *J Hand Surg [Am]* 35:566–571, 2010.

39. Ekman EF, Poehling GG: Principles of arthroscopy and wrist arthroscopy equipment. *Hand Clin* 10:557–566, 1994.

40. Feldon P, Terrono AL, Belsky MR: Wafer distal ulna resection for triangular fibrocartilage tears and/or ulna impaction syndrome. *J Hand Surg [Am]* 17:731–737, 1992.

41. Fellinger M, Peicha G, Seibert FJ, et al: Radial avulsion of the triangular fibrocartilage complex in acute wrist trauma: a new technique for arthroscopic repair. *Arthroscopy* 13:370–374, 1997.

42. Fernandes CH, Meirelles LM, Raduan Neto J, et al: Characteristics of global publications about wrist arthroscopy: a bibliometric analysis. *Hand Surg* 17(3):311–315, 2012.

43. Fontes D, Lenoble E, De Somer B, et al: Lesions ligamentaires associees aux fractures distales du radius. A propos de cinquante-huit athrographies peroperatories. *Ann Chair Main* 11:119–125, 1992.

44. Fortems Y, Mawhinney I, Lawrence T, et al: Late rupture of extensor pollicis longus after wrist arthroscopy. *Arthroscopy* 11:322–323, 1995.

45. Geissler WB, Fernandez DL: Percutaneous and limited open reductions of the articular surface of the distal radius. *J Orthop Trauma* 5:255–264, 1991.

46. Geissler WB, Savoie FH: Arthroscopic techniques of the wrist. *Medi-guide Orthop* 11:1–8, 1992.

47. Geissler WB: Arthroscopically assisted reduction of intra-articular fractures of the distal radius. *Hand Clin* 11:19–29, 1995.

48. Geissler WB, Freeland AE, Savoie FH, et al: Intercarpal soft-tissue lesions associated with an intra-articular fracture of the distal end of the radius. *J Bone Joint Surg* 78A:357–365, 1996.

49. Geissler WB, Freeland AE: Arthroscopically assisted reduction of intraarticular distal radial fractures. *Clin Orthop* 327:125–134, 1996.

50. Geissler WB, Fernandez DL, Lamey DM: Distal radioulnar joint injuries associated with fractures of the distal radius. *Clin Orthop* 327:135–146, 1996.

51. Geissler WB: Arthroscopic excision of dorsal wrist ganglia. *Tech Upper Extrem Surg* 2:196–201, 1998.

52. Geissler WB: Arthroscopic knotless peripheral ulnar-sided TFCC repair. *Hand Clin* 27(3):273–279, 2011.

53. Geissler WB, Hammit MD: Arthroscopic aided fixation of scaphoid fractures. *Hand Clin* 17:575–588, viii, 2001.

54. Geissler WB, Slade JF: Fractures of the carpal bones. In Wolfe SW, Hotchkiss RN, Peterson WC, et al, editors: *Green's operative hand surgery*, vol 1, ed 6, Philadelphia, 2010, Elsevier, pp 639–707.

55. Geissler WB: *AANA Fall Course*, Palm Springs, CA, 2014.

56. Hanker GJ: *Wrist arthroscopy in distal radius fractures*. Read at the Annual Meeting of the Arthroscopy Association of North America, Albuquerque, NM, Oct. 9, 1993.

57. Harley BJ, Werner FW, Boles SD, et al: Arthroscopic resection of arthrosis of the proximal hamate: a clinical and biomechanical study. *J Hand Surg [Am]* 29:661–667, 2004.

58. Hattori T, Tsunoda K, Watanabe K, et al: Arthroscopic mobilization for contracture of the wrist. *Arthroscopy* 22(8):850–854, 2006.

59. Hayashi K, Markel M: Thermal modification of joint capsule and ligamentous tissues. *Tech Sports Med* 6:120–125, 1998.

60. Hermansdorfer JD, Kleinman WB: Management of chronic peripheral tears of the triangular fibrocartilage complex. *J Hand Surg* 16A:340–346, 1991.

61. Hirsh L, Sodha S, Bozentka D, et al: Arthroscopic electrothermal collagen shrinkage for symptomatic laxity of the scapholunate interosseous ligament. *J Hand Surg [Br]* 30:643–647, 2005.

62. Hixon ML, Walker CW, Fitzrandolph RL, et al: Acute ligament tears of the wrist associated with Colles' fractures. *Orthop Trans* 14:164–165, 1990.

63. Ho PC: Arthroscopic partial wrist fusion. *Tech Hand Up Extrem Surg* 12:242–265, 2008.

64. Hofmeister EP, Leak RS, Culp RW, et al: Arthroscopic hemitrapeziectomy for the first metacarpal arthritis: results at seven-year follow-up. *Hand* 4(1):24–28, 2009.

65. Hollingsworth R, Morris J: The importance of the ulnar side of the wrist in fractures of the distal end of the radius. *Injury* 7:263–266, 1976.

66. Horii E, Garcia-Elias M, An KN, et al: A kinematic study of lunotriquetral dissociations. *J Hand Surg [Am]* 16:355–362, 1991.

67. Hulsizer D, Weiss AP: Akeiman E. Ulna-shortening osteotomy after failed arthroscopic debridement of the triangular fibrocartilage complex. *J Hand Surg* 22A:694–698, 1997.

68. Johnstone DJ, Thorogood S, Smith WH, et al: A comparison of magnetic resonance imaging and arthroscopy in the investigation of chronic wrist pain. *J Hand Surg* 22-B:714–718, 1997.

69. Jones CM, Grasu BL, Murphy MS: Dry wrist arthroscopy. *J Hand Surg [Am]* 40(2):388–390, 2016.

70. Knirk JL, Jupiter JB: Intra-articular fractures of the distal end of the radius in young adults. *J Bone and Joint Surg* 68A:647–659, 1986.

71. Kolkin L: *Wrist arthroscopy*. Presented at the Annual Meeting of the American Academy of Orthopaedic Surgeons, Washington, DC, Feb. 22, 1992.

72. Kreder HJ, Hanel DP, McGee M, et al: *Limited open versus standard open reduction and internal fixation of intra-articular fractures of the radius: a prospective randomized trial*. Read at the Annual Meeting of the Canadian Orthopaedic Association, Auckland, NZ, Feb. 5, 1998.

73. Larsen A, Dale K, Eek M: Radiographic evaluation of rheumatoid arthritis and related conditions by standard reference films. *Acta Radiol Diagn (Stockholm)* 18:481–491, 1977.

74. Levy HJ, Glickel SZ: Arthroscopic assisted internal fixation of volar intraarticular wrist fractures. *Arthroscopy* 9:122–124, 1993.

75. Llinas A, McKellop HA, Marshall GJ, et al: Healing and remodeling of articular incongruities in a rabbit fracture model. *J Bone Joint Surg* 75A:1508–1523, 1993.

76. Luchetti R, Atzei A, Papini-Zorli I: Arthroscopic wrist arthrolysis. *Chir Main* 25:S244–S253, 2006.

77. Mathoulin CL, Dauphin N, Wahegaonkar AL: Arthroscopic dorsal capsuloplasty in chronic scapho-lunate ligament tears: a new procedure. *Hand Clin* 27:563–572, 2011.

78. Menth-Chiari WA, Poehling GG, Wiesler ER, et al: Arthroscopic debridement for the treatment of Kienbock's disease. *Arthroscopy* 15:12–19, 1999.

79. Mitsuyasu H, Patterson RM, Shah MA, et al: The role of the dorsal intercarpal ligament in dynamic and static scapholunate instability. *J Hand Surg [Am]* 29:279–288, 2004.

80. Mohanti RC, Kar N: Study of triangular fibrocartilage of the wrist in Colles' fracture. *Injury* 11:321–324, 1980.

81. Moritomo H, Viegas SF, Elder KW, et al: Scaphoid nonunions: a 3-dimensional analysis of patterns of deformity. *J Hand Surg [Am]* 25A:520–528, 2000.

82. Moskal MJ, Savoie FH, 3rd, Field LD: Arthroscopic capsulodesis of the lunotriquetral joint. *Clin Sports Med* 20:141–153, ix–x, 2001.

83. Mudgal CS, Jones WA: Scapholunate diastasis: a component of fractures of the distal radius. *J Hand Surg* 15B:503–505, 1990.

84. Nagle DJ: *The use of lasers in wrist arthroscopy*. Read at the Annual Meeting of the Arthroscopy Association of North America, Rosemont, IL, Nov. 4, 1997.

85. Nakamura K, Patterson RM, Moritomo H, et al: Type I versus type II lunates: ligament anatomy and presence of arthrosis. *J Hand Surg [Am]* 26:428–436, 2001.

86. North ER, Thomas S: An anatomic guide for arthroscopic visualization of the wrist capsular ligaments. *J Hand Surg* 13A:815–822, 1988.

87. Oneson SR, Timins ME, Scales LM, et al: MR imaging diagnosis of triangular fibrocartilage pathology with arthroscopic correlation. *Am J Roentengol* 168:1513–1518, 1997.

88. Orellana MA, Chow JC: Arthroscopic visualization of the thumb carpometacarpal joint: introduction and evaluation of a new radial portal. *Arthroscopy* 19:583–591, 2003.

89. Osterman AL: Arthroscopic debridement of triangular fibrocartilage complex tears. *Arthroscopy* 6:120–124, 1990.

90. Osterman AL, Raphael J: Arthroscopic resection of dorsal ganglion of the wrist. *Hand Clin* 11:7–12, 1995.

91. Osterman AL, Seidman GD: The role of arthroscopy in the treatment of lunatotriquetral ligament injuries. *Hand Clin* 11:41–50, 1995.

92. Palmer AK: Triangular fibrocartilage complex lesions: a classification. *J Hand Surg* 14A:594–606, 1989.

93. Pederzini L, Luchetti R, Soragni O, et al: Evaluation of the triangular fibrocartilage complex tears by arthroscopy, arthrography, and magnetic resonance imaging. *Arthroscopy* 8:191–197, 1992.

94. Pegoli L, Ghezzi A, Cavalli E, et al: Arthroscopic assisted bone grafting for early stages of Kienbock's disease. *Hand Surg* 16(2):127–131, 2011.

95. Pell RFT, Uhl RL: Complications of thermal ablation in wrist arthroscopy. *Arthroscopy* 20(2):84–86, 2004.

96. Potter HG, Asnis-Ernberg L, Weiland AJ, et al: The utility of high-resolution magnetic imaging in the evaluation of the triangular fibrocartilage complex of the wrist. *J Bone Joint Surg* 79A:1675–1684, 1997.

97. Richards RS, Bennett JD, Roth JH, et al: Arthroscopic diagnosis of intra-articular distal radius fractures. *J Hand Surg* 22A:57–65, 1997.

98. Roth JH, Poehling GG, Whipple TL: Hand instrumentation for small joint arthroscopy. *Arthroscopy* 4:126–128, 1988.

99. Ruch DS, Smith BP: Arthroscopic and open management of dynamic scaphoid instability. *Orthop Clin North Am* 32:233–240, vii, 2001.

100. Ryu J, Fagan R: Arthroscopic treatment of acute complete thumb metacarpophalangeal ulnar collateral ligament tears. *J Hand Surg [Am]* 20:1037–1042, 1995.

101. Sagerman SD, Short W: Arthroscopic repair of radial-sided triangular fibrocartilage complex tears. *Arthroscopy* 12:339–342, 1996.

102. Sekiya I, Kobayashi M, Taneda Y, et al: Arthroscopy of the proximal interphalangeal and metacarpophalangeal joints in rheumatoid hands. *Arthroscopy* 18:292–297, 2002.

103. Short WH, Werner FW, Green JK, et al: The effect of sectioning the dorsal radiocarpal ligament and insertion of a pressure sensor into the radiocarpal joint on scaphoid and lunate kinematics. *J Hand Surg [Am]* 27:68–76, 2002.

104. Slade JF, 3rd, Geissler WB, Gutow AP, et al: Percutaneous internal fixation of selected scaphoid nonunions with an arthroscopically assisted dorsal approach. *J Bone Joint Surg Am* 85(4):20–32, 2003.

105. Slutsky DJ: Arthroscopic repair of dorsal radiocarpal ligament tears. *Arthroscopy* 18:E49, 2002.

106. Slutsky DJ: Clinical applications of volar portals in wrist arthroscopy. *Tech Hand Up Extrem Surg* 8:229–238, 2004.

107. Slutsky DJ: Distal radioulnar joint arthroscopy and the volar ulnar portal. *Tech Hand Up Extrem Surg* 11:38–44, 2007.

108. Slutsky DJ: The use of a dorsal-distal portal in trapeziometacarpal arthroscopy. *Arthroscopy* 23:1244 e1–1244 e4, 2007.

109. Slutsky DJ: The use of a volar ulnar portal in wrist arthroscopy. *Arthroscopy* 20:158–163, 2004.

110. Slutsky DJ: Wrist arthroscopy through a volar radial portal. *Arthroscopy* 18:624–630, 2002.

111. Tatebe M, Hirata H, Shinohara T, et al: Arthroscopic findings of Kienbock's disease. *J Orthop Sci* 16(6):745–748, 2011.

112. Thiru RG, Ferlic DC, Clayton ML, et al: Arterial anatomy of the triangular fibrocartilage complex of the wrist and its surgical significance. *J Hand Surg [Am]* 11(2):258–263, 1986.

113. Thomsen N, Nielsen N, Jorgensen N, et al: Arthroscopy of the proximal interphalangeal joints of the finger. *J Hand Surg [Br]* 27(3):253–255, 2002.

114. Trumble TE, Schmitt SR, Vedder NB: Factors affecting functional outcome of displaced intra-articular distal radius fractures. *J Hand Surg* 19A:325–340, 1994.

115. Trumble TE, Gilbert M, Vedder N: Isolated tears of the triangular fibrocartilage: management by early arthroscopic repair. *J Hand Surg* 22A:57–65, 1997.

116. Trumble TE, Gilbert M, Vedder N: Ulnar shortening combined with arthroscopic repairs in the delayed management of triangular fibrocartilage complex tears. *J Hand Surg* 22A:807–813, 1997.

117. Trumble TE, Culp R, Hanel DP, et al: Intra-articular fractures of the distal aspect of the radius. *J Bone Joint Surg* 80A:582–600, 1998.

118. Van Kampen RJ, Moran SL: A new volar capsulodesis for scapholunate dissociation. *J Wrist Surg* 1(2):s16–s17, 2013.

119. Vaupel GL, Andrews JR: Diagnostic and operative arthroscopy of the thumb metacarpophalangeal joint. A case report. *Am J Sports Med* 13(2):139–141, 1985.

120. Viegas SF: Midcarpal arthroscopy: anatomy and portals. *Hand Clin* 10:577–587, 1994.

121. Viegas SF, Patterson RM, Peterson PD, et al: Ulnar-sided perilunate instability: an anatomic and biomechanic study. *J Hand Surg [Am]* 15:268–278, 1990.

122. Viegas SF, Yamaguchi S, Boyd NL, et al: The dorsal ligaments of the wrist: anatomy, mechanical properties, and function. *J Hand Surg [Am]* 24:456–468, 1999.

123. Wagner WF, Jr, Tencer AF, Kiser P, et al: Effects of intra-articular distal radial depression on wrist joint contact characteristics. *J Hand Surg* 21A:554–560, 1996.

124. Wahegaonkar AL, Mathoulin CL: Arthroscopic dorsal capsule ligamentous repair in the treatment of chronic scapho-lunate ligament tears. *J Wrist Surg* 2:141–148, 2013.

125. Walsh EF, Akelman E, Fleming BC, et al: Thumb carpometacarpal arthroscopy: a topographic, anatomic study of the thenar portal. *J Hand Surg [Am]* 30:373–379, 2005.

126. Weiss APC, Akelman E, Lambiase R: Comparison of the findings of triple-injection cinearthrography of the wrist with those of arthroscopy. *J Bone Joint Surg* 78A:348–356, 1996.

127. Weiss AP, Sachar K, Glowacki KA: Arthroscopic debridement alone for intercarpal ligament tears. *J Hand Surg* 22A:344–349, 1997.

128. Weiss ND, Molina RA, Gwin S: Arthroscopic proximal row carpectomy. *J Hand Surg* 36A:577–582, 2011.

129. Whipple TL, Marotta JJ, Powell JH III: Techniques of wrist arthroscopy. *Arthroscopy* 2:244–252, 1986.

130. Whipple TL: *Arthroscopic surgery. The wrist*, Philadelphia, 1992, J. B. Lippincott, pp 103–105.

131. Whipple TL: The role of arthroscopy in the treatment of intra-articular wrist fractures. *Hand Clin* 11:13–18, 1995.

132. Whipple TL: The role of arthroscopy in the treatment of scapholunate instability. *Hand Clin* 11:37–40, 1995.

133. Wnorowki DC, Palmer AK, Werner FW, et al: Anatomic and biomechanical analysis of the arthroscopic wafer procedure. *Arthroscopy* 8:204–212, 1992.

134. Wolfe SW, Easterling KJ, Yoo HH: Arthroscopic-assisted reduction of distal radius fractures. *Arthroscopy* 11:706–714, 1995.

135. Yao J, Osterman AL: Arthroscopic techniques for wrist arthritis (radial styloidectomy and proximal pole hamate excisions). *Hand Clin* 21:519–526, 2005.

136. Yao J, Zlotolow DA, Murdock R, et al: Suture button compared with K-wire fixation for maintenance of posttrapeziectomy space height in a cadaver model of lateral pinch. *J Hand Surg [Am]* 35(12):2061–2065, 2010.

18

Fractures of the Distal Humerus

David P. Barei and Douglas P. Hanel

Fracture of the distal humerus is one of the most challenging injuries that confront the orthopedic traumatologist. Given the relative rarity of these fractures, most surgeons have only limited experience in their management.[102] Because of the complex regional anatomy, fracture comminution, and limited points for secure fixation, even experienced surgeons find it challenging to achieve stable fixation leading to early return of range of motion. Injuries of the distal humerus include extracapsular fractures in the supracondylar region, extraarticular intracapsular (transcondylar) fractures, isolated unicondylar fractures, partial or complete articular fractures, and, most commonly, combined supracondylar-intercondylar fractures. We also address infrequent patterns, which have different demands.

GENERAL CONSIDERATIONS IN DISTAL HUMERUS FRACTURES

Preoperative Evaluation

Fractures of the distal humerus occur in a bimodal age distribution, with distinct patient characteristics. Fractures that occur in physiologically young patients are typically the result of high-energy mechanisms, such as motor vehicle collisions or falls from a significant height.[39] Open wounds, other ipsilateral upper extremity injuries, and general systemic injuries frequently coexist because of the higher-energy mechanism.[39] As the elderly population increases, there is a concomitantly increasing incidence of low-energy falls resulting in fractures of the distal humerus. This distinctive version of the fracture is characterized by poor bone quality and may be associated with poor general health or preexisting arthritic changes. There is an increasing incidence of higher-energy injuries in active, higher-demand elderly patients with poor bone quality; therapeutic decisions are more difficult for the surgeon to make with these patients.

History and Physical Examination

The history should focus on the mechanism and time of injury and the identification of other sites of injury. It is also necessary to recognize prior elbow injuries or surgical procedures or preexisting medical conditions that may have affected the entire upper extremity. In addition, assessment of preexisting medical comorbidities, medication use, and function is necessary to determine optimal management. An understanding of the patient's type of employment and physical demands at work will assist in planning the goals and duration of rehabilitation, subsequently facilitating the timing and implementation of modifications at the workplace.

In addition to a complete physical examination, particularly in the setting of a high-energy mechanism, a detailed and focused examination of the injured extremity should be performed. Inspection of the limb may reveal swelling, bruising, and deformity, particularly angulation and shortening. A complete circumferential inspection of the elbow is done to avoid missing open wounds that occur most commonly on the posterior aspect.[73] Patients are typically unable to perform any significant elbow range-of-motion movements because of pain.

The distal vascular status is evaluated by inspecting the color of the distal extremity and by palpation of the radial and ulnar pulses. Poorly palpable pulses are checked using noninvasive Doppler ultrasound or pulse oximetry. If there is a questionable pulse and gross malalignment of the arm, gentle traction can often realign the limb and restore the distal pulse. Angiography or urgent operative vascular exploration is necessary in patients who continue to show an abnormal vascular examination. Any concern for vascular injury should also prompt a careful assessment for compartment syndrome and the necessary surveillance prior to and following surgery. A detailed neurologic examination of the hand and digits, including motor function, sensation, and two-point discrimination, should be performed and recorded to identify injury to the median, radial, ulnar, anterior interosseous, or posterior interosseous nerves. Gofton and coworkers[33] noted that approximately one quarter of the patients in their series exhibited incomplete ulnar neuropathy at the time of injury. These findings, particularly with two-point discrimination, are recorded for later reference in case there is a change before or after surgery. At the conclusion of the physical examination, a sterile dressing is placed over any open wounds and a lightweight above-elbow splint is applied.

Radiographic Examination

Standard anteroposterior and lateral radiographs are generally sufficient to make the diagnosis of a fracture of the distal humerus and to provide a reasonable assessment of the fracture

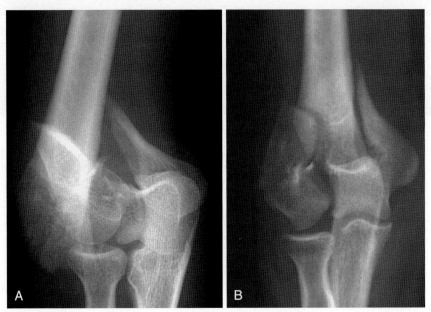

FIGURE 18.1 Resting **(A)** and traction **(B)** anteroposterior radiographs of severely displaced fracture of distal humerus. Note improved fracture comprehension obtained with traction radiograph.

pattern. Radiographs of significantly displaced fractures may be incomprehensible, however, because the normal radiographic landmarks become distorted. Gentle traction can substantially improve alignment to provide more understandable anteroposterior and lateral images. Some sedation may be needed if traction images are performed in the emergency department. Alternatively, traction images in the operating room can be obtained when complete anesthesia has been achieved. Invariably, the previously bizarre appearance of the distal humerus becomes much more understandable (Figure 18.1). Computed tomography (CT) is helpful for fractures distal to the olecranon fossa or fractures primarily occurring in the coronal plane (Figure 18.2).[53,71,101] In particular, fracture comprehension and preoperative planning seem to be improved when the CT scan is obtained with three-dimensional reconstruction.[17] CT may also be useful in older patients to assess the degree of comminution and to aid in deciding whether internal fixation or total elbow arthroplasty (TEA) should be attempted. The complexity of these fractures is underscored in a recent article that describes the number of articular fracture fragments related to fracture type as defined by three-dimensional CT. Bicolumnar patterns were associated with 19 fracture fragments; isolated capitellar and trochlear fractures were associated with 6.5 fracture fragments.[5]

ANATOMY

When viewed from an anterior or posterior position, the distal humerus appears to be shaped like a triangle. The humeral diaphysis diverges into medial and lateral bony columns in the metaphyseal portion of the distal humerus (Figure 18.3). The trochlea (a word derived from a Greek term meaning "pulley") is covered anteriorly, inferiorly, and posteriorly with articular cartilage, creating an arc of approximately 270 degrees.[70] The spatial relationships of the medial column, lateral column, and trochlea are conceptually similar to a spool of thread being held between the thumb and index finger.[55]

The blood supply to the distal humeral diaphysis is entirely dependent on a single nutrient vessel that terminates in the distal humeral metaphysis approximately 3 to 4 cm proximal to the olecranon fossa.[59,124] Vascular watersheds are areas of poor blood flow that occur between the lateral trochlea and capitellum and in the supracondylar area, specifically the olecranon, coronoid, and radial head fossa (Figure 18.4).[59] This latter finding may partially explain why this area is relatively more prone to nonunion than other regions of the distal humerus.

The posterior aspect of the lateral column is covered by the distal origin of the medial head of the triceps muscle and, distally, by the origin of the anconeus. The brachioradialis and extensor carpi radialis longus originate from the lateral supracondylar ridge. The common extensor mass, consisting of the extensor carpi radialis brevis, extensor digitorum communis, and extensor carpi ulnaris, and the cephalad portion of the anconeus muscle originate from the lateral epicondyle, immediately posterior to the origin of the lateral collateral ligament complex. The lateral ligament complex and the common extensor origin blend together and do not have discrete origins.

Most surgical exposures of the distal humerus are performed using a posterior approach; an understanding of the anatomic relationships and paths taken by the ulnar and radial nerves is essential to the safe management of these injuries (Figure 18.5). In the intact humerus, the radial nerve can be found crossing the posterior aspect of the humeral shaft approximately 20 cm proximal to the medial epicondyle (74% of the length of the humerus) to 14 cm proximal to the lateral epicondyle (51% of the length of the humerus). At the lateral aspect of the humeral shaft, the radial nerve trifurcates into a branch to the medial head of the triceps, the lower lateral brachial cutaneous nerve, and the continuation of the radial nerve into the forearm (the posterior interosseous nerve and the superficial cutaneous nerve). After the trifurcation, the posterior interosseous continuation of the radial nerve pierces the lateral intermuscular septum approximately 10 cm proximal to the lateral epicondyle (the distal 36% of the humerus) (Figure 18.6).[30]

At the level of the distal attachment of the coracobrachialis to the humerus, approximately 10 cm proximal to the medial epicondyle, the ulnar nerve courses from the anterior compart-ment to the posterior compartment of the arm by piercing the medial intermuscular septum. The nerve travels along the anteromedial border of the medial head of the triceps along the medial intermuscular septum, ultimately traveling posterior to the medial epicondyle of the distal humerus (Figure 18.7). In approximately 70% of the population, a thick fascial band (arcade of Struthers) connects the medial head of the triceps to the intermuscular septum crossing the ulnar nerve approximately 8 cm proximal to the medial epicondyle.[113] An anatomic clue to the presence of this fascial band is to identify muscle fibers of the medial head of the triceps crossing superficial to the ulnar nerve.[113] As the nerve passes posterior to the medial epicondyle, it becomes enclosed in a fibrous sheath, the roof of the cubital tunnel. As the nerve exits the cubital tunnel, it courses between the two heads of the flexor carpi ulnaris, passes beneath the fibrous origin of the flexor digitorum superficialis, and travels distally through the anterior compartment of the forearm on the anterior surface of the flexor digitorum profundus. The first branch of the ulnar nerve provides sensory inner-vation to the elbow capsule.[113] After exiting the cubital tunnel, motor branches to the flexor carpi ulnaris can be identified. The remaining branches of the ulnar nerve are encountered in the distal forearm and hand.

Classification of Distal Humerus Fractures

For decades, fractures of the distal humerus were collectively referred to as "T" or "Y" fractures, when they involved both columns, or as unicondylar fractures, when they involved only one column. With improvements and refinements in operative management over the past 30 years, a greater understanding of the complexity and variability of fracture patterns affecting the distal humerus has occurred. Ideally, a classification system should provide a basis for reporting results and permitting comparisons among surgeons and cohorts of patients. In addi-tion, the classification should guide decision making and enable some degree of prognostication for each patient. Finally, the classification system should be easy to use, widely accepted, and reproducible.

At the present time, there is no fracture classification system for the distal humerus that fulfills these objectives adequately. The problem of intraobserver and interobserver variability has been found in classification systems for many types of frac-tures; this problem does not seem to be unique to classification

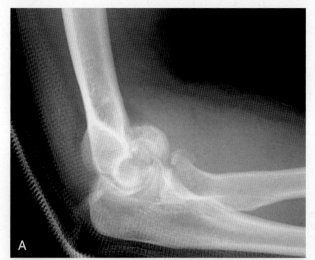

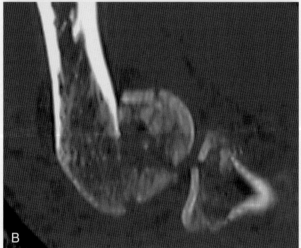

FIGURE 18.2 A, Lateral radiograph of coronal shear variant capitellar fracture. **B,** Sagittal reformation of same image more clearly identifies posterior comminu-tion of distal portion of capitellum. The preoperative plan may now require use of bone graft, changing the anticipated exposure, or use of supplemental posterolat-eral plating techniques.

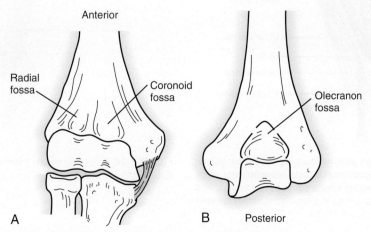

FIGURE 18.3 A and **B,** Anterior and posterior views of osseous distal humerus and important bony landmarks.

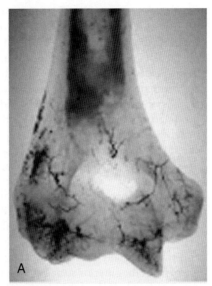
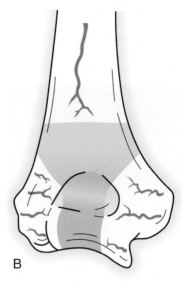

FIGURE 18.4 Actual injection study (**A**) and schematic representation (**B**) showing intraosseous blood supply of dorsal aspect of left distal humerus. Predominant blood supply to the lateral condyle is posterior; also note relative vascular watershed between medial condyle, lateral condyle, and humeral shaft. (**A,** From Kimball JP, Glowczewskie F, Wright TW: Intraosseous blood supply to the distal humerus, *J Hand Surg [Am]* 32:644, 2007.)

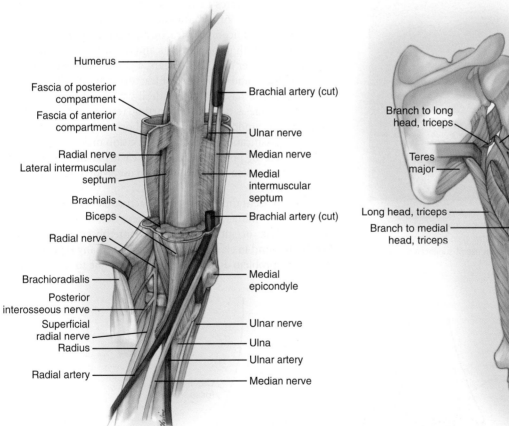

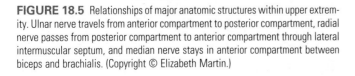

FIGURE 18.5 Relationships of major anatomic structures within upper extremity. Ulnar nerve travels from anterior compartment to posterior compartment, radial nerve passes from posterior compartment to anterior compartment through lateral intermuscular septum, and median nerve stays in anterior compartment between biceps and brachialis. (Copyright © Elizabeth Martin.)

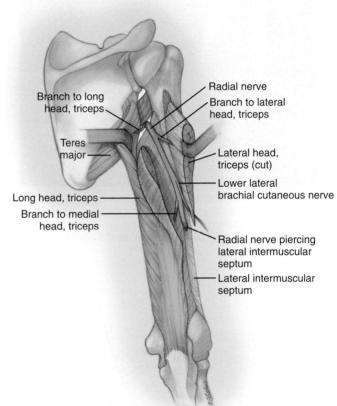

FIGURE 18.6 Posterior view of humerus focusing on midshaft to elbow joint. (Copyright © Elizabeth Martin.)

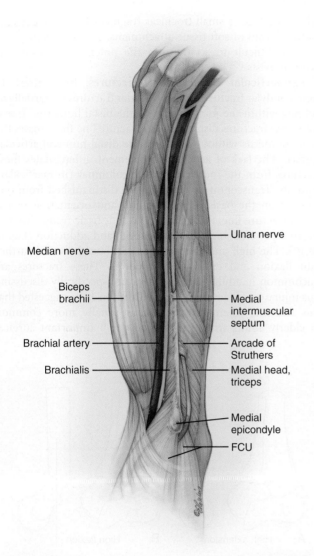

FIGURE 18.7 Course of ulnar nerve as it proceeds through medial intermuscular septum of upper extremity as it travels toward elbow. Note relationship of brachial artery to median nerve. *FCU,* Flexor carpi ulnaris. (Copyright © Elizabeth Martin.)

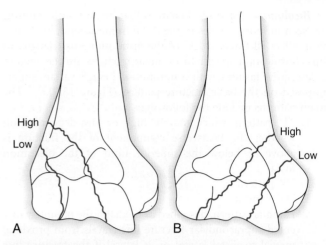

FIGURE 18.8 A, Lateral column fracture of distal humerus. **B,** Medial column fracture of distal humerus.

systems for fractures of the distal humerus. In addition, some patterns of fractures are more common in persons of a certain age than in others. Older patients often exhibit extensive comminution of the articular surface without the same pattern of column fracture described in the classification schemes (see section on fractures in elderly adults). The use of three-dimensional CT scanning may improve observer variability in the currently used distal humerus fracture classification systems.[17]

Comprehensive Classification Systems

Column Concept of Classification. Jupiter and Mehne[55] recommended that the distal humerus be described as two diverging columns supporting an intercalary articular surface, the trochlea, rather than as rounded projections known as condyles. Conceptualizing the distal humerus as medial and lateral columns more accurately describes the injury patterns and allows consistency in the general fracture categories. The Mehne and Matta classification[55,77] is based on surgical anatomic

findings and the columnar concept and helps in formulating effective preoperative surgical tactics. The basic surgical aim is to restore all three elements of the distal humerus triangle (medial column, lateral column, and intervening trochlea) with enough stability to allow early functional movement. Using this classification system, there are three basic fracture categories: intraarticular, extraarticular intracapsular, and extracapsular. Intraarticular fractures are subclassified as single-columnar or bicolumnar injuries, capitellar fractures, or trochlear fractures. Extraarticular intracapsular fractures traverse both columns of the distal humerus without involving the articular surface and are uncommon fractures more likely to be seen in pediatric patients. Extracapsular fractures include injuries to the medial or lateral epicondyles.

Intraarticular Fractures

Single-column fractures. Single-column injuries are uncommon (Figure 18.8). These injuries are divided into medial or lateral *column* fractures, rather than medial or lateral *condyle* fractures as previously described by Milch.[79] Lateral column fractures are reportedly more common than medial column fractures.[79] Rather than emphasizing the involvement of the lateral trochlear ridge, as Milch suggests,[79] this classification system differentiates two types of single-column fractures: "high" fractures and "low" fractures. High fractures have the following characteristics:

- The fractured column contains the bulk of the trochlea.
- The ulna and radius follow the displacement of the fractured column.
- Internal fixation is predictable because of the size of the fragment.

Low single-column fractures have the opposite characteristics for each of the above-mentioned items. Originally, these injuries were thought to be the result of abduction or adduction forces, with involvement of the lateral trochlear ridge being a major determinant of elbow stability.[79] Conversely, Jupiter and Mehne[55] suggested that extensive capsular injury and collateral ligament rupture are more likely to be responsible for the ultimate displacement of the fragment than involvement of the lateral trochlear ridge.

Bicolumnar fractures. Fractures that involve both columns are seen in most injuries to the distal humerus and, by definition, affect all three "sides" of the distal humerus triangle. In this classification system, bicolumnar fractures are classified in a descriptive fashion, with comminution being a variant superimposed on the basic fracture pattern (Figure 18.9).[55,77] The main patterns include the following:

1. "T" pattern, which may be high or low, depending on whether the transverse component of the fracture is above or below the superior limit of the olecranon fossa
2. "Y" pattern
3. "H" pattern
4. Lambda pattern, described as medial if the obliquely oriented supracondylar fracture line travels from proximal medial to distal lateral or as lateral if the fracture line travels from proximal lateral to distal medial

The value of this classification system is in differentiating fracture patterns that occur at or below the level of the olecranon and coronoid fossae.[100] More distal fractures produce small articular fragments that challenge secure fixation. The "H"-type injury produces a small trochlear fragment that may be completely devoid of soft tissue attachments. This fragment is frequently difficult to secure, and the potential for avascular necrosis exists.[100]

Extraarticular Intracapsular Fractures. In contrast to supracondylar fractures, transcolumnar fractures lie partially or entirely within the joint capsule of the distal humerus. Transcolumnar fractures display a main fracture line that crosses the distal humerus without involving the distal humeral articular surface. The lack of articular involvement differentiates these fractures from the more common bicolumnar (intraarticular) patterns. Transcolumnar fractures are distinguished from one another on the basis of the location and orientation of the major fracture line; this gives rise to four basic transcolumnar fracture patterns: high, low, abduction, and adduction (Figure 18.10). The high and low patterns can be subdivided further into flexion and extension subgroups. These fractures are uncommon in adults, and the literature specifically discussing this injury type is limited.[55] Several authors have suggested that this fracture, when encountered, is usually more common in elderly adults with osteopenic bone.[46] Important surgical

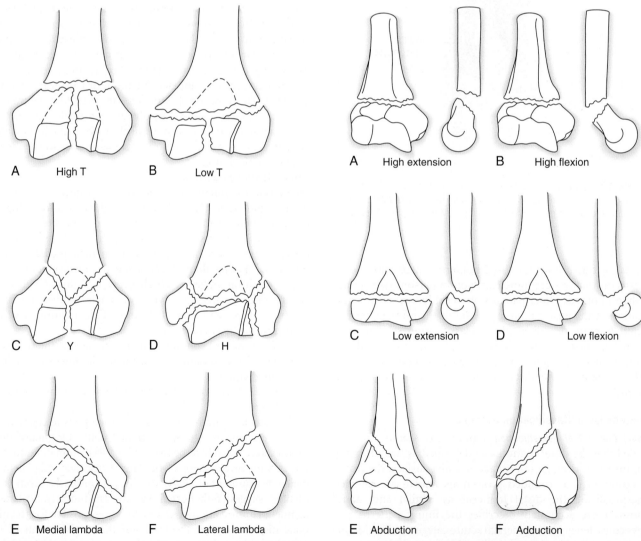

FIGURE 18.9 A to F, Bicolumnar classification of fractures of distal humerus.

FIGURE 18.10 A to F, Transcolumnar classification system.

considerations for management of this fracture type include the following:

1. The more distal the fracture is (low types), the more difficult neutralization of the articular fragment becomes. This situation is worsened in the presence of osteopenic bone.[46]

2. Fractures that are managed nonoperatively or with nonrigid fixation may develop excessive callus formation that obliterates the olecranon, coronoid, and radial fossae, resulting in a loss of motion.[46]

AO/ASIF Classification. The AO/ASIF classification is a comprehensive alphanumeric fracture classification system that distinguishes extraarticular injuries, partial articular injuries (where continuity is maintained between the shaft and a portion of the articular surface), and complete articular injuries.[90] In the three main categories, types A, B, and C, injuries are grouped according to increasing severity, intuitively suggesting that a partial articular injury is more severe than an extraarticular injury, and that a complete articular injury is more severe than a partial articular injury. Within each type, emphasis is placed on the comminution of the supracondylar metaphysis or the articular surface, or both. All three types are extensively subdivided to include most fracture patterns. Type C3 fractures are the most severe, with significant comminution of the articular surface and supracondylar area.

Classification of Fracture Patterns Unique to the Articular Surface

Although involvement of the articular surface is an integral component of most injuries of the distal humerus and a component of the classification systems already described, identification of fracture patterns unique to the articular surface continues to evolve. Conceptually, injuries of the articular surface of the distal humerus may be considered as a spectrum, rather than as discrete entities, because the components of the articular injury may be found in isolation (pure articular injury) or in association with supracondylar injury.

Fractures of the Capitellum. Fractures of the capitellum have been recognized since the mid-19th century. Despite their rarity, two types of fractures have traditionally been described.[22,76] Type I, or *Hahn-Steinthal fracture*, is a fracture of the capitellum that involves a large portion of the osseous structure of the capitellum. The fragment varies in size and usually contains a part of the adjacent ridge of the trochlea. Type II, or *Kocher-Lorenz fracture*, is superficial and mainly involves the chondral surface of the capitellum with very little bone attached. This fracture type essentially results in a shell of capitellar articular cartilage with minimal subchondral bone.[22,76] Subsequently, capitellar fractures have been classified into three types. Type I fractures are complete fractures of the capitellum (similar to the Hahn-Steinthal fracture), type II fractures are superficial (corresponding to the Kocher-Lorenz fracture), and type III fractures are comminuted. A fourth type of capitellar fracture, described by McKee and associates,[71] is termed the *coronal shear fracture*. This fracture involves the capitellum but also extends beyond the lateral trochlear ridge to include a variable, but significant, portion of the trochlea (Figure 18.11). The radiographic hallmark of the coronal shear fracture pattern is the *double-arc sign* on the lateral radiograph, which represents the subchondral bone of the capitellum and lateral trochlear ridge.[71]

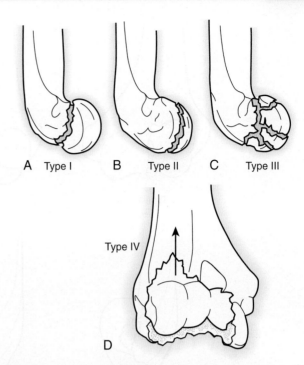

FIGURE 18.11 Four types of capitellum fractures. **A,** Type I fracture is a single fracture line of capitellum that involves a fair-sized piece of bone and anterior aspect of joint. **B,** Type II is a thin fragment, with very little bone attached to anterior cartilage. Type II fractures have much less bone attached to cartilage than seen in type I fractures. **C,** Type III is fracture of capitellum that is in multiple fragments. **D,** Type IV fracture includes capitellum but also extends medially to take off the lateral trochlear lip.

Dubberley and colleagues[21] proposed a classification system that aids with preoperative planning and the formulation of a surgical plan. Type 1 fractures primarily involve the capitellum with or without the lateral trochlear ridge, type 2 fractures involve the capitellum and trochlea as one piece, and type 3 fractures consist of fractures of the capitellum and the trochlea as separate fragments. Within each fracture type, the presence or absence of posterior condylar comminution is noted (Figure 18.12). Medial visualization and exposure are increasingly required with increasing fracture type, and the potential need for bone graft and plate fixation increases with posterior condylar comminution.

Despite the different fracture patterns and variations that exist, fractures of the capitellum are essentially shearing coronal plane injuries.[70] The mechanism of these fractures seems to be an axial load, with the final fracture configuration determined by the degree of elbow flexion at the time of loading.[71]

Fractures of the Trochlea. Isolated trochlear fractures are exceedingly rare injuries.[46,53] Although a formal classification system has not been developed, the two main patterns are fractures of the entire trochlear process and osteochondral fractures.[46,76] Jupiter and other authors[46,53] have suggested that the rarity of these injuries may be due to the trochlea lying protected within the depth of the semilunar notch of the olecranon, without capsular, muscular, or ligamentous attachments. The mechanism of injury remains speculative because of the rarity of the injury, but may involve the coronoid acting as a fulcrum when a force is applied to the flexed elbow.[53] The osteochondral

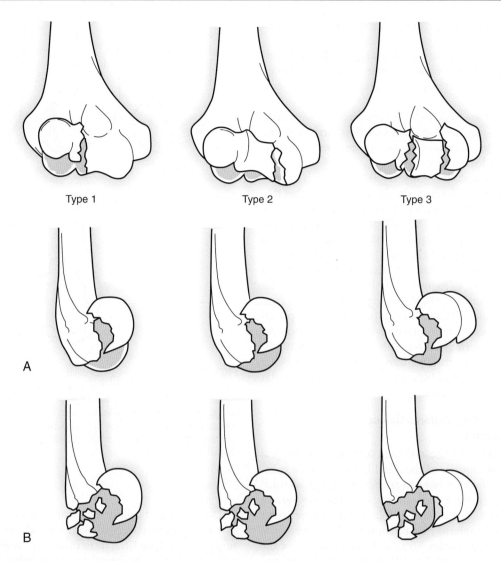

FIGURE 18.12 Type 1 fractures involve primarily capitellum with or without lateral trochlear ridge. Type 2 fractures involve capitellum and trochlea as one piece. Type 3 fractures consist of fractures of capitellum and trochlea as separate fragments. Further characterizations include absence (**A**) or presence (**B**) of posterior condylar comminution.

patterns may be associated with elbow dislocations, however, implying the involvement of a shearing force.

Other Articular Fracture Patterns. Emphasizing the fact that articular fractures of the distal humerus may represent a continuum of injury, Ring and associates[101] evaluated 21 patients with pure articular fractures of the distal humerus. The fracture fragments included and extended beyond the capitellum but did not extend above the base of the olecranon fossa. Five different patterns of injury were identified with increasing involvement of the posterolateral articular surface and medial articular surface (Figure 18.13), as follows:

Type 1 injuries are the coronal shear fractures previously described by McKee and colleagues.[71]

Type 2 fractures are type 1 fractures with involvement of the lateral epicondyle.

Type 3 fractures have associated impaction of the metaphyseal bone posterior to the capitellum.

Type 4 fractures have the additional feature of a fracture of the posterior aspect of the trochlea.

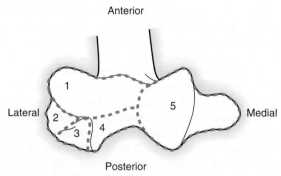

FIGURE 18.13 Classification of pure articular injuries of distal humerus.

Type 5 fractures are type 4 fractures with a fracture of the medial epicondyle.

These specific fracture types represent a progression of injury severity extending from an isolated articular component displaced in the frontal plane to combinations of shearing and

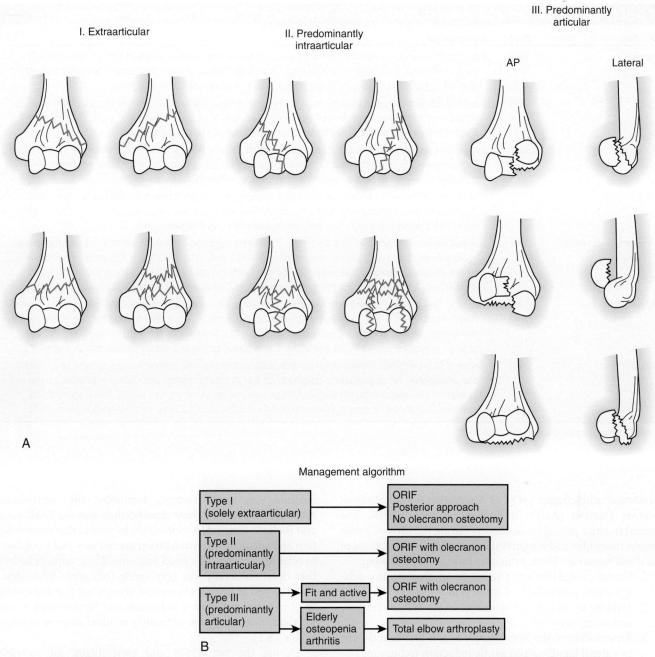

FIGURE 18.14 A, Clinically applicable classification system for fractures of distal humerus. **B,** Subsequent management algorithm using this classification as a functional tool. *AP,* Anteroposterior; *ORIF,* open reduction and internal fixation.

impaction injuries of the capitellum and trochlea with a limited zone of metaphyseal bone support. Because of the difficulty in appreciating some of the potential fracture fragments with standard radiographs, CT scanning with three-dimensional reconstructions may enhance comprehension and preoperative planning.[17,71,101]

Davies and Stanley[15] proposed a unifying classification system emphasizing clinical applicability and a management algorithm. Type I fractures are extraarticular and are analogous to AO/ASIF type A injuries. Type II injuries are single-columnar and bicolumnar fractures where the fracture lines begin in the distal humerus metaphysis and propagate into the trochlea or capitellum, or both. Type III fractures are fractures in which the fracture lines lie predominantly within the articular surface of

the distal humerus but may extend proximally into the distal metaphysis below or at the level of the olecranon fossa (Figure 18.14, *A*). This classification system was noted to be reliable and reproducible and the observer variability was superior to that of either the AO/ASIF or the Mehne classification system. Although simplistic, the proposed management algorithm when used in conjunction with the proposed classification system may be useful for determining basic therapeutic options (see Figure 18.14, *B*).

Historical Review

The history of fracture care was marked by a significant change in management philosophy during the 1960s. The group responsible for the change is known as the Arbeitsgemeinschaft

TABLE 18.1   Closed and Indirect Methods for Treatment of Distal Humerus Fractures

Author	Year	Description
Hitzrot[42]	1932	Described 25 patients treated with traction. Based on his results, Hitzrot strongly advised against open reduction, stating that anatomic reduction was of secondary importance. Eastwood would later agree, stating that perfect anatomic reduction is unnecessary to obtain a good result. Few agree with this view today.
Reich[97]	1936	Described reduction technique using ice tongs to compress condylar displacement, with portable traction to allow the patient to be ambulatory. In six patients, the results were noted to be good in three, fair in two, and poor in one. These outcomes were believed to be better than complications and results shown by ORIF.
Eastwood[23]	1937	Reviewed 14 patients treated with a collar-and-cuff support followed by early elbow mobilization (credited to Thomas). The results were so satisfactory that Eastwood believed it was unwise to use any other technique. Eastwood concluded by stating that function was more important than radiographic appearance.
Watson-Jones[121]	1944	Classic fracture textbook concluded that, "Operative reduction and internal fixation is not justified by the results." Surgical dissection, avascularity of fragments, and use of metallic implants were believed to result in dense adhesions and stiffness. Manipulative reduction, brief casting, and motion were recommended.
Riseborough and Radin[102]	1969	Unveiled Riseborough-Radin classification system. The authors suggested that this classification allowed therapeutic decision making based on amount of rotatory deformity and comminution. Despite this therapeutic classification system, Riseborough and Radin believed that ORIF was rarely indicated. This classification system was used for approximately 2 decades. The best results were obtained in 22 of 29 patients treated with casting or traction.
Brown and Morgan[6]	1971	Described "bag of bones" technique for closed management of intercondylar "T"-shaped fractures of the distal humerus. Flexion-extension arc in 6 of 10 patients was >105 degrees. Better motion seemed to be obtained in elderly patients, with younger adult patients having restricted arcs <85 degrees. These results continued to challenge the results obtained by proponents of ORIF. The role of the "bag of bones" technique in elderly patients was strengthened.
Horne[44]	1980	Review of 50 patients with supracondylar, condylar, and supracondylar/intercondylar fracture patterns. Of 29 patients treated surgically, 16 had poor results compared with 6 of 21 patients treated with casting. Inadequate internal fixation and prolonged postoperative immobilization were responsible for the poor results. Horne recommended conservative treatment for supracondylar/intercondylar distal humerus fractures, particularly when comminuted.

ORIF, Open reduction and internal fixation.

für Osteosynthesefragen (AO), or Association for the Study of Internal Fixation (ASIF) in English-speaking regions. The general fracture principles developed during the early AO days remain true today and are particularly applicable to fractures of the distal humerus. These principles include the following:

1. Fracture reduction and fixation to restore anatomic relationships, particularly of the articular surface
2. Stability by fixation or splintage, as the type of fracture and injury requires
3. Preservation of the blood supply to soft tissues and bone by careful handling and gentle reduction techniques
4. Early and safe mobilization of the part and the patient

Before the development of the AO and before their principles were widely accepted, strong opposition to operative management of distal humerus fractures existed. Reich[97] recognized, however, that open reduction was the only procedure that offered any hope of complete functional restoration. He also recognized that the unsatisfactory results seen with open treatment were due to the "frank exposure" and the difficulty in reducing and then maintaining reduction.[97] In the decades preceding the AO advances, numerous publications debated the superiority of results in patients treated with open versus conservative methods.[11,12,23,42,79,97,117] Numerous closed techniques were described, including manipulation and casting, olecranon traction, cast traction, and condylar reductions using ice tongs or clamps.[42,97,102] Influential authors such as Watson-Jones[121] and the contradictory views of the 1964 and 1966 Instructional Course Lectures from the American Academy of Orthopaedic

Surgeons on these fractures continued the controversy.[80] Although known for their classification system, Riseborough and Radin[102] concluded their article by noting that open reduction and adequate internal fixation are not easy and would seem to offer little chance of a good outcome. These authors believed that open reduction was very rarely indicated. Advocates of either closed or open management recognized that the inability to obtain and maintain a reduction and the subsequent need for rigid immobilization ultimately resulted in poor outcomes (Table 18.1).[7,23,44,50]

During the late 1960s and early 1970s, an increasing number of publications reported satisfactory results with operative reduction and fixation of distal humerus fractures.[7,11,39,53,57,74,115,119,125] A review of the operative techniques contained in these reports shows an increasing use of plate and screw fixation, rather than Kirschner wire fixation, and recommendations of early postoperative mobilization. The importance of proper technique was illustrated by Johansson and Olerud,[50] who suggested that "The osteosynthesis demands as stable fixation as possible, and in our experience this is best obtained by screws, but at the same time exact apposition of the fracture surfaces is required." They further noted that stable osteosynthesis eliminated the need for postoperative immobilization.[50]

The 1980 report by Horne[44] underscored the poor results that are obtained when the goals of open reduction and internal fixation (ORIF) are not met. Horne[44] wrote, "The availability of excellent equipment for the internal fixation of fractures is not an indication for its use," ultimately concluding that except for simple fractures and unicondylar fractures, conservative management is the recommended treatment. Shortly thereafter, Jupiter and colleagues[56] published the results of 34 intercondylar fractures of the humerus managed operatively using the techniques advanced by AO/ASIF. The high proportion of good or excellent results, using a score incorporating range of motion and pain, finally solidified the advantages of ORIF for these fractures.

The last 3 decades of the 20th century have shown tremendous advances in understanding of the various fracture patterns, the techniques used to obtain anatomic reduction and fixation, and the evaluation of these results. Improved appreciation of fracture patterns and techniques combined with substantial progress in understanding the surgical anatomy of the elbow has allowed dramatic advances in posttraumatic management of stiff or arthritic elbows. Advances in arthroplasty and newer fixation techniques are options for the management of comminuted fractures of physiologically sound but elderly patients. The optimal implant remains unknown, however. The use of tensioned-wire fixators, allograft materials, and vascularized autografts has permitted salvage of the most challenging acute high-energy injuries in younger patients. Last, outcome-scoring instruments may further assist in the assessment of treatment (Table 18.2).

OPERATIVE MANAGEMENT OF DISTAL HUMERUS FRACTURES

Operative management of specific fractures of the distal humerus requires identification of fracture and soft tissue injury and patient characteristics, including age, associated injuries, comorbidities, and functional level before injury. These considerations are used to determine the reconstructive tactics, including patient positioning, operative approach, and choice of fixation implants. Important preoperative decisions include the following:

1. Determination of whether the fracture is reconstructible or if the patient is better served by elbow arthroplasty
2. Estimation of the need for visualization of the articular surface to determine the surgical approach and handling of the extensor mechanism
3. Identification of a stable fixation construct that would allow early unrestricted range-of-motion movement

Timing of Operative Intervention

Fractures of the distal humerus are best managed early, but as with most complex intraarticular fractures, definitive treatment should be delayed until optimal surgical resources and personnel and the necessary implants are available. Preoperative planning is essential and should include imaging studies necessary to request the resources mentioned earlier. Patients with isolated injuries are managed at the discretion of the surgeon and based on readiness of the operating suite and the availability of implants. Elderly patients or patients with associated comorbidities must be stabilized before fracture reconstruction. Patients who are managed within 24 hours seem to have fewer complications associated with heterotopic ossification and elbow stiffness and may be more likely to return to work.[65]

Polytrauma Patients

Patients with trauma of multiple bones or associated multisystem trauma are managed according to their overall status and prioritization of their other injuries. This situation may result in a significant delay in definitive management ranging from days to weeks. Such delays ultimately make fracture reduction and fixation more difficult and jeopardize the long-term outcome. Close collaboration with the trauma team leader, general surgeon, or intensivist allows these team members to appreciate the importance and benefits of early fracture fixation. Similarly, the treating orthopedist should be available to proceed with fixation when the patient has been stabilized and cleared for surgery.

Open Fractures

Open fractures are managed urgently with irrigation and débridement. Definitive internal fixation should be applied when the wound is free of contamination and the general condition of the patient permits the procedure.[88] McKee and coworkers[73] reviewed the results of 26 open intraarticular supracondylar fractures managed with a posterior exposure and medial and lateral column plating. The overall infection rate in this series was 11% (3 of 26); however, only one patient developed a deep infection requiring surgical débridement.[73] Other authors have noted a deep infection rate of 28% in high-energy fractures.[34] A much larger proportion of Gustilo type III fractures was noted in the latter study compared with McKee's report (45% vs. 15.4%) and may account for the apparent discrepancy in infection rates. Not surprisingly, open fractures have been shown to have worse functional outcomes than their closed counterparts.[81]

Fractures in Elderly Adults

Successful execution of the principles of ORIF becomes increasingly more difficult in elderly patients because of fracture comminution, poor bone quality, inadequate fracture stability, and a relative intolerance of joint immobilization. Although good results have been shown in many series, complication rates approaching 30% have also been documented.[47,51,63,95,114] In response to these poor outcomes, some authors have advocated TEA as a primary treatment method.[13,58,83,89,96] Although early results of TEA for distal humerus fractures are encouraging, long-term data regarding loosening rates, periprosthetic fracture, and functional outcomes are scant. It is nearly impossible to carry out successfully a truly randomized clinical trial because often the reason for abandoning internal fixation is the practical limitation imposed by the bone quality and degree of comminution. In addition, a failed total elbow replacement in an otherwise active patient can be devastating.

Open Reduction and Internal Fixation in Elderly Adults. The ideal of stable ORIF followed by early joint mobilization and rehabilitation is usually achievable in younger patients, but elderly patients with fracture of the distal humerus may require different strategies to obtain a satisfactory result. In response to the difficulties in achieving adequate fixation in osteopenic elderly patients with distal humerus fracture, modifications to the traditional dual-plate fixation techniques have evolved, including the use of a supplemental third plate,[52,54,55] locking plates,[62,64,109] Kirschner wire augmentation,[82] and parallel plating techniques.[116] A review of ORIF in elderly patients has revealed

TABLE 18.2   Open Methods for Treatment of Distal Humerus Fractures

Author	Year	Description
Van Gorder[117]	1940	Reported eight patients with fractures of distal humerus operatively managed using posterior "triceps-turndown" approach (credited to Campbell) where an inverted "V" of the triceps aponeurosis is incised and reflected distally to gain exposure. Subsequent authors used it for open reduction of similar fractures.
Cassebaum[12]	1952	Used olecranon osteotomy for management of nine "T" and "Y" fractures of distal humerus. This is apparently the first report of the transolecranon approach for management of distal humerus fractures. The original description was credited to MacAusland[67] in 1915.
Milch[79]	1964	Classic early work on isolated fractures of humeral condyles, their injury mechanism, and their relationship with elbow dislocation. It was hypothesized that involvement of the lateral wall of the trochlea was associated with injuries that also led to elbow dislocation. In elbows with dislocations, Milch recommended open treatment.
Miller[80]	1964	This Instructional Course Lecture reviewed a 3-year experience of distal humerus fractures treated with closed means versus ORIF. In one of the first comparative series of distal humerus fractures, Miller noted that the operative group had a substantially greater elbow range of motion than the closed treatment group (111 degrees vs. 47 degrees). Miller was convinced that ORIF was the procedure of choice, but recognized the following limitation: "If the arm requires immobilization after open reduction and fixation, then the advantage of surgery is lost."
Cassebaum[11]	1969	Reported 36 distal humerus "T" and "Y" fractures treated with internal fixation using transolecranon approach. Recognized elbow arc of 50 to 165 degrees as excellent because most tasks could be completed within this range. Cassebaum's range-of-motion criteria for excellent, good, and fair were used extensively in subsequent reports.
Bryan and Bickel[7]	1971	Reviewed 25 operatively managed distal humerus fractures treated through posterior approach. Bryan and Bickel preferred screw fixation rather than Kirschner wires and recommended early mobilization after secure internal fixation. They suggested that their patients would not have done as well with closed methods but that the open technique should be done by an experienced surgeon. They also warned that occasionally the difficulties encountered during ORIF of comminuted distal humerus fractures "may be mortifying." This article was presented during a period when there was no consensus in the literature regarding the best method of treatment for these fractures.
Scharplatz and Allgower[105]	1975	Review of 105 fracture-dislocations of elbow. Principles of AO operative treatment of the distal humerus were outlined: reconstruction of the joint surface first, the trochlea being the most important part, and then connection to the shaft of the humerus.
Jupiter et al[56]	1985	Results of 34 intercondylar fractures of distal humerus treated with operative fixation using AO techniques; 27 of 34 patients obtained good to excellent results at a mean of 5.8 years. Jupiter and colleagues confirmed the ability to achieve improved and more predictable results with operative treatment even in a comminuted fracture.
Zagorski et al[125]	1986	Compared results of 42 intraarticular fractures of the distal humerus; 29 were treated operatively with screws or plate and screw constructs, and 13 were treated nonoperatively. Of patients, 76% treated with open techniques had a good to excellent result compared with 8% in the conservatively treated group. Zagorski and associates believed that final fracture reduction was related to functional end results.
Jupiter et al[57]	1988	Jupiter and coworkers managed 22 unicondylar fractures operatively; 18 had good to excellent results. This article illustrated AO principles applied to unicondylar fractures.
Helfet and Hotchkiss[36]	1990	Biomechanical study evaluated implant configurations and distal humerus fracture stability. The 90-degree orthogonal plate construct was identified and proven to be mechanically superior. Helfet and Hotchkiss could not find a difference between tubular plates, 3.5-mm reconstruction plates, or mixed plates.
John et al[51]	1994	First large series evaluating contemporary ORIF techniques in distal humerus fractures in elderly patients. Average age was 80 years (range 75 to 90 years); 85% were thought to have a functional arc of motion (>90 degrees); 66% had no pain. Implant failures were related to use of tubular plates.
Garcia et al[28]	2002	Consecutive series of 19 patients all >60 years old treated with primary TEA for nonreconstructible fracture of distal humerus. There was no associated inflammatory illness; 3-year follow-up showed 68% with no pain and a mean Mayo score of 93 (excellent). This article shows early advantages of TEA in this patient population. Long-term data are lacking, however. ORIF versus TEA in elderly patients continues to be debated.

ORIF, Open reduction and internal fixation; *TEA,* total elbow arthroplasty.

satisfactory results for the most part. Pereles and colleagues[95] showed an average arc of motion of 112 degrees, a functional Mayo Elbow Performance Score, and no difference in the SF-36 score compared with normal data in 14 patients with distal humerus fractures treated with ORIF. Good or excellent results were achieved in 12 patients, but only 25% of patients reported no pain. The mean age in this group was 70 years.

John and associates[51] evaluated 49 older patients (mean age 80 years) an average of 18 months after ORIF. Good or very good results were achieved in 85%, with 85% having a range of motion of 90 degrees or greater; 66% of these patients reported no pain. This group included extraarticular fractures (16%), unicolumnar fractures (27%), and bicolumnar fractures (57%). Huang and coworkers[47] retrospectively reviewed 19 patients older than 65 years with distal humerus fractures treated with ORIF. In this series, all fractures united with a mean time to union of 14.6 weeks, and all patients showed a good-to-excellent result based on the Mayo Elbow Performance Score.

Other more recent studies have shown far less satisfactory results, however, with higher complication rates and additional surgeries (Table 18.3).

Total Elbow Replacement in Elderly Adults. Early clinical experiences with elbow arthroplasty for various degenerative conditions showed variable results, with high rates of unsatisfactory outcomes related to loosening and instability. Advances in implant technology and surgical technique have led to predictably good outcomes in properly selected patients. The available literature evaluating elbow arthroplasty in older patients with acute distal humerus fractures shows excellent early results, with a satisfactory flexion-extension arc of approximately 110 degrees and excellent relief of pain.[13,26-28,93,96] The length of follow-up in these studies is 2 to 4 years and does not address the long-term concerns of implant loosening, mechanical failure, revision requirements, and functional implications.

More recently, Kamineni and Morrey[58] evaluated the results of 49 distal humerus fractures in 48 elderly patients treated with TEA after an average of 7 years. The authors showed high functional outcome scores, but with a relatively higher rate of postoperative complications than seen in other studies. They noted a regression of the initial flexion-extension arc by 25 degrees, ultimately still averaging a functional arc of 24 to 131 degrees. Although long-term results in patients with TEA for inflammatory arthritis do seem durable,[32,41,108,123] the results of TEA in patients with posttraumatic arthritis show lower patient satisfaction and possibly greater mechanical failure rates than in patients with inflammatory arthritis.[41,108] A patient seeking to engage in high-demand activities is a poor choice for TEA (Table 18.4).

In one of the few comparative studies, Frankle and associates[26] compared the results of TEA with ORIF in women older

TABLE 18.3 **Clinical Outcomes After Open Reduction and Internal Fixation of Distal Humerus Fractures in Elderly Patients**

Reference	No. Patients (Mean Age)	No. Good-to-Excellent Results	Mean Postoperative Flexion-Extension Arc	No./Type of Complications	No. Secondary Procedures
John et al[51]	49 (80 yr)	31/39 complete follow-up (79%)	85% with minimum of 30 to 120 degrees	10 (20%)/1 wound infection, 1 nonunion, 2 broken plates, 6 transient ulnar neurapraxias	2: 1 wound débridement for infection, 1 broken implant removal
Pereles et al[95]	18 (71 yr)	12/12 complete follow-up (100%)	18 to 130 degrees	2 (11%)/2 loose implants	1: revision for loosened implants
Huang et al[47]	19 (72 yr)	19 (100%)	17 to 128 degrees	2 (10.5%)/1 superficial wound infection, 1 ulnar nerve injury	None
Srinivasan et al[114]	21 (85 yr)	12 (57%)	22 to 100 degrees	7 (25%)/4 wound infections, 2 nonunions, 1 heterotopic ossification	1: removal of implants secondary to infection
Korner et al[63]	45 patients (73 yr)	58%	Median arc 100 degrees	13 (29%)/12 implant failure and screw loosening, 1 persistent ulnar neuropathy	7: all secondary to implant failure or loosening

Adapted from Strauss EJ, Alaia M, Egol KA: Management of distal humeral fractures in the elderly. *Injury* 38(Suppl 3):S10–S16, 2007.

TABLE 18.4 **Clinical Outcomes of Primary Total Elbow Arthroplasty for Treatment of Distal Humerus Fractures in Elderly Patients**

Reference	No. Patients (Mean Age)	No. Good-to-Excellent Results; Mean Mayo Elbow Score	Mean Postoperative Flexion-Extension Arc	No./Type of Complications	No. Secondary Procedures
Cobb and Morrey[13]	20 (72 yr)	20 (100%); 95	25 to 130 degrees	5 (25%)/1 ulnar component fracture, 3 ulnar neurapraxias, 1 reflex sympathetic dystrophy	1: revision fractured ulnar component
Ray et al[96]	7 (82 yr)	7 (100%); 92	20 to 130 degrees	1 (14%)/1 superficial wound infection	None
Gambirasio et al[27]	10 (85 yr)	10 (100%); 94	23.5 to 125 degrees	1 (10%)/1 heterotopic ossification	None
Garcia et al[28]	19 (73 yr)	16/16 complete follow-up (100%); 93	24 to 125 degrees	1 (5%)/1 superficial wound infection	None
Kamineni and Morrey[58]	49 (67 yr)	40/43 complete follow-up (93%); 93	24 to 131 degrees	17 with at least 1 complication (35%)/11 wound infections, 3 neurologic symptoms, 3 periprosthetic fractures, 3 loose implants	10: 5 wound débridements, 2 revisions for periprosthetic fracture, 3 revisions for loose components

Adapted from Strauss EJ, Alaia M, Egol KA: Management of distal humeral fractures in the elderly. *Injury* 38(Suppl 3):S10–S16, 2007.

than 65 years with distal humerus fractures. Patients treated with TEA showed significantly better results using the Mayo Elbow Performance Score than patients treated with ORIF. The authors suggested that women older than 65 years with significant associated comorbidities (e.g., rheumatoid arthritis, osteoporosis, and conditions requiring systemic steroids) and the presence of articular comminution be managed with TEA. Provided that the articular fracture components are large, however, these authors recommended ORIF as long as the patient's physiologic age is less than 90 years.

McKee and colleagues, in a prospective randomized controlled trial of ORIF versus TEA for displaced intraarticular distal humerus fractures in elderly patients, concluded that in patients who are not amenable to stable fixation with ORIF, TEA is the preferred alternative treatment modality.[75]

We agree with the previously mentioned studies of Frankle and associates[26] that successful management of these patients must take into account the patient's physiologic age, functionality, associated comorbidities, and fracture characteristics. Specific fracture characteristics in this patient population that are unreliably stabilized with internal fixation include the following:

- Significant comminution of the trochlea
- Associated coronal plane fracture patterns
- Fractures that occur almost entirely below the olecranon fossa

In these injuries, the small fragments combined with frequently coexisting osteoporosis make TEA an attractive alternative (Case Study 18.1). CT is particularly useful in assessing the presence of coronal plane fracture fragments. Patients who are unable or unwilling to refrain from strenuous physical activity must be extensively counseled regarding the risks of implant loosening and periprosthetic fracture and the potential for a poor outcome. In these patients, ORIF with techniques to obtain union of the distal humerus, including postoperative immobilization, should be strongly considered, rather than TEA.[35]

Patient Position and Anesthesia

Fractures of the distal humerus can be managed with the patient in the supine, lateral, or prone position, with the choice based on the anticipated exposure, the presence of other injuries, and surgeon preference.[38,74,92,105] The lateral and prone positions (Figure 18.15) are most commonly employed when proceeding

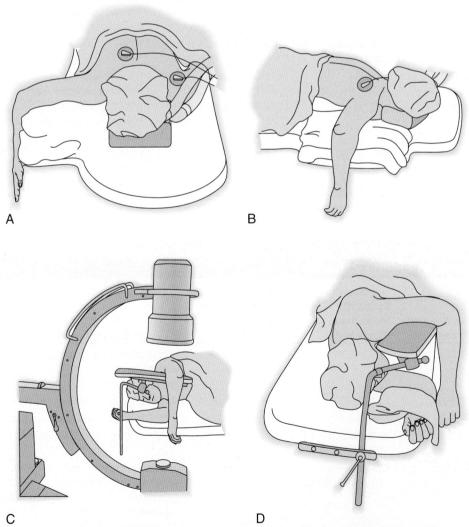

A

B

C

D

FIGURE 18.15 A and **B,** Surgical patient in prone position before open reduction and internal fixation. **C** and **D,** Same patient in lateral position. Note "C"-arm used for anteroposterior radiographs **(C).**

with posterior exposures of the elbow. The supine position is typically reserved for lateral elbow exposures or for patients with multisystem trauma that precludes lateral or prone positions.

ORIF of fractures of the distal humerus is typically a lengthy procedure requiring a general anesthetic. Postoperative pain control may include the use of selective upper extremity nerve blockades; however, the postoperative neurologic examination of the hand would be impaired for the duration of the block. Consideration should be given to postoperative block placement, which allows for examination of nerve function after completion of the case. A sterile tourniquet may be employed but is used infrequently, only if it can be placed proximal enough on the arm to avoid interference with fracture reduction and fixation.

Operative Exposures

Virtually all fractures of the distal humerus treated operatively can be approached through a midline posterior skin incision (Figure 18.16). An effort should be made to deviate the incision a full 2 cm away from the tip of the olecranon. The lateromedial plane of dissection is directed between the triceps muscle and its investing fascia. The next step in any exposure of the medial column is identification and protection of the ulnar nerve. The nerve is mobilized and protected throughout the procedure. Instruments are not attached to any loop or Penrose drain around the nerve to prevent accidental traction on the nerve. A Penrose drain is looped about the nerve and sutured to itself. No instruments should be attached to the drain to avoid accidental traction injury to the nerve. The medial intermuscular

septum is incised if fracture management requires exposure of the anteromedial elbow. Similarly, the laterally directed dissection leads to the lateral intermuscular septum.

The course of the radial nerve is less obvious than its medial counterpart but can still be reliably identified. First, the nerve crosses through the lateral intermuscular septum approximately halfway along the length of the humerus, or half the distance between the tip of the acromion and the tip of the olecranon. Second, if the dissection is directed from the lateral epicondyle proximally, the cutaneous branches to the posterior lateral arm and forearm are encountered in the dissection of the lateral intermuscular septum. These cutaneous nerves are branches of the radial nerve, and they can be followed proximally to their origin. In most distal humerus fractures treated with open reduction, the radial nerve does not need to be exposed. The lateral intermuscular septum is divided, however, for exposure to the anterolateral elbow region. This approach provides near-circumferential access to the medial and lateral columns. This posterior midline approach can be used for later reconstructive procedures, obviating the need for multiple skin incisions.

How the extensor mechanism of the elbow is subsequently managed is the key differentiating feature among the potential approaches used to expose the distal humerus and is dictated by the fracture characteristics and surgeon preference. For significant intraarticular fractures of the distal humerus requiring direct visualization of the articular surface, there are two options for management of the extensor mechanism: an olecranon osteotomy or soft tissue mobilization around the olecranon.

Paratricipital Approach

The least disruptive posterior approach is the paratricipital exposure.[1,107] This dissection entails mobilization of the triceps off the posterior aspect of the medial and lateral intermuscular septa and the posterior aspect of the humerus. Medially, the ulnar nerve is identified and protected. Laterally, the radial nerve is identified and mobilized, allowing surgical manipulation of approximately 95% of the posterior aspect of the humeral shaft.[30] At the elbow joint, the triceps can be retracted posteriorly and distally, enabling visualization of the posterior aspect of the lateral column and limited visualization of the posterior aspect of the trochlea (Figure 18.17). Supracondylar fractures, transcondylar fractures, and simple intraarticular fractures (unicolumnar or bicolumnar) without articular comminution are the main injuries that can be managed with this exposure. It is exceedingly difficult to appreciate, let alone secure, comminuted intraarticular fractures of the distal humerus through this exposure. Currently, the paratricipital approach is the authors' preferred exposure for total elbow replacement in a nonreconstructible intraarticular distal humerus fracture in an elderly patient (Case Study 18.2).

Olecranon Osteotomy

Olecranon osteotomy is the classic exposure for reduction and fixation of intraarticular fractures of the distal humerus.[11,12,67] As in the paratricipital approach, the triceps muscle is mobilized from the medial and lateral septa and followed distally. The osteotomy is performed at the deepest portion of the trochlear notch of the olecranon process and is coincident with an area devoid of articular cartilage, termed the "bare area." We favor a chevron-shaped osteotomy because of its increased

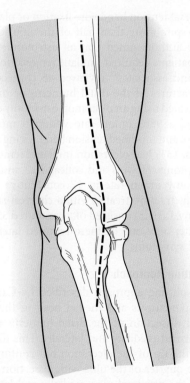

FIGURE 18.16 Posterior view of upper arm and elbow area showing location of skin incision. The ideal surgical incision is a generally straight line that gently curves laterally (or radially) to avoid tip of olecranon.

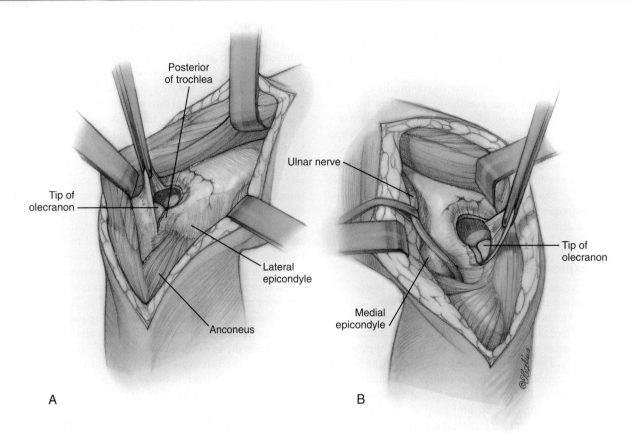

FIGURE 18.17 Paratricipital approach. **A,** Starting at lateral epicondyle, triceps is elevated from posterior aspect of humerus. More proximal dissection reveals radial nerve crossing lateral margin of humerus to enter anterior compartment of arm. Lateral column is readily identified through this dissection. Lateral aspect of trochlea is appreciated, but visualizing articular surface is difficult. **B,** Medial column and medial aspect of trochlea are exposed after mobilizing and protecting ulnar nerve. (Copyright © Elizabeth Martin.)

postfixation stability.[56] To avoid splitting the proximal olecranon fragment, the apex of the chevron points distally.[70] It is typically initiated with a fine oscillating saw and completed with a thin osteotome. The triceps muscle and the osteotomized proximal half of the olecranon are then reflected superiorly (Figure 18.18).

Techniques of olecranon osteotomy fixation include Kirschner wire and tension band constructs, screw and tension band constructs, and plate fixation.[11,12,38,39,56,57] The advantage of the olecranon osteotomy is the excellent and direct visualization of the distal humeral articular surface,[122] enabling anatomic reduction. Increased operative exposure time is a potential drawback of the olecranon osteotomy, but it may be offset by the visualization afforded for direct articular reduction. Olecranon osteotomy is most commonly used in the management of bicolumnar fractures with articular displacement. Any articular injury of the distal humerus, including unicondylar fractures, and pure articular fractures extending posterior to the capitellum or the posterior aspect of the trochlea, or both, are indications for this exposure.[56,101]

Cited complications or disadvantages of olecranon osteotomy include osteotomy nonunion, delayed union, and hardware prominence.[39] More recent evidence has suggested that these drawbacks are quite infrequent compared with previous reports. Coles and colleagues[14] reported on 70 distal humerus fractures exposed using a chevron-shaped olecranon osteotomy exposure. Osteotomies were secured with either medullary

screw and dorsal tension band wire fixation or plate fixation. In this study, despite more than half of the injuries being open fractures, the authors noted that all osteotomies united, and only 8% of patients required implant removal for local symptoms. Ring and associates[98] reviewed 45 consecutive patients with acute fractures of the distal humerus or distal humerus nonunions treated using an olecranon osteotomy exposure. The authors noted a 98% union rate within 6 months using a Kirschner wire and modified tension band wiring technique. Of these patients, 13% had olecranon implants removed for relief of local symptoms. Hewins and colleagues[40] similarly noted a 100% osteotomy union rate in 17 consecutive patients with distal humerus fracture treated with a chevron-shaped olecranon osteotomy. Repair consisted of a contoured 3.5-mm reconstruction plate; only one of these required later removal for relief of local symptoms.

Triceps-Splitting Approach

The triceps-splitting approach described by Campbell[9] splits the triceps aponeurosis and medial head in the midline.[73,126] Subperiosteal dissection of the distal humerus and proximal ulna is performed medially and laterally. This dissection does not cease at the tip of the olecranon but continues along the proximal one quarter of the ulna with dissection of the triceps insertion off the proximal ulna medially and laterally (Figure 18.19). The joint capsule is divided to allow visualization of the articular surface. At the conclusion of the procedure, the triceps

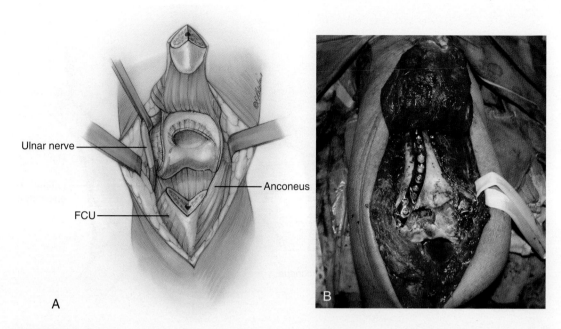

Ulnar nerve

Anconeus

FCU

A

FIGURE 18.18 Olecranon osteotomy. **A,** Entire posterior aspect of humerus is exposed, and articular surface is visualized after performing olecranon osteotomy. **B,** Intraoperative photograph after open reduction and internal fixation of comminuted open intraarticular distal humerus fracture. A portion of lateral column and posterolateral trochlea were absent at the time of ORIF. *FCU,* Flexor carpi ulnaris. (**A,** Copyright © Elizabeth Martin.)

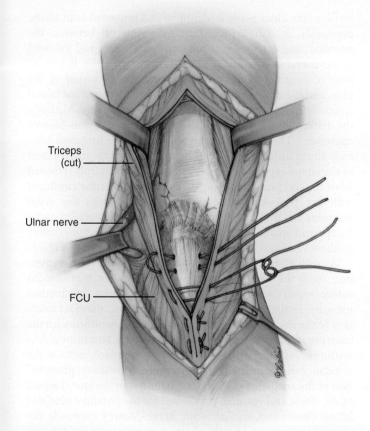

Triceps (cut)

Ulnar nerve

FCU

FIGURE 18.19 Triceps-splitting approach. Distal one third of triceps is simply split longitudinally to olecranon process. At olecranon process, split continues longitudinally, with elevation of triceps insertion sharply off bone medially and laterally. Triceps is essentially split into medial and lateral halves and retracted peripherally, allowing visualization of underlying distal humerus. *FCU,* Flexor carpi ulnaris. (Copyright © Elizabeth Martin.)

is repaired back to the proximal ulna with interrupted, nonabsorbable suture through osseous drill holes. Cited advantages of this exposure are its technical ease, the ability to use the trochlear notch as a template against which the distal humerus can be reduced, and the avoidance of hardware around the proximal ulna.[70] A potential complication of this exposure is the loss of strength of elbow extension. McKee and colleagues[74] were unable to show a difference in elbow extension strength, however, in patients treated with the triceps-splitting approach compared with patients treated with an olecranon osteotomy, making it a satisfactory alternative to olecranon osteotomy.

Although the main disadvantage of this exposure is the inability to visualize directly a significant portion of the articular surface compared with olecranon osteotomy, hyperflexion of the elbow substantially improves this limitation.[126] The main indications for this exposure have included bicolumnar intraarticular fractures of the distal humerus and extraarticular supracondylar fractures. This exposure is also indicated when the triceps aponeurosis has been transected by the distal aspect of the humeral diaphysis (Case Study 18.3); when this occurs, the fracture is typically open posteriorly.[73] In this situation, olecranon osteotomy further disrupts the integrity of the extensor mechanism, and this situation is a relative contraindication for olecranon osteotomy. McKee and colleagues[73] were able to show improved results with the triceps-splitting approach in these open injuries compared with using an olecranon osteotomy. A modification of the exposure is typically required to incorporate nonmidline traumatic disruptions of the extensor mechanism.[73,126]

Bryan-Morrey "Triceps-Sparing" Approach

The Bryan-Morrey triceps-sparing approach is commonly used for performing TEA procedures[8] but may also be used for

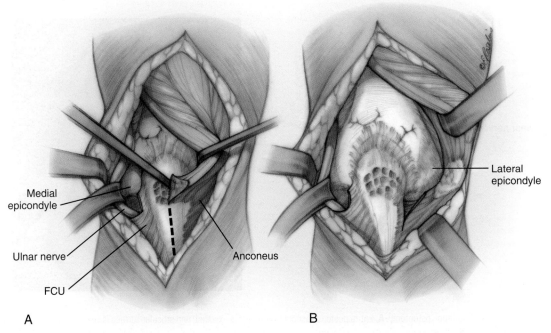

FIGURE 18.20 Bryan-Morrey "triceps-sparing" approach. **A,** Initiation of dissection on medial aspect. **B,** Entire triceps insertion taken off proximal ulna. Note view of posterior aspect of distal humerus. *FCU,* Flexor carpi ulnaris. (Copyright © Elizabeth Martin.)

fixation of fractures of the distal humerus.[24] After a midline posterior skin incision is made, the ulnar nerve is identified along the medial aspect of the triceps and is elevated from its bed. Dissection carries through the cubital tunnel and fascia over the flexor carpi ulnaris muscle until the first motor branch is identified. When the ulnar nerve is freed and protected, dissection continues with the elevation of the medial aspect of the triceps off the posterior aspect of the medial intermuscular septum and posterior aspect of the distal humerus. Distally, the fascia over the flexor carpi ulnaris is incised toward the ulna. The triceps insertion is sharply reflected directly off bone (Figure 18.20). This medial-to-lateral dissection is continued until the anconeus and triceps can be retracted over the lateral humeral condyle. Because the fascia over the proximal ulna is thin and prone to perforations during its elevation, some authors have described elevation as an osteoperiosteal flap.[94] A small osteotome can be used to elevate the fascia with small petals of bone, which aids in repositioning the triceps insertion at the conclusion of the procedure (restoring the normal length-tension relationship) and in healing of the extensor mechanism back to the proximal ulna. The triceps insertion is repaired back to the proximal ulna with nonabsorbable transosseous suture. Advantages and disadvantages of this approach are similar to the triceps-splitting procedure. This exposure is indicated in older patients undergoing ORIF of a distal humerus fracture that may require intraoperative conversion to TEA.

Triceps-Reflecting Anconeus Pedicle Approach

The triceps-reflecting anconeus pedicle (TRAP) approach, as described by O'Driscoll,[92] offers an extensile option for surgical exposure of the distal humerus without the need for olecranon osteotomy, while preserving the neurovascular supply to the anconeus muscle. After an adequate midline posterior skin

incision, the ulnar nerve is identified and protected as in all the previously described procedures. The interval between the anconeus and extensor carpi ulnaris is identified and followed to the lateral border of the ulna. Beginning distally, the anconeus is dissected subperiosteally off the lateral aspect of the ulna, and the dissection is carried proximally toward the lateral epicondyle and along the lateral supracondylar ridge. Medially, the triceps is mobilized as described in the Bryan-Morrey approach.[8] The dissection medially along the proximal ulna ends 10 cm distal to the olecranon, joining with the distal extent of the lateral exposure. The triceps insertion is sharply removed from the olecranon and carried laterally to become confluent with the previous lateral dissection. Ultimately, the distal humerus and proximal ulna are exposed subperiosteally, and a triceps and anconeus flap is created and mobilized proximally to allow visualization of the distal humerus (Figure 18.21).

As with all procedures that sharply detach the triceps insertion from the olecranon, heavy nonabsorbable transosseous suture repair is mandatory to restore extensor mechanism integrity. Similar to the Bryan-Morrey exposure, the exact insertion of the triceps into the olecranon may be identified with the incorporation of a small wafer of bone or a suture to aid in anatomic repair.[8,94] Advantages of this approach include the avoidance of complications of olecranon osteotomy; preservation of the anconeus as a dynamic stabilizer of the lateral aspect of the elbow and vascular muscle bed for the proximal ulna and lateral elbow; and, similar to the Bryan-Morrey approach, the ability to convert to TEA should fracture reduction and fixation prove to be unattainable.

Anconeus Flap Transolecranon Approach

The anconeus flap transolecranon approach, described by Athwal and colleagues,[3] combines the anconeus preservation of

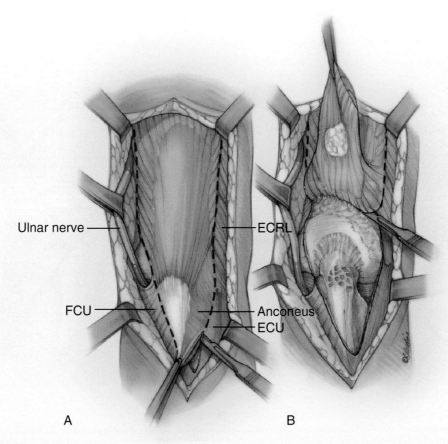

FIGURE 18.21 Triceps-reflecting anconeus pedicle (TRAP) approach. **A,** Posterior view of distal humerus after skin incision. Important features are ulnar nerve and *dotted lines* that indicate where deep dissections begin. **B,** Illustration of how triceps insertion and anconeus are taken off as single structure from proximal ulna. Extensor mechanism is reflected cephalad. *ECRL,* Extensor carpi radialis longus; *ECU,* extensor carpi ulnaris; *FCU,* flexor carpi ulnaris. (Copyright © Elizabeth Martin.)

the TRAP[92] approach with the exposure obtained from olecranon osteotomy. Using an adequate midline posterior skin incision and mobilization of the ulnar nerve, the interval between the anconeus and extensor carpi ulnaris is identified and followed to the lateral border of the ulna. The anconeus muscle is elevated from distal to proximal off the ulna to the level of the planned osteotomy, typically at the deepest portion of the trochlear notch. An apex distal chevron-shaped olecranon osteotomy is created as described earlier. The anconeus muscle flap and the olecranon fragment are elevated off the posterior aspect of the humerus, in continuity with the triceps muscle, allowing exposure of the articular surface.[3] At the conclusion of the procedure, the osteotomy is rigidly stabilized, and the anconeus flap is anatomically repaired to the extensor carpi ulnaris fascia laterally and the ulnar periosteum medially. The purported advantage of the anconeus flap transolecranon approach is the maximal articular visualization afforded by olecranon osteotomy, while preserving an innervated vascularized anconeus through the use of internervous planes (Figure 18.22).

Lateral Approach

The lateral approach may be initiated with either a lateral or a posterior skin incision.[20,94] The choice of a posterior skin incision requires the elevation of a full-thickness lateral cutaneous flap, but this may be preferred should alternative deep dissection be required, such as conversion to an olecranon osteotomy,

or if future reconstructive procedures are anticipated. The main indication for this approach and its extensile variations is in the management of significant fractures of the capitellum and other articular fracture variants.

In Kocher's lateral approach, the dissection is directed through the substance of the anconeus and the lateral capsule and then carried proximally from the exposed radial head. Hotchkiss[45] noted that this exposure disrupts a significant portion of the posterolateral capsular complex. He advocated that a better lateral approach is one that preserves this vital structure by starting proximally at the lateral condyle and proceeding distally. Using the skin incisions described earlier, the lateral epicondyle is palpated, and the muscles originating from the anterior surface of this ridge are elevated with sharp dissection. The anterior joint capsule is raised, and the capitellum is exposed. Attached to the lateral condyle are the fibers of the lateral ligament complex. Hotchkiss[45] suggested that "the articular surface of the capitellum should be bisected as one looks from the vantage point of the lateral aspect of the capitellum," and that all of the capsular structures that run anterior to this imaginary line can be elevated, whereas all of those posterior should be preserved (Figure 18.23).[45]

The anterior capsule is elevated as a single layer to the level of the radiocapitellar joint. Further distal joint exposure requires dividing the annular ligament. Still further distal dissection requires entering the common extensor compartment. The

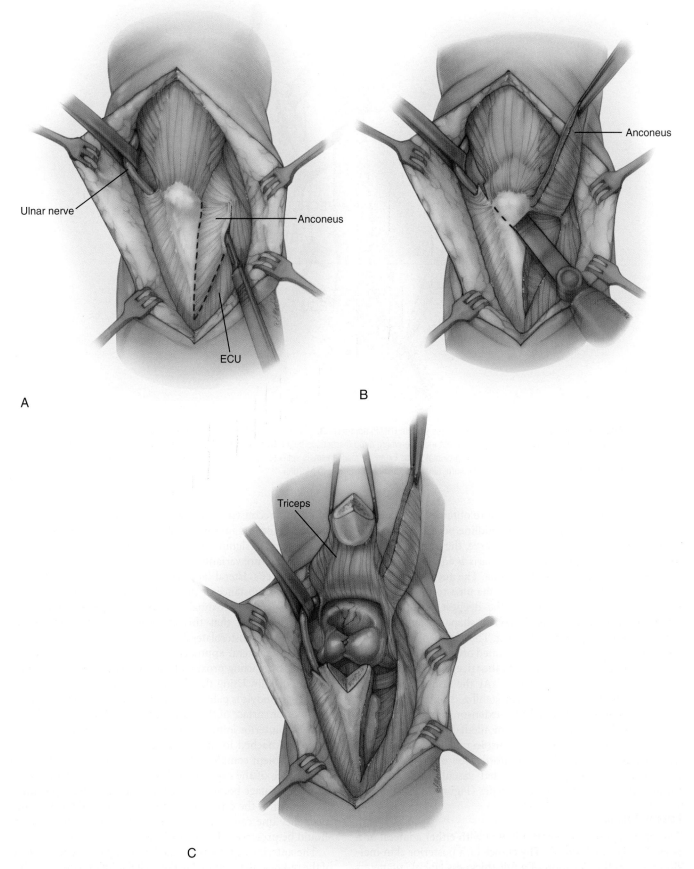

FIGURE 18.22 Anconeus flap transolecranon approach to distal humerus. **A,** The anconeus musculature is identified and elevated from the lateral aspect of the proximal ulna, preserving its neurovascular supply. **B,** With the anconeus retracted proximally, the olecranon is osteotomized. **C,** The extensor mechanism, the olecranon process, and the anconeus muscle are reflected cephalad, revealing distal humerus. *ECU,* Extensor carpi ulnaris. (Copyright © Elizabeth Martin.)

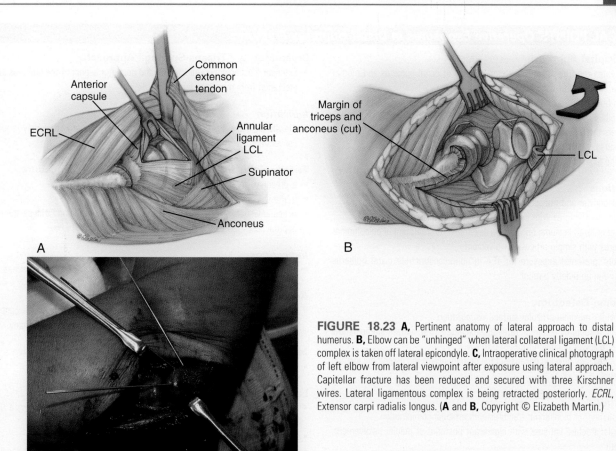

FIGURE 18.23 A, Pertinent anatomy of lateral approach to distal humerus. **B,** Elbow can be "unhinged" when lateral collateral ligament (LCL) complex is taken off lateral epicondyle. **C,** Intraoperative clinical photograph of left elbow from lateral viewpoint after exposure using lateral approach. Capitellar fracture has been reduced and secured with three Kirschner wires. Lateral ligamentous complex is being retracted posteriorly. *ECRL,* Extensor carpi radialis longus. (**A** and **B,** Copyright © Elizabeth Martin.)

posteriormost portion of this muscle mass is elevated from the septum separating it from the anconeus. As the common extensor mass is elevated, the intermuscular septum, the anconeus, and the posterior lateral ligamentous complex are left intact; this exposes the muscle fibers of the supinator muscle. The supinator muscle can be elevated from the posterior lateral margin on the ulna while holding the forearm in full pronation. This approach protects the posterior interosseous nerve while exposing the head and neck of the radius. Fractures of the lateral column and shearing fractures of the capitellum can be identified and reduced with this approach.

If the posterior aspect of the lateral column needs to be exposed, the triceps muscle is lifted from the posterior face of the lateral column and the medial edge of the triceps followed into the anconeus muscle. The posterior joint capsule can be elevated off the dorsal aspect of the lateral column, but the joint fibers that are found emanating from the distal lateral aspect of the lateral column should be left intact. They are the posterior lateral ligaments of the elbow.

In cases in which visualization of the posterior and inferior aspects of the lateral column is still inadequate, the origin of the lateral collateral ligament and the lateral margin of the triceps and anconeus can be elevated from the lateral epicondyle. At this point, the elbow can be hinged open on the intact medial collateral ligament complex.[101] At the conclusion of the procedure, the lateral collateral ligament is returned to its origin and secured to the lateral epicondyle with transosseous nonabsorbable suture or suture anchors.

Fixation Principles

The goals of operative fixation of fractures of the distal humerus are to restore articular congruity; reestablish anatomic mechanical axes; and obtain enough fracture stability to allow early, unrestricted elbow range of motion. Numerous factors contribute to making these goals difficult to reach, including the following:

1. Relatively small, cancellous distal fragments offer poor fixation potential.
2. The complex osseous anatomy makes plate contouring difficult.
3. Screws that violate the articular surfaces and the olecranon, coronoid, and radial fossae hamper motion.
4. Osteopenic bone compromises construct stability.

Despite the numerous fracture patterns possible, several fixation principles are applicable to all fracture patterns (Case Study 18.4), as follows:

1. Kirschner wires are used to provide provisional fixation before definitive plate fixation and should be placed strategically to avoid interference with the application of definitive implants. Common Kirschner wire sizes are 0.045-inch (1.14-mm), 0.054-inch (1.37-mm), and 0.062-inch (1.57-mm) wires. When Kirschner wires cannot be placed to maintain a provisional reduction reliably, small 2-mm plates secured with 2-mm screws may be used to secure a critical reduction zone. As with the placement of Kirschner wires, these small temporary plates should not interfere with definitive fixation.

CRITICAL POINTS *Operative Exposures in Distal Humerus Fractures*

Paratricipital Approach

- It elevates the triceps from posterior aspects of distal humerus and medial and lateral intermuscular septa.
- It can be converted to an olecranon osteotomy if needed.
- Laterally, it can be developed into an extensile posterior exposure.
- It offers the least visualization of the articular surface compared with other exposures.
- It is the exposure least disruptive to the extensor mechanism.

Indications

- Supracondylar and transcondylar fractures
- Bicolumnar fractures with simple articular involvement
- Medial or lateral column only can be developed for treatment of unicolumnar fractures with simple articular involvement
- Authors' preferred exposure for TEA in nonreconstructible distal humerus fracture in an elderly patient

Olecranon Osteotomy

- It provides maximal articular surface visualization.
- Historic osteotomy nonunion rates approximated 10%; current studies show markedly lower nonunion rates of 0 to 2%.
- Symptoms may develop because of the prominence of the osteotomy fixation implants.

Indications

- Unicolumnar or bicolumnar fractures with articular comminution
- Articular fracture variants with significant posterior or medial involvement, or both
- Authors' preferred exposure for fractures of distal humerus with significant articular displacement or comminution

Triceps-Splitting Approach

- Familiar exposure of the distal third of the humeral metadiaphysis is provided.
- For adequate articular visualization, the triceps insertion is dissected off the proximal one fourth of the ulna medially and laterally.

Indications

- Supracondylar and transcondylar fractures
- Bicolumnar fractures with significant disruption of the triceps aponeurosis (i.e., open fractures)
- Fractures in elderly patients that may require conversion to TEA

Bryan-Morrey "Triceps-Sparing" Approach

- Extensor mechanism is reflected off the posterior aspect of the humerus and olecranon from medial to lateral

Indication

- Classic exposure for ORIF of fractures in elderly patients that may require conversion to TEA

Triceps-Reflecting Anconeus Pedicle (TRAP) Procedure

- It preserves the neurovascular supply to the anconeus.
- It allows conversion to TEA if required.
- Articular visualization is similar to that of triceps-splitting and triceps-sparing approaches.

Indications

- Similar to indications for triceps-splitting and triceps-sparing approaches

Anconeus Flap Transolecranon Approach

- It combines the preservation of the neurovascular supply to the anconeus with the articular visualization obtained with transolecranon osteotomy.

Indications

- Similar to indications for olecranon osteotomy

Lateral Approach

- Initial dissection should be anterior to the lateral epicondyle, along a line bisecting the capitellum.
- Medial column articular injuries are not well visualized.
- Visualization is enhanced by (1) elevating the musculature and joint capsule from the anterior aspect of the supracondylar ridge of the distal humerus or (2) detaching the lateral ligamentous complex from the lateral epicondylar region.

Indication

- Isolated lateral column articular injuries (capitellar fractures and variants)

---

2. Fixation of the trochlea should achieve interfragmentary compression but avoid stenosis.[52,56] This latter situation may be encountered in patients with central sulcus comminution and functional or overt articular bone loss (Figure 18.24). Stenosis results in joint incongruity and altered cartilage loading, leading to decreased range of motion and posttraumatic arthritis. Although its use is exceedingly rare, structural corticocancellous bone graft has been recommended to bridge the defect, with satisfactory results noted.[31]

3. Whenever possible, screws placed into the distal articular segment should be placed through a plate that is subsequently attached to the diaphysis. Because of the limited space available for fixation devices within the trochlea, placement of screws through the plate allows two functions to be performed with a single implant: (1) neutralization of sagittal fracture lines within the troch-

lea and (2) attachment of the trochlea to the humeral diaphysis.

4. Smaller articular fragments can be secured with Herbert screws or independent 1.5-mm, 2-mm, or 2.4-mm screws that are countersunk below the articular surface.[71,101,115] These implants are typically placed to neutralize coronal plane articular fragments before fixation of the more common sagittally oriented trochlear fragments. These implants need to be strategically placed so as not to interfere with the trochlear fixation coming from the medial and lateral plates.

5. Medial column fractures that result in the separation of the trochlea from the medial epicondyle ("H" pattern) are particularly challenging because the trochlea has no attachment to the medial or lateral column and may be devoid of soft tissue attachments. In this situation, the medial plate can be contoured around the medial

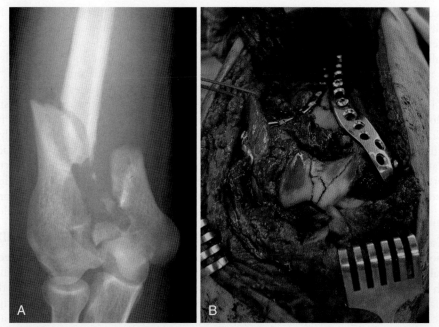

FIGURE 18.24 A, Anteroposterior injury radiograph of bicolumnar distal humerus fracture. Note central trochlear comminution. **B,** Intraoperative photograph of same injury after reduction and definitive stabilization using olecranon osteotomy exposure. Note that central trochlear comminution has been reduced and stabilized. Failure to reduce this fragment may result in overcompression of trochlea and ultimately ulnar-trochlear incongruity.

epicondyle and then distally along the medial wall of the trochlea. The most distal hole of the plate can be used additionally to secure the trochlea. Plate contouring of this area is quite difficult but can be performed on an anatomic model preoperatively to decrease operative time, or, alternatively, a precontoured periarticular distal humerus plating system that features this contour can be used. Because of the metallic bulk in this region of the cubital tunnel, the ulnar nerve is commonly transposed.

6. Secure fixation of the reconstructed articular segment to the distal humerus metadiaphysis can be enhanced with the placement of a screw that begins at the distal portion of either the medial or the lateral column plate and travels retrograde within the distal medial or lateral column, engaging the distal humerus diaphyseal cortex. These "column screws" improve the construct rigidity across the distal humerus metaphysis, but they should not jeopardize fixation of the distal articular surface to the medial or lateral plates.

7. Unicondylar fractures may be managed with single-column screw and plate implants or screw fixation alone, with both options showing satisfactory results.[57] With single-column plating techniques, the plate typically functions as an antiglide device. In unicondylar fractures with columnar comminution in the supracondylar region, the plate acts as a buttress.

Implant Biomechanics

The orthopedic community generally agrees that surgical reduction and internal fixation of distal humerus fractures show improved outcomes compared with nonoperative treatment. There is also agreement that unstable internal fixation commonly results in a poor outcome. What remains controversial is the question of which implant design and placement

would be ideal and provide optimal stability for fractures of the distal humerus. The guidelines proposed by the AO group are considered by most orthopedists to represent the standard technique for fixation of bicolumnar distal humerus fractures. Their recommended technique consists of screw fixation of the articular fragments and column stabilization with two plates at a 90-degree angle to one another. The specific recommendations for plate types have included tubular, 3.5-mm reconstruction, or combinations thereof. Subsequent to the guidelines proposed by the AO group, Helfet and Hotchkiss[36] published an influential study that confirmed that orthogonally oriented plates were much stiffer in the sagittal plane than either crossed malleolar screws or a posterior "Y"-plate. Their orthogonal plate groups consisted of medial and posterolateral 3.5-mm reconstruction plates, medial and posterolateral tubular plates, and a medial tubular plate and a posterolateral 3.5-mm reconstruction plate. No significant differences in stiffness could be detected among the orthogonal plating groups, and the authors concluded that two-plate fixation at right angles was the optimal construct for the stabilization of fractures of the distal humerus. The biomechanical properties of parallel plating constructs were not examined in this study, however, and implants were not stiffer than the 3.5-mm reconstruction plates used because these were the implants available at the time.

Jacobson and colleagues[49] examined five different distal humerus plating constructs in cadaveric specimens. They concluded that a medially applied 3.5-mm pelvic reconstruction plate and a 3.5-mm posterolateral dynamic compression plate provided the greatest sagittal plane stiffness and equivalent frontal plane and torsional stiffness compared with other constructs, including parallel-plated and triple-plated specimens. In that series, the parallel-plated specimens consisted of 3.5-mm reconstruction plates. Schemitsch and colleagues[106] evaluated the construct rigidity of distal humerus fixation with plates placed in five different configurations. These authors concluded that if maximum rigidity is required, in the absence of cortical contact between fragments, two plates applied opposite to each other are biomechanically superior in providing rigidity of fixation. Specifically, that model consisted of a medial 3.5-mm pelvic reconstruction plate and a rigid lateral, precontoured, anatomically shaped "J"-plate. They further concluded that two-plate constructs do not require placement at 90 degrees to obtain sufficient rigidity, but do require placement on separate columns and different surfaces. Schemitsch and colleagues[106] also noted that a further advantage of the lateral plate was the ability to insert long screws transversely from lateral to medial into the medial trochlea, allowing increased screw purchase.

Self and associates[110] similarly noted that a parallel plate construct consisting of a lateral "J"-plate with a medial 3.5-mm reconstruction plate showed significantly more rigidity to axial loading than orthogonal 3.5-mm reconstruction plates. Linking the parallel plates with a cross-bolt was found to stiffen and strengthen this construct further, suggesting that linking of the distal portion of the medial and lateral plates improves fixation into the distal articular segment. In a distal humerus fracture model, Arnander and coworkers[2] showed that parallel 3.5-mm reconstruction plates were significantly stronger and stiffer than perpendicular 3.5-mm reconstruction plates when they were subjected to sagittal bending forces. The strength of this study is that the only variables that changed were the plate position (from a posterolateral location to the straight lateral aspect of the lateral column) and the subsequent screw lengths that secured the lateral plate.

Despite the theoretical benefits associated with locked plate fixation in osteopenic bone, support for locking plate fixation of the distal humerus remains limited. Korner and colleagues[62] reported that locking compression plates placed in an orthogonal position showed significant improvement in sagittal bending and torsional stiffness compared with plates placed in a dorsal position. The utility of this conclusion is minimized because the use of purely dorsal plating in the management of distal humerus fractures has been abandoned. The authors further concluded, however, that the plating technique is more important for obtaining stable fracture fixation than the type of plate used because there was no significant mechanical difference between orthogonally placed conventional reconstruction plates and locking compression plates. Schuster and colleagues[109] showed improved mechanical stability of distal humerus fracture fixation with locking orthogonal plate constructs over conventional fixation in specimens with poor bone mineral density, but noted no difference in specimens with high bone mineral density. Similarly, Stoffel and colleagues[116] compared two distal humerus locking plate systems in paired cadaveric bone fracture models. These authors concluded that the parallel locking plate system provided significantly higher mechanical stability than the orthogonal system. More recently, studies comparing precontoured anatomic plates with and without locking fixation show that locking constructs provide greater fixation stiffness, with the inference that they may be more beneficial in the setting of severe comminution or poor bone quality.[48]

Despite the array of plate types, constructs, and fracture models that have been examined, some conclusions can be made regarding the mechanical stabilization of bicolumnar distal humerus fractures. First, the literature strongly continues to support two-column plating, rigid fixation, and anatomic reconstruction of the articular surface, and when properly applied, less expensive and more readily available implants can be expected to provide similar results.[10,61]

When examining plates of the same type, two parallel plates seem to offer improved mechanical stability compared with strictly orthogonal plates, particularly in the sagittal plane. As long as both columns are secured rigidly, the columnar component of the fracture is likely to heal. Limited-contact dynamic compression plates, 3.5-mm reconstruction plates, and precontoured periarticular plates all are sufficiently rigid to provide satisfactory stable fixation. Thinner one-third tubular plates used as primary column support should be avoided.[39,43]

❖ AUTHORS' PREFERRED METHOD OF TREATMENT

Fracture management requires the surgeon to be prepared with a thorough preoperative plan yet remain amenable and versatile enough to modify the initial plan as the operation proceeds. Because every fracture is unique, principles, rather than a strict series of steps, should be understood and followed. Common pitfalls should be anticipated before the patient enters the operating room. Conceptually, pitfalls may be organized as related to the fracture pattern or related to fixation problems.

General Considerations and Potential Pitfalls

Unanticipated fracture lines or comminution can pose significant problems in the execution of a preoperative plan and may require intraoperative modifications, including changing from one anticipated operative exposure to another or modifying the fracture construct, or both. Fracture patterns that are particularly troublesome are (1) coronal plane fractures of the capitellum or trochlea, or both, (2) separation of the medial aspect of the trochlea from the medial column, and (3) "low" (very distal) fracture patterns.

These fracture characteristics can be identified on plain radiographs, particularly on quality traction films. When the presence of these fractures is suspected, CT may aid in the diagnosis[71,101] and comprehension, particularly when combined with three-dimensional reconstructions.[17] When associated coronal fractures exist, they are reduced and managed before reduction of the remainder of the articular surface. Fracture of the trochlea from the medial column frequently requires distal modification of the medial column plate to ensure rigid fixation of the articular segment to the humeral shaft. Low fracture patterns result in a small distal articular segment that jeopardizes distal fixation. We believe olecranon osteotomy is required to manage these fracture patterns adequately.

Achieving adequate fixation to allow early range of motion is often crucial for successful management of fractures of the distal humerus. If the quality of fixation would not tolerate aggressive rehabilitation and motion of the elbow, preservation of the joint takes priority. Accepting some loss of motion is preferable to losing the entire articular surface of the trochlea. The articular segment is usually where fixation is most tenuous. There are techniques that may improve fixation. By placing several screws through the distal portions of medial and lateral plates across the distal articular segment, empowered fixation can be achieved through the "interference" of the screws within the segment.[91,104] The risk in this technique is the loss of reduction as the screws are forced to engage one another. A second option, particularly useful in elderly patients, is to shorten the humerus in the metaphyseal fracture area, creating enhanced bone contact and a more stable supracondylar construct. Additionally, three or more plates can be used distally to obtain orthogonal fixation within each column. These supplementary plates can provide surprisingly good stability and have been shown to be clinically effective in this setting.[33,52]

Supracondylar and Transcondylar Fractures: Proximal Patterns

Displaced extraarticular fractures of the distal humerus are managed operatively to avoid prolonged immobilization of the elbow joint and resultant stiffness. Patients may be positioned in the lateral or prone position, depending on the presence of other injuries. Because of the distal location of the fracture, stabilization generally requires the application of medial and lateral column plates, and a paratricipital approach using a posterior skin incision is used. Given the extraarticular nature of these fractures, olecranon osteotomy is rarely indicated. Occasionally, the fracture pattern results in the lateral column extending proximally to a point that sufficient distal fixation may be obtained with a single plate fixed proximally along the posterior aspect of the humeral diaphysis and, distally, along the posterior aspect of the lateral column (e.g., abduction transcondylar variant). In this situation, the extensile exposure described by Gerwin and associates[30] is used, without the need for dissection of the medial column. If at any point the stability of the fracture is in question, this approach is easily expanded to the paratricipital exposure, allowing manipulation and stabilization of the medial column.

Bicolumnar Fractures in an Active Patient With Healthy Bone

Bicolumnar fractures of the distal humerus are managed operatively with ORIF techniques using a posterior universal midline skin incision. Patients are usually placed lateral on a well-padded radiolucent table with a radiolucent arm board to support the injured upper extremity. The prone position is particularly useful for fractures that extend into the humeral diaphysis, allowing easier fluoroscopic imaging. We use the lateral position for patients who are otherwise unable to be placed prone. Definitive fixation is with medial and lateral plate and screw implants. Multiple plate constructs should be considered for significantly comminuted fractures on a case-by-case basis.

Minimally Comminuted Fractures. Preoperatively, the degree of articular comminution and displacement is assessed. Fractures with simple articular splits, with large condylar fragments, and without major displacement are exposed using the paratricipital approach. If a satisfactory reduction can be obtained along the medial or lateral column in the supracondylar region, this reduction is performed first, allowing indirect approximate reduction of the articular surface. Supracondylar reductions are provisionally stabilized with Kirschner wires. The adequacy of articular reduction is mainly confirmed fluoroscopically; with retraction of the triceps aponeurosis posteriorly and flexion of the elbow, the posterior aspect of the trochlea is also directly visualized and palpated with a small periosteal elevator, confirming or disproving fluoroscopic images. Adjustment of the

---

CRITICAL POINTS *Bicolumnar Fractures*

Preoperative Evaluation
- Obtain anteroposterior, lateral, and traction view radiographs.
- Consider CT for extreme distal (or "low") fracture patterns in elderly patients or articular fractures of variant patterns.

Pitfalls
- Unrecognized articular comminution, particularly in the coronal plane
- Fracture lines that separate the medial trochlea from the medial column
- Unanticipated poor bone quality (osteoporosis)

Operative Exposure
- Choose the exposure that best allows reduction and stabilization of the articular surface.
- With increased patient age, choose an exposure that does not compromise a TEA.
- We prefer olecranon osteotomy for managing displaced, comminuted fractures involving the articular surface. The paratricipital approach is our preferred exposure for patients who may require conversion to TEA.

Technical Points
- Medial and lateral column fixation provides the best fracture stability.
- A medial plate is usually a reconstruction-type implant and is applied directly medially; a lateral implant is frequently stiffer (dynamic compression plate) and is applied to the posterior aspect of the lateral column.
- Medial fixation is typically applied first because it is less likely to be obstructed by temporary Kirschner wires.
- Precontoured periarticular plates are available, but they may still need minor contour adjustments.
- Secure articular fragments with screws that are placed through a plate, whenever possible.
- Consider ulnar nerve transposition.
- Before wound closure, the elbow is placed through a range of motion to ensure fracture stability.

Postoperative Care
- The elbow is splinted in extension at the conclusion of the procedure.
- Range-of-motion exercises are begun within 24 to 48 hours postoperatively. The patient must understand that the initial goal of rehabilitation is to obtain motion.
- Active flexion and passive extension are performed for all exposures except for lateral and paratricipital exposures, which are allowed active extension.
- Gentle stretching and active range-of-motion exercises for extension and flexion are initiated at 6 weeks.
- Resistive and strengthening exercises begin at week 12 and should be commensurate with radiographic consolidation.
- Static progressive splinting is considered between weeks 6 and 12 if the active range of motion plateaus below a functional arc.

Athletic Participation and Manual Labor
- Consolidation of fracture lines radiographically is required.
- Strength should be approaching 75% of the contralateral uninjured extremity.

---

articular surface reduction is performed with larger-diameter Kirschner wires placed into the condyles to act as joysticks. When the articular surface is realigned, a large pointed reduction clamp is placed across the condyles, and the articular surface is compressed. The articular reduction is provisionally maintained with Kirschner wires (Case Study 18.5).

Fractures with significant comminution of the articular surface are treated using olecranon osteotomy. The reduction sequence varies, depending on the particular fracture patterns.

Multiplanar Articular Involvement. Fractures that display multiplanar involvement of the articular surface (coronal plane fragmentation) are managed first with reduction and stabilization of the anterior articular components (see Case Study 18.3). This is usually accomplished by displacing the sagittal fracture line, allowing access to the medial aspect of the capitellum and the lateral aspect of the trochlea. By allowing the metaphysis to shorten through the supracondylar fracture, visualization of the anterior components of the articular surface is facilitated. The anterior articular surface is typically definitively stabilized at this point with posterior-to-anterior minifragment screws while direct visual confirmation of secure anatomic reduction is still possible. When the anterior articular surface is secured, the sagittally oriented fracture (separating the distal articular surface into medial and lateral components) is reduced and provisionally stabilized. The metaphyseal fracture is reduced, essentially orienting the distal humerus articular segment appropriately beneath the metadiaphysis. This segment is provisionally stabilized, and intraoperative fluoroscopy is used to confirm the adequacy of reduction.

Simple Supracondylar Involvement. Intraarticular fractures that show minimal comminution in the supracondylar region have long fracture planes that are amenable to anatomic reduction (medial and lateral lambda patterns). When these features are present, we prefer to begin the reduction and temporary stabilization sequence in this supracondylar area first. The goal is to restore reliably a segment of the articular surface to the metadiaphysis and then build the remaining articular surface to this restored column. This sequence is effective, provided that the supracondylar area can be reduced and provisionally stabilized reliably.

Combined Articular and Supracondylar Comminution. Fractures with combined articular and supracondylar comminution are a significant challenge and must be individualized (Case Study 18.6). In fracture patterns where metaphyseal comminution is extensive, we initially focus on the reduction and temporary stabilization of the articular surface. The distal humerus articular surface is oriented and provisionally stabilized in the proper transverse, sagittal, and coronal planes relative to the metadiaphyseal region. In situations with marked metaphyseal comminution, this area is indirectly reduced and secured with the aid of appropriately contoured or precontoured periarticular plates; this maintains viability of the metaphyseal fragments, allowing predictable union. In an older patient undergoing ORIF, the humerus can be shortened through the comminuted metaphysis to allow intrinsic bone contact and stability of the entire construct. Shortening provides minimal functional deficits, provided that the olecranon and coronoid fossae are not obliterated, and offers improved fracture stability and union in older patients.

Technique for Olecranon Osteotomy. For maximum visualization of the articular surface of the distal humerus, we prefer to perform an olecranon osteotomy. At the conclusion of the procedure, the osteotomy is secured with a medullary screw and tension band technique. The screw is placed in a unicortical fashion with distal purchase obtained from the screw threads interacting with the endosteal ulnar surface. In many patients, a partially threaded 4.5-mm screw and washer are used; however, in older patients or patients with larger stature, a 6.5-mm lag screw is occasionally used. The technique for a 4.5-mm screw is described.

Creation of Osteotomy. Visualization of the "bare area" of the olecranon is performed by division and elevation of the medial and lateral capsular attachments along the olecranon process and corresponds to the deepest portion of the semilunar notch. Using the lateral fluoroscopic image, the olecranon is predrilled, first with a 4.5-mm glide hole to the level of the anticipated osteotomy. This is followed with a 3.2-mm drill bit. It is imperative to begin the drill hole in the center of the proximal aspect of the olecranon process relative to its medial and lateral surfaces. When the glide hole in the metaphyseal area of the olecranon is passed, the 3.2-mm drill bit is inserted to the limit of the glide hole and subsequently oscillated distally within the ulnar medullary canal. The purpose for oscillating the drill is to avoid exiting the ulnar diaphysis inadvertently. Approximately at the junction of the middle and proximal thirds, the ulna curves, presenting a convexity laterally. Drilling is stopped at this curved area, approximately 90 to 120 mm distal to the tip of the olecranon. The length of the anticipated screw is measured, and the drill hole is tapped with a 4.5-mm tap. This last step is eliminated if self-tapping screws are used.

A small sponge is placed between the articular surface of the semilunar notch and the fractured articular surface of the distal humerus. Placement of a sponge allows an assistant to provide counterpressure on the proximal ulna and avoids inadvertent injury to the distal humerus articular surface. With the aid of the lateral fluoroscopic image, a 2.5-mm drill is placed in the midline dorsal surface of the olecranon process immediately across from the "bare area." The drill is advanced to the subchondral surface, but not through it (Figure 18.25, *A*). A fine oscillating saw is used to create the osteotomy into, but not through, the subchondral bone (see Figure 18.25, *B*). The osteotomy is created in a chevron pattern, with the apex of the chevron pointing distally (see Figure 18.25, *A*). The 2.5-mm drill hole on the dorsal surface orients the operator and avoids creating an "X" at the apex of the osteotomy. A thin osteotome is inserted into the saw tract, and the osteotomy is completed by cracking the remaining osteochondral surface (see Figure 18.25, *C*). The tip of the olecranon and triceps is reflected proximally. A suture is used to hold the extensor mechanism to the skin of the proximal arm as a retraction aid. A moistened sponge is draped over the exposed triceps musculature and olecranon. Figure 18.26 provides a clinical example.

Fixation of Osteotomy. The previously placed proximal retraction suture is removed, allowing the extensor mechanism to return to its normal orientation. A 2.5-mm drill bit is used to create a bicortical drill hole from medial to lateral in the ulnar shaft approximately 3 to 4 cm distal to the osteotomy site, in anticipation of the tension band wire. A long 3.2-mm drill bit is placed by hand through the previously created drill hole in the tip of the olecranon process and delivered down the medullary canal of the ulna. This drill bit acts as a guide rail along which the olecranon process can be steered, helping to eliminate translational deformities. Medial and lateral large point-to-point reduction forceps are placed across the osteotomy and are used to fine-tune the reduction and ultimately to compress the osteotomy. Two 0.062-inch Kirschner wires are placed from the

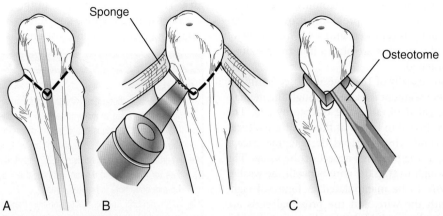

FIGURE 18.25 A, Shape of chevron osteotomy with apex pointing distally. Note drill hole at apex. B, Sponge protecting articular surface of distal humerus. C, Osteotomy with osteotome.

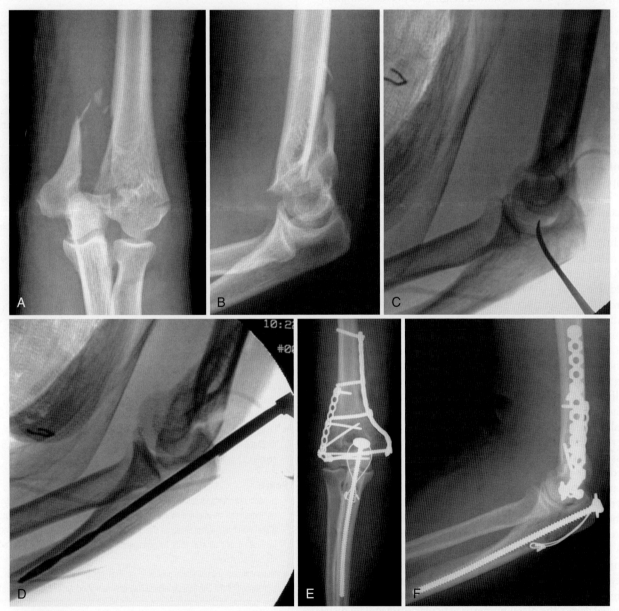

FIGURE 18.26 Anteroposterior (A) and lateral (B) injury radiographs show supracondylar/intercondylar distal humerus fracture with displacement of articular surface and very low injury of lateral column. To improve visualization of articular surface, olecranon osteotomy was chosen as preferred surgical approach. C and D, On intraoperative fluoroscopic images, a small elevator is used to show "bare area" of semilunar notch, and proximal ulna is predrilled before creation of osteotomy. E and F, Final radiographs show reduction and stabilization of distal humerus fracture and fixation of osteotomy using a 4.5-mm screw with washer and tension band wiring.

olecranon process, across the reduced osteotomy, and into the dense bone of the coronoid process, providing provisional stability. The 3.2-mm drill bit is removed, and a 4.5-mm screw of appropriate length and its washer are placed into the proximal ulna but not fully tightened.

A tension band wire, usually of 18 gauge, is subsequently cut into two segments. One segment is placed through the medial-to-lateral drill hole created distal to the osteotomy site. The second is placed from medial to lateral at the tip of the olecranon process. This second wire is placed deep to the triceps insertion and washer, at the proximal aspect of the screw. The screw is tightened enough to trap the wire beneath the washer but still allow the wire to be manipulated. A figure-of-eight pattern is created with the wire, and the proximal ends are twisted to the corresponding ends of the distal wire in a double-knot technique. The knots are placed medially and laterally, avoiding the tip of the olecranon, helping to decrease implant prominence. When the tension band wire has been fully tightened, the screw is finally fully seated and tightened. Temporary clamps and Kirschner wires are removed. The elbow is placed through a range of motion, and a secure osteotomy is ensured. Infrequently, because of inadvertent osteotomy obliquity, comminution, or olecranon fracture, stability of the osteotomy cannot be ensured with the screw and tension band technique. In these situations, we proceed with plate osteosynthesis of the osteotomy. Since the first edition of this chapter was published, various devices tailored specifically to the olecranon have been manufactured and touted for their anatomic specificity and ease of application. None to date has been demonstrated to be any more beneficial than the techniques described above.

Fixation Sequence. The fixation sequence varies depending on the individual fracture characteristics. Because most of the Kirschner wires are placed in a posterior-to-anterior direction, the medial surface of the distal humerus is usually unobstructed and free of temporary implants, allowing the medial plate to be placed first. This plate is typically a more malleable plate, such as a reconstruction plate, and is applied directly medially with attention paid to ensuring that it is accurately contoured around the medial epicondyle. The first screw inserted is usually at a point immediately proximal to the most proximal fracture line on the medial column. Slight undercontouring of the plate along the medial supracondylar ridge allows a buttressing effect distally as the screw is tightened. The orientation of the plate on the medial column is confirmed on anteroposterior and lateral intraoperative fluoroscopic studies.

Screw fixation proceeds distally with placement of screws across the distal humerus articular surface. Finally, screws are placed in the proximal portion of the plate. Because the medial implant is a malleable reconstruction plate, it tends to be contoured to the bone rather than the provisionally reduced fracture being displaced to the plate. When the medial column plate is secured to the medial column, several redundant Kirschner wires may be removed to decrease interference when the lateral column is subsequently secured. We typically use a stiff precontoured posterolateral periarticular plate to provide rigid lateral column stability while allowing screws to be placed from lateral to medial across the distal humerus articular surface. The distal lateral portion of the plate is confirmed to be in a satisfactory position clinically and fluoroscopically and is applied closely to the lateral epicondylar region to avoid plate prominence in this

area. The plate is maintained in the appropriate position with several Kirschner wires, and screws are strategically inserted beginning proximally and working distally.

CRITICAL POINTS *Olecranon Osteotomy*

Creation

- Preoperatively determine whether a 4.5-mm cortical screw or a 6.5-mm partially threaded screw will be used to secure the osteotomy.
- The choice of screw is based on the diameter of the medullary canal.
- Identify the bare area and confirm this with fluoroscopy.
- Predrill the proximal ulna using a 3.2-mm drill bit. This serves as the thread hole for 4.5-mm and 6.5-mm screws. If a 4.5-mm screw is anticipated, a 4.5-mm glide hole is created initially.
- A 2.5-mm drill hole is placed through the dorsal surface of the proximal ulna at the anticipated position of the osteotomy apex.
- An oscillating saw initiates the chevron osteotomy (apex pointing distally) at the bare area. The previously placed 2.5-mm drill hole helps orient the operator.
- A fine osteotome is used to "fracture" the articular surface, completing the osteotomy.

Fixation

- Place a 3.2-mm drill bit antegrade into the drill hole of the osteotomized fragment. Continue passing the drill bit into the medullary canal of the ulna.
- Medial and lateral pointed bone reduction clamps are placed across the osteotomy. The intramedullary drill bit helps to eliminate translational deformities during this maneuver.
- Kirschner wires are used to secure the osteotomy.
- A transverse drill hole is created in the proximal ulna, distal to the osteotomy.
- Remove the drill bit, and insert the intramedullary screw and washer.
- Before final tightening of the screw, cerclage wire is passed beneath the washer and through the transverse hole in the proximal ulna. A figure-of-eight pattern is used.
- The cerclage wire is tightened, and the screw is secured.
- Remove Kirschner wires and clamps.
- Place the elbow through a range of motion, and ensure stability of the osteotomy.

Pitfalls

- Before performing the osteotomy, the drill bit must be placed at the center of the olecranon and pass smoothly down the medullary canal of the ulna. Eccentric placement of the drill hole in the olecranon may result in translational forces and malreduction of the osteotomy during fixation.
- Osteotomies that are not perpendicular to the intramedullary screw displace with tightening.
- Long 6.5-mm screws that significantly engage the bow of the ulna may displace the osteotomy. This is less likely to occur with less stiff 4.5-mm screws.

Pearls

- If poor purchase is obtained with a 4.5-mm screw, the screw length can be increased to engage more of the curved portion of the ulna. Improved distal purchase is obtained as the screw bends to accommodate the medullary canal. If this still fails to give satisfactory purchase, a 6.5-mm screw should be used.
- Osteotomies that remain unstable or that continually displace with final tightening of the intramedullary screw are managed with plate stabilization.

Unicolumnar Fractures

The surgical tactic for management of single-column fractures of the distal humerus begins with an assessment of the degree of comminution of the articular surface and a close inspection of the opposite column to rule out subtle fracture lines that change the diagnosis to a bicolumnar injury (Case Study 18.7). Invariably, significantly displaced fractures of the lateral or medial column are approached through a universal posterior skin incision with the patient in the prone or lateral position. Depending on the involved column, the corresponding paratricipital interval is developed. Regardless of which column is fractured, the ulnar nerve is routinely mobilized and protected. If significant articular surface comminution exists, both paratricipital intervals are exposed and an olecranon osteotomy is performed. If the articular surface is not comminuted, the fractured column is mobilized, and the triceps is elevated off the posterior aspect of the distal humerus. The fracture is reduced using cortical metaphyseal fracture interdigitations, indirectly reducing the articular surface. The olecranon is gently distracted from the distal humerus articular surface, and the articular reduction is assessed under direct vision and with palpation with a blunt periosteal elevator.

If a satisfactory reduction cannot be obtained, or the articular surface is significantly comminuted, we proceed with olecranon osteotomy. In significantly displaced, or "high," unicolumnar fractures, the radius and ulna frequently follow the displaced trochlear fragment. In this situation, reduction of the fractured column is quite difficult without the aid of osteotomy because the weight of the arm continues to act as a displacing force. Lag screw fixation alone is infrequently used for these injuries; we prefer plate stabilization of the injured column.

Capitellar and Articular Variant Fractures

The elucidation of the injury spectrum that occurs in capitellar injuries of the distal humerus continues to evolve, with the realization that many of these fractures are much more complicated than originally described.[103] Associated medial collateral ligament tears, disruption of the lateral ligamentous complex, and other periarticular fractures are common. More liberal use of CT has resulted in increased identification of several additional fracture features, including (1) involvement of the adjacent trochlea, (2) comminution of the posterior aspect of the capitellum or trochlea, or both, and (3) epicondylar fractures that may destabilize the ulnohumeral articulation further.[21,71,101]

These features are important because the surgical tactic may need to include an approach that allows access to the medial aspect of the elbow, visualization of the articular surface through the use of an olecranon osteotomy, and bone graft material. For these reasons, we recommend thin-cut preoperative CT evaluation in patients whose fracture patterns show any potential involvement of the posterior aspect of the capitellum or trochlea on plain radiographs. Isolated capitellar fractures and other articular fracture variants are managed operatively in physiologically active patients. In physiologically older patients, a fracture with significant articular comminution and displacement that cannot be reconstructed with standard ORIF techniques is treated with elbow arthroplasty.

Simple Fractures of the Capitellum

Simple capitellar fractures, including those with a coronal shear pattern, are managed with the patient in the supine position. The common feature of these fractures is that they are mainly confined to the anterolateral aspect of the distal humerus and are accessible using a lateral approach.

The patient is placed supine on the operating table, and a radiolucent arm board is used to support the injured extremity. A posterior universal skin incision is made, and the anconeus and extensor carpi ulnaris interval is developed. The joint capsule is incised, and the fracture is identified, cleansed of hematoma, and assessed. Simple fractures may be reduced at this point; however, comminuted capitellar fragments or fragments that extend beyond the lateral trochlear ridge require improved visualization. To improve visualization, detaching the origins of the extensor carpi ulnaris, common extensor tendon, and a portion of the extensor carpi radialis longus from the lateral supracondylar ridge extends the proximal interval. The origin of the lateral collateral ligament is detached sharply from its origin at the lateral epicondyle, and the elbow joint capsule is incised at its origin on the distal humerus. The capitellar fracture fragments are reduced with dental picks to the intact distal humerus. Temporary fixation is performed with small Kirschner wires, and the reduction is confirmed under direct visualization and with biplanar fluorographic imaging.

There is no consensus regarding the optimal fixation method for these fractures. Early reports in the literature recommended 4-mm cancellous lag screws or Herbert screws placed in an anterior-to-posterior direction.[71,76] In a cadaveric model, Elkowitz and associates[25] showed that posterior-to-anterior cancellous screw fixation was biomechanically superior, however, suggesting that the countersinking of the anterior-to-posterior screws removed dense subchondral bone, resulting in less rigid fixation. In the same study, headless anterior-to-posterior screws showed the strongest fixation, perhaps because of the preservation of the subchondral bone. The potential detrimental effects of removing a portion of the articular surface of the capitellum to insert anterior-to-posterior screws have not been determined, however. Posterolateral plate fixations have also been described and are most useful for providing a buttress effect to support the fractures with posterolateral comminution.[21,78] In our experience, definitive fixation is individualized based on the fracture pattern. Typically, fixation is achieved with 1.5-mm, 2-mm, or 2.4-mm countersunk screws. Posterolateral minifragment plate fixation is used to buttress complex capitellar fractures with posterolateral comminution. The lateral collateral ligament is repaired to its origin using suture anchors, and the extensor origins are repaired along the lateral supracondylar ridge.

Complex Capitellar Fractures and Articular Fracture Variants

Complex capitellar fractures and articular fracture variants are considered separately from simple capitellar fractures because of the potential involvement of the posterior aspect of the capitellum, lateral epicondyle, trochlea, and medial epicondylar region (Case Study 18.8).[21,101] With increasing involvement of the posterior and medial articular surfaces, visualization, reduction, and stabilization become increasingly difficult. As described by Ring and associates,[101] the inability to reduce the anterior capitellar fragments, or a capitellar fracture involving the lateral epicondyle, suggests the presence of this associated posterior injury. As noted earlier, preoperative CT evaluation identifies these important fracture features.

In patterns that involve the capitellum and the posterior aspect of the lateral column, the posterolateral aspect of the medial head of triceps and the anconeus are elevated. The elbow is hinged open posterolaterally, allowing access to the posterior aspect of the lateral column. If the fracture begins to involve the posterior aspect of the trochlea or medial epicondyle, we prefer to use olecranon osteotomy to access the components of these challenging fractures more reliably. Stabilization is with small or minifragment screws. Fractures with significant comminution or impaction may require bone grafting or plating, or both, to help support articular segments.[21]

Distal Humerus Fractures With Extensive Related Injuries

Massive Bone Loss. Patients sustaining open injuries with massive bone loss are rarely encountered. The initial focus is on determining if the limb is viable or salvageable. A detailed vascular examination of the ipsilateral hand and digits is crucial. In situations with a salvageable injury, the open wound is thoroughly irrigated and débrided in the operating room. An intraoperative assessment of the amount of bone loss is performed and correlated with the radiographic assessment. Because of the high energy involved in the creation of these injuries, patients frequently have associated polytrauma or markedly contaminated wounds around the elbow, or both, and temporary spanning external fixation is performed acutely. This temporary fixation allows the skeleton and soft tissues to be stabilized rapidly and allows other serious injuries to be managed. A simple uniplanar external fixator is applied, with Schanz pins placed into the humeral diaphysis under direct vision (to avoid injury to the radial nerve) and into the ulna. Repeated débridements are performed until all nonviable tissue is excised. Definitive management depends on the type and amount of bone lost.

Nonarticular Bone Loss. Patients with a reconstructible articular surface and supracondylar bone loss are managed with ORIF, shortening of the humerus through the area of bone loss, and placement of antibiotic beads in the region of any residual bone defect. Delayed bone grafting is performed when the soft tissue envelope has stabilized, typically at 6 to 8 weeks. Patients are at high risk for elbow stiffness or ankylosis that may be improved with elbow mobilization procedures after fracture union is confirmed.

Articular Bone Loss. Options for patients presenting with significant articular bone loss include procedures that allow the development of a pseudarthrosis in the region of the distal humerus, elbow fusion, and allograft elbow replacements. In severely contaminated wounds or selected patients, some of these injuries are managed with a brief period of immobilization to allow soft tissue recovery, followed by active range-of-motion exercises. These patients develop a mobile pseudoarticulation that provides some mobility and function. Elbow fusions are typically reserved for patients with articular loss; overt infection; and painful, mobile residual articulations not amenable to elbow arthroplasty.[68]

In physiologically young patients with partial articular bone loss, salvage of the patient's native distal humerus should remain the goal. Giannoudis and colleagues[31] described the use of tricortical iliac crest bone graft for the primary reconstruction of the trochlea. Similarly, Spang and coworkers[112] described reconstruction of severe fractures of the lateral trochlea and capitellum using structural ipsilateral radial head autograft with excellent results (Case Study 18.9). In these situations, we have acceptable functional results with satisfactory flexion-extension and pronation-supination arcs of motion. In situations with dramatic articular bone loss, we prefer allograft replacement.[16] This option offers the ability to maintain a mobile, comfortable elbow articulation in the short term and to restore bone stock for later elbow arthroplasty if needed (Case Study 18.10).

Ballistic Injuries. Low-energy ballistic injuries usually have minor to moderate contamination and soft tissue injury and minor to moderate bone comminution. The fracture is managed according to the principles outlined earlier.

Conversely, high-energy ballistic injuries are associated with neurovascular injury, large contaminated wounds, and significant skeletal comminution with or without functional bone loss. The management of these injuries is with repeated débridements until a healthy, viable soft tissue envelope is created. Fixation is performed using the principles outlined earlier. The surgeon should anticipate some amount of bone loss (articular or nonarticular, or both) when managing these fractures. Some of these injuries have been salvaged with circular tensioned-wire fixators[60] or uniplanar external fixation as definitive treatment,[88] but we have little experience with this in the acute setting.

Postoperative Care

At the conclusion of the procedure, the surgical incisions and traumatic wounds are covered with sterile gauze bandages, and the extremity is placed into a long-arm plaster splint with the elbow in extension. Patients are managed with 24 hours of postoperative antibiotic administration. A suction drain, if used, is removed after 24 hours. Approximately 48 hours postoperatively, the splint is removed, and the surgical incision is inspected. Provided that the surgical incision is sealed, range-of-motion exercises are begun. Therapy is performed several times per day and consists of active range of motion of the shoulder, forearm, wrist, and fingers. Exercises are initially performed under the supervision of a physical therapist before discharge.

Active and active-assisted elbow flexion is permitted for all situations. Patients managed via a paratricipital approach or olecranon osteotomy are allowed active elbow extension. Patients treated with an approach that mobilizes the extensor insertion from the proximal ulna, such as the Bryan-Morrey approach, perform passive, gravity-assisted elbow extension movements for 6 weeks. Strengthening exercises, particularly resisted elbow extension, are deferred until radiographic union occurs. In situations where patients fail to make progress toward a functional arc of motion (30 to 130 degrees at the ulnohumeral joint) despite a supervised physical therapy program, the use of static progressive splinting is strongly considered. More recent reports have shown sustained improvements in the overall arc of motion, with several patients avoiding operative contracture release.[18,29] Although the optimal timing for the institution of static progressive splinting is unknown, we prefer to initiate this treatment when conventional active and active-assisted methods plateau below a functional arc of motion, typically 6 to 12 weeks after the injury.

Patients are examined in the outpatient clinic at the following intervals:

- Postoperative day 7 to 10 for examination of the surgical incision, suture removal, edema control, and reinforcement of the physical therapy regimen; patients who are unclear regarding the importance, frequency, or timing of physical therapy are seen by a therapist in the outpatient clinic area to review exercises and to arrange outpatient therapy at a convenient location

- Week 6 for motion evaluation and radiographs
- Week 12 for motion evaluation, radiographic assessment, and initiation of strengthening and stretching exercises
- Weeks 20 to 26 for motion evaluation, radiographic assessment, identification of patient concerns, and discussion of return to athletics or heavy labor
- Week 52 and as needed for final radiographic assessment and identification of any patient concerns

Expectations

Several parameters are used to assess the outcome of fractures of the distal humerus. Elbow range of motion, forearm rotation, occurrence of and time to union, and complication rates all have been reported in the literature. It is recognized, however, that these parameters may not accurately reflect the patient's perception of satisfaction. For this reason, limb-specific and disease-specific validated outcome scoring measures have been created in an attempt to assess more accurately outcomes of numerous conditions.

All fractures of the distal humerus are associated with some degree of measurable loss of range of motion, particularly extension. Despite this absolute loss of "normal" motion, most patients can expect functional results. Patients with significant associated polytrauma, high-energy injuries, or significant soft tissue injury can be expected to have worse outcomes.

Most activities of daily living require a flexion-extension arc at the elbow of approximately 100 degrees (30 to 130 degrees) and an arc of forearm rotation from 50 degrees of supination to 50 degrees of pronation.[87] In bicolumnar fractures of the distal humerus treated with bicolumnar plating, McKee and colleagues[74] showed a flexion-extension arc of approximately 108 degrees with a mean flexion contracture of approximately 25 degrees. This represents approximately 74% of the motion on the contralateral, uninjured side. Similarly, flexion and extension strength were approximately 75% that of the uninjured side.[74] Using an orthogonal plating and olecranon osteotomy approach, Gofton and associates[33] reported on 23 patients with "C"-type distal humerus fractures. At a mean follow-up of 45 months, the authors showed an average flexion-extension arc of approximately 122 degrees, but noted a reduction in flexion-extension strength of approximately 20% and a similar 20% loss of pronation-supination strength. Despite the limitations in motion and strength, most patients had minimal functional loss and low pain scores, and 93% were satisfied with their outcome.

Sanchez-Sotelo and coworkers[104] reported the results of 32 distal humerus fractures at a mean follow-up of 2 years. These fractures were treated with a parallel plating technique using various surgical approaches, most of which were soft tissue mobilizations of the extensor mechanism from the proximal ulna. Of 32 fractures, 31 united primarily, with no elbow showing failure of internal fixation. Despite the high proportion of open fractures and fractures with intraarticular comminution, the authors showed an average flexion-extension arc of 99 degrees, with an average arc of motion of 26 to 125 degrees.

Using the Mayo Elbow Performance Score, 27 patients were graded as having a good-to-excellent result. Other authors have shown similar functional motion arcs and losses of flexion and extension strength in studies done over the short term.[56]

The best long-term data examining the results of distal humerus fractures were provided by Doornberg and colleagues,[19] who evaluated 30 patients at an average of 19 years after ORIF of a distal humerus fracture. Most patients were treated with plates and screws via olecranon osteotomy, and no patient was treated with ulnar nerve transposition. The authors noted an average flexion arc of 106 degrees, with minimal disability and excellent outcome scores when measured with numerous validated functional outcome measurement systems. The findings of these studies are similar to those of shorter-term studies, suggesting that the initial results are durable over the long term. Despite most patients showing the radiographic presence of arthrosis, this variable was not predictive of disability or elbow function. A unique factor in this study was the finding that most variations in the physician-based elbow rating scores were attributable to pain, limb dominance, and flexion arc. Additionally, only one patient had signs and symptoms of ulnar nerve dysfunction at the time of follow-up; this finding makes one question the need for routine anterior subcutaneous ulnar nerve transposition, a step that is recommended by some authorities.

Expectations must be tailored to the individual patient, and the data obtained by McKee and colleagues[73,74] and Gofton and associates[33] provide a useful framework for discussion with patients and their families. In patients with isolated, closed fractures of the distal humerus or open fractures without significant contamination or soft tissue destruction, the expected results are similar to those described previously. Patients with sedentary employment are encouraged to return to part-time work when they are feeling systemically stable. Ideally, the workplace should allow for slower completion of tasks, with frequent breaks for rest or periods of physical therapy. Patients who are engaged in labor that requires more physical exertion are also encouraged to return to the workplace, but in a modified role. Patients who are active in heavy labor are assessed individually. Frequently, an independent medical examination or physical capacities review is performed to obtain an objective measure of the patient's ability to return to the same job or a similar one. These employment issues frequently are foremost on patients' minds, and discussion of the plan to return to work is initiated early in the management phase.

At our institution, a high percentage of distal humerus fractures are secondary to high-energy injuries and have associated polytrauma. Patients who sustain significant associated injuries are expected to have a worse outcome in terms of range of motion and strength.[100] In patients with polytrauma where the operative delay approaches 7 days, significant stiffness has been noted. In these patients, we still strive for anatomic reduction of the articular surface and axial realignment, planning on delayed excision of heterotopic ossification or capsular release, or both. This "staged" approach to an ultimately functional elbow is explained to the family and patient during the early phase of care. In these situations, the ultimate outcome is satisfactory, provided that the distal humerus articular anatomy is restored at the time of the initial procedure and the patient is able to participate fully in the postsurgical rehabilitation program.[118]

The functional outcome after ORIF of capitellar fractures and the coronal shear variant seems to be very satisfactory,[71,115] with several authors describing near-normal flexion-extension and pronation-supination arcs.[71,115] Most patients in these series were managed with screw fixation, with comparatively poorer results noted with Kirschner wire fixation. Because of the absence of significant soft tissue attachments to the capitellar fragment, avascular necrosis is a commonly discussed potential complication of this fracture pattern. Avascular necrosis changes noted with plain radiography seem to be relatively infrequent, however, with an incidence ranging from 0% to 20% in larger series.[66,71,115] The clinical sequelae of avascular necrosis seem to be even less frequent than sequelae seen on radiographic studies.[115]

With more of the articular surface involved, a decrease in the flexion-extension arc and lower functional outcome scores have been shown.[101] Dubberley and colleagues[21] evaluated 28 patients with capitellar and trochlear fractures managed with operative fixation. These authors noted an average flexion-extension motion arc of 119 degrees (range 19 to 138 degrees), with a high proportion of patients reporting excellent function and minimal disability. It was noted, however, that patients with isolated noncomminuted capitellar or trochlear fractures have better results than patients with more complex fractures.

Complications

Nonunion of the Distal Humerus

Nonunion of fractures of the distal humerus has been reported in 2 to 10% of cases, invariably occurring in the metadiaphyseal region.[56,111,119,125] Nonunion is primarily the consequence of inadequate fixation[39,111] that may be the result of other predisposing factors, such as high-energy injuries, extensive comminution, and poor bone quality. Patients are typically significantly disabled because of pain and loss of function. The frequent presentation is of a painful, mobile nonunion with significant motion restriction at the ulnar-humeral articulation. Associated ulnar neuropathy is common.[37]

A few of these nonunions can be treated satisfactorily in a brace; however, most require operative management to achieve a stable, comfortable, functional elbow. Surgical reconstruction is technically demanding because of the distorted local anatomy, scarring, retained or broken implants, poor bone quality of the articular component, and capsular contracture.[37,69] Despite these difficulties, operative reconstruction is the procedure of choice in active individuals.

The surgical plan involves a wide posterior surgical exposure incorporating previous skin incisions if possible. The use of olecranon osteotomy depends on the presence of significant articular malunion or nonunion and the location of the supracondylar nonunion. If osteotomy is not required, a paratricipital exposure is performed. The ulnar nerve is identified and freed from scar tissue well above and below the medial epicondyle. Substantial perineural fibrosis is often encountered. Posterior capsular adhesions and fibrosis are resected, particularly those crowding the olecranon fossa. Anterior capsular adhesions are released by working through the nonunion site or by elevating the structures from the lateral supracondylar ridge. The lateral collateral ligament origin should be preserved during this exposure, but it may be elevated and subsequently repaired if needed. The nonunion site is cleared of its fibrous material,

and the bone ends are resected to healthy, bleeding margins. Intraoperative cultures are routinely obtained. Secure fixation typically entails medial and lateral plate fixation, and bone grafting is invariably required. The elbow is placed through a range of motion, and the stability of the construct is tested. The ulnar nerve is transposed anteriorly.[37,99] Early motion is initiated when the wound is sealed.

Results of nonunion repair have been satisfactory. Helfet and coworkers[37] showed satisfactory union in 51 of 52 patients after a single procedure. The average motion arc improved from 71 degrees preoperatively to 94 degrees postoperatively; however, it is likely that the preoperative motion was a combination of ulnar-humeral and nonunion motion, giving an overestimation of the preoperative motion arc. Similarly, McKee and colleagues[69] showed an average postoperative arc of motion of 97 degrees, with ulnar nerve function improving in all cases. Excellent improvement in pain can be expected, but associated injuries can influence the ultimate functional outcome, and significant long-term disability may persist despite bony union.[37,54,69]

Total elbow replacement in nonunited fractures in elderly patients has also been described.[85,99] This procedure is particularly effective in low-demand patients with poor bone stock. Satisfactory results can be expected, provided that septic complications are minimized.[85,86] In a series of complex distal humerus nonunions, Brinker and coworkers[4] showed the effectiveness of Ilizarov treatment for infected distal humerus nonunions after failure of internal fixation. The authors noted a 100% union rate with substantial improvements in levels of disability, pain, and quality-of-life measurements. The average arc of motion was documented at 81 degrees, with all patients having at least 95 degrees of elbow flexion.

Nonunion of the Olecranon Osteotomy

Nonunion or delayed union of an olecranon osteotomy has been reported in the literature with rates of 10%.[33,38,39,43,56] Henley and associates[39] described 3 of 29 (10%) osteotomies that developed delayed unions or nonunions. More recently, Gofton and associates[33] reported 2 of 22 (9%) olecranon osteotomies with nonunions. Several factors, such as lack of inherent fracture interdigitation and suboptimal osteotomy fixation, are believed to be responsible for the development of this complication.[38,39] Olecranon osteotomy nonunions have been described with Kirschner wire and screw fixations.[39,56] The use of a chevron osteotomy, rather than a transverse osteotomy, creates increased surface area for bone union and improved rotational stability of the osteotomy and would be expected to improve union rates.

To prevent the occurrence of olecranon osteotomy nonunion, we prefer to create a chevron osteotomy. Compressive apposition of the osteotomy surfaces is performed with the application of medial and lateral clamps that are removed after the osteotomy is temporarily secured with Kirschner wires. Medullary screw fixation, rather than Kirschner wire fixation, is used for a secure definitive construct. At the conclusion of the osteotomy fixation, the elbow is placed through a range of motion to assess the stability of the osteotomy. Any significant gapping or instability should be recognized and managed. In the unusual situations where this occurs, we prefer immediate plate fixation to improve osteotomy stability and healing.

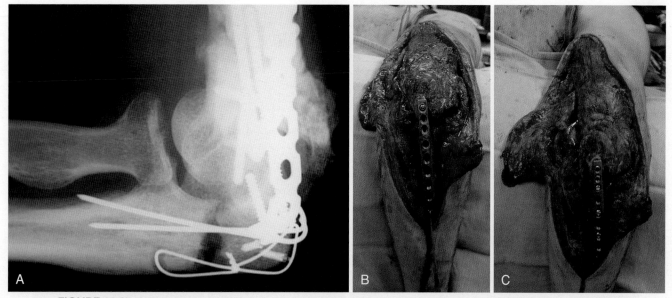

FIGURE 18.27 A, Lateral radiograph of bicolumnar distal humerus fracture managed using olecranon osteotomy. Osteotomy was secured with Kirschner wires and figure-of-eight tension band technique. Note obvious nonunion at site of osteotomy. **B,** Intraoperative photograph of posterior aspect of right elbow. The hand is located at the bottom of the image. Olecranon nonunion has been débrided to viable bone margins, and autogenous bone graft has been applied. Dynamic compression plate has been applied to dorsal surface and secured to proximal fragment. Proximal portion of this plate is narrowed and has tighter hole spacing to accommodate multiple 2.7-mm screws into smaller proximal olecranon fragment; distal aspect of plate is composed of standard 3.5-mm plate and hole specifications. Bone hook located at distal aspect of plate is used to tension plate and compress nonunion. **C,** Intraoperative photograph of posterior aspect of right elbow showing final screw placement and secure fixation of nonunion.

Current literature supports the use of multiple fixation techniques, all of which show exceptionally high union rates.[11,40,90]

Management of olecranon osteotomy nonunion is with repeat osteosynthesis using plate fixation and autogenous bone grafting (Figure 18.27). In situations where the proximal fragment is of insufficient size or quality, the fragment is excised and the triceps tendon is advanced.[70]

Infection

The deep infection rate of surgically managed fractures of the distal humerus is low despite the soft tissue dissection, prolonged operative time, and frequency of open injuries. Most deep infection rates reported range from 0 to 9%.[33,39,57,73,74] Management of acute postoperative wound infections requires débridement of nonviable tissue and an assessment of fracture stability. If the implants continue to stabilize the fracture, management is with suppressive culture-specific antibiotics until union occurs. In the setting of sepsis with fracture instability, treatment requires débridement and antibiotics with repeat osteosynthesis when the infection is controlled. Late presentations after union respond well to removal of internal fixation and antibiotic therapy. Severe deep infections with articular destruction may require salvage procedures, such as resection arthroplasty or elbow fusion.

Ulnar Neuropathy

Symptoms attributable to dysfunction of the ulnar nerve are common after fractures of the distal humerus.[56,100] Patients presenting with reconstructive issues almost invariably have ulnar nerve symptoms or signs. Factors responsible for postoperative ulnar neuropathy include injury from displaced bone fragments, excessive manipulation and retraction during the surgical procedure, and fibrosis and scarring of the tissues around the nerve in the region of the medial epicondyle and cubital tunnel.[70,100]

We use several techniques to minimize complications attributed to the ulnar nerve. When the posterior approach is used, adequate liberation of the nerve proximally and distally is performed at the beginning of the procedure, with care taken not to devascularize the nerve during mobilization. A broad Penrose drain is used for retraction purposes. To minimize traction injury to the nerve, the ends of the Penrose drain are sutured rather than clamped. At the conclusion of the procedure, anterior subcutaneous transposition of the nerve is performed for most fractures of the distal humerus. Isolated capitellar fractures and variants, lateral condyle fractures, and fractures managed using the Kocher interval do not require transposition.

Routine subcutaneous transposition of the ulnar nerve after operative fixation of a bicolumnar distal humerus fracture is very controversial. Because ulnar neuropathy is a common associated component of the complaints that may occur after distal humerus fractures, routine anterior subcutaneous transposition has evolved as a logical "preventive" measure in decreasing their incidence. Using routine transposition, Wang and colleagues[120] were unable to identify any postoperative ulnar neuropathy in 20 patients treated with dual plating. Other authors have shown similar results with routine anterior subcutaneous ulnar nerve transposition.[33,104] Although these results seem encouraging, Doornberg and associates[19] noted the rarity of ulnar nerve problems in long-term follow-up in patients after ORIF of distal humerus fractures, in whom no ulnar nerve

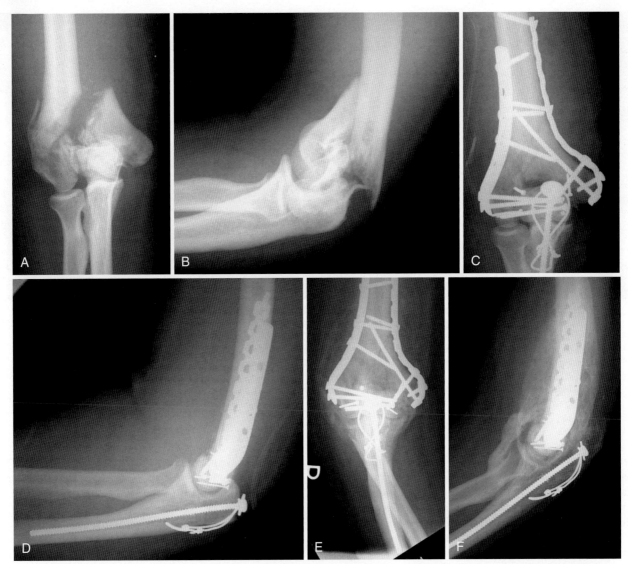

FIGURE 18.28 A 24-year-old man was involved in a high-speed motor vehicle collision. He sustained serious injuries, including severe bilateral pulmonary contusions, a closed head injury, and multiple fractures. **A** and **B,** Anteroposterior and lateral radiographs of right distal humerus show significant displacement and comminution of articular surface. Because of the patient's other injuries, operative fixation of distal humerus fracture was performed 8 days after the accident. **C** and **D,** Operative treatment consisted of medial and lateral plate fixation via olecranon osteotomy. **E** and **F,** Follow-up radiographs show maintenance of reduction and union of fracture, but also development of massive periarticular elbow heterotopic ossification resulting in complete ankylosis of elbow joint.

transposition occurred, calling into question whether routine transposition is necessary.

The successful management of ulnar neuropathy has been shown with ulnar neurolysis and anterior transposition.[69,72,118] Despite high patient satisfaction and improved objective measures, ulnar nerve function does not seem to normalize, and all efforts at minimizing complications of the ulnar nerve should be taken.[70,72]

Stiffness and Heterotopic Ossification

Most patients who undergo operative management with appropriate internal fixation usually obtain functional flexion-extension arcs. Significant contractures may be encountered in polytrauma patients, patients who undergo a significant delay before definitive management, patients who sustain high-energy injury, or patients with open fractures (Figure 18.28).[65,101,118] Kundel and coworkers[65] showed significant differences in time to return to work, ultimate range of motion, and incidence of significant heterotopic ossification in patients treated beyond 24 hours compared with patients managed within 24 hours of injury. In this same study, cases of ankylosing heterotopic ossification occurred exclusively in the delayed group. Provided that the fracture proceeds to union with satisfactory restoration of the articular surface and mechanical axes, a good result can still be obtained after capsular release and heterotopic ossification excision.

To prevent significant ankylosis, we prefer to manage fractures of the distal humerus as soon as possible, achieving secure fixation that allows early and unrestricted motion. We rarely use heterotopic ossification prophylaxis because we have found patient compliance with medical prophylaxis to be exceedingly low.

Management of a stiff elbow after operative fixation of a distal humerus fracture entails removal of internal fixation; capsulectomy; débridement of the olecranon, coronoid, and radial fossae; and excision of ectopic bone if necessary.[84,118] Management is performed after fracture union, typically 6 to 12 months after injury, and depends on complete fracture union and recovery from any other injuries that the patient may have incurred.[118] For a successful outcome after contracture release, it is vital that the patient be able to devote full attention to postoperative rehabilitation.

For Case Studies, Videos, and more, please visit ExpertConsult.com.

REFERENCES

1. Alonso-Llames M: Bilaterotricipital approach to the elbow: its application in the osteosynthesis of supracondylar fractures of the humerus in children. *Acta Orthop Scand* 43:479–490, 1972.
2. Arnander MW, Reeves A, MacLeod IA, et al: A biomechanical comparison of plate configuration in distal humerus fractures. *J Orthop Trauma* 22:332–336, 2008.
3. Athwal GS, Rispoli DM, Steinmann SP: The anconeus flap transolecranon approach to the distal humerus. *J Orthop Trauma* 20:282–285, 2006.
4. Brinker MR, O'Connor DP, Crouch CC, et al: Ilizarov treatment of infected nonunions of the distal humerus after failure of internal fixation: an outcomes study. *J Orthop Trauma* 21:178–184, 2007.
5. Brouwer KM, Bolmers A, Ring D: Quantitative 3-dimensional computed tomography measurement of distal humerus fractures. *J Shoulder Elbow Surg* 21(7):977–982, 2012.
6. Brown RF, Morgan RG: Intercondylar T-shaped fracture of the humerus: results in ten cases treated by early mobilisation. *J Bone Joint Surg Br* 53:425–428, 1971.
7. Bryan RS, Bickel WH: "T" condylar fractures of distal humerus. *J Trauma* 11:830–835, 1971.
8. Bryan RS, Morrey BF: Extensive posterior exposure of the elbow: a triceps sparing approach. *Clin Orthop Relat Res* 166:188–192, 1982.
9. Campbell WC: Incision for exposure of the elbow joint. *Am J Surg* 15:65–67, 1932.
10. Caravaggi P, Laratta JL, Yoon RS, et al: Internal fixation of the distal humerus: a comprehensive biomechanical study evaluating current fixation techniques. *J Orthop Trauma* 28(4):222–226, 2014.
11. Cassebaum WH: Open reduction of T and Y fractures of the lower end of the humerus. *J Trauma* 9:915–925, 1969.
12. Cassebaum WH: Operative treatment of T and Y fractures of the lower end of the humerus. *Am J Surg* 83:265–270, 1952.
13. Cobb TK, Morrey BF: Total elbow arthroplasty as primary treatment for distal humeral fractures in elderly patients. *J Bone Joint Surg Am* 79:826–832, 1997.
14. Coles CP, Barei DP, Nork SE, et al: The olecranon osteotomy: a six-year experience in the treatment of intraarticular fractures of the distal humerus. *J Orthop Trauma* 20:164–171, 2006.
15. Davies MB, Stanley D: A clinically applicable fracture classification for distal humeral fractures. *J Shoulder Elbow Surg* 15:602–608, 2006.
16. Dean GS, Holliger EHT, Urbaniak JR: Elbow allograft for reconstruction of the elbow with massive bone loss: long term results. *Clin Orthop Relat Res* 341:12–22, 1997.
17. Doornberg J, Lindenhovius A, Kloen P, et al: Two- and three-dimensional computed tomography for the classification and management of distal humeral fractures: evaluation of reliability and diagnostic accuracy. *J Bone Joint Surg Am* 88:1795–1801, 2006.
18. Doornberg JN, Ring D, Jupiter JB: Static progressive splinting for posttraumatic elbow stiffness. *J Orthop Trauma* 20:400–404, 2006.
19. Doornberg JN, van Duijn PJ, Linzel D, et al: Surgical treatment of intra-articular fractures of the distal part of the humerus: functional outcome after twelve to thirty years. *J Bone Joint Surg Am* 89:524–532, 2007.
20. Dowdy PA, Bain GI, King GJ, et al: The midline posterior elbow incision: an anatomical appraisal. *J Bone Joint Surg Br* 77:696–699, 1995.
21. Dubberley JH, Faber KJ, Macdermid JC, et al: Outcome after open reduction and internal fixation of capitellar and trochlear fractures. *J Bone Joint Surg Am* 88:46–54, 2006.
22. Dushuttle RP, Coyle MP, Zawadsky JP, et al: Fractures of the capitellum. *J Trauma* 25:317–321, 1985.
23. Eastwood WJ: The T-shaped fracture of the lower end of the humerus. *J Bone Joint Surg Am* 19:364–369, 1937.
24. Ek ET, Goldwasser M, Bonomo AL: Functional outcome of complex intercondylar fractures of the distal humerus treated through a triceps-sparing approach. *J Shoulder Elbow Surg* 17:441–446, 2008.
25. Elkowitz SJ, Polatsch DB, Egol KA, et al: Capitellum fractures: a biomechanical evaluation of three fixation methods. *J Orthop Trauma* 16:503–506, 2002.
26. Frankle MA, Herscovici D, Jr, DiPasquale TG, et al: A comparison of open reduction and internal fixation and primary total elbow arthroplasty in the treatment of intraarticular distal humerus fractures in women older than age 65. *J Orthop Trauma* 17:473–480, 2003.
27. Gambirasio R, Riand N, Stern R, et al: Total elbow replacement for complex fractures of the distal humerus: an option for the elderly patient. *J Bone Joint Surg Br* 83:974–978, 2001.
28. Garcia JA, Mykula R, Stanley D: Complex fractures of the distal humerus in the elderly: the role of total elbow replacement as primary treatment. *J Bone Joint Surg Br* 84:812–816, 2002.
29. Gelinas JJ, Faber KJ, Patterson SD, et al: The effectiveness of turnbuckle splinting for elbow contractures. *J Bone Joint Surg Br* 82:74–78, 2000.
30. Gerwin M, Hotchkiss RN, Weiland AJ: Alternative operative exposures of the posterior aspect of the humeral diaphysis with reference to the radial nerve. *J Bone Joint Surg Am* 78:1690–1695, 1996.
31. Giannoudis PV, Al-Lami MK, Tzioupis C, et al: Tricortical bone graft for primary reconstruction of comminuted distal humerus fractures. *J Orthop Trauma* 19:741–743, 2005.
32. Gill DR, Morrey BF: The Coonrad-Morrey total elbow arthroplasty in patients who have rheumatoid arthritis: a ten- to fifteen-year follow-up study. *J Bone Joint Surg Am* 80:1327–1335, 1998.
33. Gofton WT, Macdermid JC, Patterson SD, et al: Functional outcome of AO type C distal humeral fractures. *J Hand Surg [Am]* 28:294–308, 2003.
34. Grant SD, Gorczyca JT, Pugh KJ: *Open distal humerus fractures*, Boston, Orthopaedic Trauma Association 12th Annual Meeting, 1996.
35. Hausman M, Panozzo A: Treatment of distal humerus fractures in the elderly. *Clin Orthop Relat Res* (425):55–63, 2004.
36. Helfet DL, Hotchkiss RN: Internal fixation of the distal humerus: a biomechanical comparison of methods. *J Orthop Trauma* 4:260–264, 1990.
37. Helfet DL, Kloen P, Anand N, et al: Open reduction and internal fixation of delayed unions and nonunions of fractures of the distal part of the humerus. *J Bone Joint Surg Am* 85:33–40, 2003.
38. Henley MB: Intra-articular distal humeral fractures in adults. *Orthop Clin North Am* 10.11–23, 1987.
39. Henley MB, Bone LB, Parker B: Operative management of intra-articular fractures of the distal humerus. *J Orthop Trauma* 1:24–35, 1987.
40. Hewins EA, Gofton WT, Dubberly J, et al: Plate fixation of olecranon osteotomies. *J Orthop Trauma* 21:58–62, 2007.
41. Hildebrand KA, Patterson SD, Regan WD, et al: Functional outcome of semiconstrained total elbow arthroplasty. *J Bone Joint Surg Am* 82:1379–1386, 2000.
42. Hitzrot JM: Fractures at the lower end of the humerus in adults. *Surg Clin North Am* 12:291–304, 1932.
43. Holdsworth BJ, Mossad MM: Fractures of the adult distal humerus: elbow function after internal fixation. *J Bone Joint Surg Br* 72:362–365, 1990.
44. Horne G: Supracondylar fractures of the humerus in adults. *J Trauma* 20:71–74, 1980.
45. Hotchkiss RN: Displaced fractures of the radial head: internal fixation or excision? *J Am Acad Orthop Surg* 5:1–10, 1997.
46. Hotchkiss RN: Fractures and dislocations of the elbow. In Rockwood CA, Jr, Green DP, Bucholz RW, et al, editors: *Rockwood and Green's fractures in adults* (vol 1), ed 4, Philadelphia, 1996, Lippincott-Raven, pp 929–1024.
47. Huang TL, Chiu FY, Chuang TY, et al: The results of open reduction and internal fixation in elderly patients with severe fractures of the distal humerus: a critical analysis of the results. *J Trauma* 58:62–69, 2005.
48. Hungerer S, Wipf F, von Oldenburg G, et al: Complex distal humerus fractures: comparison of polyaxial locking and nonlocking screw configurations: a preliminary biomechanical study. *J Orthop Trauma* 28(3):130–136, 2014.
49. Jacobson SR, Glisson RR, Urbaniak JR: Comparison of distal humerus fracture fixation: a biomechanical study. *J South Orthop Assoc* 6:241–249, 1997.
50. Johansson H, Olerud S: Operative treatment of intercondylar fractures of the humerus. *J Trauma* 11:836–843, 1971.
51. John H, Rosso R, Neff U, et al: Operative treatment of distal humeral fractures in the elderly. *J Bone Joint Surg Br* 76:793–796, 1994.
52. Jupiter JB: The surgical management of intraarticular fractures of the distal humerus. In Morrey BF, editor: *The elbow*, ed 2, Philadelphia, 2002, Lippincott Williams & Wilkins, pp 65–81.
53. Jupiter JB, Barnes KA, Goodman LJ, et al: Multiplane fracture of the distal humerus. *J Orthop Trauma* 7:216–220, 1993.
54. Jupiter JB, Goodman LF: The management of complex distal humerus nonunions in the elderly by elbow capsulectomy, triple plating, and ulnar nerve neurolysis. *J Shoulder Elbow Surg* 1:37–46, 1992.

55. Jupiter JB, Mehne DK: Fractures of the distal humerus. *Orthopedics* 15:825–833, 1992.

56. Jupiter JB, Neff U, Holzach P, et al: Intercondylar fractures of the humerus: an operative approach. *J Bone Joint Surg Am* 67:226–239, 1985.

57. Jupiter JB, Neff U, Regazzoni P, et al: Unicondylar fractures of the distal humerus: an operative approach. *J Orthop Trauma* 2:102–109, 1988.

58. Kamineni S, Morrey BF: Distal humeral fractures treated with noncustom total elbow replacement. *J Bone Joint Surg Am* 86:940–947, 2004.

59. Kimball JP, Glowczewskie F, Wright TW: Intraosseous blood supply to the distal humerus. *J Hand Surg [Am]* 32:642–646, 2007.

60. Komurcu M, Yanmis I, Atesalp AS, et al: Treatment results for open comminuted distal humerus intra-articular fractures with Ilizarov circular external fixator. *Mil Med* 168:694–697, 2003.

61. Koonce RC, Baldini TH, Morgan SJ: Are conventional reconstruction plates equivalent to precontoured locking plates for distal humerus fracture fixation? A biomechanics cadaver study. *Clin Biomech (Bristol, Avon)* 27(7):697–701, 2012.

62. Korner J, Diederichs G, Arzdorf M, et al: A biomechanical evaluation of methods of distal humerus fracture fixation using locking compression plates versus conventional reconstruction plates. *J Orthop Trauma* 18:286–293, 2004.

63. Korner J, Lill H, Muller LP, et al: Distal humerus fractures in elderly patients: results after open reduction and internal fixation. *Osteoporos Int* 16(Suppl 2):S73–S79, 2005.

64. Korner J, Lill H, Muller LP, et al: The LCP-concept in the operative treatment of distal humerus fractures: biological, biomechanical and surgical aspects. *Injury* 34(Suppl 2):B20–B30, 2003.

65. Kundel K, Braun W, Wieberneit J, et al: Intraarticular distal humerus fractures: factors affecting functional outcome. *Clin Orthop Relat Res* 332:200–208, 1996.

66. Liberman N, Katz T, Howard CB, et al: Fixation of capitellar fractures with the Herbert screw. *Arch Orthop Trauma Surg* 110:155–157, 1991.

67. MacAusland WR: Ankylosis of the elbow: with report of 4 cases treated by arthroplasty. *JAMA* 64:312–318, 1915.

68. McAuliffe JA: Surgical alternatives for elbow arthritis in the young adult. *Hand Clin* 18:99–111, 2002.

69. McKee M, Jupiter J, Toh CL, et al: Reconstruction after malunion and nonunion of intra-articular fractures of the distal humerus: methods and results in 13 adults. *J Bone Joint Surg Br* 76:614–621, 1994.

70. McKee M, Jupiter JB: Fractures of the distal humerus. In Browner BD, Jupiter JB, Levine AM, et al, editors: *Skeletal trauma: basic science, management, and reconstruction* (vol 2), ed 3, Philadelphia, 2003, WB Saunders, pp 1436–1480.

71. McKee MD, Jupiter JB, Bamberger HB: Coronal shear fractures of the distal end of the humerus. *J Bone Joint Surg Am* 78:49–54, 1996.

72. McKee MD, Jupiter JB, Bosse G, et al: Outcome of ulnar neurolysis during post-traumatic reconstruction of the elbow. *J Bone Joint Surg Br* 80:100–105, 1998.

73. McKee MD, Kim J, Kebaish K, et al: Functional outcome after open supracondylar fractures of the humerus: the effect of the surgical approach. *J Bone Joint Surg Br* 82:646–651, 2000.

74. McKee MD, Wilson TL, Winston L, et al: Functional outcome following surgical treatment of intra-articular distal humeral fractures through a posterior approach. *J Bone Joint Surg Am* 82:1701–1707, 2000.

75. McKee MD, Veillette CJ, Hall JA, et al: A multicenter, prospective, randomized, controlled trial of open reduction–internal fixation versus total elbow arthroplasty for displaced intra-articular distal humeral fractures in elderly patients. *J Shoulder Elbow Surg* 18(1):3–12, 2009.

76. Mehdian H, McKee MD: Fractures of capitellum and trochlea. *Orthop Clin North Am* 31:115–127, 2000.

77. Mehne DK, Matta J: *Bicolumn fractures of the adult humerus*, New Orleans, Fifty-third Annual Meeting of the American Academy of Orthopaedic Surgeons, 1986.

78. Mighell MA, Harkins D, Klein D, et al: Technique for internal fixation of capitellum and lateral trochlea fractures. *J Orthop Trauma* 20:699–704, 2006.

79. Milch H: Fractures and fracture dislocations of the humeral condyles. *J Trauma* 15:592–607, 1964.

80. Miller WE: Comminuted fractures of the distal end of the humerus in the adult. *J Bone Joint Surg Am* 46:644–657, 1964.

81. Min W, Ding BC, Tejwani NC: Comparative functional outcome of AO/OTA type C distal humerus fractures: open injuries do worse than closed fractures. *J Trauma Acute Care Surg* 72(2):E27–E32, 2012.

82. Molloy S, Jasper LE, Burkhart BG, et al: Interference Kirschner wires augment distal humeral fracture fixation in the elderly. *J Orthop Trauma* 19:377–379, 2005.

83. Morrey BF: Fractures of the distal humerus: role of elbow replacement. *Orthop Clin North Am* 31:145–154, 2000.

84. Morrey BF: Surgical treatment of extraarticular elbow contracture. *Clin Orthop Relat Res* 370:57–64, 2000.

85. Morrey BF, Adams RA: Semiconstrained elbow replacement for distal humeral nonunion. *J Bone Joint Surg Br* 77:67–72, 1995.

86. Morrey BF, Adams RA, Bryan RS: Total replacement for post-traumatic arthritis of the elbow. *J Bone Joint Surg Br* 73:607–612, 1991.

87. Morrey BF, Askew LJ, Chao EY: A biomechanical study of normal functional elbow motion. *J Bone Joint Surg Am* 63:872–877, 1981.

88. Mostafavi HR, Tornetta P, 3rd: Open fractures of the humerus treated with external fixation. *Clin Orthop Relat Res* 337:187–197, 1997.

89. Muller LP, Kamineni S, Rommens PM, et al: Primary total elbow replacement for fractures of the distal humerus. *Oper Orthop Traumatol* 17:119–142, 2005.

90. Muller ME, Nazarian S, Koch P, et al: *The comprehensive classification of fractures of long bones*, Berlin, 1990, Springer-Verlag.

91. O'Driscoll SW: Optimizing stability in distal humeral fracture fixation. *J Shoulder Elbow Surg* 14(1 Suppl S):186S–194S, 2005.

92. O'Driscoll SW: The triceps-reflecting anconeus pedicle (TRAP) approach for distal humeral fractures and nonunions. *Orthop Clin North Am* 31:91–101, 2000.

93. Obremskey WT, Bhandari M, Dirschl DR, et al: Internal fixation versus arthroplasty of comminuted fractures of the distal humerus. *J Orthop Trauma* 17:463–465, 2003.

94. Patterson SD, Bain GI, Mehta JA: Surgical approaches to the elbow. *Clin Orthop Relat Res* 370:19–33, 2000.

95. Pereles TR, Koval KJ, Gallagher M, et al: Open reduction and internal fixation of the distal humerus: functional outcome in the elderly. *J Trauma* 43:578–584, 1997.

96. Ray PS, Kakarlapudi K, Rajsekhar C, et al: Total elbow arthroplasty as primary treatment for distal humeral fractures in elderly patients. *Injury* 31:687–692, 2000.

97. Reich RS: Treatment of intercondylar fractures of the elbow by means of traction. *J Bone Joint Surg Am* 18:997–1004, 1936.

98. Ring D, Gulotta L, Chin K, et al: Olecranon osteotomy for exposure of fractures and nonunions of the distal humerus. *J Orthop Trauma* 18:446–449, 2004.

99. Ring D, Gulotta L, Jupiter JB: Unstable nonunions of the distal part of the humerus. *J Bone Joint Surg Am* 85:1040–1046, 2003.

100. Ring D, Jupiter JB: Complex fractures of the distal humerus and their complications. *J Shoulder Elbow Surg* 8:85–97, 1999.

101. Ring D, Jupiter JB, Gulotta L: Articular fractures of the distal part of the humerus. *J Bone Joint Surg Am* 85:232–238, 2003.

102. Riseborough EJ, Radin EL: Intercondylar T fractures of the humerus in the adult: a comparison of operative and non-operative treatment in twenty-nine cases. *J Bone Joint Surg Am* 51:130–141, 1969.

103. Root CG, Meyers K, Wright T, et al: Capitellum excision: mechanical implications and clinical consequences. *J Orthop Res* 32(2):346–350, 2014.

104. Sanchez-Sotelo J, Torchia ME, O'Driscoll SW: Complex distal humeral fractures: internal fixation with a principle-based parallel-plate technique. *J Bone Joint Surg Am* 89:961–969, 2007.

105. Scharplatz D, Allgower M: Fracture-dislocations of the elbow. *Injury* 7:143–159, 1975.

106. Schemitsch EH, Tencer AF, Henley MB: Biomechanical evaluation of methods of internal fixation of the distal humerus. *J Orthop Trauma* 8:468–475, 1994.

107. Schildhauer TA, Nork SE, Mills WJ, et al: Extensor mechanism-sparing paratricipital posterior approach to the distal humerus. *J Orthop Trauma* 17:374–378, 2003.

108. Schneeberger AG, Adams R, Morrey BF: Semiconstrained total elbow replacement for the treatment of post-traumatic osteoarthrosis. *J Bone Joint Surg Am* 79:1211–1222, 1997.

109. Schuster I, Korner J, Arzdorf M, et al: Mechanical comparison in cadaver specimens of three different 90-degree double-plate osteosyntheses for simulated C2-type distal humerus fractures with varying bone densities. *J Orthop Trauma* 22:113–120, 2008.

110. Self J, Viegas SF, Buford WL, Jr, et al: A comparison of double-plate fixation methods for complex distal humerus fractures. *J Shoulder Elbow Surg* 4(1 Pt 1):10–16, 1995.

111. Sodergard J, Sandelin J, Bostman O: Mechanical failures of internal fixation in T and Y fractures of the distal humerus. *J Trauma* 33:687–690, 1992.

112. Spang JT, Del Gaizo DJ, Dahners LE: Reconstruction of lateral trochlear defect with radial head autograft. *J Orthop Trauma* 22:351–356, 2008.

113. Spinner M, Spinner RJ: Nerve decompression. In Morrey BF, editor: *The elbow*, ed 2, Philadelphia, 2002, Lippincott Williams & Wilkins, pp 265–289.

114. Srinivasan K, Agarwal M, Matthews SJ, et al: Fractures of the distal humerus in the elderly: is internal fixation the treatment of choice? *Clin Orthop Relat Res* 434:222–230, 2005.

115. Stamatis E, Paxinos O: The treatment and functional outcome of type IV coronal shear fractures of the distal humerus: a retrospective review of five cases. *J Orthop Trauma* 17:279–284, 2003.

116. Stoffel K, Cunneen S, Morgan R, et al: Comparative stability of perpendicular versus parallel double-locking plating systems in osteoporotic comminuted distal humerus fractures. *J Orthop Res* 26:778–784, 2008.

117. Van Gorder GW: Surgical approach in supracondylar "T" fractures of the humerus requiring open reduction. *J Bone Joint Surg Am* 22:278–292, 1940.

118. Viola RW, Hanel DP: Early "simple" release of posttraumatic elbow contracture associated with heterotopic ossification. *J Hand Surg [Am]* 24:370–380, 1999.

119. Waddell JP, Hatch J, Richards R: Supracondylar fractures of the humerus: results of surgical treatment. *J Trauma* 28:1615–1621, 1988.

120. Wang KC, Shih HN, Hsu KY, et al: Intercondylar fractures of the distal humerus: routine anterior subcutaneous transposition of the ulnar nerve in a posterior operative approach. *J Trauma* 36:770–773, 1994.

121. Watson-Jones R: *Fractures and joint injuries* (vol 2), ed 3, Baltimore, 1944, Williams & Wilkins.

122. Wilkinson JM, Stanley D: Posterior surgical approaches to the elbow: a comparative anatomic study. *J Shoulder Elbow Surg* 10:380–382, 2001.

123. Wright TW, Wong AM, Jaffe R: Functional outcome comparison of semiconstrained and unconstrained total elbow arthroplasties. *J Shoulder Elbow Surg* 9:524–531, 2000.

124. Yamaguchi K, Sweet FA, Bindra R, et al: The extraosseous and intraosseous arterial anatomy of the adult elbow. *J Bone Joint Surg Am* 79:1653–1662, 1997.

125. Zagorski JB, Jennings JJ, Burkhalter WE, et al: Comminuted intraarticular fractures of the distal humeral condyles: surgical vs. nonsurgical treatment. *Clin Orthop Relat Res* 202:197–204, 1986.

126. Ziran BH, Smith WR, Balk ML, et al: A true triceps-splitting approach for treatment of distal humerus fractures: a preliminary report. *J Trauma* 58:70–75, 2005.

Fractures of the Radial Head

Graham J.W. King

▶ These videos may be found at
ExpertConsult.com:
19.1 Open reduction and internal fixation of the radial head.
19.2 Radial head replacement. *(Copyright © Wright Medical Technology. Used by permission.)*

Fractures of the head of the radius are the most common fractures of the elbow. The majority occur between the ages of 20 and 60, with the incidence in females being twice that of males. Although fractures that are not displaced typically occur in isolation, displaced fractures are frequently associated with ligament injuries of the medial and lateral collateral ligaments and/or of the interosseous membrane. In more severe injuries, dislocations of the elbow and forearm may be associated with fractures of the radial head. Fractures of the coronoid, olecranon, and capitellum are commonly seen with fractures of the radial head and further impair elbow stability. The radial head is an important stabilizer for the elbow in the setting of these associated bony and ligamentous injuries.

Although undisplaced and minimally displaced fractures of the radial head usually have a favorable functional outcome with nonoperative management, there is little information demonstrating the optimal treatment of patients with displaced and/or comminuted fractures. In 1935, Jones stated: "Fracture of the head or neck of the radius with displacement is a serious injury. While the prognosis is good for recovery of a useful elbow, rarely is it a normal elbow."[105] This statement remains true today. A mechanical block to motion is an absolute indication for surgery. Concomitant injuries requiring surgical treatment, such as a large displaced coronoid fracture or elbow instability, frequently dictate the management of the radial head. Good results have been reported following open reduction and internal fixation for selected noncomminuted displaced radial head fractures. Excision of fragments, early or delayed radial head excision, and arthroplasty all have a role in the management of more comminuted displaced fractures.

EVALUATION

Clinical Assessment

A patient's history usually indicates that there was a fall onto the outstretched hand. High-energy injuries, such as a motor vehicle crash, typically have more comminuted fracture patterns and a higher incidence of associated injuries. Inspection may reveal ecchymosis along the forearm and/or medial aspect of the elbow. Tenderness over the radial head is expected and typically the most notable is anteriorly. Pain over the lateral epicondyle may represent a concomitant injury of the lateral collateral ligament. Careful palpation of the medial epicondyle and the sublime tubercle of the ulna should be performed to look for an associated medial collateral ligament injury. The interosseous membrane of the forearm and the distal radioulnar joint should be evaluated for tenderness; however, these injuries are often subtle and may not be evident even with a careful physical examination. Because associated injuries of the shoulder, forearm, wrist, and hand are common, these areas should also be examined. A careful neurologic and vascular examination of the extremity needs to be performed; however, concomitant nerve and arterial injuries are rare and usually associated with severe injuries.

Range of motion, including forearm rotation and elbow flexion–extension, should be evaluated. Palpable and auditory crepitus should be noted during movement. Forearm rotation is generally preserved but may sometimes be limited by pain or a mechanical block. In these circumstances, reevaluation a few days later may be prudent. Alternatively, aspiration of the hemarthrosis and injection of local anesthetic should be considered.[47,92,168,214] With a sterile technique and with the forearm in pronation to protect the radial nerve, a needle is introduced into the lateral soft spot located at the center of a triangle formed by the lateral epicondyle, olecranon, and radial head (Figure 19.1). After the hemarthrosis is aspirated, 10 mL of 1% lidocaine (Xylocaine) is injected. Persistent loss of rotation after pain relief suggests a mechanical block, whereas palpable grating suggests articular incongruity, both require surgical management. A mild loss of terminal elbow flexion and extension is expected as a consequence of an elbow hemarthrosis and does not necessarily indicate a mechanical block that needs surgical treatment.

Imaging

Anteroposterior, lateral, and oblique elbow radiographs usually provide sufficient information for the diagnosis and treatment of fractures of the head of the radius. The x-ray beam must be centered on the radiocapitellar joint to ensure a tangential view of the radial head. Because a hemarthrosis prevents elbow extension, two anteroposterior radiographs may be required if there is significant loss of extension: anteroposterior views of the distal humerus and the forearm. An oblique radiocapitellar view can be useful as it places the radial head in profile.[75] The elbow is positioned for a lateral radiograph but the x-ray tube is angled 45 degrees cephalad (Figure 19.2). In patients with undisplaced fractures of the radial head or neck, plain radiographs may only demonstrate elevation of the anterior or posterior fat pads (sail sign) as a consequence of a hemarthrosis (Figure 19.3). Bilateral posteroanterior radiographs of both wrists in neutral rotation should be performed to evaluate ulnar variance in patients with wrist discomfort and in those who have a comminuted fracture of the radial head as there is a higher incidence of an associated interosseous membrane injury in these patients.[44,99,209] A magnetic resonance image (MRI) or ultrasound may be considered to evaluate the presence of associated collateral ligament or interosseous membrane injuries but these investigations are uncommonly required.[56,99] Because of the cylindrical shape of the radial head, conventional elbow radiographs often underestimate the extent of articular surface involvement and magnitude of displacement.[104,115] Computed tomography (CT) is useful to quantify fracture size, location, displacement, and comminution in cases in which the indications for surgery are less clear. CT may also assist with preoperative planning with respect to the need

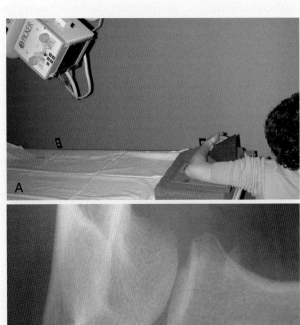

FIGURE 19.2 The radiocapitellar view can be useful because it places the radial head in profile. **A**, **B**, The elbow is positioned for a lateral radiograph, but the x-ray tube is angled 45 degrees cephalad.

FIGURE 19.1 Aspiration of the elbow. Under a sterile technique with the forearm maintained in pronation, a needle is introduced into the center of a triangle formed by the lateral epicondyle, radial head, and tip of the olecranon. The hemarthrosis is aspirated, and local anesthetic is injected. An improvement in rotation is suggestive of pain-limiting motion, whereas a persistent restriction of rotation is suggestive of a mechanical block requiring surgical management.

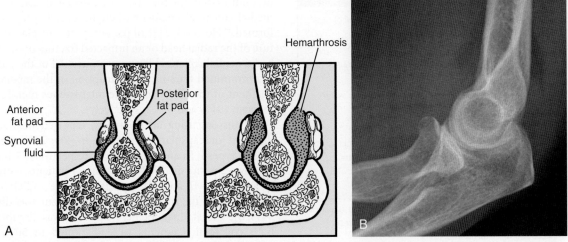

FIGURE 19.3 Fat pad sign. **A**, Normal position of fat pads in the elbow and displacement of fat pads induced by an intraarticular effusion. **B**, Lateral radiograph demonstrating anterior and posterior fat pad signs in patient with an undisplaced fracture of the radial head.

for specialized equipment for fracture fixation or prosthetic replacement.

Mason classified fractures of the radial head into three types: type I, fissure or marginal sector fractures without displacement; type II, marginal sector fractures with displacement; and type III, comminuted fractures involving the whole head (Figure 19.4).[135] One study demonstrated moderate to poor intra- and interobserver reproducibility of this classification based on plain radiographs.[146] Other authors have reported that many Mason II fractures are reclassified to type III during surgery owing to additional fracture segments being found that are not revealed on plain radiographs.[115] Johnston added a fourth type: fracture of the radial head associated with an elbow dislocation.[104] This additional category does little to direct treatment other than to emphasize that radial head excision without replacement is contraindicated in the setting of an associated elbow dislocation. Morrey has suggested that isolated fractures of the radial head be referred to as "simple or uncomplicated," while those associated with other soft tissue or bony injuries be referred to as "complex or complicated."[148]

More recently Hotchkiss developed a management-based classification with three types[93] (Table 19.1):

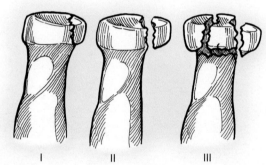

FIGURE 19.4 Mason classification. Mason described three types of fractures of the radial head: *I*, undisplaced; *II*, displaced wedge fragment(s); and *III*, comminuted.

TABLE 19.1	Hotchkiss Classification of Proximal Radial Fractures*	
Type I	Nondisplaced or minimally displaced fracture of head or neck No mechanical block to rotation Displacement > 2 mm or a marginal lip fracture	
Type II	Displaced (usually >2 mm) fracture of head or neck (angulated) May have mechanical block to motion or be incongruous Without severe comminution (technically possible to repair using open reduction and internal fixation) More than a marginal lip fracture of the radial head	
Type III	Severely comminuted fracture of the radial head or neck Judged not reconstructable on basis of radiographic or intraoperative appearance Usually requires excision for movement	

*All of these fractures may have associated injuries (e.g., a coronoid fracture, elbow dislocation, medial collateral or lateral collateral ligaments) or interosseous membrane tears.
From Hotchkiss RN: Displaced fractures of the radial head: Internal fixation or excision. *J Am Acad Orthop Surg* 5:1–10, 1997.

Type I: undisplaced or minimally displaced (<2 mm) small marginal fracture of the head or neck with no mechanical block to motion

Type II: displaced (>2 mm) fracture of the head or neck that is reconstructable with open reduction and internal fixation (ORIF). It may have a mechanical block or be incongruous; more than a marginal lip fracture

Type III: comminuted fracture of the head or neck that is unreconstructable as judged by radiographs or at surgery; usually requires excision for movement

While the Hotchkiss classification helps to direct treatment, the type of operation needed is less clear because the distinction between types II and III fractures remains problematic. The decision as to which fracture is reconstructable depends on surgeon factors (e.g., experience and implants available), patient factors (e.g., osteoporosis), and fracture factors (e.g., fragment size, comminution, and associated soft tissue injuries). The final decision as to whether a fracture is reconstructable or whether it requires radial head excision and/or replacement often can only be decided during surgery. Therefore, this classification, to some extent, may be of more use retrospectively and is less helpful in deciding which type of surgery should be performed.

Associated Injuries

Fractures of the radial head and neck commonly occur following a fall on the outstretched hand. A comminuted fracture of the radial head or neck is likely the result of failure in compression due to axial or valgus loads (Figure 19.5). In one cadaveric study, an isolated fracture of the radial head was most likely to occur when an axial load between 35 and 80 degrees of flexion is applied.[6] In 1924, Odelberg-Johnson reported that elbow subluxation was an important mechanism of wedge fractures in a series of cadaveric experiments.[157] In the author's experience posterolateral rotatory subluxation of the elbow, the first stage of an elbow dislocation, likely causes many of these anterolateral wedge fractures. This segment of the radial head shears off as the rim of the radial head dish subluxates off the capitellum with the forearm in neutral to supination.

Displaced fractures of the radial head are commonly associated with disruption of the ligaments of the elbow or forearm.[44,99,102,109,210] In one study, no patient with a minimally or undisplaced fracture had an associated disruption of the medial collateral ligament when stress radiographs were performed.[44] However, 71% of patients with a displaced shear fracture of the radial head or an impacted fracture of the radial neck had a medial collateral ligament injury. All of the patients with a comminuted fracture had disruption of the medial collateral ligament of the elbow or of the interosseous membrane of the forearm (91% and 9%, respectively).

Johansson, using arthrography, reported medial collateral ligament or capsular disruptions in 4%, 21%, and 85% of Mason types I, II, and III fractures, respectively.[102] Itamura and colleagues performed MR scans on 24 patients with displaced Mason types II and III fractures of the radial head. They reported that the medial collateral ligament was disrupted in 54%, the lateral ulnar collateral ligament was disrupted in 80%, both collateral ligaments were disrupted in 50%, capitellar osteochondral defects were present in 29%, capitellar bone bruises were evident in 96%, and loose bodies were noted in

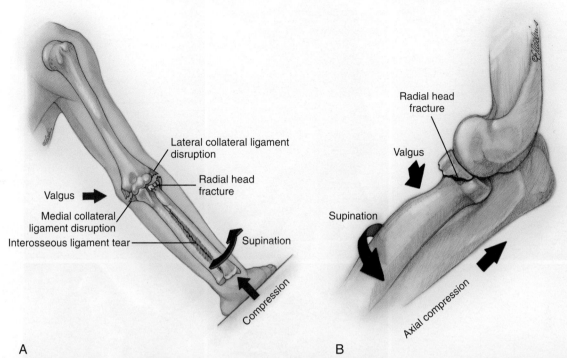

FIGURE 19.5 Mechanism of fracture of the radial head. **A**, Valgus and/or axial loading of the elbow causes failure of the radial head in compression and possible medial collateral ligament or interosseous membrane disruption. **B**, Posterolateral rotatory subluxation of the elbow causes disruption of the lateral ulnar collateral ligament and the anterolateral aspect of the radial head to shear off as it slides posterior to the capitellum with the forearm in supination. This mechanism likely explains the commonly associated lateral ligamentous injuries and chondral damage of the capitellum seen with this fracture pattern. Continued subluxation of the elbow may result in a fracture of the coronoid, disruption of the medial collateral ligament, and a complete dislocation.

92%.[99] In one series of patients with Essex-Lopresti injuries presenting for reconstruction, 15 of 20 had undergone a radial head resection without knowledge of the forearm ligamentous injury, suggesting that this uncommon injury may be easily missed in clinical practice.[206] Collectively, these data suggest that minimally displaced fractures have a low incidence of associated soft tissue disruption. More displaced and comminuted fractures are likely with higher energy, and therefore have a greater incidence of associated ligamentous injuries. Careful physical examination and intraoperative evaluation of the elbow are needed to detect these associated ligamentous injuries.

Fractures of the capitellum may be appear as chondral injuries[89] or displaced osteochondral fractures. Ward and Nunley reported that 50% of patients with fractures of the capitellum had an associated fracture of the radial head, whereas only 1% of the fractures of the radial head had a capitellar fracture.[217] For displaced fractures of the radial head treated operatively, the incidence of an associated capitellar fracture was 24%. These injuries may or may not be visible with plain radiographs or CT scans and are often only diagnosed during surgery.[31] Capitellar fractures may be responsible for a mechanical block of elbow or forearm motion in the absence of significant displacement of a fracture of the radial head seen radiographically (Figure 19.6).

Dislocations of the elbow are seen in 3 to 10% of patients with fractures of the radial head.[104,106,172] Patients with an associated elbow subluxation or dislocation may have a fracture of the coronoid as part of a "terrible triad" injury with disruption of one or both collateral ligaments of the elbow.[171] Small

coronoid fragments typically present as triangular fragments situated anteriorly in the coronoid fossa and are often mistaken as a fragment of the radial head. Larger coronoid fragments are associated with greater instability of the elbow and require specific treatment as outlined in Chapter 22. Elbow fracture–dislocations should be managed by immediate closed reduction followed by treatment of the radial head, the same as for isolated fractures.[27,61,104,106] Whereas some authors recommend urgent operative management of the radial head if needed (within 24 h) to reduce the incidence of heterotopic ossification, this practice remains controversial.[67,104] Early motion seems to improve outcome; therefore urgent, not emergent, management of the fracture is appropriate. Excision of the radial head without replacement should be avoided for patients with associated dislocations due to a high risk of another dislocation and instability.[61,106,178] Fractures of the olecranon or proximal ulna may also be seen in association with fractures of the radial head as a variant of the Monteggia fracture.[147]

ANATOMY AND BIOMECHANICS

The anatomy of the radial head and neck is complex and highly variable.[117,211] The head of the radius consists of a circular concave dish that articulates with the spherical capitellum (Figure 19.7). The dish has a greater radius of curvature than the capitellum making this articulation only moderately constrained. The articular dish is variably offset from the axis of the radial neck. The margin of the radial head that articulates with the radial notch of the ulna is slightly elliptical[14] producing a cam effect during forearm rotation that displaces the shaft

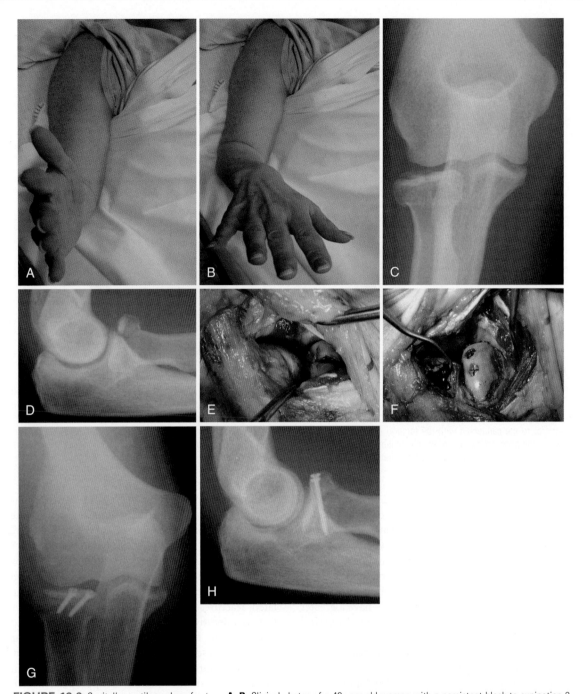

FIGURE 19.6 Capitellar cartilage shear fracture. **A, B,** Clinical photos of a 49-year-old woman with a persistent block to supination 2 weeks after a minimally displaced fracture of the radial head. **C, D,** Preoperative anteroposterior and lateral radiographs demonstrating a displaced fracture of the radial head. **E,** Intraoperative photograph of cartilage shear fracture. **F,** Intraoperative photograph demonstrating reduction of the fracture with two 2.0-mm screws and cancellous bone grafting of the radial neck from the lateral epicondyle. **G, H,** Postoperative anteroposterior and lateral radiographs after open reduction and internal fixation of the radial head and débridement of the capitellum.

somewhat radially during pronation.[58] The radial notch of the proximal ulna comprises an arc of 60 to 70 degrees and forms a relatively congruous articulation with the radial head, allowing for only modest radioulnar translation during forearm rotation. The anterolateral one-third of the articular margin of the radial head is devoid of cartilage allowing placement of internal fixation without impingement with the radial notch during forearm rotation.

A "safe zone" for internal fixation has been described as a 110-degree arc centered on a point 10 degrees anterior to the midpoint of the lateral side of the radial head as judged with the forearm in neutral rotation (Figure 19.8).[32,58,192,194] This nonarticular portion can also be identified by the rounded shape of its margin relative to the flatter surface that articulates with the proximal radioulnar joint. The rotational interval between the Lister tubercle and the radial styloid of the distal radius is another useful anatomic landmark for the nonarticular portion of the radial head.[32] Placement of plates on the nonarticular margin may be required when managing fractures involving the radial neck. The radial head is surrounded by the annular ligament; therefore, bulky internal fixation is poorly tolerated. Implants should be low profile to minimize soft tissue adherence that may impede forearm rotation.

The cancellous trabeculae are oriented perpendicular to the surface of the radial head confirming the load-bearing function of the radial head. It has been suggested that the subchondral bone is weaker in the anterolateral portion of the radial head; this was confirmed by a recent CT imaging study which demonstrated that the cancellous bone volume was lowest in the anterolateral quadrant of the radial head.[86]

The blood supply of the radial head is composed of both intra- and extraosseous sources.[72] Vessels penetrate the radial neck from the periosteum at the head–neck junction; the dorsolateral periosteum is a key area for these branches. Preservation of the periosteal attachment of displaced fragments is important during open reduction and internal fixation of fractures of the radial head and neck. Proximal radius plate fixation further compromises the vascularity of the radial head.[121]

A better understanding of the lateral ligamentous anatomy of the elbow has resulted in improvements in surgical techniques for fractures of the head of the radius. The annular ligament wraps around the radial head, attaching to the anterior and posterior margins of the radial notch, of the ulna and stabilizes the radial head in the proximal radioulnar joint. The radial collateral ligament arises from the lateral epicondyle and attaches to the annular ligament. The lateral ulnar collateral ligament arises from the lateral epicondyle and is inserted on the crista supinatoris of the proximal ulna. The lateral ulnar collateral and radial collateral ligaments are important restraints against varus and posterolateral rotational instability of the elbow (Figure 19.9).[51,155,156]

Conventional surgical approaches to the radial head through the Kocher interval (between the extensor carpi ulnaris and the anconeus) often cause iatrogenic injury to the lateral ulnar collateral ligament unless the dissection is brought more anterior such that the radial collateral and annular ligaments are divided at the midaxis of the radial head.[120] Additionally, this approach tends to expose the radial head too posteriorly to permit internal fixation of the commonly involved anterolateral portion of

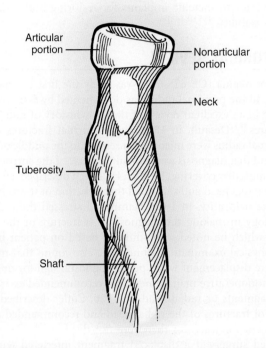

FIGURE 19.7 Anatomy of the proximal radius. The radial head is somewhat elliptical. The concave surface of the radial head that articulates with the capitellum is variably offset in a radial direction from the axis of the radial neck. The portion of the radial head that does not articulate with the radial notch of the ulna is more rounded, whereas the articulating portion is more flattened.

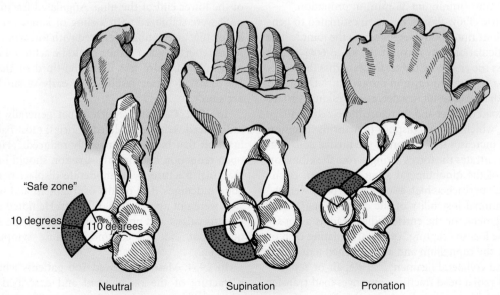

FIGURE 19.8 Nonarticular portion of the radial head. The nonarticular portion "safe zone" of the radial head can be identified as a 110-degree arc centered on a point 10 degrees anterior to the midpoint of the lateral side of the radial head with the forearm in neutral rotation.

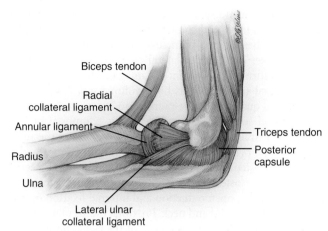

FIGURE 19.9 Lateral ligaments of the elbow. The lateral ligaments of the elbow include the radial collateral, lateral ulnar collateral, and annular ligaments. The lateral ulnar collateral ligament is an important stabilizer against posterolateral rotational and varus instability of the elbow. The annular ligament stabilizes the proximal radioulnar joint and contributes to varus and posterolateral rotatory elbow instability by virtue of its attachment to the radial collateral ligament.

the radial head. Maintaining the integrity of the lateral ulnar collateral ligament or performing a strong repair to bone is essential to prevent instability, which may be an important cause of failure of internal fixation, late pain, and arthritis.

Repair of the fascial interval between the anconeus and extensor carpi ulnaris has also been shown to further augment elbow stability.[39] For isolated fractures of the radial head without associated ligamentous or osseous injuries, a more anterior muscle–tendon splitting approach through the common extensor tendon at the midportion of the radial head should be considered. This approach allows for good visualization of the radial head and avoids detachment of the lateral ulnar collateral ligament. However, it is less extensile distally, limited by the proximity of the posterior interosseous nerve, which lies on average 33 mm (minimum 22 mm) from the capitellum in supination and 52 mm (minimum 38 mm) in pronation.[46]

Resisted isometric elbow flexion has been estimated to generate forces up to four times body weight across the joint.[4,5] The radiocapitellar articulation may account for up to 60% of the load transfer across the elbow.[79] Contact forces across this articulation are greatest with the forearm in pronation.[150] Displaced fractures of the radial head result in a decreased residual surface area available for load transfer and therefore increased cartilage contact pressures, which may predispose to arthritis. Excision of the radial head increases the tension in the medial collateral ligament and concentrates the forces acting across the elbow on the lateral aspect of the ulnohumeral joint; it has been calculated that the force can reach as high as nine times body weight.[4] Posterolateral rotational instability of the elbow is aggravated by excision of fragments or the entire radial head as a consequence of both the loss of "capture" of the articulating dish of the radial head by the capitellum and a diminished tensioning effect on the lateral collateral ligament.[16,155] Repair or replacement of displaced radial head fractures improves load transfer and elbow stability.[17,103]

The head of the radius is an important valgus stabilizer of the elbow, particularly in the setting of an incompetent medial collateral ligament.[118,149,153,165,181] In vitro biomechanical studies have shown that the kinematics and stability of the elbow are altered by radial head excision, even in the setting of intact collateral ligaments.[17,101] Replacement of the radial head with metallic prostheses has been demonstrated to improve the stability of elbows with intact and deficient medial and/or lateral collateral ligaments.[17,118] Axial forearm stability is also improved by metallic radial head prostheses in the setting of an interosseous ligament disruption.[183] Silicone radial head replacements are inferior to metallic implants for restoring both axial and valgus stability.[94,95,118,167,183]

HISTORICAL REVIEW

Paul of Aegina (CE 625-690) was likely the first to report an injury to the proximal radius, as documented by Schwartz and Young in an excellent review of the early history of radial head fractures.[182] Desault, in 1811, suggested that fractures of the proximal radius were uncommon relative to the middle or distal end and that diagnosis was difficult because of the surrounding thick muscular covering. In 1897, Helserich described a fracture of the radial head and suggested that resection of it was helpful for late deformity. In 1910, Hammond stressed the utility of radiology in making the diagnosis of a fracture of the radial head, which he noted to be difficult based on patient history and physical examination alone.[82] He also found that marked fracture displacement was a poor prognostic sign for outcome with nonoperative management and recommended excision of the fragments or radial head. In 1926, Cutler described three types of fractures of the radial head and recommended closed treatment for fractures that were not displaced.[43] He recommended surgery if a displaced fragment interfered with full motion, prevented reduction of an elbow dislocation, and in cases of malunion, ankylosis, or forearm stiffness.

Watson-Jones reported in 1930 that only a 50% good result could be obtained in the management of displaced fractures of the radial head.[218] He avoided excision of it as a result of the "inevitable" radial shortening with subluxation or dislocation of the lower end of the ulna. Angulated fractures of the radial neck were stabilized with a sling of kangaroo tendon because he felt that angulation interfered with forearm rotation. In 1935, Jones reported good results could be achieved by excising fragments that involve less than one-third of the radial head.[105] He reported better results with early-versus-late radial head excision.

In 1950, Carstam reported that generally fractures of the radial head were not isolated injuries; most had an elbow subluxation that had spontaneously reduced.[35] He suggested that open reduction and internal fixation should be considered for marginal fractures with moderate displacement and reported good outcomes. The results of fragment and whole-head excision were not appreciably different. He noted changes, such as cubitus valgus and proximal migration of the radius, were frequent but did not commonly cause symptoms, except in children.

In 1954, Mason reviewed 100 patients who had sustained a fracture of the radial head and described a classification system.[135] He recommended nonoperative treatment for undisplaced type I fractures and reported good results. Type II fractures, which he described as "marginal sector fractures with displacement," had more variable results. He recommended that conservative treatment should be pursued if the fracture fragment did not involve more than one-quarter of the articular circumference and was reasonably well aligned. In all other cases, "no matter how minimal the tilting and comminution of the fracture segment," he recommended excision of the radial head. He described the axiom of radial head fracture treatment as: "If in doubt—resect." Type III fractures were comminuted, and he advised primary radial head excision and reported good early results. In 1962, Johnston added a fourth subtype to the Mason classification: a radial head fracture associated with an elbow dislocation.[104] He considered that radial head excision was not a benign procedure and stated: "If in doubt, treat conservatively."

Subsequent to these papers, there has been an explosion of interest in radial head anatomy,[21,32,74,117] biomechanics,[5,6,14,79,101,118,149,150,152,153,165,167,183,184] and fracture management.[93] The importance of the radial head to the kinematics and load transfer of the elbow is now better understood, and there is an increasing interest in salvaging the radial head whenever possible.[8,25,54,57,64,68,69,89,93,113,115,138,161,174,179,185] Advances in screw-and-plate designs have resulted in increasing utilization of open reduction and internal fixation for displaced fractures of the radial head with excellent results for simple fracture configurations. Even though long-term follow-up studies suggest that radial head excision is generally well tolerated clinically in the absence of associated ligament injuries, the incidence of osteoarthritis has been high.[25,41,61,63,73,97,100,114,144,178,216] Implant arthroplasty has become popular for the treatment of comminuted displaced fractures of the radial head where open reduction and internal fixation is less predictable.

Speed reported the use of a metallic radial head arthroplasty in 1941.[195] Subsequently, acrylic was employed with some early success.[37] Silicone implants gained widespread use in the 1970s and early 1980s.[25,33,131,151,196,199,213] More recently there has been a resurgence of interest in metallic radial head implant arthroplasty as a result of problems with wear and failure of silicone when placed under compressive load.[34,84,85,107,108,119,147,147,189,195] The success of first-generation metallic radial head implants has led to newer modular designs to allow easier implantation and improved sizing options to provide a closer match to patients' anatomy.[21,76,78,117,127,186]

TREATMENT OPTIONS

Fractures of the head of the radius should be managed based on patient factors such as age, bone quality, associated injuries, and activity level.[81] Fracture factors that influence decision making include size, displacement and location, and the presence of a mechanical block to elbow or forearm motion. For example, an older patient with osteoporosis and a comminuted fracture of the radial head is a poor candidate for internal fixation. Arthroplasty of the radial head is the preferred option for displaced nonreconstructable fractures in the setting of an associated injury to the medial or lateral collateral ligaments or the interosseous membrane because excision further compromises instability.[94,95,118,134,165,167,183]

The influence of radial head fracture size and displacement on patient outcome is unknown due to a lack of scientific data directing clinical practice. In vitro biomechanical studies

revealed a progressive loss in radiocapitellar joint stability with increasing size of wedge defects in the radial head.[18,19] Wedge defects greater than one-third of the radial head did not contribute to stability in this model. These data suggest that, particularly in the setting of elbow instability, fixation of fragments smaller than one-third of the radial head may be advantageous. Whereas, it seems that most displaced intraarticular fractures in other joints benefit from anatomic reduction, stable fixation, and early motion; displaced fractures of the radial head historically have often been managed nonoperatively if they do not impede joint motion.

Good long-term clinical results have been reported in the majority of patients with the nonoperative treatment of isolated displaced partial articular fractures of the proximal radius.[2] Articular displacement causes abnormal joint contact pressures and may predispose one to the development of arthritis or persistent pain at either early or late follow-up. While delayed excision of the radial head is typically helpful under these circumstances, complete relief of symptoms is not assured.[26,63,216] Randomized clinical trials are needed to compare the outcomes of operative and nonoperative treatment of displaced radial head fractures without a block to motion or associated injuries requiring treatment. Fractures with a mechanical block to motion have a clear indication for surgical treatment regardless of their size. These are typically fractures that involve the articular portion of the radius or fragments that extrude into the proximal radioulnar joint.

The degree of displacement of a fracture of the neck of the radius that requires surgery in adults is unknown; a mechanical block to rotation remains the primary indication for surgical management.[10] Although most undisplaced fractures of the radial neck heal when treated with early motion, nonunions do occur.[38,57,173] Nonoperative treatment is recommended except in the setting of associated injuries requiring surgical management such as fractures of the coronoid or olecranon. Translation of the radial head on the neck produces a cam effect and often impedes forearm rotation if it is greater than 2 to 3 mm. Neck angulation of more than 20 degrees in adults commonly interferes with forearm rotation as a result of altered kinematics with the capitellum and radial notch of the ulna and should be considered for surgical management.[10]

The initial management of a fracture of the radial head associated with an elbow dislocation is a gentle closed reduction of the elbow under intravenous sedation. Repeat radiographs taken after the reduction should be obtained to better evaluate the radial head fracture for further management, either nonoperative or operative. A careful assessment for an associated fracture of the coronoid and/or capitellum is needed for patients with a fracture of the radial head, particularly those with a history of an elbow dislocation. The presence of a coronoid fracture suggests an unstable elbow for which operative management may be required to achieve an optimal outcome. The author's recommended management is the algorithm shown in Figure 19.10.

Nonoperative Management

Undisplaced or isolated displaced fractures of the radial head and neck, which do not cause a block to elbow or forearm motion, are offered nonoperative management. Depressed fractures generally do not impede forearm rotation, whereas

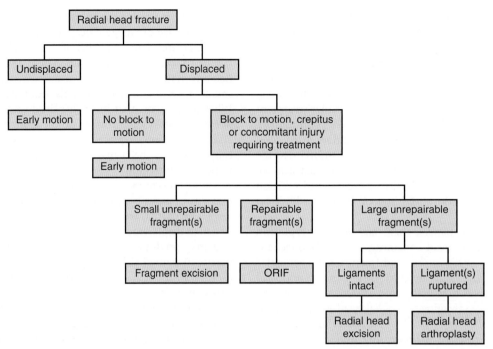

FIGURE 19.10 Author's recommended management algorithm for fracture of the head of the radius. Note the indications for surgery for isolated displaced fractures without a block to motion are controversial. Radial head excision is avoided in the setting of acute injuries due to the high incidence of associated damage to the collateral ligaments and/or interosseous membrane. *ORIF*, Open reduction and internal fixation.

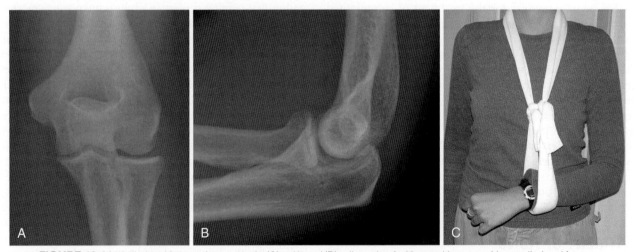

FIGURE 19.11 Undisplaced fracture. Anteroposterior (**A**) and lateral (**B**) radiographs of a 28-year-old woman with an undisplaced fracture of the radial neck. **C**, Management with a collar and cuff sling. The patient had a complete return of motion and no residual pain.

extruded fragments do, often by virtue of their impingement with the proximal radioulnar joint and annular ligament. Whereas some authors have recommended cast immobilization,[77,137] most studies have supported the concept of early motion.[36,129,136,204,207,219] Aspiration of the elbow hemarthrosis and injection of local anesthetic, as previously described, should be considered only if there is sufficient pain to prevent evaluation of forearm rotation.[47,168] In a prospective randomized clinical trial, aspiration and injection of anesthetic in the absence of a mechanical block to motion demonstrated that the final outcome was not altered.

Active motion should be initiated within one week, owing to the frequent development of elbow stiffness with longer periods of immobilization. A collar and cuff, or sling, is used for comfort between periods of active motion and should be discontinued by 4 weeks (Figure 19.11). The use of a static progressive extension splint should be considered at night if elbow extension does not progressively improve in the first 4 to 6 weeks following the injury. Although subsequent displacement is uncommon, careful clinical and radiographic follow-up is required. Late displacement may be more common with fractures involving more than one-third of the radial head.[135]

Operative Management

Open Reduction and Internal Fixation

Patients with isolated noncomminuted displaced fractures of the radial head with a mechanical block to forearm or elbow motion and those with concomitant injuries requiring surgical management (e.g., coronoid, olecranon, or capitellum fractures or complex elbow instability) are managed with ORIF if stable fracture repair is possible. Based on a lack of scientific evidence to direct management, the option of ORIF is explained to healthy active patients if they have an isolated noncomminuted fracture of the radial head that is displaced more than 2 mm and involves greater than one-third of the diameter without a mechanical block to rotation. I also explain that many patients with these fractures can do well with nonsurgical treatment, and that we are not sure what the optimal management is.[221] Mason suggested that displaced fractures greater than one-fourth of the diameter of the radial head should be treated by radial head excision.[135]

Geel and colleagues recommended ORIF of displaced (>2 mm) fractures involving more than one-fourth of the radial head.[69] Radin and Riseborough[170] suggested that displaced fractures greater than one-third of the radial head should be managed operatively. Miller and others reported that fragment size had no effect on the outcome of type II fractures.[145] Ultimately, it is best to try to help the patient make an informed decision between operative and nonoperative management.

The ability to reliably repair the radial head often can only be determined intraoperatively. ORIF of multifragmented radial head fractures can be successful if stable internal fixation is achieved so that early motion can be initiated.[25,54,69,89,93,113,115,138,158,161,164,174,179,185] One study has reported a high incidence of complications following ORIF of greater than three fragments, suggesting an alternative treatment method should be considered for more comminuted fractures.[174] Failure to achieve a congruous reduction and rigid fixation owing to comminution or osteoporosis should prompt the surgeon to intraoperatively consider excision of the radial head or replacement. Tenuous fixation in the setting of associated ligamentous injuries should be avoided because minimal residual instability following ligament repair will likely lead to fixation failure.[115,172,174] Failed surgical reconstruction usually leads to articular injury of the capitellum and the radial notch of the ulna. Stiffness and pain frequently require further surgery, often with less than satisfactory results. The outcome for patients with failed internal fixation is typically not as successful as those managed initially with excision of the radial head or replacement, suggesting that intraoperative decision making is critical to optimize treatment result.[186]

Reduction and internal fixation of displaced fractures of the radial head using arthroscopy are difficult owing to the inability to distract the radiocapitellar joint to properly evaluate the articular reduction. Furthermore, bleeding often compromises the view such that a 3- to 5-day delay before surgery is recommended. Standard elbow arthroscopic techniques and equipment are employed; however, a 70-degree arthroscope may be helpful to better visualize the joint's surface. The efficacy and indications for arthroscopic reduction of fractures of the radial head are evolving. Open surgical approaches remain the current standard of care.

Although most authors prefer a Kocher approach,[120] some have employed a lateral epicondyle osteotomy.[88] Splitting the common extensor tendon allows better access to the anterior radial head where most marginal fractures occur and avoids injuring the lateral ulnar collateral ligament which is at risk with the Kocher approach.[45]

Fixation is performed using bioabsorbable pins, headless screws, 1.5- or 2.0-mm screws, and 2.5- or 3.0-mm cannulated screws. Plate options include standard small-fixation systems or purpose-designed proximal radius precontoured locking systems. Smooth Kirschner wires are useful to reduce fragments and provide provisional fixation; however, they should not be employed for definitive fixation because of the tendency for these to migrate during the postoperative period. Screws should be countersunk to prevent impingement with the radial notch and annular ligament even if placed on the nonarticular margin.

The use of crossed cannulated 2.5- or 3.0-mm screws has been found to be effective for stabilizing the radial head on the neck in the absence of comminution.[71,190] Intramedullary fixation also has been reported.[111] Plate fixation is employed for comminuted radial neck fractures in an effort to stabilize the radial head onto the neck and achieve union. Precontoured locking plates are biomechanically superior to the standard T-plates and may yield improved clinical results.[71,160] Plates should be placed on the nonarticular portion of the radial head as previously described.[194] If bone grafting is required following elevation of a depressed fragment(s), the lateral epicondyle or proximal ulna is a convenient source. Caution should be exercised when performing ORIF of comminuted displaced fractures of the radial neck in adults as even with optimal reduction and rigid fixation, avascular necrosis and nonunion may occur due to the disruption of both the interosseous and periosteal blood supply to the head.

Excision of Fragments of the Radial Head

Fragment excision is infrequently indicated with the advent of improved fixation systems with small diameter screws. Cartilage flaps and small displaced fragments (less than one-third of the radial head) that block forearm rotation due to extrusion into the proximal radioulnar joint or loose fragments that prevent elbow flexion or extension are treated with open or arthroscopic fragment excision if ORIF is not technically feasible because of small fragment size, comminution, or osteoporosis.[36,105,154,220] Fragments that articulate with the proximal radioulnar joint should not be excised because of interference with forearm rotation.

Delayed Excision of the Radial Head

Early motion with delayed excision of the radial head may be considered for patients with displaced fractures who have no mechanical block to forearm or elbow motion. This approach may be useful in elderly low-demand patients with concomitant injuries to the medial collateral or interosseous ligaments and for patients with a delayed presentation. The radial head can be excised either open or arthroscopically if the patient remains symptomatic after healing of the fracture and any associated ligamentous injury.[1,26,63] The radial head is excised just distal to

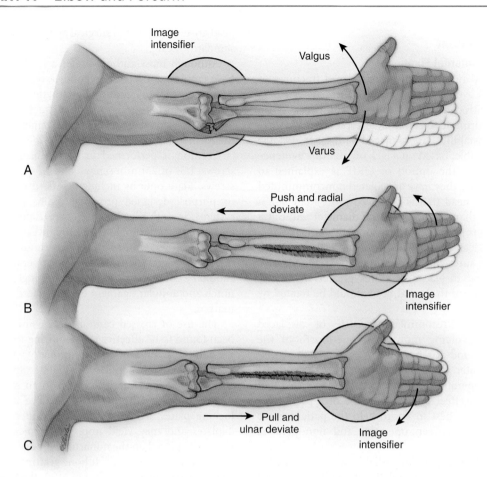

FIGURE 19.12 A, A valgus and varus stress test of the elbow should be performed to evaluate the integrity of the medial and lateral collateral ligaments using an image intensifier before excision of the radial head. **B, C,** Similarly, the axial stability of the forearm should be evaluated by alternatively applying axial traction/ulnar deviation and compression/radial deviation to the forearm and wrist while monitoring ulnar variance at the wrist with an image intensifier.

the radial notch with careful preservation of the lateral ulnar collateral ligament and repair of the annular ligament if done through an arthrotomy. To ensure replacement arthroplasty is not required; intraoperative valgus and a varus stress fluoroscopy should be obtained after radial head excision to ensure competency of the medial and lateral collateral ligaments of the elbow.[44] To evaluate for an interosseous ligament tear, perform axial loading with radial deviation of the wrist and forearm distraction with ulnar deviation of the wrist while monitoring ulnar variance with fluoroscopy (Figure 19.12). Using a serrated reduction clamp on the radial neck and applying a proximal–distal pull may be a more sensitive technique to identify axial instability after radial head excision.[191]

Excision of the Radial Head

Prior to the development of more reliable methods of internal fixation and durable prostheses, displaced fractures of the radial head, both simple and comminuted, were commonly treated by open excision of the radial head.[1,24,36,41,43,90,105,114,135,144,154,170,214,216] Although less frequently performed currently, excision of the radial head is preferable to an unstable or incongruous ORIF.[174] Should radial head reconstruction be technically impossible, associated soft tissue injuries and concomitant fractures should be evaluated because acute radial head excision is contraindi-

cated in the setting of concomitant disruption of the medial or lateral collateral ligaments, interosseous membrane, or an elbow dislocation.[1,104]

The radial head can be excised either through an arthrotomy or arthroscopically[130,143] as previously noted. If the intraoperative stress tests for varus, valgus, and axial instability described are negative, there was no associated elbow dislocation and no clinical suspicion of a ligamentous injury, acute radial head excision without implant replacement may be considered. Given the high incidence of associated ligamentous injuries with comminuted radial head fractures, and the difficulty in diagnosing these associated conditions, the author currently does not perform this procedure unless there is gross wound contamination, a nonreconstructable extension of the fracture into the radial neck, or a concomitant severe articular injury to the capitellum that precludes the use of a metallic radial head arthroplasty. Careful preservation of the lateral ulnar collateral ligament and repair of the annular ligament should be performed if the radial head is excised open. The timing of radial head excision is controversial as a result of concerns regarding the potential development of heterotopic ossification, with some authors recommending early excision (<24 h)[1,67,104,203] and others excision within 10 days.[35,135] The presence of an associated dislocation and head injury appears to be the risk factor most associated with the development of heterotopic ossification following elbow surgery.[1,66,203]

Arthroplasty of the Radial Head

Replacement arthroplasty is indicated for displaced comminuted fractures of the radial head and neck when an anatomic reduction and stable internal fixation is not achievable and there are, or are likely to be, associated soft tissue or bony injuries. These include soft tissue injuries to the medial or lateral collateral ligaments, the interosseous membrane, and/or triangular fibrocartilage and bony injuries of the coronoid or olecranon.

Silicone implants have been employed in the past.[25,33,131,151,196,199] However, they are no longer recommended as they are biomechanically inferior to metal and have a high incidence of fracture and fragmentation, sometimes with the development of silicone synovitis.[118,167,183] Recent clinical series of studies using metallic implants noted good results relative to earlier reports using silicone.[11,49,59,76,84,85,108,119,147,189,222] Earlier metallic radial head implants employed a monoblock design making size-matching suboptimal and implant insertion often difficult owing to the need to subluxate the elbow to allow for insertion of these devices.[78] Modular metallic radial head prostheses, with separate heads and stems, are now employed, allowing improved sizing options and easier implantation. The implantation techniques for the currently available implants vary somewhat; however, most employ a Kocher or common extensor tendon-splitting approach and divide the radial collateral and annular ligaments while preserving the integrity of the lateral ulnar collateral ligament when it is intact.[120] Available prostheses include smooth stem spacer implants, press-fit, or ingrowth stems, as well as cemented devices. Metallic and pyrolytic carbon articulations are also available. Most implants have a fixed head-stem but bipolar devices are available too. Although most designs are axisymmetric, there is one currently available system with a more elliptical articulation. There are no reported studies comparing the clinical outcome of the various radial head implant designs.

Even with intact ligaments, biomechanical studies have demonstrated an alteration in the kinematics and stability of the elbow following radial head excision.[17,101] These in vitro studies have also shown that metallic radial head replacement restores the kinematics and stability of the elbow similar to that with a native radial head.[15,17] Furthermore, the clinical results of radial head excision at long-term follow up have been variable[26,28,30,41,63,68,73,90,97,100,114,144,152,202] while the medium-term results of metallic radial head arthroplasty have been encouraging.[11,49,59,76,84,85,119,147,189,222] On the basis of these biomechanical and clinical studies and the known high incidence of concomitant ligamentous injuries with comminuted fractures, this author routinely replaces the radial head in the setting of a nonreconstructable fracture.

❖ AUTHOR'S PREFERRED TREATMENT

Surgical Approach. Place the patient in the supine position on the operating table and use a sandbag beneath the ipsilateral scapula to assist in positioning the arm across the chest. Alternatively, an arm table can be used with the surgeon sitting. Use a lateral decubitus position in the setting of a concomitant proximal ulna or olecranon requiring fixation. Administer pro-

phylactic intravenous antibiotics. General or regional anesthesia should be employed. I perform a fluoroscopic evaluation of the elbow prior to prepping and draping to look for associated ligament injuries and instability of it and/or forearm.

Use a sterile tourniquet. While many surgeons use a lateral incision, I prefer a midline posterior elbow incision just lateral to the tip of the olecranon and elevate a full-thickness lateral flap on the deep fascia (Figure 19.13). This extensile incision decreases the risk of cutaneous nerve injury and provides access to the radial head, coronoid, medial, and lateral collateral ligaments if needed for the management of more complex injuries.[50,159] A posterior incision is also more cosmetically acceptable than standard laterally placed incisions. Maintain the forearm in pronation to move the posterior interosseous nerve more distal and anterior during the surgical approach.[197]

In patients with known injuries to the lateral collateral ligament, such as following a dislocation or as identified using fluoroscopy, my preference is a Kocher approach to access the radial head and to facilitate ligament repair.[120] Identify the fascial interval between the anconeus and extensor carpi ulnaris by noting the diverging direction of the muscle fibers and small vascular perforators that exit at this interval (Figure 19.14). Humeral avulsion of the lateral collateral ligament and common extensor muscles from the lateral epicondyle are commonly noted in patients following fractures of the radial head; this is a consistent finding in patients with a concomitant elbow dislocation, simplifying surgical exposure of the radial head. In these circumstances the radial head is easily visualized after opening the fascia of the Kocher interval at which point a bald lateral epicondyle is evident and the deep dissection exploits this disruption to approach the radial head.[141]

If the lateral ligament is intact, elevate the extensor carpi ulnaris anteriorly off the underlying lateral ulnar collateral ligament and incise the radial collateral and annular ligaments longitudinally at the midaxis of the radial head. Elevate the humeral origin of the radial collateral ligament and the overlying extensor muscles anteriorly off the lateral epicondyle to better expose the anterior half of the radial head if required. Avoid posterior dissection in the setting of intact ligaments to preserve the integrity of the lateral ulnar collateral ligament and thereby maintain the varus and posterolateral rotatory stability of the elbow.[52,155] Release the posterior component of the lateral collateral ligament if further exposure is needed, and carefully repair the ligament at the end of the procedure. Elevate the supinator, and identify the posterior interosseous nerve if dissection is required distal to the radial tuberosity to allow fixation of a proximal radius fracture.

For patients with an intact lateral collateral ligament, I prefer a common extensor tendon-splitting approach (Figure 19.15).[45] Divide the common extensor tendon and the underlying radial collateral and annular ligaments longitudinally at the midaspect of the radial head. Keep the forearm in pronation and avoid dissection distal to the radial tuberosity to protect the posterior interosseous nerve. Elevate the radial collateral ligament and common extensor muscles anteriorly off the lateral epicondyle if needed to further improve exposure. Division of the posterior component of the lateral collateral ligament can be considered if further exposure of the radial head is needed, but a meticulous ligament repair is required. Similarly, extension distal to

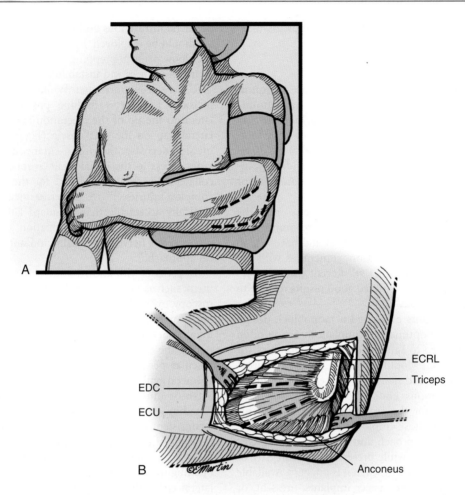

FIGURE 19.13 Superficial surgical approaches. **A,** Posterior midline skin incision is employed just lateral to the tip of the olecranon. **B,** A full-thickness lateral flap is elevated. The use of this incision allows access to the medial aspect of the elbow (if necessary) to manage associated injuries to the medial collateral ligament or coronoid, is less obvious due to its location, and has a low incidence of cutaneous nerve injury. Alternatively, lateral incision can be employed at the surgeon's discretion. Lateral extensor musculature. Exposure of the radial head can be obtained using either a Kocher approach between the anconeus and extensor carpi ulnaris or a more anterior common extensor tendon split. *ECU,* Extensor carpi ulnaris; *EDC,* extensor digitorum communis; *ECRL,* extensor carpi radialis longus.

the proximal aspect of the radial tuberosity requires identification of the posterior interosseous nerve.

Fragment Excision. If a decision can be made preoperatively that a small, displaced fragment(s) cannot be reliably fixed with ORIF, I use arthroscopy to remove the fragments. Localization of the fragment(s) is superior to what can be achieved with a limited arthrotomy, and the morbidity is low. Standard arthroscopic techniques, as described in Chapter 26, are employed. Surgery is performed 3 to 5 days after injury to avoid problematic bleeding that may occur with early surgery.

The decision that a fracture cannot be reliably fixed is most commonly made intraoperatively during an attempted open reduction (Figure 19.16). I use an image intensifier, a pituitary rongeur, and copious irrigation to extract small, displaced, unreconstructable fragments.[105,220] Avoid inadvertent removal of a coronoid fragment by noting its triangular shape and attaching it to the anterior capsule. Evaluate the remaining radial head to ensure that the deficient portion does not articulate with the radial notch in any position of forearm rotation. Ensure congruent tracking of the residual radial head with the capitellum before repairing the annular, radial, and lateral ulnar

collateral ligaments as described later. Because removal of the anterior rim of the radial head in the setting of a lateral collateral ligament injury may contribute to residual posterolateral rotatory instability,[18,19] careful lateral collateral ligament repair and rehabilitation with the forearm in pronation is essential to achieve a successful outcome.[52]

Open Reduction and Internal Fixation. In my experience, arthroscopic reduction and internal fixation of fractures of the radial head has not been rewarding because of the difficulty of obtaining a good view of the articular dish, which is obscured by the curvature of the capitellum. The inability to distract the radiocapitellar joint makes visualization of the reduction much more difficult than similar approaches at the wrist or knee. Further complicating arthroscopic reduction and internal fixation is the small working space in which the fragments can be manipulated and limited safe-approach angles for fixation devices.

One of the two open surgical approaches is used, as previously described. For displaced partial articular fractures I carefully reduce the fragments to avoid the loss of any residual periosteal attachments with its concomitant blood supply

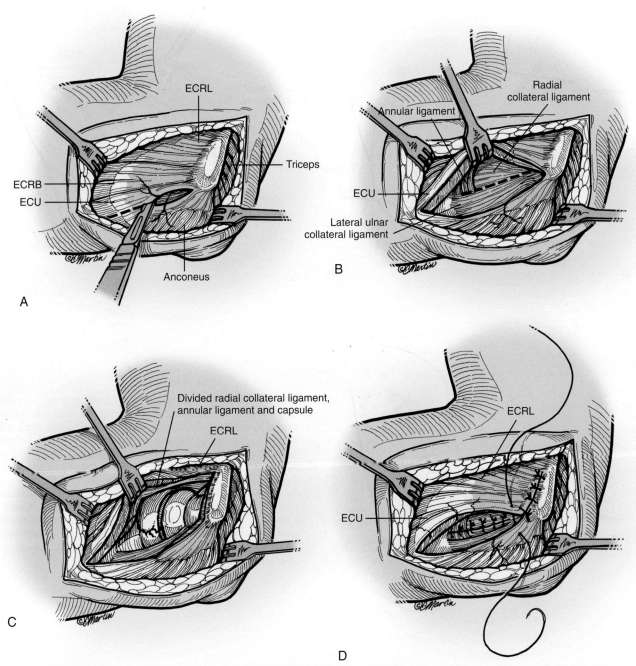

FIGURE 19.14 The Kocher approach to the radial head. **A**, The interval between the anconeus and extensor carpi ulnaris (ECU) is opened as evident by the divergent muscle fibers and vascular perforators that exit this interval. **B**, The ECU is elevated anteriorly off the lateral collateral ligament and an arthrotomy is performed at the midportion of the radial head, thereby avoiding detachment of the lateral ulnar collateral ligament. The radial collateral and annular ligaments are divided to give adequate exposure of the fracture. The radial collateral ligament and extensor muscles commonly need to be detached off the lateral epicondyle to achieve visualization of the anterior portion of the radial head (*dotted line*). **C**, The radial collateral ligament and extensor muscles are detached from the lateral epicondyle to achieve visualization of the anterior portion of the radial head. **D**, Closure of the arthrotomy is accomplished by reattaching the radial collateral ligament to the intact lateral ulnar collateral ligament. The fascia of the Kocher interval is then repaired. If the lateral ligaments are incompetent, either as a result of injury or surgical release, a careful repair is required as outlined in Figure 19.21. *ECRB,* Extensor carpi radialis brevis; *ECRL,* extensor carpi radialis longus.

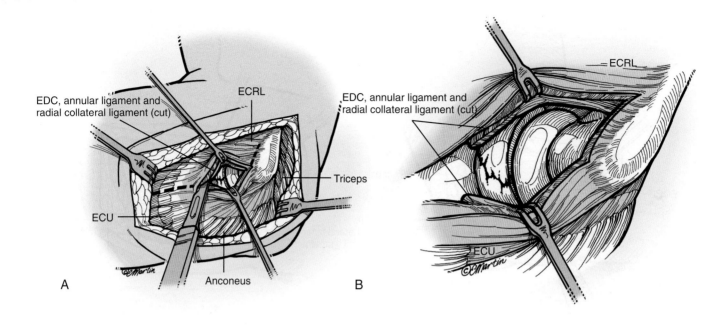

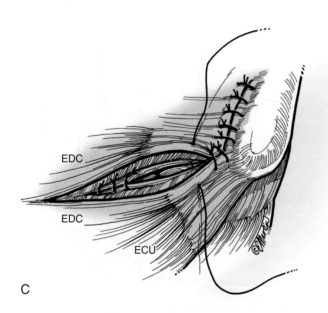

FIGURE 19.15 Common extensor tendon-splitting approach to the radial head and neck. **A,** The common extensor tendon, the radial collateral, and annular ligaments are divided longitudinally at the mid portion of the radial head as a single layer (*dotted line*). The forearm is maintained in pronation to protect the posterior interosseous nerve. **B,** Elevation of the radial collateral ligament and extensor muscles anteriorly off the lateral epicondyle is required to provide better access to anterior fragments of the radial head. This approach gives adequate access to manage most fractures of the radial head and neck and is preferred if the lateral ulnar collateral ligament is known to be intact. **C,** Closure is accomplished by repairing the common extensor tendon, radial collateral ligament, and annular ligament with a side-to-side repair. *ECRL,* Extensor carpi radialis longus; *ECU,* extensor carpi ulnaris; *EDC,* extensor digitorum communis.

CRITICAL POINTS *Fragment Excision*

Indication
- Displaced unreconstructable fragment(s) less than one-third radial head diameter that is blocking forearm or elbow motion or is interposed within the articulation.

Pearls
- Localize fragments with CT preoperatively and an image intensifier intraoperatively.
- Compare size of missing section of radial head to removed fragment(s) to ensure all fragments have been found.

Pitfalls
- Displaced medial fragments may be missed if a lateral surgical approach is used.

- Elbow instability due to deficiency of collateral ligaments is exacerbated by partial excision of the radial head.

Technical Points
- Arthroscopic fragment removal allows complete joint inspection.
- Use an open approach through a common extensor tendon split or Kocher interval.
- Consider fragment fixation if it is technically possible.
- Use pituitary rongeur and copious irrigation to remove loose unreconstructable fragments.

Postoperative Care
- Begin early range of motion exercises to avoid restricted forearm rotation as a consequence of annular ligament adherence to deficient portion of the radial head.

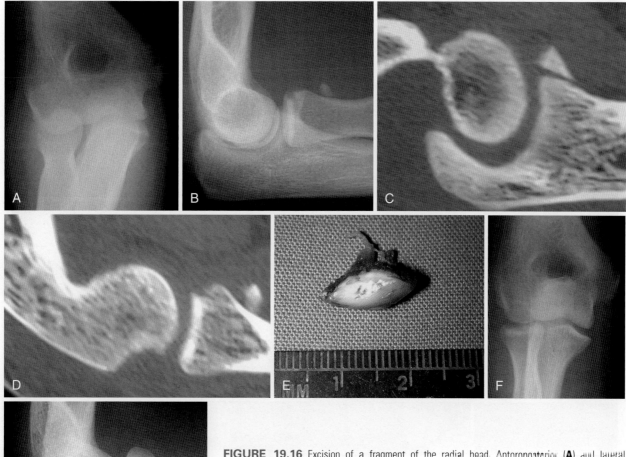

FIGURE 19.16 Excision of a fragment of the radial head. Anteroposterior (**A**) and lateral (**B**) radiographs of a 32-year-old man who fell while rollerblading; he had limited prosupination. **C, D,** CT scan demonstrated an undisplaced coronoid fracture, a posterior capitellum impression fracture, and a fragment of the radial head anterior to the radial neck. **E,** Attempts to retrieve the fragment arthroscopically failed due to its location distal to the radial head, and an arthrotomy was needed to excise the small fragment. **F, G,** After a lateral ligament repair and early range-of-motion exercises the patient recovered a full arc of forearm rotation and a functional arc of elbow motion.

(Figure 19.17).[72] Use smooth Kirschner wires as joysticks to elevate depressed fragments and to achieve provisional fixation. Fix fragments using appropriate screws, typically 1.5 or 2.0 mm. Countersink all screws to avoid impingement with the annular ligament and radial notch. Avoid perforation of the far cortex while drilling to allow for more accurate length measurements with a depth gauge. Screws that are too long should be avoided as they may interfere with forearm rotation (Video 19.1).

For complete articular fractures, in which the radial head has separated from the neck, I assemble the radial head on a back table if there are no soft tissue attachments to the fragments. After rigid fixation of the radial head has been achieved, secure the radial head to the neck using divergent cannulated 2.5-mm screws if the neck is not comminuted (Figure 19.18). The cannulated feature of the screws prevents the tips from glancing off the cortex when placed at an oblique angle. I treat most comminuted radial neck fractures with implant arthroplasty due to

the high risk of nonunion, avascular necrosis, hardware failure, and stiffness. However, if the bone quality is good and the patient is young, I perform ORIF with a fixed-angle precontoured locking plate. Secondary hardware removal is often needed to manage rotational stiffness (Figure 19.19). I no longer use small plates because, in my experience and that of others, they provide less rigid fixation than fixed-angle devices and have had a high risk of nonunion.[160] Place plates on the nonarticular portion "safe zone" of the radial head to prevent interference with the proximal radioulnar joint.[32,192] Use cancellous bone from the lateral epicondyle, the proximal ulna, or the distal radius to graft bone defects if necessary.

Check hardware placement with an image intensifier at completion of the internal fixation to ensure that screw lengths are appropriate. Plain radiographs are insufficient; imaging in multiple positions of forearm rotation is needed to confirm appropriate placement of the hardware. If an anatomic reduction and stable fixation cannot be achieved, I perform radial head

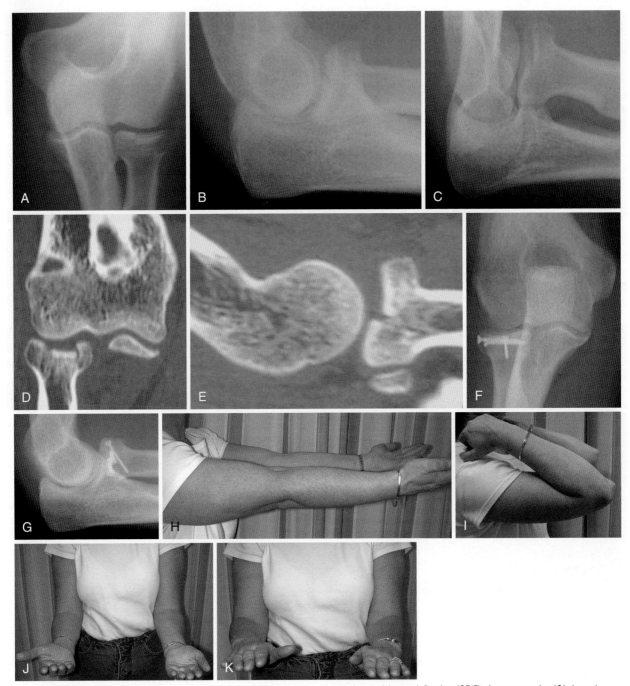

FIGURE 19.17 Partial articular fracture of the radial head: open reduction and internal fixation (ORIF). Anteroposterior (**A**), lateral (**B**), and oblique (**C**) radiographs of a 38-year-old woman who fell while ice-skating. **D, E,** CT confirmed significant fracture displacement. **F, G,** The patient underwent ORIF of the radial head with 2.0- and 1.5-mm screws. **H-K,** The patient recovered a full arc of elbow and forearm motion and had no pain 6 months following the injury.

replacement because of the high incidence of failure of ORIF under these circumstances.[115,174]

Excision of the Radial Head. I no longer perform radial head excision without replacement for acute fractures except in the setting of gross wound contamination or extensive fractures of the radial neck or capitellum that cannot be reconstructed. I use either of the two open surgical approaches described earlier depending on the integrity of the lateral collateral ligament (Figure 19.20). The excised fragments are reassembled outside of the elbow to ensure that all of the radial head has been

retrieved. Use a microsaggital saw to complete the resection until it is just distal to the radial notch. Avoid excessive removal of the radial neck to prevent proximal radioulnar impingement. Evaluate the valgus, axial, and rotational stability of the elbow, and check for residual fragments using an image intensifier.[44] If there is any suggestion or suspicion of an associated ligamentous injury (and there usually is as previously described), I perform a radial head arthroplasty. Revise the surgical approach to reduce the residual laxity induced by the loss of collateral ligament tension resulting from excision of the radial head.

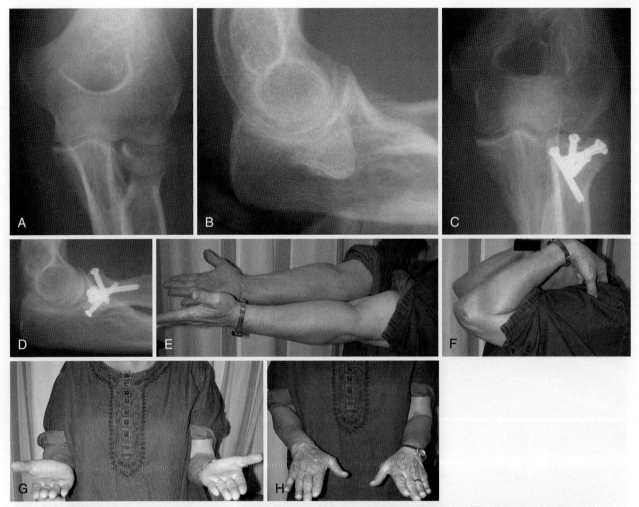

FIGURE 19.18 Complete articular fracture of the radial neck: ORIF. Anteroposterior (**A**) and lateral (**B**) radiographs of a 52-year-old woman who slipped and fell and sustained a displaced fracture of the radial neck. **C, D,** The fracture was fixed using cannulated 3.0 mm screws. **E-H,** An excellent clinical result was achieved with no evidence of avascular necrosis at 6 months.

CRITICAL POINTS *Open Reduction and Internal Fixation*

Indication
- Displaced reconstructable fragments(s) interfering with forearm or elbow motion or concomitant fractures or ligament injuries of the elbow requiring treatment

Pearls
- CT scan may be helpful in planning surgery.
- Avoid screw penetration through opposite cortex.
- Fragments are typically quite anterior; avoid posterior dissection with damage to lateral ulnar collateral ligament.

Pitfalls
- Hardware impingement with annular ligament
- Nonrigid fixation
- Fixation of comminuted fractures involving more than three fragments

Technical Points
- Use an open approach through common extensor tendon split or Kocher's interval.
- Use cross-cannulated screws for noncomminuted fractures of the radial neck.
- Use fixed-angle precontoured plates for selected comminuted fractures of the radial neck; arthroplasty preferred for most patients.
- Place plate on the nonarticular portion of radial head which presents laterally with forearm in neutral rotation.
- Perform careful ligament repair to avoid radiocapitellar subluxation with failure of fixation.

Postoperative Care
- Early range-of-motion exercises are required to avoid annular ligament adherence to hardware or fracture lines.

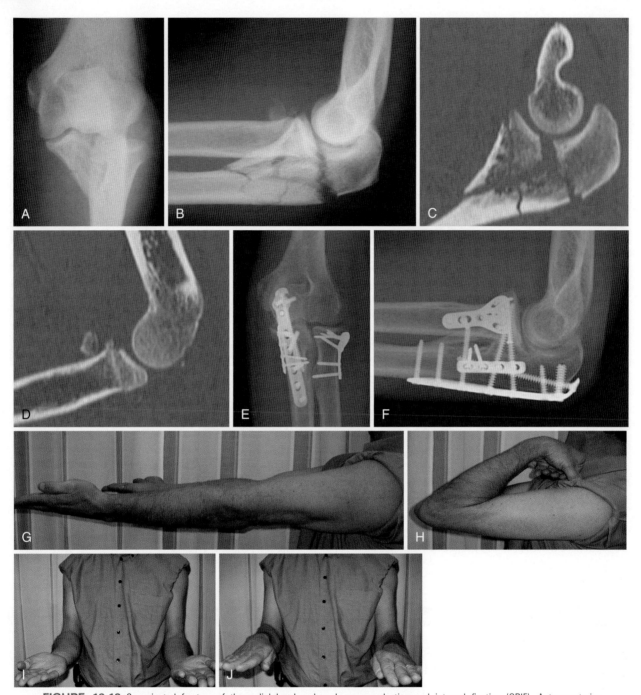

FIGURE 19.19 Comminuted fracture of the radial head and neck: open reduction and internal fixation (ORIF). Anteroposterior (**A**) and lateral (**B**) radiographs of a 35-year-old man who fell off a ladder, sustaining a comminuted fracture of the proximal ulna and radius. **C**, **D**, CT scans define the nature of the fractures more clearly. **E**, **F**, Radiographs two years postop: ORIF. A precontoured locking plate was used for fixation of the proximal radius (Wright Medical Technology, Arlington, TN). **G-J**, At 2 years the patient had no pain and near complete range of motion.

I perform arthroscopic excision of the radial head for non-unions, malunions, and posttraumatic arthritis using standard portals and instruments.[130,143] Use a high-speed bur, resectors, and pituitary rongeurs to remove the cartilaginous and osseous fragments. A tourniquet is essential to control bleeding. Use imaging to ensure that the elbow and forearm are stable, all of the fragments have been removed, and an adequate resection has been accomplished.

Implant Arthroplasty of the Radial Head. I use a common extensor tendon-splitting approach if the lateral collateral ligament is intact and a Kocher's approach if the lateral collateral ligament is deficient as described earlier. Collect the fragments of the radial head, and reconstruct it for sizing purposes and to ensure all of the radial head is excised. The implantation technique will vary slightly depending on the arthroplasty design selected. Over the last 25 years, I have employed an uncemented

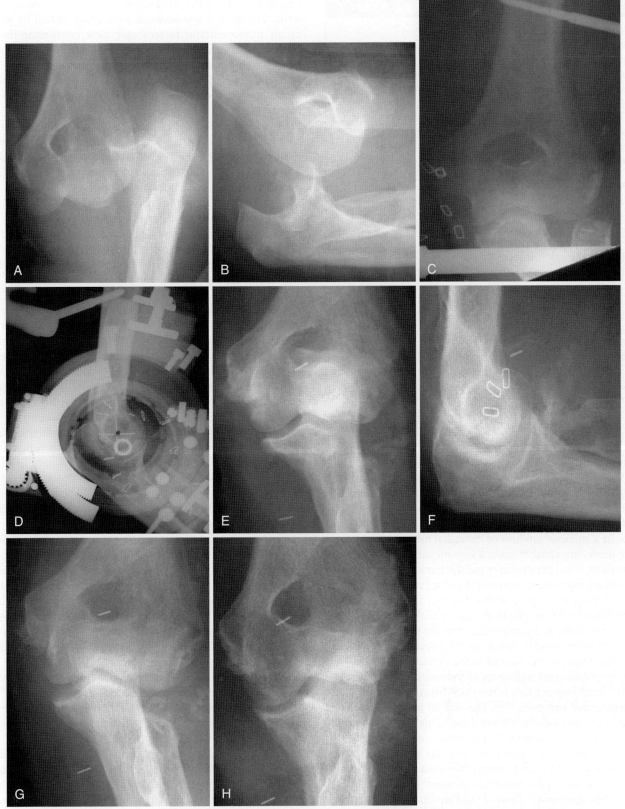

FIGURE 19.20 Comminuted fracture of the radial head and neck: excision. **A, B,** Radiographs of a 69-year-old man with a compound fracture-dislocation of the elbow and renal insufficiency. Owing to extensive contamination of the wound, delayed treatment, and chronic immunosuppression he was managed by excision of the radial head without replacement. **C, D,** An articulated external fixator (Compass Hinge, Smith and Nephew Richards) was employed to maintain a concentric reduction of the elbow. **E, F,** After fixator removal the patient had mild pain and a functional arc of motion. Stress testing disclosed significant residual valgus instability (**G**) and varus instability (**H**).

CRITICAL POINTS *Excision of the Radial Head*

Indications
- Rarely employed for acute fractures; typically for nonunions, malunions and posttraumatic arthritis
- Displaced unreconstructable fragments(s) interfering with forearm or elbow motion without a known associated or probable medial or lateral collateral ligaments or an interosseous membrane injury

Pearls
- Assemble excised fragments to ensure all are removed; intraoperative fluoroscopy is helpful.

Pitfalls
- Avoid excision with unrecognized ligamentous injuries.
- Excessive excision of the radial neck may cause proximal radioulnar impingement.

Critical Technical Points
- Use an open approach through a common extensor tendon split or the Kocher interval.
- Excise the radial head just distal to the proximal radioulnar joint.
- Use intraoperative fluoroscopy to perform varus, valgus, and axial stress tests.

Postop Management
- Early range-of-motion exercises are critical to avoid soft tissue adherence to radial neck.

metallic smooth stem implant, which functions as a spacer while healing of the soft tissue occurs[49,76,84,85,147,186] (Figure 19.21 and Video 19.2). Most implants are now modular to facilitate improved size-matching of the native radial head and neck and to allow easier placement in the setting where the lateral ligaments of the elbow are competent.[117]

Excise a minimal amount of the radial neck at a right angle to the medullary canal to make a smooth surface for seating of the implant. Select the diameter and thickness of the radial head arthroplasty from the reconstructed excised radial head (Figure 19.22). Choose an implant with a diameter that is equal to the minor diameter of the elliptical native radial head. The minor diameter typically is 2 mm smaller than the major diameter of the native radial head.[117] Select the thickness of the prosthesis using the height of the reconstructed excised radial head as a template. Avoid overlengthening of the radius by placement of a radial head implant that is too thick because this may cause capitellar wear and pain.[208,212] The lack of a gap between the radial head and capitellum is not a useful method of determining the correct thickness of the prosthesis since the lateral ligaments are often incompetent for patients undergoing radial head arthroplasty. Check to ensure that the arthroplasty articulates at the height of the proximal radioulnar joint, about 2-mm distal to the coronoid.[48] This is a valid landmark except in cases of disruption of the interosseous membrane where proximal migration of the radius may be present. Check the ulnar variance at the wrist to rule out an Essex-Lopresti injury. If the radius is overlengthened, the lateral ulnohumeral joint will be gapped open laterally; however, this is difficult to visualize intraoperatively without using a dental mirror. Using fluoroscopy, check the alignment of the distal radioulnar joint to ensure that the ulnar variance is equivalent to the opposite wrist. The medial ulnohumeral joint space should be parallel on an anteroposterior fluoroscopic view, confirming that the prosthesis is neither too thick nor too thin, resulting in a varus or valgus alignment of the elbow, respectively.

The lateral ulnohumeral joint space is often wider than the medial ulnohumeral joint radiographically so it cannot be used to evaluate prosthesis thickness unless a contralateral radiograph is available.[176,12,13] Postoperative radiographs are unreliable when evaluating the length of the radius; therefore, the most accurate technique to ensure the correct implant thickness is employed is to use an implant constructed with the same overall thickness as that of the excised radial head.[48,176,187] I use preoperative radiographic templating of the contralateral normal radial head in the setting of a secondary radial head replacement, such as a previous excision or a malunion, but not for a primary replacement for an acute fracture where the radial head is available for sizing. The capitellum diameter is also a useful parameter in the setting of a prior radial head excision.[3,123]

Deliver the radial neck laterally by placing a Hohmann retractor around the posterior aspect of the proximal radial neck and prying against the ulna. Do not use anteriorly placed Hohmann retractors owing to the risk of injury from pressure on the posterior interosseous nerve. Ream the medullary canal of the radial neck using hand reamers until cortical contact is encountered. Insert a trial stem 1 mm smaller than the size of the final reamer to achieve a nontight fit of the smooth stem. Attach a trial head of the appropriate diameter and thickness to the stem, and evaluate the congruency of the prosthesis both visually and with an image intensifier as previously described. If the prosthesis is not tracking properly on the capitellum with forearm rotation, a smaller stem size should be placed to ensure that the articulation of the radial head with the capitellum is optimal. With this spacer design, motion pathways of the radial head are controlled by the annular ligament and the articular congruency of the implant with the capitellum and radial notch. The motions of the radial head prosthesis with respect to the capitellum are not dictated by the motions of the proximal radius because the stem is smooth and able to move within the medullary canal. The spacer concept of this implant allows the use of an axisymmetric prosthesis when replacing the native radial head, which has a complex shape that is difficult to replicate with an off-the-shelf prosthesis.[117] Movement of the stem is well tolerated and lucencies around the stem are expected and have not been correlated with residual symptoms.[49,76,147,186] The concept is similar to a bipolar design without the need for a polyethylene articulation and potential concerns about wear debris and durability.[166]

Place a Hohmann retractor behind the radial neck, and pull the radius laterally by prying against the ulna to insert the assembled modular radial head prosthesis. In some patients insufficient translation of the proximal radius prevents the insertion of a preassembled modular implant, typically in the setting of reconstruction rather than acute fractures. If it is not possible to place an assembled prosthesis, insert the stem first, place the head onto the stem, and couple the implant in situ using the locking tool. Repair the annular ligament to ensure congruent tracking of the radial head implant on the capitellum. Close the lateral deep surgical approach as previously described.

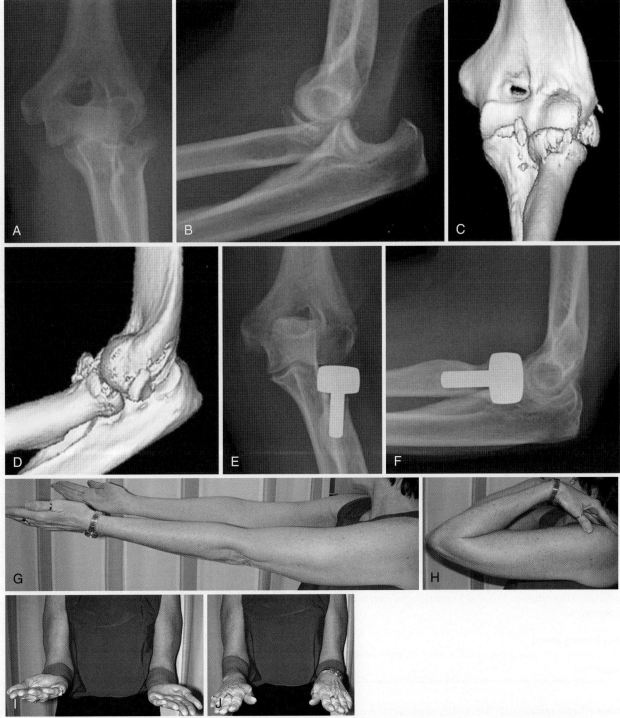

FIGURE 19.21 Comminuted fracture of the radial head and neck: replacement. Anteroposterior (**A**) and lateral radiographs (**B**) of a 55-year-old woman who slipped on the ice sustaining a posterolateral elbow dislocation and a comminuted fracture of the radial head. **C, D,** Computed tomography following a closed reduction demonstrated the extent of injury to the radial head and an associated comminuted fracture of the tip of the coronoid. **E, F,** A modular radial head arthroplasty was employed (Evolve, Wright Medical Technology, Arlington, TN), and the lateral ligaments were repaired using drill holes in the lateral epicondyle. The coronoid fracture was not fixed. Although the medial collateral ligament repair was disrupted, repair was not required to allow early motion. At 2 years postoperatively dystrophic calcification is seen in the medial collateral ligament and some typical nonprogressive lucencies are noted around the implant stem in the proximal radius. **G-J,** An excellent range of motion was achieved, and the patient was asymptomatic at 2 years.

CRITICAL POINTS *Implant Arthroplasty of the Radial Head*

Indications
- Displaced unreconstructable fracture larger than one-third of the diameter of the radial head with known or probable medial or lateral collateral ligament or interosseous membrane injury
- Nonunion, malunion, and posttraumatic arthritis of the radial head

Pearls
- Choose the diameter and thickness of radial head implant on the basis of the reconstructed excised radial head if available.
- The diameter of the radial head arthroplasty is determined from the minor diameter of the elliptical reconstructed excised radial head. This is typically 2 mm smaller than the major diameter of the native radial head.
- The radial head prosthesis should articulate at the level of proximal radioulnar joint, 2-mm distal to the coronoid.
- If radial head does not articulate well with the capitellum, downsize the stem.
- Translate the radial neck laterally to facilitate implant placement.

Pitfalls
- Choosing the size of prosthesis by evaluating the gap between the radial head and capitellum will result in overlengthening of the radius since the lateral ligaments are often incompetent in patients undergoing radial head arthroplasty.
- Avoid placing Hohmann retractors anteriorly on the radial neck because of pressure on the posterior interosseous nerve.
- Avoid excessive thickness and diameter of the radial head.

Critical Technical Points
- Open approach through common extensor tendon split or the Kocher interval
- Excise the radial head perpendicular to the radial neck.
- Using the reconstructed excised radial head as a template, select an implant thickness to restore radial length and an implant diameter similar to the minor diameter of the native radial head.
- Use intraoperative fluoroscopy to check implant thickness by evaluating whether the medial ulnohumeral joint space is parallel, the implant is at the level of proximal radioulnar joint, 2-mm distal to coronoid and that ulnar variance is corrected.
- Careful lateral ligament repair is required if damaged by the injury or surgical approach.

Postop Management
- Early range-of-motion exercises are critical to avoid soft tissue adherence to radial neck.

Closure. After fragment excision, ORIF, or excision or replacement of the radial head, repair the lateral collateral ligament and common extensor muscle origins. If the anterior half of the lateral collateral ligament and extensor origin was detached from the lateral epicondyle, repair the anterior half of the lateral collateral ligament (the annular and radial collateral ligaments) to the posterior half using interrupted absorbable sutures. If the lateral collateral ligament and extensor origin have been completely detached either by the injury or surgical exposure, repair these using drill holes through bone and nonabsorbable sutures. I use transosseous tunnels as opposed to suture anchors because the soft tissues can be drawn toward the attachment site, better tensioning the repair (Figure 19.23). Drill a single hole at the axis of motion (the center of the arc of curvature of the capitel-

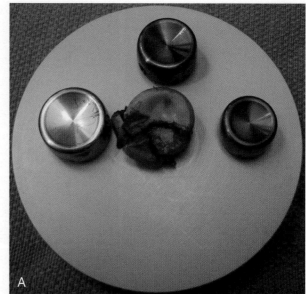

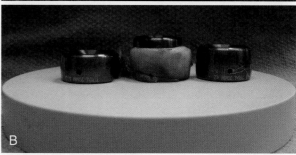

FIGURE 19.22 Sizing of the radial head prosthesis. The diameter and thickness of the prosthesis are best determined using the reconstructed excised radial head as a template. **A**, The articular dish diameter is typically 2 mm smaller than the outer diameter of the radial head and is selected as the diameter of the implant head. **B**, The overall thickness of the prosthesis should be the same as the excised radial head with care taken to avoid placing a prosthesis that is too thick.

lum), and connect this to a hole placed anterior and posterior to the lateral supracondylar ridge. Alternatively, if bone quality is good, I use two drill holes posterior to the supracondylar ridge because passing the sutures posteriorly is technically easier. Use a locking suture technique to obtain a secure hold of both the lateral collateral ligament and the common extensor muscle fascia. Pull the ligament sutures and extensor origin sutures into the holes drilled in the distal humerus using suture retrievers. Pronate the forearm, and avoid varus forces to close the lateral side of the elbow while tensioning the sutures prior to tying them. Avoid overtensioning the repair as this can pull the elbow into varus, particularly if the medial collateral ligament is deficient.[62] Place the knots anterior or posterior to the lateral supracondylar ridge to avoid prominence.

POSTOPERATIVE MANAGEMENT AND EXPECTATIONS

Outcome Data

Nonoperative Management

The outcome of undisplaced fractures of the radial head is generally favorable, with return of function within 6 to 12

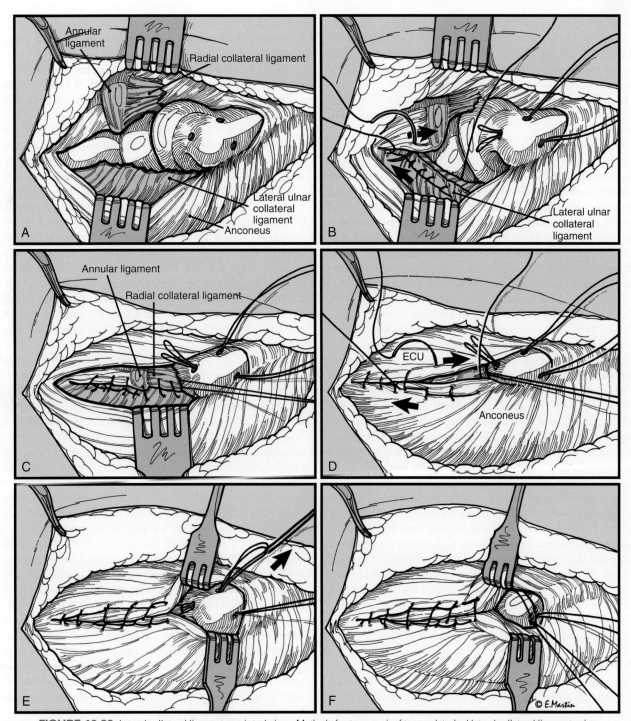

FIGURE 19.23 Lateral collateral ligament repair technique. Method of suture repair of torn or detached lateral collateral ligament using transosseous sutures in the lateral epicondyle. **A**, A single hole is drilled at the axis of motion (the center of the arc of curvature of the capitellum) and connected to a hole placed anterior and posterior to the lateral supracondylar ridge. Suture passers are placed to facilitate the repair. **B, C**, A locking suture technique is employed to gain a secure hold of the lateral ulnar collateral ligament. The interval between the radial collateral and lateral ulnar collateral ligaments and the annular ligament are closed as this suture is brought back to the lateral epicondyle. **D, E**, The common extensor muscles and fascia of the Kocher interval is closed as a separate layer in a similar fashion. **F**, The ligament and fascial sutures are pulled into the holes drilled in the distal humerus while maintaining the forearm in pronation and avoiding varus forces while tying the sutures. *ECU,* extensor carpi ulnaris.

weeks. Late displacement is uncommon but has been reported, particularly with fracture fragments that are greater than one-third of the diameter of the radial head.[135,170] Careful clinical and radiographic follow-up of these injuries is mandatory. Residual pain is uncommon. Mild residual flexion contractures

of 10 to 15 degrees are not infrequent sequelae.[129,135,136,204,207,219] Some patients develop arthrofibrosis and a more severe capsular contracture unresponsive to therapy and splinting requiring arthroscopic or open capsular release (see Chapter 24). Stiffness is more common in patients with associated injuries such as an elbow dislocation, ligamentous injury, or coronoid fracture. Overall, most study series report 85 to 95% good results for undisplaced fractures managed with early motion. An initial period of cast immobilization does not appear to be necessary, nor is it advisable, as demonstrated in one prospective randomized trial.[207] Aspiration of the elbow in the absence of a block to forearm rotation does not appear to influence ultimate outcome.[47,92]

Although successful nonoperative management has been reported for displaced fractures of the radial head, the outcome seems to be less reliable.[1,2,29,113,135,145,170] Mason reported that 9 of 15 patients had some pain at an average of 11 years following nonoperative treatment for fractures involving greater than 25% of the joint surface.[135] He advocated excision of the radial head. Radin and Riseborough reported better motion in patients with displaced radial head fractures managed with radial head excision than that achieved with nonoperative treatment.[170] Burton reported that only 2 of 9 patients with displaced radial head fractures managed nonoperatively had good results; he recommended radial head excision in such cases.[29] Khalfayan and coworkers reported on 26 patients with Mason type II radial head fractures at an average of 18 months following either open reduction and internal fixation or nonoperative treatment with early motion.[113] The operatively treated group had 90% good or excellent results while the nonoperatively treated group had 44% good or excellent results. Pain, functional limitations, and osteoarthritis were more frequent in the nonoperatively treated group. Akesson and coworkers reported on the outcome of 49 patients with moderately displaced Mason type II partial articular two-fragment fractures at an average of 19 years.[2]

At final follow up the incidence of osteoarthritis was high at 82%; however, only 6 patients had an unsatisfactory result requiring a subsequent radial head excision and only 9 of the 49 patients had subjective complaints. Collectively these studies indicate that the outcome of nonoperative treatment of isolated displaced radial head fractures can be successful for many patients provided there is no block to motion and early motion is initiated. Randomized clinical trials are needed to determine which subgroup of patients with displaced fractures of the radial head should be offered operative treatment.

Open Reduction and Internal Fixation

The clinical outcome of ORIF of the radial head has been good when an anatomic reduction and rigid internal fixation has been achieved and early motion is initiated in the postoperative period.[10,25,35,54,61,69,88,89,93,97,98,113,115,128,138,158,161,163,174,179,185,221] There has been a low incidence of nonunion, avascular necrosis or stiffness requiring further surgery. For simple partial articular fractures, success rates generally exceed 90%; however, the outcome has been worse and the complication rate has been higher in patients with more comminuted fractures, particularly fractures that completely separate the radial head and neck.

King et al reviewed the elbows of 14 patients treated with open reduction and internal fixation at an average follow up of 32 months.[115] Mason type II fractures had 100% good or excellent results. Only 33% of Mason type III fractures treated with open reduction and internal fixation had a good or excellent result. An associated elbow dislocation did not affect the results

significantly but was associated with an increased fixed-flexion deformity. Fractures were often more comminuted than suggested by plain radiographs. Excellent results were obtained provided an anatomic reduction with stable fixation and early range of motion were achieved. However, if a stable anatomic reduction cannot be obtained, alternative treatment methods should be considered.

More recently Ikeda and coworkers reported 90% good to excellent results using ORIF of comminuted Mason type III fractures treated with low-profile miniplates, suggesting that with recent advances in techniques and implants successful ORIF is possible in selected patients with comminuted fractures.[98] Ring and coworkers reviewed the results of open reduction and internal fixation of fractures of the radial head in 56 patients.[174] These authors recommended open reduction and internal fixation for partial articular fractures consisting of a single fragment and for complete articular fractures with three or less fragments. They recommended that comminuted fractures were best managed by radial head excision or replacement arthroplasty. Concomitant injuries, such as dislocations and other fractures, increased the failure rate of ORIF of the radial head.

There are no prospective randomized studies comparing ORIF with nonoperative management. The clinical and radiographic results of nonoperatively treated displaced radial head fractures were inferior for a similar group of patients treated with open reduction and internal fixation as reported by Khalfayan et al.[113] Boulas and Morrey compared the outcome of 36 patients managed with open reduction and internal fixation, excision, silastic replacement, and nonoperative management.[25] The best outcome was achieved with ORIF of displaced radial head fractures. Lindenhovius and coworkers compared the results of ORIF versus excision for unstable displaced fractures of the radial head in 28 patients at an average of 17 years' follow-up.[128] They reported that ORIF reduced the incidence of subsequent elbow dislocation and reduced the frequency and severity of osteoarthritis when compared to patients who had a primary radial head excision. Ikeda and coworkers also reported better outcomes with ORIF when compared to a matched cohort of patients who had radial head excision for comminuted Mason type III fractures.[96] In a nonrandomized comparison of partial articular radial head fractures displaced 5 mm or less performed by Yoon et al, comparing 30 patients treated with ORIF to 27 patients managed nonoperatively, the functional outcomes were similar; however, the complications were higher with surgical care.[133]

Collectively these studies demonstrate that ORIF of displaced radial head fractures leads to a successful outcome for the majority of patients and is superior to radial head excision. The indication for ORIF versus nonoperative management remains unclear and requires further study.

Fragment Excision

Although fragment excision is infrequently indicated with the advent of improved small diameter screws and surgical techniques, the outcome can be favorable in carefully selected patients. Fragment excision should be limited to small marginal fragments that are not amenable to ORIF because of comminution or osteopenia. Some authors have reported good results in more than 80% of patients, but others have reported less satisfactory results.[105,154,220] Carstam reported that only 17 of 33 patients (52%) managed with fragment excision had good or excellent results.[35] Fragment excision should be performed with caution when concomitant elbow instability is present because the loss of the stabilizing effect of the fragment may further compromise elbow stability.

Delayed Radial Head Excision

Reports in the literature are conflicting as to the success of delayed radial head excision.[1,26,35,63,170] Delayed radial head excision was often employed in the past because of a lack of sophisticated internal fixation devices and prostheses and concerns about stiffness and heterotopic ossification with early surgery.[1,26,35,67] Current thinking is that the extent of the initial trauma and presence of concomitant associated injuries are more important variables in the development of stiffness. Surgical timing is now thought to be less critical, so definitive early management of fractures of the radial head is preferred.[27,63] Delayed radial head excision is currently employed for residual symptoms from malunions and arthritis. Considerable improvement in pain and motion can be expected; however, the pain relief is variable, primarily dependent on whether arthritis has developed in the ulnohumeral joint.[1,26,63,112]

Adler and Shaftan reported good results with delayed excision (8 weeks) and recommended against early excision except in the setting of a block to motion.[1] Broberg and Morrey reported that delayed excision (1 month to 20 years after fracture) improved motion and decreased pain in 81% of the 21 patients reviewed.[26] In 77% of patients there was a good or excellent result. Osteoarthritis was common at follow-up, being mild to moderate in 77%. Fuchs and Chylarecki reported a better outcome following early (<2 weeks) versus delayed excision.[63] Sixty-nine percent of patients who underwent early excision were satisfied as compared with 44% who had a delayed excision.

Primary Resection of the Radial Head

The outcome after primary resection of the radial head without replacement is controversial in the literature with some authors reporting good clinical and radiographic results and others reporting a high incidence of pain, valgus and/or axial instability, elbow dislocation, weakness and degenerative elbow, and/or wrist arthritis, particularly at long-term follow-up.[1,41,63,73,96,97,100,105,106,128,144,145,152,202,214,216] Morrey et al reported 80% satisfactory results after resection for displaced fractures of the radial head at an average of 20 years' follow-up.[152] Mild ulnohumeral arthritis was common radiographically, but residual symptoms were uncommon and mild. Wrist pain occurred in 15% of patients but was usually mild. Proximal migration averaged 2 mm. Fuchs and Chylarecki assessed the outcome of 108 patients after radial head resection at an average of 6 years; 64% had an isolated fracture and 26% had an associated elbow dislocation.[63] Clinical outcome and strength were better for patients treated with a primary versus a secondary radial head excision.

Ikeda and Oka reviewed 15 patients treated with early radial head resection for a fracture of the radial head at an average of 10 years.[97] All of the patients had reduced elbow power and only 5 of them were pain free. Janssen and Vetger reported on a follow-up of 21 patients with a Mason type III fracture treated by excision of the radial head at between 16 and 30 years.[100] Only 4 of their patients had elbow pain. Of the 16 patients who had radiographic follow-up, 11 had degenerative arthritis of the elbow. Berger and coworkers reported good or excellent results in 10 of 30 patients at an average of 5 years.[22] Valgus deformity of the elbow was common.

Josefsson et al reported on 23 patients with an elbow dislocation associated with a displaced fracture of the radial head.[106] Nineteen patients had the radial head excised at an average of 2 days after injury. In 4 patients' elbows with an associated displaced fracture of the coronoid process, redislocation occurred. A follow-up examination performed in 19 patients between 3 and 34 years after the injury demonstrated severe osteoarthritis in 12 elbows. Reduced range of motion was the most common complaint, and reduced extension was the most common finding. To lower the risk and prevent severe instability, the authors recommended that the radial head should be preserved if possible in the setting of an associated elbow dislocation. Mikic and Vukadinovic reported on 58 patients who had been treated with excision of a radial head and who were reviewed at an average of 6.5 years.[144] Osteoarthritis was present in 52% and residual symptoms were found in 43%. Forearm rotation was limited in 58%, and 25% had symptomatic proximal migration of the radius with distal radioulnar joint symptoms. Given their 50% fair or poor results, the authors suggested that the indications for radial head excision should be relatively limited.

More recently, Antuna and coworkers reviewed 26 patients at an average follow-up of 25 years following a primary radial head excision for a displaced radial head fracture without associated elbow instability. The functional outcome was good or excellent in 92% of the patients, an increased carrying angle and osteoarthritis were present in all; however, wrist pain was only significant in 3 patients.[7]

Arthroplasty of the Radial Head

Silicone arthroplasty of the radial head, although initially successful in many patients,[22,25,33,125,131,151,196,199] has fallen out of favor due to problems with residual instability and late arthritis. Reports of implant fracture and silicone synovitis as a result of particulate debris have provided further evidence to support the use of alternative materials.[196,213] While the short- and medium-term results of metallic radial head implants are encouraging, the long-term outcome with respect to loosening, capitellar wear, and arthritis has not been reported.[11,34,49,59,76,84,85,108,119,147,166,186,189,195,222] Knight et al reported on 31 patients with comminuted fractures of the radial head treated by primary replacement with a Vitallium prosthesis at mean follow-up of 4.5 years.[119] There was reliable restoration of stability and prevention of proximal radial migration. There were no dislocations or prosthetic failures, but two implants were removed for symptomatic loosening.

Moro and coworkers reported the functional outcome of 25 patients managed with a monoblock titanium smooth stem arthroplasty of the radial head for unreconstructable fractures at an average follow-up of 3.5 years.[147] The results were rated as 7 excellent, 10 good, 5 fair, and 3 poor. The radial head prosthesis restored elbow stability when the fractured radial head occurred in combination with a dislocation of the elbow, rupture of the medial collateral ligament, fracture of the coronoid, or fracture of the proximal ulna. No patients required removal of the implant. Harrington et al reported their experience with monoblock titanium smooth stem arthroplasty of the radial head in 20 patients at an average follow-up of 12 years.[106] The results were excellent in 12, good in 4, fair in 2, and poor in 2; 4 patients had the implant removed.

Doornberg and coworkers evaluated the outcome of 27 patients treated with a modular cobalt-chrome smooth stem radial head prosthesis at an average of 3.5 years.[49] Stability was restored to all elbows and 22 patients displayed good or excellent results. Although stem lucencies were common, they did not correlate with residual elbow symptoms. Popovic and coworkers reviewed the results of 51 bipolar cemented prostheses at an average of 8 years. They reported 14 excellent, 24 good, 9 fair, and 3 poor results. They observed a high prevalence of periprosthetic osteolysis possibly due to polyethylene wear and suggested that bipolar implants should be used cautiously in young active patients. Zunkiewicz et al reported a mean Mayo elbow performance index (MEPI) of 92 at an average of 3 years following a smooth stem bipolar implant.[222] Osteolysis was not noted as an issue with this device at this early follow-up. Flinkkila et al reviewed 37 patients who had metallic press-fit prostheses at an average of 4 years.[59] Early stem loosening occurred in 12 patients and of these, 9 required removal due to pain and progressive osteolysis; the average MEPI was 86. Sarris et al reported the early results of a pyrocarbon implant, an alternative bearing surface to metal. At a mean of 27 months postoperatively they reported good clinical outcomes in 97% of patients despite two catastrophic failures at the head–neck junction and six patients with osteolysis.[180] Comparative clinical trials are needed to evaluate the outcome of the different prosthesis design concepts.

Postoperative Protocol

Following fragment excision, ORIF, excision of the radial head, or replacement arthroplasty and lateral soft tissue closure as previously described, the elbow should be placed through an arc of flexion–extension intraoperatively while carefully evaluating for elbow stability in pronation, neutral, and supination.[91] Pronation is generally beneficial if the lateral ligaments are still deficient,[52] supination is helpful if the medial ligaments are deficient,[9] and the neutral position is used if both sides have been damaged. For patients who have an associated elbow dislocation, repair of the medial collateral ligament and flexor pronator origin should be considered if the elbow subluxates at 30 degrees or more of flexion following appropriate management of the radial head, coronoid, and lateral ligament, as previously described.[60]

The elbow, with a stable osseous and ligamentous repair, should be splinted in extension and elevated for 24 to 48 h to diminish swelling, decrease tension on the posterior wound, and minimize the tendency to develop a flexion contracture. In the setting of a more tenuous ligamentous repair or the presence of some residual instability at the end of the operative procedure, the elbow should initially be splinted in 60 to 90 degrees of flexion in the optimal position of forearm rotation to maintain stability as outlined earlier.

The efficacy of indomethacin in the prevention of heterotopic ossification of the elbow remains unproven. Indomethacin 25 mg three times daily for three weeks may be considered for patients undergoing surgery on the radial head to decrease postoperative pain, reduce swelling, and potentially lower the incidence of heterotopic ossification. In patients with a concomitant dislocation, those undergoing delayed or repeat surgery and those with an associated head injury, the incidence of heterotopic ossification may be increased.[1,203] This medication should be avoided in elderly patients, those with a history of peptic ulcer disease, or those with a known allergy to the medication. Radiation should be avoided in acute injuries because it retards bone and soft tissue healing.[80]

For an isolated fracture of the radial head treated with a lateral ulnar collateral ligament-sparing approach, active range of motion should be initiated within a few days of surgery. A sling or collar and cuff with the elbow maintained at 90 degrees is employed for comfort between exercises. A static progressive extension splint is fabricated for nighttime use (Figure 19.24). This splint is adjusted weekly as extension improves and is discontinued when full extension is achieved. Strengthening commences once fracture union is secure, typically 8 weeks postoperatively.

Patients with associated fractures and ligamentous injuries should begin active range-of-motion exercises within a few days postoperatively.[201] Elbow extension is limited to a safe arc as defined by the stability of the elbow during surgery. Elbows with significant instability should begin with a rehabilitation protocol with the elbow overhead.[124] The patient is supine and the humerus is oriented 90 degrees to the bed; active motion is encouraged. Hinged braces are to be avoided. A resting splint with the elbow maintained at 90 degrees and the forearm in the appropriate rotation position is employed for 3 to 6 weeks. Active forearm rotation is performed with the elbow in flexion to minimize stress on the medial and/or lateral ligamentous injuries or repairs. A static progressive night extension splinting program is initiated as ligamentous healing progresses and stability improves, usually at 4 to 6 weeks postoperatively. Passive stretching is not permitted for 6 weeks to reduce the incidence

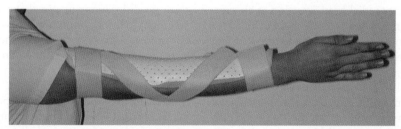

FIGURE 19.24 Static progressive extension splint. An orthosis is molded to the anterior surface of the elbow and forearm to maintain the elbow in comfortable extension. The splint is worn at night and adjusted weekly by a therapist as motion improves.

of heterotopic ossification. Strengthening exercises are initiated once the fracture and ligament injuries have adequately healed, usually at 8 weeks postoperatively.

Complications

Nerve Injury

Posterior interosseous nerve injuries are uncommon but may occur after management of fractures of the radial head. Risk factors include dissection distal to the radial tuberosity and placement of retractors anterior to the radial neck.[142,197,198,205] Prevention of these injuries can be achieved by maintaining the forearm in pronation while performing the surgical approach.[46] Placement of retractors around the radial neck should be done cautiously. Isolation and protection of the posterior interosseous nerve are recommended if dissection is required greater

than 2 cm distal to the radial head with the forearm in supination and 4 cm in pronation.[46]

Avascular Necrosis

Avascular necrosis is likely to be common after fractures of the radial head because displaced fragments typically have an absent or precarious blood supply.[72] Fortunately, it is usually asymptomatic; the fragments usually heal if stably fixed, revascularize uneventfully, and late collapse is uncommon. A temporizing approach should be taken. Avascular necrosis of the entire radial head in association with fractures of the radial neck is more problematic because this is often associated with the development of a nonunion and failure of hardware requiring radial head excision or revision to a radial head arthroplasty (Figure 19.25).

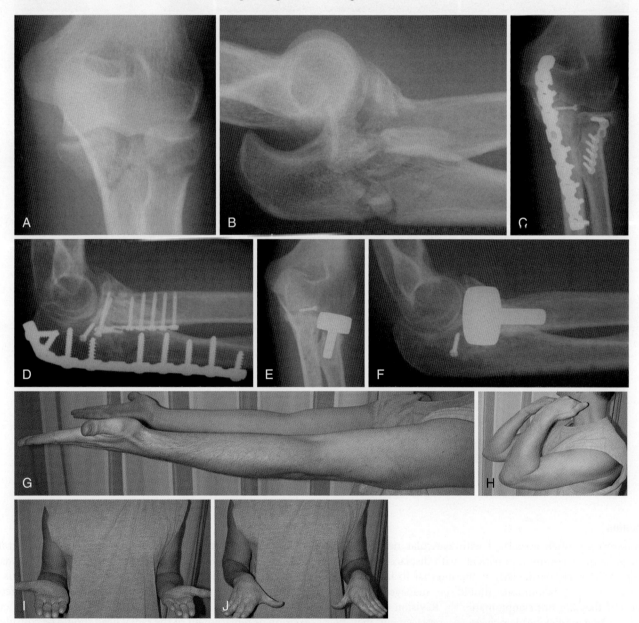

FIGURE 19.25 Avascular necrosis/nonunion of fracture of the radial neck. Anteroposterior (**A**) and lateral (**B**) radiographs demonstrating a comminuted radial head and a proximal ulnar fracture treated with ORIF of the radial head/neck and ulna. **C, D,** The patient developed a nonunion of the radial neck with associated avascular necrosis and a stiff elbow with limited forearm rotation. **E, F,** An elbow contracture release, removal of hardware, and an arthroplasty of the radial head was performed. **G-J,** An excellent range of motion was achieved postoperatively.

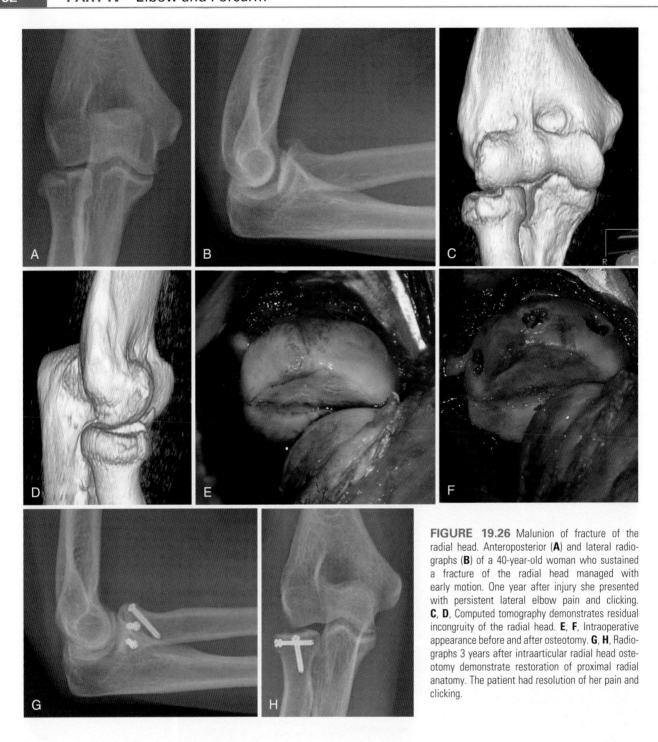

FIGURE 19.26 Malunion of fracture of the radial head. Anteroposterior (**A**) and lateral radiographs (**B**) of a 40-year-old woman who sustained a fracture of the radial head managed with early motion. One year after injury she presented with persistent lateral elbow pain and clicking. **C**, **D**, Computed tomography demonstrates residual incongruity of the radial head. **E**, **F**, Intraoperative appearance before and after osteotomy. **G**, **H**, Radiographs 3 years after intraarticular radial head osteotomy demonstrate restoration of proximal radial anatomy. The patient had resolution of her pain and clicking.

Nonunion

Nonunions are often associated with avascular necrosis and seem to be more common in patients with displaced fractures of the radial neck, particularly if the internal fixation is not secure.[38,57,115,173,174] Nonunions should be managed without surgery if they are not symptomatic.[38,173] Revision ORIF with bone grafting, radial head excision, or replacement may be employed if the nonunion is symptomatic. This author's experience with attempts to achieve union in this setting have been meager, likely owing to compromised blood supply, so revision to a radial head arthroplasty is preferred.

Malunion

Malunions are usually seen as a consequence of nonoperative treatment, unstable fracture fixation, or collapse due to avascular necrosis. Restricted motion, pain, clicking, or crepitus are typical clinical features. Extraarticular or intraarticular osteotomies (Figure 19.26) may be helpful in younger patients, whereas excision or replacement of the radial head should be considered in those who are older and of lower demand.[175] Careful preoperative planning is required if an intraarticular osteotomy is being considered. If there is significant osteoarthritis of the capitellum, excision of the radial head may be preferable.

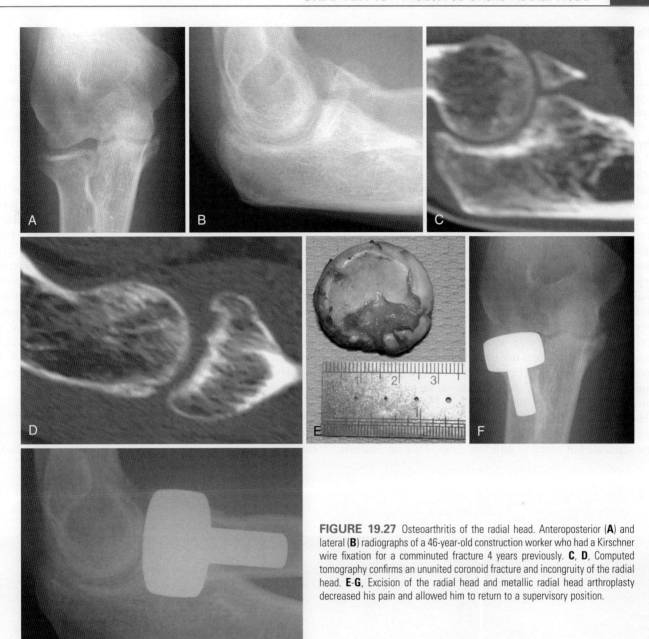

FIGURE 19.27 Osteoarthritis of the radial head. Anteroposterior (**A**) and lateral (**B**) radiographs of a 46-year-old construction worker who had a Kirschner wire fixation for a comminuted fracture 4 years previously. **C, D,** Computed tomography confirms an ununited coronoid fracture and incongruity of the radial head. **E-G,** Excision of the radial head and metallic radial head arthroplasty decreased his pain and allowed him to return to a supervisory position.

Preservation of a periosteal sleeve of the osteotomized fragment should be attempted to avoid problems with avascular necrosis and/or healing. Rigid fixation and bone grafting should be performed to promote union and early postoperative range-of-motion exercises initiated.

Osteoarthritis

Osteoarthritis is seen as a consequence of articular cartilage damage from the initial injury, articular incongruity, or persistent instability. Pain and stiffness develop as the arthritis progresses. Although typically beginning in the radiocapitellar joint, it usually progresses to involve the ulnohumeral articulation. Débridement, either open or arthroscopic, can be helpful to manage mechanical symptoms from loose bodies or osteophytes. Radial head arthroplasty can be employed in the early stages when the capitellum is not too severely arthritic (Figure 19.27).[186] Excision of the radial head, either open or arthroscopically, can be helpful if the ulnohumeral joint is not too involved and there is no residual elbow or forearm instability. In my experience, ulnohumeral arthritis tends to progress more rapidly following radial head excision, so débridement or replacement is preferred over excision. Unicompartmental radiocapitellar arthroplasty may have a role in the management of radiocapitellar arthritis when radial head replacement is contraindicated; however, the clinical outcome and durability of these new devices have not been established yet.[177] Total elbow arthroplasty may be required for more generalized posttraumatic elbow arthritis.

Stiffness and Heterotopic Bone

Stiffness is a common sequelae of fractures of the radial head and may be the result of capsular contracture, heterotopic ossification, impinging hardware, or retained cartilaginous or osseous fragments.[67,115,135,174] Loss of terminal extension is most frequent. Capsular contractures identified at 6 to 8 weeks usually respond to passive stretching under the supervision of a physical therapist.[116] Static progressive splinting using a flexion cuff and/or a resting extension splint also may be helpful in regaining terminal range. A static progressive or dynamic prosupination splint is employed for patients with loss of forearm rotation. Turnbuckle splinting initiated 12 to 16 weeks postoperatively can be useful to regain flexion or extension in patients refractory to standard therapy.[70]

Patients who fail nonoperative management and who are symptomatic due to residual stiffness can be reliably managed by open or arthroscopic capsular release, which restores a functional arc of motion in most patients.[40,132] Loss of forearm rotation tends to be less successfully treated on a delayed basis than loss of flexion–extension which can be improved even years later. I have had much better results when operating early for loss of rotation, which does not respond to therapy, typically at 6 months postoperatively (Figure 19.28).[20] This may be due to secondary contractures of the interosseous membrane or the capsule of the distal radioulnar joint.

Heterotopic bone can be excised as soon as the cortical margins are well defined and the elbow is no longer inflamed.[139] Bone scans are not useful in directing surgical timing. Patients treated with early (<6 months) excision of heterotopic bone are managed by a single dose of radiation postoperatively to prevent recurrence, typically 500 cGy. Late excision is usually managed using indomethacin, with radiation reserved for those with a contraindication or known intolerance to nonsteroidal antiinflammatory agents. Patients with residual cognitive deficits after head injuries should also be considered for radiation owing to a higher risk of recurrent heterotopic bone.[65]

Valgus Instability

Late symptomatic valgus instability is uncommon unless the radial head has been excised and not replaced. Prevention is key because late reconstruction often leads to less than satisfactory results. Medial collateral ligament reconstruction has not been reliable in restoring stability in the absence of a radial head replacement, likely owing to attenuation of the soft tissue repair. Metallic arthroplasty of the radial head may have a role to play in the resolution of these difficult clinical problems provided the capitellar cartilage is not excessively damaged and the proximal radius has not subluxated too far posteriorly such that the radial neck cannot be realigned with the capitellum. Valgus instability can be managed with metallic replacement of the radial head and reconstruction of the medial collateral ligament at the same time.[42]

Axial Instability

Morrey and Coleman and their colleagues reported that proximal radial migration averaged 2 mm in patients who had a

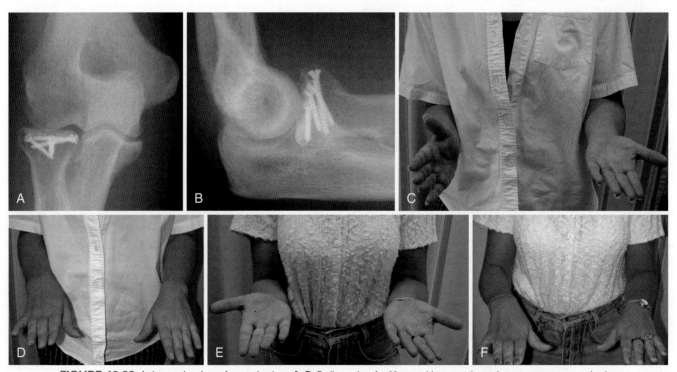

FIGURE 19.28 Arthroscopic release for rotation loss. **A, B,** Radiographs of a 36-year-old woman 4 months status-post open reduction and internal fixation of a displaced fracture of the radial head. **C, D,** Clinical appearance with loss of rotation that had persisted in spite of physiotherapy and splinting. **E, F,** At 6 weeks after arthroscopic release of arthrofibrosis there was a marked improvement in forearm supination.

radial head resection, and most were asymptomatic.[41,152] The incidence and magnitude and symptoms of proximal migration vary considerably between studies.[140,202] Lewis and Thibodeau reported this phenomenon in 7 of 8 patients who had a radial head excision; 2 of their patients were symptomatic.[126] Some patients have greater migration and may develop impingement of the proximal radial stump on the capitellum or the distal ulna on the carpus. True Essex-Lopresti injuries are uncommon[23,53,55,83,114,125]; however, they often go unrecognized[56,206] and present as a late problem.[28,30,140,193] If detected early, preservation of the radial head with ORIF or metallic radial head arthroplasty is indicated.[183] Late reconstruction of axial forearm instability remains a difficult surgical problem without a definitive solution.[30,94,169,184,193] Whereas a one bone forearm can solve the instability problem, nonunions and other complications are common.[162]

Salvage using allografts of the radial head has been reported; however, increasing experience and longer follow-up suggests a higher incidence of complications (e.g., nonunion, collapse, and resorption) such that they can no longer be recommended.[110,200] Reconstruction of the interosseous membrane combined with a metallic arthroplasty of the radial head has been proposed in biomechanical studies; however, no clinical outcome studies are available.[94,122,133,183,188,215] Ulnar shortening alone is ineffective because the correction in ulnar variance is commonly not maintained.[193] This author's preference is to reconstruct late axial instability in a staged manner using a metallic implant of the radial head. Prerequisites are a proximal radial stump that can be reduced to the capitellum and the absence of significant capitellar arthritis. The metallic arthroplasty of the radial head is performed first, avoiding overlengthening of the radius. Six months later, an ulnar shortening osteotomy is performed to restore the normal relationship of the distal radial ulnar joint. This staged reconstruction seems to allow the cartilage and bone of the capitellum to respond to reloading in a more graduated manner and avoids capitellar erosion and pain that has been seen when completing a single-stage reconstruction (Figure 19.29).[87]

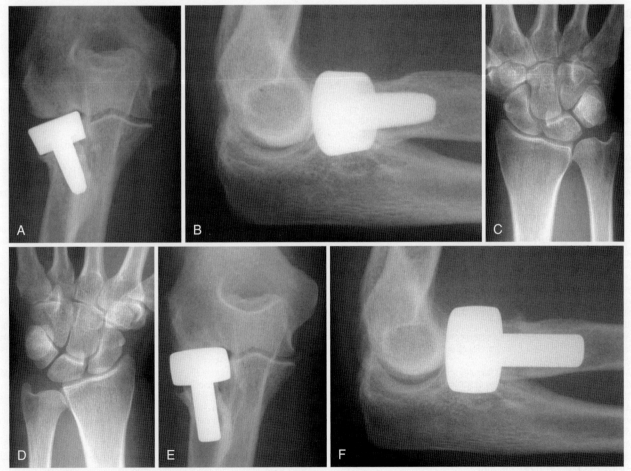

FIGURE 19.29 Essex-Lopresti prosthetic reconstruction. Anteroposterior (**A**) and lateral (**B**) radiographs of the right elbow and bilateral posteroanterior wrist radiographs (**C**, **D**) of a 47-year-old woman who had previously had two Silastic and one metallic arthroplasty for a missed Essex-Lopresti injury initially managed with excision of the radial head. She had persistent pain in both her elbow and wrist. **E**, **F**, Following revision of the malarticulated arthroplasty of the radial head to a modular design (Evolve, Wright Medical Technology, Arlington, TN).

Continued

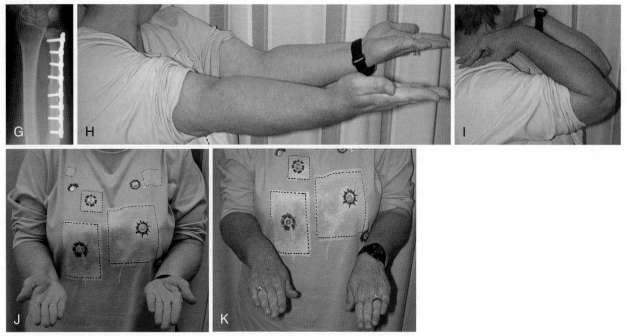

FIGURE 19.29, cont'd **G**, An ulnar shortening osteotomy was done 6 months later. **H-K**, Her wrist and elbow pain has resolved.

For Case Studies, Videos, and more, please visit ExpertConsult.com.

REFERENCES

1. Adler JB, Shaftan GW: Radial head fractures, is excision necessary? *J Trauma* 4:115–136, 1962.
2. Akesson T, Herbertsson P, Josefsson PO, et al: Primary nonoperative treatment of moderately displaced two-part fractures of the radial head. *J Bone Joint Surg Am* 88(9):1909–1914, 2006.
3. Alolabi B, Studer A, Gray A, et al: Selecting the diameter of a radial head implant: an assessment of local landmarks. *J Shoulder Elbow Surg* 22(10):1395–1399, 2013.
4. Amis AA, Miller JH, Dowson D, et al: Biomechanical aspects of the elbow: joint forces related to prosthesis design. *Eng Med* 10(2):65–68, 1981.
5. Amis AA, Dowson D, Wright V: Elbow joint force predictions for some strenuous isometric actions. *J Biomech* 13(9):765–775, 1980.
6. Amis AA, Miller JH: The mechanisms of elbow fractures: an investigation using impact tests in vitro. *Injury* 26(3):163–168, 1995.
7. Antuna SA, Sanchez-Marquez JM, Barco R: Long-term results of radial head resection following isolated radial head fractures in patients younger than forty years old. *J Bone Joint Surg Am* 92(3):558–566, 2010.
8. Arce AA, Garin DM, Garcia MV, et al: Treatment of radial head fractures using a fibrin adhesive seal. A review of 15 cases. *J Bone Joint Surg Br* 77(3):422–424, 1995.
9. Armstrong AD, Dunning CE, Faber KJ, et al: Rehabilitation of the medial collateral ligament-deficient elbow: an in vitro biomechanical study. *J Hand Surg [Am]* 25(6):1051–1057, 2000.
10. Arner O, Ekengren K, Von Schreeb T: Fractures of the head and neck of the radius: a clinical and roentgenographic stduy of 310 cases. *Acta Chir Scand* 112:115, 1957.
11. Ashwood N, Bain GI, Unni R: Management of Mason type-III radial head fractures with a titanium prosthesis, ligament repair, and early mobilization. *J Bone Joint Surg Am* 86A(2):274–280, 2004.
12. Athwal GS, Frank SG, Grewal R, et al: Determination of correct implant size in radial head arthroplasty to avoid overlengthening: surgical technique. *J Bone Joint Surg Am* 92(Suppl 1 Pt 2):250–257, 2010.
13. Athwal GS, Rouleau DM, MacDermid JC, et al: Contralateral elbow radiographs can reliably diagnose radial head implant overlengthening. *J Bone Joint Surg Am* 93(14):1339–1346, 2011.
14. Bartz B, Tillmann B, Schleicher A: Stress in the human elbow joint. II. Proximal radio-ulnar joint. *Anat Embryol (Berl)* 169(3):309–318, 1984.
15. Beingessner DM, Bennett JD, King GJ: Intraarticular radial head osteotomy. *J Shoulder Elbow Surg* 8(2):172–174, 1999.
16. Beingessner DM, Dunning CE, Beingessner CJ, et al: The effect of radial head fracture size on radiocapitellar joint stability. *Clin Biomech (Bristol, Avon)* 18(7):677–681, 2003.
17. Beingessner DM, Dunning CE, Gordon KD, et al: The effect of radial head excision and arthroplasty on elbow kinematics and stability. *J Bone Joint Surg Am* 86A(8):1730–1739, 2004.
18. Beingessner DM, Dunning CE, Beingessner CJ, et al: The effect of radial head fracture size on radiocapitellar joint stability. *Clin Biomech (Bristol, Avon)* 18(7):677–681, 2003.
19. Beingessner DM, Dunning CE, Gordon KD, et al: The effect of radial head fracture size on elbow kinematics and stability. *J Orthop Res* 23(1):210–217, 2005.
20. Beingessner DM, Patterson SD, King GJ: Early excision of heterotopic bone in the forearm. *J Hand Surg [Am]* 25(3):483–488, 2000.
21. Beredjiklian PK, Nalbantoglu U, Potter HG, et al: Prosthetic radial head components and proximal radial morphology: a mismatch. *J Shoulder Elbow Surg* 8(5):471–475, 1999.
22. Berger M, Urvoy P, Mestdagh H: [Comparative study of the treatment of fractures of the head of the radius by resection or by Swanson's silastic implant]. *Ann Chir* 45(5):418–425, 1991 [in French].
23. Bock GW, Cohen MS, Resnick D: Fracture-dislocation of the elbow with inferior radioulnar dislocation: a variant of the Essex-Lopresti injury. *Skeletal Radiol* 21(5):315–317, 1992.
24. Bohrer JV: Fractures of the head and neck of the radius. *Ann Surg* 97:204–208, 1933.
25. Boulas HJ, Morrey BF: Biomechanical evaluation of the elbow following radial head fracture. Comparison of open reduction and internal fixation vs. excision, silastic replacement, and non-operative management. *Chir Main* 17(4):314–320, 1998.
26. Broberg MA, Morrey BF: Results of delayed excision of the radial head after fracture. *J Bone Joint Surg Am* 68(5):669–674, 1986.
27. Broberg MA, Morrey BF: Results of treatment of fracture-dislocations of the elbow. *Clin Orthop* (216):109–119, 1987.
28. Brockman EP: Two cases of disability at the wrist joint following excision of the head of the radius. *Proc R Soc Med* 24:904, 1930.
29. Burton AE: Fractures of the head of the radius. *Proc R Soc Med* 35:764–765, 1942.
30. Capuano L, Craig N, Ashcroft GP, et al: Distraction lengthening of the radius for radial longitudinal instability after distal radio-ulnar subluxation and excision of the radial head: a case report. *Scand J Plast Reconstr Surg Hand Surg* 35(3):331–335, 2001.
31. Caputo AE, Burton KJ, Cohen MS, et al: Articular cartilage injuries of the capitellum interposed in radial head fractures: a report of ten cases. *J Shoulder Elbow Surg* 15(6):716–720, 2006.

32. Caputo AE, Mazzocca AD, Santoro VM: The nonarticulating portion of the radial head: anatomic and clinical correlations for internal fixation. *J Hand Surg [Am]* 23(6):1082–1090, 1998.

33. Carn RM, Medige J, Curtain D, et al: Silicone rubber replacement of the severely fractured radial head. *Clin Orthop* (209):259–269, 1986.

34. Carr CR, Howard JW: Metallic cap replacement of radial head following fracture. *West J Surg* 59:539–546, 1951.

35. Carstam N: Operative treatment of fractures of the upper end of the radius. *Acta Orthop Scand* 59:502–523, 1950.

36. Castberg T, Thing E: Treatment of fractures of the upper end of the radius. *Acta Chir Scand* 1051:62–69, 1953.

37. Cherry JC: Use of acrylic prothesis in the treatment of fracture of the head of the radius. *J Bone Joint Surg Br* 35B:70–71, 1953.

38. Cobb TK, Beckenbaugh RD: Nonunion of the radial neck following fracture of the radial head and neck: case reports and a review of the literature. *Orthopedics* 21(3):364–368, 1998.

39. Cohen MS, Hastings H: Rotatory instability of the elbow. The anatomy and role of the lateral stabilizers. *J Bone Joint Surg Am* 79(2):225–233, 1997.

40. Cohen MS, Hastings H: Operative release for elbow contracture: the lateral collateral ligament sparing technique. *Orthop Clin North Am* 30(1):133–139, 1999.

41. Coleman DA, Blair WF, Shurr D: Resection of the radial head for fracture of the radial head. Long-term follow-up of seventeen cases. *J Bone Joint Surg Am* 69(3):385–392, 1987.

42. Conway JE, Jobe FW, Glousman RE, et al: Medial instability of the elbow in throwing athletes. Treatment by repair or reconstruction of the ulnar collateral ligament. *J Bone Joint Surg Am* 74(1):67–83, 1992.

43. Cutler CW: Fractures of the head and neck of the radius. *Ann Surg* 8:267–278, 1926.

44. Davidson PA, Moseley JB, Jr, Tullos HS: Radial head fracture. A potentially complex injury. *Clin Orthop* (297):224–230, 1993.

45. Desloges W, Louati H, Papp SR, et al: Objective analysis of lateral elbow exposure with the extensor digitorum communis split compared with the Kocher interval. *J Bone Joint Surg Am* 96(5):387–393, 2014.

46. Diliberti T, Botte MJ, Abrams RA: Anatomical considerations regarding the posterior interosseous nerve during posterolateral approaches to the proximal part of the radius. *J Bone Joint Surg Am* 82(6):809–813, 2000.

47. Dooley JF, Angus PD: The importance of elbow aspiration when treating radial head fractures. *Arch Emerg Med* 8(2):117–121, 1991.

48. Doornberg JN, Linzel DS, Zurakowski D, et al: Reference points for radial head prosthesis size. *J Hand Surg [Am]* 31(1):53–57, 2006.

49. Doornberg JN, Parisien R, van Duijn PJ, et al: Radial head arthroplasty with a modular metal spacer to treat acute traumatic elbow instability. *J Bone Joint Surg Am* 89(5):1075–1080, 2007.

50. Dowdy PA, Bain GI, King GJ, et al: The midline posterior elbow incision. An anatomical appraisal. *J Bone Joint Surg Br* 77(5):696–699, 1995.

51. Dunning CE, Zarzour ZD, Patterson SD, et al: Ligamentous stabilizers against posterolateral rotatory instability of the elbow. *J Bone Joint Surg Am* 83-A(12):1823–1828, 2001.

52. Dunning CE, Zarzour ZD, Patterson SD, et al: Muscle forces and pronation stabilize the lateral ligament deficient elbow. *Clin Orthop* 388:118–124, 2001.

53. Edwards GS, Jr, Jupiter JB: Radial head fractures with acute distal radioulnar dislocation. Essex-Lopresti revisited. *Clin Orthop* 234:61–69, 1988.

54. Esser RD, Davis S, Taavao T: Fractures of the radial head treated by internal fixation: late results in 26 cases. *J Orthop Trauma* 9(4):318–323, 1995.

55. Essex-Lopresti P: Fractures of the radial head with distal radio-ulnar dislocation. *J Bone Joint Surg Br* 33B:244–247, 1951.

56. Failla JM, Jacobson J, van Holsbeeck M: Ultrasound diagnosis and surgical pathology of the torn interosseous membrane in forearm fractures/dislocations. *J Hand Surg [Am]* 24(2):257–266, 1999.

57. Faraj AA, Lively P, Branfoot T: Nonunion of fracture of the neck of the radius: a report of three cases. *J Orthop Trauma* 13(7):513–515, 1999.

58. Fischer LP, Gonon GP, Carret JP, et al: [Possibility of screwing in various simple fractures of the radial head (with anatomo-physiologic considerations of the radiocubital joint)]. *Rev Chir Orthop Reparatrice Appar Mot* 62(2 Suppl):89–96, 1976.

59. Flinkkila T, Kaisto T, Sirnio K, et al: Short- to mid-term results of metallic press-fit radial head arthroplasty in unstable injuries of the elbow. *J Bone Joint Surg Br* 94(6):805–810, 2012.

60. Forthman C, Henket M, Ring DC: Elbow dislocation with intra-articular fracture: the results of operative treatment without repair of the medial collateral ligament. *J Hand Surg [Am]* 32(8):1200–1209, 2007.

61. Frankle MA, Koval KJ, Sanders RW, et al: Radial head fractures associated with elbow dislocations treated by immediate stabilization and early motion. *J Shoulder Elbow Surg* 8(4):355–360, 1999.

62. Fraser GS, Pichora JE, Ferreira LM, et al: Lateral collateral ligament repair restores the initial varus stability of the elbow: an in vitro biomechanical study. *J Orthop Trauma* 22(9):615–623, 2008.

63. Fuchs S, Chylarecki C: Do functional deficits result from radial head resection? *J Shoulder Elbow Surg* 8(3):247–251, 1999.

64. Furry KL, Clinkscales CM: Comminuted fractures of the radial head. Arthroplasty versus internal fixation. *Clin Orthop* (353):40–52, 1998.

65. Garland DE, Hanscom DA, Keenan MA, et al: Resection of heterotopic ossification in the adult with head trauma. *J Bone Joint Surg Am* 67(8):1261–1269, 1985.

66. Garland DE, O'Hollaren RM: Fractures and dislocations about the elbow in the head-injured adult. *Clin Orthop* 49(168):38–41, 1982.

67. Gaston SR, Smith FM, Baab OD: Adult injuries of the radial head and neck: importance of time element in treatment. *Am J Surg* 78:631–635, 1949.

68. Geel CW, Palmer AK: Radial head fractures and their effect on the distal radioulnar joint. A rationale for treatment. *Clin Orthop* (275):79–84, 1992.

69. Geel CW, Palmer AK, Ruedi T, et al: Internal fixation of proximal radial head fractures. *J Orthop Trauma* 4(3):270–274, 1990.

70. Gelinas JJ, Faber KJ, Patterson SD, et al: The effectiveness of turnbuckle splinting for elbow contractures. *J Bone Joint Surg Br* 82(1):74–78, 2000.

71. Giffin JR, King GJ, Patterson SD, et al: Internal fixation of radial neck fractures: an in vitro biomechanical analysis. *Clin Biomech (Bristol, Avon)* 19(4):358–361, 2004.

72. Girard JY, Rogez JM, Robert R, et al: Vascularisation of the head of the radius in the adult. *Surg Radiol Anat* 17(1):41–45, 1995.

73. Goldberg I, Peylan J, Yosipovitch Z: Late results of excision of the radial head for an isolated closed fracture. *J Bone Joint Surg Am* 68(5):675–679, 1986.

74. Gordon KD, Duck TR, King GJ, et al: Mechanical properties of subchondral cancellous bone of the radial head. *J Orthop Trauma* 17(4):285–289, 2003.

75. Greenspan A, Norman A, Rosen H: Radial head-capitellum view in elbow trauma: clinical application and radiographic-anatomic correlation. *AJR Am J Roentgenol* 143(2):355–359, 1984.

76. Grewal R, MacDermid JC, Faber KJ, et al: Comminuted radial head fractures treated with a modular metallic radial head arthroplasty. Study of outcomes. *J Bone Joint Surg Am* 88(10):2192–2200, 2006.

77. Grossman J: Fracture of the head and neck of the radius. *New York Medical Journal* 117:472–475, 1923.

78. Gupta GG, Lucas G, Hahn DL: Biomechanical and computer analysis of radial head prostheses. *J Shoulder Elbow Surg* 6(1):37–48, 1997.

79. Halls AA, Travill A: Transmission of pressures across the elbow joint. *Anat Rec* 150:243–248, 1964.

80. Hamid N, Ashraf N, Bosse MJ, et al: Radiation therapy for heterotopic ossification prophylaxis acutely after elbow trauma: a prospective randomized study. *J Bone Joint Surg Am* 92(11):2032–2038, 2010.

81. Hammacher ER, van der Werken C: Radial head fractures: operative or conservative treatment? The Greek temple model. *Acta Orthop Belg* 62(Suppl 1):112–115, 1996.

82. Hammond R: Fracture of the head and neck of the radius. *Ann Surg* 53:207–214, 1910.

83. Hargadon EJ, Porter ML: The Essex-Lopresti injury: a variation. *J Hand Surg [Br]* 13(4):450–452, 1988.

84. Harrington IJ, Sekyi-Otu A, Barrington TW, et al: The functional outcome with metallic radial head implants in the treatment of unstable elbow fractures: a long-term review. *J Trauma* 50(1):46–52, 2001.

85. Harrington IJ, Tountas AA: Replacement of the radial head in the treatment of unstable elbow fractures. *Injury* 12(5):405–412, 1981.

86. Haverstock JP, Katchky RN, Lalone EA, et al: Regional variations in radial head bone volume and density: implications for fracture patterns and fixation. *J Shoulder Elbow Surg* 21(12):1669–1673, 2012.

87. Heijink A, Morrey BF, van Riet RP, et al: Delayed treatment of elbow pain and dysfunction following Essex-Lopresti injury with metallic radial head replacement: a case series. *J Shoulder Elbow Surg* 19(6):929–936, 2010.

88. Heim U: [Surgical treatment of radial head fracture]. *Z Unfallchir Versicherungsmed* 85(1):3–11, 1992.

89. Heim U, Trub HJ: [Experiences with primary osteosynthesis in radial head fractures]. *Helv Chir Acta* 45(1–2):63–69, 1978.

90. Hergenroeder PT, Gelberman R: Distal radioulnar joint subluxation secondary to excision of the radial head. *Orthopedics* 3:649–650, 1980.

91. Hildebrand KA, Patterson SD, King GJ: Acute elbow dislocations: simple and complex. *Orthop Clin North Am* 30(1):63–79, 1999.

92. Holdsworth BJ, Clement DA, Rothwell PN: Fractures of the radial head—the benefit of aspiration: a prospective controlled trial. *Injury* 18(1):44–47, 1987.

93. Hotchkiss RN: Displaced fractures of the radial head: internal fixation or excision? *J Am Acad Orthop Surg* 5(1):1–10, 1997.

94. Hotchkiss RN, An KN, Sowa DT, et al: An anatomic and mechanical study of the interosseous membrane of the forearm: pathomechanics of proximal migration of the radius. *J Hand Surg [Am]* 14(2 Pt 1):256–261, 1989.

95. Hotchkiss R, Weiland A: Valgus stability of the elbow. *J Orthop Res* 5(3):372–377, 1987.

96. Ikeda M, Sugiyama K, Kang C, et al: Comminuted fractures of the radial head. Comparison of resection and internal fixation. *J Bone Joint Surg Am* 87A:76–84, 2005.

97. Ikeda M, Oka Y: Function after early radial head resection for fracture: a retrospective evaluation of 15 patients followed for 3-18 years. *Acta Orthop Scand* 71(2):191–194, 2000.

98. Ikeda M, Yamashina Y, Kamimoto M, et al: Open reduction and internal fixation of comminuted fractures of the radial head using low-profile mini-plates. *J Bone Joint Surg Br* 85(7):1040–1044, 2003.

99. Itamura J, Roidis N, Mirzayan R, et al: Radial head fractures: MRI evaluation of associated injuries. *J Shoulder Elbow Surg* 14(4):421–424, 2005.

100. Janssen RP, Vegter J: Resection of the radial head after Mason type-III fractures of the elbow: follow-up at 16 to 30 years. *J Bone Joint Surg Br* 80(2):231–233, 1998.

101. Jensen SL, Olsen BS, Sojbjerg JO: Elbow joint kinematics after excision of the radial head. *J Shoulder Elbow Surg* 8(3):238–241, 1999.

102. Johansson O: Capsular and ligament injuries of the elbow joint. A clinical and arthrographic study. *Acta Chir Scand* 287(Suppl):5–71, 1962.

103. Johnson JA, Beingessner DM, Gordon KD, et al: Kinematics and stability of the fractured and implant reconstructed radial head. *J Shoulder Elbow Surg* 14(Suppl 1):195S–201S, 2005.

104. Johnston GW: A follow-up of one hundred cases of fracture of the head of the radius with a review of the literature. *Ulster Med J* 31:51–56, 1962.

105. Jones SG: Fractures of the head and neck of the radius—separation of upper radial epiphysis. *N Engl J Med* 212:914–917, 1935.

106. Josefsson PO, Gentz CF, Johnell O, et al: Dislocations of the elbow and intraarticular fractures. *Clin Orthop* (246):126–130, 1989.

107. Judet T: Results of acute excision of the radial head in elbow radial head fracture-dislocations. *J Orthop Trauma* 15(4):308–309, 2001.

108. Judet T, Garreau DL, Piriou P, et al: A floating prosthesis for radial-head fractures. *J Bone Joint Surg Br* 78(2):244–249, 1996.

109. Kaas L, van Riet RP, Vroemen JP, et al: The incidence of associated fractures of the upper limb in fractures of the radial head. *Strategies Trauma Limb Reconstr* 3(2):71–74, 2008.

110. Karlstad R, Morrey BF, Cooney WP: Failure of fresh-frozen radial head allografts in the treatment of Essex-Lopresti injury. A report of four cases. *J Bone Joint Surg Am* 87(8):1828–1833, 2005.

111. Keller HW, Rehm KE, Helling J: Intramedullary reduction and stabilisation of adult radial neck fractures. *J Bone Joint Surg Br* 76(3):406–408, 1994.

112. Key J: Treatment of fractures of the head and neck of the radius. *JAMA* 96:101–104, 1930.

113. Khalfayan EE, Culp RW, Alexander AH: Mason type II radial head fractures: operative versus nonoperative treatment. *J Orthop Trauma* 6(3):283–289, 1992.

114. King B: Resection of the radial head and neck: An end-result study of thirteen cases. *J Bone Joint Surg Br* 21:839–857, 1939.

115. King GJ, Evans DC, Kellam JF: Open reduction and internal fixation of radial head fractures. *J Orthop Trauma* 5(1):21–28, 1991.

116. King GJ, Faber KJ: Posttraumatic elbow stiffness. *Orthop Clin North Am* 31(1):129–143, 2000.

117. King GJ, Zarzour ZD, Patterson SD, et al: An anthropometric study of the radial head: implications in the design of a prosthesis. *J Arthroplasty* 16(1):112–116, 2001.

118. King GJ, Zarzour ZD, Rath DA, et al: Metallic radial head arthroplasty improves valgus stability of the elbow. *Clin Orthop* (368):114–125, 1999.

119. Knight DJ, Rymaszewski LA, Amis AA, et al: Primary replacement of the fractured radial head with a metal prosthesis. *J Bone Joint Surg Br* 75(4):572–576, 1993.

120. Kocher T: *Textbook of operative surgery*, ed 3, London, 1911, Adam and Charles Black.

121. Koslowsky TC, Schliwa S, Koebke J: Presentation of the microscopic vascular architecture of the radial head using a sequential plastination technique. *Clin Anat* 24(6):721–732, 2011.

122. Lanting BA, Ferreira LM, Johnson JA, et al: The effect of excision of the radial head and metallic radial head replacement on the tension in the interosseous membrane. *Bone Joint J* 95B(10):1383–1387, 2013.

123. Leclerc AE, Deluce S, Ferreira L, et al: Measurements of the ispilateral capitellum can reliably predict the diameter of the radial head. *J Shoulder Elbow Surg* 22(12):1724–1728, 2013.

124. Lee AT, Schrumpf MA, Choi D, et al: The influence of gravity on the unstable elbow. *J Shoulder Elbow Surg* 22(1):81–87, 2013.

125. Levin PD: Fracture of the radial head with dislocation of the distal radio-ulnar joint: case report. Treatment by prosthetic replacement of the radial head. *J Bone Joint Surg Am* 55(4):837–840, 1973.

126. Lewis RW, Thibodeau AA: Deformity of the wrist following resection of the radial head. *Surg Gynecol Obstet* 64:1079–1085, 1937.

127. Liew VS, Cooper IC, Ferreira LM, et al: The effect of metallic radial head arthroplasty on radiocapitellar joint contact area. *Clin Biomech (Bristol, Avon)* 18(2):115–118, 2003.

128. Lindenhovius AL, Felsch Q, Doornberg JN, et al: Open reduction and internal fixation compared with excision for unstable displaced fractures of the radial head. *J Hand Surg [Am]* 32(5):630–636, 2007.

129. Liow RY, Cregan A, Nanda R, et al: Early mobilisation for minimally displaced radial head fractures is desirable. A prospective randomised study of two protocols. *Injury* 33(9):801–806, 2002.

130. Lo IK, King GJ: Arthroscopic radial head excision. *Arthroscopy* 10(6):689–692, 1994.

131. Mackay I, FitzGerald B, Miller JH: Silastic replacement of the head of the radius in trauma. *J Bone Joint Surg Br* 61B(4):494–497, 1979.

132. Mansat P, Morrey BF: The column procedure: a limited lateral approach for extrinsic contracture of the elbow. *J Bone Joint Surg Am* 80(11):1603–1615, 1998.

133. Marcotte AL, Osterman AL: Longitudinal radioulnar dissociation: identification and treatment of acute and chronic injuries. *Hand Clin* 23(2):195–208, vi, 2007.

134. Markolf KL, Lamey D, Yang S, et al: Radioulnar load-sharing in the forearm. A study in cadavera. *J Bone Joint Surg Am* 80(6):879–888, 1998.

135. Mason ML: Some observations on fracture of the head of the radius with a review of one hundred cases. *Br J Surg* 42:123–132, 1954.

136. Mason JA, Shutkin NM: Immediate active motion in the treatment of fractures of the head and neck of the radius. *Surg Gynecol Obstet* 76:731–737, 1943.

137. Mathur N, Sharma CS: Fracture of the head of the radius treated by elbow cast. *Acta Orthop Scand* 55(5):567–568, 1984.

138. McArthur RA: Herbert screw fixation of fracture of the head of the radius. *Clin Orthop* (224):79–87, 1987.

139. McAuliffe JA, Wolfson AH: Early excision of heterotopic ossification about the elbow followed by radiation therapy [see comments]. *J Bone Joint Surg Am* 79(5):749–755, 1997.

140. McDougall A, White J: Subluxation of the inferior radio-ulnar joint complicating fracture of the radial head. *J Bone Joint Surg Br* 39B:278–287, 1957.

141. McKee MD, Schemitsch EH, Sala MJ, et al: The pathoanatomy of lateral ligamentous disruption in complex elbow instability. *J Shoulder Elbow Surg* 12(4):391–396, 2003.

142. Mekhail AO, Ebraheim NA, Jackson WT, et al: Vulnerability of the posterior interosseous nerve during proximal radius exposures. *Clin Orthop* (315):199–208, 1995 Jun.

143. Menth-Chiari WA, Ruch DS, Poehling GG: Arthroscopic excision of the radial head: Clinical outcome in 12 patients with post-traumatic arthritis after fracture of the radial head or rheumatoid arthritis. *Arthroscopy* 17(9):918–923, 2001.

144. Mikic ZD, Vukadinovic SM: Late results in fractures of the radial head treated by excision. *Clin Orthop* (181):220–228, 1983.

145. Miller GK, Drennan DB, Maylahn DJ: Treatment of displaced segmental radial-head fractures. Long-term follow-up. *J Bone Joint Surg Am* 63(5):712–717, 1981.

146. Morgan SJ, Groshen SL, Itamura JM, et al: Reliability evaluation of classifying radial head fractures by the system of Mason. *Bull Hosp Jt Dis* 56(2):95–98, 1997.

147. Moro JK, Werier J, MacDermid JC, et al: Arthroplasty with a metal radial head for unreconstructible fractures of the radial head. *J Bone Joint Surg Am* 83A(8):1201–1211, 2001.

148. Morrey BF: Radial head fracture. In Morrey BF, editor: *The elbow and its disorders*, ed 3, Philadelphia, 2000, W.B. Saunders, pp 341–364.

149. Morrey BF, An KN: Articular and ligamentous contributions to the stability of the elbow joint. *Am J Sports Med* 11(5):315–319, 1983.

150. Morrey BF, An KN, Stormont TJ: Force transmission through the radial head. *J Bone Joint Surg Am* 70(2):250–256, 1988.

151. Morrey BF, Askew L, Chao EY: Silastic prosthetic replacement for the radial head. *J Bone Joint Surg Am* 63(3):454–458, 1981.

152. Morrey BF, Chao EY, Hui FC: Biomechanical study of the elbow following excision of the radial head. *J Bone Joint Surg Am* 61(1):63–68, 1979.

153. Morrey BF, Tanaka S, An KN: Valgus stability of the elbow. A definition of primary and secondary constraints. *Clin Orthop* (265):187–195, 1991.

154. Murray RC: Fractures of the head and neck of the radius. *Br J Surg* 27:106–118, 1940.

155. O'Driscoll SW, Bell DF, Morrey BF: Posterolateral rotatory instability of the elbow. *J Bone Joint Surg Am* 73(3):440–446, 1991.

156. O'Driscoll SW, Morrey BF, Korinek S, et al: Elbow subluxation and dislocation. A spectrum of instability. *Clin Orthop* 74(280):186–197, 1992.

157. Odelberg-Johnsson G: On fractures of the proximal portion of the radius and their causes. *Acta Radiol* 3:45–53, 1924.

158. Odenheimer K, Harvey JP, Jr: Internal fixation of fracture of the head of the radius. Two case reports. *J Bone Joint Surg Am* 61(5):785–787, 1979.

159. Patterson SD, Bain GI, Mehta JA: Surgical approaches to the elbow. *Clin Orthop* 370:19–33, 2000.

160. Patterson JD, Jones CK, Glisson RR, et al: Stiffness of simulated radial neck fractures fixed with 4 different devices. *J Shoulder Elbow Surg* 10(1):57–61, 2001.

161. Pelto K, Hirvensalo E, Bostman O, et al: Treatment of radial head fractures with absorbable polyglycolide pins: a study on the security of the fixation in 38 cases. *J Orthop Trauma* 8(2):94–98, 1994.

162. Peterson CA, Maki S, Wood MB: Clinical results of the one-bone forearm. *J Hand Surg [Am]* 20(4):609–618, 1995.

163. Pike JM, Athwal GS, Faber KJ, et al: Radial head fractures—an update. *J Hand Surg [Am]* 34(3):557–565, 2009.

164. Pike JM, Grewal R, Athwal GS, et al: Open reduction and internal fixation of radial head fractures: do outcomes differ between simple and complex injuries? *Clin Orthop Relat Res* 471(7):2120–2127, 2014.

165. Pomianowski S, Morrey BF, Neale PG, et al: Contribution of monoblock and bipolar radial head prostheses to valgus stability of the elbow. *J Bone Joint Surg Am* 83A(12):1829–1834, 2001.

166. Popovic N, Lemaire R, Georis P, et al: Midterm results with a bipolar radial head prosthesis: radiographic evidence of loosening at the bone-cement interface. *J Bone Joint Surg Am* 89(11):2469–2476, 2007.

167. Pribyl CR, Kester MA, Cook SD, et al: The effect of the radial head excision and prosthetic radial head replacement on resisting valgus stress at the elbow. *Orthopedics* 9(5):723–726, 1986.

168. Quigley TB: Aspiration of the elbow joint in the treatment of fractures of the head of the radius. *N Engl J Med* 240:915–916, 1949.

169. Rabinowitz RS, Light TR, Havey RM, et al: The role of the interosseous membrane and triangular fibrocartilage complex in forearm stability. *J Hand Surg [Am]* 19A:385–393, 1994.

170. Radin EL, Riseborough EJ: Fractures of the radial head. A review of eighty-eight cases and analysis of the indications for excision of the radial head and non-operative treatment. *J Bone Joint Surg Am* 48(6):1055–1064, 1966.

171. Regan W, Morrey B: Fractures of the coronoid process of the ulna. *J Bone Joint Surg Am* 71(9):1348–1354, 1989.

172. Ring D, Jupiter JB, Zilberfarb J: Posterior dislocation of the elbow with fractures of the radial head and coronoid. *J Bone Joint Surg Am* 84-A(4):547–551, 2002.

173. Ring D, Psychoyios VN, Chin KR, et al: Nonunion of nonoperatively treated fractures of the radial head. *Clin Orthop* 398:235–238, 2002.

174. Ring D, Quintero J, Jupiter JB: Open reduction and internal fixation of fractures of the radial head. *J Bone Joint Surg Am* 84A(10):1811–1815, 2002.

175. Rosenblatt Y, Young C, MacDermid JC, et al: Osteotomy of the head of the radius for partial articular malunion. *J Bone Joint Surg Br* 91(10):1341–1346, 2009.

176. Rowland AS, Athwal GS, MacDermid JC, et al: Lateral ulnohumeral joint space widening is not diagnostic of radial head arthroplasty overstuffing. *J Hand Surg [Am]* 32(5):637–641, 2007.

177. Sabo MT, Shannon HL, Deluce S, et al: Capitellar excision and hemiarthroplasty affects elbow kinematics and stability. *J Shoulder Elbow Surg* 21(8):1024–1031, 2012.

178. Sanchez-Sotelo J, Romanillos O, Garay EG: Results of acute excision of the radial head in elbow radial head fracture-dislocations. *J Orthop Trauma* 14(5):354–358, 2000.

179. Sanders RA, French HG: Open reduction and internal fixation of comminuted radial head fractures. *Am J Sports Med* 14(2):130–135, 1986.

180. Sarris IK, Kyrkos MJ, Galanis NN, et al: Radial head replacement with the MoPyC pyrocarbon prosthesis. *J Shoulder Elbow Surg* 21(9):1222–1228, 2012.

181. Schwab GH, Bennett JB, Woods GW, et al: Biomechanics of elbow instability. The role of the medial collateral ligament. *Clin Orthop* 146:42–52, 1980.

182. Schwartz RP, Young F: Treatment of fractures of the head and neck of the radius and slipped radial epiphysis in children. *Surg Gynecol Obstet* 528–537, 1933.

183. Sellman DC, Seitz WH, Jr, Postak PD, et al: Reconstructive strategies for radioulnar dissociation: a biomechanical study. *J Orthop Trauma* 9(6):516–522, 1995.

184. Shepard MF, Markolf KL, Dunbar AM: Effects of radial head excision and distal radial shortening on load sharing in cadaver forearms. *J Bone Joint Surg Am* 83A(1):92–100, 2001.

185. Shmueli G, Herold HZ: Compression screwing of displaced fractures of the head of the radius. *J Bone Joint Surg Br* 63B(4):535–538, 1981.

186. Shore BJ, Mozzon JB, MacDermid JC, et al: Chronic posttraumatic elbow disorders treated with metallic radial head arthroplasty. *J Bone Joint Surg Am* 90(2):271–280, 2008.

187. Shors HC, Gannon C, Miller MC, et al: Plain radiographs are inadequate to identify overlengthening with a radial head prosthesis. *J Hand Surg [Am]* 33(3):335–339, 2008.

188. Skahen JR, III, Palmer AK, Werner FW, et al: Reconstruction of the interosseous membrane of the forearm in cadavers. *J Hand Surg [Am]* 22(6):986–994, 1997.

189. Smets S, Govaers K, Jansen N, et al: The floating radial head prosthesis for comminuted radial head fractures: a multicentric study. *Acta Orthop Belg* 66(4):353–358, 2000.

190. Smith AM, Morrey BF, Steinmann SP: Low profile fixation of radial head and neck fractures: surgical technique and clinical experience. *J Orthop Trauma* 21(10):718–724, 2007.

191. Smith AM, Urbanosky LR, Castle JA, et al: Radius pull test: predictor of longitudinal forearm instability. *J Bone Joint Surg Am* 84A(11):1970–1976, 2002.

192. Smith GR, Hotchkiss RN: Radial head and neck fractures: anatomic guidelines for proper placement of internal fixation. *J Shoulder Elbow Surg* 5(2 Pt 1):113–117, 1996.

193. Sowa DT, Hotchkiss RN, Weiland AJ: Symptomatic proximal translation of the radius following radial head resection. *Clin Orthop* (317):106–113, 1995.

194. Soyer AD, Nowotarski PJ, Kelso TB, et al: Optimal position for plate fixation of complex fractures of the proximal radius: a cadaver study. *J Orthop Trauma* 12(4):291–293, 1998.

195. Speed K: Ferrule caps for the head of the radius. *Surg Gynecol Obstet* 73:845–850, 1941.

196. Stoffelen DV, Holdsworth BJ: Excision or silastic replacement for comminuted radial head fractures. A long-term follow-up. *Acta Orthop Belg* 60(4):402–407, 1994.

197. Strachan JC, Ellis BW: Vulnerability of the posterior interosseous nerve during radial head resection. *J Bone Joint Surg Br* 53(2):320–323, 1971.

198. Strauch RJ, Rosenwasser MP, Glazer PA: Surgical exposure of the dorsal proximal third of the radius: how vulnerable is the posterior interosseous nerve? *J Shoulder Elbow Surg* 5(5):342–346, 1996.

199. Swanson AB, Jaeger SH, La Rochelle D: Comminuted fractures of the radial head. The role of silicone-implant replacement arthroplasty. *J Bone Joint Surg Am* 63(7):1039–1049, 1981.

200. Szabo RM, Hotchkiss RN, Slater RR, Jr: The use of frozen-allograft radial head replacement for treatment of established symptomatic proximal translation of the radius: preliminary experience in five cases. *J Hand Surg [Am]* 22(2):269–278, 1997.

201. Szekeres M, Chinchalkar SJ, King GJ: Optimizing elbow rehabilitation after instability. *Hand Clin* 24(1):27–38, 2008.

202. Taylor TKF, O'Connor BT: The effect upon the inferior radioulnar joint of excision of the head of the radius in adults. *J Bone Joint Surg Br* 46B:83–88, 1964.

203. Thompson HC, III, Garcia A: Myositis ossificans: aftermath of elbow injuries. *Clin Orthop* 50:129–134, 1967.

204. Thompson JD: Comparison of flexion versus extension splinting in the treatment of Mason type I radial head and neck fractures. *J Orthop Trauma* 2(2):117–119, 1988.

205. Tornetta P, III, Hochwald N, Bono C, et al: Anatomy of the posterior interosseous nerve in relation to fixation of the radial head. *Clin Orthop* (345):215–218, 1997.

206. Trousdale RT, Amadio PC, Cooney WP, et al: Radio-ulnar dissociation. A review of twenty cases. *J Bone Joint Surg Am* 74(10):1486–1497, 1992.

207. Unsworth-White J, Koka R, Churchill M, et al: The non-operative management of radial head fractures: a randomized trial of three treatments. *Injury* 25(3):165–167, 1994.

208. Van Glabbeek F, van Riet RP, Baumfeld JA, et al: Detrimental effects of overstuffing or understuffing with a radial head replacement in the medial collateral-ligament deficient elbow. *J Bone Joint Surg Am* 86A(12):2629–2635, 2004.

209. van Riet RP, Morrey BF: Documentation of associated injuries occurring with radial head fracture. *Clin Orthop Relat Res* 466(1):130–134, 2008.

210. van Riet RP, Morrey BF, O'Driscoll SW, et al: Associated injuries complicating radial head fractures: a demographic study. *Clin Orthop Relat Res* 441:351–355, 2005.

211. van Riet RP, Van Glabbeek F, Neale PG, et al: The noncircular shape of the radial head. *J Hand Surg [Am]* 28(6):972–978, 2003.

212. van Riet RP, Van Glabbeek F, Verborgt O, et al: Capitellar erosion caused by a metal radial head prosthesis. A case report. *J Bone Joint Surg Am* 86A(5):1061–1064, 2004.

213. Vanderwilde RS, Morrey BF, Melberg MW, et al: Inflammatory arthritis after failure of silicone rubber replacement of the radial head. *J Bone Joint Surg Br* 76(1):78–81, 1994.

214. Wagner CJ: Fractures of the head of the radius. *Am J Surg* 89:911–913, 1955.

215. Wallace AL, Walsh WR, Rooijen M, et al: The interosseous membrane in radio-ulnar dissociation. *J Bone Joint Surg Br* 79B:422–427, 1997.

216. Wallenbock E, Potsch F: Resection of the radial head: an alternative to use of a prosthesis? *J Trauma* 43(6):959–961, 1997.

217. Ward WG, Nunley JA: Concomitant fractures of the capitellum and radial head. *J Orthop Trauma* 2(2):110–116, 1988.

218. Watson-Jones R: Discussion of minor injuries of the elbow joint. *Proc R Soc Med* 23:323–327, 1930.

219. Weseley MS, Barenfeld PA, Eisenstein AL: Closed treatment of isolated radial head fractures. *J Trauma* 23(1):36–39, 1983.

220. Wexner SD, Goodwin C, Parkes JC, et al: Treatment of fractures of the radial head by partial excision. *Orthop Rev* 14:83–86, 1985.

221. Yoon A, King GJ, Grewal R: Is ORIF superior to nonoperative treatment in isolated displaced partial articular fractures of the radial head? *Clin Orthop Relat Res* 427(7):2105–2112, 2014.

222. Zunkiewicz MR, Clemente JS, Miller MC, et al: Radial head replacement with a bipolar system: a minimum 2-year follow-up. *J Shoulder Elbow Surg* 21(1):98–104, 2011.

20

Fractures of the Proximal Ulna

George S.M. Dyer and David Ring

Acknowledgment: The authors would like to acknowledge the contributions of Jesse Jupiter, an author of this chapter in the previous edition.

Fractures of the proximal ulna include olecranon fractures, olecranon fracture-dislocations, Monteggia fractures, and fractures of the coronoid process. Fractures of the proximal ulna may compromise the function of both the elbow and forearm articulations. Recognition of patterns and common injury characteristics is improving, and this, in turn, may improve the results of treatment.

PREOPERATIVE EVALUATION

As with other traumatic injuries, the first step in management is to perform a thorough evaluation according to the Advanced Trauma Life Support guidelines. Most fractures of the proximal ulna are associated with low-energy falls in older patients.[64] Such patients should be evaluated for medical conditions that may have contributed to the fall, for injuries related to older age (e.g., other osteoporosis-related fractures, subdural hematoma), and for the effect the injury may have on their social situation (i.e., whether they will be able to live independently while recovering).

The elbow should be checked for wounds and neurovascular injury. Anterior and lateral Monteggia fractures can be associated with injury to the posterior interosseous nerve. Fracture-dislocations can injure the ulnar nerve. High-energy complex fractures of the proximal ulna are occasionally associated with forearm compartment syndrome, especially when there is another fracture within the forearm.[27]

The initial radiographs obtained after the injury are often of low quality due to the deformity and pain in the limb. Nevertheless, it is usually possible to discern the overall pattern of the injury, which may lead one to suspect other injury components that may not be immediately obvious. For example, a posterior olecranon fracture-dislocation is often associated with fractures of the radial head and coronoid process as well as injury to the lateral collateral ligament complex,[64] whereas an anterior fracture-dislocation rarely involves injury to the radial head or collateral ligaments.[63]

Radiographs obtained after manipulative reduction and splint immobilization of the limb (when appropriate) may provide better views of the elbow and additional information about the injury (Figure 20.1, *A* and *B*). When additional information about fractures of the radial head or coronoid may influence decision making, computed tomography (CT) is useful (see Figure 20.1, *C*).[14] In particular, three-dimensional reconstructions with the distal humerus removed can provide a very accurate characterization of the injury (see Figure 20.1, *D* and *E*). Use of such images makes the preoperative planning more accurate.[32]

Additional information regarding the character of the injury can be obtained by viewing the elbow under the image intensifier once the patient is anesthetized. For some complex injuries, complete characterization of the injury pattern—and, therefore, a final treatment plan—can only be made after the injury is exposed operatively. The surgeon must therefore be comfortable with extensile exposures providing adequate access to the injury components.

◾ ANATOMY

Trochlear Notch of the Ulna

The trochlear notch of the ulna has a circumference of nearly 180 degrees, making it one of the most inherently constrained human articulations. Further enhancements of stability include (1) a central longitudinal ridge that interdigitates with a groove in the trochlear articular surface of the distal humerus and (2) a posterior tilt of the articular surface, with the angle between the tip of the coronoid and olecranon processes subtending approximately 30 degrees with a line parallel to the ulnar shaft (Figure 20.2).[37] There is a complementary anterior offset of the trochlea of the humerus from the shaft. This combination is what permits the ulnohumeral joint to flex to 140 degrees, and to extend not at all.

The articular surface has separate coronoid and olecranon areas separated by a small nonarticular transverse groove (see Figure 20.2, *B*).[36,71] Consequently, the treatment of articular fractures of the trochlear notch should focus primarily on restoring the proper relationship between the coronoid and olecranon processes; injury to the region between their articular facets has less impact than similar injuries at other articulations.[63,64]

Coronoid Process

It is useful to consider the following areas of the coronoid articular surface: the anteromedial facet, the lesser sigmoid notch region, the tip, and the base. The anteromedial facet, in particular, is now recognized as a critical stabilizer of the elbow under varus and rotational stress.[13-15]

The soft tissue attachments to the coronoid also figure prominently in the understanding of proximal ulnar fractures (Figure 20.3). The anterior band of the medial collateral ligament

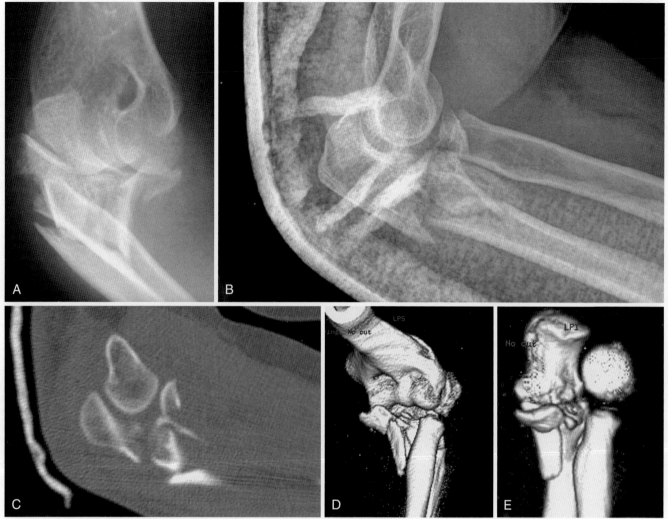

FIGURE 20.1 Imaging of complex proximal ulnar fractures. **A,** A radiograph taken immediately after the injury, before manipulative reduction, gives important information about the injury pattern and displacement. **B,** After manipulative reduction and splinting, the characteristics of the fractures may be more apparent. **C,** Two-dimensional CT scanning can show greater detail, but it can be difficult to follow specific fracture fragments between images. **D,** Three-dimensional reconstructions of CT images can be easier to interpret, particularly after the distal humerus has been removed from the image **(E)**. (Copyright © David Ring, MD.)

inserts on the base of the coronoid process.[5] Consequently, the anterior band of the medial collateral ligament is likely to be intact in complex fractures associated with large fractures of the coronoid base or anteromedial coronoid fractures, although its function will be disrupted by the bony injury and restored with stable internal fixation. Surgically, the fragment is a useful landmark for identifying the location of the medial collateral ligament.[14,17]

The brachialis has a broad insertion that extends distal to the coronoid process.[5] Even with large coronoid fractures, a substantial portion of the brachialis insertion remains on the ulnar shaft.

The lateral collateral ligament complex has a broad insertion on the lateral ulna below the radial head and neck and below the level of most coronoid fractures.[8] Traumatic failure of this complex occurs almost without exception as an avulsion of its origin from the lateral epicondyle and not as an intrasubstance tear or avulsion from the ulna.

The anterior capsule inserts a few millimeters below the tip of the olecranon process.[5] This has been interpreted to mean that very small coronoid fractures (a simple fleck, according to Regan and Morrey[53]) may represent intraarticular free fragments; however, operative treatment of these injuries discloses that coronoid tip fractures are much larger than might be guessed based on radiographs and that they always include the capsular insertion.[18,59,60]

Olecranon Process

The junction of the olecranon process with the proximal ulnar metaphysis occurs at the transverse groove of the olecranon, which is a nonarticular area with consequently less subchondral bone and which is also a relatively narrow area in the sagittal plane. These factors may increase the susceptibility to fracture at this site.[36]

The triceps has a very broad and thick insertion onto the posterior and proximal aspects of the olecranon. This is notable

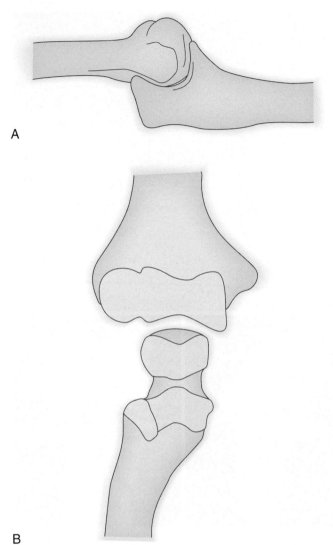

A

B

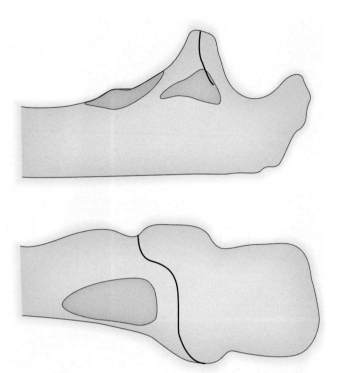

FIGURE 20.3 Soft tissue attachments to the coronoid. The brachialis has a broad and very distal insertion that goes beyond the coronoid and is therefore not disrupted by coronoid fractures. The anterior band of the medial collateral ligament inserts at the base of the coronoid process so that only a very large or medial-sided coronoid fracture will involve the medial collateral ligament insertion. The anterior elbow capsule inserts a few millimeters below the tip of the coronoid process; however, even coronoid fractures that are very small on radiographs nearly always remain attached to the capsule. (Adapted from Cage DJN, Abrams RA, Callahan JJ, Botte MJ: Soft tissue attachments of the ulnar coronoid process. *Clin Orthop Relat Res* 320:154–158, 1995.)

FIGURE 20.2 Anatomy of the trochlear notch. **A,** The trochlear notch of the ulna has a circumference of nearly 180 degrees that tilts somewhat posteriorly. A line drawn between the tips of the olecranon and coronoid processes should create a 30-degree angle with a line parallel to the ulnar shaft. **B,** The stability of the ulnotrochlear articulation is enhanced by interdigitation of a central ridge in the trochlear notch with a groove in the trochlea. The trochlear notch has separate coronoid and olecranon articular facets with an intervening nonarticular area.

during the application of a plate that contours around this portion of the bone: if the center of the triceps insertion is not split and elevated from the bone, the proximal aspect of the plate will rest well off the bone. For complex olecranon fractures this situation may sometimes be preferable to additional dissection of the soft tissue attachments. Removal of the plate is often needed after healing.

Radial Head

The anatomy of the radial head is difficult to replicate with a prosthesis. It has a slightly elliptic cross section and interdigitates precisely with both the lesser sigmoid notch and the lateral lip of the trochlea, not to mention the capitellar articular surface.[11,12,31] The slight angulation of the proximal radius with respect to the shaft further complicates attempts to reconstruct or replace the radius.

When plates are used to repair the radial head, several anatomic features are important. First, the posterior interosseous nerve runs deep to the supinator along the lateral aspect of the radial neck and is therefore at risk during operative dissection and implant application. Full pronation provides an average of approximately 5 cm of safe area for dissection and internal fixation,[9] but this is not the usual position for internal fixation, and it may be safest to routinely expose the nerve when very distal dissection is needed.[25]

Second, the radial head has a relatively small nonarticular surface, so implants placed on the articular surface must be countersunk. This is possible with plates as well as screws.[21] The nonarticular area can be determined as an arc of roughly 90 degrees with its midpoint directly lateral with the arm in neutral position, with a slightly greater margin anteriorly.[70] As a rough guide to this area, the area between the Lister tubercle and the radial styloid on the distal radius has been suggested.[6]

Finally, the vascular supply to the radial head is limited and tenuous.[72] This may be one reason for the nonunions observed after both operative and nonoperative treatment.[67]

Anatomy of Elbow Stability

The foundation of elbow stability has been increasingly well understood in recent years. The large bony notch formed by the coronoid and olecranon is an obvious source of stability in the sagittal plane, but the coronal plane anatomy of the coronoid has been elucidated as essential for varus-valgus stability as well.[10,13] Considering ligaments, attempts to quantify the contributions of various anatomic structures to elbow stability have suggested that the anterior band of the medial collateral ligament is the most important stabilizer of the elbow under valgus stress[39] and that the radial head is a secondary stabilizer under valgus stress.[40] It may be more useful to consider the roles of the medial collateral ligament and radial head as overlapping and synergistic rather than hierarchic. Throwing a baseball or javelin probably requires all of these structures.

Observations of valgus stability have had a strong influence on considerations of elbow stability overall: however, if global elbow stability or the ability to maintain a concentric reduction is considered, the complexity increases. Either subluxation or dislocation of the elbow is more directly related to injury to the lateral collateral ligament complex than to the medial collateral ligament.[46,59] Complete dislocation of the elbow can occur with the anterior band of the medial collateral ligament intact. Furthermore, most cases of recurrent elbow instability are related to lateral collateral ligament insufficiency.[44] Loss of the radial head, coronoid, or olecranon will exacerbate this posterolateral rotatory instability.[51,57]

Mechanical studies in cadavers have demonstrated a progressive loss of ulnohumeral stability with greater amounts of olecranon excision, even when all of the ligaments and the radial head are preserved.[1]

Clinical and radiograph-based studies have found that even small coronoid fractures are associated with a substantial effect on elbow stability.[13-15] Clinical experience corroborates these predictions; coronoid fracture is associated with patterns of injury that are notoriously unstable and probably reflect greater capsuloligamentous and musculotendinous injury in addition to the loss of bony buttress.[66]

The contribution of the radial head to stability may not be apparent in the laboratory until several soft tissue structures have also been divided, but in the clinical setting, when managing complex trauma of the elbow and forearm, contact between the radial head and capitellum provides substantial stability. Furthermore, some have suggested that the ulnohumeral joint is more susceptible to arthritis in the absence of radiocapitellar contact,[68] although this will be difficult to prove or disprove.

CLASSIFICATION AND PATTERNS OF INJURY

Monteggia Fractures

Fractures of the proximal ulna that do not involve the trochlear notch often have associated dislocation of the proximal radioulnar joint, the so-called Monteggia lesion.[37,64] The most commonly used classification of these injuries is that of Bado, who distinguished four lesions based on the direction of dislocation of the radial head: type 1, anterior; type 2, posterior; type 3, lateral; and type 4, any direction, associated with a diaphyseal fracture of the radius.[2] In practice, the most useful distinction is between fractures with anterior or lateral displacement of the radial head and those with posterior displacement. The management of injuries with anterior or lateral displacement centers on stable restoration of the ulnar alignment, which nearly always restores alignment and function of the proximal radioulnar joint.[52,64,65]

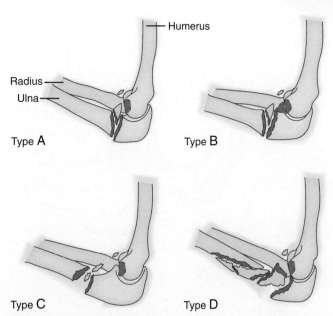

FIGURE 20.4 Illustration of a spectrum of posterior Monteggia injuries. Type A, injury at the ulnohumeral joint with fractures of the olecranon and coronoid; type B, injury at the most common location, the proximal ulnar metaphysis; type C, injury at the diaphyseal level; type D, complex fractures that involve multiple levels. (Copyright © Massachusetts General Hospital Department of Orthopaedic Surgery.)

The Bado type 2, or posterior Monteggia, lesion has long been recognized as a distinct injury that is usually associated with fracture of the radial head and often occurs in the setting of osteoporosis.[29,48,49] There is a spectrum of posterior Monteggia injuries with similar features that vary according to the location of the ulnar fracture.[29] These have been subclassified as type A when the fracture is at the level of the trochlear notch (involving the olecranon and often the coronoid processes); type B when the fracture is in the metaphysis just distal to the trochlear notch; and type C when the fracture is in the diaphysis. Type D fractures are multifragmented fractures that involve more than one region (Figure 20.4).[29] Type D fractures are inherently unstable by virtue of the associated capsuloligamentous damage, fracture and dislocation of the radial head, and morphologic situation of the ulnar fracture, which often involves a triangular or quadrangular fragment of the ulna that includes the anterior ulnar cortex and, sometimes, the coronoid process.

Olecranon Fractures

The Mayo classification of olecranon fractures distinguishes three factors that have a direct influence on treatment: (1) fracture displacement, (2) comminution, and (3) ulnohumeral instability (Figure 20.5).[37] Type 1 fractures that are nondisplaced or minimally displaced are either noncomminuted (type 1A) or comminuted (type 1B) and are treated nonoperatively. Type II fractures feature displacement of the proximal fragment without elbow instability; these fractures require operative treatment. Type IIA fractures (without comminution) are usually treated with tension band wire fixation. When the fracture is oblique, an ancillary interfragmentary compression screw can be added. Type IIB fractures are comminuted and

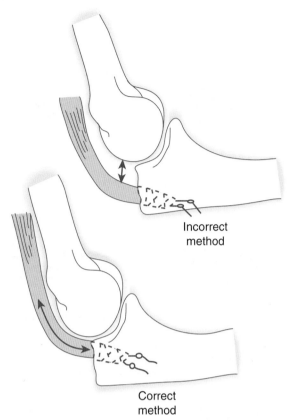

FIGURE 20.5 When the triceps is advanced and reattached to the proximal ulna after olecranon excision, it is better to insert it close to the articular margin.

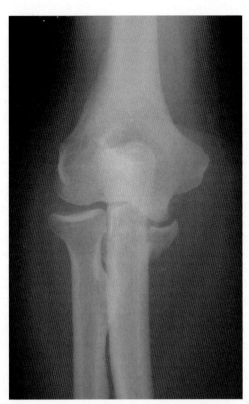

FIGURE 20.6 The posteromedial varus rotational instability–pattern injury has only recently been recognized. It is characterized by a fracture of the anteromedial coronoid facet and rupture of the origin of the lateral collateral ligament complex from the lateral epicondyle. (Copyright © David Ring, MD.)

require plate fixation. Type III fractures feature instability of the ulnohumeral joint.

Olecranon Fracture-Dislocations

Fractures of the proximal ulna can appear extremely complex. The identification of basic injury patterns can facilitate management. Even a simple fracture pattern of the olecranon can have associated injuries, which the surgeon must be careful not to miss.

Posteromedial varus rotational instability–pattern injuries (Figure 20.6) arise from fracture of the anteromedial facet of the coronoid process, resulting in varus instability.[51] There is an associated injury of either an avulsion of the lateral collateral ligament complex from the lateral epicondyle or a fracture of the olecranon, but rarely both. The radial head is rarely fractured.

On rare occasion, a simple elbow dislocation is associated with a fracture of the olecranon (Figure 20.7). The pattern of olecranon fracture may represent a bony alternative to rupture of the medial collateral ligament complex.

The majority of olecranon fracture-dislocations occur in either an anterior or a posterior direction.[4,63,64]

Anterior (transolecranon) olecranon fracture-dislocations are less common and are often caused by a high-energy direct blow to the forearm.[63] The injury is defined by a complex olecranon or proximal ulna facture, dislocation of the forearm, and *maintenance of the proximal radioulnar relationship* (see Figure 20.8).[41,42,63] This injury pattern was first referred to as a

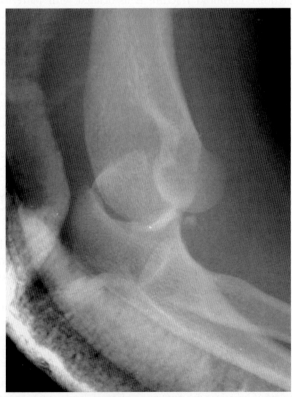

FIGURE 20.7 In this unusual case, a patient has sustained a posterior dislocation of the elbow associated with a fracture of the olecranon process on the medial aspect, essentially avulsing the posterior aspect of the medial collateral ligament complex. (Copyright © David Ring, MD.)

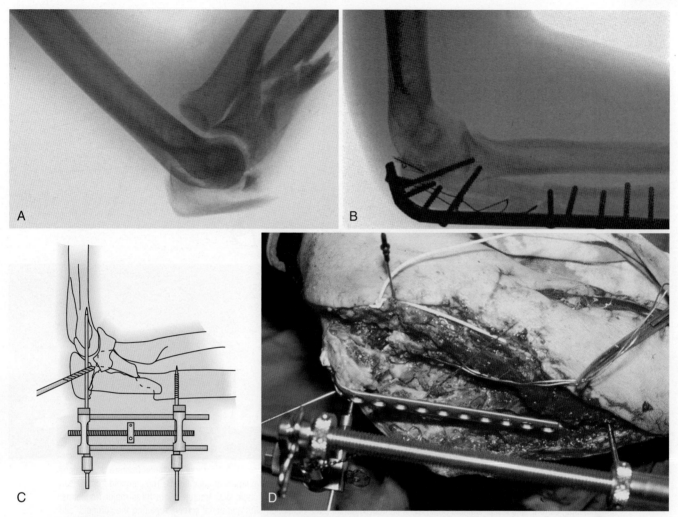

FIGURE 20.8 Anterior (transolecranon) fracture-dislocation of the elbow. **A,** The forearm is displaced anteriorly with the radioulnar relationship relatively spared. The trochlea has imploded through the proximal ulna, creating a very complex fracture with a large coronoid fracture and comminution extending into the diaphysis. The collateral ligaments are usually not injured. **B,** A long contoured dorsal plate secures the relationship between the coronoid and olecranon processes (the contour and dimensions of the trochlear notch) and bridges the comminution. A tension wire engages the fragmented olecranon process. **C,** As described by Mast, an external fixator can assist with reduction and provisional fixation. **D,** The olecranon fragment is held to the trochlea with a stout smooth Kirschner wire. Distraction between this wire and a second distal wire helps realign the intervening fragments. (Copyright © David Ring, MD.)

"trans-olecranon fracture dislocation" in 1974 by Biga and Thomine.[4] This and subsequent studies emphasized the distinction from Monteggia injuries, in which the radioulnar relationship is dissociated.[42,63] When the capsuloligamentous structures are maintained, the elbow is typically rendered stable once the proximal ulnar anatomy is reduced and secured. Associated collateral ligament injury is unusual,[4,63] and the outcomes are generally favorable.[41]

It is useful to consider posterior fracture-dislocations of the olecranon as the most proximal type of posterior Monteggia injuries.[9] Common features of posterior Monteggia injuries include an apex-posterior fracture of the ulna, posterior translation of the radial head with respect to the capitellum, fracture of the radial head, and frequent injury to the lateral collateral ligament complex. With posterior olecranon fracture-dislocations (or type A posterior Monteggia fractures, according to Jupiter and colleagues[29]), the fracture of the ulna occurs at the level of the olecranon and is nearly always associated with

a fracture of the coronoid process (Figure 20.9). When a complex olecranon fracture-dislocation is identified as being posterior, fractures of the radial head and coronoid and injury to the lateral collateral ligament should be suspected.

HISTORICAL REVIEW

Lister selected fracture of the olecranon as the first fracture to undergo internal fixation (with a silver wire) using his antiseptic surgical techniques in 1873.[22] Screws may have been used even earlier.[3] Since that time, attempts to repair fractures of the olecranon with simple wiring techniques or long screws have been associated with problems with loosening and migration (or at least prominence) of implants, leading to secondary surgeries to address symptoms and complications such as infection, malunion, and nonunion.[33] This led to a debate regarding whether to repair these fractures or simply excise them and advance the triceps.[20] With careful consideration of technical

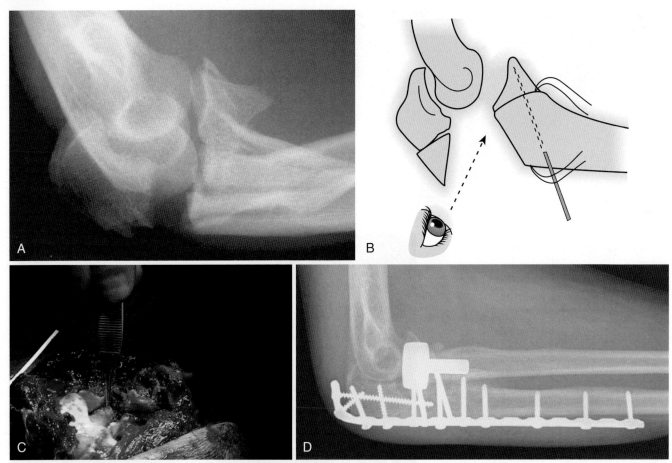

FIGURE 20.9 Posterior olecranon fracture-dislocation (posterior Monteggia fracture type A). **A,** Posterior olecranon fracture-dislocations feature fractures of the coronoid and radial head and frequent injury to the lateral collateral ligament complex. **B,** The coronoid fracture can be visualized and manipulated through the olecranon fracture. **C,** In this patient the coronoid was fractured into three major fragments: anteromedial, central, and lesser sigmoid notch. **D,** A contoured dorsal plate is applied with additional screws repairing the coronoid, and the radial head is replaced with a prosthesis. (Copyright © David Ring, MD.)

aspects of olecranon fixation, the complications have been diminished to the point that excision of the olecranon is used very rarely, and usually only in a very infirm patient.

The major advances in understanding proximal ulnar fractures have related to the recognition of the more complex injury patterns described. An elbow injury that includes a fracture of the ulna is no longer seen as just an "olecranon fracture." Bony injury to the ulna is increasingly seen as one element along a continuum of ligamentous and bony injury that may destabilize the elbow joint. O'Driscoll, Morrey, and others have better defined the mechanism of dislocation and the fracture-related anatomy of the medial collateral ligament.[45,46] Schneeberger and others elucidated the relationship between the bone and ligament stabilizers and the mechanisms of disclocation.[43,69] It is now recognized that both simple olecranon fractures associated with other fractures or ligament injuries and comminuted olecranon fractures are better treated with a plate and screws than with simpler techniques intended for simple olecranon fractures. The characterization of anterior and posterior patterns of olecranon fracture-dislocations is not new but is better recognized, and the value of these distinctions in patient management is better understood.

Our understanding of fractures of the coronoid continues to expand. The importance of a separate fracture of the anterome-

dial facet is evidence that the Regan and Morrey classification[53] may no longer be adequate to describe these injuries. Using detailed analysis of imaging, Ring, Jupiter, and Doornberg have improved our understanding of the osseous anatomy of the coronoid and called particular attention to its anteromedial facet.[13,14,55] Whereas Regan and Morrey cited large coronoid fractures as more troublesome,[54] recent work has shown that operative fixation of these fractures can be associated with good results[63,64] and that smaller fractures are often associated with more troublesome injury patterns such as the "terrible triad."[66] Many surgeons now believe that most coronoid fractures associated with complex injury patterns merit internal fixation; however, the exposures and fixation techniques are still in evolution.[61]

OPERATIVE PROCEDURE

Skin Incision

A midline posterior skin incision is used for all complex fractures of the proximal ulna. Traumatic wounds are incorporated. Some surgeons prefer that the incision not pass directly over the olecranon and so curve it slightly.[36] A direct midline incision may cut fewer cutaneous nerves.[16]

Excision and Triceps Advancement

The olecranon process is rarely so fragmented that it cannot be repaired. Tension wire techniques can gain fixation of the soft tissue attachments until healing occurs. Hence, excision of the olecranon and triceps advancement is used sparingly for primary treatment of fractures of the olecranon and occasionally for treatment of secondary complications. As primary treatment, excision of the olecranon is best suited to infirm older patients with limited functional demands. The surgeon must be certain that the collateral ligaments, radial head, and coronoid process are intact.

The fragments of the olecranon are excised. Holes are drilled starting from immediately adjacent to the articular margin of the remaining olecranon and exiting the dorsal surface of the ulna. Stout sutures are placed in the triceps using one of a variety of techniques designed to gain hold over a broad portion of the tendon. These are then passed through the drill holes in the ulna, put under tension, and tied.

The elbow is immobilized for 4 weeks, and active motion is allowed thereafter. In low-demand individuals, formal therapy is not necessary.

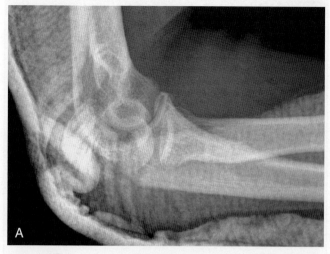

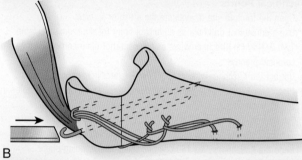

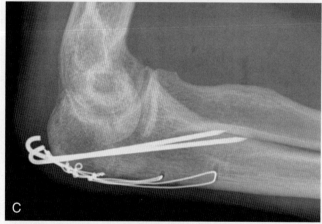

FIGURE 20.10 Tension band wiring. **A,** Tension band wiring is suitable for simple fractures without fracture of the radial head or coronoid or dislocation/subluxation of the ulnohumeral joint. **B,** A technique using anteriorly oriented Kirschner wires, impaction of the proximal ends into the olecranon beneath the triceps insertion, and two small-gauge tension wires can limit hardware-related problems. **C,** Active motion is initiated the morning after surgery. (Copyright © David Ring, MD.)

CRITICAL POINTS *Olecranon Excision and Advancement of the Triceps*

Indications
- Comminuted, osteoporotic fracture
- Older, infirm, inactive patient
- No instability or associated fractures
- Salvage of complex cases
- Rarely used today

Preoperative Evaluation
- Anteroposterior and lateral radiographs of the elbow
- Evaluation of elbow stability under anesthesia

Pearls and Pitfalls
- If the triceps is not advanced to the articular margin of the ulna, this margin may be prominent and grind against the trochlea of the distal humerus.
- Suture anchors cannot be relied on in osteoporotic metaphyseal bone, and the sutures should be passed through drill holes and tied over the dorsum of the ulna.

Postoperative Care
- Provide cast immobilization for 4 to 6 weeks.
- Allow unrestricted active use of the arm thereafter with selective use of therapy.

Athletic Participation
- Not applicable

Tension Band Wiring

Tension band wiring is appropriate for relatively simple fractures at the level of the transverse groove of the trochlear notch, without associated ligament injuries or fracture of the coronoid or radial head (Figure 20.10, *A*). Tension band wire techniques have been described using screws or Kirschner wires. The most common mistake is the failure to distinguish a simple fracture at the transverse groove from a fracture more distal,

comminuted, or complex, where a tension band technique will likely fail.

The fracture is opened and hematoma removed to be sure that comminution and articular involvement are limited. The periosteum and muscular attachments are elevated minimally, just enough to ensure accurate reduction of the fragment. A large tenaculum clamp can be used to maintain reduction of the olecranon. A hole drilled in the dorsal surface of the ulna can provide a good anchor point for the distal tine of the clamp.

CRITICAL POINTS *Tension Band Wiring*

Indications
- Simple, noncomminuted fracture
- No instability or associated fractures
- Location of the fracture must be at or proximal to the midpoint of the olecranon fossa

Preoperative Evaluation
- Anteroposterior and lateral radiographs of the elbow

Pearls
- The use of two smaller-gauge wires can limit the prominence of the knots.
- Kirschner wire engagement of the anterior ulnar cortex and olecranon can limit migration.
- Small implants placed appropriately provide adequate fixation for active motion.

Technical Points
- Open the fracture site to evaluate the articular surface.
- Use a dorsoulnar drill hole as an anchor point for the reduction clamp.
- Two 0.045-inch Kirschner wires exit the anterior ulnar cortex distal to the coronoid process.
- Retract the Kirschner wires 5 to 10 mm for later impaction.
- Place two 22-gauge stainless steel wires through separate drill holes in the ulnar diaphysis.
- Pass wires underneath the triceps insertion using a large-bore needle.
- Tension figure-of-eight wires both medially and laterally.
- Bend the Kirschner wires 180 degrees using wire-bending pliers.
- Perform impaction of the cut proximal ends of the Kirschner wires into the olecranon.
- Test the security of the fixation through full flexion.

Pitfalls
- Small (22-gauge) wires are easy to break; use tension but do not tighten.
- Wires left above the triceps insertion are prominent when swelling resolves.

Postoperative Care
- Active elbow motion initiated the morning after surgery
- Arm used for light functional activity
- Resistive exercises when early healing has been established (about 6 weeks)

Athletic Participation
- Allowed after fracture has healed and motion and strength are normal or near-normal (4 to 6 months)

Kirschner Wire Technique

Two parallel Kirschner wires are drilled across the osteotomy site. The majority of surgeons use 0.062-inch wires, but we use 0.045-inch wires with few problems. The wires are often drilled parallel to the ulnar diaphysis, but we and others favor drilling the wires obliquely so that they pass through the anterior ulnar cortex, just distal to the coronoid process.[50,56] This is intended to limit the potential for wire migration; the wires are anchored in the anterior ulnar cortex. After exiting the anterior cortex, the wires are retracted from 5 to 10 mm, anticipating subsequent impaction of the wires into the olecranon process proximally.

The extensor carpi ulnaris and flexor carpi ulnaris muscles are partly elevated from the apex of the ulna distal to the osteotomy site to expose the cortex. The appropriate distance between the fracture and this drill hole has been based on mechanical calculations, but the placement of these holes is determined more practically by transition from the flat proximal ulna to the apex posterior triangular shape of the diaphysis. Likewise, the placement of the drill holes in the anteroposterior plane is not critical, except that they should not be so dorsal as to risk breaking out of the ulna. Large drill holes (2.5 mm) facilitate wire passage.

Many surgeons use a single 18-gauge stainless steel wire for the tension wire, but we prefer to use two 22-gauge stainless steel wires, each passed through its own drill hole distally. The smaller wires are less prominent. An alternative is a size 5 metric sternal wire of the type used in cardiac surgery, which is approximately the same gauge as a 23-gauge wire and comes swedged to a large cutting needle. This facilitates passage through bone tunnels and through the triceps tendon.

The tension wires are placed in a figure-of-eight arrangement over the dorsal ulna. The proximal end of the wire is passed dorsal to the Kirschner wires through the insertion of the triceps using a large-gauge needle. The tension wires are tensioned on both the medial and lateral sides of the ulna until the wires rest flush with the ulna. Some surgeons prefer to twist the wires until they are very tight, but this cannot be done with smaller-gauge wires because they will break. The wires do not need to be tight, only free of slack. This tension is achieved by twisting the wire until it starts to bend over itself. The twisted ends are trimmed and bent into adjacent soft tissues to limit prominence.

The proximal ends of the Kirschner wires are bent 180 degrees and trimmed. The triceps insertion is incised, and impaction of the bent ends into the proximal olecranon is achieved with a bone tamp (see Figure 20.10, *B* and *C*). The strength of the fixation can be tested by completely flexing the elbow; the fracture should not separate.

Screw Technique

Some surgeons prefer to use screws instead of Kirschner wires. Some recommend using a very long screw that engages the intramedullary canal of the ulnar diaphysis distally.[26] Others recommend aiming the screw anteriorly to engage the anterior ulnar cortex. An oblique screw is particularly well suited to an oblique fracture. The remaining portion of the technique is as described for the Kirschner wire technique.

A large (6.5-mm) screw, meant to capture the distal canal of the ulna, may cause a fracture of the distal ulna on insertion. If this occurs, the tension band technique must be abandoned for the plate fixation described next.

Plate and Screws

A plate and screws are used for comminuted olecranon fractures (Figure 20.11), Monteggia fractures (Figure 20.12), and olecranon fracture-dislocations (see Figures 20.8 and 20.9).

Standard Techniques

When a plate is applied to the proximal ulna, it should be contoured to wrap around the proximal aspect of the ulna. A straight plate will have only two or three screws in the

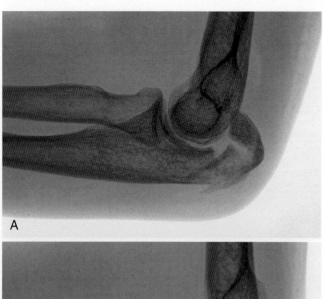

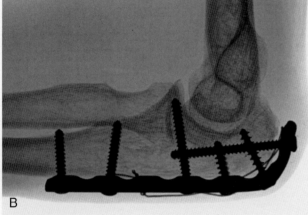

FIGURE 20.11 Plate fixation. **A,** Plate fixation is used for comminuted fractures and fracture-dislocations. **B,** The plate is applied to the dorsal surface of the ulna and contoured around the proximal olecranon. A tension wire engaging the triceps insertion can enhance fixation. (Copyright © David Ring, MD.)

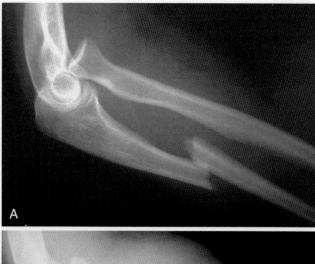

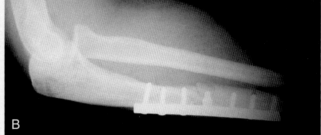

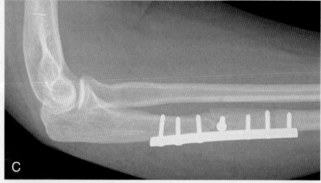

FIGURE 20.12 Anterior (Bado I) Monteggia fracture. **A,** The anterior Monteggia fracture (fracture of the ulnar diaphysis with anterior dislocation of the proximal radioulnar joint) is uncommon in adult patients. **B,** Persistent subluxation of the proximal radioulnar (and radiocapitellar) joints nearly always reflects residual malalignment of the ulna. **C,** Revision of the ulnar fixation achieved better alignment of the forearm. (Copyright © David Ring, MD.)

metaphyseal bone proximal to the fracture. Many patients with complex proximal ulnar fractures have osteopenic bone, which further compromises the strength of plate and screw fixation. Bending the plate around the proximal aspect of the olecranon provides additional screws in the proximal fragment. In addition, the most proximal screws are oriented so that they are orthogonal to more distal screws. Finally, the most proximal screws can be very long screws crossing the fracture line into the distal fragment. In some cases, these screws can be directed to engage one of the cortices of the distal fragment, such as the anterior ulnar cortex. There are now many plating systems that are precontoured to apply to the proximal ulna and may offer a technical advantage and ease of use. These systems also offer locking screws, which improve stability in osteopenic or comminuted bone.

A plate applied to the dorsal surface of the proximal ulna also has several advantages over plates applied to the medial or lateral aspect of the ulna. Placing the plate along the flat dorsal surface can assist with obtaining and monitoring reduction. The dorsal surface is in the plane of the forces generated by active elbow motion, so that the plate functions to a certain extent as a tension band. Finally, dorsal plate placement requires very limited soft tissue stripping.

Exposure of the ulna should preserve periosteal and muscle attachments. A plate contoured to wrap around the proximal ulna can be placed on top of the triceps insertion with few problems. This is particularly useful when the olecranon fragment is small or fragmented. Alternatively, the triceps insertion can be incised longitudinally and partially elevated medially and laterally enough to allow direct plate contact with bone.

Distally, a dorsal plate will lie directly on the apex of the ulnar diaphysis. This might seem unsettling to some surgeons but has not been a problem. One advantage of this situation is that the muscle needs be split only enough to gain access to this apex; there is no need to elevate the muscle or periosteum off either the medial or lateral flat aspect of the ulna. No attempt is made to precisely realign intervening fragmentation. Once the relationship of the coronoid and olecranon facets is restored and the overall alignment is regained, the remaining fragments are bridged, leaving their soft tissue attachments intact. In spite of extensive fragmentation, bone grafts[28] are rarely necessary if the soft tissue attachments are preserved.[63,64]

CRITICAL POINTS *Plate Fixation*

Indications
- Comminuted fractures of the olecranon
- Fracture-dislocations of the elbow

Preoperative Evaluation
- Anteroposterior and lateral radiographs of the elbow
- CT scan and three-dimensional reconstructions to evaluate coronoid and radial head

Pearls
- The pattern of injury can indicate the injury components and prognosis.
- Medial facet coronoid fractures may need direct medial fixation.
- Use of ancillary tension wire can enhance fixation of small, comminuted, or osteoporotic olecranon fragments.
- Restoration of the coronoid and olecranon processes is critical.
- If stripping is limited and fixation is secure, the metaphyseal bone will heal without grafting in most cases.

Technical Points
- Use a dorsal skin incision.
- Use full-thickness skin flaps.
- Access the coronoid through the olecranon fracture or a medial or lateral fascial exposure, within the same single dorsal skin incision.
- Perform provisional fixation of articular fragments to the distal humerus as needed.
- Use contoured dorsal plate fixation.

Pitfalls
- A third tubular plate may be inadequate; fixation may require a dynamic compression plate or its equivalent.
- Comminuted coronoid fractures may need to be protected with hinged fixation.

Postoperative Care
- Active elbow motion is initiated the morning after surgery when fixation is secure.
- Avoid stressing the lateral collateral ligament repair; advise the patient not to abduct the shoulder.
- The arm can be used for light functional activity.
- The arm should be protected in a splint or in hinged external fixation for complex or tenuous repairs.
- Resistive exercises can begin when early healing is established (about 6 weeks).

Athletic Participation
- Allowed after fracture has healed, and motion and strength are normal or near-normal (4 to 6 months)

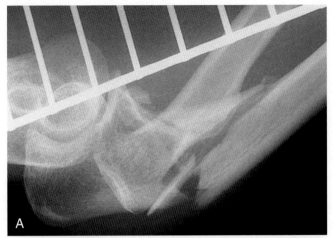

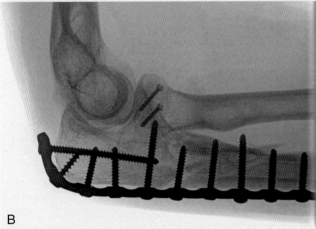

FIGURE 20.13 Metaphyseal posterior Monteggia fracture. **A,** Fractures at the level of the metaphysis often feature a triangular or quadrangular anterior fragment. **B,** Contoured dorsal plate fixation can provide adequate stability to bridge this comminuted area and prevent recurrent apex posterior deformity. (Copyright © David Ring, MD.)

Monteggia Fractures

The majority of anterior and lateral Monteggia lesions feature diaphyseal fractures of the ulna. Standard compression plate techniques with the plate applied to one of the flat surfaces of the ulna should restore forearm alignment.[64] If the radial head does not align with the capitellum after the ulna is reduced, misalignment of the ulna is the cause until proved otherwise (see Figure 20.12). Only on rare occasions is a separate open reduction of the radial head necessary. If a soft tissue block to reduction is present, the posterior interosseous nerve may be entrapped. Therefore, one should not simply divide the tissue without adequate exposure.

Posterior Monteggia injuries that do not involve the ulnohumeral joint most frequently occur at the level of the proximal ulnar metaphysis. In this location a dorsally applied plate is preferred (Figure 20.13).[65] Posterior Monteggia injuries are also associated with radial head fractures and lateral collateral ligament injuries that may need to be addressed.

Fracture-Dislocations

Fractures of the radial head and coronoid process can be evaluated and often definitively treated through the exposure provided by the fracture of the olecranon process. With little additional dissection, the olecranon fragment can be mobilized proximally, providing exposure of the coronoid through the ulnohumeral joint. If the exposure of the radial head through the posterior injury is inadequate, a separate muscle interval (e.g., Kocher or Kaplan interval[36]) can be used and approached by the elevation of a broad lateral skin flap.

If the exposure of the coronoid is inadequate through the straight dorsal skin incision, a separate deep medial or lateral fascial exposure can be developed. Posterior olecranon fracture-dislocations often require a lateral exposure to address a fracture of the radial head or coronoid or to repair the lateral

CRITICAL POINTS *Extraarticular Monteggia Fractures*

Indications
- Anterior or lateral Monteggia fractures
- Extraarticular Monteggia fractures

Preoperative Evaluation
- Anteroposterior and lateral radiographs of the elbow

Pearls
- Residual radiocapitellar malalignment nearly always reflects ulnar malalignment.
- Posterior Monteggia fractures are often associated with radial head fractures and lateral collateral ligament injury (and therefore elbow instability).

Technical Points
- Perform open reduction of the ulnar fracture.
- Perform closed reduction of the proximal radioulnar joint/radiocapitellar relationship.
- Use plate fixation of the ulna.
- Use a long plate for comminuted fractures.
- Use a contoured dorsal plate for proximal, osteoporotic fractures.
- Check forearm and elbow relationships through full motion.
- Open reduction and stabilization of the radial head is rarely necessary.

Pitfalls
- Residual malalignment of the ulna
- Ulnohumeral instability after posterior Monteggia fracture owing to inadequate treatment of the radial head and lateral collateral ligament
- Early loss of alignment of the ulna owing to an inadequate plate (often a plate placed on the medial or lateral surface of the ulna and with too few proximal screws)

Postoperative Care
- Active motion the morning after surgery
- Functional use of the arm for light tasks
- Resistive exercises when early healing is established (about 6 weeks)

Athletic Participation
- Allowed after fracture has healed, and motion and strength are normal or near-normal (4 to 6 months)

collateral ligament. When the lateral collateral ligament is injured, it is usually avulsed from the lateral epicondyle. This facilitates both exposure and repair. The lateral collateral ligament origin and common extensor musculature can be included in an anterior or posterior flap or mobilized distally.

Exposure of the coronoid can be improved by releasing the origins of the radial wrist extensors from the lateral supracondylar ridge and elevating the brachialis from the anterior humerus and by excising the fractured radial head.[18] A medial exposure, obtained between the two heads of the flexor carpi ulnaris or by splitting the flexor-pronator mass more anteriorly, may be needed to address a complex fracture of the coronoid, particularly one that involves the anteromedial facet of the coronoid process (see Figure 20.6).

The fracture of the coronoid can often be reduced directly through the elbow joint using the limited access provided by the olecranon fracture[18,24] (see Figure 20.9). Provisional fixation can be obtained using Kirschner wires to attach the fragments either to the metaphyseal or diaphyseal fragments of the ulna or to the trochlea of the distal humerus when there is extensive fragmentation of the proximal ulna.[23,34] An alternative to keep in mind when there is extensive fragmentation of the proximal ulna is the use of a skeletal distractor (a temporary external fixator)[34,63] (see Figure 20.16).

External fixation applied between a wire driven through the olecranon fragment and up into the trochlea and a second wire in the distal ulnar diaphysis can often obtain reduction indirectly when distraction is applied between the pins. Definitive fixation can usually be obtained with screws applied under the guidance of an image intensifier. The screws are placed through the plate when there is extensive fragmentation of the proximal ulna. If the coronoid fracture is very comminuted and cannot be securely repaired, the ulnohumeral joint should be protected with temporary hinged or static external fixation or with temporary pin fixation of the ulnohumeral joint, depending on the equipment and expertise available.

A long plate is contoured to wrap around the proximal olecranon. A very long plate (between 12 and 16 holes) should be considered, particularly when there is extensive fragmentation or the bone quality is poor. When the olecranon is fragmented or osteoporotic, a plate and screws alone may not provide reliable fixation. In this situation, it has proved useful to use ancillary tension wire fixation to control the olecranon fragments through the triceps insertion.

❖ AUTHORS' PREFERRED METHOD OF TREATMENT

Nondisplaced, Stable Fractures (Type I)
We use cast immobilization for stable, nondisplaced fractures of the olecranon. The elbow is immobilized at 90 degrees of flexion and neutral forearm rotation. The cast is discontinued after 3 or 4 weeks, and active-assisted elbow range-of-motion exercises are initiated. These injuries are rare, and careful surveillance for displacement must be employed.

Displaced Fractures Without Comminution and Proximal to the Midpoint of the Olecranon (Type IIA)
For simple, noncomminuted fractures without associated ligament injuries, we use tension band wiring. We use 0.045-inch Kirschner wires directed to engage the anterior ulnar cortex distal to the coronoid and bent 180 degrees and impacted into the olecranon proximally. We use two 22-gauge stainless steel tension wires, or size 5 metric sternal suture wires, each passed through its own hole to limit the prominence of the implants.[56]

Displaced Fractures With Comminution and/or Dislocation of the Elbow
For comminuted fractures and fracture-dislocations, we use a dorsal plate and screws contoured to wrap around the proximal ulna.[59,63,64] For some complex fractures, we place the proximal aspect of the plate over the triceps insertion, and otherwise we elevate the triceps insertion and place the plate directly on bone. When the proximal olecranon fragment is small, fragmented, or osteopenic, we also use a tension wire that engages the triceps insertion (see Figures 20.8 and 20.10). In our experience, plates with numerous small screws for the olecranon fragment have not been reliable in this situation. For fracture-dislocations, we use the methods described earlier.

Coronoid Fractures

For fractures of the coronoid that involve the anteromedial facet we use a medial plate unless the fragments are large enough to reliably repair with screws.[18] For nonreconstructible or very complex fractures of the coronoid, we allow 4 to 8 weeks of hinged external fixation to maintain a concentric ulnohumeral reduction and protect the healing coronoid.[7]

POSTOPERATIVE MANAGEMENT AND EXPECTATIONS

Postoperative Protocol

The goal of internal fixation of the proximal ulna is secure fixation allowing active-assisted elbow motion the day after surgery. In the unusual circumstance with more tenuous fixation (usually in an older patient with a complex, osteoporotic fracture), the elbow can be immobilized in a removable elbow splint for 4 weeks before initiating active-assisted elbow motion.

Hand exercises are critical to eliminating hand swelling and preventing hand stiffness. Passive elbow manipulation and joint mobilization are never used. Gravity-assisted and splint-assisted exercises under the control of the patient are very useful. Static progressive splints have been more useful than dynamic splints in our experience.

Resistive exercises and strengthening of the limb are delayed until early healing is established. Full activity is allowed when solid healing is apparent, usually between 3 and 4 months after injury. Plate removal is elective and should be delayed at least 12 to 18 months after injury to avoid the risk of refracture.

Expected Outcome

Intraarticular elbow injuries are commonly associated with some loss of elbow flexion. With very complex injuries, the flexion contracture may be as much as 30 to 40 degrees. Nearly full flexion should be possible in the absence of heterotopic bone or ulnar neuropathy but is also commonly restricted after complex injuries. Forearm rotation is rarely restricted with injury to the olecranon, but posterior fracture-dislocations associated with fracture of the radial head can be associated with diminished forearm rotation.

There is a moderate chance of additional surgery related to prominent or loose implants, elbow contracture with or without heterotopic ossification,[2] or ulnar neuropathy.[19]

Arthrosis is uncommon except after fracture-dislocations, particularly those that involve a coronoid fracture. In spite of arthrosis, the elbow is usually durable if the trochlear notch is restored.

COMPLICATIONS

Early Failure of Fixation

Tension band wire constructs can fail when used for complex fractures or fracture-dislocations (Figure 20.14), but they rarely fail when used for simple fractures unless the patient returns to forceful activity too soon. Plate loosening is most common in older patients with fracture-dislocations when a noncontoured plate has been placed on either the medial or the lateral side of the proximal ulna (Figure 20.15).

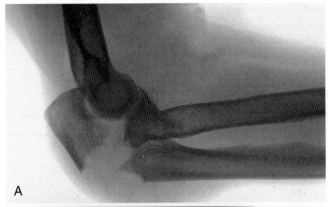

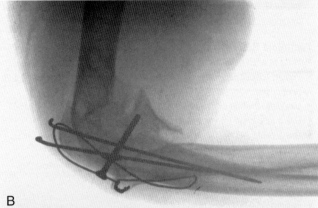

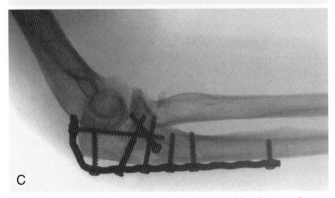

FIGURE 20.14 Failed operative fixation of a posterior olecranon fracture-dislocation. **A,** Type A posterior Monteggia fracture with fractures of the olecranon, coronoid, and radial head. **B,** Internal fixation with a tension band wire construct and a screw proved insufficient. **C,** Revision to a dorsal contoured plate achieved better alignment and more secure fixation. (Copyright © David Ring, MD.)

Failed internal fixation can be salvaged with realignment and repeat internal fixation using a dorsal contoured plate and screws (see Figures 20.14 and 20.15). If there is a bone defect or delayed union, autogenous cancellous bone graft can be applied to the fracture site.

Infection

Infection is unusual after operative treatment of a closed injury and is most often encountered after a complex open injury. In either case, if stable fixation is retained the infection can be treated without implant removal. Adequate soft tissue coverage, serial débridements, and parenteral antibiotics can often eradicate an infection and at a minimum can allow healing to become established before implant removal. For this to be successful, no

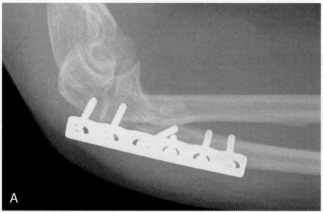

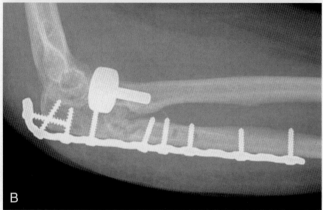

FIGURE 20.15 Plate loosening after operative treatment of a posterior Monteggia fracture. **A,** Posterior Monteggia fractures are common in older, osteoporotic patients. A plate applied to the medial or lateral surface and not contoured around the proximal ulna may have an inadequate hold on the proximal metaphyseal segment. **B,** Revision to a long contoured dorsal plate can achieve better fixation and improve elbow and forearm function. (Copyright © David Ring, MD.)

devitalized tissue can remain in the wound. If there is extensive devitalized tissue, a more thorough débridement and removal of implants may be necessary.

Instability

Elbow instability can occur after posterior olecranon fracture-dislocations and posterior Monteggia fractures.[50] It can result from one or more features, including residual posterior angulation of the proximal ulna with posterior subluxation of the radial head with respect to the capitellum; inadequate restoration of the coronoid or radial head; or lateral collateral ligament injury. Restoration of these factors along with temporary hinged external fixation can usually restore stability. The procedure is addressed more completely in Chapter 23 (Figure 20.16).

Nonunion

Nonunion after simple olecranon fractures is very unusual.[40] Proximal ulna nonunion usually occurs after a fracture-dislocation of the proximal ulna. Union can usually be achieved with contoured dorsal plate fixation and autogenous bone grafting[47,62] (Figure 20.17).

Ulnar Neuropathy

Ulnar neuropathy is an important and increasingly recognized sequel of complex elbow trauma. Patients who struggle with flexion during the postoperative period and have hypersensitivity or complaints of pain greater than expected should be carefully evaluated for symptoms and signs of ulnar neuropathy.

On occasion, a patient who initially is recovering well will lose motion and have increased pain between 4 and 6 weeks after injury concomitant with signs and symptoms of ulnar neuropathy. Patients with this type of subacute ulnar neuropathy might benefit from ulnar nerve release.[19]

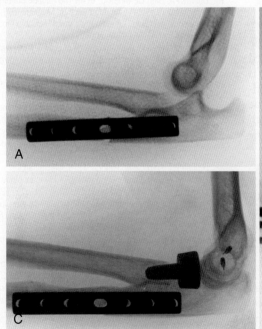

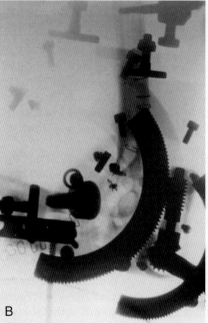

FIGURE 20.16 Ulnohumeral instability after posterior Monteggia fracture. **A,** Surgeons are occasionally surprised by ulnohumeral instability after what was perceived to be a forearm injury; however, posterior Monteggia injuries can include fracture of the radial head and injury to the lateral collateral ligament complex. **B,** Open relocation of the ulnohumeral joint, restoration of radiocapitellar contact with a radial head prosthesis, repair of the lateral collateral ligament complex, and temporary hinged fixation were used to restore stability. **C,** A stable, well-aligned elbow and forearm with good function was achieved. (Copyright © David Ring, MD.)

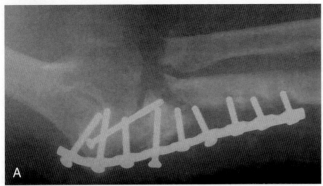

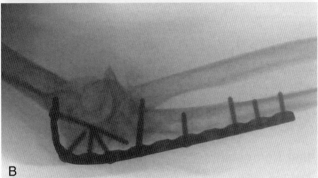

FIGURE 20.17 Nonunion of the proximal ulna. **A,** Nonunion of the proximal ulna is most common after a complex fracture and is uncommon after simple olecranon fracture. This patient has loose internal fixation and a synovial nonunion. **B,** Contoured dorsal plate fixation and autogenous cancellous bone grafting achieved union and improved elbow and forearm function. (Copyright © David Ring, MD.)

Chronic ulnar neuropathy can respond to ulnar nerve release. Even weakness and atrophy can sometimes improve after release, although it may take many years.[35]

Stiffness of Heterotopic Ossification

Stiffness is a very common complication of fractures of the proximal ulna.[2] The ulnar nerve should be carefully evaluated and addressed as just described. If heterotopic ossification is restricting motion, this can be resected as soon as radiographically mature (within 3 to 4 months) as long as the soft tissue envelope is stable and mobile.[30,58] Postoperative irradiation can serve as useful prophylaxis against recurrent heterotopic bone (see Chapter 24).

In the absence of ulnar neuropathy or heterotopic bone, capsular contracture will usually respond to active-assisted elbow mobility exercises. Dynamic or static progressive splints are also very useful in this situation. If nonoperative treatment is unsuccessful, operative capsular excision will restore motion in most patients.

Arthrosis

Severe arthrosis is uncommon after proximal ulnar fractures. With lesser grades of arthrosis, the native elbow will function better than a prosthetic or interpositional arthroplasty and should be maintained as long as possible. Older, infirm patients with severe arthrosis can be treated with semiconstrained total elbow arthroplasty.[32] Healthy active patients with stiffness and pain from arthrosis may be better treated by interpositional arthroplasty.[38]

For Case Studies, Videos, and more, please visit
ExpertConsult.com.

REFERENCES

1. An KN, Morrey BF, Chao EY: The effect of partial removal of proximal ulna on elbow constraint. *Clin Orthop Relat Res* 209:270–279, 1986.
2. Bauer AS, Lawson BK, Bliss RL, et al: Risk factors for posttraumatic heterotopic ossification of the elbow: case-control study. *J Hand Surg [Am]* 37(7):1422–1429, 2012.
3. Berenger-Feraud L, editor: *Des Fractures en V au point de vue de leur gravite et de leur traitement*, Paris, Impr, 1864, Hennuyer.
4. Biga N, Thomine JM: [Trans-olecranal dislocations of the elbow]. *Rev Chir Orthop Reparatrice Appar Mot* 60(7):557–567, 1974.
5. Cage DJ, Abrams RA, Callahan JJ, et al: Soft tissue attachments of the ulnar coronoid process. An anatomic study with radiographic correlation. *Clin Orthop Relat Res* 320:154–158, 1995.
6. Caputo AE, Mazzocca AD, Santoro VM: The nonarticulating portion of the radial head: anatomic and clinical correlations for internal fixation. *J Hand Surg [Am]* 23(6):1082–1090, 1998.
7. Cobb TK, Morrey BF: Use of distraction arthroplasty in unstable fracture dislocations of the elbow. *Clin Orthop Relat Res* 312:201–210, 1995.
8. Cohen MS, Hastings H, 2nd: Rotatory instability of the elbow. The anatomy and role of the lateral stabilizers. *J Bone Joint Surg Am* 79(2):225–233, 1997.
9. Diliberti T, Botte MJ, Abrams RA: Anatomical considerations regarding the posterior interosseous nerve during posterolateral approaches to the proximal part of the radius. *J Bone Joint Surg Am* 82(6):809–813, 2000.
10. Doornberg JN, de Jong IM, Lindenhovius AL, et al: The anteromedial facet of the coronoid process of the ulna. *J Shoulder Elbow Surg* 16(5):667–670, 2007.
11. Doornberg JN, Linzel DS, Zurakowski D, et al: Reference points for radial head prosthesis size. *J Hand Surg [Am]* 31(1):53–57, 2006.
12. Doornberg JN, Parisien R, van Duijn PJ, et al: Radial head arthroplasty with a modular metal spacer to treat acute traumatic elbow instability. *J Bone Joint Surg Am* 89(5):1075–1080, 2007.
13. Doornberg JN, Ring D: Coronoid fracture patterns. *J Hand Surg [Am]* 31(1):45–52, 2006.
14. Doornberg JN, Ring DC: Fracture of the anteromedial facet of the coronoid process. *J Bone Joint Surg Am* 88(10):2216–2224, 2006.
15. Doornberg JN, van Duijn J, Ring D: Coronoid fracture height in terrible-triad injuries. *J Hand Surg [Am]* 31(5):794–797, 2006.
16. Dowdy PA, Bain GI, King GJ, et al: The midline posterior elbow incision. An anatomical appraisal. *J Bone Joint Surg Br* 77(5):696–699, 1995.
17. Duckworth AD, Ring D, Kulijdian A, et al: Unstable elbow dislocations. *J Shoulder Elbow Surg* 17(2):281–286, 2008.
18. Dyer GSM, Ring D: Open treatment of complex traumatic elbow instability. In Lee DH, Neviaser RJ, editors: *Shoulder and elbow surgery: operative techniques*, Philadelphia, 2011, Elsevier.
19. Faierman E, Wang J, Jupiter JB: Secondary ulnar nerve palsy in adults after elbow trauma: a report of two cases. *J Hand Surg [Am]* 26(4):675–678, 2001.
20. Gartsman GM, Sculco TP, Otis JC: Operative treatment of olecranon fractures. Excision or open reduction with internal fixation. *J Bone Joint Surg Am* 63(5):718–721, 1981.
21. Geel CW, Palmer AK, Ruedi T, et al: Internal fixation of proximal radial head fractures. *J Orthop Trauma* 4(3):270–274, 1990.
22. Godlee RJ: *Lord Lister*, London, 1918, Macmillan.
23. Hastings H, 2nd, Engles DR: Fixation of complex elbow fractures. Part II: Proximal ulna and radius fractures. *Hand Clin* 13(4):721–735, 1997.
24. Heim U: [Combined fractures of the radius and the ulna at the elbow level in the adult. Analysis of 120 cases after more than 1 year]. *Rev Chir Orthop Reparatrice Appar Mot* 84(2):142–153, 1998.
25. Hotchkiss RN: Displaced fractures of the radial head: internal fixation or excision? *J Am Acad Orthop Surg* 5(1):1–10, 1997.
26. Hutchinson DT, Horwitz DS, Ha G, et al: Cyclic loading of olecranon fracture fixation constructs. *J Bone Joint Surg Am* 85(5):831–837, 2003.
27. Hwang RW, de Witte PB, Ring D: Compartment syndrome associated with distal radial fracture and ipsilateral elbow injury. *J Bone Joint Surg Am* 91(3):642–645, 2009.
28. Ikeda M, Fukushima Y, Kobayashi Y, et al: Comminuted fractures of the olecranon. Management by bone graft from the iliac crest and multiple tension-band wiring. *J Bone Joint Surg Br* 83(6):805–808, 2001.
29. Jupiter JB, Leibovic SJ, Ribbans W, et al: The posterior Monteggia lesion. *J Orthop Trauma* 5(4):395–402, 1991.
30. Jupiter JB, Ring D: Operative treatment of post-traumatic proximal radioulnar synostosis. *J Bone Joint Surg Am* 80(2):248–257, 1998.

31. Kapandji AI: *The physiology of the joints*, vol I, upper limb, ed 6, St. Louis, 2007, Churchill Livingstone–Elsevier.
32. Lindenhovius A, Karanicolas PJ, Bhandari M, et al: Interobserver reliability of coronoid fracture classification: two-dimensional versus three-dimensional computed tomography. *J Hand Surg [Am]* 34(9):1640–1646, 2009.
33. Macko D, Szabo RM: Complications of tension-band wiring of olecranon fractures. *J Bone Joint Surg Am* 67(9):1396–1401, 1985.
34. Mast J, Jakob R, Ganz R, editors: *Planning and reduction technique in fracture surgery*, Heidelberg, 1989, Springer.
35. McKee MD, Jupiter JB, Bosse G, et al: Outcome of ulnar neurolysis during post-traumatic reconstruction of the elbow. *J Bone Joint Surg Br* 80(1):100–105, 1998.
36. Morrey B, editor: Surgical exposures of the elbow. In *The elbow and its disorders*, Philadelphia, 1995, WB Saunders, pp 16–52.
37. Morrey BF: Current concepts in the treatment of fractures of the radial head, the olecranon, and the coronoid. *Instr Course Lect* 44:175–185, 1995.
38. Morrey BF, Adams RA, Bryan RS: Total replacement for post-traumatic arthritis of the elbow. *J Bone Joint Surg Br* 73(4):607–612, 1991.
39. Morrey BF, An KN: Articular and ligamentous contributions to the stability of the elbow joint. *Am J Sports Med* 11(5):315–319, 1983.
40. Morrey BF, Tanaka S, An KN: Valgus stability of the elbow. A definition of primary and secondary constraints. *Clin Orthop Relat Res* 265:187–195, 1991.
41. Mortazavi SM, Asadollahi S, Tahririan MA: Functional outcome following treatment of transolecranon fracture-dislocation of the elbow. *Injury* 37(3):284–288, 2006.
42. Mouhsine E, Akiki A, Castagna A, et al: Transolecranon anterior fracture dislocation. *J Shoulder Elbow Surg* 16(3):352–357, 2007.
43. O'Driscoll SW: Elbow instability. *Hand Clin* 0(3):405–415, 1994.
44. O'Driscoll SW, Bell DF, Morrey BF: Posterolateral rotatory instability of the elbow. *J Bone Joint Surg Am* 73(3):440–446, 1991.
45. O'Driscoll SW, Jaloszynski R, Morrey BF, et al: Origin of the medial ulnar collateral ligament. *J Hand Surg [Am]* 17(1):164–168, 1992.
46. O'Driscoll SW, Morrey BF, Korinek S, et al: Elbow subluxation and dislocation. A spectrum of instability. *Clin Orthop Relat Res* 280:186–197, 1992.
47. Papagelopoulos PJ, Morrey BF: Treatment of nonunion of olecranon fractures. *J Bone Joint Surg Br* 76(4):627–635, 1994.
48. Pavel A, Pitman JM, Lance EM, et al: The posterior Monteggia fracture: a clinical study. *J Trauma* 5:185–199, 1965.
49. Penrose JH: The Monteggia fracture with posterior dislocation of the radial head. *J Bone Joint Surg Br* 33(1):65–73, 1951.
50. Prayson MJ, Williams JL, Marshall MP, et al: Biomechanical comparison of fixation methods in transverse olecranon fractures: a cadaveric study. *J Orthop Trauma* 11(8):565–572, 1997.
51. Pribyl CR, Kester MA, Cook SD, et al: The effect of the radial head and prosthetic radial head replacement on resisting valgus stress at the elbow. *Orthopedics* 9(5):723–726, 1986.
52. Radin EL, Riseborough EJ: Fractures of the radial head. A review of eighty-eight cases and analysis of the indications for excision of the radial head and non-operative treatment. *J Bone Joint Surg Am* 48(6):1055–1064, 1966.
53. Regan W, Morrey B: Fractures of the coronoid process of the ulna. *J Bone Joint Surg Am* 71(9):1348–1354, 1989.
54. Regan W, Morrey BF: Classification and treatment of coronoid process fractures. *Orthopedics* 15(7):845–848, 1992.
55. Ring D, Doornberg JN: Fracture of the anteromedial facet of the coronoid process. Surgical technique. *J Bone Joint Surg Am* 89(Suppl 2 Pt 2):267–283, 2007.
56. Ring D, Gulotta L, Chin K, et al: Olecranon osteotomy for exposure of fractures and nonunions of the distal humerus. *J Orthop Trauma* 18(7):446–449, 2004.
57. Ring D, Hannouche D, Jupiter JB: Surgical treatment of persistent dislocation or subluxation of the ulnohumeral joint after fracture-dislocation of the elbow. *J Hand Surg [Am]* 29(3):470–480, 2004.
58. Ring D, Jupiter JB: Excision of heterotopic bone around the elbow. *Tech Hand Up Extrem Surg* 8(1):25–33, 2004.
59. Ring D, Jupiter JB: Fracture-dislocation of the elbow. *J Bone Joint Surg Am* 80(4):566–580, 1998.
60. Ring D, Jupiter JB: Operative exposure of fractures of the distal radius. *Tech Hand Up Extrem Surg* 3(4):259–264, 1999.
61. Ring D, Jupiter JB: Reconstruction of posttraumatic elbow instability. *Clin Orthop Relat Res* 370:44–56, 2000.
62. Ring D, Jupiter JB, Gulotta L: Atrophic nonunions of the proximal ulna. *Clin Orthop Relat Res* 409:268–274, 2003.
63. Ring D, Jupiter JB, Sanders RW, et al: Transolecranon fracture-dislocation of the elbow. *J Orthop Trauma* 11(8):545–550, 1997.
64. Ring D, Jupiter JB, Simpson NS: Monteggia fractures in adults. *J Bone Joint Surg Am* 80(12):1733–1744, 1998.
65. Ring D, Jupiter JB, Waters PM: Monteggia fractures in children and adults. *J Am Acad Orthop Surg* 6(4):215–224, 1998.
66. Ring D, Jupiter JB, Zilberfarb J: Posterior dislocation of the elbow with fractures of the radial head and coronoid. *J Bone Joint Surg Am* 84(4):547–551, 2002.
67. Ring D, Quintero J, Jupiter JB: Open reduction and internal fixation of fractures of the radial head. *J Bone Joint Surg Am* 84(10):1811–1815, 2002.
68. Sanchez-Sotelo J, Morrey BF, O'Driscoll SW: Ligamentous repair and reconstruction for posterolateral rotatory instability of the elbow. *J Bone Joint Surg Br* 87(1):54–61, 2005.
69. Schneeberger AG, Sadowski MM, Jacob HA: Coronoid process and radial head as posterolateral rotatory stabilizers of the elbow. *J Bone Joint Surg Am* 86(5):975–982, 2004.
70. Smith GR, Hotchkiss RN: Radial head and neck fractures: anatomic guidelines for proper placement of internal fixation. *J Shoulder Elbow Surg* 5(2 Pt 1):113–117, 1996.
71. Tillmann B: *A contribution to the functional morphology of articular surfaces*, Stuttgart, 1978, PSG.
72. Yamaguchi K, Sweet FA, Bindra R, et al: The extraosseous and intraosseous arterial anatomy of the adult elbow. *J Bone Joint Surg Am* 79(11):1653–1662, 1997.

21

Disorders of the Forearm Axis

Mark E. Baratz

Acknowledgments: I would like to acknowledge Kenneth R. Means, Jr., and Thomas J. Graham for their sixth edition version of this chapter. A special thank you goes to Alexandra Andoga, BS, for her help in the preparation of the seventh edition of this chapter.

FOREARM FUNCTIONAL ANATOMY

The elbow, forearm, and wrist act as a unified structure to provide a stable, strong, and highly mobile unit for positioning the hand in space and for performing load-bearing tasks. Understanding the relevant anatomy and biomechanics is essential for the surgeon who treats disorders of the forearm axis.[135]

The ulna is the primary "load-bearing" bone of the forearm and supports the radius as it rotates during pronation and supination. The ulna is essentially straight and suspends the radius through stabilizing ligaments at the wrist, at the elbow (proximal radioulnar joint [PRUJ]), and in the midshaft. The radius has an anterior bow allowing it to rotate around the ulna. Just proximal to the tuberosity of the radius, the bone is oriented exactly parallel to the axis of rotation of the forearm and lies at a 15-degree angle to the shaft of the radius. This configuration allows the radius to line up and articulate in a congruent fashion at the PRUJ. It is worth noting that malalignment of the PRUJ is relatively well tolerated and does not have much effect on forearm rotation. Conversely, malalignment of the distal radioulnar joint (DRUJ) has a major effect on pronation and supination. This is due to the fact that the distal radius has to swing in three planes to rotate about the ulnar head. The longitudinal axis of forearm rotation passes through the center of the radial head at the elbow and through the fovea of the ulnar head at wrist level (Figure 21.1).[135] This axis is not constant but changes slightly as the radial and ulnar heads shift on their respective articular surfaces during pronation and supination. With pronation the radial head moves into a position that is anterior and medial on the capitellum. With supination the head moves into a position that is lateral and posterior.[44]

Forearm rotation occurs between the radial head and the radial notch of the ulna proximally (PRUJ) and between the ulnar head and the sigmoid notch of the radius distally (DRUJ). These joints act as hemijoints in facilitating forearm rotation. In addition, the component parts of the interosseous membrane (IOM) act to stabilize the radius on the ulna during forearm rotation and loading (as well as presenting an expanded surface from which certain muscles take origin). The IOM has distal, middle, and proximal portions, together constituting an integrated mechanism constraining the relative movements of the radius and ulna. The condensations within the membrane that appear to have the greatest mechanical strength are the distal oblique band, the central and accessory bands, the dorsal oblique accessory cord, and the proximal oblique cord (Figure 21.2).[91] Forearm rotation is a complex motion with rotational and translational elements. Injuries and inflammatory conditions can disrupt the seamless relationship between the forearm structures.[70]

This chapter focuses on pertinent anatomy and biomechanics, as well as operative techniques for adult disorders, including radial shaft fractures, middle and distal ulnar shaft fractures, both-bone fractures of the forearm, removal of radial and ulnar shaft plates, nonunion and malunion of the radius and ulna, radioulnar synostosis, and longitudinal instability of the forearm.

RADIAL SHAFT FRACTURES

General Evaluation and Preoperative Considerations

Fractures of the radial shaft may be isolated or may be more extensive and have significant associated soft tissue involvement, as seen on radiographic views. The unique "bowed" osseous anatomy of the radius, supported between the stable PRUJ and DRUJ, makes it vulnerable to direct trauma through its diaphysis. Transmission of forces created by a fall on the outstretched hand may lead to a global forearm injury. Because of the unique anatomy, any deviation in the spatial orientation of the radius can decrease forearm rotation. Restoration of motion requires acceptable axial and rotational alignment in addition to the maintenance of the radial bow.

The concept of the forearm as a ring helps direct the evaluation and treatment of all forearm fractures. High-energy injuries can disrupt the ligaments supporting the DRUJ or PRUJ. As such, it is judicious to examine the entire extremity. This includes the neurologic and vascular systems.

Imaging should begin with frontal and lateral radiographs of the entire forearm with a low threshold to obtain views of the wrist and elbow.[8,81,122] Computed tomography (CT) or magnetic resonance imaging (MRI) is not typically necessary in the initial assessment of acute forearm shaft fractures. However, imaging with CT can be useful in evaluating the extent of healing following open reduction and plate fixation.

◆ PERTINENT ANATOMY

Neurovascular structures are vulnerable to trauma and to surgical treatment of forearm fractures and dislocations (Figure

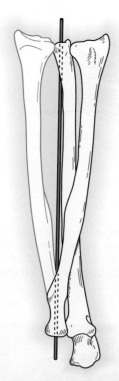

FIGURE 21.1 The axis of rotation for the forearm passes through the center of the radial head proximally and through the ulnar fovea at the base of the ulnar styloid distally.

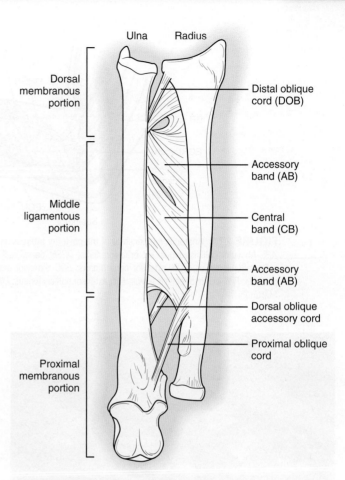

FIGURE 21.2 Diagram of the interosseous membrane (right forearm, anterior aspect). Key features include the distal oblique cord (DOB) that lies within the distal membranous portion and the proximal oblique cord that lies on the anterior surface proximally. The middle ligamentous complex contains the central band (CB) and accessory bands (AB). (Reproduced with permission of Elsevier from Noda K, Goro A, Murase T, et al: Interosseous membrane of the forearm: an anatomical study of ligament. *J Hand Surg [Am]* 34:415–422, 2009.)

21.3). As the radial nerve enters the forearm, it divides into the deep posterior interosseous nerve and the superficial sensory, or dorsal radial sensory, nerve. The posterior interosseous nerve (PIN) passes anterior to the elbow capsule and enters the supinator. The PIN crosses the proximal radius 5 to 6 cm distal to the radiocapitellar joint before exiting the supinator (Figures 21.4 and 21.5). This nerve is particularly vulnerable to injury in this region from trauma or in the course of the surgical exposure of the proximal radius (Figure 21.6). The PIN provides motor fibers, in succession, to the extensor carpi radialis brevis (ECRB), supinator, extensor digitorum communis (EDC), extensor digiti minimi, extensor carpi ulnaris, abductor pollicis longus, extensor pollicis longus (EPL), extensor pollicis brevis (EPB), and extensor indicis proprius. The nerve terminates as a proprioceptive sensory nerve to the wrist. The superficial sensory branch of the radial nerve travels beneath the brachioradialis and emerges between the brachioradialis and extensor carpi radialis longus (ECRL) tendons approximately 8 cm proximal to the radial styloid.[84,108]

After entering the forearm beneath the bicipital aponeurosis, the median nerve travels between the two heads of the pronator teres. The anterior interosseous nerve is a branch that emanates just proximal to the flexor digitorum superficialis (FDS) and then passes between the two heads of this muscle. The median nerve proper continues distally in the forearm between the FDS and flexor digitorum profundus (FDP) until it enters the carpal tunnel, passing beneath the palmaris longus. The palmar cutaneous nerve branches from the median nerve in the distal part of the forearm, approximately 8.5 cm proximal to the distal volar wrist crease. It runs between the flexor carpi radialis and palmaris longus, deep to the forearm fascia. It pierces the fascia approximately 4.5 cm proximal to the volar wrist crease.

The radial and ulnar arteries branch from the brachial artery after it exits beneath the bicipital aponeurosis. The radial artery continues into the forearm beneath the brachioradialis until it reaches the distal end of the forearm, where it immediately becomes a subfascial structure.

Understanding of the osseous morphology of the radius, especially the anterior bow in the diaphysis, helps the surgeon when treating radius fractures or malunions. This is especially true with comminuted fractures and injuries with segmental bone loss. As discussed, the radial bow is crucial to pronation and supination because it allows the radius to rotate about the ulna. The radial bow is assessed on a frontal radiograph with the forearm in neutral rotation, the shoulder abducted 90 degrees, and the elbow flexed 90 degrees. The radial bow can be defined by drawing a line between the radial tuberosity proximally and the most ulnar edge of the radius distally. A perpendicular line is drawn at the point of maximal radial bow, and the length of this line is measured (Figure 21.7).[116]

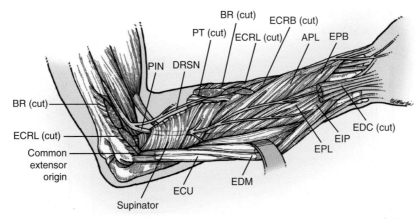

FIGURE 21.3 Anatomic relationships of the posterior interosseous and superficial sensory branches of the radial nerve in the forearm. *APL,* Abductor pollicis longus; *BR,* brachioradialis; *DRSN,* dorsal radial sensory nerve; *ECRB,* extensor carpi radialis brevis; *ECRL,* extensor carpi radialis longus; *ECU,* extensor carpi ulnaris; *EDC,* extensor digitorum communis; *EDM,* extensor digiti minimi; *EIP,* extensor indicis proprius; *EPB,* extensor pollicis brevis; *EPL,* extensor pollicis longus; *PIN,* posterior interosseous nerve; *PT,* pronator teres. (Copyright Elizabeth Martin.)

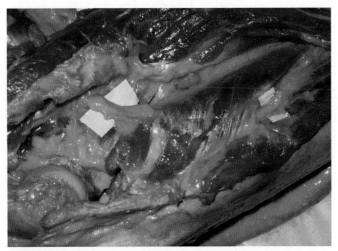

FIGURE 21.4 The posterior interosseous nerve of a right forearm is highlighted with a *light blue background* as it passes through the supinator.

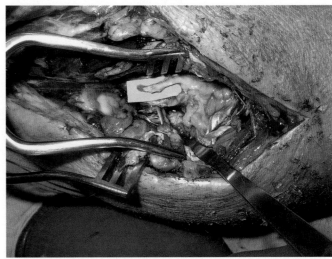

FIGURE 21.6 The posterior interosseous nerve (lying on a *light blue background*) was found to be transected following surgery to treat an elbow fracture-dislocation with a radial head fracture.

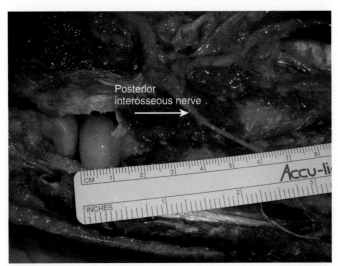

FIGURE 21.5 The posterior interosseous nerve crosses the radius approximately 5 to 6 cm from the radiocapitellar joint.

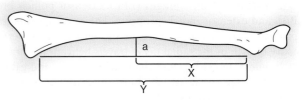

Maximum radial bow
a (mm)
Location of maximum radial bow
X/Y × 100

FIGURE 21.7 Measuring radial bow.

Surgical Approaches for Fractures of the Radial Shaft

Anterior Approach

There are several advantages to the anterior approach to the radial shaft, also known as the "volar approach of Henry." The entire radius may be exposed with this approach, from the radial head proximally to the radial styloid distally. The anterior approach to the radial shaft is indicated for practically any fracture involving the radius. There are well-defined intervals for the exposure that permit hardware to be placed on the anterior surface of the radius while still providing excellent muscle and soft tissue coverage. During the anterior approach, "blind" placement of curved retractors around the proximal radial shaft should be performed, with care taken to avoid injury to the PIN.

The patient is placed supine on the operating room table. A radiolucent arm board is placed under the injured extremity. All potential pressure areas are well padded. General or regional anesthesia is appropriate. Prophylactic intravenous antibiotics are administered when surgical implants are anticipated.[107] A nonsterile tourniquet padded with a cotton roll is applied to the upper part of the operative extremity.

An incision of varying length, determined by the longitudinal extent of the fracture, is made on the anterior and radial aspect of the forearm by using a line extending from the lateral aspect of the distal biceps tendon to the radial styloid (Figure 21.8). The incision is centered on the site of the fracture and extended proximally and distally to allow reduction and fixation without undue retraction on the skin edges or underlying structures. The fascia of the anterior forearm musculature is incised longitudinally, just ulnar to the brachioradialis, which may be seen just deep to the fascia. Once the fascia is opened,

the radial artery can be identified ulnar to the brachioradialis. The interval between the radial artery and the brachioradialis is developed (Figure 21.9), and arterial branches to the brachioradialis are ligated or cauterized. In the distal third of the forearm, the radial artery will be clearly distinct and ulnar to the brachioradialis. More proximally, the radial artery lies deep to the brachioradialis. When mobilizing the brachioradialis radially, the superficial sensory branch of the radial nerve should be identified deep to the brachioradialis and protected. It is mobilized radially with the brachioradialis (Figure 21.10).

Deep dissection differs proximally and distally. In the proximal third of the forearm, the lateral antebrachial cutaneous nerve should be identified and protected as it exits between the brachioradialis and the distal biceps muscle. One should then find the insertion of the biceps tendon. Just lateral to it, there is a small bursa. An incision is made in the bursa (the radial artery at that level is medial and superficial to the biceps tendon, so that dissection is safe lateral to the tendon). It is more difficult to mobilize the brachioradialis radially as it travels obliquely across the forearm. By staying lateral to the distal biceps tendon, the brachioradialis and radial artery are separated. The recurrent branch of the radial artery is usually seen at this level and may need to be divided to allow for adequate exposure. Supination of the forearm reveals the supinator muscle, which is elevated in a subperiosteal plane in an ulnar

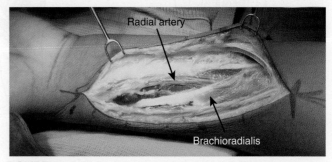

FIGURE 21.9 Clinical photograph demonstrating superficial exposure of the anterior approach to the radius and the anatomic relationships of the radial artery.

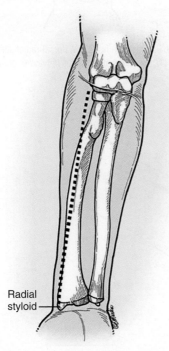

FIGURE 21.8 Incision for the anterior approach to the radial shaft. The length of the incision varies depending on exposure requirements. (Copyright Elizabeth Martin.)

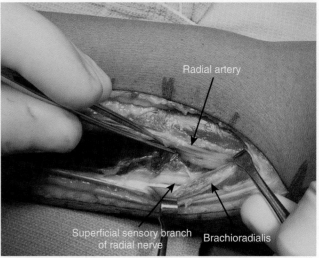

FIGURE 21.10 Clinical photograph demonstrating anatomic relationships of the radial artery, brachioradialis, and superficial sensory branch of the radial nerve.

to radial direction (Figure 21.11). Because the PIN may lie directly on the posterior aspect of the radial shaft at this level, subperiosteal dissection does not necessarily ensure that the nerve has been elevated and is protected. For this reason, the anterior portion of the radius is exposed only in a supinated position. Curved retractors or other tools should not be placed around the posterior aspect of the radial shaft at this level. Once the interval between the brachioradialis and the radial artery is developed, the pronator teres is visualized and divided at its radial insertion. The pronator is elevated in a radial to ulnar direction to expose the radial shaft. In the distal third of the forearm, the interval between the radial artery and the flexor carpi radialis may be used. The flexor pollicis longus and pronator quadratus muscles are dissected off of the radial shaft in a radial to ulnar direction to expose the shaft.

Posterior Approach for Radial Shaft Fixation

The posterior approach to the radial shaft (*Thompson approach*) is used primarily for proximal fractures. This approach requires that the surgeon identify the PIN. The entire radius can be exposed when working between muscle intervals.

The patient is placed supine on the operating table. The arm may be placed on an arm board or across the patient's chest. With the forearm pronated, an incision is made starting just anterior to the lateral epicondyle and proceeding distally toward the middle of the wrist (Figure 21.12). The incision is carried

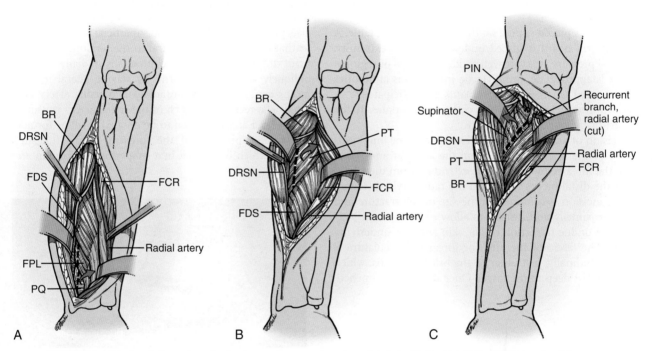

FIGURE 21.11 A to **C,** Deep dissection for the anterior approach to the radial shaft. *BR,* Brachioradialis; *DRSN,* dorsal radial sensory nerve; *FCR,* flexor carpi radialis; *FDS,* flexor digitorum superficialis; *FPL,* flexor pollicis longus; *PIN,* posterior interosseous nerve; *PQ,* pronator quadratus; *PT,* pronator teres. (Copyright Elizabeth Martin.)

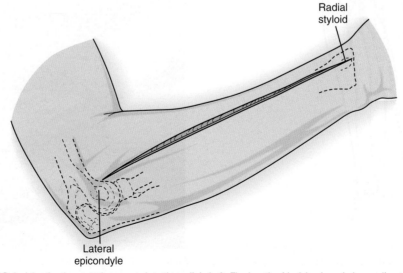

FIGURE 21.12 Incision for the posterior approach to the radial shaft. The length of incision is varied according to exposure needs.

through the subcutaneous tissue. The interval between the ECRB and the EDC is identified and developed (Figure 21.13). Once the incision is deep to those muscles, the supinator is immediately apparent. The radial nerve is within the substance of the muscle and should be dissected, mobilized, and protected. Distally, the abductor pollicis longus and EPB (first extensor compartment muscles) emerge from between the EDC and the ECRB, making the interval more identifiable at this level (Figure 21.14). Immediately deep to the EDC-ECRB interval proximally is the supinator muscle belly. The PIN is identified as it enters the supinator muscle proximally. The nerve is dissected through the length of the supinator by dividing its superficial head. Once the nerve has been identified and protected, the supinator is elevated off of the radial shaft in an anterior to posterior direction. The shaft is now exposed, and reduction and stabilization can proceed. The abductor pollicis longus and EPB cover the radius near the junction of the middle and distal third of the shaft and may be elevated proximally or distally as needed. Distal to this level, the interval is between the ECRB

and the EPL, or it can be shifted between the EPL and EDC if exposure is required more distally.

Fracture Stabilization

Conventional wisdom has suggested that optimal fixation of radial shaft fractures consists of compression plating with a 3.5-mm plate and screws engaging five or six cortices proximal and distal to the fracture ends.[18,124] Recent studies have demonstrated a high union rate (90%) with only four cortices of fixation proximal and distal to the fracture site, but often with supplemental lag screw fixation. In addition, the screws are placed in a near-far/near-far orientation relative to both sides of the fracture site.[24,75] Plates larger than 3.5 mm are not typically used, because of concern for fracture through the screw holes, cross-union of the radius and ulna, or fracture after plate removal.[11]

With regard to locking versus nonlocking plates, the evidence suggests that there is no difference in union rates or clinical outcome between these two implants for most forearm

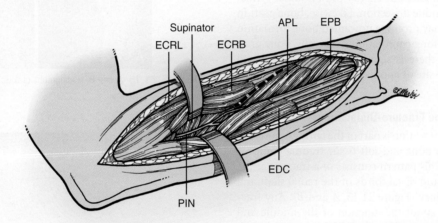

FIGURE 21.13 Superficial muscular intervals for the Thompson posterior approach to the radial shaft. *APL*, Abductor pollicis longus; *ECRB*, extensor carpi radialis brevis; *ECRL*, extensor carpi radialis longus; *EDC*, extensor digitorum communis; *EPB*, extensor pollicis brevis; *PIN*, posterior interosseous nerve. (Copyright Elizabeth Martin.)

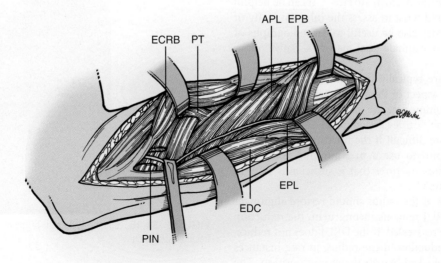

FIGURE 21.14 Distal interval. *APL*, Abductor pollicis longus; *ECRB*, extensor carpi radialis brevis; *EDC*, extensor digitorum communis; *EPB*, extensor pollicis brevis; *EPL*, extensor pollicis longus; *PIN*, posterior interosseous nerve; *PT*, pronator teres. (Copyright Elizabeth Martin.)

fractures.[7] Locking plates may help for fractures with significant comminution when the implant functions as a bridge plate and for fixation of osteoporotic bone.[43,121]

Segmental fractures require longer plates, and their use will necessitate contouring of the plate to maintain an acceptable radial bow. If significant contouring is required, reconstruction-type plates (with scallops along the sides of the plate) may be considered, but these plates are substantially weaker than compression plates. Newer prebent plates with a radial bow contour that do not have this disadvantage are available for long radial shaft fractures. Fractures with significant comminution but without proximal-distal cortical contact may need to be bridged by a plate without compression of the fracture site. In this situation, comparison radiographs from the uninjured forearm may help determine the appropriate length and radial bow.

Bone Grafting

The indications for bone grafting are somewhat controversial. Some studies suggest that grafting of comminuted fractures confers no significant benefit.[4,105,138,140] Application of bone graft should not be indiscriminate. The chance of radioulnar synostosis is increased with undue dissection. Likewise, bone graft in the interosseous space may promote unwanted bone formation that can lead to limited forearm rotation. Generally, bone graft is recommended when there is significant comminution and bone loss at the fracture site of approximately 50% of the bony diameter.

Fixation of Galeazzi-Type Fracture-Dislocations

The Galeazzi fracture-dislocation is part of the family of forearm axis injuries where both bone and soft tissue trauma compromise forearm stability. This pattern consists of a fracture at the junction of the middle and distal thirds of the radial shaft and DRUJ dislocation or injury (Figure 21.15, *A* and *B*). Any fracture of the radial shaft about the junction of the middle and distal thirds should raise suspicion of a DRUJ injury, although isolated shaft fractures remain statistically more common.[106] In one study, radial shaft fractures within 7.5 cm of the distal radial articular surface had a significantly higher likelihood of associated DRUJ instability than did those that were more than 7.5 cm away from the distal articular surface.[103] It can be helpful to examine the uninjured wrist to assess the inherent laxity of the patient's DRUJ. It may also be useful to get radiographs of the uninjured wrist to estimate that patient's native ulnar variance.

Galeazzi fractures are typically fixed with a 3.5-mm plate placed on the anterior aspect of the radius. The plate needs to be bent distally to accommodate the anterior concavity of the radius at the metadiaphyseal level (Figure 21.16). Fixation in this region may be more difficult if the fracture is more distal. In this case, it is helpful to use a precontoured volar plate designed for distal radius fractures that is sufficiently long to span the fracture proximally.

Anatomic reduction of the radius should restore alignment to the DRUJ. If the DRUJ remains incongruent, the reduction of the radius should be reassessed. If the DRUJ does not reduce, in spite of anatomic reduction of the radius, in rare instances the reduction can be blocked by soft tissue interposition. The extensor carpi ulnaris is a common culprit in this setting.[13,16,56] During the operation, one can examine the DRUJ. A "clunk"

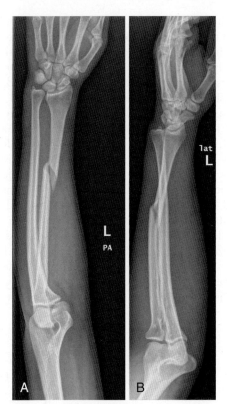

FIGURE 21.15 A and **B,** Radiographs of a Galeazzi fracture-dislocation.

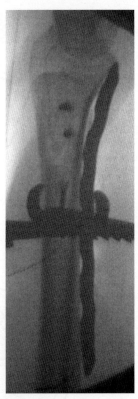

FIGURE 21.16 Lateral radiograph of proposed fixation for a Galeazzi fracture-dislocation.

with passive rotation is evidence of gross instability. Translation of the ulnar head with the forearm in full pronation, neutral rotation, and supination can also be assessed.

If the reduced DRUJ is not stable throughout a full arc of rotation, there are several options. Typically the DRUJ will be more stable in supination and can be immobilized in that position for 3 to 4 weeks. Gross laxity of the DRUJ can be managed with two 0.062-inch smooth Kirschner wires placed proximal to the DRUJ across all four cortices. Having the pin tips exit the radial aspect of the radius and the ulnar aspect of the ulna ensures that all pins can be extracted if the pins break in the interosseous space.

Some surgeons have advocated open or arthroscopic repair of the triangular fibrocartilage complex or open repair of an associated ulnar styloid fracture. In one study, van Duijvenbode and colleagues[130] reviewed the outcome of isolated diaphyseal radius fractures with and without dislocation of the DRUJ. They concluded that anatomic fixation of the radius seemed sufficient without concomitant pinning of the radius to the ulna or repair of the triangular fibrocartilage complex.

Alternative Fixation Methods for Fractures of the Radial Shaft: Intramedullary Rods and External Fixation

The forearm remains the only major diaphyseal segment in which intramedullary fixation is rarely used. Obvious advantages of intramedullary implants in the forearm include minimizing soft tissue stripping, facilitating load sharing, having a low profile design, and reducing the risk of refracture with implant removal.[64] This is particularly true in segmental injuries (Figure 21.17) and instances where the soft tissues have been compromised by severe contusion or burns. Unfortunately, this

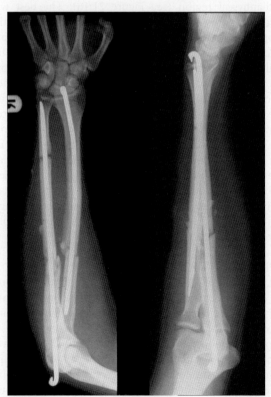

FIGURE 21.17 Intramedullary fixation of radial shaft and segmental ulnar shaft fractures associated with significant blunt soft tissue injury.

technique has been plagued by high rates of nonunion and malunion. There is also a risk of injury to neurovascular structures, especially with proximal locking screws.[125] Locked nails provide increased stability and have union rates that approach or match those of compression plating.[45,137]

One attractive indication for intramedullary nailing is the management of pathologic fractures. This is particularly true for lesions where the diagnosis is known and treatment consists of bone stabilization followed by irradiation.[77]

The contraindications for nailing of forearm fractures include active infection, previous malunion, canal diameter smaller than that of the available implant,[101] and fracture extension to the metaphysis or articular surface.[71]

The evidence for plate versus nail fixation of adult forearm fractures consists mostly of retrospective reviews of closed radius or ulna fractures and those in which bone grafting is deemed unnecessary. Lee and associates[73] reported their experience in 27 patients with 38 fractures using a contoured, locking intramedullary nail (Acumed, Hillsboro, OR). The nail has a proximal interlocking screw and a "paddle tip" to provide rotational stability. In their series, which included seven open fractures, there was one superficial infection and one nonunion. Five nails (13%) were removed, with no refractures. The average Disabilities of the Arm, Shoulder, and Hand (DASH) score was 15 (range, 5 to 61), with 92% of patients obtaining good or excellent results.

Ozkaya and coworkers[95] retrospectively compared results of treatment in 42 patients with diaphyseal forearm fractures. Twenty-two of the fractures were treated with open reduction and plate fixation, and 20 were treated with closed reduction and locked intramedullary nailing. There was no difference in fracture severity between the groups. Three fractures in the plate group were bone grafted; none was grafted in the nail group. All of the fractures healed. The plates were removed in 12 patients (55%), and the nails were removed in 5 patients (25%). There were no significant differences in outcome.

Visna and colleagues[134] reported the results of a prospective study evaluating 80 patients with 115 forearm fractures treated with either plate or nail fixation. There was one refracture following plate removal. There were two cases of incomplete synostosis and two cases of partial migration of the interlocking screw in the nail group. No significant differences in functional outcome were detected.

Finally, external fixation of fractures of the forearm is limited to temporary stabilization of complex forearm injuries and management of segmental defects associated with infection (Figure 21.18, A to C).

❖ AUTHOR'S PREFERRED METHOD OF TREATMENT: Radial Shaft Fractures

Nonoperative treatment is limited to nondisplaced or minimally displaced or angulated shaft fractures and to patients who are too sick to undergo surgical treatment.

The forearm shaft fracture "tool kit" includes 3.5-mm plates with fracture instrumentation, intraoperative fluoroscopy, and a plan for bone graft if necessary (autograft, allograft, or a bone graft substitute). The anterior approach is used for all fractures of the radius except for proximal fractures involving the radial head and/or neck that extend to the radial tuberosity. In those instances we prefer the Thompson approach. Periosteal

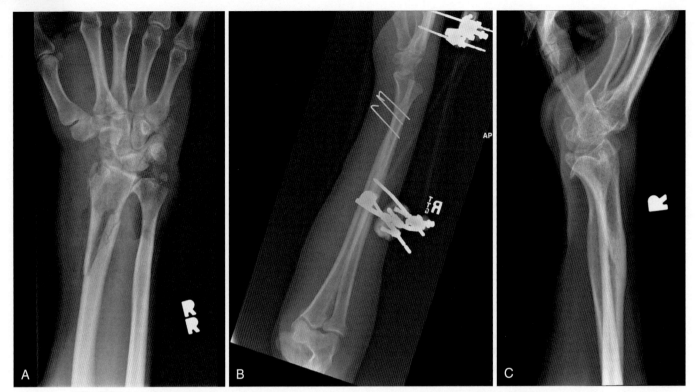

FIGURE 21.18 A to **C,** Radiographs of a patient seen in delayed fashion with a grossly contaminated distal forearm and wrist crush injury with open fractures. External fixation plus limited internal fixation was used to provide adequate initial stability to allow soft tissue and radial shaft fracture healing.

elevation is limited to the fracture site. Reduction clamps are used to grasp the shaft of the radius and raise the bone ends sufficiently to clean the fractured surfaces. Spiral and long oblique components of the fracture can be fixed with 2.7-mm lag screws and neutralized with a 3.5-mm compression plate. Transverse fractures will often interdigitate and simplify the reduction and stabilization. Short oblique fractures can be "slippery" and therefore more challenging. One can gain control of one end of the fracture by first contouring the plate replicating the radial bow and then securing this to either the proximal or the distal fragment with a single screw. Fluoroscopy is used to confirm reduction, restoration of the radial bow, and hardware position. We still strive to secure six cortices on either side of the fracture (Figure 21.19, *A* and *B*).

In instances where there is severe comminution, a "bridge plate" can be precontoured to span the defect. It is as important to re-create the correct location of maximal bow as it is to re-create the amount of maximal bow.[116] Transverse or short oblique fractures can usually be fixed with straight plates while maintaining the radial bow. It is considered safe to use a straight plate even if the radial or ulnar edge of the plate is slightly off the bone proximally or distally (as long as the screw purchase is not compromised). Plates used for longer fractures will need to be contoured. In these cases, it may be helpful to have a radiograph of the contralateral, uninjured forearm. Rotational alignment of the radius can be checked by comparing the proximal bicipital tuberosity with the distal radial styloid on a fully supinated radiograph. With an anatomic reduction, the tuberosity and styloid should be seen in profile and facing in opposite directions, that is, ulnarly and radially, respectively. With more

distal shaft fractures, an anterior bend may need to be placed in the plate to match the anterior flare of the radius in the metadiaphyseal region (see Figure 21.16). The best way to ensure re-creation of an adequate radial bow and restoration of appropriate rotational and angular alignment is to check passive rotation after provisional fixation. With full forearm rotation, it is likely that near-normal relationships have been restored.

As mentioned above, the role of bone grafting is somewhat controversial. We use bone grafting in fractures in which contact at the fracture site is 50% or less. Most commonly, cancellous autograft is harvested from either the iliac crest or the proximal tibia. The olecranon process of the ulna and the distal radius (in proximal fractures) are other options. Compressed cancellous autograft is also used for significant gaps with stable fixation. If fracture fixation is tenuous, intercalary corticocancellous grafting using the iliac crest can be considered to augment stability. Locking plates are useful in this setting and may obviate the need for structural bone graft.

Postoperative Management and Expectations

Hand stiffness and loss of forearm supination are among the most common complications of forearm trauma. A nonconstrictive dressing will help facilitate free finger motion. Immediate forearm rotation should be possible in most cases after fixation. Immobilization is typically limited to short-arm immobilization in a lightweight splint for comfort and support. Weight bearing, strengthening, and static progressive splinting are deferred until there is radiographic evidence of union. Long-arm immobilization for approximately 4 weeks is typical for patients with a Galeazzi fracture when there was instability

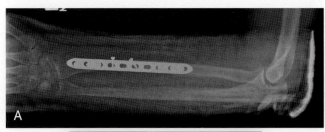

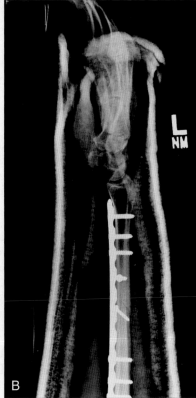

FIGURE 21.19 **A** and **B,** Posteroanterior and lateral radiographs of the DRUJ after anatomic reduction and fixation of the radial shaft in a Galeazzi fracture-dislocation.

CRITICAL POINTS *Anterior Approach for Plate Fixation of the Radial Shaft*

- Maintain a superficial interval between the brachioradialis and radial artery/flexor carpi radialis.
- Protect the dorsal radial sensory nerve beneath the brachioradialis.
- The deep interval is dependent on the proximal-distal level of the fracture.
- Use interfragmentary compression techniques (lag screws or compression plating, or both) when possible.
- Use intraoperative fluoroscopy to confirm adequate reduction and hardware placement.
- Ensure adequate passive pronation-supination after reduction and provisional fixation.

---

of the DRUJ. These patients are given a short-arm splint for 2 weeks thereafter and closely monitored for residual instability.

Union rates for uncomplicated radial shaft fractures are in excess of 95%.[30,32,48,52,121] Morrey and associates[87] defined the functional arc of forearm rotation as 50 degrees of supination and 50 degrees of pronation. This should be easily achievable

in most shaft fractures. Ultimate forearm rotation will vary with the severity of the associated soft tissue injury and the time to union. Droll and coworkers[32] noted a "moderate reduction" in the strength of the forearm, wrist, and hand.

EXPECTED OUTCOMES *Anterior Approach for Plate Fixation of the Radial Shaft*

- Near-anatomic reduction with stable fixation
- Greater than 95% union rates
- Excellent hand motion and a functional arc of forearm rotation
- Mild to moderate loss of forearm strength

Complications

Most of the untoward consequences of forearm shaft fractures are the result of soft tissue damage from the energy dissipated by the injury. In its wake lie damaged muscle, bruised or cut tendons, damaged nerves, and a swollen limb. Appropriate treatment can minimize but not eliminate the effects of this initial insult to the arm. Higher-energy injuries carry higher risks of nonunion, malunion, and residual stiffness.

DISTAL AND MIDSHAFT ULNAR FRACTURES

Preoperative Evaluation

Isolated distal and midshaft ulnar fractures are most often a result of direct trauma. One should always be wary of possible associated injuries to the wrist, forearm, and elbow. In isolation, the so-called *nightstick fracture* follows a blow to the subcutaneous border of the ulna. Closed distal and midshaft ulnar fractures can be treated successfully with nonoperative methods, such as functional bracing or short-arm casting, when the displacement or angulation is minimal.[3,6,23,46,115] A recent Cochrane review[54] included three trials comparing various methods of nonoperative treatment for isolated diaphyseal fractures of the middle and distal thirds of the ulna in adults. The review concluded that there was no evidence that immobilization of the elbow provided short-term benefit in terms of pain relief or fracture union compared with casts or braces that immobilized only the forearm. Van Leemput and colleagues[132] reviewed a total of 102 patients who were treated with a compression bandage (n = 34), a short-arm cast for 6 weeks (n = 36), or a long-arm cast for 3 weeks followed by a short-arm cast for 3 additional weeks (n = 32). At 12 weeks of follow-up, there was no significant difference in the incidence of delayed union, time to fracture union, mean pain scores, or range of motion among the three groups.

The ideal treatment of these fractures, regardless of the degree of displacement, has yet to be determined.[53] Displaced fractures with more than 10 degrees of angulation or 50% displacement are considered candidates for operative treatment.[15,100] It has been suggested that displacement of more than 50% indicates that at least partial disruption of the IOM is present.[35,94]

⬛ PERTINENT ANATOMY

The ulna is the stable post of the forearm. The radius rotates about the ulna to allow a functional arc of forearm rotation.[100] In the distal and midshaft portions, the ulna is essentially straight. The midshaft region has a narrow apex adjacent to the

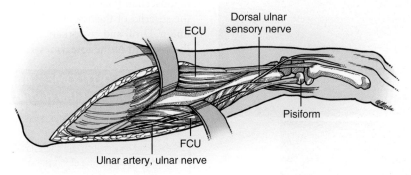

FIGURE 21.20 Pertinent anatomy relative to the surgical approach to the ulna. Note the proximity of the ulnar neurovascular structures to the incision and deep dissection and, in particular, the course of the ulnar sensory nerve through the "ulnar snuffbox." *ECU,* Extensor carpi ulnaris; *FCU,* flexor carpi ulnaris. (Copyright Elizabeth Martin.)

subcutaneous border, which makes direct ulnar placement of a plate more difficult. The ulna is triangular through most of the diaphysis, with a sharp radial border serving as the origin of the interosseous ligament. This morphologic picture affords a relatively flat volar surface where the ulna is also relatively wide, making it well suited for longitudinal implants. Volar placement also provides better soft tissue coverage, better matching of the undersurface plate structure with the underlying bone structure, and, theoretically, minimization of the need for future plate removal due to plate prominence.

The ulnar nerve and artery lie deep to the flexor carpi ulnaris muscle belly in the proximal part of the forearm and are radial and deep to its tendon. The dorsal ulnar sensory nerve may exit the deep forearm fascia anywhere from 1 to 4 cm proximal to the ulnar styloid. It courses though the "ulnar snuffbox" in a proximal volar to distal dorsal direction[84] (Figure 21.20).

Surgical Alternatives for Fractures of the Ulnar Shaft

Direct Ulnar Approach for Distal and Midshaft Ulnar Fixation

The main advantage of this approach is the ease of exposing the entirety of the ulna. Disadvantages are a potential difficulty with soft tissue coverage of the bone and implants along the subcutaneous border of the ulna.

Plate Fixation for Ulnar Shaft Fractures

The principles of plate fixation for ulnar shaft fractures are identical to those of radial shaft fractures, as outlined above. Locking plates have not been shown to improve clinical or biomechanical results for isolated, uncomplicated fractures of the ulna.[4,140] Segmental fractures and those with extensive comminution may require "bridge" plating and the use of supplemental autogenous bone grafting or bone graft substitutes. In these situations, locked plating systems may be useful.[4,105] Plates are ideally placed anterior to the subcutaneous border of the ulna to minimize plate prominence.

Intramedullary Rods for Ulnar Shaft Fractures

There has been renewed interest in intramedullary nail fixation of displaced forearm fractures. Early reports were disappointing, with high rates of nonunion.[112] It is easier to use intramedullary devices for the ulna than for the radius because of the

significant bow in the radius that must be re-created when stabilizing fractures.[27] Nails may be helpful, especially for segmental fractures.[45] Further comparative studies are needed to define the risk-benefit ratio of intramedullary fixation.

Preoperative Planning

Because isolated ulnar shaft fractures do not typically require contouring of the plate, special instrument sets and substantial preoperative planning to include contralateral imaging are not generally necessary. The ulna is primarily a cortical bone and small in caliber, so the use of supplemental bone graft is a key consideration, especially for comminuted fractures or those with bone loss.

❖ AUTHOR'S PREFERRED METHOD OF TREATMENT: Direct Ulnar Approach for Plate Fixation of Distal and Midshaft Ulnar Fractures

Operating on the ulna can be facilitated by suspending the hand in a wrist arthroscopy traction tower. An incision of appropriate length is made along the subcutaneous border of the ulna. If the incision is over the distal third of the ulna, the dorsal cutaneous branches of the ulnar nerve should be protected. This superficial sensory nerve is typically distal enough to be considered out of the operative field for the majority of forearm injuries; it may exit the deep forearm fascia anywhere from approximately 1 to 4 cm proximal to the ulnar styloid. The nerve courses in a proximal volar to distal dorsal direction and crosses the midaxis of the hand-forearm unit between the ulnar styloid and the base of the fifth metacarpal.[84] In the rare case when ulnar styloid fixation is required, the nerve must be identified and protected.

The interval between the ulnar-innervated flexor carpi ulnaris and the PIN-innervated extensor carpi ulnaris is developed. Distally, it is easier to identify this interval and rapidly expose the periosteum surrounding the ulna. As dissection proceeds proximally, the extensor carpi ulnaris is elevated dorsally. The periosteum is opened only near the fracture site, and the fracture is cleaned. Standard fixation principles are applied, depending on the orientation of the fracture (e.g., transverse, short oblique, long oblique, comminuted). Transverse and short oblique fractures are fixed with compression plating, typically with five or six cortices of fixation proximal and distal to the fracture.

We prefer placing the plate on the anterior surface of the ulna. Long oblique fractures may be amenable to interfragmentary lag screw fixation using the plate for neutralization. For fractures with comminution, if the fragments are large enough, they may first be fixed with small lag screws and then the comminution can be spanned with a neutralization plate. If the comminution is more severe, the fragments may be left with their periosteal sleeve intact and bridged with a plate. Alternatively, if the fragments have significant soft tissue stripping and are unlikely to heal, they may be removed and the fracture gap bone-grafted and bridged with a plate. The bone graft may be cancellous bone or a corticocancellous structural supporting graft when segmental bone loss compromises the stability of the fracture-plate construct. With locking plates as previously noted, structural bone graft may not be needed. After provisional fracture fixation, clinical and radiographic alignments are checked. It is important to visualize the fracture, the length of the ulna (usually best judged at the DRUJ), and the elbow and wrist to ensure that anatomic relationships have been restored.

CRITICAL POINTS *Plate Fixation of Distal and Midshaft Ulnar Fractures*

- Maintain the interval between the extensor carpi ulnaris and flexor carpi ulnaris.
- Protect the dorsal ulnar sensory nerve up to 4 cm proximal to the ulnar styloid.
- Use interfragmentary compression techniques (lag screws or compression plating, or both).
- Ensure adequate passive wrist and elbow range of motion after provisional fixation.
- Check the ulnar length relative to the radius at the wrist.

Postoperative Management and Expectations

If stable fixation is achieved in the operating room, early motion is instituted. In 7 to 10 days the surgical dressing and splint are removed and replaced with a long-wrist splint or clamshell brace. Union is expected in at least 95% of cases, and a nearly normal range of motion is typically achieved in all but complex injuries.[23] Patients are typically protected from sports and heavy use until there is evidence of radiographic consolidation.

EXPECTED OUTCOMES *Ulnar Approach for Plate Fixation of the Ulnar Shaft*

- Nearly anatomic reduction is achieved with stable fixation.
- High union rates are seen (>90% to 95% for uncomplicated fractures).
- Nearly normal pronation-supination and flexion-extension of the wrist and elbow are achieved.
- There is minor loss of strength without functional deficit.

Complications

Infection may occur after surgical treatment. This is more common in open injuries. Failure to achieve anatomic or nearly anatomic alignment of the ulna may cause incongruity and instability of the PRUJ or DRUJ, or both. This may be more frequent when considerable bone defects are encountered. Malunion and nonunion may be a result of the severity of the injury, unstable fixation, or excessive load in the postoperative period.

FRACTURES OF BOTH BONES OF THE FOREARM

Preoperative Evaluation

Preoperative evaluation of patients with both-bone forearm fractures begins with understanding that higher-energy trauma is typically required to produce this injury. The workup should be tailored to the mechanism of injury. For example, an isolated blow to the forearm does not require a general trauma evaluation. However, a fall from a height or a motor vehicle collision does require a more comprehensive evaluation. The skin envelope must be examined for skin breaks, particularly on the anterior and ulnar aspects of the forearm. The elbow and wrist are examined for tenderness and joint stability.[16] Pulses, nerve function, and compartment turgor are documented.[2,96]

Radiographs of the wrist, full forearm, and elbow are helpful in these injuries. In highly comminuted or segmental fractures, radiographs of the contralateral forearm can aid in preoperative planning and intraoperative confirmation of appropriate fracture reduction.

❖ **AUTHOR'S PREFERRED METHOD OF TREATMENT:** **Anterior Approach for Radial Shaft Fixation and Direct Ulnar Approach for Ulnar Shaft Fixation**

An anterior approach to the radius and exposure along the subcutaneous border of the ulna are the workhorses for the majority of both-bone fractures. Open fractures, even Gustilo and Anderson grade IIIA fractures, can be treated with immediate internal fixation.[52,65,83,84] Grades IIIB and IIIC open fractures are associated with worse outcomes when treated with immediate plating, although optimal treatment has not been determined for these most difficult injuries.[34] Open fractures of the radial and ulnar shafts require irrigation and débridement of contaminated or devitalized tissue, including bone. Significant soft tissue injuries may require repeat operative débridement prior to bone grafting. Only in rare instances is immediate plate fixation not advisable.

For both closed and open fractures, separate approaches to the radius and ulna help decrease the chance of a synostosis.[9,55] We typically expose both bones first and then reduce and fix the radius, followed by reduction and fixation of the ulna. If one bone is comminuted, the fracture with less comminution is reduced first. The IOM and DRUJ/PRUJ may then help with indirect reduction of the other more severely comminuted bone.[102,113,116] Fractures that are transverse and at different levels can be challenging to reduce once one of the fractures is plated. In these cases, it may be easier to reduce both prior to plating either one.

Intraoperative fluoroscopy is particularly helpful when there is comminution of both the radius and ulna. With the forearm in full supination, a frontal view should show the bicipital tuberosity and the radial styloid pointing in opposite directions

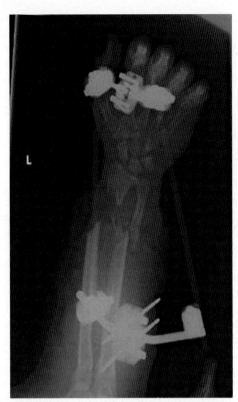

FIGURE 21.21 Radiograph of a both-bone forearm fracture with significant bone loss associated with the radial fracture. (Courtesy of Leon Nesti, MD, and Walter Reed Army Medical Center.)

(in an ulnar direction and a radial direction, respectively). The ulnar styloid should be seen in the center of the ulnar head. With the forearm in full supination, the bicipital tuberosity should not be visible on a true lateral view of the forearm. With forearm supination, the ulnar styloid should appear dorsal to the dorsal cortex of the distal radius on a lateral view of the wrist. Once clinical and radiographic assessment confirms appropriate reduction, definitive fixation of both bones is completed.

The ulnar wound is usually closed to ensure coverage of the fracture and hardware. The radial wound may be closed if there is no undue tension. When the forearm is swollen and the anterior wound cannot be closed, it can be managed with a wound vacuum. A less expensive option is the use of staples along the skin edges and a vessel loop threaded through the staples like a shoelace. The vessel loop can be subsequently tightened as the swelling subsides until the wound is narrow enough for healing by secondary intention or a return to the operating room for delayed primary closure. Fractures with significant bone loss may require bone grafting as part of the index procedure (Figure 21.21). See the Author's Preferred Methods for Radial Shaft Fractures.

Postoperative Management and Expectations

With anatomic reduction and rigid fixation of both-bone forearm fractures, patients can expect a union rate of 95% or greater and functional forearm rotation.[30,32,48,52,121] A moderate amount of objective strength loss is expected, although it is not necessarily perceived as functionally limiting by patient-rated

outcome measures such as the DASH questionnaire and the short-form health survey, 36 items (SF-36).[32,47]

EXPECTED OUTCOMES *Plate Fixation of Both-Bone Forearm Fractures*

- Anatomic reduction with stable fixation if minimal comminution exists
- High union rates (>95% for uncomplicated fractures)
- Nearly normal pronation-supination and flexion-extension of the wrist and elbow
- Minor loss of strength without functional deficit

If stable fixation is achieved intraoperatively, early range of motion may be implemented. This usually consists of flexion-extension and pronation-supination of the elbow and wrist once pain and soft tissue swelling have eased enough to allow these motions. After sufficient range of motion has been achieved and clinical and radiographic evidence has confirmed continued fracture stability, strengthening is initiated. This typically occurs at 6 to 8 weeks postoperatively. Once strength is more than 50% to 75% of the uninvolved side, resumption of normal activities is permitted. We allow patients to resume noncontact athletic activities after they have achieved this milestone and at least 3 months has elapsed since the surgery date. Contact sports are allowed in the 3- to 6-month range with use of a playing splint or brace, if feasible, and patients are permitted to play without a brace after 6 months.

Potential complications specific to these injuries include malunion, nonunion, synostosis, and compartment syndrome. Specific treatment of nonunion, malunion, and synostosis is detailed later.

REMOVAL OF HARDWARE FROM THE RADIUS AND ULNA

There is little evidence to support routine removal of forearm hardware in an asymptomatic patient. It was initially thought that plates should be removed because of concern for later insufficiency fractures as a result of stress shielding by stainless steel plates with their high modulus of elasticity.[24,88,90] Studies have shown a higher-than-expected rate of fracture after plate removal.[24,29,60,111] Some evidence suggests that the decrease in bone density beneath stiff plates resolves in approximately 2 years after insertion.[110] There is also a lower fracture rate after the removal of smaller, less stiff plates such as one-third tubular plates.[10] However, the higher incidence of nonunion and malunion associated with such plates outweighs the benefits of a decreased fracture rate after removal.[52] There is evidence to show that the use of plates of 4.5 mm or larger is associated with an unacceptably higher rate of fracture but does not confer a significant improvement in the union rate when compared with systems of 3.5 mm.[24,116]

The major concern with hardware removal remains refracture at the original fracture site or occasionally through one of the vacated screw holes.[74,82] It would be rare for a fracture to occur at a site either proximal or distal to the previously applied plate, but off-center screw application (i.e., a transcortical screw) may cause enough increased stress to precipitate refracture.

Infection and nerve complications are possible consequences of plate and screw removal.[24,72] If a patient is complaining of pain as a reason to consider hardware removal, the surgeon must determine whether there are other causes, including infection, nonunion, or malunion. CT scanning or fluoroscopic examination may assist in determining whether union has truly been achieved. Inspecting the screw holes carefully for evidence of lucency may indicate whether there is micromotion or infection.

The subcutaneous positioning of an ulnar plate and screws has a higher potential for causing skin and soft tissue irritation. It is rare for the radial shaft hardware itself to cause direct tissue irritation unless the screws are too long. Some authors believe that hardware should be removed if the patient is resuming contact or high-energy sports or other activities, whereas others do not.[116] Military service or other specialized vocations may require removal of metallic implants.

The ideal time for removal of hardware, as well as the duration of restrictions after hardware removal, is also controversial because refracture occurs most often 6 months or longer after plate removal.[59] From our experience and a review of the literature, we typically recommend that hardware remain in place unless there are specific requirements for removal. If removal is necessary, we prefer to wait 1 year or longer after implantation.[10]

Preoperative radiographs for hardware removal should include frontal, lateral, and oblique views to look for radiolucency at the initial fracture site.[82,117] If there is a question regarding fracture consolidation, a CT scan may be helpful. After plate removal, any hypertrophic bone around the plate or screw margins is removed until it is smooth, without violating the native cortex. Immediate range of motion is permitted while wearing a protective splint for sleep and activities for 6 weeks. If at 6 weeks patients have no pain or tenderness and radiographs confirm complete healing at the fracture site, patients are allowed to return to activities as tolerated.[121] Patients are counselled that there is always a chance for refracture or a new fracture in the area where hardware had been placed previously.

NONUNION AND MALUNION OF THE RADIAL AND ULNAR SHAFTS

Preoperative Evaluation

Loss of forearm rotation and the presence of wrist pain from malalignment are common presenting complaints of a patient with malunion of the radius or ulna (Figure 21.22).[20,78,89,92,114,126] The individual with an ununited fracture will have the added issue of pain at the nonunion site. Surgical treatment is dictated on the basis of clinical and radiographic findings. Pain, tenderness, and radiolucency at the fracture site are concerning for delayed union or nonunion. Screw loosening and plate fracture are obvious signs and nearly always require operative intervention. Isolated nonunion of the ulna occurs most commonly in the middle third.[46,94] Most forearm nonunions are atrophic or oligotrophic.[104] Hypertrophic nonunion is more common in fractures treated nonoperatively or with intramedullary devices. Hypertrophic nonunion of the radius or ulna may be treated with compression plating alone. Although some recommend

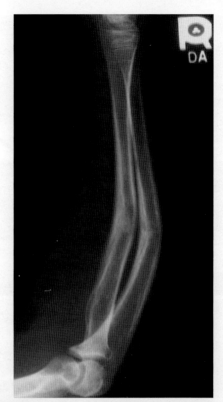

FIGURE 21.22 Malunion of a both-bone forearm fracture.

that autogenous bone graft should be applied at the nonunion site, it is typically not necessary in the hypertrophic setting.[109]

Preoperative evaluation includes an assessment of the soft tissue envelope of the forearm with an eye toward scar contractures and signs of chronic infection. Motion and stability of the elbow, forearm, and wrist are documented. Although bone alignment can typically be corrected, extensive soft tissue contractures may preclude a favorable outcome. Several studies have suggested that the length of time from the initial injury is inversely correlated with the chance of successful correction of malunion and directly correlated with the complication rate.[129,131]

Preoperative radiographs should include views of the elbow and forearm and a true PA view of the wrist to establish ulnar variance. The PA view is obtained with the shoulder abducted 90 degrees, the elbow flexed 90 degrees, and the forearm in neutral rotation (the so-called *zero rotation series*).[38] Contralateral images of an uninvolved forearm may be helpful. CT scans can be helpful to confirm union at the fracture site, document infection, or help characterize angular and rotational malunion.[12,69]

A recent study using fluoroscopy and cross-sectional MRI to assess forearm mechanics in healthy volunteers found a normal side-to-side variation in torsion profile of 20 degrees for the ulna and 35 degrees for the radius. The authors recommend considering derotational osteotomy only if the difference in the contralateral forearm exceeds these parameters.[33]

The possibility of chronic infection as a cause of nonunion is best considered prior to surgery, particularly when the initial injury was open. The preoperative workup can include a complete blood count, erythrocyte sedimentation rate, and

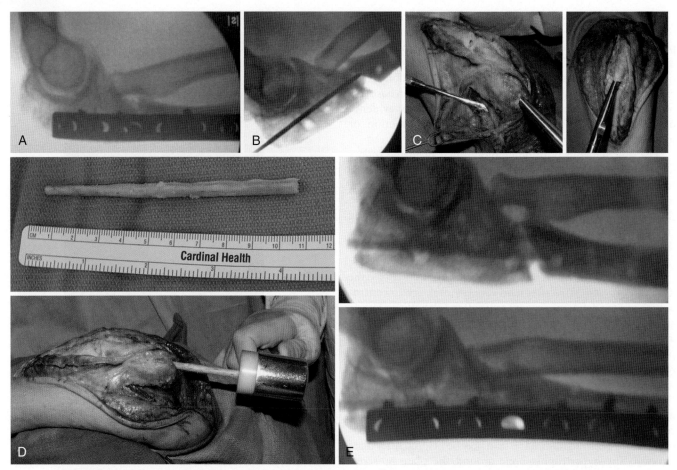

FIGURE 21.23 A, Initial radiographs of recalcitrant proximal ulna nonunion. **B,** Intraoperative fluoroscopic study of intramedullary preparation of the proximal ulnar shaft. **C,** Intraoperative photographs demonstrating preparation of the ulnar canal. **D,** Intraoperative photograph of a fibular allograft strut fashioned and being driven proximally to distally down the ulnar canal. **E,** Initial radiograph showing intramedullary fibular allograft peg fixation followed by manual compression of the proximal and distal ulnar fragments along the allograft peg, plate and screw fixation, and cancellous bone grafting.

quantitative C-reactive protein levels. MRI and a triple-phase bone scan with indium-tagged white blood cells may be useful. Unfortunately, the results of imaging studies are unlikely to change the surgical algorithm. What is most important is preparing a strategy in the event that osteomyelitis is encountered at the time of surgery. This includes a frank discussion with the patient and family that the procedure may need to be staged. On the day of surgery, preoperative antibiotics should be held until cultures are obtained, along with gram-stained smears for bacteria and fungal elements and tissue for assessment of white blood cells per high-power field. The laboratory may be unable to verify to the surgeon's satisfaction that an infection is present. In some cases, if the fracture site does not look healthy, one can débride all necrotic tissue and bone, provide temporary stabilization of the bone, and place an antibiotic-impregnated cement spacer. Empirical treatment with intravenous antibiotics should be initiated. Reconstruction of the defect can proceed if available cultures are negative or after a course of intravenous antibiotics if an infection is confirmed.

In a setting of nonunion, compression of the bone ends is the goal, but this must be balanced with the need to maintain appropriate bone length. As with acute fractures, sufficient radial bow and a straight ulna must be restored to maximize stability and the arc of pronation-supination. The nonunion is most commonly stabilized with 3.5-mm compression plates.

The range of choices for bridging gaps in forearm nonunions includes compressed cancellous autograft, corticocancellous autograft, vascularized bone transfer, and allograft.[22,28,39,67,85,86,88,100,109,120,139] (Figures 21.23 and 21.24).

❖ AUTHOR'S PREFERRED METHOD OF TREATMENT: Open Reduction and Internal Fixation of Nonunion of the Radius or Ulna

There is a spectrum of nonunions of the forearm, ranging from hypertrophic nonunion in a young, healthy patient to failure of fixation following an open, high-energy injury with the possibility of osteomyelitis. For the more complex injuries, treatment begins with an earnest discussion with the patient and family regarding the challenges they face. As discussed, the procedure may have to be staged, achieving union may be difficult, and there is a high likelihood of residual forearm dysfunction. Patients have to quit smoking or chewing tobacco. Their nutritional status is optimized. Consent is obtained for autogenous graft from either the iliac crest, the proximal tibia, or a free-vascularized fibula in rare cases. The CT scan is the single best preoperative imaging tool; it can define the location of the

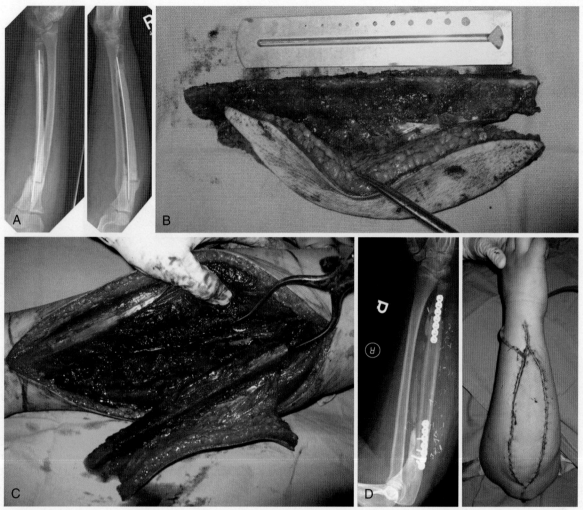

FIGURE 21.24 A, Initial radiographs of a long ulnar shaft defect secondary to osteomyelitis previously treated by resection and insertion of the antibiotic-impregnated cement spacer seen here. **B,** Clinical photograph of an osseoseptocutaneous free fibula flap. **C,** Clinical photograph of inset of the free fibular flap. **D,** Radiograph and clinical photograph after internal fixation and wound closure.

nonunion and the quality of the adjacent bone, and it may show reactive bone consistent with osteomyelitis.

The nonunion tool kit includes a 3.5-mm compression plating system, an external fixator, Steinmann pins, antibiotic-impregnated cement, and osteotomes and curets for obtaining bone graft. After exposing the fracture site, loose hardware, devitalized bone, and tissue are débrided. Multiple cultures are taken, and tissue is sent for quantification of the white blood cells per high-power field. If infection is suspected, the bone is stabilized with an external fixator or, more simply, with a Steinmann pin cut slightly longer than the defect. The pin is wrapped in antibiotic-impregnated cement, and a tip of the pin on either end is left free. Once the cement is hard, the pin-cement construct is keyed into either end of the proximal and distal bone. The wound is closed and a splint is applied. While awaiting cultures, empirical treatment with intravenous antibiotics is initiated. Treatment thereafter is based on the results of culture.

Once it is deemed safe to proceed with reconstruction, the site is again débrided and multiple specimens are sent for culture a second time. Most cases are managed with bridge plating using a 3.5-mm compression plate with eight cortices distally and eight cortices proximally. Locking implants are

useful in this setting. If the construct is stable, the gap is filled with cancellous autograft that is compressed in a syringe and laid into the defect. Using this technique, Ring and coworkers[104] reported a 100% union rate in 35 patients with atrophic nonunion of the forearm diaphysis. If the construct is not stable after using the bridge plate, stability may be enhanced by placing an intercalary corticocancellous iliac crest graft. For recalcitrant nonunions, a free-vascularized fibula may be required to span the defect and obtain union.

Rotational or Angular Osteotomies for Malunion of the Radius or Ulna

Templating of the malunion from normal contralateral forearm radiographs is helpful for preoperative planning. If rotational malunion is suspected, a CT scan with both forearms in maximal pronation and supination may aid in determining the degree of correction required.[57] Three-dimensional reconstructions of these scans can aid in visualization of the true plane of deformity. Plastic bone models derived from CT scans of malunited forearm fractures have been used to design a prebent plate and guide the corrective osteotomy. Using this technique, with a three-dimensional corrective osteotomy,

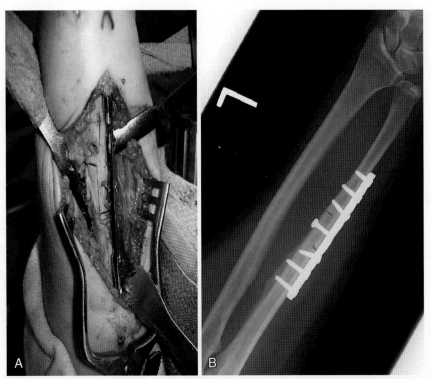

FIGURE 21.25 A, Step-cut osteotomy of the ulna. **B,** Radiograph showing step-cut osteotomy of the ulna with lag screw across the osteotomy site.

Kataoka and colleagues were able to precisely correct four forearm malunions.[69]

An anterior approach is used for the radius and an incision along the subcutaneous border for the ulna. If both bones are malunited, the more severe malunion is addressed first. Any hardware that is already in place is removed. The site of the previous fracture is localized with fluoroscopy. An 18-gauge wire can be twisted into the site if the fracture is not mature. Callous is removed from the surrounding region down to native cortical bone. Again, this is more easily performed if the fracture has not remodeled. The malunion is taken down, when possible, with osteotomes and a narrow rongeur along the course of the previous fracture. As previously discussed, it is possible to obtain a CT-generated plastic model of the malunion and prebent plates to optimize correction of the deformity. The ideal situation for this approach is a deformity in three planes, in which remodeling obliterates the path of the original fracture. If this technique is not an option, long oblique osteotomies will facilitate multiplanar correction, as well as provide a larger surface area for healing. Provisional fixation is established proximal and distal to the malunion. Passive pronation-supination is checked. Intraoperative fluoroscopy of the provisional fixation is used to determine rotational alignment of the wrist, forearm bones, and elbow by using anatomic landmarks as described previously. Once the alignment is acceptable, plate fixation with eight cortices is performed proximal and distal to the malunion. Cancellous autograft is harvested from the proximal tibia or iliac crest and placed around the osteotomy site.

If correction of the more severe malunion produces sufficiently increased intraoperative motion, the other bone may not require surgical treatment.[57] If both bones will require correction, the ulna is fixed first to re-create the stable and straight unit of the forearm. If length discrepancy is the only correction required, a long step-cut osteotomy of the ulna allows fine-tuning of the length during fixation (Figure 21.25).

There are few studies examining corrective osteotomies of forearm fracture malunion. Matthews and associates[78] did combined osteotomies of the middle thirds of the radius and ulna in cadavers and found that there was minimal loss of pronation-supination with 10 degrees of angulation but a functional loss of motion with 20 degrees of angulation. In another cadaveric study by Tarr and coworkers,[126] a 10-degree angular deformity in both bones of the forearm resulted in an average loss of pronation-supination of 13% when the fracture was in the distal third of the forearm and an average loss of 16% when it was in the middle third. The researchers also observed that rotatory deformities produced a loss of pronation and supination that was equal to the degree of deformity. Trousdale and Linscheid[129] did a retrospective review of 27 corrective osteotomies for malunited fractures of the forearm. They obtained a mean improvement of 79 degrees in forearm rotation when an osteotomy was done within 12 months of injury, compared with a gain of only 30 degrees if the corrective osteotomy was done more than 12 months after the injury. They proposed that soft tissue contractures involving the IOM may contribute to this difference and recommended that corrective osteotomies be done within 12 months of injury.[129] In contrast, Chia and colleagues[20] performed corrective osteotomies for six symptomatic adults with malunited forearm shaft fractures. The average interval between the original fracture and the corrective osteotomy was 42 months. They reported improved function despite a long delay between the injury and subsequent osteotomy.

CRITICAL POINTS *Plate Fixation of Nonunion or Malunion of the Radius or Ulna*

- Determine with plain radiographs if it is possible to follow the line of the previous fracture when taking down the malunion.
- If the fracture has completely remodeled, consider using a CT-generated model and a prebent plate.
- Preoperative templating with the contralateral forearm can serve as a guide.
- Use interfragmentary compression techniques (lag screws or compression plating, or both) when possible.
- Confirm adequate passive wrist and elbow range of motion, including pronation-supination, after provisional fixation.
- Intraoperative fluoroscopic studies can document restoration of near-normal relationship of bony landmarks.
- Graft the site with autogenous cancellous graft.

Treatment of Nonunion of Forearm Bones Using Distraction-Compression Osteogenesis

Use of a circular external frame with fine wires is effective in nonunions and malunions with deformities in multiple planes.[93] The treatment may be monofocal or bifocal. Monofocal treatment, developed by Ilizarov, involves compression (first phase) followed by distraction at the nonunion site. Bifocal treatment involves simultaneous compression at the nonunion site and lengthening at a different location within the same bone. Orzechowski and colleagues[93] presented six patients with pseudarthroses of the forearm bones with limb shortening and axis deformity, which were treated with a circular frame. Union was achieved in all patients. Normal radial length was restored in four patients, while a residual shortening of 1 cm persisted in two patients. Significant improvements in limb function and appearance were achieved in all patients.

Postoperative Management and Expectations

Union rates for malunion and nonunion of the radius and ulna are lower than those for primary fracture treatment but are still 90% or greater.[14,94] Restoration of normal motion and strength is rarely possible.[61,99,109]

The optimal time to begin postoperative motion is defined by the stability of the plate-bone construct and by the environment in which the procedure took place. A single-plane osteotomy with excellent fixation in a young, healthy patient can begin immediately. Forearm rotation is begun more cautiously following revision surgery for a recalcitrant nonunion.[50] Though the available evidence suggests that electromagnetic field stimulation may offer some benefit in the treatment of delayed union and nonunion of long bone fractures, the literature is inconclusive and cannot, by itself, guide current practice. Ultrasound has also been used to stimulate bone growth. The evidence regarding ultrasound for this application is, similarly, inconclusive.[51] When healing is in question at 3 to 4 months following operation, a CT scan may be performed.

The complications associated with treatment of forearm nonunion and malunion are similar to those associated with treatment of acute radial and ulnar shaft fractures. In the patients with nonunion or malunion, the rate of complications is higher and may be as much as 50% in some series.[25,57,109]

RADIOULNAR SYNOSTOSIS

Posttraumatic radioulnar synostosis is a relatively rare complication, estimated to occur in 1.2% to 6.6% of patients with a fracture of one or both bones of the forearm following treatment with compression plating.[47,99] The rate of synostosis is higher in persons with head injury, occurring in as many as 18%.[31] The literature consists mostly of level IV retrospective case studies and case reports. The synostosis may be located anywhere from the ulnohumeral articulation to the DRUJ. The formation of ectopic bone is not easily accommodated in the forearm, where "tolerances" are small (Figure 21.26). Risk factors include Monteggia fracture, fracture of both bones at the same level, high-energy injuries, burns, open fractures, comminuted fractures, bone fragments on the IOM, and head injury.[47,107,133] Iatrogenic risk is lessened by the use of separate incisions to approach the radius and ulna for fracture fixation.[47] In complete synostosis, the patient is free of pain, with forearm rotation completely blocked. The patient with an incomplete synostosis may have a painful block to forearm rotation.

A classification system was established to describe heterotopic ossification about the elbow and forearm (Table 21.1).[57] This system took into account the fact that any amount of ectopic bone may limit both the elbow flexion-extension arc and forearm rotation, with limitations ranging from a partial block to frank ankylosis.

Preoperative evaluation of forearm heterotopic ossification or cross-union should include plain radiographs of the forearm,

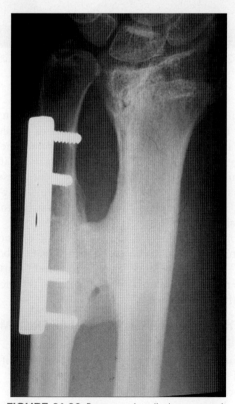

FIGURE 21.26 Posttraumatic radioulnar synostosis.

TABLE 21.1 Classification of Heterotopic Ossification

Class	Description
Class I	HO that does not cause functional limitation
Class II	HO that causes subtotal limitation of motion
Class IIA	Partial loss of elbow flexion-extension
Class IIB	Partial loss of forearm supination-pronation
Class IIC	Partial loss of both flexion-extension and supination-pronation
Class III	Complete ankylosis of the elbow or forearm, or both

From Hastings H 2nd, Graham TJ: The classification and treatment of heterotopic ossification about the elbow and forearm. *Hand Clin* 10:417–437, 1994.

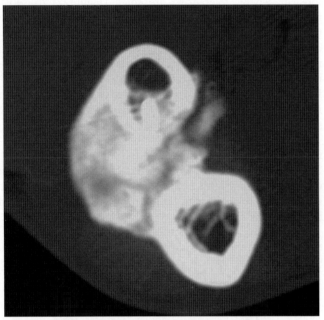

FIGURE 21.27 CT scan demonstrating the location and extent of radioulnar synostosis.

with frontal, lateral, and oblique views. A CT scan with or without three-dimensional reconstruction is invaluable in defining the site of cross-union and in planning the surgical approach (Figure 21.27). The synostosis can occur at a single site or multiple sites. Nonsurgical management is reserved for low-demand patients, those with recurrence following multiple attempts at resection, and those who are unable to tolerate additional procedures.

The optimal timing for the takedown of a synostosis is unknown. In the past, it was recommended that the bone mass "mature" prior to resection. There is no current consensus or evidence regarding timing. However, resection is typically considered after approximately 3 to 4 months.

❖ AUTHOR'S PREFERRED METHOD OF TREATMENT: Radioulnar Synostosis

Several factors help indicate whether the takedown of a synostosis will be successful:

1. Localization of the bone mass
2. Healed fracture(s) in acceptable alignment

3. Normal PRUJ and DRUJ
4. A compliant IOM and soft tissue envelope

A preoperative CT scan of the forearm, including the PRUJ and DRUJ, will show whether the first three factors are present. The presence of factor four is more difficult to assess, but skin contractures from burns or crushing and degloving injuries may hinder efforts to restore motion.

The location of the synostosis as defined by a CT scan will determine the surgical approach. Proximal synostoses may be accessible by elevating the anconeus and common extensor muscle mass. In cases where the bone extends anteriorly, it may be prudent to use an anterior approach in which the median and radial nerves can be identified and protected. Access to middiaphyseal synostoses is typically via an anterior Henry approach. Exposure along the subcutaneous border of the ulna is also an option. Distal synostoses can be reached through an anterior or dorsal approach. There may be an associated soft tissue contracture that will limit motion after bone resection (e.g., release of the anterior capsule of the DRUJ often helps recover forearm supination).

Surgical hardware may be left in place unless it is specifically limiting exposure or range of motion. Intraoperative fluoroscopy is used to localize the borders between normal cortical bone and heterotopic bone. The borders can be marked with Kirschner wires. The bone is removed with osteotomes, a bur, and/or rongeurs. Postresection fluoroscopy helps confirm the resection margins.

Various strategies have been employed to prevent reformation of the synostosis, including use of medications, irradiation, and interposed barriers.[10,11,23,56,59,82,106] There are no prospective controlled studies to suggest which, if any, intervention is best to prevent recurrence.[31,102] Our practice has been to simply cover the exposed bone with bone wax and begin early motion. There is little evidence to support the use of preoperative or postoperative irradiation.[68] The one situation in which irradiation may be indicated is the unusual case involving recurrent heterotopic bone; the patient is given a perioperative dose of 350 to 700 Gy.

Lastly, there are instances where taking down the synostosis is not feasible. One example is recurrent synostosis involving most of the proximal third of the forearm. In these instances, one can consider creating a resection arthroplasty distal to the synostosis (Figure 21.28).

Postoperative Management and Expectations

Active, active-assisted, and passive motion are begun immediately after surgery. Patients are reevaluated frequently to assess their progress. Once the wounds are healed, static progressive splinting can be added. Significant gains in rotation are expected assuming that the resection was adequate, the bones are aligned, the PRUJ and DRUJ are congruent, and the skin is supple.[41] The reported chance of recurrence is 5% to 10%, especially at the proximal and distal ends of the forearm axis.[55,58]

LONGITUDINAL INSTABILITY OF THE FOREARM AXIS

Essex-Lopresti is credited with the concept of dissociation of the forearm axis, although the actual disorder had been previously described.[26,40] It is a rare injury. Longitudinal forearm

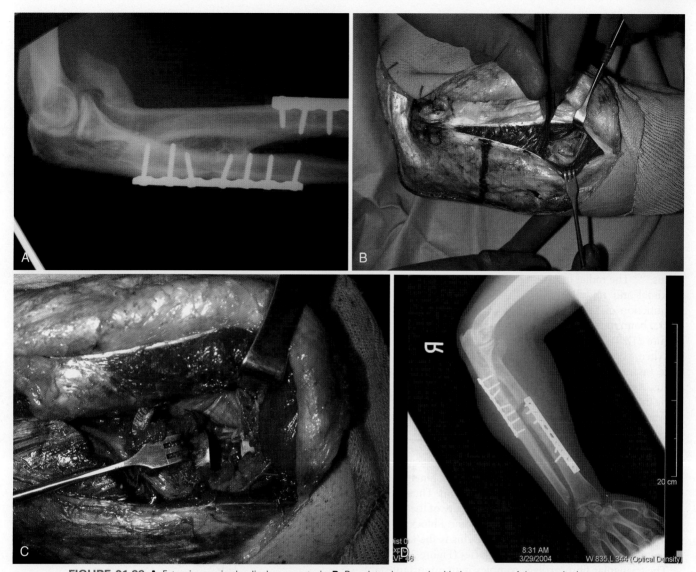

FIGURE 21.28 A, Extensive proximal radioulnar synostosis. **B,** Dorsolateral approach with the exposure of the posterior interosseous nerve. **C,** Resection of 2 cm of the radial shaft. **D,** Lateral radiograph of the forearm 2 years later. Patient had 10 degrees of supination and full pronation.

instability results from an axial load leading to fracture of the radial head and disruption of the IOM and triangular fibrocartilage complex.[80] The radiographic and clinical findings may not be immediately apparent at the time of initial evaluation.[66,49] In a series of 106 referred Essex-Lopresti injuries, the diagnosis was made only 38% of the time.[76]

Appreciation of the extent of injury often follows surgical resection of a radial head or neck fracture. Proximal migration of the radial shaft occurs, and the distal ulna abuts the carpus.[128] Longitudinal instability of the forearm axis has been seen in combination with other forearm fractures, but loss of radiocapitellar support, which uncovers the incompetence of the DRUJ stabilizers and disrupted IOM, is the classic scenario.[37]

The initial physical examination helps direct the diagnosis. Wrist pain in conjunction with a radial head fracture should raise one's suspicion. Instability of the DRUJ should further raise suspicion regarding a forearm axis injury. Radiographs of

the elbow and a neutral rotation view of the wrist are useful in evaluating the relative ulnar variance.[38] It is worthwhile to get comparison views of the contralateral wrist.

MRI can be helpful in confirming the diagnosis of an IOM disruption. It has been shown to have nearly 90% or greater sensitivity, specificity, and positive and negative predictive values.[79] Fester and colleagues[42] used a cadaver model to establish the sensitivity and specificity of MRI to diagnose central band transections of the IOM. The mean sensitivity was 93%, specificity 100%, and overall accuracy in diagnosing an IOM central third disruption 96%.[42] Ultrasound is another effective method to evaluate the integrity of the IOM; it is less expensive than MRI, can be performed quickly, and allows for a dynamic evaluation of the soft tissues. In the same model, Fester and associates evaluated the effectiveness of ultrasound to diagnose IOM disruptions. The sensitivity was 100%, specificity 89%, and overall accuracy 94%. In their comparison between ultrasound and MRI, they found no significant difference between the accuracy of the two methods.[42] CT scanning is useful in assessing concurrent articular fractures of the wrist or elbow or to help determine whether reconstructive or salvage options are appropriate in the subacute or chronic setting. Axial CT scans of both radioulnar joints in supination, pronation, and neutral position can confirm suspected DRUJ instability.

▌ PERTINENT ANATOMY

The primary structure that prevents proximal radius migration is the radial head. Secondary structures include the central band of the IOM and the structures about the triangular fibrocartilage complex and DRUJ. The IOM is a complex structure composed of five distinct bands.[91] The most mechanically stout is the central band, sometimes referred to as the interosseous ligament. The central band suspends the radius by virtue of fibers that originate on the distal ulna and insert on the proximal radius.[62,98] The radial insertion is located at the junction of the proximal and middle thirds of the radius. The origin is at the junction of the middle and distal thirds of the ulna. The central band rests at an angle of approximately 20 to 25 degrees (Figure 21.29).[17,119]

When axial forces are experienced at the wrist, most of the force (as much as 75% to 80%) is transmitted through the radius. Axial compression of the radius is converted to tension in the interosseous ligament, amplifying the magnitude of compressive forces in the ulnar column. Because of the conversion of lateral or radial compression to tension through the interosseous ligament and ultimately to ulnar compression, the normal forces recorded at the elbow demonstrate a rough equalization of the joint reactive forces between the radial and ulnar columns, slightly weighted toward the ulnotrochlear joint. Thus, excision of the radial head, in combination with rupture of the IOM and interosseous ligament, removes any mechanical block to proximal radial migration under axial loads. This is the key pathoanatomic finding in Essex-Lopresti injuries (Figure 21.30).

The triangular fibrocartilage complex is an important stabilizer of the radius and ulna at the DRUJ, preventing longitudinal instability. It is responsible for 8% of the forearm's resistance to axial load.

Types of Operations
Prevention of Longitudinal Instability of the Forearm

Preventing the downward spiral of events that result from radial head excision is the preferred approach to handling this complex problem. By recognizing the global extent of the injury and addressing each component in the acute period, it may be possible to avoid further instability. Treatment of acute injuries is associated with improved outcomes when compared with treatment of chronic instability.[97]

In the acute setting, the ideal option is to repair the radial head. When this is not possible, the integrity of the IOM is

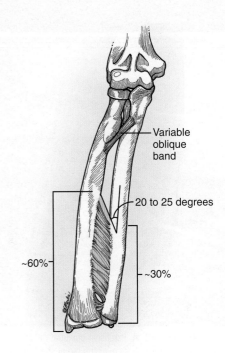

FIGURE 21.29 Illustration of the interosseous ligament and its anatomic relationships. (Copyright Elizabeth Martin.)

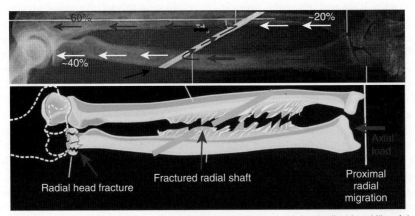

FIGURE 21.30 Illustration of biomechanics of a normal forearm and a forearm with longitudinal instability of the forearm axis.

evaluated by the pull test. The cut end of the proximal radius is secured with a towel clip. As one pulls on the radius, ulnar variance is evaluated using fluoroscopy. Two millimeters of radial excursion is within the range of normal. Three millimeters or more suggests longitudinal instability in cadaver studies. If there is evidence of longitudinal stability in the face of an unrepairable radial head, a metal radial head implant should be used. In the normal forearm, the central band shares the load with the radial head. Radial head replacement should thus, theoretically, allow the central band and the triangular fibrocartilage complex to heal.[36,38,66,76] However, there is suspicion that the ruptured IOM may not be capable of healing. This raises two issues:

1. Should an attempt be made to repair or reconstruct the central band acutely to reduce loads across the articulation of the prosthesis and capitellum?
2. Subsequent procedures should be performed with caution and with assessment of longitudinal stability of the forearm axis.[123]

After the radial head is addressed, the stability of the DRUJ is evaluated. Instability can be managed with immobilization in a position of stability, repair of the triangular fibrocartilage complex, or simple pinning of the DRUJ, as described above. There is no evidence to guide selection among these three options.

Restoration of the Length of the Radius and Ulna With Reduction of the Distal and Proximal Radioulnar Joints

Replacing the radial head and reducing and pinning the DRUJ are possible in the acute setting. In a subacute setting, this procedure can be combined with an ulnar-shortening osteotomy. Unfortunately, this approach places tremendous loads across the radiocapitellar joint.

Reconstruction of the Central Band of the Interosseous Membrane

Reconstruction of the central band of the IOM has the advantage of also attempting to restore the normal relationships between the radius and ulna, DRUJ, and PRUJ. Reconstruction of the IOM has been described using the palmaris longus, flexor carpi radialis tendon, Achilles allograft, pronator teres, synthetic materials, and bone–patellar tendon–bone graft (Figure 21.31,

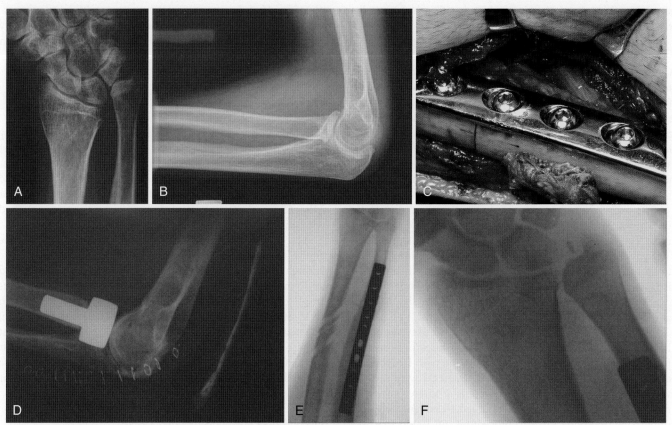

FIGURE 21.31 A and **B,** Initial radiographs showing severe proximal radial migration after radial head excision in the setting of disruption of the forearm axis. **C,** Intraoperative photograph demonstrating plate and screw fixation of the ulnar-shortening osteotomy and ulnar docking of the semitendinosus allograft. **D,** Radiograph after replacement of the radial head with a prosthesis. **E,** Anteroposterior radiograph of the forearm after ulnar-shortening osteotomy and fixation, radial head replacement, and reconstruction of the interosseous ligament with a semitendinosus allograft. **F,** Restoration of the normal relationships of the radius and ulna length. (Courtesy of Andrew Stein, MD, Anthony Deluise, MD, and Seth Levitz, MD.)

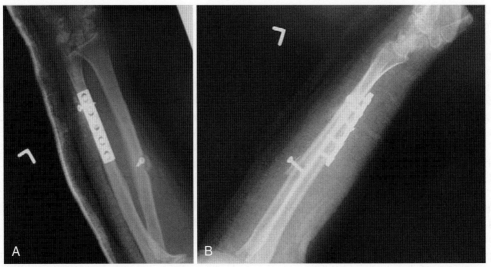

FIGURE 21.32 A and B, Anteroposterior and lateral radiographs after ulnar-shortening osteotomy and bone–patellar tendon–bone reconstruction of the interosseous ligament.

A to *F*).[21,76,118,123,127] The bone-ligament-bone reconstruction described by Marcotte and Osterman involves an ulnar-shortening osteotomy that is combined with a bone–patellar tendon–bone allograft (Figure 21.32).[76]

One-Bone Forearm Technique

Creating a one-bone forearm is considered the definitive salvage technique for the multiply operated, painful, and unstable forearm. The advantage of this procedure is that it provides a stable platform for the hand so that the shoulder and elbow may position the hand in space. The ulnohumeral joint is maintained to allow elbow flexion and extension, and wrist motion should be minimally affected. The disadvantages include complete loss of pronation-supination and the risk of nonunion, infection, and compartment syndrome.[136]

The two main techniques are transferring the radius to the ulna and creating a bridging synostosis between the radius and ulna. Typically the forearm is positioned in slight pronation. The patient can "test drive" different positions by immobilizing the forearm with a Munster-style splint or cast.[5] If supination is lacking in the contralateral forearm, the one-bone forearm can be placed in slight supination because the shoulder can abduct to compensate for a deficit in pronation.

Allende and Allende[1] reported that seven of seven patients in their series who underwent a one-bone forearm procedure for posttraumatic instability had a stable and pain-free forearm at an average follow-up of 9 years. All patients were satisfied with the position, function, and cosmesis of the reconstructed forearm. Jacoby and colleagues[63] studied 10 patients who had undergone one-bone forearm procedures but found that they experienced poor functional outcomes. The largest case series to date was reported by Peterson and associates,[97] who presented the outcomes of 19 patients. The authors categorized their patients into two groups based on the cause of injury: those who underwent one-bone forearm surgery because of posttraumatic instability and those who underwent the surgery

because of instability after oncologic resection or a congenital deformity. The authors noted that nearly all of the major complications after surgery occurred in patients with acquired posttraumatic instability and concluded that the higher-energy injuries had worse results regardless of the reconstruction technique.

❖ AUTHOR'S PREFERRED METHODS OF TREATMENT

Acute Injuries

The initial evaluation begins with a history of a high-energy axial load to the forearm with complaints of elbow and wrist pain. The physical examination includes palpation and stress testing of the DRUJ for tenderness or instability. If an IOM injury is suspected, the forearm is studied with ultrasound or MRI. A neutral-rotation PA of the contralateral wrist is obtained with and without grip.

The surgical procedure begins with a lateral approach to the elbow. The radial head is repaired if the construct appears stable enough to support axial loads. If not, the radial head is resected and a pull test is performed as described previously. If the radius translates 3 mm or more or if there is a high suspicion of an IOM injury, a radial head arthroplasty is inserted. The lateral ligament complex of the elbow must be repaired to prevent posterolateral rotatory instability. If the DRUJ is unstable, our preference is to place two 0.062-inch pins across the distal ulna and radius proximal to the DRUJ. The pins should exit the far cortex of the radius. This facilitates retrieval if the pins break.

Interosseous Ligament Reconstruction

We have modified the technique using a bone-ligament-bone graft as described by Marcotte and Osterman.[76] The distal ulna is exposed along its subcutaneous border. The origin of the central band is estimated at the junction of the distal and middle thirds of the ulna. A 2.5-mm drill hole is created on an angle of around 25 degrees in a medial to lateral direction. The extensor carpi ulnaris is elevated, and two No. 5 braided, non-absorbable sutures are passed through the hole from lateral to medial. This is facilitated by first passing a bent 24-gauge dental wire through the hole from medial to lateral and using it as a suture retriever. A counterincision is made on the dorsoradial aspect of the forearm at the approximate junction of the middle and proximal thirds of the radius. The proximal radius is accessed between the ECRB and ECRL, with care taken to protect the radial sensory nerve. A 2.5-mm drill hole is made at the insertion of the central band and angled 25 degrees toward the ulna. Wrist extension and elbow flexion will help relax the extensor mass. Starting from the radial incision, a large, curved Kelly hemostat is used to gently create a path along the dorsal surface of the radius and ulna, aiming for the drill holes in the ulna. The two No. 5 sutures are retrieved and passed through the drill hole in the proximal radius. The bone-ligament-bone allograft is fashioned so that it spans the radius and ulna along the course of the native IOM. The bone is trimmed so that the bone blocks do not sit directly over the drill holes. This is intended to protect the suture when a screw is used to secure the block. A shallow notch for the bone block is created on the dorsal surface of the radius and ulna with a barrel bur. The bone-ligament-bone graft is passed beneath the extensors.

Once the reconstruction is "teed-up," the elbow is accessed by a lateral approach. The integrity of the lateral collateral ligament complex is confirmed by extending the elbow and retracting the common extensors. The status of the articular cartilage of the capitellum is evaluated and documented. A gauze pad is placed on the capitellum, and a lamina spreader is used to distract the proximal radius. Intraoperative fluoroscopy is used to confirm reduction of the DRUJ. The distal ulna is pinned to the radius with two 0.062-inch wires placed proximal to the DRUJ. With the length of the radius restored, a radial head prosthesis is placed in the proximal radius. This implant is intended to prevent convergence of the proximal radius and ulna. It need not and should not have a tight fit against the capitellum.

The reconstruction is completed by tying the two ends of the suture over a button on the proximal radius. The sutures are tensioned at the distal ulna and tied over a button. The bone block is fixed to the radius proximally using a single lag screw. The graft is tensioned and fixed to the ulna with a single lag screw distally.

The arm is immobilized in a long-arm splint. This can be converted to a Munster splint in 2 weeks. The pins are removed at 6 weeks following operation. At that time, active forearm rotation is allowed. At 3 months, the patient can begin light resistance exercises and, if necessary, participate in passive forearm rotation and static progressive splinting.

One-Bone Forearm Technique

We have no personal experience creating a one-bone forearm. The previous authors of this chapter recommended a bridging synostosis technique as opposed to the actual transfer of the radius to the ulna. Unless previous incisions or specific post-traumatic soft tissue concerns dictate otherwise, the radius is approached anteriorly. An osteotomy of the radius is made near the midshaft level. The distal radial shaft is pushed proximally or distally as needed to correct any length mismatch of the distal radius and ulna. The opposing cortices of the radius and ulna at the sites of planned cross-union are prepared by decortica-tion with a bur. The radius is pinned to the ulna proximally and distally with temporary Kirschner wires, and intraoperative fluoroscopy is used to confirm anatomic positioning of the radius and ulna at the wrist and elbow. At least three quadri-cortical screws are placed proximal *and* distal to the radial shaft osteotomy. The screws are directed from the radius, across the interosseous space, and into the ulna. Cancellous autograft is placed in the interosseous space. Only the subcutaneous tissues and skin are closed. The fascia is left open, and a drain is used. Patients are monitored overnight. Elbow and wrist motion is allowed while bracing the forearm to prevent pronation-supination. Resistive exercises and weight bearing are restricted until clinical and radiographic healing is present.

A one-bone forearm can also be created with the aid of a vascularized free fibula graft if additional length or stability is needed.[5,22]

Postoperative Expectations

Following reconstruction of the IOM, the goal is a stable forearm with minimal pain and a functional arc of forearm rotation. Marcotte and Osterman reviewed a series of 16 patients who had been treated by bone-ligament-bone reconstruction and ulnar-shortening osteotomy since 1992 with an average follow-up of 78 months.[76] They reported that 15 of these patients had improvement in wrist pain and required no further surgery for longitudinal instability. Grip strength improved from 59% preoperatively to 86% postoperatively relative to the contralateral limb.

Following creation of a one-bone forearm, patients can expect little to no pain, a stable forearm, and no forearm rotation. Patients must understand the severity of their injury, realize the complexity of the reconstruction involved, and have reasonable expectations of being "functional" but not "normal."

Complications

Complications resulting from the initial injury include arthrosis at the wrist or elbow, or both, pain, lost range of motion, and lost function. Complications as a result of the IOM reconstruction also include persistent pain, recurrent instability, and progressive arthritis. The one-bone forearm technique carries with it a concern for compartment syndrome. Malunion and non-union are also potential complications. Because the procedure is done infrequently, the true incidence of nonunion is unknown, but it has been reported to be up to 30%.[19,97]

REFERENCES

1. Allende C, Allende B: Posttraumatic one-bone forearm reconstruction: a report of seven cases. *J Bone Joint Surg Am* 86:364–369, 2004.
2. al-Qattan MM, Clarke HM, Zimmer P: Radiological signs of entrapment of the median nerve in forearm shaft fractures. *J Hand Surg [Br]* 19:713–719, 1994.
3. Altner PC, Hartmann JT: Isolated fractures of the ulnar shaft in the adult. *Surg Clin North Am* 52:155–170, 1972.
4. Anderson LD, Sisk TD, Tooms RE, et al: Compression-plate fixation in acute diaphyseal fractures of the radius and ulna. *J Bone Joint Surg Am* 57:287–297, 1975.
5. Arai K, Toh S, Yasumura M, et al: One-bone forearm formation using vascularized fibula graft for massive bone defect of the forearm with infection: case report. *J Reconstr Microsurg* 17:151–155, 2001.
6. Atkin DM, Bohay DR, Slabaugh P, et al: Treatment of ulnar shaft fractures: a prospective, randomized study. *Orthopedics* 18:543–547, 1995.

7. Azboy I, Demirtas A, Uçar BY, et al: Effectiveness of locking versus dynamic compression plates for diaphyseal forearm fractures. *Orthopedics* 36(7):e917–e922, 2013.

8. Barquet A: Posterior dislocation of the ulna at the elbow with associated fracture of the radial shaft. *Injury* 15:390–392, 1984.

9. Bauer G, Arand M, Mutschler W: Post-traumatic radio-ulnar synostosis after forearm fracture osteosynthesis. *Arch Orthop Trauma Surg* 110:142–145, 1991.

10. Beaupre GS, Csongradi JJ: Refracture risk after plate removal in the forearm. *J Orthop Trauma* 10:87–92, 1996.

11. Bednar DA, Grandwilewski W: Complications of forearm-plate removal. *Can J Surg* 35:428–431, 1992.

12. Bindra RR, Cole RJ, Yamaguchi K, et al: Quantification of the radial torsion angle with computerized tomography in cadaver specimens. *J Bone Joint Surg Am* 79:833–837, 1997.

13. Borens O, Chehab EL, Roberts MM, et al: Bilateral Galeazzi fracture-dislocations. *Am J Orthop* 35:369–372, 2006.

14. Boyd HB, Lipinski SW: Causes and treatment of non-union of the shafts of the long bones with a review of 741 patients. *Instr Course Lect* 17:165–183, 1960.

15. Brakenbury PH, Corea JR, Blakemore ME: Non-union of the isolated fracture of the ulnar shaft in adults. *Injury* 12:371–375, 1981.

16. Bruckner JD, Lichtman DM, Alexander AH: Complex dislocations of the distal radio-ulnar joint. Recognition and management. *Clin Orthop Relat Res* 275:90–103, 1992.

17. Chandler JW, Stabile KJ, Pfaeffle HJ, et al: Anatomic parameters for planning of interosseous ligament reconstruction using computer-assisted techniques. *J Hand Surg [Am]* 28:111–116, 2003.

18. Chapman MW, Gordon JE, Zissimos AG: Compression-plate fixation of acute fractures of the diaphyses of the radius and ulna. *J Bone Joint Surg Am* 71:159–169, 1989.

19. Chen F, Culp RW, Schneider LH, et al: Revision of the ununited one-bone forearm. *J Hand Surg [Am]* 23:1091–1096, 1998.

20. Chia DS, Lim YJ, Chew WY: Corrective osteotomy in forearm fracture malunion improves functional outcome in adults. *J Hand Surg Eur Vol* 36(2):102–106, 2011.

21. Chloros GD, Wiesler ER, Stabile KJ, et al: Reconstruction of Essex-Lopresti injury of the forearm: technical note. *J Hand Surg [Am]* 33(1):124–130, 2008.

22. Choudry UH, Bakri K, Moran SL, et al: The vascularized medial femoral condyle periosteal bone flap for the treatment of recalcitrant bony nonunions. *Ann Plast Surg* 60:174–180, 2008.

23. Corea JR, Brakenbury PH, Blakemore ME: The treatment of isolated fractures of the ulnar shaft in adults. *Injury* 12:365–370, 1981.

24. Crow BD, Mundis G, Anglen JO: Clinical results of minimal screw plate fixation of forearm fractures. *Am J Orthop* 36:477–480, 2007.

25. Cullen JP, Pellegrini VD, Jr, Miller RJ, et al: Treatment of traumatic radio-ulnar synostosis by excision and postoperative low-dose irradiation. *J Hand Surg [Am]* 19:394–401, 1994.

26. Curr JF, Moe WA: Dislocation of the inferior radio-ulnar joint. *Br J Surg* 34:74–77, 1946.

27. De Pedro JA, Garcia-Navarrete F, Garcia De Lucas F, et al: Internal fixation of ulnar fractures by locking nail. *Clin Orthop Relat Res* 283:81–85, 1992.

28. Dell PC, Sheppard JE: Vascularized bone grafts in the treatment of infected forearm nonunions. *J Hand Surg [Am]* 9:653–658, 1984.

29. Deluca PA, Lindsey RW, Ruwe PA: Refracture of bones of the forearm after the removal of compression plates. *J Bone Joint Surg Am* 70:1372–1376, 1988.

30. Dodge HS, Cady GW: Treatment of fractures of the radius and ulna with compression plates. *J Bone Joint Surg Am* 54:1167–1176, 1972.

31. Dohn P, Khiami F, Rolland E, et al: Adult post-traumatic radioulnar synostosis. *Orthop Traumatol Surg Res* 98(6):709–714, 2012.

32. Droll KP, Perna P, Potter J, et al: Outcomes following plate fixation of fractures of both bones of the forearm in adults. *J Bone Joint Surg Am* 89:2619–2624, 2007.

33. Dumont CE, Nagy L, Ziegler D, et al: Fluoroscopic and magnetic resonance cross-sectional imaging assessments of radial and ulnar torsion profiles in volunteers. *J Hand Surg [Am]* 32:501–509, 2007.

34. Duncan R, Geissler W, Freeland AE, et al: Immediate internal fixation of open fractures of the diaphysis of the forearm. *J Orthop Trauma* 6:25–31, 1992.

35. Dymond IW: The treatment of isolated fractures of the distal ulna. *J Bone Joint Surg Br* 66:408–410, 1984.

36. Edwards GS, Jr, Jupiter JB: Radial head fractures with acute distal radioulnar dislocation. Essex-Lopresti revisited. *Clin Orthop Relat Res* 234:61–69, 1988.

37. Eglseder WA, Hay M: Combined Essex-Lopresti and radial shaft fractures: case report. *J Trauma* 34:310–312, 1993.

38. Epner RA, Bowers WH, Guilford WB: Ulnar variance: the effect of wrist positioning and roentgen filming technique. *J Hand Surg [Am]* 7:298–305, 1982.

39. Esser RD: Treatment of a bone defect of the forearm by bone transport. A case report. *Clin Orthop Relat Res* 326:221–224, 1996.

40. Essex-Lopresti P: Fractures of the radial head with distal radio-ulnar dislocation: report of two cases. *J Bone Joint Surg Br* 33:244–247, 1951.

41. Failla JM, Amadio PC, Morrey BF: Post-traumatic proximal radio-ulnar synostosis. Results of surgical treatment. *J Bone Joint Surg Am* 71:1208–1213, 1989.

42. Fester E, Murray P, Sanders T, et al: The efficacy of magnetic resonance imaging and ultrasound in detecting disruptions of the forearm interosseous membrane: a cadaver study. *J Hand Surg [Am]* 27:418–424, 2002.

43. Fulkerson E, Egol KA, Kubiak EN, et al: Fixation of diaphyseal fractures with a segmental defect: a biomechanical comparison of locked and conventional plating techniques. *J Trauma* 60:830–835, 2006.

44. Galik K, Baratz ME, Butler AL, et al: The effect of the annular ligament on kinematics of the radial head. *J Hand Surg [Am]* 32(8):1218–1224, 2007.

45. Gao H, Luo CF, Zhang CQ, et al: Internal fixation of diaphyseal fractures of the forearm by interlocking intramedullary nail: short-term results in eighteen patients. *J Orthop Trauma* 19:384–391, 2005.

46. Gebuhr P, Hölmich P, Orsnes T, et al: Isolated ulnar shaft fractures. Comparison of treatment by a functional brace and long-arm cast. *J Bone Joint Surg Br* 74:757–759, 1992.

47. Goldfarb CA, Ricci WM, Tull F, et al: Functional outcome after fracture of both bones of the forearm. *J Bone Joint Surg Br* 87:374–379, 2005.

48. Grace TG: Eversmann WW, Jr: Forearm fractures: treatment by rigid fixation with early motion. *J Bone Joint Surg Am* 62:433–438, 1980.

49. Green JB, Zelouf DS: Forearm instability. *J Hand Surg [Am]* 34(5):953–961, 2009.

50. Griffin XL, Costa ML, Parsons N, et al: Electromagnetic field stimulation for treating delayed union or non-union of long bone fractures in adults. *Cochrane Database Syst Rev* (4):CD008471, 2011.

51. Griffin XL, Smith N, Parsons N, et al: Ultrasound and shockwave therapy for acute fractures in adults. *Cochrane Database Syst Rev* (2):CD008579, 2012.

52. Hadden WA, Reschauer R, Seggl W: Results of AO plate fixation of forearm shaft fractures in adults. *Injury* 15:44–52, 1983.

53. Handoll HH, Pearce PK: Interventions for isolated diaphyseal fractures of the ulna in adults. *Cochrane Database Syst Rev* (2):CD000523, 2004.

54. Handoll HHG, Pearce P: Interventions for treating isolated diaphyseal fractures of the ulna in adults. *Cochrane Database Syst Rev* (6):CD000523, 2012.

55. Hanel DP, Pfaeffle HJ, Ayalla A: Management of posttraumatic metadiaphyseal radio-ulnar synostosis. *Hand Clin* 23:227–234, vi-vii, 2007.

56. Hanel DP, Scheid DK: Irreducible fracture-dislocation of the distal radio-ulnar joint secondary to entrapment of the extensor carpi ulnaris tendon. *Clin Orthop Relat Res* 234:56–60, 1988.

57. Hastings H, 2nd, Graham TJ: The classification and treatment of heterotopic ossification about the elbow and forearm. *Hand Clin* 10:417–437, 1994.

58. Henket M, van Duijn PJ, Doornberg JN, et al: A comparison of proximal radioulnar synostosis excision after trauma and distal biceps reattachment. *J Shoulder Elbow Surg* 16:626–630, 2007.

59. Hertel R, Pisan M, Lambert S, et al: Plate osteosynthesis of diaphyseal fractures of the radius and ulna. *Injury* 27:545–548, 1996.

60. Hidaka S, Gustilo RB: Refracture of bones of the forearm after plate removal. *J Bone Joint Surg Am* 66:1241–1243, 1984.

61. Hong G, Cong-Feng L, Hui-Peng S, et al: Treatment of diaphyseal forearm non-unions with interlocking intramedullary nails. *Clin Orthop Relat Res* 450:186–192, 2006.

62. Hotchkiss RN, An KN, Sowa DT, et al: An anatomic and mechanical study of the interosseous membrane of the forearm: pathomechanics of proximal migration of the radius. *J Hand Surg [Am]* 14:256–261, 1989.

63. Jacoby SM, Bachoura A, Diprinzio EV, et al: Complications following one-bone forearm surgery for posttraumatic forearm and distal radioulnar joint instability. *J Hand Surg [Am]* 38(5):976–982, 2013.

64. Jones DB, Jr, Kakar SJ: Adult diaphyseal forearm fractures: intramedullary nail versus plate fixation. *J Hand Surg [Am]* 36(7):1216–1219, 2011.

65. Jones JA: Immediate internal fixation of high-energy open forearm fractures. *J Orthop Trauma* 5:272–279, 1991.

66. Jungbluth P, Frangen TM, Muhr G, et al: A primarily overlooked and incorrectly treated Essex-Lopresti injury: what can this lead to? *Arch Orthop Trauma Surg* 128:89–95, 2008.

67. Jupiter JB, Gerhard HJ, Guerrero J, et al: Treatment of segmental defects of the radius with use of the vascularized osteoseptocutaneous fibular autogenous graft. *J Bone Joint Surg Am* 79:542–550, 1997.

68. Jupiter JB, Ring D: Operative treatment of post-traumatic proximal radioulnar synostosis. *J Bone Joint Surg Am* 80(2):248–257, 1998.

69. Kataoka T, Oka K, Miyake J, et al: Three-dimensional prebent plate fixation in corrective osteotomy of malunited upper extremity fractures using a real-sized plastic bone model prepared by preoperative computer simulation. *J Hand Surg [Am]* 38(5):909–919, 2013.

70. Kei O, Matsuki KM, Shang M, et al: In vivo 3D kinematics of normal forearms: analysis of dynamic forearm rotation. *Clin Biomech* 25:979–983, 2010.

71. Knight RA, Purvis GD: Fractures of both bones of the forearm in adults. *J Bone Joint Surg Am* 31(4):755–764, 1949.

72. Langkamer VG, Ackroyd CE: Removal of forearm plates. A review of the complications. *J Bone Joint Surg Br* 72:601–604, 1990.

73. Lee YH, Lee SK, Chung MS, et al: Interlocking contoured intramedullary nail fixation for selected diaphyseal fractures of the forearm in adults. *J Bone Joint Surg Am* 90:1891–1898, 2008.

74. Leung F, Chow SP: A prospective, randomized trial comparing the limited contact dynamic compression plate with the point contact fixator for forearm fractures. *J Bone Joint Surg Am* 85:2343–2348, 2003.

75. Lindvall EM, Sagi HC: Selective screw placement in forearm compression plating: results of 75 consecutive fractures stabilized with 4 cortices of screw fixation on either side of the fracture. *J Orthop Trauma* 20:157–162, discussion 162–163, 2006.

76. Marcotte AL, Osterman AL: Longitudinal radioulnar dissociation: identification and treatment of acute and chronic injuries. *Hand Clin* 23:195–208, vi, 2007.

77. Martin W, Field J, Kulkarni M: Intramedullary nailing of pathological forearm fractures. *Injury* 33(6):530–532, 2002.

78. Matthews LS, Kaufer H, Garver DF, et al: The effect on supination-pronation of angular malalignment of fractures of both bones of the forearm. *J Bone Joint Surg Am* 64:14–17, 1982.

79. McGinley JC, Roach N, Hopgood BC, et al: Forearm interosseous membrane trauma: MRI diagnostic criteria and injury patterns. *Skeletal Radiol* 35:275–281, 2006.

80. McGlinn EP, Sebastin SJ, Chung KC: A historical perspective on the Essex-Lopresti injury. *J Hand Surg [Am]* 38(8):1599–1606, 2013.

81. Mehara AK, Bhan S: Ipsilateral radial head dislocation with radial shaft fracture: case report. *J Trauma* 35:958–959, 1993.

82. Mih AD, Cooney WP, Idler RS, et al: Long-term follow-up of forearm bone diaphyseal plating. *Clin Orthop Relat Res* 299:256–258, 1994.

83. Moed BR, Kellam JF, Foster RJ, et al: Immediate internal fixation of open fractures of the diaphysis of the forearm. *J Bone Joint Surg Am* 68:1008–1017, 1986.

84. Mok D, Nikolis A, Harris PG: The cutaneous innervation of the dorsal hand: detailed anatomy with clinical implications. *J Hand Surg [Am]* 31:565–574, 2006.

85. Moroni A, Caja VL, Sabato C, et al: Composite bone grafting and plate fixation for the treatment of nonunions of the forearm with segmental bone loss: a report of eight cases. *J Orthop Trauma* 9:419–426, 1995.

86. Moroni A, Rollo G, Guzzardella M, et al: Surgical treatment of isolated forearm non-union with segmental bone loss. *Injury* 28:497–504, 1997.

87. Morrey BF, Askew LJ, Chao EY: A biomechanical study of normal functional elbow motion. *J Bone Joint Surg Am* 63:872–877, 1981.

88. Muller ME, Allgower M, Willenegger H: *Technique of internal fixation of fractures*, Berlin, 1963, Springer-Verlag.

89. Nagy L, Jankauskas L, Dumont CE: Correction of forearm malunion guided by the preoperative complaint. *Clin Orthop Relat Res* 466(6):1419–1428, 2008.

90. Naiman PT, Schein AJ, Siffert RS: Use of ASIF compression plates in selected shaft fractures of the upper extremity: a preliminary report. *Clin Orthop Relat Res* 71:208–216, 1970.

91. Noda K, Goro A, Murase T, et al: Interosseous membrane of the forearm: an anatomical study of ligament. *J Hand Surg [Am]* 34:415–422, 2009.

92. Oda T, Wada T, Isogai S, et al: Corrective osteotomy for volar instability of the distal radio-ulnar joint associated with radial shaft malunion. *J Hand Surg Eur Vol* 32:573–577, 2007.

93. Orzechowski W, Morasiewicz L, Dragan S, et al: Treatment of non-union of the forearm using distraction-compression osteogenesis. *Orthop Traumatol Rehabil* 9(4):357–365, 2007.

94. Ostermann PA, Ekkernkamp A, Henry SL, et al: Bracing of stable shaft fractures of the ulna. *J Orthop Trauma* 8:245–248, 1994.

95. Ozkaya U, Kiliç A, Ozdoan U, et al: Comparison between locked intramedullary nailing and plate osteosynthesis in the management of adult forearm fractures [in Turkish]. *Acta Orthop Traumatol Turc* 43:14–20, 2009.

96. Pai VS: Unusual arterial injury following a fracture of the forearm bones: a case report. *J Orthop Surg (Hong Kong)* 8:15–17, 2000.

97. Peterson CA, 2nd, Maki S, Wood MB: Clinical results of the one-bone forearm. *J Hand Surg [Am]* 20:609–618, 1995.

98. Poitevin LA: Anatomy and biomechanics of the interosseous membrane: its importance in the longitudinal stability of the forearm. *Hand Clin* 17:97–110, vii, 2001.

99. Posman CL, Little RE: Radio-ulnar synostosis following an isolated fracture of the ulnar shaft. A case report. *Clin Orthop Relat Res* 213:207–210, 1986.

100. Ray RD, Johnson RJ, Jameson RM: Rotation of the forearm: an experimental study of pronation and supination. *J Bone Joint Surg Am* 33:993–996, 1951.

101. Rehman S, Sokunbi G: Intramedullary fixation of forearm fractures. *Hand Clin* 26(3):391–401, 2010.

102. Reilly TJ: Isolated and combined fractures of the diaphysis of the radius and ulna. *Hand Clin* 18:179–194, 2002.

103. Rettig ME, Raskin KB: Galeazzi fracture-dislocation: a new treatment-oriented classification. *J Hand Surg [Am]* 26:228–235, 2001.

104. Ring D, Allende C, Jafarnia K, et al: Ununited diaphyseal forearm fractures with segmental defects: plate fixation and autogenous cancellous bone-grafting. *J Bone Joint Surg Am* 86:2440–2445, 2004.

105. Ring D, Rhim R, Carpenter C, et al: Comminuted diaphyseal fractures of the radius and ulna: does bone grafting affect nonunion rate? *J Trauma* 59:438–441, discussion 442, 2005.

106. Ring D, Rhim R, Carpenter C, et al: Isolated radial shaft fractures are more common than Galeazzi fractures. *J Hand Surg [Am]* 31:17–21, 2006.

107. Rizvi M, Bille B, Holtom P, et al: The role of prophylactic antibiotics in elective hand surgery. *J Hand Surg [Am]* 33:413–420, 2008.

108. Robson AJ, See MS, Ellis H: Applied anatomy of the superficial branch of the radial nerve. *Clin Anat* 21:38–45, 2008.

109. Rosen H: Compression treatment of long bone pseudarthroses. *Clin Orthop Relat Res* 138:154–166, 1979.

110. Rosson JW, Petley GW, Shearer JR: Bone structure after removal of internal fixation plates. *J Bone Joint Surg Br* 73:65–67, 1991.

111. Rosson JW, Shearer JR: Refracture after the removal of plates from the forearm. An avoidable complication. *J Bone Joint Surg Br* 73:415–417, 1991.

112. Sage FP, Smith H: Medullary fixation of forearm fractures. *J Bone Joint Surg Am* 39:91–98, 1957.

113. Salvi AE: Forearm diaphyseal fractures: which bone to synthesize first? *Orthopedics* 29:669–671, discussion 671, 2006.

114. Sarmiento A, Ebramzadeh E, Brys D, et al: Angular deformities and forearm function. *J Orthop Res* 10:121–133, 1992.

115. Sarmiento A, Kinman PB, Murphy RB, et al: Treatment of ulnar fractures by functional bracing. *J Bone Joint Surg Am* 58:1104–1107, 1976.

116. Schemitsch EH, Richards RR: The effect of malunion on functional outcome after plate fixation of fractures of both bones of the forearm in adults. *J Bone Joint Surg Am* 74:1068–1078, 1992.

117. Schweitzer G: Refracture of bones of the forearm after the removal of compression plates. *J Bone Joint Surg Am* 72:152, 1990.

118. Sellman DC, Seitz WH, Jr, Postak PD, et al: Reconstructive strategies for radio-ulnar dissociation: a biomechanical study. *J Orthop Trauma* 9:516–522, 1995.

119. Skahen JR, 3rd, Palmer AK, Werner FW, et al: Reconstruction of the interosseous membrane of the forearm in cadavers. *J Hand Surg [Am]* 22:986–994, 1997.

120. Smith WR, Elbatrawy YA, Andreassen GS, et al: Treatment of traumatic forearm bone loss with Ilizarov ring fixation and bone transport. *Int Orthop* 31:165–170, 2007.

121. Snow M, Thompson G, Turner PG: A mechanical comparison of the locking compression plate (LCP) and the low contact-dynamic compression plate (DCP) in an osteoporotic bone model. *J Orthop Trauma* 22:121–125, 2008.

122. Soon JC, Kumar VP, Satkunanartham K: Elbow dislocation with ipsilateral radial shaft fracture. An unusual outcome. *Clin Orthop Relat Res* 329:212–215, 1996.

123. Sowa DT, Hotchkiss RN, Weiland AJ: Symptomatic proximal translation of the radius following radial head resection. *Clin Orthop Relat Res* 317:106–113, 1995.

124. Stern PJ, Drury WJ: Complications of plate fixation of forearm fractures. *Clin Orthop Relat Res* 175:25–29, 1983.

125. Tabor OB, Jr, Bosse MJ, Sims SH, et al: Iatrogenic posterior interosseous nerve injury: is transosseous static locked nailing of the radius feasible? *J Orthop Trauma* 9:427–429, 1995.

126. Tarr RR, Garfinkel AI, Sarmiento A: The effects of angular and rotational deformities of both bones of the forearm. An in vitro study. *J Bone Joint Surg Am* 66:65–70, 1984.

127. Tomaino MM, Pfaeffle J, Stabile K, et al: Reconstruction of the interosseous ligament of the forearm reduces load on the radial head in cadavers. *J Hand Surg [Br]* 28:267–270, 2003.

128. Trousdale RT, Amadio PC, Cooney WP, et al: Radio-ulnar dissociation. A review of twenty cases. *J Bone Joint Surg Am* 74:1486–1497, 1992.

129. Trousdale RT, Linscheid RL: Operative treatment of malunited fractures of the forearm. *J Bone Joint Surg Am* 77:894–902, 1995.

130. van Duijvenbode DC, Guitton TG, Raaymakers EL, et al: Long-term outcome of isolated diaphyseal radius fractures with and without dislocation of the distal radioulnar joint. *J Hand Surg [Am]* 37(3):523–527, 2012.

131. van Geenen RC, Besselaar PP: Outcome after corrective osteotomy for malunited fractures of the forearm sustained in childhood. *J Bone Joint Surg Br* 89:236–239, 2007.

132. Van Leemput T, Mahieu G: Conservative management of minimally displaced isolated fractures of the ulnar shaft. *Acta Orthop Belg* 73:710–713, 2007.

133. Vince KG, Miller JE: Cross-union complicating fracture of the forearm. Part I: adults. *J Bone Joint Surg Am* 69:640–653, 1987.

134. Visna P, Vicek M, Valcha M, et al: Management of diaphyseal forearm fractures using LCP angle stable fixation devices and intramedullary nailing. *Rozhl Chir* 88:708–715, 2009.

135. Lees VC: The functional anatomy of forearm rotation. *J Hand Microsurg* 1(2):92–99, 2009.

136. Wang AA, Jacobson-Petrov J, Stubin-Amelio L, et al: Selection of fusion position during forearm arthrodesis. *J Hand Surg [Am]* 25:842–848, 2000.

137. Weckbach A, Blattert TR, Weisser CH: Interlocking nailing of forearm fractures. *Arch Orthop Trauma Surg* 126:309–315, 2006.

138. Wei SY, Born CT, Abene A, et al: Diaphyseal forearm fractures treated with and without bone graft. *J Trauma* 46:1045–1048, 1999.

139. Wood MB: Upper extremity reconstruction by vascularized bone transfers: results and complications. *J Hand Surg [Am]* 12:422–427, 1987.

140. Wright RR, Schmeling GJ, Schwab JP: The necessity of acute bone grafting in diaphyseal forearm fractures: a retrospective review. *J Orthop Trauma* 11:288–294, 1997.

22

Complex Traumatic Elbow Dislocation

George S.M. Dyer and Jesse B. Jupiter

Acknowledgment: We wish to thank Dr. Jawa and Dr. Hotchkiss for their excellent chapter in the last edition of Green's Operative Hand Surgery *and their generosity in permitting much of their text and many of their illustrations to be reused.*

The elbow is one of the most constrained and inherently stable joints in the body, owing to numerous bony and soft tissue structures.[66,68] Therefore even simple elbow dislocation, where there is no fracture, indicates substantial soft tissue injury with disruption of the capsule and ligaments.[45,48] It is unusual, however, to observe chronic elbow instability or arthrosis after a stable reduction of a simple dislocation.[47,65,83]

In contrast, complex elbow dislocations are defined by capsuloligamentous disruption in association with fracture of one or more of the major bony stabilizers: the radial head, coronoid, or olecranon.[8,94] These fractures make the dislocation inherently unstable and almost always necessitate operative intervention to restore anatomic alignment and elbow stability.[46,108] The risk of recurrent instability and late arthrosis increases with the complexity of the injury and the number of stabilizers that are injured.[38,94,98] Understanding of the pathoanatomy of these injuries is still developing, and many questions exist about the best treatment algorithm. Successful evaluation and treatment require an understanding of the importance, function, and relationship of each major element of bony and soft tissue anatomy and its contribution to elbow stability.

FUNCTIONAL ANATOMY

Ulnar-Humeral Joint

The primary contributor to elbow stability is the ulnar-humeral joint. It is highly constrained: 180 degrees of the trochlea articulates with the proximal ulna.[1,66,68] The distal humerus tilts 30 degrees anteriorly, and the semilunar notch tilts posteriorly.[105,118] This reciprocal relationship increases the prominence of the coronoid and makes it a key stabilizer of the ulnar-humeral joint. The intact coronoid resists the posteriorly directed moments of the biceps and the triceps (Figure 22.1).[4,19,68] The coronoid is also important because the anterior band of the medial collateral ligament (MCL) inserts at its base. The MCL is the primary stabilizer to valgus moments.[9] More recently, the anteromedial facet of coronoid has been recognized as important for resisting varus moments as well[15,19,89,108] (Figure 22.2).

The olecranon is less important as a bony stabilizer. In cadaveric studies, resistance to posterior translation decreases linearly with olecranon excision, although 50% of the olecranon can be resected without affecting elbow stability.[1] The intact olecranon is important, however, in resistance to valgus moments.[67]

Radiocapitellar Joint

The radial head, along with the coronoid, resists posterior subluxation of the ulna.[103] With other osseous and ligamentous components of the elbow intact, the radiocapitellar articulation contributes minimally to valgus stability.[44,68] With MCL or coronoid injury, the radial head becomes the primary stabilizer to valgus stress and prevents subluxation or dislocation of the elbow.[69]

Capsuloligamentous Components

The MCL and the lateral collateral ligament (LCL) are the main capsuloligamentous stabilizers of the elbow.[74,75] The MCL is composed of anterior, posterior, and transverse bundles. The posterior and transverse bundles are subtle thickenings of the capsule, whereas the anterior bundle is a robust, identifiable structure that is crucial to resist valgus moments.[29,67,107] The anterior bundle originates from the medial epicondyle and inserts on the sublime tubercle at the base of the coronoid process.[27,77] Medial epicondyle fracture, large coronoid fracture, and MCL tear all are injury variants that can cause valgus elbow instability.[75]

The LCL complex comprises the radial collateral ligament, annular ligament, and posterior band, or lateral ulnar collateral ligament (LUCL).[104] The LUCL originates from the lateral epicondyle and inserts on the supinator crest of the proximal ulna where it is confluent with the annular ligament. The LUCL is the prime restraint to posterolateral rotatory instability.[23,72,76,79] Additional lateral soft tissues, including the extensor origin and the annular ligament, contribute to resisting posterolateral instability.[13,24,78]

Musculotendinous Components

The osseous and ligamentous structures all provide static stability for the elbow, whereas the muscles crossing the elbow joint provide dynamic stability.[94] The biceps, brachialis, and triceps muscles help maintain the trochlea in the semilunar notch with posteriorly directed forces.[29] The flexor and extensor masses are secondary stabilizers of the medial and lateral sides.[13,23]

PREOPERATIVE EVALUATION

Clinical Assessment

Acute Injury

As in all acute fractures, especially high-energy elbow fracture-dislocations, the patient should be evaluated first according to the Advanced Trauma Life Support guidelines. Associated head trauma has an effect on management and outcome of the elbow

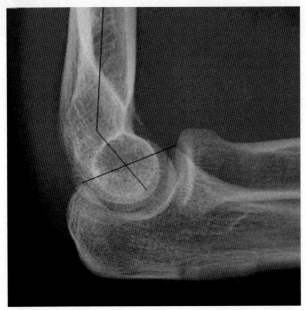

FIGURE 22.1 The elbow is highly constrained; 180 degrees of the articulating surface of trochlea is in contact with proximal ulna. The distal humerus tilts approximately 30 degrees anteriorly, and semilunar notch tilts posteriorly in a reciprocal relationship.

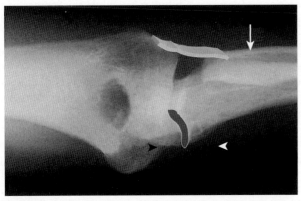

FIGURE 22.2 The elbow joint experiences varus stress *(arrow)* when shoulder abduction occurs. Resistance to varus load comes from tension in posterior lateral collateral ligament and load across medial facet of coronoid and distal humerus *(arrowheads)*. (Copyright Robert N. Hotchkiss.)

because of increased incidence of heterotopic bone formation.[30,32] Additionally, concomitant fractures, dislocations, and injuries in the ipsilateral upper extremity occur in 10% to 20% of cases.[108] Distal radioulnar joint tenderness may represent an interosseous ligament disruption and should alert the examiner to the possibility of an Essex-Lopresti injury.[34,108,111]

Fracture-dislocations are notable for significant swelling, pain, and visible deformity. A thorough neurovascular examination before and after any reduction or manipulation is mandatory because of the high-energy nature of these injuries. Most nerve injuries are secondary to traction. The ulnar nerve is the most vulnerable and commonly injured because of its positioning directly medial to the joint.[60,106] Median nerve and radial nerve injuries are rare but have been reported, including entrapment of both nerves in the joint.[58,115] Stretching and tearing of other anterior structures, including the brachial artery, have

been reported and rarely can lead to ischemia and compartment syndrome.[109] These injuries are seen more often in pediatric patients.[39]

Monitoring of the soft tissue swelling is essential because forearm compartment syndrome must always be suspected in high-energy injuries. A "floating forearm" injury, where a more distal radius fracture occurs together with an elbow fracture, is particularly associated with forearm compartment syndrome.[43]

Delayed Treatment or Previous Surgery

For patients who present for delayed treatment or who may have had previous surgery, a careful assessment of their range of motion, pain, and nerve function should be recorded. Ulnar nerve function may be already diminished without the patient being aware, overshadowed by the pain and overall impact of the elbow injury.[26] Flexion and extension and forearm rotation should be checked.

Imaging
Acute Injury

Anteroposterior and lateral radiographs of the elbow are necessary; however, it is often difficult to evaluate these complex injuries fully with the initial radiographs. Trauma films may be inadequate because of pain, deformity, bandages, and splinting material. Radiographs of the shoulder, wrist, and hand should also be included to rule out ipsilateral injuries. Two-dimensional and three-dimensional reformatted computed tomography (CT) scans of the elbow after closed reduction are extremely helpful for understanding the injury pattern and for preoperative planning. CT scans identify and help quantify injuries of the coronoid, radial head, or olecranon that may have been missed on plain radiographs. Lastly, fluoroscopic examination under anesthesia is useful while making operative decisions for treatment.[55]

Delayed Treatment or Previous Surgery

In cases in which the patient has undergone previous treatment but has an elbow that remains either dislocated or unstable, imaging must be tailored to the individual circumstances. Plain radiographs are mandatory, but because the joint is often stiff and the patient is unable to change its position, this situation requires some creativity and collaboration with the radiology staff for nonstandard views. The goal of plain radiographs is to document the integrity and alignment of the articulating surfaces of the distal humerus, radial head, and proximal ulna. Displaced articular fragments may be difficult to see. Internal fixation and radial head implants can obscure the joint surfaces and alignment. In these cases, magnetic resonance imaging (MRI) can be more valuable than CT because the scatter from the metal can be effectively reduced.

CLASSIFICATION AND PATTERNS OF INJURY

Posterolateral Rotational Injury

Most complex dislocations occur from a high-energy injury, such as a fall on an outstretched hand or motor vehicle accident. In 90% of dislocations, the injury is a combination of valgus, supination, and axial directed moments that combine to cause a posterior or posterolateral displacement of the proximal ulna from the trochlea.[14,75,76,108] Sequential and predictable injury starts from the lateral side and moves anteriorly and posteriorly to the medial side. This pattern of disruption is commonly referred to as the Horii circle.[40,78] The LCL complex is one of the first injured structures and is usually avulsed from the lateral epicondyle. The anterior band of the MCL is the last structure injured, and experimentally the elbow may dislocate with it intact. The flexor and extensor origins have a variable degree of injury.[25,45] Depending on how the energy is dissipated, the injury may result in pure capsuloligamentous disruption and a simple elbow dislocation or a complex dislocation with fractures of the radial head or coronoid or both.[25,46,94]

Dislocation With Radial Head Fracture

Ulnar-humeral dislocation is seen in less than 10% of radial head fractures[46] (Figure 22.3). These are higher-energy injuries than simple dislocations and involve greater instability and a higher risk of arthrosis. Hotchkiss' modification of the Mason classification (see Chapter 19) provides a useful scheme for evaluation. In the context of a fracture-dislocation, type I fractures do not require operative intervention, type II fractures require fixation, and type III fractures require replacement arthroplasty.[41] The LCL is typically avulsed from its origin at

the lateral epicondyle and must be addressed surgically; conversely, although the MCL is sometimes disrupted, it rarely causes persistent instability.[28]

Dislocation With Radial Head and Coronoid Fracture ("Terrible Triad")

These injuries have an increasing threat of persistent instability and posttraumatic arthrosis[12,84,98] (Figure 22.4). Coronoid fractures may be classified by their location and size into tip fractures, anteromedial fractures, and basal fractures (Figure 22.5). Subtype I tip fractures are 2 mm or smaller in size. Subtype II fractures are greater than 2 mm in size, but do not extend into the sublime tubercle.[18,108] The distinction between the two subtypes is arbitrary, however, and does not seem to affect treatment. The anterior capsule is usually still attached to the coronoid piece and must be considered when treating this fracture.[18] Anteromedial and basal fractures are typically seen with varus posteromedial rotational injuries and olecranon fracture-dislocations and are discussed in the next sections. The LCL and MCL are disrupted, although sometimes the anterior bundle of the MCL may remain intact. Ultimately, elbow stability is proportional to the size and location of the coronoid fracture, the extent of radial head comminution, and the severity of ligamentous disruption.[20,87]

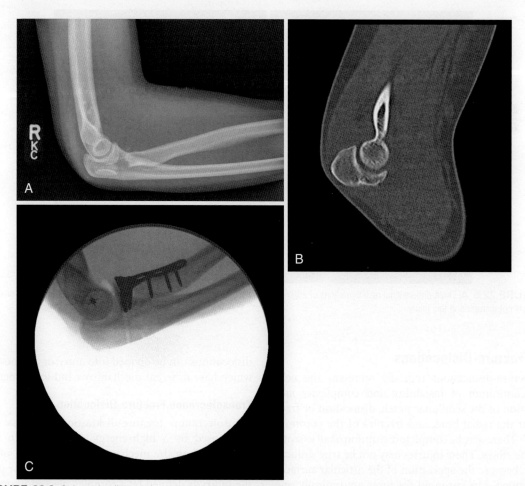

FIGURE 22.3 A, Lateral radiograph in a 16-year-old girl with a radial head fracture associated with elbow dislocation. The elbow is shown here reduced, but the incarcerated radial head fragment, the malalignment of the radial neck and capitellum, and the fleck from the coronoid are clues to instability. **B,** Sagittal CT showing telltale coronoid fracture. **C,** Reconstructed elbow. The anterior instability has been repaired with transosseous suture, the radial head has been repaired, and the LCL repaired with a suture anchor.

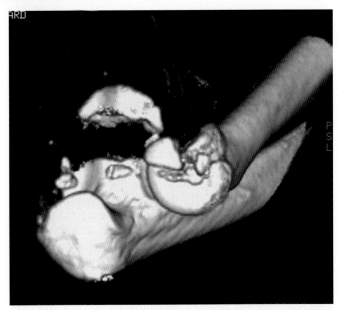

FIGURE 22.4 A 3D CT scan shows a coronoid fracture that is typical for a terrible triad injury: a single transverse fragment that includes the insertion of the anterior capsule. Notice that the radial head fracture involves only 40% of the articular surface but is too complex to repair. (Courtesy David Ring, MD, PhD)

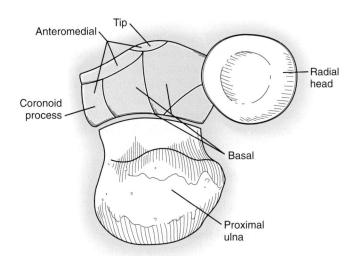

FIGURE 22.5 Coronoid fracture classification as described in O'Driscoll and colleagues.[78] Tip fractures have two subtypes: Subtype I involves <2 mm of coronoid height, and subtype II involves >2 mm of coronoid height. Anteromedial fractures have three subtypes: Subtype I involves the anteromedial rim, subtype II involves the anteromedial rim and tip, and subtype III involves the anteromedial rim and sublime tubercle. Basal fractures have two subtypes: Subtype I involves the coronoid body, indicated by at least 50% of the height of the coronoid, and subtype II is associated with olecranon fractures.

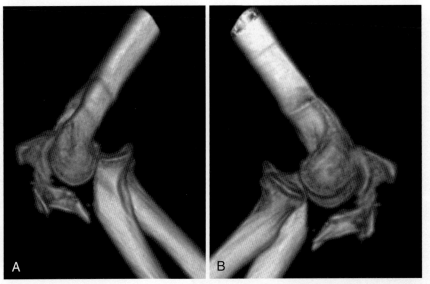

FIGURE 22.6 A, Three-dimensional reconstructions of anterior transolecranon fracture-dislocation. **B,** Proximal radioulnar joint relationship is not disrupted in this injury.

Olecranon Fracture-Dislocations

Olecranon fracture-dislocations typically represent the next stage in the continuum of instability and complexity and include disruption of the semilunar notch, dislocation or fracture or both of the radial head, and fracture of the coronoid process.[49,94,96,113] There may be complete disruption of all osseous stabilizers of the elbow. These injuries may not be true dislocations, however, because the apposition of the articular surfaces may be maintained. The coronoid fractures are typically one large piece (>50% height), but may also be comminuted; the basal subtype II fractures are most commonly associated with olecranon fractures[18,89] (see Figure 22.5). These fracture-

dislocations can be divided into anterior and posterior injuries, which have different mechanisms and injury patterns.

Transolecranon Fracture-Dislocation

Transolecranon fracture-dislocations are less common and are caused by a high-energy direct blow to the forearm.[96] Depending on the mechanism and direction of the blow, the forearm may be dislocated either anteriorly or posteriorly, but the injury is defined by a complex olecranon or proximal ulna facture, dislocation of the forearm, and maintenance of the proximal radioulnar relationship[70,71,96] (Figure 22.6). This injury pattern was first described and named "trans-olecranal fracture dislocation" in 1974 by Biga and Thomine.[6] This and subsequent studies emphasized the distinction from Monteggia fractures, in which the radioulnar relationship is dissociated.[71,97] When the capsuloligamentous structures are maintained, the elbow is typically rendered stable once the proximal ulna anatomy is reduced and fixed. Even when ligamentous repair is required, outcomes are often favorable. This is because the forearm is not disrupted, so good recovery of forearm rotation can be expected.[70]

Posterior Monteggia Lesion

Chapter 21 explores the Monteggia lesion in detail, so that injury is covered here only briefly. Penrose[81a] proposed that the posterior Monteggia lesion is a type of fracture-dislocation of the elbow[49,81,97,100] (Figure 22.7). The injury is usually seen in older osteopenic women after a low-energy fall onto the elbow. The injury is characterized by a posterior radial head dislocation, a proximal ulna fracture, a coronoid fracture (basal subtype II), and ulnar-humeral instability.[73,93,108] The coronoid fracture is more variable than with anterior injuries, may involve the tip or the anteromedial facet, and may be comminuted. The

radial head is fractured in two-thirds of injuries. The LCL may be injured, but the MCL is typically spared. In contrast to anterior olecranon fracture-dislocations, instability may persist after restoration of the bony stabilizers.[98] Posterior Monteggia injuries can be classified as follows[49,117]:

Type A: Fractures including the coronoid process
Type B: Fractures of the ulnar metaphysis
Type C: Fractures of the ulnar diaphysis
Type D: Complex, comminuted fractures of the entire proximal ulna

Varus Posteromedial Rotational Injury

Varus posteromedial rotational injury is a less common variant.[18,19] Similar to olecranon fracture-dislocations, these injuries may not be true dislocations in that the relationship of the articular surfaces is maintained[89] (Figure 22.8). In these injuries, a fall on an outstretched arm with the shoulder in flexion and abduction creates a varus posteromedial rotational force on the forearm. This force causes the LCL complex to tear from the lateral epicondyle in tension. Simultaneously, the medial coronoid process is forced against the medial trochlea and sometimes results in an anteromedial facet fracture of the coronoid. The coronoid fracture can just involve the anteromedial rim (subtype I), extend to involve the tip with comminution (subtype II), or involve the sublime tubercle and the attachment of the anterior band of the MCL (subtype III) (see Figure 22.5). Anteromedial facet fractures are seen in combination with elbow dislocation, sometimes with an olecranon fracture, but rarely with an associated radial head fracture.[19] This fracture pattern of instability may show only subtle joint incongruity and may be missed, leading to rapid development of arthrosis.[4,5,15,28]

HISTORICAL REVIEW

In 1927, McWhorter[64] reported on his indications and techniques for treatment of olecranon and coronoid fractures. His technique of exposure to the coronoid and proposed fixation with suture or a screw is very similar to what we do today. He recognized almost 90 years ago that coronoid fractures associated with dislocations and radial head fractures had poor outcomes. He encouraged operative fixation of displaced fractures and early motion—concepts that we are currently rediscovering.

After McWhorter's work, the diagnosis and treatment of elbow fracture-dislocations progressed slowly for several decades. Poor outcomes were acknowledged, but the critical components of elbow instability were not recognized. It was not until the 1980s that Josefsson and colleagues[46,47] made the clear distinction between the excellent long-term outcomes of simple elbow dislocations and the poor outcomes of fracture-dislocations.

Subsequently, understanding of the patterns of injury and treatment of complex elbow dislocations continued to expand rapidly. Regan and Morrey[86,87] classified and recognized the importance of the coronoid fracture to stability, whereas Hotchkiss[41] formally recognized the terrible triad injury pattern, which McWhorter described 80 years earlier.

Since 2000 there has been steady improvement in understanding of the pathoanatomy of elbow fracture-dislocations

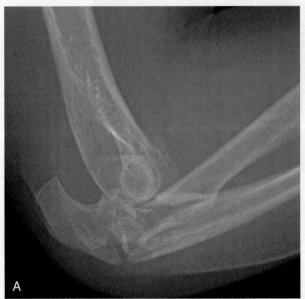
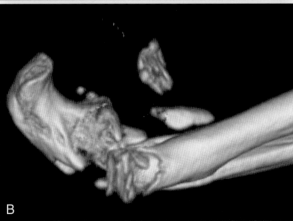

FIGURE 22.7 A, Lateral radiograph of posterior Monteggia fracture-dislocation. **B,** Three-dimensional reconstruction of posterior Monteggia injury. Note posterior position of radial head and loss of normal proximal radioulnar relationship. Also note coronoid fracture that is typically seen with these injuries.

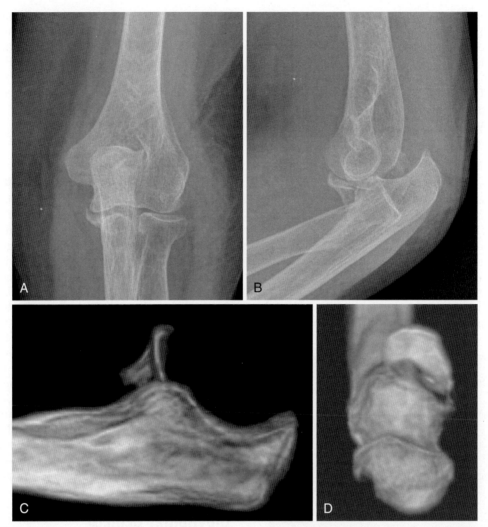

FIGURE 22.8 Posteroanterior (**A**) and lateral (**B**) radiographs of acute, isolated anteromedial facet coronoid fracture. Note ulnar-humeral instability in this fracture pattern. **C** and **D,** Three-dimensional reconstructions of fracture.

and the development of standard ways of approaching them surgically. O'Driscoll, Morrey and others have better defined the mechanism of dislocation and the fracture-related anatomy of the MCL.[77,78] Schneeberger and others elucidated the relationship between the bone and ligament stabilizers and the mechanisms of dislocation.[74,103] Using detailed analysis of imaging, Ring, Jupiter, and Doornberg have improved our understanding of the osseous anatomy of the coronoid and called particular attention to its anteromedial facet.[15,92,94] McKee and colleagues published what they called a "standard protocol" for addressing the terrible triad injury, with systematic management of coronoid and anterior capsule injury, radial head fracture, and LCL injury, in that order.[62] These advances have led to substantially better outcomes for patients with these injuries. Yet problems remain including stiffness,[91] associated nerve injury,[26,106] and heterotopic ossification.[3]

TREATMENT OPTIONS

Acute Injuries (Less Than 2 Weeks)

Treatment of acute injuries is done with the intention of establishing sufficient stability to allow for early active motion. The first step is to restore osseous stability by anatomically aligning

and stabilizing the articular surface of the semilunar notch.[95] Next, the radial head and the radiocapitellar contact need to be restored. Finally, the ligaments need to be repaired. The LCL complex is more important to stability in the setting of complex traumatic dislocations than the MCL. The MCL rarely needs to be repaired and heals with restoration of bony anatomy and with active motion.[28]

Dislocation

Simple dislocations should be managed by immediate closed reduction. Reduction requires adequate relaxation and analgesia, but can be readily performed in the emergency department with conscious sedation and intravenous medication. The reduction maneuver requires placing firm pressure on the olecranon tip to push the ulna distal to allow the trochlea to fall into the semilunar notch. Successful reduction is accompanied by a clunking sensation. The elbow should be tested for stability at this point by taking it through a range of motion. Most elbows are stable after reduction, but may have a tendency for redislocation in extension or with valgus stress. Radiographs should confirm a concentric reduction, and the elbow should be splinted in approximately 90 degrees of flexion for 1 week, at which time repeat radiographs should confirm reduction.

Splinting can help reduce swelling and pain, but should not be prolonged. Motion should be started in the first week, although splinting for 2 weeks does not seem to affect long-term outcomes. Splinting beyond 3 weeks increases the risk of persistent flexion contracture and pain and may predispose to heterotopic ossification.[65,102]

Sometimes, slight postreduction subluxation of the elbow is identified on radiographs and is known as the "drop sign." This is analogous to pseudosubluxation of the shoulder after closed reduction and can be treated with exercises and avoidance of varus stress.[22] Infrequently, simple elbow dislocations are unstable after reduction and require operative intervention with ligamentous repairs or skeletal fixation. This topic is discussed further in Chapter 23.

Fracture-Dislocation (Radial Head)

Closed reduction of the elbow dislocation is performed as described earlier. Fracture of the radial head with an associated ulnar-humeral dislocation creates an additional potential cause of elbow instability. CT scan is useful to rule out a subtle, but important, coronoid fracture that may necessitate operative intervention. The radial head generally should not be resected (without replacement) in the setting of dislocation because the injured ligaments must heal at the correct length and tension. Maintenance of radiocapitellar contact is important in the early postinjury period.

Nonoperative Management. In the absence of a coronoid fracture, a radial head fracture with an elbow dislocation can be treated nonoperatively. Josefsson and colleagues[45] and Broberg and Morrey[8] reported good results in patients treated with closed reduction with or without radial head excision and cast immobilization. The best results were obtained in patients with Mason type II fractures treated with closed reduction and Mason type III fractures treated with excision.[83] None of these patients had an associated coronoid fracture and many of the patients treated nonoperatively required delayed radial excisions for pain or stiffness.[7] Additionally, there is some risk of instability if fractures are treated nonoperatively. Motivated patients who understand the risks who choose nonoperative treatment should be seen within 1 week after injury for radiographs to show maintenance of reduction. Although Broberg and Morrey[8] treated patients in a cast for 1 month, it is reasonable to treat patients in a splint with early range of motion and close follow-up. The reader is referred to Chapter 19 for a more detailed discussion of radial head fractures.

Operative Treatment: Repair, Arthroplasty, and Lateral Collateral Ligament Complex Repair. Restoration of the native anatomy of the lateral column contributes to elbow stability and prevention of late arthrosis, so the radial head should be fixed when possible and the LCL complex repaired.[34,51,85] One- or two-part partial articular fractures and fractures that separate the entire head in one piece with a clean break are generally amenable to repair. It is advisable to replace the head when struggling to reconstruct it in situations that would either greatly extend the length of the operation, when the resulting construct would be too delicate to withstand early motion, or when the complexity and deformity portend a poor prognosis in terms of union or forearm rotation.[88,90] For fractures that have three or more articular fragments or cannot be repaired with confidence, resection and replacement with a metal radial head arthroplasty

are appropriate (see Chapter 20).[37,99,119] Silicone replacements should not be used.[10,82,116] Short-term results appear similar whether the radial head is replaced or repaired.[54] Oversizing the radial head should be avoided because it may cause capitellar arthrosis and pain.[1] The reconstructed articular surface should end up no more than 1 mm proud of the corner of the lesser sigmoid notch[16] (Figure 22.9).

After radial head repair or replacement, the LCL and extensor musculature origin commonly require repair (especially if there is disruption or persistent instability).[13,63] This can be done with suture anchors or transosseous drill holes placed through the lateral epicondyle. MCL repair is rarely required, but needs to be evaluated if instability remains after radial head and LCL repair and reconstruction.[28]

Technique of Lateral Collateral Ligament Repair. If the LCL is avulsed off the epicondyle, it is repaired with suture anchors or heavy suture (usually No. 2 nonabsorbable suture) passed through drilled bone tunnels or by simply driving a stout suture needle through the bone in the desired direction. A locking weave using a Krackow-type loop is used to secure the LCL complex. The suture anchor or the bone tunnels should be placed at the isometric point of the lateral ligamentous complex. This point is located at the central axis of the capitellar circumference and is surprisingly distal and anterior to the lateral epicondyle, typically 2 or 3 mm anterior and distal. The two tunnels should exit posteriorly and should be separated by a sufficient bony bridge over which the suture is tied. The sutures are passed and tied over bone after bony fixation is completed with the joint reduced.

Fracture-Dislocation (Coronoid)

The understanding of elbow dislocations with isolated coronoid fractures has been rapidly developing. Despite the often small size of the fracture, the injury may be unstable and require operative intervention.[4,19] The initiation of active range of motion, without coronoid fixation, may result in chronic subluxation and the rapid development of arthrosis.[18,20,80,89,92,108]

Examination Under Anesthesia. Stress radiographs have been suggested, but in the setting of an acute trauma this may be impractical. Examining these patients under anesthesia with image intensification is often useful to reveal subtle ulnar-humeral subluxation as the elbow is taken through a range of motion. Varus stress may elucidate LCL injury with opening of the radiocapitellar joint. In the unusual circumstance that no instability exists under anesthesia, nonoperative treatment may be appropriate, but this should be done with great caution and frequent clinical and radiographic follow-up.

Technique: Open Reduction and Internal Fixation. The patient is placed in a supine position with an arm table. The arm can be draped free with either a sterile or a nonsterile tourniquet. Either a posterior midline incision with elevation of a medial skin flap or a direct medial approach can be used. If a medial approach is used, the medial antebrachial cutaneous nerve should be protected. The ulnar nerve should always be found and protected. The ulnar nerve can be held and protected anteriorly by suturing the skin flap to the forearm fascia. At the end of the procedure, the ulnar nerve may be transposed subcutaneously but some authors have found that moving the nerve increases the incidence of palsy.[106] The coronoid fracture is exposed between the two heads of flexor carpi ulnaris, where

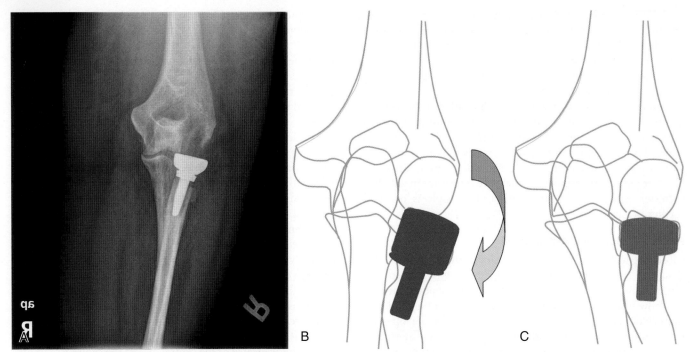

FIGURE 22.9 Oversizing the radial head may "stabilize" the elbow by placing the entire lateral soft tissue complex on tension, but this is an error. **A,** Anteroposterior radiograph showing excessive lateral ulnohumeral joint space and medial ulnohumeral translation due to overstuffing of the radial head prosthesis. **B,** The anatomical relationships with a radial head prosthesis that is too large. **C,** A sketch showing the appropriate anatomical relationships.

the ulnar nerve lies; through elevation of the entire flexor pronator mass; or through the over-the-top approach described by Hotchkiss.[41] Details of this description can be found in Chapter 24.

The anterior band of the MCL, which lies below the flexor pronator mass, should be protected to prevent injury and further instability. After the fracture is exposed and reduced, various options for fixation exist, including transosseous sutures, Kirschner wires, lag screws, and plate fixation. Isolated coronoid fractures with elbow dislocation and without a radial head fracture are typically anteromedial facet fractures and require stable, anatomic fixation. Threaded 0.062-inch Kirschner wires may be passed through the ulna into the coronoid fragment, or lag screws, small T-plates, or special coronoid buttress plates can be used for fixation. Generally, large anteromedial coronoid fragments are best stabilized with lag screws or buttress plates, whereas small tip fragments may be best treated with Kirschner wire fixation or transosseous sutures. If LCL complex injury is present, the lateral skin flap should be elevated or a separate lateral incision should be made and the ligament repaired as detailed earlier. Failure to repair the LCL may result in persistent instability. The elbow should be taken through a range of motion under image intensification to assess stability.

❖ AUTHORS' PREFERRED TECHNIQUE

We prefer a posterior skin incision, then isolating and protecting the ulnar nerve. The coronoid fracture is exposed directly through the heads of the flexor carpi ulnaris, where the nerve lies before transposition. The MCL is protected, and the fracture is fixed with a T-plate or a specially designed buttress plate. Stability of the elbow is tested after fixation with gravity

extension. If instability persists, a separate lateral exposure is used through the same skin incision to repair the LCL with suture anchors. The LCL typically needs to be repaired with this fracture pattern. Postoperatively, active and active-assisted motion may begin 1 to 2 days after surgery.

Dislocation With Radial Head and Coronoid Fractures (Terrible Triad Injuries)

The addition of a coronoid fracture, regardless of size, to an elbow dislocation with a radial head fracture substantially increases the chances of acute and chronic instability and posttraumatic elbow arthrosis.[98] CT scans are helpful for preoperative planning, specifically for evaluating coronoid fractures. The coronoid fragment should be fixed by suture repair of the anterior capsule, screw fixation, or plate and screws to restore elbow stability.

Nonoperative Management. A small subset of terrible triad injuries with small coronoid and radial head fractures that remain concentrically reduced can be treated effectively without surgery. Patients must be able to avoid shoulder abduction and must be willing to flex their elbow actively with confidence. The patients we have treated nonoperatively were seen a few days or a week after injury and were either out of the splint moving well or were very motivated to avoid surgery. As a rule, however, virtually all terrible triad injuries should be considered to require surgery.

Operative Management. The patient is placed in a supine position with an arm table. The arm should be draped free with either a sterile or a nonsterile tourniquet. The injury can be repaired with a lateral approach to the elbow if the radial head is going to be excised and replaced. A posterior midline approach, elevating a lateral skin flap, can be used, however, if

CRITICAL POINTS *Coronoid Repair*

Indications
- Coronoid fracture with elbow instability

Preoperative Evaluation
- Posteroanterior and lateral radiographs of elbow
- CT scan with three-dimensional reconstructions

Pearls
- The LCL typically needs to be repaired.
- The ulnar nerve can be held and protected anteriorly by suturing the skin flap to the forearm fascia.

Technical Points
- Release and protect the ulnar nerve.
- Expose the fracture through the flexor carpi ulnaris heads.
- Remain superficial to the MCL.
- A small T-plate or a specially designed buttress plate is preferred for fixation.
- Test elbow stability with image intensification.
- If instability persists, a separate lateral deep exposure should be made to repair the LCL.
- If instability persists after LCL repair, a hinged external fixator (see Chapter 24) should be used.

Pitfalls
- Ulnar neuropathy can occur because of excessive retraction on the nerve.
- Excision of a seemingly small coronoid piece can lead to persistent instability and arthrosis.
- Anteromedial facet fractures require anatomic, stable reduction; otherwise, instability may persist.

Postoperative Care
- Active range of motion is begun 1 to 2 days after surgery.
- Avoid shoulder abduction, which stresses the LCL repair.
- Check the elbow frequently in the early postoperative period for maintenance of reduction.

a medial approach is contemplated. A traumatic rent in the fascia is almost always present and may be developed for exposure. Otherwise, the supracondylar ridge is identified, and the extensor origins are elevated anteriorly. At this point, it is often noted that the LCL and the extensor musculature are traumatized or pulled off of the ridge and epicondyle.

Distally, an incision is made that extends from the tip of the lateral epicondyle and bisects the radial head and neck. The traumatic rent in the extensor musculature can usually be exploited to gain exposure to the radial head. The dissection should stay anterior to the midline of the capitellum to preserve residual soft tissue attachments. Distally, dissection should be unnecessary beyond the radial neck, and caution should be used because the posterior interosseous nerve is at risk. Keeping the forearm in pronation minimizes risk to the nerve.

At this point, a decision to repair or replace the radial head is made. If the radial head is to be repaired, the coronoid tip fracture can be fixed after resection of the radial head because this greatly improves exposure. To further improve access to the coronoid, the elbow can be hinged open on the intact medial structures. Deep retractors, such as Z-knee retractors, are helpful to gain exposure to the coronoid. If access is still

difficult, a medial skin flap can be raised from the posterior incision, or a separate medial incision can be made to expose the coronoid fracture. Medial exposure should also be used when the coronoid fracture includes a portion or all of the medial facet. In these cases, screw or plate and screw fixation should be used as detailed above.

After identifying the coronoid tip fracture fragment, two tunnels for suture can be made with a small drill bit or a 0.062-inch Kirschner wire from the subcutaneous border of the ulna into the base of the coronoid fracture. One tunnel should be medial and one lateral in the fracture base. The dorsal exit points should be positioned 1 cm apart to create a bone bridge to tie over and may be placed slightly off the very ridge of the ulna to reduce knot prominence. The transtibial guide used in cruciate ligament reconstruction of the knee is helpful for this step. The tip fragment itself may be resected if it is tiny, or it may be included in the suture repair to reduce and fix it. Heavy nonabsorbable suture (No. 2 or No. 5) is passed through the anterior capsule or brachialis insertion. The suture is passed through the drill holes with a suture passer or a Keith needle from the dorsal ulna. Exact anatomic reduction is unnecessary; instead, the goal is to restore the anterior capsular attachment to the proximal ulna. The suture should not be tied until after the radial head replacement has been completed to avoid disrupting the coronoid fixation.

If the LCL complex is avulsed off the epicondyle, it must be repaired with suture anchors or heavy suture (usually No. 2) passed through transosseous drilled bone tunnels (as previously described). After the repair is complete, stability should be checked visually and under image intensification through an arc of motion. If instability persists, thought should be given to repair of the MCL, application of a hinged external fixator (see Chapter 24), or both (Figure 22.10).

The MCL is repaired through a separate deep medial exposure. The ulnar nerve is found and released from the intermuscular septum to the Osborne fascia. The nerve is protected and transposed into the subcutaneous tissue anteriorly. The avulsed MCL origin and common flexor origin are identified and repaired using suture anchors or sutures passed through bone tunnels (as described for the LCL complex repair in Chapter 20).

If the elbow continues to be unstable despite the surgeon's best efforts, an external fixator can be applied. Alternatively, the joint can be cross pinned. After manipulation under fluoroscopy, two large Kirschner wires (0.078 in) are drilled through the ulnar-humeral joint. The wires are directed posteriorly through the posterior humeral cortex to prevent pin migration. After reduction is confirmed, the wires are cut and bent at the skin, and a well-padded cast is applied. The wires are removed at 3 or 4 weeks, and active motion is initiated.

❖ AUTHORS' PREFERRED TECHNIQUE

We treat the injury from inside out, first fixing the coronoid, then the radial head, and then the LCL. The LCL typically needs to be repaired back to the lateral epicondyle with a suture anchor or through bone tunnels. The elbow is tested with gravity extension with the forearm in neutral. If the ulnar-humeral joint remains reduced from full flexion to 45 degrees of flexion, MCL repair is unnecessary. Otherwise, the MCL should be repaired or extension should be limited postoperatively for up to 4 weeks by a splint or hinged elbow brace while

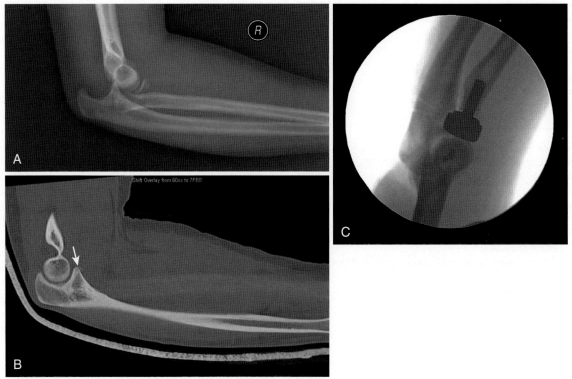

FIGURE 22.10 A, Lateral radiograph of an acute terrible triad injury in a 32-year-old man. **B,** Postreduction, preoperative CT scan showing fleck from coronoid is the only clue to anterior instability. **C,** Reconstructed elbow. The anterior instability was repaired with transosseous suture, the radial head has been replaced, and the LCL repaired with a suture anchor. The elbow was still unstable so the medial collateral ligament was also repaired.

CRITICAL POINTS *Terrible Triad Repair*

Indications
- Virtually all terrible triad injuries require operative repair.

Preoperative Evaluation
- Posteroanterior and lateral radiographs of elbow
- CT scan with three-dimensional reconstructions

Pearls
- Most repairs can be done from the lateral side.
- Z-knee or deep retractors help with exposure medially from the lateral side.

Technical Points
- Elevate the extensors off the supracondylar ridge.
- Expose the radial head, preserving the LCL posteriorly.
- Excise the radial head if it is not repairable for better exposure of the coronoid.
- Fix the coronoid with the suture technique, replace the radial head, and repair the LCL.

- Make a separate medial approach if exposure to the coronoid is difficult because of a largely intact, repairable radial head.
- Test elbow stability with image intensification.

Pitfalls
- Instability may result from failure to fix a small coronoid fracture.
- Failure to use an external fixator if instability persists.
- Resection of the radial head without replacement leads to persistent instability.

Postoperative Care
- Active range of motion is begun 1 to 2 days after surgery.
- Avoid shoulder abduction, which stresses the LCL repair.
- Check the elbow frequently in the early postoperative period for maintenance of reduction.
- Strengthening begins after evidence of bony healing at 6 to 8 weeks.

---

the MCL heals. Stability is usually obtained, however, without the need for MCL repair, hinged external fixation, or cross pinning of the elbow. If the MCL requires repair, a separate medial exposure is used. Postoperatively, active and active-assisted motion should begin 1 to 2 days after surgery.

Olecranon Fracture-Dislocations

The critical element in the treatment of proximal ulna fractures is the restoration of the semilunar notch with anatomic alignment of the coronoid and olecranon. Anterior fracture-dislocations rarely involve the radial head and LCL, whereas posterior injuries often do. For this reason, instability may persist after restoration of bony stabilizers for posterior fracture-dislocations. A distractor may be helpful in reducing the fracture. The details of surgical repair and technique are provided in Chapter 21, although we briefly review our experience here.

Operative Technique. In our experience, these fractures can usually be treated entirely through the olecranon fracture,

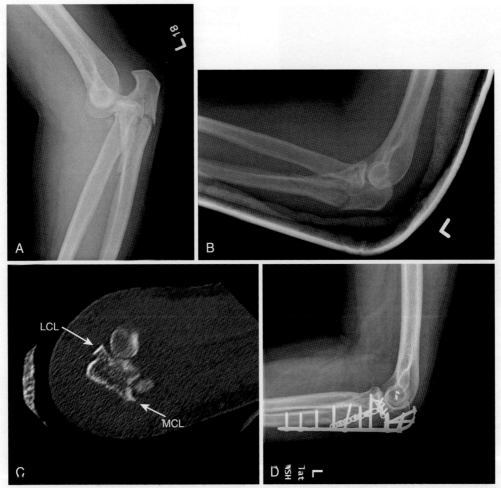

FIGURE 22.11 A, Lateral radiograph of an unstable transolecranon fracture-dislocation in a 24-year-old man. **B,** The same injury after reduction. **C,** Axial CT showing characteristic bony fragments corresponding to the attachments of the medial collateral ligament (*MCL*) and lateral collateral ligament (*LCL*). **D,** Postoperative construct. The proximal ulna was reconstructed with a medial buttress plate and a dorsal bridging plate. Anterior stability was restored using sutures passed through an empty screw hole that lined up with the coronoid. The LCL and MCL were repaired with suture anchors.

which is exposed through a midline posterior skin incision. The radial head is typically replaced because of comminution, and the LCL needs to be exposed and repaired. The coronoid fractures can be quite comminuted and difficult to repair. There are usually large fragments associated with the attachment points of the LCL (the crista supinatoris) and the MCL (the sublime tubercle). This consistent pattern is useful for orienting and understanding the jumbled fragments (Figure 22.11). A distractor may be helpful to attain reduction, and a hinged external fixator may be needed to maintain the reduction. The addition of a tension band to plate fixation may help in stabilizing a comminuted olecranon fracture. The keys to maintaining stability are repair of the torn LCL and stable coronoid fixation.

Hinged External Fixation

After reconstruction of the bony and ligamentous structures, the elbow should be tested with image intensification for stability. The elbow is tested by gravity extension with the forearm in neutral position from full flexion until reaching 45 to 60 degrees of flexion. Some authors recommend testing the elbow in pro-

nation because it enhances elbow stability. Slight subluxation may be seen radiographically and may be acceptable.[21] If the elbow seems unstable and vulnerable to redislocation after fixation, we also recommend the use of an external fixator that stabilizes the joint and allows immediate mobilization.[50,84,112] The goal of the hinged external fixator is to allow concentric ulnar-humeral motion, while protecting the bony and ligamentous repairs.[110,114] With external fixation, the patient starts moving the elbow from the first postoperative day, gradually increasing the range of motion and preventing stiffness. If a hinged external fixator is not available, it is acceptable to use a static frame or pin the ulnohumeral joint with a large K-wire or Steinmann pin.

The external fixator is removed 6 to 8 weeks later, and the patient starts strengthening exercises. The patient returns to his or her previous activities approximately 4 to 6 months after the repair when full strength of the arm is regained.

Successful treatment of complex elbow fracture-dislocations demands facility with the indications and application of the hinged external fixator. The extra operative time and technical difficulties may make surgeons reluctant to use the device. A

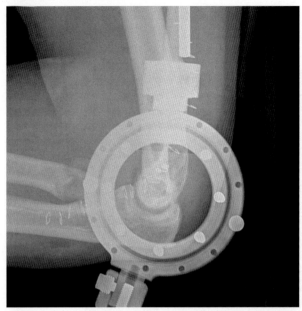

FIGURE 22.12 Lateral radiograph showing that the hinged external fixator is built around a temporary axis pin placed through the trochlea and capitellum at the center of ulnar-humeral rotation. The center of the external fixator ring corresponds with the center of the trochlea.

stiff, unstable elbow is an even larger problem to manage, however.

Operative Technique. Surgical application of a hinged fixator is demanding and requires knowledge and experience with one of the commercially available devices. There are two types of devices used: unilateral, which are generally easier to place, or multiplanar, which provide more rigid fixation. The placement of an axis pin around which the frame is built (Figure 22.12) is crucial to each device. Slight misalignment of the pin can increase the energy of motion significantly.[59,110]

The temporary axis pin is placed under fluoroscopic guidance and must be colinear with axis of rotation at the center of trochlea and capitellum. This line is slightly distal to the lateral epicondyle and slightly distal and anterior to the medial epicondyle. Care should be taken not to disrupt bony fixation or collateral ligament repair while placing the pin, although this can be technically challenging. If a multiplanar frame is used, the pin penetrates the medial cortex and the ulnar nerve needs to be protected. Based on the axis pin, half pins are placed on the humerus and ulna, although typically the humeral pins are placed first. The radial nerve should be identified and retracted through an open incision before placement of the lateral humeral pins. It is equally important to identify and protect the ulnar nerve while placing the medial humeral pins. The most distal humeral pin should be placed proximal to the metaphyseal flare. When the humeral pins are fixed, the joint can be reduced and the ulnar pins can be placed. Joint reduction can be facilitated by the use of gravity to align the joint and, if needed, by temporary cross wire fixation of the joint. The ulnar pins are placed lateral to medial or dorsal to volar. After the frame is placed, concentric elbow motion should be checked with image intensification. The axis pin is removed to prevent septic arthritis. Active mobilization should be initiated the day after surgery, and the fixator should be removed at 6 to 8 weeks.

CRITICAL POINTS *Hinged External Fixation*

Indications
- Persistent instability after attempted bony and ligamentous repair in the acute setting
- Chronic elbow instability in delayed treatment or failed previous treatment

Evaluation
- Intraoperative gravity extension with image intensification

Technical Points
- Different commercial external fixators are available that are either unilateral or multiplanar.
- A joint axis pin must be placed colinear with the axis of rotation.
- The line of rotation is slightly distal to the lateral epicondyle and slightly anterior and distal to the medial epicondyle.
- Find the radial nerve before placing the lateral humeral pins and the ulnar nerve if placing medial humeral pin.
- Reduce the joint and temporarily hold it reduced with smooth 0.078-inch wires.
- Place the distal pins with direct visualization.

Pearls and Pitfalls
- The work of elbow motion is increased fourfold with 5 degrees of misalignment of the axis pin.
- Ligamentous repair failure or loss of fracture reduction can occur with placement of the fixator.
- Avoid impaling muscle or tendon because this limits motion.
- All pins should be placed with direct visualization to prevent nerve injury.

Postoperative Care
- Active range of motion is begun soon after surgery.
- The fixator is removed at 6 to 8 weeks.
- Therapy with dynamic or static splinting is begun to improve range of motion after removal.

Delayed Treatment

The challenges of precise restoration of bony alignment and soft tissue stability for elbow fracture-dislocations are compounded by a delay in treatment. Additional difficulties may include extensive scar, partially or nonunited bone fragments, poor skin cover, and a subluxated or dislocated joint. For patients who present for treatment several weeks or months after the original injury, the difficulty of the case is often intensified by damage to the articular surfaces.

❖ AUTHORS' PREFERRED TECHNIQUE

Positioning and Incision. The best position for delayed operative treatment may be either the lateral or the prone position. These positions permit a simple posterior incision and a wide exposure of the joint. This position also makes application of the hinged fixator simpler because there is a tendency for the joint to rest in a position of reduction rather than dislocation.

The skin incisions are dictated by previous incisions and the particular problem. Generally, previous incisions should be used to avoid loss of skin coverage in the postoperative period. We prefer either a single posterior or separate medial or lateral incisions to permit access to the lateral and medial joint surfaces, the ulnar nerve, and the posterior ulna. The first structure that must be identified and protected is the ulnar nerve.

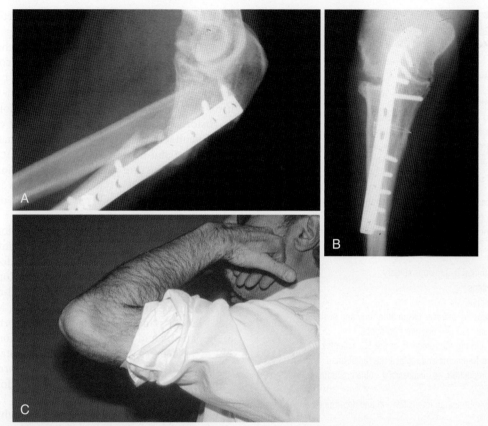

FIGURE 22.13 A, Lateral radiograph of a 64-year-old patient 3 weeks after initial open treatment of posterior Monteggia fracture-dislocation. The radial head is dislocated posteriorly and the proximal ulna is malaligned. **B,** Postoperative radiograph after replating ulna. **C,** Postoperative motion showing loss of extension and adequate flexion.

Dissection of the nerve must be done carefully, usually starting proximal to the previous dissection. We free the nerve gently and transpose it to an anterior subcutaneous location with adequate mobilization to perform the open reduction.

Reconstruction. When the nerve is free, the next task is to reduce the joint and expose the fracture fragments for fixation. The thickened capsule on the anterior and posterior surfaces must be completely excised to permit the joint to be reduced. The posterior olecranon fossa and the coronoid fossa are also gently excavated down to the original surfaces so that the ulna can track properly. The articular surfaces on both sides of the joint are usually covered with thickened scar tissue, and this layer must be carefully lifted away without damaging the underlying remaining articular cartilage. A small blunt elevator is often useful at this point in the case. The condition of these surfaces is unpredictable, and it is common to find extensive delamination and damage.

During the exposure, the lateral collateral ligament complex should be identified and isolated for later reattachment and repair. We do not routinely repair or reconstruct the medial ligaments; however, if there is tissue that can be approximated on the medial side after reduction of the joint, it should be prepared for repair.

When the joint has been completely dissected free of restraining scar and it can be held in a reduced position through an acceptable range of motion, the bone work can be done. Occasionally, malalignment of the ulna must also be addressed before the joint is stable, and the surgeon should be prepared for these situations (Figure 22.13). Nonetheless, with the joint now reduced, the radial head can be prepared for replacement. In cases of delayed treatment, we have not found repair to be likely or possible.

The lateral ligament complex is reattached as in the acute situation. It is important not to tie the ligament repairs if a hinged fixator is to be used. At this stage, the joint is grossly unstable, and we prefer to secure the joint into position with hinged fixation and with the sutures in place but not tied. After the fixator is in place, we tie them securely, without fear of dislodging the repair while applying the fixator. Additional bone anchors can be used to secure the posterior tissues to the anterior lateral capsule, further improving varus stability.

We often use a hinged external fixator in these complex and delayed reconstructions.[10,16,40,116] There is often only one more chance to achieve stable and useful elbow function; if persistent painful dislocation recurs, the only remaining options are to accept the situation or consider a distraction-interposition arthroplasty, total elbow replacement, or arthrodesis.

POSTOPERATIVE MANAGEMENT AND OUTCOME

Postoperative Management

For all elbow fracture-dislocations, postoperative management is based on the same principles. Gentle active and active-assisted range of motion exercises are started several days after surgery.

CRITICAL POINTS *Delayed Treatment or Previous Repair*

Indications
- Instability more than 2 weeks after injury or after previous repair

Preoperative Evaluation
- Posteroanterior and lateral radiographs of elbow
- CT scan with three-dimensional reconstructions
- Other imaging tailored to the individual circumstances and previous surgery
- Assessment of ulnar, median, and radial nerve function

Pearls
- Prone positioning can help with the placement of a hinged external fixator.
- An osteotomy may be required to obtain fixation.
- Tie down the ligamentous repairs after placement of the external fixator.

Technical Points
- Incisions are determined by previous surgery.
- Elevate large skin flaps.
- Identify the ulnar nerve.
- Excise thickened capsule and scar tissue anteriorly and posteriorly.
- Clear the articular surface and fracture fragments.
- Identify, preserve, and tag the remnants of the LCL complex.
- Reduce the fracture fragments and replace the radial head.
- If ulnar-humeral reduction is impossible, ulna osteotomy may be necessary.
- Test elbow stability with image intensification and determine the need for external fixation.
- Place a hinged external fixator or tie ligament repairs.

Pitfalls
- Instability may result from failure to place an external fixator.

Postoperative Care
- Active range of motion is begun soon after surgery.
- The hinged fixator is removed in 6 to 8 weeks.

For anteromedial facet fractures of the coronoid, a hinged brace may be helpful in resisting gravitational varus stresses that may stress the fracture fixation. If the fixation is tenuous, especially in osteoporotic bone, immobilization in 90 degrees of flexion may be advisable until the first postoperative visit at 1 to 2 weeks, before movement is started. Stiffness occurs if motion is not initiated soon after fixation. If a choice needs to be made between joint stability and early mobility, stability takes precedence. It is easier to correct a stiff congruent joint than a chronically unstable one.

Expected Outcomes

Outcomes after elbow fracture-dislocations are directly related to the degree of soft tissue and bony injury. Because understanding and treatment of these injuries are still evolving, there are few data to know the long-term outcomes for many treatments. Some degree of stiffness and arthrosis often results.

The outcomes for simple radial head fractures treated with open reduction and internal fixation or comminuted fractures treated with radial head replacement have been favorable.[2,17,28,51,52] Some decreased forearm rotation and elbow extension can be expected. Less favorable outcomes have been reported after open reduction and internal fixation of radial

head fractures that have more than three articular fragments.[88] Ring and colleagues[99] showed that 13 of 14 patients with Mason type III fractures characterized by more than three articular fragments had unsatisfactory results. In contrast, of the 12 patients with Mason type III fractures with two or three simple fragments, none had early failure, one had a nonunion, and all had greater than 100 degrees of forearm motion.

Historically, outcomes for treatment of coronoid fractures are difficult to interpret because the pathoanatomy was not fully understood and the fractures were often combined with other injuries.[86] As fracture patterns have been more clearly appreciated and appropriately stabilized, outcomes are generally favorable and residual instability is rare. Some degree of arthrosis and stiffness is expected.

Terrible triad injuries have historically done poorly because of recurrent instability and the development of arthrosis.[8,46,98] With improved understanding and standardization of operative protocols as described in this chapter,[62] postoperative results are significantly improved, however. Few well-documented large series of these injuries have been reported. McKee and associates[62] used a standardized algorithm for terrible triad injuries in 36 patients and showed an average flexion-extension arc of 112 ± 11 degrees, an average forearm rotation of 136 ± 16 degrees, and an average Mayo elbow performance score of 88 (range 45-100) out of 100 at an average follow-up of nearly 3 years.

Olecranon fracture-dislocations, although high-energy injuries, have better results than terrible triad injuries with decreased incidence of postoperative instability and arthrosis.[71,96] As a rule, treatment of posterior dislocations is much less predictable than anterior dislocations. Posterior Monteggia injuries have higher rates of recurrent instability and poor outcomes.[49,97,100] The crucial factor for success of these injuries seems to be anatomic reduction of the ulna and the greater semilunar notch.

Delayed treatment and failed previous treatment have less predictable outcomes and depend on the individual fracture patterns and the skill and experience of the surgeon. Some reports incorporating a protocol of hinged external fixation have had success in maintaining stability and gaining satisfactory results.[50,61,93,101] In four studies that used hinged external fixation, the average flexion arc ranged from 84 to 123 degrees of motion. Functional forearm rotation was maintained in all studies. Three studies used the Mayo elbow performance index and showed an average score greater than 84 points, indicating a "good" outcome.[50,61,93,101]

COMPLICATIONS

Recurrent Instability

Failure to recognize or treat a fracture or ligament injury is the most common cause of recurrent instability. As described earlier, salvage may involve reconstruction of disrupted or attenuated ligamentous structures, osteotomies or grafting for osseous malunions or bone loss, and hinged external fixation.

Heterotopic Ossification

Heterotopic ossification increases with higher levels of injury and soft tissue damage, brain injury, infection, delay to surgery, and burns.[3,30,32,35,113] It is most often seen anteriorly between the capsule and brachialis and posteriorly between the capsule and triceps. There is no consensus on the ideal timing for resection, but many surgeons resect the heterotopic bone when trabeculae are seen on plain radiographs. This typically occurs 3 to 4 months after the initial insult. Prophylaxis with indomethacin (Indocin) or radiation is unproven for traumatic elbow injuries and may impair fracture healing.[30] A prospective randomized study suggests radiation therapy should not be used acutely for prophylaxis after elbow trauma because of the increased rate of fracture or olecranon osteotomy nonunion.[36]

Stiffness

Some loss of motion after elbow fracture-dislocation is expected. Typically, patients lose more extension than flexion. The amount of stiffness increases with the energy of the initial injury, the amount of heterotopic bone formed, and delay of motion after repair.[83,87] Treatment includes static or dynamic splinting, heterotopic bone excision, and capsular release.[33,35,42,56,91]

Posttraumatic Arthritis

Arthritis is common after high-energy injuries and is likely attributable to a combination of the initial chondral impact and the degree of recurrent instability. Fascial arthroplasty is an option for younger patients, whereas total elbow replacement is an option for older, less active patients.[11,53]

REFERENCES

1. An KN, Morrey BF, Chao EY: The effect of partial removal of proximal ulna on elbow constraint. Clin Orthop Relat Res (209):270–279, 1986.
2. Bain GI, Ashwood N, Baird R, et al: Management of Mason type-III radial head fractures with a titanium prosthesis, ligament repair, and early mobilization. Surgical technique. J Bone Joint Surg Am 87(Suppl 1 Pt 1):136–147, 2005.
3. Bauer AS, Lawson BK, Bliss RL, et al: Risk factors for posttraumatic heterotopic ossification of the elbow: case-control study. J Hand Surg [Am] 37(7):1422–1429, e1–6, 2012.
4. Beingessner DM, Dunning CE, Stacpoole RA, et al: The effect of coronoid fractures on elbow kinematics and stability. Clin Biomech (Bristol, UK) 22(2):183–190, 2007.
5. Beingessner DM, Stacpoole RA, Dunning CE, et al: The effect of suture fixation of type I coronoid fractures on the kinematics and stability of the elbow with and without medial collateral ligament repair. J Shoulder Elbow Surg 16(2):213–217, 2007.
6. Biga N, Thomine JM: [Trans-olecranal dislocations of the elbow]. Rev Chir Orthop Reparatrice Appar Mot 60(7):557–567, 1974.
7. Broberg MA, Morrey BF: Results of delayed excision of the radial head after fracture. J Bone Joint Surg Am 68(5):669–674, 1986.
8. Broberg MA, Morrey BF: Results of treatment of fracture-dislocations of the elbow. Clin Orthop Relat Res 216:109–119, 1987.
9. Cage DJ, Abrams RA, Callahan JJ, et al: Soft tissue attachments of the ulnar coronoid process. An anatomic study with radiographic correlation. Clin Orthop Relat Res 320:154–158, 1995.
10. Carn RM, Medige J, Curtain D, et al: Silicone rubber replacement of the severely fractured radial head. Clin Orthop Relat Res 209:259–269, 1986.
11. Cheng SL, Morrey BF: Treatment of the mobile, painful arthritic elbow by distraction interposition arthroplasty. J Bone Joint Surg Br 82(2):233–238, 2000.
12. Cobb TK, Morrey BF: Use of distraction arthroplasty in unstable fracture dislocations of the elbow. Clin Orthop Relat Res 312:201–210, 1995.
13. Cohen MS, Hastings H, 2nd: Rotatory instability of the elbow. The anatomy and role of the lateral stabilizers. J Bone Joint Surg Am 79(2):225–233, 1997.
14. Deutch SR, Jensen SL, Olsen BS, et al: Elbow joint stability in relation to forced external rotation: An experimental study of the osseous constraint. J Shoulder Elbow Surg 12(3):287–292, 2003.
15. Doornberg JN, de Jong IM, Lindenhovius AL, et al: The anteromedial facet of the coronoid process of the ulna. J Shoulder Elbow Surg 16(5):667–670, 2007.
16. Doornberg JN, Linzel DS, Zurakowski D, et al: Reference points for radial head prosthesis size. J Hand Surg [Am] 31(1):53–57, 2006.
17. Doornberg JN, Parisien R, van Duijn PJ, et al: Radial head arthroplasty with a modular metal spacer to treat acute traumatic elbow instability. J Bone Joint Surg Am 89(5):1075–1080, 2007.
18. Doornberg JN, Ring D: Coronoid fracture patterns. J Hand Surg [Am] 31(1):45–52, 2006.
19. Doornberg JN, Ring DC: Fracture of the anteromedial facet of the coronoid process. J Bone Joint Surg Am 88(10):2216–2224, 2006.
20. Doornberg JN, van Duijn J, Ring D: Coronoid fracture height in terrible-triad injuries. J Hand Surg [Am] 31(5):794–797, 2006.
21. Duckworth AD, Kulijdian A, McKee MD, et al: Residual subluxation of the elbow after dislocation or fracture-dislocation: treatment with active elbow exercises and avoidance of varus stress. J Shoulder Elbow Surg 17(2):276–280, 2008.
22. Duckworth AD, Ring D, Kulijdian A, et al: Unstable elbow dislocations. J Shoulder Elbow Surg 17(2):281–286, 2008.
23. Dunning CE, Zarzour ZD, Patterson SD, et al: Ligamentous stabilizers against posterolateral rotatory instability of the elbow. J Bone Joint Surg Am 83-A(12):1823–1828, 2001.
24. Dunning CE, Zarzour ZD, Patterson SD, et al: Muscle forces and pronation stabilize the lateral ligament deficient elbow. Clin Orthop Relat Res 388:118–124, 2001.
25. Durig M, Muller W, Ruedi TP, et al: The operative treatment of elbow dislocation in the adult. J Bone Joint Surg Am 61(2):239–244, 1979.
26. Faierman E, Wang J, Jupiter JB: Secondary ulnar nerve palsy in adults after elbow trauma: a report of two cases. J Hand Surg [Am] 26(4):675–678, 2001.
27. Floris S, Olsen BS, Dalstra M, et al: The medial collateral ligament of the elbow joint: anatomy and kinematics. J Shoulder Elbow Surg 7(4):345–351, 1998.
28. Forthman C, Henket M, Ring DC: Elbow dislocation with intra-articular fracture: the results of operative treatment without repair of the medial collateral ligament. J Hand Surg [Am] 32(8):1200–1209, 2007.
29. Fuss FK: The ulnar collateral ligament of the human elbow joint. Anatomy, function and biomechanics. J Anat 175:203–212, 1991.
30. Garland DE: Clinical observations on fractures and heterotopic ossification in the spinal cord and traumatic brain injured populations. Clin Orthop Relat Res 233:86–101, 1988.
31. Garland DE, Blum CE, Waters RL: Periarticular heterotopic ossification in head-injured adults. Incidence and location. J Bone Joint Surg Am 62(7):1143–1146, 1980.
32. Garland DE, O'Hollaren RM: Fractures and dislocations about the elbow in the head-injured adult. Clin Orthop Relat Res 168:38–41, 1982.
33. Gates HS, 3rd, Sullivan FL, Urbaniak JR: Anterior capsulotomy and continuous passive motion in the treatment of post-traumatic flexion contracture of the elbow. A prospective study. J Bone Joint Surg Am 74(8):1229–1234, 1992.
34. Geel CW, Palmer AK, Ruedi T, et al: Internal fixation of proximal radial head fractures. J Orthop Trauma 4(3):270–274, 1990.
35. Green DP, McCoy H: Turnbuckle orthotic correction of elbow-flexion contractures after acute injuries. J Bone Joint Surg Am 61(7):1092–1095, 1979.
36. Hamid N, Ashraf N, Bosse MJ, et al: Radiation therapy for heterotopic ossification prophylaxis acutely after elbow trauma: a prospective randomized study. J Bone Joint Surg Am 92(11):2032–2038, 2010.
37. Harrington IJ, Sekyi-Otu A, Barrington TW, et al: The functional outcome with metallic radial head implants in the treatment of unstable elbow fractures: a long-term review. J Trauma 50(1):46–52, 2001.
38. Heim U: [Combined fractures of the radius and the ulna at the elbow level in the adult. Analysis of 120 cases after more than 1 year]. Rev Chir Orthop Reparatrice Appar Mot 84(2):142–153, 1998.
39. Hofammann KE, 3rd, Moneim MS, Omer GE, et al: Brachial artery disruption following closed posterior elbow dislocation in a child: assessment with intravenous digital angiography. A case report with review of the literature. Clin Orthop Relat Res 184:145–149, 1984.
40. Horii E, Nakamura R, Watanabe K, et al: [Posterolateral rotatory instability of the elbow—a case report and anatomical study of the lateral collateral ligament]. Nihon Seikeigeka Gakkai Zasshi 67(1):34–39, 1993.
41. Hotchkiss RN: Displaced fractures of the radial head: internal fixation or excision? J Am Acad Orthop Surg 5(1):1–10, 1997.
42. Husband JB, Hastings H, 2nd: The lateral approach for operative release of post-traumatic contracture of the elbow. J Bone Joint Surg Am 72(9):1353–1358, 1990.
43. Hwang RW, de Witte PB, Ring D: Compartment syndrome associated with distal radial fracture and ipsilateral elbow injury. J Bone Joint Surg Am 91(3):642–645, 2009.
44. Jensen SL, Deutch SR, Olsen BS, et al: Laxity of the elbow after experimental excision of the radial head and division of the medial collateral ligament. Efficacy of ligament repair and radial head prosthetic replacement: a cadaver study. J Bone Joint Surg Br 85(7):1006–1010, 2003.
45. Josefsson PO, Gentz CF, Johnell O, et al: Surgical versus non-surgical treatment of ligamentous injuries following dislocation of the elbow joint. A prospective randomized study. J Bone Joint Surg Am 69(4):605–608, 1987.

46. Josefsson PO, Gentz CF, Johnell O, et al: Dislocations of the elbow and intraarticular fractures. *Clin Orthop Relat Res* 246:126–130, 1989.

47. Josefsson PO, Johnell O, Gentz CF: Long-term sequelae of simple dislocation of the elbow. *J Bone Joint Surg Am* 66(6):927–930, 1984.

48. Josefsson PO, Johnell O, Wendeberg B: Ligamentous injuries in dislocations of the elbow joint. *Clin Orthop Relat Res* 221:221–225, 1987.

49. Jupiter JB, Leibovic SJ, Ribbans W, et al: The posterior Monteggia lesion. *J Orthop Trauma* 5(4):395–402, 1991.

50. Jupiter JB, Ring D: Treatment of unreduced elbow dislocations with hinged external fixation. *J Bone Joint Surg Am* 84-A(9):1630–1635, 2002.

51. King GJ, Evans DC, Kellam JF: Open reduction and internal fixation of radial head fractures. *J Orthop Trauma* 5(1):21–28, 1991.

52. Knight DJ, Rymaszewski LA, Amis AA, et al: Primary replacement of the fractured radial head with a metal prosthesis. *J Bone Joint Surg Br* 75(4):572–576, 1993.

53. Lee DH: Posttraumatic elbow arthritis and arthroplasty. *Orthop Clin North Am* 30(1):141–162, 1999.

54. Leigh WB, Ball CM: Radial head reconstruction versus replacement in the treatment of terrible triad injuries of the elbow. *J Shoulder Elbow Surg* 21(10):1336–1341, 2012.

55. Lindenhovius A, Karanicolas PJ, Bhandari M, et al: Interobserver reliability of coronoid fracture classification: two-dimensional versus three-dimensional computed tomography. *J Hand Surg [Am]* 34(9):1640–1646, 2009.

56. Lindenhovius AL, Doornberg JN, Brouwer KM, et al: A prospective randomized controlled trial of dynamic versus static progressive elbow splinting for posttraumatic elbow stiffness. *J Bone Joint Surg Am* 94(8):694–700, 2012.

57. Lindenhovius AL, Jupiter JB: The posttraumatic stiff elbow: a review of the literature. *J Hand Surg [Am]* 32(10):1605–1623, 2007.

58. Liu GS, Jupiter JB: Posterolateral rotatory elbow subluxation with intra-articular entrapment of the radial nerve. A case report. *J Bone Joint Surg Am* 86-A(3):603–606, 2004.

59. Madey SM, Bottlang M, Steyers CM, et al: Hinged external fixation of the elbow: optimal axis alignment to minimize motion resistance. *J Orthop Trauma* 14(1):41–47, 2000.

60. Malkawi H: Recurrent dislocation of the elbow accompanied by ulnar neuropathy: a case report and review of the literature. *Clin Orthop Relat Res* 161:270–274, 1981.

61. McKee MD, Bowden SH, King GJ, et al: Management of recurrent, complex instability of the elbow with a hinged external fixator. *J Bone Joint Surg Br* 80(6):1031–1036, 1998.

62. McKee MD, Pugh DM, Wild LM, et al: Standard surgical protocol to treat elbow dislocations with radial head and coronoid fractures. Surgical technique. *J Bone Joint Surg Am* 87(Suppl 1 Pt 1):22–32, 2005.

63. McKee MD, Schemitsch EH, Sala MJ, et al: The pathoanatomy of lateral ligamentous disruption in complex elbow instability. *J Shoulder Elbow Surg* 12(4):391–396, 2003.

64. McWhorter G: Fracture of both the coronoid and the olecranon process of the ulna: indications for operation and treatment. *J Bone Joint Surg Am* 9:767–777, 1965.

65. Mehlhoff TL, Noble PC, Bennett JB, et al: Simple dislocation of the elbow in the adult. Results after closed treatment. *J Bone Joint Surg Am* 70(2):244–249, 1988.

66. Morrey BF, An KN: Articular and ligamentous contributions to the stability of the elbow joint. *Am J Sports Med* 11(5):315–319, 1983.

67. Morrey BF, An KN: Functional anatomy of the ligaments of the elbow. *Clin Orthop Relat Res* 201:84–90, 1985.

68. Morrey BF, An KN: Stability of the elbow: osseous constraints. *J Shoulder Elbow Surg* 14(1 Suppl S):174S–178S, 2005.

69. Morrey BF, Tanaka S, An KN: Valgus stability of the elbow. A definition of primary and secondary constraints. *Clin Orthop Relat Res* 265:187–195, 1991.

70. Mortazavi SM, Asadollahi S, Tahririan MA: Functional outcome following treatment of transolecranon fracture-dislocation of the elbow. *Injury* 37(3):284–288, 2006.

71. Mouhsine E, Akiki A, Castagna A, et al: Transolecranon anterior fracture dislocation. *J Shoulder Elbow Surg* 16(3):352–357, 2007.

72. Nestor BJ, O'Driscoll SW, Morrey BF: Ligamentous reconstruction for posterolateral rotatory instability of the elbow. *J Bone Joint Surg Am* 74(8):1235–1241, 1992.

73. Nsouli AZ, Makarem RR, Nsouli TA: Fracture-dislocation of the coronoid and olecranon processes of the ulna with posterolateral dislocation of the head of the radius: case report. *J Trauma* 37(5):855–857, 1994.

74. O'Driscoll SW: Elbow instability. *Hand Clin* 10(3):405–415, 1994.

75. O'Driscoll SW: Elbow instability. *Acta Orthop Belg* 65(4):404–415, 1999.

76. O'Driscoll SW, Bell DF, Morrey BF: Posterolateral rotatory instability of the elbow. *J Bone Joint Surg Am* 73(3):440–446, 1991.

77. O'Driscoll SW, Jaloszynski R, Morrey BF, et al: Origin of the medial ulnar collateral ligament. *J Hand Surg [Am]* 17(1):164–168, 1992.

78. O'Driscoll SW, Morrey BF, Korinek S, et al: Elbow subluxation and dislocation. A spectrum of instability. *Clin Orthop Relat Res* 280:186–197, 1992.

79. Olsen BS, Vaesel MT, Sojbjerg JO, et al: Lateral collateral ligament of the elbow joint: anatomy and kinematics. *J Shoulder Elbow Surg* 5(2 Pt 1):103–112, 1996.

80. Papandrea RF, Morrey BF, O'Driscoll SW: Reconstruction for persistent instability of the elbow after coronoid fracture-dislocation. *J Shoulder Elbow Surg* 16(1):68–77, 2007.

81. Pavel A, Pitman JM, Lance EM, et al: The posterior Monteggia fracture: a clinical study. *J Trauma* 5:185–199, 1965.

81a. Penrose JH: The Monteggia fracture with posterior dislocation of the radial head. *J Bone Joint Surg [Br]* 33(1):65–73, 1951.

82. Pribyl CR, Kester MA, Cook SD, et al: The effect of the radial head and prosthetic radial head replacement on resisting valgus stress at the elbow. *Orthopedics* 9(5):723–726, 1986.

83. Protzman RR: Dislocation of the elbow joint. *J Bone Joint Surg Am* 60(4):539–541, 1978.

84. Pugh DM, Wild LM, Schemitsch EH, et al: Standard surgical protocol to treat elbow dislocations with radial head and coronoid fractures. *J Bone Joint Surg Am* 86-A(6):1122–1130, 2004.

85. Ramon Soler R, Paz Tarela J, Soler Minores JM: Internal fixation of fractures of the proximal end of the radius in adults. *Injury* 10(4):268–272, 1979.

86. Regan W, Morrey B: Fractures of the coronoid process of the ulna. *J Bone Joint Surg Am* 71(9):1348–1354, 1989.

87. Regan W, Morrey BF: Classification and treatment of coronoid process fractures. *Orthopedics* 15(7):845–848, 1992.

88. Ring D: Open reduction and internal fixation of fractures of the radial head. *Hand Clin* 20(4):415–427, vi, 2004.

89. Ring D: Fractures of the coronoid process of the ulna. *J Hand Surg [Am]* 31(10):1679–1689, 2006.

90. Ring D: Radial head fracture: open reduction-internal fixation or prosthetic replacement. *J Shoulder Elbow Surg* 20(2 Suppl):S107–S112, 2011.

91. Ring D, Adey L, Zurakowski D, et al: Elbow capsulectomy for posttraumatic elbow stiffness. *J Hand Surg [Am]* 31(8):1264–1271, 2006.

92. Ring D, Doornberg JN: Fracture of the anteromedial facet of the coronoid process. Surgical technique. *J Bone Joint Surg Am* 89(Suppl 2 Pt 2):267–283, 2007.

93. Ring D, Hannouche D, Jupiter JB: Surgical treatment of persistent dislocation or subluxation of the ulnohumeral joint after fracture-dislocation of the elbow. *J Hand Surg [Am]* 29(3):470–480, 2004.

94. Ring D, Jupiter JB: Fracture-dislocation of the elbow. *J Bone Joint Surg Am* 80(4):566–580, 1998.

95. Ring D, Jupiter JB: Reconstruction of posttraumatic elbow instability. *Clin Orthop Relat Res* 370:44–56, 2000.

96. Ring D, Jupiter JB, Sanders RW, et al: Transolecranon fracture-dislocation of the elbow. *J Orthop Trauma* 11(8):545–550, 1997.

97. Ring D, Jupiter JB, Simpson NS: Monteggia fractures in adults. *J Bone Joint Surg Am* 80(12):1733–1744, 1998.

98. Ring D, Jupiter JB, Zilberfarb J: Posterior dislocation of the elbow with fractures of the radial head and coronoid. *J Bone Joint Surg Am* 84-A(4):547–551, 2002.

99. Ring D, Quintero J, Jupiter JB: Open reduction and internal fixation of fractures of the radial head. *J Bone Joint Surg Am* 84-A(10):1811–1815, 2002.

100. Ring D, Tavakolian J, Kloen P, et al: Loss of alignment after surgical treatment of posterior Monteggia fractures: salvage with dorsal contoured plating. *J Hand Surg [Am]* 29(4):694–702, 2004.

101. Ruch DS, Triepel CR: Hinged elbow fixation for recurrent instability following fracture dislocation. *Injury* 32(Suppl 4):SD70–SD78, 2001.

102. Schippinger G, Seibert FJ, Steinbock J, et al: Management of simple elbow dislocations. Does the period of immobilization affect the eventual results? *Langenbecks Arch Surg* 384(3):294–297, 1999.

103. Schneeberger AG, Sadowski MM, Jacob HA: Coronoid process and radial head as posterolateral rotatory stabilizers of the elbow. *J Bone Joint Surg Am* 86-A(5):975–982, 2004.

104. Seki A, Olsen BS, Jensen SL, et al: Functional anatomy of the lateral collateral ligament complex of the elbow: configuration of Y and its role. *J Shoulder Elbow Surg* 11(1):53–59, 2002.

105. Shiba R, Sorbie C, Siu DW, et al: Geometry of the humeroulnar joint. *J Orthop Res* 6(6):897–906, 1988.

106. Shin R, Ring D: The ulnar nerve in elbow trauma. *J Bone Joint Surg Am* 89(5):1108–1116, 2007.

107. Sojbjerg JO, Ovesen J, Nielsen S: Experimental elbow instability after transection of the medial collateral ligament. *Clin Orthop Relat Res* 218:186–190, 1987.

108. Sotereanos DG, Darlis NA, Wright TW, et al: Unstable fracture-dislocations of the elbow. *Instr Course Lect* 56:369–376, 2007.

109. Squires NA, Tomaino MM: Brachial artery rupture without median nerve dysfunction after closed elbow dislocation. *Am J Orthop (Belle Mead NJ)* 32(6):298–300, 2003.

110. Stavlas P, Jensen SL, Sojbjerg JO: Kinematics of the ligamentous unstable elbow joint after application of a hinged external fixation device: a cadaveric study. *J Shoulder Elbow Surg* 16(4):491–496, 2007.

111. Szabo RM, Hotchkiss RN, Slater RR, Jr: The use of frozen-allograft radial head replacement for treatment of established symptomatic proximal translation of the radius: preliminary experience in five cases. *J Hand Surg [Am]* 22(2):269–278, 1997.

112. Tan V, Daluiski A, Capo J, et al: Hinged elbow external fixators: indications and uses. *J Am Acad Orthop Surg* 13(8):503–514, 2005.

113. Teasdall R, Savoie FH, Hughes JL: Comminuted fractures of the proximal radius and ulna. *Clin Orthop Relat Res* 292:37–47, 1993.

114. Tomaino MM, Sotereanos DG, Plakseychuk A: Technique for ensuring ulnohumeral reduction during application of the Richards compass elbow hinge. *Am J Orthop (Belle Mead NJ)* 26(9):646–647, 1997.

115. Tropet Y, Menez D, Brientini JM, et al: [Entrapment of the median nerve after dislocation of the elbow]. *Acta Orthop Belg* 55(2):217–221, 1989.

116. Vanderwilde RS, Morrey BF, Melberg MW, et al: Inflammatory arthritis after failure of silicone rubber replacement of the radial head. *J Bone Joint Surg Br* 76(1):78–81, 1994.

117. Vichard P, Tropet Y, Dreyfus-Schmidt G, et al: Fractures of the proximal end of the radius associated with other traumatic lesions of the upper limb. A report of seventy-three cases. *Ann Chir Main* 7(1):45–53, 1988.

118. Wadstrom J, Kinast C, Pfeiffer K: Anatomical variations of the semilunar notch in elbow dislocations. *Arch Orthop Trauma Surg* 105(5):313–315, 1986.

119. Watters TS, Garrigues GE, Ring D, et al: Fixation versus replacement of radial head in terrible triad: is there a difference in elbow stability and prognosis? *Clin Orthop Relat Res* 472(7):2128–2135, 2014.

23

Chronic Elbow Instability
Ligament Reconstruction

Mark S. Cohen

The elbow is one of the most congruous joints in the body. Joint stability is provided by a combination of the bony architecture and the collateral ligaments and muscles. The lateral collateral ligament (LCL) complex plays a key role in elbow stability, preventing the proximal ulna and radius from subluxating as the supinated forearm is axially loaded.[14] Trauma, usually dislocation, is the most frequent cause of disruption of the LCL complex.[54,56] However, chronic varus load and steroid injections for epicondylitis have been described as possible causes of LCL insufficiency.[44,52] After trauma has occurred, restoration of lateral soft tissue support can usually be accomplished by a direct repair of the lateral ligament and extensor tendon origins to the humeral epicondyle. In instances of recurrent dislocation or subluxation, temporally remote from the initial injury, a tendon graft may be needed.

The medial collateral ligament (MCL) resists valgus force and supports the ulnohumeral joint. Medial collateral instability is most commonly due to chronic attenuation of the medial ligament complex resulting from overhead throwing motions. It can also occur in javelin throwers, gymnasts, quarterbacks, and other athletes who use overhead throwing motions and exert a repetitive valgus stress across the elbow.[23,24,33,41] When medial instability limits athletic participation and conservative care fails, a free tendon graft reconstruction is typically required.

CHRONIC LATERAL INSTABILITY

Preoperative Evaluation

Chronic LCL insufficiency varies in its presentation. A patient may report a painful clunking and/or snapping of the elbow.[3] Others will describe apprehension or weakness when reaching for an object with an outstretched hand, in varus load. Some may have episodes of frank giving way or apprehension, especially when the elbow is axially loaded in extension and supination. This can occur, for example, when one is pushing up from a chair. In this setting, the supinated radius and proximal ulna rotate laterally off of the distal humerus in a pattern termed *posterolateral rotatory instability (PLRI)*. Occasionally, unremitting lateral elbow pain is the patient's chief complaint.

Physical Examination

Physical examination in patients with chronic PLRI is characteristically benign. Grip strength and range of motion are usually unaffected, although some extension deficit may be present. In the setting of chronic instability, minor discomfort may be present on palpation of the lateral elbow. Occasionally, a synovial fistula can be observed as a fluid collection about the lateral elbow.[44]

Due to apprehension and guarding in a patient who is awake, it is often difficult to elicit frank posterolateral instability in the office, especially in muscular individuals. Subluxation of the elbow can be appreciated, however, with the appropriate provocative maneuvers. The elbow may be examined with a patient sitting or lying supine on a table. In the sitting position, one hand stabilizes the adducted humerus, with the fingers placed along the lateral ulnohumeral joint. While the elbow is partially flexed 40 to 45 degrees, the examiner's contralateral hand loads the proximal forearm in supination with slight axial and valgus force applied. Instability is appreciated as gapping at the ulnohumeral articulation as the radius and ulna subluxate. This results in a posterolateral prominence as the radial head subluxates away from the capitellum. The ulnohumeral articulation can be reduced by pronation of the forearm and slight flexion of the joint. Reduction is occasionally accompanied by a palpable clunk.

Alternatively, the *posterolateral rotatory apprehension (pivot shift)* and *drawer tests* are performed with the patient in the supine position. The patient's arm is brought overhead while the examiner stands at the head of the patient. By maximally flexing and externally rotating the shoulder, the humerus is "locked" into a fixed position. For the *pivot shift test*, the forearm is held in maximal supination while a valgus moment and axial compression is applied through the elbow at 40 to 70 degrees of flexion. In the relaxed patient with PLRI, this maneuver will lead to dimpling of the skin overlying the radiocapitellar joint, which occurs when the ulna and radius rotate off of the distal humerus. The subluxated elbow is reduced with flexion, frequently causing a palpable and visible (and sometimes audible) clunk.[54] The *posterolateral rotatory drawer test* is performed in the same position. A posteriorly directed force is applied onto the proximal radius while holding the forearm and elbow in the same position as for the apprehension test. Dimpling of the skin around the radiocapitellar joint at 40 to 70 degrees of flexion confirms PLRI. The amount of instability should decrease with greater elbow flexion.

In addition, in our practice, we routinely examine patients with suspected PLRI under image intensification. The clinical suspicion can in many cases be confirmed radiographically, aiding in establishing an appropriate treatment plan. In addition to the aforementioned rotatory tests, the extended elbow

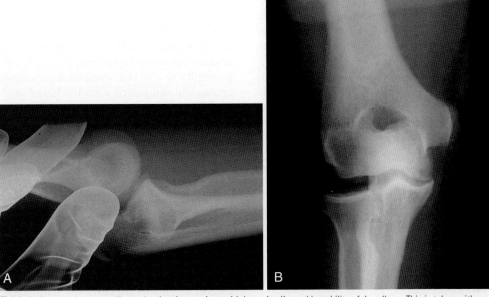

FIGURE 23.1 A, Lateral stress radiograph taken in a patient with lateral collateral instability of the elbow. This is taken with provocative stress applied using the rotatory instability test (supination with axial and valgus force applied). Note the gapping at the ulnohumeral articulation and posterior translation of the radial head now projecting posterior to the center of the capitellum. **B,** Anteroposterior stress radiograph in a patient with lateral collateral instability of the elbow. This is taken with varus stress applied to the joint. Note the gross gapping of the lateral joint between the radial head and the capitellum, confirming the diagnosis. (Copyright © Mark S. Cohen, Chicago.)

can be simply loaded in varus. Pathologic gapping at the radiocapitellar joint confirms instability laterally. This can be readily compared with the contralateral, unaffected side (see the following).

Patients with PLRI characteristically actively resist provocative maneuvers that stress the joint, which in and of itself can be interpreted as a "positive apprehension sign." However, in the cooperative patient, a successful examination can be performed with careful manipulation. As one would expect, the most reliable examination is performed under anesthesia. The recommendation is to always perform these maneuvers as the first step in evaluation of a patient for surgical reconstruction. It is also advisable to include these examination maneuvers prior to elective surgery for lateral epicondylitis.

Diagnostic Imaging

Plain radiographs of the elbow are frequently negative in patients with PLRI. However, small avulsion fragments or ossification at the humeral origin of the LCL can frequently be visualized. If PLRI is suspected, a lateral stress or varus stress view of the elbow can be obtained in the office using image intensification. The elbow is maximally supinated and axially loaded. Instability is confirmed by widening of the ulnohumeral joint and posterior subluxation of the radial head (Figure 23.1). Anteroposterior radiographs or fluoroscopy under varus load can often reveal pathologic gapping of the radiocapitellar joint (see Figure 23.1). As noted, imaging of the contralateral elbow is recommended to help confirm asymmetric gapping or displacement. Magnetic resonance imaging can aid in confirming the diagnosis. Signal changes are commonly seen at the epicondyle, revealing disruption of the lateral collateral and tendinous origins at the humeral epicondyle (Figure 23.2).

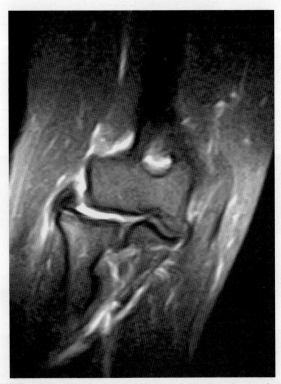

FIGURE 23.2 Magnetic resonance image of the elbow in a patient with chronic lateral collateral ligament insufficiency. Fluid is seen between the collateral ligament and extensor tendon origins and the lateral epicondyle. Magnetic resonance scanning can help confirm the diagnosis and rule out other pathologic processes about the lateral elbow. (Copyright © Mark S. Cohen, Chicago.)

◊ PERTINENT ANATOMY

The LCL complex originates at the base of the lateral epicondyle and lateral aspect of the capitellum. The isometric origin of the LCL is located at the geometric center of the capitellum.[50] In the reduced elbow, the isometric origin is located at the intersection of a distal projection of the anterior cortex of the humerus and the longitudinal axis of the radial head.[16] Distally, the LCL blends with the annular ligament to form a broad common insertion onto the proximal ulna (Figure 23.3).[16,18]

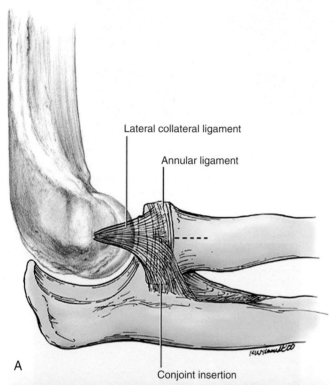

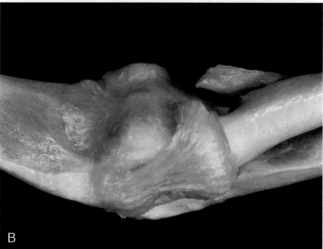

FIGURE 23.3 Schematic drawing **(A)** and cadaveric specimen **(B)** depicting anatomy of the lateral collateral and annular ligament complex. The overlying extensor muscles and supinator fibers have been removed. The collateral ligament originates at the base of the lateral epicondyle and fans out, blending with the annular ligament. These form a broad conjoined insertion onto the proximal ulna along the supinator crest just posterior to the proximal radioulnar joint. (Copyright © Mark S. Cohen, Chicago.)

The posterior fibers, which extend over 2 cm along the supinator crest from the proximal border of the radial head distally, have been termed the "lateral ulnar collateral ligament."[52] The LCL complex is covered anteriorly by the supinator muscle, which originates off the lateral epicondyle, supinator crest, and annular ligament. Posteriorly, the anconeus muscle is in close proximity to the LCL complex as it originates off the lateral epicondyle and inserts onto the lateral aspect of the proximal ulna.[38]

Both ligamentous and musculotendinous restraints provide stability to the elbow. The LCL complex, along with the anterior bundle of the MCL and the ulnohumeral joint, has been shown to act as a primary stabilizer of the elbow. Clinically, lateral elbow instability requires insufficiency of both ligamentous and musculotendinous stabilizers. The most common mechanism involves proximal attenuation or avulsion of these structures from their humeral original.[17,18,43,70] Occasionally, the distal insertion of the LCL may become compromised either as an avulsion injury or as a fracture of the supinator crest.[7,68]

The contribution of the LCL complex and overlying extensor tendon origins to lateral elbow joint stability have been well described in ex vivo studies.[18,27] The LCL complex represents the primary lateral stabilizer of the elbow, maintaining the ulnohumeral and radiocapitellar joints in a reduced position when the elbow is axially loaded with the forearm in supination. The extensor muscles, along with their fascial bands and intermuscular septae, assume a role as secondary restraints.[18] The extensor muscles serve to independently support the forearm unit from laterally rotating away from the humerus. In supination, these muscles provide a static and dynamic force supporting the lateral joint. The extensor carpi ulnaris is the most proximal of the extensor muscles and thus has the best mechanical advantage in supporting the proximal forearm. This muscle has a consistent fascial band on its undersurface, which originates at the inferior aspect of the lateral epicondyle and inserts onto the ulna approximately 5 cm distal to the radial head. The fascial band of the extensor carpi ulnaris becomes taut in supination and, along with the extensor tendon origins and septae, provides secondary resistance to lateral rotatory instability.[18]

Disruption of the LCL complex occurs in most instances as a consequence of an acute elbow dislocation mechanism. Although more than one pattern exists, dislocations frequently occur as the elbow is loaded with a combination of axial compressive, external rotatory, and valgus forces, in which the body internally rotates with respect to the affected extremity.[54,56] In this setting, disruption of elbow stabilizers proceeds in a circular path from lateral to medial.[58] Less frequently, instability may result as a consequence of a varus-deforming force applied to the extended elbow.[52] LCL insufficiency should be kept in mind as a differential diagnosis in patients with nonremitting lateral epicondylitis, with or without a history of previous local steroid injections.[44] Patients with chronic cubitus varus deformity, a prior history of failed surgery for lateral epicondylitis, or prior surgery of the radial head may have underlying iatrogenic lateral elbow instability.[48,59]

Indications

Primary repair of the LCL is required in the setting of fracture-dislocations of the elbow. The so-called *terrible triad of the elbow* indicates a fracture of the coronoid process and radial head with an associated injury to the LCL. In this setting, LCL repair is an integral part of the treatment algorithm. In chronic PLRI of the elbow, some authors have shown favorable outcomes with simple repair of the LCL complex, but reconstruction is typically required to restore lateral joint stability.

Contraindications

LCL repair or reconstruction requires an intact buttress at the proximal radius. In cases of radial head insufficiency, operative reduction and fixation of the radial head or prosthetic replacement should accompany the reconstruction. Patient compliance with postoperative rehabilitation plays a key role in achieving adequate outcomes. Patients who are unable or unwilling to follow rehabilitation guidelines should not undergo reconstruction, especially as an elective procedure.

Technique

❖ AUTHOR'S PREFERRED TECHNIQUE

In the setting of chronic PLRI of the elbow, reconstruction is typically performed with tendon graft augmentation. Allograft hamstring and ipsilateral palmaris longus tendon grafts are most commonly used. If autograft is chosen for reconstruction, patients should be examined for the presence of a palmaris longus tendon. Frequently, the palmaris autograft is found to be suboptimal (too small or too short) to use for reconstruction. Alternative autograft options include the contralateral palmaris, flexor carpi radialis, and gracilis tendons. We favor hamstring allografts when the palmaris is not of sufficient quality, and the gracilis seems to be most optimal in terms of diameter and length.

Surgical equipment required for ligament reconstruction includes standard retractors and elevators for the elbow, drill bits and drill sleeves for the bone tunnels (typically 3.2 mm and 4.5 mm in diameter), a cannulated 4.5-mm drill, and strong braided nonabsorbable suture material. Optional equipment includes a tendon stripper for autograft harvest, ligature passers and/or fine monofilament wire (e.g., 26-gauge) to aid graft passage through the bone tunnels, and a cortical button.

The procedure is commonly performed under regional anesthesia with a long-acting block. Examination under anesthesia is recommended to confirm the diagnosis of PLRI. An extended Kocher incision is used beginning along the supracondylar humeral ridge and passing distally over the lateral epicondyle toward the ulna.[34] Deep dissection is continued along the lateral supracondylar ridge, beneath the epicondyle and distally between the anconeus and the extensor carpi ulnaris. The anconeus is reflected posteriorly with the triceps and the extensor carpi ulnaris is retracted anteriorly, revealing the deep collateral and annular ligament layer overlying the radial head. The capsule over the so-called soft spot of the elbow is maintained to provide a layer between the joint and the graft.

In preparation for the humeral tunnel, a separate arthrotomy at the midline of the radiocapitellar joint exposes the epicondyle and the radiocapitellar joint. To reach this, the extensor carpi ulnaris and part of the extensor digitorum tendons are carefully elevated tangentially from posterior to anterior off of the deep ligament layer to the midline of the radiocapitellar joint. A transverse arthrotomy allows for direct inspection of

the joint to visualize the curvature of the capitellum and identify its geometric center where the isometric origin of the LCL will be located (Figure 23.4). Additionally, localization of the radiocapitellar joint will allow accurate placement of the ulnar tunnels. Not uncommonly, one will visualize wear and flattening on the rim of the radial head due to chronic subluxation.

It is important to have a clear understanding of the insertion of the lateral collateral and annular ligament complex when fashioning the ulnar tunnels. An entry hole is made in the lateral cortex of the ulna at the proximal margin of the radial head and just several millimeters posterior to the joint using sequential drill bits. Typically, a 3.2-mm drill bit is used followed by a 4.5-mm drill bit. An exit hole is created approximately 2 cm distally along the supinator crest (see Figure 23.4). Theoretically, more distally placed tunnels provide a graft that better resists varus stress and more proximal tunnels provide greater resistance to joint subluxation in supination. Curets are used to create a path within the ulna between the drill holes.

For the humeral graft attachment, we favor a single tunnel. This is easiest to create with a cannulated drill because the angle is quite "flat." A 0.062-inch guide pin is started for a 4.5-mm drill bit so that the posterior and distal periphery of the hole will be located at the isometric origin of the LCL (see Figure 23.4). It is important to avoid placing the tunnel posterior to the isometric point, as this will lead to laxity of the graft in extension where it is needed most. Once adequate placement of this pin into the posterior aspect of the lateral humeral column has been confirmed, the 4.5-mm cannulated drill is advanced from distal to proximal without penetrating the far cortex. The far cortex is perforated using a 3.2-mm drill. This will allow for ideal fixation using the cortical button.

The tendon graft is obtained either by harvesting an autograft or by thawing an allograft. The graft is prepared by placing a running, locking nonabsorbable suture on one end (typically, the distal tendon.) A double-armed suture attached to a Keith needle (#2 FiberLoop, Arthrex, Naples, FL) can be used to facilitate this. The suture ends are shuttled through the ulnar tunnel using a bent suture passer or fine monofilament wire. Care must be taken to clear the tunnel adequately to allow passage of the graft. Prior to securing the tendon in the humerus, the lateral capsulotomy that had been made at the midline of the radiocapitellar joint is repaired. In addition, we have found it useful to reattach the origin of the native collateral ligament and extensor tendon origins to reinforce the reconstruction. To this end, a stout nonabsorbable running, locking suture is placed starting at the tendon and ligament origin on the humerus, run distally into the common extensor tendon down toward the ulna, and run back to the entry point. These sutures are passed into the humeral tunnel prior to the graft with the help of a straight suture retriever or wire. A hemostat helps maintain these proximally.

The prepared end of the graft is placed into the humeral entry hole with the sutures exiting posteriorly. Although the original description of the technique suggested the use of a four-ply graft,[52] most surgeons now use a "docking" technique popularized on the medial side of the elbow for ligament reconstruction in the throwing athlete (see Figure 23.4). The goal of this method is for both arms of the free graft to be "docked" within the humeral tunnel, with only the two sets of sutures

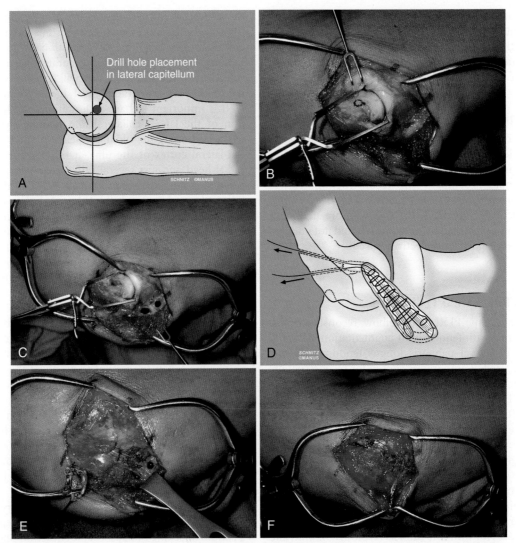

FIGURE 23.4 A, Schematic drawing depicting appropriate position for the humeral tunnel origin. Note how the tunnel begins anterior to the center of the capitellum (isometric point). In this way, the posteriormost margin of the tunnel will define isometry. **B,** Intraoperative photograph depicting the starting point for the humeral tunnel. **C,** Intraoperative photograph after the humeral and ulnar tunnels have been created. Note that the proximal ulnar tunnel is drilled just posterior to the proximal aspect of the radial head to re-create normal ligament anatomy. **D,** Schematic drawing depicting "docking" technique used to secure the free tendon graft. A triangular graft configuration is created by cutting the graft length so that both tendon arms end in a single humeral tunnel. In this diagram, the sutures alone are passed through separate bone tunnels posteriorly. Tension is provided, and the graft is secured by tying the sutures over a humeral bone bridge. Alternatively, a cortical button can be used. **E,** Intraoperative photograph depicting final graft position after being passed through the humeral tunnels. Note how the arms of the graft have been sutured to one another and the underlying native soft tissue to reinforce the reconstruction. **F,** The anconeus and extensor carpi ulnaris fascia have been closed over this free tendon graft, completing the procedure. (**A** and **D,** Courtesy of Hill Hastings II, MD, and The Indiana Hand Center. **B, C, E,** and **F,** Copyright © Mark S. Cohen, Chicago.)

exiting out of the posterior humerus. Once approximately 10 to 15 mm of the graft is within the humeral tunnel, the second arm of the graft is cut at the appropriate length that will allow it to end within the humerus. Care is taken not to cut the graft too short. The second end of the graft is prepared with a separate running, locking suture. Tails of this suture are passed out of the humeral tunnel. Traction on the two sets of graft sutures should allow the two-ply graft to become taut as it advances within the humerus. When using this technique with one humeral tunnel, the suture ends are threaded through the eyelets of an endobutton behind the lateral humeral column.

The forearm is flexed to approximately 45 to 60 degrees and fully pronated, reducing any residual posterolateral sublux-

ation. The forearm is lifted off of the table to remove any varus stress. First, the two ends of the suture that have been placed in the native tissue are tied over the posterior humeral bone bridge or endobutton. The tendon graft is pulled taut, and the four suture strands are tied, completing the reconstruction. The arms of the free tendon graft spanning the elbow joint can be sutured to one another and to the underlying collateral and annular complex to reinforce and tension the reconstruction if necessary. The elbow can be taken through a range of motion once the graft is secured. One will now appreciate the function of the graft, which acts as a reinforcement to the radial collateral and annular ligament complex. It holds up the proximal ulna to the humeral trochlea and, in addition, provides a lateral restraint to the radial head, not allowing it to subluxate laterally from the capitellum in supination.

For closure, the split in the anconeus and extensor fascia is repaired, sealing the reconstruction, and the skin is sutured in layers (see Figure 23.4). A compressive dressing is applied, with a splint maintaining the elbow in at least 90 degrees of flexion and the forearm in neutral rotation or slight pronation.

Postoperative Management and Expectations

Motion may be started at 7 to 10 days after surgery. However, motion may be delayed for 2 to 3 weeks without significant morbidity, as stiffness is not typically a problem in this patient population.[15] A progressive range-of-motion program is subsequently started, with interval splinting for protection and support. Initially, all motion is performed with the arm at the patient's side, avoiding shoulder abduction. Supination is allowed only with the elbow maximally flexed, which helps lock the ulnohumeral joint, thereby protecting the lateral soft tissue structures. Patients gradually gain elbow extension over the first 6 to 8 weeks. At that time, the protective splint is weaned and full extension should be safely achieved. Isometric strengthening can begin at 8 to 10 weeks. More vigorous strengthening or loading of the elbow is not started until closer to 4 to 6 months after surgery. Unrestricted use of the extremity is delayed until at least 6 months postoperatively, to allow time for the graft to incorporate and mature.

Expected Outcomes

Several surgical techniques have been described for management of PLRI. Most recently, Daluiski and colleagues[20] reported on primary repair of the LCL complex in patients undergoing surgery within 30 days of injury versus more than 30 days after dislocation; the results were similar. In their cohort of 34 patients, only 2 had recurrent instability; both had undergone operation in the early postoperative period.[20] Lee and associates reported excellent or good results in 8 of 10 patients who underwent either tendon graft reconstruction (6 patients) or humeral reattachment (4 patients). All patients treated with graft reconstruction had an excellent result.[46] Nestor and coworkers reported on 11 patients who underwent either advancement or reconstruction of the lateral elbow. Of the five patients who underwent reconstruction with a palmaris longus graft, three were graded as having an excellent result and two as having a fair result, based on a scale that evaluates stability, range of motion, and pain.[52] Lin and colleagues reported on 14 patients who underwent ligament reconstruction using either a palmaris or gracilis autograft. Reconstruction was performed in 11 patients with only lateral instability and 3 with concomitant medial instability. Excellent and good results based on the scale of Nestor and associates was reported in patients with lateral instability only, whereas of the patients with associated medial instability 2 had a good result and 1 a fair result.[47] Using a docking technique for reconstruction of eight purely ligamentous PLRIs, Jones and coworkers reported a mean Mayo Elbow Performance Score of 88 (range, 75 to 100) at a mean follow-up of 7 years. Complete resolution of instability was achieved in six patients, while two had occasional instability.[42] In a previous article, the senior author reported the results of reconstruction on 16 patients with documented chronic PRLI using the technique described in this paper. Symptoms of instability resolved

in all patients, with elbow range of motion returning to baseline at 3 months after surgery. Loss of range of motion consisted of 5 to 10 degrees of terminal extension in 7 patients, but it did not affect final elbow function.

In a recent systematic review of the literature, Anakwenze and colleagues analyzed eight studies that included a total of 130 patients who underwent LCL reconstruction for PLRI. Ninety-one percent of patients had good or excellent results. However, complications occurred in 11% of patients, with recurrent instability occurring in 8%.[4]

Complications

Recurrent instability is the most frequent complication after LCL reconstruction. This is reported to occur in up to 25% of cases.[42] Revision surgery poses special challenges because of bone loss from a prior attempted reconstruction. Baghdadi and associates assessed 11 patients who underwent revision surgery for PLRI over an 11-year period. Although instability was corrected in 8 patients, only 6 patients achieved good or excellent outcomes according to the Mayo Elbow Performance Score.[9]

CHRONIC MEDIAL INSTABILITY

Preoperative Evaluation

Physical Examination

Physical examination of an individual with presumed medial joint insufficiency should focus on palpation of the course of the MCL. The patient may have pain at its origin (humeral epicondyle) or insertion site (sublime tubercle of the ulna). Irritation of the ulnar nerve, with symptoms of ulnar neuritis, may be present secondary to inflammation of the ligamentous complex.[13] Valgus stress testing of the elbow should be performed with the examiner stabilizing the forearm and supporting the proximal arm at the axilla. The elbow is flexed past 30 degrees and a valgus stress is applied across the elbow joint. Provocative maneuvers have been described to help confirm the diagnosis of medial ligamentous insufficiency. The "milking" maneuver consists of static traction placed on the thumb with the elbow flexed beyond 90 degrees and the shoulder externally rotated. The moving valgus stress test involves a similar load applied to the elbow while the joint is taken through a range of motion. Pain at approximately 70 to 120 degrees (the position of late cocking and early acceleration of throwing) characteristically occurs in patients with symptomatic medial ligament insufficiency.[57,69]

Diagnostic Imaging

Plain films are commonly negative in these individuals, although a small fragment of bone can occasionally be seen along the medial joint line. Stress anteroposterior radiographs can be used with a valgus load applied to the joint, but especially in the awake patient, these are often normal. Magnetic resonance imaging can be used to confirm pathologic conditions of the ligament.[73] Most commonly, the medial ligament fails distally at its ulnar insertion, but proximal ligament failure and midsubstance attenuation can also occur (Figure 23.5). The use of magnetic resonance arthrography has been suggested to be more sensitive, allowing the identification of undersurface tears in the ligament.[36] However, it is now clear that in a subset of patients with symptomatic medial ligament pathologic conditions, MRI scans are relatively normal. In these cases, the diagnosis is confirmed by the history and physical examination findings.

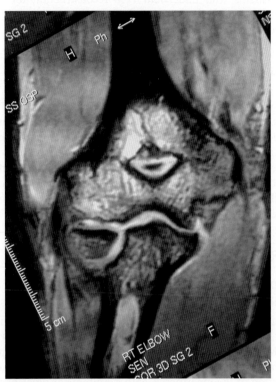

FIGURE 23.5 Magnetic resonance image of the elbow in a patient with chronic medial collateral ligament insufficiency. Fluid is seen between the collateral ligament and its insertion point on the ulna. Magnetic resonance scanning can help confirm the diagnosis of ligament disruption and identify any associated intraarticular pathologic conditions. (Copyright © Mark S. Cohen, Chicago.)

PERTINENT ANATOMY

The MCL of the elbow can be divided into three components, the anterior, posterior, and transverse bundles (Figure 23.6).[12,30,32,50] The anterior bundle originates on the central 65% of the anteroinferior surface of the medial epicondyle, just posterior to the axis of the elbow joint,[50,53,55] with a footprint that is approximately 10 mm wide. Previously it was believed that the ulnar collateral ligament inserted on a small area of the sublime tubercle (a protuberance off of the medial coronoid) of the proximal ulna, but recent evidence demonstrates that the ulnar collateral ligament inserts in a broad fashion over a span of 25 mm.[29] The anterior bundle is composed of two functional components.[12,30,66] The anterior band of the anterior bundle is taut from full extension to 60 degrees of flexion, while the posterior component is taut from 60 to 120 degrees of flexion.[12,61,66] There is a distinct ridge on the sublime tubercle that separates the anterior and posterior band attachments.[26,29]

The anterior bundle of the MCL is the strongest and stiffest of the elbow collateral ligaments, with an average load to failure of 260 Newtons.[61] Certain activities such as throwing have been estimated to generate up to 290 Newtons of tensile force on the medial elbow, highlighting the importance of dynamic stability provided by the flexor-pronator muscle group.[76] Ochi and colleagues determined that the deep middle portion of the anterior band is isometric during elbow flexion.[53] They further demonstrated that this deep middle bundle is positioned along the ulnohumeral joint axis.

The posterior bundle of the MCL is a less well-defined thickening of the posterior elbow joint capsule.[10,43] The transverse bundle, also known as the Cooper ligament, is variably present.[30,45,50] It is composed of fibers running along the medial joint capsule from the tip of the olecranon to the medial ulna, just distal to the coronoid.[10,50] The transverse fibers have little role in elbow joint stability because they originate and insert on the ulna (see Figure 23.6).

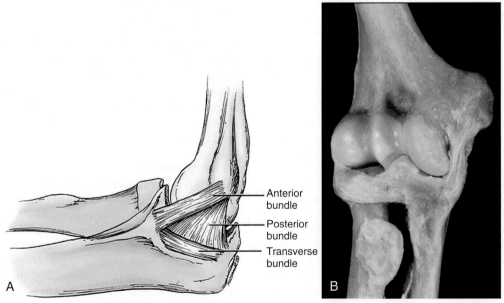

FIGURE 23.6 Schematic diagram (**A**) and cadaveric specimen (**B**) depicting the anatomy of the medial collateral ligament complex of the elbow, including the three bundles. The stout anterior bundle is the main stabilizer of the elbow to valgus stress. (Copyright © Mark S. Cohen, Chicago.)

The principal function of the MCL complex is to maintain medial joint stability with applied valgus stress. As noted, the anterior band of the anterior bundle is the most important component of the ligamentous complex, as it primarily stabilizes the elbow from 30 to 120 degrees of flexion.[12,30,37,49-51,71] The posterior band of the anterior bundle functions equally as a corestraint with the anterior band at terminal elbow flexion. The radial head functions as a secondary ulnohumeral joint stabilizer to valgus loads.[37,51] The flexor-pronator muscles originate at the medial epicondyle and provide additional static and dynamic support to the medial elbow.[2] The flexor carpi ulnaris and flexor digitorum superficialis are the most effective in this regard.[21]

A subset of patients with MCL injury present with ulnar nerve symptoms or positive cubital tunnel findings on physical examination. The ulnar nerve lies along the medial joint line just posterior to the anterior bundle of the MCL. As such, the nerve is predisposed to local trauma and inflammation when ligament attenuation has occurred. Aoki and associates measured the strain on the ulnar nerve during overhead throwing. They found that the strain recorded during the acceleration phase of throwing approximated the elastic limit of the ulnar nerve.[6] This suggests that the repetitive strain of throwing can lead to intraneural ischemia and deformation and ulnar nerve symptoms, especially when the ligament is incompetent.

The most common mechanism of MCL insufficiency is chronic attenuation, as seen in athletes who perform overhead throwing. Patients typically report a single episode of severe pain with throwing, although on careful questioning most report that low-grade symptoms had been present earlier. Following the development of pain, vigorous throwing is typically not possible and reproduces medial joint symptoms. Although not as common, the medial elbow ligament can also fail in a posttraumatic setting, usually following a fall on an outstretched arm. A combination of valgus and external rotation force has been proposed.[8,19,40,45,66] Associated injuries following trauma may include fractures of the radial head, olecranon, or medial humeral epicondyle.[45,66] Finally, MCL injury can be iatrogenic, secondary to excessive medial epicondylectomy for cubital tunnel syndrome.[31,35]

Indications

The indication for operative reconstruction of the medial elbow ligament is failure of conservative measures; a subset of patients with these injuries will heal without reconstruction.[24,62] Treatment for early symptoms of MCL injury includes rest with cessation of throwing or valgus loading for 8 to 12 weeks, physical therapy modalities, and nonsteroidal antiinflammatory medication. Strengthening of the flexor-pronator mass (the flexor carpi ulnaris and flexor digitorum superficialis in particular) may facilitate rehabilitation.[21] These muscles provide a secondary restraint to valgus stress and protect the underlying ligamentous complex. Because the medial ligament's function is important mainly in throwing motions, elbow reconstruction is warranted only in patients who want to play sports that involve throwing. In some patients, activity modification is a reasonable alternative to surgery. Valgus laxity has been shown to cause minimal functional impairment with normal activities of daily living.[45] In addition, unlike chronic lateral ligament insufficiency, there is little long-term detrimental effect of medial ligament pathology on elbow motion or function.

Contraindications

Patients must be compliant and willing to undergo the rehabilitation necessary for a proper surgical outcome. Because throwing is delayed for many months, patients must be willing to wait for the lengthy recovery needed.

Technique

Dr. Frank Jobe first published his initial ulnar collateral ligament reconstruction technique in 1986, which involved elevation of the flexor pronator mass, a figure-of-eight graft configuration, and tunnels on both the ulnar and humerus.[40] Over the years there have been several modifications of this technique, including the "modified Jobe technique" (a flexor-pronator muscle-splitting approach with a figure-of-eight graft configuration), the "docking technique" (the use of a triangular graft configuration through a single humeral tunnel), the "DANE-TJ technique" (the use of an interference screw for ulnar graft fixation), and the "ASMI technique" (a more posterior approach to the sublime tubercle working through the cubital tunnel).[5,22,63,72] These surgical modifications include differences in relation to graft configuration, fixation, and management of the flexor pronator mass. At present, no consensus has been reached in the literature regarding the optimal technique for reconstruction.[1,60,67]

❖ AUTHOR'S PREFERRED TECHNIQUE

In chronic cases, operative treatment typically involves a reconstruction with a free tendon graft. Several options exist for the graft, including a palmaris longus or hamstring autograft or a hamstring or Achilles allograft. No study to date has demonstrated the superiority of any one graft.[11,65] Because the palmaris tendon is often of insufficient width or length, a back-up tendon is necessary even when the palmaris is present. We favor the semitendinosis, either as autograft or allograft, which is the largest hamstring tendon.

The surgical equipment required for ligament reconstruction includes standard elbow instruments, drill bits and sleeves of 3.2 mm and 4.5 mm in diameter for the bone tunnels, a 4.5-mm cannulated drill, and a strong braided nonabsorbable suture. Optional equipment includes a tendon stripper for autograft harvest, ligature passers and/or fine monofilament wire (e.g., 26-gauge) to aid graft passage through the bone tunnels, and a cortical button.

Some authors elect to perform routine elbow arthroscopy prior to ulnar collateral ligament reconstruction to remove posteromedial osteophytes and to assess the overall status of the elbow joint. We do not routinely perform elbow arthroscopy unless concomitant pathologic change exists that is most amenable to arthroscopic treatment.

The procedure is commonly performed under regional anesthesia. A medial approach to the elbow is used, and the medial antebrachial cutaneous sensory branches are dissected out and protected. For this procedure, the entire flexor-pronator musculotendinous origin needs to be exposed. The ulnar nerve is identified and released proximally to expose the medial humeral column beneath the triceps muscle. This nerve dissection can be carried down to the proximal aspect of the cubital tunnel.

The nerve can be simply left in situ or formally transposed into a subcutaneous position after the reconstruction has been completed. We tend to only transpose the ulnar nerve in patients with preoperative ulnar nerve symptoms or signs of nerve involvement (a positive Tinel sign or elbow flexion test). Occasionally, patients with MCL insufficiency have a symptomatic posteromedial osteophyte. Simple elevation of the triceps allows direct access to the posteromedial olecranon tip if spur débridement is necessary.

As noted above, although the original description of the technique involved elevation of the flexor-pronator muscle mass from the humerus (Figure 23.7),[39,40] we prefer a muscle-splitting approach. This allows identification of the anterior band of the medial ligament with less morbidity. The posterior aspect of the flexor-pronator fascia is opened along the line of its fibers, usually through a white fibrous raphe along the anterior margin of the humeral head of the flexor carpi ulnaris. The flexor-pronator muscle is bluntly split down to the ligament. The ligament is defined as a stout, white structure coursing from the epicondyle to the sublime tubercle of the ulna. The tubercle can often be palpated distally, and it guides the plane of the muscle split. Of note, the sublime tubercle is always more distal than one would think. Deep retractors are placed, and an Army-Navy retractor placed distally is especially useful for exposure. The ligament is split longitudinally. This allows visualization of the medial ulnohumeral joint. Forced supination and valgus load commonly demonstrate insufficiency of the ligament, which manifests as gapping of the medial ulnohumeral joint. Distally, limited subperiosteal dissection allows identification of the sublime tubercle, which is palpable as a prominence with a central ridge. This has a triangular configuration tapering distally.

In the past, we used anterior and posterior bone tunnels in the ulna analogous to the lateral side. However, this does require significant stripping to expose the anterior and posterior slopes of the sublime tubercle. In addition, in this area an adequate bone bridge can be challenging to preserve. Furthermore, posteriorly it must be appreciated that the ulnar nerve lies very near to the ligament edge. As such, for safety and simplicity, we now use a single tunnel in the ulna similar to the humerus (a double-docking technique). Without a bone bridge in the ulna, a single-strand graft may be used. For the ulna, a 4.5-mm drill hole is made in the center of the sublime tubercle perpendicular to its surface beginning approximately 3 mm distal to the joint (Figure 23.8). It may be easiest to start this with a 3.2-mm drill and enlarge the hole with the bigger drill. A curet can be used to create a cavity in which to seat the graft. Through this tunnel, divergent holes can be made exiting the posterolateral cortex of the ulna for the tendon sutures. A 0.062-inch Kirschner wire with a drill sleeve to protect the soft tissues is useful for this purpose. Care is taken to leave at least a 1-cm separation between the two exit points. These can usually be exposed through the same incision by elevating a full-thickness skin flap posteriorly and dissecting in a subperiosteal fashion along the ulna posteriorly and laterally. A ligature passer that has the tendon loop proximally (nitinol wire) allows easiest passage of the ultimate sutures (see Figure 23.8).

The isometric point for the humerus is important and is defined by the midpoint of the medial epicondyle height (from base to tip) on the face of the anteroinferior epicondyle.[26,30,55] Enough epicondyle is exposed to allow for identification of this origin (Figure 23.9). Typically, the tunnel is started just superficial to this point to allow for closure of the native ligament beneath the tendon graft. As was the case laterally, it is easiest to create the medial humeral tunnel with a cannulated 4.5-mm drill. A 0.062-inch guide pin is placed at the tunnel starting point, exiting the posteromedial column of the humerus. Care is taken to leave an adequate medial cortical bone bridge without aiming too far laterally toward the posterior ulnohumeral joint. Once the pin is properly placed, the tunnel is created with the cannulated drill, with care taken to retract and protect the ulnar nerve posteriorly at the tunnel's exit.

The tendon graft is prepared in a fashion similar to that described laterally. Because this technique uses a single-strand graft, if the palmaris longus is chosen it is folded upon itself (two-ply). For the semitendinosis, a running, locking stitch is simply placed into one end. If there is any concern that the tendon graft may not fit within the tunnels, the graft can be passed through the 4.5-mm drill sleeve to confirm proper sizing (and trimmed accordingly).

The graft is now seated in the ulna. Both suture ends are pulled through the transosseous tunnels using the nitinol wire ligature passer. Traction placed on the sutures brings the tendon edge to the tunnel entry. Manual placement of the graft end into the tunnel can be helpful to aid in seating of the graft. The sutures are tied over the cortical bone bridge of the ulna. The knot can be pushed laterally, beneath the extensor carpi ulnaris, and the fascia can be repaired posteriorly over the ulna to complete the closure.

Next the graft is reflected distally and the native medial ligament is repaired, closing the longitudinal split (see Figure 23.8). Care is taken to carefully suture the ligament distally to cover the medial ulnohumeral joint. It may be easiest to place the most distal sutures in the native ligament (without tightening them) before the graft is seated to allow free access to both the

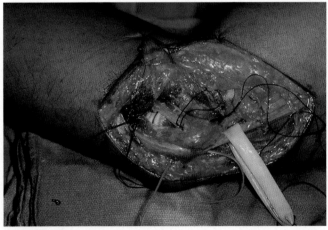

FIGURE 23.7 Intraoperative photograph in a patient undergoing a medial ligament reconstruction. In this case, the origin of the flexor-pronator muscles has been elevated and retracted distally to allow exposure of the ligament. Note the protection of the ulnar nerve posteriorly (Penrose drain) and the longitudinal split in the ligament, revealing the medial aspect of the ulnohumeral joint. This approach has been replaced by the more popular technique in which the muscle is split in line with its fibers to expose the underlying ligament. (Copyright © Mark S. Cohen, Chicago.)

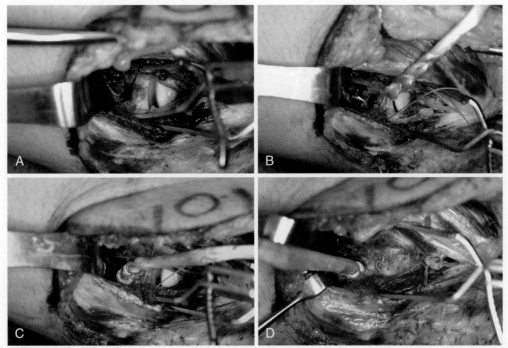

FIGURE 23.8 A, Intraoperative photograph depicting a single ulnar tunnel in the center of the sublime tubercule. Note the two ligature passers which are positioned to thread the tendon sutures through the ulna. **B,** A single semitendinosis hamstring autograft is now being advanced into the tunnel. **C,** Final graft seating with the sutures tied over bone bridge on the posterolateral cortex of the ulna. **D,** The tendon has been reflected distally, revealing the repair of the native ligament. Note how this completely covers the ulnohumeral joint. (Copyright © Mark S. Cohen, Chicago, IL.)

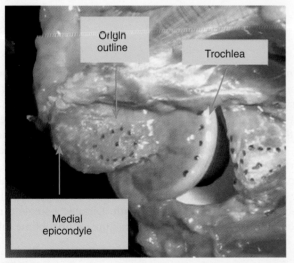

FIGURE 23.9 Cadaveric specimen depicting the origin of the anterior bundle of the medial collateral ligament on the medial epicondyle. Note how the ligament originates on the inferior face of the epicondyle at the center of its height (base to tip). One can also see the outline of the distal ligament attachment on the sublime tubercle of the ulna *(outlined with dots).* (Dugas JR, Ostrander RV, Cain EL, et al: Anatomy of the anterior bundle of the ulnar collateral ligament. *J Shoulder Elbow Surg* 16:657–660, 2007. Reproduced with permission from Elsevier.)

ligament edge and the tunnel. Proximally, the ligament is repaired up to the humerus without completely blocking the tunnel entry point.

For the humerus, a docking technique is used as it was for the lateral reconstruction. Care is taken not to make the graft too short. Once the proximal running, locking suture is placed, the suture is guided through the humerus and threaded through an endobutton (Figure 23.10). During graft tightening, care is taken to lift the elbow off of the table to remove any valgus stress. In addition, the elbow is placed in maximum supination, which closes down the medial ulnohumeral joint. The elbow can be moved from 30 to 90 degrees of its range of motion several times to pretension the graft, at which time the sutures are tied over the endobutton. The suture knot is pushed laterally, and the medial triceps fascia can typically be closed, protecting the ulnar nerve from the endobutton and suture knot if it is not to be transposed.

Once secured, the arms of the graft can be sutured down to the underlying native ligament to reinforce the reconstruction. This is often unnecessary, and again it must be appreciated that the ulnar nerve rests just posterior to the native ligament and graft. The flexor-pronator muscle split is repaired, and the ulnar nerve is either maintained or transposed anteriorly into a subcutaneous position. A compressive dressing is applied, with a splint maintaining the elbow in approximately 90 degrees of flexion.

Postoperative Management and Expectations

The elbow is immobilized in a splint for the first week after operation. Following this, rehabilitation begins, initially concentrating on the recovery of elbow motion. A long-arm splint is used between exercises for comfort and support. Gentle isometric strengthening is initiated at 6 to 8 weeks. A light under-hand medicine ball toss and light bench press exercises are begun at 12 to 20 weeks. At 20 weeks (5 months), light throwing on a flat ground is allowed at 45 feet every other day and can

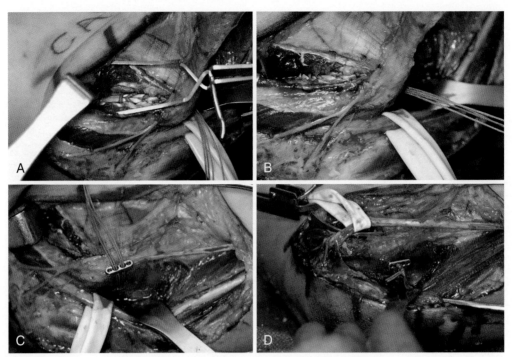

FIGURE 23.10 A, Intraoperative view of a patient undergoing medial ligament reconstruction. The graft has been seated distally, and the sutures have been passed through the humeral tunnel. Note the ulnar nerve (Penrose drain) and the medial antebrachial cutaneous sensory nerve branch beneath and distal to the epicondyle, respectively. These have been identified and protected. **B,** The sutures that have been placed in a running, locking fashion in the tendon ends have been passed through the humeral tunnel, exiting the posterior humeral column. **C,** With the ulnar nerve retracted, the sutures are passed through an endobutton, which functions as a washer for the suture knot. This simplifies the humeral tunnel configuration. **D,** Final tightening and seating of the sutures and the endobutton, completing the tendon graft reconstruction. In this case, the ulnar nerve has been completely dissected out in preparation for anterior transposition. (Copyright © Mark S. Cohen, Chicago.)

be slowly increased to 60 feet by the 6-month mark. Proper pitching mechanics have to be monitored, and strengthening is focused on the flexor-pronator muscle mass. Athletes who use overhead throwing can begin to throw off of a mound at 50% speed and effort at 7 to 8 months with no special pitches. Intensity is gradually increased, and lower-extremity weight training (including squats and lunges with weight) may be initiated. Playing in a game, including batting, is allowed at 8 to 10 months postoperatively; however, a full return to effective play may not be successful for several additional months.

Expected Outcomes

Several series have documented the success of reconstruction in returning athletes to competitive throwing. One of the earliest series reported a return to a high level of throwing of 68%.[19] More recent series quote a higher percentage of success of between 82% and 93%.[8,11,25,28,64,72,74] The further along the athlete is in the level of play (e.g., a high school athlete versus a professional athlete), the higher the percentage of success.

Complications

Complications of the procedure most commonly include ulnar nerve embarrassment, fracture of the ulnar bone bridge, or fracture of the medial epicondyle.[75] Identification and protection of the ulnar nerve is paramount during this procedure. The nerve is always dissected out and protected proximally during exposure of the posterior aspect of the medial humeral column.

It must be retracted when drilling the humeral tunnel. In addition, in early cases, it may be prudent to first identify the ulnar nerve distally between the two heads of the flexor carpi ulnaris. The muscle split for ligament exposure will then be just anterior to this level. It cannot be overemphasized how close the nerve lies relative to the medial ligament. Even retractors placed during the flexor-pronator muscle split can compromise the nerve. To avoid postoperative humeral fracture, we have found the described cannulated drill technique to be helpful. It allows precise planning for the tunnel path. Distally, a single tunnel also minimizes the potential for a fracture of the sublime tubercle bone bridge.

REFERENCES

1. Ahmad CS, Lee TQ, El Attrache NS: Biomechanical evaluation of a new ulnar collateral ligament reconstruction technique with interference screw fixation. *Am J Sports Med* 31(3):332–337, 2003.
2. An KN, Zobitz ME, Morrey BF: Biomechanics of the elbow. In Morrey BF, editor: *The elbow and its disorders*, ed 4, St. Louis, 2009, WB Saunders, pp 39–63.
3. Anakwenze OA, Kancherla VK, Iyengar J, et al: Posterolateral rotatory instability of the elbow. *Am J Sports Med* 42(2):485–491, 2014.
4. Anakwenze OA, Kwon D, O'Donnell E, et al: Surgical treatment of posterolateral rotatory instability of the elbow. *Arthroscopy* 30(7):866–871, 2014.
5. Andrews JR, Timmerman LA: Outcome of elbow surgery in professional baseball players. *Am J Sports Med* 23(4):407–413, 1995.
6. Aoki M, Takasaki H, Muraki T, et al: Strain on the ulnar nerve at the elbow and wrist during throwing motion. *J Bone Joint Surg Am* 87:2508–2514, 2005.
7. Athwal GS, Faber KJ, King GJ, et al: Crista supinatoris fractures of the proximal part of the ulna. *J Bone Joint Surg Am* 96(4):326–331, 2014.

8. Azar FM, Andrews JR, Wilk KE, et al: Operative treatment of ulnar collateral ligament injuries of the elbow in athletes. *Am J Sports Med* 28:16–23, 2000.
9. Baghdadi YM, Morrey BF, O'Driscoll SW, et al: Revision allograft reconstruction of the lateral collateral ligament complex in elbows with previous failed reconstruction and persistent posterolateral rotatory instability. *Clin Orthop Relat Res* 472(7):2061–2067, 2014.
10. Berg EE, DeHoll D: Radiography of the medial elbow ligaments. *J Shoulder Elbow Surg* 6:528–533, 1997.
11. Cain EL, Jr, Andrews JR, Dugas JR, et al: Outcome of ulnar collateral ligament reconstruction of the elbow in 1281 athletes: results in 743 athletes with minimum 2-year follow-up. *Am J Sports Med* 38(12):2426–2434, 2010.
12. Callaway GH, Field LD, Deng XH, et al: Biomechanical evaluation of the medial collateral ligament of the elbow. *J Bone Joint Surg Am* 79:1223–1231, 1997.
13. Ciccotti MG, Jobe FW: Medial collateral ligament instability and ulnar neuritis in the athlete's elbow. *Instr Course Lect* 48:383–391, 1999.
14. Cohen MS: Lateral collateral ligament instability of the elbow. *Hand Clin* 24(1):69–77, 2008.
15. Cohen MS: Lateral collateral ligament reconstruction. In Baker CL, Plancher KD, editors: *Operative Treatment of Elbow Injuries*, New York, 2002, Springer-Verlag, pp 101–108.
16. Cohen MS, Bruno RJ: The collateral ligaments of the elbow: anatomy and clinical correlation. *Clin Orthop Relat Res* 383:123–130, 2001.
17. Cohen MS, Hastings H: Acute elbow dislocation: evaluation and management. *J Am Acad Orthop Surg* 6(1):15–23, 1998.
18. Cohen MS, Hastings H: Rotatory instability of the elbow: the role of the lateral stabilizers. *J Bone Joint Surg Am* 79:225–233, 1997.
19. Conway JE, Jobe FW, Glousman RE, et al: Medial instability of the elbow in throwing athletes: treatment by repair or reconstruction of the ulnar collateral ligament. *J Bone Joint Surg Am* 74:67–83, 1992.
20. Daluiski A, Schrumpf MA, Schreiber JJ, et al: Direct repair for managing acute and chronic lateral ulnar collateral ligament disruptions. *J Hand Surg [Am]* 39(6):1125–1129, 2014.
21. Davidson PA, Pink M, Perry J, et al: Functional anatomy of the flexor pronator muscle group in relation to the medial collateral ligament of the elbow. *Am J Sports Med* 23:245–250, 1995.
22. Dines JS, El Attrache NS, Conway JE, et al: Clinical outcomes of the DANE TJ technique to treat ulnar collateral ligament insufficiency of the elbow. *Am J Sports Med* 35(12):2039–2044, 2007.
23. Dinoo JS, Jones KJ, Kahlenberg C, et al: Elbow ulnar collateral ligament reconstruction in javelin throwers at a minimum 2-year follow-up. *Am J Sports Med* 40(1):148–151, 2012.
24. Dodson CC, Slenker N, Cohen SB, et al: Ulnar collateral ligament injuries of the elbow in professional football quarterbacks. *J Shoulder Elbow Surg* 19(8):1276–1280, 2010.
25. Dodson CC, Thomas A, Dines JS, et al: Medial ulnar collateral ligament reconstruction of the elbow in throwing athletes. *Am J Sports Med* 34(12):1926–1932, 2006.
26. Dugas JR, Ostrander RV, Cain EL, et al: Anatomy of the anterior bundle of the ulnar collateral ligament. *J Shoulder Elbow Surg* 16:657–660, 2007.
27. Dunning CE, Zarzour ZDS, Patterson SD, et al: Ligamentous stabilizers against posterolateral rotatory instability of the elbow. *J Bone Joint Surg Am* 83:1823–1828, 2001.
28. El Attrache NS, Bast SC, David T: Medial collateral ligament reconstruction. *Tech Shoulder Elbow Surg* 2:38–49, 2001.
29. Farrow LD, Mahoney AJ, Stefancin JJ, et al: Quantitative analysis of the medial ulnar collateral ligament footprint and its relationship to the ulnar sublime tubercle. *Am J Sports Med* 39(9):1936–1941, 2011.
30. Floris S, Olsen BS, Dalstra M, et al: The medial collateral ligament of the elbow joint: anatomy and kinematics. *J Shoulder Elbow Surg* 7:345–351, 1998.
31. Froimson AI, Anouchi YS, Seitz WH, et al: Ulnar nerve decompression with medial epicondylectomy for neuropathy at the elbow. *Clin Orthop Relat Res* 265:200–206, 1991.
32. Fuss FK: The ulnar collateral ligament of the human elbow joint: anatomy, function and biomechanics. *J Anat* 175:203–212, 1991.
33. Grumet RC, Friel NA, Cole BJ: Bony avulsion of the medial ulnar collateral ligament in a gymnast: a case report. *J Shoulder Elbow Surg* 19(7):e1–e6, 2010.
34. Hastings HH, Cohen MS: General deep approaches to the elbow: lateral approaches. *Tech Shoulder Elbow Surg* 3(1):10–15, 2002.
35. Heithoff SJ, Millender LH, Nalebuff EA, et al: Medial epicondylectomy for the treatment of ulnar nerve compression at the elbow. *J Hand Surg [Am]* 15:22–29, 1990.
36. Hill NB, Bucchieri JS, Shon F, et al: Magnetic resonance imaging of injury to the medial collateral ligament of the elbow: a cadaveric model. *J Shoulder Elbow Surg* 9:18–22, 2000.
37. Hotchkiss RN, Weiland AJ: Valgus stability of the elbow. *J Orthop Res* 5:372–377, 1987.
38. Imatani J, Ogura T, Morito Y, et al: Anatomic and histologic studies of lateral collateral ligament complex of the elbow joint. *J Shoulder Elbow Surg* 8(6):625–627, 1999.
39. Jobe FW, Kvitne RS: Reconstruction of the ulnar collateral ligament of the elbow. *Tech Orthop* 6:39–42, 1991.
40. Jobe FW, Stark H, Lombardo SJ: Reconstruction of the ulnar collateral ligament in athletes. *J Bone Joint Surg Am* 68:1158–1163, 1986.
41. Jones KJ, Conte S, Patterson N, et al: Functional outcomes following revision ulnar collateral ligament reconstruction in major league baseball pitchers. *J Shoulder Elbow Surg* 22(5):642–646, 2013.
42. Jones KJ, Dodson CC, Osbahr DC, et al: The docking technique for lateral ulnar collateral ligament reconstruction: surgical technique and clinical outcomes. *J Shoulder Elbow Surg* 21(3):389–395, 2012.
43. Josefsson PO, Johnell O, Wendeberg B: Ligamentous injuries in dislocations of the elbow joint. *Clin Orthop Relat Res* 221:221–225, 1987.
44. Kalainov DM, Cohen MS: Posterolateral rotatory instability of the elbow in association with lateral epicondylitis. *J Bone Joint Surg Am* 87:1120–1125, 2005.
45. Kuroda S, Sakamaki K: Ulnar collateral ligament tears of the elbow joint. *Clin Orthop Relat Res* 208:266–271, 1986.
46. Lee BP, Teo LH: Surgical reconstruction for posterolateral rotatory instability of the elbow. *J Shoulder Elbow Surg* 12(5):476–479, 2003.
47. Lin KY, Shen PH, Lee CH, et al: Functional outcomes of surgical reconstruction for posterolateral rotatory instability of the elbow. *Injury* 43(10):1657–1661, 2012.
48. Morrey BF: Re-operation for failed tennis elbow surgery. *J Shoulder Elbow Surg* 1:47–49, 1992.
49. Morrey BF, An KN: Articular and ligamentous contributions to the stability of the elbow joint. *Am J Sports Med* 11:315–319, 1983.
50. Morrey BF, An KN: Functional anatomy of the ligaments of the elbow. *Clin Orthop Relat Res* 201:84–90, 1985.
51. Morrey BF, Tanaka S, An KN: Valgus stability of the elbow: a definition of primary and secondary constraints. *Clin Orthop Relat Res* 265:187–195, 1991.
52. Nestor BJ, O'Driscoll SW, Morrey BF: Ligamentous reconstruction for posterolateral rotatory instability of the elbow. *J Bone Joint Surg Am* 4:1235–1241, 1992.
53. Ochi N, Ogura T, Hashizume H, et al: Anatomic relation between the medial collateral ligament of the elbow and the humero-ulnar joint axis. *J Shoulder Elbow Surg* 8:6–10, 1999.
54. O'Driscoll SW, Bell DF, Morrey BF: Posterolateral rotatory instability of the elbow. *J Bone Joint Surg Am* 73:440–446, 1991.
55. O'Driscoll SW, Jaloszynski R, Morrey BF, et al: Origin of the medial ulnar collateral ligament. *J Hand Surg [Am]* 17:164–168, 1992.
56. O'Driscoll SW, Jupiter JB, Cohen MS, et al: Difficult elbow fractures: pearls and pitfalls. *Instr Course Lect* 52:113–136, 2003.
57. O'Driscoll SW, Lawton RL, Smith AM: The "moving valgus stress test" for medial collateral ligament tears of the elbow. *Am J Sports Med* 33:231–239, 2005.
58. O'Driscoll SW, Morrey BF, Korinek S, et al: Elbow subluxation and dislocation. A spectrum of instability. *Clin Orthop Relat Res* 280:186–197, 1992.
59. O'Driscoll SW, Spinner RJ, McKee MD, et al: Tardy posterolateral rotatory instability of the elbow due to cubitus varus. *J Bone Joint Surg Am* 83:1358–1369, 2001.
60. Paletta GA, Jr, Klepps SJ, Difelice GS, et al: Biomechanical evaluation of 2 techniques for ulnar collateral ligament reconstruction of the elbow. *Am J Sports Med* 34(10):1599–1603, 2006.
61. Regan WD, Korinek SL, Morrey BF, et al: Biomechanical study of ligaments around the elbow joint. *Clin Orthop Relat Res* 271:170–179, 1991.
62. Rettig AC, Sherrill C, Snead DS, et al: Nonoperative treatment of ulnar collateral ligament injuries in throwing athletes. *Am J Sports Med* 29:15–17, 2001.
63. Rohrbough JT, Altchek DW, Hyman J, et al: Medial collateral ligament reconstruction of the elbow using the docking technique. *Am J Sports Med* 30(4):541–548, 2002.
64. Deleted in review.
65. Savoie FH, 3rd, Morgan C, Yaste J, et al: Medial ulnar collateral ligament reconstruction using hamstring allograft in overhead throwing athletes. *J Bone Joint Surg Am* 95(12):1062–1066, 2013.
66. Schwab GH, Bennett JB, Woods GW, et al: Biomechanics of elbow instability: the role of the medial collateral ligament. *Clin Orthop Relat Res* 146:42–52, 1980.
67. Shah RP, Lindsey DP, Sungar GW, et al: An analysis of four ulnar collateral ligament reconstruction procedures with cyclic valgus loading. *J Shoulder Elbow Surg* 18(1):58–63, 2009.
68. Shukla DR, O'Driscoll S: Atypical etiology of lateral collateral ligament disruption and instability. *J Orthop Trauma* 27(6):e144–e146, 2013.
69. Smith AM, O'Driscoll SW: Diagnosing medial elbow pain in throwers. *J Musculoskeletal Med* 22:305–316, 2005.
70. Sojbjerg JO, Helmig P, Kjaersgaard-Anderson P: Dislocation of the elbow: an experimental study of the ligamentous injuries. *Orthopedics* 12:461–463, 1989.
71. Sojbjerg JO, Ovesen J, Nielsen S: Experimental elbow instability after transection of the medial collateral ligament. *Clin Orthop Relat Res* 218:186–190, 1987.

72. Thompson WH, Jobe FW, Yocum LA, et al: Ulnar collateral ligament reconstruction in athletes: muscle-splitting approach without transposition of the ulnar nerve. *J Shoulder Elbow Surg* 10:152–157, 2001.

73. Timmerman LA, Schwartz ML, Andrews JR: Preoperative evaluation of the ulnar collateral ligament by magnetic resonance imaging and computed tomography arthrography. Evaluation in 25 baseball players with surgical confirmation. *Am J Sports Med* 22(1):26–31, 1994.

74. Vitale MA, Ahmad CS: The outcome of elbow ulnar collateral ligament reconstruction in overhead athletes: a systematic review. *Am J Sports Med* 36:1193–1205, 2008.

75. Watson JN, McQueen P, Hutchinson MR: A systematic review of ulnar collateral ligament reconstruction techniques. *Am J Sports Med* 42(10):2510–2516, 2014.

76. Werner SL, Fleisig GS, Dillman CJ, et al: biomechanics of the elbow during baseball pitching. *J Orthop Sports Phys Ther* 1:274–278, 1993.

24

Treatment of the Stiff Elbow

Robert N. Hotchkiss

Although this text carries the title *Operative Hand Surgery* and was originally conceived as a compilation of techniques for surgery of the hand, attention to the problem of the stiff elbow is warranted for three reasons. First, loss of motion of the elbow directly restricts the ability to place the hand in space to and from the body, thereby disabling the function of the entire upper limb. Second, surgeons skilled in operations on the hand are increasingly called on to evaluate and treat stiff elbows following trauma or caused by arthritis and other conditions. Surgical release of a contracted elbow often requires meticulous dissection of neurovascular structures at the elbow, an area of anatomy that usually falls most comfortably under the purview of the hand surgeon. Finally, in the past 20 years, development of more dependable methods and techniques has made contracture release more reliable and clinically possible.

Before the 1990s, the published literature, including textbooks on orthopedics, reflected a general reluctance to treat the stiff elbow surgically. The condition was seldom discussed in textbooks; Wilson[78] was one of the few who wrote about the subject in the 1940s. The terms that were applied in the literature, such as *contracture, stiff elbow, posttraumatic elbow*, and *arthrolysis,* were not precise enough for comparative purposes. Since then, operative treatment has become more common and results more predictable, although the lack of uniformity in reporting for evidence-based comparison persists. In general, reported results reflect a consensus that open capsulectomy, carefully performed on a willing patient, using a medial, lateral, or mediolateral approach to the elbow joint, results in a consistent and notable improvement in motion with only a small risk of serious complications.* The use of arthroscopy alone remains controversial,[21,32,57,64] and the need for hinged external fixation seems more limited.[60,71] For further reading, I recommend the well-written summaries of King,[33] Modabber and Jupiter,[44] and Sojbjerg.[68]

CAUSES AND PREVENTION OF THE STIFF AND CONTRACTED ELBOW

Our understanding of what creates a stiff joint is limited. We do know that an intraarticular effusion causes the joint to assume a position of flexion to maximize the volume of the capsule and minimize pressure. This may explain the position of flexion assumed for comfort immediately after injury.[7] In addition, there are biologic factors that help explain this process.[25] Once in a flexed position, the flexors and extensors tend to contract together, perhaps to minimize pain, leading to a cycle of increasing stiffness. More research is needed to understand the neuromuscular response to pain and trauma.[3,5,55] Before injury and capsular scarring has occurred, the elbow has adequate clearance for full extension and flexion, and the capsule is thin and usually transparent. After trauma, the capsule thickens, limiting flexion and extension as a "block" and a "tether," respectively. The thickness of the capsule that requires excision, even after minimal trauma, may exceed 5 mm (Figure 24.1).

It is important to institute active motion with gentle passive assistance as soon as is practical after injury, although there are times when rehabilitation must be tempered owing to tenuous fixation of intraarticular fractures. Often, unfortunately, motion is not started until 6 weeks or longer after a simple fracture or dislocation, and by that time it is often too late.[66] Even with attentive, supervised therapy that is initiated early, however, many patients will not regain optimal motion after trauma.

Our tools for minimizing contracture after injury are generally limited to physical therapy and splinting. Manipulation has been reported as useful but should be approached with caution after fracture or in the presence of internal fixation. Undoubtedly, as we begin to understand more about protective or overactive muscle reflexes and pain, as well as the molecular biology of scar formation, we will have better tools to minimize pathologic contractures.

It is helpful to remember a few guidelines when discussing a stiff elbow with a patient and the family, especially after trauma:

1. Unless evidence of gross malpractice exists, the contracture is seldom caused by the method of internal fixation or technical performance of the surgeon.
2. The therapist usually has not *failed to improve* the patient's motion. Many therapists have minimal experience with stiff elbows following trauma and are appropriately timid. However, blaming a therapist for using a dynamic splint for 9 months with little success (which is not uncommon) serves no purpose. The therapist is often caught between the frustration of the patient and the hidden worry of the surgeon, both of whom see the failure to regain motion as a defeat.
3. The patient is usually not at fault, either. It is not uncommon for a patient to state that both the surgeon and the therapist have told the patient "You didn't work hard enough." Patients respond to treatment differently, and those with a traumatized elbow demonstrate a wide range of responses. It is helpful to listen carefully to the patient and family. Most will tell of weeks and months of visits

---

*See references 22, 29, 41, 49, 67, 74, and 76.

to the therapist, painful dynamic splints, and, finally, frustration. Any patient on whom one is considering operative treatment must be brought into the team and made to feel an integral part of the solution.

In summary, there is usually little value in spending time laying blame for a stiff or contracted elbow. A more productive use of time can be discussing your evaluation and plans to improve the situation and your rationale for treatment.

PREOPERATIVE ASSESSMENT

It is helpful to categorize the contracture as severe, moderate, or minimal (Table 24.1). This classification permits a starting point for assessment, operative planning, postoperative management, and expectations. As the surgeon gains experience, the arbitrary categories become a continuum and consequently less valuable.

Operative treatment of a stiff elbow begins with an understanding of the probable cause of the patient's contracture and the patient's functional requirements, both vocationally and recreationally. Other factors such as the patient's age and the time since injury must be considered (discussed in more detail later). These factors, taken together, determine not only the indications for surgery but also which surgical approach and type of postoperative treatment are likely to produce a successful result. The checklist in Table 24.1 is intended to help guide patient selection, operative approach, and regimen of postoperative rehabilitation. However, the need for midcourse corrections in the operating room and during the postoperative period is a constant and fundamental feature of operative treatment for a stiff elbow. To make these adjustments, the surgeon and therapist must have all of the resources for assessment and treatment available.

Patient History

Age of the Patient

The group of patients with the highest success rate in my practice is from 18 to 50 years old. These are generally people with high motivation who are capable of understanding their disability and seek to change it. The results reported in the

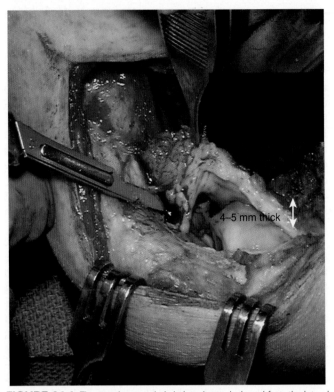

FIGURE 24.1 The anterior capsule is being elevated, viewed from the lateral exposure. The capsule is approximately 5 mm thick.

4–5 mm thick

TABLE 24.1	**Categories of Posttraumatic Stiffness**			
Category	**Range of Motion**	**Associated Findings and Characteristics**	**Likely Treatment**	**Likely Outcome**
Minimal	Less than 30 degrees of motion loss (usually extension)	Single isolated injury Single previous surgery Near-normal joint Identifiable cause of motion loss	Open release with limited exposure Possible arthroscopic release Outpatient PT	Nearly complete recovery of motion
Moderate	40 to 100 degrees of total motion	Moderately severe injury More than one previous operation Ulnar nerve at risk Moderate HO present, both anteriorly and posteriorly Minor joint surface injury	Ulnar nerve release (transposition) Open release with medial and lateral exposure Coordinated PT Inpatient CPM with indwelling catheter	Seldom regain full extension
Severe	Less than 30 degrees total motion	Severe injury Several previous operative procedures "Enveloping fibrosis" Joint surface injury may be present Nerve entrapment or risk Often, all three of above findings Massive HO Potential joint surface incongruity Triceps may be adherent to midhumerus	Complete dissection/protection of all nerves Resection of HO from all blocking locations Triceps tenolysis Possible hinged external fixation Protection of posterolateral ligament Comprehensive-coordinated PT (indwelling catheter)	30° to 130° of motion achieved Prolonged rehabilitation Strength and power often limited

CPM, Continuous passive motion; *HO*, heterotopic ossification; *PT*, physical therapy.

pediatric population are more varied.[2,41,43,69] Despite this, my success rate has improved with careful selection and better management. I have reviewed 30 patients with open elbow contracture release at a mean age of 13.9 years (range, 5 to 18 years). In a somewhat arbitrary fashion, I separated the patients into three groups. Seven patients were younger than 10 years of age, 9 were between 10 and 14 years, and 14 were between 15 and 18 years at the time of surgery. The net improvement in the total arc of elbow motion ranged from approximately 70 degrees to 125 degrees and did not vary significantly between groups. A child with joint injury and cartilage damage is still very challenging, and surgery should be contemplated with caution. This is especially true in adolescents who are in a rebellious phase or who lack the maturity for cooperation.[2] Occasionally, parents will bring an unwilling and uncooperative teenager for consideration of operative contracture release. Such patients will generally not participate in the postoperative therapy program and fail to regain motion. Some may even worsen after operative treatment. However, some individuals in this age group can also be quite rewarding to treat, especially those injured during participation in organized sports (such as gymnastics and wrestling), who are anxious to return to the team. They are usually highly motivated and will follow instructions to the letter.

Lower rates of success are generally achieved with the elderly.[41] Elderly patients with a stiff elbow may have significant associated swelling of the hand and stiffness of the shoulder, both of which limit the possibility of success and the impact of improved elbow mobility. In addition, the quality of the joint may be so poor that the only reasonable option is total elbow replacement. In these cases, the long-standing dysfunction, usually caused by protracted immobilization of the entire limb, makes for prolonged and often incomplete restoration of function.

Duration of Contracture and Timing of Operative Release

There has been much speculation about the timing of contracture release, especially when considering excision of heterotopic ossification (HO)[75] (Figure 24.2). Although the use of technetium bone scans was touted in the past for predicting the "activity" and, therefore, the probability of recurrence of HO, this test should be completely discarded as irrelevant because the scan sometimes remains "hot" for many years.

The optimal timing of intervention depends on the source of the contracture. If the loss of motion is due to a fracture that has fallen apart because of failed internal fixation or a persistently dislocated elbow, waiting serves no purpose.[39] These patients should have the joint surfaces and congruity restored as soon as is practical in the hope of preserving some function. These cases are the most difficult and require both contracture release and restoration of the architecture, followed by immediate motion. Often, external fixation, hinged or fixed, is required (see Chapter 22).

For patients who have normal or nearly normal articulation, the timing of intervention should be based on documented failure of physical therapy and progressive splinting to improve motion. Although there is increased interest in earlier operative intervention, it is important to be certain that all nonoperative methods have been exhausted. In general, most patients do not improve beyond 4 to 6 months after injury (except children with supracondylar fractures). At the 6-month mark, unless there is significant brain injury, intervention can be considered. In cases with HO, the process has usually matured and can safely be removed at this time as well without fear of recurrence (see Fig. 24.2). Some have reported that contracture release after more than 1 year after injury has been associated with a lesser gain in motion.[22] For patients who have had a significant loss of motion for more than 10 years, regaining substantial motion may be impossible without humeral shortening and ulnohumeral arthroplasty because of changes in length of the median nerve and brachial artery.

Pain and the Stiff Elbow

Most uncomplicated posttraumatic contractures are not very painful. There may be some discomfort at the end range of motion, but within the zone of limited motion, the patient is generally comfortable. If this is not the case, one should suspect posttraumatic arthrosis or joint incongruity. Patients who have had excessively forceful manipulations or passive mobilization in a misguided attempt to restore motion at a late date may have reactive pain and swelling. However, as the scar matures and tissue equilibrium is regained, this inflammatory response usually abates.

Ipsilateral shoulder pain is common with flexion contractures over 40 degrees as the patient attempts to position the hand at the side while walking or carrying, causing the shoulder to extend. In the patient with long-standing stiffness, an examination of the shoulder is helpful, because limited rotation or abduction may decrease access during surgery of the elbow.

Another source of pain may be ulnar nerve entrapment.[13] Patients with a sensitive or trapped ulnar nerve after trauma may not exhibit the usual symptoms and signs of cubital tunnel syndrome. Instead of a definitive loss of sensibility in the distribution of the ulnar nerve, these patients may only exhibit resistance and reluctance to flexion in the first 2 months and tenderness along the medial elbow. They may describe "tightness" or "soreness" in the ulnar digits without frank sensory changes or weakness. As the contracture matures, the ulnar nerve is not under tension and therefore may not exhibit dysfunction.

In primary arthritis of the elbow associated with anterior and posterior osteophyte formation, pain is usually present at the end range of flexion and extension. That is where the osteophytes impinge. The middle range is usually comfortable and without crepitation. However, as the condition progresses and further deterioration of the trochlear surface of the humerus and other cartilage loss occurs, the pain may be more constant, severe, and present in all positions.

Assessment of Motion Loss and the Effect on Function

What Degree of Motion Is Necessary?

Morrey and colleagues studied normal subjects by electrogoniometry and determined that most tasks of daily living could be performed in a range of 30 to 130 degrees of flexion and extension.[50] This study was helpful in defining what most normal people use throughout the course of daily activity, but it did not ask the question, *what is required for these tasks.*

With the assistance of our therapy department, my colleagues and I studied 52 patients with decreased elbow motion and recorded the tasks that they could perform with and

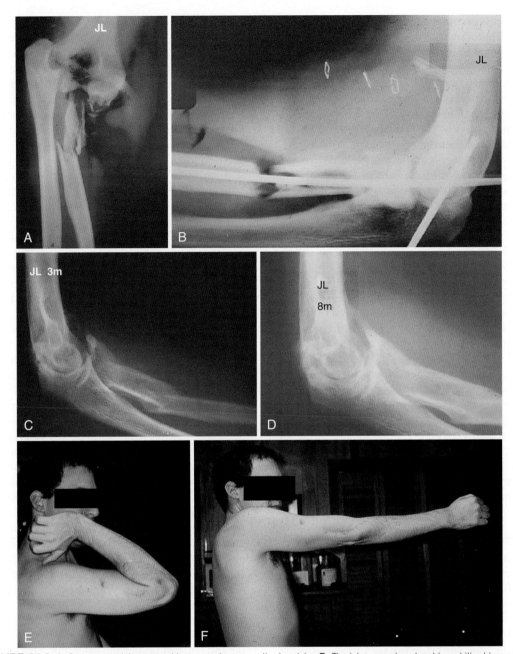

FIGURE 24.2 A, Severe open injury caused by a motorboat propeller in a lake. **B,** The joint was pinned and immobilized in a reduced position. Plates were not used for fear of infection and soft tissue stripping. **C,** Three months after the injury, wispy immature heterotopic ossification can be seen forming along the anterior surface of the joint. **D,** At 8 months, both sides of the joint are enveloped by bone. The patient has no motion in the elbow. **E** and **F,** Two years after open release and hinged external fixation with a Compass Hinge, the patient has nearly full extension and flexion without pain or deterioration of the joint. This excellent result was possible because the initial treating surgeon kept the joint reduced. Despite the ensuing stiffness, the reduced joint protected cartilage and ligaments. (Copyright © Robert N. Hotchkiss.)

without specified adaptations. Twenty elbow-dependent tasks ranging from buttoning a collar to reaching for a lower drawer were evaluated. The goal was to examine which tasks could be performed and, of those performed, which required a significant postural or spatial adaptation. The study found that patients lacking flexion of more than 110 degrees were unlikely to be able to button a collar, shave the face, place an earring, or tie a scarf or necktie. Loss of elbow flexion limits using eating utensils and self-care of the hair, face, and neck. In our study, patients could not compensate for loss of flexion; the neck and

wrist are limited in their capacity to flex to assist the hand in reaching the neck, face, head, or ears. Although loss of flexion is generally ignored in the published literature, every effort should be made to improve flexion, especially when there is less than 105 degrees present.

Patients with lack of extension, however, can much more easily accommodate for the loss. In our study, flexion contracture of greater than 40 degrees required positional adaptation, but the tasks could still be accomplished. Reaching the feet or toes was possible with increased knee, hip, and trunk flexion.

For opening low drawers, the patient could kneel to pull them open bimanually. In other words, positioning the hand in space, away from the body or to the feet, is limited with loss of extension, but the patient can accommodate for this by moving the trunk (and hand) closer to the object of interest.

An important conclusion from our study was that if improved extension is sought, it should not be obtained at the expense of flexion. This is not a "trade" that patients will want to make.

In the preoperative assessment it is helpful for patients to detail what tasks they have difficulty performing because of limitation of motion. Patients may be functional with a 40-degree flexion contracture but simply not like the appearance. Given the complexity of the surgery and the postoperative effort usually required, I generally do not recommend contracture release for the improvement of appearance only.

Elbow motion must be carefully documented by goniometry and a standardized technique. I have found the interobserver error in trained personnel to be about ±10 degrees. My own intraobserver error is about 5 degrees when using a large goniometer. Given these numbers, I doubt the value of reporting elbow measurements in increments of less than 5 degrees. It is important for the surgeon to measure the angles personally and not merely rely on measurements recorded by others.

Indications for Contracture Release

It is impossible to set absolute indications for operative contracture release. Generally, any patient with a 40-degree loss of extension or with less than 105 degrees of flexion will benefit from improved motion and should be considered for contracture release. It is seldom possible to guarantee full extension, irrespective of the operative approach or postoperative management. This point is especially important to discuss with patients such as gymnasts, who require full extension, or even hyperextension, to "lock out" the arms during handstands or floor exercises. Occasionally, patients with posttraumatic contractures of 30 degrees or less, despite being very functional, seek nearly full extension for sports, especially for the throwing arm. If the contracture is simple and uncomplicated by joint incongruity, these patients can often be improved by either arthroscopic release or a release from the lateral approach alone.

Physical Examination of the Ulnar Nerve

The ulnar nerve is vulnerable to injury, scarring, and dysfunction after trauma, distal humeral internal fixation, and complex dislocations.[6] Hence, careful preoperative assessment of the nerve is mandatory. In many cases it is not possible to be certain whether the nerve has been transposed. Even if the previous operative note is available and states that a transposition was performed, the nerve may have slipped back into a more posterior position.

If the ulnar nerve is entrapped or shows signs of significant dysfunction, neurolysis and transposition at the time of contracture release can restore sensibility and strength in the proximal muscles innervated by the ulnar nerve. The more distal intrinsic muscles of the hand are less likely to recover, although occasionally in younger patients dramatic improvement may be seen.

Most patients with loss of flexion require ulnar nerve transposition at the time of surgery, and this point should be discussed with the patient. Patients with primary osteoarthritis of the elbow often demonstrate osteophytes extending into the cubital tunnel. These patients, usually middle-aged men, may have a subclinical, indolent course. When carefully examined, the intrinsic weakness may be subtle and the loss of sensibility discovered only with threshold measurements or two-point discrimination. If there is doubt, preoperative electrophysiologic testing, with special attention to electromyography, should be performed.

Patients may have temporary postoperative ulnar nerve dysfunction, especially if the nerve is already symptomatic. Most improve with neurolysis and transposition, but recovery is often slow if the dysfunction has been present for a long time.

When dissecting the ulnar nerve, there is seldom any reason to perform an internal neurolysis or intrafascicular or even epineural dissection. Instead, the goal is to free the nerve from the entrapment posterior to the axis of the joint and allow it to be transposed to the anterior position. Leaving a cuff of soft tissue, especially in a setting of reoperation, poses less threat to nerve function than trying to strip all soft tissue from the nerve.

Assessment of the Ulnohumeral Joint Surface After Trauma

The most challenging reconstructive problem is elbow stiffness with concomitant cartilage loss in the ulnohumeral joint. Hence, assessment of this surface either by computed tomography (CT) or magnetic resonance imaging (MRI) is paramount if the joint surface is suspected to be of poor quality. Ultimately, however, the articular surface must be inspected at the time of surgery to determine whether there is adequate cartilage in the functional zone of motion. The radiocapitellar surface can be sacrificed with radial head resection or excision of the capitellum. In some cases, the end-bearing surface of the radial head is devoid of cartilage, but patients are not symptomatic during forearm rotation. In these patients, typically middle-aged men with osteoarthritis, the radial head does not need to be addressed. However, if incongruity or poor cartilage surfaces in the ulnohumeral joint are present, a contracture release alone is not likely to be beneficial. I have made the mistake of improving motion but inducing pain by performing a contracture release in degenerated joints.

In the older patient with limited demand, total elbow replacement may be the optimal choice (see Chapter 27). In the younger patient with severe incongruity, interposition arthroplasty is sufficiently unpredictable that I seldom perform this procedure following trauma.

Imaging the Stiff Elbow

Many radiologic features need to be assessed before surgery is considered:

- What is the quality of the joint and relative health of the cartilage?
- Where is the hardware, and is it impeding motion? (Is removal necessary?)
- Where is the HO or impingement located?
- Are the fractures healed?

A significant flexion contracture may preclude visualization of the distal humeral articular surface with standard radiographic techniques. Typically, the technician places the film plate perpendicular to the joint at midrange. An anteroposterior view with the distal humerus lying flat on the cassette is a helpful additional view. A true lateral view is also mandatory. In some cases I also obtain true lateral views in maximal active flexion and maximal active extension. Technicians find these difficult at first because the humerus tends to internally or externally rotate at the extremes of position and the "true lateral" view is lost.[37] These additional views may show subtle shifts of the joint, as well as previously unseen projections of heterotopic bone.

As noted previously, the quality of the articular surfaces in a stiff posttraumatic elbow is of paramount importance. The ulnohumeral joint is probably more important than the radiocapitellar joint, although having both intact and functional is optimal. Assessing this joint and the quality of the cartilage is best done with plain radiographs. If this is insufficient, CT scans with thin slices in the sagittal and coronal planes may be needed. I recommend 0.8-mm–thick contiguous slices with overlap. This acquisition method permits multiplanar reconstruction and other manipulations. Three-dimensional surface reconstructions can be helpful in preoperative planning.

For fracture cases, it is sometimes difficult to determine whether union has been achieved, especially when plates and screws overlie the area in question. CT is problematic because of "noise" from the metal; however, CT radiologists continue to improve their ability to suppress this effect, especially with titanium implants. MRI techniques are improving to better assess fragment healing, viability, and perfusion, even in the presence of metallic hardware.[15,36]

At no time have I used bone scans to assess a contracted elbow, finding them of no use in patients with posttraumatic contracture with or without heterotopic bone.

The Preoperative Discussion

Once you have determined that a surgical release *could* be performed, it is important to discuss expectations, the surgery, and the potential complications with the patient. From this discussion alone, the patient may shy away and appropriately conclude that it is possible to live quite well with the limitation of motion.

Much like rehabilitation after flexor tendon repair, without the full cooperation and dedication of the patient, surgery may not succeed. In fact, given the complexity of some cases, the attempted release may worsen motion.

As detailed later, each contracture requires at least two operative plans. If the first approach does not succeed in achieving the expected goal during surgery, the second option should be employed. If you believed that a medial approach to the joint would permit a complete capsulectomy but at surgery find the lateral structures both limiting and out of safe reach, then a concomitant lateral approach should be considered. Likewise, postoperative management varies greatly, depending on each patient's individual response. It is important to explain the variability in response to operative release. Fortunately, most patients with contractures understand this because they have already been told that this was in some way their fault or the fault of their "muscles." Some require very little supervised therapy, even little continuous passive motion (CPM); others need serial static progressive bracing (flexion and extension) and occasionally a carefully administered manipulation. For massive HO with long-standing contractures, I also explain the use of dynamic hinged external fixation. As a matter of

disclosure, I helped design and patent the Compass Elbow Hinge (manufactured by Smith and Nephew, UK). However, for 15 years I have received no compensation in any form.

If during any of the discussion with the patient you detect unwillingness or wariness, waiting may be warranted. I also encourage patients to discuss their questions with other patients, and I keep a list of former patients willing to discuss their operative experience.

Patients should also be informed about the possibility of transient increased ulnar nerve symptoms.

Classifying the Contracture and Matching the Operative Plan

After deciding to proceed with contracture release, it is helpful to classify the contracture as minimal, moderate, or severe (see Table 24.1). This general guide may help in planning what is needed to succeed. The most common reason for a failed contracture release, in my opinion, is a failure on the part of the surgeon to abandon an orthodox method in favor of a less assured technique (arthroscopy) or to use a single anatomic approach to the joint when the potential gain in motion is not achieved at the time of surgery. The operative contracture release requires a progressive, adaptive surgical approach, and the surgeon must safely increase the exposure in order to excise the offending fibrosis on nearly all aspects of the joint, anteroposterior and mediolateral.[41,72] If an uncomplicated, simple dislocation has caused a 30-degree flexion contracture, arthroscopic capsular excision might be sufficient; however, this technique has little role in moderate stiffness and none in severe cases.

The operative tools needed for successful contracture release range from arthroscopy to hinged external fixation to total elbow arthroplasty. Deciding which one you need depends on the patient's age, the cause of the stiffness, the quality of the joint, and, in some ways, the patient's personality. As we have gained experience with both the different causes of contracture and different types of patients, we have also had access to new tools and methods of treatment. The best care for a given patient with a contracture is the most minimal necessary surgery, including minimal anatomic exposure, and rehabilitation to achieve the desired result. For instance, a patient with a range of 40 to 105 degrees and HO will usually require exposure of the capsule for complete excision from both the medial and lateral approaches but not necessarily hinged fixation. Although in this situation the use of hinged fixation may potentially improve extension (from 20 degrees achieved with capsulectomy alone to perhaps 5 additional degrees with hinged fixation), I do not believe that this is worth the cost, potential complications, or aggravation to the patient.

In a different circumstance with more massive HO, hinged external fixation may be necessary to stabilize the elbow postoperatively and permit immediate motion with intermittent passive stretch.

I set out to perform the operation most likely to achieve the goal, but I am always prepared to change methods, extend the exposure, or approach the joint from an additional direction, and I explain this to the patient preoperatively. In other words, if I think that an arthroscopic release is likely to be sufficient, I also plan for the possibility of an open release if full passive motion is not achieved on the operating table. In cases in which I am reasonably certain that a dual-approach, anteroposterior release will suffice, I may plan for hinged fixation in case there is unexpected muscle-tendon tightness and failure to regain extension or flexion on the table or the joint is surprisingly or excessively worn and requires interposition. Having now performed more than 400 contracture releases, I have found the need for hinged fixation to be less likely.[60,71] In older patients with suspected cartilage damage or avascular bone, total elbow replacement should be available and discussed before surgery.

Predicting what you need and what will succeed is an iterative process that comes from your own experience and the seasoned opinions of others. It is important to be prepared to change and not be wedded to any single approach.[33] Orthodoxy here should only be a dedication to optimizing your patient's motion and not to a single exposure, approach, or device.

ANESTHESIA FOR CONTRACTURE RELEASE

Regional blocks are preferred[39] and are in fact the only method I have used for contracture release over the past 20 years. At my institution, ultrasound-guided infraclavicular blocks have become standard for contracture release; an indwelling catheter is often used so that additional dosing can occur 24 to 72 hours postoperatively.[52] Long-acting agents are the norm. Bupivacaine may leave the patient blocked for 24 to 48 hours. Although this may cause the surgeon concern, especially regarding the inability to check the status of the nerve, the pain relief and slow return of sensation are helpful as the patient begins motion the next day.

If the infraclavicular (or supraclavicular) technique or catheter is not available, axillary blocks may be used, but these may leave the upper end of the medial incision with sensibility. A small amount of local anesthetic in this area is usually all that is needed.

General anesthesia with endotracheal intubation may be used if regional blocks are unsuccessful or the anesthesia staff is unwilling to do regional blocks. More narcotics may be needed in the immediate postoperative period.

In children, I use infraclavicular indwelling catheters combined with general anesthesia. This is the "best of both worlds" for this challenging age group.

OPERATIVE TECHNIQUES AND APPROACHES

Arthroscopic Release

Arthroscopic elbow release is becoming more applicable as the techniques and instruments are improved and experience is gained.[28] This method works best in a young athlete with loose bodies or a history of a hyperextended elbow and a resultant minimal but annoying contracture. The anterior capsule can safely be released under direct arthroscopic visualization.

Two groups should be approached with great caution. The first group includes patients with a posttraumatic stiff elbow, in whom the capsule may be quite thick, sometimes 0.5 to 1 cm thick, and adherent to the anterior humerus. Because of this envelope of fibrotic tissue, arthroscopic release fails to excise the restraining tissue and puts the ulnar, median, and radial nerves at risk.[21,31,56]

The other group "at risk" is typified by a 45- to 55-year-old with primary osteoarthritis and simple osteophytes projecting from the coronoid and the tip of the olecranon.[37] In my opinion,

arthroscopic release *should not* be performed if the patient requires ulnar nerve transposition or if there are large osteophytes in the posteromedial corner, which is the floor of the cubital tunnel.[4] I have treated two patients in whom the ulnar nerve had accidentally been débrided with an arthroscopic shaver. Other injuries have also been reported.[21] The surgeon should resist the temptation to use the shaver in this region unless the ulnar nerve is mobilized. Open techniques are safe and relatively simple, permitting visualization of the relevant neurovascular structures as needed. It is my firm belief that one should understand and be able to perform an open capsulectomy (described in the following) using both medial and lateral approaches before using the arthroscope as the primary tool of visualization and capsulectomy. Furthermore, adequate experience and skill in elbow arthroscopy is required because this is technically a difficult arthroscopic operation.

Open Release

When an open release is planned, the location of the potential pathologic condition and the nature of the contracture should determine the approach to the joint. One should not feel constrained to use one approach over another because of an unfounded allegiance to a given method. If the patient has a simple flexion contracture related to a radial head fracture, the lateral approach is usually sufficient and is relatively simple to perform.[7,8,27,35,40] In more complex cases in which the ulnar nerve requires exposure, I usually begin with the medial "over-the-top" exposure.[30,45,76] I am always prepared to use a supplementary lateral approach in these cases if there is HO located on the lateral side, if I am concerned about the position and safety of the radial nerve, or if there is an impinging osteophyte behind the capitellum. It is therefore important to understand both the medial and lateral approaches and be able to use them as needed in the operating room. Both a transhumeral and a transolecranon approach have been described, but I have not used either.[23,79] I also no longer use the Outerbridge-Kashiwagi procedure[48] (transhumeral trephination), which is designed to treat patients with primary arthritis of the elbow. If there is a significant lack of flexion (limited to <90 degrees), evidence of ulnar nerve dysfunction, or osteophytes in the posteromedial joint line, I prefer the medial "over-the-top" approach. As described in the next section, this approach permits exposure of the ulnar nerve and access to the anterior and posterior osteophytes. If flexion is minimally limited and the ulnar nerve is palpable and mobile, I prefer arthroscopic débridement and contracture release.

Only rarely can contracture be treated with anterior capsulectomy alone. Of the more than 400 contractures that I have treated operatively over the past 10 years, only a handful were adequately freed by incising the anterior capsule alone. In most instances, you should always plan to have access to the posterior joint surface, whether from the medial or lateral side of the joint. The olecranon fossa must be free of bone and soft tissue for full terminal extension to be achieved.

The advantage of knowing and using both the medial and lateral approaches is that you can protect the anterior medial ligament on the medial side by using the medial "over-the-top" approach. From the lateral exposure, the lateral ligaments described as noted by Husband and Hastings[27] and others[7,40] can be protected.

Medial "Over-the-Top" Approach

The principal advantages of this approach are as follows:
- Allows exposure, protection, and transposition of the ulnar nerve
- Preserves the anterior medial collateral ligament
- Preserves the posterolateral ulnohumeral ligament complex
- Permits both anterior and posterior access to the joint
- Allows access to the coronoid and anterior osteophytes with an intact radial head
- Can be easily converted to the triceps-sparing exposure of Bryan-Morrey, which permits complete dislocation of the joint and a more extensile approach (for total elbow replacement)

The disadvantages are as follows:
- Difficult to remove heterotopic bone or osteophytes on the lateral side of the joint
- Poor access to the radial head

Patient Position and Preparation. The patient is usually supine with the arm supported by a hand table (Figure 24.3, *A*). It is helpful to bring as much of the patient as possible onto the hand table. The patient's head may require support with a small foam ring because a standard pillow projects too far toward the shoulder and impedes the skin preparation. Two folded towels should be placed under the ipsilateral scapula to lift the shoulder away from the surgical table. The preparation should include the axilla to allow a sterile tourniquet to be applied. For the surgeon to visualize the anterior and posterior surfaces of the distal humerus, the patient should have fairly free external rotation of the shoulder.

Skin Incision and Superficial Exposure. The skin incision for this exposure can vary between the boundaries of a pure posterior skin incision and a midline medial incision (see Figure 24.3, *B*). The key to this exposure is identification of the medial supracondylar ridge of the humerus (see Figure 24.3, *C*). At this level one can locate the medial intermuscular septum, the origin of the flexor-pronator muscle mass, and the ulnar nerve. This location also serves as the point to begin the subperiosteal extracapsular dissection of the joint for both the anterior and posterior surfaces.

Once the subcutaneous skin is elevated, the first structure to identify is the medial intermuscular septum. If the skin incision is more posterior, the medial intermuscular septum can be found by locating the aponeurosis of the triceps tendon 2 to 3 cm proximal to the medial epicondyle and gently spreading with scissors anteriorly. Anterior to the septum and running immediately on top of the fascia (and not in the subdermal tissue) is the medial antebrachial cutaneous nerve, which usually has several branches. Generally this nerve can be traced distally and protected in this approach, but the branching pattern varies. It is occasionally necessary to divide this nerve to gain full exposure and adequately mobilize the ulnar nerve, especially in revision surgery. If nerve excision is required, the nerve should be divided as far proximally as the skin incision will allow while ensuring that the cut nerve end lies in the subcutaneous fat. If the patient has had previous surgery, the ulnar

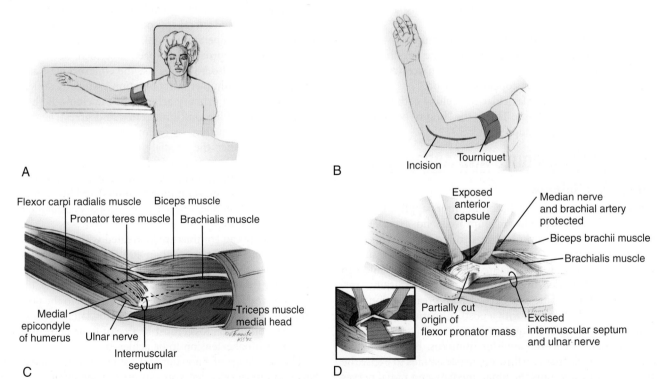

FIGURE 24.3 Medial "over-the-top" approach. **A,** The supine position is the most useful. Two folded towels should be placed under the ipsilateral scapula. **B,** The skin incision may vary according to previous incisions. If the incision is made along the posterior surface, larger flaps are needed. **C,** The intermuscular septum should be recognized as a landmark and excised for adequate mobilization of the ulnar nerve. **D,** The anterior capsule is first exposed by splitting fibers between the flexor carpi ulnaris and the pronator. The anterior portion of the medial collateral ligament is protected.

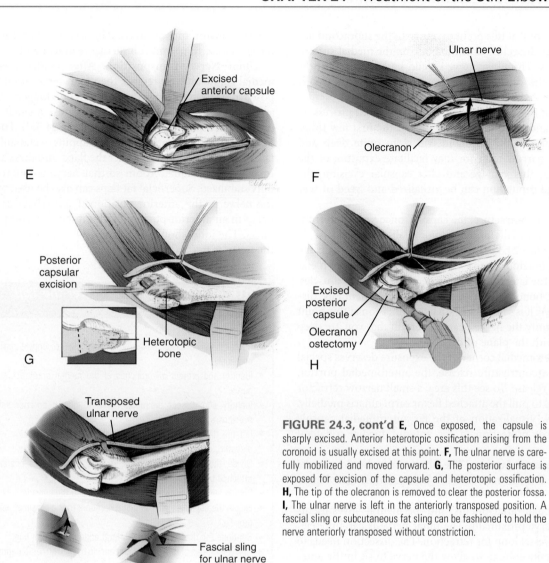

E, Excised anterior capsule

F, Ulnar nerve / Olecranon

G, Posterior capsular excision / Heterotopic bone

H, Excised posterior capsule / Olecranon ostectomy

I, Transposed ulnar nerve / Fascial sling for ulnar nerve

FIGURE 24.3, cont'd E, Once exposed, the capsule is sharply excised. Anterior heterotopic ossification arising from the coronoid is usually excised at this point. **F,** The ulnar nerve is carefully mobilized and moved forward. **G,** The posterior surface is exposed for excision of the capsule and heterotopic ossification. **H,** The tip of the olecranon is removed to clear the posterior fossa. **I,** The ulnar nerve is left in the anteriorly transposed position. A fascial sling or subcutaneous fat sling can be fashioned to hold the nerve anteriorly transposed without constriction.

nerve should be identified proximally before proceeding distally. If a previous anterior transposition has been performed, the nerve should be fully identified and mobilized before proceeding. In this setting, the nerve is flattened over the medial flexor-pronator muscle mass. Great care is needed to dissect the nerve in this location.

Once the medial intermuscular septum has been identified proximally, the surface of the origin of the flexor-pronator muscle mass can be found by dissecting at this same level and sweeping the subcutaneous tissue laterally. In most cases the medial antebrachial cutaneous nerve will be in this flap of subcutaneous tissue. The nerve will generally cross to the posterior aspect of the elbow distal to the epicondyle and can be elevated with the flap and retracted out of harm's way.

The medial intermuscular septum can now be excised from its insertion on the supracondylar ridge to the proximal extent of the wound, usually about 5 cm. There are many veins and perforating arteries at the most distal portion that require cautery. The septum can be cleared of muscle by using a small Cobb elevator along the posterior surface above the ulnar nerve.

Anterior Capsular Exposure. The supracondylar ridge is located, and the anterior muscle is elevated with a wide Cobb elevator (see Figure 24.3, *D*). All the anterior structures in the distal humeral region are elevated sufficiently subperiosteally to allow placement of a wide Bennett retractor. The median nerve, brachial vein, and brachial artery are superficial to the brachialis muscle. Once the septum is excised, the flexor-pronator muscle mass is divided parallel to its fibers, with a span of approximately 1.5 cm of flexor carpi ulnaris tendon left attached to the epicondyle. A tag stitch can be used to help align the tissues at closure. A small cuff of fibrous tissue of the origin can be left on the supracondylar ridge as the muscle is elevated. This facilitates reattachment when closing. A proximal transverse incision in the lacertus fibrosus may also be needed to adequately mobilize this layer of muscle. The flexor-pronator origin should be dissected down to the level of bone but superficial to the joint capsule. As this plane is developed, the brachialis muscle will be encountered from the underside. This muscle should be kept anterior and elevated from the capsule and anterior surface of the distal humerus.

It is often helpful at this point to return to the supracondylar ridge by sharply dissecting down to bone on the medial surface of the humerus. The ulnar nerve should be lying posteriorly. Dissection of the capsule to separate it from the brachialis muscle can proceed both laterally and distally.

At this point it is helpful to feel for the coronoid process by gently flexing and extending the elbow. For the first few times using this approach the coronoid will seem quite deep and distal. A deep, narrow retractor may facilitate exposure of the coronoid. From this vantage and after capsular excision, the radial head and capitellum can be visualized and freed of scar as needed.

In the case of contracture, the capsule, once separated from the overlying brachialis and brachioradialis, can be sharply excised (see Figure 24.3, *E*). The radial nerve lies between the brachialis and brachioradialis. Care should be taken when elevating over to the lateral side to stay deep to these two muscles. If heterotopic bone or previous surgery has potentially displaced the nerve, it is safer to make a lateral incision at this point and either identify the nerve or make certain that you are deep to the nerve with the plane of dissection.

The far anteromedial corner of the exposure deserves special comment. In a contracture release, the anteromedial portion often requires release. To see this area, a small narrow retractor can be inserted to pull the attached flexor carpi ulnaris medially. This will allow visualization of the far anteromedial capsule and also affords protection of the anterior medial collateral ligament.

Posterior Capsular Exposure. The ulnar nerve should now be fully mobilized to permit anterior transposition (see Figure 24.3, *F*). Because the intermuscular septum has been excised, only the vascular attachments and perineural investments confine the nerve proximally. The ulnar nerve is carefully elevated using a vessel loop for retraction. The dissection needs to be carried distally enough to allow the nerve to sit in the anterior position without kinking distal to the epicondyle.

The posterior capsule of the joint is exposed in a fashion analogous to that for the anterior capsule. The supracondylar ridge is again identified. With a Cobb elevator the triceps is elevated from the posterior distal surface of the humerus. The exposure should be proximal enough to permit the use of a Bennett retractor.

The posterior capsule can be separated from the triceps as the elevator sweeps in a proximal-to-distal direction. The medial joint line should also be identified (see Figure 24.3, *G*). In contracture release, the posterior capsule and posteromedial ligaments should be excised. The medial joint line, up to the anterior medial ligament, should also be exposed and the capsule excised. Along this line there is usually heterotopic bone on the olecranon or posterior medial osteophytes. More olecranon needs to be excised than one would expect (see Figure 24.3, *H*). The posterior fossa must be completely clear of impinging soft tissue or bone. If not, maximal extension will be limited.

Structures That Require Repair
Flexor-Pronator Muscle Origin. The flexor-pronator mass should be reattached to the supracondylar ridge with nonabsorbable braided 1-0 or 0 suture. If enough fibrous tissue was left behind, no holes in bone are needed. If not, holes can be drilled in the edge of the supracondylar ridge to secure the

flexor-pronator muscle mass. The lacertus fibrosus often requires release to permit full medial reattachment.

Ulnar Nerve Transposition. After reattachment to the medial supracondylar region, the ulnar nerve should be transposed and left in the anterior position. I no longer routinely use a fascial sling, but I will occasionally raise a small fat flap to prevent posterior subluxation (see Figure 24.3, *I*). The sling can be fashioned by elevating two overlapping rectangular flaps of fascia. The nerve is placed under the flaps, and these are approximated with adequate room so that nerve is not compressed, only stabilized. Superficial fat flaps can also be used to maintain the nerve in the anterior position. I use whatever keeps the nerve in an anterior position without tension, compression, or kinks. The joint should be flexed and extended to ensure that the nerve is free to move.

CRITICAL POINTS *Medial "Over-the-Top" Approach*

Anterior Joint
- Center the skin incision posterior to the medial epicondyle (may be directly posterior).
- Identify and protect all branches of the medial antebrachial cutaneous nerve.
- Identify and dissect the ulnar nerve to permit anterior subcutaneous transposition.
- Lift the flexor-pronator off the medial supracondylar ridge with a Cobb elevator.
- Divide the flexor carpi ulnaris, leaving 1 cm of the posterior portion attached to the epicondyle.
- Bluntly separate the anterior muscle, leaving the capsule behind.
- Excise the capsule from the distal humerus to the proximal ulna (coronoid process).
- Continue the dissection to the lateral edge of the joint line.
- Check for areas of remaining taut capsule by gently manipulating the elbow into extension and flexion.

Posterior Joint
- Complete mobilization of the ulnar nerve for anterior transposition.
- Starting at the medial supracondylar ridge, lift the triceps off with a Cobb elevator.
- Continue the dissection distally, lifting the triceps tendon, leaving the posterior capsule behind.
- Excise the posterior capsule, including the posteromedial corner.
- Remove the posterior olecranon, usually about 1 cm (depends on the size of the osteophytes).
- Check for posterior impingement and deepen the olecranon fossa as necessary.
- Check for areas of remaining taut capsule by gently manipulating the elbow into extension and flexion.
- If there are still soft tissue limitations along the lateral joint line, these can be incised, but beware of the radial nerve; if uncertain, approach it from the lateral column.

Lateral Approach

Patient Position, Preparation, and Skin Incision. In the lateral approach,[7,27,40] the patient is usually in the supine position and the arm supported by a hand table. A sterile tourniquet for the upper arm is useful because it permits proximal exposure if needed. The skin incision is centered over the lateral epicondyle.

The proximal extent of the skin incision depends on the needs of the case. For contracture release or treatment of fractures of the distal humerus, the skin incision may extend from 4 to 8 cm proximal to the lateral epicondyle, as needed. For simple contracture release, the incision may need to be extended only to the supracondylar ridge. For exposure of the radial head, the proximal extension may need to be only 5 cm. Extension of the exposure to 10 cm proximal to the lateral epicondyle may risk injury to the radial nerve. If proximal extension to 10 cm or more above the lateral epicondyle is planned, the radial nerve should be identified in the interval between the brachioradialis and brachialis.

The skin incision does not need to be over the lateral epicondyle but may also begin in the posterior midline. If this incision is used, a longer skin incision will be needed and larger flaps developed to gain access to the lateral joint.

The anterolateral approach to the elbow remains anterior to the anconeus. Once full-thickness skin flaps have been elevated, the key to this exposure is identification of the lateral supracondylar ridge of the distal humerus and the posterior border of the wrist extensor muscle mass. The flare of the ridge is palpated just superior to the lateral epicondyle, anterior to the triceps and posterior to the brachioradialis. The plane of the anterior dissection will continue anterior to the midline of the epicondyle, especially distally. The posterior dissection will continue between the anconeus and the extensor carpi ulnaris. In this way, the central origin of the extensor mass and the collateral ligament are preserved.

Anterior Capsular Exposure. After subperiosteal dissection of the distal humerus, a Bennett retractor can be inserted beneath the brachioradialis to retract the anterior tissues. When this exposure is used for contracture release, an elevator is used to bluntly separate the brachioradialis and the capsule as the dissection proceeds distally. In this interval the radial nerve is more vulnerable because the plane of dissection is more superficial. However, if the elevator is carefully advanced on top of the capsule and the muscle fibers pushed anteriorly, the radial nerve will be protected by muscle. If in doubt, find the nerve between the brachioradialis and brachialis proximally. With the Bennett retractor in place, sharp division of the more distal capsule, down to bone, will expose the articular portion of the distal humerus. The capsule should be excised at the level of the joint, across to the medial side.

The joint should be gently manipulated to test whether sufficient release has been achieved. If not, a decision needs to be made about whether to switch to the medial joint exposure or to expose the posterior joint from the lateral side while protecting the posterolateral ligament complex.

Posterior Capsular Exposure From the Lateral Side. As described by Husband and Hastings[27] and others,[7,40] the posterior capsule can be safely excised from the lateral side, and even HO can be removed from the posterior surface. If the ulnar nerve has not been exposed, remember that it is vulnerable, trapped in scar tissue, and located at the very edge of the posteromedial extent of the exposure, so that it will be difficult to see.

The posterolateral ligament complex is identified distally between the anconeus and extensor carpi ulnaris and is *not* incised. An elevator is introduced near the supracondylar flare of the distal humerus and swept distally along the posterior surface. It is helpful to leave the capsule attached before excising

it. The tip of the olecranon usually requires excision to clear the posterior fossa for adequate extension.

Immediate Postoperative Care

Closed Suction Drainage. Although I have heard surgeons remark that they do not routinely use closed suction drainage, I believe that this is vital in almost all cases after open release. Occasionally, a simple lateral approach with anterior-only release is associated with minimal postoperative bleeding and drains are not required. However, as the complexity of the surgery and the severity move up the scale, postoperative hematoma must be avoided. Retained blood and hematoma cause pain, inflammation, and occasional temporary nerve dysfunction, all of which retard progress toward improved motion. If hinged fixation or CPM is planned for the immediate postoperative period, I secure the drains with sutures. Because these drains are left in place for 2 to 3 days after surgery, they can easily be dislodged either during placement of the hinged external fixator or during CPM. The elbow is usually splinted in maximal extension following surgery. These splints are left in place until CPM begins the following day.

The First 24 Hours. Many surgeons prefer to begin CPM immediately after surgery. However, I now use the first 12 to 18 hours for rest, application of ice, and elevation of the extremity. If a hinge fixator is used, the device is set in maximal tolerable extension and ice bags are placed around the elbow.

CRITICAL POINTS *Contracture Release: Technical Tips and Suggestions*

- Wait to remove hardware until the end of the procedure and after any manipulation that may be required.
- Secure the suction drains with sutures and plan to leave them in place as the postoperative CPM is under way.
- Seldom, if ever, does the range of motion improve from what is gained in the operating room.
- Honestly measure and dictate in the operative note the degree of motion achieved with light pressure applied in both flexion/extension and supination/pronation.
- Splint the patient in the position of greatest "challenge" before beginning CPM. In general, this is in extension.
- If splinting in flexion, inspect the posterior skin over the olecranon. Occasionally this will blanch and lead to skin breakdown if not progressively flexed.

Special Circumstances

Fracture of the Distal Humerus After Open Reduction and Internal Fixation

After fracture of the distal humerus, the stiffness of the joint can come from intraarticular malunion, HO, or capsular contracture. CT is helpful for visualizing the distal humerus and specifically the ulnohumeral joint. In thin patients, the plates on the medial and lateral columns of the distal humerus may feel superficial, and the patient often requests their removal. The fracture must be solidly healed if the hardware is to be removed. If there is uncertainty, the surgeon must be prepared to replate and bone graft a nonunion while performing the contracture release. If the fracture is healed and the hardware is to be removed, the contracture release is done first, followed by hardware removal. If the hardware is removed first, refracture may occur even with gentle manipulation during the contracture release. This complication can be avoided by releasing the contracture, performing the intraoperative manipulation, and then removing the hardware if indicated.

In elderly patients, if there is a nonunion or if avascular necrosis of the articular surface is suspected, total elbow replacement with a semiconstrained linked implant is the best option (see Chapter 27).

Nonunion of the Distal Humerus

Most nonunions of the distal humerus are associated with joint contracture. This finding is especially true in patients with failed attempts at internal fixation, in whom the elbow is often immobilized in the slim hope that union may occur despite the presence of mechanical failure. To treat the nonunion, the contracture of the joint must be completely relieved. If not, the newly plated nonunion site will experience continued excessive torque and be prone to repeated failure. If the joint contracture is released, stress is minimized at the distal humeral fixation.

Head Trauma and Brain Injury

Patients with head trauma and associated residual spasticity have two strikes against them (Figure 24.4).[1,16,54,62] First, they tend to have exuberant HO and are often prevented from seeking care for excision in the first year. Therefore, the ankylosis is usually complete and the surrounding tissue thickened and unyielding. Second, voluntary control of the elbow is difficult to judge. After the brain injury has stabilized, I have tried to assess effective volitional control in these patients by both physical examination and surface electromyography. At a minimum, patients must be able to fire the biceps and triceps on command before contracture release is considered. Unfortunately, the capacity to contract these muscles volitionally while the joint is ankylosed does not guarantee the ability to flex and extend with strength once passive motion is achieved. I have unfortunately seen patients regain remarkable passive motion after the excision of massive HO only to watch them gradually lose mobility over a period of months because of a lack of active strength and effective control over the entire arc of motion. In addition, the hand, wrist, and forearm may also be spastic and of little use beyond simple positioning. The goals and expectations of the patient (and the family) must be carefully weighed before proceeding with contracture release. Nonetheless, this is also a group of patients who are extremely grateful if they can regain some motion for positioning their hands for transfer, the use of motorized devices, and self-care.

It is important to allow the patient with brain injury to recover. This may mean waiting 12 to 24 months. Recovery of volitional muscle control and strength will occur in adjacent muscles and should be viewed as a positive prognosis. During this time, the family and patient will become more realistic about the goals of contracture release. In addition, the patient's capacity for rehabilitation and social setting will generally improve, permitting a more reasoned assessment of the patient's and family's capacity for postoperative care and rehabilitation.

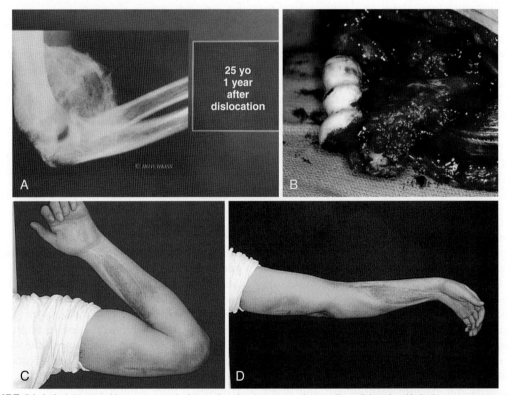

FIGURE 24.4 A, A 25-year-old man presented with previous head trauma and open elbow dislocation. He had no permanent spasticity and had complete volitional control. **B,** Because of extensive heterotopic ossification 1 year after dislocation, the distal humerus required complete exposure and excision of ligaments. This degree of intraoperative instability required hinged external fixation. This patient wore the hinge for 10 weeks. **C** and **D,** Three years after surgery he retained excellent motion and strength. (Copyright © Robert N. Hotchkiss.)

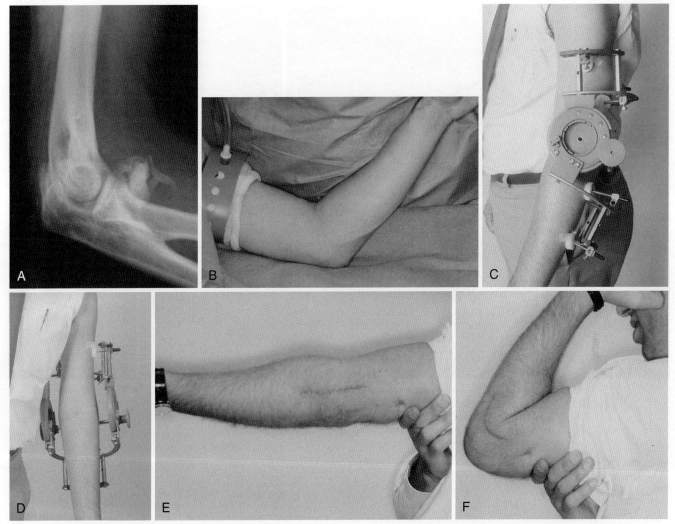

FIGURE 24.5 A, Heterotopic bone is seen on both the front and the back of the joint in this radiograph following treatment for a fracture-dislocation. A previous attempt at contracture release was unsuccessful. **B,** Maximal extension under anesthesia. **C** and **D,** Patient wearing the hinged external fixator. **E** and **F,** Range of motion approximately 2 years after treatment. No degenerative changes developed in the joint. (Copyright © Robert N. Hotchkiss.)

Hinged Fixation After Contracture Release

Indications for the use of hinged external fixation* are (1) instability after contracture release, (2) excessive muscle-tendon tightness noted at the time of complete capsular release (Figure 24.5), and (3) distraction arthroplasty (with or without interposition).†

Each type of hinged fixator requires a detailed understanding of the principles of use, method of application, and problems that may be encountered. I believe that the primary surgeon must be familiar with one type of fixator and the specific techniques required for successful application. Each of the companies that manufacture these devices provides instructional materials and courses. It may be useful to visit someone with experience. The assisting surgeon should also be familiar

with the device and its application. During placement, one set of eyes is often needed to place a half-pin properly while the primary surgeon makes certain that the overall alignment of the device is maintained.

In addition to the technical challenges, these cases can be of long duration, exceeding 4 hours. For inexperienced operators, a difficult contracture release, requiring extensive dissection with careful protection of all nerves, can be tiring. The application of the hinged fixator cannot be viewed as an afterthought. If the pins are misaligned or care is not taken to ensure that the joint is completely reduced, all the work is for naught.

Instability After Release

Instability after release is common and has been noted by many authors, especially in patients with severe joint involvement or those with more massive HO.[16] In these cases, the stabilizing ligaments are often trapped in the HO and cannot be protected during release. Even if the ligaments are not completely released, a wide area of capsular excision and stripping is often needed

---

*See references 14, 18, 30, 53, 59, 61, and 63.

†See references 14, 18, 30, 34, 46, 53, and 73.

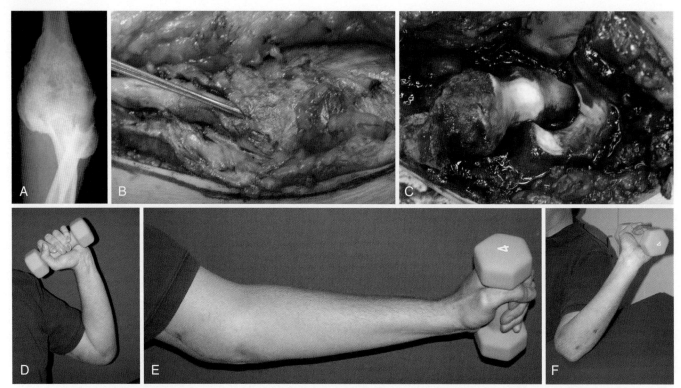

FIGURE 24.6 A, An ankylosed elbow after combined head and elbow trauma in a 45-year-old man confined to a wheelchair. Note the faint hint of a joint line in the ulnohumeral joint. **B,** The ulnar nerve is covered by bone during neurolysis. (A Freer elevator is under a shelf of bone.) **C,** Intraoperative instability from radical resection of medial heterotopic ossification that included medial ligaments, requiring the use of hinged fixation. **D** and **E,** At 6 months there is good mobility and he is able to transfer using his left arm. **F,** Even without reconstruction of the medial collateral ligament, there is no valgus instability. (Copyright © Robert N. Hotchkiss.)

to free the joint. In this circumstance, especially if there has been a long-standing limitation (>18 months), the patient has a very difficult time regaining motion and maintaining that motion in the first 8 weeks after surgery. Hinged fixation is used in those settings where acute and gross instability is created after contracture release (Figure 24.6). In general, as one gains experience, there is less need for the use of hinged fixation after contracture release.

Excessive Muscle Tightness

In a long-standing contracture with excessive muscle tightness, some have recommended lengthening of the biceps, brachialis, or triceps tendons.[10] In my opinion this should be avoided if at all possible. The muscle-tendon unit is undoubtedly shortened in the case of a long-standing contracture, but lengthening these structures in a nonspastic patient risks loss of strength and requires some protection of the repair during rehabilitation.

Distraction (Interposition) Arthroplasty

For interposition arthroplasty, there are several devices that provide stability and distraction of the joint. A fixator is used to temporarily stabilize the joint after resurfacing of the joint with fascia or cutis (skin with the epidermal layer removed). The fixator replicates the flexion/extension axis of the elbow, permitting motion. One device uses hinged fixators with a passive drive mechanism, and another device uses hinged fixators without a passive drive mechanism. The axis of rotation, centered at the distal humerus, is located by several methods, depending on which device is used. External fixation pins, usually two in the humerus and two in the ulna, are applied. The axis pin is then removed so that there is less chance of infection during the postoperative period. The passive drive mechanism in the Compass Elbow Hinge (Smith and Nephew, Memphis, TN) allows passive mobilization, but most surgeons consider it to be more complicated to apply. All devices require an understanding of the anatomy and kinematics of the elbow in addition to the use of the particular device. For most commercially available devices, technique manuals are available online.

If hinged fixation is used, the device must be left on for at least 6 to 8 weeks while maximizing motion and allowing the soft tissues to regain stability. Further information about both of these devices is available from the manufacturers. Familiarity with one or both devices is essential for complex reconstructive surgery on the elbow.

The clinical results from distraction arthroplasty for posttraumatic contracture are not stellar. Often the patient feels instability. The distal humerus may also undergo bony dissolution over months, resulting in more laxity and instability. I use interposition arthroplasty with hinged fixation very sparingly in the posttraumatic patient. The goals should be limited to some pain relief and a notable gain in motion (especially flexion). Few if any patients achieve a high-performance elbow with heavy lifting capacity and full mobility.

POSTOPERATIVE MANAGEMENT

Use of Intravenous Dexamethasone for Postoperative Swelling

Intravenous dexamethasone has been quite helpful in reducing the associated swelling in the perioperative period. We routinely give adult patients 8 mg intravenously before the incision is made and continue with a dose of 8 mg intravenously every 8 hours while the patient is in the hospital, usually for 48 hours. The impact of this strategy was first noted by maxillofacial surgeons, who realized that it avoided the untoward effects of infection or other problems associated with long-term steroid use.[77] In patients with diabetes, caution and judgment must be used.

Adjuvant Therapy for Heterotopic Ossification

The efficacy of nonsteroidal medication or irradiation for the prevention of HO has *not* been studied using randomized double-blind trials. Nonetheless, there are numerous reports that support the use of indomethacin or low-dose irradiation for the prevention of recurrent growth of HO.* Jupiter and colleagues reported abandoning the use of any nonsteroidal agents and reported no pathologic recurrence of HO.[29] I no longer prescribe antiinflammatory agents for this purpose and have noted no increase in the recurrence of HO. Patients who have undergone major organ transplantation are especially vulnerable to HO formation and usually are not permitted to take oral antiinflammatory agents.[51] In adults who have widespread HO and tend to form osteophytes with only minor trauma, I use radiation therapy at a single dose of 700 cGy within 72 hours of surgery. The use of gentle CPM, passive turnbuckle splinting, or dynamic external hinged fixation has undoubtedly diminished the incidence of HO, irrespective of adjuvant therapy.*

In the aforementioned last 450 cases, I have employed irradiation on six occasions.

Physical Therapy and Splinting

A knowledgeable therapy department is a valuable and perhaps crucial asset for success in treatment of stiff elbows. Once the contracture is released, patients may benefit from therapy to overcome the spasm and pain associated with immediate motion. As with many conditions, the frequency of visits to the therapist varies from patient to patient. However, the need for splints is nearly universal. Several texts and articles describe the fabrication and use of these devices.[20,26,38,80] There will undoubtedly be continued improvement in the design, comfort, and effectiveness as materials and technology improve. I do not use any dynamic splints for elbow contractures; I have found that patients do not tolerate these splints and compliance is very low. The constant torque applied by the dynamic splints is painful and poorly tolerated, which often lowers compliance. The splints described here rely instead on intermittent passive and static progressive positioning. These splints apply an incremental displacement to the joint, followed by stress relaxation of the muscle and soft tissue. For reasons that are unclear, this

approach, much like an Ilizarov lengthening, is more effective with my patients.

The splints I use regularly are designed to maintain the gains made in the operating room. Seldom if ever can a surface splint (as opposed to hinged external fixation) increase the motion that was achieved on the operating table.[19]

Static Splints

Resting Extension Splint. After 24 to 48 hours following operation, we employ resting extension splints when not using CPM. At 24 to 48 hours after surgery, in conjunction with CPM, we use static extension splints to maintain maximal tolerated extension. After swelling decreases days later, a static flexion splint is also added, again, to maintain maximal flexion at end range. The splints are worn usually at night to maintain position after removal of the CPM device. A slight extension moment applied by tightening the splint's strap is most effective at maintaining the position of the elbow at or near full extension.

Turnbuckle Splint (for Extension or Flexion). If the elbow is tending toward a flexion contracture of 30 degrees or more, a turnbuckle splint should be considered (Figure 24.7). The turnbuckle splint, as first reported by Green and McCoy,[20] is invaluable in static progressive splinting. In my view, this splint is most helpful for patients with a 25- to 40-degree flexion contracture that requires mechanical assistance to increase extension. We have used the Aircast Mayo Clinic Elbow Brace (DonJoy Orthopedics, Vista, CA) with modifications and success.[36] There are many commercially fabricated splinting systems available to provide a "serial static" mode of patient-controlled displacement. There is no single manufacturer or design that fits all.

These splints are generally required for 8 to 12 weeks after surgery, following the period of acute postoperative swelling and pain. The duration of wear must be tailored to the individual. Most patients cannot wear them all the time, especially when a significant displacement force is applied. However, even if these splints only help maintain the position gained in the operating room during the early phase, they are worth using. Later, the splint will help regain the motion that has been temporarily lost during the acute postoperative period.

"Come-Along" Flexion Splint. Patients highly value improvement in flexion, more so than gains of extension. I have found that a static progressive splint, fabricated from D-rings and straps, is well tolerated and not as limiting or as complicated to construct as a turnbuckle device. The patient simply pulls the straps on each side in a sequential fashion, pulling the elbow into more flexion, as tolerated (Figure 24.8).

Continuous Passive Motion (or Slow Intermittent Passive Positioning) Device

CPM devices have been used by many authors and are reported to assist in maintaining the motion gained after surgical release.[17,34] I use CPM in all patients who have undergone open release but were not fitted with a dynamic hinged fixator. After arthroscopic release, a supervised outpatient program usually suffices with end-range splinting.

CPM is helpful when used according to a different principle than continuous motion. Rather than having the device flexing and extending the elbow on a continuous basis, I use the

---

*See references 12, 24, 29, 42, 61, and 65.

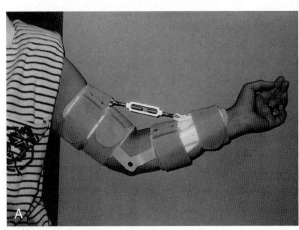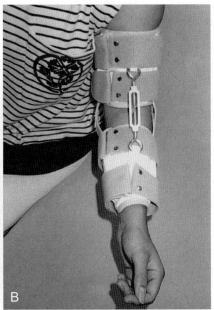

FIGURE 24.7 A and **B,** The turnbuckle splint is especially effective with flexion contractures of more than 40 degrees. Once the patient achieves more extension, other splinting devices may be more effective. (Courtesy of S. Davila, San Antonio, Texas.)

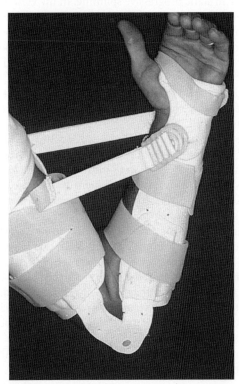

FIGURE 24.8 A "come-along" splint designed to increase flexion of the elbow. The patient advances each successive ring onto a hook placed on both the dorsal and palmar surfaces of the distal portion of the forearm section. Once the soft tissues have relaxed, the next ring is hooked into place. (Copyright © Robert N. Hotchkiss.)

device as *slow intermittent passive positioning.* My patients begin slow intermittent passive positioning the day after release, the first 12 to 24 hours being used for rest and elevation. The machine is initially set at the maximal tolerable positions of extension and flexion. It is important to remove the

bandages in the antecubital fossa because they will block flexion. The patient (or parent) is taught to use the button that stops the machine. The rate of displacement is set at the absolute minimum. The patient is instructed to allow the device to move the elbow to maximal extension and then stop and hold it at that position for 20 to 30 minutes. The button is clicked to resume motion to the point of maximally tolerated flexion. Again, the position is held for 20 to 30 minutes. In this way the joint is held at the extremes of position from the beginning of rehabilitation, which is the goal. Cycling the joint faster and more frequently has no advantage and may increase the amount of swelling. If the CPM evokes significant guarding, the indwelling catheter (see anesthesia section previously) can be used to administer anesthesia to relieve pain and relax the muscular guarding.

EXPECTATIONS AND RESULTS

The results of most reports and my personal experience are gratifying, with significant improvement in over 90% of patients. The published literature, as mentioned in the first section of this chapter, is filled with inconsistent inclusion criteria, different methods of operative exposure, and variance in postoperative management. This lack of standardization reflects the varied nature of the condition; differences among patients; and continued enhancements in surgical technique, postoperative devices, and management. As with all complex surgical procedures, there are complications, disappointments, and failures.

For a minimal uncomplicated flexion contracture (<30 to 40 degrees), extension will usually improve to 5 to 10 degrees of residual contracture without loss of flexion.

For more moderate contractures with localized HO and motion limited in both flexion and extension (50 to 105 degrees), a final range of motion of 20 to 130 degrees is a reasonable expectation.

For patients with less than 30 degrees of total motion, a reasonable goal is 25 to 130 degrees. However, the results of this group of patients are variable. Some patients do surprisingly well and can achieve even better results despite starting with a completely ankylosed joint (see Figure 24.6).[61]

COMPLICATIONS AND OBSTACLES

Acute Recurrent Stiffness: "Gelling"

The primary reason to carefully follow patients in the first 2 to 3 weeks after surgery is to assess their range of motion. In my experience with the last 400 contracture releases, nearly 25% of patients experience a temporary setback in their progress, many commonly losing the gains in flexion made in the operating room. It is critical to record their motion in the operating room and immediately after surgery while in the hospital. A critical parameter is *failure to achieve 105 to 110 degrees* of flexion between the second and third week after surgery. The usual source seems to be pain in the distal triceps against the surface of the posterior humerus. In these cases with stalled progress, the patient undergoes a *gentle* closed manipulation under regional anesthesia. The procedure is done in a procedure room or a monitored setting using an infraclavicular block and as little sedation as possible to allow the patient to witness and visualize the amount of motion achieved. Often the elbow will be splinted in the flexed position for 4 to 6 hours followed by immediate resumption of therapy and splinting.

It is less common to lose extension in the early recovery phase, but the same level of scrutiny should be applied.

Nerve Palsy

The ulnar nerve, as noted earlier, is particularly vulnerable because of entrapment, previous injury, and intraoperative surgical manipulation. Care must be taken to painstakingly mobilize and protect the nerve during contracture release, especially if hinged fixation is used. Even with these precautions, I have found that about 10% of patients will have dysfunction of the nerve after release. Most of these resolve over a period of days, weeks, or months. Often there is preoperative ulnar nerve dysfunction that may not be evident. It is therefore important to document ulnar nerve function preoperatively and warn patients that nerve function may temporarily worsen and may not necessarily improve to normal after release. As mentioned earlier, arthroscopic release may pose an even greater risk of permanent damage.[21]

The radial and posterior interosseous nerves are also vulnerable, especially if excessive retraction is applied through the lateral approach. If there is abundant HO at the lateral joint, the posterior interosseous nerve should be carefully exposed and protected during excision of the HO. In most cases the HO lifts the nerve and muscle away from the joint. In nonreduced dislocations with HO or in more proximal fractures, the radial nerve may be entrapped in bone and require meticulous, painstaking dissection from the surrounding bone. I have had two patients with temporary radial nerve palsies after contracture release. Both palsies resolved completely.

Heterotopic Ossification

Recurrent pathologic HO (i.e., ossification that blocks motion) after contracture release has become rare since the advent of

better methods of restoration of motion in the early postoperative period. It is not uncommon to see HO along the ligamentous structures or edge of the capsule. As a reflection of the benignity of these flecks of bone, this condition is sometimes referred to as "ectopic calcification" as opposed to true HO. This bone usually does not restrict motion. In the more dramatic cases of ankylosis, the use of hinged external fixation has eliminated the need for temporary casting or splinting in a flexed position for instability, thus minimizing the risk of recurrent HO.

Pin Tract Infections

The risk of pin tract infection is significant with the use of hinged external fixation. There is a 50-50 chance that the patient will need to take oral antibiotics for the duration of treatment. The actual incidence of pin redness and erythema is 60% for the elbow. I treat each of these patients with a 5- to 7-day course of an oral cephalosporin. In no patient has pin tract–related osteomyelitis developed.

Joint Infection

A far more worrisome and potentially devastating infection may occur in the joint itself. The most vulnerable patient is one with poor soft tissue coverage and a history of previous infection. Another risk factor is distraction interposition arthroplasty in a patient with poorly vascularized bone. (The majority of infections in my practice have come after this procedure.) In these cases, the distal humerus often has a poor blood supply, and the material inserted as interposition is avascular and a foreign body. Additionally, external pins either at the joint or nearby may act as a nidus for spread into the joint. If these pins become infected, the joint should be débrided of all foreign material and stabilized by using different pin sites. Although my experience with these patients is fortunately limited, the joint often performs surprisingly well despite the travail.

Soft Tissue Deficiencies or Wound Necrosis

Patients with burns or long-standing contractures may lack sufficient soft tissue to permit mobilization or may develop skin necrosis over the tip of the olecranon, especially as they attempt to regain flexion.[9,11,58,61,70] If one predicts the need for additional soft tissue, it is usually better to perform the soft tissue reconstruction as a separate procedure before contracture release. Depending on the amount of tissue needed, the flaps I most commonly use are either a gracilis free flap with a split-thickness skin graft or, for smaller defects over the olecranon, a radial forearm flap as an island pedicle. The radial forearm flap, using the distal skin and fascia at the distal forearm, causes a donor defect that bothers some patients. Nonetheless, the coverage over the olecranon is ideal in thickness and mobility. A flexor carpi ulnaris pedicle flap has also been described for this region. The delayed recognition of skin loss after contracture release may temporarily stall progress, but acting quickly to cover the wound with sufficient soft tissue will usually rescue the contracture release and permit the flexion gained in the primary contracture release. In other words, one should not simply wait and hope that the posterior ulceration will simply get better, especially if there is exposed bone (Figure 24.9). (See Chapter 44 for a more detailed discussion of coverage of elbow defects.)

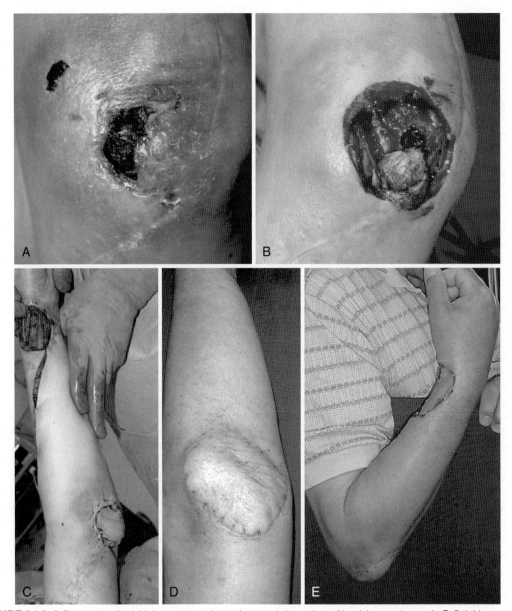

FIGURE 24.9 A, Two weeks after initial contracture release, the wound shows signs of breakdown and necrosis. **B,** Débridement reveals a larger wound than was initially thought. **C,** Intraoperative photo of a radial forearm flap. Note the distal harvest site. **D** and **E,** Postoperative flap of a different patient with a similar defect approximately 2 weeks after surgery. **E,** Note the degree of flexion permitted. (Copyright © Robert N. Hotchkiss.)

Failure to Achieve Improved Motion

Three percent to 8% of patients will completely fail to achieve the goals of improved motion, sustained painless function, and stability. The usual cause of failure is articular surface destruction that is either underappreciated or progressive. Morrey refers to this as "intrinsic contracture."[47] The only option in these cases is to resurface the elbow. In older patients, a total elbow arthroplasty is the optimal choice. Distraction interposition arthroplasty may be an option in younger patients but must be carefully considered, and in my hands it remains unpredictable.

Finally, approximately 1% to 2% of patients seem to experience a pathologic arthrofibrosis. Despite careful dissection, relatively routine operative release, and attentive rehabilitation, these patients develop recurrent contracture without any notable HO. In these rare cases,[2] I have returned to excise the contracted capsule and used hinged fixation with the passive drive (i.e., Compass Elbow Hinge) with success.

REFERENCES

1. Ada L, Canning CG, Low SL: Stroke patients have selective muscle weakness in shortened range. *Brain* 126:724–731, 2003.
2. Bae DS, Waters PM: Surgical treatment of posttraumatic elbow contracture in adolescents. *J Pediatr Orthop* 21:580–584, 2001.
3. Bankov S: A test for differentiation between contracture and spasm of the biceps muscle in post-traumatic rigiditis of the elbow joint. *Hand* 7:262–265, 1975.

4. Blonna D, Wolf JM, Fitzsimmons JS, et al: Prevention of nerve injury during arthroscopic capsulectomy of the elbow utilizing a safety-driven strategy. *J Bone Joint Surg Am* 95(15):1373–1381, 2013.

5. Chantelot C, Fontaine C, Migaud H, et al: [Retrospective study of 23 arthrolyses of the elbow for post-traumatic stiffness: result predicting factors]. *Rev Chir Orthop Reparatrice Appar Mot* 85:823–827, 1999.

6. Chen NC, Liu A: The role of prophylactic ulnar nerve release during elbow contracture release. *J Hand Surg [Am]* 39(9):1837–1839, 2014.

7. Cohen MS, Hastings H: Post-traumatic contracture of the elbow: operative release using a lateral collateral ligament sparing approach. *J Bone Joint Surg Br* 80:805–812, 1998.

8. Cohen MS, Hastings H: Operative release for elbow contracture: the lateral collateral ligament sparing technique. *Orthop Clin North Am* 30:133–139, 1999.

9. Dias DA: Heterotopic para-articular ossification of the elbow with soft tissue contracture in burns. *Burns Incl Therm Inj* 9:128–134, 1982.

10. Duke JB, Tessler RH, Dell PC: Manipulation of the stiff elbow with patient under anesthesia. *J Hand Surg [Am]* 16:19–24, 1991.

11. El Khatib HA, Mahboub TA, Ali TA: Use of an adipofascial flap based on the proximal perforators of the ulnar artery to correct contracture of elbow burn scars: an anatomic and clinical approach. *Plast Reconstr Surg* 109:130–136, 2002.

12. Ellerin BE, Helfet D, Parikh S, et al: Current therapy in the management of heterotopic ossification of the elbow: a review with case studies. *Am J Phys Med Rehabil* 78:259–271, 1999.

13. Faierman E, Wang J, Jupiter JB: Secondary ulnar nerve palsy in adults after elbow trauma: a report of two cases. *J Hand Surg [Am]* 26:675–678, 2001.

14. Fox RJ, Varitimidis SE, Plakseychuk A, et al: The Compass Elbow Hinge: indications and initial results. *J Hand Surg [Br]* 25:568–572, 2000.

15. Ganapathi M, Savage R, Jones AR: MRI assessment of the proximal pole of the scaphoid after internal fixation with a titanium alloy Herbert screw. *J Hand Surg [Br]* 26:326–329, 2001.

16. Garland DE: Surgical approaches for resection of heterotopic ossification in traumatic brain-injured adults. *Clin Orthop Relat Res* 263:59–70, 1991.

17. Gates HS, III, Sullivan FL, Urbaniak JR: Anterior capsulotomy and continuous passive motion in the treatment of post-traumatic flexion contracture of the elbow: a prospective study. *J Bone Joint Surg Am* 74:1229–1234, 1992.

18. Gilbert MS, Radomisli TE: Management of fixed flexion contracture of the elbow in haemophilia. *Haemophilia* 5(Suppl 1):39–42, 1999.

19. Glynn JJ, Niebauer JJ: Flexion and extension contracture of the elbow: surgical management. *Clin Orthop Relat Res* 117:289–291, 1976.

20. Green DP, McCoy H: Turnbuckle orthotic correction of elbow-flexion contractures after acute injuries. *J Bone Joint Surg Am* 61:1092–1095, 1979.

21. Haapaniemi T, Berggren M, Adolfsson L: Complete transection of the median and radial nerves during arthroscopic release of post-traumatic elbow contracture. *Arthroscopy* 15:784–787, 1999.

22. Heirweg S, De Smet L: Operative treatment of elbow stiffness: evaluation and outcome. *Acta Orthop Belg* 69:18–22, 2003.

23. Hertel R, Pisan M, Lambert S, et al: Operative management of the stiff elbow: sequential arthrolysis based on a transhumeral approach. *J Shoulder Elbow Surg* 6:82–88, 1997.

24. Heyd R, Strassmann G, Schopohl B, et al: Radiation therapy for the prevention of heterotopic ossification at the elbow. *J Bone Joint Surg Br* 83:332–334, 2001.

25. Hildebrand KA, Zhang M, Salo PT, et al: Joint capsule mast cells and neuropeptides are increased within four weeks of injury and remain elevated in chronic stages of posttraumatic contractures. *J Orthop Res* 26:1313–1319, 2008.

26. Hotchkiss RN, Davila S: Rehabilitation of the elbow contracture. In Nickel VL, editor: *Orthopaedic rehabilitation*, New York, 1992, Churchill Livingstone, pp 746–773.

27. Husband JB, Hastings H: The lateral approach for operative release of posttraumatic contracture of the elbow. *J Bone Joint Surg Am* 72:1353–1358, 1990.

28. Jones GS, Savoie FH, III: Arthroscopic capsular release of flexion contractures (arthrofibrosis) of the elbow. *Arthroscopy* 9:277–283, 1993.

29. Jupiter JB, O'Driscoll SW, Cohen MS: The assessment and management of the stiff elbow. *Instr Course Lect* 52:93–111, 2003.

30. Kasparyan NG, Hotchkiss RN: Dynamic skeletal fixation in the upper extremity. *Hand Clin* 13:643–663, 1997.

31. Katolik LI, Cohen MS: Anterior interosseous nerve palsy after open capsular release for elbow stiffness: report of 2 cases. *J Hand Surg [Am]* 34:288–291, 2009.

32. Kim SJ, Kim HK, Lee JW: Arthroscopy for limitation of motion of the elbow. *Arthroscopy* 11:680–683, 1995.

33. King GJ: Stiffness and ankylosis of the elbow. In Norris TR, editor: *Orthopedic knowledge update: shoulder and elbow*, Rosemont, IL, 1997, American Academy of Orthopaedic Surgeons, pp 325–336.

34. King GJ, Faber KJ: Posttraumatic elbow stiffness. *Orthop Clin North Am* 31:129–143, 2000.

35. Kraushaar BS, Nirschl RP, Cox W: A modified lateral approach for release of posttraumatic elbow flexion contracture. *J Shoulder Elbow Surg* 8:476–480, 1999.

36. Libicher M, Freyschmidt J: [Radiological diagnosis in contracted elbow joint: value of CT and MRI]. *Orthopade* 30:593–601, 2001.

37. London JT: Kinematics of the elbow. *J Bone Joint Surg Am* 63:529–535, 1981.

38. MacKay-Lyons M: Low-load, prolonged stretch in treatment of elbow flexion contractures secondary to head trauma: a case report. *Phys Ther* 69:292–296, 1989.

39. Mahaisavariya B, Laupattarakasem W, Supachutikul A, et al: Late reduction of dislocated elbow: need triceps be lengthened? *J Bone Joint Surg Br* 75:426–428, 1993.

40. Mansat P, Morrey BF: The column procedure: a limited lateral approach for extrinsic contracture of the elbow. *J Bone Joint Surg Am* 80:1603–1615, 1998.

41. Marti RK, Kerkhoffs GM, Maas M: Progressive surgical release of a posttraumatic stiff elbow: technique and outcome after 2-18 years in 46 patients. *Acta Orthop Scand* 73:144–150, 2002.

42. McAuliffe JA, Wolfson AH: Early excision of heterotopic ossification about the elbow followed by radiation therapy. *J Bone Joint Surg Am* 79:749–755, 1997.

43. Mih AD, Wolf FG: Surgical release of elbow-capsular contracture in pediatric patients. *J Pediatr Orthop* 14:458–461, 1994.

44. Modabber MR, Jupiter JB: Reconstruction for post-traumatic conditions of the elbow joint. *J Bone Joint Surg Am* 77:1431–1446, 1995.

45. Moritomo H, Tada K, Yoshida T: Early, wide excision of heterotopic ossification in the medial elbow. *J Shoulder Elbow Surg* 10:164–168, 2001.

46. Morrey BF: Post-traumatic contracture of the elbow: operative treatment, including distraction arthroplasty. *J Bone Joint Surg Am* 72:601–618, 1990.

47. Morrey BF: Posttraumatic stiffness: distraction arthroplasty. *Orthopedics* 15:863–869, 1992.

48. Morrey BF: Primary degenerative arthritis of the elbow: treatment by ulnohumeral arthroplasty. *J Bone Joint Surg Br* 74:409–413, 1992.

49. Morrey BF: Surgical treatment of extraarticular elbow contracture. *Clin Orthop Relat Res* 370:57–64, 2000.

50. Morrey BF, Askew LJ, Chao EY: A biomechanical study of normal functional elbow motion. *J Bone Joint Surg Am* 63:872–877, 1981.

51. Munin MC, Balu G, Sotereanos DG: Elbow complications after organ transplantation: case reports. *Am J Phys Med Rehabil* 74:67–72, 1995.

52. Neidhardt A, Neidhardt-Audion M, Mourand JL, et al: [Subclavicular brachial plexus anesthesia: Apropos of 200 cases. Anatomical and clinical justification]. *Cah Anesthesiol* 32:651–655, 1984.

53. Nielsen D, Nowinski RJ, Bamberger HB: Indications, alternatives, and complications of external fixation about the elbow. *Hand Clin* 18:87–97, 2002.

54. O'Dwyer NJ, Ada L, Neilson PD: Spasticity and muscle contracture following stroke. *Brain* 119(Pt 5):1737–1749, 1996.

55. Page C, Backus SI, Lenhoff MW: Electromyographic activity in stiff and normal elbows during elbow flexion and extension. *J Hand Ther* 16:5–11, 2003.

56. Park JY, Cho CH, Choi JH, et al: Radial nerve palsy after arthroscopic anterior capsular release for degenerative elbow contracture. *Arthroscopy* 23:1360.e1–1360.e3, 2007.

57. Phillips BB, Strasburger S: Arthroscopic treatment of arthrofibrosis of the elbow joint. *Arthroscopy* 14:38–44, 1998.

58. Prakash V, Bajaj SP: A new concept for the treatment of postburn contracture of the elbow. *Ann Plast Surg* 45:339, 2000.

59. Regan WD, Reilly CD: Distraction arthroplasty of the elbow. *Hand Clin* 9:719–728, 1993.

60. Ring D, Hotchkiss RN, Guss D, et al: Hinged elbow external fixation for severe elbow contracture. *J Bone Joint Surg Am* 87:1293–1296, 2005.

61. Ring D, Jupiter JB: Operative release of complete ankylosis of the elbow due to heterotopic bone in patients without severe injury of the central nervous system. *J Bone Joint Surg Am* 85:849–857, 2003.

62. Roberts JB, Pankratz DG: The surgical treatment of heterotopic ossification at the elbow following long-term coma. *J Bone Joint Surg Am* 61:760–763, 1979.

63. Rodriguez-Merchan EC: Therapeutic options in the management of articular contractures in haemophiliacs. *Haemophilia* 5(Suppl 1):5–9, 1999.

64. Sahajpal D, Choi T, Wright TW: Arthroscopic release of the stiff elbow. *J Hand Surg [Am]* 34:540–544, 2009.

65. Schaeffer MA, Sosner J: Heterotopic ossification: treatment of established bone with radiation therapy. *Arch Phys Med Rehabil* 76:284–286, 1995.

66. Schippinger G, Seibert FJ, Steinbock J: Management of simple elbow dislocations. Does the period of immobilization affect the eventual results? *Langenbecks Arch Surg* 384:294–297, 1999.

67. Schrumpf MA, Lyman S, Do H, et al: Incidence of postoperative elbow contracture release in New York State. *J Hand Surg [Am]* 38(9):1746–1752.e1-3, 2013.

68. Sojbjerg JO: The stiff elbow. *Acta Orthop Scand* 67:626–631, 1996.

69. Stans AA, Maritz NG, O'Driscoll SW: Operative treatment of elbow contracture in patients twenty-one years of age or younger. *J Bone Joint Surg Am* 84:382–387, 2002.

70. Stern PJ, Law EJ, Benedict FE: Surgical treatment of elbow contractures in postburn children. *Plast Reconstr Surg* 76:441–446, 1985.

71. Tan V, Daluiski A, Capo J: Hinged elbow external fixators: indications and uses. *J Am Acad Orthop Surg* 13:503–514, 2005.

72. Tan V, Daluiski A, Simic P: Outcome of open release for post-traumatic elbow stiffness. *J Trauma* 61:673–678, 2006.

73. Tomaino MM, Sotereanos DG, Plakseychuk A: Technique for ensuring ulnohumeral reduction during application of the Richards compass elbow hinge. *Am J Orthop* 26:646–647, 1997.

74. Vardakas DG, Varitimidis SE, Goebel F, et al: Evaluating and treating the stiff elbow. *Hand Clin* 18:77–85, 2002.

75. Viola RW, Hanel DP: Early "simple" release of posttraumatic elbow contracture associated with heterotopic ossification. *J Hand Surg [Am]* 24:370–380, 1999.

76. Wada T, Ishii S, Usui M, et al: The medial approach for operative release of post-traumatic contracture of the elbow. *J Bone Joint Surg Br* 82:68–73, 2000.

77. Weber CR, Griffin JM: Evaluation of dexamethasone for reducing postoperative edema and inflammatory response after orthognathic surgery. *J Oral Maxillofac Surg* 52(1):35–39, 1994.

78. Wilson PD: Capsulectomy for the relief of flexion contractures of the elbow following fracture. *Clin Orthop Relat Res* 370:3–8, 2000.

79. Wu CC: Posttraumatic contracture of elbow treated with intraarticular technique. *Arch Orthop Trauma Surg* 123:494–500, 2003.

80. Zander CL, Healy NL: Elbow flexion contractures treated with serial casts and conservative therapy. *J Hand Surg [Am]* 17:694–697, 1992.

Elbow Tendinopathies and Tendon Ruptures

Julie E. Adams and Scott P. Steinmann

> These videos may be found at
> *ExpertConsult.com:*
> **25.1** Endobutton single-incision repair of the distal biceps tendon.

LATERAL EPICONDYLITIS

History

In 1873, Runge described a condition associated with lateral humeral condylar tenderness and difficulty writing; Morris referred to it in 1882 as "lawn tennis arm." Eventually, this entity became known as "tennis elbow" or lateral epicondylitis.[45]

Multiple treatments have been proposed for epicondylitis affecting the elbow, ranging from benign neglect to physiotherapy, bracing modalities, injection of various substances, and surgery; the optimal treatment remains controversial. Boyer and Hastings[28] suggested that "there is much witchcraft and pseudoscience involved in the treatment of patients with lateral tennis elbow." In 1936, Cyriax[46] suggested "that the condition usually clears up in eight to twelve months without any treatment except perhaps avoidance of the painful movements for a time," although cases ". . . lasting much longer . . . are encountered." Few conditions elicit as much frustration and controversy regarding cause, treatment, and outcomes among patients and physicians.

Etiology, Associations, and Pathophysiology

Boyer and Hastings[28] reported that "lateral tennis elbow is most commonly an idiopathic or a work-related condition. A distinct pathoetiology has not been definitively identified." Lateral epicondylitis likely represents a multifactorial condition with elements of repetitive microtrauma in a physiologically susceptible individual.

The pathology associated with lateral epicondylitis is believed to involve the attachment of the extensor carpi radialis brevis (ECRB) at the lateral epicondyle. It is suggested that the extensor digitorum communis (EDC) is involved in approximately one third of cases, and rarely the extensor carpi radialis longus (ECRL) or extensor carpi ulnaris (ECU) is involved.[29,118] The ECRB and EDC origins are indistinguishable at the level of the lateral epicondyle. They only visibly become separate muscle-tendon units several centimeters distal at the elbow.

Lateral epicondylitis has been associated with forceful repetitive activities and smoking.[96,134,143] The peak prevalence is at age 45 years, with most patients 35 to 54 years old[75,143] and the dominant arm usually affected.[75] There is an equal distribution between the genders.[75] Of patients followed for 18 months after initial presentation to a general practitioner with the diagnosis of lateral epicondylitis, more than half exhibited a recurrence of symptoms.[75]

It is now recognized that lateral epicondylitis is a degenerative tendinopathy or tendinosis, rather than an inflammatory tendinitis.[3,4,29,64,88,99,112,118,130,133,158] Nirschl[118] described the histologic findings as an angiofibroblastic tendinosis, with a gross appearance of a gray friable edematous tendon structure.[29,118,120] The first three stages of epicondylitis include an inflammatory stage that is restricted to the early course of the disease, followed by angiofibroblastic degeneration in stage II and structural failure in stage III. The fourth stage has a hallmark of fibrosis or calcification in the setting of components of stage II or III.[36,119]

Repetitive contraction of the extensors is believed to cause microtrauma to the tendons, eventually resulting in lateral epicondylitis.[4,42,91,135] Other authors have suggested that impingement of the ECRB tendon against the lateral edge of the capitellum causes abrasion and wear of the tendon during elbow motion, which eventually results in the condition.[30]

In the diseased state, the normally avascular tendon attempts to repair itself with fibroblastic elaboration of collagen and fibrovascular proliferation.[3,4,29,99] Continued mechanical trauma in the setting of an inadequate healing response leads to tendinosis.

Histopathologic findings include fibrocartilaginous formation[64,88,158] or mucoid or hyaline degeneration,[64,88,130,133] fibrovascular proliferation,[64,88,130,133,158] and focal calcifications.[64,88,112,130,158] Milz and colleagues[112] investigated the gross and histologic and molecular features of the common flexor and extensor origins in cadaveric specimens to attempt to describe the ranges of normal and pathologic findings at these locations. The tendon insertions medially and laterally showed confluence with the underlying collateral ligaments, resulting in a complex integrated structure. Fibrocartilage, which had previously been thought to represent a pathologic condition, was found frequently in all age groups, suggesting that it may be present under normal conditions. In addition, degeneration of tendon structure at the epicondylar insertions was present in elderly specimens, indicating that the presence of degenerative changes at the epicondyle may be associated with age.

Presentation

In lateral epicondylitis, patients typically complain of pain localized to the lateral epicondyle and at the ECRB origin, just slightly distal and anterior to the lateral epicondyle; the pain is exacerbated by wrist extension. On clinical examination, pain is elicited with resisted wrist extension with the forearm pronated and elbow fully extended. Additionally, resisted supination with the wrist flexed can precipitate the pain of lateral epicondylitis. The "chair test," in which the patient is asked to lift a chair with the arm in forearm pronation and wrist flexion, typically causes pain.[66] There is an overlap with radial tunnel syndrome in patient complaints and physical findings with use of provocative tests.[155] Pain occurs with resisted finger extension and resisted forearm supination in both processes, so these are not definitive tests for either diagnosis.

If the history is vague and pain is poorly localized or unrelated to activity, other conditions should be considered. This is especially true if the physical examination fails to localize the area of tenderness as described previously. Chondromalacia, periarticular tumors, loose bodies, plica, osteochondral defects, cervical radiculopathy, or ligamentous instability should be considered. Radial tunnel syndrome (supinator syndrome) may also be present (with an estimated incidence of 5%).[63,155]

Diagnosis

The diagnosis of lateral epicondylitis is based on the clinical history and examination findings of pain centered over the origin of the common extensor mechanism, particularly the area of the ECRB and EDC. Radiographic evaluation of the elbow is typically not helpful in lateral epicondylitis but may exclude other disease entities. There might occasionally be some ossification of the soft tissues, but whether this is a result of treatment from multiple injections or is a natural process of the disease is uncertain.

Frequently, magnetic resonance imaging (MRI) studies are obtained in patients with elbow pain, often ordered by the referring physician or requested by the patient. MRI findings consistent with lateral epicondylitis include increased signal on T1 and T2 sequences.[108,130] MRI can show frank tearing and separation of muscle from the bone,[130,158] and it has been suggested that there is good correlation between MRI findings and intraoperative findings.[130]

Frequently, asymptomatic patients have false-positive findings with signal enhancement,[108,139] however, and enhancement may persist even after clinical resolution of symptoms.[139]

In practice, just about every patient with mild pain over the lateral aspect of the elbow seems to have positive changes on MRI, particularly if the patient has had a series of injections. MRI is not significantly helpful in making the diagnosis or dictating treatment but can be used as an adjunct to look for other causes of potential pain around the elbow.

MEDIAL EPICONDYLITIS

Presentation

Medial epicondylitis is much less common than lateral epicondylitis, with a prevalence of 0.4% compared with 1.3% in one study.[143] Other studies have found an estimated prevalence of 3.2% to 8.2% in patients employed in repetitive labor tasks.[51,105,134] Medial epicondylitis is suggested to constitute 10% to 20% of all epicondylitis cases.[35,98,153]

Risk factors are similar to those in lateral epicondylitis and seem to include obesity, physical loads, and smoking; some studies suggest a female preponderance, whereas others do not.[51,74,96,143]

There seems to be an association of medial epicondylitis with other work-related or overuse musculoskeletal disorders.[51,124] As in lateral epicondylitis, patients are typically middle-aged (fourth to fifth decades) and the dominant arm is usually involved.[35,124] An exception is young throwing athletes who may experience medial-sided elbow pain.[111]

The history typically involves an insidious onset of pain at the medial aspect of the elbow. Tenderness exists at the medial epicondyle and distally over the pronator teres (PT) and flexor carpi radialis (FCR). Pain is worsened with resisted pronation and resisted wrist flexion.[35]

Etiology and Pathogenesis

It has been suggested that the cause is related to overuse or repetitive motions leading to microtrauma to the muscular origins at the medial epicondyle; most commonly, to the PT and FCR, but also occasionally to the palmaris longus, flexor digitorum superficialis, and flexor carpi ulnaris origins.[23,29,36,98,110,118,124] As implied by the layperson's term *golfer's elbow*, repetitive use and microtrauma can precipitate the condition, and it has been associated with repetitive valgus loads in golf, racquet sports, football, baseball, weight lifting, and archery, in addition to occupational exposures requiring repetitive motions of the hand, wrist, elbow, or forearm.[35,65,89,98,124,168] One of the oldest references is that of Morris,[116] who described a condition in rowers occurring after "long and vigorous sculling," with pain at the "inner part of the elbow," which resolved with rest and avoidance of pronosupination. Although usually associated with a chronic overuse type of phenomenon, occasionally a single sudden traumatic episode can cause avulsion of the flexor pronator origin and lead to this condition.[36]

As in lateral epicondylitis, pathologic findings include a degenerative tendinosis rather than an inflammatory tendinitis, and it has been suggested that this is due to the repetitive microtears in the setting of an inadequate healing response and, eventually, altered biomechanics of the elbow joint.[110] In pitchers, the stresses are conferred to the medial structures of the elbow, including the flexor pronator muscles and medial collateral ligament (MCL).[110]

Acceleration and valgus forces may exceed the tensile strength of the medial constraints of the elbow, leading to tears with a spectrum of pathologic findings ranging from epicondylitis to MCL insufficiency.[35,124]

The pathologic change found in medial epicondylitis is indistinguishable from that found in lateral epicondylitis with angiofibroblastic tendinosis.[124]

In 23 to 60% of patients, ulnar neuritis is present.[62,97,110,124,168] The pathophysiologic mechanism has been suggested to be a combination of traction injury with entrapment and compression.[35]

Diagnosis

The differential diagnosis includes neurologic conditions (ulnar nerve neuritis, cervical radiculopathy, pronator syndrome); intraarticular pathologic conditions such as elbow synovitis, arthritis, or osteochondral defects; and ligamentous deficiency (MCL insufficiency).[110] Typically, the diagnosis is made on clinical grounds. Radiographs may reveal calcification adjacent to the medial epicondyle or traction spurs or calcifications, particularly in throwing athletes.[36,110] As in lateral epicondylitis, radiographs are not typically necessary for the diagnosis, but they may exclude alternative causes of elbow pain. Some authors have investigated use of other imaging modalities, and ultrasonography has been noted to be highly specific and sensitive. Typically, a focal hypoechogenic or anechogenic area is shown,[127] although ultrasound is usually not necessary to make the diagnosis.

MRI may be useful to rule out other conditions, such as MCL insufficiency or intraarticular pathologic conditions such as osteochondral defects. In the setting of medial epicondylitis, MRI may show increased signal intensity on T1 and T2 series,[89] but it is again typically not required to make the diagnosis and it is not specific, because signal changes can be seen in asymptomatic individuals.[89] It has been suggested that these signal changes in asymptomatic patients may represent senescent changes or prior epicondylitis that has become quiescent.[89]

Because of a high rate of concomitant ulnar neuritis, the clinical examination should include evaluation of the ulnar nerve, including provocative maneuvers such as a cubital tunnel Tinel sign, a cubital tunnel compression test, and an elbow flexion test.[35,110] Electromyography is of limited utility because it is normal in 90% of patients with ulnar nerve symptoms.[110]

The status of the MCL should be assessed to rule out insufficiency. Valgus stress should be applied to the elbow in a position of 30 degrees short of full extension. Potential compensatory action of the flexor pronator group can be eliminated by placing the pronated forearm in a position of wrist flexion and 30 degrees of elbow extension before stress is applied. The *milking maneuver*, in which the examiner pulls on the patient's thumb, generating a valgus stress when the forearm is supinated in a position of elbow flexion, also tests for MCL insufficiency. In both tests, pain and instability are typically absent in pure medial epicondylitis, and their presence may represent MCL injury.[35,110]

TREATMENT OF MEDIAL AND LATERAL EPICONDYLITIS

Treatment considerations for medial and lateral epicondylitis are similar and are considered together. The treatment of epicondylitis is controversial. There are multiple reports advocating different techniques for treatment, but many are flawed studies.[43]

Nonoperative Treatment

Nonoperative therapy is the main treatment option for medial and lateral epicondylitis.[36] It has been suggested that more than 85 to 90% of patients respond to nonoperative treatment,[42,73,124] but some series suggest more modest results, with 40% of patients with lateral epicondylitis having some residual discomfort.[25]

Activity modification is one of the mainstays of treatment, with avoidance of precipitating activities. Several studies have noted that tennis players who use a two-handed backstroke are less likely to develop tennis elbow, perhaps because of altered biomechanics and dissipation of the forces experienced at ball contact.[68,98,135] Likewise, other modifications of equipment and action can help symptoms resolve.

Three phases of treatment have been proposed for epicondylitis. Phase one involves activity modification to avoid precipitating activities and use of icing several times daily. Nonsteroidal antiinflammatory drugs may be used to diminish any accompanying elbow synovitis. Night splinting and corticosteroid injections may be considered,[35,124] and counterforce bracing may be considered during phase one to limit contraction of the muscles, although use of these treatment options has been questioned and efficacy of injections, bracing, therapy, and oral or topical medications remains uncertain.[35,128]

Phase two involves starting a rehabilitation program after the acute symptoms are diminished with restoration of full painless wrist and elbow motion. A program of isometric exercises and stretching is initiated, followed by resistive exercises and sports or work hardening.[35]

The third phase is a maintenance phase involving equipment and technique modification for sports or work and continued conditioning to prevent recurrence.[35] Injection of various substances has been suggested as a treatment for lateral and medial epicondylitis. Nevertheless, review of the literature demonstrates conflicting and inconclusive evidence upon which to base recommendations for injections as treatment of lateral epicondylitis.[93]

Botulinum toxin injection has been suggested for lateral epicondylitis, with some benefit shown in some but not all series, although muscle weakness may be seen as an expected side effect.[82,174] Injection of autologous blood has been suggested to be beneficial for epicondylitis.[40,54,83] One series showed a beneficial effect of dry needling and injection of autologous blood in medial epicondylitis,[160] and another showed a beneficial effect in lateral epicondylitis.[54] Platelet-rich plasma injections have also been reported, with mixed results.[70,94,113,163]

Corticosteroid injection has historically been suggested to decrease pain and early inflammation or joint synovitis and in some series has been found to be beneficial, particularly in the short term.[7,164] Despite short-term improvement, corticosteroid injection does not seem to influence the outcome at 3 or 12 months.[131,146,148,154,169] A more recent study suggests that there is no difference between injection with corticosteroid and local anesthetic versus local anesthetic alone at 1 or 6 months; the presence of concomitant depression or poor coping skills was a better predictor of outcome than treatment modality.[102]

Finally, a recent study and subsequent metaanalysis should provoke caution in the use of corticosteroid injections. Coombes and colleagues found that injection of corticosteroid resulted in poorer outcomes relative to placebo at 1 year.[41] A metaanalysis suggests that despite short-term beneficial effects of corticosteroid injection, the intermediate-term results show a negative effect and the long-term effects are uncertain, with conflicting data.[123] Other studies have suggested that the technique of injection plays a larger role than the substance injected. These theories center on the ability to induce a vascular healing response by a "peppering" technique in which the needle is redirected multiple times to puncture the epicondylar region at multiple sites. This idea is supported by studies in which lateral epicondylitis was injected with either corticosteroid, autologous blood, or lidocaine, with equivalent good results at follow-up.[6,94,173]

Corticosteroid injection is better than physiotherapy and modalities in most,[25,131,154,169] but not all, series.[90,117,148]

Physiotherapy has equivocal long-term results.[117,148] Modalities such as ultrasound or iontophoresis have been suggested to provide benefit, but their efficacy and role in treatment remain controversial. One study showed that ultrasound therapy for lateral epicondylitis has no benefit.[48] Pulsed electromagnetic field therapy is suggested to be more beneficial than placebo for treatment of lateral epicondylitis; however, results across series are conflicting.[167] In addition, extracorporeal shock-wave therapy has shown some benefit in medial and lateral epicondylitis,[60,136,142,151,171] but most studies have failed to find any advantage for it over control groups and it is not routinely recommended.[26,34,78,92,100,142,152,156,157,170]

Surgical Treatment

Surgical indications for medial or lateral epicondylitis include failure of a nonoperative treatment course of 6 or more months and, in medial epicondylitis, tendon disruption in a throwing athlete or progressive ulnar neuritis.[35,110,120,124]

Surgical treatment typically involves excision of the area of tendinosis, débridement of the local tissue bed, and reattachment of the tendon origin as indicated. Reported success rates are 97% in primary lateral epicondylitis, 83% in revision cases, and 87 to 100% in primary medial epicondylitis.[52,61,111,120,124,125]

The area of pathologic change may extend beyond the visibly abnormal area, and concern exists regarding the need to débride all affected tissue while preserving normal structures. This concern is particularly relevant because gross appearance of the tendon and patients' symptoms do not always correlate with the degree of histopathology, with grossly degenerative tissue having minimal histologic findings in some cases.[29] Some authors have proposed the "scratch test" to differentiate between normal and abnormal tissue, suggesting that normal tendon would not be removed by scraping with a No. 10 knife blade.[29]

In the setting of medial epicondylitis, it is important to query the patient about symptoms and examine the patient specifically for ulnar nerve pathologic conditions, as failure to address this at the time of surgery may lead to persistent discomfort.

Lateral Epicondylitis Surgery

Choices in lateral epicondylitis surgery include open or percutaneous procedures that release the extensor origin from the lateral epicondyle, procedures in which tendinosis is removed from the lateral epicondyle and the ECRB origin is released or repaired, denervation of the lateral epicondyle, intraarticular procedures, and arthroscopic débridement or release of the ECRB origin. Outcomes after open release or débridement are generally good to excellent in 70 to 97% of patients; however, a prolonged recovery and unsatisfactory results can be seen in 15 to 20% of cases.[39,52] Percutaneous release of the common extensor origin from the lateral epicondyle has been described using a small incision. Reported success rates are 70 to 91%.[20,73,175,176]

Several cadaver and clinical studies have evaluated the safety and efficacy of arthroscopic lateral epicondylitis surgery and have suggested it is a safe and reliably reproducible procedure.[16,17,95,126,149] A classification system based on arthroscopic findings has shown three types, although outcomes do not correlate with classification type.[17] Arthroscopic treatment has been suggested to have benefits over open treatments, including easier and faster recovery, earlier return to work, and provision of a surgical means for evaluating and treating intraarticular

pathologic conditions, which in some series are present in 69% of cases.[16,17,72,81,126,129] Likewise, selective release of the involved ECRB with preservation of the uninvolved common extensor origin can be achieved.[17]

Cohen and colleagues[39] described the anatomic relationships of the extensor tendon origins and made specific recommendations from their cadaveric study for arthroscopic ECRB release. The bony origin of the ECRB was reliably found just anterior to the distalmost tip of the lateral supracondylar ridge, with a diamond-shaped footprint. Proximally, the ECRB arose from a longitudinal line paralleling the long axis of the humerus, and the superior margin was at the superior capitellum, whereas the inferior margin was at the midpoint of the radiocapitellar joint or capitellum. The ECRB was intimate but easily distinguishable from the joint capsule deep to it. Based on these dissections, the authors performed arthroscopic release of the ECRB. A standard anteromedial portal was established first, and a modified lateral portal was made from an inside-out technique 2 to 3 cm proximal and anterior to the lateral epicondyle. A monopolar thermal device was used to expose the ECRB by ablation of the capsule, and then release of the ECRB was performed.

Cohen and colleagues[39] noted that the capsule must be resected to gain access to the ECRB, which can be identified and released from the top of the capitellum to the midportion of the radiocapitellar joint; care is taken not to release it posterior to the midline of the joint so as to protect the ligament, and care is also taken to preserve the extensor aponeurosis lying superficial to the ECRB tendon.

Smith and coworkers[149] noted that inadvertent injury to the lateral ulnar collateral ligament could be avoided by using the anterior half of the radial head as a landmark for the safe region for débridement of the extensor tendon origin.

With regard to outcomes, results comparable to those of open procedures have been seen with maintained success at a mean follow-up of 130 months.[16] Superiority over open procedures has not been shown,[129] however, and some authors have suggested that arthroscopic procedures can be associated with residual tendinopathy and symptoms because of the inability to visualize and treat the area of pathologic change fully.[28,44] Likewise, elbow arthroscopy generally has a high learning curve and has been associated with neurovascular injuries, with the potential to destabilize the lateral ligamentous structures even in the most experienced of hands.[1,17,159,165]

One study comparing effectiveness and a Cochrane Database review concluded that there is no evidence to suggest one procedure over another and recommended surgeon experience and preference in deciding which procedure, open versus arthroscopic versus percutaneous, to perform.[103,161]

Surgery for Recurrent Lateral Epicondylitis

Revision surgery for failed tennis elbow surgery has been reported to have a greater than 80% success rate.[5,104,125,140] Common findings include inadequate or incomplete resection of tendinosis in 97% of cases.[125] More thorough resection of tissue and repair of the extensor aponeurosis resulted in an 83% success rate.[125] In addition, for recurrent or primary lateral epicondylitis in which a wide degenerative tendon has been seen intraoperatively, anconeus muscle flap transposition has been used with good results and a patient satisfaction rate of 94% in one series.[5,104,140]

Surgical Treatment for Medial Epicondylitis

Surgical treatment of medial epicondylitis is performed in a manner similar to that for surgery on the lateral side. The interval between the PT and FCR is developed, revealing the deep tissues that are diseased, and they are sharply excised.[62,110,124]

Caution is needed to avoid injury to the ulnar nerve and the anterior bundle of the MCL. Injury to the medial antebrachial cutaneous nerve may result in a bothersome numb patch or a painful neuroma.[124]

Expected Outcomes

Good to excellent results have been achieved in 83 to 96% of patients using variations in technique,[20,62,124,168] with poorer outcomes reported in patients with ulnar nerve symptoms.[62] Little information is available in the literature regarding optimal treatment for recurrent medial epicondylitis or failed prior surgery.

❖ AUTHORS' PREFERRED METHOD OF TREATMENT: Elbow Epicondylitis

Variable opinions exist regarding the cause and natural history of epicondylitis. Even more controversial is the subject of the optimal treatment of this condition, including the role of benign neglect, therapy, injections, modalities, and surgery.[43]

When patients present for evaluation and treatment of epicondylitis, they often expect some active intervention. Based on the available evidence, most cases resolve with patience and minimal intervention within 18 months; the probable best recommendation for treatment is oral analgesics for symptom relief, activity modification (at work and at play), and an overall plan of "waiting things out" for up to 18 months. It may be unrealistic, however, to expect most patients to accept the intellectual explanation that "lateral elbow pain is a harmless rite of passage into middle age"[102] that often resolves on its own, and that "leaving things be" and allowing significant time for healing is sufficient treatment.

Based on available evidence in the literature, corticosteroid injection, although commonly used by physicians and frequently requested by patients, has little, if any, benefit over placebo. Likewise, such injections usually do not change the natural history of the disease, although recent data suggest that poorer results are seen in the intermediate and long term following corticosteroid injections relative to placebo. With respect to corticosteroid injection and short-term relief of symptoms, there is some evidence to suggest improvement, although injection with local anesthetic or saline may fulfill the same role.[102,131,146,148,154,169]

In our practice, we attempt to have a frank, complete discussion with the patient about the pathologic conditions and explain the available evidence suggesting that with a significant amount of time (≤2 years), the process tends to be self-limiting and dissipates.[147] Some patients will find this reassuring, but many do not. There is evidence in the literature to suggest that poorer outcomes are seen in patients who complain of severe pain, have concomitant neck pain, are involved in workers' compensation claims, have concomitant depression, or have poor coping skills.[102,147] Patients who are inclined to reject the notion that this is a benign, albeit frustrating, self-limited process and want "something done" may request and be offered an injection with local anesthetic or corticosteroid, although the

recent data again suggest that long-term outcomes are poorer with corticosteroid injection. We encourage patients to modify activity to avoid sports and work-related extension of the elbow with wrist extension and flexion.

If a patient continues to have symptoms beyond 6 to 9 months despite activity modification, surgical intervention is offered if the patient desires further treatment. Surgical treatment of lateral epicondylitis can be performed either by open procedures or arthroscopically. The literature confirms that outcomes between the two procedures are comparable. We discuss with the patient the minimally invasive nature of arthroscopic treatment; however, we also explain that arthroscopy is accompanied by an increased risk of neurovascular injury and instability compared with open release of the elbow.[1,17] Surgical treatment of medial epicondylitis is by open procedures only; there is no arthroscopic option.

Open release of lateral epicondylitis is performed under tourniquet control for visualization or "wide-awake" anesthesia with local anesthesia combined with epinephrine. A lateral incision of approximately 4 cm is made overlying the epicondyle or just anterior to it (Figure 25.1). The ECRL-EDC interface is identified and incised, and the ECRL is retracted anteriorly (Figure 25.2). The degenerated tissue at the ECRB origin is identified, usually appearing as a white-gray friable abnormal tissue. This tissue is sharply excised (Figure 25.3). Typically, the joint is not opened. It is also important to protect the lateral ulnar collateral ligament by restricting the excision of the degenerated tissue to the anterolateral epicondyle. As discussed in Chapter 23, some surgeons have inadvertently excised the

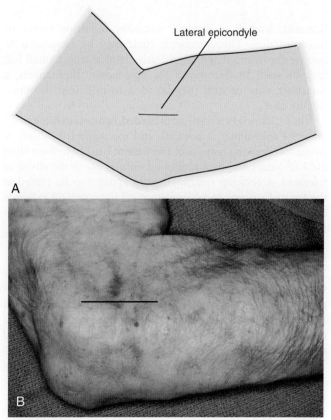

FIGURE 25.1 Skin incision is based just distal to lateral epicondyle.

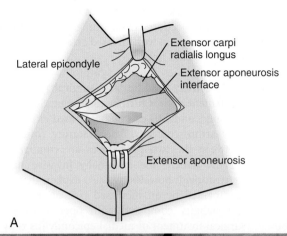

A

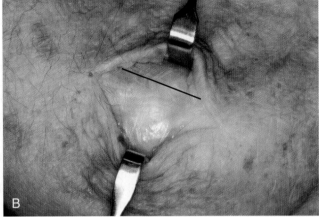

B

FIGURE 25.2 Extensor carpi radialis longus–extensor digitorum communis interface is identified.

ligament, leading to chronic instability requiring repair or reconstruction. The epicondyle itself may be rongeured to remove the diseased and degenerative tendon, and a small bur may be used to decorticate the epicondyle; alternatively, a Kirschner wire or drill may be used to drill into the bone (Figure 25.4).

The ECRL origin is repaired as needed, hemostasis is obtained after the tourniquet is released, and the wound is closed. A sterile soft dressing is applied. The patient is asked to use a sling for 2 to 3 days and then is allowed normal use of the elbow as tolerated. A cock-up removable wrist splint may be placed at the time of surgery to take pressure off the common extensor origins and can be worn for 1 to 2 weeks until the wound is healed and elbow motion has returned to normal.

Arthroscopic Technique

The patient is positioned in the lateral position, and the arm is secured in a dedicated arm holder. Regional anesthesia is generally avoided, so that an accurate neurovascular examination can be performed after completion of the procedure. The elbow is examined to rule out a subluxating ulnar nerve, and all portal sites and bony landmarks are marked before joint insufflation. The joint is distended with 30 mL of saline introduced via an 18-gauge needle into the anterolateral portal. Arthroscopic treatment of lateral epicondylitis is achieved through two portals, with viewing from the anteromedial portal and working through the anterolateral portal. We prefer to start the arthros-

copy from the anterolateral portal, with a subsequent antero-medial portal made under direct visualization and using a switching stick to swap viewing portals; however, establishing the anteromedial portal first is acceptable as well. The antero-lateral portal should be placed slightly more distally and anteriorly than the standard anterolateral portal, just distal to the radiocapitellar joint. If the portal is placed directly over the radiocapitellar joint, it can be difficult to address the area of the ECRB.

Diagnostic arthroscopy is performed to rule out any other articular pathologic findings, such as loose bodies, plicae, or thickening of the annular ligament. A shaver or radiofrequency probe is used to débride the capsule through the anterolateral portal.[17] This débridement exposes the undersurface of the white tendinous ECRB-EDC conjoined tendon origins, which have a clearly visible demarcation from the muscular, more anterior ECRL. The ECRB (and part of the EDC) is released from its origin with a shaver or a radiofrequency probe. A radiofrequency probe is useful to elevate the ECRB, which may then be released from the lateral epicondyle. Release posterior to the midline of the radiocapitellar joint should be avoided to prevent instability. A shaver or bur may be used to decorticate the lateral epicondyle, especially in chronic cases, to promote vascularity and healing.[17]

The instruments are withdrawn, and no suturing or closure, other than of the skin portals, is required. A sterile dressing is applied, and the arm is placed into a sling. Within 24 to 48 hours, the patient is allowed to use the arm for gentle activities. A removable cock-up wrist splint, as used with the open procedure, is helpful.

Surgical Technique for Treatment of Medial Epicondylitis

Surgical treatment for medial epicondylitis is rarely required; most patients respond to nonoperative treatment. Failure to respond to activity modifications and other nonoperative means for more than 6 to 9 months may represent an indication for surgical management, however. A procedure similar to what is done on the lateral side is performed. There is no current arthroscopic treatment for this condition.

A tourniquet is used on the upper arm to facilitate visualization. The incision is made from 2 cm proximal to the medial epicondyle and extends distally parallel to the epicondyle for 4 to 5 cm (Figure 25.5). The medial antebrachial cutaneous nerve and its branches are preserved; inadvertent injury may lead to a bothersome numbness or a painful neuroma. The interval between the PT and FCR is developed (Figure 25.6).[62,124] The PT is retracted anteriorly and the FCR is retracted posteriorly to reveal the deep tissues that are diseased in this condition; these are sharply excised (Figure 25.7).[110] Care is taken to preserve the anterior bundle of the MCL; otherwise, iatrogenic instability may ensue. Abnormal tissue is removed, and the medial epicondyle is prepared by cutting away fibrous tissue with a rongeur and placing small drill holes through the cortex to improve vascularity (Figure 25.8).

The PT-FCR interval is closed with running 2-0 braided suture (Figure 25.9); this is adequate in simple cases of medial epicondylitis without concomitant MCL injury. For the latter condition, the PT-FCR interval is developed further, and the common flexor origin is split along its fibers. The MCL is

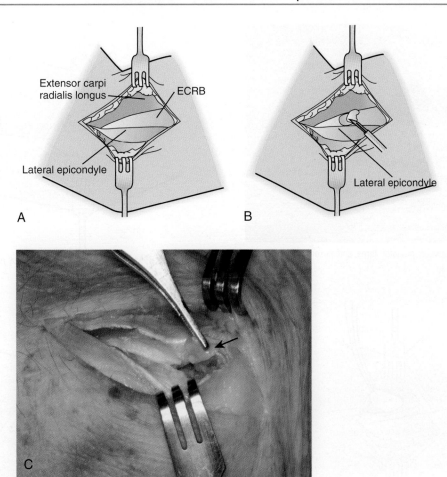

FIGURE 25.3 A to **C,** Degenerated tissue at extensor carpi radialis brevis (ECRB) is identified and incised.

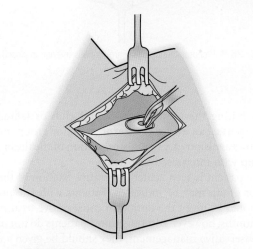

FIGURE 25.4 A bur is used to decorticate bone.

exposed, the anterior bundle of the MCL is reconstructed as indicated, and drilling and reattachment of the origin are performed as described earlier. If ulnar nerve symptoms are present preoperatively, the ulnar nerve should be decompressed in situ or transposed.

Postoperatively, the arm is placed in a sling for comfort for 1 to 2 weeks until sutures are removed. Range of motion and gentle use of the arm are allowed. Resisted wrist flexion or pronation is avoided for 4 to 6 weeks for simple medial epicondylitis; more restrictions are required if reconstruction of the MCL has been performed.

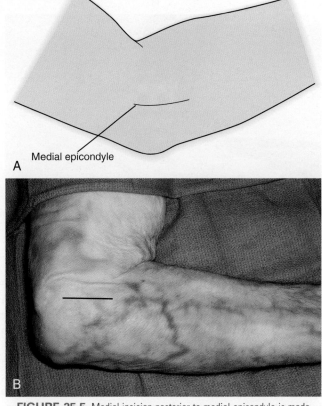

FIGURE 25.5 Medial incision posterior to medial epicondyle is made.

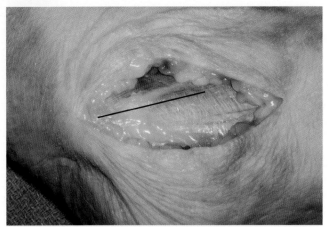

FIGURE 25.6 Interval between pronator teres and flexor carpi radialis is identified and developed.

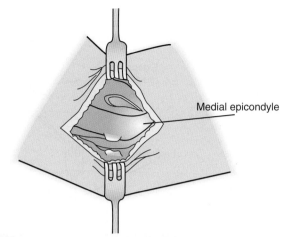

FIGURE 25.8 Medial epicondyle is prepared by removing fibrous tissue with rongeur.

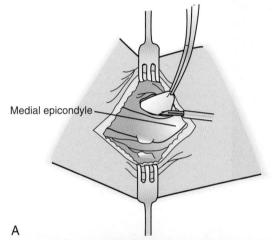

A

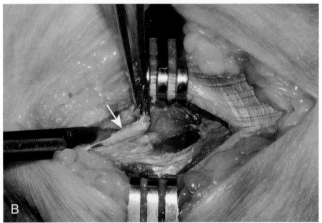

FIGURE 25.7 A and **B,** Area of tendinosis is identified and excised.

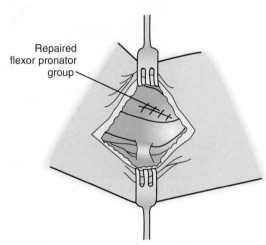

FIGURE 25.9 Pronator teres–flexor carpi radialis interval is closed with 2-0 suture.

Avulsion of the flexor pronator origin is important to rule out in the evaluation of medial elbow pain. This condition can commonly occur in golfers who hit the ground instead of the ball or in individuals after a fall, conferring a sudden injury to the medial elbow. In this instance, this is not medial epicondylitis but rather true avulsion of the flexor pronator origin. This avulsion can often be mistaken for medial epicondylitis; however, flexor pronator avulsion does not tend to improve with conservative treatment. It is surprising how trivial injuries,

such as hitting the ground with a golf club or falling while playing sports, can avulse the flexor pronator group; however, MRI shows avulsion of a significant portion of the flexor pronator group with interposed scar tissue.

If the patient is seen acutely, operative fixation of the flexor pronator group may be indicated. Patients with late presentations should be given the option of conservative treatment for 3 to 6 months, however. Although most patients do not improve with conservative management, they should be given a chance.

Operative treatment of a flexor pronator avulsion involves a posterior incision with full-thickness flaps developed to expose the medial side or a direct medial approach. Often chronic cases have interposed scar at the edge of the flexor pronator group; this must be débrided to a healthy muscular origin. The origin is repaired with No. 0 braided nonabsorbable suture to the medial epicondyle through drill holes (or, alternatively, suture anchors may be used). The wound is closed in the usual fashion. The patient is placed in a long-arm splint in neutral rotation and neutral wrist position until he or she returns for suture removal at 7 to 14 days. Subsequently, the patient is protected from forced extension of the wrist or powerful active flexion of the wrist for 4 to 6 weeks with a removable splint.

CRITICAL POINTS *Lateral and*
Medial Epicondylitis

- In lateral and medial epicondylitis, most patients respond to nonoperative therapy (activity modifications with or without adjunctive measures) within 18 months.
- Little evidence exists regarding the efficacy of adjunctive nonoperative therapies over placebo; however, they are widely used and may give the patient satisfaction and some subjective benefit in pursuing an "active" treatment.
- Operative treatment may be considered after more than 6 to 9 months of recalcitrant symptoms; in medial epicondylitis, the presence of acute avulsion of the flexor pronator origin, worsening ulnar neuritis, or MCL insufficiency in a throwing athlete are also indications for surgery.
- In open lateral epicondylitis surgery and medial epicondylitis surgery, the abnormal tissue is identified as a gray, friable, edematous tendon and is excised.
- The origins are repaired as indicated, and resisted wrist motion is avoided postoperatively.
- Arthroscopic lateral epicondylitis surgery requires familiarity and competency with arthroscopic elbow procedures and anatomy.

DISTAL BICEPS RUPTURE

Ruptures of the distal biceps tendon are readily diagnosed by the history in most cases. The patient is typically a middle-aged man (fifth or sixth decade) who relates a history of lifting an object or a forced extension of a flexed and loaded forearm.[114] It is exceedingly unusual for distal biceps pathologic conditions to occur in women. There have been anecdotal reports of distal biceps rupture in women[19,172]; however, our personal experience involves only two female patients who had partial tearing and tendinopathy involving the distal biceps that was unresolved and responded well to operative treatment of débridement and reinsertion of the biceps tendon. Commonly, a middle-aged man experiences a sudden "pop" or giving way in the antecubital fossa after flexing and supinating the elbow against a form of resistance. If the patient is seen a few days after this episode, there is ecchymosis present over the elbow and proximal forearm, and the patient often points out the asymmetry and the "Popeye" deformity in the biceps muscle belly. This makes the diagnosis quite easy to make, and with this classic history, the diagnosis can also be made over the telephone. Partial biceps tendon tears may result from an acute event or tearing in conjunction with chronic degeneration.[14,50] Clinical complaints and findings are similar to those of complete rupture, with pain in the antecubital fossa and weakness of supination. In contrast, the biceps may still be palpable, and MRI findings suggest a partial tear.[14]

In some patients, the diagnosis is less clear. These patients frequently have a partial tear of a chronic and slowly degenerative nature and complain of nonspecific elbow pain that is worsened with daily activities. They may not complain specifically of pain while supinating the forearm. On physical examination, patients often point to the anterior middle aspect of the antecubital fossa but do not specifically point to the posterolateral aspect of the elbow or the area of the radial tuberosity. This presentation can make the diagnosis less obvious, and other pathologic changes around the elbow, such as lateral epicondylitis, plica, or elbow arthritis, may be considered. On examination, full range of motion is present, but frequently there is exacerbation of symptoms with resisted elbow flexion and supination and with deep palpation of the biceps and antecubital fossa. In addition, deep palpation of the radial tuberosity from the posterolateral aspect while passively pronating the forearm sometimes elicits pain. This finding of pain noted with palpation over the radial tuberosity is a very good indication of tendinopathy involving the insertion of the distal biceps.

The pathologic changes that occur with distal biceps tendinopathy may be similar to those of tendinopathies elsewhere in the body, such as in the shoulder or wrist. The insertion site of the tendon on the radial tuberosity undergoes degenerative changes that are visible and begin with partial tearing of the tendon. This process can be painful, but it also clearly can be asymptomatic. We have treated many patients with distal biceps ruptures that showed, in addition to the acute rupture for which they were undergoing surgical treatment, signs of significant chronic degeneration with partial tearing before rupture. Many of these patients deny having any symptoms referable to their distal biceps insertion before the acute event (rupture) that caused them to present for treatment.

Diagnosis

On clinical examination, a patient with biceps pathologic conditions exhibits pain and weakness in flexion and supination and sometimes ecchymoses in the antecubital fossa or an abnormal muscle contour of the biceps. Also, with the elbow at 90 degrees of flexion, one may ask the patient to rotate the pronated forearm into supination; normally, the examiner can hook the tip of his or her thumb around the biceps tendon in the cubital fossa (Figure 25.10).[122] With distal avulsion of the tendon, this may be impossible.

Occasionally, some fibers or a fascial sleeve may remain intact, giving an appearance of an intact tendon. The examiner must discriminate between the normal lacertus fibrosus, which often remains intact even with biceps rupture, and the biceps tendon.

Imaging studies are of mixed benefit in the workup of a patient with suspected distal biceps pathologic findings. Plain film radiographs should be obtained, but are most commonly normal and do not show pathologic changes. Biceps ruptures typically do not involve bony ruptures, and minimal changes are seen on standard radiographs of the elbow.

MRI may show rupture, but it is unnecessary in most cases and occasionally may be read as falsely negative, although some authors suggest a 100% correlation with intraoperative findings.[58] MRI may be useful to exclude alternative diagnoses and to evaluate the extent of suspected partial rupture; it also may be useful in cases in which the history suggests a biceps rupture but the clinical examination is unclear.[56,58] MRI findings suggestive of complete rupture include absence of the tendon insertion or a fluid-filled sheath, whereas partial ruptures are typically seen as high signal intensity, fluid within the tendon sheath, or thinning or thickening of the tendon distally.[56,69] Positioning of the prone patient with the shoulder abducted over the head and the elbow in 90 degrees of flexion and the forearm in supination (the so-called FABS view) (Figure 25.11)[32] has been suggested to improve visualization of the distal biceps insertion into the radial tuberosity.[69] Ultrasound is a lower-cost diagnostic tool that is also usually unnecessary but has been

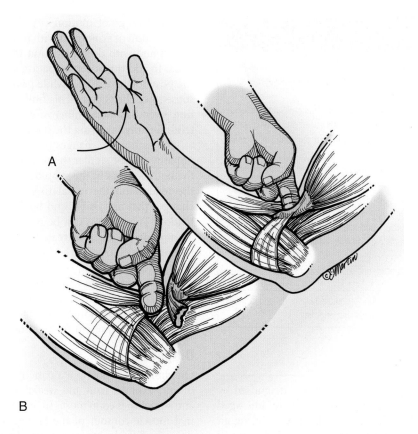

FIGURE 25.10 A and **B,** Hook test described by O'Driscoll and colleagues involves assessment for intact biceps tendon by "hooking" examiner's finger around biceps with elbow at 90 degrees and in supination. (From O'Driscoll SW, Goncalves LB, Dietz P: The hook test for distal biceps tendon avulsion, *Am J Sports Med* 35:1865-1869, 2007. Redrawn by Elizabeth Martin.)

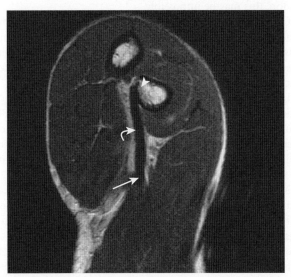

FIGURE 25.11 Forearm in supination view by magnetic resonance imaging shows insertion of biceps tendon into radial tuberosity (*arrows,* biceps tendon; *arrowhead,* biceps insertion into radial tuberosity). (From Giuffrè BM, Moss MJ: Optimal positioning for MRI of the distal biceps brachii tendon: flexed abducted supinated view, *AJR Am J Roentgenol* 182:944-946, 2004.)

shown to be accurate in the diagnosis of complete or partial tears.[22] Findings suggestive of complete rupture include tendon absence, fluid, and mass in the antecubital fossa; incomplete rupture may be represented by a focal hypoechogenic area or thinning of the tendon.[22]

Treatment

Treatment of partial or complete biceps ruptures may be nonoperative; however, an estimated loss of 40% to 60% of supination power and 30% of flexion power can be anticipated in the setting of untreated complete distal biceps ruptures. Despite this, some patients may compensate well and even regain substantial supination strength over time.[21,33,59,115,141] Although functional difficulties may persist and one series has suggested that a high rate of residual pain and weakness may persist at 4.5 years of follow-up after nonoperative treatment,[15,33,67] other series have suggested that many patients compensate well, with a high rate of satisfactory outcomes scores and only a modest loss of supination strength at a median follow-up of 38 months.[59] If operative treatment is elected, it should ideally proceed within 7 to 10 days of injury, before tissue can become retracted and scarred. In addition, complications of early repairs are less likely, although a recent series challenges this thought, with no higher complication rate seen in patients up to 4 weeks following rupture.[8,27,38,84]

Primary repair is almost certainly possible 4 weeks after injury and as late as 9 months in our experience. Commonly, the lacertus fibrosus is partially intact, which serves to anchor the biceps distally and prevent proximal retraction to some extent. The biceps can be mobilized and repaired to the tuberosity even with the elbow in some flexion, which universally stretches out over time, yielding nearly full extension at final follow-up. Rarely, augmentation, as with Achilles tendon allograft, is required.[138] Using a graft extension does not restore the proper muscle tendon length, just as adding a tendon graft to a profundus tendon rupture does not restore finger flexion. Although it is tempting to add a graft to restore continuity of the muscle-tendon unit, it does little to restore elbow active function. A better alternative to repair with graft in chronic cases is tenodesis of the distal biceps to the brachialis, although results in postoperative strength may be less satisfactory.[21] Good results can be seen with operative treatment of partial tears.[50,84] In surgical treatment, issues that remain unclear include optimal fixation technique of the tendon to bone and whether a two-incision versus one-incision surgical approach has fewer complications or better outcome.[24,31]

PERTINENT ANATOMY

Anatomic studies have shown that the insertion site of the tendon onto the radial tuberosity occurs through a long, thin, ribbon-like insertion. The advantage of this long, thin insertion, primarily on the medial aspect of the tuberosity, is that the tendon can wrap around the tuberosity, which acts as a cam, giving mechanical advantage to rotation of the radius (Figure 25.12). In addition, it has become apparent that the distal biceps tendon represents continuations of the short and long heads of the muscle distally. The short head, which is more significant, inserts distal to the radial tuberosity and functions as a flexor of the elbow, whereas the long head inserts away from the axis of rotation, to function in supination (Figure 25.13).[12,53,80,109] Restoring the correct anatomic alignment is crucial for optimal function of the biceps.[12,53,80,109]

The anatomy of the radial tuberosity varies widely; it is similar to retroversion of the humeral head. This can range from 30 degrees off of the radial tuberosity to almost 90 degrees. Repair techniques using a single anterior incision may be unable to accurately restore the correct insertion point of the tendon if the medially oriented angle of insertion is closer to 90 degrees. Detailed anatomic studies of the footprint of the biceps insertion have revealed that the biceps inserts on the posterior ulnar portion of the radial tuberosity, suggesting that an anatomic

repair through a single anterior approach may be difficult, particularly if forearm supination is limited preoperatively.[12,80]

Two-incision techniques offer the ability to limit the size of the anterior exposure and decrease the risk of neurovascular injury, and if a muscle-splitting approach is used, there is no higher risk of radioulnar synostosis (Figure 25.14). El-Hawary and associates[55] compared complications after a single-incision technique and after a modified Boyd-Anderson two-incision technique. Complication rates were 44% versus 10% in the single-incision and two-incision techniques, respectively; patients undergoing the two-incision technique had a slightly more rapid recovery of flexion strength. At final follow-up, differences between the two groups were minimal. Other series have suggested a 7% synostosis rate with a two-incision technique.[27] Although a two-incision technique is said to be associated with heterotopic ossification, a single-incision technique may also be complicated by this problem.[87]

Grewal and colleagues[71] evaluated patients who were prospectively randomized to either a single-incision repair with suture anchors or a two-incision technique with bony tunnels. Outcomes were similar, with two exceptions: there was a significantly increased risk of complications (mostly related to neurapraxia of the lateral antebrachial cutaneous nerve) associated with the single-incision technique, and there was a significant increase of 10% in flexion strength in the two-incision group over the single-incision group. Technique of repair to bone is also variable. Options include direct repair to bone through bony tunnels and use of interference screws, suture anchors, or other devices. Although fixation with a button device is strongest in biomechanical testing in vitro, it seems from clinical series and biomechanical testing that fixation with transosseous sutures and suture anchors is sufficient to withstand forces in vivo exerted during rehabilitation.[27,31,77,85,86] Transosseous sutures are also less costly and biologically provide a bone-to-tendon interface for robust healing. Comparison of transosseous fixation two-incision techniques with suture anchor techniques or tie-on button techniques shows satisfactory

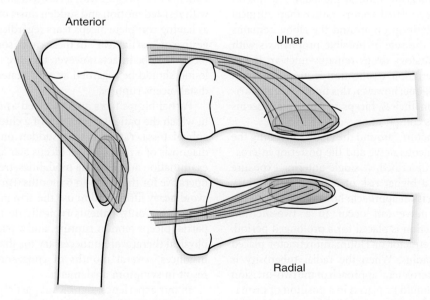

FIGURE 25.12 Biceps insertion occurs in long, ribbon-like fashion onto ulnar aspect of radial tuberosity. (From Mazzocca AD, Cohen M, Berkson E, et al: The anatomy of the bicipital tuberosity and distal biceps tendon, *J Shoulder Elbow Surg* 16:122-127, 2007.)

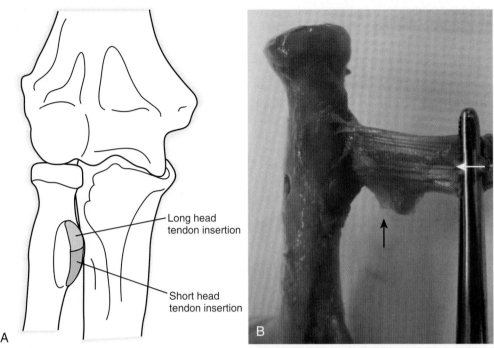

FIGURE 25.13 A and **B,** Long and short heads of biceps have distinct anatomic insertions at radial tuberosity. (From Athwal GS, Steinmann SP, Rispoli DM: The distal biceps tendon: footprint and relevant clinical anatomy, *J Hand Surg [Am]* 32:1225-1229, 2007.)

outcomes in all groups. Practically speaking, all techniques in common practice today have an acceptable complication risk and nearly comparable results.

Complications

Risks of surgery include recurrence of rupture; heterotopic ossification; injury to neurovascular structures, especially the lateral antebrachial cutaneous nerve and the posterior interosseous nerve; and persistent anterior elbow pain. Recurrence of rupture is exceedingly rare, with most series reporting a rate of 0 to 4%.

Heterotopic ossification is uncommon and likely depends on patient-related and injury-related factors rather than surgical technique. Heterotopic ossification around the elbow remains poorly understood, and the role of possible prophylaxis with nonsteroidal antiinflammatory drugs remains unclear. It has been suggested that heterotopic ossification is more common with a two-incision technique; however, this finding seems variable across series.[31,55] Nonetheless, biceps repair surgery seems particularly prone to this complication.

Injury to vascular structures around the elbow, including the lateral antebrachial cutaneous nerve and the posterior interosseous nerve, have been described. A single anterior exposure may be associated with a higher risk of neurovascular injury compared with a two-incision approach; however, injury to the posterior interosseous nerve can occur in a two-incision approach if excessive traction is placed for a prolonged period, as with a self-retaining retractor or Hohmann retractor placed over the neck of the radius. When the radial tuberosity is exposed through the posterolateral approach of the two-incision technique, the forearm should be placed in a position of pronation to allow the posterior interosseous nerve to fall further away from the surgical field.[1]

Expected Outcomes

Postoperatively, most patients are satisfied and experience a full return to flexion-extension motion. Rotation motion may be limited in some, but not all, cases, and strength and endurance in flexion can be expected to return to nearly normal. Supination strength and endurance in most series returns to normal or nearly normal, although it may be less than normal in some cases, particularly in the nondominant arm.[2,15,18,47,49]

❖ AUTHORS' PREFERRED METHOD OF TREATMENT: Partial Biceps Tears

Patients who present with a classic history of a "pop" in the arm with resisted motion and sudden onset of pain should be treated as having complete biceps tears regardless of MRI findings suggestive of "partial tear." In these cases, some strands of the distal biceps may be intact; however, they are not functional, and this lesion should be regarded as and treated as an acute complete distal biceps rupture.

Partial biceps tears are described as a chronic tendinopathy in which the patient complains of a chronic aching in the antecubital fossa, rather than a sudden onset of pain. When the diagnosis of a partial distal biceps tear is made through clinical examination and imaging modalities, treatment should be nonoperative for the first 3 to 6 months. Patients are encouraged to avoid heavy lifting and to use the arm primarily for activities of daily living only. Patients typically do not lose motion with a partial biceps tendon rupture, and strengthening exercises and physical therapy are unnecessary for these individuals. In some instances, several months of conservative management may result in symptom abatement.

In our experience, significant partial distal biceps tears commonly do not improve after even 6 months of nonoperative treatment. In this situation, operative treatment, which involves

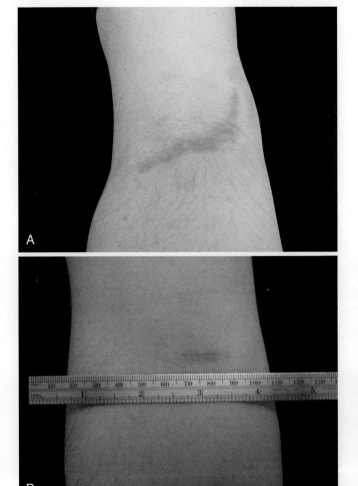

FIGURE 25.14 **A,** Large incision is required to perform repair safely via single anterior approach. **B,** Two-incision approach allows use of smaller cosmetic anterior incision. (From Hartman MW, Merten SM, Steinmann SP: Mini-open 2-incision technique for repair of distal biceps tendon ruptures, *J Shoulder Elbow Surg* 16:616-620, 2007.)

taking down the remaining fibers of the distal biceps and repair to the insertion site, has been found to be satisfactory with restoration of function and resolution of symptoms through a single posterior incision.

Treatment of Acute Complete Biceps Ruptures

Acute distal biceps ruptures are commonly seen in middle-aged men, and operative and nonoperative treatments have been advocated for these individuals. Proponents of nonoperative treatment point out the fact that patients have full flexion and extension of the elbow and are able to pronate and supinate even when seen shortly after an acute injury. Long-term studies of nonoperative treatment of biceps tendon ruptures show that with time, patients experience resolution of pain and continue to have full flexion and extension and good pronation and supination, but may continue to have functional deficits. Studies performed at the Mayo Clinic on chronic tears showed a loss of supination strength of 40% and loss of flexion strength of 30%.[21,33,115]

In our experience, many patients are told that they should be treated nonoperatively, often by a primary care provider or

family member. Quite often, these patients come to orthopedic attention because they find nonoperative care to be unsatisfactory, with functional difficulties, cosmetic complaints owing to the "Popeye muscle," and a sense of achiness and cramping in the biceps muscle itself. Although studies after nonoperative treatment show a small loss of flexion and supination strength, they cannot put a "number" on the achiness and cramping that patients often experience because the muscle-tendon unit (the biceps) has been detached and is nonfunctional. It is common to have a patient complain of a cramping and aching in the biceps that takes several hours to resolve after a vigorous day of work or play.

Operative treatment of acute distal biceps ruptures is preferred in most cases. Operative treatment tends to involve either a single anterior incision or dual incisions, one in an anterior location and one in a posterolateral location. Essentially, the literature supports use of either approach, and the individual surgeon should use the one that he or she is most comfortable with and yields the best results in his or her hands.

Single-Incision Technique

The single-incision approach typically involves either a large longitudinal (see Figure 25.14) or a boat-race type of incision that mirrors the River Thames from Putney to Mortlake as it makes an "S" shape up the arm. It is important when doing a single anterior approach to have good visualization of the radial tuberosity, which is deep in the forearm, and this involves a significant operative exposure to visualize the radial tuberosity safely. The surgery is performed under tourniquet control for this purpose.

During the exposure, the lateral antebrachial cutaneous nerve is at risk as it enters the antecubital area between the biceps and the brachialis laterally. There are multiple veins in this area that must be ligated as needed, and the radial nerve, although not directly in the area of dissection, is within a few centimeters. The significant neurovascular structures on the medial aspect of the elbow, the median nerve, and the brachial artery can be palpated and are located more medially than the biceps itself. The stump of the tendon is identified in the antecubital fossa wound or retrieved proximally if it has retracted. Dissection proceeds distally to identify the bicipital tuberosity on the radius, which can be palpated by pronating and supinating the forearm. It is cleared of tendon debris and fibrous tissue and prepared for reinsertion of the biceps tendon.

Multiple techniques have been proposed for securing the tendon to bone; essentially all have been shown to provide sufficient in vivo strength of repair. Through an anterior incision, suture anchors or endobutton devices typically are used according to the manufacturer's instructions (Video 25.1). The postoperative regimen is described subsequently in the two-incision technique. Because of the large and noncosmetic incision needed to perform this procedure safely and the difficulty in restoring the anatomic insertion site via anterior incision techniques, we prefer the two-incision technique.

Two-Incision Repair

In our hands, advantages of a two-incision technique include a more cosmetic and smaller (<2 cm) scar anteriorly (Figure 25.15; see also Figure 25.14) and the ability to restore the biceps insertion site more anatomically through the second

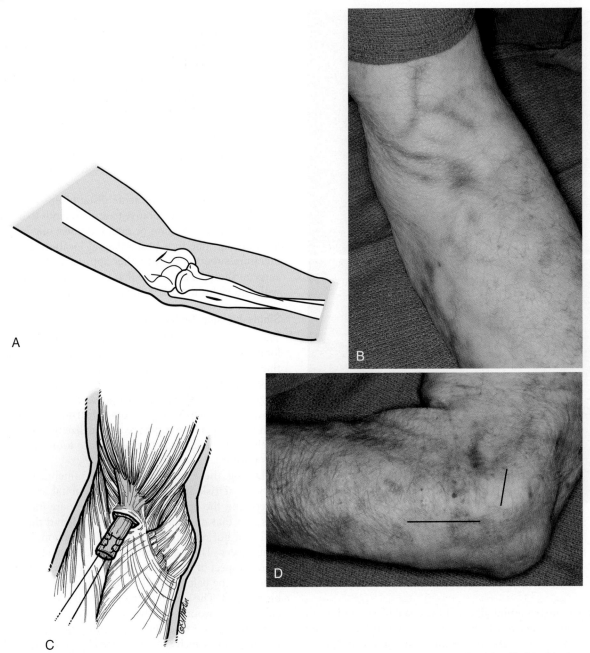

FIGURE 25.15 **A** to **D,** Two-incision approach involves short anterior transverse incision and posterolateral incision. (**C,** Copyright © Elizabeth Martin.)

posterolateral incision. The surgery is performed with the patient in the supine position, with an arm board. A sterile tourniquet is applied, and just distal to the cubital crease, a transverse incision of 2 to 3 cm is made centered over the cubital fossa (Figure 25.16; see also Figure 25.15, *B, D*). Dissection proceeds, with care taken to identify and preserve the lateral antebrachial cutaneous nerve, which lies lateral to the biceps tendon (Figure 25.17). The unwary surgeon may mistake the brachialis for an untorn biceps tendon.

The biceps tendon often retracts proximally, and blunt exploration with the surgeon's finger can retrieve the stump into the surgical wound. The end of the tendon is typically bulbous and thickened. This is débrided, and the end is

freshened up to healthy tissue and trimmed so that it fits into the tuberosity. A Krackow stitch is used with No. 2 nonabsorbable braided suture, with the tails exiting through the center of the tendon distally (Figure 25.18).

After the tendon is prepared, attention is turned to the insertion site. Multiple techniques have been proposed for securing the tendon to bone; essentially, all have been shown to provide sufficient in vivo strength of repair. We prefer a bony tunnel technique. By pronating and supinating the forearm, the biceps tuberosity can be palpated in all but the most muscular or obese patients. Intraoperative fluoroscopy can be useful in larger individuals for this purpose. An incision is made over this region (see Figure 25.15, *D*), with dissection proceeding down to the

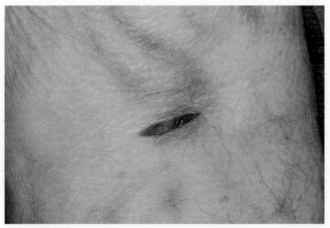

FIGURE 25.16 A 2-cm incision is made in antecubital fossa.

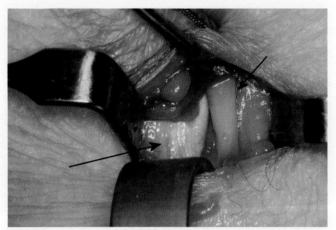

FIGURE 25.17 Lateral antebrachial cutaneous nerve *(short arrow)* lies in close proximity to biceps tendon *(long arrow)*.

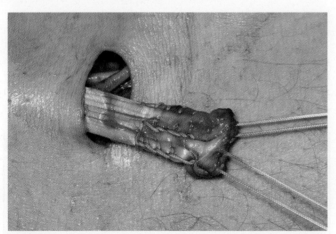

FIGURE 25.18 Krackow stitch is placed in preparation for fixation to bone. (From Hartman MW, Merten SM, Steinmann SP: Mini-open 2-incision technique for repair of distal biceps tendon ruptures, *J Shoulder Elbow Surg* 16:616-620, 2007.)

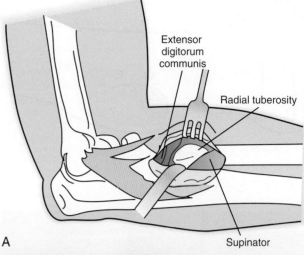

Extensor digitorum communis

Radial tuberosity

Supinator

A

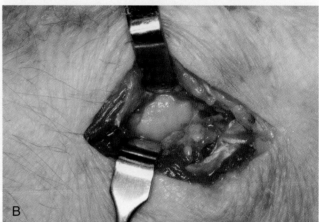

B

FIGURE 25.19 **A** and **B,** Incision is made over tuberosity, and muscle-splitting approach is made to expose tuberosity.

tuberosity, splitting the common extensors and supinator (Figure 25.19). The forearm is placed in a position of full pronation, and the tuberosity is prepared. Usually, there is retained soft tissue and tendon debris on the tuberosity; this is excised, and a bur is used to create a cancellous trough for the tendon

(Figure 25.20). The forearm is supinated slightly, bringing the radial edge of the trough into view, and two small drill holes are placed exiting into the trough. Care should be taken to allow for a sufficient bony bridge.

The suture tails of the prepared biceps stump are passed distally into the posterolateral wound (Figure 25.21). Care should be taken to exit through the muscle-splitting approach rather than exposing the ulna. The sutures are passed through the bony tunnels such that the biceps tendon is delivered into the tuberosity trough; this is facilitated by supinating the forearm slightly and may be done with the Hewson suture passer, 26-gauge wire, or a free needle. The sutures are drawn taut, and the forearm is gently supinated and pronated to seat the tendon into the tuberosity trough (Figure 25.22). Finally, the sutures are tied over the bony bridge with the forearm slightly supinated (Figure 25.23). The elbow is gently ranged in pronation-supination and flexion-extension. One can fully pronate to document seating of the tendon end into the bony cavity. The wounds are closed in layers, with a running subcuticular stitch for the skin.

Postoperative Treatment Protocol

Historically, patients have been immobilized in a cast or splint for 2 to 4 weeks before initiation of motion. More recently, early

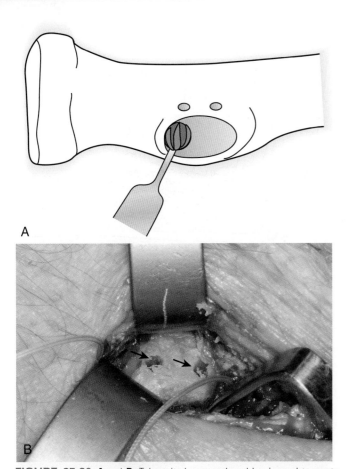

FIGURE 25.20 **A** and **B,** Tuberosity is exposed, and bur is used to create trough.

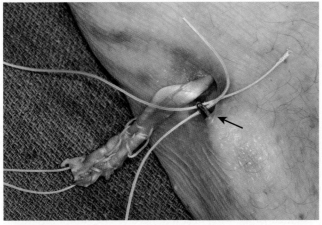

FIGURE 25.21 Tails of sutures are passed into posterolateral wound.

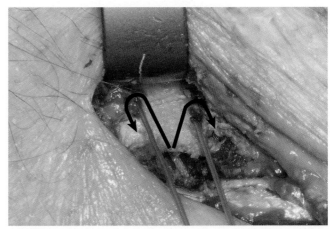

FIGURE 25.22 Sutures are drawn taut, and forearm is gently supinated and pronated to seat tendon into tuberosity.

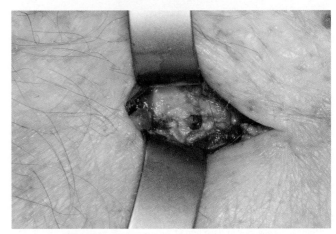

FIGURE 25.23 Sutures are tied over bony bridge.

mobilization has become more widespread, and in our experience, after a standard repair, patients can be allowed full active motion of the elbow with no resistance at 2 days postoperatively with no splinting.[77] Patients are allowed to use the arm for activities of daily living with no "lifting heavier than a telephone receiver." Passive supination and pronation with the elbow at 90 degrees of flexion are initiated within days of surgery.

With this motion protocol, at 2 to 3 weeks patients typically have a full range of motion in flexion-extension and by the end of 1 month have full pronation and supination of the elbow. Although good results in general and a high percentage of intact repairs have been reported in series where patients have been immobilized for 4 weeks or more, it has been shown that earlier mobilization of the elbow allows for high patient satisfaction and, most importantly, continuity of the repaired tendon.[77]

CRITICAL POINTS *Distal Biceps Rupture*

- Patients with the classic history of a "pop" while lifting objects and pain in the antecubital fossa almost inevitably have an acute complete distal biceps rupture.
- In most cases, acute complete distal biceps ruptures are treated operatively in younger, more active individuals.
- Chronic tendinopathy may ultimately require surgical management.
- The available literature supports either a single anterior incision or a two-incision technique.
- Most techniques have sufficient strength at the time of repair to permit early gentle active motion during the initial postoperative period.

TRICEPS AVULSIONS AND RUPTURE

Injury to the triceps may occur at the osseous insertion, at the musculotendinous junction, or as an intrasubstance muscle rupture. Avulsion from the osseous insertion is the most common pattern of injury, whereas intrasubstance rupture is the least common.[144,145,162]

Although the terms *rupture* and *avulsion* are often used interchangeably, Tarsne[162] suggested that *avulsion* be used for disruption at the osseous insertion and *rupture* be used for intrasubstance or musculotendinous disruption. It must be noted that "complete" rupture typically involves both the long and lateral tendinous heads of the triceps, with some of the deeper muscular insertion of the medial head remaining intact.

Spontaneous injury of the triceps tendon other than that associated with prior total elbow arthroplasty is rare.* At the Mayo Clinic, over a 25-year period, only 14 patients were seen with 16 triceps avulsions.[144] Of 1014 tendon injuries in one review, less than 0.8% were triceps injuries, and half of those represented open lacerations.[10]

The pathogenesis usually involves direct or indirect trauma in association with forced eccentric contraction.[10,57,79,144,145] Typically, the defect occurs at the osseous insertion. Diagnosis is usually clinical, with a palpable defect and lack of forceful active extension function. Partial ruptures may occur and are marked by decreased extension strength against resistance. Radiographs are indicated and are useful to rule out olecranon fracture or bony avulsion.[57,79,144] In addition, radial head fracture has been reported in association with this lesion.[101] MRI or ultrasound may be useful to show the pathologic changes and help differentiate between partial and complete lesions (Figure 25.24).[76,106,107,144]

Much has been speculated about predisposing factors, including enthesiopathies, medication associations, renal failure with or without hyperparathyroidism, and anabolic steroid

*References 9, 10, 13, 79, 132, 144, 145, 162, 166.

usage.[13,57,144,150,166] It seems that intrasubstance rupture is not associated with steroid use or chronic medical conditions, in contrast to avulsion or musculotendinous rupture.[11,107,121,145]

Early surgical repair is indicated for acute complete avulsions. This involves repair with locking nonabsorbable sutures attaching the tendon to the olecranon through drill holes. If a large bony fragment is present, use of hardware to fix bone to bone may facilitate earlier rehabilitation, but prominent hardware sometimes mandates later reoperation for hardware removal.[9,57,76,79,107,132,144] The arm is immobilized for approximately 3 to 4 weeks in 30 to 45 degrees of flexion, followed by gentle mobilization and, finally, active extension beginning at 6 weeks. Weight bearing or lifting should be avoided for 4 to 6 months.[9,57,144]

The treating physician should differentiate between complete avulsions and partial avulsions by assessing active elbow extension. It has been suggested that incomplete avulsions may be treated nonoperatively with close follow-up to ensure that they do not become complete.[57] In addition, some patients with partial triceps avulsions treated nonoperatively have residual weakness or functional defects, or both, and come to surgical management.[106] Chronic lesions in which local tissue is inadequate or in which retraction of the muscle tendon makes primary repair difficult may require augmentation using allograft or reconstruction with triceps aponeurosis or fascia or a local rotational anconeus flap.[37,137,140]

Intramuscular ruptures of the triceps or ruptures at the musculotendinous junction are even more rare, and the literature is mixed regarding the need for operative therapy. It has been suggested that nonoperative treatment is effective, particularly in patients who have only partial rupture and do not require full elbow extension strength.[121,145] This lesion is more likely to be seen in young patients without significant comorbidities and may be associated with sports injury.[11,121,145]

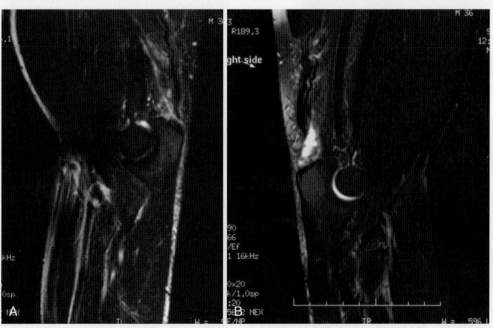

FIGURE 25.24 A and **B**, Magnetic resonance images showing avulsion of triceps with proximal retraction of musculotendinous units. (From Sierra RJ, Weiss NG, Shrader MW, et al: Acute triceps ruptures: case report and retrospective chart review, *J Shoulder Elbow Surg* 15:130-134, 2006.)

❖ AUTHORS' PREFERRED METHOD OF TREATMENT: Repair of Complete Avulsion Injuries

The surgery is performed with the patient in the supine position with the arm across the chest. A midline posterior incision is used to expose the triceps tendon (Figure 25.25). Commonly, there is a significant partial tear with a portion of the deep muscular fibers of the triceps still attached to the olecranon. Sometimes this is a delaminating tear in which the triceps splits along superficial and deep planes; similar to the situation in rotator cuff tears, the dorsal portion may have a superficially benign appearance. MRI and surgical exposure show a deeper injury to the tendon, however, than had been initially apparent.

After the tear has been exposed (Figure 25.26), any fibrous tissue or scar tissue is excised to "freshen up" the tendon edges.

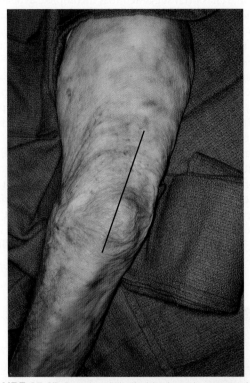

FIGURE 25.25 Posterior midline incision is used to expose triceps.

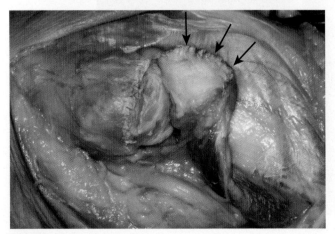

FIGURE 25.26 Triceps is exposed and prepared for reattachment to bone. *Arrows* indicate the triceps tendon.

A heavy nonabsorbable braided No. 5 suture is placed with a Krackow stitch through the triceps to prepare for reattachment to bone (Figure 25.27). The tip of the olecranon is decorticated to bleeding bone, and a 2-mm drill or Keith needle is used to create bony tunnels to pass the sutures. The sutures are passed and tied over a bony bridge (Figure 25.28). The patient is placed in a sling, and gentle motion is initiated in 1 to 2 weeks. If the repair occurs late or if myotendinous contracture has occurred, the arm should be splinted in extension for the initial 2 weeks after surgery and then slowly allowed to regain motion over the ensuing 4 to 6 weeks.

Partial tears of the triceps may sometimes present a diagnostic and therapeutic dilemma. The typical history is one in which the patient sustains an eccentric load to the elbow and presents with point tenderness over the posterior humerus and elbow. There is often tenderness at the triceps insertion. Active elbow extension is intact, however, and MRI reveals a partial triceps tear. In our experience, many patients do poorly with nonoperative therapy; however, some respond. Patients should be given a trial of conservative treatment and followed for 3 to 6 months; they may be offered surgical intervention if improvement is not seen. Of note, it is important to differentiate what can be read as a "partial triceps rupture." As discussed, in a partial rupture, no tendon has been torn and retracted proximally. A complete rupture of the long and lateral heads with some deep triceps muscle remaining intact is not a "partial" injury.

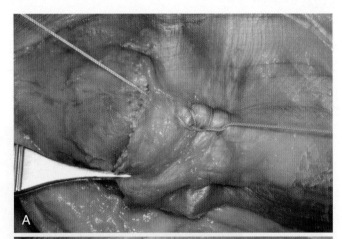

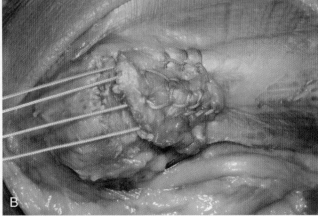

FIGURE 25.27 A and **B,** Krackow stitches are placed to secure triceps to bone.

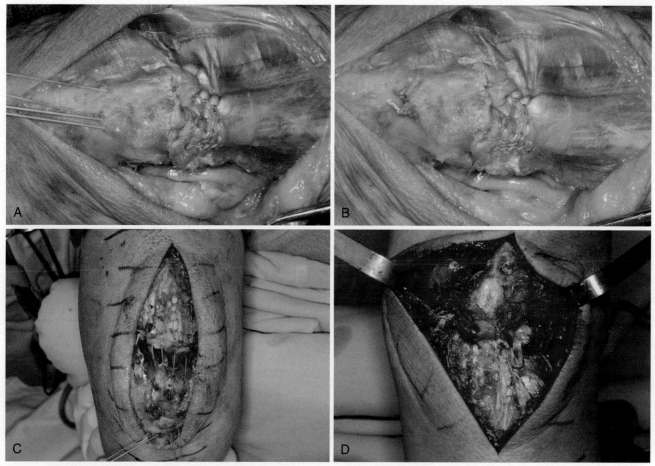

FIGURE 25.28 A to **D**, Sutures are passed through bony tunnels and tied. (**C** and **D**, From Sierra RJ, Weiss NG, Shrader MW, et al: Acute triceps ruptures: case report and retrospective chart review, *J Shoulder Elbow Surg* 15:130-134, 2006.)

CRITICAL POINTS *Triceps Avulsions and Ruptures*

- Triceps injuries are rare.
- Injuries may occur at the tendinous insertion (avulsion), as a rupture at the musculotendinous junction, or as an intramuscular rupture.
- Early repair of avulsions is generally preferred.

For Case Studies, Videos, and more, please visit ExpertConsult.com.

REFERENCES

1. Adams JE, Steinmann SP: Nerve injuries about the elbow. *J Hand Surg [Am]* 31:303–313, 2006.
2. Agins HJ, Chess JL, Hoekstra DV, et al: Rupture of the distal insertion of the biceps brachii tendon. *Clin Orthop Relat Res* 234:34–38, 1988.
3. Almekinders LC: Tendinitis and other chronic tendinopathies. *J Am Acad Orthop Surg* 6:157–164, 1998.
4. Almekinders LC, Temple JD: Etiology, diagnosis, and treatment of tendonitis: an analysis of the literature. *Med Sci Sports Exerc* 30:1183–1190, 1998.
5. Almquist EE, Necking L, Bach AW: Epicondylar resection with anconeus muscle transfer for chronic lateral epicondylitis. *J Hand Surg [Am]* 23:723–731, 1998.
6. Altay T, Gunal I, Ozturk H: Local injection treatment for lateral epicondylitis. *Clin Orthop Relat Res* 398:127–130, 2002.
7. Alvarez-Nemegyei J, Canoso JJ: Evidence-based soft tissue rheumatology: epicondylitis and hand stenosing tendinopathy. *J Clin Rheumatol* 10:33–40, 2004.
8. Anakwenze OA, Baldwin K, Abboud JA: Distal biceps tendon repair: an analysis of timing of surgery on outcomes. *J Athl Train* 48(1):9–11, 2013.
9. Anderson KJ, Lecocq JF: Rupture of the triceps tendon. *J Bone Joint Surg Am* 39:444–446, 1957.
10. Anzel SH, Covey KW, Weiner AD, et al: Disruption of muscles and tendons: an analysis of 1,014 cases. *Surgery* 45:406–414, 1959.
11. Aso K, Torisu T: Muscle belly tear of the triceps. *Am J Sports Med* 12:485–487, 1984.
12. Athwal GS, Steinmann SP, Rispoli DM: The distal biceps tendon: footprint and relevant clinical anatomy. *J Hand Surg [Am]* 32:1225–1229, 2007.
13. Bach BR, Jr, Warren RF, Wickiewicz TL: Triceps rupture: a case report and literature review. *Am J Sports Med* 15:285–289, 1987.
14. Bain GI, Johnson LJ, Turner PC: Treatment of partial distal biceps tendon tears. *Sports Med Arthrosc* 16:154–161, 2008.
15. Baker BE, Bierwagen D: Rupture of the distal tendon of the biceps brachii: operative versus non-operative treatment. *J Bone Joint Surg Am* 67:414–417, 1985.
16. Baker CL, Jr, Baker CL, 3rd: Long-term follow-up of arthroscopic treatment of lateral epicondylitis. *Am J Sports Med* 36:254–260, 2008.
17. Baker CL, Jr, Murphy KP, Gottlob CA, et al: Arthroscopic classification and treatment of lateral epicondylitis: two-year clinical results. *J Shoulder Elbow Surg* 9:475–482, 2000.
18. Balabaud L, Ruiz C, Nonnenmacher J, et al: Repair of distal biceps tendon ruptures using a suture anchor and an anterior approach. *J Hand Surg [Br]* 29:178–182, 2004.
19. Bauman JT, Sotereanos DG, Weiser RW: Complete rupture of the distal biceps tendon in a woman: case report. *J Hand Surg [Am]* 31:798–800, 2006.
20. Baumgard SH, Schwartz DR: Percutaneous release of the epicondylar muscles for humeral epicondylitis. *Am J Sports Med* 10:233–236, 1982.
21. Bell RH, Wiley WB, Noble JS, et al: Repair of distal biceps brachii tendon ruptures. *J Shoulder Elbow Surg* 9:223–226, 2000.
22. Belli P, Costantini M, Mirk P, et al: Sonographic diagnosis of distal biceps tendon rupture: a prospective study of 25 cases. *J Ultrasound Med* 20:587–595, 2001.
23. Bennett JB: Lateral and medial epicondylitis. *Hand Clin* 10:157–163, 1994.
24. Berlet GC, Johnson JA, Milne AD, et al: Distal biceps brachii tendon repair: an in vitro biomechanical study of tendon reattachment. *Am J Sports Med* 26:428–432, 1998.

25. Binder AI, Hazleman BL: Lateral humeral epicondylitis—a study of natural history and the effect of conservative therapy. *Br J Rheumatol* 22:73–76, 1983.

26. Bisset L, Paungmali A, Vicenzino B, et al: A systematic review and meta-analysis of clinical trials on physical interventions for lateral epicondylalgia. *Br J Sports Med* 39:411–422, discussion 411–422, 2005.

27. Bisson L, Moyer M, Lanighan K, et al: Complications associated with repair of a distal biceps rupture using the modified two- incision technique. *J Shoulder Elbow Surg* 17(1 Suppl):67S–71S, 2008.

28. Boyer MI, Hastings H, 2nd: Lateral tennis elbow. "Is there any science out there?" *J Shoulder Elbow Surg* 8:481–491, 1999.

29. Budoff JE, Hicks JM, Ayala G, et al: The reliability of the "scratch test." *J Hand Surg Eur Vol* 33:166–169, 2008.

30. Bunata RE, Brown DS, Capelo R: Anatomic factors related to the cause of tennis elbow. *J Bone Joint Surg Am* 89:1955–1963, 2007.

31. Chavan PR, Duquin TR, Bisson LJ: Repair of the ruptured distal biceps tendon: a systematic review. *Am J Sports Med* 36:1618–1624, 2008.

32. Chew ML, Giuffre BM: Disorders of the distal biceps brachii tendon. *Radiographics* 25:1227–1237, 2005.

33. Chillemi C, Marinelli M, De Cupis V: Rupture of the distal biceps brachii tendon: conservative treatment versus anatomic reinsertion—clinical and radiological evaluation after 2 years. *Arch Orthop Trauma Surg* 127:705–708, 2007.

34. Chung B, Wiley JP: Effectiveness of extracorporeal shock wave therapy in the treatment of previously untreated lateral epicondylitis: a randomized controlled trial. *Am J Sports Med* 32:1660–1667, 2004.

35. Ciccotti MC, Schwartz MA, Ciccotti MG: Diagnosis and treatment of medial epicondylitis of the elbow. *Clin Sports Med* 23:693–705, xi, 2004.

36. Ciccotti MG, Ramani MN: Medial epicondylitis. *Tech Hand Up Extrem Surg* 7:190–196, 2003.

37. Clayton ML, Thirupathi RG: Rupture of the triceps tendon with olecranon bursitis: a case report with a new method of repair. *Clin Orthop Relat Res* 184:183–185, 1984.

38. Cohen MS: Complications of distal biceps tendon repairs. *Sports Med Arthrosc* 16:148–153, 2008.

39. Cohen MS, Romeo AA, Hennigan SP, et al: Lateral epicondylitis: anatomic relationships of the extensor tendon origins and implications for arthroscopic treatment. *J Shoulder Elbow Surg* 17:954–960, 2008.

40. Connell DA, Ali KE, Ahmad M, et al: Ultrasound-guided autologous blood injection for tennis elbow. *Skeletal Radiol* 35:371–377, 2006.

41. Coombes BK, Bisset L, Brooks P, et al: Effect of corticosteroid injection, physiotherapy, or both on clinical outcomes in patients with unilateral lateral epicondylalgia: a randomized controlled trial. *JAMA* 309(5):461, 2013.

42. Coonrad RW, Hooper WR: Tennis elbow: its course, natural history, conservative and surgical management. *J Bone Joint Surg Am* 55:1177–1182, 1973.

43. Cowan J, Lozano-Calderon S, Ring D: Quality of prospective controlled randomized trials: analysis of trials of treatment for lateral epicondylitis as an example. *J Bone Joint Surg Am* 89:1693–1699, 2007.

44. Cummins CA: Lateral epicondylitis: in vivo assessment of arthroscopic debridement and correlation with patient outcomes. *Am J Sports Med* 34:1486–1491, 2006.

45. Cyriax JH: Tennis elbow. *BMJ* 559:1937.

46. Cyriax JH: The pathology and treatment of tennis elbow. *J Bone Joint Surg Br* 18:921–940, 1936.

47. D'Alessandro DF, Shields CL, Jr, Tibone JE, et al: Repair of distal biceps tendon ruptures in athletes. *Am J Sports Med* 21:114–119, 1993.

48. D'Vaz AP, Ostor AJ, Speed CA, et al: Pulsed low-intensity ultrasound therapy for chronic lateral epicondylitis: a randomized controlled trial. *Rheumatology (Oxf)* 45:566–570, 2006.

49. Davison BL, Engber WD, Tigert LJ: Long term evaluation of repaired distal biceps brachii tendon ruptures. *Clin Orthop Relat Res* 333:186–191, 1996.

50. Dellaero DT, Mallon WJ: Surgical treatment of partial biceps tendon ruptures at the elbow. *J Shoulder Elbow Surg* 15:215–217, 2006.

51. Descatha A, Leclerc A, Chastang JF, et al: Medial epicondylitis in occupational settings: prevalence, incidence and associated risk factors. *J Occup Environ Med* 45:993–1001, 2003.

52. Dunn JH, Kim JJ, Davis L, et al: Ten- to 14-year follow-up of the Nirschl surgical technique for lateral epicondylitis. *Am J Sports Med* 36:261–266, 2008.

53. Eames MH, Bain GI, Fogg QA, et al: Distal biceps tendon anatomy: a cadaveric study. *J Bone Joint Surg Am* 89:1044–1049, 2007.

54. Edwards SG, Calandruccio JH: Autologous blood injections for refractory lateral epicondylitis. *J Hand Surg [Am]* 28:272–278, 2003.

55. El-Hawary R, Macdermid JC, Faber KJ, et al: Distal biceps tendon repair: comparison of surgical techniques. *J Hand Surg [Am]* 28:496–502, 2003.

56. Falchook FS, Zlatkin MB, Erbacher GE, et al: Rupture of the distal biceps tendon: evaluation with MR imaging. *Radiology* 190:659–663, 1994.

57. Farrar EL, 3rd, Lippert FG, 3rd: Avulsion of the triceps tendon. *Clin Orthop Relat Res* 161:242–246, 1981.

58. Fitzgerald SW, Curry DR, Erickson SJ, et al: Distal biceps tendon injury: MR imaging diagnosis. *Radiology* 191:203–206, 1994.

59. Freeman CR, McCormick KR, Mahoney D, et al: Nonoperative treatment of distal biceps tendon ruptures compared with a historical control group. *J Bone Joint Surg Am* 91(10):2329, 2009.

60. Furia JP: Safety and efficacy of extracorporeal shock wave therapy for chronic lateral epicondylitis. *Am J Orthop* 34:13–19, discussion 19, 2005.

61. Gabel GT: Acute and chronic tendinopathies at the elbow. *Curr Opin Rheumatol* 11:138–143, 1999.

62. Gabel GT, Morrey BF: Operative treatment of medical epicondylitis: influence of concomitant ulnar neuropathy at the elbow. *J Bone Joint Surg Am* 77:1065–1069, 1995.

63. Gabel GT, Morrey BF: Tennis elbow. *Instr Course Lect* 47:165–172, 1998.

64. Galliani I, Burattini S, Mariani AR, et al: Morpho-functional changes in human tendon tissue. *Eur J Histochem* 46:3–12, 2002.

65. Galloway M, DeMaio M, Mangine R: Rehabilitative techniques in the treatment of medial and lateral epicondylitis. *Orthopedics* 15:1089–1096, 1992.

66. Gardner RC: Tennis elbow: diagnosis, pathology and treatment. Nine severe cases treated by a new reconstructive operation. *Clin Orthop Relat Res* 72:248–253, 1970.

67. Geaney LE, Brenneman DJ, Cote MP, et al: Outcomes and practical information for patients choosing nonoperative treatment for distal biceps ruptures. *Orthopedics* 33(6):391, 2010.

68. Giangarra CE, Conroy B, Jobe FW, et al: Electromyographic and cinematographic analysis of elbow function in tennis players using single- and double-handed backhand strokes. *Am J Sports Med* 21:394–399, 1993.

69. Giuffre BM, Moss MJ: Optimal positioning for MRI of the distal biceps brachii tendon: flexed abducted supinated view. *AJR Am J Roentgenol* 182:944–946, 2004.

70. Gosens T, Peerbooms JC, van Laar W, et al: Ongoing positive effect of platelet-rich plasma versus corticosteroid injection in lateral epicondylitis: a double-blind randomized controlled trial with 2-year follow-up. *Am J Sports Med* 39(6):1200, 2011.

71. Grewal R, Athwal GS, MacDermid JC, et al: Single vs double incision technique for the repair of acute distal biceps ruptures: a randomized clinical trial. *J Bone Joint Surg Am* 94(13):1166–1174, 2012.

72. Grifka J, Boenke S, Kramer J: Endoscopic therapy in epicondylitis radialis humeri. *Arthroscopy* 11:743–748, 1995.

73. Grundberg AB, Dobson JF: Percutaneous release of the common extensor origin for tennis elbow. *Clin Orthop Relat Res* 376:137–140, 2000.

74. Hales TR, Bernard BP: Epidemiology of work-related musculoskeletal disorders. *Orthop Clin North Am* 27:679–709, 1996.

75. Hamilton PG: The prevalence of humeral epicondylitis: a survey in general practice. *J R Coll Gen Pract* 36:464–465, 1986.

76. Harris PC, Atkinson D, Moorehead JD: Bilateral partial rupture of triceps tendon: case report and quantitative assessment of recovery. *Am J Sports Med* 32:787–792, 2004.

77. Hartman MW, Merten SM, Steinmann SP: Mini-open 2-incision technique for repair of distal biceps tendon ruptures. *J Shoulder Elbow Surg* 16:616–620, 2007.

78. Ho C: Extracorporeal shock wave treatment for chronic lateral epicondylitis (tennis elbow). *Issues Emerg Health Technol* 96(Pt 2):1–4, 2007.

79. Holleb PD, Bach BR, Jr: Triceps brachii injuries. *Sports Med* 10:273–276, 1990.

80. Hutchinson HL, Gloystein D, Gillespie M: Distal biceps tendon insertion: an anatomic study. *J Shoulder Elbow Surg* 17:342–346, 2008.

81. Jerosch J, Schunck J: Arthroscopic treatment of lateral epicondylitis: indication, technique and early results. *Knee Surg Sports Traumatol Arthrosc* 14:379–382, 2006.

82. Kalichman L, Bannuru RR, Severin M, et al: Injection of botulinum toxin for treatment of chronic lateral epicondylitis: systematic review and meta-analysis. *Semin Arthritis Rheum* 40(6):532, 2011.

83. Kazemi M, Azma K, Tavana B, et al: Autologous blood vs corticosteroid local injection in the short term treatment of lateral elbow tendinopathy: a randomized clinical trial of efficacy. *Am J Phys Med Rehabil* 89(8):660–667, 2010.

84. Kelly EW, Steinmann S, O'Driscoll SW: Surgical treatment of partial distal biceps tendon ruptures through a single posterior incision. *J Shoulder Elbow Surg* 12:456–461, 2003.

85. Kettler M, Lunger J, Kuhn V, et al: Failure strengths in distal biceps tendon repair. *Am J Sports Med* 35:1544–1548, 2007.

86. Kettler M, Tingart MJ, Lunger J, et al: Reattachment of the distal tendon of biceps: factors affecting the failure strength of the repair. *J Bone Joint Surg Br* 90:103–106, 2008.

87. Khan AD, Penna S, Yin Q, et al: Repair of distal biceps tendon ruptures using suture anchors through a single anterior incision. *Arthroscopy* 24:39–45, 2008.

88. Khan KM, Cook JL, Bonar F, et al: Histopathology of common tendinopathies: update and implications for clinical management. *Sports Med* 27:393–408, 1999.

89. Kijowski R, De Smet AA: Magnetic resonance imaging findings in patients with medial epicondylitis. *Skeletal Radiol* 34:196–202, 2005.

90. Korthals-de Bos IB, Smidt N, van Tulder MW, et al: Cost effectiveness of interventions for lateral epicondylitis: results from a randomised controlled trial in primary care. *Pharmacoeconomics* 22:185–195, 2004.

91. Kraushaar BS, Nirschl RP: Tendinosis of the elbow (tennis elbow): clinical features and findings of histological, immunohistochemical, and electron microscopy studies. *J Bone Joint Surg Am* 81:259–278, 1999.

92. Krischek O, Hopf C, Nafe B, et al: Shock-wave therapy for tennis and golfer's elbow—1 year follow-up. *Arch Orthop Trauma Surg* 119(1–2):62–66, 1999.

93. Krogh TP, Bartels EM, Ellingsen T, et al: Comparative effectiveness of injection therapies in lateral epicondylitis: a systematic review and network meta-analysis of randomized controlled trials. *Am J Sports Med* 41(6):1435, 2013.

94. Krogh TP, Fredberg U, Stengaard-Pedersen K, et al: Treatment of lateral epicondylitis with platelet rich plasma, glucocorticoid, or saline: a randomized, double-blind, placebo controlled trial. *Am J Sports Med* 41(3):625, 2013.

95. Kuklo TR, Taylor KF, Murphy KP, et al: Arthroscopic release for lateral epicondylitis: a cadaveric model. *Arthroscopy* 15:259–264, 1999.

96. Kurppa K, Viikari-Juntura E, Kuosma E, et al: Incidence of tenosynovitis or peritendinitis and epicondylitis in a meat-processing factory. *Scand J Work Environ Health* 17:32–37, 1991.

97. Kurvers H, Verhaar J: The results of operative treatment of medial epicondylitis. *J Bone Joint Surg Am* 77:1374–1379, 1995.

98. Leach RE, Miller JK: Lateral and medial epicondylitis of the elbow. *Clin Sports Med* 6:259–272, 1987.

99. Leadbetter WB: Cell-matrix response in tendon injury. *Clin Sports Med* 11:533–578, 1992.

100. Lebrun CM: Low-dose extracorporeal shock wave therapy for previously untreated lateral epicondylitis. *Clin J Sport Med* 15:401–402, 2005.

101. Levy M, Fishel RE, Stern GM: Triceps tendon avulsion with or without fracture of the radial head—a rare injury? *J Trauma* 18:677–679, 1978.

102. Lindenhovius A, Henket M, Gilligan BP, et al: Injection of dexamethasone versus placebo for lateral elbow pain: a prospective, double-blind, randomized clinical trial. *J Hand Surg [Am]* 33:909–919, 2008.

103. Lo MY, Safran MR: Surgical treatment of lateral epicondylitis: a systematic review. *Clin Orthop Relat Res* 463:98–106, 2007.

104. Luchetti R, Atzei A, Brunelli F, et al: Anconeus muscle transposition for chronic lateral epicondylitis, recurrences, and complications. *Tech Hand Up Extrem Surg* 9:105–112, 2005.

105. Luopajarvi T, Kuorinka I, Virolainen M, et al: Prevalence of tenosynovitis and other injuries of the upper extremities in repetitive work. *Scand J Work Environ Health* 5(Suppl 3):48–55, 1979.

106. Madsen M, Marx RG, Millett PJ, et al: Surgical anatomy of the triceps brachii tendon: anatomical study and clinical correlation. *Am J Sports Med* 34:1839–1843, 2006.

107. Mair SD, Isbell WM, Gill TJ, et al: Triceps tendon ruptures in professional football players. *Am J Sports Med* 32:431–434, 2004.

108. Martin CE, Schweitzer ME: MR imaging of epicondylitis. *Skeletal Radiol* 27:133–138, 1998.

109. Mazzocca AD, Cohen M, Berkson E, et al: The anatomy of the bicipital tuberosity and distal biceps tendon. *J Shoulder Elbow Surg* 16:122–127, 2007.

110. McCluskey GM: Open treatment of medial epicondylitis. In Yamaguchi K, King GW, McKee MD, et al, editors: *Advanced reconstruction elbow*, Chicago, 2007, American Academy of Orthopaedic Surgeons, pp 137–142.

111. McCluskey GM, Merkley MS: Lateral and medial epicondylitis. In Baker CL, Jr, Plancher KD, editors: *Operative treatment of elbow injuries*, New York, 2002, Springer.

112. Milz S, Tischer T, Buettner A, et al: Molecular composition and pathology of entheses on the medial and lateral epicondyles of the humerus: a structural basis for epicondylitis. *Ann Rheum Dis* 63:1015–1021, 2004.

113. Mishra AK, Skrepnik NV, Edwards SG, et al: Efficacy of platelet-rich plasma for chronic tennis elbow: a double-blind prospective, multi center, randomized controlled trial of 230 patients. *Am J Sports Med* 42(2):463–471, 2014.

114. Morrey BF: Tendon injuries about the elbow. In Morrey BF, editor: *The elbow and its disorders*, Philadelphia, 1993, WB Saunders, pp 492–504.

115. Morrey BF, Askew LJ, An KN, et al: Rupture of the distal tendon of the biceps brachii: a biomechanical study. *J Bone Joint Surg Am* 67:418–421, 1985.

116. Morris H: Lawn tennis elbow. *BMJ* 2:557, 1883.

117. Newcomer KL, Laskowski ER, Idank DM, et al: Corticosteroid injection in early treatment of lateral epicondylitis. *Clin J Sport Med* 11:214–222, 2001.

118. Nirschl RP: Elbow tendinosis/tennis elbow. *Clin Sports Med* 11:851–870, 1992.

119. Nirschl RP: Prevention and treatment of elbow and shoulder injuries in the tennis player. *Clin Sports Med* 7:289–308, 1988.

120. Nirschl RP, Pettrone FA: Tennis elbow: The surgical treatment of lateral epicondylitis. *J Bone Joint Surg Am* 61:832–839, 1979.

121. O'Driscoll SW: Intramuscular triceps rupture. *Can J Surg* 35:203–207, 1992.

122. O'Driscoll SW, Goncalves LB, Dietz P: The hook test for distal biceps tendon avulsion. *Am J Sports Med* 35:1865–1869, 2007.

123. Olaussen M, Holmedal O, Lindbaek M, et al: Treating lateral epicondylitis with corticosteroid injections or non-electrotherapeutical physiotherapy: a systematic review. *BMJ Open* 3(10):29, 2013.

124. Ollivierre CO, Nirschl RP, Pettrone FA: Resection and repair for medial tennis elbow: a prospective analysis. *Am J Sports Med* 23:214–221, 1995.

125. Organ SW, Nirschl RP, Kraushaar BS, et al: Salvage surgery for lateral tennis elbow. *Am J Sports Med* 25:746–750, 1997.

126. Owens BD, Murphy KP, Kuklo TR: Arthroscopic release for lateral epicondylitis. *Arthroscopy* 17:582–587, 2001.

127. Park GY, Lee SM, Lee MY: Diagnostic value of ultrasonography for clinical medial epicondylitis. *Arch Phys Med Rehabil* 89:738–742, 2008.

128. Pattanittum P, Turner T, Green S, et al: Non-steroidal anti-inflammatory drugs (NSAIDs) for treating lateral elbow pain in adults. *Cochrane Database Syst Rev* 5:CD003686, 2013.

129. Peart RE, Strickler SS, Schweitzer KM, Jr: Lateral epicondylitis: a comparative study of open and arthroscopic lateral release. *Am J Orthop* 33:565–567, 2004.

130. Potter HG, Hannafin JA, Morwessel RM, et al: Lateral epicondylitis: correlation of MR imaging, surgical, and histopathologic findings. *Radiology* 196:43–46, 1995.

131. Price R, Sinclair H, Heinrich I, et al: Local injection treatment of tennis elbow—hydrocortisone, triamcinolone and lignocaine compared. *Br J Rheumatol* 30:39–44, 1991.

132. Rajasekhar C, Kakarlapudi TK, Bhamra MS: Avulsion of the triceps tendon. *Emerg Med J* 19:271–272, 2002.

133. Regan W, Wold LE, Coonrad R, et al: Microscopic histopathology of chronic refractory lateral epicondylitis. *Am J Sports Med* 20:746–749, 1992.

134. Ritz BR: Humeral epicondylitis among gas- and waterworks employees. *Scand J Work Environ Health* 21:478–486, 1995.

135. Roetert EP, Brody H, Dillman CJ, et al: The biomechanics of tennis elbow: an integrated approach. *Clin Sports Med* 14:47–57, 1995.

136. Rompe JD, Decking J, Schoellner C, et al: Repetitive low-energy shock wave treatment for chronic lateral epicondylitis in tennis players. *Am J Sports Med* 32:734–743, 2004.

137. Sanchez-Sotelo J, Morrey BF: Surgical techniques for reconstruction of chronic insufficiency of the triceps: Rotation flap using anconeus and tendon Achilles allograft. *J Bone Joint Surg Br* 84:1116–1120, 2002.

138. Sanchez-Sotelo J, Morrey BF, Adams RA, et al: Reconstruction of chronic ruptures of the distal biceps tendon with use of an Achilles tendon allograft. *J Bone Joint Surg Am* 84:999–1005, 2002.

139. Savnik A, Jensen B, Norregaard J, et al: Magnetic resonance imaging in the evaluation of treatment response of lateral epicondylitis of the elbow. *Eur Radiol* 14:964–969, 2004.

140. Schmidt CC, Kohut GN, Greenberg JA, et al: The anconeus muscle flap: its anatomy and clinical application. *J Hand Surg [Am]* 24:359–369, 1999.

141. Schmidt CC, Brown BT, Sawardeker PJ, et al: Factors affecting supination strength after a distal biceps rupture. *J Shoulder Elbow Surg* 23(1):68, 2014.

142. Sems A, Dimeff R, Iannotti JP: Extracorporeal shock wave therapy in the treatment of chronic tendinopathies. *J Am Acad Orthop Surg* 14:195–204, 2006.

143. Shiri R, Viikari-Juntura E, Varonen H, et al: Prevalence and determinants of lateral and medial epicondylitis: a population study. *Am J Epidemiol* 164:1065–1074, 2006.

144. Sierra RJ, Weiss NG, Shrader MW, et al: Acute triceps ruptures: case report and retrospective chart review. *J Shoulder Elbow Surg* 15:130–134, 2006.

145. Singh RK, Pooley J: Complete rupture of the triceps brachii muscle. *Br J Sports Med* 36:467–469, 2002.

146. Smidt N, Assendelft WJ, van der Windt DA, et al: Corticosteroid injections for lateral epicondylitis: a systematic review. *Pain* 96(1–2):23–40, 2002.

147. Smidt N, Lewis M, van der Windt DA, et al: Lateral epicondylitis in general practice: course and prognostic indicators of outcome. *J Rheumatol* 33:2053–2059, 2006.

148. Smidt N, van der Windt DA, Assendelft WJ, et al: Corticosteroid injections, physiotherapy, or a wait-and-see policy for lateral epicondylitis: a randomised controlled trial. *Lancet* 359:657–662, 2002.

149. Smith AM, Castle JA, Ruch DS: Arthroscopic resection of the common extensor origin: anatomic considerations. *J Shoulder Elbow Surg* 12:375–379, 2003.

150. Sollender JL, Rayan GM, Barden GA: Triceps tendon rupture in weight lifters. *J Shoulder Elbow Surg* 7:151–153, 1998.

151. Spacca G, Necozione S, Cacchio A: Radial shock wave therapy for lateral epicondylitis: a prospective randomised controlled single-blind study. *Eura Medicophys* 41:17–25, 2005.

152. Speed CA, Nichols D, Richards C, et al: Extracorporeal shock wave therapy for lateral epicondylitis—a double blind randomised controlled trial. *J Orthop Res* 20:895–898, 2002.

153. Spencer GE, Jr, Herndon CH: Surgical treatment of epicondylitis. *J Bone Joint Surg Am* 35:421–424, 1953.

154. Stahl S, Kaufman T: The efficacy of an injection of steroids for medial epicondylitis: a prospective study of sixty elbows. *J Bone Joint Surg Am* 79:1648–1652, 1997.

155. Stanley J: Radial tunnel syndrome: a surgeon's perspective. *J Hand Ther* 19:180–184, 2006.

156. Staples MP, Forbes A, Ptasznik R, et al: A randomized controlled trial of extracorporeal shock wave therapy for lateral epicondylitis (tennis elbow). *J Rheumatol* 35:2038–2046, 2008.

157. Stasinopoulos D, Johnson MI: Effectiveness of extracorporeal shock wave therapy for tennis elbow (lateral epicondylitis). *Br J Sports Med* 39:132–136, 2005.

158. Steinborn M, Heuck A, Jessel C, et al: Magnetic resonance imaging of lateral epicondylitis of the elbow with a 0.2-T dedicated system. *Eur Radiol* 9:1376–1380, 1999.

159. Steinmann SP: Elbow arthroscopy: where are we now? *Arthroscopy* 23:1231–1236, 2007.

160. Suresh SP, Ali KE, Jones H, et al: Medial epicondylitis: is ultrasound guided autologous blood injection an effective treatment? *Br J Sports Med* 40:935–939, discussion 939, 2006.

161. Szabo SJ, Savoie FH, 3rd, Field LD, et al: Tendinosis of the extensor carpi radialis brevis: an evaluation of three methods of operative treatment. *J Shoulder Elbow Surg* 15:721–727, 2006.

162. Tarsney FF: Rupture and avulsion of the triceps. *Clin Orthop Relat Res* 83:177–183, 1972.

163. Thanasas C, Papadimitriou G, Charalambidis C, et al: Platelet-rich plasma vs autologous whole blood for the treatment of chronic lateral elbow epicondylitis: a randomized controlled clinical trial. *Am J Sports Med* 39(10):2130–2134, 2011.

164. Tonks JH, Pai SK, Murali SR: Steroid injection therapy is the best conservative treatment for lateral epicondylitis: a prospective randomised controlled trial. *Int J Clin Pract* 61:240–246, 2007.

165. Tseng V: Arthroscopic lateral release for treatment of tennis elbow. *Arthroscopy* 10:335–336, 1994.

166. Tsourvakas S, Gouvalas K, Gimtsas C, et al: Bilateral and simultaneous rupture of the triceps tendons in chronic renal failure and secondary hyperparathyroidism. *Arch Orthop Trauma Surg* 124:278–280, 2004.

167. Uzunca K, Birtane M, Tastekin N: Effectiveness of pulsed electromagnetic field therapy in lateral epicondylitis. *Clin Rheumatol* 26:69–74, 2007.

168. Vangsness CT, Jr, Jobe FW: Surgical treatment of medial epicondylitis: results in 35 elbows. *J Bone Joint Surg Br* 73:409–411, 1991.

169. Verhaar JA, Walenkamp GH, van Mameren H, et al: Local corticosteroid injection versus Cyriax-type physiotherapy for tennis elbow. *J Bone Joint Surg Br* 78:128–132, 1996.

170. Wang CJ: An overview of shock wave therapy in musculoskeletal disorders. *Chang Gung Med J* 26:220–232, 2003.

171. Wang CJ, Chen HS: Shock wave therapy for patients with lateral epicondylitis of the elbow: a one- to two-year follow-up study. *Am J Sports Med* 30:422–425, 2002.

172. Wilson BP, Kocheta AA, Forgacs B: Two-level complete rupture of the distal biceps tendon in a woman: a case report. *J Shoulder Elbow Surg* 17:e1–e3, 2008.

173. Wolf JM, Ozer K, Scott F, et al: Comparison of autologous blood, corticosteroid, and saline injection in the treatment of lateral epicondylitis: a prospective, randomized, controlled, multi center trial. *J Hand Surg [Am]* 36(8):1269, 2011.

174. Wong SM, Hui AC, Tong PY, et al: Treatment of lateral epicondylitis with botulinum toxin: a randomized, double-blind, placebo-controlled trial. *Ann Intern Med* 143:793–797, 2005.

175. Yerger B, Turner T: Percutaneous extensor tenotomy for chronic tennis elbow: an office procedure. *Orthopedics* 8:1261–1263, 1985.

176. Zhu J, Hu B, Xing C, et al: Ultrasound-guided, minimally invasive, percutaneous needle puncture treatment for tennis elbow. *Adv Ther* 25:1031–1036, 2008.

26

Elbow Arthroscopy

George S. Athwal

Acknowledgment: The author would like to acknowledge Dr. Laura Kember for her assistance with the preparation of this manuscript.

Arthroscopy of the elbow, as with arthroscopy of other joints, has undergone a transition from simple diagnostic procedures to complex advanced procedures for the management of stiffness, fractures, and arthritis. The technical advances in elbow arthroscopy have been possible because of an improved understanding of anatomy, the use of safe portals, and the development of improved instruments and motorized tools specific to arthroscopy. In addition, transitional techniques have been developed, such as miniopen procedures and the use of arthroscopic retractors to improve visualization and protect adjacent neurovascular structures. Presently, the accepted indications[46] for elbow arthroscopy include the treatment of rheumatoid arthritis, degenerative arthritis, lateral epicondylitis, synovitis, osteochondritis dissecans, loose bodies, symptomatic plica, infection, contracture, instability, and fractures of the coronoid, capitellum, trochlea, and radial head. Unfortunately, as the complexity of elbow arthroscopy procedures increases, so does the risk of complications. Complications encountered with elbow arthroscopy include nerve injury, vascular injury, infection, instability, and stiffness. The purpose of this chapter is to describe the various techniques of elbow arthroscopy for the management of the aforementioned disorders. Specifically, débridement of an osteoarthritic elbow with hypertrophic osteophytes requiring a capsulectomy will be used as a representative example.

PREOPERATIVE EVALUATION

The detailed disease-specific evaluation of the patient who may benefit from elbow arthroscopy is beyond the scope of this chapter. A comprehensive history is mandatory, detailing the location of injury or disease; the hand dominance; the symptoms, such as pain or numbness, and situations that exacerbate symptoms; the mechanism of injury; the patient's medical history, including medications taken and prior nonoperative and operative treatments; the patient's occupation; and the presence of allergies. Signs and symptoms specific to the disease process should be sought. For example, with rheumatoid arthritis, the history would include questions about pain and swelling affecting multiple joints, cervical spine involvement, and the use of biologic agents.

Symptoms specifically of the elbow should be documented, such as impingement pain at the extremes of flexion and extension, joint locking or snapping, instability, numbness, and the location of pain (in the anterior, medial, lateral, or posterior elbow).

Physical Examination

Examination of the elbow should take a general approach consisting of inspection, palpation, and evaluation of active and passive range of motion and the neurovascular status. Tests for specific diseases should be conducted as indicated.

Inspection of the elbow should include an assessment of deformities, muscle bulk, swelling, masses, and scarring from past surgical incisions. The elbow has several discrete bony and soft tissue landmarks that should be palpated for tenderness, such as the epicondyles, biceps and triceps tendons, ulnar nerve, collateral ligaments, and joint lines. Active and passive range of motion of the elbow, including flexion, extension, supination, and pronation, should be measured with a long-arm goniometer and documented. Patients with a limited range of motion should have the end range assessed for bony or soft tissue end points. Anterior and posterior bony impingement tests[12] for symptomatic impinging osteophytes should be conducted.

A standard neurovascular examination is appropriate. The ulnar nerve, however, does require special attention. Ulnar neuritis or neuropathy is commonly associated with elbow disorders. Also, the location of the ulnar nerve is important when considering arthroscopic portals, especially the anteromedial portals. In situ release or transposition of the ulnar nerve may be indicated as an associated procedure in the arthroscopic management of the stiff elbow, especially in patients with limited flexion or those who have preoperative symptoms related to ulnar nerve disorders.

A prior ulnar nerve transposition or a subluxating nerve is not an absolute contraindication to elbow arthroscopy; however, particular attention must be directed to identifying the location of the nerve via palpation, ultrasound studies, or a miniopen procedure. Alternatively, if the elbow disorder allows, anterior joint arthroscopy may be conducted via two laterally based portals, avoiding the anteromedial portals altogether.

The elbow arthroscopist should be familiar with several tests for specific diseases of the elbow. Common elbow disorders for which special tests may be performed are posterolateral rotatory instability, medial collateral ligament insufficiency, lateral epicondylitis, and radiocapitellar plica syndrome.[12] Examination of the elbow should conclude with an examination of the hand, shoulder, and cervical spine. In many cases, ipsilateral joint involvement may have an effect on the elbow. For example, patients with rheumatoid arthritis may have profound shoulder stiffness, which may influence ideal positioning during the surgical setup for elbow arthroscopy.

Diagnostic Imaging

In preparation for elbow arthroscopy, standard anteroposterior, oblique, and lateral elbow radiographs are indicated. The radiographs should be scrutinized for alignment, deformity, arthritic changes, osteophytes, heterotopic ossification, loose bodies, and fractures. In patients with osteoarthritis, rheumatoid arthritis, posttraumatic arthritis, bony deformity, posteromedial impingement, osteochondritis dissecans, or loose bodies, computed tomography (CT) is recommended. Three-dimensional reconstructions are particularly helpful in preoperative planning. These predictably allow for a much more rapid assessment of bony architecture. For osteoarthritis, three-dimensional CT reconstructions allow for visualization of the orientation, size, and location of impinging osteophytes. Typically, with osteoarthritis of the elbow (Figure 26.1), posterior osteophytes are identified within the olecranon fossa and along the medial and lateral aspects of the olecranon process.[28] Anteriorly, osteophytes are usually located on the coronoid tip and within the radial fossa and coronoid fossae. Additionally, occult osteophytes may be found along the posterior aspect of the capitellum that may impinge against the radial head in extension (see Figure 26.1, *E*).

CT scanning is useful for characterizing fractures that are amenable to arthroscopic fixation, such as fractures of the coronoid, capitellum, distal humerus, and radial head. Additionally, the size, orientation, and depth of osteochondritis dissecans lesions can be appreciated, along with characterization of the osteochondritis dissecans fragment to determine its size and reparability. If loose bodies are present, many may be cartilaginous, and therefore a CT arthrogram or magnetic resonance imaging (MRI) study may be beneficial if standard imaging techniques are normal.

MRI is useful if required to assist with the diagnosis of disorders of soft tissue. Many soft tissue disorders can be diagnosed on clinical examination, such as tears of the medial collateral ligament, lateral epicondylitis, medial epicondylitis, triceps tears, and distal biceps tears. MRI is also helpful in intraarticular disorders, such as radiocapitellar plica (Figure 26.2), osteochondritis dissecans lesions, or cartilaginous loose bodies.

ANESTHESIA AND POSITIONING

Elbow arthroscopy may be performed under a general anesthetic or a regional anesthetic. A general anesthetic has the advantage of muscle relaxation and ease of patient positioning. For arthroscopy, patients may be positioned in either the lateral decubitus or prone position, either of which is poorly tolerated in a patient who is awake. Regional anesthetic techniques, such as supraclavicular and interscalene blocks, are commonly used; patients should be educated about the length of the procedure and the requirement to remain still, however. In addition to regional blocks, intravenous sedation may be beneficial for patient relaxation.

After appropriate anesthesia, patient positioning and the arthroscopy setup are important early steps in a successful procedure. If a patient is poorly positioned, portal identification and creation and joint instrumentation may be challenging and visualization may be limited. Patients are typically placed in the prone or lateral position. Supine positioning is a less common option. Positioning typically depends on surgeon preference; certain disorders may lend themselves to one form of positioning over another, however.

The supine position was first reported by Andrews and Carson[4] and involves abducting the extremity to 90 degrees and flexing the elbow to 90 degrees. The wrist and/or forearm are secured to an overhead traction device. The advantage of this arrangement is that it is well known to anesthesiologists and nurses, airway access is routine, and there is a lower risk of complications related to positioning, such as compressive neuropathies. Another advantage of supine positioning is that the arthroscopic procedure can be easily converted to an open procedure. Disadvantages of supine positioning include the need for overhead traction and the increased difficulties in obtaining access to the posterior elbow compartment.

Prone positioning was described by Poehling and colleagues.[34] It involves placing the patient flat on chest bolsters. The arm is abducted to 90 degrees and the elbow is flexed over an elbow positioner. An advantage of prone positioning is that the posterior compartment of the elbow and the ulnar nerve are easily accessible and a traction device or holder is not required. Disadvantages typically include a longer setup time, limited airway access, and susceptibility to compression-related complications. Prone positioning is poorly tolerated with regional anesthetic techniques.

The author prefers lateral positioning, in which the patient is placed operative side up on a beanbag. The nonoperative arm is placed in 90 degrees of forward elevation and 90 degrees of elbow flexion and rested on an arm board. A well-padded axillary roll is placed slightly distal in the nonoperative axilla to decrease pressure on the contralateral brachial plexus. Additionally, pillows and pads are placed between the legs and beneath the malleoli and fibular head of the lower leg. The operative arm is elevated forward to 90 degrees and internally rotated at the shoulder, and the elbow is flexed over an arm positioner (Figure 26.3). Advantages of lateral positioning over prone positioning include better access to the posterior compartment, better access to the airway, and, generally, better positioning of the patient. Additionally, when regional anesthesia is used and the patient is awake, the patient tolerates the lateral position better than the prone position. Disadvantages include a longer time to set up lateral positioning than supine positioning, a risk of compression-related complications, and the possible need for repositioning if conversion to open débridement is required.

▧ PERTINENT ANATOMY AND PORTALS

The elbow, fortunately, has several subcutaneous bony landmarks that can be used to orient the surgeon, locate neurovascular structures, and create safe portals. The neurovascular structures are of special importance due to their close proximity to arthroscopic portals and the joint capsule (Figure 26.4). The median nerve and brachial artery are located just superficial to the anteromedial joint capsule and brachialis muscle. On the anterolateral side of the elbow, the radial nerve splits into the superficial sensory branch and the posterior interosseous nerve. The posterior interosseous nerve is just superficial to the anterior joint capsule, and at the level of the radiocapitellar joint, it courses longitudinally along the medial side of the capitellum.[32] At the level of the joint, a thin layer of brachialis lies between

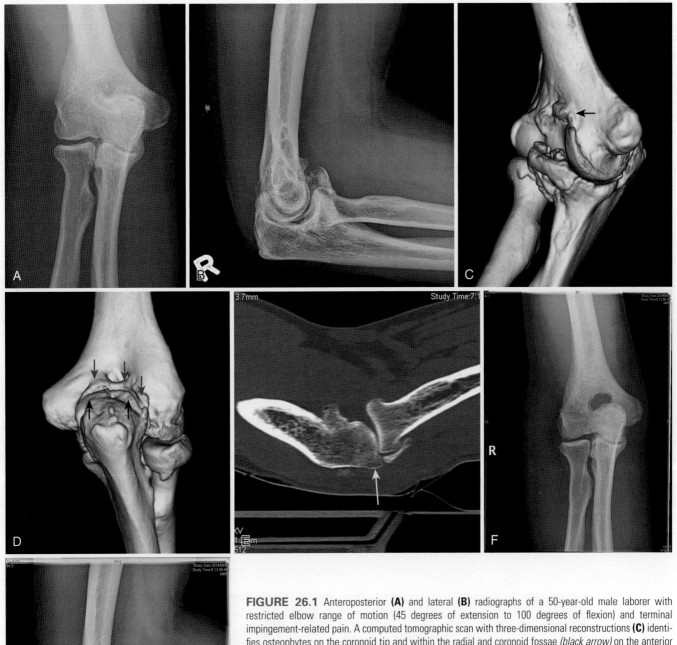

FIGURE 26.1 Anteroposterior **(A)** and lateral **(B)** radiographs of a 50-year-old male laborer with restricted elbow range of motion (45 degrees of extension to 100 degrees of flexion) and terminal impingement-related pain. A computed tomographic scan with three-dimensional reconstructions **(C)** identifies osteophytes on the coronoid tip and within the radial and coronoid fossae *(black arrow)* on the anterior humerus. A posterior view **(D)** of the olecranon identifies osteophytes on the medial and lateral aspects of the olecranon process *(black arrows)*, which are impinging against osteophytes in the olecranon fossa *(red arrows)*. In addition to osteophytes on the olecranon and in the olecranon fossa, restriction in extension may also be caused by osteophytes present on the posterior portion of the capitellum *(yellow arrow)*, which impinge against the radial head in extension **(E)**. After an arthroscopic débridement, olecranon fossa fenestration, and capsulectomy, as described in the Débridement for Osteoarthritis section (see Figures 26.9 to 26.11), the patient has functional range of motion, with postoperative radiographs demonstrating osteophyte removal **(F and G)**.

the posterior interosseous nerve and the capsule; distally, at the level of the radial neck, the nerve may come into direct contact with the capsule, however. Capsular resection at the level of the radial neck should be avoided or conducted with extreme caution because the nerve may be adhering to the joint capsule.[32] The ulnar nerve is located just superficial to the posteromedial joint capsule and should be identified and assessed for anterior subluxation with palpation. Alternatively, if any concerns exist with respect to the ulnar nerve, it can be identified via arthroscopic exposure or by a miniopen incision.

The locations of the above nerves can be predicted based on an assessment of surface anatomy. Typically, landmarks that are marked on the elbow prior to starting arthroscopy are the medial epicondyle, ulnar nerve, olecranon, lateral epicondyle, and radial head. Special care is taken to draw out the path of the ulnar nerve.

Three compartments are used in arthroscopy of the elbow joint, the anterior, posterior, and posterolateral (posterior radiocapitellar) compartments. Several portals may be used to address pathologic findings within a compartment. It is not unusual to use four to six portals for a simple elbow arthroscopy and up to seven or eight for more complex cases.

Anterior Compartment Portals

There are five commonly described anterior joint arthroscopy portals. On the medial side of the elbow, two portals are commonly used, the anteromedial and proximal anteromedial portals. On the lateral side, three portals are described, the proximal anterolateral, midanterolateral, and distal anterolateral portals. All portals are typically created with the elbow flexed to 90 degrees. Before the portals are created, a sterile tourniquet is inflated to 250 mm Hg and 20 to 40 mL of saline is injected into the joint for distention. The saline is injected with a syringe through either the soft spot (triangle between the lateral epicondyle, radial head, and olecranon) or percutaneously through the triceps tendon into the olecranon fossa.

Anteromedial Portals

Proximal Anteromedial Portal. The proximal anteromedial portal is likely the most frequently used anteromedial portal (Figure 26.5). It was described by Poehling and associates[34] to be located approximately 2 cm proximal to the medial epicondyle and just anterior to the medial intermuscular septum. To create this portal, the medial intermuscular septum is palpated and a surgical marker is used to mark a location approximately 2 cm proximal to the medial epicondyle. The location of this portal in the proximal-distal direction will vary according to patient size. The purpose of this portal is to allow entry into the joint just proximal to the level of the superior aspect of the medial trochlea. Before the skin is incised, the location of the ulnar nerve, posterior to the medial epicondyle, is confirmed. After the skin is incised, a portal can be created by using a blunt trocar or by carrying dissection down to the capsule with a hemostat. It is the author's preference to use a dull switching stick to enter the joint, aiming toward the capitellum while staying in contact

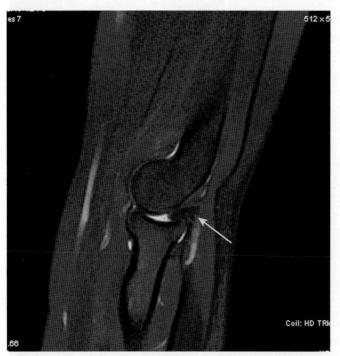

FIGURE 26.2 A sagittal magnetic resonance image depicting a symptomatic posterior radiocapitellar plica *(yellow arrow)*.

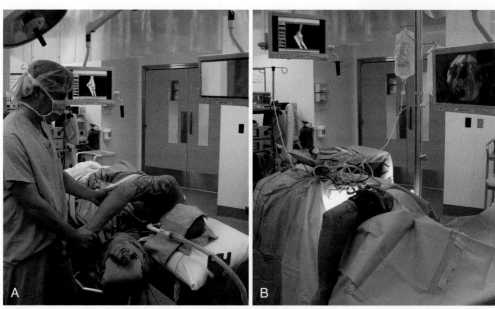

FIGURE 26.3 Lateral positioning on a beanbag with use of an elbow-positioning device prior to surgical preparation **(A)** and after preparation and draping **(B)**.

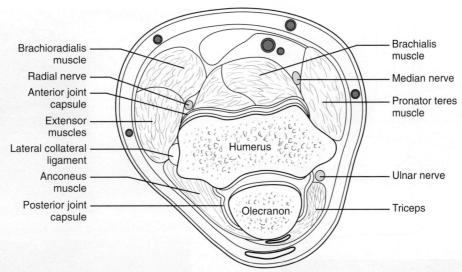

FIGURE 26.4 The three major nerves to the hand all cross the elbow and are in close proximity to arthroscopic portals and the joint capsule.

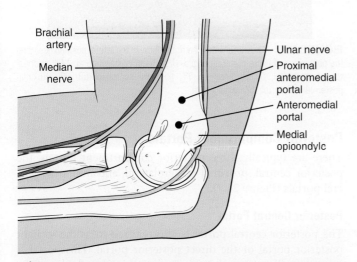

A

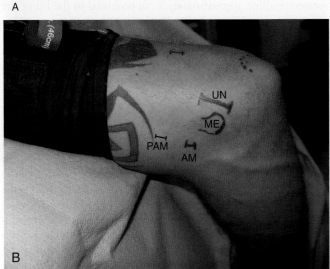

B

FIGURE 26.5 A medical illustration **(A)** and intraoperative markings **(B)** on a right elbow in the lateral position depicting medial portals. *AM,* Anteromedial portal; *ME,* medial epicondyle; *PAM,* proximal anteromedial portal; *UN,* ulnar nerve.

with the anterior humerus. Inserting a standard 30-degree arthroscope through this portal will allow visualization of the entire anterior joint compartment, including the radial head, capitellum, trochlea, and coronoid.

Anteromedial Portal. The standard anteromedial portal is described as 2 cm distal and 2 cm anterior to the medial epicondyle. This portal enters the elbow at the level of the anteromedial joint line. The portal is created by directing the trocar laterally, which places the portal in close proximity to the median and medial antebrachial cutaneous nerves. The standard anteromedial portal, although described in the literature, is not recommended by the author because the proximal anteromedial portal affords better visualization and is farther away from local nerves.

Anterolateral Portals

There are three commonly described anterolateral portals for anterior compartment arthroscopy, the proximal anterolateral, midanterolateral, and distal anterolateral portals (Figure 26.6).

Proximal Anterolateral Portal. The proximal anterolateral portal has been described by several authors.[11,40] It is templated 2 cm proximal to and 1 to 2 cm anterior to the lateral epicondyle. The portal is directed toward the center of the joint, with the tip of the trocar maintaining contact with the anterolateral humerus (see Figure 26.6). This portal has been described as the safest of the anterolateral portals.[11] Through this portal, the entire anterior compartment can be visualized, and especially good visualization can be obtained of the anteromedial joint structures, such as the medial trochlea and anteromedial coronoid. When working through this portal, there is good access to the capitellum, radial head, radial fossa, anterolateral joint capsule, and extensor tendon origin. When one is looking from the medial side, this portal can be made using a spinal needle for localization and an outside-in technique.

Midanterolateral Portal. The midanterolateral portal is also known as the anterosuperior lateral portal. This portal is landmarked 1 cm anterior to the lateral epicondyle (see Figure 26.6). The portal can be made via an outside-in or inside-out

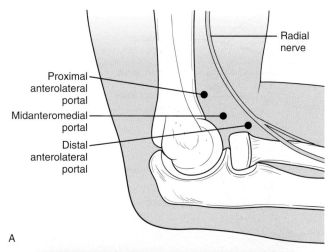

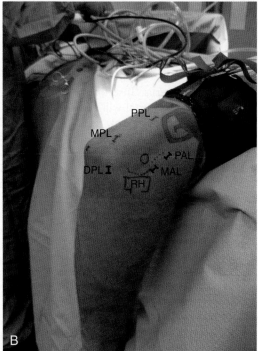

FIGURE 26.6 A medial illustration **(A)** and intraoperative markings **(B)** on a right elbow in the lateral position depicting the lateral portals. *DPL*, Distal posterolateral portal; *MAL*, midanterolateral portal; *MPL*, midposterolateral portal; *PAL*, proximal anterolateral portal; *PPL*, proximal posterolateral portal; *RH*, radial head.

technique. The portal enters the elbow joint at the superior aspect of the radiocapitellar joint. It has several purposes; it can be used as a viewing portal, an instrumentation portal, or an accessory portal.

Distal Anterolateral Portal. The distal anterolateral portal is also known as the original anterolateral portal. This portal was described by Andrews and Carson[4] and is located 3 cm distal to and 1 cm anterior to the lateral epicondyle. This portal is quite close to the radial nerve and the posterior antebrachial cutaneous nerve.[23] Because of the proximity of this portal to neurologic structures and because the midanterolateral and proximal anterolateral portals offer similar capabilities, most surgeons do not recommend using the distal anterolateral portal.

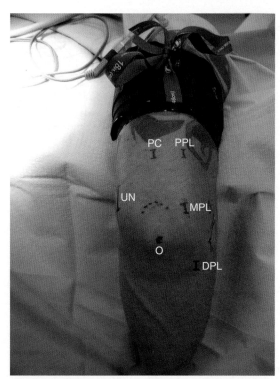

FIGURE 26.7 A posterior view of a right elbow in the lateral position depicting the posterior and posterolateral portals. *DPL*, Distal posterolateral; *MPL*, midposterolateral portal; *O*, olecranon tip; *PC*, posterior central portal; *PPL*, proximal posterolateral portal; *UN*, ulnar nerve.

Posterior Compartment Portals

There are typically three posterior compartment portals, the posterior central, proximal posterolateral, and midposterolateral portals (Figure 26.7).

Posterior Central Portal

The posterior central portal is also referred to as the straight posterior portal or the direct posterior portal. This portal is located midline approximately 3 cm proximal to the tip of the olecranon (see Figure 26.7). The orientation of the portal is obliquely directed through the musculotendinous junction of the triceps mechanism to the olecranon fossa. This portal functions as both a working portal and a viewing portal.

Proximal Posterolateral Portal

The proximal posterolateral portal is located adjacent to the posterior central portal along the lateral margin of the triceps (see Figure 26.7). The portal is typically made with an outside-in technique using a spinal needle or trocar. It typically functions as a viewing portal because it provides good visualization of the olecranon process, olecranon fossa, and medial gutter of the elbow joint. When conducting a medial gutter débridement with the camera in the proximal posterolateral portal, a retractor may be introduced through the posterior central portal to protect the medial gutter capsule and the immediately adjacent ulnar nerve.

Midposterolateral Portal

The midposterolateral portal is usually used for viewing at the beginning of posterior joint arthroscopy. This portal is located in the proximal aspect of the lateral gutter as it enters the olecranon fossa. The landmarks for this portal require drawing a line from the subcutaneous olecranon tip to the lateral epicondyle. The midpoint of this line is typically located over the posterolateral ulnohumeral joint (lateral gutter). The midposterolateral portal is made approximately 1 cm farther proximal, and the portal trajectory is to the olecranon fossa (see Figure 26.7). By placing the portal 1 cm proximal to the lateral gutter, a 30-degree scope can be used to visualize the area past the olecranon tip and down the medial gutter. Any instruments inserted through this portal can be used in the medial gutter.

Posterolateral Compartment Portals

The posterolateral compartment is composed of the posterior aspect of the radiocapitellar joint and the distal lateral aspect of the ulnohumeral joint. The posterolateral compartment can be visualized and instrumented by several portals, the midposterolateral, distal posterolateral, and distal ulnar portals (see Figure 26.7).

Midposterolateral Portal

The midposterolateral portal is described above as a posterior compartment portal. This portal can be used to visualize the posterolateral elbow compartment. By advancing the scope distally along the lateral margin of the ulnohumeral joint, the posterolateral compartment can be reached.

Distal Posterolateral Portal

The distal posterolateral portal is also referred to as the midlateral, direct lateral, or soft spot portal. This portal is formed at the center of a triangle created by the olecranon tip, radial head, and lateral epicondyle. This portal traverses through the anconeus muscle. This portal can be used as a working portal with visualization obtained from the midposterolateral portal. In larger individuals and in some conditions such as osteochondritis of the capitellum, a second distal posterolateral portal can be made adjacent to the first one. This allows direct visualization of the inferior hemisphere of the capitellum and the radial head. With side-by-side distal posterolateral portals, one portal is used for visualization and the other for instrumentation (see Figure 26.7).

Distal Ulnar Portal

The distal ulnar portal is described as located 3 to 4 cm distal to the posterior aspect of the radiocapitellar joint and just lateral to the palpable subcutaneous border of the ulna.[43] The trajectory of the portal is directed deep and obliquely toward the posterior radiocapitellar joint. This portal is usually used as a viewing portal, which leaves the standard distal posterolateral portal available for a working portal.

INSTRUMENTATION

Fluid management techniques for elbow arthroscopy include gravity inflow versus commercially available arthroscopic pumps. In general, it is the author's preference to use gravity inflow with two 3-L bags of normal saline placed to a height of approximately 5 feet. The gravity method is cheap and easy to use, but vigilance is required to monitor the elbow for swelling.

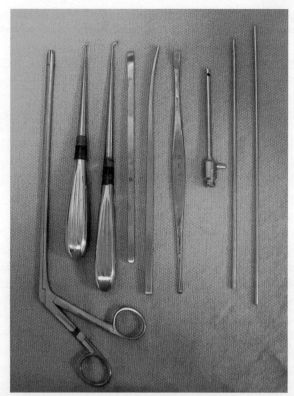

FIGURE 26.8 Standard arthroscopy instruments that may be useful when conducting elbow arthroscopy. From left to right, a large pituitary grasper, two angled curets, straight and curved osteotomes, a Howarth retractor, a standard metal cannula, a dull pointed switching stick, and a standard switching stick.

It is the author's preference to use a sterile tourniquet; however, a nonsterile tourniquet may also be used.

In general, a standard 4-mm, 30-degree arthroscope is used; however, smaller scopes may be required for smaller elbows or to visualize tight areas. Cannulas may or may not be used, depending on surgeon preference. Standard arthroscopic instruments include a dull switching stick, a pointed switching stick, an arthroscopic grasper (or a pituitary grasper), a motorized arthroscopic shaver, and a motorized arthroscopic bur (Figure 26.8). Other instruments that may be beneficial during elbow arthroscopy include a Howarth retractor, which is used to retract tissues such as the joint capsule or to protect neurovascular structures. Curved and/or straight osteotomes of 5 to 8 mm may be useful for removing osteophytes. Additionally, curved curets may be useful to clear out spaces, such as the coronoid fossa and the radial fossa along the anterior aspect of humerus.

Specialized instrumentation may be required depending on the case being conducted. For example, arthroscopic fixation of fractures may require cannulated screws, fracture reduction clamps, and intraoperative fluoroscopy. The treatment of osteochondritis dissecans with osteochondral grafts will require specialized arthroscopic harvest and insertion instruments.

HISTORICAL REVIEW

In 1931, the elbow was described as a joint that was not suitable for arthroscopic examination. Only 1 year later, the elbow was described as arthroscopically appropriate. Table 26.1 lists the historically important advancements in elbow arthroscopy.

TABLE 26.1 **Contributions to Elbow Arthroscopy**

Author	Publication Date	Main Area of Contribution	Significance
Burman	1932	Technique	Reported that elbow arthroscopy was technically feasible
Andrews and Carson	1985	Technique	Described the initial technique of diagnostic arthroscopy and loose body removal
Guhl	1985	Technique and indications	Described the technique; established indications for inflammatory synovectomy, débridement of osteochondritis dissecans, excision of osteophytes, and treatment of fractures
Lynch et al	1986	Neurovascular anatomy	Described the proximity of neurovascular structures to portals
Clarke	1988	Plica	Described the arthroscopic features of a radiocapitellar plica
O'Driscoll et al	1990	Anatomy	Reported the intraarticular volume of the elbow joint
O'Driscoll et al	1992	Risks	Reported on the complications associated with elbow arthroscopy
Jones et al	1993	Contractures	Described the arthroscopic release of elbow flexion contractures
Lo and King	1994	Indications	Reported on arthroscopic excision of the radial head
Ogilvie-Harris et al	1995	Indications	Described posterior joint débridement for osteoarthritis
Baker et al	2000	Anatomy	Reported the arthroscopic appearance and classification of lateral epicondylitis
Hardy et al	2002	Indications	First report of arthroscopic management of capitellar fractures
Smith et al	2003	Anatomy	Defined the safe zone for arthroscopic tennis elbow release to be anterior to an intraarticular line bisecting the radial head
Adams et al	2007	Fractures	Arthroscopic fixation of coronoid fractures is described
Athwal et al	2009	Triceps tendon	Described the technique of arthroscopic triceps tendon repair
Yeoh et al	2012	Indications	Reported the evidence-based indications for elbow arthroscopy
O'Brien et al	2014	Ligament repair	An arthroscopic repair of the lateral collateral ligament is described

TYPES OF OPERATIONS

Loose Body Removal

Loose bodies frequently are found in the elbow, causing symptoms such as joint locking, clicking, pain, and limited range of motion. The arthroscopic removal of loose bodies is an established procedure that is safe and effective. There are several advantages to removing elbow loose bodies arthroscopically, such as a reduced surgical insult compared with open arthrotomy, the ability to better visualize all compartments of the elbow, and possible reduction of postoperative scarring and stiffness as compared with open techniques. The only disadvantage of arthroscopic loose body removal is related to the inherent risks of elbow arthroscopy. The surgeon planning to conduct elbow arthroscopy should be experienced and familiar with the anatomy, location of neurovascular structures, and described safe portals.

In patients presenting with symptoms of loose bodies, imaging studies should be examined to confirm the presence of loose bodies and the potential underlying cause that resulted in the loose bodies. Standard radiographs may be able to visualize bony loose bodies, but loose bodies may be cartilaginous and also hidden in the elbow gutters. MRI or CT arthrogram studies are better able to visualize the numbers and locations of loose bodies. These imaging studies should also be examined to identify the potential cause, such as osteoarthritis, fractured osteophytes, osteochondritis dissecans, or synovial chondromatosis.

Indications and Contraindications

The primary indication for arthroscopic removal of loose bodies is a symptomatic patient who has failed nonoperative management. Symptoms may include joint locking, crepitus, pain, catching, and stiffness. The contraindications to arthroscopic removal include elbow conditions that preclude arthroscopy, such as extensive postoperative scarring, altered anatomy, and deformity. When an elbow condition does not allow accurate assessment of the local anatomy to determine predictably safe portal locations, this is a contraindication to arthroscopy unless miniopen portals are created to ensure that neurovascular structures are not at risk. A prior ulnar nerve transposition or nerve subluxation is a relative contraindication; unless arthroscopy is conducted via lateral portals only, a miniopen technique is used for the medial portals, or intraoperative ultrasound is used to confirm the location of the ulnar nerve.

Preoperative Planning

Imaging studies should be scrutinized to assess the location and approximate number of loose bodies. No specific special instruments are required, other than a large pituitary grasper or an arthroscopic grasper. Hemostats of various sizes are also helpful. For larger loose bodies, the surgeon should be prepared to expand the working portal to ensure complete removal.

Technique

For isolated loose body removal, standard arthroscopic techniques are used. The bone and soft tissue landmarks are marked on the skin, antibiotics are administered, the tourniquet is inflated, the joint is insufflated with saline via a syringe, and the standard portals are used. Surgeon preference and the location of the loose bodies on preoperative imaging will determine which elbow compartment is examined first. However, it is essential that all three compartments be visualized, including the medial and lateral gutters, to ensure complete removal of loose bodies and for diagnostic purposes.

For anterior compartment loose body removal, the arthroscope is introduced via the proximal anteromedial portal, and the proximal or midanterolateral portals are used for loose body removal. The camera is switched to an anterolateral portal to ensure that there are no loose bodies in the anteromedial gutter adjacent to the anteromedial facet of the coronoid. For posterior compartment arthroscopy, the posterior central and midposterolateral portals are typically used. The posteromedial gutter must be visualized, and this can usually be accomplished with the camera in the midposterolateral portal; if visualization is incomplete, however, the camera should be switched to the posterior central portal. The posterolateral compartment can be accessed with the camera in the midposterolateral portal, and work can proceed through the distal posterolateral portal (soft spot portal).

When loose bodies are encountered, they can be removed with pituitary or arthroscopic grasping instruments. Larger loose bodies can be removed by crushing them into fragments or via a dilated portal. If loose bodies are difficult to grasp because they are swirling in eddies of fluid, the arthroscopic fluid inflow can be temporarily turned off to decrease turbulence, making it easier to capture moving loose bodies.

Postoperative Management

Arthroscopy is usually conducted as an outpatient procedure. Patients are discharged to go home with a light surgical bandage that does not restrict range of motion and a sling for comfort. Patients are encouraged to start elbow range-of-motion exercises immediately following surgery. Formal physiotherapy may be started within the first week following operation if required. If range-of-motion recovery is incomplete at 3 to 4 weeks following operation, flexion and extension splinting is recommended.

Outcomes

Arthroscopic loose body removal has been reported as safe and effective.[29,31,46] However, when patients have other concomitant pathologic conditions such as osteoarthritis, removal of loose bodies in isolation is ineffective in resolving symptoms.

Débridement for Osteoarthritis

Elbow osteoarthritis can present with pain and restricted range of motion. Typically, nonoperative management is initially recommended to address symptoms. In patients with symptoms that are refractory to nonoperative treatment modalities, surgery is offered. The type of surgery depends on the patient's symptoms, age, activity level, degree of joint degeneration, and bony deformity. Depending on the above factors, surgical options include arthroscopic débridement, open débridement, interposition arthroplasty, elbow arthroplasty, and fusion.

Arthroscopic débridement of the osteoarthritic elbow, which is also termed *arthroscopic osteocapsular arthroplasty*, has gained increasing acceptance as arthroscopic techniques have advanced. However, arthroscopic débridement has not demonstrated any clinical superiority over traditional open débridement procedures. Arthroscopic débridement is best suited to patients with a relatively well-preserved joint space and symptoms stemming from peripheral osteophytes and capsular contracture that restrict range of motion and cause terminal motion impingement pain. The primary goal of arthroscopic management of the osteoarthritic elbow is to remove osteophytes, remove loose bodies, improve the impingement-free range of motion, and possibly release the capsule if it is restricting motion.

Indications and Contraindications

The indications for proceeding to arthroscopic débridement are failure of nonoperative management, the presence of a relatively well-preserved ulnohumeral joint space, and a compliant patient. The relative contraindications include bone loss, joint deformity, instability, and ankylosis. A patient who has undergone multiple prior open procedures may also be a relatively poor candidate. If an open operation has already been performed in an elbow, arthroscopic procedures for the elbow should be approached with caution because structures such as the ulnar nerve may have been transposed, resulting in altered anatomy.

Preoperative Planning

Standard elbow radiographs are required to make the diagnosis of elbow arthritis. When planning a complete arthroscopic débridement, however, a CT scan is helpful in identifying the sizes and locations of impinging osteophytes (see Figure 26.1). Additionally, a three-dimensional reconstruction of the joint can greatly enhance preoperative planning because osteophyte locations, orientations, and sizes are easier to visualize.

Disposable arthroscopic instruments typically used when conducting an osteocapsular arthroplasty include a 5.5-mm soft tissue motorized shaver, a 5- to 6-mm motorized bur, and possibly a radiofrequency ablation device. Additional instruments that are helpful include a No. 11 scalpel blade, a switching stick, a dull pointed switching stick, and an arthroscopic grasper (or a pituitary grasper). A Howarth retractor, which is used to retract tissues such as the joint capsule, may also be helpful (see Figure 26.8). Curved and/or straight 5- to 8-mm osteotomes may be convenient for removing osteophytes. Curved curets may be helpful in débriding bony spaces such as the coronoid fossa and the radial fossa along the anterior aspect of the humerus. Because some osteocapsular arthroplasties are conducted with a limited in situ ulnar nerve decompression, tenotomy scissors, small angled retractors, and a bipolar cautery unit may be useful.

Technique

Patients are typically placed in the lateral decubitus position on a beanbag, and the affected elbow is flexed over an elbow-positioning stand (see Figure 26.3). A viewing monitor is placed at eye level across from the elbow, and another monitor is used to display the three-dimensional CT scan. To prevent instruments and motorized devices from falling on the floor, a Mayo stand is brought over the patient to serve as a flat surface on which to place instruments when they are not being used (see Figure 26.3, *B*). A sterile tourniquet is used with gravity inflow for the arthroscopy fluid.

In patients undergoing osteocapsular arthroplasty who will be starting continuous passive motion postoperatively, it is the author's practice to conduct a limited in situ ulnar nerve decompression to decrease the potential for delayed onset of ulnar neuritis.[6,7]

In preparation for arthroscopy, the relevant arthroscopy portals are marked and fluid is injected into the elbow joint, as described earlier. It is the author's preference to create the standard anteromedial portal first, to function as a fluid drainage portal. A No. 11 scalpel blade is used to incise the skin only. Following skin incision, a dull-tipped switching stick is pushed through the soft tissues from the anteromedial portal and directed into the anterior elbow joint, aiming toward the capitellum. Once the anterior elbow joint is entered from the anteromedial portal, a small-diameter metal cannula is inserted over the switching stick to allow fluid drainage. Once a drainage portal is established in patients with tricompartmental osteoarthritis, it is the author's preference to conduct the posterior compartment débridement first, followed by débridement of the posterolateral radiocapitellar compartment and then the anterior joint compartment.

Arthroscopic débridement of the posterior compartment is started by placing the camera through the midposterolateral portal and the shaver and radiofrequency ablation device through the posterior central portal (Figure 26.9, *A*). The olecranon fossa fat pad is débrided to allow visualization of the arthritic olecranon fossa and olecranon tip (see Figure 26.9, *B*). Typically, the olecranon fossa contains a transverse ridge of osteophytes, which function as a mechanical block to extension. The ridge of osteophytes is removed with a bur (see Figure 26.9, *C* and *D*), which can also be used to remove osteophytes present on the lateral and central portions of the olecranon tip in extension. Once the central portion of the posterior compartment is débrided, attention is directed to the posteromedial gutter.

The posteromedial gutter is safely viewed by placing the camera into the proximal posterolateral portal (see Figure 26.9, *E*). A Howarth retractor can be inserted from the posterior central portal and used to safely retract the posteromedial joint capsule to protect the ulnar nerve. With the posteromedial capsule retracted, the shaver, bur, or osteotome can be used to remove osteophytes from the medial aspect of the olecranon and the posteromedial trochlea (see Figure 26.9, *F* and *G*). At the completion of osteophyte removal from the medial gutter, the posterior bundle of the medial collateral ligament may rarely require release to obtain further flexion. If necessary (rarely), a duckbill tissue resector can be used to carefully release the posteromedial capsule and the ligament. This should be done with extreme caution because the ulnar nerve is in close proximity. Alternatively, if a miniopen ulnar nerve release is being done, the posteromedial capsule can be released through the open incision with gentle retraction of the ulnar nerve.

A direct central view of the olecranon tip can be obtained by inserting the camera into the posterior central portal for viewing in a distal direction (see Figure 26.9, *H*). With the camera in the posterior central portal, a bur can be brought into the posterior compartment via the proximal posterolateral portal or the midposterolateral portal. The bur is used to complete osteophyte removal from the olecranon fossa and the central and lateral aspects of the olecranon. If needed, the olecranon fossa can be arthroscopically fenestrated, as is done during the *Outerbridge-Kashiwagi procedure*. An advantage of fenestration of the olecranon fossa is that it provides an additional portal option for viewing the anterior compartment (see Figure 26.9, *I* and *J*).

The posterolateral radiocapitellar compartment is viewed by inserting the camera through the midposterolateral portal and sliding it distally along the lateral gutter. The lateral gutter terminates at the posterior aspect of the radiocapitellar joint. A working portal is typically established through the soft spot (distal posterolateral portal), and the motorized instruments are used to resect soft tissues and débride osteophytes (Figure 26.10). At times, an osteophyte may be present along the posterior aspect of the capitellum and should be removed if it is functioning to block full extension by impinging on the radial head.

Anterior compartment arthroscopy requires switching the camera and instruments between the medial and lateral portals to allow ideal visualization and instrument trajectory for débriding and resecting impinging bone. It is the author's preference to insert the camera through the anteromedial drainage portal that has already been created. With the camera view directed toward the anterolateral capsule, a standard midanterolateral portal is created using an outside-in technique. Using a combination of burs, shavers, radiofrequency ablation devices, osteotomes, and angled curets, the radial fossa on the anterolateral distal humerus and the coronoid fossa on the anteromedial distal humerus are re-created; soft tissue, osteophytes, and loose bodies are removed. In most cases, the coronoid tip can be débrided or osteotomized with the camera remaining in the anteromedial portal (Figure 26.11). The osteotome is typically brought in from the lateral portal to osteotomize the coronoid tip. To excise osteophytes on the anteromedial coronoid facet, the camera is switched to a lateral portal and the bur is brought in through the anteromedial portal. Once the bony débridement is done in the anterior compartment, the elbow is placed through a range of motion. If an extension deficit related to the soft tissue exists, because of an anterior capsular tether, the anterior capsule is released or excised. It is the author's preference to use a duckbill resector to begin the capsulotomy and develop a plane between the anterior capsule and the overlying brachialis muscle. The capsulotomy is done with great care because the radial nerve is adjacent to the anterolateral capsule[32] at the level of the medial capitellum. Additionally, on the anteromedial side of the elbow, the median nerve is at risk. The more proximal the capsulotomy, the safer it is. Once the capsulotomy has been conducted, the residual capsule is resected using a soft tissue shaver. Alternatively, the anterior capsular tether can be bluntly released from its attachment on the humerus using a Howarth retractor or elevator-type instrument.

Upon completion of the tricompartmental débridement, the elbow is placed through a gentle range of motion. If substantial blocks to motion exist, the arthroscope is reintroduced to the various compartments to assess for any areas of impingement or soft tissue contracture. When complete, the tourniquet is deflated and a drain is typically placed into the posterior compartment. The portals are closed with a nonabsorbable monofilament suture, and the elbow is placed into nearly full extension.

Postoperative Management

Once the patient has recovered from the anesthetic and has been transferred to a hospital room, continuous passive motion is typically initiated within a few hours. Patients are monitored

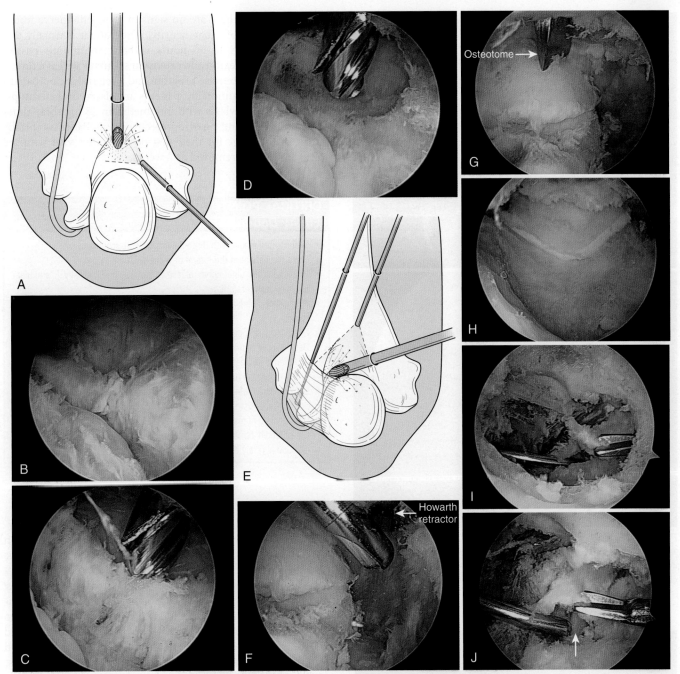

FIGURE 26.9 Arthroscopic débridement for osteoarthritis of the posterior compartment is started with the camera in the midposterolateral portal and the shaver/bur in the posterior central portal (**A**). The osteophytes in the olecranon fossa and olecranon tip are removed with a bur (**B** to **D**). The posteromedial gutter is safely viewed by placing the camera into the proximal posterolateral portal (**E**); a Howarth retractor can be inserted from the posterior central portal to retract the posteromedial joint capsule and protect the ulnar nerve. The posteromedial gutter is cleared of osteophytes using a bur and/or osteotomes (**F** and **G**). By placing the camera into the posterior central portal (**H**), a direct view of the olecranon process and the medial and lateral gutters can be obtained. To resect remaining osteophytes in the olecranon fossa and on the olecranon process, the bur is used via the midposterolateral portal. If needed, the olecranon fossa can be arthroscopically fenestrated to prevent impingement and to function as an accessory-view portal. The camera can be placed through the posterior central portal and driven through the fenestrated olecranon fossa to view the anterior joint (**I**). If the camera is held by the assistant, the surgeon can dissect anterior structures bimanually with instruments inserted via both the anteromedial and anterolateral portals (**J**). **J** depicts the view from the arthroscope when it is inserted from the posterior central portal and directed through the olecranon fenestration. The switching stick is used to retract the posterior interosseous nerve *(arrow)* as the duckbill punch is used to remove the anterior capsule.

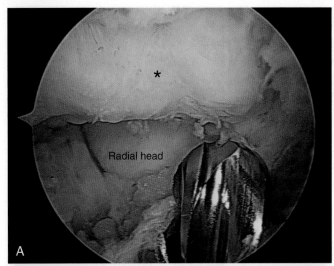

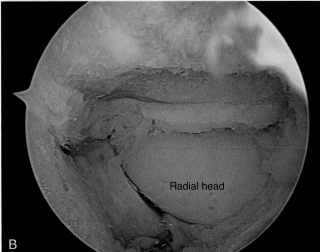

FIGURE 26.10 Posterolateral radiocapitellar joint débridement is conducted with the camera in the midposterolateral portal **(A)** and the radiofrequency/bur inserted through the distal posterolateral (soft spot) portal. Osteophytes present along the posterior aspect of the capitellum *(star)* are resected **(B)**.

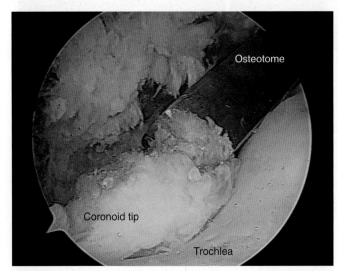

FIGURE 26.11 An osteotome is used to osteotomize the coronoid tip osteophyte. Additionally, a bur can be used to resect any remaining osteophytes present on the coronoid or in the radial or coronoid fossae.

closely to ensure there are no signs of iatrogenic nerve injury or delayed onset of ulnar neuritis. The patient is usually discharged within 24 to 36 hours without continuous passive motion but with flexion and extension splints as well as a range-of-motion home exercise program and a referral for outpatient physiotherapy. Additionally, patients are placed on heterotopic ossification prophylaxis with indomethacin 25 mg three times daily for 3 weeks and a gastroprotective agent. Patients typically return to the clinic for their first postoperative visit within a week. Sutures are removed at 2 weeks.

CRITICAL POINTS *Arthroscopic Elbow Débridement*

- Examine the elbow with three-dimensional CT scanning.
- Place the patient in the lateral or prone position.
- Be prepared for ulnar nerve release or transposition (typically, in situ ulnar nerve decompression).
- On the skin, mark the position of the portals and the location of the ulnar nerve.
- Use gravity or a pump to manage joint distention by fluid.
- Débridement of the posterior joint is performed first in the olecranon fossa and then in the medial gutter, olecranon tip, and lateral gutter; fenestration of the olecranon fossa is performed if needed.
- During posterolateral radiocapitellar joint débridement, remove the posterior capitellar osteophytes and assess for plicae.
- Débridement of the anterior joint focuses on the radial and coronoid fossae; the coronoid tip is excised; capsulotomy is done if needed; radial head excision is rarely done.

Outcomes

The outcomes of arthroscopic débridement for elbow osteoarthritis are generally good.[46] Adams and colleagues[3] reported on 42 elbows with osteoarthritis that underwent arthroscopic débridement, which consisted of removal of loose bodies, resection of osteophytes, and release of contracted capsular tissues. At a minimum of 24 months of follow-up, there were statistically significant improvements in range of motion and Mayo Elbow Performance scores, with 81% of patients reporting good to excellent outcomes. The complications were acceptable and included heterotopic ossification and ulnar nerve dysesthesias.

Cohen and associates[9] conducted a comparative study between open and arthroscopic débridement in a heterogeneous cohort, which consisted mostly of patients with osteoarthritis. In most of these patients, even though they were treated before some of the newer, more advanced arthroscopic techniques were available, the outcomes were good. The authors found that the group who had undergone open procedures had better flexion range of motion and the group who had undergone arthroscopy had better pain control. Savoie and coworkers[39] reported on 24 patients undergoing arthroscopic débridement and found substantial improvements in pain and range of motion. The complication rate was similar to that reported with open débridement.

In summary, there is a robust amount of literature supporting the effectiveness of arthroscopic débridement for elbow osteoarthritis. In their systematic review, Yeoh and colleagues[46] stated that there is poor-quality evidence for, rather than against, the arthroscopic treatment of degenerative arthritis. In their review of the literature, they found the most common complications were transient neurologic injuries and heterotopic ossification.

Synovectomy for Rheumatoid Arthritis

Arthroscopic techniques are well suited for conducting débridement of a synovitic elbow. The arthroscope and resection instruments are able to view all compartments of the elbow to allow for a thorough synovectomy. Overall, the incidence of surgical intervention for recalcitrant rheumatoid disease is on the decline because of the widespread use of disease-modifying agents and biologics. However, in patients with synovitis recalcitrant to rheumatologic medications, arthroscopic synovectomy of the elbow is effective and safe. It does, however, often require advanced arthroscopic skill.

Indications and Contraindications

The indications for arthroscopic synovectomy are a painful, stiff, inflamed elbow due to synovitis that has failed medical management. Typically, the elbow is described as boggy and swollen. Patients with limited joint destruction (Larsen grade 2 or less) have better outcomes than those with altered bony architecture. The goals of surgery are to decrease pain, improve the range of motion, and potentially provide joint preservation by removal of the aggressive inflammatory panus. Contraindications to arthroscopic synovectomy are severe bone loss with instability, a "dry" rheumatoid elbow without synovitis, and bony ankylosis.

Preoperative Planning

Radiographs of the involved elbow are examined for joint space abnormalities, bone loss, erosions, and instability. An MRI may be helpful to visualize the degree and location of the synovitis. In preparation for surgical intervention, patients with inflammatory arthritis typically undergo a cervical spine examination to rule out instability. Consultation with an anesthesiologist for airway assessment can be considered as well. In patients with gross cervical instability, cervical stabilization surgery may supersede elective elbow surgery.

Technique

The patient is positioned as previously described. In patients with cervical spine disease, supine positioning may be preferable. The technical aspects and viewing portals are similar to those described in the section on débridement for osteoarthritis. In patients with active rheumatoid arthritis, however, synovitis may obscure the typical landmarks inside of the joint. In addition, the capsular tissue in these individuals is typically much thinner and more friable than in patients with osteoarthritis. Therefore, when conducting the synovectomy with a motorized soft tissue resector, great care must be taken to avoid perforating the capsule and injuring adjacent critical neurovascular structures. Two areas in the rheumatoid elbow where specific caution should be observed are the anterolateral capsule above the radial head and neck (radial nerve) and the posteromedial gutter (ulnar nerve). Methods that may be used to minimize damage to the capsule in high-risk areas include limiting the use of suction, directing the aperture of the resecting instruments away from the capsule, and using soft tissue retractors.

Ideally, a complete synovectomy should be conducted, resecting inflamed synovium from the anterior joint, posterior joint, posterolateral radiocapitellar compartment, and medial and lateral gutters. Resection of bone is not usually required in rheumatoid arthritis. If some bone removal is required, the surgeon should remember that rheumatoid bone is typically softer than osteoarthritic bone and, therefore, burs should be used cautiously. Finally, if one of the goals of surgery is to restore the range of motion, manipulation of the elbow after synovectomy and arthroscopic release should be minimized or done very gently, because there is a greater risk of iatrogenic fracture in individuals with this disorder.

Postoperative Management

Patients typically start range-of-motion movements in the immediate postoperative period. Flexion and extension splints may be used under the guidance of a physiotherapist. Continuous passive motion protocols may also be used. However, there is no high-level evidence to support the additional costs.

Outcomes

The outcomes of arthroscopic elbow synovectomy for rheumatoid arthritis are generally good. Tanaka and associates[41] conducted a prospective cohort study comparing arthroscopic synovectomy with open synovectomy in patients with rheumatoid arthritis of Larsen grade 2 or less. Overall, all patients benefited from the synovectomy procedure, with improved pain control and function. There were no statistically significant differences between groups. The authors observed better pain relief in the arthroscopic group and better function in the open group, however.

Nemoto and coworkers[27] reported on 11 elbows that were treated with arthroscopic synovectomy. The authors divided the cohort into group A, patients with Larsen grade 1 to 3 disease, and group B, patients with Larsen grade 4 disease. Overall, the authors reported substantial improvement in pain relief and function. When comparing groups, pain relief occurred in both, but range of motion improved more in group A. The authors concluded that arthroscopic synovectomy of the elbow is a beneficial procedure, even in patients with Larsen grade 4 changes.

Yeoh and colleagues,[46] in their systematic review, concluded that arthroscopic synovectomy should be given a "B" recommendation. The authors stated that consistent findings across multiple studies showed that arthroscopic synovectomy for rheumatoid arthritis is beneficial.

Arthroscopy for Lateral Epicondylitis

Lateral epicondylitis, or *tennis elbow*, is one of the most common conditions involving the elbow. The cause is debatable; most believe it is a degenerative condition of the origin of the extensor tendons, specifically the extensor carpi radialis brevis tendon. Traditionally, treatment is nonsurgical, with rest, activity modification, splints, physiotherapy, and steroid injections. In cases recalcitrant to nonoperative management, surgery may be considered, consisting of release and débridement of the extensor carpi radialis brevis tendon origin. Historically, surgery has consisted of an open procedure; over the past 2 decades, however, arthroscopic techniques have gained popularity.

Cohen and colleagues[10] conducted an anatomic study that outlined the insertional footprint of the extensor carpi radialis brevis tendon on the lateral epicondyle. The authors reported a discrete origin site of the extensor carpi radialis brevis that was approximately 13 mm in length and 7 mm in width, located at the distalmost extent of the supracondylar ridge between the midline of the radiocapitellar joint and the top of the capitellum. The tendon footprint was described as diamond shaped. The authors concluded that this footprint could be effectively released and débrided using arthroscopic techniques.[10]

Indications and Contraindications

Arthroscopic tennis elbow release is indicated in patients who have failed nonoperative management. The precise duration of nonoperative management that should be instituted before surgical treatment is offered is controversial. Most believe a patient should have recalcitrant symptoms for a minimum of 6 to 12 months before surgery is considered. Lateral elbow pain, unfortunately, is common and may be due to other pathologic conditions, such as a synovial plica, osteochondritis dissecans, radiocapitellar arthritis, or posterolateral rotatory instability.

Preoperative Planning

Preoperative planning for lateral elbow pain includes a detailed history, physical examination, and imaging that corroborates the diagnosis of lateral epicondylitis. Typically, if the history and physical examination are clear without any red flags, the only imaging studies required are plain radiographs. Elbow films are usually normal in patients with lateral epicondylitis, although some may show signs of lateral calcific deposits at the epicondyle (Figure 26.12). In patients with atypical findings, advanced imaging may be helpful.

Technique

The patient is positioned in the lateral decubitus position, as described earlier. An examination under anesthesia is conducted to ensure that the elbow has a full range of motion and is stable. Kalainov and Cohen[18] have reported on the association of posterolateral rotatory instability with lateral epicondylitis treatment.

It is the author's practice to examine the posterior compartment and the medial and lateral gutters first with a scope to identify any loose bodies or other pathologic conditions. Following posterior compartment arthroscopy, the camera is driven into the posterior radiocapitellar joint. The radiocapitellar joint is viewed to rule out a posterolateral radiocapitellar plica, which is excised if identified.

Following posterior compartment diagnostic arthroscopy, the camera is introduced through the anteromedial portal. At times, disruption of the extensor origin can be visualized (see Figure 26.12, *B*). For the midanterolateral portal, it is the author's preference to create this portal higher than normal. Creating this portal slightly more anterior and proximal will allow a better trajectory for the arthroscopic instruments in approaching the extensor carpi radialis brevis origin. Initially, an arthroscopic shaver or ablation device is used to detach the capsule. The ablation device (preferred) or shaver is then used to detach the extensor carpi radialis brevis tendon origin on the distal aspect of the lateral supracondylar ridge, as described by Cohen and associates.[10] During release of the tendon origin, dissection remains above the midequator of the capitellum to avoid disruption of the lateral collateral ligament origin.

Postoperative Management

Following operation, patients are placed into a light dressing and immobilized in a sling for less than 1 week. Early range of motion is encouraged. It is the author's preference to place patients into a removable wrist splint to limit forced wrist extension. As pain subsides, patients are encouraged to use the arm as tolerated.

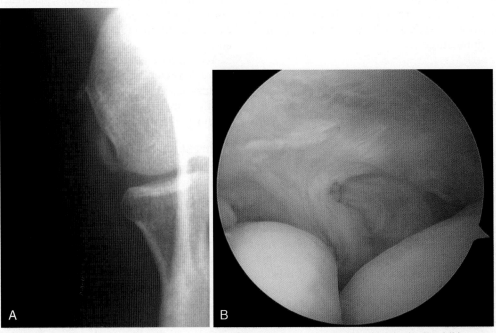

FIGURE 26.12 Calcific tendonitis within the extensor carpi radialis brevis tendon in a patient with lateral epicondylitis symptoms **(A)**. An intraoperative view of a right elbow demonstrating an avulsion of the extensor origin **(B)**.

Outcomes

The literature on arthroscopic management of lateral epicondylitis demonstrates outcomes similar to those of open techniques.[46] Peart and colleagues[33] conducted a comparative cohort study between open and arthroscopic techniques. At follow-up, all patients had relief of pain and improvement of function; however, there was an earlier return to work in the arthroscopic group. Rubenthaler and associates,[36] in a similar study, found no difference between arthroscopic and open techniques with respect to pain, functional scores, surgical time, and range of motion.

Lattermann and coworkers[22] conducted a retrospective review of 36 patients treated for recalcitrant lateral epicondylitis with arthroscopic débridement. At a mean of 3.5 years of follow-up, patient-rated pain and elbow scores were significantly improved from the preoperative scores. Interestingly, approximately 30% of patients still described mild pain with strenuous activities. Overall, the authors concluded that arthroscopic techniques were safe and effective and allowed for identification and treatment of other associated intraarticular pathologic conditions. Preoperative education is essential, however. As with all procedures for epicondylitis, there is a subset of patients who will fail and others who still have symptoms during loading.

Fracture Management by Arthroscopic Fixation

Articular fracture of the distal humerus, radial head, or coronoid can be managed with arthroscopic techniques. The advantage of arthroscopically assisted fracture fixation is that it allows visualization of the intraarticular anatomy without an extensive open surgical approach. Fractures that are amenable to arthroscopic reduction and internal fixation are those of the capitellum-trochlea, coronoid, and radial head and a limited subset of distal humerus injuries.[14,16,25,35,44] The suitability of fractures for arthroscopic techniques should be individualized based on the degree of comminution, associated injuries, timing of the fracture, fracture characteristics, and patient factors. The literature on arthroscopic techniques for elbow fracture fixation is limited to case reports and small case series. For the purposes of this chapter, we will discuss arthroscopic techniques for the management of capitellar fractures, coronoid fractures, and radial head fractures.

Indications and Contraindications

It is beyond the focus of this chapter to discuss the various fracture-specific indications for reduction and internal fixation. Fractures should meet the operative indications for arthroscopic techniques and should have characteristics amenable to screw fixation. Plate fixation, for example, for a bicolumnar distal humerus fracture, is likely best managed with open techniques.

Preoperative Planning

It is the author's preference to obtain three-dimensional CT scans for most patients undergoing arthroscopically assisted fracture reduction and fixation. The scans can provide good characterization of fracture patterns and identify fracture comminution. Typically, fracture comminutions or multiple fracture fragments are much more difficult to manage arthroscopically than with open techniques. It is the author's preference to place patients in the lateral decubitus position on a beanbag using an elbow positioner. Intraoperative fluoroscopy is also essential.

Technique for Arthroscopic Fixation of Capitellar Fractures

Simple displaced capitellar fractures can be effectively managed arthroscopically (Figure 26.13). The presence of comminution or impaction of the lateral column increases the complexity of the procedure, however, and therefore these patterns are better suited to more experienced arthroscopists.

For capitellar shear fractures, it is the author's preference to start the arthroscopy in the posterior compartment. The hematoma is evacuated and the arthroscope is directed into the posterolateral radiocapitellar compartment via the midposterolateral portal. A distal posterolateral portal is used to débride and clear the fracture bed of hematoma and debris. An angled curet may be useful in débriding the fracture bed and also in elevating any depressed bony fragments of the lateral column. Typically, displaced capitellar fractures are hinged open anteriorly by the radial head. Following preparation of the fracture bed, a reduction maneuver is conducted by extending the elbow with the forearm in supination and applying a gentle varus force. If this is unsuccessful, the surgeon can apply external manual pressure on the displaced capitellum. If this fails, a midanterolateral portal can be used to introduce a dental pick or a Howarth retractor to manipulate the capitellum inferiorly and posteriorly for reduction.

Once a reduction is obtained, it is examined from the posterolateral compartment and the anterior compartment. The arthroscope may now be introduced into the anterior compartment through the anteromedial portal. If the reduction is anatomic, the elbow is maintained in 90 degrees of flexion to allow the radial head to engage and compress the fractured capitellum. Fluoroscopy may also be used to assess the reduction. Once deemed appropriate, guidewires from a cannulated screw system are introduced from the posterior aspect of the lateral column into the capitellum. The guidewires can be passed into the radiocapitellar joint to assist with ideal screw position and length. It is the author's preference to place a hemostat clamp on the guidewire tip through the midanterolateral portal to prevent it from backing out during drilling. Two, or preferably three, posterior-to-anterior partially threaded cannulated screws are typically inserted into the capitellum for internal fixation. Direct arthroscopic visualization and fluoroscopy are used to confirm the reduction and appropriate screw lengths.

Postoperatively, if stable fixation has been attained, a splint is applied at 90 degrees of elbow flexion for 2 to 5 days. At the patient's first follow-up visit, the splint is removed and elbow radiographs are obtained. If the radiographs demonstrate appropriate reduction and stability, early active range of motion may be initiated.

Technique for Arthroscopic Fixation of Coronoid Fractures

Coronoid fractures rarely occur in isolation and are typically associated with complex elbow fracture-dislocations. In many cases, coronoid fractures are associated with severe triad-type injuries, Monteggia fractures, and transolecranon fracture-dislocations. In these sorts of injuries, open approaches are required to appropriately address the associated injuries, such as radial head arthroplasty for comminuted radial head

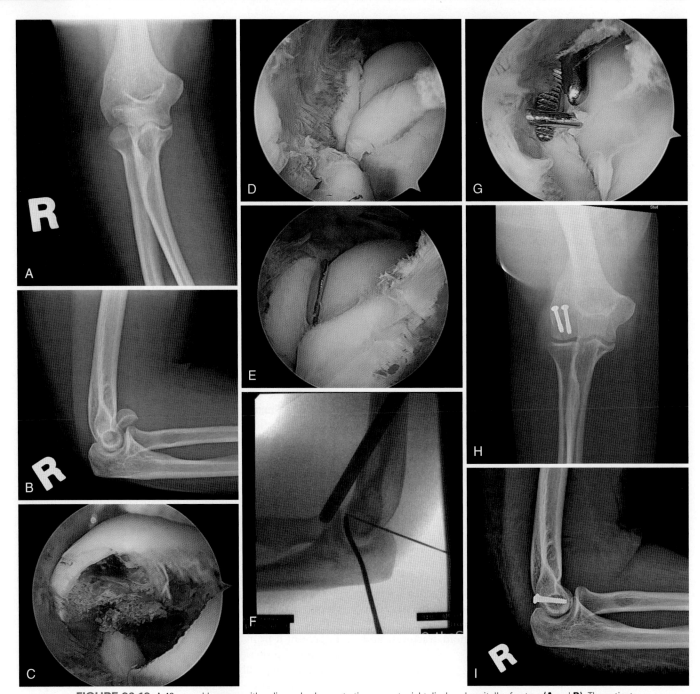

FIGURE 26.13 A 43-year-old woman with radiographs demonstrating an acute right displaced capitellar fracture **(A** and **B)**. The patient was managed with arthroscopic reduction and internal fixation with cannulated screws. An arthroscopic view from the anteromedial portal demonstrates the displaced fracture **(C)**. After provisional reduction **(D)**, an anatomic reduction is obtained by inserting a Howarth retractor through the soft spot portal to compress the capitellum **(E)**. Guide pins from a cannulated screw system are inserted in a retrograde manner with fluoroscopic assistance **(F** and **G)**. Radiographs at 6 months after cannulated screw fixation demonstrate anatomic healing **(H** and **I)**.

fractures and plate fixation for proximal ulnar fractures. Arthroscopically assisted techniques for the coronoid in these circumstances provide little added benefit and may actually increase the complexity of treatment. At present, our indications for arthroscopic fixation of coronoid fractures are isolated displaced basilar coronoid fractures, displaced Regan-Morrey type 2 fractures with Mason type 1 or 2 radial head fractures where the radial head fracture is amenable to nonoperative

management or arthroscopic fixation, and larger anteromedial coronoid fractures that are not comminuted.

For coronoid fractures, the patient is placed in the lateral decubitus position and fluoroscopy is used. It is the author's preference to use a scope in the posterior and posterolateral compartments of the elbow initially to evacuate hematomas and assess for any associated injuries or osteochondral loose fragments. Following posterior compartment arthroscopy, the

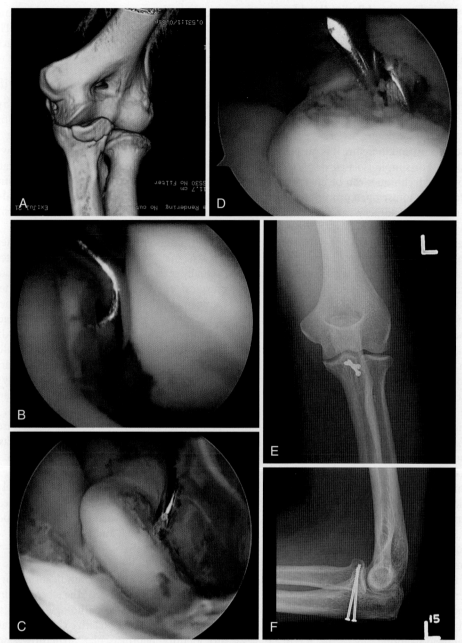

FIGURE 26.14 A 19-year-old male wrestler sustained a left displaced coronoid fracture **(A)**. The patient underwent arthroscopic reduction and internal fixation with two cannulated screws. An angled curet **(B)** and an arthroscopic shaver were used to débride the fracture site of hematoma. Once débridement had been done, an AO reduction forceps was used to provisionally reduce the fracture **(C)** until a guide pin was inserted in a retrograde manner **(D)**. Radiographs after 6 months demonstrate healing of the fracture **(E** and **F)**.

camera is introduced into the anterior compartment (Figure 26.14). Reduction of the coronoid fragment is obtained by use of a dental pick. To provisionally maintain the reduction, one tine of a pointed AO large reduction forceps can be brought in through a portal and used to clamp down on the fracture, with the other tine percutaneously placed on the subcutaneous border of the ulna. It is the author's preference to insert two or three guidewires with fluoroscopic guidance from the subcutaneous border of the ulna directed into the coronoid tip. Alternatively, an anterior cruciate ligament (ACL)-type targeting device can be used to direct the guidewires into the coronoid tip. Ideally, two partially threaded 2.7- to 3.5-mm cannulated screws are inserted from posterior to anterior. In smaller coronoid factures, however, it may be possible to insert only a single screw. After arthroscopic reduction and internal fixation of the coronoid fracture, other associated injuries are addressed, such as radial head fixation or lateral collateral ligament repair. Although lateral collateral ligaments can be repaired arthroscopically, it is the author's preference to repair them via a miniopen incision placed directly over the isometric point of the lateral epicondyle. Prior to completion of the surgical procedure, fluoroscopy is used to ensure an anatomic reduction and appropriate screw lengths and to assess elbow stability. Postoperative immobilization and rehabilitation are conducted based on an assessment of the stability of the fixation and also based on the associated injuries.

Technique for Arthroscopic Fixation of Radial Head Fractures

Arthroscopic techniques can be used for fixation of displaced radial head fractures. The advantages of arthroscopic techniques are better visualization of the entire joint, with less soft tissue disruption than in an open approach. The indications for arthroscopically assisted fixation are few, because in most patients with displaced radial head fractures, associated injuries are present that may preclude arthroscopy. Additionally, displaced and separated radial head fragments are typically difficult to reduce arthroscopically, and therefore it is my preference to use an open approach. For simple isolated displaced radial head fractures, arthroscopic techniques can be effective. At the present time, my preference is to use open procedures for most radial head fractures that require surgery.

It is my preference to start the arthroscopy in the posterior compartment. The hematoma is evacuated and the arthroscope is directed into the lateral gutter and posterior radiocapitellar joint. If the radial head fracture was associated with a dislocation, an impression fracture caused by the once dislocated radial head may be visible on the posterior aspect of the capitellum. The radial head is viewed from the midposterolateral portal. The radial head is placed through a full arc of prosupination to determine the best viewing and working portals for reduction and internal fixation. If the radial head fracture fragment is accessible from the posterior approach, a dental pick or elevator is placed through the distal posterolateral portal and used to elevate the depressed fragment. It is our experience that elevation of impacted radial head fracture fragments is difficult and typically requires more force than expected. Once a reduction is obtained, percutaneous guide pins are inserted into the fracture fragment. If fracture visualization or mobilization is poor through the posterior portals, the arthroscope can be introduced through the midanteromedial portal, with the midanterolateral portal functioning as a working portal. Cannulated screws of 2.7, 3, or 3.5 mm are typically used for internal fixation. Fluoroscopy is used to ensure an anatomic reduction and appropriate screw lengths.

Prior to closure, the elbow is placed through a range of motion to ensure there are no blocks to motion and stability is maintained. Postoperatively, range-of-motion movements can be initiated immediately because internal fixation typically results in stable radial head fixation.

Outcomes

The peer-reviewed outcome literature on the arthroscopic management of elbow fractures is limited. Kuriyama and colleagues[21] reported on two patients undergoing arthroscopic fixation of capitellar-trochlear fractures with good outcomes. Adams and associates[1a] reported on seven patients with coronoid fractures treated with arthroscopic techniques. The authors state that all patients had good function and a pain-free result after arthroscopic treatment. Hausman and coworkers[15] also reported on patients with coronoid fractures treated with arthroscopic techniques. In their series, four patients underwent arthroscopic reduction and fixation and were evaluated at a minimum of 1 year following surgery. All patients achieved a functional range of motion, and the authors concluded that arthroscopic techniques allow for excellent fracture visualization that enables anatomic repair without extensive open soft tissue dissection. For the radial head, Michels and colleagues[25] reported on 14 patients who underwent arthroscopic management for displaced partial articular head fractures. The authors reported that all patients had good to excellent outcomes. They caution, however, that the technique is technically demanding.

Arthroscopic Release of Elbow Stiffness Caused by Trauma or Developing Following Surgery

Arthroscopic management of elbow stiffness caused by subacute trauma or developing following surgery should be reserved for the highly experienced elbow arthroscopist. Stiffness may be due to intrinsic or extrinsic causes. Intrinsic causes include articular damage or malunion, intraarticular hardware, and loose bodies; extrinsic causes include a contracted joint capsule and ligaments, heterotopic ossification, prominent hardware, and skin contracture.

Although in theory the technical steps for arthroscopic release may be similar to those for osteoarthritis, there are actually several important differences. A posttraumatic or postsurgical contracture is typically associated with a damaged, abnormally thickened joint capsule and the potential for altered anatomy. The joint space is usually contracted, and the capsule is scarred down to the bones, making it difficult to even enter the elbow joint. The anatomy can be visually confusing once the joint is entered because adhesions and scarring may be present. Because the anterior soft tissues are usually contracted, the locations of the median and radial nerves may be altered. In some cases, endoscopic nerve identification may be required to safely conduct an arthroscopic contracture release. For this reason, the major disadvantage of arthroscopic release of postsurgical or posttraumatic stiffness is damage to the adjacent neurologic structures (and/or the articular cartilage). The major advantage of the procedure, if it is conducted safely by an experienced arthroscopist, is effective contracture release without the possible complications associated with an open approach, such as hematoma, seroma, and skin flap issues.

Indications and Contraindications

The indications and contraindications for arthroscopic release of nonarthritic stiffness of the elbow are individualized to each patient, the associated pathologic findings, and the experience of the arthroscopist. Relative contraindications are an inability to identify neurovascular structures safely, the presence of extensive heterotopic ossification or myositis ossificans, or the presence of a large amount of hardware, removal of which would require an extensive open approach.

Preoperative Planning

Preoperative planning is individualized to the patient's particular pathologic condition. Along with radiographs, CT scans are typically helpful to identify heterotopic ossification, locate hardware or screws, and define the articular pathologic findings. Ultrasound or MRI may also be helpful if the locations of nerves are unknown, for example, to identify an ulnar nerve transposition.

Technique

The major technical steps of contracture release of a stiff elbow are similar to those for release in osteoarthritis. However, the execution of the steps is technically much more challenging and should be reserved for the highly experienced arthroscopist.

The surgery progresses through all of the elbow compartments in a systematic fashion, with pathologic structures being excised or released as required. It is beyond the scope of this chapter to outline the techniques for endoscopic nerve neurolysis or extracapsular arthroscopic releases (outside-in arthroscopic release).[19] It is the author's recommendation that posttraumatic or postsurgical stiffness of the elbow be cautiously approached with arthroscopy.

Outcomes

Cefo and Eygendaal[8] reported on 27 patients undergoing arthroscopic release for posttraumatic stiffness. At follow-up, the patients' range of motion was significantly better, with the mean total arc of motion improving from 99 degrees preoperatively to 125 degrees postoperatively. The elbow function assessment scores improved significantly from 69 preoperatively to 91 postoperatively. The authors concluded that arthroscopic release is safe and reliable. However, it is a technically challenging procedure.

Timmerman and Andrews[42] reported on 19 cases of posttraumatic stiffness from elbow fracture or fracture-dislocation. In their series, good to excellent results were obtained in 79% of patients. The extension range of motion improved from 29 to 11 degrees, and flexion improved from 123 to 134 degrees. The authors stated that although good outcomes can be expected in most patients, recovery of full range of motion is unlikely.

Although the literature cited previously demonstrates good outcomes with arthroscopic techniques for posttraumatic stiffness, results should be interpreted with caution because the cohorts are likely biased. The papers are authored by expert arthroscopists who also conduct open procedures for cases deemed too risky for arthroscopy. The patients in the two series cited did not have high-grade contractures or ankylosis as evidenced by the preoperative range-of-motion values. Each patient with posttraumatic or postsurgical stiffness should be evaluated individually for suitability for an arthroscopic release. Furthermore, if arthroscopic release is attempted, one must be ready to convert to an open approach if necessary.

Advanced Arthroscopic Procedures

In addition to the previously mentioned procedures, several other pathologic conditions may be managed arthroscopically. Unfortunately, it is beyond the scope of this chapter to specifically address all of the conditions that can be managed with elbow arthroscopy. O'Brien and colleagues[28a] have described an arthroscopic technique for repair of the lateral collateral ligament after acute and subacute elbow dislocations in high-demand patients. Fourteen patients were reviewed at a mean of 30 months following surgery. All patients were described as satisfied with their outcome, and the authors concluded that the procedure is safe and effective at restoring elbow stability and allowing patients to return to activities.

Arthroscopic techniques can also be used to repair partial and complete triceps tendon injuries. Athwal and associates[5] described arthroscopic repair of isolated avulsions of the medial head of the triceps insertion in two patients with good outcomes. Heikenfeld and coworkers[17] described the endoscopic repair of partial triceps tendon insertional tears in 14 patients. The authors described the endoscopic repair of superficial triceps tears as leading to excellent outcomes at 1 year of follow-up.

Zonno and colleagues[47] conducted a cadaveric study to examine the technique of arthroscopic medial epicondylitis surgery. The authors concluded that arthroscopic medial epicondylar débridement can be performed with minimal risk of injury to the ulnar nerve or medial collateral ligament. In their cadaveric study, the mean distance between the débridement site and the ulnar nerve or medial collateral ligament was 21 mm and 8 mm, respectively.

COMPLICATIONS

As with any surgical procedure, complications do occur with elbow arthroscopy. The greatest concern is injury to the adjacent nerves. The literature has demonstrated that all major nerves around the elbow are at risk for injury.[1,2,20,24,26,37,38,45] The overall incidence of nerve injury after elbow arthroscopy is likely underestimated; however, the literature reports a rate of between 1 and 14%. Nerve injuries are most frequently reported as neurapraxias; with elbow arthroscopy, however, the risk of nerve transection is higher than normal. Nerve transection can occur with the insertion of sharp trocars through portals and inadvertently with motorized soft tissue resectors. Factors that may be associated with an increased risk of nerve injury include rheumatoid arthritis, severe contractures, ankylosis, postsurgical contractures, and posttraumatic stiffness. Any condition that results in altered anatomy may place the nerves at risk. With rheumatoid arthritis, the risk is believed to be higher due to the thin capsular tissue that is easily resected, with resultant injury to the adjacent nerves.

Superficial portal site infection or localized stitch abscesses are common following arthroscopy and can be managed with local wound care and oral antibiotics. Deep infection following arthroscopy is rare and typically should be managed with surgical débridement and intravenous antibiotics. Other complications that are reported to occur after elbow arthroscopy are compartment syndrome, heterotopic ossification, thromboembolism, arthrofibrosis, and fracture.[1,9,13,38-40,44-47]

REFERENCES

1. Adams JE, King GJ, Steinmann SP, et al: Elbow arthroscopy: indications, techniques, outcomes, and complications. *J Am Acad Orthop Surg* 22(12):810–818, 2014.
1a. Adams JE, Merten SM, Steinmann SP: Arthroscopic-assisted treatment of coronoid fractures. *Arthroscopy* 23(10):1060–1065, 2007.
2. Adams JE, Steinmann SP: Nerve injuries about the elbow. *J Hand Surg [Am]* 31(2):303–313, 2006.
3. Adams JE, Wolff LH, 3rd, Merten SM, et al: Osteoarthritis of the elbow: results of arthroscopic osteophyte resection and capsulectomy. *J Shoulder Elbow Surg* 17(1):126–131, 2008.
4. Andrews JR, Carson WG: Arthroscopy of the elbow. *Arthroscopy* 1(2):97–107, 1985.
5. Athwal GS, McGill RJ, Rispoli DM: Isolated avulsion of the medial head of the triceps tendon: an anatomic study and arthroscopic repair in 2 cases. *Arthroscopy* 25(9):983–988, 2009.
6. Blonna D, Huffmann GR, O'Driscoll SW: Delayed-onset ulnar neuritis after release of elbow contractures: clinical presentation, pathological findings, and treatment. *Am J Sports Med* 42(9):2113–2121, 2014.
7. Blonna D, O'Driscoll SW: Delayed-onset ulnar neuritis after release of elbow contracture: preventive strategies derived from a study of 563 cases. *Arthroscopy* 30(8):947–956, 2014.
8. Cefo I, Eygendaal D: Arthroscopic arthrolysis for posttraumatic elbow stiffness. *J Shoulder Elbow Surg* 20(3):434–439, 2011.

9. Cohen AP, Redden JF, Stanley D: Treatment of osteoarthritis of the elbow: a comparison of open and arthroscopic debridement. *Arthroscopy* 16(7):701–706, 2000.

10. Cohen MS, Romeo AA, Hennigan SP, et al: Lateral epicondylitis: anatomic relationships of the extensor tendon origins and implications for arthroscopic treatment. *J Shoulder Elbow Surg* 17(6):954–960, 2008.

11. Field LD, Altchek DW, Warren RF, et al: Arthroscopic anatomy of the lateral elbow: a comparison of three portals. *Arthroscopy* 10(6):602–607, 1994.

12. Gammon B, Bicknell RT, Athwal GS: Physical examination of the shoulder and elbow. In Boyer MI, editor: *AAOS comprehensive orthopaedic review 2*, ed 2, Rosemont, IL, 2014, American Academy of Orthpaedic Surgeons, pp 899–912.

13. Gofton WT, King GJ: Heterotopic ossification following elbow arthroscopy. *Arthroscopy* 17(1):E2, 2001.

14. Hardy P, Menguy F, Guillot S: Arthroscopic treatment of capitellum fracture of the humerus. *Arthroscopy* 18(4):422–426, 2002.

15. Hausman MR, Klug RA, Qureshi S, et al: Arthroscopically assisted coronoid fracture fixation: a preliminary report. *Clin Orthop Relat Res* 466(12):3147–3152, 2008.

16. Hausman MR, Qureshi S, Goldstein R, et al: Arthroscopically-assisted treatment of pediatric lateral humeral condyle fractures. *J Pediatr Orthop* 27(7):739–742, 2007.

17. Heikenfeld R, Listringhaus R, Godolias G: Endoscopic repair of tears of the superficial layer of the distal triceps tendon. *Arthroscopy* 30(7):785–789, 2014.

18. Kalainov DM, Cohen MS: Posterolateral rotatory instability of the elbow in association with lateral epicondylitis. A report of three cases. *J Bone Joint Surg Am* 87(5):1120–1125, 2005.

19. Kamineni S, Savoie FH, 3rd, ElAttrache N: Endoscopic extracapsular capsulectomy of the elbow: a neurovascularly safe technique for high-grade contractures. *Arthroscopy* 23(7):789–792, 2007.

20. Kelly EW, Morrey BF, O'Driscoll SW: Complications of elbow arthroscopy. *J Bone Joint Surg Am* 83(1):25–34, 2001.

21. Kuriyama K, Kawanishi Y, Yamamoto K: Arthroscopic-assisted reduction and percutaneous fixation for coronal shear fractures of the distal humerus: report of two cases. *J Hand Surg [Am]* 35(9):1506–1509, 2010.

22. Lattermann C, Romeo AA, Anbari A, et al: Arthroscopic debridement of the extensor carpi radialis brevis for recalcitrant lateral epicondylitis. *J Shoulder Elbow Surg* 19(5):651–656, 2010.

23. Lynch GJ, Meyers JF, Whipple TL, et al: Neurovascular anatomy and elbow arthroscopy: inherent risks. *Arthroscopy* 2(3):190–197, 1986.

24. Marti D, Spross C, Jost B: The first 100 elbow arthroscopies of one surgeon: analysis of complications. *J Shoulder Elbow Surg* 22(4):567–573, 2013.

25. Michels F, Pouliart N, Handelberg F: Arthroscopic management of Mason type 2 radial head fractures. *Knee Surg Sports Traumatol Arthrosc* 15(10):1244–1250, 2007.

26. Nelson GN, Wu T, Galatz LM, et al: Elbow arthroscopy: early complications and associated risk factors. *J Shoulder Elbow Surg* 23(2):273–278, 2014.

27. Nemoto K, Arino H, Yoshihara Y, et al: Arthroscopic synovectomy for the rheumatoid elbow: a short-term outcome. *J Shoulder Elbow Surg* 13(6):652–655, 2004.

28. Nishiwaki M, Willing R, Johnson JA, et al: Identifying the location and volume of bony impingement in elbow osteoarthritis by 3-dimensional computational modeling. *J Hand Surg [Am]* 38(7):1370–1376, 2013.

28a. O'Brien MJ, Lee Murphy R, Savoie FH, 3rd: A preliminary report of acute and subacute arthroscopic repair of the radial ulnohumeral ligament after elbow dislocation in the high-demand patient. *Arthroscopy* 30(6):679–687, 2014.

29. O'Driscoll SW: Elbow arthroscopy for loose bodies. *Orthopedics* 15(7):855–859, 1992.

30. O'Driscoll SW, Morrey BF: Arthroscopy of the elbow. Diagnostic and therapeutic benefits and hazards. *J Bone Joint Surg Am* 74(1):84–94, 1992.

31. Ogilvie-Harris DJ, Schemitsch E: Arthroscopy of the elbow for removal of loose bodies. *Arthroscopy* 9(1):5–8, 1993.

32. Omid R, Hamid N, Keener JD, et al: Relation of the radial nerve to the anterior capsule of the elbow: anatomy with correlation to arthroscopy. *Arthroscopy* 28(12):1800–1804, 2012.

33. Peart RE, Strickler SS, Schweitzer KM, Jr: Lateral epicondylitis: a comparative study of open and arthroscopic lateral release. *Am J Orthop (Belle Mead NJ)* 33(11):565–567, 2004.

34. Poehling GG, Whipple TL, Sisco L, et al: Elbow arthroscopy: a new technique. *Arthroscopy* 5(3):222–224, 1989.

35. Rolla PR, Surace MF, Bini A, et al: Arthroscopic treatment of fractures of the radial head. *Arthroscopy* 22(2):233 e1–233 e6, 2006.

36. Rubenthaler F, Wiese M, Senge A, et al: Long-term follow-up of open and endoscopic Hohmann procedures for lateral epicondylitis. *Arthroscopy* 21(6):684–690, 2005.

37. Ruch DS, Poehling GG: Anterior interosseus nerve injury following elbow arthroscopy. *Arthroscopy* 13(6):756–758, 1997.

38. Savoie FH, 3rd, Field LD: Arthrofibrosis and complications in arthroscopy of the elbow. *Clin Sports Med* 20(1):123–129, ix, 2001.

39. Savoie FH, 3rd, Nunley PD, Field LD: Arthroscopic management of the arthritic elbow: indications, technique, and results. *J Shoulder Elbow Surg* 8(3):214–219, 1999.

40. Stothers K, Day B, Regan WR: Arthroscopy of the elbow: anatomy, portal sites, and a description of the proximal lateral portal. *Arthroscopy* 11(4):449–457, 1995.

41. Tanaka N, Sakahashi H, Hirose K, et al: Arthroscopic and open synovectomy of the elbow in rheumatoid arthritis. *J Bone Joint Surg Am* 88(3):521–525, 2006.

42. Timmerman LA, Andrews JR: Arthroscopic treatment of posttraumatic elbow pain and stiffness. *Am J Sports Med* 22(2):230–235, 1994.

43. van den Ende KI, McIntosh AL, Adams JE, et al: Osteochondritis dissecans of the capitellum: a review of the literature and a distal ulnar portal. *Arthroscopy* 27(1):122–128, 2011.

44. Van Tongel A, Macdonald P, Van Riet R, et al: Elbow arthroscopy in acute injuries. *Knee Surg Sports Traumatol Arthrosc* 20(12):2542–2548, 2012.

45. Verhaar J, van Mameren H, Brandsma A: Risks of neurovascular injury in elbow arthroscopy: starting anteromedially or anterolaterally? *Arthroscopy* 7(3):287–290, 1991.

46. Yeoh KM, King GJ, Faber KJ, et al: Evidence-based indications for elbow arthroscopy. *Arthroscopy* 28(2):272–282, 2012.

47. Zonno A, Manuel J, Merrell G, et al: Arthroscopic technique for medial epicondylitis: technique and safety analysis. *Arthroscopy* 26(5):610–616, 2010.

27

Total Elbow Arthroplasty

Mark S. Cohen and Neal C. Chen

Acknowledgments: We would like to acknowledge the contributions of prior author Leonid Katolik, MD, for his contributions to earlier editions and his insights in developing the current text.

Total elbow arthroplasty (TEA) is increasingly used for the treatment of debilitating elbow arthropathies. Although clinical outcomes following TEA were initially disappointing, modifications in surgical technique and implant design have improved reliability; however, durability with normal loading (>10 pounds) is uncertain. Prosthetic replacement of the elbow relieves pain and typically provides a functional arc of motion, thereby permitting patients to better perform low-load activities of daily living. The longevity of implants in younger patients (those younger than 70 years) is often short, and revision options are limited. Long-term follow-up studies report high rates of revision relative to arthroplasties of the hip, knee, and shoulder.[15,30] Because of the high potential for mechanical failure and loosening, this procedure should be limited to low-demand elderly patients or those terribly debilitated by pain and instability. It is hoped that improvements in materials, implant design, and surgical technique will one day extend the suitability of TEA to a wider array of pathologic conditions and a broader demographic spectrum.

RHEUMATOID ARTHRITIS

Twenty percent of patients with rheumatoid arthritis have arthritic changes in the elbow.[45] As with other major joints affected by rheumatoid arthritis, the elbow undergoes a predictable pattern of intraarticular degeneration of the ulnohumeral and radiocapitellar surfaces, ultimately leading to functional loss in advanced cases. Rheumatoid arthritis has been divided into four stages, based on the physical examination and plain radiographs.[21] Stage I reveals osteoporosis and active synovitis with normal radiographs. Stage II demonstrates chronic synovitis with mild arthritic changes and some loss of joint space. In these early stages, arthroscopic synovectomy can be effective and seems to be more long-lasting in combination with the newer systemic agents. However, regardless of treatment, some patients proceed to complete loss of cartilage with associated pain and loss of strength (stage III). The most severe form (stage IV) demonstrates extensive loss of bone and gross instability (Figure 27.1). It is this last group of patients that derives the greatest benefit from TEA.

Preoperative Evaluation

Multiple Joint Involvement

Before considering TEA in a rheumatoid patient, the patient's overall status must be considered. If lower extremity joint replacements are planned, use of the affected limb may be needed for assisted ambulation. If shoulder replacement is being considered, this should generally be performed before TEA; surgical access to the elbow will be simpler, and the elbow replacement will not be stressed during shoulder replacement surgery. The cervical spine should be evaluated preoperatively, with special attention placed on atlantoaxial instability.

Physical Examination

Nerve Status. The status of the radial, ulnar, and median nerves should be assessed and documented before surgery. Rheumatoid arthritis of the elbow can lead to secondary compressive neuropathies of the upper extremity. Antecubital cysts and proliferative synovitis may extend through the joint, compressing the posterior interosseous nerve in the region of the proximal radioulnar joint. Similarly, the ulnar nerve lies along the medial ulnohumeral joint and may be compromised by bony deformity, instability, and direct soft tissue compression from synovitis. A careful neurologic evaluation is thus required in all patients before elbow replacement surgery.

If unconstrained arthroplasty is being considered, it is important to evaluate the integrity of the collateral ligaments. Ligamentous laxity or insufficiency may lead one to consider using a convertible or semiconstrained arthroplasty instead.

Medications. Patients with rheumatoid arthritis are now being treated with a variety of medications that require management in the perioperative period. It is wise to consult with the patient's rheumatologist before surgery. Methotrexate can generally be continued during the perioperative period, in the hope of avoiding a flare of inflammation. In contrast, the biologic drugs (anti–tumor necrosis factor agents) are withheld for at least one cycle before surgery and resumed after suture or staple removal. Patients who have been receiving long-term corticosteroid treatment may require stress dosing in the perioperative period. Further study is needed to determine the relative risk of infection and poor wound healing versus stimulating an inflammatory flare by withholding these valuable medications.

Preoperative Planning

Preoperative radiographs should include multiple views of the elbow as well as long-length humerus and forearm films. Views of the contralateral elbow may be helpful for templating if there

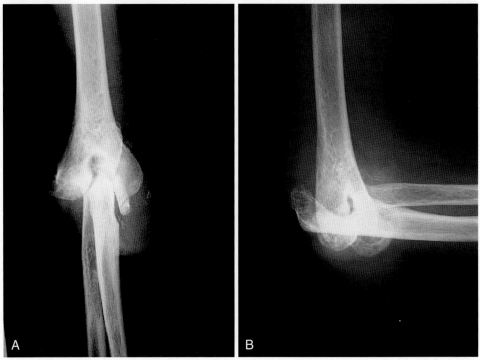

FIGURE 27.1 Anteroposterior **(A)** and lateral **(B)** radiographs of a severe stage IV rheumatoid elbow. The loss of bone support and ligamentous integrity leads to gross joint instability.

are large areas of bony destruction in the affected joint. Any arthroplasties of adjacent joints are evaluated for stem length, mode of fixation, and any cement defects. Any areas of cortical thinning should also be noted. For all elbow arthroplasties, preoperative templating should be performed to anticipate stem length and size.

POSTTRAUMATIC ARTHRITIS

Posttraumatic arthritis is an increasingly common indication for replacement arthroplasty.[39] The treatment of posttraumatic arthritis must take into account the age and activity level of the patient, degree of impairment, and joint pathologic findings involved. Given the lack of durability of TEA and the propensity for implant failure, techniques such as internal fixation for nonunion and malunion, joint release and débridement, and interposition arthroplasty should be considered in younger, more active adults. Evaluation of the deformity and the quality of the articular surface may require additional radiographic studies in these patients, such as computed tomography. Replacement arthroplasty should be considered when the ulnohumeral joint is no longer salvageable (Figure 27.2). This option is typically limited to individuals older than approximately 60 to 65 years with lower physical demands. However, there may be circumstances in which the impairment and pain warrant the consideration of TEA. Any history of infection after fracture treatment requires careful consideration and may require a staged approach.

Preoperative Assessment
Soft Tissue Envelope
Some patients have had multiple surgeries or flap coverage and incisions should be evaluated carefully. In general, attempts are made to incorporate prior incisions into the approach. If a flap is present, Doppler identification of the flap pedicle may be considered and incisions can be designed to preserve it.

Preoperative Planning
Prior hardware should be noted and preparations for hardware removal should be made, taking into account the hardware manufacturer and the possibility that screws may be difficult to remove, especially if they are made of titanium. Preoperative templating should be used in order to bypass the most proximal humeral or distal ulnar screw hole by two diaphyseal widths if possible.

FRACTURES OF THE DISTAL HUMERUS

TEA may be indicated for elderly patients with displaced and comminuted fractures of the distal humerus.[5,11,34] In the past, the so-called bag-of-bones treatment was recommended because the fracture fragments were too small and the bone too osteoporotic to permit rigid internal fixation. However, this treatment of hopeful neglect frequently resulted in significant pain, stiffness, and decreased function of the hand. TEA after a fracture beyond repair may permit a more rapid return to function. TEA should also be considered in patients with fracture when there is preexisting joint destruction (Figure 27.3). Again, elbow arthroplasty should be limited to older, lower-demand individuals.

Preoperative Assessment
Radiographs
Radiographs of the shoulder and wrist should be performed to screen for other fractures. Radiographs of the elbow should be scrutinized for any extension into the humeral diaphysis that

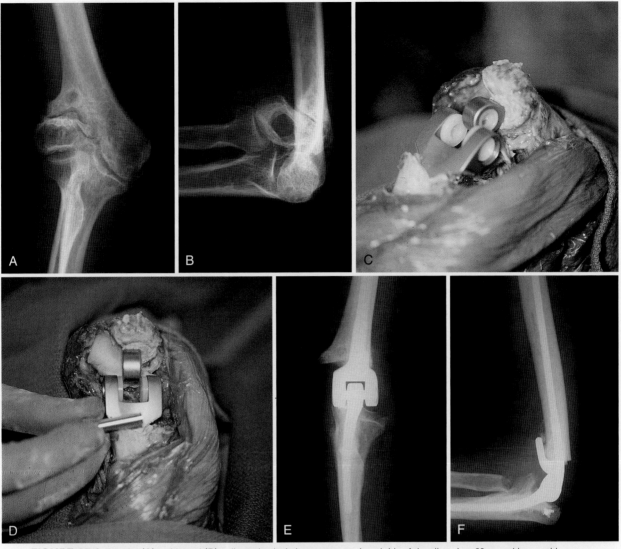

FIGURE 27.2 Anterior **(A)** and lateral **(B)** radiographs depicting posttraumatic arthritis of the elbow in a 66-year-old man with severe deformity and loss of function. **C,** Intraoperative view with the triceps reflected, showing humeral and ulnar components cemented in place. The remaining humeral condyles have been resected. **D,** Semiconstrained arthroplasty uses an axis pin to unite the components. Final anteroposterior **(E)** and lateral **(F)** radiographs of total elbow arthroplasty.

may affect arthroplasty placement. Advanced imaging (computerized tomography) may be used in this regard. It is important to understand the morphologic status of the distal humerus fracture. Injuries with low supracondylar involvement and osteoporotic bone with comminution may be amenable to TEA. Internal fixation is preferred for more proximal fractures, for example, when the transverse limb is proximal to the olecranon fossa.

PRIMARY OSTEOARTHRITIS

Primary osteoarthritis of the elbow affects middle-aged and older individuals, primarily men in the fifth decade of life or later; it is rare in women. Most cases involve the dominant side, and many patients report a lifetime of heavy loading. The most common presenting complaint in this population is pain at the extremes of motion, with loss of terminal flexion and extension.

Loss of forearm rotation is less common. Intermittent "locking" and pain may be due to loose bodies within the joint.

Individuals with primary arthritis of the elbow typically have bony overgrowth and osteophytes at the coronoid and olecranon processes. Fluffy densities may be observed filling the olecranon and coronoid fossae, and loose bodies can be seen. Narrowing at the radiocapitellar joint is a common finding, although it is not typically symptomatic. The central aspect of the ulnohumeral joint is characteristically spared in this patient population. Pain throughout the entire arc of elbow motion usually signifies synovitis or articular cartilage degeneration in the central ulnohumeral articulation. This is rare and is seen only in late disease.

It must be emphasized that up to 20% of patients with primary osteoarthritis of the elbow have some degree of ulnar neuropathy. The signs and symptoms can be quite insidious and may go unnoticed by the patient until there is substantial nerve

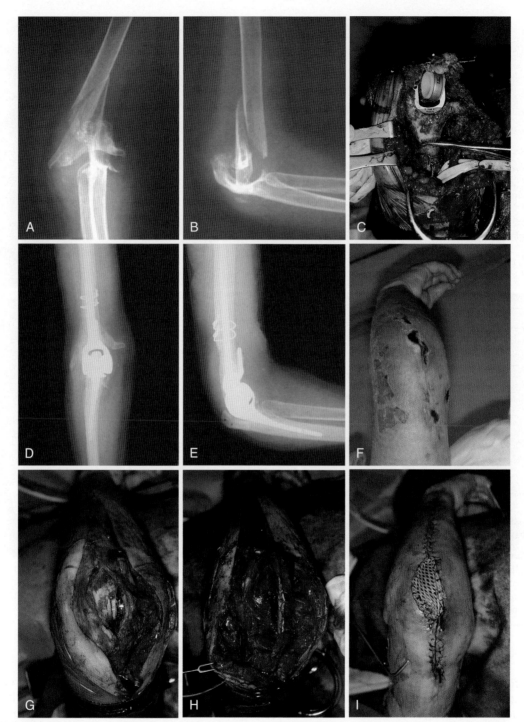

FIGURE 27.3 Anteroposterior **(A)** and lateral **(B)** radiographs of a 64-year-old woman with rheumatoid arthritis and an unstable distal humerus fracture above a severely arthritic joint. Note the presence of osteopenia. **C,** Intraoperative photograph depicts open reduction and internal fixation of the fracture with cerclage wires and cemented arthroplasty components. Postoperative anteroposterior **(D)** and lateral **(E)** radiographs. Note reduction of the humerus fracture. **F,** Unfortunately, the patient exhibited wound dehiscence, which failed to heal with local wound care. She was taking several immunosuppressive agents. **G,** Intraoperative view once the skin has been opened. The component is visible and communicates with the wound owing to partial triceps subluxation laterally. **H,** Joint and component coverage is obtained with a flexor carpi ulnaris muscle pedicle flap. **I,** Final coverage with a split-thickness skin graft over muscle. The joint cultures grew several organisms. The patient received 6 weeks of intravenous antibiotics and is taking chronic oral suppression therapy. At 3 years' follow-up, she has not had a recurrent infection.

dysfunction. The close association of the nerve to the postero-medial joint capsule leaves it susceptible to impingement from osteophytes or from medial joint synovitis expanding the capsule. Early cubital tunnel syndrome in these patients often manifests as pain at the medial elbow. It is thus important to examine these individuals for ulnar nerve irritability and traction signs.

Initial management of primary elbow arthritis consists of activity modification, antiinflammatory medication, intraarticular injection, and, occasionally, therapy. When these modalities prove unsuccessful and symptoms are troublesome, surgical intervention may be warranted. Given the generally young age and high functional demand of patients with primary osteoarthritis at the elbow, prosthetic replacement is usually not recommended. Arthroscopic or open joint débridement and release have traditionally been the primary surgical options because the central ulnohumeral joint space is typically maintained. TEA is reserved for individuals with more advanced arthrosis and lower functional demands who are older than 60 to 65 years. The mechanical failure of TEA in this group of patients has been well documented, so this treatment should be reserved for patients who are willing to reduce their level of activity.

HEMOPHILIC ARTHROPATHY

Patients with hemophilia may present with severe joint destruction as a result of hemophilic arthropathy. Involvement is commonly multiarticular, affecting the shoulders, elbows, hips, knees, and ankles. Potentially severe functional deficits may result. Surgical intervention for hemophilic arthropathy requires a coordinated, multidisciplinary approach. Factor VIII must be supplemented during the perioperative period. Furthermore, the prevalence of human immunodeficiency virus (HIV) in this population predisposes patients to considerable risks, including an increased incidence of secondary infection and a more rapid progression to acquired immunodeficiency syndrome (AIDS) in those with low CD4 counts.[18] Further investigation is needed to define the role of total elbow replacement in treating hemophilic arthropathy.

Preoperative Considerations

Perioperative Management of Blood Clotting

Perioperative management of hemophilia depends on the cause of the clotting disorder. It is important to have the patient's hematologist involved in blood product management and factor replacement throughout the preoperative and postoperative periods. In classic hemophilia, factor VIII must be supplemented during the perioperative period. In patients with von Willebrand disease, DDAVP or cryoprecipitate may be needed. Preparations with the inpatient blood bank are crucial to ensure adequate blood products are available at the time of surgery. At surgery, careful attention to hemostasis is important to avoid postoperative hematoma. Postoperative drain placement may be considered.

CONTRAINDICATIONS TO TOTAL ELBOW ARTHROPLASTY

There are several absolute and relative contraindications to TEA.

Presence of Infection at the Elbow

Any suspicion of infection in the skin, soft tissue, or bone should cause a postponement of the surgery.[53] Patients with rheumatoid arthritis and poor skin quality who are taking immunosuppressive drugs are especially prone to catastrophic postoperative infections. Other sources of bacteria, such as urinary tract infections, should also be screened. If an attempt at internal fixation for fracture has failed, deep infection at the site should be considered, and cultures should be obtained while the patient is free of any antibiotic treatment. The organisms can be quite indolent, especially *Staphylococcus epidermidis* species.

If active infection is present or even suspected, full débridement of all infected or compromised tissue is required, including all hardware. Trustworthy cultures must be obtained and the proper antibiotics administered through a peripherally inserted central catheter (PICC) line typically for a minimum of 6 weeks. Often a follow-up culture and biopsy of the elbow are obtained after the patient has stopped taking all antibiotics for 6 or more weeks. TEA is considered only after these studies confirm the absence of infection and acute inflammation.

Complete Ankylosis of the Neuropathic Joint

In patients with complete and painless ankylosis of the elbow, implant arthroplasty may not improve overall function. Although a considerable improvement in functional arc of motion has been reported following the conversion of elbow arthrodesis to prosthetic replacement,[24] the nature of the underlying pathologic condition leads to frequent postoperative complications and a less predictable outcome. Total elbow replacement is contraindicated in patients with neuropathic joint destruction owing to their inherent inability to comply with postoperative restrictions.

Poor-Quality Soft Tissue at the Elbow

Severely contracted, scarred, or burned skin needs to be assessed before considering total elbow replacement. For the implant to function properly, the skin and soft tissue need to be pliable enough to permit manipulation for placement of the implant. If there is inadequate soft tissue, a muscle flap should be considered before arthroplasty (see Chapter 44 on soft tissue coverage about the elbow).

HISTORICAL REVIEW OF TOTAL ELBOW ARTHROPLASTY

Elbow arthroplasty has evolved from attempts at resurfacing of the distal humerus or ulna with various materials. Constrained TEA, using a rigid hinge, led to rapid failures. Attempts at distal humeral and proximal ulna resurfacing were commonly complicated by component failure. These prototypes have evolved into the designs used currently (Table 27.1).

TYPES OF IMPLANTS

There are two general types of implants for the arthritic elbow: linked and unlinked. An unlinked or nonconstrained prosthesis relies on adequate bony support and collateral ligaments for stability. This theoretically decreases loosening at the

TABLE 27.1 **Historical Review of Elbow Arthroplasty**

Device and Era	Year of Notable Development	Author	Significance
Hemiarthroplasty, 1920 to 2000s	1952	Venable[48]	Metal distal humerus replacement
	1965	Barr and Eaton[2]	Vitallium replacement of distal humerus
	1970	Johnson and Schlein[16]	Vitallium replacement of proximal ulna
	1971	Peterson and Janes[31]	Vitallium ulnar "saddle" interposition; limited arc of motion; acceptable longevity
	2011	Burkhart et al[3]	Convertible hemiarthroplasty for distal humerus fracture
Constrained Arthroplasty, 1970 to 1980s	1972	Dee[7]	Hinged total elbow arthroplasty
	1982	Dee[8]	Recognition that rigid hinge has high rate of implant loosening
Surface Replacement Arthroplasty, 1970 to 1990s	1984	Rydholm et al[35]	Wadsworth prosthesis had high rates of humeral component loosening
	1990	Kudo and Iwano[19]	70% of surface replacements had humeral subsidence
Stemmed Unconstrained Arthroplasty, 1970s to 1990s	1983	Pritchard[32]	Early experience with stemmed resurfacing arthroplasty of ulna, radius, and distal humerus
	1994	Kudo et al[20]	Titanium-stemmed unconstrained arthroplasty: failures observed at humeral stem junction
	1999	Trail et al[47]	Souter-Strathclyde unconstrained arthroplasty: flanges into medial and lateral columns for added stability
Stemmed Semiconstrained Arthroplasty, 1970 to Present	1977	Schlein[38]	Introduction of semiconstrained prosthesis
	1982	Morrey and Bryan[26]	Recognition that semiconstrained prosthesis has better survivorship than tightly constrained hinge
	1992	O'Driscoll et al[28]	Anterior flange limits stress on cement interface

bone-cement interface but carries a greater risk of instability, especially in the rheumatoid population. Many unlinked designs have been discontinued but may be encountered in the revision setting. These include the Kudo/Instrumented Bone Preserving (Biomet Europe), Souter-Strathclyde (Wright, Arlington, TN; Figure 27.4), and Pritchard ERS (Depuy, Warsaw, IN).

Currently, linked designs involve stemmed implants with a semiconstrained articulation. Semiconstrained devices have the advantage over unlinked devices with respect to stability. However, even with several degrees of varus-valgus laxity, the most popular sloppy hinge mechanisms allow only a small area of contact between the humeral and ulnar components, leading to high contact stresses. Polyethylene wear of the bushings, osteolysis, and subsequent failure remain clinical problems.[21] Commonly used semiconstrained designs include the Coonrad-Morrey (Zimmer, Warsaw, IN) and Solar (Stryker, Mahwah, NJ).

In practice, reports of pain relief and functional gains appear to be similar for linked and unlinked designs. In an effort to improve on polyethylene wear, several new implants have been introduced. Some do not depend on a true hinge for stability and theoretically lead to decreased wear, as seen in prior hinge

designs (Discovery, Biomet, Warsaw, IN). Other prostheses have the capacity to be inserted in either a linked or an unlinked fashion (Latitude, Tornier, Saint-Ismier, France). No long-term data exist on these newer designs. It is hoped that continued advances in biomaterials and better anatomic designs will lead to improved and more durable implant options in the future.

❖ AUTHORS' PREFERRED METHOD OF TREATMENT

We currently use a semiconstrained linked prosthesis with either a loose hinge or a spherical articulation for the majority of elbow replacement surgeries. Although the unlinked designs should theoretically have lower loosening rates, this has not been proven clinically. The procedure is typically performed in a laminar flow room. The patient is positioned in a semilateral decubitus position on a beanbag, and the affected arm is rested across the chest on a bolster. A sterile tourniquet is applied. A posterior skin incision is made and taken down to the fascia, raising full-thickness fasciocutaneous flaps medially and laterally. The ulnar nerve is carefully dissected, transposed anteriorly into a subcutaneous pocket, and protected throughout the procedure.

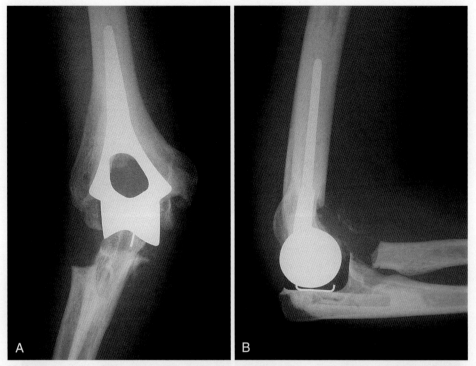

FIGURE 27.4 Anteroposterior **(A)** and lateral **(B)** radiographs of a Souter-Strathclyde unconstrained implant. The ulnar component consists of polyethylene, which is radiolucent.

Several options exist for reflecting the triceps mechanism to expose the joint. In the traditional approach, described by Bryan and Morrey, the triceps is elevated from medial to lateral in continuity with the anconeus to expose the distal humerus and elbow. One problem with this approach is postoperative triceps insufficiency, presumed to be related to failure of the repair. One of us (MSC) uses a straight triceps-splitting approach as described by Gschwend, in which the triceps muscle and tendon are split longitudinally and sharply elevated off the proximal ulna down the midline (Figure 27.5).[4,14] This may allow for a more secure repair of the triceps muscle and tendon at the completion of the procedure, with less theoretical tendency for the triceps to slide back off the olecranon process laterally. It is yet to be determined whether the rate of triceps insufficiency is reduced with this method.

Another option is a triceps-preserving approach.[33] The entirety of the triceps insertion is left intact while bone preparation, provisional assembly, and final prosthesis implantation are performed through medial and lateral windows. This approach allows immediate active triceps rehabilitation. However, it limits exposure and makes broaching of the ulnar canal and prosthesis assembly somewhat more challenging in situ. Furthermore, exposure of the humerus requires complete release of both collateral ligaments. It is unclear whether this soft tissue release adds morbidity with respect to implant longevity, such as by increasing stress on the polyethylene owing to a loss of ligamentous support.

Whichever approach is chosen to reflect the triceps mechanism, it is important to carefully dissect the Sharpey fibers off the olecranon process in a subperiosteal fashion. This can be very tedious, especially in the rheumatoid population. A knife should be used for this purpose, not a monopolar cautery. The latter can lead to tissue necrosis and may inhibit tendon healing following repair. The insertion point of the triceps on the tip of the olecranon should be tagged to allow a more anatomic repair following implantation. This may help decrease triceps dysfunction postoperatively.

In cases with deficient distal humeral columns, including fractures and nonunions, one can use a true triceps-sparing approach. In this technique, the distal humerus is excised, and one can work through either side of the triceps insertion while preserving its attachment to the olecranon (Figure 27.6). As noted, this does compromise visualization, especially for the ulna. Because triceps insufficiency is not uncommon following arthroplasty, and because humeral condyle resection does not affect the ultimate strength or functional outcome when using semiconstrained devices,[25] one may consider resecting the distal humerus at the proximal aspect of the trochlea in selected cases (e.g., elderly patients with rheumatoid arthritis). This approach necessitates complete release of the collateral ligaments and flexor-pronator and extensor muscle origins from the humerus. Rehabilitation is simplified, and this may improve elbow extension power and control. The amount of distal humerus resected also depends on the type of articulation of the implant arthroplasty.

Once the joint surfaces are exposed, including the trochlea, humeral columns, and olecranon process, the bony work is initiated. Exposure is facilitated by hyperflexion and subluxation of the elbow with external rotation of the shoulder. The tip of the olecranon and the tip of the coronoid process are resected to decrease the potential for impingement. Bony impingement of the olecranon or coronoid should be checked

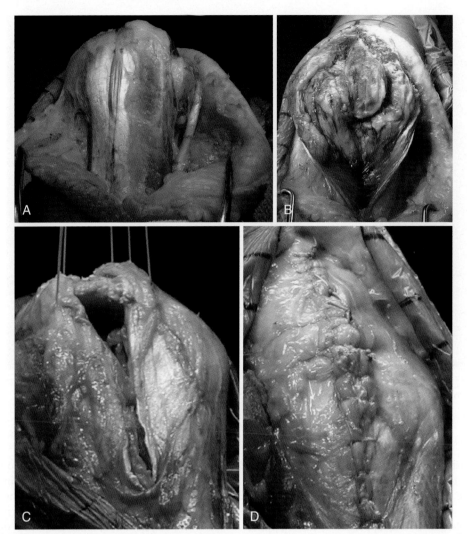

FIGURE 27.5 A, Intraoperative view of the Gschwend triceps-splitting approach to the elbow. Note that the ulnar nerve has been dissected out and protected. The split occurs in the tendinous portion of the triceps. **B,** Joint exposure is obtained with full-thickness medial and lateral flaps. **C,** Sutures are in place for repair and closure of the split. **D,** Final repair, with several sutures placed through drill holes in the olecranon.

both during trial implant insertion and after the permanent implant is placed. Unless the arthritis is limited to the ulnohumeral articulation, the radial head is commonly excised. Care should be taken to place retractors around the neck of the radius to protect the posterior interosseous nerve, which lies just anterior to the radial head outside the elbow capsule. Next, the central aspect of the trochlea is resected, and the humeral canal is entered with a bur. The entry point is typically more posterior than initially appreciated. Once the canal is defined, cutting guides are typically used to prepare the distal humerus and trial implants can be evaluated. Complete seating of the prosthesis can be blocked by the anterior cortex, which occasionally has to be deepened to accept the anterior flange of the implant.

The ulna is more difficult to prepare than the humerus. The ulnar canal is commonly entered with a bur, and the opening is enlarged with a bur and rasps. It is important to open the proximal ulna widely. A common technical error is to make an ulnar aperture that is too small. This makes seating of the rasps difficult. A second technical error is to seat the ulnar component too distally into the ulna, causing impingement of the coronoid against the remaining distal humerus in flexion. Care must be taken not to perforate the thin cortices of the proximal ulna, especially in patients with rheumatoid arthritis. If the alignment is in question, intraoperative fluoroscopy may be helpful to confirm the direction of the rasp, bur, and stem. One must appreciate the 4- to 5-degree valgus angulation of the shaft of the ulna relative to the greater sigmoid notch. When there is difficulty seating a rasp, bone at the canal entry is most commonly the limiting factor. In addition, a trough is commonly required in the posterior olecranon to avoid placing the ulnar component in flexion. Once component sizes are chosen, one should insert trial implants to ensure an adequate arc of motion without impingement.

During insertion of the trial components, the range of motion should be carefully examined. Elbow joints that were quite stiff before surgery may require an extensive release of the anterior capsule from the humerus and a more generous

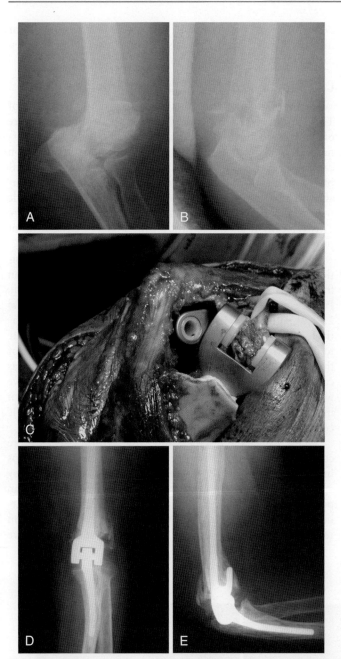

FIGURE 27.6 Anteroposterior **(A)** and lateral **(B)** radiographs of a severe distal humerus fracture in an 89-year-old woman with osteopenia. Note the high degree of comminution and osteopenia. **C,** Intraoperative view shows the triceps-preserving approach, with exposure of the humerus by working on each side of the triceps mechanism without distal detachment. This approach is possible in fractures or nonunions when the distal humerus is resected. Postoperative anteroposterior **(D)** and lateral **(E)** films, with the cemented semiconstrained arthroplasty in place. Note the condylar resection. (**C,** Courtesy of Graham King, MD.)

antibiotic-laden cement in a retrograde fashion using a cement gun with thin tubing. It is helpful to cool the cement and inject it in a more liquid state because it may be difficult to deliver viscous cement down the long, thin tube. Once placing the components, if the design allows, the joint may be cycled to theoretically help with component alignment. The elbow is then held in extension until the polymerization is complete. If the triceps is intact, cementing both components simultaneously may be more challenging. Excess cement is removed during this process.

Hemostasis is obtained once the tourniquet is deflated and the triceps mechanism is meticulously repaired. We use a running, locking, Kevlar-reinforced suture passed through drill holes in the olecranon tip for reattachment. This aspect of the procedure is very important, and care must be taken to complete a secure and anatomic repair. Tension after reattachment of the triceps needs to be checked so that full flexion can be achieved without detachment. If the Gschwend splitting approach is chosen, the running, locking stitch can be placed several millimeters away from the tendon edge, and additional side-to-side sutures can be placed centrally. More than one transosseous suture is commonly used with either method. The soft tissues are closed in a routine fashion, and the ulnar nerve is maintained in a subcutaneous position anterior to the epicondyle. A suction drain may be used depending on surgeon preference.

POSTOPERATIVE MANAGEMENT AND EXPECTATIONS

In rheumatoid patients with thin and friable skin, we immobilize the elbow for 10 to 14 days to allow soft tissue healing before motion is instituted. If the triceps was released from the ulna during exposure, the repair must be protected by restricting active extension for 6 to 8 weeks postoperatively. Initially, we often prescribe a sling during the day and a nighttime elbow orthosis in maximal extension to decrease the potential for flexion contracture. A removable long-arm orthosis for comfort and support between exercises may also be considered. At follow-up, patients are counseled on the importance of protecting the joint from excessive loads. Empirically, a 5-pound limit when lifting with the operated arm is recommended. Yearly clinical and radiographic evaluations are arranged, regardless of clinical symptoms.

At follow-up, frontal and lateral radiographs should be evaluated carefully, paying particular attention to the cement mantle and any signs of osteolysis. The ulnar component is at greatest risk for loosening. The bearing should be evaluated carefully for signs of wear on a true anteroposterior film with the elbow in full extension. In a Coonrad-Morrey semiconstrained prosthesis, partial wear is defined as greater than 7 degrees of ulnar component angulation relative to the humeral yoke.[12] Complete wear is defined as greater than 10 degrees of ulnar component angulation relative to the humeral yoke.[12] In cases of advanced osteolysis, lucencies may be seen at either the bone-cement or prosthetic-cement interface. The expected outcome following uncomplicated surgery is a nearly painless and functional arc of elbow motion. Patients commonly do not recover terminal elbow extension but ultimately regain full flexion within several months. Overall functional scores and satisfaction are generally

resection of the distal humerus, shortening the bone and permitting greater extension of the joint.

We currently use polyethylene cement restrictors in both the humeral and ulnar canals. As the humeral canal gets larger proximally, standard restrictors often do not allow a seal; umbrella designs are more effective (e.g., Tornier, Saint-Ismier, France). Alternatively, a small piece of cancellous bone can be used in the ulna. The canals are lavaged, dried, and injected with higher and long-term complications are lower in rheumatoid patients than in those with posttraumatic arthritis.[12] This likely relates to the lower demands of the rheumatoid population. Although pain relief is almost uniformly excellent in rheumatoid individuals, range of motion often improves only modestly. This is especially true in patients with very limited elbow function preoperatively, such as that seen in juvenile rheumatoid disease. These individuals often remain quite stiff even after successful arthroplasty.

For posttraumatic arthritis, results are less uniform. One study reported that 69 of 85 joints were functional at a mean follow-up of 9 years with the use of a semiconstrained prosthesis for posttraumatic dysfunction. Sixty-eight percent of patients had a good to excellent Mayo Elbow Performance Score. However, 29 elbows had complications, including infection, component fracture, and bushing wear.[46]

When arthroplasty is used for acute trauma following distal humerus fracture, successful results can be obtained in selected patients. The largest study reviewed 49 cases with an average follow-up of 7 years. Many of the patients (62%) had coexistent conditions, with nearly 40% suffering from rheumatoid arthritis.[17] It was therefore difficult to generalize to patients with only fractures. Although 93% of patients had a satisfactory outcome, 29% reported complications. These included wound problems, transient nerve dysfunction, component fracture, and component loosening. The authors stressed the need for strict inclusion criteria when using arthroplasty in this setting.

Prosthesis Longevity

The national registries of Scotland and Finland report 10-year survivorship rates of TEA at 90% and 83%, respectively.[15] Other studies have reported an overall 5-year survivorship rate as low as 72%.[41] TEA in patients with rheumatoid arthritis has superior longevity, with a survival rate of 92% at 10 years.[12] TEA performed for posttraumatic arthritis has a 70% 15-year implant survival rate, with a significant association between earlier age at time of arthroplasty and implant failure.[46]

Complications of Total Elbow Arthroplasty

When the world literature is reviewed, the complication rate of TEA varies between 20% and 45%.[14] Intraoperatively, fracture of a humeral condyle can be treated with simple excision. Alternatively, if the fragment is large, reduction and internal fixation can be considered (Figure 27.7). The risk of intraoperative complications due to bone loss is significantly increased in individuals with advanced rheumatoid arthritis.[23] Late humeral condyle fracture can occur, most commonly along the medial column. This typically heals uneventfully with a short period of joint protection.

Regardless of the care taken during dissection and transposition of the ulnar nerve, sensory dysfunction is not uncommon following arthroplasty. Ulnar motor weakness is less common. Postoperative ulnar neuropathy has been reported in up to 25% of patients.[14,27] Excessive traction on the nerve perioperatively, hematoma, constricting dressings, thermal damage due to polymerization of methylmethacrylate, and devitalization of the nerve during translocation have all been implicated as causative factors. Incomplete sensory deficits typically improve with time, but normal subjective sensation does not return in all cases, especially in an elderly person with multiple comorbidities.

Elbow extension weakness following arthroplasty is more common than is typically appreciated, especially if the triceps insertion was detached using the traditional Bryan-Morrey approach. Although the cause of triceps insufficiency is unclear, possible explanations include alteration of the joint level, affecting triceps tension, and failure of reattachment, with tendon retraction or subluxation. We believe the latter to be more

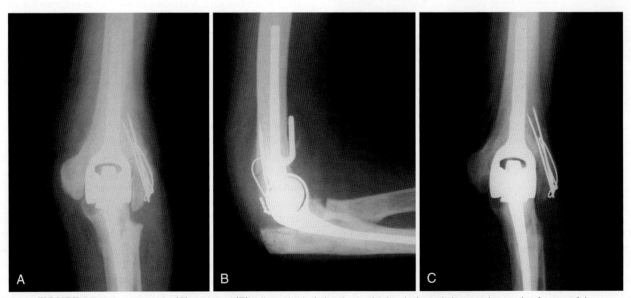

FIGURE 27.7 Anteroposterior **(A)** and lateral **(B)** radiographs depicting the tension band wire technique used to repair a fracture of the lateral column that occurred intraoperatively. Most commonly, these fragments are excised. Internal fixation was chosen in this case because of the patient's young age and the proximal extent of the fracture. This preserves bone stock as well as the extensor muscle origin at the epicondyle. **C,** Healing of the fracture at 3 months' follow-up.

probable and have observed this mode of tendon failure during revision surgery for loosening. Fortunately, even with detachment of the triceps from its insertion on the olecranon tip, some extensor function typically remains. Because elbow extension weakness is reasonably well tolerated using gravity assistance, there is usually little indication for triceps repair or reconstruction owing to insufficiency following arthroplasty.

Instability following TEA is largely limited to unlinked designs. Prevention of instability with a nonlinked prosthesis depends on meticulous technique, with restoration of proper tension to the soft tissues following implantation. Ligamentous insufficiency is a relative contraindication for these designs. Furthermore, implants that sacrifice the radial head decrease lateral joint support and impart a greater load to the collateral ligaments. Finally, axial malalignment of either component may compromise stability.[44] Limiting elbow extension in the immediate postoperative period may minimize the incidence of dislocation.[43,44] If a dislocation occurs, immobilization of the elbow at 90 degrees for 3 to 6 weeks is recommended. Recurrent symptomatic instability is addressed with soft tissue reconstruction when possible or revision to a linked design.

Disassembly of a linked prosthesis may occur. This was a particular problem with the earlier designs, such as the GSB III.[17] It was thought that an overly extensive soft tissue release, as well as component malposition, might lead to gradual overload of the linkage mechanism until disassembly ultimately occurred.

Mechanical Failure

Mechanical failure, loosening, and osteolysis underscore the fact that arthroplasty is relatively contraindicated in patients who anticipate strenuous physical activity or are not expected to comply with the postoperative protocol. Arthroplasty candidates must be willing to adhere to postoperative limitations of not lifting anything heavier than approximately 5 to 10 pounds and no repetitive lifting of any object heavier than 2 to 3 pounds. Optimal cementing technique may help minimize loosening. This includes careful canal preparation, use of a cement restrictor, and application of low-viscosity cement with pressurization. These methods are thought to improve the initial fixation of the humeral component and perhaps decrease the incidence of aseptic loosening.[6,9]

Unfortunately, wear debris and osteolysis can be seen relatively early, even in lower-demand individuals (Figure 27.8). This may be secondary to stress concentration and mechanical wear of the bushings in the current semiconstrained designs. Suboptimal positioning of the prosthesis may affect its longevity. For example, it has been shown that if the humeral component of the Coonrad-Morrey prosthesis is inserted in more than 10 degrees of malrotation, the varus and valgus laxity during the flexion and extension arc follow the structural limits of the hinge.[40] This neutralizes the advantages of the sloppy hinge mechanism and leads to increased stresses on the polyethylene and the bone-cement interface. Excessively tight soft tissues, such as those following inadequate release, may also contribute to wear.

If progressive osteolysis is noted on serial radiographs, even in the absence of symptoms, consideration must be given to revision surgery. If the components are stable and positioned appropriately, débridement, bone grafting, and replacement of the polyethylene bushings may be all that are indicated. Consideration can also be given to oral diphosphonates, which slow osteolytic progression. If the components are found to be loose intraoperatively, implant revision is required.

Osteolysis and aseptic loosening are increasingly recognized complications of TEA. This is likely due to multiple modes of wear, including asymmetric thinning of the humeral bushings and unintended metal-on-metal wear between bearing and nonbearing surfaces or between two nonbearing surfaces. Wear between the stem and cement mantle is typically observed in most ulnar components at the time of revision. The histopathologic status of the periprosthetic tissues at the time of revision surgery has been found to be similar in character to that observed in association with osteolysis and loosening of total hip and knee replacements.[13,22,50]

The potential for component fracture is inherent to any implantable device. For the elbow, a resultant force vector of up to three times body weight is directed anteriorly in flexion and posteriorly in extension. Approximately 1 million compression-distraction loading cycles are generated per year. In spite of these tremendous stresses, advanced metallurgy and modifications in prosthetic design make ulnar or humeral stem fracture an uncommon event, cited in 0.6 to 12% of cases.[14,39] The most common cause of implant fracture is periarticular osteolysis, leading to cantilever bending and fatigue fracture of the prosthetic stem (see Figure 27.8). Notch sensitivity and component design are postulated to further contribute to component fracture. When implant fracture occurs, revision is indicated. This can be accomplished by techniques such as cement-within-cement reimplantation. These techniques have been shown to be reliable for relieving pain and restoring function in revision surgery.[1]

Periprosthetic fractures of the humerus and ulna following TEA can be very challenging to treat. They can be related to significant trauma to the upper extremity or represent pathologic fractures from osteolysis and bone loss at the tip of the stem (Figures 27.9 and 27.10). The cited incidence is between 3% and 5%.[29] These fractures are managed based on their location, the quality of prosthetic fixation, and the quality of the remaining bone stock. Experience with periprosthetic fractures in the lower extremity has been extrapolated and applied to the upper extremity.[29,36] Periprosthetic humeral fractures have been classified as H1-fractures around the condyles or column, H2-fractures around the stem, and H3-fractures proximal to the implant.[36] Periprosthetic ulna fractures have been classified as U1-fractures of the olecranon, U2-fractures around the stem, and U3-fractures distal to the implant. Fractures around the stem are subclassified as 1-well fixed, 2-loose with acceptable bone stock, or 3-loose with severe bone loss.[10]

Unfortunately, uncemented stems, which account for the bulk of revision fixation options in the lower extremity, are not available in revision TEAs. When the components are stable, standard fracture treatment is typically indicated, including internal fixation with or without the incorporation of allograft struts. Periprosthetic fractures around a loose humeral component can be treated with revision cemented arthroplasty using strut allograft augmentation to improve bone stock, with predictable union rates.[10,36] Large cavitary defects have been treated with impaction grafting and massive defects have been treated

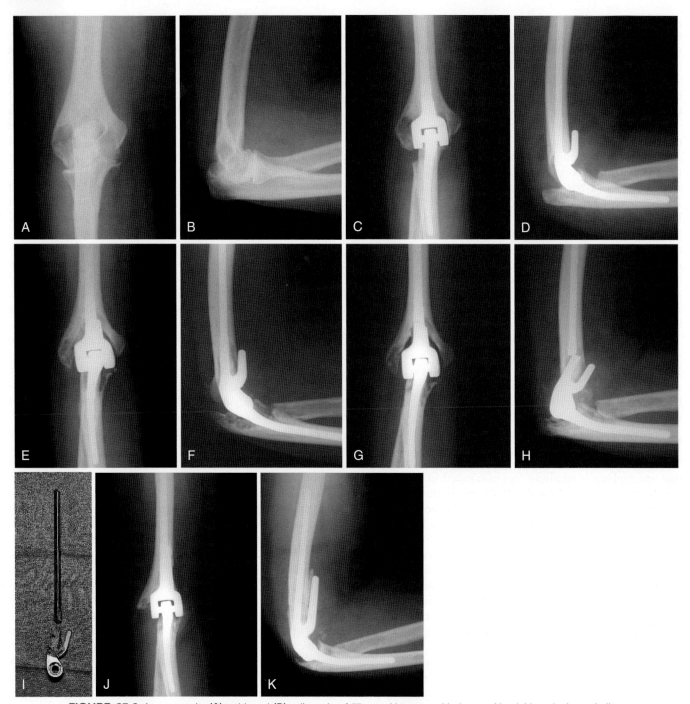

FIGURE 27.8 Anteroposterior **(A)** and lateral **(B)** radiographs of 57-year-old woman with rheumatoid arthritis and advanced elbow arthritis who failed conservative measures. Immediate postoperative anteroposterior **(C)** and lateral **(D)** radiographs depict the semiconstrained device. On the 3-year follow-up anteroposterior **(E)** and lateral **(F)** films, note osteolysis involving the distal humerus and proximal ulna adjacent to the hinge. Anteroposterior **(G)** and lateral **(H)** views 2 years later when the patient presented with acute pain after lifting a box of detergent at home. Progressive osteolysis has placed excessive stress on the component, leading to implant fracture. Intraoperative photograph **(I)** of the broken implant at revision surgery. Anteroposterior **(J)** and lateral **(K)** radiographs after revision surgery. Note the humeral component's long anterior flange. The ulnar component was well fixed, so the proximal ulnar canal was débrided and bone-grafted.

with allograft prosthetic composites. When exposure of the humeral diaphysis is necessary, it is important to identify and protect the radial nerve. In certain cases, for example, when large humeral allografts are necessary, the radial nerve can be transposed anterior to the humeral shaft to facilitate future revision surgery.

Infection

Finally, infection is a potentially devastating complication of TEA.[49] The reported rate of infection is between 1% and 11%, with approximately half being superficial infections and half deep infections.[14,49,52] Risk factors include immunosuppressive therapy or immune compromise, diabetes mellitus, poor

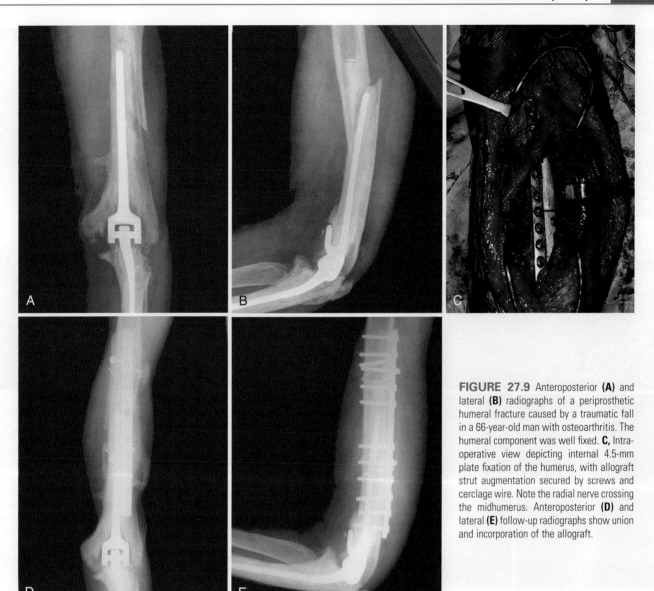

FIGURE 27.9 Anteroposterior **(A)** and lateral **(B)** radiographs of a periprosthetic humeral fracture caused by a traumatic fall in a 66-year-old man with osteoarthritis. The humeral component was well fixed. **C,** Intraoperative view depicting internal 4.5-mm plate fixation of the humerus, with allograft strut augmentation secured by screws and cerclage wire. Note the radial nerve crossing the midhumerus. Anteroposterior **(D)** and lateral **(E)** follow-up radiographs show union and incorporation of the allograft.

nutrition, obesity, multiple prior surgical interventions, prior infection, and prolonged wound drainage. Infection rates may be reduced with proper prophylactic measures, such as the use of intravenous antibiotics, antibiotic-impregnated cement, care and preservation of a robust soft tissue envelope, laminar flow operating rooms, and exhaust suits.[52]

When a deep infection occurs, a decision must be made regarding implant preservation. Patient factors, the duration of symptoms, bacteriologic factors, the quality of component fixation, the presence of a sinus, and a history of preceding bacteremia are important considerations in treatment planning. Options include surgical débridement (with or without polyethylene exchange) combined with chronic suppressive antibiotic therapy versus implant removal with or without a second-stage reimplantation. *Staphylococcus aureus* infections may be more amenable to repeat débridement and component retention.[27,52] Although less virulent, *S. epidermidis* has an increased propensity for adherence and biofilm formation and

has been associated with a higher failure rate with attempted prosthetic retention.[52] Early irrigation and débridements with component retention may be possible for well-fixed components, symptom duration of less than 30 days, infection with a low-virulence organism, and medically fit patients.[49] The overall success of irrigation and débridement ranges from 22 to 70%.[49,52]

Staged exchange is another treatment alternative for an infected TEA. Much of the experience with staged exchange is derived from its successful use in the lower extremities. In a medically fit patient with a loose component and a duration of infection longer than 21 days, this may be a viable option for TEA salvage. It requires meticulous cement removal, which may involve extended osteotomies of the ulna and humerus. This is followed by placement of an antibiotic-laden cement spacer and intravenous antibiotics used typically for 6 weeks; clearance of infection is demonstrated by negative tissue biopsy prior to reimplantation.

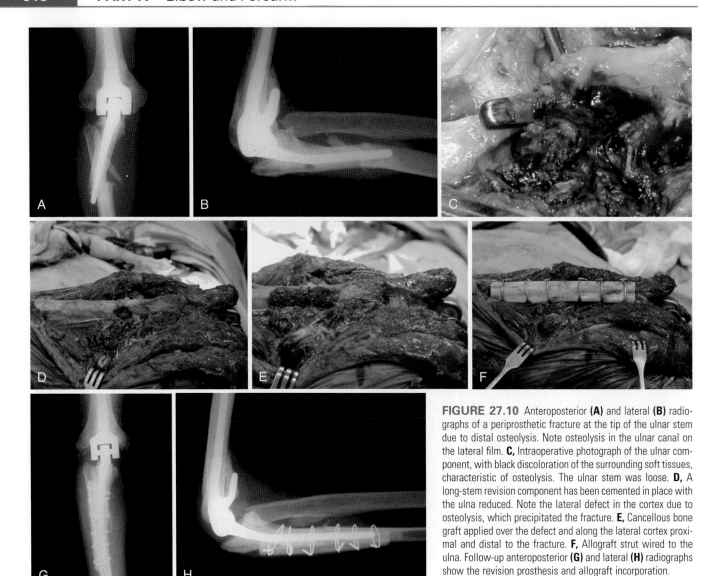

FIGURE 27.10 Anteroposterior **(A)** and lateral **(B)** radiographs of a periprosthetic fracture at the tip of the ulnar stem due to distal osteolysis. Note osteolysis in the ulnar canal on the lateral film. **C,** Intraoperative photograph of the ulnar component, with black discoloration of the surrounding soft tissues, characteristic of osteolysis. The ulnar stem was loose. **D,** A long-stem revision component has been cemented in place with the ulna reduced. Note the lateral defect in the cortex due to osteolysis, which precipitated the fracture. **E,** Cancellous bone graft applied over the defect and along the lateral cortex proximal and distal to the fracture. **F,** Allograft strut wired to the ulna. Follow-up anteroposterior **(G)** and lateral **(H)** radiographs show the revision prosthesis and allograft incorporation.

In the setting of infected TEA, soft tissue coverage in the face of ongoing disease and multiple surgeries may pose additional treatment challenges. Regional or free tissue transfer may be required to provide a stable soft tissue envelope and maximize the potential for preserving elbow function. We have found the flexor carpi ulnaris pedicle flap to be effective in providing vascularized coverage for the posterior elbow (see Figure 27.3).[51] Larger defects can be treated with a scapular flap, periscapular flap, or pedicled latissimus flap. It is important to educate the patient about protecting the flap as it is insensate and susceptible to pressure injuries.

For chronic deep infections following TEA, resection arthroplasty is probably the only viable option. It is clearly the treatment of choice for severely debilitated or medically compromised patients, including those who are severely immunocompromised. If the medial and lateral humeral columns are left intact and contoured to encircle the remaining ulna, the patient will likely be left with reasonable stability and a limited pain-free range of motion. An exception to this approach may be elderly, debilitated patients with multiple medical problems and well-fixed components who are asymptomatic and have no systemic signs of infection. These individuals often develop draining sinuses, which decompress the joint. When it is decided to leave an infected prosthesis in place in this specific clinical setting, chronic oral suppressive antibiotics and local wound care are continued indefinitely.

Mortality Rates

Perioperative mortality has been extensively explored with regard to lower extremity arthroplasty but has not been well researched in TEA. With advancements in prosthetic design and a broadening of operative indications for arthroplasty, such information is vital to the process of informed consent for all arthroplasty patients. The 90-day mortality rate following TEA has been estimated at approximately 0.64%.[37] Risk factors include age older than 60 years, multiple comorbidities, and arthroplasty for the treatment of trauma or nonunion.

CRITICAL POINTS *Total Elbow Arthroplasty*

Indications

Pain, stiffness, and loss of function associated with:

- Rheumatoid arthritis
- Posttraumatic arthritis
- Primary osteoarthritis
- Hemophilic arthropathy
- Comminuted fracture of the distal humerus in an elderly person when osteosynthesis is not possible

Contraindications

- Neuropathic joint
- Poor soft tissue coverage
- Presence of infection at the elbow

Technical Points

Exposure Through Full-Thickness Fasciocutaneous Flaps Posteriorly

- Transpose ulnar nerve
- Reflect triceps
- Carefully dissect the Sharpey fibers off the olecranon in a subperiosteal fashion
- Bryan-Morrey approach: elevate triceps from medial to lateral in continuity with anconeus
- Gschwend approach: split triceps muscle and tendon longitudinally and elevate them off of the proximal ulna in the midline
- Triceps-sparing approach (insertion left intact): useful in patients with deficient distal humeral columns (fractures, nonunions)

Humeral Preparation

- Resect the central aspect of the trochlea
- Enter the humeral canal with a bur
- Use cutting guides to prepare the distal humerus
- Evaluate trial implants
- Anterior cortex may need to be deepened to accept the anterior flange of the implant and allow complete seating of the prosthesis

Ulnar Preparation

- Resect tips of olecranon and coronoid process
- Enter canal with a bur, and enlarge it with rasps
- Must appreciate 5 degrees of valgus of the ulnar shaft relative to the sigmoid notch
- Bone at canal entry often limits complete component seating

Trial Components

- Evaluate range of motion
- Use capsular release if needed

Cement

- Thoroughly lavage and dry canals
- Use restrictors in humerus and ulna
- Use thin flexible tubing for retrograde filling
- Use low-viscosity cement (consider antibiotic-laden cement)
- Use cement early in the polymerization process

Repair of Extensor Mechanism

- Use multiple transosseous sutures distally

Closure

- Wound is closed in layers after hemostasis is achieved
- Ulnar nerve is transposed anteriorly
- Drains are optional with adequate hemostasis
- Compressive dressing is applied, and arm is splinted in partial extension

Postoperative Care

- Elevate the elbow and begin intravenous antibiotic therapy
- Begin active and gentle passive range-of-motion exercises at 7 to 10 days (in immunosuppressed or rheumatoid patients with thin, friable skin, the elbow can be immobilized for a longer period to allow soft tissue healing before motion is initiated)
- Protect triceps (if detached) for 6 to 8 weeks
- Use nighttime elbow extension splint in maximal extension to limit potential flexion contracture
- Limit lifting to 5 pounds with operated extremity, indefinitely[23,42]

REFERENCES

1. Athwal GS, Morrey BF: Revision total elbow arthroplasty for prosthetic fractures. *J Bone Joint Surg Am* 88:2017–2026, 2006.
2. Barr JS, Eaton RG: Elbow reconstruction with a new prosthesis to replace the distal end of the humerus. A case report. *J Bone Joint Surg Am* 47:1408–1413, 1965.
3. Burkhart KJ, Nijs S, Mattyasovszky SG, et al: Distal humerus hemiarthroplasty of the elbow for comminuted distal humeral fractures in the elderly patient. *J Trauma* 71:635–642, 2011.
4. Cheung EV, Steinmann SP: Surgical approaches to the elbow. *J Am Acad Orthop Surg* 17:325–333, 2009.
5. Cobb TK, Morrey BF: Total elbow arthroplasty as primary treatment for distal humeral fractures in elderly patients. *J Bone Joint Surg Am* 79:826–832, 1997.
6. Danter MR, King GJ, Chess DG, et al: The effect of cement restrictors on the occlusion of the humeral canal: an in vitro comparative study of 2 devices. *J Arthroplasty* 15:113–119, 2000.
7. Dee R: Total replacement arthroplasty of the elbow for rheumatoid arthritis. *J Bone Joint Surg Br* 54:88–95, 1972.
8. Dee R: Reconstructive surgery following total elbow endoprosthesis. *Clin Orthop Relat Res* 196–203, 1982.
9. Faber KJ, Cordy ME, Milne AD, et al: Advanced cement technique improves fixation in elbow arthroplasty. *Clin Orthop Relat Res* 334:150–156, 1997.
10. Foruria AM, Sanchez-Sotelo J, Oh LS, et al: The surgical treatment of periprosthetic elbow fractures around the ulnar stem following semiconstrained total elbow arthroplasty. *J Bone Joint Surg Am* 93:1399–1407, 2011.
11. Gambirasio R, Riand N, Stern R, et al: Total elbow replacement for complex fractures of the distal humerus. An option for the elderly patient. *J Bone Joint Surg Br* 83:974–978, 2001.
12. Gill DR, Morrey BF: The Coonrad-Morrey total elbow arthroplasty in patients who have rheumatoid arthritis. A ten- to fifteen-year follow-up study. *J Bone Joint Surg Am* 80:1327–1335, 1998.
13. Goldberg SH, Urban RM, Jacobs JJ, et al: Modes of wear after semiconstrained total elbow arthroplasty. *J Bone Joint Surg Am* 90:609–619, 2008.
14. Gschwend N, Simmen BR, Matejovsky Z: Late complications in elbow arthroplasty. *J Shoulder Elbow Surg* 5:86–96, 1996.
15. Jenkins PJ, Watts AC, Norwood T, et al: Total elbow replacement: outcome of 1,146 arthroplasties from the Scottish Arthroplasty Project. *Acta Orthop* 84:119–123, 2013.
16. Johnson EW, Jr, Schlein AP: Vitallium prosthesis for the olecranon and proximal part of the ulna. Case report with thirteen-year follow-up. *J Bone Joint Surg Am* 52:721–724, 1970.
17. Kamineni S, Morrey BF: Distal humeral fractures treated with noncustom total elbow replacement. *J Bone Joint Surg Am* 86:940–947, 2004.
18. Kjaersgaard-Andersen P, Christiansen SE, Ingerslev J, et al: Total knee arthroplasty in classic hemophilia. *Clin Orthop Relat Res* 256:137–146, 1990.
19. Kudo H, Iwano K: Total elbow arthroplasty with a non-constrained surface-replacement prosthesis in patients who have rheumatoid arthritis. A long-term follow-up study. *J Bone Joint Surg Am* 72:355–362, 1990.
20. Kudo H, Iwano K, Nishino J: Cementless or hybrid total elbow arthroplasty with titanium-alloy implants. A study of interim clinical results and specific complications. *J Arthroplasty* 9:269–278, 1994.

21. Larsen A, Dale K, Eek M: Radiographic evaluation of rheumatoid arthritis and related conditions by standard reference films. *Acta Radiol Diagn (Stockh)* 18:481–491, 1977.
22. Lee BP, Adams RA, Morrey BF: Polyethylene wear after total elbow arthroplasty. *J Bone Joint Surg Am* 87:1080–1087, 2005.
23. Lehtinen JT, Kaarela K, Kauppi MJ, et al: Bone destruction patterns of the rheumatoid elbow: a radiographic assessment of 148 elbows at 15 years. *J Shoulder Elbow Surg* 11:253–258, 2002.
24. Mansat P, Morrey BF: Semiconstrained total elbow arthroplasty for ankylosed and stiff elbows. *J Bone Joint Surg Am* 82:1260–1268, 2000.
25. McKee MD, Pugh DM, Richards RR, et al: Effect of humeral condylar resection on strength and functional outcome after semiconstrained total elbow arthroplasty. *J Bone Joint Surg Am* 85:802–807, 2003.
26. Morrey BF, Bryan RS: Complications of total elbow arthroplasty. *Clin Orthop Relat Res* 170:204–212, 1982.
27. Morrey BF, Bryan RS: Revision total elbow arthroplasty. *J Bone Joint Surg Am* 69:523–532, 1987.
28. O'Driscoll SW, An KN, Korinek S, et al: Kinematics of semi-constrained total elbow arthroplasty. *J Bone Joint Surg Br* 74:297–299, 1992.
29. O'Driscoll SW, Morrey BF: Periprosthetic fractures about the elbow. *Orthop Clin North Am* 30:319–325, 1999.
30. Park SE, Kim JY, Cho SW, et al: Complications and revision rate compared by type of total elbow arthroplasty. *J Shoulder Elbow Surg* 22:1121–1127, 2013.
31. Peterson LF, Janes JM: Surgery of the rheumatoid elbow. *Orthop Clin North Am* 2:667–677, 1971.
32. Pritchard RW: Anatomic surface elbow arthroplasty. A preliminary report. *Clin Orthop Relat Res* 179:223–230, 1983.
33. Prokopis PM, Weiland AJ: The triceps-preserving approach for semiconstrained total elbow arthroplasty. *J Shoulder Elbow Surg* 17:454–458, 2008.
34. Ray PS, Kakarlapudi K, Rajsekhar C, et al: Total elbow arthroplasty as primary treatment for distal humeral fractures in elderly patients. *Injury* 31:687–692, 2000.
35. Rydholm U, Tjornstrand B, Pettersson H, et al: Surface replacement of the elbow in rheumatoid arthritis. Early results with the Wadsworth prosthesis. *J Bone Joint Surg Br* 66:737–741, 1984.
36. Sanchez-Sotelo J, O'Driscoll S, Morrey BF: Periprosthetic humeral fractures after total elbow arthroplasty: treatment with implant revision and strut allograft augmentation. *J Bone Joint Surg Am* 84:1642–1650, 2002.
37. Sanchez-Sotelo J, Sperling JW, Morrey BF: Ninety-day mortality after total elbow arthroplasty. *J Bone Joint Surg Am* 89:1449–1451, 2007.
38. Schlein AP: Semiconstrained total elbow arthroplasty. *Clin Orthop Relat Res* 121:222–229, 1976.
39. Schneeberger AG, Adams R, Morrey BF: Semiconstrained total elbow replacement for the treatment of post-traumatic osteoarthrosis. *J Bone Joint Surg Am* 79:1211–1222, 1997.
40. Schuind F, O'Driscoll S, Korinek S, et al: Loose-hinge total elbow arthroplasty. An experimental study of the effects of implant alignment on three-dimensional elbow kinematics. *J Arthroplasty* 10:670–678, 1995.
41. Shi LL, Zurakowski D, Jones DG, et al: Semiconstrained primary and revision total elbow arthroplasty with use of the Coonrad-Morrey prosthesis. *J Bone Joint Surg Am* 89:1467–1475, 2007.
42. Sneppen O, Fredensborg N, Karle A, et al: Lateral dislocation of the patella following Marmor and Guepar arthroplasty of the knee. *Acta Orthop Scand* 49:291–294, 1978.
43. Soni RK, Cavendish ME: A review of the Liverpool elbow prosthesis from 1974 to 1982. *J Bone Joint Surg Br* 66:248–253, 1984.
44. Stokdijk M, Nagels J, Garling EH, et al: The kinematic elbow axis as a parameter to evaluate total elbow replacement: A cadaver study of the iBP elbow system. *J Shoulder Elbow Surg* 12:63–68, 2003.
45. Tanaka E, Saito A, Kamitsuji S, et al: Impact of shoulder, elbow, and knee joint involvement on assessment of rheumatoid arthritis using the American College of Rheumatology Core Data Set. *Arthritis Rheum* 53:864–871, 2005.
46. Throckmorton T, Zarkadas P, Sanchez-Sotelo J, et al: Failure patterns after linked semiconstrained total elbow arthroplasty for posttraumatic arthritis. *J Bone Joint Surg Am* 92:1432–1441, 2010.
47. Trail IA, Nuttall D, Stanley JK: Survivorship and radiological analysis of the standard Souter-Strathclyde total elbow arthroplasty. *J Bone Joint Surg Br* 81:80–84, 1999.
48. Venable CS: An elbow and an elbow prosthesis; case of complete loss of the lower third of the humerus. *Am J Surg* 83:271–275, 1952.
49. Wolfe SW, Figgie MP, Inglis AE, et al: Management of infection about total elbow prostheses. *J Bone Joint Surg Am* 72:198–212, 1990.
50. Wright TW, Hastings H: Total elbow arthroplasty failure due to overuse, C-ring failure, and/or bushing wear. *J Shoulder Elbow Surg* 14:65–72, 2005.
51. Wysocki RW, Gray RL, Fernandez JJ, et al: Posterior elbow coverage using whole and split flexor carpi ulnaris flaps: a cadaveric study. *J Hand Surg [Am]* 33:1807–1812, 2008.
52. Yamaguchi K, Adams RA, Morrey BF: Infection after total elbow arthroplasty. *J Bone Joint Surg Am* 80:481–491, 1998.
53. Yamaguchi K, Adams RA, Morrey BF: Semiconstrained total elbow arthroplasty in the context of treated previous infection. *J Shoulder Elbow Surg* 8:461–465, 1999.

28

Compression Neuropathies

Susan E. Mackinnon and Christine B. Novak

Acknowledgment: We would like to acknowledge Robert M. Szabo, MD, and William W. Eversmann, Jr., MD, for their contributions to the chapter on this subject in previous editions of this textbook.

▶ These videos may be found at *ExpertConsult.com*:

28.1 Carpal tunnel release—standard *(Courtesy Washington University of St. Louis, School of Medicine.)*

28.2 Carpal tunnel release—extended *(Courtesy Washington University of St. Louis, School of Medicine.)*

28.3 Median nerve forearm decompression—standard *(Courtesy Washington University of St. Louis, School of Medicine.)*

28.4 Median nerve release in the forearm *(Courtesy Washington University of St. Louis, School of Medicine.)*

28.5 Guyon canal and carpal tunnel release—standard *(Courtesy Washington University of St. Louis, School of Medicine.)*

28.6 Submuscular ulnar nerve transposition—standard *(Courtesy Washington University of St. Louis, School of Medicine.)*

28.7 Transmuscular ulnar nerve transposition *(Courtesy Washington University of St. Louis, School of Medicine.)*

28.8 Posterior interosseous nerve release *(Courtesy Washington University of St. Louis, School of Medicine.)*

28.9 Revision carpal tunnel release *(Courtesy Washington University of St. Louis, School of Medicine.)*

28.10 Revision carpal tunnel release, part I *(Courtesy Washington University of St. Louis, School of Medicine.)*

Compression neuropathies in the upper extremity are common and are being recognized with increasing frequency. The rising prevalence of obesity in North America coupled with an aging population suggests that the problems of upper extremity compression neuropathy will likely increase in the next decade. The etiologic relationship between nerve compression disorders and occupation was extremely controversial in the 1990s.[31,68] The existence of multiple levels of nerve compression is now generally recognized, although the contributions of work-related issues of these problems is still debated.[90] Except for significant exposure to vibration and some specific occupations with a high prevalence of carpal tunnel syndrome, it is generally accepted that work is just one component of many factors that contribute to and aggravate compression neuropathy.[6,90] When compared with other compression neuropathies in the upper extremity, carpal tunnel syndrome is, in general, managed less successfully with nonoperative treatment.

Surgeons treating nerve compression in the upper extremity must be aware of other neurologic problems, such as brachial plexus neuritis, Parsonage-Turner syndrome, mononeuritis, and motor neuropathies that can mimic entrapment neuropathies and will not respond to surgical intervention. Similarly, there exists a group of individuals who are genetically sensitive to the development of nerve compression. The prevalence of genetic predisposition is unknown but may help to explain some clinical manifestations of entrapment neuropathy, as do systemic factors such as obesity, diabetes, and thyroid disease.

PATHOPHYSIOLOGY OF CHRONIC NERVE COMPRESSION

The clinical findings in patients with chronic nerve compression are variable and reflect the broad spectrum of histopathologic changes that occur in the nerve. Because of associated morbidity, biopsy of neural tissue is not performed, and much of the information known about the histopathology of human nerve compression has been extrapolated from animal models. Some studies have suggested neural ischemia as contributing to compression neuropathies.[26,54] Many of these studies, however, reflect acute changes that occur with compression. Several animal models have been described in which different techniques are used to induce chronic nerve compression.[62,87] Although there is some concern about the potential for silicone tubes to induce reactive effects on a nerve, the histologic changes seen in the silicone tube cuff model are essentially identical to those noted in the few histologic studies of chronic nerve compression that have been published. Studies have shown limited tissue reaction around the tubes 1 year after human nerve repair.

The continuum of neural changes that will take place depends on the force and duration of the compression. The histopathologic changes that occur with chronic nerve compression begin with breakdown of the blood-nerve barrier, followed by endoneurial edema and, subsequently, perineurial thickening (Figure 28.1).[62,87] Increased endoneurial pressure will result in changes in the microneural circulation and render

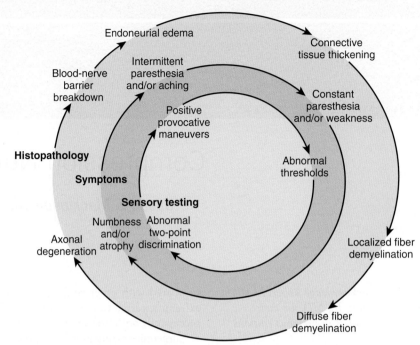

FIGURE 28.1 The histopathologic findings of chronic nerve compression span a spectrum of changes that begins with breakdown of the blood-nerve barrier and, with continued compression, progression to axonal degeneration. The patient's signs and symptoms and sensory testing will parallel the histopathologic changes occurring in the nerve.

the nerve susceptible to dynamic ischemia. With increased compression, there will be localized demyelination, followed by more diffuse demyelination and finally axonal degeneration. Neural changes may not occur uniformly across the nerve and may vary depending on the distribution of compressive forces across the nerve. Superficial fascicles will undergo changes sooner and may result in varying patient symptoms within a single nerve distribution.[52] For example, in early carpal tunnel syndrome the superficial fascicles to the long finger and ring finger are usually affected before the fascicles to the thumb and radial side of the index finger.

Patient sensory complaints will generally parallel the histopathologic neural changes and will progress from intermittent paresthesia to persistent numbness (see Figure 28.1). Sensory testing will also vary with the degree of nerve compression. Initially, patients will have altered threshold measures, and with more severe nerve compression, they will progress to deficits in two-point discrimination.

Double-Crush Mechanism

First introduced by Upton and McComas,[111] the double-crush mechanism is an important concept in nerve compression. In their clinical review of 115 patients with median or ulnar nerve compression, 81 had evidence of a cervical root lesion, and they concluded that compression of a nerve at one level will make the nerve more susceptible to damage at another level. The authors hypothesized that axoplasmic flow would be compromised by proximal compression on the nerve and then be further compromised by the distal compression site. The reverse double-crush syndrome was described by Lundborg.[52] He hypothesized that a distal site of compression would decrease the flow of neurotrophic substances back to the neuron and

thus decrease the production of substances to be transported distally. Other clinical studies have supported the double-crush mechanism with associations between the cervical spine, thoracic outlet, and distal sites of compression, including the carpal and cubital tunnels. Hurst and associates reported on 1000 cases of carpal tunnel syndrome in 888 patients and noted a significant relationship between bilateral carpal tunnel syndrome and patients with cervical arthritis and diabetes.[37] Other studies have reported similar findings with cervical radiculopathy, thoracic outlet syndrome, and distal nerve entrapment in the arm.

Animal models demonstrating the double-crush mechanism have been described.[20,79] Using a canine model, Nemoto and colleagues placed compression clamps on the sciatic nerve and evaluated conduction velocity.[79] Placement of a second clamp at a proximal site reduced motor conduction velocity to a value less than that in both the normal state and the clamped state. This study also evaluated the effect of removing the sequential compression clamps 3 weeks later. Removal of both clamps improved motor conduction velocity to 65% of the original value, whereas removal of only one clamp improved conduction velocity to a lesser amount. Dellon and Mackinnon developed a rodent model that simulated sciatic nerve compression with silicone tubes.[20] In one of three groups of animals the silicone tube was placed proximal to the sciatic nerve trifurcation (group 1), in the second group the tube was placed on the tibial nerve distal to the trifurcation (group 2), and in the third group, tubes were placed simultaneously on the sciatic nerve and the peroneal nerve. In groups 1 and 2 after 7 months, a second tube was placed on the nerve (on the tibial nerve in group 1 and proximal to the sciatic nerve trifurcation in group 2) and no surgery was performed on the double-banded group. After 5 more months, the final electrodiagnostic studies were performed. The addition of a second band either proximally or distally resulted in a decrease in conduction velocity equal to that in the group that received the double bands initially. Because both the proximal and distal second band compromised conduction velocity equally, this study supports the double-crush and the reverse double-crush mechanisms of nerve compression.

Systemic Conditions and Personal Factors

Other medical conditions and personal factors have been associated with carpal tunnel syndrome, including diabetes mellitus, hypothyroidism, excessive alcohol use, obesity, and tobacco use.[39,77,78] When compared with a control group without symptoms of carpal tunnel syndrome, patients with carpal tunnel syndrome demonstrated a higher prevalence of hypothyroidism, diabetes, and obesity.[39] These findings supported previous reports of an increased prevalence of these conditions in patients with carpal tunnel syndrome. In a retrospective case-control study, smoking history did not result in an increased incidence of carpal tunnel syndrome.[39]

Hereditary motor-sensory neuropathy consists of a group of inherited disorders that affect the motor and sensory nerves of the peripheral nervous system, including Charcot-Marie-Tooth disease and hereditary neuropathy with liability to pressure palsies (HNPP). HNPP is an autosomal dominant demyelinating motor-sensory neuropathy. It is characterized by underexpression of the peripheral myelin protein-22 gene on chromosome 17 and is manifested as recurrent, multifocal nerve compression. Patients may have rapid-onset neuropathies after minor trauma with decreased nerve conduction (motor and sensory) in the affected and unaffected nerves. In most cases, recovery is complete without surgery. In the upper extremity, the ulnar nerve is most commonly affected, and in the lower extremity the peroneal nerve is affected. The presence of HNPP should be considered in patients with multiple recurrent neuropathies.

Longitudinal Nerve Mobility

Longitudinal nerve mobility is important for normal nerve function. Although some longitudinal movement is permitted via the plexus formation within a nerve and via the loose attachment of its mesoneurium, damage may occur with excessive or prolonged traction. Venous obstruction has been shown with acute stretching of 8% of a nerve's resting length, and ischemia occurred when it was stretched 15% of its resting length.[55] Watanabe and colleagues investigated nerve strain in a rat model.[114] The authors used the same amount of strain in the continuous and the repetitive strain groups and reported abnormalities in the repetitive strain group as determined by histologic, electrophysiologic, and functional evaluation. They concluded that a small amount of repetitive strain on neural tissue may result in neural dysfunction, particularly in cases with underlying subclinical nerve pathologic findings.

Studies have shown evidence of strain on the median and ulnar nerves during median and ulnar nerve tension tests and reported restriction of median nerve excursion in patients with carpal tunnel syndrome. Nerve compression may induce connective tissue and synovial thickening that may secondarily result in restriction of neural mobility with joint motion.[76,105]

Authors' Opinion

Much of the controversy associated with nerve compression is related to patients with diffuse symptoms and to the relationship of occupation to nerve compression disorders. Certain postures and positions may contribute to nerve compression. It is well accepted that wrist positions of moderate flexion and extension will increase pressure within the carpal canal, and this is hypothesized to contribute to carpal tunnel syndrome.[25,117] Similarly, elbow flexion will increase pressure within the cubital tunnel and thereby compromise the ulnar nerve.[26,93] However, these postures and positions will not only have an impact on the nerve but may also affect the surrounding musculature (Figure 28.2).[67] We believe that prolonged or extreme postures

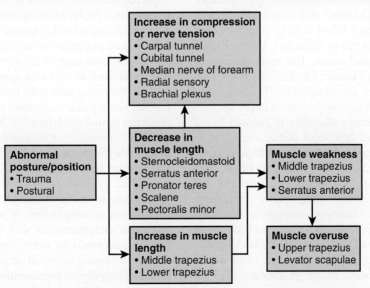

FIGURE 28.2 Abnormal postures or positions will have three main effects: (1) nerves may be compressed or placed on tension and progress to chronic nerve compression, (2) muscles may be placed in shortened positions and then secondarily compress nerves, or (3) muscles in elongated or shortened positions will be weakened and thus underused. Other muscles will compensate for the weakness and be overused, thereby establishing a pattern of muscle imbalance.

or positions will affect the nerves and soft tissues in the upper extremity and cervicoscapular region and that multifocal nerve compression and muscle imbalance can contribute to diffuse upper quadrant patient symptoms.

EVALUATION OF COMPRESSION NEUROPATHIES

To develop an effective treatment plan, it is necessary to identify all sites of nerve compression and the musculoskeletal disorders that are contributing to a patient's symptoms. Different diagnostic tests will yield important information at different stages of nerve compression (see Figure 28.1). Not all tests will be positive at all stages; therefore, it is important to use the assessment tools that will give the most accurate information for identifying a pathologic change or determining the grade severity. A complete sensory and motor evaluation, including electrodiagnostic studies, can determine the severity of nerve compression. In patients with work-related symptoms, detailed consideration should be given to determine the involvement of work as a contributing factor. Use of a subjective pain evaluation questionnaire is helpful to identify all symptomatic areas and other factors that may contribute to a patient's symptoms.[40,47,74] We have found the use of a pain evaluation questionnaire that includes a body diagram, a subjective questionnaire, and visual analog scales to be very useful in the evaluation of patients with nerve compression or diffuse symptoms, or with both (Figure 28.3).

Self-report questionnaires are useful to capture the patient's perception of physical impairment, impact of the condition, and level of disability. A number of validated questionnaires to assess both global upper extremity and specific nerve-related symptoms and disability have been used in the assessment of nerve compression. The carpal tunnel syndrome questionnaire is a disease-specific measure that allows specific items related to carpal tunnel syndrome to be assessed from the patient's perspective and has been shown to be reliable, valid, and sensitive to change.[2,23,30,34,45,47] The carpal tunnel syndrome questionnaire assesses symptom severity (11 items) and functional status (8 items). Each item is ranked on a Likert scale (1 is the low level and 5 is the high level of symptoms or difficulty), and the higher mean values indicate decreased status. The most commonly used generic upper extremity measure for disability is the Disabilities of the Arm, Shoulder, and Hand (DASH) score; using a standardized 30 items allows for comparison of upper extremity conditions.[35] Upper extremity disability is assessed based upon physical symptoms and functional status; each item is ranked from 1 to 5. Scores are calculated, and higher scores indicate higher levels of disability. The Michigan Hand Outcomes Questionnaire (MHQ) is a longer questionnaire (67 items) and has the capability of addressing specific domains of overall hand function, physical function, cosmesis, and satisfaction.[15] Similar to the DASH, each item is scored on a Likert scale (1 to 5), but in contrast to the DASH, the MHQ assesses function of each upper extremity (independent use, hand dominance, and bilateral involvement). Although standardized item questionnaires provide the opportunity to compare scores and answers between patients and conditions, these generic questionnaires may not reflect specific changes in each patient or the items that are most important to each patient. Question-

naires such as the Patient-Specific Functional Scale (PSFS) assesses items that are identified by each patient. In this assessment each patient identifies three activities or tasks that the patient finds difficult or impossible to perform.[102] Each item is ranked on a scale from 0 to 10 and anchored based on perceived ability to perform these separate activities. Good validity, reliability, and responsiveness have been shown in patients with upper extremity disorders.[33,73] Although the PSFS allows patients to select items that are specifically relevant, comparison between patients is more challenging. Combined use of generic questionnaires such as the DASH, MHQ, and our pain evaluation questionnaire in combination with the PSFS may provide a more comprehensive self-report evaluation.

For successful management, evaluation and treatment should be directed at all levels of nerve compression and any soft tissue disorders that are present.

Use of Provocation Tests

Many signs and provocation tests have been described for clinical evaluation of carpal tunnel syndrome.[57,94,95] The concept of increasing tension or compression on a nerve to assess for nerve compression at the carpal tunnel may be extrapolated to other sites of nerve compression in the upper extremity. The concept of the double-crush mechanism is important in the assessment of patients with suspected upper extremity nerve compression. Because one site of nerve compression may affect other sites of nerve compression, all potential entrapment sites of nerve compression should be evaluated.

Provocation tests involving direct pressure or joint movement to increase compression on the nerve can be performed (Table 28.1). Beginning at the more distal sites and advancing proximally, a *Tinel sign* or a *nerve percussion test* is performed by applying repeated digital percussion at each potential entrapment site (carpal tunnel, median nerve in the forearm, cubital tunnel, radial sensory nerve, brachial plexus). The test is considered positive with radiation of a tingling sensation into the affected nerve's sensory neural distribution. In patients who are hyperresponsive to stimuli or have positive nerve percussion test results at multiple entrapment sites, it is helpful to perform a nerve percussion test at points where nerves are not anatomically located as a negative control. Similarly, all provocative tests are done in both upper extremities in all patients, even in those with symptoms in only one upper extremity.

The *Phalen test* uses wrist flexion to increase pressure on the median nerve and is a common provocation test for assessment of carpal tunnel syndrome.[94,95] Since first described in 1966, a number of provocation tests using position or pressure, or both, to increase compression on the nerve have been reported.[18,57,120] Provocation tests should be maintained for 1 minute and are considered positive when symptoms are reproduced in the appropriate neural distribution. To correctly identify a site of chronic nerve compression, it is important to compress only one nerve entrapment site with each test. Pressure provocation can be performed to assess the median nerve at the carpal tunnel by placing the wrist in either flexion or extension and then applying digital pressure just proximal to the carpal tunnel. In patients with restricted wrist movement, the pressure provocative test can be done with the wrist in a neutral position. Because the median nerve and the ulnar nerve can be compressed in this position, sensory alteration in the median and

Pain Questionnaire

Name:_____ Date:_____

Age:___ Sex: Male_ Female_ Dominant hand: Right_ Left_ Diagnosis:_____

1. Pain is difficult to describe. Circle the words that best describe your symptoms.

Burning	Throbbing	Aching	Stabbing	Tingling	Twisting	Squeezing
Cramping	Cutting	Shooting	Numbing	Vague	Stinging	Indescribable
Pulling	Smarting	Pressure	Coldness	Dull	Other: _____	

Level of symptoms: place a mark through the line to indicate the level of your pain, if zero is no pain and the end of the line is the most severe pain you can imagine having.

For Example:

No pain ——————————|—————————— Most severe pain

2. Mark your average level of pain in the last month

No pain ———————————————————— Most severe pain

3. Mark your worst level of pain in the last week

Right

No pain ———————————————————— Most severe pain

Left

No pain ———————————————————— Most severe pain

4. Where is your pain? (draw on diagram)

L   R   L   R

5. Mark your average level of stress in the last month.

at home 0 ———————————— 10

at work 0 ———————————— 10

6. How well are you able to cope with that stress?

at home Very well ———————————— Not at all

at work Very well ———————————— Not at all

7. How did the pain that you are now experiencing occur?
   a. Sudden onset with accident or definable event
   b. Slow progressive onset
   c. Slow progressive onset with acute exacerbation without an accident or definable event
   d. A sudden onset without an accident or definable event

8. How many surgical procedures have you had **in order to eliminate the cause of your pain**?
   a. None or one
   b. Two surgical procedures
   c. Three or four surgical procedures
   d. Greater than four surgical procedures

9. Does movement have any effect on your pain?
   a. The pain is always worsened by use or movement
   b. The pain is usually worsened by use and movement
   c. The pain is not altered by use and movement

10. Does weather have any effect on your pain?
   a. The pain is usually worse with damp or cold weather.
   b. The pain is occasionally worse with damp or cold weather.
   c. Damp or cold weather has no effect on the pain.

11. Do you ever have trouble falling asleep or awaken from sleep?
   a. No - Proceed to Question 12 b. Yes - Proceed to 11A & 11B

   11A. How often do you have trouble falling asleep?
      a. Trouble falling asleep every night due to pain
      b. Trouble falling asleep due to pain most nights of the week
      c. Occasionally having difficulty falling asleep due to pain
      d. No trouble falling asleep due to pain
      e. Trouble falling asleep which is not related to pain

   11B. How often do you awaken from sleep?
      a. Awakened by pain every night
      b. Awakened from sleep by pain more than 3 times per week
      c. Not usually awakened from sleep by pain
      d. Restless sleep or early morning awakening with or without being able to return to sleep, both unrelated to pain

12. Has your pain affected your intimate personal relationships?
   a. No   b. Yes

13. Are you involved in any legal action regarding your physical complaint?
   a. No   b. Yes

14. Is this a Workers' Compensation case?
   a. No   b. Yes

15. Are you presently receiving psychiatric treatment?
   a. No   b. Yes   c. Previous psychiatric treatment

16. Have you ever thought of suicide?
   a. No   b. Yes   c. Previous suicide attempts

17. Are you a victim of emotional abuse?
   a. No   b. Yes   c. No comment

18. Are you a victim of physical abuse?
   a. No   b. Yes   c. No comment

19. Are you a victim of sexual abuse?
   a. No   b. Yes   c. No comment

20. Are you presently a victim of abuse?
   a. No   b. Yes   c. No comment

21. If you are retired, a student, or a homemaker, proceed to Question 21B.
   21A. Are you still working?
      a. Working every day at the same job I had before pain developed
      b. Working every day but the job is not the same as the job I had before pain developed; I now have reduced responsibility and physical activity
      c. Working occasionally
      d. Not presently working
   21B. Are you able to do your household chores?
      a. Do same level of household activities without discomfort
      b. Do same level of household chores with discomfort
      c. Do a reduced amount of household chores
      d. Most household chores are now performed by others

22. What medications have you used in the past month?
   a. No medications
   b. List medications:_____
   _____
   _____

23. If you had three wishes for anything in the world, what would you wish for?
   1._____
   2._____
   3._____

   0% ———————————————————— 100%

FIGURE 28.3 The pain evaluation questionnaire consists of pain adjectives, a body diagram, a questionnaire, and visual analog scales scored from 0 to 10 for pain, stress, and coping. Patients who select more than three adjectives, draw a pain pattern that does not follow a known anatomic pattern, or score more than 20 on the questionnaire are considered positive for that component. Patients who score positive in more than two components are considered for psychological or psychiatric evaluation before any surgical intervention. (Modified from Hendler N, Viernstein M, Gucer P, et al: A preoperative screening test for chronic back pain patients, *Psychosomatics* 20:801–808, 1979; Mackinnon SE, Dellon AL: *Surgery of the peripheral nerve*, New York, Thieme Medical, 1988; and Melzack R: The McGill pain questionnaire: major properties and scoring methods, *Pain* 1:277–299, 1975.)

Continued

PAIN EVALUATION SCORE SHEET

Name: _____   Date: _____

DOB: _____ Age: _____ Sex: M __ F __   Dominant Hand: R __ L __

Diagnosis: _____

1. Number of Descriptors: ___

2. Pain Level: on average ___   3. Pain level: worst   right ___   left ___

4. Body Diagram: _____

5. Stress Level: home ___ work ___   6. Coping Level: home ___ work ___

7. a. 0	8. a. 0	9. a. 0	10. a. 0	11. a. 3	11A. a. 0	11B. a. 0
b. 0	b. 2	b. 2	b. 2	b. 0	b. 1	b. 1
c. 3	c. 3	c. 3	c. 3		c. 2	c. 3
d. 4	d. 4				d. 3	d. 4
					e. 4	

12. a. 0	13. a. 0	14. a. 0	15. a. 0	16. a. 0	17. a. 0	18. a. 0
b. 2	b. 3	b. 2	b. 4	b. 2	b. 5	b. 5
			c. 2	c. 5	c. 3	c. 3

19. a. 0	20. a. 0	21A. a. 0	21B. a. 0	22. a. 0	23. a. 0 No pain only wish
b. 5	b. 5	b. 0	b. 0	b. 1 Valium	b. 1 No pain one of wishes
c. 3	c. 3	c. 2	c. 2	c. 2 Narcotic	c. 2 Wishes only of personal nature
		d. 3	d. 3	d. 3 Psychotropic or antidepressant drugs	d. 3 Wishes of nonpersonal nature (i.e., world peace)

Total: _____

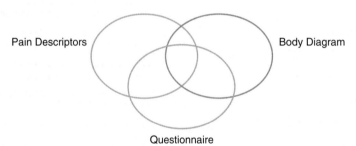

Pain Descriptors   Body Diagram

Questionnaire

FIGURE 28.3, cont'd

TABLE 28.1	**Provocative Tests for Nerve Compression**		
Nerve	**Entrapment Site**	**Provocative Test**	**Conservative Management**
Median	Carpal tunnel	Pressure proximal to the carpal tunnel Phalen test Reverse Phalen test (hyperextension of the wrist)	Splint the wrist in neutral position at night
	Proximal forearm	Pressure over the proximal forearm in the region of the pronator teres with the forearm in supination Resisted elbow flexion, pronation, and finger flexion	Use stretching exercises for the pronator teres
Ulnar	Guyon canal	Pressure proximal to Guyon canal Reverse Phalen test	Splint the wrist in neutral position at night
	Cubital tunnel	Elbow flexion and pressure proximal to the cubital tunnel	Educate about the elbow pad, positioning in elbow extension, and decreasing direct pressure on the nerve
Radial (posterior interosseous)	Arcade of Fröhse	Pressure over the supinator Resisted supination Resisted long-finger and wrist extension	Position in supination and avoid repetitive pronation and supination activities
Radial (sensory)	Forearm	Pressure over the junction of the brachioradialis/extensor carpi radialis tendon Forearm pronation with wrist ulnar flexion	Avoid repetitive pronation and supination activities
Brachial plexus	Supraclavicular	Elevation of arms above the head Pressure over the brachial plexus in the interscalene region	Avoid provocative positions Stretch shortened muscles and strengthen weakened scapular stabilizers

ulnar nerve distribution may be reported and should be documented. To evaluate the median nerve in the forearm, the patient's forearm is placed in full supination with full elbow extension, and digital pressure is applied to the median nerve in the region of the pronator teres muscle. A positive response is noted with sensory alteration in the median nerve distribution. To evaluate the cubital tunnel, the elbow is placed in full flexion with neutral forearm rotation and the wrist in neutral. Digital pressure is placed on the ulnar nerve just proximal to the cubital tunnel.[80] The position of the ulnar nerve should also be evaluated because subluxation of the ulnar nerve over the medial epicondyle may occur in some patients. The radial sensory nerve is evaluated by placing the wrist in flexion and ulnar deviation and the forearm in a pronated position. Compression of the brachial plexus at the thoracic outlet should also be screened by having the patient raise both arms overhead and noting reproduction of the patient's symptoms in the hands.[83] Pain in the shoulder region is not considered predictive of brachial plexus nerve compression, and further evaluation of the shoulder is indicated.

Cervical nerve root impingement is assessed clinically with the *Spurling test*.[108] This foraminal nerve root encroachment test is performed by placing the patient's cervical spine in slight extension and lateral flexion. Axial compression is then applied to the patient's head, and if a "spray" of symptoms into the arm is reported, it is considered positive for nerve root compression. The test is repeated with lateral flexion to the contralateral side. Tong and colleagues evaluated 255 patients and found the Spurling test to have a sensitivity of 30% and a specificity of 93%.[108] This study would suggest that the test correctly identifies patients with no cervical radiculopathy but is not an effective screening test to identify patients with cervical radiculopathy. Therefore, in a patient with symptoms suggesting involvement of the cervical spine and a negative response to the Spurling test, further cervical spine radiologic investigation may be indicated.

The *scratch collapse test* is another clinical test that may be used to identify a site of nerve compression and has been shown to have good psychometric properties.[9,13,28] This test is unique in that it uses a response independent of the sites of compression in the upper extremity. A positive response relies on the loss of muscle strength (shoulder external rotation) and therefore provides an outcome unrelated to the site of nerve compression. This test has been shown to have good positive and negative predictive value in the assessment of patients with carpal and cubital tunnel syndrome with abnormal nerve conduction studies.[13] However, this test is particularly useful in patients with diffuse symptoms, multiple levels of nerve compression, and normal nerve conduction studies. For examination with the scratch collapse test, the examiner is positioned in front of the patient with arms in neutral shoulder rotation, 90 degrees of elbow flexion, wrists in neutral position, and fingers extended. The examiner assesses isometric shoulder external rotation strength by applying a force to both forearms, and the patient applies an equal resisted force of external shoulder rotation to maintain the arms in a static position. The skin over the site of nerve compression to be assessed is lightly scratched and a similar force is applied to the forearms to resist isometric shoulder external rotation. A loss of shoulder external rotation strength will result in "collapse" of the arm toward the abdomen.

This is a positive response and indicative of nerve compression at the site of provocation. Each site of nerve compression may be assessed independently.

Shoulder and Scapular Movement Examination

Examination of the shoulder and evaluation of scapular movement patterns are important components of the physical examination of patients complaining of upper extremity pain.[41,67,99] Abnormal postures of the neck, shoulder, and scapular region are frequently associated with muscle imbalance, especially weakness of the serratus anterior and middle/lower trapezius muscles. To evaluate the strength of the serratus anterior muscles, the patient is asked to flex the shoulders forward while raising the arms above the head. Scapular position and movement are noted with the movement and at end range of motion. As the arms are slowly lowered, the examiner looks for any winging of the scapula to evaluate for serratus anterior strength. Similarly, to evaluate trapezius muscle strength, the patient is asked to abduct the shoulders and raise the arms above the head and then slowly lower the arms (in the coronal plane) as the examiner looks for winging of the scapula.

Compression of the mixed motor/sensory nerves in the upper extremity will produce symptoms of paresthesia and numbness. By contrast, aching pain and arm fatigue symptoms are associated more with muscle imbalance. Pure motor nerve compression (e.g., long thoracic, suprascapular, dorsal scapular, spinoaccessory nerve) can present with the above symptoms and atrophy. In patients with these symptoms, if examination of the scapular position and movement indicates weakness of the serratus anterior and middle/lower trapezius muscles, this should be further evaluated and treated. Similarly, if the patient has associated rotator cuff tendinitis or shoulder impingement, the symptoms will also be reflected in upper extremity discomfort. Examination of the shoulder for these problems is likewise important.

Sensory Evaluation

Even though provocation of the nerve can help identify sites of nerve compression, it does not quantify sensory function. Many instruments and assessment devices have been described for evaluation of sensibility, but no single test has been accepted as the gold standard. This in part relates to the varying capacities of the sensory tests to evaluate different parameters of nerve function.

The four sensory receptors that are found in the glabrous skin of the hand are categorized by differing receptive field size and response qualities. The slowly adapting receptors (Merkel cell neurite complex and Ruffini end-organs) respond to static touch, whereas the quickly adapting receptors (Meissner and Pacinian corpuscles) respond to moving touch. The threshold and tactile discrimination of the quickly and slowly adapting receptors can be evaluated. Threshold is the minimum stimulus required to elicit a response and is assessed with vibration thresholds (quickly adapting receptors) and with cutaneous pressure thresholds (slowly adapting receptors). Tactile discrimination reflects the number of innervated sensory receptors and is assessed with moving and static two-point discrimination. Vibration and cutaneous pressure thresholds will permit quantification of the early changes that occur with chronic nerve compression. Changes in sensory receptor innervation density will occur in the later stages of chronic nerve compression, and therefore two-point discrimination measures will become abnormal only in the more severe stages of nerve compression.

Light Moving Touch

Quick screening of the large A-beta fibers can be performed with the *ten test*.[103] Introduced by Strauch and coworkers, the ten test allows patients to rank their sensation of light moving touch on a scale from 0 to 10 in comparison with the normal contralateral area.[103] Good reliability and validity were reported when compared with Semmes-Weinstein monofilament testing. In patients with carpal tunnel syndrome, Patel and Bassini reported the ten test to be more sensitive than the Weinstein Enhanced Sensory Test and two-point discrimination.[92] For assessment with the ten test, the examiner applies a light touch and moves the stimulus with a finger to an area of normal sensation on the contralateral digit. A similar stimulus is applied simultaneously to the affected area, and the patient is asked to rank the sensation on a scale from 0 to 10, with 10 being perfect sensation and 0 being no sensation. Although this has proved to be an excellent screening test, it has limited use in patients with systemic sensory neuropathy and bilateral upper extremity nerve compression.

Vibration Thresholds

Vibration can be used to assess the thresholds of quickly adapting receptors. Qualitatively, vibration thresholds may be evaluated with a tuning fork. The tuning fork is applied to the affected and contralateral digit pulp, and the patient is asked to compare the stimuli. Limitations of this test include patient subjective assessment in recalling the applied stimuli and lack of consistent application of the tuning fork by the examiner.

A number of fixed-frequency and variable-frequency vibrometers have been described that permit quantification of vibration thresholds. Although good reliability has been reported with single-frequency vibrometers, the greatest limitation is that only one frequency is assessed. In a study of 130 factory workers, Werner and colleagues did not find single-frequency vibrometry useful as a screening tool for median nerve pathologic conditions.[118] In those with nerve compression, it is hypothesized that perception of the higher frequencies is affected earlier; therefore, evaluation at multiple frequencies may permit earlier identification of sensory loss.[53] However, in a study of patients with brachial plexus nerve compression, vibration thresholds measured at multiple frequencies were not useful in identifying these patients.[17]

Cutaneous Pressure Thresholds

Pressure thresholds of the slowly adapting receptors are commonly evaluated with Semmes-Weinstein monofilaments. These nylon monofilaments vary in diameter and thus differ in application force and produce different pressure thresholds. The set of Semmes-Weinstein monofilaments increases in diameter on a logarithmic scale ($\log_{10}$ force of 0.1 mg). The examiner applies pressure with each successive nylon filament until the filament just begins to bend. The smallest monofilament that the patient can perceive is documented as the pressure threshold. Each monofilament size is associated with a grading of sensory impairment (e.g., normal, diminished light touch, diminished protective sensation). Consistency in monofilament diameter and the testing procedure is necessary to ensure reliability.[46,112] Pressure thresholds have been shown to be sensitive in testing for carpal tunnel syndrome.

Two-Point Discrimination

Two-point discrimination reflects the number of innervated sensory receptors. Initially measured with a paper clip, other instruments such as the Disk-Criminator (Patterson Medical/Sammons Preston, Bolingbrook, IL) have been described for the measurement of static and moving two-point discrimination. Although good reliability has been shown with the Disk-Criminator,[85] alterations in two-point discrimination occur only with advanced nerve compression. Therefore, this is not a very sensitive test for patients with mild chronic nerve compression and may be more appropriate for assessment of recovery after nerve repair. In our clinical experience, two-point discrimination of greater than 8 mm is essentially nonfunctional, and we therefore classify this as "no two-point discrimination." Consequently, in the upper extremity, we have standardized our measurement of moving and static two-point discrimination to include two-point discrimination up to 8 mm.

Electrodiagnostic Studies

Electrodiagnostic studies include electromyography and nerve conduction studies. The tests are not a substitute for a detailed clinical examination by an experienced clinician. Unfortunately, some physicians rely on these studies without recognizing the major limitations of electrodiagnostic examination.[119] A well-performed electromyogram (EMG) and nerve conduction study can complement the clinical evaluation by helping to localize the level and severity of the injury and predict the likelihood of spontaneous regeneration and recovery.

A major limitation of the nerve conduction portion of the electrodiagnostic study is that it evaluates only the large myelinated fibers. This includes the motor axons and sensory axons relaying vibration and light touch but not the smaller axons conveying pain or temperature sensation. The determination of nerve latency reflects the conduction of the best myelinated fibers rather than the most severely affected axons, and normal latency may still be present even when many nerve fibers are affected. In chronic nerve compression, the first alterations that occur in the nerve fiber population are changes in unmyelinated nerve fibers, which cannot be evaluated with electrodiagnostic studies.[63] For example, early symptoms of pain and paresthesia cannot be assessed objectively with electrodiagnostic studies. Another limitation of nerve conduction studies relates to the location of the nerve injury in the extremity. Nerve problems occurring very distally or very proximally in the extremity are difficult to assess. Dynamic changes in blood flow that may produce intermittent alterations in peripheral nerve function may not be detected with electrodiagnostic studies. The timing of nerve conduction studies also influences their utility because even complete nerve transection will not become apparent for 2 to 6 weeks after injury. In situations with more than one level of injury or when a systemic polyneuropathy is present, nerve conduction studies may be less reliable. Although electrodiagnostic studies provide the surgeon with quantifiable values, they are extremely dependent on the expertise of the examiner who performs them.

Electromyography

For the EMG component of the study, needle recording electrodes are inserted into the muscles to evaluate either spontaneous or volitional electrical activity. Muscle response with needle insertion at rest and during activation is noted. A normal muscle will respond with a brief burst of electrical activity on needle insertion (insertional activity). Abnormal insertional activity can include insertional positive sharp waves, as seen with early denervation, or electrical silence, which is associated with chronic muscle degeneration without reinnervation. In the rest phase there will normally be electrical silence, but after nerve injury, spontaneous activity with fibrillation potentials is noted. Fibrillation potentials are the earliest sign of muscle denervation and are generated by muscles after denervation of at least 2 weeks' duration. A single motor axon innervates hundreds to thousands of muscle fibers; thus, fibrillation potentials are the most sensitive indicator of motor axon loss and can be seen in nerve compression syndromes long before there is any clinical evidence of muscle weakness. During the muscle activation portion of the EMG, the patient is instructed to contract the muscle to elicit voluntary motor unit potentials (MUPs). In a normal muscle, because numerous MUPs are activated, individual MUPs cannot be seen and a full interference pattern is noted. With nerve injury, incomplete MUP activation and reduced MUP recruitment are seen. Patients responding with pain or decreased effort can show incomplete MUP activation, but the rate will be slow to moderate. With reduced MUP recruitment because of a peripheral nerve problem, the firing rate will be faster and the configuration will be of increased duration and amplitude. The neurologist doing the EMG will be able to determine chronic neurogenic MUP changes from incomplete MUP activation as seen with upper motor neuron disease or decreased patient effort. MUPs associated with reinnervation will initially be of very low amplitude and extremely polyphasic, and they will fire at a slow to moderate rate. Eventually, they will remodel so that the duration and number of phases decrease and the amplitude increases.

Nerve Conduction Studies

Nerve conduction studies can be used to study motor, sensory, and mixed nerves. Surface electrodes are used to stimulate and record from the nerve. During motor nerve conduction studies, electrodes are placed over the muscle and the motor axons are stimulated proximal to the surface electrode. Motor axons are *indirectly* assessed by the size and configuration of the compound muscle action potentials (CMAPs) that are generated in response to nerve stimulation. Motor nerve conduction studies are characterized by a large-amplitude response, in contrast to sensory nerve conduction studies, in which the sensory axons themselves are directly assessed and the sensory nerve action potential (SNAP) is very small. Sensory nerve function can be assessed in antegrade (orthodromic) or retrograde (antidromic) fashion by placing the recording electrode either proximal or distal to the stimulating electrode, respectively. Because of their small size and low amplitude, SNAPs may be adversely affected by technical problems or by factors such as skin or room temperature. The parameters of nerve conduction studies include wave amplitude, duration, latency, the area of the recorded response, and conduction velocity. Laboratories have their own set of normal values based on age. It is customary for individuals with unilateral neurologic problems to have a drop in amplitude of 50% or more on the symptomatic side as compared with the normal extremity.

Latency is an indirect measure of the speed of impulse conduction along the fastest conducting fibers and is expressed in milliseconds. Sensory nerves are stimulated at one point and recorded at a surface electrode, and the recorded latency is defined as the time elapsed until onset of the peak deflection. Motor latency is defined as the time elapsed between a supramaximal stimulus over the involved nerve and the onset of deflection at the motor point of the innervated muscle.

Amplitude is the height of the action potential expressed in millivolts for motor nerve conduction studies and in microvolts for sensory nerve conduction studies. The amplitude provides an assessment of the number of conducting axons. Amplitudes are more difficult to assess, but because they reflect the number of functioning axons, they may give more information about muscle weakness and paresthesia than latency measurements, which reflect only the fastest conducting fibers. Conduction velocity is calculated by stimulating the nerve at two measured distances and determining the rate of conduction in meters per second between the two points. It is useful when comparing results between subjects with different limb lengths. Diffusely slowed conduction velocity across several nerves may also indicate a systemic peripheral neuropathy. However, conduction velocity reflects the speed of the fastest conducting fibers and, unlike amplitude, does not give any information regarding the number of conducting axons. Area beneath the curve is a function of amplitude and duration of response and more accurately reflects the number of axons, but like amplitude, it is technically more difficult to assess.

Electrodiagnostic Studies and Nerve Compression

Nerve conduction studies give information about axon and myelin pathologic conditions, and each component is important to properly identify such conditions of nerves. Latency and conduction velocity should not be viewed in isolation, because the speed of conduction relates only to the "healthiest surviving" myelinated nerve fibers. Similarly, even though amplitude is a reflection of the number of functioning axons, amplitude may also be affected by other pathologic situations, such as myopathy. In moderate cases of nerve compression, EMG studies may demonstrate scarce fibrillation potentials, and if the axonal problem is more severe, reduced MUP recruitment will be present. In rare cases, the examiner may identify fibrillation potentials on the EMG with maintenance of normal nerve latencies. With progression, the number of fibrillation potentials will increase and action potential amplitudes will decrease. SNAP amplitudes are affected before CMAP amplitudes. Eventually, MUP recruitment will decrease. With a complete injury, nerve conduction motor and sensory responses will be absent, fibrillation potentials will be marked, and no MUPs will be identified.

The early stage of nerve compression is associated with dynamic ischemic events involving the nerve. Thus, the results of electrodiagnostic studies for the most part are normal. As the nerve compression progresses, demyelination will occur and conduction velocity will slow across the site of compression. Axonal loss does not usually take place until late in the course of the neuropathy. With carpal tunnel syndrome, nerve conduction study latencies may be prolonged, but the EMG is generally normal until late in the disease. Demyelination and focal conduction slowing are typical of most patients with carpal tunnel syndrome and at least half of those with cubital tunnel syndrome, with axonal changes being found much later in the course of the disease.

Electrodiagnostic studies are useful in ruling out other associated problems such as cervical disk disease, motor neuron problems, myopathy, or superimposed polyneuropathies. They are particularly useful in the investigation of symptoms related to the ulnar nerve, which can sometimes herald the presence of other, more sinister diagnoses. Patients with isolated motor deficits and spared sensory function must have a motor neuropathy ruled out before an entrapment neuropathy can be diagnosed. Electrodiagnostic studies can also help rule out problems that are "functional." Muscles that are weak or atrophic because of disuse will show no EMG abnormalities other than poor voluntary MUP generation, in keeping with submaximal effort by the patient. If the muscle is weak or atrophic because of a peripheral nerve problem, the CMAP will be of low amplitude, MUP recruitment will be reduced, and fibrillation potentials will be noted, unless the process is extremely chronic. Electrodiagnostic studies are not generally helpful in confirming a diagnosis of thoracic outlet syndrome because of its proximal location at the brachial plexus and the often dynamic nature of the compression.

COMPRESSION OF THE MEDIAN NERVE

Median Nerve Compression at the Wrist: Carpal Tunnel Syndrome

Carpal tunnel syndrome refers to compression of the median nerve at the wrist and is the most commonly diagnosed site of nerve compression in the upper extremity. Symptoms include paresthesia or numbness (or both) in the median nerve distribution (thumb, index finger, middle finger, and radial side of the ring finger). Nocturnal paresthesias in the radial three digits of the hand are nearly pathognomonic for carpal tunnel syndrome. Paresthesias also occur characteristically in "fixed wrist activities" such as reading a book or a newspaper, driving, or use of a keyboard or mouse. Patients may describe aching in the thenar eminence and, with advanced nerve compression, weakness and atrophy of the abductor pollicis brevis and opponens pollicis. Carpal tunnel syndrome is a clinical diagnosis based on a combination of symptoms and characteristic physical findings; its presence may be subsequently confirmed with electrodiagnostic studies.[38,96] Electrodiagnostic studies are useful to stage the degree of nerve compression and may therefore assist the surgeon and patient in anticipating the time needed for recovery of nerve function. Patients with long-standing symptoms, severe atrophy of the thenar musculature, and dense sensory loss should be cautioned that release can only arrest the progression of the disorder and will not lead to complete recovery of sensation or thenar strength.

◣ ANATOMY

The roof of the carpal canal is the flexor retinaculum, which extends from the hamate and triquetrum on the ulnar side to the scaphoid and trapezium on the radial side. The median

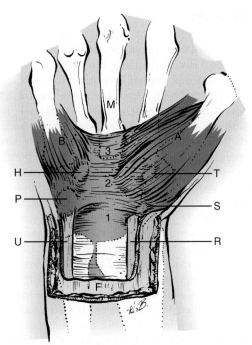

FIGURE 28.4 Anatomy of the three portions of the flexor retinaculum. The distal portion of the flexor retinaculum (3) consists of a thick aponeurosis between the thenar (A) and hypothenar (B) muscles. The thenar muscles attach to the radial half of the classic flexor retinaculum, which is composed of the distal portion of the flexor retinaculum (3) and the transverse carpal ligament (2). Bony attachments of the transverse carpal ligament—pisiform (P), hamate (H), tubercle of the trapezium (T), and tubercle of the scaphoid (S)—are also shown. The proximal portion of the flexor retinaculum (1) courses deep to the flexor carpi ulnaris (U) and flexor carpi radialis (R). The flexor carpi radialis tendon is shown as it pierces the flexor retinaculum at the junction of the proximal and middle portions to enter its fibroosseous canal. F, Antebrachial fascia; M, third metacarpal. (From Cobb TK, Dalley BK, Posteraro RH, et al: Anatomy of flexor retinaculum, *J Hand Surg [Am]* 18:91–99, 1993. Redrawn by Elizabeth Martin.)

nerve and flexor tendons (flexor pollicis longus tendon, four flexor digitorum superficialis tendons, and four flexor digitorum profundus tendons) pass through this tunnel. Although the carpal tunnel is open at its proximal and distal ends, it maintains distinct tissue fluid pressure levels. The diameter of the carpal tunnel is narrowest at a point approximately 2 cm from its leading edge (Figure 28.4), and this corresponds to the site of morphologic changes in the nerve in patients with carpal tunnel syndrome. The median nerve lies just beneath the flexor retinaculum. At the distal end of the flexor retinaculum, the median nerve gives off the recurrent motor branch to innervate the abductor pollicis brevis muscle, superficial head of the flexor pollicis brevis muscle, and opponens pollicis muscles and then divides into the digital nerves that provide sensation to the thumb and index finger, middle finger, and radial half of the ring finger.

Knowledge of variations in the branching pattern of the median nerve is important, particularly during surgical decompression.[61] Lanz has classified variations of the recurrent motor branch into four subgroups (Figures 28.5 to 28.7).[43] In most cases, the motor branch divides from the median nerve distal to the flexor retinaculum in an extraligamentous pattern (46-90%). Less common variations include the subligamentous pattern (31%) and transligamentous pattern (23%). There have

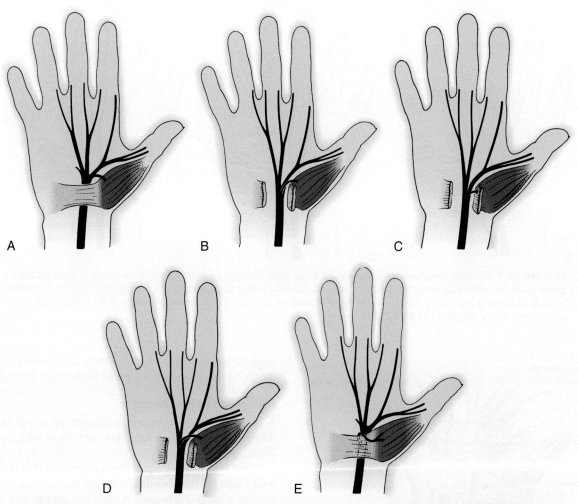

FIGURE 28.5 Variations in median nerve anatomy in the carpal tunnel. **A,** The most common pattern of the motor branch is extraligamentous and recurrent. **B,** Subligamentous branching of a recurrent median nerve. **C,** Transligamentous course of the recurrent branch of the median nerve. **D,** The motor branch can uncommonly originate from the ulnar border of the median nerve. **E,** The motor branch can lie on top of the transverse carpal ligament. (From Lanz U: Anatomical variations of the median nerve in the carpal tunnel, *J Hand Surg [Am]* 2:44–53, 1977.)

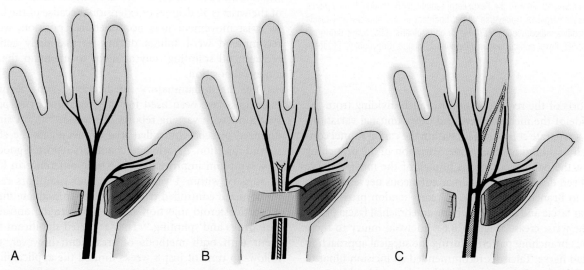

FIGURE 28.6 Variations in median nerve anatomy in the carpal tunnel. Group III variations include high divisions of the median nerve **(A)** that may be separated by a persistent median artery **(B)** or an aberrant muscle **(C)**. (From Lanz U: Anatomical variations of the median nerve in the carpal tunnel, *J Hand Surg [Am]* 2:44–53, 1977.)

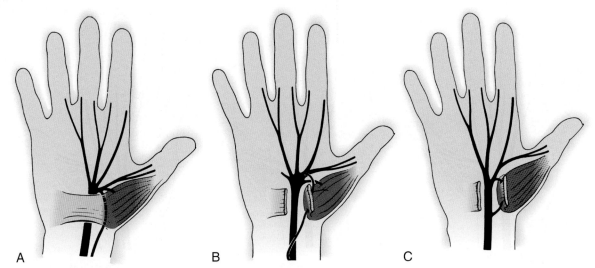

FIGURE 28.7 Variations in median nerve anatomy in the carpal tunnel. Group IV variations include rare instances in which the thenar branch leaves the median nerve proximal to the carpal tunnel: **A,** accessory branch; **B,** accessory branch from the ulnar aspect of the median nerve; **C,** accessory branch running directly into the thenar musculature. (From Lanz U: Anatomical variations of the median nerve in the carpal tunnel, *J Hand Surg [Am]* 2:44–53, 1977.)

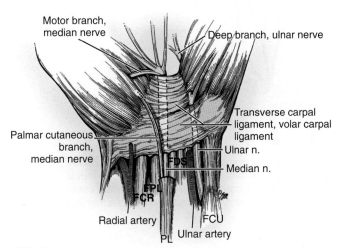

FIGURE 28.8 The palmar cutaneous branch of the median nerve lies radial to the median nerve and ulnar to the flexor carpi radialis (FCR) tendon. It may pierce either the volar carpal or transverse carpal ligament or the antebrachial fascia before it becomes subcutaneous. *FCU,* Flexor carpi ulnaris; *FDS,* flexor digitorum superficialis; *FPL,* flexor pollicis longus; *PL,* palmaris longus. (Copyright © Elizabeth Martin.)

been reports of the recurrent motor branch dividing from the medial side of the median nerve and other unusual variations in which a separate compartment within the carpal tunnel contained half of a bifid median nerve. Variation in the branching pattern of the palmar cutaneous branch of the median nerve has also been described. The palmar cutaneous nerve has been reported to branch through the palmaris tendon proximal to the palmar fascia and also through the antebrachial fascia proximal to the wrist crease (Figure 28.8). To avoid injury to these anomalous branching patterns during the surgical approach to the median nerve, Taleisnik recommended an incision ulnar to the axis of the flexed ring finger.[106] Although considerable variation in the length and location of the surgical incision used for carpal tunnel release exists among hand surgeons,[48] consider-

ation of the anatomy of the palmar cutaneous and recurrent motor nerves is essential to avoid inadvertent nerve injury.

Nonoperative Management

A number of nonoperative treatments of carpal tunnel syndrome have been described that vary from wrist splinting to corticosteroid injection.

Wrist splinting is frequently recommended for nonoperative treatment.[12,116] Prefabricated wrist splints are often used and can present a unique problem if they are placed in a functional position of 30 degrees of extension. Carpal canal pressures have been shown to be elevated in patients with carpal tunnel syndrome, and pressure is further elevated when the wrist is in a position of extension.[25] To control symptoms related to nerve compression at the wrist, wrist splints are most effective in a neutral position.[8] Maintaining the wrist in a neutral position will minimize carpal canal pressure, but the functional position of the wrist is 30 degrees of extension. Because of the limitation of wrist movement in a nonfunctional position, we do not recommend wrist splints during normal daily activity. We recommend splinting only at night to maintain the wrist in a neutral position.

Oral antiinflammatory medications and corticosteroid injections have been used for the treatment of carpal tunnel syndrome with varying reports of success.[4,12,24,116] Using a randomized placebo-controlled trial to investigate the efficacy of steroid injection, Atroshi and coauthors reported good temporary symptom improvement but little difference in likelihood of surgery within 1 year.[4] Celiker and coauthors reported a randomized controlled trial conducted to evaluate the efficacy of corticosteroid injection versus nonsteroidal antiinflammatory drugs and splinting.[12] They reported significant improvement with both methods of treatment; however, the brief follow-up time of just 8 weeks limited the applicability of the study. Green[29] reported that temporary relief after carpal tunnel injection was an excellent prognostic factor for successful carpal tunnel surgery. Complications with steroid injection have been reported, including injury to the median nerve. In a study evaluating the effects of steroid nerve injection in a rodent model, dexamethasone was found to have no deleterious effects on the nerve, even when injected directly into the nerve.[65] All other corticosteroids caused varying degrees of nerve injury when directly injected into the rodent sciatic nerve. However, given its temporary relief of symptoms and finite risk for nerve injury, in our practice corticosteroid injection is not indicated routinely.

More recently, nerve gliding exercises have been used to alleviate symptoms of nerve compression.[10,98,100] Rozmaryn and associates used nerve and tendon gliding exercises to treat a group of patients with carpal tunnel syndrome and noted less surgical intervention in this group than in a historical control group.[98] Seradge and coauthors reported good symptomatic relief and avoidance of surgery in up to 80% of patients with mild or moderate compression treated with nerve gliding and stretching exercises who were monitored for 18 months.[100]

Operative Treatment

When a regimen of conservative treatment fails to relieve the patient's symptoms, surgical decompression of the median nerve is usually recommended. The first carpal tunnel release was reportedly performed by Herbert Galloway in 1924. Numerous approaches for carpal tunnel release have been described that range from an open technique to a small incision to endoscopic release. The controversy regarding open versus endoscopic carpal tunnel release continues and the decision is largely dependent on surgeon preference and patient selection. A meta-analysis was published in 2008 to evaluate outcomes related to endoscopic and open carpal tunnel release. The authors concluded that the data related to symptom relief and return to work are inconclusive and there is increased likelihood of reversible nerve injury with endoscopic release.[107] A study using a randomized controlled design evaluated one compared to two incisions and found no long-term differences between these surgical techniques.[11] Although release of the median nerve is the goal of treatment, injury to even a few fascicles of the nerve can have devastating consequences for the patient. Therefore, the surgeon should choose the surgical method that offers the best visualization of the median nerve to avoid nerve injury.

Minimal incision and endoscopic techniques were introduced to decrease the length of the incision and thus potentially decrease postoperative incisional discomfort. A number of endoscopic systems have been described, but the risk for complications, including iatrogenic nerve injury, poor visualization, inability to identify anatomic variations, incomplete release, and apparent beneficial cost savings, is still debated. Those who support endoscopic carpal tunnel release also advocate specialized training in cadaveric courses before performance of endoscopic carpal tunnel release. Others have introduced surgical releases with smaller incisions termed "minimally invasive" to decrease postoperative incisional pain and thus minimize postoperative morbidity. In this chapter, we have reviewed the original endoscopic techniques as introduced by Chow and Agee, but others have also introduced variations of endoscopic approaches.[32]

Chow Two-Portal Endoscopic Technique. A two-portal endoscopic technique was introduced by Chow.[14] A tourniquet is placed but not inflated. Local anesthesia with 1% lidocaine without epinephrine is used, with or without intravenous sedation. The entry portal is located by drawing a line 1 to 1.5 cm radially from the proximal pole of the pisiform and a second line 0.5 cm proximally from the first line. A 1-cm transverse incision is made through the skin radially from the end of the second line. A longitudinal incision is made through the fascia. A curved dissector-obturator slotted cannula assembly is inserted through the distal edge of the entry portal incision along the long axis of the forearm. It is used to free synovial tissue from the inferior surface of the flexor retinaculum. The assembly tip touches the hook of the hamate, the hand is lifted off the table, and the wrist and fingers are hyperextended. At 1 cm proximal to a line drawn that bisects the angle formed by the distal border of the fully abducted thumb and the third web space, a 0.5-cm exit portal incision is made. The slotted cannula assembly is advanced distally and the tip palpated at the exit portal in the palm. The assembly is passed through, and the hand is stabilized in a custom hand-holding device. The endoscope is inserted into the proximal tube opening, and a probe is inserted distally to identify the distal edge of the flexor retinaculum. The probe knife is used to release the distal edge of the flexor retinaculum in a distal to proximal direction. The triangle knife is then used to release the midsection of the flexor retinaculum, and the retrograde knife is positioned in the second cut and drawn distally to join the first cut to release the distal part of the flexor retinaculum. The endoscope is withdrawn and replaced in the distal tube opening, and the probe knife is used to release the proximal edge of the flexor retinaculum. The retrograde knife is inserted into the midsection and drawn proximally to complete release of the flexor retinaculum. The trocar is reinserted and the cannula removed. The antebrachial fascia is released through the proximal incision with tenotomy scissors, and the skin is sutured.

Agee Single-Portal Endoscopic Technique. A single-incision technique was described by Agee and associates.[1] A tourniquet is used for this procedure. The authors recommend that initially a general or regional anesthetic be used, and with more surgeon experience, they recommend local anesthesia. A 2- to 3-cm transverse skin incision is made in the distal wrist flexion crease between the flexor carpi radialis and flexor carpi ulnaris tendons. With the use of spreading longitudinal dissection, the cutaneous nerves are protected and the forearm fascia is identified. A "U"-shaped, distally based flap of forearm fascia is incised and elevated in a palmar direction. A probe is passed down the ulnar side of the carpal tunnel, radial to the hook of the hamate. The wrist is placed in slight extension, and the blade assembly is inserted with the viewing window toward the inner aspect of the flexor retinaculum. The tip of the blade assembly is palpated with the surgeon's contralateral hand. The distal edge of the flexor retinaculum is located by video, ballottement, and light touch through the skin. When the correct position is ensured, the blade is deployed upward from within the device, the device is withdrawn, and the distal aspect of the flexor retinaculum is incised. The blade is retracted, the assembly is reinserted, the flexor retinaculum division is inspected, and additional cuts are made to release the remaining flexor retinaculum. Using tenotomy scissors, the antebrachial forearm fascia is released proximal to the skin incision. The skin incision is closed, and splinting is performed at the discretion of the surgeon. Agee and colleagues strongly recommend that if complete visualization is not obtained, the endoscopic technique should be abandoned and the carpal tunnel released with an open technique.

❖ AUTHORS' PREFERRED METHOD OF TREATMENT: Open Carpal Tunnel Release

We prefer the classic open carpal tunnel release with intravenous regional anesthesia (Bier block) for the treatment of carpal tunnel syndrome (Videos 28.1 and 28.2). General anesthesia is rarely indicated; more recently there has been a trend toward increased use of local and regional anesthesia. Axillary blocks have been associated with nerve injection injuries, and although this complication is exceedingly rare, when it does occur, it may be devastating for the patient. Many surgeons use local anesthesia, but we believe that patients are more comfortable with some sedation and tolerate the tourniquet better with an intravenous regional block (250 mm Hg). In the rare cases in which use of a tourniquet is contraindicated, anesthetic nerve blocks of the median, radial, and ulnar nerves at the elbow can be used as an alternative to general anesthesia or brachial plexus blocks. As a preemptive action against the sympathetic nervous system, dexmedetomidine hydrochloride is usually included with the intravenous regional anesthetic. A double tourniquet on the upper part of the arm is used, and the tourniquets are changed at 10 minutes so that patients do not experience tourniquet pain. A forearm tourniquet is used for obese patients because the upper arm tourniquet can sometimes be less reliable and result in a venous tourniquet. In thin patients with small hands when the tourniquet time is going to be exceedingly short, a forearm tourniquet is used. Less volume of anesthetic is needed and no dexmedetomidine hydrochloride is used, and the tourniquet can be released earlier.

The incision is marked about 6 mm ulnar to the thenar crease to ensure that any scarring is away from the median nerve and that the incision is well ulnar to the palmar cutaneous branch of the median nerve, which is located in the thenar crease (Figure 28.9). A curvilinear incision is made that parallels the thenar crease, 2 or 3 cm in length, and ends just distal to the transverse wrist crease. If more exposure is necessary to release the antebrachial fascia, the incision is extended proximally in a zigzag fashion across the wrist in an ulnar direction. With the increased prevalence of obesity, use of a longer incision should be considered in these patients to provide adequate visualization. Two double hooks are used for retraction, and dissection is carried out through the soft tissue. About 15% of the time, a crossing cutaneous branch from the ulnar nerve will be identified in the distal portion of the incision and protected. Senn retractors are used to retract through the fatty tissue to expose the proximal portion of the flexor retinaculum and the distal portion of the antebrachial fascia. A No. 15 blade is used, and very carefully, slowly, and with control, the proximal portion of the flexor retinaculum and distal portion of the antebrachial fascia are opened. A different color of the darker synovium around the flexor tendons will be seen once the ligament has been cut. The blunt end of a Freer retractor can be placed gently into the carpal canal if desired. The rake portions of the two Senn retractors are used to retract the soft tissue above the flexor retinaculum, and tenotomy scissors are used to spread the fatty tissue for identification of the flexor retinaculum. The carpal ligament is carefully released along the ulnar side. The flexor retinaculum is released as far distally as the fat

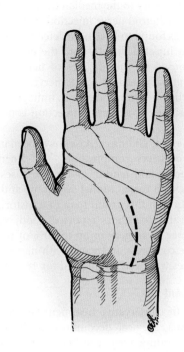

FIGURE 28.9 Authors' preferred carpal tunnel incision. A curved longitudinal incision is made so that it parallels the thenar crease and crosses the wrist crease obliquely in an ulnar direction at a point in line with the long axis of the flexed ring finger or just on the ulnar side of the palmaris longus tendon. (Copyright © Elizabeth Martin.)

around the superficial arch. With observation of the fat, one knows that the distal ligament has been released completely. In obese individuals or people with very large hands, the incision may need to be extended more distally to ensure that the entire ligament has been released and to identify the fatty tissue signaling the end of the ligament. Proximally, using the down-curved portion of two Senn retractors, the fatty tissue is retracted above the antebrachial fascia. The surgeon is positioned at the end of the hand table to ensure excellent visualization. With the use of pick-ups, one edge of the antebrachial fascia is pulled distally. With slight volar wrist flexion, the median nerve will drop away from the antebrachial fascia. Under direct vision, the antebrachial fascia is released with the tenotomy scissors or a No. 15 blade. If difficulty releasing this antebrachial fascia under direct vision is encountered, the incision must be extended proximally above the wrist to ensure that the antebrachial fascia has been adequately released and that there is no injury to the median nerve. The rake end of the Senn retractor is used to retract the radial side of the divided flexor retinaculum up or anteriorly. The median nerve is visualized. Rarely, before operation, some patients will describe a deep, aching thenar pain or present with significant thenar wasting with minimal sensory complaints, findings indicating that specific exploration of the recurrent motor branch of the median nerve is warranted. The rake end of the Senn retractor is used to pull up on the radial side of the divided ligament, and the median nerve is carefully retracted toward the surgeon. This will cause the recurrent motor branch of the median nerve to tent up as it enters the thenar muscle mass and allow identification of the recurrent motor branch as it curves toward the thenar muscle. In patients with deep, aching thenar pain or thenar muscle wasting (or both), the recurrent motor branch will often enter the thenar musculature through its own tendinous tunnel. (Similarly, in these patients, the thenar motor branch may come off of the ulnar side of the median nerve, exposing it to more compression as it travels across the top of the nerve and directly under the ligament.) This maneuver of pulling up on the flexor retinaculum and pulling the median nerve medially toward the surgeon will help with easy identification of the recurrent motor branch. The floor of the carpal canal can be visualized by retracting the flexor tendons to evaluate for any pathologic conditions such as ganglions. We believe that neurolysis of the median nerve during primary carpal tunnel release is not indicated.[66] Studies have also reported no benefit with epineurotomy.[7] Similarly, synovectomy is not indicated during primary carpal tunnel decompression. The tourniquet is deflated, and bupivacaine (Marcaine) is injected into the incision under careful direct vision for postoperative comfort. Microbipolar cautery is used for hemostasis. The incision is closed with interrupted 4-0 nylon suture, and a bulky dressing is applied while keeping the wrist in neutral, with fiberglass casting incorporated into the dressing. A sling may be used for the early postoperative period, but the patient is cautioned against unnecessary elbow flexion, which may result in flare-up of an associated cubital tunnel syndrome, and against shoulder immobilization, which may result in shoulder stiffness.

In cases of severe carpal tunnel syndrome with thenar muscle atrophy, opponensplasty may be considered. In this patient population, a palmaris longus (Camitz) transfer is the ideal transfer for improved thenar abduction because of its minimal donor deficit and immediate availability in the same surgical incision. In the authors' opinion, it is rarely required, as patients have adapted to the slow progressive loss associated with the chronic neuropathy. Because this is an in-continuity nerve lesion, there is also the potential for muscle reinnervation and motor recovery, as is the case with sensory recovery. Finally, the older population that presents with severe thenar atrophy may not desire or tolerate the requisite cast immobilization after tendon transfer.

Expected Outcome After Carpal Tunnel Decompression

Following carpal tunnel decompression for mild or moderate compression, there will be return of "painless" sensation to the digits innervated by the median nerve in mild or moderate compression. Reinnervation of the thenar muscles will also occur, and there will be full range of motion at the wrist.

Postoperative Care

Immobilization after decompression of the carpal tunnel was historically used to protect the wound and immobilize the wrist to prevent the flexor tendons from bowstringing. However, because of advancing knowledge in the importance of postoperative tendon and nerve gliding, such postoperative immobilization has been dramatically decreased.[36,44] After carpal tunnel decompression, a bulky dressing is used to restrict wrist range of motion during the first 2 postoperative days for patient comfort and is then removed. The patient is instructed in range-of-motion exercises for the fingers, wrist, and arm. A splint in a wrist neutral position is used at night for 2 to 3 weeks for patient comfort or until the patient has regained comfortable

full range of motion of the wrist. The sutures are removed 12 to 14 days postoperatively. At 1 month after surgery patients are allowed to return to work with a 2-pound weight restriction, and at 6 to 8 weeks after surgery they are allowed full activity without restrictions.

CRITICAL POINTS *Carpal Tunnel Release*

Indications
- Failed night splinting with the wrist in neutral position

Preoperative Evaluation
- Electrodiagnostic studies to "stage" the degree of nerve compression for helping to predict the anticipated rate and degree of recovery

Pearls
- Document preoperative pain distribution.
- Document preoperative examination of the entire upper extremity.
- Use dexmedetomidine hydrochloride in a Bier block.
- Postoperatively, begin early movement.

Technical Points
- Make an incision ulnar to the thenar crease and extend it proximally in obese patients.
- Avoid the ulnar cutaneous branch (15%) in the distal portion of the incision.
- Release the flexor retinaculum in a proximal to distal direction.
- Release the ligament distally to the fat pad.
- Release the antebrachial fascia under direct vision.
- Provide hemostasis after release of the tourniquet.
- Use bupivacaine in the incision.

Pitfalls
- In obese patients, use a forearm tourniquet to avoid a "venous" tourniquet.
- Failure to adequately release the distal ligament or the proximal antebrachial fascia may occur.

Postoperative Care
- Remove the dressing on day 2 or 3.
- Use night splinting in a wrist neutral position for 2 to 3 weeks for patient comfort.
- Begin range-of-movement exercises on day 2 or 3.
- Avoid unnecessary elbow flexion because it may result in irritation of the ulnar nerve.
- Begin strengthening exercises after 4 weeks.
- There are no restrictions after the second month.

Median Nerve Compression at the Elbow and Forearm

A rare and very proximal site of median nerve compression in the upper extremity occurs under the ligament of Struthers in patients who have a supracondylar process (Figure 28.10). An accessory bicipital aponeurosis that can cause an anterior interosseous nerve palsy has also been identified. Sensory disturbance in the median nerve by a snapping brachialis tendon has been reported. Fibrous bands between the deep and superficial heads of the pronator teres are frequently cited as the cause of compression in cases of anterior interosseous nerve palsy and pronator teres syndrome. Compression may result from a fibrous arch between the two heads of the pronator teres, from

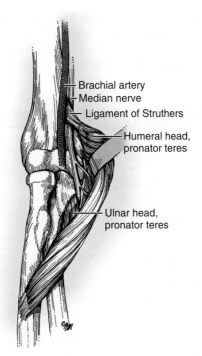

FIGURE 28.10 The median nerve lies deep and the brachial artery lies superficial to the ligament of Struthers, which forms an accessory origin for the pronator teres. (Copyright © Elizabeth Martin.)

Labels in figure:
- Brachial artery
- Median nerve
- Ligament of Struthers
- Humeral head, pronator teres
- Ulnar head, pronator teres

a tendinous deep head of the pronator teres, from the flexor digitorum superficialis arch, or from other bands in the distal part of the forearm. Other accessory and anomalous muscles, including the accessory head of the flexor pollicis longus (Gantzer muscle), the palmaris profundus, and the flexor carpi radialis brevis, have been identified as compressive structures. The Gantzer muscle was found to be present in 45% in one cadaveric study. Cadaveric dissections to identify the anatomic variations and fibrous arches that may contribute to compression in the forearm revealed that the superficial head of the pronator teres was always present, the flexor digitorum superficialis varied in origin size, and the median nerve may be crossed by one or two fibrous aponeurotic arches. The fibrous arch of the pronator teres has been found to be located 3 to 7.5 cm distal to the humeral epicondylar line and the fibrous arch of the flexor digitorum superficialis to be 6.5 cm distal to the humeral epicondylar line in its most proximal position.

Compression of the median nerve in the forearm is less common than carpal tunnel syndrome. Compression in the forearm can produce sensory disturbance in the median nerve distribution or motor dysfunction of the muscles innervated by the anterior interosseous nerve and median nerve, or both sensory and motor dysfunction. Parsonage and Turner described spontaneous paralysis of the flexor pollicis longus and flexor digitorum profundus to the index finger, which they termed "neuralgic amyotrophy."[91,110] The pathologic findings of this mononeuritis is related to the anterior horn cell and most commonly occurs after a viral illness. Parsonage-Turner neuritis is not confined to the anterior interosseous nerve; the periscapular and shoulder muscles may be affected as well. Anterior interosseous nerve palsy can also occur after a surgical procedure in the ipsilateral upper extremity, which makes the etiologic

picture more confusing. There is almost always complete recovery without surgical intervention, although this recovery may take many months.

ANATOMY

The median nerve is formed from branches of the medial and lateral cords of the brachial plexus. It receives its sensory contribution predominantly from the lateral cord and its motor fibers predominantly from the medial cord. The median nerve crosses over the brachial artery to lie on the medial side in contact with the brachialis muscle. It continues distally between the brachialis muscle and the medial intermuscular septum and then passes through the antecubital fossa and under the lacertus fibrosus (bicipital aponeurosis). The nerve travels between the deep and superficial heads of the pronator teres and in some cases posterior to the pronator teres. Before the nerve divides into the main median nerve and the anterior interosseous nerve, the fascicles remain separate within the median nerve.[104] Before passing through the pronator teres, there are branches exiting to the palmaris longus, flexor carpi radialis, flexor digitorum superficialis, and, rarely, flexor digitorum profundus. In a cadaveric anatomic study by Tung and Mackinnon, the pronator teres muscle received more than one branch in 73% of cases and the flexor digitorum superficialis received two or more branches in 94% of cases.[109] After exiting the pronator teres, the median nerve courses deep to the fibrous arch of the flexor digitorum superficialis and becomes more superficial in the distal part of the forearm.

The anterior interosseous nerve provides innervation to the flexor digitorum profundus of the index and middle fingers, the flexor pollicis longus, and the pronator quadratus. The nerve provides sensory fibers to the radiocarpal, intercarpal, carpometacarpal, and radioulnar joints. The anterior interosseous nerve is relatively tethered as it separates from the main median nerve, which makes it relatively more susceptible to traction injuries. A Martin-Gruber anastomosis (connection between the median and ulnar nerves in the forearm) is found in 15% of the population, and in half of the cases the communicating branch originates from the anterior interosseous nerve.

The palmar cutaneous nerve branches from the median nerve approximately 5 cm proximal to the proximal wrist crease. It separates from the median nerve and enters a tunnel immediately medial to the flexor carpi radialis tendon and then innervates the skin of the thenar eminence. Evaluation of thenar sensation is helpful in differentiating median nerve compression in the carpal canal from more proximal sites of compression.

Pronator Syndrome

Pronator syndrome is defined as compression of the median nerve in the forearm that results in isolated sensory alteration in the median nerve distribution in the digits and thenar eminence. This syndrome is much less common than carpal tunnel syndrome and has been reported in individuals who do repetitive upper extremity activity. Provocation tests should reproduce symptoms in affected patients. These tests include resisted forearm pronation, with the forearm in full supination and elbow extended, and also in some cases resisted elbow flexion or flexion of the middle finger flexor digitorum superficialis. If the forearm is placed in maximum supination with the wrist in a neutral position, pressure over the leading edge of the pronator teres will produce paresthesias in the median sensory distribution. Also in patients with median nerve compression at the pronator teres, the scratch collapse test is positive with deep digital pressure over the leading edge of pronator teres and not with scratching the skin over this region. In the majority of patients, electrodiagnostic testing is negative. Radiographs of the distal end of the humerus can identify the rare supracondylar process and alert the physician to the probability of the presence of a ligament of Struthers.

Anterior Interosseous Nerve Syndrome

Anterior interosseous nerve syndrome is manifested as weakness or motor loss of the flexor pollicis longus, the flexor digitorum profundus to the index finger, the pronator quadratus, and, occasionally, the flexor digitorum profundus to the middle finger. In a true anterior interosseous nerve syndrome, the weakness or loss of motor function usually occurs spontaneously. Patients may describe clumsiness with fine motor skills, such as writing and pinching. Because the anterior interosseous nerve does not innervate the skin, the syndrome is not associated with sensory loss.

Parsonage-Turner mononeuritis should be considered in the differential diagnosis in patients with an anterior interosseous nerve palsy. These patients typically have a history of severe pain for several days or weeks. The pain may follow a viral illness. High doses of corticosteroids and antiviral medications such as acyclovir are recommended if the neuritis is diagnosed early. In a neuritis involving the anterior interosseous nerve, spontaneous recovery usually occurs, although up to 1 year may be needed for full recovery. In patients with a spontaneous anterior interosseous nerve palsy and no electrodiagnostic evidence of reinnervation, consideration should be given to nerve exploration or nerve transfer (or both) at 7 to 10 months.[69] In patients with concomitant nerve compression, local decompression in those with Parsonage-Turner syndrome may accelerate recovery.

Operative Technique

The operative technique for decompression of the median nerve in the forearm is the same for pronator syndrome and compression of the anterior interosseous nerve; all potential compressive sites should be released.

❖ AUTHORS' PREFERRED METHOD OF TREATMENT

Preoperatively, significant compression points on the median nerve are determined by physical examination, either with stress on a particular tendon or muscle unit or with elicitation of pain by direct palpation. A padded tourniquet is applied to the arm several centimeters above the cubital crease and inflated after exsanguination. The incision begins at the antecubital fossa and continues distally in a lazy-"S" direction for about 10 cm (Figure 28.11 and Videos 28.3 and 28.4). The dissection is carried down through soft tissue to identify and preserve any cutaneous sensory branches. The bicipital aponeurosis (lacertus fibrosus) is identified and divided (Figure 28.12). The tendon of the superficial head of the pronator teres is identified, which is best done in the distal portion of the surgical exposure just radial to the radial vessels. A step-lengthening incision is made in the tendon by performing the "up" cut distally where visualization

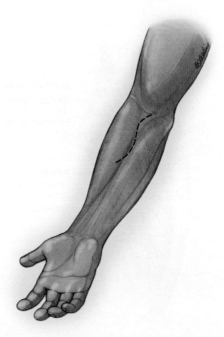

FIGURE 28.11 The incision to explore the median nerve and anterior interosseous nerve in the proximal part of the forearm begins at least 5 cm above the elbow crease. (Copyright © Elizabeth Martin.)

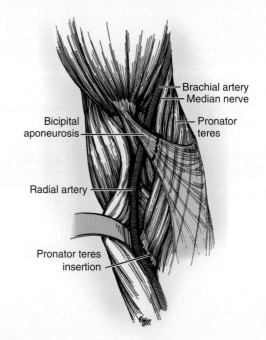

FIGURE 28.12 The bicipital aponeurosis may act as a compressive band across the flexor muscle in pronation; it should be divided during any exploration of the median nerve. A step-lengthening tenotomy of the tendon of the superficial head of the pronator teres is necessary to allow exposure of the median nerve. (Copyright © Elizabeth Martin.)

is more difficult. The "down" cut is done proximally (Figure 28.13). Lengthening will take tension off the superficial (radial) head of the pronator teres muscle and allow better visualization of the median nerve. The median nerve is identified proximally, just medial to the brachial artery and vein. The nerve is intimate with the pronator muscle and can be found just distal to the

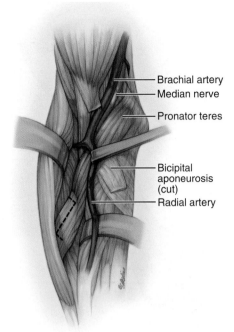

FIGURE 28.13 Exposure of the median nerve and anterior interosseous nerve by reflection of the humeral (the superficial head of the pronator teres also exposes the arch of the superficialis) and the deep head of the pronator teres (ulnar head). The step-lengthening tenotomy facilitates the exposure. (Copyright © Elizabeth Martin.)

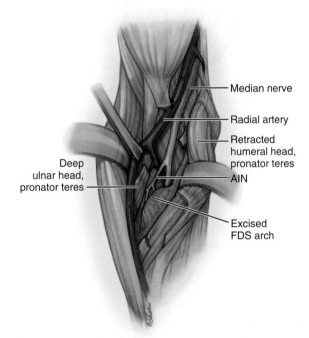

FIGURE 28.14 The proximal tendinous attachment of the deep head (ulnar) of the pronator teres and the proximal tendinous arch of the superficialis are excised to completely release the median nerve. *AIN,* Anterior interosseous nerve; *FDS,* flexor digitorum superficialis. (Copyright © Elizabeth Martin.)

cubital crease, adjacent to if not just within the flexor pronator muscle mass (Figure 28.14). The median nerve is followed distally to identify the deep head of the pronator teres where it blends with the leading tendinous edge of the flexor digitorum superficialis. The proximal tendinous attachment of the deep head is about 2 cm in length. It arches around the median nerve

and attaches at the deep ulnar head of the pronator teres onto the ulna. There is muscle attached to the tendinous tissue, and the tendinous portion is excised. The tendinous portion of the arch from the leading edge of the flexor digitorum superficialis tendons is divided to completely release the median nerve. The surgeon can run a finger proximally along the median nerve, and if a ligament of Struthers is identified, the incision is extended above the elbow crease. During dissection, care is taken to obtain complete hemostasis. The vessels in this area are very thin walled and will "stain" the tissues if good hemostasis is not achieved with microbipolar cautery or ligature ties as necessary. Internal neurolysis or epineurotomy techniques are not indicated. There is no need to reconstruct the tendon lengthening of the superficial head of the pronator teres because the deep head has been left intact. The incision is closed with 3-0 absorbable suture in the subcutaneous tissue and 4-0 subcuticular suture with adhesive strips. Bupivacaine is placed in the incision for postoperative comfort. In rare cases in which the patient had extreme pain preoperatively, a bupivacaine infusion pump can be used. Fiberglass casting is incorporated into the dressing to keep the elbow slightly flexed and the wrist in a neutral position.

Postoperative Care

The bulky dressing is removed 2 days after surgery. The patient is instructed in range-of-motion exercises for the fingers, wrist, and arm. A sling may be used at night for patient comfort to prevent full elbow extension. However, the patient is encouraged to begin exercises to regain full elbow extension with forearm supination. Patients are allowed full activity and can return to work without restrictions 6 to 8 weeks after surgery.

COMPRESSION OF THE ULNAR NERVE

The ulnar nerve is most commonly compressed at the elbow in the region of the cubital tunnel and less frequently at the wrist in the Guyon canal. With compression of the ulnar nerve, patient complaints will include paresthesia or numbness, or both, in the small or the ring finger, or in both. In more severe cases, ulnar nerve motor dysfunction will lead to weakness, atrophy, and hand clumsiness.[72]

Compression of the Guyon Canal

Guyon in 1861 first described the space in the hypothenar region of the wrist where the ulnar nerve divides and suggested that ulnar nerve compression could occur in this region. Compression in the Guyon canal may result from a number of causes, including acute or repetitive trauma, hamate hook nonunion, anomalous muscles, or space-occupying lesions, including ganglions, thrombosis, and pseudoaneurysms.

The unique anatomy of the Guyon canal will influence the symptoms. The nerve can be compressed proximal to its bifurcation (zone I), thereby yielding a mix of both motor and sensory deficits; along the course of the deep motor branch (zone II), characterized by pure motor loss; or along its superficial sensory branch (zone III), which is associated with pure sensory changes. If the compression produces intrinsic weakness, the functional motor loss in the hand can be profound, manifested by a strongly positive Froment sign, clawing of the ring and small digits, and severe interosseous atrophy. Because

CRITICAL POINTS *Median Nerve Release in the Proximal Forearm*

Indications
- Rare as a pain syndrome
- Anterior interosseous nerve palsy localizing to the forearm
- De novo anterior interosseous nerve palsy is most likely a neuritis and not caused by mechanical compression.
- Patients with median nerve sensory complaints localizing to the level of the pronator teres are usually treated successfully with forearm flexor muscle stretching exercises.
- Patients with associated carpal tunnel syndrome generally require only carpal tunnel release.

Preoperative Evaluation
- Without motor symptoms, electrodiagnostic studies are usually normal.
- Persistent median nerve symptoms are reproduced by provocation at the forearm.

Pearls
- The tendon of the superficial head of the pronator teres is located just lateral to the radial vessels in the distal part of the surgical exposure.
- The median nerve is located just medial to the vessels in the proximal portion of the surgical field and is intimate with the flexor pronator muscle mass.

Technical Points
- Use a lazy "S" incision in the proximal part of the forearm.
- Release the lacertus fibrosus.
- Identify the superficial tendon of the pronator teres lateral to vessels.
- Use a step-lengthening tenotomy of the superficial tendon of the pronator teres.
- Identify the median nerve in the proximal part of the forearm medial to vessels.
- Identify and excise the deep head of the pronator teres.
- Release the superficial tendinous arch of the flexor digitorum superficialis.
- Ensure that no compressive bands are located proximally over the median nerve.
- Use bupivacaine in the incision and consider suction drainage.
- Immobilize the elbow and wrist in a bulky dressing.

Pitfall
- Beware of inadequate release of the median nerve compression points of the arch of the pronator teres muscles and the flexor digitorum superficialis.

Postoperative Care
- Remove the dressing on day 2 or 3.
- Begin early range-of-motion exercises on day 2 or 3.
- Begin strengthening exercises in the second month.

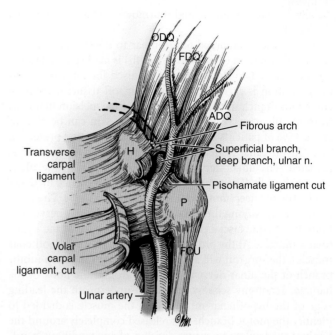

FIGURE 28.15 The ulnar nerve courses through the Guyon canal between the volar carpal ligament and the transverse carpal ligament. *ADQ,* Abductor digiti quinti; *FCU,* flexor carpi ulnaris; *FDQ,* flexor digiti quinti; *H,* hamate; *ODQ,* opponens digiti quinti; *P,* pisiform. (Copyright © Elizabeth Martin.)

on the dorsal and volar sides of the fifth digit can only occur in compression proximal to the wrist, as the dorsal sensory branch exits the ulnar nerve several centimeters proximal to the wrist crease. Motor weakness confined to the intrinsic muscles, particularly when unassociated with sensory symptoms, focuses any compressive cause on zone II of the Guyon canal. Because of the unopposed force of the normal flexor digitorum profundus, clawing from distal entrapment is paradoxically worse than compression at more proximal sites, which weaken the ulnar flexor digitorum profundus symmetrically.

ANATOMY

After passing anterior to the flexor retinaculum, the ulnar nerve divides into superficial and deep branches. The superficial branch innervates the palmaris brevis muscle and then supplies sensory innervation to the small finger and the medial side of the ring finger. The deep branch of the ulnar nerve innervates the hypothenar muscle, the medial two lumbricales, the interosseous muscles, the adductor pollicis muscle, and half of the flexor pollicis brevis (Figure 28.15).

Nonoperative Management

Nonoperative treatment is recommended with acute cases of localized closed trauma (i.e., long-distance cycling). A wrist splint in neutral position for a few weeks may be helpful. Electrodiagnostic studies may be used to monitor improvement.

Operative Technique

❖ AUTHORS' PREFERRED METHOD OF TREATMENT

The incision used for carpal tunnel release is appropriate for release of the ulnar nerve in the Guyon canal, except that it will need to be extended slightly more proximally and

of the propensity for space-occupying lesions within the Guyon canal, the preoperative workup should include appropriate imaging studies in addition to electrodiagnostic studies, particularly when an isolated motor palsy is identified.

It is critical that the examiner differentiate ulnar nerve compression at the wrist from more proximal sites in the upper limb. The localization of numbness and paresthesias to the arm or forearm should alert the examiner to more proximal sites, including the plexus and thoracic outlet. Similarly, paresthesias distally. Similar anesthetic and tourniquet techniques are used (Video 28.5).

The incision is marked 6 mm ulnar to the thenar crease. A curvilinear incision (3 to 4 cm in length) is made parallel to the thenar crease. Two double hooks are used for retraction, and the dissection is carried down through soft tissue. A crossing cutaneous branch in the distal portion of the incision that runs from the ulnar nerve up to the overlying skin can be seen in about 15% of patients and needs to be identified and protected. The Guyon canal is opened, and the hook of the hamate is palpated. The ulnar nerve lies deep and medial to the ulnar vascular bundle. The neurovascular bundle is retracted medially to identify the deep motor branch of the ulnar nerve. The technique for identifying the motor branch of the ulnar nerve is to note the oblique fascial pattern along the surface of the hypothenar muscles. At the proximal leading edge of the hypothenar muscles, the surgeon will see just 1 or 2 mm of the deep motor branch of the ulnar nerve as it curves around the hook of the hamate. Tenotomy scissors are placed underneath the leading edge of the hypothenar muscles, and the muscle is divided to identify the motor branch. It is released completely around the hook of the hamate to ensure division of any tendinous bands within the hypothenar muscles distally that can compress the ulnar nerve. There are also small, thin-walled vessels running with the motor branch that should be protected so that the surgeon does not need to subsequently obtain hemostasis with cautery deep in the wound in proximity to the nerve. The ulnar nerve proper is released through the Guyon canal, and the incision is usually extended in a zigzag fashion proximal to the wrist to release the distal extent of the antebrachial fascia. The tourniquet is deflated, and microbipolar cautery is used for hemostasis. Bupivacaine is infiltrated into the incision for postoperative comfort. The incision is closed with interrupted 4-0 nylon suture and a bulky dressing is applied while keeping the wrist in a neutral position, with fiberglass casting being incorporated into the dressing. If a carpal tunnel release has also been done, night splinting with the wrist in neutral is maintained for 3 weeks; otherwise, night splinting is continued for patient comfort.

Postoperative Care

A bulky dressing is applied to maintain a wrist neutral position, and this dressing is removed 2 days after surgery. The patient is instructed in range-of-motion exercises for the fingers, wrist, and arm. A splint in a wrist neutral position is used at night for patient comfort. The sutures are removed 12 to 14 days postoperatively. Patients are allowed full activity and return to work without restrictions 6 to 8 weeks after surgery.

Cubital Tunnel Syndrome

Chronic compression of the ulnar nerve at the cubital tunnel may occur as a result of ischemia or mechanical compression by repeated elbow flexion, posttraumatic scarring, anomalous musculature, or direct compression, although the exact cause may be difficult to identify. Acute trauma to the ulnar nerve from periarticular elbow fractures or subsequent surgery may compromise ulnar nerve function. Ulnar nerve subluxation may also contribute to cubital tunnel syndrome, in addition to the slack region and restricted mobility of the ulnar nerve.[86] The area within the cubital tunnel is decreased with elbow flexion,

---

CRITICAL POINTS *Guyon Canal Release*

Indications
- Uncommon
- Ulnar nerve symptoms and signs localizing to Guyon canal on physical examination

Preoperative Evaluation
- Electrodiagnostic studies are often helpful in localizing the compression point to Guyon canal.
- Preoperative imaging studies are needed if a space-occupying lesion is suspected.

Pearls
- Only 1 or 2 mm of the deep motor branch can be seen diving beneath the hypothenar muscles.
- Look for the deep motor branch at the free edge of the hypothenar muscles.

Technical Points
- Same incision as for a carpal tunnel release, but extend it both proximally and distally.
- Avoid the ulnar cutaneous communicating branch in the distal portion of the incision.
- Open the Guyon canal.
- Palpate the hook of the hamate.
- Dissect the neurovascular bundle ulnarward along its length through the Guyon canal.
- Visualize the leading tendinous edge of the hypothenar muscles.
- Release the deep motor branch of the ulnar nerve, which is located just below the leading tendinous edge of the hypothenar muscle origin.

Pitfall
- Failure to identify and release the deep motor branch of the ulnar nerve

Postoperative Care
- Remove the dressing on day 2 or 3.
- Splint the wrist in neutral for 2 weeks at night.
- Begin range-of-motion exercises on day 2 or 3.
- Begin strengthening exercises after 4 weeks.
- If the carpal tunnel has also been released, use a night splint in a wrist neutral position for 3 weeks.

---

and this can increase pressure on the cubital tunnel. Apfelberg and Larson reported a 55% decrease in cubital tunnel area with elbow flexion.[3] Pechan and Julis reported increased pressure within the cubital tunnel with elbow flexion, and this pressure was further compromised with wrist extension or shoulder abduction (or with both).[93] Gelberman and colleagues reported increased intraneural ulnar nerve pressure and decreased cubital tunnel volume with elbow flexion.[26]

Compression of the ulnar nerve at the cubital tunnel is extremely common and second in incidence only to carpal tunnel syndrome. The diagnosis is a clinical one because electrodiagnostic testing is frequently negative. Complaints often include paresthesia and numbness in the small and ring fingers with aching in the medial aspect of the elbow and forearm. The Tinel sign is usually positive over the nerve at or proximal to the cubital tunnel, but the test is overly sensitive and usually bilaterally positive. Provocative testing for cubital tunnel syndrome consisting of combined elbow flexion with digital pressure placed on the ulnar nerve proximal to the cubital tunnel has good sensitivity and specificity.[80] With severe ulnar nerve compression, patients may exhibit clawing of the small and ring fingers, atrophy of the ulnar nerve–innervated intrinsic muscles, and positive Froment and Wartenberg signs. These motor changes will not identify the level of ulnar nerve compression. However, many patients are initially seen in the early stages of nerve compression and will have no obvious motor deficit. Careful sensory testing as outlined previously can help quantify changes in sensibility. In the early stages of nerve compression, provocation testing may be the only positive sign, followed by alteration of threshold testing (vibration and Semmes-Weinstein monofilaments). In the later stages, two-point discrimination will become abnormal.[51,80] McGowan described a classification system for ulnar neuropathy at the elbow that is based predominantly on the loss of ulnar nerve motor function and does not include sensory changes.[72] This classification system is widely quoted in the literature, although it is limited in clinical applicability. In the McGowan classification, grade I neuropathies have no muscle weakness, grade II neuropathies have muscle weakness with no atrophy, and grade III neuropathies have muscle atrophy.

Although clinical diagnosis of cubital tunnel syndrome remains the gold standard, electrodiagnostic studies may be used to confirm the diagnosis. Nerve conduction studies and EMG are useful in localizing the level of nerve compression, in addition to identifying other sites of nerve compression or other disease processes that may be present (i.e., upper motor neuron disease, peripheral neuropathy). To confirm the diagnosis of cubital tunnel syndrome with nerve conduction studies, many reports support the use of a decreased motor conduction velocity across the elbow.[51] Ulnar nerve motor conduction velocity across the elbow of less than 50 m/sec is considered confirmatory of cubital tunnel syndrome.

Unlike carpal tunnel syndrome, there are other sinister diagnoses that can mimic cubital tunnel syndrome, such as motor neuron disease or Guillain-Barré syndrome. The surgeon must be alert for the common problem of cervical disk disease and the rare but devastating problem of amyotrophic lateral sclerosis when evaluating patients with ulnar motor complaints, particularly if the motor findings exceed the sensory findings (severe motor loss with minimal sensory changes).

ANATOMY

The ulnar nerve is derived from the C8 and T1 nerve roots and is a terminal branch of the medial cord. In the upper part of the arm, the ulnar nerve is posteromedial to the brachial artery, posterior to the intermuscular septum, and anterior to the medial head of the triceps muscle (Figure 28.16). The intermuscular septum is continuous from the humeral medial epicondyle to the coracobrachialis muscle. The arcade of Struthers is a band of deep brachial fascia that attaches to the intermuscular septum and covers the ulnar nerve approximately 8 cm proximal to the medial epicondyle (Figure 28.17). The medial antebrachial cutaneous nerve passes posterior to the ulnar nerve at or proximal to the epicondyle in 90% of cases.[71] The proximal branch of the medial antebrachial cutaneous nerve often runs with the medial intramuscular septum.[50] The ulnar nerve passes posterior to the medial epicondyle and medial to the olecranon. The ulnar nerve then enters the cubital tunnel, which is defined by a taut fascial layer extending from the flexor carpi ulnaris

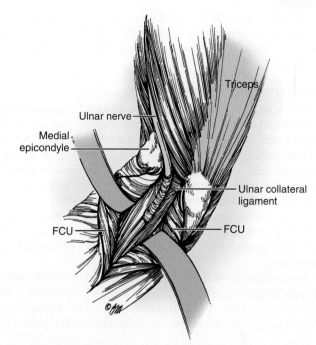

FIGURE 28.16 The ulnar nerve lies on the medial head of the triceps muscle, enters the cubital tunnel behind the medial epicondyle, and continues distally beneath the arcade of fascia, where it joins the heads of the flexor carpi ulnaris (FCU). (Copyright © Elizabeth Martin.)

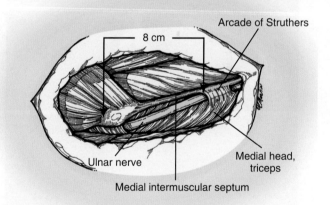

FIGURE 28.17 The arcade of Struthers arises 8 cm proximal to the medial humeral epicondyle. (From Spinner M: Nerve decompression. In Morrey BF, editor: *The elbow*, New York, Raven Press, 1994, and by permission of Mayo Foundation. Redrawn by Elizabeth Martin.)

muscle and the arcuate ligament of Osborne. After passing through the cubital tunnel, the ulnar nerve travels deep into the forearm between the ulnar and humeral heads of the flexor carpi ulnaris muscle.

A number of sites within the region of the cubital tunnel can contribute to ulnar nerve compression, including the arcade of Struthers, the intermuscular septum, the flexor carpi ulnaris fascia, the anconeus epitrochlearis, the Osborne ligament, and fascial bands within the flexor carpi ulnaris distally. The cause is variable among affected individuals. The superficial position of the ulnar nerve at the cubital tunnel and the increase in tension and traction that it experiences with elbow flexion probably combine to make it susceptible to compression neuropathy.

Nonoperative Management

Cubital tunnel syndrome can often be managed conservatively, with education of the patient to avoid positions and activities that combine elbow flexion with pressure over the ulnar nerve, such as while driving or speaking on the telephone or during sleep. Postural modifications may be necessary for several months before the symptoms resolve, and occasionally surgery will be needed to relieve the symptoms. Unfortunately, the incidence of poor outcomes after surgical management of cubital tunnel syndrome far exceeds that of carpal tunnel syndrome, and when surgery fails, the consequences for patients can be devastating.

Demonstration of the changes in skin tension can be useful in explaining the tightness that occurs in the ulnar nerve with elbow flexion (Figure 28.18). Decreasing elbow flexion and direct pressure on the nerve may help alleviate symptoms in

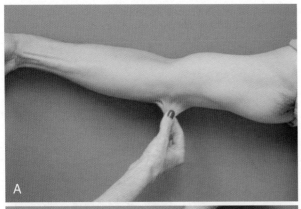

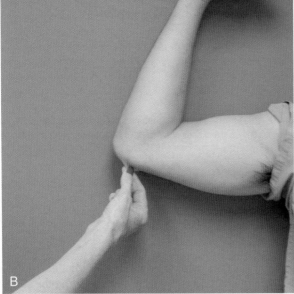

FIGURE 28.18 A, The effect of elbow flexion in increasing tension on the ulnar nerve is illustrated to the patient by noting that when the elbow is extended, just as when the skin is loose, the ulnar nerve is loose. **B,** By contrast, when the elbow is flexed, just as when the skin is tight, the nerve is stretched and tight.

patients with a mild or moderate degree of nerve compression. Recommendations for nonoperative treatment have included static night splinting of the elbow in extension. Rigid night splints are often ineffective because of patient discomfort and noncompliance. Soft elbow pads can be used to protect the ulnar nerve from direct compression. We recommend wearing these pads up to 24 hours per day; both to protect the ulnar nerve from direct compression and also to remind the patient about positions that may be eliciting symptoms. Because the ulnar nerve can be compressed between the two heads of the flexor carpi ulnaris muscle during hand and wrist activities, patients are instructed in specific stretching and nerve gliding exercises.

In our experience, many patients with mild cubital tunnel syndrome can be managed successfully with 2 to 4 months of nonoperative treatment. We use motor conduction velocity across the elbow as a guide to management and treat all patients with a conduction velocity of 40 m/sec or greater with a minimum of 2 to 3 months of nonoperative treatment. If this approach is unsuccessful or if the initial conduction velocity is less than 40 m/sec, the patient will likely require surgical intervention. A number of surgical approaches have been described for the treatment of cubital tunnel syndrome and include simple decompression, medial epicondylectomy, and anterior transposition of the ulnar nerve in a subcutaneous, submuscular, intramuscular, or transmuscular position. More recently, minimally invasive and endoscopic approaches have been introduced as a surgical option for decompression of the ulnar nerve at the cubital tunnel.[16]

Operative Treatment

The fact that there are several techniques currently recommended by experienced hand surgeons for the surgical management of cubital tunnel syndrome speaks to the ongoing controversy regarding its treatment. Surgical options range from simple decompression to medial epicondylectomy to various anterior transposition techniques.[82] The ideal operative technique should address the mechanism of cubital tunnel syndrome. The superficial position of the nerve at the elbow renders it susceptible to mechanical compression, and its position behind the medial epicondyle causes it to undergo increased tension with elbow flexion. In theory, only a transposition procedure would substantially change the tension on the nerve as the elbow is flexed. A comprehensive review concluded that with more advanced cubital tunnel syndrome, simple decompression was unlikely to be successful.[19] In a metaanalysis of the treatment of cubital tunnel syndrome that included 30 studies over a period of 5 decades, Mowlavi and colleagues concluded that the recurrence rate was highest in nonoperated patients.[75] In patients with moderate nerve compression, relief was achieved most often with a submuscular transposition, and in severely affected patients, all treatments produced similarly poor results.[75] In contrast, a review by Bartels and coworkers determined that patients with severe compression had the best outcome with subcutaneous transposition.[5] These authors recommended simple decompression for the surgical treatment of mild to moderate cubital tunnel syndrome unless ulnar nerve subluxation or severe compression is present, in which case anterior subcutaneous transposition is performed. To investigate the outcome predictors following anterior ulnar nerve transposition, a systematic review was conducted and found conflicting results across the 26 studies included in the review. The authors concluded that higher-quality studies needed to be performed to identify the predictors of surgical outcome.[101] A metaanalysis was performed to compare outcomes following simple decompression and submuscular transposition of the ulnar nerve. Combining data from 10 studies (published from 1979 to 2006), the authors found no statistical differences between procedures.[56]

In our opinion, the indications for in situ decompression of the ulnar nerve are limited because mild cases of cubital tunnel syndrome in patients with a short duration of symptoms can usually be managed conservatively. Furthermore, if simple decompression fails to relieve the symptoms, any secondary surgery needed to transpose the nerve will be significantly more difficult because of scar tissue formation in the previously operated region.

Technique of in Situ Decompression. An intravenous or regional anesthetic technique is used, and a 6- to 10-cm incision is made along the course of the ulnar nerve midway between the medial epicondyle and the olecranon. Care is taken to avoid injury to the medial antebrachial cutaneous nerve. The intramuscular septum is palpated proximally, and the ulnar nerve is identified just below this septum. The ulnar nerve is decompressed from well above the medial epicondyle distally through the cubital tunnel. The nerve is exposed between the two heads of the flexor carpi ulnaris muscle, and the leading tendinous edge of the flexor carpi ulnaris muscle is released. The ulnar nerve need not be disturbed in its bed, and neurolysis is not performed. Care is taken to ensure that good distal and proximal release of the ulnar nerve has been achieved. The elbow is moved through a range of movement, and any points that might compress the ulnar nerve either proximally or distally are evaluated. The intramuscular septum and the brachial fascia where it might compress the ulnar nerve proximally are excised. If the ulnar nerve subluxates over the medial epicondyle when the elbow moves into flexion, consideration should be given to medial epicondylectomy or anterior transposition to avoid postoperative discomfort. At the conclusion of the procedure, the tourniquet is deflated and hemostasis is obtained. Bupivacaine may be placed in the incision and the subcutaneous layer closed with a subcuticular skin closure. A bulky dressing with or without fiberglass support is applied. The postoperative dressing is removed 2 to 3 days after surgery, and active range of motion is started at that time. A sling may be used at night during sleep for patient comfort until full elbow range of motion is achieved.

Medial Epicondylectomy for Ulnar Neuritis. In 1950, King and Morgan described removal of the medial epicondyle in 16 patients with ulnar neuritis and reported their long-term outcomes in 1959. Most patients in the series had posttraumatic injuries and were not typical of those with idiopathic cubital tunnel syndrome. Other surgeons have expanded this technique to treat nontraumatic causes of cubital tunnel syndrome and believe that it allows some degree of anterior transposition with less dissection. A potential complication of this technique is medial elbow instability, which can occur with "overzealous resection" of the epicondyle. O'Driscoll and associates demonstrated that only approximately 20% of the overall depth of the epicondyle can be removed without violating a portion of the anterior medial collateral ligament and described a safer plane

for removal that would avoid the anteroinferior origin of the ligament from the epicondyle.[88]

An intravenous or regional anesthetic is used and the ulnar nerve is decompressed as for a simple decompression. The ulnar nerve is not disturbed in its bed. It is not necessary to perform internal or external neurolysis. The medial epicondyle is exposed subperiosteally, with the flexor-pronator origin being left in continuity with the periosteal sleeve (Figure 28.19). A 2.5-cm osteotome is used to score the leading edge of the epicondyle. To avoid detachment of the anterior medial band of the ulnar collateral ligament, a plane is chosen between the sagittal and coronal planes of the humerus, not along the medial margin of the trochlea as traditionally described. A portion of the epicondyle along with the attached medial intramuscular septum is removed (Figure 28.20). Care should be taken not to enter the

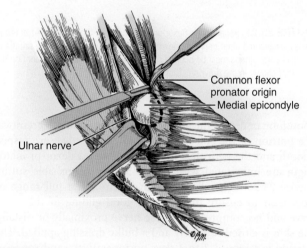

FIGURE 28.19 Medial epicondylectomy is begun by protecting the ulnar nerve and elevating the common flexor pronator origin from the medial epicondyle. The arcade of the flexor carpi ulnaris must be incised to the midportion of the proximal third of the forearm (not shown in the drawing). (Copyright © Elizabeth Martin.)

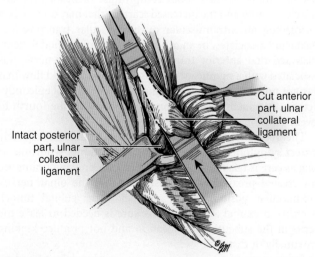

FIGURE 28.20 The guide for the proper plane of osteotomy for the medial epicondyle is the plane between the sagittal and coronal planes. The sharp posterior edge of the osteotomy must be smoothed and rounded. (Copyright © Elizabeth Martin.)

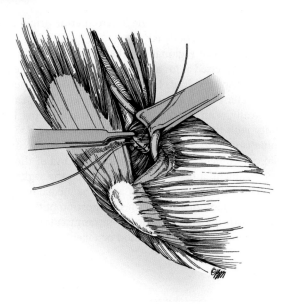

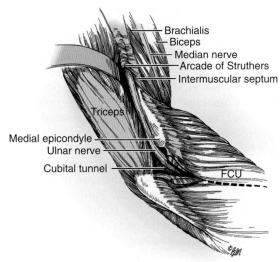

FIGURE 28.22 Mobilization of the ulnar nerve and any associated vessels necessitates decompression of the cubital tunnel, fasciotomy of the flexor carpi ulnaris (FCU), and dissection along the ulnar nerve, at least 8 cm proximal to the medial epicondyle. (Copyright © Elizabeth Martin.)

FIGURE 28.21 Repair of the flexor-pronator origin to the humerus. After repair of the muscles, the ulnar nerve is allowed to seek its own position. The arcade of the flexor carpi ulnaris must be opened sufficiently to prevent impingement on the nerve (not shown in the drawing). (Copyright © Elizabeth Martin.)

elbow joint or detach the ulnar collateral ligament. After removal of a portion of the epicondyle, the raw bone edges are rasped smooth and the periosteal flaps with attached flexor-pronator origin are imbricated with buried 3-0 nonabsorbable suture (Figure 28.21). The elbow is moved through a full range of movement to ensure that there is good gliding of the ulnar nerve and no compression of the nerve proximally or distally. The skin is closed routinely and a bulky dressing applied. The dressing is removed 2 to 3 days postoperatively, and range of motion is started.

Subcutaneous Anterior Transposition of the Ulnar Nerve. Proponents of the anterior transposition of the ulnar nerve believe that the procedure further reduces tension on the ulnar nerve during elbow flexion. Some advocates of subcutaneous transposition are concerned about compromise of flexor-pronator muscle strength and the increased scarring that may occur when performing an intramuscular or submuscular transposition. Ogata and associates, in an experimental primate model, demonstrated that anterior transposition of the ulnar nerve was associated with a significant decrease in regional blood flow that was not noted with simple decompression or medial epicondylectomy. Intraneural circulation was restored by the fourth to seventh postoperative day.[89]

Theoretically, anterior transposition should adequately correct symptoms associated with cubital tunnel syndrome as long as care is taken to ensure that new compression points are not created proximally and distally. Given the ulnar nerve's submuscular position above and below the cubital tunnel, extensive proximal and distal exposure is needed to leave the nerve in the subcutaneous location and not produce kinking proximally or distally.

Intravenous or regional anesthesia is used and the procedure begins as a simple decompression. A longer incision is necessary (≈15 cm in length) to accommodate the transposition. The distal medial antebrachial cutaneous nerve crosses the incision

about 3.5 cm distal to the medial epicondyle. The proximal branch of this nerve crosses the incision 1.5 cm proximal to the medial epicondyle and often runs with the medial intramuscular septum. These sensory nerves are protected throughout the procedure. The ulnar nerve is identified posterior to the medial intramuscular septum. After removal of the medial intramuscular septum, the ulnar nerve is released through the cubital tunnel and followed between the two heads of the flexor carpi ulnaris muscle. The motor branches to the flexor carpi ulnaris and the flexor digitorum profundus are preserved. The nerve is then carefully lifted from its bed with its accompanying longitudinal vascular supply intact by using a small Penrose drain to prevent constriction. Segmental feeding vessels are identified and ligated to prevent tethering. Neurolysis can be performed as necessary to separate the posterior motor branches from the main ulnar nerve to allow adequate anterior transposition without tension.[115] These motor branches can also be followed into the flexor carpi ulnaris muscle to allow mobilization of the ulnar nerve and protection of these posterior motor branches. The ulnar nerve is moved anteriorly to a subcutaneous position (Figure 28.22). The ulnar nerve should be examined proximally and especially distally to ensure that it lies loosely with no proximal or distal compression points (Figure 28.23). Even very thin fascial bands distally will compress the nerve and lead to a suboptimal result. To keep the ulnar nerve in its anterior position and prevent it from returning to its original position, some of the soft tissue of the anterior skin flap can be sutured to the fascia over the medial epicondyle. Care is taken to exclude any branches of the medial antebrachial cutaneous nerve. One recommendation has been to elevate a 1- to 1.5-cm² flap of flexor pronator fascia based on the medial epicondyle and then sew it to the overlying dermis to create a barrier that maintains the nerve in its anterior transposed position. Care must be taken to ensure that the fascial flap does not compress the ulnar nerve and cause a new compression point. Closure, dressing, and postoperative care are as previously described for the other cubital tunnel surgeries.

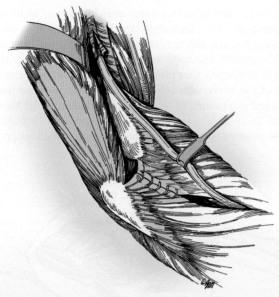

FIGURE 28.23 At the completion of a subcutaneous transposition, the arcade of Struthers does not bind the ulnar nerve and there is adequate release of the flexor carpi ulnaris for the ulnar nerve to reenter the forearm. (Copyright © Elizabeth Martin.)

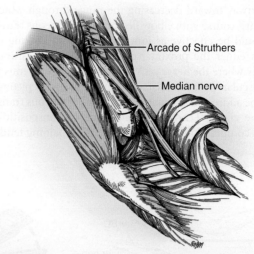

FIGURE 28.24 After submuscular transposition, care must be taken to prevent angulation of the ulnar nerve at the arcade of Struthers. The branches to the flexor carpi ulnaris should be preserved. (Copyright © Elizabeth Martin.)

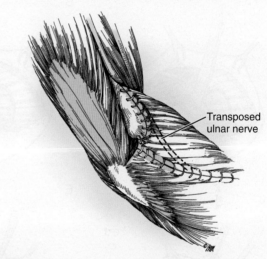

FIGURE 28.25 Completion of the submuscular transposition by repair of the flexor muscles to the medial epicondyle. (Copyright © Elizabeth Martin.)

Intramuscular Transposition of the Ulnar Nerve. In 1918, Adson described intramuscular transposition of the ulnar nerve, and this is the technique also used by Kleinman and Bishop.[42] Proponents of this method believe that it is an improvement over subcutaneous transposition because the nerve lies in a straighter position as it moves from the arm to the forearm and in a more protected position than with the subcutaneous location. Critics suggest that dissection into the muscle will cause more scarring.

The procedure is the same as for subcutaneous transposition except that a groove is dissected in the muscle in line with the location of the ulnar nerve in its transposed position. Fibrous septa within the pronator teres muscle are removed to provide a soft vascularized muscle bed. A fascial flap or a subcutaneous flap is created as for a subcutaneous transposition to keep the nerve in its anterior location. Proponents of this procedure recommend 3 weeks of immobilization and do not allow unrestricted activity until 10 weeks after this procedure.

Submuscular Transposition of the Ulnar Nerve. In 1942, Learmonth described his classic submuscular transposition (Video 28.6). Proponents advocate submuscular transposition as being the "definitive" procedure and the technique of choice in throwing athletes and after previously failed cubital tunnel surgery. Critics cite the extensive dissection and concern for the longitudinal blood supply of the ulnar nerve, as well as the potential for new compression or heterotopic bone under the incised flexor-pronator muscle mass.

The ulnar nerve is exposed and transposed as described earlier for subcutaneous anterior transposition. The incision, however, will be longer (15 to 20 cm). The extent of the flexor-pronator muscle mass is identified. A plane is developed distal to the medial epicondyle and beneath the flexor-pronator muscle mass. The flexor-pronator muscle mass is then incised 1 to 2 cm distal to the medial epicondyle, and a periosteal elevator is used to reflect the muscle distally. Care is taken not to disrupt the ulnar collateral ligament. The median nerve is

exposed at the point where it lies on the brachialis muscle by dividing the lacertus fibrosus and dissecting lateral to the elevated flexor-pronator muscle mass. The ulnar nerve is transposed anteriorly, adjacent and parallel to the median nerve (Figure 28.24). The flexor-pronator muscle mass is anatomically reattached with nonabsorbable suture (Figure 28.25). Alternatively, the flexor-pronator mass can be divided in a stepcut fashion and lengthened by 1 to 2 cm during closure to decrease compression on the transposed nerve. The elbow is maintained at 90 degrees with a plaster-reinforced bulky dressing. Range of movement is started 5 to 10 days after surgery.

❖ AUTHORS' PREFERRED METHOD OF TREATMENT

Optimal surgical management of cubital tunnel syndrome is controversial. Because the mechanism of cubital tunnel syndrome is related to the position of the nerve behind the axis of the elbow joint and because elbow flexion increases tension on the nerve, procedures that do not transpose the nerve may not consistently correct the condition. A medial epicondylectomy goes partway toward decreasing the range through which the nerve must course with elbow flexion. Subcutaneous transposition should be effective as long as there is no kinking of the nerve in either the proximal or the distal transposition site, especially where the nerve moves from the subcutaneous to the intramuscular position distally. Any associated epicondylitis cannot be addressed adequately with a subcutaneous transposition. The classic Learmonth submuscular transposition can result in compression of the nerve by any remaining tendinous bands within the flexor-pronator muscle mass or at its distal transposition site. Associated medial epicondylitis is not addressed because the tension on the flexor-pronator muscle origin is actually increased as it is reset tighter when the flexor origin is reattached. Our preferred method is anterior transposition of the nerve with release of the flexor-pronator muscle origin and positioning of the nerve in a transmuscular location (Figure 28.26 and Video 28.7).[51,59] Transposition through the muscle places no tension on the nerve in any direction and

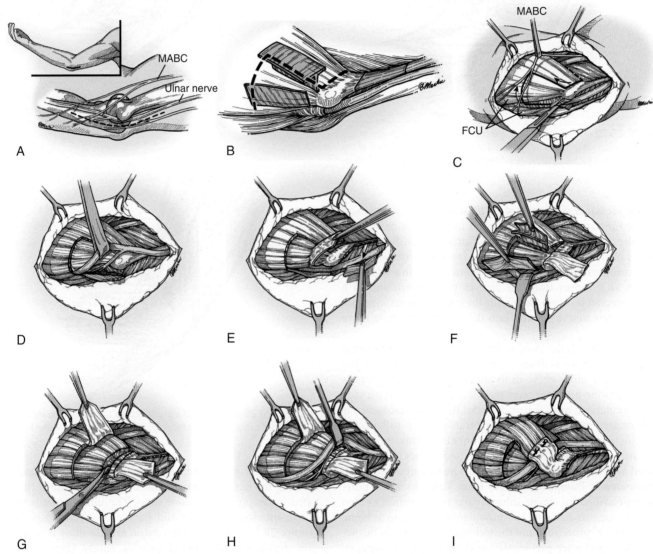

FIGURE 28.26 Authors' preferred technique of transmuscular transposition of the ulnar nerve. **A,** Avoid injury to the branches of the medial antebrachial cutaneous nerve (MABC). **B,** A series of three-dimensional fascial planes underlie the skin and subcutaneous tissues at the elbow: the intermuscular septum above the elbow, the cubital tunnel fascia overlying the ulnar nerve, the "T"-shaped fascia within the pronator teres muscle, the septum separating the pronator teres from the flexor carpi ulnaris muscle, and the leading edge of the flexor carpi ulnaris musculature. These structures must be released or excised to allow mobilization and transposition of the ulnar nerve. **C,** The flexor-pronator origin is identified, and the fascia overlying the muscle is incised in half along its obliquity. A perpendicular incision connects the fascia-splitting incision, with the incision dividing the leading edge of the flexor carpi ulnaris (FCU) to create a distal fascial flap. A second perpendicular incision connects the initial fascia-splitting incision with the free proximal border of the flexor-pronator muscle origin to create a proximal flap. **D,** The posterior motor branch is neurolyzed proximally. **E,** The intermuscular septum is removed. **F,** With elevation of the distal pronator fascia flap, a "T"-shaped fascial structure composed of a horizontal plate overlying a vertical plate is exposed. The flexor-pronator muscle is dissected from these fascial edges. This fascial structure is sharply excised. The fascial septum separating the pronator teres from the FCU is excised. **G,** The proximal flap is elevated from the flexor-pronator muscle origin. The muscle is dissected to the level of the brachialis muscle proximally, but distally some flexor-pronator muscle is left intact. **H,** The ulnar nerve is transposed with no tension either proximally or distally. **I,** The fascia flaps are sutured very loosely. After adequate hemostasis, a Jackson-Pratt drain and a bupivacaine (Marcaine) infusion pump are placed in the wound. The wound is closed in dermal and subcuticular layers. (Copyright © Elizabeth Martin.)

shortens the distance that the ulnar nerve must traverse in all ranges of elbow movement. Identification and removal of all potential tendons, bands, and fascial septum ensure that no new compression points on the nerve will occur. Release of the flexor-pronator muscle origin treats any associated medial epicondylitis. Leaving some flexor-pronator muscle intact facilitates earlier return of strength. The results of this procedure have been extremely satisfactory.[21,84]

The procedure is performed with the patient under general anesthesia and a single tourniquet, augmented by a Bier block with dexmedetomidine hydrochloride and lidocaine. The incision is placed behind the medial epicondyle (10 to 12 cm). Complete release of all points of ulnar nerve compression is performed as described earlier, and care is taken to identify and protect branches of the medial antebrachial cutaneous nerve.[50] The soft tissue above the flexor-pronator muscle origin is elevated, and then the fascial flaps are marked for elevation and transposition (see Figure 28.26, B and C). The flexor-pronator muscle origin is marked in half, and the first incision is made along this line. Distally, the flap is connected to the incision that was made in the fascia of the flexor carpi ulnaris overlying the ulnar nerve. The proximal edge of the proximal flap is the free border of the flexor-pronator muscle fascia. The distal fascial flap is elevated by sharp dissection. The proximal flap elevates easily with some muscle attached. The fascial bands are identified within the flexor-pronator muscle origin. The muscle attachments are released in a proximal to distal direction to preserve muscle innervation. The "T"-shaped tendinous fascia (about 4 cm in length) is removed. The ulnar nerve is identified as it courses through the proximal portion of the flexor carpi ulnaris muscle. There is another fascial septum here that needs to be removed. This septum is located between the median nerve–innervated flexor-pronator muscle and the ulnar nerve–innervated flexor carpi ulnaris muscle and curves around distally and over the ulnar nerve (see Figure 28.26, B). Just like the proximal medial intramuscular septum, if left intact, it will kink the ulnar nerve at the distal location of the transposition. Proximally, the flexor-pronator muscle is released for a short distance down to the level of the brachialis. Distally, the flexor-pronator muscle is released only as necessary to transpose the ulnar nerve anteriorly without tension. It is important to ensure that the ulnar nerve, when transposed, lies in a straight line with no compression proximally or distally. If necessary, the proximal motor branch of the ulnar nerve (branches to the flexor carpi ulnaris) can be neurolyzed from the main trunk with loupe magnification and microinstrumentation so that the branch does not tether the ulnar nerve when it is moved anteriorly. The fascial flaps are closed loosely over the ulnar nerve with two nonabsorbable sutures. It should be possible to put at least a finger between the fascial flaps and the nerve below so that there is no pressure on the ulnar nerve from these flaps. The nerve should be evaluated again to ensure that no kinking of the nerve is present either proximally or distally. The more anterior the nerve is transposed, the more distal in the forearm that possible "kinking" sites will be located. If inadvertently a branch of the medial antebrachial cutaneous nerve has been injured, the distal end should be cauterized and transposed well above the elbow and away from the scar. To assist in pain control, bupivacaine is placed in the incision and a continuous infusion pump can also be used.

A 2-mL infusion pump is used, and the catheter is placed anteriorly over the ulnar nerve. A Jackson-Pratt drain is placed in the ulnar groove. The incision is closed with 3-0 absorbable subcutaneous and 4-0 monofilament intradermal suture with Steri-Strips. The arm is immobilized with 4-inch light casting material in a padded dressing while keeping the wrist in neutral, the forearm pronated, and the elbow flexed.

Expected Outcome After Anterior Transposition of the Ulnar Nerve With Release of the Flexor-Pronator Muscle Origin for Cubital Tunnel Syndrome

In mild to moderate cases, there is return of "painless" functional sensation to the digits innervated by the ulnar nerve. There is also reinnervation of the muscles innervated by the ulnar nerve distal to the cubital tunnel. The elbow and forearm have full range of motion.

Postoperative Care

The bulky dressing, bupivacaine infusion pump, and Jackson-Pratt drain are removed 2 days after surgery. The patient is instructed in range-of-motion exercises for the fingers, wrist, forearm, elbow, and shoulder. For patient comfort, a sling is used at night to limit elbow extension until full elbow extension with forearm supination is achieved. The patient is restricted from heavy lifting for 1 month after surgery. Patients who do not regain full active range of motion within the first 2 to 3 weeks after surgery are referred for therapy. Most patients, however, begin therapy for strengthening exercises 4 weeks after surgery. Patients are allowed full activity and return to work without restrictions 8 weeks after surgery.

In a follow-up study of 119 operated cases at least 2 years after anterior transmuscular transposition of the ulnar nerve, 75% of patients who underwent unilateral procedures reported improvement and 68% of patients with bilateral surgery reported improvement.[84] There were no significant differences in patients with workers' compensation/litigation, obesity, concomitant carpal tunnel syndrome, or abnormal preoperative nerve conduction studies. However, nonsmokers had significantly better outcomes than smokers. Patients with severe and chronic compression, atrophy and dense sensory loss should be cautioned that surgery will arrest the progression and improve their symptoms but will not return normal strength or sensation.

COMPRESSION OF THE RADIAL NERVE

Superficial Radial Nerve Compression

In 1932, Wartenberg described five cases of compression neuropathy of the radial sensory nerve in the forearm and coined the term *cheiralgia paresthetica*. The superficial location of the radial sensory nerve in the forearm renders it susceptible to external compression. Tight wristwatch bands or handcuffs have been described in this compression neuropathy. Work-related repetitive activity requiring significant pronation or supination of the forearm or ulnar wrist flexion has also been associated with compression of the radial sensory nerve. It has been suggested that anatomically the radial sensory nerve is relatively susceptible to increased compression and traction. In pronation, the tendons of the brachioradialis and extensor carpi radialis longus approximate, and as the wrist moves from radial

CRITICAL POINTS *Cubital Tunnel Surgery*

Indications
- Failure to relieve symptoms with the use of an elbow pad and avoidance of elbow flexion and activity modification
- Ulnar intrinsic muscle atrophy

Preoperative Evaluation
- Electrodiagnostic studies to "stage" the degree of nerve compression to help predict the anticipated rate of recovery

Pearls
- Document the preoperative pain distribution.
- Document preoperative examination of the entire upper extremity.
- Use dexmedetomidine hydrochloride and a Bier block.
- Use a bupivacaine infusion pump.
- Begin early movement (postoperative day 2 or 3).

Technical Points
- Avoid injury to all branches of the medial antebrachial cutaneous nerve.
- Remove the intramuscular septum.
- Elevate fascial flaps.
- Remove tendinous bands in the flexor-pronator muscle mass.
- Remove the distal intermuscular septum between the flexor carpi ulnaris and the flexor-pronator muscles.
- Dissect enough flexor-pronator muscle to allow the ulnar nerve to run in a straight line anterior to the medial epicondyle.
- Close the fascial flaps above the ulnar nerve extremely loosely.
- Most importantly, ensure that the ulnar nerve is not kinked at the distal transposition site.
- Place bupivacaine in the incision.
- Use a suction drain and an infusion bupivacaine pump.
- Begin early range of motion postoperatively.

Pitfalls
- Kinking of the ulnar nerve may occur distally as it moves from its position within the flexor carpi ulnaris to its position anterior to the medial epicondyle.
- Do not immobilize the arm for more than 2 or 3 days postoperatively.

Postoperative Care
- Remove the dressing on postoperative day 2 or 3.
- Begin range-of-motion exercises within the patient's comfort level starting on postoperative day 2 or 3.
- Use a sling at night for 3 weeks.
- Begin strengthening exercises in the second month.
- Restrict weight lifting to 5 pounds at 1 month.
- There are no restrictions after the second month.

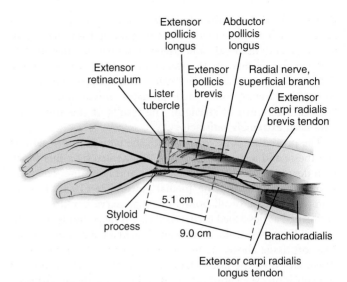

FIGURE 28.27 The most common pattern of the superficial branch of the radial nerve. (From Abrams RA, Brown RA, Botte MJ: The superficial branch of the radial nerve: an anatomic study with surgical implications, *J Hand Surg [Am]* 17:1037–1041, 1992.)

extension to ulnar flexion, the nerve becomes stretched, and these tendons may compress the nerve. Over time, edema and fibrosis can cause chronic nerve compression. This compression neuropathy has been described histopathologically to range from subperineurial edema or fibrosis to segmental demyelination to Wallerian degeneration.[63,64]

ANATOMY

The radial sensory nerve branches from the main radial nerve at the lateral humeral epicondyle below the brachioradialis and enters the subcutaneous tissue between the tendons of the brachioradialis and the extensor carpi radialis longus in the mid-

forearm. In 3 to 10% of individuals, the superficial branch of the radial nerve will become subcutaneous by actually piercing the tendon of the brachioradialis. It bifurcates into two main branches 5 cm proximal to the radial styloid, and the major palmar branch continues to innervate the dorsal radial aspect of the thumb. The major dorsal branch continues to innervate the dorsal ulnar aspect of the thumb and the dorsal radial aspect of the index finger. A third branch continues to become the dorsoulnar and dorsoradial digital nerves of the index and long fingers (Figure 28.27). The lateral antebrachial cutaneous nerve has a significant overlap pattern with the radial sensory nerve.[60]

Patients with radial sensory nerve compression typically describe paresthesia, pain, or numbness in the radial sensory nerve distribution. The diagnosis of radial sensory nerve entrapment is suspected when symptoms are reproduced by forearm pronation and ulnar wrist flexion. A positive nerve percussion sign is identified over the radial sensory nerve at the point where it exits the deep fascia in the forearm. The differential diagnosis of radial sensory nerve entrapment should include de Quervain disease; conversely, the Finkelstein sign can also be positive in patients with Wartenberg syndrome. It has been reported that both conditions can coexist because entrapment of the first dorsal compartment tendons can cause scarring or neuritis of the distal branch of the superficial radial nerve. Patients with de Quervain disease should demonstrate normal sensory testing in the dorsal radial aspect of the hand, in contrast to patients with radial sensory nerve compression, in whom sensation may be decreased. Patients with de Quervain disease tend to have pain with percussion over the first extensor compartment and do not have a typical Tinel sign that reproduces symptoms in the radial sensory nerve distribution. Electrodiagnostic studies are rarely if ever useful in diagnosing this condition.

Rarely, the lateral antebrachial cutaneous nerve, which partially or completely overlaps the sensory territory of the radial sensory nerve, may be entrapped.[60] Differential nerve blocks and positive nerve percussion testing will help distinguish these two nerve entrapments, but in our experience it is relatively rare. Patients who describe paresthesia, numbness, or pain in the radial sensory nerve distribution should be examined to rule out cervical disk disease. If findings localize to the forearm and the cervical spine is excluded as a source of pathologic findings, the patient is instructed to modify inciting activities and to maintain the forearm in a more supinated position whenever possible. Modification of activities to avoid excessive pronation and supination and a local corticosteroid injection at the entrapment site between the tendons of the extensor carpi radialis longus and brachioradialis are generally successful, and surgical release is rarely necessary. Splinting is not usually successful because of the difficulty of splinting in forearm supination.

❖ AUTHORS' PREFERRED METHOD OF TREATMENT:
Radial Sensory Nerve Decompression

The radial sensory nerve is released at its point of compression between the tendons of the extensor carpi radialis longus and brachioradialis (Figure 28.28). Preoperatively, the most intense site of the Tinel sign is determined. An intravenous regional block is used with dexmedetomidine hydrochloride and lidocaine, and a padded above-elbow tourniquet is inflated after exsanguination of the limb. A longitudinal incision (2 to 3 cm) is marked just volar to the musculotendinous junction of the brachioradialis muscle. Loupe magnification is used to identify and protect the crossing branches of the lateral antebrachial cutaneous nerve. The musculotendinous junction of the brachioradialis is identified, and the fascia between the tendons of the brachioradialis and the extensor carpi radialis longus is opened. The fascia above the radial sensory nerve is released to identify the radial sensory nerve. The nerve is followed proxi-

mally and distally for a distance of about 10 cm. A portion of the tendon of the brachioradialis can be resected to completely decompress the radial sensory nerve. With proximal and distal retraction, the radial sensory nerve can be released over a long distance. Neurolysis is not performed. The tourniquet is deflated, and good hemostasis is obtained. Bupivacaine is placed in the incision. The incision is closed over a plastic angiocatheter, and 2 mL of dexamethasone is injected along the course of the radial sensory nerve through the angiocatheter, with removal of the angiocatheter when the wound is closed. A bulky dressing is applied while keeping the wrist in neutral.

Postoperative Care

The dressing is removed on the second postoperative day, and early movement of the upper extremity is encouraged. Desensitization of the radial sensory distribution on the dorsum of the hand is also started. Patients should avoid heavy lifting for the first month and then start strengthening exercises at the end of the first month.

POSTERIOR INTEROSSEOUS NERVE SYNDROME AND RADIAL TUNNEL SYNDROME

Compression of the radial nerve in the proximal forearm region can result in the posterior interosseous nerve palsy or radial tunnel syndrome. In posterior interosseous nerve palsy, the muscles innervated by the nerve are affected, including the extensor carpi radialis brevis, supinator, extensor carpi ulnaris, extensor digitorum communis, extensor digiti quinti, extensor indicis proprius, abductor pollicis longus, and extensor pollicis longus and brevis. The onset of symptoms may occur after trauma, or an insidious onset may be reported. Other causes can include proliferative rheumatoid synovitis and mononeuritis or Parsonage-Turner syndrome. Rarely, iatrogenic injury

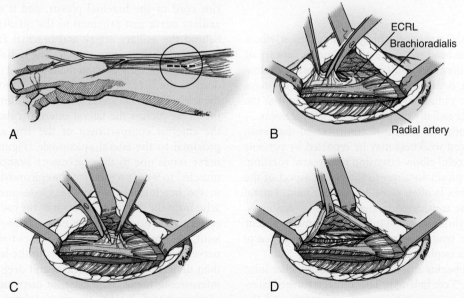

FIGURE 28.28 Radial sensory nerve decompression. **A,** The incision is made on the flexor aspect of the forearm and centered on the radial sensory nerve. The fascia between the brachioradialis and extensor carpi radialis longus tendons is divided distally **(B)** and then proximally **(C). D,** The nerve is freed from its underlying bed. *ECRL,* Extensor carpi radialis longus. (From Dellon AL, Mackinnon SE: Radial sensory nerve entrapment in the forearm, *J Hand Surg [Am]* 11:199–205, 1986. Redrawn by Elizabeth Martin.)

CRITICAL POINTS *Radial Sensory Nerve Release*

Indications
- Rare
- Failure of supination posture to relieve radial sensory symptoms

Preoperative Evaluation
- Tinel sign over the entrapment point in the forearm
- Electrodiagnostic studies

Pearls
- Encouragement of a palm-up position or corticosteroid injection (or both) usually relieves the symptoms without surgery.
- Rule out C7 cervical disk disease and thoracic outlet syndrome.

Technical Points
- Preoperatively identify the muscle-tendon junction of the brachioradialis.
- Make a longitudinal lazy-"S" incision just volar to the muscle-tendon junction of the brachioradialis.
- Take care to avoid injury to the lateral antebrachial cutaneous nerve.
- Open the fascia between the brachioradialis and extensor carpi radialis longus.
- Remove a portion of the tendon of the brachioradialis to adequately release the radial sensory nerve.
- Release the radial sensory nerve proximally and distally to ensure the absence of compressive fascial bands.
- Instill corticosteroid around the nerve and place Seprafilm over it.
- Place bupivacaine in the incision.

Pitfalls
- Confusion with cervical disk disease
- Injury to the lateral antebrachial cutaneous nerve
- Failure to diagnose associated de Quervain disease

Postoperative Care
- Remove the dressing on day 2 or 3.
- Begin range-of-motion exercises on day 2 or 3.
- Begin strengthening exercises in the second month.

can occur during elbow surgery for biceps reattachment, elbow arthroscopy, or radial head reconstruction. Tendon rupture or masses at the elbow may also result in loss of posterior interosseous nerve function. Because the extensor carpi radialis longus is innervated by the radial nerve proximal to the injury, the wrist tends to deviate radially during active wrist extension.

Radial tunnel syndrome is a more controversial diagnosis. Symptoms of pain and weakness may be reported by patients after activities of forceful elbow extension or forearm rotation. The forearm pain typically localizes to the lateral aspect of the forearm, and weakness is often secondary to the pain. Lateral epicondylitis must be considered in the differential diagnosis. Both lateral epicondylitis and radial tunnel syndrome can occur simultaneously. The tendinous origin of the extensor carpi radialis brevis can be implicated in both conditions.

The radial tunnel begins anterior to the radiocapitellar joint and is approximately 5 cm in length. The tunnel is formed laterally by the extensor carpi radialis longus and brevis and the brachioradialis muscles, medially by the biceps tendon and brachialis, and posteriorly by the radiocapitellar joint capsule. The brachioradialis muscle passes over the nerve in a lateral to anterior direction to form the roof of the tunnel. Although the tunnel was originally described as ending at the arcade of Fröhse, compressive tendinous bands have been described that extend to the distal end of the supinator muscle.

Radial tunnel syndrome is a clinical diagnosis based on tenderness over the radial tunnel, pain at the origin of the extensor carpi radialis brevis with resistance of middle finger extension, and pain with resisted forearm supination. Electrodiagnostic studies are not particularly useful in this condition. Because reproduction of pain with deep palpation is important in making this diagnosis, it is important to test the contralateral asymptomatic arm for comparison. Pressure is placed over the posterior interosseous nerve in the interval between the brachioradialis and extensor carpi radialis brevis muscles, and the patient's response is compared between the two forearms. Pressure over the supinator may be quite painful. To determine whether a concomitant problem exists over the radial nerve, pressure is exerted between the brachioradialis and brachialis muscles just above the elbow. Because this is a subjective diagnosis, it is important to check the patient's pain response at nonentrapment sites and to reexamine the patient on a few occasions. The scratch collapse test is also useful in the physical examination to identify radial tunnel compression. Some physicians find it helpful to use sequential diagnostic injections of lidocaine into the lateral epicondyle and then the supinator (to effect a posterior interosseous nerve block) to help differentiate nerve entrapment from lateral epicondylitis.

There is no specific nonoperative treatment of radial tunnel syndrome. However, nerve gliding exercises may be useful. In patients with concomitant lateral epicondylitis, therapy may ameliorate the symptoms associated with lateral epicondylitis. Tennis elbow straps are not recommended for patients with radial tunnel syndrome because of the increased pressure that may be placed on the radial nerve.

ANATOMY

The radial nerve is one of two terminal branches of the posterior cord of the brachial plexus, and it splits away from the axillary nerve just proximal to the quadrangular space. It lies behind the axillary artery and brachial artery anterior to the long head of the triceps muscle. The radial nerve courses laterally and posteriorly deep to the long head of the triceps and lies deep to the lateral head and superficial to the medial head of the triceps near the spiral groove. After innervating the triceps, the nerve pierces the lateral intermuscular septum and enters the anterior compartment of the arm approximately 10 cm proximal to the lateral epicondyle (Figure 28.29). The radial nerve sends one to three accessory branches to the brachialis muscle 3 to 9 cm proximal to the epicondyle and a larger branch to the brachioradialis muscle. Occasionally, this branch can arise from the superficial branch of the radial nerve distal to the epicondyle. The anconeus muscle is innervated proximal to the joint, followed by the extensor carpi radialis longus. The radial nerve enters the forearm anterior to the lateral epicondyle and then divides into the superficial and deep branches (posterior interosseous nerve). The extensor carpi radialis brevis is generally innervated distal to the elbow joint from either the posterior interosseous nerve or the superficial radial nerve. The posterior interosseous nerve passes under the arcade of Fröhse before passing between the two heads of the supinator. The

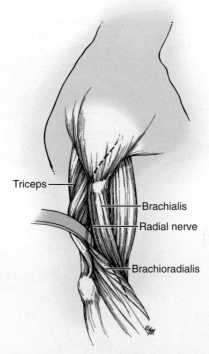

FIGURE 28.29 The radial nerve pierces the lateral intermuscular septum 10 cm above the lateral humeral condyle and courses in a groove between the brachialis and brachioradialis muscles. (Copyright © Elizabeth Martin.)

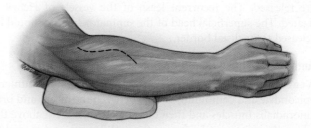

FIGURE 28.30 Extended approach to the posterior interosseous nerve through the brachioradialis-splitting approach. (Copyright © Elizabeth Martin.)

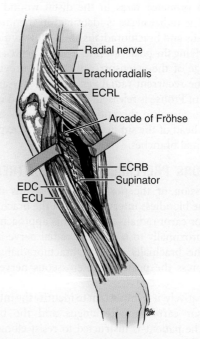

FIGURE 28.31 Extension of the posterior Thompson approach to the radial tunnel. *ECRB*, Extensor carpi radialis brevis; *ECRL*, extensor carpi radialis longus; *ECU*, extensor carpi ulnaris; *EDC*, extensor digitorum communis. (Copyright © Elizabeth Martin.)

arcade of Fröhse is a fibrous arch that originates from the lateral epicondyle and in a number of cases has a tendinous consistency. Fibrous bands within the supinator muscle or hypertrophy of the superficial head may cause compression in this location. After exiting the supinator muscle, the posterior interosseous nerve divides into deep and superficial branches. The superficial branch innervates the extensor carpi ulnaris, extensor digitorum communis, and extensor digiti quinti muscles. The deep branch innervates the abductor pollicis longus, extensor pollicis longus, extensor pollicis brevis, and, finally, the extensor indicis proprius muscle.

Operative Techniques

Several approaches (anterior, posterior, and transmuscular brachioradialis splitting) have been described for release of the posterior interosseous nerve based on the relationship of the incision to the brachioradialis muscle (Video 28.8).

Transmuscular Brachioradialis-Splitting Approach

With the use of regional or intravenous block anesthesia, a longitudinal or "S"-shaped incision is made beginning proximal to the radial head and 3 cm lateral to the biceps tendon (Figure 28.30). The fascia over the brachioradialis muscle is incised and the muscle belly is split bluntly while aiming for the radial head until the fat overlying the radial nerve is seen. The brachioradialis muscle split is lengthened over the radial tunnel. Transverse vessels are coagulated, and the fibrous bands overlying the posterior interosseous nerve and the fibrous edge of the extensor carpi radialis brevis are divided. Recurrent radial vessels are ligated and the superficial head of the supinator muscle is divided completely.

Posterior (Henry or Thompson) Approach

The forearm is pronated and a 10-cm straight skin incision is made along an imaginary line extending from the lateral epicondyle to the Lister tubercle. The incision can be extended proximally onto the lateral ridge of the epicondyle as necessary (Figure 28.31). The posterior cutaneous nerve of the forearm is identified and protected. The forearm fascia is incised in the interval between the extensor digitorum communis and the extensor carpi radialis longus. Dissection begins at a point where the two tendons can be identified distally and is extended proximally to the lateral epicondyle. The extensor carpi radialis brevis lies deep to the extensor carpi radialis longus, and its tendon of origin can safely be detached from the lateral epicondyle as needed for exposure. The extensor digitorum communis muscle can be partially detached from the lateral epicondyle anteriorly. The supinator is identified deep to the extensor muscles in the proximal third of the incision. The posterior interosseous nerve can then be found at the proximal edge of the supinator, and the fibrous leading edge of the extensor carpi radialis brevis and the tendinous leading edge of the supinator are released. The recurrent leash of the vessels of Henry is ligated. The superficial head of the supinator muscle should be released to its distal border.

Anterior (Modified Henry) Approach

A curvilinear incision is made starting above the lateral humeral epicondyle and continuing distally between the biceps and brachioradialis muscles and then curving laterally 2 cm above the elbow flexion crease, back over the mobile wad, and medial to the ulnar border of the brachioradialis muscle. The cutaneous nerves are identified and protected and the fascia divided along the brachioradialis muscle, which is retracted laterally while the biceps and pronator teres in the distal wound are retracted medially. The radial nerve is identified in the interval between the brachialis and brachioradialis and followed distally. Fibrous bands overlying the posterior interosseous nerve and the fibrous leading edge of the extensor carpi radialis brevis muscles are divided. The recurrent radial vessels of Henry are ligated and the arcade of Fröhse is released. The mobile wad is elevated and retracted to visualize the entire length of the supinator. The superficial head of the supinator is divided to expose the nerve to its terminal branches.

❖ AUTHORS' PREFERRED METHOD OF TREATMENT

Decompression of the posterior interosseous nerve is done through the bloodless interval between the brachioradialis and the extensor carpi radialis longus. This approach can easily be extended proximally to release the radial nerve in the interval between the brachialis and the brachioradialis and distally to decompress the posterior interosseous nerve through the supinator.

Preoperatively, it is important to identify the interval between the extensor carpi radialis longus and the brachioradialis muscles. The patient is instructed to resist elbow flexion, and the planned incision is marked along the posterior border of the brachioradialis muscle. Intravenous regional or general anesthesia is used, as are loupe magnification and microbipolar cautery. A straight 10-cm incision is made along the posterior border of the brachioradialis muscle. The posterior cutaneous nerve of the forearm is small, but it is always located exactly at the junction between the fascia of the brachioradialis muscle and the extensor carpi radialis longus muscle. There is a color distinction between the fascia of these two muscles. The brachioradialis muscle is a more intense red color because the fascia is thinner. By contrast, the fascia of the extensor carpi radialis longus is thicker and appears lighter. This fascial interval is sharply divided with a No. 15 blade, and the dissection is deepened by blunt finger dissection down to the region of the arcade of Fröhse (Figure 28.32, A). If the dissection is not an easy finger dissection, the surgeon is not in the correct plane. Deep retractors are used to retract the brachioradialis muscle and the extensor carpi radialis longus muscle. The crossing vessels are identified and carefully ligated and divided. The surgeon can then easily identify the radial sensory nerve, the small nerve to the extensor carpi radialis brevis, and the posterior interosseous nerve (see Figure 28-32, B). The tendon of the extensor carpi radialis brevis is divided from its origin on the lateral epicondyle. This effectively treats any component of the symptoms that may be attributed to lateral epicondylitis. Both the tendinous part and the underlying muscle of the

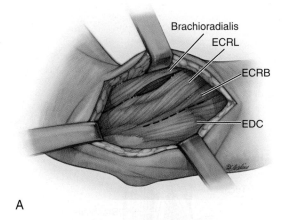

A

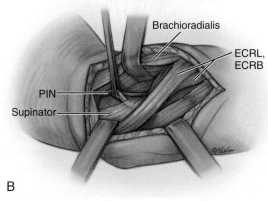

B

FIGURE 28.32 Extended approach to the posterior interosseous nerve (PIN) through the brachioradialis/extensor carpi radialis longus (ECRL) interval. **A,** Superficial exposure. **B,** Deep exposure. *ECRB,* Extensor carpi radialis brevis; *EDC,* extensor digitorum communis. (Copyright © Elizabeth Martin.)

superficial head of the supinator are divided to release the posterior interosseous nerve completely. Occasionally, there will be tendinous bands compressing the posterior interosseous nerve distally within the supinator, and thus the division should proceed to its distal edge. The surgeon should run a finger along the proximal portion of the radial nerve above the elbow; if any bands are encountered, a second incision may be needed above the elbow along the anterior border of the brachioradialis muscle. Deep dissection is performed bluntly between the brachioradialis muscle and the brachialis muscles. If the dissection is difficult or through muscle fibers, the surgeon is in the wrong plane. The radial nerve proper is easily identified and followed proximally to release any tendinous bands up to the level of the lateral intermuscular septum. Bupivacaine is placed in the incision or incisions. The tourniquet is deflated, and hemostasis is achieved with bipolar electrocautery. A drain is rarely needed. The incisions are closed in layers with absorbable suture. A bulky dressing immobilizes the arm with the wrist in neutral and the elbow flexed.

Postoperative Care

The dressing is removed 2 to 3 days postoperatively, and the patient is encouraged to begin full range-of-motion exercises. The sutures are removed 10 to 14 days after surgery. In the second month, strengthening exercises are begun. The patient is returned to light duty work at the end of the first month and released to full and unrestricted duty after 2 months.

CRITICAL POINTS *Posterior Interosseous and Radial Tunnel Nerve Release*

Indications
- Localized pain over the posterior interosseous nerve in the region of the arcade of Fröhse
- Failure to respond to physical therapy and treatment of possible concomitant lateral epicondylitis

Preoperative Evaluation
- Document discrete significant pain at the junction of the brachioradialis and extensor carpi radialis longus.

Pearls
- Preoperatively mark the incision just dorsal to the brachioradialis muscle.
- Use dexmedetomidine hydrochloride and a Bier block.
- Note that the fascia of the brachioradialis is redder than the lighter fascia of the extensor carpi radialis longus.
- Release the tendon of the extensor carpi radialis brevis across the forearm to treat for any potential associated lateral epicondylitis.
- Ensure complete hemostasis.
- Begin early movement.
- If the patient preoperatively had localized pain over the radial nerve above the elbow, a second incision is made to decompress the main radial nerve above the elbow.

Technical Points
- Make an incision along the junction between the brachioradialis and extensor carpi radialis longus.
- Identify and protect the posterior cutaneous nerve of the forearm.

- Use blunt dissection in the interval between the brachioradialis and the extensor carpi radialis longus down to the arcade of Fröhse.
- Preserve the nerve to the extensor carpi radialis brevis.
- Ligate the crossing vessels.
- Release the tendon of the extensor carpi radialis brevis over the posterior interosseous nerve and across the forearm.
- Release the superficial head of the supinator to completely decompress the posterior interosseous nerve.
- Use finger palpation proximally to feel for any fibrous bands over the radial head.
- Make a proximal incision above the elbow between the brachioradialis and brachialis if any fibrous bands are palpated from the distal incision.
- Place bupivacaine in the incision.

Pitfalls
- Failure to identify and protect the posterior cutaneous nerve of the forearm and the radial sensory nerve
- Failure to adequately excise the extensor carpi radialis brevis tendon and the entire superficial head of the supinator
- Failure to achieve meticulous hemostasis

Postoperative Care
- Remove the dressing on postoperative day 2 or 3.
- Begin range-of-motion exercises on day 2 or 3.
- Continue range-of-motion exercises throughout the first month.
- Start strengthening exercises in the second month.
- If patient has undergone an associated procedure on the lateral epicondyle, use a soft sling for 1 or 2 weeks.

PROXIMAL RADIAL NERVE COMPRESSION

Compression of the radial nerve proximal to the elbow is uncommon. A fibrous arch from the lateral head of the triceps has been associated with radial nerve compression, and cases have been reported after strenuous muscular activity. A bony exostosis of the humerus has also been associated with this problem. Patients will have variable degrees of radial nerve dysfunction. Typically it is not painful, and spontaneous recovery usually occurs. Patients may provide a history of alcohol or drug abuse that suggests prolonged positioning with pressure over the radial nerve in the spiral groove. If there is no clinical evidence of recovery in 3 months, electrodiagnostic studies should be done. If these do not show evidence of reinnervation, surgical release of the radial nerve can be considered. In chronic, recurrent, or painful cases of radial nerve compression related to sports or exertion, decompression is occasionally indicated despite normal electrodiagnostic studies.

Operative Technique

With the patient under general anesthesia, the entire arm is prepared and draped. Although distal dissection can be performed with the use of a sterile tourniquet, the procedure cannot be completed under tourniquet control because of the proximal exposure required. A long lateral incision is made between the deltoid and the lateral head of the triceps muscle, extends distally along the lateral margin of the biceps, and ends in the interval between the brachioradialis and brachialis muscles just proximal to the cubital crease. The radial nerve is first identified by blunt dissection in the interval between the

brachioradialis and brachialis muscles. The nerve is then followed proximally and the lateral intermuscular septum divided to follow the nerve proximally under the lateral head of the triceps. Care is taken to protect the cutaneous radial branches. If necessary, intraoperative electrodiagnostic studies can be done to confirm the area of conduction block. If the long head of the triceps and the tendons of the teres major and latissimus dorsi are divided, these tendons must be reattached at the conclusion of the procedure. The incision is closed in layers, and a bulky dressing is applied along with an arm sling.

If the surgeon believes that proximal decompression will be likely, the modified posterior approach of Gerwin and colleagues enables exposure of the radial nerve along 94% of the humerus by elevating the medial and lateral heads of the triceps without detachment after dividing the entire intermuscular septum.[27]

Postoperative Care

The dressing is removed 2 to 3 days after surgery, and general range-of-motion exercises are started. The sling can be used at night for comfort for 3 weeks after surgery. If a triceps, teres major, and latissimus dorsi release and repair have been performed, active shoulder exercises are delayed 3 to 4 weeks.

SURGERY FOR PREVIOUSLY FAILED PROCEDURES

In carefully selected patients, well-performed surgery with good postoperative patient compliance should adequately decompress or take tension off a nerve such that symptoms from the compression neuropathy resolve and further surgery is not needed. As extremity surgeons become experienced in the management of patients with compression neuropathies, they are likely to be referred patients who have undergone previous decompression surgeries with less than favorable results. Management of this patient population is much more challenging than that of patients with primary compressive neuropathies.[58,121] These patients often have a very significant pain component. Our pain evaluation form (see Figure 28.3) is critical in helping to identify ongoing symptoms and to determine potential surgical candidates. The assistance of a pain management physician may also be required. Pregabalin or nortriptyline, or both, can be recommended. If surgery is suggested, informed consent will emphasize the possibility of incomplete relief of pain and even decreased neurologic function. In general, if the patient has undergone more than two surgical attempts to correct a nerve compression problem, it is less likely that a third operation to relieve symptoms and improve function will be helpful. In patients with a motor deficit, nerve graft, nerve transfer, or tendon transfers are considered. If pain is the primary problem, a peripheral nerve stimulator or dorsal column stimulator should be considered.[81]

In general, after a failed procedure to treat nerve compression, patients can be classified into three groups: (1) patients may describe the same symptoms postoperatively as they had preoperatively with no relief of symptoms; (2) they may describe a period of relief of compression symptoms, followed at 6 months or later by recurrence of the same symptoms; or (3) they may describe an entirely new symptom complex after the decompression surgery. This last group is the most challenging to manage because it typically includes patients with substantial pain and nerve injury, either to the affected nerve and/or to a nearby cutaneous nerve.

Recurrent Carpal Tunnel Syndrome

The most common reasons for persistent symptoms are failure to adequately decompress the carpal tunnel. In our recent review, the most common intraoperative findings were incomplete release of the flexor retinaculum and median nerve adherence to surrounding tissue.[121] In obese patients, failure to make an incision of adequate length may have led to insufficient decompression of the median nerve, especially at the proximal and distal sites of the surgical exposure. The Phalen test will be positive in these patients, and no other significant sites of compression neuropathy along the course of the median nerve will be noted. Electrodiagnostic studies to evaluate recurrent carpal tunnel syndrome may not be particularly helpful given that patients with successful carpal tunnel surgery will frequently have persistent electrical changes.[22] A second common cause of persistent symptoms after primary carpal tunnel release is the likelihood that carpal tunnel syndrome was not the correct diagnosis or that it was causing an insignificant component of the patient's symptom complex. These patients may demonstrate compression on the median nerve in the forearm or cervical disk disease or may have a sensory neuropathy resistant to surgical decompression. Similarly, patients with sensory complaints on the dorsal aspect of the thumb and the index and long fingers will obviously not respond to carpal tunnel release.

In patients who have definite relief of symptoms for 6 months or longer and then have a recurrence of the same symptoms, a secondary traction neuritis of the median nerve has probably developed as a result of scar formation. Incisions that are placed directly over the median nerve are susceptible to the development of scar between the median nerve and the overlying flexor retinaculum at a later period. In these patients, the Phalen test is positive and there are no other sites of significant proximal median nerve compression.

The most challenging patient management group consists of patients in whom completely new symptoms develop after carpal tunnel release, and this development is usually accompanied by very significant pain dysfunction. Although reflex sympathetic dystrophy or complex regional pain syndrome is uncommon after carpal tunnel release, minor injuries to the median nerve or the palmar cutaneous branch of the median nerve are unfortunately well-recognized complications of carpal tunnel release. A patient's history and physical examination will allow the surgeon to determine which component or components of the median nerve or nearby cutaneous nerves have been injured. A proximal percussion test may help determine this; beginning 2 to 3 inches proximal to the surgical incision, gentle digital percussion is made along the course of the median nerve and its palmar cutaneous branch. At this level, the patient may describe painful paresthesia in the distribution of the involved nerve or nerve branches. By contrast, if digital percussion is done exactly over the area of nerve injury, it may be so painful that the patient cannot be specific about what components (fascicles) of the median nerve have been injured. Typically, the more superficial branch to the third web space (radial side of the ring finger and ulnar side of the long finger) is injured or entrapped in scar tissue. In cases of nerve injury, nonoperative treatment will be unsuccessful.

Patients are referred for therapy to decrease pain, increase range of motion, and increase strength. Medications such as pregabalin or nortriptyline may be helpful in decreasing neuropathic pain. After an appropriate trial of nonoperative treatment, revision surgery is recommended for patients with continued or recurrent symptoms in the median nerve distribution that localize with provocation to the level of the carpal tunnel or with identification of a partial median nerve injury or one to the palmar cutaneous branch of the median nerve.

Revision Surgery

The surgical management of persistent and recurrent carpal tunnel syndrome requires an incision well ulnar to the thenar crease regardless of the first incision and extends this proximal and distal to the area of the previous surgery. Dissection begins proximally to identify the median nerve and is then followed distally through the surgical site. The median nerve is usually found to be densely adherent to the underside of the flexor retinaculum. Micro-internal neurolysis is almost always necessary in recurrent cases but is never indicated for primary carpal tunnel syndrome. Microsurgical instruments are used to perform a longitudinal epineurotomy. Frequently, however, there will be tension on the nerve both transversely and longitudinally, and thus a second epineurotomy going circumferentially around the nerve is also performed. The external epineurium is reflected and neurolysis performed until bands of Fontana are noted in the fascicles. These bands represent redundancy in the peripheral nerves and are thus an "endpoint" for the neurolysis technique. Rarely, an abductor digiti minimi flap is used to provide soft tissue coverage over the nerve. Alternatively, the nerve can be covered with fat transposed from the neighboring Guyon canal. If the patient has a neuroma of the palmar cutaneous branch of the median nerve, neurolysis of the injured fascicle is performed well proximal to its branching point, and the transected nerve is transposed proximally to lie in the muscle interface between the deep and superficial flexors of the forearm. Injuries to the median nerve itself are treated as for the management of a neuroma in continuity; that is, injuries to the fascicles of the median nerve innervating the third web space can be reconstructed with a short nerve graft, or this fascicular group can be easily separated from the main median nerve for a very long distance and transposed proximally into the forearm between the two flexor masses.[97] The distal end of the common digital nerve to the third web space can be transferred in an end-to-side fashion to the second common digital nerve to recover some sensibility in the third web space.[113] With motor branch deficits and no thumb opposition, local tendon transfers are recommended (Videos 28.9 and 28.10).

Recurrent Cubital Tunnel Syndrome

A review of 100 patients after repeat cubital tunnel surgery and a survey of the operative procedures have led us to a hypothesis regarding the operative management of cubital tunnel syndrome.[70,82] Discussion and debates on the "best" operative procedure have resulted in numerous publications that support various procedures with claims of "excellent results." It is our hypothesis that an understanding of the etiologic factors inherent in the development of cubital tunnel syndrome and an understanding of the potential for surgery to create *new* problems will yield optimal outcomes. Therefore, any of the operative procedures described for cubital tunnel syndrome can result in an excellent outcome if the basic principles related to cubital tunnel syndrome are followed. However, without adherence to these principles, a poor result can occur with any of the standard cubital tunnel procedures. An understanding of the etiologic factors that result in cubital tunnel syndrome is necessary, and, most importantly, it is essential that the surgical procedure does not create any new areas of compression on the ulnar nerve.

Surgical failures are more frequent in cases of cubital tunnel syndrome than in cases of carpal tunnel syndrome, and management of such failures is made exceedingly difficult by the previous surgical procedure and resultant scarring of the nerve. The classification of failed cubital tunnel syndrome is similar to that for carpal tunnel syndrome. Patients may have persistence of the same preoperative symptoms with no change at all in their clinical status. They may have relief of symptoms for several months to years and then have recurrent problems. Finally, they may exhibit new symptoms of neurologic loss or pain (or both) after the cubital tunnel surgery.

Many conditions can mimic cubital tunnel syndrome, and the surgeon needs to be well aware of these. Amyotrophic lateral sclerosis or Pancoast tumors can be accompanied by ulnar nerve symptoms. It is important to be alert for a situation in which the sensory loss and motor loss are decidedly different. If the sensory loss far exceeds the motor complaints, a sensory neuropathy should be considered. By contrast, if the motor complaints exceed the sensory complaints, compression in the Guyon canal should be considered, especially if the proximal extrinsic hand muscles are normal and there is no thenar atrophy. If there is additional thenar atrophy, compression in the thoracic outlet with the very rare Gilliatt "true" neurogenic thoracic outlet syndrome should be considered. If the extrinsic motors are equally involved, brachial plexus neuritis can be considered or upper motor neuron disease if the deep tendon reflexes are increased. Electrodiagnostic studies by an experienced examiner are critical in the differential diagnosis and localization of the level of compression.

Failure to relieve symptoms may imply an incomplete decompression with the primary surgical procedure or an incorrect diagnosis. Recurrence of symptoms after a period of 6 months or more after initial relief of the symptoms usually implies a new site of ulnar nerve compression in the previous surgical field. Severe causalgia-type pain at the elbow radiating into the medial aspect of the forearm suggests a neuroma of the medial antebrachial cutaneous nerve. Severe causalgia-type pain in the ulnar nerve distribution suggests an injury to the ulnar nerve itself. A proximal percussion test above the area of the previous surgical site along the course of the basilic vein will result in pain and/or paresthesia, in the distribution of the medial antebrachial cutaneous nerve if there is a neuroma of this nerve. Similarly, percussion along the course of the ulnar nerve above the area of the previous surgery will result in paresthesia and pain in the ulnar nerve distribution if there is a problem with the ulnar nerve itself. Palpation along the course of the ulnar nerve in the distal forearm progressing to the region of the surgical site will result in deep pain distal to the previous surgical site if a new compression point has developed at the site of the distal surgical exposure. This finding is common if great care has not been taken to ensure smooth transposition of the ulnar nerve from its position in the forearm underneath the flexor carpi ulnaris to the transposition site at the elbow.

Revision Surgery

Surgical management of secondary cubital tunnel syndrome has been reviewed.[49] In a recent review of the operative findings during reoperation for cubital tunnel syndrome, the most common patient complaints after the primary surgery included new symptoms in the ulnar nerve distribution and pain in the medial antebrachial cutaneous nerve distribution.[70] Operative findings included a medial antebrachial cutaneous neuroma and distal kinking of the ulnar nerve as it was moved into the transposed position anterior to the medial epicondyle.[70]

If the patient previously underwent simple decompression, the finding is usually scar around the ulnar nerve in the surgical site or a tendency for the ulnar nerve to sublux over the medial epicondyle (or both). In both cases the ulnar nerve must be mobilized, and a transmuscular transposition is performed as described previously. Similar findings and management are used if the patient has previously had an unsuccessful medial epicondylectomy. If the patient has previously undergone a subcutaneous transposition, the nerve is usually found to be scarred along its course within the surgical site, either to the anterior surface of the medial epicondyle or distally where the ulnar nerve moves from its transposition site to the flexor carpi ulnaris muscle mass. Occasionally, a retained medial intermuscular septum will cause compression on the nerve proximally. In all cases, the ulnar nerve is mobilized, the distal and proximal compression sites are released, and a transmuscular procedure is performed.

If the patient has previously undergone an intramuscular procedure, the nerve is generally scarred along its entire surgical course, or a tight fascial or suture band can be identified at the medial epicondyle, where the surgeon has created a sling to prevent subluxation. Typically, there is also compression of the ulnar nerve at the distal transposition site by fascia of the flexor carpi ulnaris muscle and the tendinous fascia between the pronator muscle and the flexor carpi ulnaris muscle. The ulnar nerve is mobilized, and fascial flaps are marked on the flexor-pronator muscle origin as described for a primary transmuscular transposition, except in this situation the flaps are based more anteriorly and just in front of the previous surgical intramuscular trough.

If the patient has undergone the classic Learmonth submuscular transposition, the ulnar nerve may be found to be compressed by the tendinous "T" fascia septum within the flexor-pronator muscle origin. The nerve typically takes a right-angled turn when it goes from its submuscular position in front of the medial epicondyle near the median nerve to its posterior location within the flexor carpi ulnaris muscle. The distal fascial septum between the pronator and the flexor carpi ulnaris is also usually intact and may compress the nerve. In these situations, the dissection starts proximally out of the area of the previous surgical site. The dissection carefully follows the ulnar nerve into the area of the previous surgery. The ulnar nerve is found distal to the previous surgical site and followed proximally along its course into the region of the previous surgery. Because a Learmonth submuscular transposition has previously been performed, it is usually possible to leave some overlying muscle intact and remove the tendinous fascial septa that are compressing the ulnar nerve. Thus, no fascial flaps are needed to prevent the ulnar nerve from relocating posteriorly because the overlying flexor-pronator muscle accomplishes this. All tendinous bands and septa that are compressing the nerve are released under the muscle and proximally and distally.

When operating for recurrent cubital tunnel syndrome and particularly in patients who have undergone multiple procedures, extreme care must be taken to preserve the vascular supply to the nerve. The profound intrinsic blood supply of the normal ulnar nerve may become more dependent on the extrinsic blood supply, and ischemia of the nerve can occur if excessive neurolysis is performed. An external epineurotomy and cautious external neurolysis are preferred only to ensure that the ulnar nerve fascicles and bands of Fontana are visualized. In all situations of secondary cubital tunnel surgery, care must be taken to identify the medial antebrachial cutaneous nerve and follow the two main branches distally to make sure that they have been protected. If the branches have been injured, the neuromas are excised and these nerves are transposed proximally to lie well away from the elbow and overlying scar. The distal end of the transposed nerve is cauterized to "cap" the nerve endings with connective tissue and placed either in a muscular bed or in subcutaneous tissue, depending on the patient's body habitus.

Recurrent Guyon Canal Compression

Patients who have persistent ulnar intrinsic atrophy after the release of Guyon canal need to be evaluated to ensure that there is not another cause of the ulnar intrinsic atrophy, as described previously. If not, reexploration can be considered. In our experience, the majority of surgeons do not adequately release the deep motor branch of the ulnar nerve as it curves around the hook of the hamate below the hypothenar muscles. Review of the previous operative notes should provide insight about whether that portion of the procedure had been performed.

For Case Studies, Videos, and more, please visit ExpertConsult.com.

REFERENCES

1. Agee JM, Peimer CA, Pyrek JD, et al: Endoscopic carpal tunnel release: A prospective study of complications and surgical experience. *J Hand Surg Am* 20A:165–172, 1995.
2. Amadio PC, Silverstein MD, Ilstrup DM, et al: Outcome assessment for carpal tunnel surgery: The relative responsiveness of generic, arthritis-specific, disease-specific and physical examination measures. *J Hand Surg Am* 21A:338–346, 1996.
3. Apefelberg DB, Larson SJ: Dynamic anatomy of the ulnar nerve at the elbow. *Plast Reconstr Surg* 51(1):76–81, 1973.
4. Atroshi I, Flondell M, Hofer M, et al: Methylprednisolone injections for the carpal tunnel syndrome: a randomized, placebo-controlled trial. *Ann Intern Med* 159(5):309–317, 2013.
5. Bartels RHMA, Menovsky T, Van Overbeeke JJ, et al: Surgical management of ulnar nerve compression at the elbow: an analysis of the literature. *J Neurosurg* 89:722–727, 1998.
6. Bernard BP: *Musculoskeletal disorders and workplace factors. DHHS(NIOSH) Publication No. 97-141*, Cincinnati, 1997, U.S. Department of Health and Human Services.
7. Blair WF, Goetz DD, Ross MA, et al: Carpal tunnel release with and without epineurotomy: A comparative prospective trial. *J Hand Surg Am* 21A:655–661, 1996.
8. Brininger TL, Rogers JC, Holm MB, et al: Efficacy of a fabricated customized splint and tendon and nerve gliding exercises for the treatment of carpal tunnel syndrome: A randomized controlled trial. *Arch Phys Med Rehabil* 88:1429–1435, 2007.
9. Brown JM, Mohktee D, Evangelista MS, et al: Scratch collapse test localizes Osborne's band as the point of maximal nerve compression in cubital tunnel syndrome. *Hand* 4:50–54, 2009.
10. Butler DS: *Mobilisation of the nervous system*, Melbourne, 1991, Churchill Livingstone.
11. Castillo TN, Yao J: Prospective randomized comparison of single-incision and two-inciison carpal tunnel release outcomes. *Hand* 9:36–42, 2014.
12. Celiker R, Arslan S, Inanici F: Corticosteroid injection vs nonsteroidal antiinflammatory drug and splinting in carpal tunnel syndrome. *Am J Phys Med Rehabil* 81(3):182–186, 2002.
13. Cheng CJ, Mackinnon-Patterson B, Beck JL, et al: The scratch collapse test for evaluation of carpal and cubital tunnel syndrome. *J Hand Surg Am* 33A:1518–1524, 2008.
14. Chow JC: Endoscopic carpal tunnel release: Two-portal technique. *Hand Clin* 10:637–646, 1994.
15. Chung KC, Pillsbury MS, Walters MR, et al: Reliability and validity testing of the Michigan Hand Outcomes Questionnaire. *J Hand Surg Am* 23A(4):575–587, 1998.
16. Cobb TK: Endoscopic cubital tunnel release. *J Hand Surg Am* 35A:1690–1697, 2010.
17. Dale A, Novak CB, Mackinnon SE: Utility of vibration thresholds in patients with brachial plexus nerve compression. *Ann Plast Surg* 42(6):613–618, 1999.
18. de Krom MCTFM, Knipschild PG, Kester ADM, et al: Efficacy of provocative tests for diagnosis of carpal tunnel syndrome. *Lancet* 335:393–395, 1990.
19. Dellon AL: Review of treatment results for ulnar nerve entrapment at the elbow. *J Hand Surg Am* 14A(4):688–700, 1989.
20. Dellon AL, Mackinnon SE: Chronic nerve compression model for the double crush hypothesis. *Ann Plast Surg* 26(3):259–264, 1991.
21. Ebersole GC, Davidge K, Damiano M, et al: Validity and responsiveness of the DASH questionnaire as an outcome measure following ulnar nerve transposition for cubital tunnel syndrome. *Plast Reconstr Surg* 132:81e–90e, 2013.
22. Faour-Martin O, Martin-Ferrero MA, Almaraz-Gomez A, et al: The long-term postoperative electromyographic evaluation of patients who have undergone carpal tunnel decompression. *J Bone Joint Surg* 94B(7):941–945, 2012.
23. Gay RE, Amadio PC, Johnson JC: Comparative responsiveness of the Disabilities of the Arm, Shoulder and Hand, the Carpal Tunnel Questionnaire, and the SF-36

to clinical change after carpal tunnel release. *J Hand Surg Am* 28A(2):250–254, 2003.

24. Gelberman RH, Aronson D, Weisman MH: Carpal tunnel syndrome. Results of a prospective trial of steroid injection and splinting. *J Bone Joint Surg* 62A:1181–1184, 1980.
25. Gelberman RH, Hergenroeder PT, Hargens AR, et al: The carpal tunnel syndrome: A study of carpal canal pressures. *J Bone Joint Surg* 63A:380–383, 1981.
26. Gelberman RH, Yamaguchi K, Hollstien SB, et al: Changes in interstitial pressure and cross-sectional area of the cubital tunnel and of the ulnar nerve with flexion of the elbow. *J Bone Joint Surg* 80A(4):492–501, 1998.
27. Gerwin M, Hotchkiss RN, Weiland AJ: Alternative operative exposures of the posterior aspect of the humeral diaphysis with reference to the radial nerve. *J Bone Joint Surg* 78A(11):1690–1695, 1996.
28. Gillenwater J, Cheng J, Mackinnon SE: Evaluation of the scratch collapse test in peroneal nerve compression. *Plast Reconstr Surg* 128(4):933–939, 2011.
29. Green DP: Diagnostic and therapeutic value of carpal tunnel injection. *J Hand Surg Am* 9A:850–854, 1984.
30. Greenslade JR, Mehta RL, Belward P, et al: Dash and Boston questionnaire assessment of carpal tunnel syndrome outcome: what is the responsiveness of an outcome questionnaire? *J Hand Surg Am* 29B(2):159–164, 2004.
31. Hadler NM: Repetitive upper extremity motions in the workplace are not hazardous. *J Hand Surg Am* 22A(1):19–29, 1997.
32. Hansen TB, Majeed HG: Endoscopic carpal tunnel release. *Hand Clin* 30:47–53, 2014.
33. Hefford C, Abbot JH, Arnold R, et al: The patient-specific functional scale: validity, reliability, and responsiveness in patients with upper extremity musculoskeletal problems. *J Orthop Sports Phys Ther* 42:56–65, 2012.
34. Heybeli N, Kutluhan S, Demirci S, et al: Assessment of outcome of carpal tunnel syndrome: a comparison of electrophysiological findings and a self-administered Boston Questionnaire. *J Hand Surg Am* 27B(3):259–264, 2002.
35. Hudak PL, Amadio PC, Bombardier C: Development of an upper extremity outcome measure: The DASH (Disabilities of the Arm, Shoulder and Hand). *Am J Ind Med* 29(6):602–608, 1996.
36. Huemer GM, Koller M, Pachinger T, et al: Postoperative splinting after open carpal tunnel release does not improve functional and neurological outcome. *Muscle Nerve* 36:528–531, 2007.
37. Hurst LC, Weissberg D, Carroll RE: The relationship of the double crush to carpal tunnel syndrome. *J Hand Surg Am* 10B(2):202–204, 1985.
38. Jablecki CK, Andary MT, So YT, et al: Literature review of the usefulness of nerve conduction studies and electromyography for the evaluation of patients with carpal tunnel syndrome. *Muscle Nerve* 16(12):1392–1414, 1993.
39. Karpitskaya Y, Novak CB, Mackinnon SE: Prevalence of smoking, obesity, diabetes mellitus and thyroid disease in patients with carpal tunnel syndrome. *Ann Plast Surg* 48:269–273, 2002.
40. Katz JN, Stirrat CR, Larson MG, et al: A self-administered hand symptom diagram for the diagnosis and epidemiologic study of carpal tunnel syndrome. *J Rheumatol* 17(11):1495–1498, 1990.
41. Kendall FP, McCreary EK, Provance PG: *Muscles: testing and function*, Baltimore, 1993, Williams & Wilkins.
42. Kleinman WB, Bishop AT: Anterior intramuscular transposition of the ulnar nerve. *J Hand Surg Am* 14A(6):972–979, 1989.
43. Lanz U: Anatomic variations of the median nerve in the carpal tunnel. *J Hand Surg Am* 2A:44–53, 1977.
44. Leinberry CF, Rivlin M, Maltenfort M, et al: Treatment of carpal tunnel syndrome by members of the American Society for Surgery of the Hand: A 25-year perspective. *J Hand Surg Am* 37A:1997–2003, 2012.
45. Leite JC, Jerosch-Herold C, Song F: A systematic review of the psychometric properties of the Boston Carpal Tunnel Questionnaire. *BMC Musculoskelet Disord* 7(78):1–9, 2006.
46. Levin S, Pearsall G, Ruderman RJ: Von Frey's methods of measuring pressure sensibility in the hand: An engineering analysis of the Weinstein-Semmes pressure aesthesiometer. *J Hand Surg Am* 3A:211–216, 1978.
47. Levine DW, Simmons BP, Koris MJ, et al: A self-administered questionnaire for the assessment of severity of symptoms and functional status in carpal tunnel syndrome. *J Bone Joint Surg* 75A(11):1585–1592, 1993.
48. Levis CM, Tung TH, Mackinnon SE: Variations in incisions and postoperative management in carpal tunnel surgery. *Can J Plast Surg* 10:63–67, 2002.
49. Lowe JB, Mackinnon SE: Management of secondary cubital tunnel syndrome. *Plast Reconstr Surg* 113:1e–16e, 2004.
50. Lowe JB, Maggi S, Mackinnon SE: The position of crossing branches of the medial antebrachial cutaneous nerve during cubital tunnel surgery in humans. *Plast Reconstr Surg* 114:692–696, 2004.
51. Lowe JB, Novak CB, Mackinnon SE: Current approach to cubital tunnel syndrome. *Neurosurg Clin N Am* 12(2):267–284, 2001.
52. Lundborg G: *Nerve injury and repair: regeneration, reconstruction, and cortical remodeling*, ed 2, New York, 2004, Elsevier.

53. Lundborg G, Lie-Stenstrom A, Stromberg T, et al: Digital vibrogram: A new diagnostic tool for sensory testing in compression neuropathy. *J Hand Surg Am* 11A:693–699, 1986.
54. Lundborg G, Myers R, Powell H: Nerve compression injury and increased endoneurial fluid pressure: A miniature compartment syndrome. *J Neurol Neurosurg Psychiatry* 46:1119–1124, 1983.
55. Lundborg G, Rydevik BL: Effects of stretching the tibial nerve of the rabbit: Preliminary study of the intraneural circulation of the barrier function of the perineurium. *J Bone Joint Surg* 55B:390–401, 1973.
56. Macadam SA, Gandhi R, Bezuhly M, et al: Simple decompression versus anterior subcutaneous and submuscular transposition of the ulnar nerve for cubital tunnel syndrome: a meta-analysis. *J Hand Surg Am* 33A:1314–1324, 2014.
57. MacDermid J: Accuracy of clinical tests used in the detection of carpal tunnel syndrome: A literature review. *J Hand Ther* 4:169–176, 1991.
58. Mackinnon SE: Secondary carpal tunnel syndrome. *Neurosurg Clin N Am* 2:75–91, 1991.
59. Mackinnon SE: Submuscular transposition of the ulnar nerve at the elbow. In Rengachary SS, Wilkins RH, editors: *Neurosurgical operative atlas*, Park Ridge, IL, 1995, American Association of Neurological Surgeons, pp 225–233.
60. Mackinnon SE, Dellon AL: The overlap pattern of the lateral antebrachial cutaneous nerve and the superficial branch of the radial nerve. *J Hand Surg Am* 10A:522–526, 1985.
61. Mackinnon SE, Dellon AL: Anatomic investigations of nerves at the wrist: I. Orientation of the motor fascicle of the median nerve in the carpal tunnel. *Ann Plast Surg* 21:32–35, 1988.
62. Mackinnon SE, Dellon AL, Hudson AR, et al: A primate model for chronic nerve compression. *J Reconstr Microsurg* 1:185–195, 1985.
63. Mackinnon SE, Dellon AL, Hudson AR, et al: Chronic human nerve compression: a histological assessment. *Neuropathol Appl Neurobiol* 12:547–565, 1986.
64. Mackinnon SE, Dellon AL, Hudson AR, et al: Histopathology of chronic nerve compression of the superficial radial nerve in the forearm. *J Hand Surg Am* 11A:206–210, 1986.
65. Mackinnon SE, Hudson AR, Gentili F, et al: Peripheral nerve injection injury with steroid agents. *Plast Reconstr Surg* 69:482–489, 1982.
66. Mackinnon SE, McCabe S, Murray JF: Internal neurolysis fails to improve the results of primary carpal tunnel decompression. *J Hand Surg Am* 16A:211–218, 1991.
67. Mackinnon SE, Novak CB: Clinical commentary: Pathogenesis of cumulative trauma disorder. *J Hand Surg Am* 19A(5):073–003, 1994.
68. Mackinnon SE, Novak CB: Repetitive strain in the workplace. *J Hand Surg Am* 22A:2–18, 1997.
69. Mackinnon SE, Novak CB: Nerve Transfers. *Hand Clin* 15(4):643–666, 1999.
70. Mackinnon SE, Novak CB: Operative findings in reoperation of patients with cubital tunnel syndrome. *Hand* 2(3):137–142, 2007.
71. Masear VR, Meyer RD, Pichora DR: Surgical anatomy of the medial antebrachial cutaneous nerves. *J Hand Surg Am* 14A:267–271, 1989.
72. McGowan AJ: The results of transposition of the ulnar nerve for traumatic ulnar neuritis. *J Bone Joint Surg* 32B(3):293–301, 1950.
73. McMillan CR, Binhammer PA: Which outcome measure is the best? Evaluating responsiveness of the Disabilities of the Arm, Shoulder and Hand questionnaire, the Michigan Hand Questionnaire and the Patient-Specific Functional Scale following hand and wrist surgery. *Hand* 4(3):311–318, 2009.
74. Melzack R: The McGill pain questionnaire: Major properties and scoring methods. *Pain* 1(3):277–299, 1975.
75. Mowlavi A, Andrews K, Lille S, et al: The management of cubital tunnel syndrome: A meta-analysis of clinical studies. *Plast Reconstr Surg* 106(2):327–334, 2000.
76. Nakamichi K, Tachibana S: Restricted motion of the median nerve in carpal tunnel syndrome. *J Hand Surg Am* 20B(4):460–464, 1995.
77. Nathan PA, Keniston RC, Lockwood RS, et al: Tobacco, caffeine, alcohol and carpal tunnel syndrome in American industry. A cross-sectional study of 1464 workers. *J Occup Environ Med* 38(3):290–298, 1996.
78. Nathan PA, Keniston RC, Myers LD, et al: Obesity as a risk factor for slowing of sensory conduction of the median nerve in industry. *J Occup Med* 34:379–383, 1992.
79. Nemoto K, Matsumoto N, Tazaki K, et al: An experimental study on the "double crush" hypothesis. *J Hand Surg Am* 12A(4):552–559, 1987.
80. Novak CB, Lee GW, Mackinnon SE, et al: Provocative testing for cubital tunnel syndrome. *J Hand Surg Am* 19A(5):817–820, 1994.
81. Novak CB, Mackinnon SE: Outcome following implantation of a peripheral nerve stimulator in patients with chronic nerve pain. *Plast Reconstr Surg* 105(6):1967–1972, 2000.
82. Novak CB, Mackinnon SE: Selection of operative procedures for cubital tunnel syndrome. *Hand* 4(1):50–54, 2009.
83. Novak CB, Mackinnon SE, Patterson GA: Evaluation of patients with thoracic outlet syndrome. *J Hand Surg Am* 18A(2):292–299, 1993.

84. Novak CB, Mackinnon SE, Stuebe AM: Patient self-reported outcome after ulnar nerve transposition. *Ann Plast Surg* 48(3):274–280, 2002.

85. Novak CB, Mackinnon SE, Williams JI, et al: Establishment of reliability in the evaluation of hand sensibility. *Plast Reconstr Surg* 92(2):311–322, 1993.

86. Novak CB, Mehdian H, von Schroeder HP: Laxity of the ulnar nerve during elbow flexion and extension. *J Hand Surg Am* 37A:1163–1167, 2012.

87. O'Brien JP, Mackinnon SE, MacLean AR, et al: A model of chronic nerve compression in the rat. *Ann Plast Surg* 19(5):430–435, 1987.

88. O'Driscoll SW, Jaloszynski R, Morrey BF, et al: Origin of the medial ulnar collateral ligament. *J Hand Surg Am* 17A:164–168, 1992.

89. Ogata K, Manske PR, Lesker PA: The effects of surgical dissection on regional blood flow to the ulnar nerve in the cubital tunnel. *Clin Orthop Relat Res* 193:195–198, 1985.

90. Panel on Musculoskeletal Disorders and the Workplace: *Musculoskeletal disorders and the workplace*, Washington, D.C., 2001, National Academy Press.

91. Parsonage MJ, Turner JW: Neuralgic amyotrophy: The shoulder-girdle syndrome. *Lancet* 254:974–978, 1948.

92. Patel MR, Bassini L: A comparison of five tests for determining hand sensibility. *J Reconstr Microsurg* 15(7):523–526, 1999.

93. Pechan J, Julis I: The pressure measurement in the ulnar nerve. A contribution to the pathophysiology of the cubital tunnel syndrome. *J Biomech* 8:75–79, 1975.

94. Phalen GS: The carpal tunnel syndrome: Seventeen years experience in diagnosis and treatment of six hundred and fifty four hands. *J Bone Joint Surg* 48A(2):211–228, 1966.

95. Phalen GS: The carpal tunnel syndrome. Clinical evaluation of 598 hands. *Clin Orthop Relat Res* 83:29–40, 1972.

96. Rempel D, Evanoff BA, Amadio PC, et al: Consensus criteria for the classification of carpal tunnel syndrome in epidemiologic studies. *Am J Public Health* 88(10):1447–1451, 1998.

97. Ross DC, Mackinnon SE, Chang YL: Intraneural anatomy of the median nerve provides "third web space" donor nerve graft. *J Reconstr Microsurg* 8:225–232, 1992.

98. Rozmaryn LM, Dovelle S, Rothman ER, et al: Nerve and tendon gliding exercises and the conservative management of carpal tunnel syndrome. *J Hand Ther* 11:171–179, 1998.

99. Sahrmann SA: *Diagnosis and treatment of movement impairment syndromes*, St. Louis, 2002, Mosby.

100. Seradge H, Parker W, Baer C, et al: Conservative treatment of carpal tunnel syndrome: an outcome study of adjunct exercises. *J Okla State Med Assoc* 95:7–14, 2002.

101. Shi Q, MacDermid JC, Santaguida PL, et al: Predictors of surgical outcomes following anterior transpostion of ulnar nerve for cubital tunnel syndrome: a systematic review. *J Hand Surg Am* 36A(12):e1–e6, 2011.

102. Stratford P, Gill C, Westaway M, et al: Assessing disability and change on individual patients: A report of a patient specific measure. *Physiotherapy Canada* 47(4):258–262, 1995.

103. Strauch B, Lang A, Ferder M, et al: The Ten Test. *Plast Reconstr Surg* 99(4):1074–1078, 1997.

104. Sunderland S: *Nerve and nerve injuries*, ed 2, Edinburgh, 1978, Churchill Livingstone.

105. Szabo RM, Bay BK, Sharkey NA: Median nerve displacement through the carpal tunnel. *J Hand Surg Am* 19A:901–906, 1994.

106. Taleisnik J: The palmar cutaneous branch of the median nerve and the apporach to the carpal tunnel: An anatomical study. *J Bone Joint Surg* 55A:1212–1217, 1973.

107. Thoma A, Veltri K, Haines T, et al: A meta-analysis of randomized controlled trials comparing endoscopic and open carpal tunnel decompression. *Plast Reconstr Surg* 114(5):1137–1146, 2008.

108. Tong HC, Haig AJ, Yamakawa K: The Spurling test and cervical radiculopathy. *Spine* 27:156–159, 2002.

109. Tung TH, Mackinnon SE: Flexor digitorum superficialis nerve transfer to restore pronation: Two case reports and anatomic study. *J Hand Surg Am* 26A:1065–1072, 2001.

110. Turner JW, Parsonage MJ: Neuralgic anyotrophy (paralytic brachial neuritis) with special reference to prognosis. *Lancet* 273:209–211, 1957.

111. Upton ARM, McComas AJ: The double crush in nerve-entrapment syndromes. *Lancet* 2:359–362, 1973.

112. van Vliet D, Novak CB, Mackinnon SE: Duration of contact time alters cutaneous pressure threshold measurements. *Ann Plast Surg* 31(4):335–339, 1993.

113. Vernadakis AJ, Koch H, Mackinnon SE: Management of neuromas. *Clin Plast Surg* 30:247–268, 2003.

114. Watanabe M, Yamaga M, Kato T, et al: The implication of repeated versus continuous strain on nerve function in a rat forelimb model. *J Hand Surg Am* 26A:663–669, 2001.

115. Watchmaker GP, Lee GW, Mackinnon SE: Intraneural topography of the ulnar nerve in the cubital tunnel facilitates anterior transposition. *J Hand Surg Am* 19A(6):915–922, 1994.

116. Weiss AP, Sachar K, Gendreau M: Conservative management of carpal tunnel syndrome: A reexamination of steroid injection and splinting. *J Hand Surg Am* 19A:410–415, 1994.

117. Weiss ND, Gordon L, Bloom T, et al: Position of the wrist associated with the lowest carpal-tunnel pressures: Implications for splint design. *J Bone Joint Surg* 77A(11):1695–1699, 1995.

118. Werner R, Franzblau A, Johnston E: Comparison of multiple frequency vibrometry testing and sensory nerve conduction measures in screening for carpal tunnel syndrome in an industrial setting. *Am J Phys Med Rehabil* 74(2):101–106, 1995.

119. Wilbourn AJ: The electrodiagnostic examination with peripheral nerve injuries. *Clin Plast Surg* 30:139–154, 2003.

120. Williams TM, Mackinnon SE, Novak CB, et al: Verification of the pressure provocative test in carpal tunnel syndrome. *Ann Plast Surg* 29(1):8–11, 1992.

121. Zieske L, Ebersole GC, Davidge K, et al: Revision carpal tunnel surgery: a 10-year review of intraoperative findings and outcomes. *J Hand Surg Am* 38A(8):1530–1539, 2013.

29

Thoracic Outlet Compression Syndrome

Richard Meyer

Acknowledgment: The author would like to thank and acknowledge the work of Dr. Karen Johnson Jones in previous versions of this chapter.

> These videos may be found at
> *ExpertConsult.com:*
> 29.1 Resection with improved pulse: Complete mobilization of the subclavian artery is required to visualize the lower trunk, and this includes ligation of the deep transverse cervical artery when present. Note the presence of sutures. Complete decompression also requires excision of anterior and medial scalene muscles; note the pleura and lung deep to the vessel. © Scott W. Wolfe, MD.

Treatment of peripheral nerve compression in the upper extremity is one of the main components of a hand surgeon's practice; however, most of them shy away from treatment of thoracic outlet syndrome (TOS). Seeing that objective electrodiagnostic studies of TOS can confirm clinical suspicions, refute them, or determine the stage of disease, there is little controversy about treatment regimens for carpal tunnel, cubital tunnel, and other entrapment neuropathies. Because TOS is a compressive neuropathy that may include all of the nerves to the upper extremity, neck, shoulder, upper back, and chest, it may share the characteristics of or mimic the other compressive neuropathies. For most surgeons who do not regularly operate on the upper extremity, and for many who do, there are few disorders as difficult to diagnose or as frustrating to treat as TOS. Diagnosis of it is by exclusion and suspicion, which often are based on clinical diagnostic criteria alone, because there is no definitive electrodiagnostic test that can verify the surgeon's opinion. Most TOS patients have seen an average of 4.7 doctors before a diagnosis is established.[40]

Although hand surgeons see many patients with vague upper-extremity pain, few have received training in recognition and treatment of TOS. In major texts that describe TOS, there are no chapters by hand surgeons. Because the area of compression lies in "expensive real estate," even fewer treat TOS surgically, and still fewer operate without collaborating with a vascular or thoracic surgeon. In an email survey of the American Society for Surgery of the Hand (ASSH) membership regarding TOS, 60% of respondents reported that they treat patients, but only 19% perform surgery for TOS, and only 10 of the 255 hand surgeons who responded treat more than 10 cases per year. A third of respondents operate with a vascular or thoracic surgeon present; this may be appropriate because the typical fellowship-trained hand surgeon may not be prepared to handle the potential risks. Interestingly, almost 20% of the respondents did not believe TOS exists as a legitimate diagnosis.[110]

HISTORY

Historically significant events in the early recognition of TOS as a clinical entity are detailed in the text by Sanders and Haug, *Thoracic Outlet Syndrome: A Common Sequela of Neck Injuries*.[91] These authors note three important historical periods, and the reader is referred to that text for a comprehensive discussion of the individual historical events. A second excellent source of historical information and state-of-the-art treatment is available as a monograph published as an edition of *Hand Clinics*.[109]

CLASSIFICATION

The two basic types of TOS are vascular and neurogenic. The vascular type is further divided into arterial and venous subtypes, and the neurogenic type has been subdivided into "true" and "disputed" neurogenic. The subclassification and distinction of true versus disputed neurogenic TOS are attributed to Wilbourn.[111]

Patients with the arterial, venous, and electrically positive neurogenic TOS present with an obvious mechanical obstruction to blood flow, or have positive nerve conduction study results, rarely have secondary concerns (e.g., workers' compensation issues, litigation) that cloud the issue. Diagnosis by physical examination, routine diagnostic imaging, or testing for neurogenic TOS is straightforward, and surgical treatment, when indicated, is relatively successful.

The fourth subtype (i.e., disputed neurogenic), however, has been more difficult for some patients to accept. Although the classification was described first in 1984, it is time to drop this nomenclature and adopt the term *electrically negative neurogenic TOS*. This is because patients with it account for up to 97% of all those diagnosed and treated for TOS. It is only a disputed entity for those clinicians who must do objective diagnostic studies or imaging. So far there have been no definitive studies or means by which one can make the diagnosis; therein lies the problem.

Arterial Thoracic Outlet Syndrome

Arterial TOS is uncommon, accounting for only 1 to 2% of all cases of TOS. There is almost always an osseous anomaly such as a cervical rib, an anomalous first rib, or a history of fracture

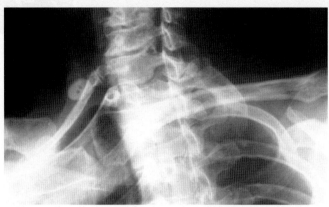

FIGURE 29.1 An oblique radiograph of the cervical spine of a patient with a complete right cervical rib and true thoracic outlet syndrome ("button marks" on the rib). (From the Christine M. Kleinert Institute for Hand and Microsurgery, Inc., with permission).

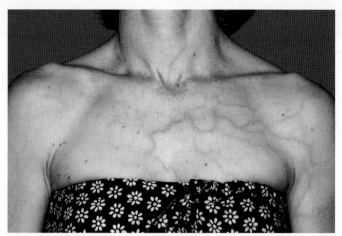

FIGURE 29.2 Photograph of venous collaterals in a patient's left anterior chest with subclavian thrombosis (i.e., Paget-Schroetter syndrome).

(Figure 29.1). Arterial TOS may present as a limb-threatening condition. The subclavian artery can become stenotic or develop an aneurysm because of compression between the rib and the clavicle or because of traction over the cervical rib. In addition, it can ulcerate, become occluded, or become thrombotic.[26,42] There can be fingertip ulcerations, Raynaud's symptoms, pain, and claudication. The arterial type is more commonly indolent and has a history that suggests intermittent complete or partial arterial occlusion. Symptoms may be brought on by sports activities that place the upper extremity in an extended and hyperabducted position. Clavicle nonunion, malunion, post-traumatic subluxation of the sternoclavicular joint, and rib fractures also have been identified as causes.[26]

Venous Thoracic Outlet Syndrome

Venous TOS is slightly more common than the arterial type and represents 2 to 3% of all cases. These patients may have a sudden, effort-induced thrombosis (i.e., Paget-Schroetter syndrome) or, less commonly, a thrombosis that occurs at rest with the extremity in a compromised position for a prolonged time. There may be intermittent venous compression alone or intermittent compression that precedes a sudden event. With time, large venous collaterals around the shoulder, chest, or breast may develop (Figure 29.2).

In acute thrombosis, pain, edema, and cyanosis are dramatic. In contrast, in patients who have a history of intermittent compression, collateral venous drainage minimizes the signs of distal swelling and cyanosis. In the intermittent compression group, however, fullness in the supraclavicular and infraclavicular areas may make the clavicle difficult to discern. Most acute venous TOS is seen in muscular young males with symptoms that develop after vigorous exercise or physical exertion. Throwing athletes and swimmers have been recognized as "at risk" owing to repetitive extremity positioning in postures that occlude the subclavian vein.[19] Hypercoagulable states put these people at risk as well.

Neurogenic Thoracic Outlet Syndrome

True or electrically positive neurogenic TOS is also rare, occurring in 1 out of 1 million patients with TOS.[27] These patients have objective physical evidence of chronic nerve compression

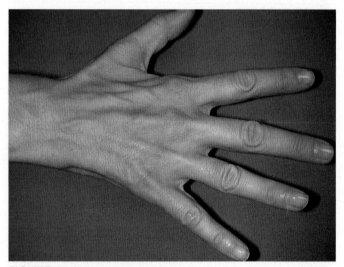

FIGURE 29.3 Photograph of a patient with true thoracic outlet syndrome; it demonstrates intrinsic atrophy of the right hand.

(e.g., hypothenar atrophy, decreased grip, and sensory deficits), usually in the C8-T1 distribution (Figure 29.3). The pain and paresthesias seen in the other subtypes also may occur. In true neurogenic TOS there may be a bony anomaly causing the compression, such as a rudimentary or fully developed cervical rib[76] (Figures 29.4 and 29.5), although most patients I have seen with this just have compressive bands.

Electrically Negative Neurogenic Thoracic Outlet Syndrome

This type of TOS is by far the most commonly encountered (>95% of cases). These patients have a wide variety of upper extremity complaints, and usually no objective findings are found on electrodiagnostic testing, Doppler imaging, pulse volume recordings, or radiographs. Even though there may be some ambiguity of symptoms, most patients have numbness in the hand and pain in the arm, hand, and especially the shoulder and neck. Frequently there is activity-related or positional exacerbation. Most TOS surgeons would agree that physical complaints reproduced by provocative testing alone, in the absence

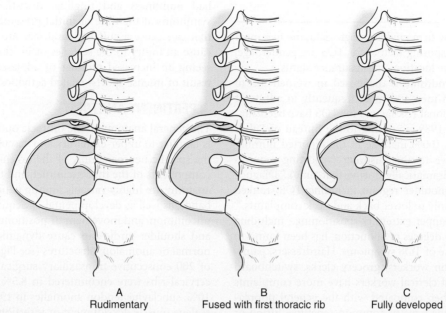

FIGURE 29.4 Three common variants of cervical ribs: **A,** rudimentary; **B,** fused with first thoracic rib; **C,** fully developed. (Redrawn from the Christine M. Kleinert Institute for Hand and Microsurgery, Inc., with permission).

A
Rudimentary

B
Fused with first thoracic rib

C
Fully developed

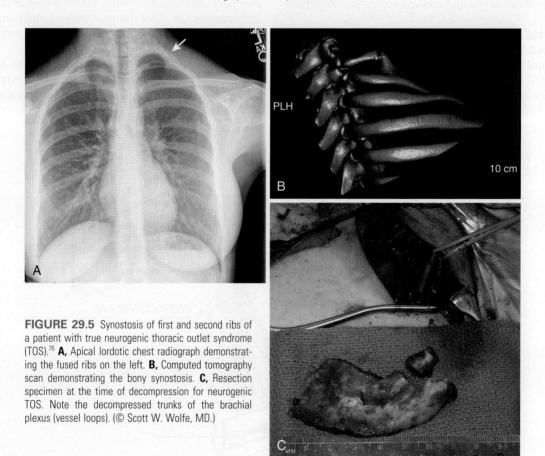

FIGURE 29.5 Synostosis of first and second ribs of a patient with true neurogenic thoracic outlet syndrome (TOS).[76] **A,** Apical lordotic chest radiograph demonstrating the fused ribs on the left. **B,** Computed tomography scan demonstrating the bony synostosis. **C,** Resection specimen at the time of decompression for neurogenic TOS. Note the decompressed trunks of the brachial plexus (vessel loops). (© Scott W. Wolfe, MD.)

of another explanation for the patient's complaints, are sufficient to justify a working diagnosis of neurogenic TOS. In our practice, numbness in the ulnar nerve distribution of a patient with clinical symptoms suggestive of TOS, but with negative electrodiagnostic studies, is indicative of TOS until proven otherwise.

In 1982, Roos classified TOS according to the segment of the brachial plexus involved.[82] Categories of compression include upper trunk, lower trunk, and combined. Symptoms attributable to the lower- and combined-compression groups are found in 85 to 90% of all patients with TOS. Electrical studies are of no value for this classification scheme.

EPIDEMIOLOGY

Although there are few firm epidemiologic data, the five most frequently cited predisposing factors for TOS are gender, age, occupation, geographic location, and insurance status.

Thoracic outlet syndrome is diagnosed in women 3.5 to 4 times as often as in men and most frequently in adults of working age. Occupational risk factors for TOS have been suggested. From 1987 to 1989, according to the Bureau of Labor Statistics, there was a 100% increase in the reported number of cases of cumulative trauma disorder (reporting requirements also changed dramatically during that time).[9] Diagnoses reported in the shoulder region, including TOS, ranked second in frequency only to lower back and neck complaints.[96] Awkward or static upper-extremity positioning, including holding the arm in 45 degrees of abduction, has been found to increase the prevalence of TOS symptoms. Hairdressers, painters, heavy construction workers, grocery clerks, switchboard operators, nurses, and clerical workers have more complaints of TOS symptoms when compared with the general population. These occupations have in common repetitive lifting or repetitive, uninterrupted arm movements with the hand at or above the shoulder level, and awkward or static extremity posture.[41,78,96]

The reported incidence of TOS in the general population is 1% or 2%, and it may be this low because TOS is underdiagnosed and undertreated.[3,83] In my series of several hundred patients with TOS, 25% of them had previously had shoulder surgery on the same side. Also, in the same group of patients with rotator cuff and shoulder injuries, a significant number had numbness and tingling, dysesthesias, and neurogenic symptoms at the time of initial presentation. The same forces that can cause a cuff or labral tear are certainly sufficient to cause an injury to the scalenes or brachial plexus. We are now seeing an increased number of adolescent TOS patients as a result of intense sports–related activities.

▶ PERTINENT ANATOMY

The general anatomy of the thoracic outlet and brachial plexus is familiar to upper-extremity and vascular surgeons. However, the specific neuroanatomy of the brachial plexus, the vascular components of the thoracic outlet, and the bony and muscular anatomy are highly variable among patients. Fibrous or fascial bands, as well as developmental or acquired variations, are not uncommon, and movement or positioning of the neck, thorax, and shoulder girdle can cause dynamic compression against normal or anomalous structures (see Figure 29.4). In one series of 200 consecutive transaxillary surgical approaches for TOS, cervical ribs were encountered in 8.5%, scalenus minimus in 10%, subclavius tendon anomalies in 19.5%, and anomalies of scalene muscle development or insertion in 43%.[53] The limited exposure of the plexus afforded by the transaxillary approach may have obscured additional anomalies. In another study of 250 cadavers (i.e., 500 thoracic outlets), anatomic anomalies were noted in 46%.[75] In a study of 40 aborted fetuses, anomalies were found in 60%.[24,74]

The anatomic corridor in the thoracic outlet has been partitioned into three sections: the interscalene triangle, the costoclavicular triangle, and the subcoracoid or pectoralis minor space (Figure 29.6).

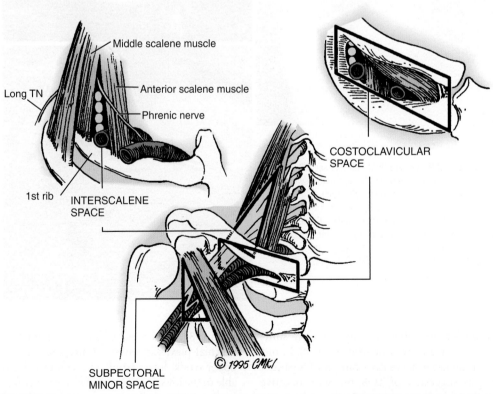

FIGURE 29.6 The three anatomic triangles of the thoracic outlet. *TN,* Thoracic nerve. (From the Christine M. Kleinert Institute for Hand and Microsurgery, Inc., with permission.)

Interscalene Triangle

The interscalene triangle (the most common site for compression) is defined anteriorly by the anterior scalene muscle, posteriorly by the middle scalene muscle, and inferiorly by the first rib. The subclavian vein passes anterior to the anterior scalene and just inferior and lateral to the costocoracoid or costoclavicular ligament.[53] The subclavian artery passes with the plexus between the anterior and middle scalenes. The anterior scalene originates from the anterior tubercles of the transverse processes of C3 to C6. The middle scalene originates from the posterior tubercles of the transverse processes of C2 to C7.[67]

A wide range of anatomic variation can predispose to pathology. Actual crossing, or "intercostalization," of the scalene insertions has been found in 15% of cadaver dissections. It is not uncommon to find slips of the middle scalene penetrating between the upper and middle, or middle and lower, trunks causing direct compression with every contracture. This also may produce a "V"-shaped deformity at the base that can have a scissoring effect on the neural and vascular structures. Alternatively, a "U"-shaped formation can create a sling effect that places pressure on the structures from below.[3]

The scalenus minimus muscle comes up from C6 to C7 and inserts on the deep fascia between the subclavian artery and lower trunk, where it can produce a wedge effect on the lower

trunk.[3] It also may wrap around the subclavian artery and pull it against pleural bands, causing positional changes in flow. The downward slope of the first rib, when increased (more commonly seen in women), may drive the neurovascular structures into the angle formed by the lateral edge of the anterior scalene tendon and the first rib (see Figure 29.6, A).[67]

Cervical ribs, a commonly cited etiology for TOS, have been identified in 0.5 to 0.6% of the population and are bilateral in 50 to 80% of those affected. Because cervical rib growth is developmentally suppressed by a full contribution of the lower spinal nerve root (T1) to the plexus, there is an association between cervical ribs and a prefixed plexus.[53] Many cervical ribs will be incomplete but have a taut fibrous band, or "anlagen," connecting the bony tip to the first rib or deep fascia (see Figure 29.4, B). Such a fibrous band represents only one of many types or locations of fibrous bands that cause nerve compression in TOS patients.[99]

Roos[80,86] described nine different patterns of fibrous bands seen in clinical and cadaveric specimens, and Poitevin[71] reported three additional types of bands a decade later (Figure 29.7). The most frequently found bands were those seen to bowstring across the anterior concavity of the first rib, the "scalenus minimus" muscle band, and the fascial attachments between the anterior and middle scalene muscle groups, crossing the nerve roots of the brachial plexus in either an oblique or a perpendicular manner.

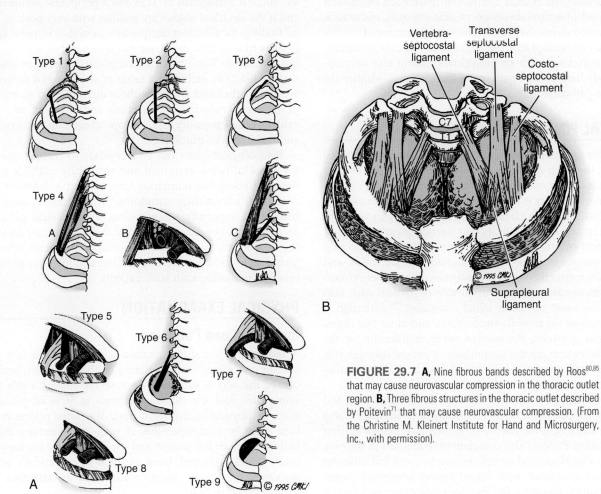

FIGURE 29.7 A, Nine fibrous bands described by Roos[80,85] that may cause neurovascular compression in the thoracic outlet region. **B,** Three fibrous structures in the thoracic outlet described by Poitevin[71] that may cause neurovascular compression. (From the Christine M. Kleinert Institute for Hand and Microsurgery, Inc., with permission).

Costoclavicular Triangle

The costoclavicular space is bounded anteriorly by the clavicle, subclavius muscle, and costocoracoid ligament; posteromedially by the first rib; and posterolaterally by the superior border of the scapula (see Figure 29.6). Physiologic narrowing of this space with limb movement is enhanced by the mobility of joints at both ends of the space's boundaries. A hypertrophied subclavius tendon insertion can apply compression specifically to the subclavian vein, as in Paget-Schroetter syndrome. Although there is little in the literature regarding the costocoracoid (or coracocostal) ligament, it can occasionally be much larger than the coracoacromial ligament and may firmly compress the plexus against the chest wall.

Subcoracoid or Pectoralis Minor Space

The subcoracoid space allows compression via three mechanisms. With arm abduction, the neurovascular bundle stretches around the coracoid, and external rotation of the scapula accentuates this pulley effect. Abduction also tenses the pectoralis minor tendon and, in some instances, the tendon and/or muscle belly may compress the plexus.

Histologic study of operative specimens from patients with TOS has demonstrated an increased amount of connective tissue in the scalene muscles, supporting theories of muscle imbalance or developmental abnormality that can lead to problems.[89] The influence of posture, repetitive strain, muscle imbalance, and eccentric muscle contraction have been extensively studied, and objective effects on muscle strength, endurance, and decreased sarcomere length have been documented.[23,25,88] It should be emphasized that the presence of these abnormalities must be correlated with an individual's growth and development, body habitus, and patterns of limb usage to identify the particular pathoanatomy.

CLINICAL FINDINGS

Because the vast majority of symptomatic patients are classified as having the electrically negative neurogenic type of TOS, the diagnosis is usually made by physical examination and provocative maneuvers. There is no substitute for experience in evaluating patients. Although clinical symptoms are highly variable, there are certain commonalities that warrant mention.

The most commonly reported complaints are chronic pain of insidious onset involving the shoulder girdle, neck, and upper back in association with paresthesias of the upper extremity. Paresthesias are present in up to 95% of patients with TOS and are the most common initial complaint.[106] Although it usually involves the medial arm, forearm, and ulnar two digits, paresthesias involving the median nerve distribution or the entire hand or arm are not uncommon. A patient may describe the pain as dull, nagging, or throbbing. Fatigue of the extremity when used in a provocative position is typical.

As in carpal tunnel syndrome, symptoms while driving and grooming are common. Women typically have difficulty doing their hair and frequently have to bend their heads down to limit arm deviation. Patients also complain of tenderness at the base of their necks. Nocturnal complaints are frequent but different from those associated with carpal tunnel syndrome. Some patients request narcotics, but they are rarely prescribed preoperatively. Tricyclic antidepressants, neurotropics, or benzodiazepines may help patients sleep. The clinician should exercise considerable caution when dispensing medications.

An association between distal nerve compression and TOS has been attributed to a form of double-crush syndrome.[45,49,56] Advocates of a double-crush theory have described carpal tunnel syndrome in 21 to 45% of patients with TOS; cubital tunnel syndrome in up to 10%; and, more rarely, radial tunnel syndrome, pronator syndrome, or cervical radiculopathy.[49,59] Critics believe that these "associations" are not actually separate areas of pathology but rather misdiagnoses.

Carroll and Hurst were the first to publish a large patient series with variable symptoms that they attributed to nerve compression at only one site.[10] Although in their study patients did have multiple areas of surgery, in-depth review of their symptoms revealed that relief was obtained by one procedure in each instance. These authors emphasized the difficulty of diagnosing carpal tunnel syndrome and differentiating it from TOS in patients with a primary complaint of shoulder pain. They also emphasized the importance of diagnosing and treating distal compression neuropathies in patients suspected of having TOS. These distal sites of compression are typically simpler and more economical to treat, with less risk to the patient.[51]

Others characterize TOS as a great mimicker and cite patients in whom the diagnosis of it is delayed because of multiple prior surgeries on distal nerves without relief.[72] In our practice, if we feel there is a diagnosis of TOS *and* a peripheral compression, and if the electrical studies are positive with very positive clinical findings for a distinct compression, and they respond appropriately to a discrete block, we will do a separate release of the involved nerve. Vague vascular complaints are very common in neurogenic TOS, including a sense of swelling and differential coolness of the hand, with or without discoloration. Complaints of migraine headaches are extremely common and, to a lesser extent, vertigo, memory loss, syncope, chest pain, eye irritation, and facial pain or numbness.[3,7,41,52,64,67]

Psychological issues can be secondary to chronic pain and the stress of being examined and treated by multiple practitioners, undergoing numerous tests without a definitive diagnosis, and unremitting symptoms.[32,47] Depression, anger, and frustration, especially when dealing with medical personnel, become more prevalent the longer the symptoms persist. For this reason, the concept of a multispecialty team approach, including psychological testing and therapy, may play an important role in dealing with such patients.

PHYSICAL EXAMINATION

Inspection and Palpation

A thorough physical examination with the patient in a gown and all concealing or constricting clothing, jewelry, and hair out of the way is essential. Because the history tends to be nonspecific and the clinical diagnosis in 97% of patients is made by physical examination alone, the initial patient evaluation must be comprehensive. A pain questionnaire may be helpful for both the patient and the clinician. Many unspoken issues can be gleaned from analysis of a patient's written responses on a pain questionnaire and an anatomic pain diagram (Figure 29.8).

The general appearance of the patient both standing and sitting should be noted, as follows:
- Does the patient slouch with the head in a forward position?
- Is the female patient particularly large breasted?
- Are there thick grooves in the shoulders from an "industrial-strength" brassiere?
- Is the neck held to one side?
- Is one shoulder drooping?
- Is there scapular asymmetry at rest or when moving the arms? If so, one must determine whether it is related to

shoulder pathology or to muscle imbalance with or without neurologic deficit.

Important clues to muscle imbalance should be sought. The skin and contour of the anterior and posterior chest wall should be inspected.

Masses, fullness, and, in particular, tenderness in the supra-clavicular and infraclavicular area, and venous engorgement or collaterals should be noted (see Figure 29.2). Most patients with TOS have moderate to significant tenderness in the anterior triangle and/or infraclavicular area as well. Dysesthesias and reproduction of radicular pain, when palpating these areas, is

---

Cervical Brachial Symptom Questionnaire ("CBSQ")

NAME _____ DATE _____

READ INSTRUCTIONS FIRST. This form is important for measuring the outcome of treatment.
Based on your experiences in the PAST WEEK, answer the following questions regarding how often symptoms would be likely to increase if you were to engage in certain activities.
Circle the number corresponding to how likely it would be for symptoms to increase during an activity so much that you would have to stop or modify the activity.
DO NOT LEAVE ANY BLANKS.
If a CONSTANT ongoing symptom would not be more noticeable during the activity, mark the answer "0."
If a symptom would increase during half of the instances of the activity, mark the answer "5."
Only mark "10" if your symptoms would increase during EVERY instance of the activity.

1. Pain going down the arm increases with neck movement, as in turning, flexing, or extending the neck.

    0   1   2   3   4   5   6   7   8   9   10
It would NEVER happen this past week   This past week, it would happen ALWAYS

2. Pain in the arm or shoulder increases instantly with brief shoulder movement as in throwing something or in reaching behind the body.

    0   1   2   3   4   5   6   7   8   9   10
It would NEVER happen this past week   This past week, it would happen ALWAYS

3. Hand or arm aches or fatigues with arm exercise, particularly with overhead or outstretched positioning.

    0   1   2   3   4   5   6   7   8   9   10
It would NEVER happen this past week   This past week, it would happen ALWAYS

4. Hand or arm swells after arm exercise, including after any activities that require repetitive arm movements.

    0   1   2   3   4   5   6   7   8   9   10
It would NEVER happen this past week   This past week, it would happen ALWAYS

5. Sensations of tingling or numbness in the hand or arm increase when reaching overhead or outwards. Examples include brushing hair or blow-drying hair, reaching for an overhead shelf, or working with arms overhead as in painting a ceiling or screwing in light bulbs.

    0   1   2   3   4   5   6   7   8   9   10
It would NEVER happen this past week   This past week, it would happen ALWAYS

6. Sensations of tingling or numbness increase in hand or arm when awakening from sleep.

    0   1   2   3   4   5   6   7   8   9   10
It would NEVER happen this past week   This past week, it would happen ALWAYS

FIGURE 29.8 Example of 3-page pain questionnaire. (From Jordan SE, Ahn SS, Gelabert HA: Differentiation of thoracic outlet syndrome from treatment-resistant cervical brachial pain syndromes: development and utilization of a questionnaire, clinical examination and ultrasound evaluation. *Pain Physician* 10:441–452, 2007. Official Journal of the American Society of Interventional Pain Physicians, Issue 3.)

Continued

7.   Sensations of tingling or numbness increase in the hand or arm with repetitive finger movements as in writing, typing, sewing, playing musical instruments, or assembling objects.

    0   1   2   3   4   5   6   7   8   9   10
It would NEVER happen this past week   This past week, it would happen ALWAYS

8.   Sensations of tingling or numbness increase with prolonged or forceful grasping as in holding a steering wheel to drive, using tools, handling office instruments, or controlling industrial equipment.

    0   1   2   3   4   5   6   7   8   9   10
It would NEVER happen this past week   This past week, it would happen ALWAYS

9.   Sensations of tingling or numbness increase while bending the elbow or leaning on the elbow, for example, while holding a telephone receiver or leaning on a desk.

    0   1   2   3   4   5   6   7   8   9   10
It would NEVER happen this past week   This past week, it would happen ALWAYS

10.   Hand is clumsy or weak while trying to hold onto objects or while attempting to open jars, use keys to open a lock, pull zippers, or button clothing.

    0   1   2   3   4   5   6   7   8   9   10
It would NEVER happen this past week   This past week, it would happen ALWAYS

11.   Pain is caused by experiences that ordinarily are not painful. Examples include a light touch to the hand, arm, or neck, such as a light draft, the rub and tug of clothing, or the touch of something moderately hot or cold.

    0   1   2   3   4   5   6   7   8   9   10
It would NEVER happen this past week   This past week, it would happen ALWAYS

12.   Disabling pain that can last into the next day is caused by activities that ordinarily produce only mild discomfort. Examples include a light exercise session, a physical therapy treatment, or physical examination.

    0   1   2   3   4   5   6   7   8   9   10
It would NEVER happen this past week   This past week, it would happen ALWAYS

13.   Symptoms have occurred with the above activities in the past without recurrence in the past week.

    Yes No   (circle your answer) If the answer is "yes," please list by number and explain on back.

14.   Hand becomes blue, red, swollen, sweaty, or hot.   Yes No   (circle answer)   If "yes" explain on back.

FIGURE 29.8, cont'd

extremely important. The tone and bulk of the muscles of the neck, upper back, shoulder, arm, forearm, and hand need to be inspected by palpation and against resistance; two-point testing has not been particularly helpful. Provocative testing to assess distal sites of compression should be conducted before provocative testing for TOS; this is because once a provocative TOS test is conducted, a patient may complain of symptoms with just about every maneuver from that point forward during the examination. The examiner should start distally and work proximally, looking for carpal tunnel syndrome, tendinitis, cubital tunnel syndrome, rotator cuff problems, and cervical radiculopathy before testing for TOS.

Provocative Tests for Thoracic Outlet Syndrome

There are several standard provocative maneuvers for TOS. In general, the patient's symptoms must be reproduced or the radial pulse diminished or obliterated for a test to be considered positive. Older literature mentions the Adson, Wright, and Halstead tests, but they are frequently positive in the normal population and are neither sensitive nor specific enough, especially for neurogenic TOS. Anterior scalene bands that wrap around the subclavian artery are generally causative in this situation.

The Roos Test

This test is also called the 90-degree abduction external rotation test, the stick-up test, and the elevated arm stress test (EAST). The patient holds the arm(s) in the abducted, externally rotated position and pumps the hands open and closed quickly and repetitively for 3 minutes. A positive test requires reproduction of symptoms or rapid fatigue of the extremity (Figure 29.9). Patients with positional nerve compression can tolerate this

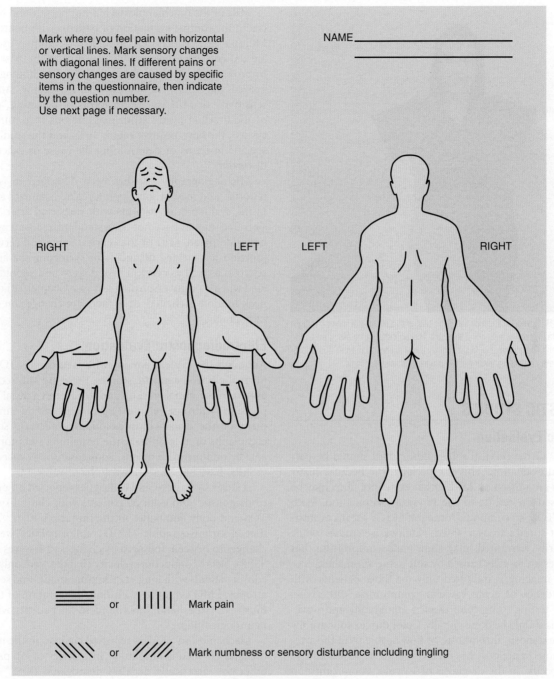

Mark where you feel pain with horizontal or vertical lines. Mark sensory changes with diagonal lines. If different pains or sensory changes are caused by specific items in the questionnaire, then indicate by the question number.
Use next page if necessary.

NAME_____

RIGHT   LEFT   LEFT   RIGHT

≡≡≡ or ||||| Mark pain

\\\\ or ///// Mark numbness or sensory disturbance including tingling

FIGURE 29.8, cont'd

position for 1 minute or less. This maneuver is thought by many to be the most sensitive and reproducible provocative maneuver for the patient with TOS.[81,84] The degree to which symptoms occur also indicates the severity of the compression, in a manner similar to Phalen's sign at the wrist. Changes in the radial pulse also should be noted at this time.

Upper-Limb Tension Test

In this test, the arms are elevated out to the sides with the elbows straight and the head facing forward. Next, with the arms still out, the wrists are dorsiflexed. Finally, the head is tilted away from the side being evaluated (Figure 29.10). In a patient with TOS, each subsequent maneuver elicits increasing discomfort

and/or paresthesias as the tension on the plexus increases. This is Sanders' modification of the test described by Elvey.[90]

Scalene Injection

Although some physicians advocate diagnostic injection of the scalenes[89] with lidocaine during one of the initial encounters, this is perhaps best done under ultrasound guidance.[34,35] As an adjuvant to physical therapy, scalene injection with a long-acting anesthetic and corticosteroid has been advocated for the patient with palpable spasm of the scalenes. If the injection helps, it is highly diagnostic; if it makes no difference, it has not determined anything. If it helps, the injection may be worth repeating.

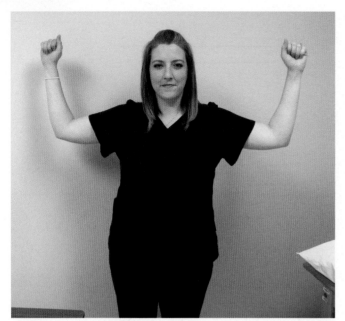

FIGURE 29.9 Demonstration of the Roos test with the patient making a tight fist and then relaxing repeatedly for 3 minutes. The arm should be elevated to the shoulder level and the elbow should be slightly more extended than in this photograph to eliminate conflicting ulnar nerve compression at the elbow.

DIAGNOSTIC STUDIES

Radiologic Evaluation

Radiographs of the cervical spine and/or chest should be part of the initial evaluation. This is especially true because many cervical ribs are missed on MRI. Other extremity films may be justified based on results of the physical examination. With neurogenic TOS, no computed tomography (CT) scans or invasive vascular studies are warranted. Noninvasive studies, while not necessarily warranted, may show mild compromise, but these changes are usually caused by soft tissue anomalies.

Vascular imaging is indicated only for those patients with physical evidence of acute vascular compromise. Otherwise, noninvasive testing using color duplex sonography and waveform analysis should be done initially. Color duplex sonography can visualize stenosis, thrombosis, or flow problems in the arterial and venous systems. It has been found to be 92% sensitive and 95% specific in the diagnosis of vascular compromise in patients with TOS.[46] Photoplethysmography (i.e., pulse volume recordings) can suggest arterial compression, which then can be followed by MR or CT angiography or arteriography, if the clinical situation warrants.[21]

Angiography remains the "gold standard" for evaluation of arterial TOS and provides the best visualization of arterial anatomy as well as the potential for therapeutic thrombolysis in the acute situation. Special attention should be given to evaluation of the bony structures in the thoracic outlet of any patient with suspected arterial compression because this is the most common cause of it, and any bone anomalies need to be surgically addressed. Conventional arteriography and venography (Figure 29.11) may demonstrate the presence of extrinsic compression. Unfortunately, they do not allow a clear depiction of the impinging anatomic structure and tend to be replaced by less invasive procedures (e.g., CT, MRI, sonography).

MRI of the brachial plexus has not been found to be beneficial in the routine evaluation of patients with neurogenic TOS. Multiple case reports describing MR techniques used to evaluate patients have been published during the past decade.[15,66] Improvements in software and magnet technology have improved the ability to identify pathoanatomy. Although the sensitivity of MRI is 79% in terms of detecting "distortions" of the brachial plexus from mass lesions (e.g., tumors, aneurysms), the false-positive rate is 10%, and the studies were not specific in terms of determining the cause or exact site of the distortion.[66]

MR angiography also has been described in isolated case reports[65] and may, at some point, replace standard angiography in the evaluation of patients with suspected arterial compression. Techniques have not been standardized, and availability is not widespread. MRI of the cervical spine and cervicothoracic junction has yielded diagnoses of syringomyelia and multiple sclerosis as well as cervical disk disease and should be considered when a positive Spurling test (see Chapter 28) or pain with neck motion is elicited, or if there are changes on the cervical radiographs.

Electrodiagnostic Evaluation

Although the typical patient with neurogenic TOS can have normal electrodiagnostic studies, these are still recommended as part of the initial workup and to rule out a distal nerve compression syndrome (e.g., carpal tunnel, cubital tunnel). Treatment of the distal compression may alleviate some of the complaints or at least make the remaining symptoms manageable by nonoperative means. Somatosensory-evoked potentials (SSEPs) have not been shown to be of value.[38,107]

A study by Passero and colleagues reported on positive electrodiagnostic studies in 30 patients with clinical symptoms of TOS and bony anomalies in the thoracic outlet.[68] They found that electromyographic (EMG) abnormalities were the first changes to be seen, followed by changes in F waves and, finally, SSEPs. Nerve conduction velocity changes were only seen belatedly in patients with long-standing anomalies and severe muscle atrophy. EMG evidence of chronic denervation of the intrinsic muscles of the hand was found in all patients with obvious neurologic findings.

Machanic and Sanders reported changes in the medial antebrachial cutaneous amplitude in a series of 41 patients with otherwise electrically negative neurogenic TOS.[48] From these studies, one may conclude that abnormalities in medial antebrachial cutaneous amplitude or distal sensory nerve action potential (SNAP) from the wrist to the digits in patients with lower trunk compression may be useful early findings in neurogenic TOS. EMG findings in the intrinsic muscles of the hand actually may be the earliest findings in TOS patients but are frequently dismissed by the neurologist.

TREATMENT

Nonoperative Treatment

There is universal agreement in the literature that nonoperative management is the first line of treatment for all patients with neurogenic TOS. Increased risk factors for failure of nonoperative treatment include obesity (based on BMI), poor cardiovascular condition, and failure to comply with a multimodality

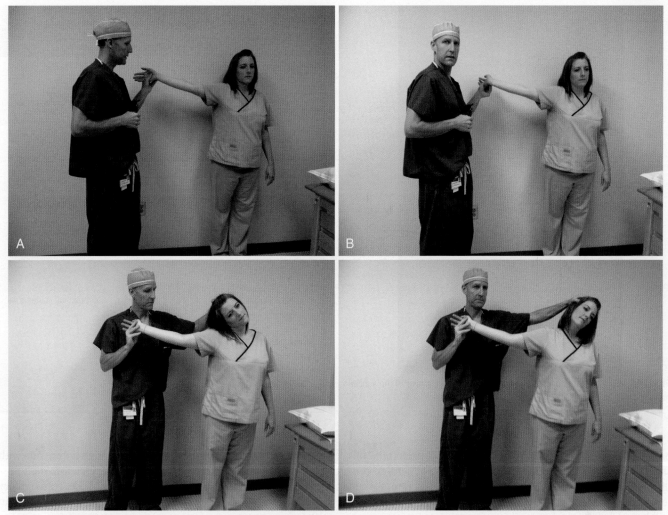

FIGURE 29.10 Upper-limb tension test: **A-D,** The head is brought to the affected side. If there is significant pain with just the abduction or wrist extension, the author considers it highly positive. If the patient has pain with the wrist hyperextended and the head away, which is relieved by bringing the head to the affected side, this is also very positive.

treatment program that addresses poor posture and exacerbating activities, both at work and at home. Patients not compliant with conservative measures are not likely to comply with mandatory postop protocols either. These patients must commit themselves to significant lifestyle and workplace modifications to have any hope of a good outcome. Nutritional counseling, diet, and exercise programs must start simultaneously with treatment.

A conservative therapy program should consist of four stages. The first goal is to relieve pain and control progression of symptoms. Thus, stage I focuses on identification and treatment of myofascial trigger points, local areas of spasm, and tendinitis or bursitis. Moderate use of muscle relaxants, antidepressants, antiinflammatories, or sleeping aids may be necessary; however, the anticonvulsant gabapentin (Neurontin) or pregabalin (Lyrica) is the drug of choice. Most therapists advocate the use of moist heat or ice, transcutaneous electrical nerve stimulation, ultrasound, and other modalities at this stage; on the other hand, Novak argues that overuse of these modalities may encourage dependence on therapy.[61] Trigger-point injections and scalene muscle injections can be beneficial in the appropriate clinical setting.

Stage II is generally instituted concurrently and consists of using stretching, relaxation, breathing, and myofascial manipulation to restore normal mobility and a balanced posture to the cervical spine, shoulder girdle, and cervicothoracic region. Strengthening of the scalenes and deep tissue massage of the scalene area are to be avoided, as this will aggravate the condition. Cardiovascular conditioning and weight-loss programs should be instituted at this stage and are continued throughout the program. Pathologic postures, such as the head-forward position, lead to decreased overall flexibility of the cervicothoracic unit and compensatory cervical lordosis, thoracic flexion, internal shoulder rotation, and scapular abduction. Such postures are thought to lead to tightening of the anterior muscle groups and compensatory elongation of the posterior muscles. This pathologic muscle imbalance has been cited by MacKinnon, Novak, and others as being one of the key pathologic entities to identify and correct.[50,52,61-63,69] Attention to lumbar lordosis, leg-length discrepancy, and other dysfunctional postures is necessary.

Stage III consists of parascapular and core muscle strengthening (except for the scalenes), increasing endurance, and restoration of the patient to presymptomatic levels of function

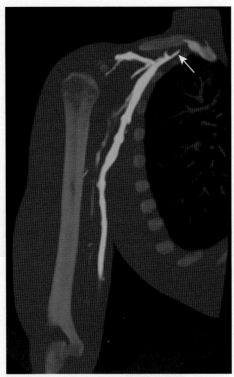

FIGURE 29.11 Venography of a patient with acute thrombosis of the subclavian and internal jugular (*arrow*).

CRITICAL POINTS *Initial Physical Examination, Diagnostic Evaluation, and Nonoperative Treatment*

Initial Physical Examination
• Initial comprehensive exam and patient history
• Patient must be undressed from the waist up so as to search for atrophy, swelling, venous engorgement, and scapular asymmetry

Sequence of Examination
• Observation
• Peripheral nerve examination
• Cervical spine evaluation
• TOS examination (the Roos, upper-limb tension test, anterior triangle tenderness, the Tinel, dysesthesias, infraclavicular tenderness)

Diagnostic Evaluation
• Radiographs of cervical spine or chest and other areas if indicated by history and physical exam
• Noninvasive vascular testing, if warranted
• Electrodiagnostic studies, including medial antebrachial cutaneous amplitude

Nonoperative Treatment
Neurogenic TOS
• Initiate four-stage physical therapy program, including postural and activity modification
• Nutritional counseling, as indicated

both at work and at home. The therapist must undertake this stage carefully because too vigorous an exercise or aerobic conditioning program can exacerbate symptoms.[102] It is important to establish realistic goals and understand that not all patients will be rendered pain-free.

If a patient graduates through the first three stages of treatment, stage IV consists of establishing a home program and returning the patient to the workplace. Analysis of the job site is frequently beneficial before return to work. Lifestyle changes and proper "work hygiene," consisting of taking breaks as necessary for stretching, breathing, and relaxation are important in the maintenance program. Necessary ingredients of the home exercise program include scalene stretching, cervical protraction and retraction, diaphragmatic exercises, pectoralis stretching, and shoulder circumduction exercises. The exercises should be done 10 times each, 3 times per day.[30,108] Some have advocated using custom-made scapular retraction harnesses, but these are rarely used.

The results of nonoperative treatment are variable and difficult to objectify, considering the lack of firm findings or diagnostic criteria. Reports of successful treatment range from 50 to 100%. Success is usually defined as avoidance of surgery, satisfactory pain relief, and return to work.

Operative Treatment

Operative treatment of TOS has evolved significantly during the past 70 years. Although Coote excised a cervical rib in 1860,[16] it was not until the next century that surgical management of TOS became accepted. In 1927, Adson and Coffey described their diagnostic maneuver for scalenus anticus syndrome and recommended anterior scalenotomy as a means of operative

treatment.[2] In 1962, Clagett documented a high failure rate with scalenotomy alone and advocated first-rib resection via a posterior approach for patients with TOS.[14] The transaxillary approach to first-rib resection was introduced by Roos in 1966.[79]

During the 1980s, a combined transaxillary and supraclavicular approach was introduced as a means of resecting the first rib and releasing the scalenes.[73] Current approaches differ among surgeons and their subspecialties of surgery. The two most popular surgical approaches are the transaxillary and the supraclavicular. Atasoy recommends transaxillary resection of the first rib followed by transcervical anterior and middle scalenectomy.[4] Others use this technique for the "failed" or "recurrent" TOS patient. The isolated supraclavicular approach for anterior and middle scalenectomy without first-rib resection has been advocated as well.[12,77,93]

Although some surgeons prefer more limited procedures,[18] the most widely performed method for neurogenic TOS currently includes (1) excision or release of anomalous anatomy, (2) resection of the first rib if it is compressing the plexus or causing traction on the plexus, (3) excision of the anterior and middle scalene muscles, (4) neurolysis of the involved portions of the supraclavicular brachial plexus, and (5) possible release of the pectoralis minor tendon and or coracocostal ligament. Recently, Merele reported on a complete excision of the middle scalene and any compressive bands or ligaments alone, and does not resect the rib or anterior scalene (personal communication, Merele, M., Club Narakas, France, 2013).

Reported surgical results are similar as long as the first rib is removed, the scalenes are divided, and any anomalies are adequately decompressed. Some advocate the transaxillary approach for safety because the brachial plexus and vessels do not need to be manipulated, although the intercostobrachial nerve is at risk. Others advocate the supraclavicular approach, even though the plexus and vessels have to be retracted, and injuries to the phrenic nerve have been reported. Which approach to use is largely a matter of surgeon preference.

For patients with vascular TOS and arterial compression, early or urgent decompression is favored, with removal of the responsible bony anomaly and arterial reconstruction as necessary. If no emboli or ulcerations in the vessel wall are present, simple arteriolysis may suffice. In patients with venous compression or Paget-Schroetter syndrome, early thrombolysis followed by first-rib resection is recommended; the procedures do not need to be done concomitantly. A workup for clotting disorders must be done. Once the area is decompressed, long-term anticoagulation is not thought to be necessary unless the patient has a thrombotic predisposition.

In neurogenic TOS, a patient who has failed to complete 3 months of physical therapy and other conservative measures and who has no evidence for a peripheral nerve compression is a candidate for surgery. Upper-extremity surgeons who surgically decompress the thoracic outlet may choose to collaborate with a vascular surgeon, depending on their experience and training. For neurogenic TOS, it is certainly reasonable for an upper-extremity surgeon who is knowledgeable in this area to proceed without a vascular surgeon depending on the requirements of the case.

❖ AUTHOR'S PREFERRED METHOD OF TREATMENT:
Neurogenic Thoracic Outlet Syndrome

I obtain the informed consent for surgery from each patient. A thorough discussion of potential complications should include the major ones: death, major bleeding requiring vascular reconstruction, pneumothorax and placement of a chest tube, increased pain, plexus or peripheral nerve injury, phrenic nerve injury, stellate ganglion injury, and periincisional numbness. We draw the proposed incision points on the patient at the preoperative visit. The supraclavicular approach (Figure 29.12) is used for all neurogenic types and most vascular ones as well. Surgery is performed under loupe magnification with the patient in a barber-chair position. We have found that sandbags and turning or twisting the head increase tension in the plexus and therefore avoid them. Long-acting paralytic agents also should be avoided to allow for intraoperative nerve stimulation.

The incision used is slightly modified from that for doing an open reduction of the clavicle, located 1 to 2 cm above it. We curve it more posteriorly as we go laterally. It starts at the lateral border of the sternocleidomastoid muscle, and if the plexus can be palpated, we extend the incision slightly lateral (Figure 29.13). The greatest number of supraclavicular nerves are lateral, so staying as medial as possible can avoid some of them, although several must be sacrificed. The platysma and some of the sternocleidomastoid are divided and retracted with the skin flaps to maximize exposure. The external jugular vein should be retracted if possible, and the omohyoid should be divided (Figure 29.14). At this point the supraclavicular fat pad is mobilized from inferiorly and is retracted superiorly or laterally. Great care should be taken when elevating the fat pad to look

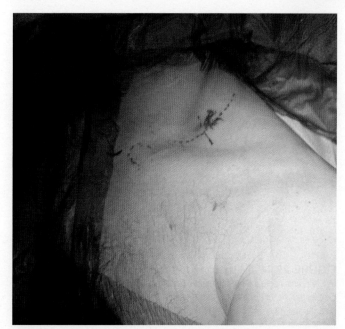

FIGURE 29.12 Preparation and draping should cross the midline; the sternal notch is the small solid medial mark. The incision (*dotted posterior line*) is centered on the plexus (*vertical solid line next to initials*); it curves more posterior than an incision for a clavicular repair.

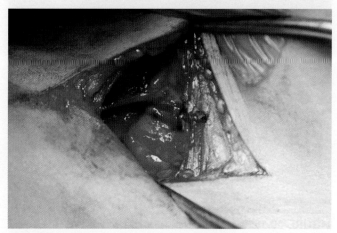

FIGURE 29.13 Any supraclavicular nerves have been divided along with the platysma and omohyoid muscles, exposing the anterior triangle fat overlying the plexus. The fat pad should be dissected bluntly and carefully because the suprascapular nerve may be encased within it.

for the suprascapular and long thoracic nerves and elevate the pad off and superior to it.

With the plexus now visible, we expose and define the posterior border of the plexus consisting of the long thoracic and suprascapular nerves. The dorsal–scapular nerve or large cervical sensory nerves may appear here and should be looked for and avoided. A nerve stimulator can be helpful to define and positively identify the various nerves. The long thoracic nerve is mobilized proximally well into the middle scalene, and the branch coming from the middle trunk can be identified, decompressed, and preserved (Figure 29.15). The suprascapular nerve is now mobilized proximally and, if necessary, distally to the notch. Often branches of the deep transverse cervical artery or

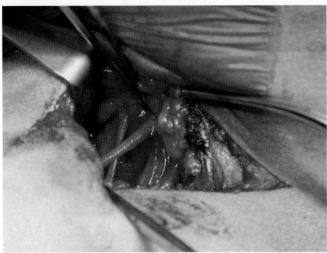

FIGURE 29.14 The posterior border of the plexus is defined here; note the long thoracic nerve exiting the middle scalene (forceps). Mobilize it proximally and distally to look for discrete compression in the scalene. In addition, look for a large contribution from C7. It is easy to mobilize the suprascapular nerve all the way to the scapular notch.

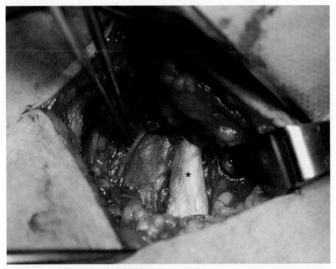

FIGURE 29.15 The anterior border is identified in this left-sided exposure. Note the phrenic nerve lying on the scalene (forceps), although it is rarely in this "classic" position. It should be looked for and carefully protected. Note that only the upper trunk is visible at this time (*asterisk*), but there is a space between the upper trunk and the scalene.

vein are entrapping the long thoracic nerve; these should be tied off with suture ligatures and divided. If vascular branches at the posterior border of the plexus are large, we divide them now, making mobilization of the subclavian artery easier. When the posterior border is defined, we move to the anterior aspect.

From the anterior aspect, we look for the phrenic nerve (Figure 29.15). It rarely lies on the scalene muscle as depicted in anatomy books. Frequently, it is very proximal on the scalene and has crossed medially well proximal to the rib. Sometimes it is very anterior and never touches the scalene, and sometimes it is actually lateral to the anterior scalene. If it is not easily found, the superficial surface of the anterior scalene is cleaned, and we find the medial border and elevate the internal jugular

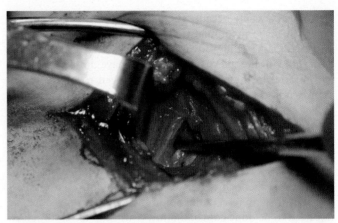

FIGURE 29.16 The space between the plexus and scalene is cleaned and opened. In a primary TOS there is always some fat and space between the artery, pleura, and scalene. Note the suction tip displacing the artery and going behind the scalene. It is not necessary to place anything here when dividing the scalene from the rib.

vein and other structures with a retractor and keep them anterior.

The subclavian artery is now identified and cleaned superficially for exposure, and the interval between the scalene and the artery is identified (Figure 29.16). This space is always present in patients who have not undergone previous surgery. Starting laterally and next to the artery, we divide the anterior scalene off the first rib. Usually, there is fat and space between the muscle and the pleura. The tendon at the rib insertion can be quite thick or very thin, and simply going slowly until the pleura is reached will avoid a pneumothorax. Once the anterior scalene is divided at the rib, it is excised as proximal as possible.

Again, care should be taken to avoid the phrenic nerve if it is coming across the muscle more proximally. Once the scalene has been excised, the subclavian artery is visible for a long way medially. Frequently, it has scalene bands around it either from the anterior scalene or from the middle scalene or scalene minimus. These bands are the cause of most of the vascular findings unless there is a definable skeletal abnormality. These bands and any tether should be excised.

Simple resection allows the artery to balloon up and have a better pulse (Figure 29.17) (see Video 29.1). If there was no deep transverse artery and vein on the posterior border, the subclavian artery should be mobile now and can be taken anterior and medial and away from the anterior border of the lower trunk. If the deep transverse vessels were there posteriorly, the artery is tightly tethered to the lower trunk and the deep vessels must be divided from the subclavian with ligatures (Figure 29.18). Once this is done the artery becomes mobile and can be taken away from the lower trunk. Orthopedists and hand surgeons breathe easier at this point.

Next, the first rib is cleaned of ligamentous structures and pleura. Frequently, a very thick pleural band is found coming from the posterior part of the rib or from a transverse process and discretely compresses the lower trunk; occasionally a neuroma can be seen or felt at this level (Figure 29.19). Now that the plexus is free and mobile anteriorly, the trunks can be mobilized easily and separated into upper, middle, and lower trunks. The middle scalene is incised from the first rib and the

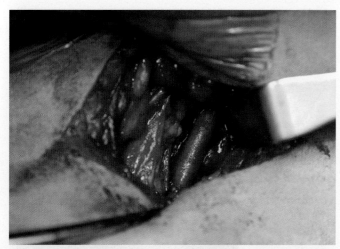

FIGURE 29.17 Once the anterior scalene has been completely excised, the subclavian artery is completely visible and can be cleaned of fibrous bands and scalene minimus that may wrap around it. If the subclavian artery is not mobile, the deep transverse cervical artery must be divided. (See also Video 29.1.)

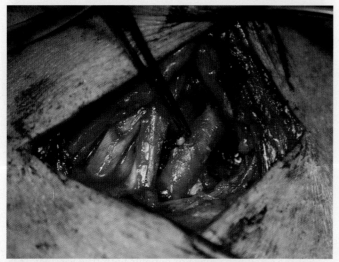

FIGURE 29.18 The deep transverse artery has been divided; if present, it lies between the middle and lower trunks and may be a source of lower trunk compression. Once it has been divided, access to the lower trunk and entire plexus is ensured.

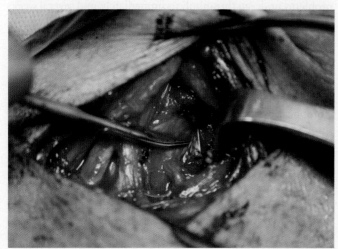

FIGURE 29.19 With the subclavian artery taken anterior and medially, the lower trunk behind the scissors is seen visibly compressed by a pleural band. Hourglass nerve constrictions and neuromas in continuity are frequently seen when these bands are excised.

vast majority or it resected, with care taken to avoid the long thoracic and dorsal–scapular nerves. The plexus is now completely free and mobile.

The C8 and T1 nerve roots are mobilized so that they are lying free across the top of the lung and rib. The arm is abducted and externally rotated now, and several items are evaluated with respect to the first rib. If the plexus is compressed between the clavicle and the first rib and if the lower trunk gets more tension with abduction and external rotation, or the C8—T1 roots are very short—the first rib is removed. Pressure is determined by placing a finger between the rib and clavicle, and if there is pressure on the finger with abduction and external rotation, the rib is removed.

Frequently, there is no pressure and the lower trunk actually has less tension with this position. If there are no further compressive elements or tension, the rib is left in place. Some surgeons routinely remove the first rib. Cervical ribs are easily and safely excised using this approach, and they are excised to the extent that all compressive elements are removed. It may be necessary to excise some of the transverse process of C7 as well, even in the absence of cervical ribs.

Should the surgeon elect to excise the rib, a microsaw is used and a cut made through the rib well anterior to the artery and medial to the posterior facet joint (Figure 29.20). The microsaw requires much less space than rib cutters, so the plexus is retracted much less. The intercalated piece is then gently dissected free and removed (Figure 29.21); this can be done without excessive traction on the plexus if the arm is supported during this portion of the process.

Now all compressive elements have been removed and the incision is closed after checking for air leaks (Figure 29.22). Positive pressure is maintained while the wound is filled with saline and any air bubbles are looked for. This step is repeated twice, and all fluid is carefully sucked out each time while the lung is expanded to lessen postoperative pain with respiration. The wound also is inspected for bleeding at this time.

Closure is done over a red rubber drain left in the lung's apex and another drain is placed subcutaneously. After closure, all air

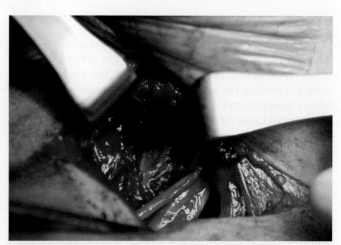

FIGURE 29.20 The pleura can now be taken off the rib, the plexus completely mobilized, and the rib excised. Note the posterior portion of the rib ready to be cut across. The plexus is easily retracted as the arm and shoulder are elevated, putting slack in the nerves. A small microoscillating saw requires much less space and retraction than a standard rib cutter.

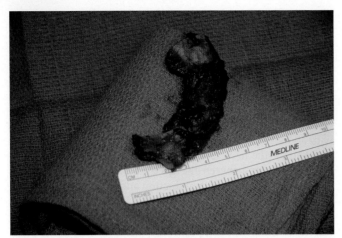

FIGURE 29.21 Similarly, the plexus and artery are retracted away from the anterior portion of the rib; the rib is cut across here and then gently excised and removed. The majority of the rib can be easily excised in this manner. Note rib medial to the facet joint that should be removed if taking the rib.

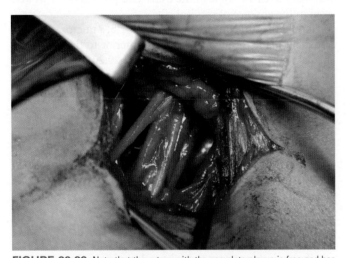

FIGURE 29.22 Note that the artery with the complete plexus is free and has nothing to further compress it. The lung is seen deep. The pleura is left open and closure done after checking for air leaks by maintaining positive pressure, covering the lung with saline, and looking for air bubbles.

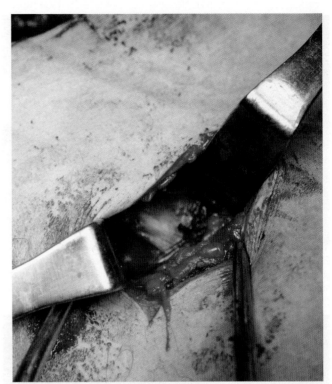

FIGURE 29.23 The infraclavicular incision on the medial border of the coracoid. Note the large coracocostal ligament arising from the medial border of the coracoid and inserting on the first or second rib and compressing the plexus underneath. It can be as large or larger than the CA ligament and should be divided.

is sucked out through the red drain, then it is removed. Patients who stay in the barber-chair position do not get air other than at the apex, and if there is no injury to the visceral pleura, simply removing the air this way has not presented any problems. During closure it is important to pull the fat pad back to the infraclavicular fat or fascia so that it covers the plexus. Skin closure method is the surgeon's choice.

The approach to use now routinely includes an infraclavicular incision, which is made in the skin lines medial to the coracoids; dissection is taken down to the coracoid in the interval between the deltoid and pectoralis major. The pectoralis minor tendon is identified and the plexus is examined deep into it. It is easy to sweep the area with a finger to check for any fibrous bands or constrictions. The arm is then abducted and externally rotated, and if the tendon compresses the plexus, it is incised from the medial border of the coracoid.

Next, look for any coracocostal ligaments, and if present, incise (Figure 29.23). The plexus is then mobilized off the chest

wall. If no further entrapments are found, the wound is closed in a similar manner but without additional drains. Postoperatively, chest radiographs are taken in the recovery room. When awake, the patient is started on active abduction and external rotation. An arm sling is used for comfort only for a few days, then the patient begins physical therapy.

For the small percentage of patients with true vascular TOS, we also use a supraclavicular approach. Arterial reconstruction is done by a vascular surgeon, and neural decompression is done by an upper-extremity surgeon. Patients with venous problems undergo thrombolysis immediately, and several weeks later decompression is done by either team, depending on whether the remaining symptoms are neurogenic or vascular. An in-depth discussion of this is beyond the scope of this chapter.

Complications

Complications of nonoperative treatment are few and relatively minor, except in the rare case of a patient with electrically positive neurogenic or vascular TOS who refuses surgical intervention and experiences progression of the disease. Most patients report exacerbations of the symptoms if their physical therapy regimen emphasizes a vigorous strengthening program instead of stretching. There is also a risk of drug dependency, severe depression, or other psychiatric disorders if care is not taken to manage the patient's chronic pain and associated psychosocial issues. Certainly if emboli occur, significant peripheral problems may occur.

In contrast, complications of surgical treatment for TOS can be significant. Problems related to surgery were recognized as early as the late 1800s, as recorded by Keen in his 1907 review of the subject.[36] It was not until a review by Dale in 1982 that some representation of the true incidence and extent of brachial plexus injuries was recognized.[17] His survey of the members of the International Cardiovascular Society revealed that 52% of the surgeons who responded had seen some sort of brachial plexus injury, and the numbers indicated that 273 injuries of varying degree had occurred. From this point forward it seems that clinicians began to take a more serious look at the signs for surgery and technique.

Although surgical treatment is deemed "successful" in approximately 80% of cases when careful patient selection is done, 20% of them end up with unsatisfactory outcomes.[101,105] Reported surgical complications include injuries to the subclavian artery or vein that have led to exsanguination and subsequent death, transection of phrenic or long thoracic nerves, and division of the medial cord or C8 nerve root.[37]

Additional surgical complications include hemothorax, pneumothorax, chylothorax, causalgia, and traction injuries to the plexus, including total paralysis and complete sensory loss.[29] Horner syndrome rarely occurs because of manipulation of the C8 and/or T1 nerve roots. Traction injuries are more common with the axillary approach. Although many brachial plexus injuries are transient, in unusual cases they require surgical treatment. Cutaneous nerve dysesthesias involving the intercostobrachial nerves, posterior cutaneous nerves, and supraclavicular nerves also have been known to occur almost universally. Although these dysesthesias generally resolve within 6 months, some may be present for a long time, and there will be an area of permanent numbness below the clavicle with the supraclavicular approach. It is extremely rare for these to be a significant problem because this approach is used for clavicular fractures with minimal reported difficulties.

Although the aforementioned complications account for some surgical failures, other patients have unsatisfactory outcomes with no surgical problems. Some believe that one of the largest reasons for "failed" TOS surgery is an incorrect diagnosis. A report by Kostic and Kulka analyzed reasons for failed surgery in 142 operations on 124 patients.[39] Missed diagnoses included glenohumeral or cervical arthritis and cervical disk herniation. Another patient had a Pancoast (i.e., pulmonary sulcus) tumor that was missed during the initial evaluation. For 13 patients, an additional operation was necessary because of inadequate or failed first-rib resection.

As experience with the surgical treatment of patients with TOS of all types increases, complications have decreased, and careful analysis of complications, failed surgery, and recurrent or persistent symptoms have been recognized and investigated. The majority of carefully selected patients with neurogenic TOS do well with surgical treatment.

Results

The results of operative and nonoperative treatment of TOS are difficult to objectively assess because there is no standardized means of patient diagnosis or assessment. Many patients in the electrically negative neurogenic TOS category have short-term symptoms precipitated by an isolated event, activity, or accident. These patients have symptoms that can be self-limited and improve with short courses of physical therapy, activity modification, and medication.

For patients with more persistent or severe symptoms, nonoperative treatment, such as the four-stage rehabilitation program advocated by Novak and colleagues, is recommended and successful, at least in the short term.[62] In one study, 44 patients with symptoms of TOS were followed for 12 months, and none was reported to be worse in terms of symptoms, lifestyle, or work activities. Of these patients, 4 of 44 were "not improved" and only 3 of 44 were "completely" improved. Most of them (i.e., 35 of 44) were either "partially" or "almost completely" better. Another report detailed 100% complete relief of symptoms in the short term with a multimodality therapy program.[97] The long-term outcome for these patients is not known and requires further study.

The literature that reviews surgical treatment is abundant and demonstrates a high degree of variability, with good to excellent results achieved in 24 to 100%.[8,28,31,44,57,64,89,92,112] This variability can be attributed to many factors, including the lack of objective outcome measures, diagnostic criteria, follow-up periods, and widely variable surgical techniques and training. Early results (at 3 months) show improvement, with a 90% or better success rate, and long-term results (>5 years) indicate an approximately 70% success rate (Figure 29.24).

A review by Sanders provides the most extensive summary of the literature to date.[89] This paper demonstrates that the combination of anterior and middle scalenectomies and first-rib resection yields the best results when compared with scalenotomy alone (99% vs. 57% satisfied). In Sanders' own series, in which subtotal scalenectomy alone was compared with first-rib resection and combined scalenectomy and rib resection, no difference between early and long-term results was noted.[87,89] Despite this, Sanders' current surgical technique includes a "complete" scalenectomy, and he believes that the combination of rib resection and scalenectomy yields "slightly" better results than either procedure alone.[54]

Patients with vascular or true neurogenic TOS are thought to have a better outcome with surgical treatment than those with the electrically negative type of TOS. However, in one of the few studies with disabilities of the arm, shoulder and hand (DASH) and the 12-Item Short Form Health Survey (SF-12) comparisons, Chang and colleagues reported that there was no difference in ability to return to work between the venous and neurogenic groups of patients.[11] The main variation was in the time required before returning to work. Interestingly, these authors' preoperative assessment identified low scores on the physical component scale, on par with patients with chronic congestive heart failure, and they did not return to normal baseline scores until 2 years postoperatively.[11] Similarly, there are supportive data to demonstrate that patients with work-related claims or litigation do worse than others, whether treated surgically or nonsurgically.[8,22,28,72,89] Sanders notes that patients with workers' compensation claims had 13 to 15% lower rates of success than all others.

Recurrent Symptoms After Surgical Treatment. Failure of surgical decompression of the thoracic outlet should be carefully scrutinized to determine whether there was a symptom-free interval. Failure to improve after adequate decompression or first-rib resection implies either incorrect diagnosis or other issues, including the potential for secondary gain. The rate of true recurrent symptoms is reported to be between 5% and 25%, and the symptoms tend to occur within 4 to 6 months

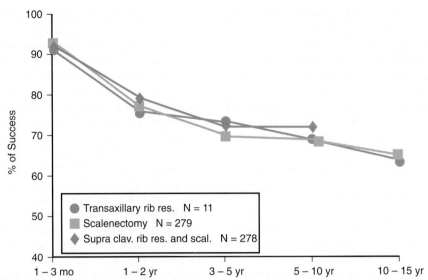

FIGURE 29.24 Results of three primary operations for thoracic outlet syndrome: transaxillary rib resection, scalenectomy, and supraclavicular rib resection and scalenectomy (supra clav. rib res. and scal.).

postoperatively.[4,5,55,57,58,70,89,92,94,98,104] Although patients undergoing anterior scalenotomy (now rarely performed) alone have a higher likelihood of recurrent symptoms, the recurrence rate for patients undergoing combined anterior and middle scalenectomies (14%) is similar to that of transaxillary first-rib resection alone (19%). Patients undergoing a combined first-rib resection and scalenotomy have the lowest recurrence rate (6%).[87,92]

In several reviews, the cause of recurrent symptoms was most frequently scar tissue around the brachial plexus or a retained or unstable segment of the first rib.[13,43,87,92,94] The supraclavicular approach seems to be the most popular one for revision surgery because it allows better access to the brachial plexus. It also allows access to supraclavicular fat, which can be used to wrap the plexus after neurolysis in an attempt to prevent recurrence of adhesions between the plexus and the scalenes.

The complication rate for secondary procedures is higher than that for primary procedures, with the incidence of pleural tears or pneumothorax as high as 62% in one series.[13] Results of reoperation for recurrent symptoms demonstrate early "improvement" or "success" in 74 to 90% of patients after surgery (3 months). Recurrence of symptoms and "surgical failure," however, occur in up to 59% of patients after 10 to 15 years. Surgical results correlate directly with the identification of residual anomalous anatomy, such as retained bone, periosteum, or an unstable residual rib, and are worse for patients in whom only scar tissue around the brachial plexus is found at the time of another operation.

Sympathectomy at the time of reoperation has been recommended to improve results but is not commonly performed.[81] Comparative analysis of reoperation techniques is impossible because of the small number of patients and the lack of a standardized objective means of preoperative or postoperative assessment.

CONCLUSION

Most upper-extremity surgeons perform few, if any, surgical procedures for TOS. A surgeon with a thorough understanding of and ability to recognize the problem can identify a large number of affected patients in a typical upper-extremity practice. Careful attention to details about the patient's history and physical examination is the key to diagnosis. The practitioner must recognize this and schedule appropriate time for the initial examination. Patients who demonstrate vascular or electrically positive neurogenic TOS should be considered early on for surgery or referred for operative consultation.

For those without obvious vascular compromise or electrical findings, conservative treatment can be successful in controlling symptoms in most patients, at least in the short term. Psychological assessment and support are essential on initial recognition of TOS, as are lifestyle and workplace modifications. Persistent symptoms warrant thorough radiographic evaluation, electrodiagnostic studies, and specialized diagnostic testing to identify bony or soft tissue anomalies and to rule out other treatable afflictions.

Selected patients who have failed to improve after several months of nonoperative treatment, and continue to have significant or progressive symptoms, may warrant surgical decompression.[60] Great care should be exercised in patient selection, especially in workers' compensation cases. A comprehensive approach that allows for complete plexus decompression, resection of anterior and middle scalene muscles, and first-rib resection should be used.

For patients who require operative treatment, careful consideration should be given to referral of them to a surgeon or surgical team that routinely performs TOS surgery. The treatment is best handled by a hand or upper-extremity surgeon who understands nerve compression because that is the underlying problem of TOS. There are several major centers in the United States that perform TOS surgery, and results of treatment of patients in them are predictably superior to the results of surgeons who perform <10 procedures a year. The ones who do perform operative treatment should have hands-on, individual training in the procedure to be used. They should be able to manage potential complications themselves or have a vascular or thoracic surgeon immediately available. Once learned, the procedure is not that difficult. If TOS is recognized early on and treated properly, treatment results can be extremely satisfactory.

For Case Studies, Videos, and more, please visit ExpertConsult.com.

REFERENCES

1. Adams JT, DeWeese JA, Mahoney EB, et al: Intermittent subclavian vein obstruction without thrombosis. *Surgery* 63:147–165, 1968.
2. Adson AW, Coffey JR: Cervical rib: a method of anterior approach. *Ann Surg* 85:839–856, 1927.
3. Atasoy E: Thoracic outlet compression syndrome. *Orthop Clin North Am* 27:265–303, 1996.
4. Atasoy E: Combined surgical treatment of thoracic outlet syndrome: transaxillary first-rib resection and transcervical scalenectomy. *Hand Clin* 20:71–82, 2004.
5. Axelrod DA, Proctor MC, Geisser ME, et al: Outcomes after surgery for thoracic outlet syndrome. *J Vasc Surg* 33:1220–1225, 2001.
6. Bilbey JH, Muller NL, Connell DG, et al: Thoracic outlet syndrome: evaluation with CT. *Radiology* 171:381–384, 1989.
7. Bingham DH: Thoracic outlet syndrome: a misunderstood and potentially devastating problem. *Nebr Med J* 79:145–150, 1994.
8. Bredenburg C, Dardik H, Green RM, et al: Discussion of Green R, et al. Long-term follow-up after thoracic outlet decompression: an analysis of factors determining outcome. *J Vasc Surg* 14:745–746, 1991.
9. Bureau of Labor Statistics: *Annual survey of occupational injuries and illnesses (abstract)*, Washington, DC, 1990, US Government Printing Office.
10. Carroll RE, Hurst LC: The relationship of thoracic outlet syndrome and carpal tunnel syndrome. *Clin Orthop* 164:149–153, 1982.
11. Chang DC, Rotellini-Coltvet MA, Mukherjee D, et al: Surgical intervention for thoracic outlet syndrome improves patient's quality of life. *J Vasc Surg* 49:630–635, 2009.
12. Cheng SWK, Reilly LM, Nelken NA, et al: Neurogenic thoracic outlet decompression: rationale for sparing the first rib. *Cardiovasc Surg* 3:617–623, 1995.
13. Cheng SWK, Stoney RJ: Supraclavicular reoperation for neurogenic thoracic outlet syndrome. *J Vasc Surg* 19:565–572, 1994.
14. Clagett OT: Presidential Address: Research and prosearch. *J Thorac Cardiovasc Surg* 44:153, 1962.
15. Collins JD, Disher AC, Miller TQ: The anatomy of the brachial plexus as displayed by magnetic resonance imaging: technique and application. *J Natl Med Assoc* 87:489–498, 1995.
16. Coote H: Pressure on the axillary vessels and nerve by an exostosis from cervical rib; interference with the circulation of the arm, removal of the rib and exostosis; recovery. *Med Times Gazette* 2:108, 1861.
17. Dale WA: Thoracic outlet compression syndrome. *Arch Surg* 117:1437–1445, 1982.
18. Dellon AL: The results of supraclavicular brachial plexus neurolysis (without first rib resection) in management of post-traumatic "thoracic outlet syndrome." *J Reconstr Microsurg* 9:11–17, 1993.
19. Dugas JR, Weiland AJ: Vascular pathology in the throwing athlete. *Hand Clin* 16:477–485, 2000.
20. Durham JR, McIntyre KE: Complications following surgical treatment of the thoracic outlet syndrome. In Bernared VM, Towne JB, editors: *Complications in vascular surgery*, Orlando, 1985, Grune & Stratton, pp 111–120.
21. Dymarkowski S, Bosmans H, Marchal G, et al: Three-dimensional MR angiography in the evaluation of thoracic outlet syndrome. *AJR Am J Roentgenol* 173:1005–1008, 1999.
22. Ellison DW, Wood VE: Trauma-related thoracic outlet syndrome. *J Hand Surg [Br]* 19:424–426, 1994.
23. Faulkner JA, Brooks SV, Opiteck JA: Injury to skeletal muscle fibers during contractions: conditions of occurrence and prevention. *Phys Ther* 73:911–921, 1993.
24. Fodor M, Fodor L, Cluce C: Anomalies of thoracic outlet in human fetuses: anatomical study. *Ann Vasc Surg* 25(7):961–968, 2011.
25. Friden J, Sjöstrom M, Ekblom B: Myofibrillar damage following intense eccentric exercise in man. *Int J Sports Med* 4:170–176, 1983.
26. Fujita K, Matsuda K, Sakai Y, et al: Late thoracic outlet syndrome secondary to malunion of the fractured clavicle: case report and review of the literature. *J Trauma* 50:332–335, 2001.
27. Gilliatt RW: Thoracic outlet syndrome. In Dyck PJ, Thomas PK, Lambert EH, et al, editors: *Peripheral neurology*, Philadelphia, 1984, WB Saunders, p 1409.
28. Green RM, McNamara J, Ouriel K: Long-term follow-up after thoracic outlet decompression: an analysis of factors determining outcome. *J Vasc Surg* 14:739–745, 1991.
29. Horowitz SH: Brachial plexus injuries with causalgia resulting from transaxillary rib resection. *Arch Surg* 120:1189–1191, 1985.
30. Howell J: Evaluation and management of thoracic outlet syndrome. In Donatelli R, editor: *Physical therapy of the shoulder*, New York, 1991, Churchill Livingstone.
31. Jamieson WG, Chinnick B: Thoracic outlet syndrome: fact or fancy? A review of 409 consecutive patients who underwent operation. *Can J Surg* 39:321–326, 1996.
32. Jamieson WG, Merskey H: The representation of the thoracic outlet syndrome as a problem in chronic pain and psychiatric management. *Pain* 22:195–200, 1985.
33. Johnson CR: Treatment of thoracic outlet syndrome by removal of first rib and related entrapments through posterolateral approach: a 22-year experience. *J Thorac Cardiovasc Surg* 68:536–545, 1977.
34. Jordan SE, Ahn SS, Gelabert HA: Differentiation of thoracic outlet syndrome from treatment-resistant cervical brachial pain syndromes: development and utilization of a questionnaire, clinical examination and ultrasound evaluation. *Pain Physician* 10:441–452, 2007.
35. Jordan SE, Ahn SS, Gelabert HA: Combining ultrasonography and electromyography for botulinum chemodenervation treatment of thoracic outlet syndrome: comparison with fluoroscopy and electromyography guidance. *Pain Physician* 10:541–546, 2007.
36. Keen WW: The symptomatology, diagnosis and surgical treatment of cervical ribs. *Am J Med Sci* 133:173–218, 1907.
37. Kline DG, Hackett ER, Happel LH: Surgery for lesions of the brachial plexus. *Arch Neurol* 43:170–181, 1986.
38. Komanetsky RM, Novak CB, Mackinnon SE, et al: Somatosensory evoked potentials fail to diagnose thoracic outlet syndrome. *J Hand Surg [Am]* 21:662–666, 1996.
39. Kostic S, Kulka F: Reasons behind surgical failures in thoracic outlet syndrome. *Int Surg* 75:159–161, 1990.
40. Landry GJ, Moneta GL, Taylor LM, Jr, et al: Long term functional outcome of neurogenic thoracic outlet syndrome in conservatively and surgically treated patients. *J Vasc Surg* 33:292–297, 2001.
41. Leffert RD: Thoracic outlet syndromes. *Hand Clin* 8:285–297, 1992.
42. Lindgren K: Thoracic outlet syndrome with special reference to the first rib. *Ann Chir Gynaecol* 82:218–230, 1993.
43. Lindgren K, Leino E, Lepantalo M, et al: Recurrent thoracic outlet syndrome after first rib resection. *Arch Phys Med Rehabil* 72:208–210, 1991.
44. Lindgren K, Oksala I: Long-term outcome of surgery for thoracic outlet syndrome. *Am J Surg* 169:358–360, 1995.
45. Lishman WA, Russell WR: The brachial neuropathies. *Lancet* 2:941–946, 1961.
46. Longley DG, Yedlicka JW, Molina EJ, et al: Thoracic outlet syndrome: evaluation of the subclavian vessels by color duplex sonography. *AJR Am J Roentgenol* 158:623–630, 1992.
47. Luoma A, Nelems B: Thoracic outlet syndrome: thoracic surgery perspective. *Neurosurg Clin N Am* 2:187–226, 1991.
48. Machanic BI, Sanders RJ: Medial antebrachial cutaneous nerve measurements to diagnose neurogenic thoracic outlet syndrome. *Ann Vasc Surg* 22:248–254, 2008.
49. MacKinnon SE: Double and multiple "crush" syndromes—double and multiple entrapment neuropathies. *Hand Clin* 8:369–390, 1992.
50. MacKinnon SE, Novak CB: Evaluation of the patient with thoracic outlet syndrome. *Semin Thorac Cardiovasc Surg* 8:190–200, 1996.
51. MacKinnon SE, Novak CB: Thoracic outlet syndrome. *Curr Probl Surg* 39:1070–1145, 2002.
52. MacKinnon SE, Patterson GA, Novak CB: Thoracic outlet syndrome: a current overview. *Semin Thorac Cardiovasc Surg* 8:176–182, 1996.
53. Makhoul RG, Machleder HI: Discussion of Makhoul RG, Machleder HI: Developmental anomalies at the thoracic outlet: an analysis of 200 consecutive cases. *J Vasc Surg* 16:542–545, 1992.
54. Matsumura JS, Rilling WS, Pearce WH, et al: Helical computed tomography of the normal thoracic outlet. *J Vasc Surg* 26:776–783, 1997.
55. Maxwell-Armstrong CA, Noorpuri BS, Haque SA, et al: Long-term results of surgical decompression of thoracic outlet syndrome. *J R Coll Surg Edinb* 46:35–38, 2001.
56. McCarthy WJ, Yao JST, Schafer MF, et al: Upper extremity arterial injury in athletes. *J Vasc Surg* 9:297–327, 1989.
57. Mingoli A, Feldhaus RJ, Farina C, et al: Long-term outcome after transaxillary approach for thoracic outlet syndrome. *Surgery* 118:841–844, 1995.
58. Molina JE: Regarding "Long-term functional outcome of neurogenic thoracic outlet syndrome in surgically and conservatively treated patients." *J Vasc Surg* 34:760–761, 2001.
59. Narakas AO: The role of thoracic outlet syndrome in the double crush syndrome. *Ann Hand Surg* 9:329–340, 1990.
60. Nasim A, Sayers RD, Healey PA, et al: Surgical decompression of thoracic outlet syndrome: is it a worthwhile procedure? *J R Coll Surg Edinb* 42:299–323, 1997.
61. Novak CB: Conservative management of thoracic outlet syndrome. *Semin Thorac Cardiovasc Surg* 8:201–207, 1996.

62. Novak CB, Collins ED, Mackinnon SE: Outcome following conservative treatment management of thoracic outlet syndrome. *J Hand Surg [Am]* 20:542–548, 1995.

63. Novak CB, Mackinnon SE, Patterson AG: Evaluation of patients with thoracic outlet syndrome. *J Hand Surg [Am]* 18:292–299, 1993.

64. Oates SD, Daley RA: Thoracic outlet syndrome. *Hand Clin* 12:705–718, 1996.

65. Ohkawa Y, Isoda H, Hasegawa S, et al: MR angiography of thoracic outlet syndrome. *J Comput Assist Tomogr* 16:475–477, 1992.

66. Panegyres PK, Moore N, Gibson R, et al: Thoracic outlet syndromes and magnetic resonance imaging. *Brain* 116:823–841, 1993.

67. Pang D, Wessel HB: Thoracic outlet syndrome. *Neurosurgery* 22:105–121, 1988.

68. Passero S, Paradiso C, Giannini F, et al: Diagnosis of thoracic outlet syndrome: relative value of electrophysiological studies. *Acta Neurol Scand* 90:179–185, 1994.

69. Peet RM, Henriksen JD, Anderson TP, et al: Thoracic outlet syndrome: evaluation of a therapeutic exercise program. *Proc Staff Meet Mayo Clin* 29:281–287, 1956.

70. Pietre R, Spiliopoulos A, Megevand R: Transthoracic approach in the thoracic outlet syndrome: an alternate operative route for removal of the first rib. *Surgery* 106:856–860, 1989.

71. Poitevin L: Proximal compression of the upper limb neurovascular bundle: an anatomic research study. *Hand Clin* 4:575, 1988.

72. Poole GV, Thomae KR: Thoracic outlet syndrome reconsidered. *Am Surg* 62:287–291, 1996.

73. Qvarfordt PG, Ehrenfeld WK, Stoney RJ: Supraclavicular radical scalenectomy and transaxillary first rib resection for the thoracic outlet syndrome. *Am J Surg* 148:111–116, 1984.

74. Ranney D: Thoracic outlet: an anatomical redefinition that makes sense. *Clin Anat* 9:50–52, 1996.

75. Redenbach DM, Nelems B: A comparative study of structures comprising the thoracic outlet in 250 human cadavers and 72 surgical cases of thoracic outlet syndrome. *Eur J Cardiothorac Surg* 13:353–360, 1998.

76. Reidler JS, Das DS, Schreiber JJ, et al: Thoracic outlet syndrome caused by synostosis of the first and second thoracic ribs: Two case reports and review of the literature. *J Hand Surg [Am]* 39(12):2444–2447, 2014.

77. Reilly LM, Stoney RJ: Supraclavicular approach for thoracic outlet decompression. *J Vasc Surg* 8:329–334, 1988.

78. Ribbe E, Norgren L, Hamrin A: Etiological factors in thoracic outlet syndrome. *Int Angiol* 3:113, 1984.

79. Roos DB: Transaxillary approach for the first rib resection to relieve thoracic outlet syndrome. *Ann Surg* 163:354, 1966.

80. Roos DB: Congenital anomalies associated with thoracic outlet syndrome: anatomy, symptoms, diagnosis and treatment. *Am J Surg* 132:771–778, 1976.

81. Roos DB: Sympathectomy for the upper extremities: anatomy, indications and techniques, new concepts in etiology, diagnosis and surgical treatment for thoracic outlet syndrome. In Greep DM, et al, editors: *Pain syndromes in the shoulder and arm: an integrated view*, The Hague, 1979, Martinus Nijhoff Publishers.

82. Roos DB: The place for scalenotomy and first rib resection in thoracic outlet syndrome. *Surgery* 92:1077–1085, 1982.

83. Roos DB: The thoracic outlet syndrome is underrated. *Arch Neurol* 47:327–330, 1990.

84. Roos DB: Thoracic outlet syndrome is underdiagnosed. *Muscle Nerve* 22:126–137, 1990.

85. Roos DB: Historical perspectives and anatomic considerations. *Semin Thorac Cardiovasc Surg* 8:183–189, 1996.

86. Roos DB, Owens JC: Thoracic outlet syndrome. *Arch Surg* 93:71–74, 1966.

87. Roos DB, Sanders R, Stoney RP: Discussion concerning Sanders RJ et al. Recurrent thoracic outlet syndrome. *J Vasc Surg* 12:398–400, 1990.

88. Sahrmann SA: *Diagnosis and treatment of movement impairment syndromes*, St. Louis, 2002, Mosby.

89. Sanders RJ: Results of the surgical treatment for thoracic outlet syndrome. *Semin Thorac Cardiovasc Surg* 8:221–228, 1996.

90. Sanders RJ, Hammond SL, Rao NM: Diagnosis of thoracic outlet syndrome. *J Vasc Surg* 46:601–604, 2007.

91. Sanders RJ, Haug CE: *Thoracic outlet syndrome: a common sequela of neck injuries*, Philadelphia, 1991, JB Lippincott.

92. Sanders RJ, Haug CE, Pearce WH: Recurrent thoracic outlet syndrome. *J Vasc Surg* 12:390–398, 1990.

93. Sanders RJ, Pearce WH: The treatment of thoracic outlet syndrome: a comparison of different operations. *J Vasc Surg* 10:626–634, 1989.

94. Sessions RT: Reoperation for thoracic outlet syndrome. *J Cardiovasc Surg* 30:434–444, 1909.

95. Smith T, Trojaborg W: Diagnosis of thoracic outlet syndrome: value of sensory and motor conduction studies and quantitative electromyography. *Arch Neurol* 44:1161–1163, 1987.

96. Sommerich CM, McGlathlin JD, Marras WS: Occupational risk factors associated with soft tissue disorders of the shoulder: a review of recent investigations in the literature. *Ergonomics* 36:697–717, 1993.

97. Thompson JF, Webster JHH: First rib resection for vascular complications of thoracic outlet syndrome. *Br J Surg* 77:555–557, 1990.

98. Thompson RW, Petrinec D, Toursakissian B: Surgical treatment of thoracic outlet compression syndromes: II. Supraclavicular exploration and vascular reconstruction. *Ann Vasc Surg* 11:442–451, 1997.

99. Troeng T: The anatomy of the thoracic outlet and the causes of thoracic outlet syndrome. *Vasa* 16:149–152, 1987.

100. Urschel HC, Jr: The transaxillary approach for treatment of thoracic outlet. *Semin Thorac Cardiovasc Surg* 8:214–220, 1996.

101. Urschel HC, Jr, Razzuk MA: The failed operation for thoracic outlet syndrome: the difficulty of diagnosis and management. *Ann Thorac Surg* 42:523–528, 1986.

102. Urschel HC, Jr, Razzuk MA: Improved management of the Paget-Schroetter syndrome secondary to thoracic outlet compression. *Ann Thorac Surg* 52:1217–1221, 1991.

103. Urschel HC, Jr, Razzuk MA: Upper plexus thoracic outlet syndrome: optimal therapy. *Ann Thorac Surg* 63:935–939, 1997.

104. Urschel HC, Jr, Razzuk MA: Neurovascular compression in the thoracic outlet: changing management over 50 years. *Ann Surg* 228:609–617, 1998.

105. Urschel HC, Jr, Razzuk MA, Albers JE, et al: Reoperation for recurrent thoracic outlet syndrome. *Ann Thorac Surg* 21:19–25, 1976.

106. Urschel HC, Jr, Razzuk MA, Hyland JW, et al: Thoracic outlet syndrome masquerading as coronary artery disease (pseudoangina). *Ann Thorac Surg* 16:239–248, 1973.

107. Veilleux M, Stevens JC, Campbell JK: Somatosensory evoked potentials: lack of value for diagnosis of thoracic outlet syndrome. *Muscle Nerve* 11:571–575, 1988.

108. Walsh MT: Therapist management of thoracic outlet syndrome. *J Hand Ther* 7:129–144, 1994.

109. Wehbe MA: Thoracic outlet syndrome. *Hand Clin* 20:1–130, 2004.

110. Wehbe MA, Leinberry CF: Current trends in treatment of thoracic outlet syndrome. *Hand Clin* 20:119–121, 2004.

111. Wilbourn AJ: Thoracic outlet syndrome. In Coutse D, editor: *Controversies in entrapment neuropathies*, Rochester, MN, 1984, American Association of Electromyography and Electrodiagnosis, p 28.

112. Wood VE, Ellison DW: Results of upper plexus thoracic outlet syndrome operation. *Ann Thorac Surg* 58:458–461, 1994.

113. Wood VE, Frykman GK: Winging of the scapular as a complication of first-rib resection: a report of 6 cases. *Clin Orthop* 149:160–163, 1980.

Page numbers followed by "*f*" indicate figures, "*t*" indicate tables, "*b*" indicate boxes, and "*e*" indicate online content.